Textbook of Neurological Surgery

PRINCIPLES AND PRACTICE

Volume 2
Chapters 98–213

Editors

H. HUNT BATJER, M.D., F.A.C.S.

Michael Marchese Professor and Chair
Department of Neurological Surgery
Northwestern University Feinberg School of Medicine
Chair
Department of Neurological Surgery
Northwestern Memorial Hospital
Chicago, Illinois

CHRISTOPHER M. LOFTUS, M.D., F.A.C.S.

Esther and Ted Greenberg Professor and Chairman
Department of Neurological Surgery
The University of Oklahoma College of Medicine
Oklahoma City, Oklahoma

Illustrations by Thomas H. Weinzerl

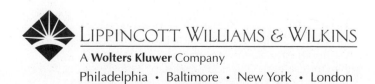

LIPPINCOTT WILLIAMS & WILKINS
A **Wolters Kluwer** Company
Philadelphia • Baltimore • New York • London
Buenos Aires • Hong Kong • Sydney • Tokyo

Acquisitions Editor: R. Craig Percy
Developmental Editor: Maureen Iannuzzi
Production Editors: Deirdre Marino and Rosemary Palumbo
Manufacturing Manager: Benjamin Rivera
Cover Designer: Christine Jenny
Compositor: Maryland Composition Company, Inc.
Printer: Quebecor World/Taunton

Library of Congress Cataloging-in-Publication Data

Textbook of neurological surgery : principles and practice / editors, H. Hunt Batjer,
Christopher M. Loftus ; illustrations by Thomas H. Weinzerl.
  p. ; cm.
  Includes bibliographical references and index.
  ISBN 0-7817-1271-8 (set)
  1. Nervous system—Surgery. I. Batjer, H. Hunt. II. Loftus, Christopher M.
  [DNLM: 1. Nervous System Diseases—surgery. 2. Nervous System
Diseases—diagnosis. 3. Neurosurgical Procedures. WL 368 T3547 2002]
RD593 .T473 2002
617.4'8—dc21

                                                                2002066108

Care has been taken to confirm the accuracy of the information presented
and to describe generally accepted practices. However, the authors, editors,
and publisher are not responsible for errors or omissions or for any
consequences from application of the information in this book and make no
warranty, expressed or implied, with respect to the currency, completeness, or
accuracy of the contents of the publication. Application of this information in a
particular situation remains the professional responsibility of the practitioner.

The authors, editors, and publisher have exerted every effort to ensure that
drug selection and dosage set forth in this text are in accordance with current
recommendations and practice at the time of publication. However, in view of
ongoing research, changes in government regulations, and the constant flow of
information relating to drug therapy and drug reactions, the reader is urged to
check the package insert for each drug for any change in indications and
dosage and for added warnings and precautions. This is particularly important
when the recommended agent is a new or infrequently employed drug.

Some drugs and medical devices presented in this publication have Food
and Drug Administration (FDA) clearance for limited use in restricted research
settings. It is the responsibility of the health care provider to ascertain the FDA
status of each drug or device planned for use in their clinical practice.

10 9 8 7 6 5 4 3 2 1

Contents

III. Principles of Clinical Neurosurgery
Section Editors: H. Hunt Batjer, Christopher M. Loftus, and Stephen J. Haines

IV. Pediatric Neurosurgery
Section Editor: Frederick A. Boop

VOLUME 2

V. *Neuro-oncology*
Section Editor: Ian E. McCutcheon

VOLUME 3

VII. Peripheral Nerves
Section Editor: Eric L. Zager

VIII. Cerebrovascular Disorders
Section Editor: Robert E. Harbaugh

IX.   *Stereotactic and Functional Surgery*
Section Editor: Jeffrey S. Schweitzer

X. Cranial and Cerebral Trauma
Section Editor: Brian T. Andrews

VOLUME 4

XI. Pain Syndromes and Chronic Pain
Section Editor: Kenneth A. Follett

XII. Neurosurgical Infections
Section Editor: Richard K. Osenbach

XIII. Nonclinical Issues Relevant
to the Neurosurgeon
Section Editors: H. Hunt Batjer and
Christopher M. Loftus

V. Neuro-oncology

Section Editor
Ian E. McCutcheon

98. Basic Brain Tumor Biology: Invasion, Angiogenesis, and Proliferation

Carlos G. Carlotti, Jr.,
Peter B. Dirks, and James T. Rutka

In the past four decades, our understanding of the basic biology of brain tumors has been revolutionized by the application of knowledge in molecular biology to the study of the human genome. When one considers that the structure of deoxyribonucleic acid (DNA) was first determined in 1953 by Watson and Crick, the advances that have taken place in molecular genetics have been no less than meteoric. By 1965, the genetic code had been deciphered such that the information encoded by DNA could be determined at the protein level. Restriction endonucleases, chemical "knives" that cut large segments of DNA into smaller, more manageable fragments, were described by 1968. Techniques of gene transfer were introduced by 1973, and have been greatly improved upon over the past 20 years. Today, gene transfer is readily accomplished using retroviral, adenoviral, and adenoviral-associated vectors. The polymerase chain reaction (PCR) was described in 1983 facilitating the amplification of minute quantities of nucleic acids. By 1986, tumor suppressor genes were described as an important family of genes that protect the host from neoplastic transformation of its normal cellular constituents. Examples of important tumor suppressor genes in brain tumors include p53, p16, neurofibromatosis type 1 (NF1) and NF2. Finally, in the past 5 years, more than 1,000 patients with genetically linked syndromes and cancer have been treated on approved gene therapy protocols illustrating the therapeutic potential of the techniques in molecular biology. In this chapter, we will review the basic biology of human brain tumors. The areas to be covered include cellular proliferation, invasion, and angiogenesis. It can be argued cogently that if we had a greater understanding of these three areas of tumor biology, then we could design novel strategies with which brain tumors could be more effectively treated than is currently possible.

Invasion

Brain invasion has long been recognized as a histopathological hallmark of brain tumors within the central nervous system (CNS) by neurosurgeons and neuropathologists (1). In the past decade, the molecular basis of brain tumor invasion has been elucidated for several different tumor types. Novel pharmacotherapeutic strategies that target the invasiveness of CNS tumors are evolving (2,3). If we had effective treatments that either eliminated or neutralized the migratory tumor cell, one could argue cogently that we would have greater success in treating patients with malignant brain tumors, and preventing local or distant treatment failures.

Brain tumor invasion is a particularly germane pathological process for tumors of the astrocytic lineage. High-grade (glioblastoma multiforme and anaplastic astrocytoma) and low-grade diffuse astrocytomas infiltrate into regions of normal brain rendering complete surgical extirpation difficult, and localized radiation therapy ineffective (4). Glioblastoma multiforme (GBM) is characterized by an area of central necrosis surrounded by a highly cellular rim of viable tumor cells which infiltrate adjacent brain tissue. GBM appears fairly well circumscribed on imaging examinations such as magnetic resonance imaging (MRI) and computed tomography (CT). At the time of surgical resection, however, stereotactic biopsies taken from areas beyond contrast-enhancing tumor have not only showed invading tumor cells, but tissue cultures of these specimens have yielded viable neoplastic cells (1). In addition, there is a high rate of recurrence of GBM along the borders of the resection cavity. Interestingly, in stark contrast to neoplasms that arise outside the CNS, anaplastic astrocytomas rarely, if ever, metastasize systemically. Astrocytoma invasion typically follows a path laid down by blood vessels, basement membrane structures, and myelinated axons (5–7). The high affinity of astrocytoma cells for myelinated tracts explains their spread along the optic radiation, across the corpus callosum or through the anterior commissure.

In general terms, the invasion of normal brain by astrocytoma cells is a complex biological process. It includes (a) the binding of specific cell-surface molecules on the plasma membrane to the extracellular matrix (ECM); (b) the synthesis and depositing of a permissive ECM by tumor cells; (c) the release by the tumor cells of proteases which can degrade ECM components, the interactions between the ECM, cell surface receptors, and the cytoskeleton; and (d) the active translocation of astrocytoma cells through the cerebral ECM (6,8–10) (Fig. 1). The salient contributions of the different elements implicated in brain invasion are described in detail below.

THE ROLE OF THE EXTRACELLULAR MATRIX. The ECM is found in the interstitial spaces of all organs. Its composition varies in different tissues, but it largely comprises a complex set of collagens, noncollagenous glycoproteins, and proteoglycans that help regulate cell migration, survival, differentiation, and axonal pathfinding in the CNS (11–13).

In the CNS, the ECM can vary considerably depending on the anatomical site studied (11,14). In the adult normal brain, a "classic" ECM is limited to the basal lamina of the cerebral vasculature, the glial limitans externa—a well-defined external membrane—which invests the entire cortical surface and separates astrocytic foot processes from the pia-arachnoid cells (11) and the basal lamina which supports choroid plexus epithelial and ependymal cells. In the brain parenchyma, the white and

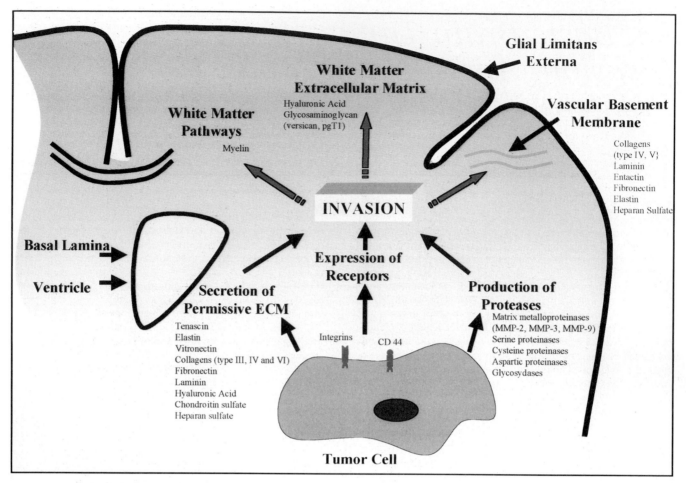

Fig. 1. Schematic of brain tumor invasion throughout the central nervous system (CNS). The CNS is enriched in glycosaminoglycans such as hyaluronic acid and versican. In the white matter, myelin is abundant. A true basal lamina exists at the glial limitans externa, and within vascular basement membranes comprised of collagen types, noncollagenous glycoproteins, and proteoglycans. Brain tumor invasion of normal brain is a function of the production of proteolytic enzymes by tumor cells, the deposition of a permissive matrix through which tumor cells can migrate, and the expression of intrinsic cell surface receptors which recognize extracellular matrix ligands. Inhibiting the process of brain tumor invasion may provide a novel strategy for controlling the spread of tumor cells in the brain.

gray matter are largely free of structural proteins and are mainly composed of glycosaminoglycans (GAGs), of which hyaluronic acid (HA) is the most abundant species (15). GAGs are highly hydrated compounds that are permissive for tumor cell migration.

The interaction between astrocytoma cells and components of the ECM has been studied in some detail. Although astrocytoma cells typically fail to penetrate the vascular basal lamina, they adhere to it and propel themselves along the vascular channels. In other ways, astrocytoma cells create a microenvironment conducive to invasion by synthesizing and depositing a permissive ECM (12). Some of the more commonly found ECM macromolecules found in human astrocytomas includes tenascin, elastin, vitronectin, collagen (III, IV, and VI), fibronectin, laminin, HA, chondroitin sulfate, and heparan sulfate proteoglycans (13,16,17). Laminin, tenascin, and collagen have been shown to serve as permissive substrates for glioma cell migration, whereas fibronectin and vitronectin do not (5).

MYELIN AS A SUBSTRATE FOR INVASION. One well-known pathway of astrocytoma invasion is along white matter tracts (5). Interestingly, myelin has been shown to be a very

inhibitory substrate for neurite outgrowth as well as for spreading and migration of astrocytoma cells. A high–molecular-weight myelin protein (NI-220/250/IN-1 antigen) plays a crucial role for this inhibitory property of myelin (18). Recently MT1-MMP, a membrane-type metalloproteinase, has been shown to play an important role in remodeling the nonpermissive CNS myelin substrate into a permissive one thus allowing for infiltration of astrocytoma cells (18).

CELL SURFACE RECEPTORS RECOGNIZE KEY EXTRA-CELLULAR MATRIX MACROMOLECULES. Cell surface adhesion molecules are crucial for the migratory process, as they couple interactions with the ECM proteins on the extracellular face of the cell membrane to the cytoskeletal apparatus inside the cell (19). The most important molecules involved in this process are the integrins (20,21), HA-binding proteins such as CD44 and RHAMM, elastin binding protein (EBP), and cell adhesion molecules such as N-CAM and I-CAM (9).

The integrins are a family of transmembrane proteins that contain a large extracellular domain, a hydrophobic membrane spanning segment, and a short cytoplasmic domain. Each integrin is composed of one of 16 α subunits variously associated with one of the 8 β subunits to form more than 20 receptors with distinct ligands (22). Integrins recognize specific peptide regions within various ECM macromolecules, of which the best characterized is the arginine-glycine-aspartic (RGD) sequence of fibronectin. Upon binding to extracellular ligands, integrins cluster on the plane of the plasma membrane and promote the assembly of molecular complexes containing both cytoskeletal and signaling elements. Although the integrin signaling pathways have not been completely characterized, many involve phosphorylation of neighboring proteins such as focal adhesion kinase (FAK), protein kinase C (PKC), Src, and mitogen-activated protein kinase (MAPK) (22–24).

CD44 is a membrane glycoprotein implicated in cell–cell adhesion, cell attachment to ECM, cell migration, tumor growth, and metastasis (19). It is the principal cell surface receptor for HA. CD44 is highly expressed in astrocytomas and astrocytoma cell lines (25). Expression of CD44 has been shown to correlate with the invasiveness of astrocytoma tumor cells. Interestingly, unlike metastatic tumors to the brain that express predominantly variant forms of CD44, astrocytomas typically express the standard form.

THE CYTOSKELETON: THE MOTOR FOR ASTROCYTOMA MIGRATION. The morphological appearance of normal human astrocytes is in part due to the structure imposed by the cytoskeleton. The cytoskeleton of the astrocyte contains all three major protein networks described in eukaryotic cells including the actin microfilaments (6 nm), the glial-specific intermediate filaments (8 to 12 nm), and the microtubules (20 nm). Glial fibrillary acidic protein (GFAP), a glial-specific intermediate filament, is the most specific marker for cells of astrocytic lineage under normal and pathological conditions. With increasing astrocytic malignancy, there is progressive loss of GFAP production (26). GFAP maintains astrocyte cell shape through interactions between glial filaments, the nuclear membrane, and the plasma membrane (27).

Cell motility is a function of the development of pseudopodia and lamellae, which adhere to the ECM and provide traction forces that propel the cell forward. These structures are intimately related to actin filament formation and dissolution, and require the interaction between actin, actin binding proteins, and cell surface receptors such as the integrins and cell adhesion molecules.

PROTEINASES. The proteolytic degradation of the ECM by proteases is an important step for tumor cell invasion in physiological and pathological processes. Several proteases are involved in the degradation of ECM including the matrix metalloproteinases (MMPs), serine proteinases (urokinase and tissue plasminogen activators), cysteine proteinases (cathepsin B and S), aspartic proteinases (cathepsin D), and glycosidases (28,29). MMPs require the binding of a zinc ion at the active site, hence the "metallo" prefix. The other proteases are characterized by specific amino acid sequences that are critical to their catalytic function (10).

MMPs play a major role in the process of invasion by human brain tumors (10,30,31). The cysteine and serine proteinases have also been implicated. At least 14 members of the MMP family have been identified and can be named and classified either according to their substrate specificity (e.g., collagenases, gelatinases, stromelysins, and membrane-type MMPs), or according to standard nomenclature forms (e.g., MMP-1, MMP-2). The regulation of MMPs is complex, but at least three mechanisms have been described including control at the transcriptional level, proenzyme activation by selective proteolysis, and

inhibition by tissue inhibitors of metalloproteinase (TIMPs) (32).

In tumors of the CNS, relatively high levels of MMPs have been identified in high-grade astrocytomas and much lower levels in low-grade astrocytomas. In high-grade astrocytomas, MMP-2 (gelatinase-A), MMP-9 (gelatinase-B), and MMP-3 (stromelysin-1) are upregulated (33–36). The TIMPs are also upregulated in high-grade gliomas, probably due to the excess action of the MMPs. Interestingly, overexpression of TIMP-1 in an invasive astrocytoma cell line has been shown to inhibit astrocytoma invasiveness (37).

Cathepsin B, a cysteine proteinase, is also expressed in astrocytomas. Expression appears to correlate with the degree of invasiveness of these cells. Cathepsin B is seen in the infiltrating tumor cells and proliferative vascular endothelium at the tumor margin (38).

Plasminogen activators (PAs) are a group of serine proteinases that convert plasminogen into the active proteolytic enzyme plasmin. This system plays an important role in tumor invasion by initiating pericellular proteolysis of the ECM. There is a high level of expression of the urokinase-type plasminogen activator (u-PA) in human gliomas and this correlates with tumor grade (39,40).

Angiogenesis

During embryogenesis, blood vessels develop by two processes: vasculogenesis, whereby endothelial cells are derived from progenitor cell types; and angiogenesis, in which new capillaries sprout from existing vessels (41–44). In the fully differentiated adult state, it was previously thought that new vessels were produced only through angiogenesis. However, it is now known that vasculogenesis can also occur by the recruitment of endothelial progenitor cells from the peripheral circulation in the adult to contribute to neovascularization (45,46). In general, the vascular bed is fairly quiescent in the normal adult mammal, except in some physiological situations such as the female reproductive cycle including ovulation, menstruation, implantation, and pregnancy, and in pathological processes such as wound healing, neovascular glaucoma, arthritis, diabetic retinopathy, and neoplasia (42,43). Interestingly, endothelial cells are among those with the longest life in the body outside the CNS (41). Yet, in response to an appropriate stimulus, this quiescent vasculature can become activated to grow new capillaries (42).

This process of angiogenesis is complex. The basement membrane that surrounds the endothelial cell tube is locally degraded, and the endothelial cells underlying this regional disruption in the barrier change shape and invade into surrounding stroma. Platelets adhere to tumor vessels and release angiogenesis stimulators (47). Degradation of the ECM is an essential component of the new vessel invasion, and it is facilitated by an alteration in the balance between proteolytic enzymes and their known endogenous inhibitors. Cell substrate receptors such as the integrins promote vascular cell migration through interactions with proteins of the ECM including collagen types and fibronectin. This process of endothelial cell invasion is accompanied by proliferation of endothelial cells at the leading edge of what becomes a migrating column. A region of differentiation trails behind the advancing front where the endothelial cells cease proliferating, change shape, and tightly adhere to each other to form a lumen of a new capillary tube. Finally, sprouting tubes fuse and coalesce into loops, circulating the blood into this newly vascularized region (Fig. 2). The pericytes

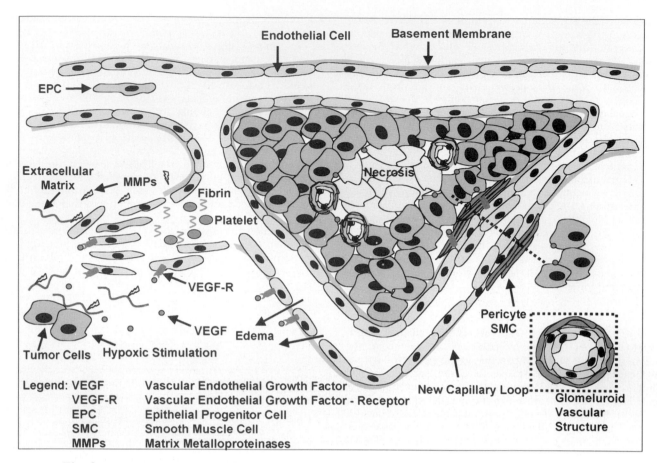

Fig. 2. The process of tumor angiogenesis. Tumor cells secrete vascular endothelial growth factor (VEGF) and attract epithelial progenitor cells following hypoxic stimulation and surrounding areas of necrosis. Newly formed vascular channels form glomeruloid structures that grow and coalesce to provide a network of vasculature to the tumor. The spread of tumor cells to surrounding regions sets up another focus of neovascularization. The roles of vascular VEGF, VEGF receptors, matrix metalloproteinases, smooth muscle cells, and the hematogenous elements are shown.

and smooth muscle cells are formed by differentiation of mesenchymal cells (42,43).

Growth of a tumor beyond 2 to 3 mm³ requires development of a microvessel network to facilitate delivery of nutrients and oxygen, and removal of catabolites (48). This is made possible by continuous growth of new blood vessels. The study of angiogenesis in experimental models of multistage tumorigenesis shows that angiogenesis occurs in early stages of tumor development (43,49), including brain tumors (50,51). Angiogenesis is regulated by well-characterized inducers and inhibitors. The first inducer to be discovered was basic fibroblast growth factor (FGF-2). Since its discovery, many others have been reported and studied such as acidic fibroblast growth factor (FGF-1), vascular endothelial growth factor (VEGF), VEGF-B, and VEGF-C. These inducers, in a paracrine mechanism, bind to receptors on endothelial cells that are transmembrane tyrosine kinases and thus are coupled through the signal transduction cascade to the cellular regulatory network.

Several endogenous angiogenic inhibitors have been described, the first of which were α-interferon and platelet factor-4. These compounds can inhibit endothelial cell chemotaxis and proliferation, respectively. The single most important discovery in this field was the identification of cryptic angiogenesis inhibitors within larger proteins. The first was a 29-kd fragment of fibronectin. Two new inhibitors have received special attention. The first was angiostatin, described in 1994 as a fragment

of plasminogen with a molecular weight of 38 kd (52). The second was endostatin, described by the same group, as a fragment of collagen XVIII with a molecular weight of 20 kd (53). Interestingly, angiostatin and endostatin were found using the same strategy within different tumor types. Angiostatin was discovered as a circulating tumor inhibitor that was identified after it was determined that the removal of certain primary tumors is often followed by the growth of distant metastases (52). Endostatin was isolated from a murine hemangioendothelioma cell line (53).

Based on the known mechanisms of angiogenesis, several therapeutic approaches have been developed to block the process of angiogenesis in neoplasia. These include blocking the release of angiogenic factors (54), inactivation of angiogenic factors or their receptors (55,56), inhibition of degradation of the basement membrane (57), inhibition of degradation of the ECM (57), inhibition of migration and proliferation of the endothelial cells (58,59), inhibition of the three-dimensional organization of microvessels (41), and various combined strategies (60).

ANGIOGENESIS IN HUMAN BRAIN TUMORS. Research in angiogenesis in the field of neuro-oncology has focused primarily on astrocytomas (61–63) and meningiomas (64–66). With respect to the astrocytomas, diffuse astrocytomas, classified as low-grade diffuse astrocytoma (World Health Organization, or WHO, grade II), anaplastic astrocytoma (WHO grade III), and GBM (WHO grade IV) have been the most commonly studied.

Interestingly, characteristics of the tumor microvasculature have often been used by neuropathologists to grade astrocytomas. With the progression from low-grade to high-grade astrocytic neoplasms, one observes an increased vessel density. In GBM, a robust microvascular proliferation occurs. This often takes the form of glomeruloid vascular structures, which are most commonly located in the vicinity of necrosis and in the peripheral infiltration zone (1).

The paradigm of the balance of angiogenic factors with activators and inhibitors has been investigated in some detail in human brain tumors. VEGF is considered one of the most important mediators of neovascularization and edema formation in human gliomas (67–72). In the normal human brain, VEGF has either not been detected or has been detected only in scattered astroglial cells (73,74). In low-grade gliomas, low levels of VEGF have been observed, and a quantitative assessment of VEGF expression in these tumors shows correlation with future malignant transformation of the tumor and the survival time of the patients (75). In glioblastoma, strong expression of VEGF is found in tumor cells but not in endothelial cells. Interestingly, high levels of VEGF are also observed in regions of pseudopalisading tumor cells surrounding areas of necrosis (74) as well as in glioma cells infiltrating into regions of normal brain (73). Some of these patterns of VEGF expression likely reflect stimulation by regional ischemia.

With respect to the VEGF receptors (VEGFR), little or no VEGFR-1 is detected in normal brain, or in low-grade gliomas. However, VEGFR-1 is significantly upregulated in the vasculature of high-grade gliomas, particularly GBM (67,73,74). VEGFR-2 is not detected in normal brain or low-grade astrocytomas, but is upregulated in anaplastic astrocytoma and GBM (67). Both receptors have been found expressed at the infiltrating margin of the tumor.

Tie-1 and Tie-2 (tek) are members of the other family of endothelial cell-specific receptors (76). The ligand for the Tie-1 receptor has not yet been found. However, angiopoetin-1 and angiopoetin-2 have been shown to be ligands for Tie-2. While Tie-2 is expressed in vascular endothelial cells of normal brain, it is upregulated in endothelial cells of astrocytomas. Angiopoetin-1 has either faint or no expression in normal brain and low-grade gliomas and is upregulated in high-grade gliomas. Angiopoetin-2 is either weakly expressed or not expressed at all in normal brain but is expressed in endothelial cells within GBM. These findings suggest that angiopoetin-1 acts synergistically with angiopoetin-2 to promote glioblastoma angiogenesis (77).

Other angiogenic stimulatory factors important in gliomagenesis include basic FGF (78) which is expressed at the same level in low-grade and high-grade gliomas (79), platelet-derived endothelial cell growth factor (PD-ECGF) (80), endothelin-1 (81), and hepatocyte growth factor/scatter factor (HGF/SF) which is upregulated in high-grade gliomas (79,82).

In meningiomas, VEGF is also upregulated (73,83), but the levels are lower than in GBM. Meningiomas with strong VEGF expression show a significantly higher peritumoral edema and also an increased vascularity in both leptomeningeal and cerebral vessels. These discoveries can be explained by VEGF induction of proliferation across the arachnoid barrier into the tumor and increased permeability of cerebral vessels around the tumor (64–66). VEGFR-1, VEGFR-2, and Tie have also been detected, but again at lower levels than in GBM.

The synthetic glucocorticoid dexamethasone, which is used to treat peritumoral edema in brain tumors has been shown to significantly downregulate VEGF expression *in vitro* (84). The inhibition of angiogenesis in brain tumors is a potentially exciting new avenue of therapy for GBM. The inhibition of angiogenesis in brain tumors has been done not only *in vitro* but also *in vivo*. Glioma cells implanted subcutaneously or intracranially in nude mice are suppressed by antibodies against basic FGF (56) or by angiostatin (85). As encouraging as these data seem, these results should be interpreted with caution because in animal glioma models, diffuse infiltration by tumor cells is rarely observed, and there is a theoretical increased rate of angiogenesis compared to the original human astrocytoma.

Proliferation

During the lifetime of an individual, cell proliferation normally occurs in different physiological situations, but the loss of control over this process becomes pathological in neoplasia. Indeed, one of the hallmarks of neoplasia is unregulated cell proliferation. Other hallmark features of neoplasia include loss of the differentiated phenotype, tumor cell invasion, angiogenesis, and metastasis. To understand the alterations in the proliferation of tumors of the CNS, it is necessary to first have a basic knowledge of the normal cell cycle. In the past decade, there has been a tremendous increase in knowledge of the regulation of the molecular cell-cycle machinery. Many of the genes involved in cell-cycle regulation have perturbed expression in cancer suggesting that they may also function as oncogenes or tumor suppressor genes (86–89). Studies of the function of these genes *in vivo* in transgenic mice or in knockout mice supports the notion that proper regulation of the cell cycle is essential for suppression of neoplasia.

THE NORMAL CELL CYCLE. A proliferating cell passes through an orderly unidirectional sequence of phases that comprise the cell cycle (Fig. 3) (90–95). Cell-cycle phases are exquisitely regulated to ensure that two identical daughter cells are produced with identical DNA content. In this way, a cell is instructed to replicate its chromosomal material only once and to complete DNA synthesis before mitosis. Any mistakes in the fidelity of the highly ordered cell cycle could lead to errors causing death of the cell or propagation of those errors into the daughter cells (90–97). Cell-cycle transitions are dependent in part upon the activity of enzymes called cyclin-dependent kinases (see the following section) (98–101). Intrinsic and extrinsic signals which determine whether a cell is to proliferate or stop proliferating are integrated through the activity of the cell cycle-regulated cyclin-dependent kinases.

The terminal phase of differentiation of a cell or the state of quiescence is called G_0. Quiescent cells can reenter the cell cycle when given appropriate stimuli such as growth factors. Terminally differentiated cells are refractory to proliferative induction by growth factor stimulation. When a cell enters the cell cycle, there is initially a phase of increase in cell size and protein synthesis (G_1 phase). During G_1 phase, the cell is still capable of responding to environmental signals (such as the presence of extracellular growth factors or proper adhesion to the ECM) which help the cell to determine whether the situation is favorable for division into two daughter cells (87,88,98–103). Inhibition of protein synthesis, withdrawal of growth factors, loss of cell adhesion to ECM, or the presence of close cell–cell contact can cause a cell in G_1 to revert back into a quiescent state, or can prevent a cell in a quiescent state from entering into the cell division cycle. Late in G_1 phase, the cell passes a point called the restriction point after which a cell will irreversibly progress through mitosis in the absence of growth factors or cell adhesion (91,103,104).

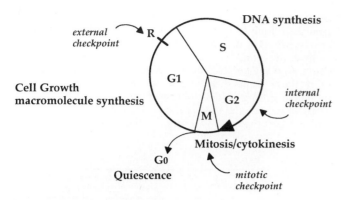

Fig. 3. A proliferating cell passes through an ordinary sequence of phases that comprise the cell cycle. Cell cycle phases are exquisitely regulated to ensure that two identical daughter cells are produced with identical DNA content. The terminal phase of differentiation of a cell or the state of quiescence is called G_0. Quiescent cells can reenter the cell cycle when given appropriate stimuli such as growth factors. When a cell enters the cell cycle, there is initially a phase of increase in cell size and protein synthesis (G_1 phase). Late in G_1 phase the cell passes a point called the restriction point. This is an important checkpoint, where the cell ensures that extracellular conditions are adequate for the generation of two daughter cells. In G_1 the cell also checks for and repairs DNA damage. The cell will arrest in G_1 if conditions are not appropriate. If the cell passes through the G_1 restriction point, it will irreversibly progress through mitosis in the absence of growth factors or cell adhesion. After G_1 phase, a phase of DNA synthesis known as S phase occurs. The entire complement of the cell's DNA is duplicated in preparation for segregation into two daughter cells. G_2 phase is the short gap that precedes mitosis, and during this phase the fidelity of DNA replication is checked. During mitosis, the DNA and cytoplasmic material is separated. Another important checkpoint ensures that the chromosomes are properly attached to the spindle apparatus prior to anaphase when chromosomes are actually separated. Mitotic phase is completed when division of the cytoplasm in cytokinesis occurs.

Aberrant signals that lead to a bypass of the restriction point can allow a cell to acquire some features of a cancer cell, such as the ability to proliferate in absence of growth factors and the loss of contact inhibition of cell proliferation (96,97,105). After G_1 phase, a phase of DNA synthesis known as S phase occurs. The entire complement of the cell's DNA is duplicated in preparation for segregation into two daughter cells. G_2 phase is the short gap that precedes mitosis, and during this phase the fidelity of DNA replication is checked (106). During mitosis, the DNA and cytoplasmic material are separated (107,108). Another important checkpoint ensures that the chromosomes are properly attached to the spindle apparatus prior to anaphase, when chromosomes are actually separated (103). Mitotic phase is completed when division of the cytoplasm in cytokinesis occurs.

CYCLINS AND CYCLIN-DEPENDENT KINASES. Cyclins are a group of proteins that share a conserved 100 amino-acid domain (called the cyclin box) and were discovered to participate in cell-cycle control because their levels oscillate dramatically with specific phases of the cell cycle (Fig. 4) (100,101, 109–111). The cyclins are a regulatory subunit of proteins called cyclin-dependent kinases (CDKs), which cause phosphorylation of specific substrates. Cyclins bind to CDKs as well as to some CDK substrates determining timing of CDK activity as well as substrate specificity. Cyclin protein levels are determined by activation of gene transcription as well as precisely controlled proteolytic degradation. There are two main classes of cyclins,

G_1 cyclins and mitotic cyclins. G_1 cyclins consist of D-cyclins (D1, D2, D3) and cyclin E which are expressed during G_1 phases of the cell cycle, and when assembled with their CDK partners contribute to control of passage through the critical G_1 restriction committing a cell to divide. Cyclin A plays a role in the initiation and continuation of DNA synthesis. Mitosis is regulated by a combination of cyclin A and cyclin B.

The D-type cyclins in particular are induced in response to a diversity of mitogenic signals, suggesting that they play a special role in transducing extracellular growth stimulatory signals to the cell-cycle machinery (102,109,112). Growth factors exert their proliferative effects via altering the activity of cyclins and CDKs. Cyclin D1 has been shown to be an important transcriptional target for growth factor signals mediated by receptor tyrosine kinases and the Ras pathway but also is activated by proliferative signals mediated by steroid receptors and G-proteins (Fig. 5) (113). Cyclin D1 expression is induced in response to mitogenic stimulation and it is then assembled with a CDK. Cyclin D1-CDK activity allows for progression through G_1 phase of the cell cycle. Cyclin E expression is sharply associated with G_1-S transition, and together with cyclin A, it allows for initiation of DNA synthesis. D-cyclins complex mainly with the cyclin-dependent kinases CDK4 or CDK6 and their activity precedes that of cyclin E-CDK2 and cyclin A-CDK2 at G_1-S transition (Fig. 6). The mitotic cyclins, cyclins A and B, are involved in the initiation of mitosis through interaction with CDK1. The dual function of cyclin A in S and M phases may be important for sequentially linking these two phases together. Most cyclins have been found to be aberrantly expressed in some types of cancer.

The particular substrates of cyclin–CDK complexes are determined by the cyclins (99). Cyclin D-associated complexes have few substrates (pRb-family proteins, see below) but the other G_1 cyclins E and A are more promiscuous in their ability to phosphorylate cellular proteins (114–116). Cyclin E-CDK complexes phosphorylate proteins involved in DNA replication, p27 CDK inhibitor, and E2F transcription factors in addition to pRb family members. The main targets of G_1 cyclin–CDK complexes are thought to be the retinoblastoma family proteins (pRb, p107, and p130). pRb is the protein product of the tumor suppressor gene initially discovered in familial retinoblastomas, whose dys-

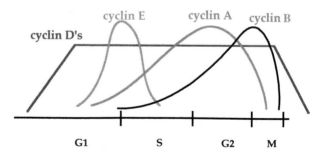

Fig. 4. Cyclins are a group of proteins discovered to participate in cell-cycle control because their levels oscillate dramatically with specific phases of the cell cycle. The cyclins are a regulatory subunit of cyclin-dependent kinases (CDKs), which cause phosphorylation of specific substrates. Cyclins bind to CDKs as well as to some CDK substrates and determine timing of CDK activity as well as substrate specificity. Cyclin protein levels are determined by activation of gene transcription as well as precisely controlled proteolytic degradation. There are two main classes of cyclins, G_1 cyclins and mitotic cyclins. G_1 cyclins consist of D-cyclins (D1, D2, D3) and cyclin E which are expressed during G_1 phases of the cell cycle. D- and E-cyclins contribute to control of passage through the critical G_1 restriction committing a cell to divide. Cyclin A plays a role in the initiation and continuation of DNA synthesis. Mitosis is regulated by a combination of cyclin A and cyclin B.

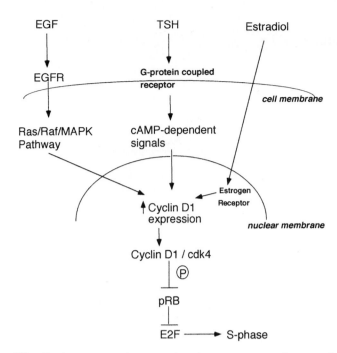

Fig. 5. The D-type cyclins are induced in response to a diversity of mitogenic signals, suggesting that they play a special role in transducing extracellular growth stimulatory signals to the cell-cycle machinery. Cyclin D1 has been shown to be an important transcriptional target for growth factor signals mediated by receptor tyrosine kinases and the Ras pathway but also is activated from proliferative signals mediated by steroid receptors and G-proteins.

function also plays an important role in many other human cancers. pRb restrains cell proliferation in part by binding to and inhibiting transcription factors known as E2Fs (discussed subsequently) (115,117–119). Sequential phosphorylation of pRb family proteins by cyclin D-CDK4 or CDK6 followed by cyclin E-CDK2 and cyclin A-CDK2 complexes impairs the ability of pRb to bind to E2F, which is then free to activate transcription of genes critical for the onset of S phase (Fig. 7).

Overexpression of cyclin D1 and cyclin E in cell cultures or in transgenic mice contributes to neoplastic transformation of the cultured cells and tumor formation in mice, supporting the hypothesis that loss of cell-cycle control, through dysregulated expression of critical cell-cycle genes, contributes to tumor formation (120,121). Also, overexpression of cyclin A in some cell types *in vitro* leads to loss of dependence on cell adhesion for continued cell proliferation, enabling the cell to acquire another characteristic of a neoplastic cell (122,123). Mitotic cyclin–CDK complexes phosphorylate structural proteins in the cell allowing for segregation of replicated DNA material and cytoplasm into two new daughter cells (124–126).

CYCLIN-DEPENDENT KINASE INHIBITORS. The activity of cyclin–CDK complexes is precisely regulated through a complex combination of processes and feedback mechanisms involving gene transcription, protein phosphorylation (stimulatory or inhibitory), protein degradation (mainly dependent on ubiquitin-dependent proteolysis), protein compartmentalization (by shuttling from cytoplasm to nucleus), and association with specific inhibitory proteins called cyclin-dependent kinase inhibitors (CKIs) (116,124–128). The CKIs bind to cyclin–CDK complexes and inhibit their ability to phosphorylate their substrates and as a result arrest cell proliferation. This property has made all these proteins potential tumor suppressor genes, as

inactivation of the CKIs is associated with tumor formation. There are two families of CKIs, the p21^{Cip1}-like family (Cip-Kip family), which also includes p27^{Kip1} and p57^{Kip2}, that regulates multiple cyclin–CDK complexes (including those containing CDK1, CDK2, CDK4, CDK6), and the p16^{Ink4a}-like Ink family, which includes p15^{Ink4b}, p18^{Ink4c}, and p19^{Ink4d}, that is more restricted to inhibition of cyclin–CDK4 or cyclin–CDK6 complexes (Fig. 8). These two families of CKIs transduce intrinsic or extrinsic growth inhibitory signals to the cell-cycle machinery. p21^{Cip1} is induced by the tumor suppressor protein p53 following DNA damage (an intrinsic inhibitory signal), and p27^{Kip1} or p15^{Ink4b} are induced after treatment of cells with the extracellular factor, tumor growth factor-β. p27^{Kip1} is also induced as a result of contact inhibition. It is not clear what signals are transduced by the CKI p16^{Ink4a}. p16^{Ink4a} may play an important role in slowing of proliferation in aged cells as it is highly expressed in senescent cells. It may also play a role in cell-cycle arrest after DNA damage (129).

Loss of expression of some of the CKIs has been demonstrated in human cancers, particularly p16^{Ink4a}, which is homozygously deleted in many different human tumors, including melanomas, pancreatic adenocarcinomas. and malignant astrocytomas (130). p16^{Ink4a} is mutated in the germline in some families with hereditary melanoma. p21^{Cip1} expression is diminished with loss of function of the tumor suppressor gene p53. Knockout of expression of the CKIs p16^{Ink4a}, p18^{Ink4c}, and p27^{Kip1} leads to tumor formation in mice and knockout of p27^{Kip1}7 and p57^{Kip2} also profoundly affects tissue growth and development (131–136). Clearly, CKIs play an important role in normal tissue development and in proper restraint of cell proliferation in normal cells, and loss of their activity contributes to tumor formation. Loss of CKI expression in cancer is thought to lead to enhanced cyclin–CDK function, enabling cells to progress unimpeded through the cell cycle.

RETINOBLASTOMA AND E2F-DP FAMILY. pRb is the most well-known and best understood gene in a family composed of two other related genes, p107 and p130 (117,137,138). Each protein binds to E2F proteins, each is phosphorylated by cyclin–CDK complexes, and each is a target for binding and inactivation by DNA tumor virus oncoproteins (such as large T anti-

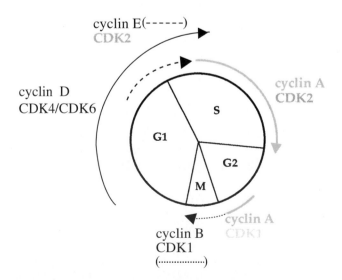

Fig. 6. Cyclins associate with different cyclin-dependent kinases (CDKs) at different phases of the cell cycle. Cyclins determine the timing and the substrate specificity of the CDK.

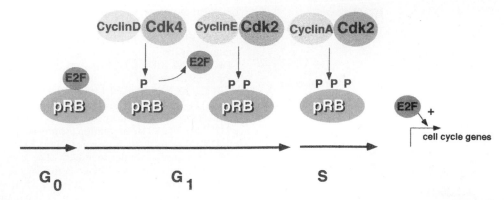

Fig. 7. The main targets of G_1 cyclin-dependent kinase (CDK) complexes are thought to be the retinoblastoma family proteins. pRb restrains cell proliferation in part by binding to and inhibiting transcription factors known as E2Fs (see text). Sequential phosphorylation of pRb family proteins by cyclin D-CDK4 followed by cyclin E-CDK2 and cyclin A-CDK2 complexes impairs the ability of pRb to bind to E2F which is then free to activate transcription of genes critical for the onset of S-phase and cell-cycle progression.

gen from SV40 virus and E7 from human papilloma virus). pRb is mutated in the germline of patients with hereditary retinoblastoma, but mutations of the other pRb family proteins have not been identified in human cancer. Heterozygous knockout of the pRb gene leads to tumor formation in mice (139).

As stated, phosphorylation of pRb family proteins by cyclin–CDKs is thought to be important for emergence of cells from quiescence and progression through G_1 phase of the cell cycle (115,118). In a hypophosphorylated form, the pRb family proteins have very high affinity for the transcription factor E2F. Hypophosphorylated pRb-E2F complexes actively inhibit transcription of genes for cell-cycle progression. The phosphorylation of pRb proteins by cyclin–CDKs alters their ability to bind to E2F, enabling "free E2F" to drive the cell through G_1 phase into S phase. Free E2F acts as a timely transcriptional activator, inducing expression of genes involved in cell proliferation and

DNA replication (Fig. 9). Efficiency of E2F transcriptional activation is improved by binding to a partner protein called DP. To date, six E2F genes and two DP genes have been found. Loss of pRb function through mutation or through binding of proteins from tumor promoting viruses (via specific binding to an LxCxE amino-acid sequence on pRb) leads to inappropriate free E2F activity which stimulates cell-cycle progression.

In cell culture, E2F overexpression alone enables a cell to progress into S phase in the absence of mitogenic signals, suggesting that the regulation of E2F activity is at the heart of a cell's commitment to DNA replication and cell division (140–143). E2F overexpression also enhances neoplastic transformation suggesting that these factors can behave as oncoproteins (141,144). However, knockout of E2F1 in transgenic mice surprisingly leads to tumor formation, suggesting that pRb-E2F function is highly complex, and E2F factors are also required for

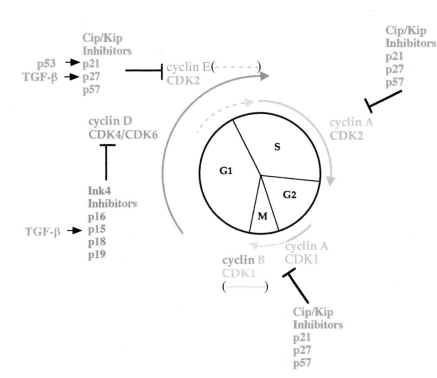

Fig. 8. The activity of cyclin–cyclin-dependent kinase (CDK) complexes is regulated in part by association with specific inhibitory proteins called cyclin-dependent kinase inhibitors (CKIs). The CKIs bind to cyclin–CDK complexes and inhibit their ability to phosphorylate their substrates and as a result arrest cell proliferation. This property has made all these proteins potential tumor suppressor genes, as inactivation of the CKIs is associated with tumor formation. There are two families of CKIs—the p21[Cip1]-like family (Cip-Kip family) which also includes p27[Kip1] and p57[Kip2], that regulates multiple cyclin–CDK complexes (including those containing CDK1, CDK2, CDK4, CDK6) and the p16[Ink4a]-like Ink family, which includes p15[Ink4b], p18[Ink4c], and p19[Ink4d], that is more restricted to inhibition of cyclin–CDK4 or cyclin–CDK6 complexes. These two families of CKIs transduce intrinsic or extrinsic growth inhibitory signals to the cell-cycle machinery. p21[Cip1] is induced by the tumor suppressor protein p53 following DNA damage (an intrinsic inhibitory signal), and p27[Kip1] or p15[Ink4b] are induced after treatment of cells with the extracellular factor tumor growth factor-β. p27[Kip1] is also induced as a result of contact inhibition. It is not clear what signals are transduced by the CKI p16[Ink4a].

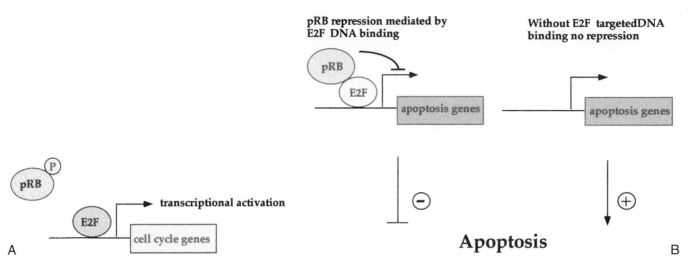

pRB repression mediated by
E2F DNA binding

Without E2F targetedDNA
binding no repression

Fig. 9. The function of pRb is regulated by phosphorylation. The state of pRb phosphorylation also determines whether there is repression or activation of transcription at E2F promoter sites. **A:** The phosphorylation of pRb proteins by cyclin–cyclin-dependent kinases alters their ability to bind to E2F, enabling "free E2F" to drive the cell through the cell cycle. Free E2F acts as a timely transcriptional activator, inducing expression of genes involved in cell proliferation and DNA replication. **B:** Hypophosphorylated pRb-E2F complexes actively inhibit transcription of genes for cell-cycle progression or inhibit genes that promote cell death.

proper pRb-mediated repression of gene expression of tumor promoting factors (145,146).

THE SPECIAL CASE OF THE INK4A LOCUS IN GROWTH CONTROL. Homozygous deletion or loss of heterozygosity at chromosome locus 9p21 is a frequent occurrence in many types of human tumors (130,147). p16^{Ink4a} is found at this locus as well as the related CKI p15^{Ink4b} (separated by 35 kilobases). Both genes may be the targets for genetic alterations at this locus. In addition, it has recently been found that the p16^{Ink4a} locus has an unusual genomic structure that encodes for a separate unrelated cell-cycle inhibitor (p19^{ARF}—ARF stands for alternate reading frame) through alternative splicing of a single exon (148–150). p16^{Ink4a} is encoded by three exons 1α, 2, and 3. A separate exon 13 to 20 kilobases upstream, called 1β, is spliced to the shared exons 2 and 3 of p16 and results in a different reading frame for exons 2 and 3, specifying a completely distinct protein, p19^{ARF} (Fig. 10). Induction of expression of p19^{ARF} causes a G_1 and G_2 cell-cycle arrest not associated with CDKs. It is now known that p19^{ARF} functions to stabilize p53 through direct interaction or via inhibition of a protein called mdm2 which functions to degrade p53. p19^{ARF} can be induced by oncoproteins such as c-myc, adenoviral E1a, or E2F-1 to cause p53-dependent cell-cycle arrest and induction of apoptosis. In this way an aberrant proliferative signal provided by an oncoprotein can be held in check through a p53-dependent pathway. Knockout of p19^{ARF} has also been shown to cause tumor formation in mice suggesting that it also is a true tumor suppressor (151).

Thus, the Ink4a locus, which encodes for two distinct proteins, functions in growth control mediated by two different pathways (Fig. 10) (150). p16^{Ink4a}, through CDK inhibition allows pRb to properly function and restrain the activity of E2Fs, and p19^{ARF} through stabilization of the p53 protein enables cell-cycle arrest and induction of cell death. Genetic alterations in tumors at the 9p21 locus therefore disrupts cell-cycle control through two different mechanisms. A pathway involving p16-cyclin D-CDK4-pRb-E2F enables proper growth restraint in G_1 phase of the cell cycle. The importance of this pathway is high-

lighted by the fact that alteration in the expression of a single member of this pathway is found in almost every cancer, through deletion of p16^{Ink4a} or pRb, or overexpression of cyclin D1 and CDK4. Loss of p16^{Ink4a} through deletion at the Ink4a locus leads to unrestrained cyclin D-CDK4 function leading to increase phosphorylation of pRb and unrestrained E2F transcriptional activity causing cell-cycle progression. However, in addition, loss at the Ink4a locus leads to loss of protection from the growth-promoting signals of oncogenes through p19^{ARF}. Loss of p19^{ARF} allows mdm2 to promote p53 degradation, diminishing the protective apoptotic effects (and tumor-suppressing ability) of p53 in response to aberrant growth-promoting signals.

P53. p53 is a tumor-suppressor gene and one of the most intensely studied human genes in the last decade. p53 mutations are found in approximately 50% of all human cancers, including brain tumors (152,153). Germline mutation of p53 occurs in the hereditary cancer syndrome described by Li and Fraumeni and knockout of the gene causes tumor formation in mice (1,139, 154,155). The p53 protein, like pRb-family proteins, is also a target for inactivation by viral oncoproteins such as SV40 large T-antigen, human papilloma virus E6 protein, and adenovirus E1a (156). Thus, p53 is also an important target for these tumor-promoting viruses to allow them to harness the cell's proliferative and survival machinery.

The p53 protein is normally present at low levels in the cell, but can be upregulated by a diverse array of insults to the cell such as DNA damage (from irradiation), hypoxia, or deregulated cell-cycle progression caused by activated oncogenes (157,158) (Fig. 11). In response to these stresses, p53 induces the transcription of genes leading to cell-cycle arrest and/or cell death. p53 thus has a role as a sensor, transducing the many different inputs into adaptive processes preventing propagation of DNA damage to daughter cells. p53 also plays a role in sensing damage to the mitotic spindle and preventing subsequent re-replication of DNA (159,160). A recent study suggests that it is likely that p53 has many other effects, such as alteration of cell adhesion and of the cell cytoskeleton, induction of secretion

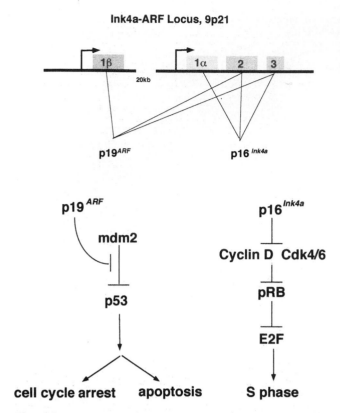

Ink4a-ARF Locus, 9p21

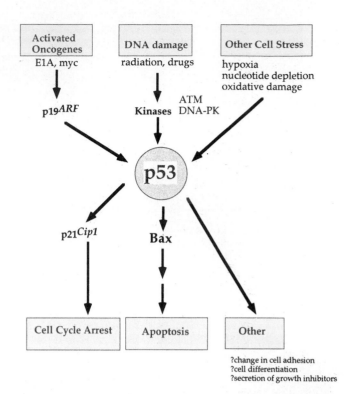

?change in cell adhesion
?cell differentiation
?secretion of growth inhibitors

Fig. 10. Homozygous deletion or loss of heterozygosity at chromosome locus 9p21 is a frequent occurrence in many human tumors. The 9p21 locus has an unusual genomic structure in that it encodes for a separate unrelated cell-cycle inhibitor (p19^{ARF}—ARF, alternate reading frame) through alternative splicing of a single exon in addition to the cyclin kinase inhibitor p16^{Ink4a}. p16^{Ink4a} is encoded by three exons 1α, 2, and 3. A separate exon 13 to 20 kilobases upstream, called 1β, is spliced to the shared exons 2 and 3 of p16 and results in a different reading frame for exons 2 and 3, specifying a completely distinct protein, p19^{ARF}. p19^{ARF} functions to stabilize the tumor suppressor p53 through direct interaction or via inhibition of a protein called mdm2 which functions to degrade p53. p53 is thus allowed to function to induce cell-cycle arrest and cell death. p16^{Ink4a} inhibits cyclin D–cyclin-dependent kinase activity to allow pRb to restrain E2F activation of expression of genes for cell-cycle progression. Thus, the Ink4a-ARF locus, which encodes for two distinct proteins, functions in growth control mediated by two different pathways.

Fig. 11. p53 is a suppressor gene and one of the most intensely studied human genes as mutations are found in about 50% of all human cancers. The p53 protein is normally present at low levels in the cell, but can be upregulated by a diverse array of insults to the cell such as DNA damage (from irradiation) hypoxia, or deregulated cell-cycle progression caused by activated oncogenes. In response to these stresses, p53 induces the transcription of genes leading to cell-cycle arrest and/or cell death. p53 thus has a role as a sensor, transducing the many different inputs into adaptive processes preventing propagation of DNA damage to daughter cells. A recent study has suggested that it is likely that p53 has many other effects, such as alteration of cell adhesion and of the cell cytoskeleton, induction of secretion of extracellular factors, and promotion of differentiation.

of extracellular factors, and promotion of differentiation (161). The discovery of two related genes, p63 and p73, suggests that a p53 family of genes with both overlapping and complementary functions may exist analogous to the pRb family (153,162).

p53 induces cell-cycle arrest by inducing the expression of the CKI p21^{Cip} and it induces apoptosis by activating the expression of a protein called Bax (152,156). p53 function is regulated by control of protein stability, protein modification by phosphorylation or acetylation, and alteration of subcellular location (158). One of the most important mechanisms of regulation of p53 gene is made by interaction with the product of mdm2 gene, which has been found to be amplified in a number of different cancers. When mdm2 binds to p53, it targets p53 for degradation and possibly also promotes the transport of p53 protein out of the nucleus (where it is transcriptionally active) and into the cytoplasm (163).

GROWTH FACTORS AND THEIR RECEPTORS. Growth factors (GFs) are polypeptides that are secreted into the extra-

cellular space and transmit their signals by binding to specific receptor proteins, the GF receptors. Signals from the GF receptor are then transduced to the nucleus where transcription factors are activated leading to the expression of genes that alters cell behavior. The process by which a signal received at the cell membrane is converted into a change in nuclear gene expression is called signal transduction. Many of the GF receptors are also tyrosine kinases and are called receptor tyrosine kinases (RTKs). The RTKs are located on the cell membrane and typically possess three domains: an extracellular domain that binds to the GFs; a hydrophobic membrane-spanning portion; and a cytoplasmic catalytic domain (164). The binding of the GFs to their cognate RTKs results in receptor activation and initiation of intracellular signaling through a diverse number of pathways (Fig. 12) (165,166). The cross-linking (dimerization) of RTKs by their specific ligands causes activation of kinase activity of the cytoplasmic portions of the receptors themselves leading to their reciprocal phosphorylation of tyrosine residues on the cytoplasmic portions of the receptor (164). Phosphorylated tyrosines act as a bait for recruitment of other signaling molecules to the activated receptor leading to the initiation of the intracellular signaling cascade which ultimately affects gene expression in the nucleus.

Extracellular factors such as GFs cause alteration in cell proliferation but also in cell differentiation, cell migration, or cell

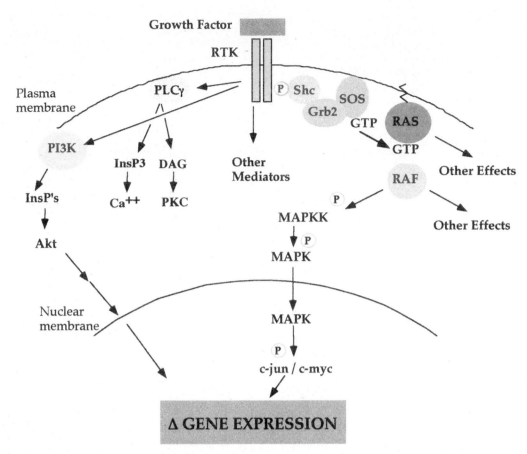

Fig. 12. Growth factors (GFs) are polypeptides that are secreted into the extracellular space and transmit their signals by binding to specific receptor proteins, the GF receptors. Signals from the GF receptor are then transduced to the nucleus where transcription factors are activated leading to the expression of genes that alter cell behavior, particularly cell proliferation. The process by which a signal received at the cell membrane is converted into a change in nuclear gene expression is called signal transduction. Many of the GF receptors are also tyrosine kinases and are called receptor tyrosine kinases (RTKs). The binding of the GFs to their cognate RTKs results in receptor activation and initiation of intracellular signaling through a diverse number of pathways, many involving phosphorylation cascades and specific protein–protein interactions (see text for details).

survival. A cell is constantly receiving many different signals at the surface from many sources including GFs, hormones, cell surface proteins attached to adjacent cells, and ECM proteins. These signals activate specific receptors but then can activate a number of intracellular signal transduction pathways whose effects are integrated in a complex and poorly understood manner leading to a change in the behavior of the cell. Cell proliferative signals from the extracellular environment are not just transduced by soluble growth factors and RTKs but are also transduced through serine-threonine kinase receptors (such as tumor GF-β or bone morphogenic protein receptors), sevenpass transmembrane receptors or G–protein-coupled receptors which transduce signals from hormones or neurotransmitters, steroid hormonal receptors which are involved in binding steroids in the nucleus, and integrin receptors which bind to ECM proteins such as collagen and fibronectin. GF signaling mechanisms are presently the best understood and will be the focus of further discussion. Mutations in a variety of different GFs lead to inappropriate cell signaling and are associated with cancer formation.

GROWTH FACTOR SIGNALING. GF signals are transduced intracellularly through Ras-dependent and Ras-independent pathways. Ras molecules function as molecular binary switches shuttling between an inactive mannose-1-phosphate guanylyltransferase (GDP) bound state and an active guanosine 5'-triphosphate (GTP) bound state (167–169). In the GTP bound state Ras is competent to initiate intracellular signals. Ras is activated by guanidine nucleotide exchange factors, such as SOS which exchanges GDP for GTP, and is inactivated by Ras GTPase-activating proteins (Ras-GAPs) through GTP hydrolysis. Ras-GAPs include the protein product of the neurofibromin gene, which is mutated in neurofibromatosis 1. Mutation of neurofibromin impairs its ability to inactivate Ras-GTP. Ras is associated with the inner plasma membrane and is a point of convergence for many different signaling events. Activation of Ras occurs after RTK activation by GFs such as EGF (epidermal growth factor), as well as through signaling from other extracellular factors through other non-RTK pathways. Phosphorylation of tyrosines on the cytoplasmic tails of RTKs creates binding sites for molecules with Src-homology 2 domains (SH2) such as Shc (170). An adaptor molecule called Grb2 then links Shc to SOS, ultimately leading to conversion of Ras GTP to Ras GDP. Activation of Ras ultimately leads to the activation of a complex series of serine-threonine kinases such as Raf and MAPK. This signaling pathway culminates in translocation of an activated MAPK from the cytoplasm to the nucleus where it activates transcription factors important for cell proliferation, such as cyclin D1 (168,171). Ras activates many parallel pathways affecting cell proliferation, cell survival, cell morphology, and cell motility, some of which are not mediated by the MAPK pathway (169). Ras-mediated intracellular signals can also be activated by other non-RTKs, such as G–protein-regulated serpentine cell receptors. Mutations in Ras leading to aberrant activation is associated with many cancers.

RTKs also activate intracellular signals through Ras-independent pathways. Again, activation of the RTK induces phosphorylation on specific tyrosine residues on the cytoplasmic domains which then serve as docking sites for other proteins containing SH2 domains. RTKs activate intracellular signaling pathways involving activation of phospholipase Cγ (PLC-γ) leading to changes in intracellular calcium, and phosphatidylinositol-3-kinase (PI3K) which activates a proto-oncogene called Akt via the production of inositol-phosphate intermediates (166). PLCγ converts phosphatidylinositol and phosphate into inositol-3-phosphate (InsP3) and diacylglycerol (DAG). InsP3 acts as a second messenger causing release of calcium from the endoplasmic reticulum into the cytoplasm and DAG induces protein kinase C. Activation of these two pathways leads to the transmission of a signal to the nucleus leading to an alteration in gene expression. PI3K phosphorylates lipids leading to production of inositol phosphate species which lead to the activation of Akt (also called protein kinase B) (172–174). Akt is a serine-threonine kinase implicated as a proto-oncogene and its expression promotes cell proliferation and cell survival. Presently, its substrates have not been extensively characterized, but it has been linked to indirect activation of β-catenin, a proto-oncogene involved in Wnt developmental signaling and in cancer (166,175). Clearly there is extensive crosstalk between different signaling pathways and the complexity of signal transduction from extracellular factors is only beginning to be understood.

Conclusion

We are in an era in which the techniques of molecular biology can be used not only to further our understanding of the basic science of human brain tumors, but also to treat patients with malignant brain tumors. The best example of this bench-to-bedside transition has been with gene therapy. Several gene therapy protocols have been put forth and are in progress for patients with malignant gliomas. While it is still too early to know whether these early trials will show promise in the long run, the fact remains that advances in molecular biology have led to some novel treatments for this difficult patient population. One of the major difficulties with all gene therapy trials to date has been that of efficient tumor targeting. Accordingly, improvements in gene delivery to target tissues will be forthcoming as the technology improves. We can expect to see developments in vector design with increased usage of liposomes and novel viral vectors. Elimination of gene overexpression in tumors may be accomplished using antisense ribonucleic acid/DNA techniques. A whole new cadre of drugs may be developed based on our knowledge of cell-cycle and angiogenesis pathways. Finally, inhibition of glioma cell invasion into normal brain by molecular methods may convert a diffuse tumor to a focal tumor, which could then be treated more effectively by local therapies. We are on the threshold of making great changes in the way we manage patients with gliomas. As we move forward, the information and techniques described in this chapter and their application to neurosurgical disorders such as brain tumors will become even more apparent than they are at the present time.

References

1. Kleihues P, Burger PC, Plate KH, et al. Glioblastoma. In: Kleihues P, Cavanne WK, eds. *Pathology and genetics of tumors of the nervous system*. Lyon: International Agency for Research on Cancer, 1997: 16–24.
2. Khoshyomn S, Penar PL, Rossi J, et al. Inhibition of phospholipase C-gamma1 activation blocks glioma cell motility and invasion of fetal rat brain aggregates. *Neurosurgery* 44:568–577; discussion 577–578, 1999.
3. Hinek A, Jung S, Rutka JT. Cell surface aggregation of elastin receptor molecules caused by suramin amplified signals leading to proliferation of human glioma cells. *Acta Neuropathol (Berl)* 97: 399–407, 1999.
4. Cavanee WK, Bigner DD, Newcomb EW, et al. Diffuse astrocytomas. In: Kleihues P, Cavanne WK, eds. *Pathology and Genetics of tumors of the nervous system*. Lyon: International Agency for Research on Cancer, 1997:16–24.
5. Giese A, Kluwe L, Laube B, et al. Migration of human glioma cells on myelin. *Neurosurgery* 38:755–764, 1996.
6. Giese A, Laube B, Zapf S, et al. Glioma cell adhesion and migration on human brain sections. *Anticancer Res* 18:2435–2347, 1998.
7. Ohnishi T, Matsumura H, Izumoto S, et al. A novel model of glioma cell invasion using organotypic brain slice culture *Cancer Res* 58: 2935–2940, 1998.
8. Giese A, Westphal M. Glioma invasion in the central nervous system. *Neurosurgery*, 39:235–250; discussion 250–252, 1996.
9. Ruoslahti E, Obrink B. Common principles in cell adhesion. *Exp Cell Res* 227:1–11, 1996.
10. Uhm, JH, Dooley NP, Villemure JG, et al. Mechanisms of glioma invasion: role of matrix-metalloproteinases. *Can J Neurol Sci* 24: 3–15, 1997.
11. Rutka JT, Apodaca G, Stern R, et al. The extracellular matrix of the central and peripheral nervous systems: structure and function. *J Neurosurg* 69:155–170, 1988.
12. Giese A, Loo MA, Rief MD, et al. Substrates for astrocytoma invasion. *Neurosurgery* 37:294–301; discussion 301–302, 1995.
13. Enam SA, Rosenblum ML, Edvardsen K. Role of extracellular matrix in tumor invasion: migration of glioma cells along fibronectin-positive mesenchymal cell processes. *Neurosurgery* 42:599–607; discussion 607–608, 1998.
14. Rutka JT, Myatt CA, Giblin JR, et al. Distribution of extracellular matrix proteins in primary human brain tumours: an immunohistochemical analysis. *Can J Neurol Sci* 14:25–30, 1987.
15. Venstrom KA, Reichardt LF. Extracellular matrix. 2: role of extracellular matrix molecules and their receptors in the nervous system. *FASEB J* 7:996–1003, 1993.
16. Jung S, Hinek A, Tsugu A, et al. Astrocytoma cell interaction with elastin substrates: implications for astrocytoma invasive potential. *Glia* 25:179–189, 1999.
17. Jung S, Rutka JT, Hinek A. Tropoelastin and elastin degradation products promote proliferation of human astrocytoma cell lines. *J Neuropathol Exp Neurol* 57:439–448, 1998.
18. Belien AT, Paganetti PA, Schwab ME. Membrane-type 1 matrix metalloprotease (MT1-MMP) enables invasive migration of glioma cells in central nervous system white matter. *J Cell Biol* 144: 373–384, 1999.
19. Rosales C, O'Brien V, Kornberg L, et al. Signal transduction by cell adhesion receptors, *Biochim Biophys Acta* 1242:77–98, 1995.
20. Paulus W, Tonn JC. Basement membrane invasion of glioma cells mediated by integrin receptors. *J Neurosurg* 80:515–519, 1994.
21. Paulus W, Baur I, Beutler AS, et al. Diffuse brain invasion of glioma cells requires beta 1 integrins. *Lab Invest* 75:819–826, 1996.
22. Clark EA, Brugge JS. Integrins and signal transduction pathways: the road taken. *Science* 268:233–239, 1995.
23. Hanks SK, Polte TR. Signaling through focal adhesion kinase. *Bioessays* 19:137–145, 1997.
24. Rutka JT, Muller M, Hubbard SL, et al. Astrocytoma adhesion to extracellular matrix: functional significance of integrin and focal adhesion kinase expression. *J Neuropathol Exp Neurol* 58:198–209, 1999.
25. Okamoto I, Kawano Y, Tsuiki H, et al. CD44 cleavage induced by a membrane-associated metalloprotease plays a critical role in tumor cell migration. *Oncogene* 18:1435–1446, 1999.

26. Rutka JT, Hubbard SL, Fukuyama K, et al. Effects of antisense glial fibrillary acidic protein complementary DNA on the growth, invasion, and adhesion of human astrocytoma cells. *Cancer Res* 54:3267–3272, 1994.

27. Rutka JT, Ackerley C, Hubbard SL, et al. Characterization of glial filament-cytoskeletal interactions in human astrocytomas: an immuno-ultrastructural analysis. *Eur J Cell Biol* 76:279–287:1998.

28. Rooprai HK, McCormick D. Proteases and their inhibitors in human brain tumours: a review. *Anticancer Res* 17:4151–4162, 1997.

29. MacDonald TJ, DeClerck YA, Laug WE. Urokinase induces receptor mediated brain tumor cell migration and invasion. *J Neurooncol* 40:215–226, 1998.

30. Wick W, Wagner S, Kerkau S, et al. BCL-2 promotes migration and invasiveness of human glioma cells. *FEBS Lett* 440:419–424, 1998.

31. Itoh T, Tanioka M, Yoshida H, et al. Reduced angiogenesis and tumor progression in gelatinase A-deficient mice. *Cancer Res* 58:1048–1051, 1998.

32. Nagase H. Activation mechanisms of matrix metalloproteinases. *Biol Chem* 378:151–160, 1997.

33. Nakano A, Tani E, Miyazaki K, et al. Matrix metalloproteinases and tissue inhibitors of metalloproteinases in human gliomas. *J Neurosurg* 83:298–307, 1995.

34. Nakagawa T, Kubota T, Kabuto M, et al. Production of matrix metalloproteinases and tissue inhibitor of metalloproteinases-1 by human brain tumors. *J Neurosurg* 81:69–77, 1994.

35. Matsuzawa K, Fukuyama K, Dirks PB, et al. Expression of stromelysin 1 in human astrocytoma cell lines. *J Neurooncol* 30:181–188, 1996.

36. Nakada M, Nakamura H, Ikeda E, et al. Expression and tissue localization of membrane-type 1, 2, and 3 matrix metalloproteinases in human astrocytic tumors. *Am J Pathol* 154:417–428, 1999.

37. Matsuzawa K, Fukuyama K, Hubbard SL, et al. Transfection of an invasive human astrocytoma cell line with a TIMP-1 cDNA: modulation of astrocytoma invasive potential. *J Neuropathol Exp Neurol* 55:88–96, 1996.

38. Mikkelsen T, Yan PS, Ho KL, et al. Immunolocalization of cathepsin B in human glioma: implications for tumor invasion and angiogenesis. *J Neurosurg* 83:285–290, 1995.

39. Hsu DW, Efird JT, Hedley-Whyte ET. Prognostic role of urokinase-type plasminogen activator in human gliomas. *Am J Pathol* 147:114–123, 1995.

40. Yamamoto M, Sawaya R, Mohanam S, et al. Expression and localization of urokinase-type plasminogen activator receptor in human gliomas. *Cancer Res* 54:5016–5020, 1994.

41. Andre T, Chastre E, Kotelevets L, et al. Angiogenese tumorale: physiopathologie, valeur pronostique et perspectives therapeutiques. *Rev Med Interne* 19:904–913, 1998.

42. Folkman J, D'Amore PA. Blood vessel formation: what is its molecular basis? *Cell* 87:1153–1155, 1996.

43. Hanahan D, Folkman J. Patterns and emerging mechanisms of the angiogenic switch during tumorigenesis. *Cell* 86:353–364, 1996.

44. Jensen RL. Growth factor-mediated angiogenesis in the malignant progression of glial tumors: a review. *Surg Neurol* 49:189–195; discussion 196, 1998.

45. Klagsbrun M. Angiogenesis and cancer: AACR special conference in cancer research. American Association for Cancer Research. *Cancer Res* 59:487–490, 1999.

46. Plate KH. Mechanisms of angiogenesis in the brain. *J Neuropathol Exp Neurol* 58:313–320, 1999.

47. Pinedo HM, Verheul HM, D'Amato RJ, et al. Involvement of platelets in tumour angiogenesis? *Lancet* 352:1775–1777, 1998.

48. McNamara DA, Harmey JH, Walsh TN, et al. Significance of angiogenesis in cancer therapy [published erratum appears in *Br J Surg* 85:1449, 1998]. *Br J Surg* 85:1044–1055, 1998.

49. Bolontrade MF, Stern MC, Binder RL, et al. Angiogenesis is an early event in the development of chemically induced skin tumors. *Carcinogenesis* 19:2107–2113, 1998.

50. Yoshimura F, Kaidoh T, Inokuchi T, et al. Changes in VEGF expression and in the vasculature during the growth of early-stage ethylnitrosourea-induced malignant astrocytomas in rats. *Virchows Arch* 433:457–463, 1998.

51. Theurillat JP, Hainfellner J, Maddalena A, et al. Early induction of angiogenetic signals in gliomas of GFAP-v-src transgenic mice. *Am J Pathol* 154:581–590, 1999.

52. O'Reilly MS, Holmgren L, Shing Y, et al. Angiostatin: a novel angiogenesis inhibitor that mediates the suppression of metastases by a Lewis lung carcinoma [see comments]. *Cell* 79:315–328, 1994.

53. O'Reilly MS, Boehm T, Shing Y, et al. Endostatin: an endogenous inhibitor of angiogenesis and tumor growth. *Cell* 88:277–285, 1997.

54. Oku T, Tjuvajev JG, Miyagawa T, et al. Tumor growth modulation by sense and antisense vascular endothelial growth factor gene expression: effects on angiogenesis, vascular permeability, blood volume, blood flow, fluorodeoxyglucose uptake, and proliferation of human melanoma intracerebral xenografts. *Cancer Res* 58:4185–4192, 1998.

55. Millauer B, Shawver LK, Plate KH, et al. Glioblastoma growth inhibited in vivo by a dominant-negative Flk-1 mutant. *Nature* 367:576–579, 1994.

56. Stan AC, Nemati MN, Pietsch T, et al. In vivo inhibition of angiogenesis and growth of the human U-87 malignant glial tumor by treatment with an antibody against basic fibroblast growth factor. *J Neurosurg* 82:1044–1052, 1995.

57. Brooks PC, Silletti S, von Schalscha TL, et al. Disruption of angiogenesis by PEX, a noncatalytic metalloproteinase fragment with integrin binding activity. *Cell* 92:391–400, 1998.

58. Lund EL, Spang-Thomsen M, Skovgaard-Poulsen H, et al. Tumor angiogenesis—a new therapeutic target in gliomas. *Acta Neurol Scand* 97:52–62, 1998.

59. Lucas R, Holmgren L, Garcia I, et al. Multiple forms of angiostatin induce apoptosis in endothelial cells. *Blood* 92:4730–4741, 1998.

60. Lode HN, Moehler T, Xiang R, et al. Synergy between an antiangiogenic integrin alphav antagonist and an antibody-cytokine fusion protein eradicates spontaneous tumor metastases. *Proc Natl Acad Sci USA* 96:1591–1596, 1999.

61. Chan AS, Leung SY, Wong MP, et al. Expression of vascular endothelial growth factor and its receptors in the anaplastic progression of astrocytoma, oligodendroglioma, and ependymoma. *Am J Surg Pathol* 22:816–826, 1998.

62. Machein MR, Kullmer J, Fiebich BL, et al. Vascular endothelial growth factor expression, vascular volume, and, capillary permeability in human brain tumors. *Neurosurgery* 44:732–740; discussion 740–741, 1999.

63. Nagashima G, Suzuki R, Hokaku H, et al. Graphic analysis of microscopic tumor cell infiltration, proliferative potential, and vascular endothelial growth factor expression in an autopsy brain with glioblastoma. *Surg Neurol* 51:292–299, 1999.

64. Provias J, Claffey K, delAguila L, et al. Meningiomas: role of vascular endothelial growth factor/vascular permeability factor in angiogenesis and peritumoral edema. *Neurosurgery* 40:1016–1026, 1997.

65. Bitzer M, Opitz H, Popp J, et al. Angiogenesis and brain oedema in intracranial meningiomas: influence of vascular endothelial growth factor. *Acta Neurochir* 140:333–340, 1998.

66. Yoshioka H, Hama S, Taniguchi E, et al. Peritumoral brain edema associated with meningioma: influence of vascular endothelial growth factor expression and vascular blood supply. *Cancer* 85:936–944, 1999.

67. Plate KH, Risau W. Angiogenesis in malignant gliomas. *Glia* 15:339–347, 1995.

68. Plate KH, Breier G, Millauer B, et al. Up-regulation of vascular endothelial growth factor and its cognate receptors in a rat glioma model of tumor angiogenesis. *Cancer Res* 53:5822–5827, 1993.

69. Plate KH, Breier G, Weich HA, et al. Vascular endothelial growth factor is a potential tumour angiogenesis factor in human gliomas in vivo. *Nature* 359:845–848, 1992.

70. Plate KH, Warnke PC. Vascular endothelial growth factor. *J Neurooncol* 35:365–372, 1997.

71. Wesseling P, Ruiter DJ, Burger PC. Angiogenesis in brain tumors; pathobiological and clinical aspects. *J Neurooncol* 32:253–265, 1997.

72. Tsai JC, Goldman CK, Gillespie GY. Vascular endothelial growth factor in human glioma cell lines: induced secretion by EGF, PDGF-BB, and bFGF. *J Neurosurg* 82:864–873, 1995.

73. Hatva E, Kaipainen A, Mentula P, et al. Expression of endothelial cell-specific receptor tyrosine kinases and growth factors in human brain tumors. *Am J Pathol* 146:368–378, 1995.

74. Plate KH, Breier G, Weich HA, et al. Vascular endothelial growth factor and glioma angiogenesis: coordinate induction of VEGF receptors, distribution of VEGF protein and possible in vivo regulatory mechanisms. *Int J Cancer* 59:520–529, 1994.

75. Abdulrauf SI, Edvardsen K, Ho KL, et al. Vascular endothelial growth factor expression and vascular density as prognostic markers of survival in patients with low-grade astrocytoma. *J Neurosurg* 88:513–520, 1998.

76. Sato TN, Tozawa Y, Deutsch U, et al. Distinct roles of the receptor tyrosine kinases Tie-1 and Tie-2 in blood vessel formation. *Nature* 376:70–74, 1995.

77. Stratmann A, Risau W, Plate KH. Cell type-specific expression of angiopoietin-1 and angiopoietin-2 suggests a role in glioblastoma angiogenesis [see Comments]. *Am J Pathol* 153:1459–1466, 1998.

78. Segal DH, Germano IM, Bederson JB. Effects of basic fibroblast growth factor on in vivo cerebral tumorigenesis in rats. *Neurosurgery* 40:1027–1033, 1997.

79. Schmidt, N. O, Westphal, M, Hagel, C, et al. Levels of vascular endothelial growth factor, hepatocyte growth factor/scatter factor and basic fibroblast growth factor in human gliomas and their relation to angiogenesis. *Int J Cancer* 84:10–18, 1999.

80. Nakayama Y, Sueishi K, Oka K, et al. Stromal angiogenesis in human glioma: a role of platelet-derived endothelial cell growth factor. *Surg Neurol* 49:181–187; discussion 187–188, 1998.

81. Stiles JD, Ostrow PT, Balos LL, et al. Correlation of endothelin-1 and transforming growth factor beta 1 with malignancy and vascularity in human gliomas. *J Neuropathol Exp Neurol* 56:435–439, 1997.

82. Lamszus K, Schmidt NO, Jin L, et al. Scatter factor promotes motility of human glioma and neuromicrovascular endothelial cells. *Int J Cancer* 75:19–28, 1998.

83. Samoto K, Ikezaki K, Ono M, et al. Expression of vascular endothelial growth factor and its possible relation with neovascularization in human brain tumors. *Cancer Res* 55:1189–1193, 1995.

84. MacHein MR, Kullmer J, Ronicke V, et al. Differential downregulation of vascular endothelial growth factor by dexamethasone in normoxic and hypoxic rat glioma cells. *Neuropathol Appl Neurobiol* 25:104–112, 1999.

85. Kirsch M, Strasser J, Allende R, et al. Angiostatin suppresses malignant glioma growth in vivo. *Cancer Res* 58:4654–4659, 1998.

86. Hall M, Peters G. Genetic alterations of cyclins, cyclin-dependent kinases, and Cdk inhibitors in human cancer. *Adv Cancer Res* 68:67–108, 1996.

87. Sherr C. Cell cycle control. Presented at: Twelfth Annual Meeting on Oncogenes; 1996; Frederick, MD.

88. Sherr CJ. Cancer cell cycles. *Science,* 274:1672–1677, 1996.

89. Dirks PB, Rutka JT. Current concepts in neuro-oncology: the cell cycle—a review. *Neurosurgery* 40:1000–1013; discussion 1013–1015, 1997.

90. Divac, I, Lavail, JH, Rakic, P, et al. Heterogeneous afferents to the inferior parietal lobule of the rhesus monkey revealed by the retrograde transport method. *Brain Res* 123:197–207, 1977.

91. Pardee AB. G1 events and regulation of the cell proliferation. *Science* 246:603–608, 1990.

92. Murray A. *The cell cycle.* New York: WH Freeman and Company, 1993.

93. King RW, Deshaies RJ, Peters JM, et al. How proteolysis drives the cell cycle. *Science* 274:1652–1659, 1996.

94. Nasmyth K. Viewpoint: putting the cell cycle in order. *Science* 274:1643–1645, 1996.

95. Stillman B. Cell cycle control of DNA replication. *Science* 274:1659–1664, 1996.

96. Paulovich AG, Hartwell LH. A checkpoint regulates the rate of progression through S phase in *S. cerevisiae* in response to DNA damage. *Cell* 82:841–847, 1995.

97. Paulovich AG, Toczyski DP, Hartwell LH. When checkpoints fail. *Cell* 88:315–21, 1997.

98. Newton RA. Balance abilities in individuals with moderate and severe traumatic brain injury. *Brain Injury* 9:445–451, 1995.

99. Nigg EA. Cyclin-dependent protein kinases: key regulators of the eukaryotic cell cycle. *Bioessays* 17:471–480, 1995.

100. Pines J. Cyclins and cyclin-dependent kinases: a biochemical view. *Biochem J* 308:697–711, 1995.

101. Roberts JM. Evolving ideas about cyclins. *Cell* 98:129–132, 1999.

102. Sherr CJ. G1 phase progression: cycling on cue. *Cell* 4:551–555, 1994.

103. Elledge SJ. Cell cycle checkpoints: preventing an identity crisis. *Science* 274:1664–1672, 1996.

104. Zetterberg A, Larsson O, Wiman KG. What is the restriction point? *Curr Opin Cell Biol* 7:835–842, 1995.

105. Hunter T. Oncoprotein networks. *Cell* 88:333–346, 1997.

106. Nurse P. Ordering S phase and M phase in the cell cycle [Comment]. *Cell* 79:547–550, 1994.

107. McIntosh JR, Koonce MP. Mitosis. *Science* 246:622–628, 1989.

108. Koshland D. Mitosis: back to basics. *Cell* 77:951–974, 1994.

109. Hunter T, Pines J. Cyclins and cancer II: cyclin D and CDK inhibitors come of age. *Cell* 4:573–582, 1994.

110. Morgan DO. Principles of CDK regulation. *Nature* 374:131–134, 1995.

111. Koepp DM, Harper JW, Elledge SJ. How the cyclin became a cyclin: regulated proteolysis in the cell cycle. *Cell* 97:431–434, 1999.

112. Sherr CJ. Mammalian G1 cyclins. *Cell* 73:1059–1065, 1993.

113. Lukas J, Parry D, Aagaard L, et al. Retinoblastoma-protein-dependent cell-cycle inhibition by the tumour suppressor p16. *Nature* 375:503–506, 1995.

114. Nevins JR, Chellappan SP, Mudryj M, et al. E2F transcription factor is a target for the RB protein and the cyclin A protein. *Cold Spring Harb Symp Quant Biol* 56:157–162, 1991.

115. Mittnacht S. Control of pRB phosphorylation. *Curr Opin Genet Dev* 8:21–27, 1998.

116. Sherr CJ, Roberts JM. CDK inhibitors: positive and negative regulators of G1-phase progression. *Genes Dev* 13:1501–1512, 1999.

117. Sidle A, Palaty C, Dirks P, et al. Activity of the retinoblastoma family proteins, pRB, p107, and p130, during cellular proliferation and differentiation. *Crit Rev Biochem Mol Biol* 31:237–271, 1996.

118. Dyson N. The regulation of E2F by pRB-family proteins. *Genes Dev* 12:2245–2262, 1998.

119. Helin K. Regulation of cell proliferation by the E2F transcription factors. *Curr Opin Genet Dev* 8:28–35, 1998.

120. Wang TC, Cardiff RD, Zuckerberg L, et al. Mammary hyperplasia and carcinoma in MMTV-cyclin D1 transgenic mice. *Nature* 369:669–671, 1994.

121. Bortner DM, Rosenberg MP. Induction of mammary gland hyperplasia and carcinomas in transgenic mice expressing human cyclin E. *Mol Cell Biol* 17:453–459, 1997.

122. Guadagno TM, Ohtsubo M, Roberts JM, et al. A link between cyclin A expression and adhesion-dependent cell cycle progression. *Science* 262:1572–1575, 1993.

123. Guadagno TM, Ohtsubo M, Roberts JM, et al. A link between cyclin A expression and adhesion–dependent cell cycle progression [published erratum appears in *Science* 263:455, 1994]. *Science* 262:1572–1575, 1993.

124. Lewin B. Driving the cell cycle: M phase kinase, its partners, and substrates. *Cell* 61:743–752, 1990.

125. Lewin B. Commitment and activation at pol II promoters: a tail of protein-protein interactions. *Cell* 61:1161–1164, 1990.

126. Moreno S, Nurse P. Substrates for p34^{cdc2}: in vivo veritas? *Cell* 61:549–551, 1990.

127. Elledge SJ, Harper JW. CDK inhibitors: on the threshold of checkpoints and development. *Curr Opin Cell Biol* 6:847–852, 1994.

128. Sherr CJ, Roberts JM. Inhibitors of mammalian G1 cyclin-dependent kinases. *Genes Dev* 9:1149–1163, 1995.

129. Shapiro GI, Edwards CD, Ewen ME, et al. p16INK4A participates in a G1 arrest checkpoint in response to DNA damage. *Mol Cell Biol* 18:378–387, 1998.

130. Ruas M, Peters G. The p16INK4a/CDKN2A tumor suppressor and its relatives, *Biochim Biophys Acta* 1378:F115–F177, 1998.

131. Fero ML, Rivkin M, et al. A syndrome of multiorgan hyperplasia with features of gigantism, tumorigenesis, and female sterility in p27^{Kip1}-deficient mice. *Cell* 85:733–744, 1996.

132. Kiyokawa H, Kineman RD, Manova-Todorova KO, et al. Enhanced growth of mice lacking the cyclin-dependent kinase inhibitor function of p27Kip1. *Cell* 85:721–732, 1996.

133. Nakayama K, Ishida N, Shirane M, et al. Mice lacking p27^{Kip1} display increased body size, multiple organ dysplasia, retinal dysplasia and pituitary tumors, *Cell* 85:707–720, 1996.

134. Franklin DS, Godfrey VL, Lee H, et al. CDK inhibitors p18(INK4c) and p27(Kip1) mediate two separate pathways to collaboratively suppress pituitary tumorigenesis. *Genes Dev* 12:2899–2911, 1998.

135. Zhang Y, Xiong Y, Yarbrough WG. ARF promotes MDM2 degradation and stabilizes p53: ARF-INK4a locus deletion impairs both the Rb and p53 tumor suppression pathways. *Cell* 92:725–734, 1998.

136. Zhang Y, Ramsay ES, Mock BA. Cdkn2a, the cyclin-dependent kinase inhibitor encoding p16INK4a and p19ARF, is a candidate for the plasmacytoma susceptibility locus, Pctr1, *Proc Natl Acad Sci USA* 95:2429–2434, 1998.

137. Mulligan G, Jacks T. The retinoblastoma gene family: cousins with overlapping interests. *Trends Genet* 14:223–229, 1998.

138. Nevins JR. Toward an understanding of the functional complexity of the E2F and retinoblastoma families. *Cell Growth Differ* 9:585–593, 1998.

139. Macleod KF, Jacks T. Insights into cancer from transgenic mouse models. *J Pathol* 187:43–60, 1999.

140. Johnson DG, Schwarz JK, Cress WD, et al. Expression of transcription factor E2F1 induces quiescent cells to enter S phase. *Nature* 365:349–352, 1993.

141. Johnson DG, Cress WD, Jakoi L, et al. Oncogenic capacity of the E2F1 gene. *Proc Natl Acad Sci USA* 91:12823–12827, 1994.

142. Qin X, Livingston DM, Kaelin WG, et al. Deregulated expression of E2F-1 in low serum leads to S-phase entry and p53-dependent apoptosis. In: *The cell cycle*. Cold Spring Harbor Laboratories, 1994: 106.

143. Qin XQ, Livingston DM, Kaelin WG Jr, et al. Deregulated transcription factor E2F-1 expression leads to S-phase entry and p53-mediated apoptosis. *Proc Natl Acad Sci USA* 91:10918–10922, 1994.

144. Schneider JW, Gu W, Zhu L, et al. Reversal of terminal differentiation mediated by p107 in Rb−/− muscle cells. *Science* 264:1467–1471, 1994.

145. Field SJ, Tsai FY, Kuo F, et al. E2F-1 functions in mice to promote apoptosis and suppress proliferation. *Cell* 85:549–561, 1996.

146. Yamasaki L, Jacks T, Bronson R, et al. Tumor induction and tissue atrophy in mice lacking E2F-1. *Cell* 85:537–548, 1996.

147. Serrano M. The tumor suppressor protein p16INK4a. *Exp Cell Res* 237:7–13, 1997.

148. Haber DA. Splicing into senescence: the curious case of p16 and p19ARF. *Cell* 91:555–558, 1997.

149. Sherr CJ. Tumor surveillance via the ARF-p53 pathway. *Genes Dev* 12:2973–2983, 1998.

150. Sharpless NE, DePinho RA. The INK4A/ARF locus and its two gene products. *Curr Opin Genet Dev* 9:22–30, 1999.

151. Kamijo T, Zindy F, Roussel MF, et al. Tumor suppression at the mouse INK4a locus mediated by the alternative reading frame product p19ARF. *Cell* 91:649–659, 1997.

152. Levine AJ. p53, the cellular gatekeeper for growth and cell division. *Cell* 88:323–331, 1997.

153. Prives C, Hall PA. The p53 pathway. *J Pathol* 187:112–126, 1999.

154. Malkin D. p53 and the Li-Fraumeni syndrome. *Biochim Biophys Acta* 1198:197–213, 1994.

155. Kleihues P, Schauble B, zur Hausen A, et al. Tumors associated with p53 germline mutations: a synopsis of 91 families. *Am J Pathol* 150:1–13, 1997.

156. Ko LJ, Prives C. p53: Puzzle and paradigm. *Genes Dev* 10:1054–1072, 1996.

157. Agarwal ML, Taylor, WR, Chernov, MV, et al. The p53 network. *J Biol Chem* 273:1–4, 1998.

158. Giaccia AJ, Kastan MB. The complexity of p53 modulation: emerging patterns from divergent signals. *Genes Dev.* 12:2973–2983, 1998.

159. Bunz F, Dutriaux A, Lengauer C, et al. Requirement for p53 and p21 to sustain G2 arrest after DNA damage. *Science* 282:1497–1501, 1998.

160. Lanni JS, Jacks T. Characterization of the p53-dependent postmitotic checkpoint following spindle disruption. *Mol Cell Biol* 18:1055–1064, 1998.

161. Almog N, Rotter V. An insight into the life of p53: a protein coping with many functions! Review of the 9th p53 Workshop, Crete, May 9–13, 1998. *Biochim Biophys Acta* 1378:R43–R54, 1998.

162. Kaelin WG Jr. The emerging p53 gene family. *J Natl Cancer Inst* 91:594–598, 1999.

163. Prives C. Signaling to p53: breaking the MDM2-p53 circuit. *Cell* 95:5–8, 1998.

164. Heldin CH. Dimerization of cell surface receptors in signal transduction. *Cell* 80:213–23, 1995.

165. Weiss FU, Daub H, Ullrich A. Novel mechanisms of RTK signal generation. *Curr Opin Genet Dev* 7:80–86, 1997.

166. Porter AC, Vaillancourt RR. Tyrosine kinase receptor-activated signal transduction pathways which lead to oncogenesis. *Oncogene* 17:1343–1352, 1998.

167. Katz ME, McCormick F. Signal transduction from multiple Ras effectors. *Curr Opin Genet Dev* 7:75–79, 1997.

168. Khosravi-Far R, Der CJ. The Ras signal transduction pathway. *Cancer Metastasis Rev* 13:67–89, 1994.

169. Campbell SL, Khosravi-Far R, Rossman KL, et al. Increasing complexity of Ras signaling. *Oncogene* 17:1395–1413, 1998.

170. Pawson T. Protein modules and signalling networks. *Nature* 373:573–580, 1995.

171. Khosravi-Far R, Campbell S, Rossman KL, et al. Increasing complexity of Ras signal transduction: involvement of Rho family proteins. *Adv Cancer Res* 72:57–107, 1998.

172. Franke TF, Kaplan DR, Cantley LC. PI3K: downstream AKTion blocks apoptosis. *Cell* 88:435–437, 1997.

173. Franke TF, Kaplan DR, Cantley LC, et al. Direct regulation of the Akt proto-oncogene product by phosphatidylinositol-3,4-bisphosphate [see Comments]. Science. 275:665–8, 1997.

174. Klippel, A, Kavanaugh, WM, Pot, D, et al. A specific product of phosphatidylinositol 3-kinase directly activates the protein kinase Akt through its pleckstrin homology domain. *Mol Cell Biol* 17:338–344, 1997.

175. Cadigan KM, Nusse R. Wnt signaling: a common theme in animal development. *Genes Dev* 11:3286–3305, 1997.

99. *The Molecular Genetics of Intracranial Gliomas*

Eric C. Holland

The fact that some reproducible differences are at last beginning to be seen between normal and cancer cells tells us that the study of cancer at the molecular level is no longer a premature Don Quixotic science that only exists because the responsible people never ask what their cancer research money is buying. On the other hand, we must not deceive ourselves that, because we can measure the amount of cAMP and, if we are more clever, that of cGMP, we are in any sense close to being on top of the cancer problem. Compared to *E. coli*, our knowledge of the structural organization and biochemistry of normal eucaryotic cells is still pitifully meager; and unless this situation changes, much cancer research will continue to resemble a search for a coin lost along a path only occasionally illuminated by street lights. Of necessity we look under the lighted regions for, no matter how long you look into the dark, the search will never be successful. Thus, as long as most components of the normal cell membrane remain essentially black boxes, the biochemistry of cancer may remain a mystery for some still future generation to understand (1).

Black boxes hiding the secrets of cell biology are fewer today because molecular biology has rapidly unlocked one after another, revealing the mysteries within. Advances in molecular genetics have provided new ways of asking and answering the age-old question—what makes a malignant cell different from surrounding normal tissues? Why does one brain cell function normally, contributing to "memory, desire, impulse, reflective capacity, power of association, even consciousness—to say nothing of sight and hearing, muscular movement and voice" (2) while an adjacent cell gives rise to a mass of cells growing unchecked, leading eventually to the patient's demise? Cell growth and differentiation and the regulation of these normal functions are dependent on molecular signals that a cell receives either from within itself (*autocrine*) or from neighboring cells or tissues (*paracrine*). The production and function of all protein molecules responsible for directing the cellular machinery—the same machinery that is dysfunctional in cancer—are determined directly or indirectly at the gene level.

Cancer results when one or more mistakes, or *mutations*, occur in a cell's *deoxyribonucleic acid (DNA)*, leading to disruption of normal signaling pathways and regulatory mechanisms. One mutation is generally not sufficient to cause cancer, as eukaryotic cells possess elaborate DNA repair mechanisms and built-in "alternate" pathways. Most tumors, therefore, contain genetic alterations at several points, often affecting several different pathways. Understanding the molecular basis for the events that regulate oncogenesis is critical in assigning the most accurate diagnoses and prognoses, and in designing the most effective therapeutic strategies for the various types of cancer. Molecular genetics, rather than persisting as a tool for laboratory scientists, has rapidly evolved into clinical usefulness—as a diagnostic tool, a prognostic indicator and, more recently, a form of therapy.

Molecular Technologies and Terminologies

GENES AND GENE PRODUCTS

Chromosomes and DNA Structure. In 1866, Gregor Mendel wrote that inheritance occurs in "units" that can be predicted based on parental characteristics. It was not until 1900, however, that Mendel's 1866 manuscript, originally published in an obscure journal, was found and correlated with contemporary discoveries. This work concluded that particulate hereditary material actually existed—inheritance was not a mystical occurrence after all—and its transmission from one generation to the next could be predicted.

A century later, we can precisely describe the molecular structure of the "particulate" hereditary material found in the cell nucleus. Chromosomes, of which there are 23 pairs in humans, are each made up of two strands of the linear polymer DNA twisted around one another into a helical structure and then folded into a compact package. A single strand of DNA is made up of a linear sequence of four possible *nucleotides*, each of which consists of a phosphate group, a sugar moiety, and one of four possible *bases*—adenine, guanine, cytosine, or thymine. Two single strands of DNA bind together via chemical interactions between bases, forming *base pairs*. Adenine and thymine residues bind to one another, as do cytosine and guanine. Once the helix is unwound and the two strands separate, DNA can replicate itself using enzymes to assemble thymine opposite adenine and guanine opposite cytosine, eventually resulting in a new strand which is a mirror image of, or is *complementary* to, the original *template*. The natural chemical reaction which takes place when bases pair with the help of enzymes is the mechanism on which much of molecular genetic technology depends.

Genes to Proteins. Genes are defined regions of chromosomes carrying inheritable genetic material in the form of specific nucleotide sequences. A gene is the blueprint for the assembly of a protein molecule out of free amino acids. The specific linear sequence of nucleotides constituting DNA determines the order of the amino acids and therefore, the identity of the final protein product of a gene. Specific nucleotide sequences also dictate whether or not the gene will actually be active, or *expressed*, in a particular cell. The protein resulting from expression of a gene is the *gene product*.

A gene is defined by a number of characteristics and can be broken down into several units (Fig. 1). Each gene contains a *promoter* site, a nucleotide sequence which encodes the message to initiate transcription and, therefore, controls the activity of the gene. Second, there is a region containing the protein coding sequence and finally, a region composed of repetitions of the nucleotide adenosine, called the *poly A sequence*, which terminates transcription.

Genetic information in the form of DNA is archived in the nucleus. Temporary copies of gene sequences are produced in the form of *ribonucleic acid (RNA)* through a process called *transcription*. The structure of RNA is similar to that of DNA, except that it is single stranded and contains the nucleotide uracil rather than adenine. Eukaryotic gene sequences often also include regions called *introns* which, although transcribed into RNA, are removed during the processing of RNA to mature messenger RNA (mRNA) in the cytoplasm.

Once the protein coding sequence of DNA has been transcribed into mRNA, it is transferred to the cytoplasm where it is *translated* into a linear sequence of amino acids making up polypeptide chains and proteins. A second type of RNA, *transfer RNA (tRNA)*, binds to free amino acids in the cytoplasm and transfers them to the site of protein synthesis, the ribosome. At the ribosome, mRNA serves as a template for protein synthesis. Each set of three nucleotides in an mRNA sequence is called a *triplet* or *codon*, and "codes" for a particular amino acid. Transfer RNA contains a complementary triplet sequence, or *anticodon*, which sticks to the mRNA codon, effectively lining up the tRNA's passenger amino acid for attachment to the polypeptide under construction.

Although nearly every cell in an organism contains a complete set of genetic material inherited from both parents, and all are therefore of identical *genotype*, each cell will express only a subset of possible genes, depending primarily on each gene's promoter sequence. In addition to general promoters, there are also tissue-specific promoter sequences and, for example, it is the summation of general and astrocyte-specific gene expression that makes a cell an astrocyte. Gene expression depends on regulatory elements, acting at the level of transcription or translation, which determine whether or not a gene will be activated or repressed in a particular cell at a particular time. The expression of the appropriate set of genes in a tissue ultimately results in production of the appropriate functional proteins. The *phenotype* of a cell is determined by the subset of genes that are actually expressed and proteins can be thought of as the "intermediaries between gene and phenotype" (3).

Gene Mutations. Because the ultimate structure of a functional cellular protein depends on the nucleotide sequence of DNA, any damage to DNA that disrupts the nucleotide sequence may cause the gene not to be expressed, to be turned on inappropriately, or to produce a nonfunctional protein. *Mutations* can occur in a variety of different ways. Insertion or deletion of nucleotides can cause the triplet code to be "misread" at the insertion/deletion point or *downstream* because the change at the insertion/deletion point shifts the *reading frame* for translation, effectively changing the amino acid sequence. These are called *frame shift* or *reading frame mutations*. Some mutations cause a necessary protein not to be expressed, while other mutations, if they are in the regulatory region of the gene, might

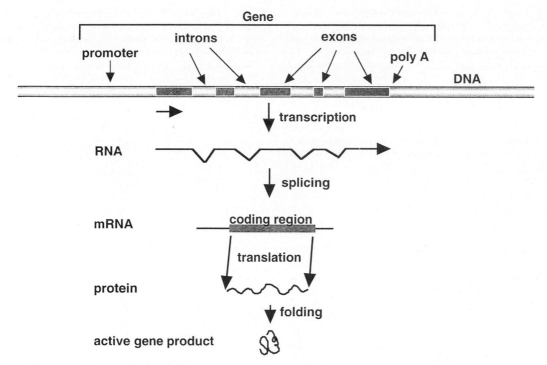

Fig. 1. From gene-to-gene product. The structure of the gene is shown. Processes involved in converting DNA sequences to protein structure: transcription, splicing, translation, and folding are diagrammed.

allow transcription and translation to occur in a gene that is normally repressed. This type of mutation results in *constitutive* expression, or continuous expression in the absence of induction.

One copy of each chromosome, and therefore of each gene, is inherited per parent, resulting in two *alleles* in each *diploid* (containing two sets of chromosomes) cell. When mutations occur in a gene, either by *deletion* or by *point mutation*, they can occur in either one or both alleles. The loss of one allele, a *heterozygous mutation*, results in a 50% reduction in gene expression. *Homozygous mutation*, or loss of both copies of a gene, results in 100% loss of gene function (4).

CLONING AND DNA ANALYSIS

Manipulation of DNA. Molecular genetic technology is entirely dependent on the fact that it is possible to isolate a segment of DNA, determine its nucleotide sequence, and then, using enzymes called *restriction endonucleases,* precisely cut the DNA at specific sites between nucleotides (3). Restriction endonucleases recognize small stretches of distinct nucleotide sequences in double-stranded DNA and break both strands, leaving unpaired bases at the ends; hundreds of these enzymes with different sequence specificities have been isolated from bacteria. Cutting DNA at a specific sequence of nucleotides results in a characteristic pattern of DNA fragments of various sizes. When these small *restriction fragments* are forced to migrate through a gel matrix by electrical currents, they migrate at different speeds depending on size, generating a unique sequence-specific pattern of bands. This restriction pattern, or *DNA fingerprint,* can be visualized using dyes and compared to that generated from a different DNA source using the same restriction enzymes. This technology provides for both qualitative and quantitative comparisons between DNA samples.

POLYMERASE CHAIN REACTION. Another technique currently emerging as an important clinical tool is beautifully simple in its theory, yet powerful enough to revolutionize molecular genetics. The *polymerase chain reaction (PCR)* permits identification and amplification of DNA sequences from nearly any source, as long as a part of the sequence is known. Therefore, any known DNA sequence can be detected in any sample of genetic material, including tumors (5).

Initially, two *oligonucleotide primers* (short pieces of DNA with sequences designed to stick to regions flanking the DNA sequence to be amplified) are designed and chemically synthesized. Template DNA is mixed together with the synthetic oligonucleotide primers (often referred to as *oligos*), free nucleotides, and an enzyme—*tac polymerase.* A heat stable version of the enzyme *DNA polymerase,* tac was originally isolated from bacteria capable of DNA synthesis at temperatures nearing the boiling point of water. The enzyme, using the bound primer as a foundation on which to add free nucleotides, builds a new strand of DNA with a complementary sequence to the original. Each PCR cycle consists of heating the mixture to *melt* double-stranded DNA into two single strands, cooling to *anneal* or "stick" primers to the DNA to be amplified, *synthesis* of a new complementary strand from free nucleotides, and then again *melting* to separate the new and old strands of DNA, resulting in a doubling of the available template. After 10 cycles of PCR the original DNA sequence is amplified approximately 1,000 times, and after 20 cycles, approximately 1 million times.

PCR is an example of a technology built on the restricted chemical interaction between bases. The annealing of primers, as well as the addition of free nucleotides during synthesis, is dependent on the formation of nucleotide base pairs. As discussed previously, thymine binds to adenine residues in the template, adenine to thymine, guanine to cytosine, and cytosine to guanine. The heating and cooling cycles critical to the success of PCR are carried out in automated *thermocyclers,* designed to precisely control reaction conditions. Once a PCR *product* is separated on a gel, DNA fragments of expected size are collected and the nucleotide sequence is checked to verify amplification of the correct target. PCR can be used to detect or quantify particular DNA sequences in a sample—for example, to detect the presence of viral sequences or to determine whether a tumor sample contains a known genetic alteration. PCR products are also used to generate purified DNA of known sequence for use in construction of novel DNA molecules.

DNA Construction. Restriction enzymes also provide a means by which unrelated DNA sequences can be combined to generate novel recombinant DNA molecules. Novel molecules can be copied and then inserted back into the same organism under control of a different promoter, to be expressed in a different cell type, or even cloned into a different species.

Such manipulation of DNA first requires replication of the *target sequence* by splicing it into the DNA of a *cloning vector*, such as a *plasmid*. Plasmids are small, circular pieces of double-stranded DNA which replicate in bacteria and can be cut open with restriction enzymes at specific sites designed to leave "sticky ends." Upon mixing with the target DNA fragment, the "sticky ends" of the plasmids bind, or *anneal,* to complementary sequences of the chosen DNA fragment, allowing the target sequence to drop into the plasmid like a cassette. Another enzyme, *DNA ligase,* seals the nicks in the DNA strands, resulting in a new plasmid containing the gene of interest. Plasmids infect, or *transfect* bacteria and replicate quickly using the bacterial machinery, giving rise to millions of copies of the target sequence. DNA sequences from unrelated sources can be inserted, or cloned, into the same plasmid, resulting in *recombinant DNA molecules* or "designer genes." After replication, plasmid DNA is isolated and purified and the insert sequence is removed using restriction enzymes appropriate for cutting at the ends of the desired sequence. The insert DNA fragment is then separated, based on size, from remaining plasmid DNA and finally purified.

DNA constructs have various forms and functions. One type of recombinant DNA construct is designed to modify the *expression pattern* of a gene. In this case, a tissue-specific promoter sequence isolated from one gene is spliced together with the protein coding region of a second gene. The resulting construct or transgene, when inserted back into the host genome, can be expressed in a novel cell type.

Other DNA constructs modify the structure of the final protein, often altering its functional activity. For example, a protein normally anchored to the cell membrane might be altered at the gene level so that it is expressed without the anchoring sequence. Although still translated, the protein is expressed as a soluble protein. Genetically engineered soluble receptor molecules might be used to competitively inhibit triggering of a cell surface receptor. Similarly, a sequence can be inserted into the protein coding region of a gene, which will cause it to "fold" into a different shape when expressed by the cell, thereby altering its function. Alternatively, the portion of a protein that transmits a signal to another molecule in the cytoplasm (the "cytoplasmic tail") might be left off in order to study where in a transduction pathway that protein functions. A similar technology gives rise to *fusion proteins*. A region of DNA coding for an entire protein, or a portion of one protein, is spliced together with the coding region for an entirely unrelated protein. The ultimate result, once transcription and translation take place, is the production of a novel protein with combined functions. For example, combining the coding sequence of gene X with that of a reporter protein that emits green fluorescence results in a fluorescent gene product, providing a means by which to monitor the expression of gene X.

Gene Transfer. Before the effects of these "designer genes" can be determined, they must be incorporated into the cell in which they are to be active, and this can be accomplished by several methods.

TRANSFECTION. Transfection is the process of incorporating DNA into cells growing in culture. Cells are mixed together with a large quantity of purified recombinant DNA, which is taken up into some percentage of cells and integrated into the host chromosome. The most frequent integration mechanism observed is *nonhomologous recombination*, in which the new sequence bears no sequence similarity to the piece of chromosome that it is integrating with. *Homologous recombination* occurs when a portion of the sequence of the new gene construction is identical to sequences within the chromosome into which it integrates. Once integrated into the chromosome, by either homologous or nonhomologous means, the new genetic material becomes part of the host genome, and as these cells proliferate, the new genes are copied and passed along as part of the natural DNA sequence. All daughter cells express the new *phenotype* designated by expression of the foreign DNA sequence.

VIRAL VECTORS. Incorporation of target DNA into *viral vectors* is another common method for transferring DNA sequences. This technology exploits the ability of viruses to adsorb to and infect eukaryotic cells, efficiently transporting the passenger DNA constructs into the cells. Viral vectors often contain powerful promoters that drive gene expression. The three most commonly used viral vectors are *retroviral vectors, herpes vectors,* and *adenoviral vectors.* Retroviruses integrate into the host genome and become permanent to all progeny. The other vectors, herpesviruses and adenoviruses, do not; they maintain their DNA episomally, or separate from the cell's own chromosomes. Episomal DNA may be passed on to daughter cells through several passages, but is eventually lost. These vectors are, however, able to infect a higher percentage of cells and, for that reason, they have been useful in gene therapy.

MOUSE TECHNOLOGY. Evaluation of the *in vivo* biological function of specific genes requires technology that alters the genetic makeup of entire organisms. During the past 15 years, the manipulation of the genome of the laboratory mouse has evolved into a routine tool for molecular biologists studying human genes. *Transgenic mice* overexpress a particular gene in a specified tissue or tissues, and *knockout mice*, as the name implies, are created by causing a specific mutation that will ablate the function of a gene. Similarly *knock-in* mice are the result of replacement of one gene by another functional gene sequence (5).

Transgenic Mice. Transgenic mice are created by introducing the desired DNA sequence, called a *transgene,* into fertilized mouse eggs, which are subsequently placed in the oviducts of pseudopregnant female mice. Progeny conceived through this process are derived from the altered oocyte and contain the transgene in all cells in their bodies. Transgenes contain promoter and regulatory sequences that direct expression in one or more tissues. Transgenes may also include inducible promoter regions, so that expression of the transgene can be controlled by administration of an inducing agent. Normally a few hundred copies of the desired foreign DNA sequence are injected into a fertilized mouse egg, where 1 to 50 copies integrate in a non-homologous fashion into random breaks in chromosomes. In most cases, the foreign DNA will not disrupt cellular function, and expression of the transgene occurs only in those tissues that use the transgene promoter sequence. Progeny are screened individually by analyzing a small amount of tissue (usually the tip of the tail) for the presence of the desired gene. Animals with the gene, called *founders*, are heterozygous for the passenger DNA sequence. Heterozygous founders are bred together, eventually resulting in a line homozygous for the transgene.

Using this technology, DNA can be transferred from one species to another. Moreover, by linking the gene of interest with a tissue-specific promoter, expression in a particular organ or cell type can be chosen. In this way one can target gene expression in certain organ systems specifically or in the animal as a whole. Analysis of transgenic mice for expression of a particular gene of interest is a *gain of function assay*. In comparing a normal mouse to the mouse expressing the transgene, one can answer the question "what is the morphological or biological outcome of expression of this gene?"

Knockout Mice. Creation of knockout mice, in which genes are mutated or disrupted, results in a *loss of function*. The technology is similar to, but more elaborate than, transgenic protocols because the gene to be ablated, along with its flanking regions, must be characterized. A new DNA construct, or *targeting vector,* is designed to have sequence homology with the flanking regions and/or one or more exons of the target gene. In addition to the homologous sequences, the new construct usually includes a gene encoding drug resistance and/or sensitivity. Once a construct is generated, it is transfected into murine embryonic stem cells (ES cells; derived from mouse embryos) and then selected for expression of the foreign DNA using the appropriate drug-based selection strategy. Because of the homology between the vector and the gene being targeted, some cells will incorporate the foreign DNA construct via *homologous recombination*, with the complementary sequences either disrupting or completely replacing the target gene.

Transfected ES cells are propagated in culture, analyzed to verify presence of the desired DNA construct, and then injected into developing mouse blastocysts. Once implanted into a pseudopregnant female, blastocysts continue to develop normally, resulting in *chimeric* progeny, in which some cells and tissues are derived from the original blastocyst and others from the genetically altered ES cells. All ES-derived cells, including some gametes, have the gene of interest disrupted or replaced with a nonfunctional sequence. Matings between these genetically manipulated animals and wild-type mice result in a few offspring heterozygous for the disrupted gene. Subsequent mating of two heterozygotes results in one-fourth of the progeny being homozygous for the mutation, and therefore deficient in the expression of the targeted gene.

Knockout mice provide a definitive method of establishing *in vivo* gene function; loss of a function after deleting a gene is direct evidence that the gene is responsible for that function. Unlike the transgenic situation, in which the DNA construct is in every cell but only expressed in certain cell types, the gene of interest is missing from every cell of a "knock-out" mouse—but only those cells/tissues in which the gene in question would normally be expressed are affected. With this technology one can ask the question, "What is the morphological or biological outcome of loss of this gene?"

Knock-in Mice. A "knock-in" is a more technically sophisticated version of the knockout. Rather than replacing the gene of interest with a nonfunctional sequence or drug-resistant gene, the target is actually replaced with a sequence coding for a modified functional gene. This can be a modification of the original gene or a completely different gene. The new gene, however, is always expressed according to the organ pattern of the original protein. In short, using homologous recombination and similar DNA constructs to those used in knockout technology, gene X is driven off of its promoter and replaced with a modified gene X or a completely different gene, which will be expressed in the same organ pattern as gene X.

Molecular Genetics of Brain Tumors

INTRODUCTION AND OVERVIEW. During the 1980s and 1990s, each of the tools of molecular biology described above played a substantial role in advancing the many branches of biology, including cancer research. Our current understanding of the biology of gliomas and recent advancements in diagnosis and treatment of these tumors became possible only once the basics of molecular genetics were known.

Cancer is caused by mutations in the DNA of single cells with subsequent *transformation* of the cell into a more proliferative, invasive, and progenitor-like phenotype. Mutations are acquired sequentially over time, resulting in many mutations in each tumor and giving altered cells a growth advantage over neighboring cells. Point mutations, along with gene amplifications or deletions ultimately alter the production of proteins required for normal cellular function. Molecular genetic analysis of excised tumors and human tumor cell lines has revealed a number of gene alterations that arise frequently. In the case of glial tumors, many mutations and gene alterations are consistently observed and tend to be found in genes encoding proteins involved in signal transduction and cell-cycle control pathways. Subsequent alterations in gene expression and enzyme activity, secondary to the original mutations, occur in proteins governing angiogenesis, invasion, and apoptosis.

In the following sections we will introduce the mechanisms cells use to regulate gene expression, cell growth, and cell proliferation, and then discuss how failure of these interrelated pathways leads to tumor formation, progression, and invasiveness. Defects in signal transduction and cell-cycle arrest pathways can, for the most part, be used to divide gliomas into two distinct categories, which will be discussed subsequently.

SIGNAL TRANSDUCTION. Cells are not self-sufficient—normal cells communicate with one another extensively. The currency of communication is the group of molecules known as *growth factors and growth factor receptors*, chemical messengers that interact on the molecular level to transmit signals from the outside of the cell to the nucleus, ultimately resulting in phenotypic change. Alterations in expression of growth factors and their receptors are commonly observed in tumors of glial origin.

Most receptors are composed of three general "regions" or domains. An extracellular domain contains the *ligand binding site,* the specific amino acid sequence which binds the signal transmitting growth factor, or *ligand*. A transmembrane region anchors the protein in the fluid-like cell membrane, and an intracellular domain with enzyme activity projects into the cytoplasm where it can, when activated, modify intracellular proteins

When the appropriate ligand binds to its receptor, the three-dimensional structure of the receptor protein is altered into a form that effects a signal to intracellular molecules. In the case of many growth factor receptors, modification of receptor structure involves *dimerization,* the process by which two single protein molecules, or *monomers,* bind together to form a *dimer* with two identical subunits. The dimer has enzymatic activity and can trigger multiple subsequent biochemical interactions within the cell, leading to a "cascade" of information. Eventually this "cascade" is transmitted to the nucleus where activation of DNA-binding *transcription factors* alter the expression of genes, thereby altering the functional program of the cell. Myriad cascades or "pathways" interact with one another in a tangled web resulting in instructions to the cell, via its genetic machinery, as to its ultimate function or fate. Some pathways are ubiquitous in nature, found in almost every living cell, while others are unique to a particular cell lineage.

Activation of growth factor receptors results in the expression of enzymatic activity, which catalyzes downstream interactions in various signal transduction pathways. The signals that seem to be most critical in gliomas are members of the tyrosine kinase receptor family, specifically epidermal growth factor receptor (EGFR), platelet-derived growth factor receptor (PDGFR), basic fibroblast growth factor receptor (b-FGFR), and many others. These receptors are related in that, upon complexing with their respective ligands, they form dimers, resulting in activation of the tyrosine kinase activity of the cytoplasmic portion of the molecule. Tyrosine kinases phosphorylate tyrosine residues on intracellular or membrane bound proteins, thereby activating a cascade of downstream interactions. One of the most critical and well-described pathways is initiated by Shc and Grb2, ultimately cascading through Ras and finally Jun and Fos, transcription factors that modify gene expression in the nucleus (Fig. 2)(6).

Another pathway activated by tyrosine kinase receptors involves phophatidylinositol-3-kinase (PI3K) which is brought to the membrane by the tyrosine kinase activity of the receptor molecule. PI3K signals by recruiting other cytoplasmic proteins, such as Akt, to the membrane where they can be activated by lipid intermediates. Subsequent signaling downstream of Akt drives cells away from apoptosis (programmed cell death) and toward proliferation (7,8).

Other pathways that incorporate proteins such as Src, protein kinase C (PKC), and Stat are also activated in this process. In short, there are multiple pathways that can be activated by a variety of messengers, and many of these pathways are common among the various receptors (9).

The importance of signal transduction pathways in tumorigenesis can be readily observed in experimental systems. For example, the potent transforming viral oncogene, Polyomavirus middle T antigen (MTA), activates three of the pathways outlined previously—Src, Shc, and PI3K (10,11). MTA is known to cause tumors in many cell types, including astrocytes, either by direct infection into animals or by injection of cells previously infected in culture (12).

Signal Transduction Alterations in Gliomas. Because modifications of the same growth factor receptors are observed frequently in the gliomas, it follows that at least some of the pathways activated by these receptors, whether singly or in combination, might be responsible for or required for tumor behavior. One common alteration in gliomas is the overproduction of growth factors, such as fibroblast growth factor (FGF). In this example, a mutation in the gene coding for the growth factor has not occurred, however there is too much growth factor or receptor being made. As a result, pathways downstream of these receptors exhibit increased activity (13). Actual mutations however have been identified in the genes coding for cellular receptors for several growth factors. For example, in somewhere between 30% and 50% of gliomas, the EGFR gene is amplified or mutated in such a way that it is constitutively active in the absence of the EGF ligand, resulting in increased signaling (14). EGFR gene amplification has been implicated in rapid regrowth kinetics in gliomas postsurgery (15).

Yet another piece of data supporting the conclusion that these signal transduction pathways are central to glioma biology is a recently discovered tumor suppressor called PTEN, a phosphatase and tensin homologue on chromosome 10. Loss of expression of this particular gene, located on chromosome 10, is found in the majority of glioblastomas. The normal function of PTEN is to prevent PI3K activation of Akt, therefore loss of PTEN function provides an oncogenic signal resulting in the activation of Akt (16,17).

CELL-CYCLE CONTROL. Regulation of the cell cycle is critical to normal development. Mechanisms exist to direct cells to proliferate when appropriate and to halt cell division when growth is inappropriate. Several pathways interact to provide cells with control over this important physiological event, however in cancer, these regulatory controls are often disrupted, leading to uncontrolled proliferation of transformed cells. Cell-cycle regulatory pathways have been extensively investigated, and several critical cell-cycle alterations have been identified in gliomas.

Overview of the Cell Cycle. Normal cells cycle through several phases (Fig. 3), each of which serves a specific function in either cell growth or cell division. During the *G_1 phase*, genes are expressed and protein synthesis occurs, but cells contain the normal complement of chromosomes with two copies each (2n; *diploid*). Some of the proteins synthesized in G_1 contribute to cell function and growth, and others are necessary prerequisites for DNA synthesis, which occurs in the next phase, *S* (for synthesis). During S phase, the cell replicates its DNA so that

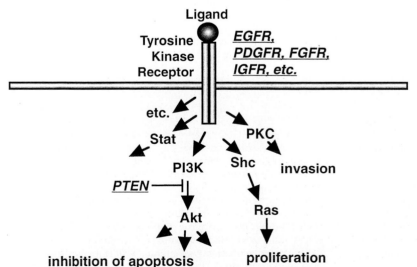

Fig. 2. Signal transduction pathways. A simplified diagram of pathways activated by tyrosine kinase receptors involved in gliomagenesis. Proteins encoded by genes mutated, amplified, or deleted in human gliomas are underlined. The result of these mutations is increased signaling through the common pathways illustrated.

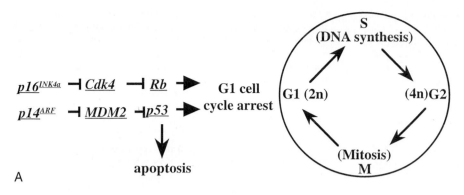

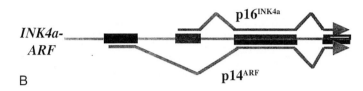

Fig. 3. Control of the cell cycle. **A:** Diagram of the cell cycle and pathways leading to G_1 cell-cycle arrest. Proteins encoded by genes either mutated, amplified, or deleted in human gliomas are underlined. The overall effect of these mutations is to inhibit the ability of a cell to maintain itself in the G_1 phase of the cell cycle, resulting in inappropriate progression into S phase and proliferation. **B:** The structure of the INK4a-ARF gene that encodes two gene products controlling the pathways outlined in **A**.

it contains two complete copies of genetic material, resulting in a doubled chromosome number (4n). The subsequent G_2 *phase* is characterized by growth and additional protein synthesis, resulting in a cell with sufficient protein and DNA content to support two daughter cells. This cell then proceeds into *M*, or mitosis, where it polarizes, and the two sets of identical chromosomes migrate to opposite poles. After the cell cleaves in the center, each of the resulting daughter cells contains 2n DNA. At this point the cells can either begin the cycle anew at G_1 or enter a quiescent phase called G_0, during which the cell is essentially at rest.

Normal cells spend most of their time in G_0 and G_1 due to regulatory mechanisms called G_1 arrest pathways, which inhibit cycling and prohibit continuous cell division. The two regulatory pathways that normally maintain G_1 status have been extensively investigated and are interwoven (18,19).

One pathway, *the Rb pathway*, is initiated by the protein p16INK4a (18,20,21). The indirect function of p16INK4a is to arrest cells in the G_1 phase by phosphorylating the protein product of the retinoblastoma gene, *Rb*. The Rb protein becomes activated when phosphorylated by cyclin-dependent kinase 4 (CDK4) in association with cyclin D1. This activation leads to the cell's progression through the cell cycle. In the absence of p16INK4a, activity of CDK4 rises, Rb is phosphorylated, and the cell progresses inappropriately to S phase.

The second pathway, designated the *p53 pathway*, (22–25) begins with a protein called p19ARF in mice and p14ARF in humans. The gene that codes for this protein was discovered in mice and the gene product name is based on the size (molecular weight) of the active mouse protein (19 kd). The human protein is smaller (14 kd) and is therefore designated p14ARF. Expression of p14ARF/p19ARF (henceforth referred to as p14ARF) regulates levels of the protein Mdm2, which in turn regulates the transcription factor p53 (26–28). In the absence of p14ARF, levels of Mdm2 rise and inhibit the normal function of p53, which is to recognize damaged DNA and regulate transcription of other genes. Normally, activated p53 either directs the arrest of the cell cycle by activating p21 or directs the cell to undergo apoptosis or programmed cell death. In the absence of p53 activity, cells with damaged DNA are permitted to proliferate, promoting mutations in cells. Similarly, the absence of p14ARF results in overexpression of Mdm2, suppression of p53 activity, and subsequently, unregulated cell proliferation.

The Rb and p53 pathways are inherently interwoven in that the initiating regulatory proteins, p16INK4a and p14ARF, are encoded by the same gene locus, *INK4a-ARF* (19,29). Expression of the two gene products, however, is under the control of separate promoter sequences and the genes are read in different reading frames, hence the designation "ARF" for *alternate reading frame*. Each uses a separate first exon and, although they share the second and third exons, the variation in reading frame at the start of the second results in completely different amino acid sequences. Although they are products of the same gene locus and have regions of sequence identity at the nucleic acid level, there is no similarity in amino acid sequence between the p16INK4a and p14ARF proteins. Nonetheless, these two gene products do exert their influence on the same phase of the cell cycle G_1, helping to inhibit cell division. Production of these two gene products is coordinately regulated, and together they control the two main pathways involved in G_1 cell-cycle arrest.

Deletions and mutations in INK4a-ARF usually generate simultaneous loss of both gene products. Rare tumors have been examined that have mutations affecting only p16INK4a (30), but more often deletions in the INK4a-ARF gene results in loss of both p16INK4a and p14ARF and dysregulation of both of these pathways upstream of cell-cycle arrest. No tumors have been found with an alteration in p14ARF alone (29). Both G_1 arrest pathways can also be simultaneously disrupted due to alterations in expression levels of other proteins in these pathways, for example, a combination of mutation in *p53* and overexpression of CDK4 would result in unregulated cell proliferation. Mice in which the INK4a-ARF locus has been deleted are viable, however, they develop spontaneous tumors at an early age and are highly sensitive to carcinogenic treatments (31), directly demonstrating the importance of the INK4a-ARF locus in suppression of neoplastic growth.

In summary, simultaneous disruption of both G_1 arrest pathways can result either from a mutation or deletion of INK4a-ARF, or from two or more independent alterations in genes encoding proteins downstream of the INK4a-ARF gene products. It is striking that this single gene, coding for two entirely different proteins, appears to, as described by Haber (29), "reside at the crossroad of regulation for both Rb and p53, through the use, unprecedented in mammalian cells, of overlapping distinct reading frames."

Effect of Cell-Cycle Disruption: Immortalization and Chromosomal Instability

IMMORTALIZATION. Under normal circumstances, cells can be isolated from an organism and grown in culture for a short time. Once placed in a culture vessel with the appropriate growth medium, they grow to confluence (the point at which cells have covered the surface of the culture vessel or are touching one another) and then stop. If the culture is divided into several new culture vessels with reduced cell density and fresh growth medium, cell division begins again and the new cultures grow to confluence. Eventually, after a number of culture divisions or "passages," growth slows and the cells reach *senescence*—they stop proliferating and die, regardless of the cell density and nutritional content of their growth medium.

An *immortalized* cell line, however, perpetuates for as long as nutrients and space are available. These cells never develop the "senescence" phenotype and do not undergo cell death. This phenotype results from disruption of G_1 arrest pathways. Analysis of DNA from many immortalized cell lines leads to the conclusion that these mutations are connected to the mechanism of immortalization—the inability to control G_1 arrest pathways. Interestingly, though, when astrocytes with disrupted G_1 arrest pathways reach confluence (i.e., come in contact with one another or essentially run out of space) they do stop dividing, therefore functional G_1 arrest pathways are not required for contact inhibition of growth (32).

Mutations in G_1 arrest pathways do not directly give rise to tumors. Mice deficient in p53 and those lacking INK4a-ARF develop and reproduce (31,33). In spite of the presence of the mutation in the DNA of every cell, only isolated cells of specific types transform and generate tumors later in life. Nonetheless, cells isolated from these mice grow immortally in culture (31, 32). In summary, disruption of the cell cycle is obviously important in formation and maintenance of glioblastoma and other cancers, but cell-cycle regulation defects are not the underlying cause of the disease.

CHROMOSOMAL INSTABILITY. Certain combinations of mutations in these pathways lead to a second consequence of cell-cycle dysregulation—disruption of chromosome stability. Under normal circumstances a cell is *diploid*, meaning that it contains two copies of each chromosome, one inherited from each parent. Mutation downstream of INK4a-ARF results in cells that eventually become *aneuploid*, meaning they have between three and ten copies of each chromosome. This is a common finding in tumors of all types including glioblastoma and the assumption is that, because G_1 arrest is also commonly effected in all of these tumors, there is a connection between the disruption of the pathways and the development of aneuploidy. For example, in astrocytes gene alterations downstream of INK4a-ARF, such as CDK4 overexpression (32), mutation in p53 (34), or overexpression of Mdm2 (35), all result in proliferating cells exhibiting aneuploidy. Alterations in the tumor suppressor gene p53 have been implicated as a major cause of "genetic instability" leading to higher grades of malignancy (36), and some investigators consider p53 to be the "guardian of the genome" (37). Overexpression of Myc, a transcription factor which plays a role downstream of signal transduction, or loss of critical Myc antagonists also result in immortalization of cells and dysregulation of chromosome number (38).

Cell-Cycle Defects in Gliomas.

It is undisputed that disruption of cell-cycle arrest pathways, although not the underlying "cause" of disease, is critical to the behavior of glial tumors in humans. Nearly all gliomas possess deletions in INK4a-ARF (39, 40) or mutation in p53 (usually associated with CDK4 overexpression or Rb loss) (41–43). Results of studies suggest that loss of p53 function promotes accelerated growth and malignant transformation in astrocytes (34). In most gliomas for which molecular genetic alterations have been pinpointed, there is an aberration in the G_1 arrest pathway. Approximately 30% of glial tumors contain a deletion or disruption of the p53 gene, and in a mostly nonoverlapping 60% of glial tumors the INK4a-ARF gene is mutated. Other genes involved in the same pathway, such as CDK4 and Rb are also well represented (43).

GLIOBLASTOMA SUBTYPES DEFINED BY SIGNAL TRANSDUCTION AND CELL-CYCLE ALTERATIONS. When the various types of mutations and alterations observed in glial tumors are analyzed, it is apparent that they are not scattered randomly. In fact, there are two apparent subtypes of glioblastoma (44). One subtype presents in older patients *de novo* as a grade IV glioma and tends to possess knockouts in the cell-cycle–related INK4a-ARF genes, p16^INK4A and p14^ARF. At the signal transduction level, these tumors tend to have EGFR gene amplifications, making them constitutively active (15,39, 41,42,45–47). The second subtype of glioma tends to arise in younger patients, usually as a lower grade glioma which progresses eventually to a higher grade. Rather than possessing INK4a-ARF deletions, these tumors typically have mutations in p53, along with either amplification of CDK4 or loss of Rb, all of which affect cell cycling downstream of the INK4a-ARF locus. Tumors of this younger group of patients also tend to express a different signal transduction alteration—amplification or overexpression of PDGF (36,48–50). According to Lang, gliomas of the second subtype discussed, which progress gradually to higher grades, can proceed by many paths, but may be "caused" by genetic instability resulting from p53 protein accumulation. Gliomas that appear to arise quickly via the *de novo* pathway, do not appear to arise due to p53 alterations, but seem to undergo genetic changes which immediately confer the malignant phenotype.

Because of this apparent pattern of genetic alterations in gliomas, a better understanding of the cell cycle, signal transduction pathways, and their respective regulatory mechanisms is critical for clinicians who wish to use new diagnostic and therapeutic modalities.

PROGRAMMED CELL DEATH: APOPTOSIS. When DNA is damaged beyond repair by radiation or chemicals, cell "suicide" normally destroys the cell before it can divide and give rise to genetically defective progeny (51–53). The previous section mentioned cell death as a possible downstream event following cell-cycle arrest. Whether a cell will undergo programmed cell death, or *apoptosis,* or be resistant to this event is controlled by a family of genes which can be divided on the basis of their "pro-apoptotic" and "anti-apoptotic" activity. Apoptosis, a specialized mechanism of cell death, is characterized by cell membrane changes, cytoplasmic and nuclear condensation, cell shrinkage, DNA fragmentation, and finally, formation of packages of cellular debris which can be easily phagocytized and cleared. Apoptosis is also an important factor in maintaining genetic stability in adult cells—by destroying cells with damaged DNA—and is a pivotal mechanism during embryonic development as the tissues take form.

Activation of an antiapoptotic gene product results in a cell that is resistant to apoptosis and therefore progresses through the cell cycle. Antiapoptotic genes are therefore, in a sense, oncogenes. As tumors increase in size, a balancing act transpires between cell proliferation and cell death. When the proliferative signal is greater than the apoptotic signal, due to activation of antiapoptotic genes, the tumor burden expands. Increasing tumorigenicity or size of the lesion can therefore be due to either enhanced proliferation or reduced apoptosis.

Antiapoptotic genes include the forerunner of this gene family, *Bcl-2*, which was first identified in a B cell lymphoma (54). Activation of this gene results in cells that do not die when appropriate, which makes it an oncogene. Two other antiapoptotic genes are *Bcl-x* and *Bcl-xl*. Proapoptotic family members—genes that force cells into apoptosis—include *Bad, Bax,* and *Bak.* When proapoptotic signals outweigh antiapoptotic signals, apoptosis progresses with mitochondrial dysfunction, caspase (protease) activity, chromosomal breakdown (DNA damage), and cell death.

Apoptosis as a mechanism of cell death fits neatly into the regulatory pathways for cell cycling and signal transduction already discussed. The transcription factor p53, which is downstream in the $p14^{ARF}$ pathway ($p14^{ARF}$ inactivates Mdm-2, subsequently inactivating p53 and permitting progression through the cell cycle), functions to assess DNA damage (e.g., due to radiation) and to either arrest the cell cycle at G_1 long enough for repair or to direct the cell to undergo apoptosis. In order to generate G_1 arrest, p53 activates p21, which in turn causes arrest. On the other hand, if the amount of DNA damage is too great to be repaired, the signal for apoptosis is generated by p53 through activation of proapoptotic gene family members including Bax and possibly Bak (55). The proapoptotic signal from p53, when it is functioning properly, is an "anti-tumor" signal. In the many tumors possessing mutations in p53, of course, including many gliomas, apoptosis dependent on a signal from p53 is not going to occur.

Several signal transduction pathways discussed previously feed into apoptotic pathways, directly or indirectly, by modifying proapoptotic and antiapoptotic activities and altering the balance between proliferation and cell death. For example, as previously described, the protein Akt, which normally functions downstream of PI3K, is inactivated by PTEN and is clearly involved in gliomagenesis (56). The function of Akt in apoptosis is to phosphorylate, and inactivate, Bad. The signal from Akt, when activated, is therefore a "pro-tumor" signal. When Bad is inactivated, the balance of proliferation versus cell death shifts toward proliferation. Additional evidence for the importance

of antiapoptotic pathways in cancer comes from recent work indicating that the EGFR may influence these pathways by activation of Bcl-xl (57).

Why is it important to understand the balance between apoptosis and proliferative signals? Some tumors are inherently resistant to apoptosis triggered by DNA damage from radiation, chemicals, and so forth, and there are other tumors that are very sensitive and can actually be cured by radiation. The reason for this probably lies in the balance between cell death and proliferation—between inhibition of proapoptotic pathways and activation of antiapoptotic pathways. Given a minor shift in that balance, a similar degree of DNA damage could be either curative or completely ineffective.

ANGIOGENESIS. Without a blood supply to carry oxygen and nutrients to rapidly proliferating cells, tumors would be essentially self-limiting. During early neoplastic growth, tumor cells are fed by the same capillaries that serve surrounding normal tissues. As tumors grow and require additional blood supply for survival, they send out signals to neighboring blood vessels, telling the endothelial cells to proliferate and to form new vessels. The endothelial cells, which make up these blood vessels, are not neoplastic themselves; they are simply responding to recruitment messages from the tumor cells. The study of *angiogenesis*, reviewed by Jensen (58), is the study of how tumor cells and endothelial cells communicate to give rise to new blood vessels. Not surprisingly, the language of this communication is growth factor/growth factor receptor interactions and signal transduction pathways (59). Tumor cells produce a number of powerful angiogenic factors (Fig. 4) including *vascular endothelial growth factor (VEGF)*. Two other factors, interleukin (IL)-8 (60,61) and b-FGF (62) are produced by both tumor cells and endothelial cells.

Endothelial cells express surface receptors for angiogenic factors. Signal transduction pathways downstream of a number of angiogenic receptors, including VEGF receptors (VEGFR), b-FGFR, and IL-8R, are the focus of current studies to determine whether receptor activation triggers changes in gene expres-

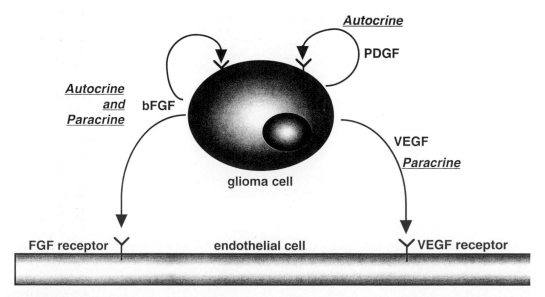

Fig. 4. Autocrine and paracrine signaling pathways controlling proliferation and angiogenesis. Vascular endothelial growth factor, basic fibroblast growth factor, and plasma-derived growth factor signaling mechanisms involved in glioma cell growth and the development of tumor vessels are diagramed and illustrate the connection between signal transduction and angiogenesis.

sion, proliferation of endothelial cells, production of blood vessels, or migration and invasion of vessels into the tumor.

Angiogenic signals are triggered in several ways. Activation of a tumor cell's VEGF gene occurs via signaling through PDGF/PDGFR (63) and possibly through other tyrosine kinase receptors as well. In astrocytoma cell lines, VEGF secretion has been shown to be mediated by Ras (64). VEGF activation is also triggered by hypoxia; as the tumor grows in size and the blood and oxygen supply becomes limiting, angiogenic factors are automatically triggered to bring in additional blood vessels. Subsequent signaling through VEGF and VEGFR is a "one way" communication from the tumor to the endothelial cell.

The mechanism of action of b-FGF differs somewhat. Basic-FGF is produced by tumor cells and b-FGF receptors are present on the surfaces of endothelial cells; in contrast to the VEGF/VEGFR situation, however, there are also receptors for b-FGF on tumor cells, leading to an *autocrine* signal (62). In short, there exists a complicated "conversation" between tumor cells and blood vessels, initiated by growth-promoting factors like PDGF and by hypoxia, resulting in proliferation of blood vessels and their spread into the growing tumor.

INVASION. As discussed previously, mutations cause cancer. Additional genetic alterations cause a cell to divide until a tumor forms. What prevents the surgeon from curing the disease is *invasion*—the process by which tumor cells move away from the initial lesion. Gliomas are especially difficult to treat surgically because glioblastoma cells appear to wander unimpeded throughout the brain, at one extreme (gliomatosis) developing into nothing more than individual cells scattered over a large area of tissue with no focal point at all. These tumor cells use protein destroying enzymes or *proteases* to "chew" their way through the extracellular matrix (ECM) which normally holds healthy brain cells together (65).

The molecular mechanisms responsible for invasion through brain tissue are currently being studied. Investigators have described migration of glial progenitor cells through the brain during normal development and their findings have shed light on the genetic pathways that may be involved in invasion by tumor cells. Interestingly, the effector molecules in invasion are also critical to nonpathological processes like embryogenesis, bone growth and remodeling, and ovulation. Several signal transduction pathways already discussed are responsible for directing tumor cells, or, in the case of normal development, progenitor cells, to migrate; one critical signal appears to be transduced via the b-FGF/b-FGFR pathway which is also active in angiogenesis. Receptors on the migrating cell first interact with ligands present in the ECM. Matrix metalloproteinases (MMPs) (65), a type of protease produced by tumor cells, digest the protein matrix and facilitate migration through the disrupted tissue. Along with MMPs, other proteases, including serine proteases and cysteine proteases, have been implicated in invasion of normal brain by glioma cells.

As discussed previously, many of the mutations observed in gliomas are in genes coding for growth factors and growth factor receptors, many of which are tyrosine kinases. Data on the effects of the overactivity of these signaling systems demonstrates that signal transduction via the ubiquitous tyrosine kinase receptors allows, or actually promotes, invasion by activating proteases (65). EGFR is a commonly amplified gene in glioblastoma, and expression appears to correlate with increasing tumor grade. Its ligand, EGF, has been shown to support invasion of tumor cells into aggregates of brain cells *in vitro* (66). Mechanistically, the connection between the growth factor receptors and invasion appears to signal through protein kinase C (PKC). PKC expression, which is upregulated downstream of

EGFR and PDGFR, has been shown to activate the expression of genes encoding the metalloproteinases (65).

CONCLUSION: A TANGLED WEB. All phenomena described in the previous pages—signal transduction, cell-cycle regulation, apoptosis, angiogenesis, and invasion—are interconnected. Downstream of all receptors that initiate signal transduction are positive as well as negative signals that feed into the molecular web which controls cell physiology. For example, functional signal transduction pathways are critical in regulation of the cell cycle. The transcription factor p53 is central to the cell cycle and apoptosis. Apoptosis is linked to both the cell cycle and signal transduction via Akt, which inactivates the proapoptotic protein Bad. The mechanisms for angiogenesis and invasion involve the same genes, so when one pathway is inhibited, so is the other. Angiogenesis depends on several signal transduction pathways, including VEGF/VEGFR, which require PDGF signaling, and invasion is potentiated by the activity of many of the tyrosine kinase receptors in these pathways. These pathways, via PKC, activate the proteases that digest migration paths between normal cells. Overexpression of Myc, a downstream target of signal transduction, or loss of Myc antagonists, results in immortalization of cells and dysregulation of chromosome number—a phenotype very similar to that observed after disruption of the cell cycle by INK4a-ARF deficiency or CDK4 overexpression. Another important link between signal transduction and the cell cycle involves the Ras pathway. Ras causes an increase in the activation of CDK4—an oncogenic activation. CDK4 is downstream of p16^{INK4a} and, once activated, inactivates Rb—one more link between signal transduction and cell-cycle control.

In short, cancer is caused by the dysregulation of multiple interacting pathways. Gene alterations result in net proliferation of the tumor cell population and overexpression of factors that promote construction of an elaborate blood supply to nourish the burgeoning tumor. Ensuing chromosomal instability and loss of senescence leaves affected cells unable to regulate their own growth. As if that were not enough, activation of some of these pathways actually promotes production of substances that can chew through the cement between cells to allow tumor cells to migrate further into tissues.

The pathways leading to these characteristics are interwoven, making cause-and-effect determinations difficult at best. However, because of our newfound ability to look into the cell and manipulate its machinery using molecular genetic technology, science and medicine have rapidly elucidated much of the structure of the tangled web of cancer biology. Through further exploitation of new molecular genetics tools at our disposal, we are approaching the day when we will unweave the tangled web in tumor cells and completely describe the molecular origins of this disease.

References

1. Watson JD. The awful incompleteness of eucaryotic cell biochemistry. In: Watson JD, ed. *Molecular biology of the gene*. Reading, MA: WA Benjamin, 1977:584.
2. Gunther J. *Death be not proud*. New York: Harper and Row Publishers, 1949.
3. Old RW, Primrose SB. Principles of gene manipulation: an introduction to genetic engineering. In: Carr N, Ingraham J, Rittenberg S, eds. *Studies in microbiology*. Vol. 2, 4th ed. Oxford: Blackwell Scientific, 1989:437.

4. Strickberger M. *Genetics.* New York: MacMillan Publishing Co, 1976.
5. Abbas A, Pober J, Lichtman A. *Cellular and molecular immunology,* 2nd ed. Philadelphia: WB Saunders, 1994:457.
6. Guha A, et al. Proliferation of human malignant astrocytomas is dependent on Ras activation. *Oncogene* 1997;15:2755–2765.
7. Jiang B, et al. Myogenic signaling of phosphatidylinositol 3-kinase requires the serine-threonine kinase Akt/protein kinase B. *Proc Natl Acad Sci USA* 1999;96(5):2077–2081.
8. Aoki M, et al. The akt kinase: molecular determinants of oncogenicity. *Proc Natl Acad Sci USA* 1998;95:14950–14955.
9. Hunter T. Protein kinases and phosphatases: the yin and yang of protein phosphorylation and signaling. *Cell* 1995;80(2):225–236.
10. Dilworth S, et al. Transformation by polyoma virus middle T antigen involves the binding and tyrosine phosphorylation of Shc. *Nature* 1994;367:87–90.
11. Summers S, Lipfer L, Birnbaum M. Polyoma middle T antigen activates the Ser/Thr kinase Akt in a PI3-kinase-dependent manner. *Biochem Biophys Res Commun* 1998;246:76–81.
12. Aguzzi A, Wagner EF, Williams RL, et al. Sympathetic hyperplasia and neuroblastomas in transgenic mice expressing polyoma middle T antigen. *New Biol* 1990;6:533–543.
13. Gross J, et al. Basic fibroblast growth factor: a potential autocrine regulator of human glioma cell growth. *J Neurosci Res* 1990;4:689–696.
14. Ekstrand A, et al. Functional characterization of an EGF receptor with a truncated extracellular domain expressed in glioblastomas with EGFR gene amplification. *Oncogene* 1994;9:2313–2330.
15. Schlegel J, et al. Amplification of the epidermal-growth-factor-receptor gene correlates with different growth behaviour in human glioblastoma. *Int J Cancer* 1994;56:72–77.
16. Li J, et al. The PTEN/MMAC1 tumor suppressor induces cell death that is rescued by the AKT/protein kinase B oncogene. *Cancer Res* 1998;58:5667–5672.
17. Wu X, et al. The PTEN/MMAC1 tumor suppressor phosphatase functions as a negative regulator of the phosphoinositide 3-kinase/Akt pathway. *Proc Natl Acad Sci USA* 1998;1998(95):26.
18. Serrano M, Hannon GJ, Beach D. A new regulatory motif in cell-cycle control causing specific inhibition of cyclin D/CDK4. *Nature* 1993;366:704–707.
19. Quelle DE, et al. Alternative reading frames of the INK4a tumor suppressor gene encoding two unrelated proteins capable of inducing cell cycle arrest. *Cell* 1995;83:993–1000.
20. Robens J. The Rb pathway. Available at: *http://www.geocities.com/CollegePark/Lab/1580/rb.html.* Accessed December 27, 2001.
21. Weinberg RA. The retinoblastoma protein and cell cycle control. *Cell* 1995;81:323–330.
22. Levine AJ. The tumor suppressor genes. *Annu Rev Biochem* 1993;62:623–651.
23. Levine A. p53, the cellular gatekeeper for growth and division. *Cell* 1997;88:323–331.
24. Thut C, Goodrich J, Tijan R. Repression of p53-mediated transcription by MDM2: a dual mechanism. *Genes Dev,* 1997;11:1974–1986.
25. Robens J. p53 Pathway. Available at: *http://www.geocities.com/CollegePark/Lab/1580/p53.html.* Accessed December 27, 2001.
26. Kamijo T, et al. Tumor suppression at the mouse INK4a locus mediated by the alternative reading frame product p19^{ARF}. *Cell* 1997;91:649–69.
27. Pomerantz J, et al. The Ink4a tumor suppressor gene product, p19^{ARF}, interacts with MDM2 and neutralizes MDM2's inhibition of p53. *Cell* 1998;92:713–723.
28. Zhang Y, Xiong Y, Yarbrough WG. ARF promotes MDM2 degradation and stabilizes p53: ARF-INK4a locus deletion impairs both the Rb and p53 tumor suppression pathways. *Cell* 1998;92:725–734.
29. Haber DA. Splicing into senescence: the curious case of p16 and p19^{ARF}. *Cell* 1997;91:555–558.
30. Quelle DE, et al. Cancer-associated mutations at the INK4a locus cancel cell cycle arrest by p16INK4a but not by the alternative reading frame protein p19ARF. *Proc Natl Acad Sci. USA* 1997;94:669–673.
31. Serrano M, Lee H, Chin L, et al. Role of the INK4a locus in tumor suppression and cell mortality. *Cell* 1996;85:27–37.
32. Holland EC, et al. Overexpression of cdk4 but not loss of INK4a-ARF induces hyperploidy in cultured mouse astrocytes, modeling mutations in the G1 arrest pathway in human gliomas. *Genes Dev* 1998;12:3644–3649.
33. Donehower LA, et al. Mice deficient for p53 are developmentally normal but susceptible to spontaneous tumours. *Nature* 1992;356:215–221.
34. Yahanda AM, et al. Astrocytes derived from p53-deficient mice provide a multistep in vitro model for development of malignant gliomas. *Mol Cell Biol* 1995;15(8):4249–4259.
35. Hively W, Holland E, Varums H. Unpublished observations.
36. Lang FF, et al. Pathways leading to glioblastoma multiforme: a molecular analysis of genetic alterations in 65 astrocytic tumors. *J Neurosurg* 1994;81:427–436.
37. Lane D. p53, the guardian of the genome. *Nature* 1992;358:15–17.
38. Zindy F, et al. Myc signaling via the ARF tumor suppressor regulates p53-dependent apoptosis and immortalization. *Genes Dev* 1998;12:2424–2433.
39. Schmidt E, et al. CDKN2 (p16/MTS1) gene deletion or cdk4 amplification occurs in the majority of glioblastomas. *Cancer Res* 1994;54:6321–6324.
40. Jen J, et al. Deletion of p16 and p15 genes in brain tumors. *Cancer Res* 1994;54:6353–6358.
41. He J, et al. CDK4 amplification is an alternative mechanism to p16 gene homozygous deletion in glioma lines. *Cancer Res* 1994;54:5804–5807.
42. He J, Olson JJ, James CD. Lack of p16INK4 or retinoblastoma protein (pRb) or amplification-associated overexpression of Cdk4 is observed in distinct subsets of malignant glial tumors and cell lines. *Cancer Res* 1995;55:4833–4836.
43. Ichimura K, et al. Human glioblastomas with no alterations of the CDKN2A (p16^{INK4A},MTS1) and CDK4 genes have frequent mutations of the retinoblastoma gene. *Oncogene* 1996;13:10655–1072.
44. von Deimling A, et al. Subsets of glioblastoma multiforme defined by molecular genetic analysis. *Brain Pathol* 1993;3:19–26.
45. Louis DN, et al. Comparative study of p53 gene and protein alterations in human astrocytic tumors. *J Neuropathol Exp Neurol* 1993;52(1):31–38.
46. Ono Y, et al. Malignant astrocytomas with homozygous CDKN2/P16 gene deletions have higher K1-67 proliferation indices. *J Neuropathol Exp Neurol* 1996;55(10):1026–1031.
47. Hayashi Y, et al. Association of EGFR gene amplification and CDKN2 (p16/MTS1) gene deletion in glioblastoma multiforme. *Brain Pathol* 1997;7:871–875.
48. Rasheed BKA, et al. Alterations of the TP53 gene in human gliomas. *Cancer Res* 1994;54:1324–1330.
49. van Meyel DJ, et al. P53 mutation, expression and DNA ploidy in evolving gliomas: evidence for two pathways of progression. *J Natl Cancer Inst* 1994;86:1011–1017.
50. Watanabe K, et al. Overexpression of the EGF receptor and p53 mutations are mutually exclusive in the evolution of primary and secondary glioblastomas. *Brain Pathol* 1996;6:217–224.
51. Robens J. Apoptosis. Available at: *http://www.geocities.com/CollegePark/Lab/1580/apoptosis.html.* Accessed December 27, 2001.
52. Hengartner M. Apoptosis. Death by crowd control. *Science* 1998;281:1298–1299.
53. Adams J, Cory S. Bcl-2 protein family: arbiters of cell survival. *Science* 1998;281:1322–1326.
54. Tsujimoto Y, et al. Involvement of the bcl-2 gene in human follicular lymphoma. *Science* 1985;228:1440–1443.
55. Bennett M. Mechanisms of p53-induced apoptosis. *Biochem Pharmacol* 1999;58(7):1089–1095.
56. Stambolic V, et al. Negative regulation of PKB/Akt-dependent cell survival by the tumor suppressor PTEN. *Cell* 1998;95(1):29–39.
57. Nagane M, et al. Drug resistance of human glioblastoma cells conferred by a tumor-specific mutant epidermal growth factor receptor through modulation of Bcl-XL and caspase-3-like proteases. *Proc Natl Acad Sci USA* 1998;95(10):5724–5729.
58. Jensen R. Growth factor-mediated angiogenesis in the malignant progression of glial tumors: a review. *Surg Neurol* 1998;49(2):189–195.
59. Schmidt N, et al. Levels of vascular endothelial growth factor, hepatocyte growth factor/scatter factor and basic fibroblast growth factor in human gliomas and their relation to angiogenesis. *Int J Cancer,* 1999;84(1):10–18.
60. Desbaillets I, et al. Upregulation of interleukin 8 by oxygen-deprived cells in glioblastoma suggests a role in leukocyte activation,

chemotaxis, and angiogenesis. *J Exp Med* 1997;186(8):1201–1212.

61. Desbaillets I, et al. Regulation of interleukin-8 expression by reduced oxygen pressure in human glioblastoma. *Oncogene* 1999;18(7):1447–1456.
62. Takahashi J, et al. Correlation of basic fibroblast growth factor expression levels with the degree of malignancy and vascularity in human gliomas. *J Neurosurg* 1992;76(5):792–798.
63. Wang D, et al. Induction of vascular endothelial growth factor expression in endothelial cells by platelet-derived growth factor

through the activation of phosphatidylinositol 3-kinase. *Cancer Res* 1999;59(7):1464–1472.
64. Feldkamp M, et al. Normoxic and hypoxic regulation of vascular endothelial growth factor (VEGF) by astrocytoma cells is mediated by Ras. *Int J Cancer* 1999;81(1):118–124.
65. Uhm JH, et al. Mechanisms of glioma invasion: role of matrix-metalloproteinases. *Can J Neurol Sci* 1997;24(1):3–15.
66. Engerbraaten O, et al. Effects of EGF, bFGF, NGF, and PDGF(bb) on cell proliferative, migratory and invasive capacities of human brain-tumor biopsies in vivo. *Int J Cancer* 1993;53:209–214.

100. Immunobiology of Intracranial Gliomas

Kevin O. Lillehei

Significant advancements have been made in our understanding of the complex nature of the immune system in the last several decades. This understanding has had a tremendous impact on our understanding of health and disease. In particular, this knowledge has revolutionized our understanding of the interactions occurring between the immune system and cancer. In this chapter we review our current understanding of the immune system, particularly as it relates to intracranial gliomas.

The concept of manipulating the immune system to eradicate tumor is not new. Over 100 years ago (in 1893), William Coley first reported on the ability to induce tumor regressions by nonspecific activation of the immune system in response to bacterial toxins (1). Coley, a young general surgeon, first recognized the occurrence of profound tumor regression in a man with advanced metastatic sarcoma who developed a concurrent erysipelas infection. From this observation, he developed a strategy for antitumor treatment, initially inoculating patients with the *Streptococcus erysipelas (S. pyogenes)* bacteria (a bold venture in the era preceding the discovery of penicillin), and later inoculating patients with the filtered or heat-treated combined cell culture supernatants of *S. pyogenes* and *Serratia marcescens* (previously called *Bacillus prodigiosus*). The overall benefit of "Coley's toxin" remains controversial, but clearly there were patients who showed tumor regression with prolonged survival. Coley's heroic efforts earned him the title of "father of immunotherapy," long before the principles of immunology were recognized. As Coley stated at the time of his discovery, "Nature often gives us hints to her profoundest secrets, and it is possible that she has given us a hint which, if we will but follow, may lead us on to the solution of this difficult problem (1)."

Despite Coley's beginnings, efforts to reliably manipulate the immune system to promote tumor regression have been universally disappointing. The concept of immunotherapy as a useful therapeutic intervention for the treatment of cancer is becoming a reality with recent advances in our understanding of the immune system and the identification and availability of numerous growth promoting and growth-suppressing cytokines. Immunology is a field that historically has been foreign to the practicing neurosurgeon. As progress in this field is being made, however, it will become increasingly important for the neurosurgeon to have a better understanding of tumor immunology as it relates to the treatment of his or her patients. This chapter discusses the current understanding of the immune system as it relates to tumor recognition, review the current knowledge concerning tumor-induced immunosuppression, and discuss current strategies of immunotherapy treatment.

Evidence Supporting the Existence of an Intracranial Local Immune Response

Pathologists have long debated the significance of local lymphocyte infiltration into high- and low-grade glioma specimens. Bertrand and Mannen in 1960 first demonstrated the presence of lymphoid infiltrates in astrocytomas (2). Since then, approximately 30% to 60% of gliomas have been shown to exhibit a mononuclear cell infiltrate. The exact role of this mononuclear infiltrate remains unclear, however. In 1971, Ridley and Cavanagh, after studying a large postmortem series of gliomas, suggested that these lymphocytes were evidence of the body's attempt to mount an antitumor immune response (3). Later, studies by Palma (4) and Brooks (5), looking at surgical biopsy specimens, demonstrated a distinct survival advantage for patients with high-grade gliomas who had evidence of lymphoid infiltrates. In Brooks' series, the most significant finding, correlating with increased patient survival was the presence of a mononuclear cell invasion into the perivascular spaces surrounding the tumor. Surprisingly, lymphocyte invasion into the tumor parenchyma itself was of less importance. The overall survival advantage, however, was small (approximately 4 months) compared to similar reports examining lymphocyte infiltration into tumors outside the central nervous system (CNS). In breast cancer it has been shown that the degree of lymphocyte invasion provides an index of prognosis equal to the histological grade of dedifferentiation (6), with the intensity of the lymphocyte infiltration directly correlating with the presence or absence of metastases (7). In malignant gliomas, it has been demonstrated that the predominant mononuclear cell in the infiltrate is the T lymphocyte, with the majority of these cells being the CD8+ suppressor/cytotoxic T lymphocyte (8).

The CD4+ helper/inducer T lymphocyte is seen less frequently, with B lymphocytes seen only rarely. The presence of this T-cell infiltrate in gliomas argues for the existence of glioma tumor-specific and -associated antigens capable of generating an immune response, albeit weak. The presence of B-cell–mediated humoral immunity in glioma patients does exist (9), but its role in tumor rejection appears limited. This T-cell immune response seems to be most prevalent in the perivascular spaces along the advancing border of the tumor, suggesting an attempt by the body to control tumor infiltration into normal brain. More recently, Miescher has shown that tumor-infiltrating lymphocytes (TILs) isolated from high-grade gliomas are significantly immunosuppressed, having virtually lost their ability to actively proliferate (10). When these same cells are cloned, however, they demonstrate clear cytotoxic activity against autologous tumor; therefore, it appears that the immune system can recognize glioma cells as foreign and the body attempts to mount an antitumor response. This response appears to be inhibited, however. The suppressed state of the T-cell–mediated immune response is felt to be secondary to immunoinhibitory factors produced by the glioma cells themselves.

Analysis of the Brain as an "Immunoprivileged" Site

For many years the brain, like the anterior chamber of the eye, was viewed as an immunoprivileged site. This was based on experimental observations demonstrating the ability of major histocompatibility complex (MHC) mismatched tissues transplanted into the brain to survive (11), the fact that animals sensitized to a foreign antigen demonstrated a delayed or incomplete immune response when challenged intracranially yet rejected the antigen systemically (12), and a number of experimental vaccine strategies showing efficacy against transplanted tumors systemically but failing intracranially (13). Factors possibly responsible for this immune isolation of the brain from the rest of the body include the absence of a conventional lymphatic drainage system, the presence of the blood–brain barrier (BBB), and the observed paucity of immune cells trafficking within the brain parenchyma. Recent evidence examining these three factors, in fact, argues against them being significant deterrents to intracranial immunoresponsiveness. We examine each of these factors individually.

LACK OF A LYMPHATIC DRAINAGE SYSTEM. Lack of a conventional lymphatic drainage system within the brain was previously thought to be important in blocking the afferent limb of the immune response. Experimental studies in mammals, in fact, have demonstrated firm physiologic evidence for the lymphatic drainage of interstitial fluid and cerebrospinal fluid (CSF) from the brains of rats, rabbits, and cats. Although the bulk of CSF within the white matter appears to drain into the ventricles and ultimately through the venous sinuses into the systemic circulation, tracer studies in gray matter show that interstitial fluid in this region passes along perivascular spaces to the surface of the brain and ultimately into the deep cervical lymph nodes. Once fluid reaches the surface of the brain, it communicates with the perivascular CSF compartments in the subarachnoid space, following the course of major arterial branches to the circle of Willis and then along ethmoidal arteries to the cribriform plate. Particulate tracers have then been shown to enter channels in the arachnoid beneath the olfactory bulbs and connect directly with the nasal lymphatics. This drainage then proceeds into the deep cervical lymph nodes, through channels that pass through holes in the cribriform plate (14). In a study using radiolabeled albumin injected into brain tissue, the protein was seen to appear in the deep cervical lymph node at about 2 hours, reaching a maximal concentration in 15 to 20 hours (15).

THE BLOOD–BRAIN BARRIER. The BBB is formed by the presence of tight junctions between cerebral capillary endothelial cells and the astrocytic processes that surround the capillary. These tight junctions prevent the passage of intravital dyes, immunoglobulins, and neuroactive compounds from normally passing between the bloodstream and brain. This barrier, however, can be disrupted during inflammation, as seen with infection, autoimmune disease, trauma, or tumor. Cells close to the cerebral capillaries, on activation, elaborate cytokines (e.g., tumor necrosis factor, TNF) that upregulate adhesion molecules promoting immune cell binding. Several cell adhesion molecules, such as RANTES, selectins, α-4, MCP-1, MIP-1α, ICAM-1, ICAM-2, VCAM-1, and LFA-3 are expressed on cerebral endothelium. Overexpression of LFA-1, α-4, CD44, and CD2 molecules on activated T lymphocytes contributes to their adhesion and their ultimate migration through the BBB (16). Inflammation by itself also is known to lead to a loosening of the tight endothelial junctions, leading to passage of lymphocytes, monocytes, and macrophages from the systemic circulation into the brain.

LYMPHOCYTE TRAFFICKING IN THE BRAIN. Finally, although the presence of lymphocytes in the brain of normal individuals is rare, their presence during pathologic conditions, such as multiple sclerosis, is now widely recognized (17). Hickey (18) and coworkers demonstrated that C14-labeled CD4+ myelin basic protein-specific T-cell lines, when activated either by the presentation of specific antigen or by concanavalin A, migrate to the brain through an intact BBB. The first phase of entry occurs within 24 hours of injection, with the second phase occurring after 96 hours. How long these lymphocytes persist within the CNS is dependent on the recognition of T-lymphocyte–specific antigens.

With the current interest in tumor vaccines for the treatment of intracranial glioma, the use of tumor homogenates containing normal glial antigens, such as myelin basic protein, carry the potential of inducing experimental allergic encephalomyelitis (EAE). EAE is a potentially devastating autoimmune, inflammatory, demyelinating process mediated by CD4+ T cells. This syndrome was first reported in 1885, when patients were vaccinated against rabies with spinal cord tissue derived from rabbits infected with the rabies virus. Subsequently it was reproduced experimentally in primates following repeated inoculations with normal brain tissue. Clearly it appears to be promoted by the use of immune adjuvants. The possibility of creating an EAE-type immune reaction always must be kept in mind in pursuing immune therapy and is of particular concern with the current use of tumor vaccine strategies employing strong immune adjuvants, such as dendritic cell stimulation.

Brain Tumor Heterogeneity

One of the major stumbling blocks to the application of immunotherapy in the treatment of gliomas has been the identification of a consistently expressed, universal tumor antigen. Well-documented genetic alterations occur within gliomas, which include the loss, gain, or amplification of different chromosomes. These alterations lead to changes in the expression of proteins that play important roles in the regulation of cell proliferation. Common genetic alterations seen at the chromosomal level in gliomas include loss of chromosomes 17p, 13q, 9p, 19, 10, 22q, and 18q, and amplification of chromosomes 7 and 12q. These alterations subsequently lead to changes in the expression of multiple genes during the genesis and progression of human gliomas. The genes affected include p53 mutations, epidermal growth factor receptor (EGFR) amplification, inactivation of the CDKN2A gene (9p21), overexpression of platelet-derived growth factor, and p16 deletion. Abnormalities have also been noted in the following genes; RB, INF α/B, MMAC1, DCC, MDM2, GLI, CDK4, SAS, MET, MYC, TGF α, CD44, VEGF, hNr-CAM, NCAM L1, p21, trkA, MMRs, C4-2, and D2-2 (19). Resultant abnormalities in protein production include the cathepsins, tenascin, matrix metalloproteases, tissue inhibitors of metalloproteases, nitric oxide synthetase, integrins, IL-13 receptor, connexin 43, uPARs, extracellular matrix proteins, and heat-shock proteins (20,21).

These findings point to a vast array of abnormalities occurring within the tumor cell, all of which could serve as targets for immunotherapy. Difficulty, however, arises in isolating changes in the tumor cell that are critical to cell survival and specifically unique to the tumor cell alone.

Major Histocompatibility Complex Expression within the Central Nervous System

The interaction of tumor antigen with local MHC Class I and II molecules is critical to the development of an antitumor immune response. T-lymphocyte activation by a specific tumor antigen requires the presentation of the antigen, along with the MHC molecule, to the appropriate receptor site on the naïve T lymphocyte. Both MHC Class I and II molecules can be detected within the CNS of most species; however, their distribution is irregular and their expression is under strict regulatory control, being limited to specific cell types. MHC Class I expression *in vivo,* within the normal CNS, is concentrated on the endothelial and parenchymal cells, with no definitive Class I staining associated with normal neurons (22). Induced or occasional Class I staining has been identified on microglia or ependymal and stromal cells (23). MHC Class II molecule expression in the normal CNS is limited to subsets of microglial cells (especially in white matter), and CNS dendritic cells (24). Although there is general agreement that neurons and oligodendrocytes do not express MHC Class II molecules under normal conditions, disagreement remains as to whether endothelial cells and astrocytes might express the Class II molecule, especially under pathologic conditions such as multiple sclerosis and EAE (25, 26). *In vitro,* all major CNS cell types except neurons have demonstrated a capacity to express MHC Class I molecules; this expression can be upregulated by exposure to interferon-γ (27). MHC Class II expression also has been demonstrated in astrocytes and oligodendrocytes under various conditions. This expression, however, remains below that usually found in microglia *in vivo* (28). Although MHC Class I or II molecule expression is not a prominent feature of glial tumors, expression of both classes of molecules on a small subset of malignant astrocytes has been demonstrated convincingly. Various methods of increasing MHC expression within the CNS, to optimize tumor antigen recognition, represent one of the goals of tumor immunotherapy.

Current Understanding of the Immunodeficiency Seen in Brain Tumor Patients

Patients with malignant gliomas have evidence of a generally suppressed immune responsiveness, particularly of cell-mediated immunity. These patients have been shown to exhibit the following deficiencies: cutaneous anergy with an abnormal delayed hypersensitivity for common recall and tumor antigens *(Mycobacterium tuberculosis, Candida albicans)*; a reduced number of circulating T lymphocytes; a depressed lymphocyte proliferative response to mitogens such as phytohemagglutinin, Concanavalin A, or phorbol ester; a decreased antibody response to tetanus toxoid, influenza virus, or other antigens; and a deficient antibody-mediated and T-cell–mediated cytotoxicity *in vitro.* The primary cause of this immune deficiency appears to reside in the CD4(+) T-lymphocyte subset. Work by Elliot has implicated a defect in IL-2 secretion and in the expression of the high-affinity IL-2 receptor in the CD4(+) T-cell subpopulation (29). Interestingly, this defect is not amenable to exogenous administration of IL-2, and is likely caused by immunosuppressive substances secreted by the glioma cells (30). This immunosuppression is partially relieved by surgical removal of the tumor (31). The responsible immunosuppressive factors currently isolated include: transforming growth factor-B (TGF-B), interleukin-10 (IL-10), insulin-like growth factor-1 (IGF-1), and prostaglandin E-2 (PGE-2).

Immunosuppressive Cytokines

Cytokines are soluble proteins secreted by cells of the immune system, either lymphocytes or monocytes, which then exert their regulatory action on other target cells. Cytokines may function to enhance or suppress the local immune response and, may act to promote or inhibit tumor cell growth depending on the particular cytokine and local environment.

TGF-B is the most well characterized immunosuppressive cytokine secreted by gliomas. TGF-B has been shown to have potent immunosuppressive effects on several immune functions such as IL-2 dependent T cell proliferation and IL-2 expression, interferon (IFN) boosting of natural killer (NK) cell activity, cytotoxic T cell development, LAK cell development, IL-1 dependent lymphocyte proliferation, IFN-γ induced MHC class II antigen expression on tumor cells, and B-cell proliferation (32). The TGF-B isoform found in the supernatant of human glioblastoma cells is TGF-B2. TGF-B2 is secreted as a large and inactive precursor, becoming biologically active only after cleavage by proteases such as plasmin or cathepsin. Normal brain astrocytes in culture express three TGF-B isoforms (TGF-B1, 2, 3) but secrete TGF-B2 only in its inactive latent form (33). Glioblastoma cell lines, however, have been shown to secrete TGF-B2 mainly in its active cleaved form. Protease inhibitors, blocking the activation of TGF-B2 by glioma-derived proteolytic enzymes, have been shown to inhibit the T-cell suppression normally produced by glioblastoma cell lines (34).

A second soluble factor produced by malignant gliomas and implicated in local immunosuppression is prostaglandin E2 (PGE2). PGE2 activates a diverse family of receptor subtypes, downregulates the generation of LAK cell activity, and has the capacity to suppress T-cell proliferation induced by mitogenic anti-CD3 antibodies *in vitro* (35). PGE2 also has been shown to downregulate the expression of the class II antigen HLA-

DR, possibly contributing to the tumor cells' ability to escape immune surveillance. Prostaglandin inhibitors such as aspirin or the nonsteroidal antiinflammatory drugs (i.e., sulindac and indomethacin) have shown a beneficial effect on the immune system, with aspirin use associated with a 50% reduction in the incidence of colon cancer when used prophylactically (36).

A third factor produced by malignant gliomas and implicated in local immunosuppression is the cytokine IL-10. It has been suggested, through indirect studies, that IL-10 acts to inhibit the release of IFN-γ by lymphocytes and to partially inhibit MHC class II expression by monocytes (37). It is not clear, however, how significant a role IL-10 plays in tumor-induced immunosuppression. IL-10 has actually been shown to enhance the antitumor immune response in some animal models.

More recently, insulin-like growth factor-1 (IGF-1), IGF-2, and their receptors (IGF-1R and IGF-2R), have been shown to act as local immunosuppressive factors. Both IGF-1 and IGF-2, along with their respective receptor mRNAs, have been demonstrated in primary human astrocytomas and meningiomas. Control, nonmalignant, human brain has been shown to express only low levels of IGF-1, IGF-1R, and IGF-2R. IGF-1 is a polypeptide crucially involved in the normal growth and development of many tissues and cell types, including fibroblasts, epithelial cells, smooth muscle cells, osteoclasts, and bone marrow stem cells. It is believed that in tumor cells, IGF-1 and its receptor may be involved in promoting continuous cell proliferation through an autocrine stimulatory loop, driving the tumorigenic phenotype. Trojan and co-workers have shown that a nonsyngeneic C6 glioma cell line can be induced to express a highly immunogenic phenotype resulting in tumor rejection by blocking IGF-1 expression through use of IGF-1 antisense RNA

(38). The immune response generated consists predominantly of CD8+ lymphocytes.

Generation of an Immune Response

It is now clearly evident that T lymphocytes play a critical role in the body's ability to generate an antitumor response. The initiation or priming of a specific T-cell response requires the recognition of a specific tumor antigen (usually presented with the aid of a professional antigen presenting cell, APC), the generation of a CD4+ (helper/inducer) T-cell response through the aid of costimulatory molecules and MHC type II antigens, and a CD8+ (suppressor/cytotoxic) T-cell response aided by local IL-2 cytokine secretion and the presence of MHC type I antigens.

The T-Cell–Mediated Immune Response

The generation of an effective T-cell–mediated immune response requires the activation of both the cytotoxic (CD8+) and helper (CD4+) T-lymphocyte subsets. As shown in Figure 1, the CD8+ cytotoxic T lymphocytes are activated by the pres-

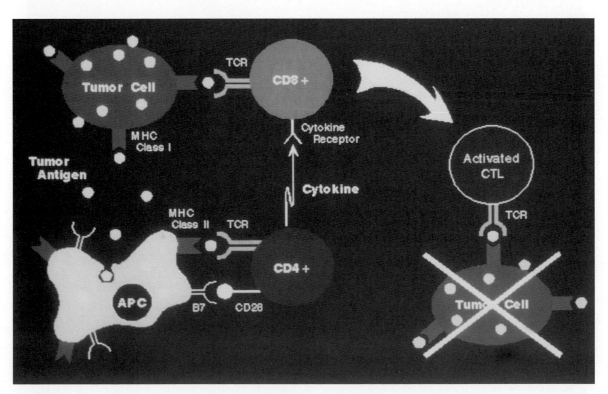

Fig. 1. The T-cell–mediated immune response. *Circles,* tumor antigen; *APC,* antigen-presenting cell; *CTL,* cytotoxic T-lymphocyte, capable of tumor antigen-specific cell lysis.

ence of tumor antigen coupled to a major histocompatibility complex (MHC) class I peptide, synthesized within the cytoplasm of the tumor cell. Nearly all cells in the body express MHC class I antigen, with the antigen binding to tumor peptides 8 to 10 amino acids long. This tumor antigen–MHC class I peptide complex then binds to the antigen specific T-cell receptor (TCR) on the CD8+ T lymphocyte, stimulating T-cell activation. However, full activation of the CD8+ T lymphocyte into a cytotoxic T lymphocyte (CTL) capable of tumor cell lysis requires the presence of cytokine as well. This cytokine secretion is provided through CD4+ helper T-cell activation. Helper T-cell activation is a more complex process than CD8+ T-cell activation and contributes to tumor cell kill in a more indirect way. For CD4+ T-lymphocyte activation, tumor antigen (in the form of peptides 13 amino acids long) must be presented to the CD4+ T lymphocyte in conjunction with an MHC class II peptide. MHC class II peptides, unlike MHC class I peptides, are not ubiquitous, but are found only on a number of specialized cells called antigen-presenting cells (APCs). APCs are cells capable of processing foreign antigen and presenting it to the CD4+ T lymphocyte in conjunction with their own MHC class II peptide. "Professional" APCs express a costimulatory molecule (e.g., B7) that engages receptors on helper T cells (e.g., CD 28) concomitant with antigen recognition by the T-cell receptor. Presentation of an antigen to the T-cell receptor in the absence of a costimulatory signal can lead to T-cell anergy, a mechanism potentially responsible for the induction of tolerance to self-antigens and possibly some tumor antigens. Common APCs in

the body include macrophages, B-lymphocytes, dendritic cells, Langerhans cells of the skin, and human endothelial cells. In the brain, candidate APCs include microglia, endothelial cells, capillary pericytes, and occasionally astrocytes themselves. Microglia are the most attractive candidates for APCs within the brain, accounting for 5% to 15% of the total cellular composition of the brain and being distributed throughout the CNS (39). Binding of antigen and MHC class II peptide to the helper T-cell receptor, usually in the presence of a costimulatory molecule such as B7, results in activation of the CD4+ helper T cell. These cells then produce a variety of cytokines (interferon-γ, IL-2, IL-4, IL-7, IL-12, etc.), which serve to amplify the immune response and fully activate the CD8+ cytotoxic T lymphocyte.

Once activated, a CTL is programmed to kill target cells that bear the same MHC class I–associated antigen that triggered pre-CTL differentiation. CTL killing is dependent on T-cell recognition of a specific antigen, which differentiates this from the less specific non–antigen dependent natural killer (NK) cell killing. CTL killing requires direct cell contact, with the CTL not being injured during the target cell lysis. Target cell kill by CTLs occurs by two parallel mechanisms, without a bystander effect (Fig. 2). The first mechanism involves the concentration of endoplasmic granules, which contain a pore-forming protein called "perforin," within the cytoplasm of the CTL, in an area adjacent to the target cell. Perforin is then secreted (exocytosed) into the extracellular milieu, where it comes into contact with calcium and undergoes polymerization. This polymerization occurs preferentially in the lipid bilayer of the plasma mem-

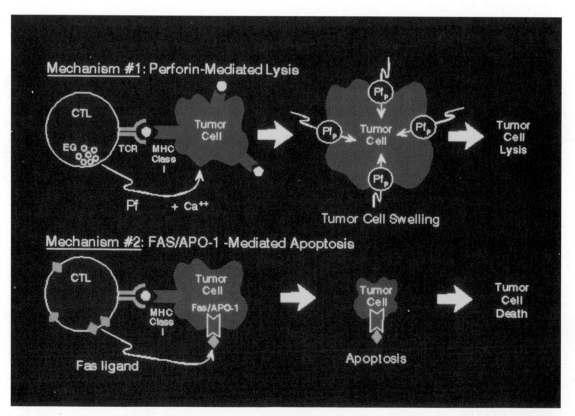

Fig. 2. Cytotoxic T-lymphocyte (CTL)–mediated tumor cell killing. *Circles,* tumor antigen; *EG,* endoplasmic granules; *Fas/APO-1,* a member of the nerve growth factor/TNF receptor superfamily that is a receptor for the cytotoxic cytokine Fas ligand. This receptor is expressed in human glioma cells but not in the normal adult brain. Fas ligand is a cytotoxic cytokine found on the surface and possibly also secreted by activated CTL; *Pf,* perforin; *Pfp,* polymerized perforin within the tumor cell lipid bilayer cell membrane; *TCR,* T-cell receptor.

brane of the target cell. This polymerized protein then acts as an ion-permeable channel in the target cell plasma membrane. If enough of these channels are present, it leads to osmotic target cell swelling and ultimate lysis. The second mechanism of target cell lysis is less well understood, and involves the activation of enzymes within the target cell to digest its own DNA. This may occur through the activation of the Fas/APO-1 receptor on the target cell surface, leading to nuclear DNA fragmentation and cell death by the process of apoptosis.

As noted, CTLs themselves are not killed by either of these two processes and disengage themselves from the target cell surface after delivery of their lethal hit. Therefore, they are capable of further migration through tissue and subsequent target cell kills.

Immunotherapy Strategies for the Treatment of Glioma

Based on our working knowledge of immune stimulation and specifically T-cell–mediated immunity, there are numerous means by which gliomas and tumors in general can escape immune surveillance (Table 1). Current strategies for immune therapy have concentrated on overcoming one or more of these deficiencies either by enhancing tumor cell antigen recognition, enhancing the processing of tumor antigen by professional APCs, or enhancing lymphocyte responsiveness. The latter can be accomplished by the inhibition of local immunosuppressive factors or the promotion of immunostimulatory cytokines and costimulatory molecules. Some of the more promising strategies in each of these areas are outlined in the following.

ENHANCING TUMOR CELL ANTIGEN RECOGNITION. In gliomas, the absence of a well-defined tumor antigen has been a major stumbling block in the generation of tumor specific immunotherapy vaccines. Most vaccination strategies to date have involved the use of irradiated intact tumor cells or tumor cell lysates with or without adjuvant. Initially, these adjuvants consisted of nonspecific immune stimulants such as BCG, *Corynebacterium parvum,* or levamisole with little definable, reproducible responses. More recently, use of the cytokines

Table 1. Potential Mechanisms of Immune-Escape by Gliomas

Defect of antigen presentation
  Failure of tumor antigen to be presented to immune cells
    Lack of tumor antigen
    Lack of major histocompatibility complex class I or class II
      molecules to process the antigen
    Lack of antigen presenting cells in the local glioma environment
  Tumor antigen presented, but not able to elicit an immune response
    Tumor peptide density below the threshold level required for T-
      cell activation
    Oncofetal antigen for which immune tolerance has already been
      established
    Lack of or inhibition of a costimulatory signal
Defect of T-cell function
  Inefficacy of the immune response
    Limited access of immune cells to the central nervous system
    Inappropriate immune stimulation
  Immunosuppressive microenviornment
    Soluble factors; TGF-B2, IL-10, PGE2
    Intracellular factors: IGF-1, IGF-2, IGF-1R, IGF-2R

such as IFN-γ and TNF-α, which increase tumor antigen expression through the upregulation of MHC class I and II molecules, has been promising (40). These studies have demonstrated clear tumor regression in the glioma animal model but their benefit in humans as an adjunct to tumor cell vaccine therapy remains unproved.

ENHANCING THE PROCESSING OF TUMOR ANTIGEN BY PROFESSIONAL ANTIGEN-PRESENTING CELLS. Although tumor specific CD8+ cytotoxic T lymphocytes are an important effector arm in antitumor immunity, the priming of the full CTL response (as outlined in the preceding) is dependent on CD4+ stimulation as well. This response requires the interaction of the MHC class II positive APCs, complete with their costimulatory molecules.

The most potent APC currently identified is the dendritic cell. Dendritic cells, which arise from bone marrow precursors, are found in small numbers in most tissues of the body and have been shown to stimulate not only a helper T-cell–dependent antibody response, but also an effective primary and secondary T-cell response to tumor-associated antigen. Recently, methods have been developed to generate large numbers of pure dendritic cells in humans and animals by culturing bone marrow progenitor cells in the presence of granulocyte-macrophage colony stimulating factor (GM-CSF) (41). Several clinical studies are currently ongoing, examining the benefit of the use of dendritic cells, pulsed with autologous or allogeneic tumor cell antigen, for the treatment of malignant glioma (42).

ENHANCING IMMUNE RESPONSIVENESS. The most intense activity in generating tumor cell vaccines has been in the area of local cytokine delivery to the tumor site. High concentrations of locally administered cytokines have been shown to upregulate antigen expression, enhance T-cell function, and augment antigen presentation. In most cases this has been achieved by introducing the cytokine gene directly into the tumor cell or into fibroblasts that are then implanted into the tumor and coadministered with irradiated tumor cells peripherally. This approach has been termed immunogene therapy. Cytokines that have been shown to enhance the immune response include: INF-γ, GM-CSF, IL-2, IL-3, IL-4, IL-6, IL-7, TNF-α, and IL-12. Yu in 1993 demonstrated significant tumor inhibition in a nude mouse model when IL-4 secreting plasmacytoma cells were coimplanted subcutaneously with a rat or human glioma cell line (43). In addition, he demonstrated enhanced survival when the glioma cells, mixed with the IL-4 secreting cells, were implanted intracranially. Histopathological analysis in the latter case revealed a dramatic eosinophil cell infiltrate in regions of necrotic tumor, suggesting that an antitumor immune response was possible within the CNS. Somewhat to the contrary, Ram in 1994, using the rat 9L glioma model, transduced tumor cells *in vitro* with the human IL-2 gene and demonstrated growth inhibition of transduced 9L glioma cells when implanted subcutaneously, but they showed no growth inhibition when implanted intracranially (44). Glick and colleagues demonstrated a significant increase in survival in the mouse glioma model when tumor cells mixed with IL-2 or IL-2/IFN-γ gene transfected fibroblasts were injected subcutaneously or intracerebrally (45). Animals treated with the IL-2/IFN-γ double cytokine secreting allogeneic fibroblasts demonstrated the greatest antiglioma immune response, mediated predominantly by NK and LAK cells. Tjuvajev explored the therapeutic potential of direct intratumoral transduction of the IL-2 or IFN-γ cytokine gene by coimplanting RG2 rat glioma cells with retroviral cytokine vector producer cells (46). He found that local intratumoral production of IL-2 or IFN-γ generated a cell-mediated antitumor response *in vivo,* but local production of IL-2 and IFN-γ appeared to cause severe CNS toxicity. Wakimoto, using a mouse glioma model to test use of various cytokines in combination, found that vaccination with irradiated glioma cells transduced with the combination of GM-CSF and IL-4 produced the greatest antitumor immunity (47). Finally, Sampson, using a B16 intracerebral melanoma mouse model, examined the most effective cytokine used in conjunction with irradiated B16 tumor cells, injected subcutaneously, to develop an antitumor vaccine (48). Irradiated tumor cells genetically modified to produce IL-3, IL-6, or GM-CSF increased survival of mice challenged with viable B16 tumor cells into the brain. IL-4 and IFN-γ producing tumor cells had no effect. Vaccination with IL-2 producing cells actually shortened survival. In animals showing a prolonged survival, they demonstrated that the immune response was dependent on the CD8+ immune cell, and not so much on the CD4+ immune cells.

Very innovative approaches have been used to deliver cytokines locally as outlined in the preceding. These approaches have been successful in creating both a local as well as systemic T-cell immune response. Although these studies have been very effective in creating an antitumor immune response prior to tumor cell challenge, few have been successful in treating already established intracranial gliomas (49).

A second approach to enhancing the lymphocyte immune responsiveness has been to block the effect of glioma secreted immunosuppressive factors. The best example of this work is by Fakhrai and associates using the antisense transforming growth factor-B (TGF-B) gene transfected into glioma tumor cells (50). Using a rat 9L glioma model, viable 9L glioma cells were implanted intracranially, followed by twice-weekly subcutaneous vaccinations of the irradiated antisense TGF-B glioma cells. Vaccinations were initiated 5 days after intracranial tumor implantation. Results showed 100% animal survival at 12 weeks, with no histological evidence of residual intracranial tumor. A clinical trial based on this treatment strategy currently is in progress.

Finally, a third approach to enhancing lymphocyte responsiveness to glioma cells has been the use of antisense technology to inhibit tumor derived insulin-like growth factor-1 (IGF-1). IGF-1 and its related polypeptide, IGF-2, are expressed in many tissues including the brain. In the brain it is felt to be involved in the proliferation of neuronal and glial precursors. IGF-1 and -2 have been shown to be expressed in high levels in some CNS tumors, including gliomas and meningiomas, where its expression has been correlated with continuous tumor cell proliferation in culture, suggesting its involvement in an autocrine stimulatory loop. Work by Trojan and associates demonstrated that a C6 glioma cell line stably transfected with antisense IGF-1, elicited a highly immunogenic phenotype when introduced into the immunocompetent syngeneic rat (38). The transfected cell line was capable of generating a host immune response consisting predominantly of CD8+ T lymphocytes. They demonstrated not only that the transduced antisense C6 cell line failed to grow subcutaneously, but also inhibited growth of nontransfected C6 cells injected simultaneously at the same or a distant site. In addition, they demonstrated regression of previously implanted, nontransduced tumors following subcutaneous injection of antisense IGF-1–transduced cells. They were able to demonstrate that this inhibition of growth was specific to the C6 glioma cell and did not cross react with a coimplanted neuroblastoma cell line.

The immune strategies described in the preceding, along with numerous others, are a start to unraveling the complex interactions occurring between the immune system and brain. With time, we hope to better understand the intracranial antitumor immune response and use it to our advantage as an adjuvant in the treatment of malignant brain tumors.

Conclusion

This chapter has provided an overview of our current understanding of the complex interrelationship between the immune system and malignant gliomas. Our understanding of the key elements involved in generating an immune response and the factors responsible for local and systemic immunosuppression have greatly increased over the last decade. Although an effective immunotherapeutic regimen in humans has yet to be developed, we now have numerous strategies that have proven effective in animal models, waiting only to be proven in humans. What role immunotherapy ultimately will play in the treatment of brain tumors is unknown. Undoubtedly, however, it will serve as an adjunct to our current treatment modalities, possibly being employed at a time when the tumor burden is low, thereby minimizing the inherent immunosuppressive effects caused by the tumor itself.

References

1. Coley WB. The treatment of malignant tumors by repeated inoculations of erysipelas: with a report of ten original cases. *Am J Med* 1893;105:487–511.
2. Bertrand I MH. Study of the vascular reaction seen in astrocytomas. *Rev Neurol* 1960;102:3–19.
3. Ridley A, Cavanagh JB. Lymphocytic infiltration in gliomas: evidence of possible host resistance. *Brain* 1971;94:117–124.
4. Palma L, Di Lorenzo N, Guidetti B. Lymphocytic infiltrates in primary glioblastomas and recidivous gliomas. Incidence, fate, and relevance to prognosis in 228 operated cases. *J Neurosurg* 1978;49: 854–861.
5. Brooks WH, Markesbery WR, Gupta GD, et al. Relationship of lymphocyte invasion and survival of brain tumor patients. *Ann Neurol* 1978;4:219–224.
6. Hamblin IME. Possible host resistance in carcinomas of the breast: a histological study. *Br J Cancer* 1968;22:383–401.
7. Husby G, Hoagland PM, Strickland RG, et al. Tissue T and B cell infiltration of primary and metastatic cancer. *J Clin Invest* 1976;57: 1471–1482.
8. Rossi ML, Hughes JT, Esiri MM, et al. Immunohistological study of mononuclear cell infiltrate in malignant gliomas. *Acta Neuropathol (Berlin)* 1987;74:269–277.
9. Coakham HB, Kornblith PL, Quindlen EA, et al. Autologous humoral response to human gliomas and analysis of certain cell surface antigens: *in vitro* study with the use of microcytotoxicity and immune adherence assays. *J Natl Cancer Inst* 1980;64:223–233.
10. Miescher S, Whiteside TL, de Tribolet N, et al. *In situ* characterization, clonogenic potential, and antitumor cytolytic activity of T lymphocytes infiltrating human brain cancers. *J Neurosurg* 1988;68: 438–448.
11. Murphy JB SE. Conditions determining the transplantability of tissues in the brain. *J Exp Med* 1923;38:183–194.
12. Medawar PB. Immunity to homologous grafted skin. III. The fate of skin homografts transplanted to the brain, to subcutaneous tissue, and to the anterior chamber of the eye. *Br J Exp Pathol* 1948;29: 58–69.
13. Kida Y, Cravioto H, Hochwald GM, et al. Immunity to transplantable nitrosourea-induced neurogenic tumors. II. Immunoprophylaxis of tumors of the brain. *J Neuropathol Exp Neurol* 1983;42:122–135.
14. Weller RO, Kida S, Zhang ET. Pathways of fluid drainage from the brain—morphological aspects and immunological significance in rat and man. *Brain Pathol* 1992;2:277–284.
15. Yamada S, DePasquale M, Patlak CS, et al. Albumin outflow into deep cervical lymph from different regions of rabbit brain. *Am J Physiol* 1991;261:H1197–H1204.
16. Weller RO, Engelhardt B, Phillips MJ. Lymphocyte targeting of the central nervous system: a review of afferent and efferent CNS-immune pathways. *Brain Pathol* 1996;6:275–288.

17. Paterson PY, Day ED. Current perspectives of neuroimmunologic disease: multiple sclerosis and experimental allergic encephalomyelitis (1,2). *Clin Immunol Rev* 1981;1:581–697.

18. Hickey WF, Hsu BL, Kimura H. T-lymphocyte entry into the central nervous system. *J Neurosci Res* 1991;28:254–260.

19. Sehgal ABM. Basic concepts of immunology and neuroimmunology. *Neurosurg Focus* 2000;9:1–6.

20. Cavenee WK, Furnari FB, Nagane M, et al. Astrocytic tumours: diffusely infiltrating astrocytomas. In: Kleihues P, Cavenee WK, ed. *Pathology and genetics: tumors of the nervous system*. Lyon, France: International Agency for Research on Cancer, 2000:10–21.

21. von Deimling A, Louis DN, Wiestler OD. Molecular pathways in the formation of gliomas. *Glia* 1995;15:328–338.

22. Lampson LA. Interpreting MHC class I expression and class I/class II reciprocity in the CNS: reconciling divergent findings. *Microsc Res Technol* 1995;32:267–285.

23. Vass K, Lassmann H. Intrathecal application of interferon gamma. Progressive appearance of MHC antigens within the rat nervous system. *Am J Pathol* 1990;137:789–800.

24. McMenamin PG FJ. Dendritic cells in the central nervous system and eye and their associated supporting tissues. In: Lotze MTTA, ed. *Dendritic cells: biology and clinical applications*, 1st ed. New York: Academic Press, 1999:205–248.

25. Lee SC, Moore GR, Golenwsky G, et al. Multiple sclerosis: a role for astroglia in active demyelination suggested by class II MHC expression and ultrastructural study. *J Neuropathol Exp Neurol* 1990; 49:122–136.

26. Hickey WF, Osborn JP, Kirby WM. Expression of Ia molecules by astrocytes during acute experimental allergic encephalomyelitis in the Lewis rat. *Cell Immunol* 1985;91:528–535.

27. Wong GH, Bartlett PF, Clark-Lewis I, et al. Interferon-gamma induces the expression of H-2 and Ia antigens on brain cells. *J Neuroimmunol* 1985;7:255–278.

28. Satoh J, Kim SU, Kastrukoff LF, et al. Expression and induction of intercellular adhesion molecules (ICAMs) and major histocompatibility complex (MHC) antigens on cultured murine oligodendrocytes and astrocytes. *J Neurosci Res* 1991;29:1–12.

29. Elliott L, Brooks W, Roszman T. Role of interleukin-2 (IL-2) and IL-2 receptor expression in the proliferative defect observed in mitogen-stimulated lymphocytes from patients with gliomas. *J Natl Cancer Inst* 1987;78:919–922.

30. Dietrich P dN. Immune response against malignant astrocytic tumors and related therapy. In: Raffel CHG, ed. *The molecular basis of neurological disease*, 1st ed. Baltimore: Williams & Wilkins, 1996: 211–237.

31. Brooks WH, Latta RB, Mahaley MS, et al. Immunobiology of primary intracranial tumors. Part 5: Correlation of a lymphocyte index and clinical status. *J Neurosurg* 1981;54:331–337.

32. Kuppner MC, Hamou MF, Sawamura Y, et al. Inhibition of lymphocyte function by glioblastoma-derived transforming growth factor B 2. *J Neurosurg* 1989;71:211–217.

33. Dietrich PY, Walker PR, Saas P, et al. Immunobiology of gliomas: new perspectives for therapy. *Ann NY Acad Sci* 1997;824:124–140.

34. Huber D, Philipp J, Fontana A. Protease inhibitors interfere with the transforming growth factor-B-dependent but not the transforming growth factor-B-independent pathway of tumor cell-mediated immunosuppression. *J Immunol* 1992;148:277–284.

35. Wojtowicz-Praga S. Reversal of tumor-induced immunosuppression: a new approach to cancer therapy [see comments]. *J Immunother* 1997;20:165–177.

36. Marnett LJ. Aspirin and related nonsteroidal anti-inflammatory drugs as chemopreventive agents against colon cancer. *Prev Med* 1995; 24:103–106.

37. Hishii M, Nitta T, Ishida H, et al. Human glioma-derived interleukin-10 inhibits antitumor immune responses *in vitro*. *Neurosurgery* 1995;37:1160–1166.

38. Trojan J, Johnson TR, Rudin SD, et al. Treatment and prevention of rat glioblastoma by immunogenic C6 cells expressing antisense insulin-like growth factor I RNA [see comments]. *Science* 1993;259: 94–97.

39. Davis EJ, Foster TD, Thomas WE. Cellular forms and functions of brain microglia. *Brain Res Bull* 1994;34:73–78.

40. Gansbacher B, Bannerji R, Daniels B, et al. Retroviral vector-mediated gamma-interferon gene transfer into tumor cells generates potent and long lasting antitumor immunity. *Cancer Res* 1990;50: 7820–7825.

41. Sallusto F, Lanzavecchia A. Efficient presentation of soluble antigen by cultured human dendritic cells is maintained by granulocyte/macrophage colony-stimulating factor plus interleukin 4 and down-regulated by tumor necrosis factor α. *J Exp Med* 1994;179: 1109–1118.

42. Vandenabeele S LLAD. Dendritic cell immunotherapy for brain tumors. In: Liau LM, Becker DP, Cloughesy TF, et al., eds. *Brain tumor immunotherapy*, 1st ed. Totowa, NJ: Humana Press, 2001:307–325.

43. Yu JS, Wei MX, Chiocca EA, et al. Treatment of glioma by engineered interleukin 4-secreting cells. *Cancer Res* 1993;53:3125–3128.

44. Ram Z, Walbridge S, Heiss JD, et al. *In vivo* transfer of the human interleukin-2 gene: negative tumoricidal results in experimental brain tumors. *J Neurosurg* 1994;80:535–540.

45. Glick RPLTCE. Cytokine-based immuno-gene therapy for brain tumors. In: Liau LM, Becker DP, Cloughesy TF, et al., eds. *Brain tumor immunotherapy*, 1st ed. Totowa, NJ: Humana Press, 2001:273–288.

46. Tjuvajev J, Gansbacher B, Desai R, et al. RG-2 glioma growth attenuation and severe brain edema caused by local production of interleukin-2 and interferon-gamma. *Cancer Res* 1995;55:1902–1910.

47. Wakimoto H, Abe J, Tsunoda R, et al. Intensified antitumor immunity by a cancer vaccine that produces granulocyte-macrophage colony-stimulating factor plus interleukin 4. *Cancer Res* 1996;56:1828–1833.

48. Sampson JH, Archer GE, Ashley DM, et al. Subcutaneous vaccination with irradiated, cytokine-producing tumor cells stimulates CD8 + cell-mediated immunity against tumors located in the "immunologically privileged" central nervous system. *Proc Natl Acad Sci USA* 1996;93:10399–10404.

49. Lillehei KO, Liu Y, Kong Q. Current perspectives in immunotherapy. *Ann Thorac Surg* 1999;68:S28–S33.

50. Fakhrai H GSS. Downregulation of transforming growth factor B as therapeutic approach for brain tumors. In: Liau LM, Becker DP, Cloughesy TF, et al., eds. *Brain tumor immunotherapy*, 1st ed. Totowa, NJ: Humana Press, 2001:289–305.

101. Methods for Imaging Tumors within the Brain: CT, MRI, and Functional Imaging

Russell R. Margraf,
Jeffrey R. Petrella, Linda Gray,
J.C. Leveque, and Michael M.
Haglund

In a contemporary neurosurgical practice, most patients with a suspected intracranial lesion present with an imaging study in hand. Computed tomography (CT), magnetic resonance imaging (MRI), and, to an increasing degree, functional MR imaging (fMRI) are common modalities seen on a daily basis by neurosurgeons and neurologists. Given advancing technology and the expanding number of image sequences and protocols, an understanding of modern imaging is important in the diagnosis and management of neurosurgical patients. In this chapter, current and future roles of CT, MRI, and fMRI are reviewed.

CT Imaging

The development of CT in 1973 by Godfrey Hounsfield provided a major imaging advance from conventional radiographs for examining intracranial pathology (1). Hounsfield's clinical colleague, James Ambrose, worked with the first diagnostic EMI machine at Atkinson Morley's Hospital in Wimbledon, England and soon after that the technology was introduced in the United States by Professor Bull at the Albert Einstein Medical Center. Pneumoencephalography, once the convention for detection of mass lesions, disappeared within 6 years as every major hospital acquired CT scan units (2).

CT is a basic imaging tool used in all disciplines of medicine. In the head, CT is used to diagnose and localize hemorrhage, plan treatment, and aid in prognosis (Fig. 1). High-resolution CT detects subtle subarachnoid and parenchymal hemorrhage, and is a sensitive method for detecting intracranial calcium, and subtle skull lesions not seen on conventional radiography. Anatomical assessment of aneurysms obscured during angiography by bone or large vascular branches is provided by three-dimensional (3D) reconstruction of spiral CT images (3D CT angiography) and is increasingly helpful in diagnosis and management (Fig. 2). Regarding tumors within the brain, CT is a useful, noninvasive method of monitoring the progression of tumors and the presence of calcium or hemorrhage, and is used by neurosurgeons and neurologists in postoperative or postprocedural follow-up. CT imaging provides important information about the size, location, and often etiology of intracranial lesions. In addition to assessment of tumors and other lesions with conventional CT, Xenon CT provides quantitative information about regional blood flow and tumor vascularity. Regional cerebral blood volume and blood/tissue partition coefficient (lambda) is calculated following inhalation of xenon gas. Xenon CT is more precise than conventional contrast-enhanced MRI and has the potential to provide earlier detection of vascular dysplastic alteration in supratentorial gliomas (3).

CT is limited, however, in its ability to distinguish subtle differences in tissue characteristics. In these instances, MRI is more sensitive and specific. CT and MRI have the potential to be used together to provide accurate information about intracranial tumor size and location (4). CT-MRI fusion software (Picker International, St. David, PA) electronically integrates MRI data into a CT-based 3D planning system for tumor localization and volumetric analysis.

MRI

MRI is recognized as a more sensitive and specific imaging modality compared to CT in identifying precise anatomical structures, and has had its biggest application to the brain and spine. MR has the added benefit of multiplanar imaging, using axial, sagittal, and coronal planes for better localization and definition of lesions and their relationship to adjacent structures.

MRI is a dynamic discipline within the field of neuroradiology focusing on the response of protons contained in water and fat to an applied magnetic field. Pulse sequences constantly evolve, and it is important to critically evaluate and understand their clinical utility. Frequent MRI sequences used for imaging tumors within the brain include T1-weighted spin echo with and without the use of gadolinium chelates as intravenous contrast material, T2-weighted and proton density (PD) weighted spin echo or fast spin echo, and fast FLAIR sequences. More advanced MRI techniques are increasingly common in the evaluation of intracranial tumors. For example, perfusion and diffusion MRI is used with increasing frequency to investigate brain tumors and associated changes in regional cerebral blood volume. Measurements of capillary blood volume are used to differentiate high- from low-grade tumors, and radiation necrosis from recurrent disease. Similarly, permeability or dynamic MRI measures the rate of transit across the blood–brain barrier, and is potentially beneficial in noninvasively differentiating histopathologic types of gliomas. Functional MRI (fMRI) has become increasingly popular for preoperative planning and mapping of eloquent cortex associated with speech and sensorimotor activity.

T1- and T2-weighted MRI

The infiltrative nature of malignant gliomas and white matter changes associated with increased cellularity are shown well on proton density (PD) or T2 imaging as hyperintense signal and correlates with increased water content. Most tumors and associated surrounding edema have long T2 relaxation times, and are visible as hyperintense signal (Fig. 3). T2 images have long repetition times (TR) and long echo times (TE) and PD

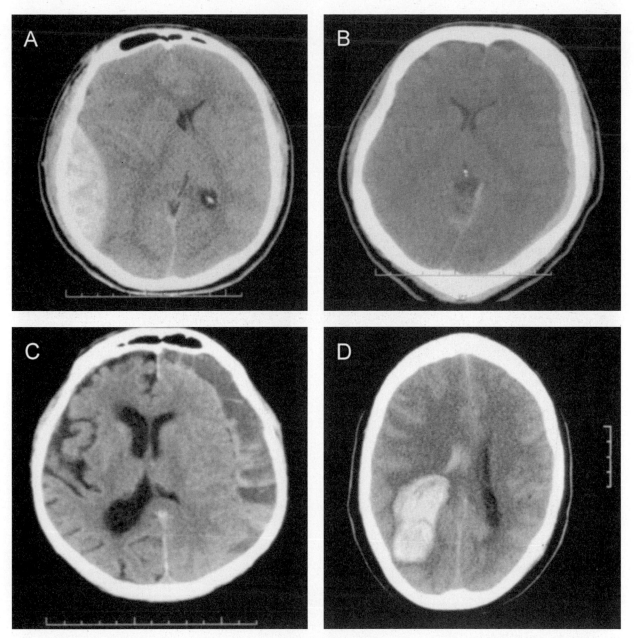

Fig. 1. Conventional computed tomographic (CT) imaging. **A:** An 18-year-old man fell from the back of a pickup truck and presented to the emergency department after a lucid interval. CT shows a large, right temporal/parietal epidural hematoma. The lens-shaped high-density fluid collection effaces the gray–white matter interface and there is subfalcine herniation of the lateral ventricles. **B:** A 55-year-old man suffered a fall and subsequent seizure. CT shows an acute left subdural hematoma. The high-density crescent-shaped fluid collection spreads diffusely over the underlying hemisphere. **C:** A 79-year-old woman with a history of falls and recent change in mental status. CT shows left acute on chronic subdural hematoma. The sulcal pattern of the underlying hemisphere is effaced, and there is mass effect on the ipsilateral lateral ventricle. **D:** A 67-year-old woman with hypertension. CT showing a right thalamic intraparenchymal hemorrhage with intraventricular extension.

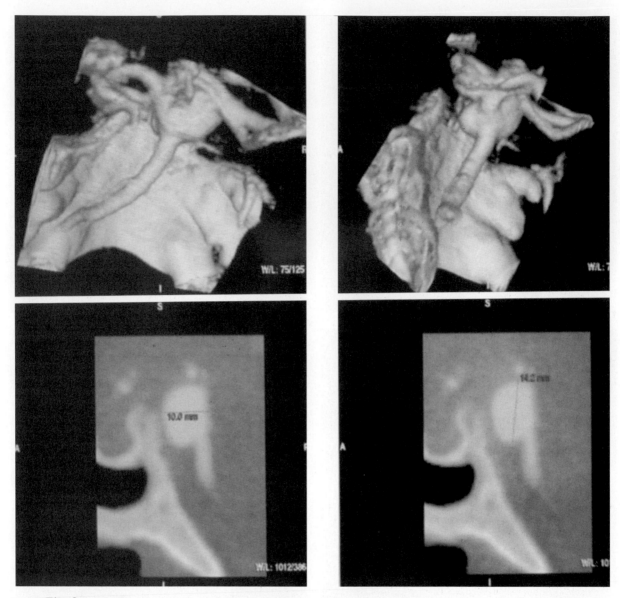

Fig. 2. Three-dimensional computed tomography angiography of a basilar artery aneurysm. Relevant vascular anatomy and the relationship of the origin of the superior cerebellar and posterior cerebral arteries to the dome of the aneurysm are shown on oblique views *(above)*. The size and relationship of the aneurysm to the clivus and posterior clinoid is shown on sagittal images *(below)*.

images have long TR and short TE. T1-weighted images have both a short TR and short TE.

Hyperintense lesions can be seen with both spin echo (SE) and fast spin echo (FSE) images. FSE, and other faster imaging techniques such as echo-planar imaging (EPI), and hybrid imaging techniques were developed as methods for obtaining T2-weighted images while reducing scan time. Scan time becomes increasingly important for permeability or dynamic imaging where the scan must be fast enough to stop motion such as arterial pulsation, or to follow intravascular contrast, vascular flow, or cerebral spinal fluid pulsation. Faster scan time is often achieved at the expense of decreased lesion conspicuity and increased partial-volume effects. Consequently, FSE images are less sensitive for the detection of intracranial hemorrhage and brain iron compared to SE, and are thus limited in their detec-

tion of cavernous hemangiomas, capillary telangiectasias, hemorrhagic infarcts, and certain tumors.

Heavily T2-weighted images are advantageous in that lesion conspicuity is increased, and shown as an area of hyperintense signal; an exception is at brain–cerebrospinal fluid (CSF) interfaces around ventricles and cisterns where lesions may be masked because of partial-volume effects and motion from adjacent CSF. Fast fluid-attenuated inversion recovery (FLAIR) sequence (discussed in the following) was developed to help overcome such disadvantages. Low T2 signal, shown as an area of hypointense signal, also increases lesion conspicuity and may be diagnostic. One example is the ring of hypointense T2 signal surrounding cerebral abscesses (Fig. 4C).

Glial tumors have a diffuse and infiltrative nature. The gross appearance and consistency of the tumor margins at the time

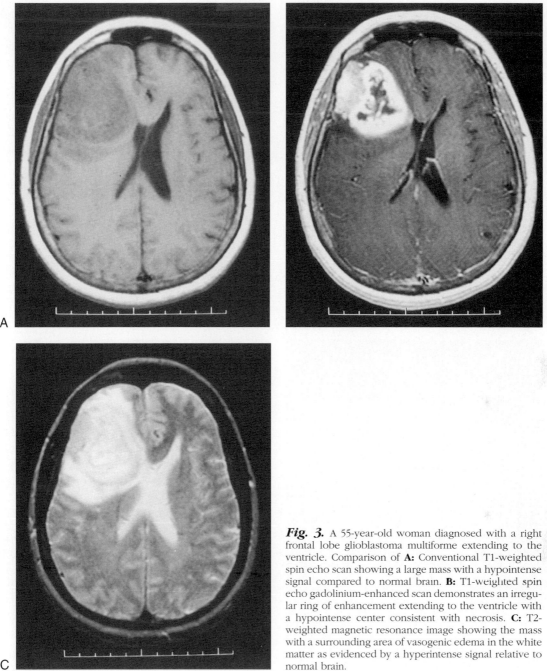

Fig. 3. A 55-year-old woman diagnosed with a right frontal lobe glioblastoma multiforme extending to the ventricle. Comparison of **A:** Conventional T1-weighted spin echo scan showing a large mass with a hypointense signal compared to normal brain. **B:** T1-weighted spin echo gadolinium-enhanced scan demonstrates an irregular ring of enhancement extending to the ventricle with a hypointense center consistent with necrosis. **C:** T2-weighted magnetic resonance image showing the mass with a surrounding area of vasogenic edema in the white matter as evidenced by a hyperintense signal relative to normal brain.

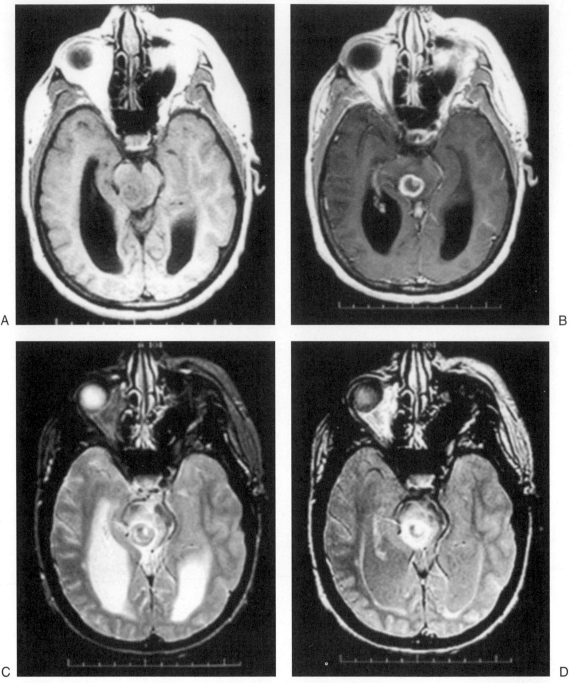

Fig. 4. An immunocompromised 48-year-old woman with signs and symptoms of hydrocephalus, left-sided weakness, and anisocoria. **A:** T1-weighted spin echo scan. **B:** T1-weighted with gadolinium showing a 1.5-cm ring-enhancing lesion in the dorsal midbrain with a central area of hypointense signal. **C:** T2-weighted image through the same area showing a nodular component anteriorly, an area of hypointense signal surrounding the rim of the lesion, and vasogenic edema. **D:** Fluid-attenuated inversion recovery sequence with suppression of cerebrospinal fluid signal in the ventricles and basilar cisterns resulting in increased lesion conspicuity. Surgical pathology consistent with abscess.

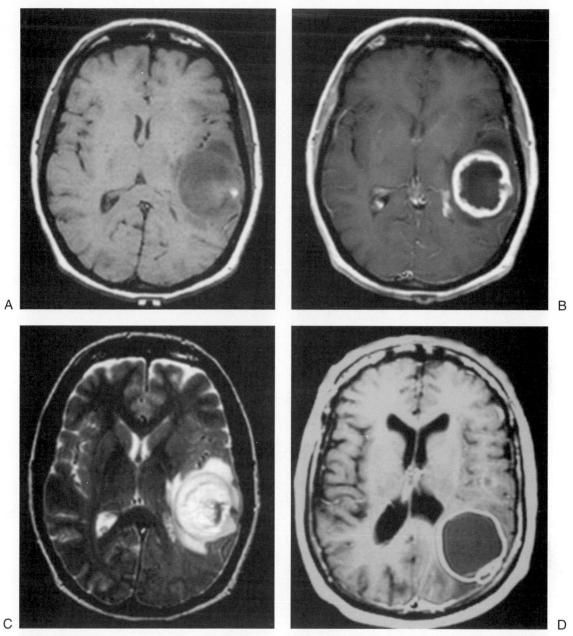

Fig. 5. A 55-year-old woman with left temporal glioblastoma multiforme **(A–C),** and a 75-year-old woman with left posterior temporal cerebral abscess **(D)**. **A:** T1-weighted spin echo scan and **B:** T1-weighted image with gadolinium showing a 4-cm irregular ring enhancing lesion in the left temporal lobe with a central area of hypointense signal. **C:** T2-weighted image through the same area showing increased lesion conspicuity and surrounding vasogenic edema. Also noted is an area of hypointense signal surrounding the rim of the lesion as often found with cerebral abscess. **D:** Different patient demonstrating the smooth, regular ring enhancement typically found in cerebral abscess.

of operation rarely provides sufficient information to achieve radical resection. The majority of glioblastomas and anaplastic astrocytomas show enhancement on T1-weighted scans following administration of gadolinium contrast and often have a marked but irregular peripheral ring-like enhancement (Figs. 3B and 5B). Ring enhancement surrounding cerebral abscesses generally has a smooth contour (Fig. 5D). Contrast enhancement is relatively uncommon in low-grade gliomas (5).

Frequently there is discrepancy between intraoperative observations of glial tumor margins and diagnostic imaging studies. For example, malignant cells have been found in stereotac-

tically obtained tissue several centimeters beyond contrast-enhancing lesions shown on CT or MRI in patients with high-grade glioma, and beyond the area of hyperintense signal on T2-weighted MRI in patients with low-grade astrocytic gliomas (6). Methods to enhance tumor localization preoperatively and intraoperatively may improve assessment of tumor margins and patient outcome. Many investigators have attempted to correlate the clinical grade of CNS gliomas with T1 and T2 appearance (7–9), or with the maximum rate of contrast change during dynamic MRI scanning (10,11). Enhanced optical imaging is another recently introduced technique that has the potential to grade astrocytomas, identify residual tumor in the resection cavity, and improve the diagnosis, surgery, and management of patients with primary brain tumors (6,12,13).

Fast Fluid-Attenuated Inversion Recovery

Fast fluid-attenuated inversion recovery (FLAIR) MRI employs a suppression pulse, and produces a heavily T2-weighted image with CSF suppression. As a result, signal abnormalities adjacent to CSF filled structures are often more conspicuous than with conventional T2-weighted imaging (14). The principal advantage is the ability to null CSF, decreasing its signal intensity. This produces greater gray–white differentiation, and decreased flow artifacts. Applications of FLAIR MRI include qualitative evaluation of intraaxial brain tumors and the delineation of enhancing and nonenhancing tumor parts (15). Fast FLAIR is superior in showing lesions located at the periphery of the brain, around the basal cisterns, in the brainstem (Fig. 4C) at the gray–white junction, and adjacent to some portions of the lateral ventricles (Fig. 6D). It is more limited in identifying le-

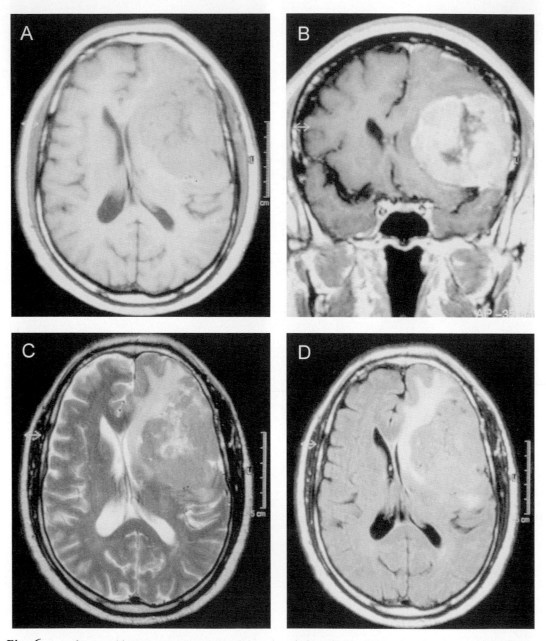

Fig. 6. **A:** A 62-year-old man presenting with subtle right-sided weakness, personality changes, and memory loss. **A:** T1-weighted spin echo scan and **B:** T1-weighted image with gadolinium showing a 6-cm inhomogeneously enhancing lesion in the left frontal lobe with a central area of hypointense signal consistent with necrosis. **C:** T2-weighted image through the same area showing mixed areas of hyperintensity and isointensity compared to normal brain, and surrounding vasogenic edema in the white matter. **D:** Fluid-attenuated inversion recovery sequence with cerebrospinal fluid (CSF) suppression in the lateral ventricles. A CSF cleft is noted along the anterior–medial border consistent with an extraaxial lesion. Surgical pathology revealed meningioma.

sions adjacent to the ventricles given that normal high signal is often seen outlining the third and fourth ventricles, and capping the frontal and occipital horns of the lateral ventricles (Fig. 5D).

Magnetization Transfer Imaging

Magnetization transfer (MT) is an MRI technique where tissue contrast is determined by interactions between tissue macromolecules and tissue water. An RF pulse several hundred hertz away from the resonance frequency of free water has the effect of saturating protons associated with macromolecules, and results in an overall decrease in signal of stationary tissues. Contrast between vessels and stationary tissues is increased. Further, conspicuity of enhancing lesions is increased because MT causes suppression of normal brain tissue. This causes increased contrast between intraparenchymal lesions or leptomeningeal lesions and normal brain tissue. MT effects are prominent in normal cerebral white matter, appearing as low signal intensity on FSE images as compared to SE images. White matter lesions and pathological processes of myelin have low MT, and consequently appear more conspicuous with FSE versus SE because of contrast differences. Overall, the utility of the technique is to improve visualization of blood vessels and intracranial enhancing lesions, as well as quantifiably measure pathological processes in the brain using a parameter known as the magnetization transfer ratio (MTR). In addition to improving visualization gadolinium enhancing lesions, MT imaging also may be used to identify microscopic changes not seen using standard MRI. Clinically, MT is used for characterization of intracranial mass lesions, including tumor tissue, ischemic brain, wallerian degeneration, and demyelinating diseases. Compared to normal brain, the MTR for brain tumors is low, and the MTR for meningioma is higher than other brain tumors (16). The MTR of physically soft tumors is significantly lower than the MTR of hard tumors, suggesting that MT may be useful in presurgical planning (16). Other investigators also have found MT to be a superior method of assessing histological grade compared to quantitative measures of T1 and T2 relaxation times (17–19).

Advanced MRI

PERFUSION-WEIGHTED IMAGING OF BRAIN TUMORS. Perfusion weighted imaging (PWI) is used with increasing frequency for evaluating regional cerebral hemodynamics. This is of particular interest given the dysplastic vascular changes observed in association with high-grade gliomas demonstrated by Xenon-CT. Compared to Xenon-CT, perfusion MRI provides quantitative measure of local cerebral hemodynamics in addition to high-resolution MR anatomy (20).

PERMEABILITY MRI. Permeability or dynamic MR imaging is a technique for evaluating the rate of contrast uptake in a lesion of interest by performing a series of images in rapid succession after a bolus injection of contrast. The early phase of contrast uptake is related to the intravascular distribution of contrast. The late phase results from diffusion of contrast into adjacent interstitial space. Given the profuse vascular proliferation associated with malignant gliomas, dynamic MRI measurements of contrast uptake may be an indirect measure of tumor vascular-

ity, and be used to differentiate high-grade tumors from benign lesions or radiation necrosis. Maximum rate of uptake of gadolinium in dynamic MRI can be a prognostic measure for patients with malignant glioma (10,11). Unlike PET, dynamic MRI requires no radioactive tracer.

DIFFUSION-WEIGHTED IMAGING OF BRAIN TUMORS. Diffusion-weighted MR imaging (DWI) has the potential to investigate biologic tissues and measure the displacement of water molecules at a microscopic level. Proton displacement is expressed by an apparent diffusion coefficient (ADC) in units of square millimeters per second over a given observation time. DWI is most commonly used clinically to identify areas of acute infarction or ischemia following total or near total perfusion deficit (21). Ischemic or infarcted regions can be identified within minutes of insult as an area of increased signal abnormality or decreased ADC. The central portions of abscesses also demonstrate high signal on DWI, and this method may be useful in discriminating necrotic or cystic brain tumors from brain abscess (22). Other entities with low signal or nonrestricted diffusion include reversible encephalopathy syndromes. DWI is less commonly used in the evaluation of brain tumors, but there are some useful applications. For example, high ADC values may be used to separate vasogenic edema from tumor margins that have lower ADC values. DWI has the potential for monitoring early response of brain tumors to therapy (23,24). DWI is useful for distinguishing epidermoids from arachnoid cysts, and cystic from solid components of tumors (25). Extraaxial cysts demonstrate increased ADCs, whereas epidermoids have ADCs similar to brain parenchyma. Some tumors and cysts contain fluid high in protein. With such lesions, differentiating between cystic and solid is difficult on T1- and T2-weighted images, and diffusion may be of benefit.

FUNCTIONAL MRI. Functional MRI (fMRI) may be used to measure brain activation during various cognitive tasks to identify primary motor, sensory, visual, and language areas of the cerebral cortex by asking the patient to perform various tasks alternating with rest periods. fMRI plays a role in preoperative planning for lesions located near areas of functionally eloquent cortex. Brain activation is measured by a process that generates images based on variations in blood oxygen content as a result of cerebral activation (Color Plate 25). The aim of most fMRI studies is to help select patients who are candidates for craniotomy and the addition of intraoperative mapping of motor, sensory, or language areas (13). fMRI localization of motor/sensory cortex is advancing rapidly; however, the use of fMRI to identify essential language areas that must be preserved is still in its infancy. Whether the areas identified by fMRI are critical areas as determined by the gold standard of intraoperative electrical stimulation mapping remains to be elucidated.

In addition to preoperative planning using fMRI, MRI also has been adapted to differentiate high from low-grade tumors (Color Plates 26 and 27, respectively) and recurrent tumor from radiation necrosis (Color Plate 28).

fMRI also may assist neurosurgeons in the operating room. Recently, advanced methods of image acquisition and processing have allowed for accurate planning, target definition, and trajectory optimization for interactive MR-guided biopsies of brain tumors (26). Such procedures allow the operator good visualization of the target along with real time feedback and control of the procedure, and may improve the diagnostic yield of brain biopsies (27). Real time imaging techniques also may be used in providing accurate intraoperative information regarding anatomy. Improving visualization using improved image acquisition and processing will reduce incision length, patient and surgical team exposure to radiation in cases requiring intraoperative x-ray, operative time, and postoperative hospitalization.

MAGNETIC RESONANCE SPECTROSCOPY. High-resolution magic angle spinning protons (HRMAS 1H) magnetic resonance spectroscopy is an imaging modality producing highly resolved spectra of metabolites from intact tissue specimens, and may have the potential to characterize tumor types and biochemical characteristics (28). MR spectroscopy may be used as a supportive diagnostic tool to differentiate clinically stable brain tumors from those undergoing malignant transformation. In one study, the interval measurement of percent change in choline signal intensity is used to segregate stable cerebral gliomas from those with malignant degeneration (29). In that study, tumors progressing as a result of low- to high-grade malignant transformation or posttherapeutic recurrence showed a choline signal increase of more than 45%, whereas stable cases showed statistically less elevation, no change, or a decrease in signal intensity.

Positron Emission Tomography Imaging

Although conventional and advanced MRI are sensitive techniques for evaluating intracranial tumors, they are sometimes limited in distinguishing between tumor recurrence and post-treatment radiation necrosis. Metabolic imaging with positron emission tomography (PET) using the glucose analogue [^{18}F]-fluorodeoxyglucose (FDG-PET) is useful in this regard (30). PET allows for both quantitative and qualitative investigation of cerebral physiologic and biochemical processes. Physiologic variables frequently evaluated include cerebral glucose metabolism with FDG, cerebral blood flow with ^{15}O-labeled CO_2 or H_2O, rate of protein synthesis with ^{11}C-labeled amino acids, and cerebral blood volume with ^{11}C- or ^{15}O-labeled CO.

Early studies of cerebral glucose metabolism with FDG-PET in patients with brain tumors described an association between the rate of metabolism and growth rate of malignant cells. Subsequently, FDG-PET has been widely used clinically to differentiate low- and high-grade gliomas, residual postoperative tumor, and posttreatment radiation necrosis from recurrence (31,32).

Language mapping using measurements of relative cerebral blood flow with ^{15}O-labeled water PET is a noninvasive method of identifying primary language-related cortex (33). This technique, developed prior to fMRI, is still useful for surgical planning in patients with various lesions in and surrounding primary eloquent cortex, and in determining hemispheric language dominance. This technique is best used with anatomical evaluation performed with conventional MRI, ideally with coregistration of images.

In conclusion, CT and MRI have become increasingly important to neurosurgeons, neurologists, and clinical science researchers. This is in part because modern imaging is safe, noninvasive, and provides excellent soft-tissue resolution. There also is an expanded awareness of the clinical and scientific utility, and a growing need for better imaging technology for both preoperative and intraoperative management of patients.

References

1. Hounsfield GN. Computerized transverse axial scanning (tomography). I. Description of system. *Br J Radiol* 1973;46:1016–1022.
2. Heinz ER. History of neuroradiology. In: Wilkins RH, Rengachary SS, eds. *Neurosurgery,* vol 1. New York: McGraw-Hill, 1996:20.
3. Nasel C, Schindler E. Xenon-CT and perfusion MRI in the diagnosis of cerebral gliomas. *Radiologe* 1998;38:930–934.
4. Lattanzi JP, Fein DA, McNeeley SW, et al. Computed-tomography-magnetic resonance image fusion: a clinical evaluation of an innovative approach for improved tumor localization in primary central nervous system lesions. *Radiat Oncol Invest* 1997;5:195–205.
5. Osborn AG. Astrocytomas and other glial neoplasms. In: Osborn AG. *Diagnostic neuroradiology.* Philadelphia: Mosby–Year Book, 1994;535–543.
6. Haglund MM, Hochman DW, Spence AM, et al. Enhanced optical imaging of rat gliomas and tumor margins. *Neurosurgery* 1994;35:930–941.
7. Englund E, Brun A, Larsson EM, et al. Tumours of the central nervous system. Proton magnetic resonance relaxation times T1 and T2 and histopathologic correlates. *Acta Radiol Diag* 1986;27:653–659.
8. Kjaer L, Thomsen C, Gjerris F, et al. Tissue characterization of intracranial tumors by MR imaging. In vivo evaluation of T1- and T2-relaxation behavior at 1.5 T. *Acta Radiol* 1991;32:498–504.
9. Kjaer L, Ring P, Thomsen C, et al. Texture analysis in quantitative MR imaging. Tissue characterisation of normal brain and intracranial tumours at 1.5 T. *Acta Radiol* 1995;36:127–135.
10. Wong ET, Jackson EF, Hess KR, et al. Correlation between dynamic MRI and outcome in patients with malignant gliomas. *Neurology* 1998;50:777–781.
11. Hazle JD, Jackson EF, Schomer DF, et al. Dynamic imaging of intracranial lesions using fast spin echo imaging: differentiation of brain tumors and treatment effects. *J MRI* 1997;7:1084–1093.
12. Haglund MM, Berger MS, Spence AM, et al. Optical imaging of tumors in rat and human gliomas. *Br J Neurosurg* 1993;7:158.
13. Haglund MM, Hochman DW, Spence AM, et al. Enhanced optical imaging of rat gliomas and tumor margins. *Neurosurgery* 1994;35:930–940; discussion 940–941.
14. Mathews VP, Greenspan SL, Caldemeyer KS, et al. FLAIR and HASTE imaging in neurologic diseases. *MRI Clin North Am* 1998;6:53–65.
15. Essig M, Hawighorst H, Schoenberg SO, et al. Fast fluid-attenuated inversion recovery (FLAIR) MRI in the assessment of intraaxial brain tumors. *J MRI* 1998;8:789–798.
16. Okumura A, Takenaka K, Nishimura Y, et al. The characterization of human brain tumor using magnetization transfer technique in magnetic resonance imaging. *Neurol Res* 1991;21:250–254.
17. Kurki T, Lundbom N, Kalimo H, et al. MR classification of brain gliomas: value of magnetization transfer and conventional imaging. *MRI* 1995;13:501–511.
18. Kurki T, Lundbom N, Valtonen S. Tissue characterisation of intracranial tumours: the value of magnetisation transfer and conventional MRI. *Neuroradiology* 1995;37:515–521.
19. Kurki T, Lundbom N, Komu M, et al. Tissue characterization of intracranial tumors by magnetization transfer and spin-lattice relaxation parameters in vivo. *J MRI* 1996;6:573–579.
20. Hagen T, Bartylla K, Piepgras U. Correlation of regional cerebral blood flow measured by stable xenon CT and perfusion MRI. *J Comp Assist Tomogr* 1999;23:257–264.
21. Gray L, MacFall J. Overview of diffusion imaging. *MRI Clin North Am* 1998;6:125–138.
22. Kim YJ, Chang KH, Song IC, et al. Brain abscess and necrotic or cystic brain tumor: discrimination with signal intensity on diffusion-weighted MR imaging. *Am J Roentgenol* 1998;171:1487–1490.
23. Ostergaard L, Hochberg FH, Rabinov JD, et al. Early changes measured by magnetic resonance imaging in cerebral blood flow, blood volume, and blood-brain barrier permeability following dexamethasone treatment in patients with brain tumors. *J Neurosurg* 1999;90:300–305.
24. Chenevert TL, McKeever PE, Ross BD. Monitoring early response of experimental brain tumors to therapy using diffusion magnetic resonance imaging. *Clin Cancer Res* 1997;3:1457–1466.
25. Tsuruda JS, Chew WM, Moseley ME, et al. Diffusion-weighted MR imaging of the brain: value of differentiating between extraaxial cysts and epidermoid tumors. *AJNR* 1990;11:925–931.
26. Kollias SS, Bernays R, Marugg RA, et al. Target definition and trajectory optimization for interactive MR-guided biopsies of brain tumors in an open configuration MRI system. *J MRI* 1998;8:143–159.

27. Hall WA, Martin AJ, Liu H, et al. Brain biopsy using high field strength interventional magnetic resonance imaging. *Neurosurgery* 1999;44:807–813.
28. Cheng LL, Chang IW, Louis DN, et al. Correlation of high-resolution magic angle spinning proton magnetic resonance spectroscopy with histopathology of intact human brain tumor specimens. *Cancer Res* 1998;58:1825–1832.
29. Tedeschi G, Lundbom N, Raman R, et al. Increased choline signal coinciding with malignant degeneration of cerebral gliomas: a serial proton magnetic resonance spectroscopy imaging study. *J Neurosurg* 1997;87:516–524.
30. Asensio C, Perez-Castejon MJ, Maldonado A, et al. The role of PET-FDG in questionable diagnosis of relapse in the presence of radionecrosis of brain tumors. *Rev Neurol* 1998;27:447–452.
31. Glantz MJ, Hoffman JM, Coleman RE, et al. Identification of early recurrence of primary central nervous system tumors by [18F]fluoro-deoxyglucose positron emission tomography. *Ann Neurol* 1991;29:347–355.
32. Deshmukh A, Scott JA, Palmer EL, et al. Impact of fluorodeoxyglucose positron emission tomography on the clinical management of patients with glioma. *Clin Nucl Med* 1996;21:720–725.
33. Thiel A, Herholz K, von Stockhausen HM, et al. Localization of language-related cortex with 15O-labeled water PET in patients with gliomas. *Neuroimaging* 1998;7:284–295.

102. Low-grade Glial Neoplasms

Andrew H. Kaye and David G. Walker

Low-grade gliomas are a diverse group of neoplasms which, as the name implies, are thought to arise from glial cells. Hence this groups includes astrocytomas, oligodendrogliomas, ependymomas, and mixed gliomas. They are diverse in terms of epidemiology, clinical presentation, pathology, and prognosis. Some are eminently curable and others are prone to recur and progress to more malignant lesions. In general, using the World Health Organization (WHO) classification, low-grade gliomas are either grade I or II tumors.

The term "low-grade glioma" encompasses not only low-grade astrocytomas, but other neuroepithelial tumors including oligodendrogliomas, oligoastrocytomas, ependymomas, and pilocytic astrocytomas, as well as rare tumors, such as pleomorphic xanthoastrocytomas and subependymal giant cell astrocytomas. Among these, low-grade astrocytomas are the most common low-grade gliomas and occasionally, though incorrectly, the terms are used interchangeably.

Astrocytomas

Low-grade astrocytomas (LGAs) are common brain neoplasms that primarily affect young adults. Although these patients often have a reasonably long survival, most will ultimately succumb to their tumors. The best management plan for these tumors is controversial and ranges from observation to macroscopic excision and radiotherapy. The evidence for each of these approaches is presented in this chapter and a management algorithm is provided.

LGAs are slow-growing astrocytic neoplasms with a high degree of cellular differentiation that diffusely infiltrate nearby brain. These lesions generally affect young adults and have a tendency to progress to higher grade astrocytomas. The management of LGAs, in terms of making a diagnosis, the timing and extent of surgery, and the benefits of adjuvant therapy, remains controversial.

The term astrocytoma, unless otherwise specified, usually refers to low-grade diffuse astrocytomas of adulthood. Some authors refer to these as "well-differentiated astrocytomas," or "fibrillary astrocytomas" (1), but this latter designation is more commonly used for the respective histological subtypes of LGAs. LGAs must be differentiated from pilocytic astrocytomas, which have a different age distribution, location, and biology.

PATHOLOGICAL GRADING. The most widely used pathological grading systems in current use are the WHO and the St. Anne/Mayo systems. LGAs correspond to WHO grade II (2). WHO grade I astrocytomas include pilocytic astrocytomas, pleomorphic xanthoastrocytomas, and subependymal giant cell astrocytomas (2). This is somewhat confusing since these tumors do not, as a rule, progress to higher grade astrocytomas as the designation WHO grades I to IV would suggest. The St. Anne/Mayo grading system (3) generally classifies LGAs as astrocytoma grade 2, which requires one histological criterion, usually nuclear atypia. Rarely LGAs without nuclear atypia occur and these are designated as astrocytoma grade 1 using the St. Anne/Mayo system. The various grading systems for astrocytomas are summarized in Table 1.

EPIDEMIOLOGY. LGAs represent approximately 15% of gliomas in adults and 25% of all gliomas of the cerebral hemispheres in children (4). The average incidence of these tumors has been calculated at slightly less than 1 per 100,000 population per year for both children and adults (5,6). The peak incidence is in young adults between age 30 and 40 (25% of all cases) (7). Approximately 10% occur below the age of 20, 60% between age 20 to 45, and about 30% over age 45. There is a slight predominance in males, constituting approximately 60% of cases (4,8).

LOCATION. LGAs may develop in any region of the central nervous system (CNS) but most commonly develop supratentorially in the cerebrum of both children and adults. The brainstem is the next most common site, while these tumors are distinctly uncommon in the cerebellum. Within the cerebrum, they arise roughly in proportion to the relative mass of the different lobes, hence the frontal lobe is the most common location, followed by the temporal lobe (8).

Table 1. Astrocytoma Grading Systems in Common Use

Kernohan, et al. (158) (1949)	Ringertz (159) (1950)	St. Anne/ Mayo (3) (1988)	WHO (2) (1993)
Astrocytoma grade 1		Astrocytoma grade 1	
	Astrocytoma	Astrocytoma grade 2	Astrocytoma (WHO grade II)
Astrocytoma grade 2			
	Intermediate type	Astrocytoma grade 3	Anaplastic astrocytoma (WHO grade III)
Astrocytoma grade 3			
	Glioblastoma multiforme	Astrocytoma grade 4	Glioblastoma multiforme (WHO grade IV)
Astrocytoma grade 4			

WHO, World Health Organization.

MACROSCOPIC APPEARANCE. Because of their infiltrative nature, LGAs usually show blurring of anatomical boundaries. Generally there is distortion but not destruction of the invaded structures (9). Mass lesions may be present, both in gray or white matter but they are indistinct and changes such as cysts, and areas of firmness or softening may be seen. Cystic change commonly appears as a focal spongy area, with multiple cysts of varying size, occasionally causing a gelatinous appearance. Occasionally, a single large cyst filled with clear fluid may be present, particularly in gemistocytic subtypes. Focal calcification may occasionally be present and extension into contralateral structures, particularly the frontal lobes, is often observed (8,10).

HISTOLOGICAL SUBTYPES. It is beyond the scope of this chapter to describe the detailed microscopic pathology of LGAs. Nonetheless, a brief description of astrocytoma subtypes is worthwhile.

Fibrillary Astrocytomas. Fibrillary astrocytomas are the most frequent variant of LGAs. They are predominantly composed of fibrillary neoplastic astrocytes. The occasional or regional occurrence of gemistocytic astrocytes is also compatible with this diagnosis (Fig. 1A).

Gemistocytic Astrocytomas. This variant is predominantly composed of gemistocytic neoplastic astrocytes. The histological picture is dominated by plump, eosinophilic, glassy cell bodies of angular shape. This variant appears particularly prone to progression to higher grades (11) and, hence, is thought to have a worse prognosis.

Protoplasmic Astrocytomas. This is a rare variant composed of astrocytes showing a small cell body with few flaccid processes with a low content of glial filaments. Mucoid degeneration and microcyst formation are common and tend to occur in the cortex of adults (12) (Fig. 1B). In the largest series published thus far, Prayson and Estes (12) describe 16 patients with protoplasmic astrocytoma with a mean age of 21 years. Twelve were males and four were females. Tumors mostly occurred in the temporal and frontal lobes. It is not possible to ascertain whether the prognosis is any different to that of LGAs based on this small series.

Oligoastrocytomas. These tumors are composed of a mixture of both astrocytoma and oligodendroglioma cells, as the name suggests. They correspond to WHO grade II. During the past decade, these have been increasingly recognized (2). Their recognition and differentiation from pure LGAs is important since they have a better prognosis and are more conducive to adju-

vant chemotherapy (13,14). They are discussed in more detail under "Mixed Gliomas" later in this chapter (Fig. 1C).

Pilocytic Astrocytomas. Pilocytic astrocytomas should not be confused with LGAs. They are the most common glioma of childhood with most presenting in the first two decades of life. They typically occur in the cerebellum, though can occur at other sites such as the optic nerve, optic chiasm/hypothalamus, thalamus and basal ganglia, cerebral hemispheres, and brainstem ("dorsally exophytic brainstem glioma"). They may be curable by complete excision, although this may be impossible in tumors of the optic nerve and third ventricle region. Optic nerve glioma is a synonym for pilocytic astrocytoma of the optic nerve. These are associated with the inherited condition, neurofibromatosis 1 (von Recklinghausen disease) (Fig. 1D).

CLINICAL PRESENTATION AND IMAGING FINDINGS. Common presenting symptoms of LGAs include epilepsy, headache, mental changes, and focal neurological deficit. Epilepsy is the presenting symptom in more than half of all cases (15, 16). Headache and focal neurological deficit occur less often, and signs of raised intracranial pressure with papilledema are uncommon (15).

In recent years the diagnostic procedures of choice have become computed tomography (CT) and magnetic resonance imaging (MRI). MRI is the most sensitive test available to diagnose LGAs. CT scanning in a typical case reveals a nonenhancing lesion whose density is lower than that of the surrounding brain. A mass effect upon surrounding ventricular structures is common. If enhancement does occur, it is generally faint and homogeneous. On the MRI, the lesion typically presents as a low-intensity area of the T1-weighted images whereas there is almost always an increase in signal intensity corresponding with an increased relaxation time on T2-weighted images (Figs. 2A and B). The area of increased signal is usually homogeneous and well circumscribed with no evidence of hemorrhage or necrosis (17). Enhancement on MRI may also sometimes occur. Overall, enhancement on CT or MRI occurs in between 8% and 15% of cases (18–20). Daumas-Duport and colleagues (9) have shown that tumor cells are likely to extend beyond the CT- and MRI-defined abnormalities. It has been suggested that dynamic, contrast-enhanced T2-weighted MRI may identify more malignant areas within an astrocytoma (21).

There may be a role for positron emission tomography (PET) in the diagnosis and treatment of these patients. An LGA will be hypometabolic and therefore "cold" on PET scanning. However, when dedifferentiation occurs to a more malignant state, this area will be hypermetabolic and will appear as a "hot" spot on PET scanning. This information may be valuable in determining a site for biopsy and perhaps determining the aggressiveness of therapy (22,23). MR spectroscopy may also pro-

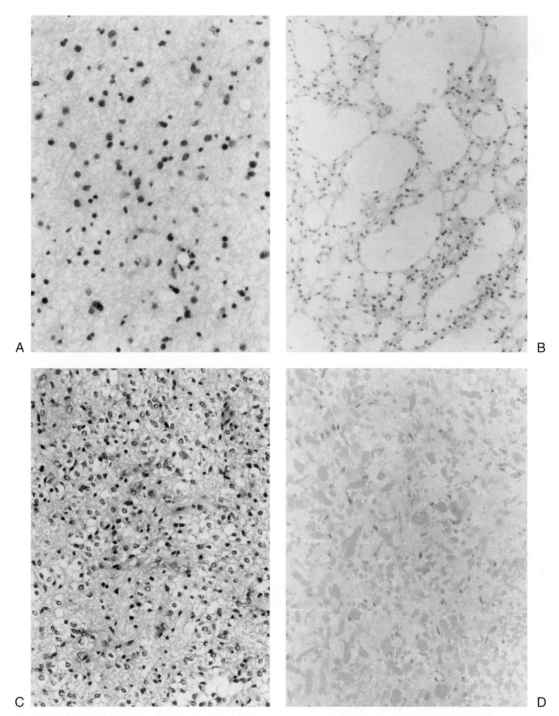

Fig. 1. Photomicrographs of astrocytoma subtypes. (Hematoxylin and eosin, ×100.) **A:** Fibrillary astrocytoma, characterized by neoplastic astrocytes with enlarged, irregular, hyperchromatic nuclei. **B:** Protoplasmic astrocytomas, as illustrated here, are characterized by neoplastic astrocytes with a small cell body and few, flaccid cell processes. Mucoid degeneration and microcyst formation are a common feature. **C:** Oligoastrocytoma, with distinct areas of oligodendroglioma, characterized by small round cells with typical perinuclear halos, admixed with typical fibrillary astrocytoma cells. **D:** Pilocytic astrocytoma, with scattered neoplastic astrocytes, often with a characteristic piloid ("hairlike") shape. In this section there are abundant Rosenthal fibers (glassy, eosinophilic masses), which are also typical of pilocytic astrocytoma.

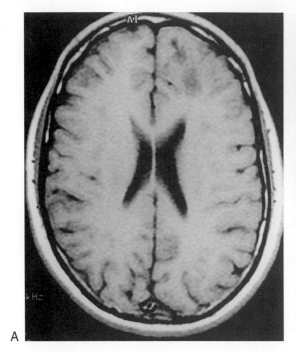

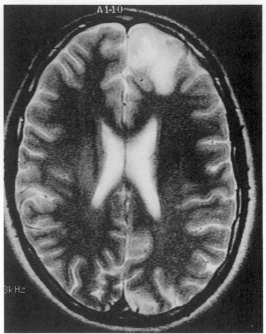

Fig. 2. Magnetic resonance images of astrocytomas. T1-weighted images **(A)**, and T2-weighted images **(B)** of a low-grade astrocytoma of the left frontal lobe showing the characteristic pattern of hypodensity on T1 imaging and hyperdensity on T2 imaging. Proton density image **(C)** showing a hypodense cortical lesion of the left temporal lobe. There was no enhancement after gadolinium. Although the lesion was asymptomatic, it was resected. Histology revealed an anaplastic astrocytoma.

vide additional information with regard to the grade of astrocytic tumor (24).

PROGNOSTIC FACTORS

Clinical and Surgical Factors. The median survival time after surgical intervention is in the range of 6 to 8 years, with marked variation. Many studies have been published on the subject of prognostic factors for LGAs (Table 2). Laws and associates (7) found the following factors important to prolonged survival:

- gross total surgical removal
- lack of preoperative neurological deficit
- long duration of symptoms prior to surgery
- seizures as a presenting symptom
- surgery in recent decades

Almost all would agree young age at the time of diagnosis is by far the most important factor that correlates with long survival (7,25–31). Seizures are correlated with a better prognosis while focal deficit and change in personality are indicative of a worse prognosis (7,31,32). The beneficial effect of a good

Table 2. Summary of Independent Prognostic Factors in Studies of Low-Grade Astrocytomas

Study	No. of Patients	Tumor Grade	Performance Status	Age	Extent of Surgery	Radiotherapy
Laws, et al. (7)	461	S	S	S	S	S
Garcia, et al. (82)	86	S	NS	ND	S	S
Piepmeier, et al. (18)	60	ND	S	ND	S	NS
Medbery, et al. (87)	50	ND	S	ND	NS	S
Shaw, et al. (63)	126	S	S	ND	S	S
Soffietti, et al. (31)	85	ND	NS	S	S	NS
North, et al. (28)	77	NS	S	S	S	NS
Kaye, et al. (73)	78	S	S	S	S	NS

S, satistically significant; NS, not significant; ND, no data.

clinical condition at diagnosis is well documented (7,19,26). Hence, patients who present with a focal neurological deficit (31) or with evidence of raised intracranial pressure with papilledema have a worse outlook than those presenting with epilepsy (7,18).

The extent of surgery may predict survival, but not all studies have agreed. Soffieti and co-workers (31) found a longer survival in those with gross surgical removal, but others have not found that the extent of surgical resection corresponds with the length of survival (18,33). In our series of 78 patients, there was a slight advantage for surgical excision (Table 2). Most, but not all (19,20), studies have indicated that patients who receive only a biopsy have a worse survival compared to resection.

Tumor and Biological Factors

PREOPERATIVE TUMOR VOLUME. An important finding of the recent randomized trial on radiation in the treatment of LGAs (34) has been the discovery that tumor volume is an important predictor both of overall survival and progression-free survival. Others have also demonstrated that large tumors behave less favorably (35,36).

CELL PROLIFERATION MARKERS. Several studies have shown that tumors identified as having a higher mitotic activity have a poorer prognosis. LGAs with a BUdR labeling index greater than 1% (37,38), or an MIB-1 labeling index of greater than 8% (39) represent a subset with a poorer prognosis. Ki-67 labeling, however, was not found to correlate with prognosis (40). Deoxyribonucleic acid ploidy as determined by flow cytometry has not been able to identify patients with worse outcomes (38).

GENETIC CHARACTERISTICS. The genetic composition of LGAs is variable. It is likely that the tendency for progression of LGAs and ultimately patient survival is dependent on the genetic makeup of the tumor. Few genetic characteristics of astrocytomas have been as thoroughly explored in this respect as that of the p53 gene and its protein product. Mutations of this tumor suppressor gene are frequent genetic aberrations in astrocytomas (41), but their predictive value is incompletely understood. Neoplasms with p53 gene mutations appear to progress to higher grades earlier and more often (42,43), though the evidence is not convincing (44). Some studies have shown a worse prognosis for patients whose tumors showed immunoreactivity for p53 protein (indicative of a mutation) (45) but others have not (40,46). In the future, it seems likely that a genetic profile of a tumor will be determinable, which will enable more accurate prediction of natural history and response to treatment than currently available. This is a valid reason to obtain a tissue diagnosis of all suspected cases at presentation, since future technologies may be applicable to today's patients, especially if samples of their tumor are available for analysis.

PROGRESSION OF LOW-GRADE ASTROCYTOMAS. The cause of death in the majority of patients with an LGA is progression to higher grade tumors (18). Progression to higher grades occurs more rapidly in older patients—in one study "age at diagnosis" showed a strong negative correlation with "interval to anaplastic progression" (47). As in other neoplasms, the development of astrocytomas and their progression to higher grades is characterized by a multistep progression and accumulation of genetic abnormalities (48). The genetic changes involved in the progression of LGAs to higher grades are summarized in Fig. 3. There is also a considerable body of evidence to suggest that more than one genetic type of diffuse astrocytoma exists (49,50). Intratumoral genetic heterogeneity is likely to be a prominent feature of astrocytoma molecular genetics (51) being reflected by well-described histological variability within individual astrocytomas (1). Within a given tumor, multiple subpopulations are likely to have evolved and those subpopulations that progress will have acquired a growth advantage (52). Eventually one would expect these more active cell populations to overtake the more indolent cells of the LGA and thus lead

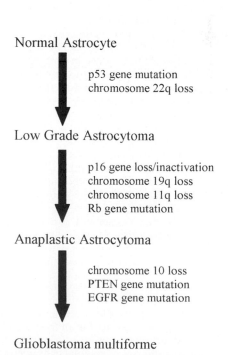

Fig. 3. Summary of the major genetic changes that occur during progression of astrocytomas.

to a higher grade tumor. Muller and colleagues (53), studying LGAs that had recurred, found that 14% of tumors were unchanged, 55% were anaplastic astrocytomas, and 30% were glioblastoma multiformes (GBMs). The authors concluded that approximately two-thirds of tumors will progress, but it was not possible to predict histologically which tumors would progress. Progression to higher grade tumors has been well documented in other series as well (7,16,19,27,31). It is difficult to predict what influences this phenomenon, although tumor volume is clearly an important parameter (30,36). The implication of these studies may be that one should attempt to remove as many of the LGA cells as possible. These tumor cells have minimal genetic alterations and if left *in situ*, they may accumulate further genetic changes over time that could allow them to become more malignant; for example, loss of the CDKN2 gene on chromosome 9p (54).

METHODS OF TREATMENT

Delayed Treatment. The option of observation or nontreatment of a patient with an LGA may be justified if the risks of treatment (surgery and/or radiation) are greater than the risks of medical treatment of the presenting symptom, usually seizures (55,56). This course, however, depends on an accurate diagnosis on clinical and imaging grounds excluding other treatable conditions and that the outcome is ultimately independent of the timing of treatment.

Patients selected for observation usually have good prognostic features—they are often young, have no or minimal neurological deficits, and usually present with seizures. The attraction of a period of observation in such patients is in avoiding the possible untoward effects of treatment of surgery and/or radiation. Although the risks of surgery have decreased with the advent of recent technological advances, morbidity and mortality are still related to tumor location (57). Patients with deep tumors or tumors in eloquent cortex are at significant risk of neurological deterioration from surgical resection or biopsy (58). These risks need to be balanced against the chance of obtaining an accurate diagnosis.

Risks of radiotherapy include neurocognitive impairment in long-term survivors of LGA (59). Radiation at moderate doses (45 to 59 Gy) is unlikely to produce severe side effects in the short term (60), yet the long-term results are uncertain. The European Organization for Research and Treatment of Cancer (EORTC) trial clearly demonstrates a worse outcome in terms of quality of life in patients who received 59.4 Gy over 6 weeks compared to those who received 45 Gy over 5 weeks (61). Other studies have also suggested that radiation therapy is associated with anaplastic changes in LGAs in children (62). Shaw and co-workers (63), on the other hand, showed a significantly better survival in patients who received high-dose postoperative radiotherapy (greater than 53 Gy) compared to low-dose (less than 53 Gy) or no radiotherapy.

If a decision is made to observe a patient with suspected LGA, a strategy must be in place to detect progressive disease, which would then require more aggressive therapy. Progression is generally heralded by new onset of seizures or worsening of seizures or impairment of neurological function (22).

Although from an oncological perspective surgery should be carried out as soon as possible in the course of a malignancy, it has never been proven that earlier treatment of LGA produces an increase in survival as measured from the time of diagnosis (64). There is a risk of misdiagnosis on imaging data (65), but in studies addressing this question, a delay in making management decisions has not seemed to affect the outcome. For example, Rajan and associates (66) did not find any difference in

outcome between patients with verified and unverified LGAs. Additionally, since many patients present with no neurological deficits and because operative intervention in some locations carries a significant risk of postoperative morbidity, delayed surgery may be more desirable. Recht and others (56) compared a group of patients who had an imaging diagnosis of LGA and no surgery to those who had immediate surgical intervention. They found no difference in survival or the incidence of progression between the groups and thus concluded that deferring surgery did not worsen outcome.

The risk of wrongly selecting a young patient with a nonenhancing, high-grade tumor for observation (65) may be offset by the fact that the survival of younger patients with high-grade tumors is better than older patients with low-grade tumors. Hence, age may be more important in predicting outcome when other factors are equal (small size, no mass effect, lack of raised intracranial pressure, and normal neurological function) (67). Yet it seems unlikely that in those individuals who are young and are wrongly selected for a period of observation, that their individual outcomes would have been as good had they received early aggressive treatment.

Imaging studies are not always accurate in the diagnosis of LGAs (65). In addition, a minority of cases of anaplastic astrocytoma and even GBM do not show enhancement on imaging (68) (Fig. 2C). Adjuvant therapy is recommended in higher grade tumors and therefore it seems justified to obtain a precise pathological diagnosis, if possible. The van Veelen group (69) came to a similar conclusion.

In another series, Afra and colleagues (16) describe a worse prognosis in patients with a shorter preoperative history and who were reoperated on, and therefore determined that dedifferentiation to higher grades may be delayed by early radical surgery.

Surgical Options

STEREOTACTIC BIOPSY. Stereotactic biopsy is an accurate and safe method for the diagnosis of LGAs (20). Framed or frameless stereotactic techniques can be used, with either CT or MRI guidance. Since MRI is more sensitive in detecting LGAs, this is probably the investigation of choice. The use of contrast is essential if previous images have shown enhancement. Multiple biopsies should be taken to increase the accuracy and these can usually be done using a single trajectory (20,70). The addition of PET scanning may guide the biopsy of more suspicious areas (22).

Lunsford and associates (20) advocate stereotactic biopsy followed by radiotherapy as the treatment of choice for LGAs. The overall median survival of their series of 35 cases was 9.8 years, which compares favorably with other series where cytoreductive surgery was employed (7,27,31). Also, their rates of mortality and morbidity were significantly lower than those of surgical series (18,27,28,32,57). Their series, however, is small.

Because astrocytomas are heterogeneous in nature, stereotactic biopsy, theoretically at least, may be inaccurate by underestimating the malignancy of a mass lesion. In addition, since even high-grade astrocytomas may not enhance on imaging studies (68), the more anaplastic areas of a tumor may not be biopsied. Stereotactic biopsy may also misdiagnose oligoastrocytoma as a pure LGA. The accurate diagnosis of oligoastrocytoma is important since these tumors respond favorably to chemotherapy (71). Sampling error, therefore, may be a significant problem.

Stereotactic biopsy is clearly not the treatment of choice in the presence of mass effects, either clinically or radiologically. Craniotomy and debulking is more appropriate in this instance.

CYTOREDUCTIVE SURGERY. Most but not all retrospective studies indicate that gross total removal of LGAs results in a longer survival for patients compared to those who have not had cytoreductive surgery (17). For instance, Janny and colleagues (15) show a respective 5- and 10-year survival of 87.5% and 68.2% in LGAs completely resected compared to 57% and 31.2% with incomplete or no surgical resection. Berger and co-workers (36) show that the patients most at risk of tumor recurrence and malignant progression are those with larger preoperative tumors and residual tumor postoperatively. However, such studies are often flawed since in cases where gross total removal was not attempted, the tumor may well have been infiltrating into deep and important structures, and this may have affected survival more so than the extent of surgery itself. Despite this, the general oncological principle of trying to remove as many neoplastic cells as possible would seem appropriate where this can be done with minimal risk of producing a postoperative neurological deficit. Another review, however, failed to demonstrate a survival advantage with a greater extent of resection (72). In our own series of 78 patients, there was an overall median survival of 8.1 years (Table 3) (73). There appeared to be a slight survival advantage following macroscopic surgical excision with a 10-year survival of 70% compared to 42% in patients who received only biopsy.

There is a clear benefit to the patient in the short term in respect of neurological function and quality of life in the presence of mass effects and raised intracranial pressure. Debulking is recommended particularly if the tumor is in an accessible position. This approach may also avoid chronic steroid use and its inherent side effects.

Cytoreductive surgery has the advantage of providing more tumor specimen for histological analysis. The likelihood of underestimating the grade of the tumor or missing an oligoastrocytoma is therefore much less. With a greater amount of tumor available, genetic analysis may also be possible. Theoretically, the less number of cells present after surgery, the less chance of genetic progression of the remaining tumor cells and the more effective adjuvant radiotherapy may be. These theoretical advantages, however, have been questioned (20,70).

If cytoreductive surgery is to be attempted, it may be difficult to localize the tumor and then obtain a clear interface between tumor and normal brain (9). Localization may be aided by intraoperative ultrasound (74) or the use of framed or frameless stereotaxy (75,76). Resection may be made easier using an ultrasonic aspirator or laser. Other adjuncts that may be useful include the use of framed or frameless stereotaxy with volumetric resection and electrophysiological monitoring.

Among low-grade gliomas, Daumas-Duport and colleagues (9) have described three structural types. Type I tumors are solid tumors with little or no invasion of surrounding brain. These include pilocytic astrocytomas, pleomorphic xanthoastrocytomas, subependymal giant cell astrocytomas, and gangli-

ogliomas. They can theoretically be completely excised. Type II tumors are solid tumors with surrounding isolated invasive tumor cells. Resection of the tumor and surrounding infiltrated brain may be possible in noneloquent brain. Type III tumors are those that are diffusely infiltrative, with no discernible solid tumor mass. Excision of these lesions is problematic.

Stereotactic volumetric resection has been pioneered by Kelly (75). Briefly, it involves the preoperative acquisition of imaging and the computer-assisted calculation of three-dimensional data. It allows not only for localization of lesions, but also for the preoperative simulation of surgical trajectory planning for selection of the safest and most effective surgical approach to the lesion. Intraoperatively, it allows for delineation of tumor boundaries and avoidance of critical areas of brain. Frameless technologies have proven similarly applicable to the resection of LGAs (77,78).

Intraoperative physiological mapping may be used to achieve the maximal safe resection of LGAs. The regions of particular interest for functional mapping encompass the dominant hemisphere temporal, posterior frontal and anterior parietal lobes for language, as well as the motor pathways (i.e., the motor cortex, corona radiata, internal capsule, and cerebral peduncles) and the sensory cortex. Any lesion located adjacent to these areas (e.g., supplementary motor area, insula, or thalamus) is a good target for mapping. The details for these techniques can be found elsewhere (79). Briefly, techniques that may be used include functional stimulation mapping of motor areas (the patient may be asleep or awake), sensory stimulation, and stimulation for language mapping (both with the patient awake). Preoperative and intraoperative mapping of epileptogenic foci may also be employed and may improve seizure control postoperatively (80). Preoperative functional MRI may be a useful adjunct in LGAs of the motor cortex (81).

The Role of Postoperative Radiation Therapy. The role of radiation therapy in the treatment of LGA remains controversial. Although the majority of studies have found that radiation therapy is beneficial when added to surgery in the treatment of LGA (7,31,63,82–84) and that radioresponsiveness can be demonstrated (20,85,86), properly conducted trials were just begun in the mid-1990s (34). Indeed, radiological response may not be associated with a better outcome (86). The retrospective studies available show no uniformity of patients, tumor pathologies, or pathological classifications; nor of radiation dose or volume or in the extent of surgical removal. Virtually no control group of patients exists.

The series of Laws and co-workers (7) is probably the largest group study of LGAs, with 461 patients. The authors interpret their data as showing a beneficial effect of radical surgery and a beneficial effect of radiation therapy only in those patients with an otherwise poor prognosis. Piepmeier and associates (18) reviewed the results of radiation therapy of 60 patients with LGA, and failed to demonstrate a beneficial effect. However, with a mean time of just under 5 years, this may not have been long enough to demonstrate an effect. Medbery and others (87) compared a group of 50 patients who received postoperative radiotherapy with 10 who did not. There appeared to be a slight survival advantage in those incompletely resected tumors receiving radiotherapy postoperatively. In 1989, Shaw and colleagues (63) reviewed the data of 167 patients from the Mayo Clinic. The 5-year survival for those receiving high-dose radiotherapy (greater than 53 Gy) was 68%, whereas the survival rate was 47% for those who received low-dose radiotherapy (less than 53 Gy) and 38% for those who did not receive radiotherapy. The 10-year survival rates were 39%, 21%, and 11%, respectively.

Whitton and Bloom (88) were unable to conclude whether postoperative radiotherapy was effective in the treatment of

Table 3. Summary of Studies of Median Survival of Patients with Astrocytoma

Series Survival	No. of Patients	Study Interval	Median (Years)
Soffietti, et al. (31)	85	1950–1982	3.2
Shaw, et al. (63)	167	1976–1983	4.5
Piepmeier, et al. (18)	60	1975–1985	7.5
Medbery, et al. (87)	50	1960–1986	4.0
Vertosick, et al. (19)	25	1978–1987	8.2
Philippon, et al. (32)	179	1978–1987	9.0
McCormack, et al. (27)	53	1977–1988	7.25
Lunsford, et al. (20)	35	1982–1992	9.8
Iwabuchi, et al. (26)	56	1967–1993	5.0
Kaye, et al. (73)	78	1983–1993	8.1

LGAs, after reviewing the results of 88 adult patients treated at the Royal Marsden Hospital, as were Janny and co-workers (15) in a French series. In the series of Vertosick and associates (19), the median survival of the entire group was 8.2 years, but there was no significant difference between the patients who received radiotherapy and those who did not. Selective radiotherapy has been advocated for cases in which partial resection only was performed (89).

In the EORTC study, no difference in outcome could be found between low-dose (45 Gy over 5 weeks) and high-dose radiation of LGAs (59.4 Gy over 6 weeks) (34). A later follow-up showed those in the higher dose group had a lower quality of life (61). Further follow-up of this trial will help elucidate whether early or delayed radiotherapy is best.

Stereotactic radiosurgery has been used in the treatment of LGAs by Pozza and colleagues (90). They demonstrated a radiological response in 12 of 14 patients. Also, re-irradiation has been reported in a patient with an LGA with an interval period of 8.5 years (91). Apparently no ill effects were caused by the second course of radiotherapy.

Radiation therapy is not without side effects (92). Careful consideration should be given prior to its administration.

DELAYED RADIATION THERAPY. Deferring radiation therapy until recurrence or progression is a viable option in patients with an otherwise good prognosis after early histological diagnosis with either stereotactic biopsy or cytoreductive surgery (18,93). This delays any potential side effects of radiation until it is clearly necessary. Patients with a good prognosis may benefit from this approach (93). The second randomized EORTC trial on radiation therapy is designed to address the issue of early or delayed radiation therapy (34).

The Role of Chemotherapy. Although some studies have shown a survival benefit for patients treated with adjuvant chemotherapy (94), a prospective, randomized trial has shown that there was no benefit (95) and therefore presently there is no proven role for chemotherapy in the treatment of LGAs. Studies have shown, however, that chemotherapy is of use in treating patients with oligodendrogliomas or oligoastrocytomas (14,96).

OUTCOME AND CONCLUSIONS. Before the MRI era, studies would indicate that a typical 5-year survival rate was approximately 40% to 50% and a 10-year survival rate was about 20% to 30% (7). Two studies may indicate that early diagnosis with CT and MRI may improve survival, with a median survival now of 7.5 years, a 5-year survival of 65%, and a 10-year survival of 40% (19,27). The experience at the Royal Melbourne Hospital in recent years is similar (Tables 2 and 3).

The management of LGAs is controversial and outcome is dependent on multiple factors, not only on the management instituted but also the variable intrinsic biology of the tumors themselves. We would recommend tissue diagnosis in all cases of suspected LGA. In patients with surgically accessible tumors, or those with mass effect on imaging and clinical grounds, craniotomy and cytoreductive surgery should be instituted. Stereotactic biopsy only is a viable option in tumors in eloquent regions with no mass effect or enhancement on imaging. In general, radiation therapy is delayed until there is evidence of progressive or recurrent disease. A more aggressive early approach is recommended for those who are over 40 years of age, who clinically have neurological impairment or raised intracranial pressure, or who have enhancing tumors on CT or MRI (Fig. 4).

Other Forms of Astrocytomas

PLEOMORPHIC XANTHOASTROCYTOMAS. Pleomorphic xanthoastrocytomas (PXAs) were originally described in 1979

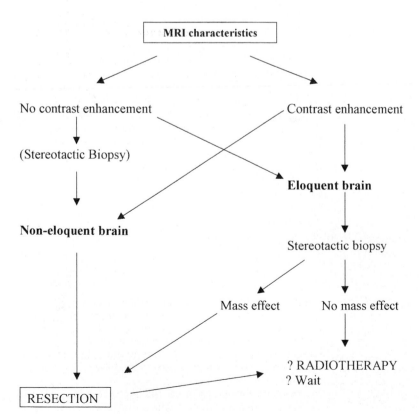

Fig. 4. Suggested protocol for the management of low-grade astrocytomas.

by Kepes and others (97). They are rare tumors that generally affect children and young adults who present with epilepsy. Two-thirds of patients are under 18 years old (98). The tumors are often superficial and affect the temporal lobe in approximately 50% of cases (99). Cases involving the spinal cord, cerebellum, and retina have been described (100–103). There is characteristically leptomeningeal involvement (97), and in keeping with their WHO grade I classification, they overall have a good prognosis.

Pathology. Using the WHO grading system, PXAs are grade I lesions. They are not included in the St. Anne/Mayo system (3). Macroscopically PXAs appear as large, cortical, well-circumscribed lesions, but there may be no distinction from normal brain on the deep surface of the tumor (1). A mural nodule of yellow-red tissue with a surrounding proteinaceous cyst is often found (104). Microscopically, there is striking pleomorphism, a reticulin meshwork, and frequent xanthomatous change of tumor cells. Characteristically, tumor cells are glial fibrillary acidic protein (GFAP)-positive. As distinct from high-grade diffuse astrocytomas, there is typically no necrosis and few mitotic figures. Because this is the characteristic difference between PXA and GBM, the distinction between the two entities may not be made with complete confidence on small samples, for example, from stereotactic biopsy. If mitotic activity is seen, progression to a higher grade is likely to have occurred (98).

Clinical Presentation and Imaging Findings. PXAs usually occur in young adults or children who present with epilepsy (99). Rarely, symptoms and signs of raised intracranial pressure or even intracranial hemorrhage are present (97,105,106). With CT or MRI scanning, the lesions appear as a superficial cortical or meningocerebral mass or nodule with an underlying cyst (107–109). On T1-weighted images tumor nodules are generally isodense, and hyperdense on T2-weighted images. Marked enhancement occurs after gadolinium (109). They can occasionally mimic meningiomas (110). Cerebral angiography demonstrates an avascular or mildly vascular nodule with a meningeal vascular supply (109). Tumors that should be considered in the differential diagnosis of a peripheral, enhancing lesion in a child or young adult, apart from PXA, would include pilocytic astrocytoma, GBM, metastasis, ganglioglioma, gangliosarcoma, meningioma, and oligodendroglioma (109).

Treatment and Prognosis. Treatment should be aimed at gross resection and radiological follow-up. There is no evidence for a role of adjuvant radiotherapy or chemotherapy. PXAs generally have a favorable prognosis with an extended survival after surgery often with improvement in seizure outcome (105). A minority of cases do recur early and may progress to higher grade tumors, and although this may represent misdiagnosis of the initial specimen in a few cases, true progression of PXAs has been documented (105). Upon recurrence or progression, further surgery and/or adjuvant therapies may be indicated. Prognosis has been associated with extent of resection and mitotic index, and the presence of necrosis has not been found to be significant (99).

SUBEPENDYMAL GIANT CELL ASTROCYTOMAS. Subependymal giant cell astrocytomas (SEGAs) are rare tumors that occur almost exclusively in the setting of tuberous sclerosis (111). They occur in approximately 10% of confirmed cases of tuberous sclerosis, generally presenting in the first two decades of life (111). Although their glial nature is sometimes in dispute, they are thought to arise from subependymal nodules and are generally classified with other astrocytomas. In the WHO system, they are grade I tumors, along with pilocytic astrocytomas

and PXAs, as a result of their indolent behavior and good prognosis compared to invasive astrocytomas.

Pathology. SEGAs tend to occur in the region of the foramen of Monro as well-demarcated, broad-based, firm and gray masses. They have a variable microscopic appearance, but characteristically have a uniform cellularity and a vasocentric cellular pattern. Cells are larger than gemistocytic astrocytes but not truly "giant." The cells are phenotypically astrocytic with a fibrillary background (1).

Clinical Presentation and Imaging Features. SEGAs may be asymptomatic, cause seizures, or lead to raised intracranial pressure from hydrocephalus. On CT or MRI, they appear as large, bulky, heterogeneous masses with variable amounts of calcification and are isodense to gray matter on T1-weighted images and hyperdense on T2-weighted images (112). They often coexist with small subependymal hamartomas but enhance uniformly and vividly with contrast, which hamartomas do not (113). The differential diagnosis would include ependymoma, subependymoma, astrocytoma, central neurocytoma, and choroid plexus papilloma (114).

Treatment and Prognosis. Patients with asymptomatic lesions need to be followed radiologically and clinically, since these lesions can grow (115). Symptomatic tumors should be resected either by a transcallosal or transcortical route. SEGAs have a favorable outlook even if they are not totally resected (116) and in the presence of mitoses and necrosis (117). Some authors advise resecting asymptomatic lesions if they are demonstrated to increase in size since they may result in a more favorable surgical outcome and have less likelihood of recurrence (118). Any attempt at surgery in children should be preceded by a thorough cardiac evaluation to exclude potentially fatal cardiac anomalies (119). Adjuvant radiotherapy or chemotherapy probably has no role in the treatment of SEGAs.

Oligodendrogliomas

After astrocytomas, oligodendrogliomas are the next most common form of glioma in adults. They represent neoplastic transformation of oligodendrocytes, which form myelin within the CNS. Oligodendrogliomas have a predilection for the frontal lobes, are often calcified, often present with seizures, and have a characteristic "fried egg" appearance on microscopy.

EPIDEMIOLOGY. Oligodendrogliomas were originally thought to comprise approximately 4% of primary brain tumors (120). However, current immunohistochemical techniques have demonstrated that many tumors with the histological appearance of astrocytoma lack GFAP staining, partly or completely, and as such are now diagnosed as either mixed oligoastrocytomas or oligodendrogliomas, respectively. Using these criteria, the incidence of oligodendrogliomas has increased (121). They have a slight male preponderance with a peak incidence of around 40 years of age, with a smaller peak at around 10 years of age (122,123).

CLINICAL PRESENTATION AND IMAGING FINDINGS. Seizures are the presenting symptom in 50% to 80 % of cases (120,122). Other symptoms include raised intracranial pressure and focal signs, both of which are less common. Many imaging characteristics of oligodendroglioma are similar to those of astrocytoma. Most often, they are seen as deep white matter lesions that infiltrate widely. On CT and even plain radiographs, calcification is often seen. Particularly characteristic is a gyriform or ribbonlike pattern of calcification. MRI is not dissimilar to that of astrocytomas (Fig. 2).

PATHOLOGY. Oligodendrogliomas occur most often in the frontal lobes (104), but may occur anywhere within the CNS, including the spinal cord (124,125). Macroscopically, these tumors are often pink to red, friable masses. There may be an apparent plane between the tumor and normal brain at surgery, more so than diffuse astrocytomas (1). Focally, the neoplasm is often extremely cellular, gray, and fleshy and therefore simulates a more anaplastic lesion. Oligodendrogliomas may visibly alter the cerebral cortex since they diffusely infiltrate gray matter.

The microscopic recognition of a typical oligodendroglioma is not difficult given an appearance of uniform sheets of cells with similar cell shape and size. Calcification is frequent, both in the tumor itself and the surrounding cerebral cortex. A helpful diagnostic feature is the appearance of perineuronal satellitosis, subpial accumulation, and perivascular aggregation (1). Often present are delicate angulated segments of capillaries, giving a "chicken wire" appearance. Oligodendrogliomas also have a tendency for intratumoral hemorrhage. The "fried egg" artifact is a distinctive feature of many oligodendrogliomas, created by autolytic imbibition of water accompanying delayed fixation, forming clear perinuclear halos (Fig. 1C).

Grading of Oligodendrogliomas. Several attempts at pathological grading of oligodendrogliomas have been made. A number of studies have confirmed the prognostic significance of certain histological features, although not all identified the same factors as being relevant (1). These features include increased cellularity, cytological atypia, mitotic activity, vascular hypertrophy, vascular proliferation, pleomorphism, and necrosis (126–130). It is unclear whether a two-, three-, or four-tiered system should be used (1). The association of age and anaplasia on one hand and prognosis on the other has been shown but this is not as pronounced as in diffuse astrocytomas (126,128). Many authorities employ a two-tiered system, classifying these tumors as either well-differentiated oligodendrogliomas or anaplastic lesions (1,123). The WHO system also recognizes two grades—oligodendroglioma (WHO grade II) and anaplastic (malignant) oligodendroglioma (WHO grade III) (2). Oligodendroglioma may also progress to GBM. It is likely that these lesions have a better prognosis than pure GBMs.

PROGNOSIS. Oligodendrogliomas are generally not considered completely resectable due to their infiltrative nature. Most ultimately result in the patient's demise, though this may be many years after the initial diagnosis. Overall, prognosis is better than for LGAs. For instance, in the Mayo Clinic experience of 82 patients, the median survival time and the 5-, 10-, and 15-year survival rates were 7.1 years, 54%, 34%, and 24%, respectively (123). Small lesions probably have a better outlook, and age may (88,127,131) or may not (120) be significant. In any case, the association of age and prognosis is probably not as strong as it is with astrocytomas. Prognosis has also been related to proliferation-associated markers PCNA and Ki-67 (132,133). As in LGAs, p53 staining by immunohistochemistry may be associated with a worse prognosis (134,135).

TREATMENT. Historically, treatment of oligodendrogliomas has been based on gross surgical resection followed by radio-

therapy. Many of the controversies that apply to the definitive management of LGAs also apply to oligodendrogliomas in terms of the role of surgery, its timing and extent, and the role of postoperative radiotherapy.

The extent of surgery correlates with survival in most series (88,120,123). For example, in the Mayo Clinic experience, Shaw and others (123) show that in patients with gross resection there is a median survival of 12.6 years and a 5- and 10-year survival of 74% and 59%, compared to a median survival of 4.9 years and a 5- and 10-year survival of 48% and 26% in those undergoing subtotal resection. However, as with LGAs, the evidence that the extent of surgery itself results in improved survival, as opposed to other patient and tumor-related factors, is lacking. Some studies have not shown a beneficial effect of extent of surgical resection on survival for oligodendroglioma (136).

The role of radiotherapy is controversial. Although often considered standard therapy, some studies have shown no or marginal survival benefit for patients given postoperative irradiation (123,137). Wallner and associates (138) show a distinct advantage for patients who received greater than 45 Gy of postoperative radiotherapy. In other series, a survival advantage has also been shown, particularly for patients who had undergone subtotal resection (139,140). Lindegaard and co-workers (139), however, show no advantage for those who had total macroscopic resection. They, in fact, believe that it is detrimental in these patients who otherwise have a good prognosis. They also show no benefit from 50 to 60 Gy as opposed to 40 to 50 Gy, and therefore recommend the lower dose regimen. On the basis of these and similar series, postoperative radiotherapy is generally recommended (141) yet the evidence for its efficacy, as for LGAs, is not well substantiated.

Recent reports have shown that oligodendrogliomas are chemosensitive (96,142–144). PCV (procarbazine, lomustine, and vincristine) is most widely used, though melphalan and thiotepa may be equally effective (143). Chemotherapy should therefore be given in patients with subtotal resection, or in those who have anaplastic or otherwise aggressive tumors (i.e., large, mass effects, extensive radiological appearance). In those with stable, nonenhancing disease who are clinically well, a period of observation before chemotherapy is probably justified.

Mixed Gliomas

Mixed gliomas are composed of more than a single type of neoplastic glial cell. Criteria for their diagnosis are difficult to define, but it is generally accepted that the essential characteristic is phenotypic heterogeneity, not necessarily biphasic tumors. By far the most common are oligoastrocytomas.

OLIGOASTROCYTOMAS. Oligoastrocytomas are defined as tumors with geographically distinct areas of unequivocal, coexisting oligodendroglioma and astrocytoma (1). They are WHO grade II lesions. Varying opinions for the minimum astroglial component for the diagnosis exist, including at least 1% (145), 25% (129), and 50% (146). It has been suggested that the microscopic presence of at least 1 per 100× field of oligodendroglioma is sufficient for the diagnosis of oligoastrocytoma, rather than astrocytoma (147).

The epidemiology, clinical presentation, and imaging findings are similar to that of pure oligodendroglioma. The prognostic significance of this tumor is uncertain. Shaw and colleagues (148) show a median survival of 6.3 years and a 5- and 10-year survival rate of 58% and 32%, respectively, in their series from the Mayo Clinic. It is likely that overall the outlook is somewhere between LGA and pure oligodendroglioma (96). Both pure oligodendroglioma and oligoastrocytoma respond to chemotherapy (96,144). Pure tumors are likely to be more chemosensitive (96) and given this, the degree to which the tumor has oligodendroglioma cells, probably dictates its chemosensitivity and hence its prognosis.

Gangliogliomas

Gangliogliomas are uncommon tumors that occur throughout the neuraxis (149,150). In general they are benign lesions that occur in children and young adults. They are composed, as the name suggests, of a mixture of neuronal and glial cells.

Gangliogliomas are most common in the temporal and frontal lobes. Most patients present with a progressive seizure disorder (151). Symptoms may be present for months to years. CT scan usually demonstrates a hypodense or isodense lesion with poor contrast enhancement (152). Tumors may be solid or cystic, with solid tumors more frequent in the temporal lobe (153). Calcification may also be seen. Most are hypodense relative to gray matter in T1-weighted MRI and hyperdense relative to gray matter in T2-weighted scans. Enhancement with gadolinium occurs in most cases.

Macroscopically, gangliogliomas are firm but may have cystic components. Microscopically, both neuronal and astrocytic components are readily seen. Anaplastic degeneration, if it occurs, is usually seen in the glial component (154). In two series (155,156), the average age of patients was 18 years and 31 years, respectively. Overall it seems that factors of prognostic significance for gangliogliomas are the degree of resection and tumor grade. The degree of surgical resection seems particularly important for anaplastic lesions. In the series of Selch and associates (155), the 4-year progression-free survival was 78% for low-grade lesions totally excised and 63% for low-grade lesions not totally resected. This compares to a 4-year progression-free survival for high-grade lesions of 75% after total resection and 25% for subtotal resection. Postoperative radiotherapy was recommended after partial resection of high-grade lesions. Rumana and co-workers (156) show that age at diagnosis was a significant negative prognosticator, but that the extent of surgery was not a statistically significant prognostic factor.

In summary then, the treatment for accessible gangliogliomas is surgical excision. This offers the best chance for cure, but long-term survival is possible even after partial excision (154). Radiotherapy may be considered in cases of partial excision, especially in the presence of anaplastic change (157).

References

1. Burger PC, Scheithauer BW. *Tumors of the central nervous system.* Washington DC: Armed Forces Institute of Pathology, 1994.
2. Kleihues P, Burger PC, Scheithauer BW. *Histological typing of tumours of the central nervous system.* Berlin: Springer-Verlag, 1993.
3. Daumas-Duport C, Scheithauer B, O'Fallon J, et al. Grading of astrocytomas. A simple and reproducible method. *Cancer* 1988; 62(10):2152–2165.
4. Guthrie BL, Laws ER Jr. Supratentorial low-grade gliomas. *Neurosurg Clin North Am* 1990;1(1):37–48.
5. Radhakrishnan K, Bohnen NI, Kurland LT. Epidemiology of brain tumors. In: Morantz RA, Walsh J, eds. *Brain tumors: a comprehensive text.* New York: Marcel Dekker, 1993.
6. Morantz RA. Low grade astrocytomas. In: Kaye AH, Laws ER Jr.,
7. Laws ER Jr., Taylor WF, Clifton MB, et al. Neurosurgical management of low-grade astrocytoma of the cerebral hemispheres. *J Neurosurg* 1984;61(4):665–673.
8. Kleihues P, Davis RL, Ohgaki H, et al. Low-grade diffuse astrocytomas. In: Kleihues P, Cavenee WK, eds. *Tumors of the nervous system: pathology and genetics.* Lyon: International Agency for Research on Cancer, 1997:10–14.
9. Daumas-Duport C, Scheithauer B, Kelly P. A histologic and cytologic method for the spatial definition of gliomas. *Mayo Clin Proc* 1987;62:435–449.
10. Burger PC, Vogel S. *Surgical pathology of the central nervous system and its coverings.* New York: Churchill Livingston, 1982.
11. Krouwer HG, Davis RL, Silver P, et al. Gemistocytic astrocytomas: a reappraisal. *J Neurosurg* 1991;74(3):399–406.
12. Prayson RA, Estes ML. Protoplasmic astrocytoma. A clinicopathologic study of 16 tumors. *Am J Clin Pathol* 1995;103(6):705–709.
13. Soffietti R, Ruda R, Bradac GB, et al. PCV chemotherapy for recurrent oligodendrogliomas and oligoastrocytomas. *Neurosurgery* 1998;43(5):1066–1073.
14. Schiffer D, Dutto A, Cavalla P, et al. Prognostic factors in oligodendroglioma. *Can J Neurol Sci* 1997;24(4):313–319.
15. Janny P, Cure H, Mohr M, et al. Low grade supratentorial astrocytomas. Management and prognostic factors. *Cancer* 1994;73(7):1937–1945.
16. Afra D, Osztie E, Sipos L, et al. Preoperative history and postoperative survival of supratentorial low-grade astrocytomas. *Br J Neurosurg* 1999;13:299–305.
17. Morantz RA. Low-grade astrocytomas. In: Wilkins RH, Rengachary SS, eds. *Neurosurgery.* New York: McGraw-Hill, 1996:789–798.
18. Piepmeier J, Christopher S, Spencer D, et al. Variations in the natural history and survival of patients with supratentorial low-grade astrocytomas. *Neurosurgery* 1996;38(5):872–878.
19. Vertosick FT Jr., Selker RG, Arena VC. Survival of patients with well-differentiated astrocytomas diagnosed in the era of computed tomography. *Neurosurgery* 1991;28(4):496–501.
20. Lunsford LD, Somaza S, Kondziolka D, et al. Survival after stereotactic biopsy and irradiation of cerebral nonanaplastic, nonpilocytic astrocytoma. *J Neurosurg* 1995;82(4):523–529.
21. Knopp EA, Cha S, Johnson G, et al. Glial neoplasms: dynamic contrast-enhanced T2*-weighted MR imaging. *Radiology* 1999; 211(3):791–798.
22. Francavilla TL, Miletich RS, Di Chiro G, et al. Positron emission tomography in the detection of malignant degeneration of low-grade gliomas. *Neurosurgery* 1989;24(1):1–5.
23. Worthington C, Tyler JL, Villemure JG. Stereotaxic biopsy and positron emission tomography correlation of cerebral gliomas. [Published erratum appears in Surg Neurol 1987;27(5):511.] *Surg Neurol* 1987;27(1):87–92.
24. Meyerand ME, Pipas JM, Mamourian A, et al. Classification of biopsy-confirmed brain tumors using single-voxel MR spectroscopy. *AJNR* 1999;20(1):117–123.
25. Franzini A, Leocata F, Cajola L, et al. Low-grade glial tumors in basal ganglia and thalamus: natural history and biological reappraisal. *Neurosurgery* 1994;35(5):817–820.
26. Iwabuchi S, Bishara S, Herbison P, et al. Prognostic factors for supratentorial low grade astrocytomas in adults. *Neurol Med Chir (Tokyo)* 1999;39(4):273–279.
27. McCormack BM, Miller DC, Budzilovich GN, et al. Treatment and survival of low-grade astrocytoma in adults—1977–1988. *Neurosurgery* 1992;31(4):636–642.
28. North CA, North RB, Epstein JA, et al. Low-grade cerebral astrocytomas. Survival and quality of life after radiation therapy. *Cancer* 1990;66(1):6–14.
29. Scanlon PW, Taylor WF. Radiotherapy of intracranial astrocytomas: analysis of 417 cases treated from 1960 through 1969. *Neurosurgery* 1979;5(3):301–308.
30. Shibamoto Y, Yamashita J, Takahashi M, et al. Supratentorial malignant glioma: an analysis of radiation therapy in 178 cases. *Radiother Oncol* 1990;18(1):9–17.
31. Soffietti R, Chio A, Giordana MT, et al. Prognostic factors in well-differentiated cerebral astrocytomas in the adult. *Neurosurgery* 1989;24(5):686–692.
32. Philippon JH, Clemenceau SH, Fauchon FH, et al. Supratentorial

eds. *Brain tumors.* Edinburgh: Churchill Livingstone, 1995:433–446.

low-grade astrocytomas in adults. *Neurosurgery* 1993;32(4): 554–559.

33. Weir B, Grace M. The relative significance of factors affecting post-operative survival in astrocytomas, grades one and two. *Can J Neurol Sci* 1976;3(1):47–50.

34. Karim AB, Maat B, Hatlevoll R, et al. A randomized trial on dose-response in radiation therapy of low-grade cerebral glioma: European Organization for Research and Treatment of Cancer (EORTC) Study 22844. *Int J Radiat Oncol Biol Phys* 1996;36(3):549–556.

35. Bahary JP, Villemure JG, Choi S, et al. Low-grade pure and mixed cerebral astrocytomas treated in the CT scan era. *J Neurooncol* 1996;27(2):173–177.

36. Berger MS, Deliganis AV, Dobbins J, et al. The effect of extent of resection on recurrence in patients with low grade cerebral hemisphere gliomas. *Cancer* 1994;74(6):1784–1791.

37. Ito S, Chandler KL, Prados MD, et al. Proliferative potential and prognostic evaluation of low-grade astrocytomas. *J Neurooncol* 1994;19(1):1–9.

38. Struikmans H, Rutgers DH, Jansent GH, et al. Prognostic relevance of cell proliferation markers and DNA-ploidy in gliomas. *Acta Neurochir (Wien)* 1998;140:140–147.

39. Schiffer D, Cavalla P, Chio A, et al. Proliferative activity and prognosis of low-grade astrocytomas. *J Neurooncol* 1997;34(1):31–35.

40. Hilton DA, Love S, Barber R, et al. Accumulation of p53 and Ki-67 expression do not predict survival in patients with fibrillary astrocytomas or the response of these tumors to radiotherapy. *Neurosurgery* 1998;42(4):724–729.

41. Louis DN. The p53 gene and protein in human brain tumors. *J Neuropathol Exp Neurol* 1994;53(1):11–21.

42. Watanabe K, Sato K, Biernat W, et al. Incidence and timing of p53 mutations during astrocytoma progression in patients with multiple biopsies. *Clin Cancer Res* 1997;3(4):523–530.

43. Reifenberger J, Ring GU, Gies U, et al. Analysis of p53 mutation and epidermal growth factor receptor amplification in recurrent gliomas with malignant progression. *J Neuropathol Exp Neurol* 1996;55(7):822–831.

44. Rasheed BK, McLendon RE, Herndon JE, et al. Alterations of the TP53 gene in human gliomas. *Cancer Res* 1994;54(5):1324–1330.

45. Chozick BS, Pezzullo JC, Epstein MH, et al. Prognostic implications of p53 overexpression in supratentorial astrocytic tumors. *Neurosurgery* 1994;35(5):831–837.

46. al Sarraj S, Bridges LR. p53 immunoreactivity in astrocytomas and its relationship to survival. *Br J Neurosurg* 1995;9(2):143–149.

47. Shafqat S, Hedley-Whyte ET, Henson JW. Age-dependent rate of anaplastic transformation in low-grade astrocytoma. *Neurology* 1999;52(4):867–869.

48. Walker DG, Lavin M. Molecular genetics of astrocytoma: a review. *J Clin Neurosci* 1997;4:114–121.

49. von Deimling A, von Ammon K, Schoenfeld D, et al. Subsets of glioblastoma multiforme defined by molecular genetic analysis. *Brain Pathol* 1993;3:19–26.

50. Lang FF, Miller DC, Koslow M, et al. Pathways leading to glioblastoma multiforme: a molecular analysis of genetic alterations in 65 astrocytic tumors. *J Neurosurg* 1994;81(3):427–436.

51. Coons SW, Johnson PC, Shapiro JR. Cytogenetic and flow cytometry DNA analysis of regional heterogeneity in a low grade human glioma. *Cancer Res* 1995;55(7):1569–1577.

52. Sidransky D, Mikkelsen T, Schwechheimer K, et al. Clonal expansion of p53 mutant cells is associated with brain tumour progression. *Nature* 1992;355(6363):846–847.

53. Muller W, Afra D, Schroder R. Supratentorial recurrences of gliomas. Morphological studies in relation to time intervals with astrocytomas. *Acta Neurochir (Wien)* 1977;37(1–2):75–91.

54. Walker DG, Duan W, Popovic EA, et al. Homozygous deletions of the multiple tumor suppressor gene 1 in the progression of human astrocytomas. *Cancer Res* 1995;55(1):20–23.

55. Smith DF, Hutton JL, Sandemann D, et al. The prognosis of primary intracerebral tumours presenting with epilepsy: the outcome of medical and surgical management. *J Neurol Neurosurg Psychiatry* 1991;54(10):915–920.

56. Recht LD, Lew R, Smith TW. Suspected low-grade glioma: is deferring treatment safe? *Ann Neurol* 1992;31(4):431–436.

57. Fadul C, Wood J, Thaler H, et al. Morbidity and mortality of craniotomy for excision of supratentorial gliomas. *Neurology* 1988;38(9): 1374–1379.

58. Cabantog AM, Bernstein M. Complications of first craniotomy for intra-axial brain tumour. *Can J Neurol Sci* 1994;21(3):213–218.

59. Gregor A, Cull A, Traynor E, et al. Neuropsychometric evaluation of long-term survivors of adult brain tumours: relationship with tumour and treatment parameters. *Radiother Oncol* 1996;41(1): 55–59.

60. Vigliani MC, Sichez N, Poisson M, et al. A prospective study of cognitive functions following conventional radiotherapy for supratentorial gliomas in young adults: 4-year results. *Int J Radiat Oncol Biol Phys* 1996;35(3):527–533.

61. Kiebert GM, Curran D, Aaronson NK, et al. Quality of life after radiation therapy of cerebral low-grade gliomas of the adult: results of a randomised phase III trial on dose response (EORTC trial 22844). EORTC Radiotherapy Co-operative Group. *Eur J Cancer* 1998;34(12):1902–1909.

62. Dirks PB, Jay V, Becker LE, et al. Development of anaplastic changes in low-grade astrocytomas of childhood. *Neurosurgery* 1994;34(1):68–78.

63. Shaw EG, Daumas-Duport C, Scheithauer BW, et al. Radiation therapy in the management of low-grade supratentorial astrocytomas. *J Neurosurg* 1989;70(6):853–861.

64. Bampoe J, Bernstein M. The role of surgery in low grade gliomas. *J Neurooncol* 1999;42(3):259–269.

65. Kondziolka D, Lunsford LD, Martinez AJ. Unreliability of contemporary neurodiagnostic imaging in evaluating suspected adult supratentorial (low-grade) astrocytoma. *J Neurosurg* 1993;79(4): 533–536.

66. Rajan B, Pickuth D, Ashley S, et al. The management of histologically unverified presumed cerebral gliomas with radiotherapy. *Int J Radiat Oncol Biol Phys* 1994;28(2):405–413.

67. Vecht CJ. Effect of age on treatment decisions in low-grade glioma. *J Neurol Neurosurg Psychiatry* 1993;56(12):1259–1264.

68. Chamberlain MC, Murovic JA, Levin VA. Absence of contrast enhancement on CT brain scans of patients with supratentorial malignant gliomas. [Published erratum appears in *Neurology* 1988; 38(11):1816.] *Neurology* 1988;38(9):1371–1374.

69. van Veelen ML, Avezaat CJ, Kros JM, et al. Supratentorial low grade astrocytoma: prognostic factors, dedifferentiation, and the issue of early versus late surgery. *J Neurol Neurosurg Psychiatry* 1998;64(5): 581–587.

70. Kondziolka D, Lunsford LD. The role of stereotactic biopsy in the management of gliomas. *J Neurooncol* 1999;42(3):205–213.

71. Lazareff JA, Bockhorst KH, Curran J, et al. Pediatric low-grade gliomas: prognosis with proton magnetic resonance spectroscopic imaging. *Neurosurgery* 1998;43(4):809–817.

72. Berger MS, Rostomily RC. Low grade gliomas: functional mapping resection strategies, extent of resection, and outcome. *J Neurooncol* 1997;34:85–101.

73. Kaye AH, Walker DG. Low grade astrocytomas: controversies in management. *J Clin Neurosci* 2000;7:475–483.

74. LeRoux PD, Winter TC, Berger MS, et al. A comparison between preoperative magnetic resonance and intraoperative ultrasound tumor volumes and margins. *J Clin Ultrasound* 1994;22(1):29–36.

75. Kelly P. Volumetric stereotactic surgical resection of intra-axial brain mass lesions. *Mayo Clin Proc* 1988;63:1186–1198.

76. Fountas KN, Kapsalaki EZ, Smisson HF III, et al. Results and complications from the use of a frameless stereotactic microscopic navigator system. *Stereotact Funct Neurosurg* 1998;71(2):76–82.

77. Iwata S, Nakagawa K, Harada H, et al. Endothelial nitric oxide synthase expression in tumor vasculature is correlated with malignancy in human supratentorial astrocytic tumors. *Neurosurgery* 1999;45(1):24–28.

78. Berger MS. The impact of technical adjuncts in the surgical management of cerebral hemispheric low-grade gliomas of childhood. *J Neurooncol* 1996;28(2–3):129–155.

79. Berger MS, Ojemann GA, Lettich E. Neurophysiological monitoring during astrocytoma surgery. *Neurosurg Clin North Am* 1990;1: 65–80.

80. Berger MS, Ghatan S, Haglund MM, et al. Low-grade gliomas associated with intractable epilepsy: seizure outcome utilizing electrocorticography during tumor resection. *J Neurosurg* 1993;79(1): 62–69.

81. Roux FE, Boulanouar K, Ranjeva JP, et al. Usefulness of motor functional MRI correlated to cortical mapping in Rolandic low-grade astrocytomas. *Acta Neurochir (Wien)* 1999;141(1):71–79.

82. Garcia DM, Fulling KH, Marks JE. The value of radiation therapy in addition to surgery for astrocytomas of the adult cerebrum. *Cancer* 1985;55(5):919–927.

83. Leibel SA, Sheline GE, Wara WM, et al. The role of radiation therapy in the treatment of astrocytomas. *Cancer* 1975;35(6):1551–1557.

84. Sheline GE. The role of radiation therapy in the treatment of low-grade gliomas. *Clin Neurosurg* 1986;33:563–574.

85. Fisher BJ, Bauman GS, Leighton CE, et al. Low-grade gliomas in children: tumor volume response to radiation. *J Neurosurg* 1998;88(6):969–974.

86. Bauman G, Pahapill P, MacDonald D, et al. Low grade glioma: a measuring radiographic response to radiotherapy. *Can J Neurol Sci* 1999;26(1):18–22.

87. Medbery CA III, Straus KL, Steinberg SM, et al. Low-grade astrocytomas: treatment results and prognostic variables. *Int J Radiat Oncol Biol Phys* 1988;15(4):837–841.

88. Whitton AC, Bloom HJ. Low grade glioma of the cerebral hemispheres in adults: a retrospective analysis of 88 cases. *Int J Radiat Oncol Biol Phys* 1990;18(4):783–786.

89. Morantz RA. Radiation therapy in the treatment of cerebral astrocytoma. *Neurosurgery* 1987;20(6):975–982.

90. Pozza F, Colombo F, Chierego G, et al. Low-grade astrocytomas: treatment with unconventionally fractionated external beam stereotactic radiation therapy. *Radiology* 1989;171(2):565–569.

91. Silbergeld DL, Griffin BR, Ojemann GA. Reirradiation for recurrent cerebral astrocytoma. *J Neurooncol* 1992;12(2):145–151.

92. Imperato JP, Paleologos NA, Vick NA. Effects of treatment on long-term survivors with malignant astrocytomas. *Ann Neurol* 1990;28(6):818–822.

93. Leighton C, Fisher B, Bauman G, et al. Supratentorial low-grade glioma in adults: an analysis of prognostic factors and timing of radiation. *J Clin Oncol* 1997;15(4):1294–1301.

94. Watne K, Hannisdal E, Nome O, et al. Combined intra-arterial chemotherapy followed by radiation in astrocytomas. *J Neurooncol* 1992;14(1):73–80.

95. Eyre HJ, Crowley JJ, Townsend JJ, et al. A randomized trial of radiotherapy versus radiotherapy plus CCNU for incompletely resected low-grade gliomas: a Southwest Oncology Group study. *J Neurosurg* 1993;78(6):909–914.

96. Soffietti R, Ruda R, Bradac GB, et al. PCV chemotherapy for recurrent oligodendrogliomas and oligoastrocytomas. *Neurosurgery* 1998;43(5):1066–1073.

97. Kepes JJ, Rubinstein LJ, Eng LF. Pleomorphic xanthoastrocytoma: a distinctive meningocerebral glioma of young subjects with relatively favorable prognosis. A study of 12 cases. *Cancer* 1979;44(5):1839–1852.

98. Giannini C, Scheithauer BW. Classification and grading of low-grade astrocytic tumors in children. *Brain Pathol* 1997;7(2):785–798.

99. Giannini C, Scheithauer BW, Burger PC, et al. Pleomorphic xanthoastrocytoma: what do we really know about it? *Cancer* 1999;85(9):2033–2045.

100. Herpers MJ, Freling G, Beuls EA. Pleomorphic xanthoastrocytoma in the spinal cord. Case report. *J Neurosurg* 1994;80(3):564–569.

101. Wasdahl DA, Scheithauer BW, Andrews BT, et al. Cerebellar pleomorphic xanthoastrocytoma: case report. *Neurosurgery* 1994;35(5):947–950.

102. Lim SC, Jang SJ, Kim YS. Cerebellar pleomorphic xanthoastrocytoma in an infant. *Pathol Int* 1999;49(9):811–815.

103. Zarate JO, Sampaolesi R. Pleomorphic xanthoastrocytoma of the retina. *Am J Surg Pathol* 1999;23(1):79–81.

104. Russell DSRLJ. *Pathology of tumors of the nervous system*, 5th ed. Baltimore: Williams & Wilkins, 1989.

105. Whittle IR, Gordon A, Misra BK, et al. Pleomorphic xanthoastrocytoma. Report of four cases. *J Neurosurg* 1989;70(3):463–468.

106. Levy RA, Allen R, McKeever P. Pleomorphic xanthoastrocytoma presenting with massive intracranial hemorrhage. *AJNR* 1996;17(1):154–156.

107. Blom RJ. Pleomorphic xanthoastrocytoma: CT appearance. *J Comput Assist Tomogr* 1988;12(2):351–352.

108. Kros JM, Vecht CJ, Stefanko SZ. The pleomorphic xanthoastrocytoma and its differential diagnosis: a study of five cases. *Hum Pathol* 1991;22(11):1128–1135.

109. Yoshino MT, Lucio R. Pleomorphic xanthoastrocytoma. *AJNR* 1992;13(5):1330–1332.

110. Pierallini A, Bonamini M, Di Stefano D, et al. Pleomorphic xanthoastrocytoma with CT and MRI appearance of meningioma. *Neuroradiology* 1999;41(1):30–34.

111. Shepherd CW, Scheithauer BW, Gomez MR, et al. Subependymal giant cell astrocytoma: a clinical, pathological, and flow cytometric study. *Neurosurgery* 1991;28(6):864–868.

112. Braffman BH, Bilaniuk LT, Naidich TP, et al. MR imaging of tuberous sclerosis: pathogenesis of this phakomatosis, use of gadopentetate dimeglumine, and literature review. *Radiology* 1992;183(1):227–238.

113. Martin N, Debussche C, De Broucker T, et al. Gadolinium-DTPA enhanced MR imaging in tuberous sclerosis. *Neuroradiology* 1990;31(6):492–497.

114. Nishio S, Fujiwara S, Tashima T, et al. Tumors of the lateral ventricular wall, especially the septum pellucidum: clinical presentation and variations in pathological features. *Neurosurgery* 1990;27(2):224–230.

115. Morimoto K, Mogami H. Sequential CT study of subependymal giant-cell astrocytoma associated with tuberous sclerosis. Case report. *J Neurosurg* 1986;65(6):874–877.

116. Nagib MG, Haines SJ, Erickson DL, et al. Tuberous sclerosis: a review for the neurosurgeon. *Neurosurgery* 1984;14(1):93–98.

117. Chow CW, Klug GL, Lewis EA. Subependymal giant-cell astrocytoma in children. An unusual discrepancy between histological and clinical features. *J Neurosurg* 1988;68(6):880–883.

118. Torres OA, Roach ES, Delgado MR, et al. Early diagnosis of subependymal giant cell astrocytoma in patients with tuberous sclerosis. *J Child Neurol* 1998;13(4):173–177.

119. Painter MJ, Pang D, Ahdab-Barmada M, et al. Connatal brain tumors in patients with tuberous sclerosis. *Neurosurgery* 1984;14(5):570–573.

120. Mork SJ, Lindegaard KF, Halvorsen TB, et al. Oligodendroglioma: incidence and biological behavior in a defined population. *J Neurosurg* 1985;63(6):881–889.

121. Holt RM, Maravilla KR. Supratentorial gliomas: imaging. In: Wilkins RH, Rengachary SS, eds. *Neurosurgery*. New York: McGraw-Hill, 1996:753–775.

122. Chin HW, Hazel JJ, Kim TH, et al. Oligodendrogliomas. I. A clinical study of cerebral oligodendrogliomas. *Cancer* 1980;45(6):1458–1466.

123. Shaw EG, Scheithauer BW, O'Fallon JR, et al. Oligodendrogliomas: the Mayo Clinic experience. *J Neurosurg* 1992;76(3):428–434.

124. Merchant TE, Nguyen D, Thompson SJ, et al. High-grade pediatric spinal cord tumors. *Pediatr Neurosurg* 1999;30(1):1–5.

125. Ushida T, Sonobe H, Mizobuchi H, et al. Oligodendroglioma of the "widespread" type in the spinal cord. *Childs Nerv Syst* 1998;14(12):751–755.

126. Burger PC, Rawlings CE, Cox EB, et al. Clinicopathologic correlations in the oligodendroglioma. *Cancer* 1987;59(7):1345–1352.

127. Kros JM, Troost D, van Eden CG, et al. Oligodendroglioma. A comparison of two grading systems. *Cancer* 1988;61(11):2251–2259.

128. Kros JM, van Eden CG, Vissers CJ, et al. Prognostic relevance of DNA flow cytometry in oligodendroglioma. *Cancer* 1992;69(7):1791–1798.

129. Mork SJ, Halvorsen TB, Lindegaard KF, et al. Oligodendroglioma. Histologic evaluation and prognosis. *J Neuropathol Exp Neurol* 1986;45(1):65–78.

130. Smith MT, Ludwig CL, Godfrey AD, et al. Grading of oligodendrogliomas. *Cancer* 1983;52(11):2107–2114.

131. Wilkinson IM, Anderson JR, Holmes AE. Oligodendroglioma: an analysis of 42 cases. *J Neurol Neurosurg Psychiatry* 1987;50(3):304–312.

132. Heegaard S, Sommer HM, Broholm H, et al. Proliferating cell nuclear antigen and Ki-67 immunohistochemistry of oligodendrogliomas with special reference to prognosis. *Cancer* 1995;76(10):1809–1813.

133. Kros JM, Hop WC, Godschalk JJ, et al. Prognostic value of the proliferation-related antigen Ki-67 in oligodendrogliomas. *Cancer* 1996;78(5):1107–1113.

134. Kros JM, Godschalk JJ, Krishnadath KK, et al. Expression of p53 in oligodendrogliomas. *J Pathol* 1993;171(4):285–290.

135. Pavelic J, Hlavka V, Poljak M, et al. p53 immunoreactivity in oligodendrogliomas. *J Neurooncol* 1994;22(1):1–6.

136. Sun ZM, Genka S, Shitara N, et al. Factors possibly influencing

the prognosis of oligodendroglioma. *Neurosurgery* 1988;22(5):886–891.

137. Reedy DP, Bay JW, Hahn JF. Role of radiation therapy in the treatment of cerebral oligodendroglioma: an analysis of 57 cases and a literature review. *Neurosurgery* 1983;13(5):499–503.

138. Wallner KE, Gonzales M, Sheline GE. Treatment of oligodendrogliomas with or without postoperative irradiation. *J Neurosurg* 1988;68(5):684–688.

139. Lindegaard KF, Mork SJ, Eide GE, et al. Statistical analysis of clinicopathological features, radiotherapy, and survival in 170 cases of oligodendroglioma. *J Neurosurg* 1987;67(2):224–230.

140. Shimizu KT, Tran LM, Mark RJ, et al. Management of oligodendrogliomas. *Radiology* 1993;186(2):569–572.

141. Plunkett SR. Conventional radiotherapy for specific central nervous system tumours. In: Wilkins RH, Rengachary SS, eds. *Neurosurgery.* New York: McGraw-Hill, 1996:1849–1865.

142. Cairncross JG, Macdonald DR. Successful chemotherapy for recurrent malignant oligodendroglioma. *Ann Neurol* 1988;23(4):360–364.

143. Cairncross JG, Macdonald DR, Ramsay DA. Aggressive oligodendroglioma: a chemosensitive tumor. *Neurosurgery* 1992;31(1):78–82.

144. Glass J, Hochberg FH, Gruber ML, et al. The treatment of oligodendrogliomas and mixed oligodendroglioma—astrocytomas with PCV chemotherapy. *J Neurosurg* 1992;76(5):741–745.

145. Kim L, Hochberg FH, Thornton AF, et al. Procarbazine, lomustine, and vincristine (PCV) chemotherapy for grade III and grade IV oligoastrocytomas. *J Neurosurg* 1996;85(4):602–607.

146. Hart MN, Petito CK, Earle KM. Mixed gliomas. *Cancer* 1974;33(1):134–140.

147. Coons SW, Johnson PC, Scheithauer BW, et al. Improving diagnostic accuracy and interobserver concordance in the classification and grading of primary gliomas. *Cancer* 1997;79(7):1381–1393.

148. Shaw EG, Scheithauer BW, O'Fallon JR, et al. Mixed oligoastrocytomas: a survival and prognostic factor analysis. *Neurosurgery* 1994;34(4):577–582.

149. Kalyan-Raman UP, Olivero WC. Ganglioglioma: a correlative clinicopathological and radiological study of ten surgically treated cases with follow-up. *Neurosurgery* 1987;20(3):428–433.

150. Miller G, Towfighi J, Page RB. Spinal cord ganglioglioma presenting as hydrocephalus. *J Neurooncol* 1990;9(2):147–152.

151. Diepholder HM, Schwechheimer K, Mohadjer M, et al. A clinicopathologic and immunomorphologic study of 13 cases of ganglioglioma. *Cancer* 1991;68(10):2192–2201.

152. Rommel T, Hamer J. Development of ganglioglioma in computed tomography. *Neuroradiology* 1983;24(4):237–239.

153. Castillo M, Davis PC, Takei Y, et al. Intracranial ganglioglioma: MR, CT, and clinical findings in 18 patients. *AJNR* 1990;11(1):109–114.

154. Zentner J, Wolf HK, Ostertun B, et al. Gangliogliomas: clinical, radiological, and histopathological findings in 51 patients. *J Neurol Neurosurg Psychiatry* 1994;57(12):1497–1502.

155. Selch MT, Goy BW, Lee SP, et al. Gangliogliomas: experience with 34 patients and review of the literature. *Am J Clin Oncol* 1998;21(6):557–564.

156. Rumana CS, Valadka AB, Contant CF. Prognostic factors in supratentorial ganglioglioma. *Acta Neurochir (Wien)* 1999;141(1):63–68.

157. Silver JM, Rawlings CE III, Rossitch E Jr, et al. Ganglioglioma: a clinical study with long-term follow-up. *Surg Neurol* 1991;35(4):261–266.

158. Kernohan JW, Mabon RF, Svien HJ, et al. A simplified classification of gliomas. *Proc Staff Mtg Mayo Clin* 1949;24:71–74.

159. Ringertz N. Grading of gliomas. *Acta Path Micro Scand* 1950;27:51–65.

103. Aggressive Glial Neoplasms

Devin K. Binder, G. Evren Keles, Kenneth Aldape, and Mitchel S. Berger

High-grade glial tumors, in particular anaplastic astrocytoma and glioblastoma multiforme, are the most frequent primary brain tumors in adults (1,2). They usually occur sporadically without identifiable familial tendency or environmental risk factors. Commonly arising in the deep white matter of the cerebral hemispheres, their removal without damage to eloquent brain areas poses a surgical challenge. Typically, these tumors present with headache, seizures, mental status or personality changes, signs and symptoms of increased intracranial pressure, hemiparesis, or other neurological deficit. Despite optimal current therapy, including surgery, radiation therapy, chemotherapy, and brachytherapy, high-grade gliomas are associated with a poor overall prognosis. The aim of clinical management is to achieve a longer progression-free interval and overall survival with preserved quality of life.

Epidemiology

Several domestic and foreign epidemiologic studies are in general agreement that the incidence of primary intracranial tumors in adults is between seven and 16 per 100,000 population (3–5). About half of these are primary tumors and half are metastatic. Neuroepithelial tumors, tumors arising from glial and/or neuronal elements, account for 50% to 60% of primary intracranial neoplasms in adults, and the vast majority of these are glial tumors (5). Of the neuroepithelial tumors, glioblastoma multiforme and anaplastic astrocytoma account for the vast majority, approximately 50% and 30%, respectively. In descending order, oligodendrogliomas (including anaplastic oligodendrogliomas), nonanaplastic astrocytomas, ependymal tumors, medulloblastomas and other less common tumors account for the other 20% of neuroepithelial tumors in adults. Thus, high-grade gliomas are the most common intracranial neoplasms in adults.

This chapter encompasses the pathology, clinical signs and symptoms, radiologic diagnosis, medical, surgical, and adjuvant (chemotherapeutic and radiotherapeutic) management of aggressive glial neoplasms. Included are the tumor types glioblastoma multiforme, anaplastic astrocytoma, anaplastic oligodendroglioma, anaplastic ependymoma, and mixed high-grade glial tumors (anaplastic oligoastrocytomas). In addition, novel agents and therapeutic modalities are discussed.

Pathology

Macroscopic features of high-grade glial tumors reflect their aggressiveness. The gross cut surface of glioblastomas shows a usually circumscribed appearance but often with ill-defined borders. The tumor itself is heterogeneous, with mottled areas of hemorrhage and necrosis (moth-eaten appearance). Often, there is marked necrosis and degeneration, which corresponds to the central area of low attenuation on computed tomography (CT) images. This central area is often surrounded by an irregular zone of denser, whiter tissue that corresponds to the area of higher attenuation and contrast enhancement on CT. Finally, there is a peripheral zone of lesser cell density, edema, and microscopic tumor infiltration that may be seen on T2-weighted magnetic resonance imaging (MRI) but often not on CT. This peripheral zone may vary in contour, with fingerlike projections extending from the main bulk tumor.

Anaplastic astrocytomas (WHO grade III) exhibit considerable variation in cellularity as well as morphologic heterogeneity (6). As a rule, compared to astrocytomas (WHO grade II), anaplastic astrocytomas exhibit greater cellularity, atypia, and the presence of multiple mitotic figures with a high degree of cellular pleomorphism but without necrosis or microvascular proliferation (Color Plate 29A). A subset of anaplastic astrocytomas show so-called "gemistocytes," or tumor cells with eccentrically placed pink cytoplasm on hematoxylin and eosin (H&E) staining.

Glioblastoma multiforme (WHO grade IV) has particular histological characteristics that differentiate it from lower-grade glial tumors (6): (a) hypercellularity; (b) mitoses; (c) nuclear atypia/pleomorphism; (d) pseudopalisading necrosis (i.e., curvilinear arrangement of tumor cells around a zone of necrosis); and (e) proliferation of vascular elements (microvascular proliferation). Importantly, marked variation in cellularity often is seen in different parts of the tumor, which can lead to misdiagnosis owing to incomplete sampling of the tumor. The primary characteristics distinguishing glioblastoma from anaplastic astrocytoma are necrosis and microvascular proliferation. A typical glioblastoma is shown in Color Plate 29B.

Anaplastic oligodendrogliomas comprise a subset of oligodendrogliomas with aggressive biologic behavior. These tumors, like anaplastic astrocytomas, appear either to arise from well-differentiated oligodendrogliomas or arise *de novo*. Hypercellularity, nuclear pleomorphism, high mitotic index, vascular proliferation, and necrosis characterize these tumors, like glioblastomas (7,8) (Color Plate 29C). The nuclei of oligodendrogliomas in general are more round and compact than the typically elongate nuclei of astrocytic tumors. GFAP-immunoreactive cells are seen in malignant oligodendrogliomas, but these cells lack the fine, GFAP-reactive processes of astrocytic tumors (9). Proliferative activity appears to be related to survival (10), as does the presence of specific genetic alterations. Mixed high-grade tumors can occur, with varying proportions of oligodendroglial and astroglial elements (anaplastic oligoastrocytoma) (Color Plate 29D).

Anaplastic progression of ependymomas is rare. Ependymomas show a characteristic pattern of perivascular rosetting, whereby tumor cells appear to encircle vessels, leaving a zone of processes between the vessel and the tumor nuclei. Anaplastic ependymomas (WHO grade III) are distinguished from ependymomas (WHO grade II) by hypercellularity, numerous mitoses, endothelial proliferation, and nuclear atypia (Color Plate 29E). Like anaplastic oligodendrogliomas, prognosis and time to tumor progression appear to be inversely correlated with mitotic and proliferative indices (11).

LOCAL INVASIVENESS. Aside from high mitotic activity, the main cellular behavior of malignant glial cells is local tissue invasion. Macroscopic and microscopic infiltration of glioblastoma cells tends to occur along the path of deep white matter tracts, such as the corpus callosum (forming the "butterfly glioma"), anterior commissure, fornix, and internal capsule (12, 13).

Microscopic evidence of malignant cells can be found well beyond the gross radiographic margins of the tumor (14). Following surgical resection or radiation therapy, such microscopic tumor foci lead to eventual local recurrence, usually within 2 cm of the original lesion (1,15). Thus, even a wide margin of resection beyond the enhancing lesion seen on imaging studies may not encompass all of the neoplastic tissue (16).

Clinical Signs and Symptoms

High-grade glial tumors arise from elements of brain parenchyma (glial cells) and are thus intraaxial tumors. Most are intraparenchymal, but occasionally can have intraventricular or subarachnoid extension.

Two basic mechanisms account for clinical manifestations of glial tumors. First, regional parenchymal changes including compression, invasion, destruction, hypoxia, electrolyte derangements, and release of cytokines and free radicals alter the tissue microenvironment, disrupting the function of local normal tissue. The clinical correlate may take the form of irritation (e.g., tumor-associated epilepsy) often arising in a focus around the site of the tumor, or depression (e.g., focal neurological deficits related to the topographic functional brain area affected).

Tumors also lead to more diffuse intracranial changes, most commonly elevated intracranial pressure resulting from either the tumor volume itself but more commonly from secondary effects on brain, blood, or cerebrospinal fluid (CSF) volume. High-grade glial tumors in particular induce significant peritumoral vasogenic edema (17), which increases local brain volume. They may also cause venous obstruction or impairment of CSF flow or absorption depending on their size, location, and mass effect.

The clinical presentation of malignant gliomas commonly is divided into general neurological findings and focal neurological findings. General neurological symptoms and signs include headache, seizures without apparent focal onset, nausea, emesis, dysequilibrium, and changes in mental status. Headache, especially during the early morning hours, is the most common symptom, seen in over 70% of patients with brain tumors (18, 19). Second most common is seizures, found in approximately one third of patients (20,21). Tumor-associated emesis and dysequilibrium are probably related to increased intracranial pressure. Alteration in mental status is variable, from minor cognitive deficits to wholesale personality and cognitive changes with depression of consciousness. Papilledema, the most common sign of increased intracranial pressure, occurs in the majority of patients with intracranial neuroepithelial tumors and usually is bilateral. Other findings indicating increased intracranial pressure include abducens palsy and diplopia. Significant increased intracranial pressure may lead to subfalcine, transtentorial, uncal, or tonsillar herniation.

Localizing or focal neurological findings also can result from regional pathological alteration of brain function by a growing tumor. Focal signs include seizures and focal neurological deficits. The type of seizure (e.g., simple partial, complex partial, or generalized) can give a clue to the location of the tumor. Focal neurological deficits can result from interruption or destruction of nearly any pathway or nucleus depending on tumor location, and the presence of such a deficit can be of significant localizing value.

Imaging Studies

If clinical history, symptoms, and signs are suggestive of an intracranial tumor, then the next step in diagnosis is to obtain an imaging study with intravenous contrast enhancement. Important imaging characteristics include signal intensity; number of lesions; location, size, and shape; character of margins; pattern of contrast enhancement; and change over time with serial scans. These all help to determine the type and components of the lesion.

CT. CT scans of high-grade glial tumors are often distinctive. CT of glioblastoma multiforme (GBM) often shows a central area of low attenuation corresponding to necrosis. An area of high attenuation that enhances with contrast and corresponds to actively dividing, proliferating tumor cells surrounds this area. A third low-attenuation area around the tumor often is seen, representing tumor-associated vasogenic edema but also containing tumor cells (14,22).

There are several lesions that must be distinguished from gliomas on CT, including infarct, plaque, abscess, arteriovenous malformation (AVM), hematoma, and glial scar. Often these can be distinguished on imaging characteristics alone. For example, infarction appears as a sharply demarcated, wedge-shaped area of low attenuation that does not enhance. However, some lesions, such as demyelination plaques, may enhance with contrast. In addition, abscesses can appear as sharply demarcated regions of low attenuation surrounded by a contrast-enhancing wall, and thus may mimic the appearance of a glial tumor. Intraparenchymal contusions or resolving hematomas may have irregular shape and attenuation, and may enhance with contrast. Although clinical context should distinguish some of the possibilities, in some cases serial scans or MRI may be necessary.

Modern CT scanners can detect tumors less than 1 cm in diameter. However, false-negative CT scans in patients eventually shown to have tumors on follow-up scans have been reported (23,24); therefore, if there is still clinical evidence of possible tumor despite a negative CT scan, an MRI should be performed. It is also important to note that CT scan does not necessarily define the margin of neoplasm. High-grade astrocytomas may not enhance on CT scans, and tumor cells may extend outside the area of contrast enhancement on serial scans (14).

MRI. MRI is more sensitive than CT in the detection of intracranial mass lesions; therefore, it is the gold standard for detecting intracranial tumors. Several factors account for the superiority of MRI over CT: high contrast, lack of bone artifact (especially in posterior fossa lesions), resolution of tumor margins, and greater differentiation of discrete histological tumor components. Technical advantages of MRI over CT include multiplanar imaging, absence of iodinated contrast agents, and absence of radiation exposure; disadvantages include incompatibility with ferromagnetic medical devices and longer study time.

Most high-grade glial tumors are detectable as a hyperintense region of signal abnormality on T2-weighted MRI images. Most neuroepithelial tumors are visible on noncontrast T2-weighted MRI scans before they can be seen on contrast-enhanced T1-weighted images (25). Tumor-associated edema is hypointense on T1- and hyperintense on T2-weighted images. MRI may show a larger area of signal abnormality than CT for the same tumor because of the superior tissue contrast characteristics of MRI; however, tumor cells beyond areas of increased signal intensity on T2-weighted scans remain undetected.

Contrast enhancement is an important tool for distinguishing other pathologies seen on T2-weighted scans from intraaxial tumors. As with CT, tumor enhancement with contrast results from leakage of the contrast agent from tumor capillaries and accumulation in the extracellular space. Gadolinium-diethylenetriamine pentaacetic acid (Gd-DTPA) is the most commonly used contrast agent in MR imaging. A paramagnetic compound, it changes the MR relaxation times of adjacent protons, making areas of contrast accumulation bright on T1- or T2-weighted images. High-grade malignant gliomas usually enhance intensely with gadolinium, whereas less rapidly growing tumors, such as fibrillary astrocytomas, may not enhance (Fig. 1).

As for CT, other processes must be differentiated from tumor on MRI. Because many nonneoplastic lesions are also hyperintense on T2-weighted images, contrast enhancement on T1-weighted images provides more specific evidence of tumor. Hemorrhage is initially low-intensity on both T1- and T2-weighted images; as deoxyhemoglobin is converted to methemoglobin, several days later the area of hemorrhage becomes hyperintense on both sequences, followed by a chronic phase with T1-hypointensity and a rim of T2-hyperintensity.

The ability to follow a lesion over time with serial scans is of critical importance to the diagnosis of intracranial lesions on imaging studies. Enlargement and/or changes in imaging characteristics of a mass in association with clinical signs and symptoms may be pivotal in determining the nature of an intracranial mass lesion.

MAGNETIC RESONANCE SPECTROSCOPY AND FUNCTIONAL IMAGING. An adjunct to conventional neuroimaging techniques is proton magnetic resonance spectroscopy (MRS), which can be obtained during the same MR examination with little additional time. This technique allows detection of metabolite levels in specific brain voxels, thereby providing local physiological data in addition to anatomical imaging (Color Plate 30). MRS has shown potential in differentiating neoplasms from inflammatory and demyelinating lesions (26), as well as detecting progression of neoplastic disease and evaluation of response to radiation therapy (27).

The advent of functional magnetic resonance imaging (fMRI) provides additional information helpful in planning tumor resection tailored to individual patients. The ability to detect the small changes in blood volume and in intrinsic T2-weighted signal that occur in eloquent cortex during physiological activation (28) provides the potential for preoperative functional mapping of eloquent cortex (Color Plate 31). This information integrated with the anatomical information obtained from conventional MRI and intraoperative stimulation mapping data can allow for more precise and complete resection of tumor and the ability to avoid adjacent eloquent brain areas (29).

Another functional imaging modality is magnetic source imaging (MSI), which combines the temporal and spatial accuracy of magnetoencephalography (MEG) with the anatomical and pathological specificity of MRI (30). The resulting magnetic source image gives accurate knowledge of cortical functional organization, such as the late neuromagnetic field elicited by simple speech sounds (31). Like fMRI, this technique is useful for preoperative mapping of rolandic cortex and determining hemispheric language dominance (Color Plate 31).

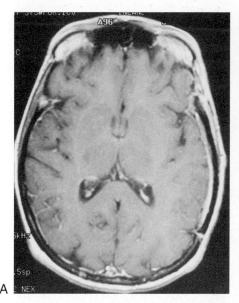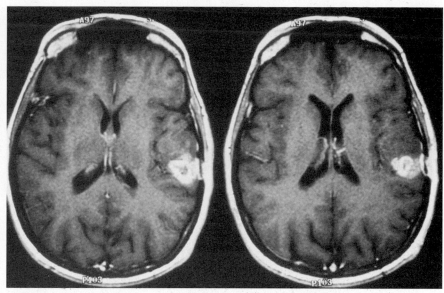

Fig. 1. T-1 weighted axial images without **(A)** and with **(B)** contrast showing marked contrast enhancement of a dominant hemisphere glioblastoma multiforme.

Medical Therapy

The role for medical management of high-grade glial tumors is quite limited. Other than cytotoxic chemotherapy (see the following), medical therapy is only used for palliation of tumor-induced neurological symptoms. The use of corticosteroids often provides rapid and dramatic symptomatic improvement (32). Neurological improvement after steroid therapy results from reduction of tumor-associated cerebral edema and mass effect (33). One proposed mechanism of steroid-induced reduction of peritumoral edema involves reduction in permeability of the capillary–endothelial cell junctions in the blood–brain barrier (BBB); however, steroid therapy palliates neurological symptoms but does not halt or slow tumor growth. In addition to steroids, patients presenting with tumor-induced seizures are placed on anticonvulsant medications. The use of prophylactic anticonvulsants in patients with no previous history of seizures undergoing surgery is common but controversial (34,35).

Surgical Therapy

Principles guiding appropriate surgical treatment of gliomas include tumor biopsy for the purpose of histological diagnosis, cytoreduction of tumor mass to the maximal extent consistent with optimal preservation of neurological function, and judicious implementation of adjuvant therapies tailored to the specific clinical situation.

BIOPSY. Diagnostic biopsy is most often accomplished by a closed stereotactic procedure performed with local anesthesia. Using image-guided stereotactic biopsy techniques, optimal acquisition of diagnostic tissue material can be obtained with a low rate of morbidity and mortality. In series from Toronto, Bernstein and colleagues have found that stereotactic brain biopsies are associated with a 6% overall complication rate, a

2% mortality rate (36), an 8% risk of failed biopsy owing to inadequate material for diagnosis (37), and a high rate of clinically silent hemorrhage postoperatively (38). These data are similar to other series (39–42). The diagnostic yield from stereotactic biopsies is likely to continue to improve as modern neuroimaging techniques permit targeting the most representative portions of intracranial tumors.

CHOICE OF PROCEDURE. The choice of operative procedure for resection of a neuroepithelial tumor depends on its location, size, gross characteristics, histological characteristics, radiosensitivity, and the preoperative neurological and medical condition of the patient. Contemporary neurosurgical methods, including frameless navigational systems, intraoperative imaging, ultrasonography, and functional mapping enable the neurosurgeon to achieve optimal cytoreduction of the tumor with minimal postoperative neurological morbidity.

NAVIGATIONAL SYSTEMS AND INTRAOPERATIVE IMAGING. The use of neuronavigation systems and intraoperative imaging modalities are of increasing importance in the treatment of malignant gliomas. A variety of neuronavigation systems have been developed to register the surgical target preoperatively with respect to surrounding brain structures and physical space using external fiducial markers. The intraoperative integration of a localization device with the stored preoperative registration information via a computer-based interface allows for frameless stereotaxy. The primary advantage is the ability to determine target trajectory independent of direct visualization. However, the success of intraoperative navigation is based on its accuracy in real-time mapping of tissue anatomy. Intraoperative changes involving displacement of brain and tumor tissue caused by surgical retraction, resection, and CSF leakage alter the accuracy of stereotactic localization based solely on preoperative imaging studies (43). Quantitative analysis of intraoperative cortical shift suggests that there may be a discrepancy of at least 1 cm in the registration of preoperative imaging studies to the surgical field (44).

Thus, in recent years intraoperative imaging using CT and

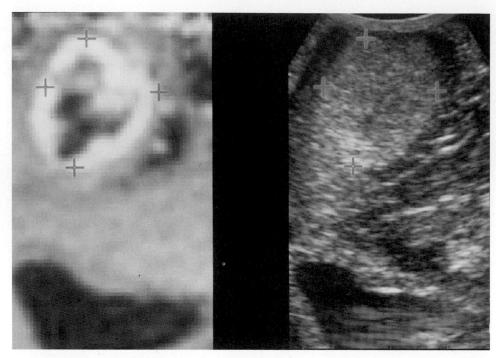

Fig. 2. (+) Signs outline the tumor margins as seen in intraoperative preresection real-time ultrasound imaging *(right)* and the Stealth navigation system *(left)*.

MRI has been developed at a few centers (45–48). The real-time images generated via intraoperative MRI allow the surgeon to assess intraoperative anatomy and thereby determine the extent of resection and/or modify the surgical approach, and eliminates the problem of brain shift. The use of intraoperative MR necessitates the use of MR-compatible surgical instruments made of ceramic or titanium.

Intraoperative ultrasonography also provides real-time intraoperative data and is helpful in detecting the tumor; delineating its margins; and differentiating tumor from peritumoral edema, cyst, necrosis, and adjacent normal brain. Although its use is limited by artifact from blood and surgical trauma at the margin of resection, it has been shown that postresection tumor volumes based on intraoperative ultrasound are significantly correlated with those determined by postoperative MRI (49). The most important use of intraoperative ultrasound may become real-time re-registration of preoperative images to correct for intraoperative brain shift (50,51) (Fig. 2).

INTRAOPERATIVE STIMULATION MAPPING. Intraoperative functional brain mapping using cortical stimulation also provides important real-time data to guide the surgeon in identifying eloquent cortical and subcortical areas (52), allowing preservation of function during tumor resection, thus minimizing morbidity (52,53) (Fig. 3). This is especially important given the marked interindividual differences in localization of function (54). Cortical stimulation mapping is accomplished by placing a bipolar electrode (5-mm spacing) on the surface for several seconds with current amplitude of 2 to 16 mA. Cold Ringer's lactate should be available for immediate irrigation of the stimulated cortex should focal motor seizures arise (55). Mapping of both cortical and subcortical sites can provide critical information regarding localization of motor, sensory, and language tracts (53).

EXTENT OF RESECTION. The degree of cytoreduction achieved as measured by extent of resection appears to correlate with outcome. Patients with gross total resection live longer than those with partial resection who in turn live longer than those who have biopsy only (56,57). A further consideration is that partial resection often is accompanied by significant postoperative edema surrounding residual tumor tissue along with increased neurological morbidity (58).

The association between extent of resection and longer survival for patients with high-grade malignant gliomas is controversial, similar to low-grade gliomas for which the prognostic effect of extensive surgery is not well defined but appears to have a positive effect on outcome (59–61). The controversy is mainly caused by lack of randomized studies addressing the issue and the inconsistent and less than objective methodology used in determining extent of resection. In a retrospective study of preoperative and postoperative tumor volumes in 92 patients with GBM, extent of tumor removal and residual tumor volume were significantly correlated with median time to tumor progression and median survival (62). In this study, greater resections did not compromise the quality of life and patients without any residual disease had a better postoperative performance status than those patients who received less than total resections.

REOPERATION. Reoperation for recurrent tumor growth after operative and adjuvant therapy often is necessary. Clinical deterioration or tumor progression on serial imaging studies despite surgery and postoperative adjuvant therapy constitutes treatment failure, and these cases should be considered for reoperation.

The goal of reoperation remains maximal cytoreduction with minimal neurological morbidity (63). Early studies showed poor outcome in patients who underwent reoperation for malignant gliomas; one study of patients with anaplastic astrocytoma or

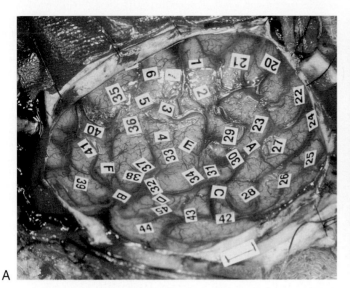 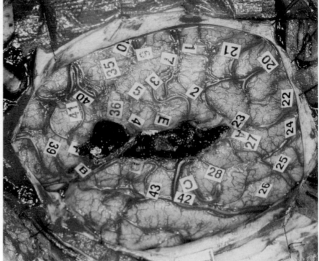

A   B

Fig. 3. Preresection (**A**) and postresection (**B**) intraoperative view of the case described in Fig. 1. Intraoperative stimulation of *25* and *28* resulted in anomia.

glioblastoma multiforme reported median survival after reoperation of only 14 weeks with a median total survival of 62 weeks (64). However, a more recent study showed a median survival of 37 weeks after reoperation and median total survival of 91 weeks (65). Reoperation is clinically reasonable when lengthened survival of acceptable quality is the likely result of surgery. Thus, it should be performed when a patient whose tumor characteristics, age, and preoperative performance status suggest the potential for a favorable outcome; of note also is that studies of patients who survive longer than 5 years nearly all have undergone reoperation as a cornerstone of therapy (66).

Adjuvant Therapies

Adjuvant therapies are defined as postsurgical therapies designed to decrease the likelihood of recurrence after operative treatment of tumors or those used to treat recurrences that arise. Chemotherapy, external beam radiation therapy, and brachytherapy are the three principal types of adjuvant therapy. Currently, most protocols for the treatment of aggressive glial neoplasms in adults combine surgery with postoperative external beam radiation therapy and carmustine or vincristine chemotherapy.

RADIATION THERAPY. Radiation therapy has been the adjuvant therapy of choice for the treatment of malignant gliomas for many years (67). In the past, patients were treated with large fields of low-energy x-rays with poor penetration, leading to substantial irradiation to normal tissue. Today, three-dimensional treatment planning based on modern CT and MRI techniques permits delivery of a full dose of radiation to the tumor with minimal irradiation of normal tissue.

EXTERNAL BEAM RADIATION THERAPY. External beam radiation therapy for brain tumors is carried out with high-energy, or megavoltage x-rays produced by a linear accelerator. These x-rays deliver increasing dose with depth up to a few

centimeters and the dose decays thereafter in approximately exponential fashion. Various beam configurations are analyzed with respect to their isodose configurations at the target site and optimal dosimetry is calculated. Radiation is thought to kill cells primarily by means of DNA damage. As the intent of radiation therapy is to destroy tumor tissue with minimal effect on normal tissue, in practice the dose-limiting factor is always the susceptibility of normal tissue to radiation damage. Radiation injury to normal brain tissue may be manifest as acute or delayed neurological sequelae, cognitive dysfunction, diffuse white matter injury, or outright radiation necrosis. These adverse effects may be limited by fractionation of the overall dose into multiple sessions. Multiple clinical trials have demonstrated improved survival for patients receiving radiation therapy, and current data support treating malignant glioma with conformal stereotactic external beam radiotherapy to a total dose of 60 Gy in 30 fractions (68). Higher doses have not demonstrated increases in survival (68). Optimal outcome is obtained with close cooperation between the radiation oncologist, neurosurgeon, and neuroradiologist.

RADIATION SENSITIZERS. Chemicals that modify radiation sensitivity have been used in the attempt to increase the therapeutic effect of standard radiation therapy. One example is the halogenated pyrimidine bromodeoxyuridine (BrdU), which incorporates into DNA of cycling cells in place of thymidine, enhances DNA strand breaks caused by radiation therapy and inhibits DNA repair (69). However, despite encouraging phase 2 results with BrdU (70), in phase 3 trials no survival advantage was seen and the study was closed (71).

Oxygen-mimetic radiosensitizers have been developed because areas of tumor hypoxia are thought to convey radioresistance. The nitroimidazole etanidazole (72) and cytotoxic sensitizer tirapazamine (73) have been studied in phase I and II trials, respectively, but no clear evidence of efficacy has been established yet.

BRACHYTHERAPY. Interstitial or intracavitary implantation of radioactive sources (brachytherapy) permits local delivery of high doses of radiation. Brachytherapy has been used primarily in the control of recurrent malignant gliomas (74), which are likely to recur locally (15). Isotopes commonly used for brachytherapy include iridium-192, iodine-125, and phosphorus-32. The rationale for use of brachytherapy is that local sources can deliver a larger radiation dose to the tumor volume while sparing surrounding tissue. Modern stereotactic techniques permit accurate placement of radioactive sources, and combined with computer-based planning systems allow for manipulation of isodose distributions to minimize dose to surrounding normal tissue. Median survival of GBM patients treated with brachytherapy at two centers is approximately 19 months (75,76). Hyperthermia is another possible local treatment as an adjunct to interstitial brachytherapy (77).

STEREOTACTIC RADIOSURGERY. Stereotactic radiosurgery has evolved considerably since its introduction by Leksell (78). Radiosurgery involves the use of numerous narrow collimated beams of radiation stereotactically directed to converge at a specific intracranial target. Three types of radiation have been used: gamma rays, produced by the radioactive decay of ^{60}Co ("gamma knife" radiosurgery); high-energy x-rays produced by linear accelerators; and charged particles such as protons produced by cyclotrons. Radiosurgery usually involves attaching a stereotactic frame on the patient, delineating the target on radiologic images, treatment planning by displaying isodose contours on these images, registering the frame and patient, and irradiating the target. Doses delivered during radiosurgery typically are lower than those delivered by fractionated radiation therapy but have greater effect because the entire dose is delivered in a single session to a highly limited target field.

Results of several long-term retrospective studies support the idea that the addition of radiosurgery prolongs median survival in the postoperative treatment of GBM (79–81). In general, radiosurgery may be used as adjuvant therapy following resection and for recurrences or disease under a certain size (e.g., <3 cm). Prospective, randomized trials are underway to help define more precisely the role of radiosurgery in the treatment of patients with GBM.

RADIOIMMUNOTHERAPY. Another approach is to deliver radiolabeled monoclonal antibodies directed at tumor-specific antigens to increase the tumor-specific radiation dose. Several groups have investigated this technology using either intravenous or intracavitary routes of administration of immunoglobulins. One study delivered intravenous ^{125}I-labeled antiepidermal growth factor antibodies, with a median survival of 13.5 months in the treatment group (82). A recent study using intracavitary delivery of ^{131}I-labeled antibodies to tenascin via Ommaya reservoir demonstrated a promising outcome in a subset of patients (83).

CHEMOTHERAPY. Many trials of cytotoxic chemotherapy for malignant brain tumors have been reported over the last three decades. The primary group of chemotherapeutic agents currently used for malignant gliomas are the nitrosoureas, including carmustine and lomustine. Nitrosoureas are lipid-soluble and readily cross the BBB. Their mode of action is incompletely understood, but their antitumor activity is likely related primarily to the formation of DNA interstrand crosslinks. Like other alkylating agents, nitrosoureas are myelosuppressive, and platelet and leukocyte counts must be closely monitored. Dosage adjustments are based on nadir blood cell counts. Other agents shown to have at least some activity against human glio-

mas include procarbazine, vincristine, hydroxyurea, carboplatin, etoposide, cyclophosphamide, and high-dose tamoxifen (84). The following is a summary of evidence regarding chemotherapy for each histological subtype of malignant glioma, for recurrent gliomas, and a discussion of novel therapies.

Glioblastoma Multiforme. An early outcome review of a large series of patients with glioblastomas treated from 1950s to 1980s demonstrated that median survival in the chemotherapy and radiation group was only 3 weeks longer than the group treated with radiation therapy alone (85). However, routine use of the nitrosoureas increased survival in the 1980s (86). Although use of nitrosoureas alone is inferior to radiation therapy alone (67), a recent metaanalysis of 16 studies published between 1975 and 1989 involving more than 3,000 patients concluded that combined therapy with radiation and chemotherapy increased survival compared to radiation therapy alone (86).

Standard therapy usually includes carmustine (BCNU) or procarbazine (Matulane), lomustine (CCNU), and vincristine (Oncovin) together (PCV). Studies comparing BCNU versus PCV in the treatment of glioblastoma multiforme have failed to consistently demonstrate a survival advantage to the three-drug regimen (87,88).

Anaplastic Astrocytoma. Specific information regarding efficacy of adjuvant chemotherapy for anaplastic astrocytoma is limited because most studies of chemotherapy for malignant glioma include both anaplastic astrocytoma and glioblastoma multiforme. However, the standard adjuvant therapy for patients with newly diagnosed anaplastic astrocytoma is nitrosourea-based. Some evidence indicates that PCV (procarbazine, lomustine, vincristine) chemotherapy may be superior to carmustine alone in treating anaplastic astrocytomas but this is controversial (87–89).

Anaplastic Oligodendroglioma and Mixed Oligodendroglial Tumors. Anaplastic oligodendrogliomas and anaplastic mixed oligoastrocytomas have been shown to respond especially well to PCV chemotherapy (90,91). Cairncross and colleagues demonstrated that the allelic loss of chromosomes 1p and 19q predicted response to chemotherapy and longer survival in patients with anaplastic oligodendrogliomas (92), establishing a molecular marker for chemosensitivity in these tumors. Indeed, increasingly neoadjuvant (i.e., preradiation) chemotherapy with PCV is being used in treating pure or mixed anaplastic oligodendrogliomas since up to 70% of patients may respond (93,94). In addition, salvage therapy with PCV may be effective in patients progressing after radiotherapy (93).

Anaplastic Ependymoma. The role of chemotherapy in ependymal tumors is poorly defined. Although some evidence suggests that there may be better response with platinum-based than with nitrosourea-based regimens for intracranial ependymoma (95), little data exist on the role of chemotherapy in anaplastic ependymomas.

Recurrent Glioma. The optimal treatment for recurrent glioma (anaplastic astrocytoma and glioblastoma) is unclear. The difficulty in evaluating efficacy of treatments in this patient population is emphasized in a recent systematic metaanalysis of 1,415 patients with recurrent gliomas (96). Temozolomide, an imidazotetrazine derivative that exerts its antitumor effect by DNA methylation, has shown good response in patients with recurrent anaplastic astrocytoma (97) and has received recent approval by the FDA for treatment of recurrent anaplastic astrocytomas. Temozolomide is also under study as therapy for recurrent glioblastoma multiforme (98) and as neoadjuvant therapy for patients with newly diagnosed AA (99). Carmustine-impregnated biodegradable polymers (Gliadel wafers) have shown some efficacy in prolonging survival in patients undergoing repeat surgical resection (100), and based on this have received FDA approval for treatment of recurrent glioblastoma multiforme. A recent study also suggests that carmustine polymers may prolong survival when given at the time of primary operation (101).

STRATEGIES TO IMPROVE CHEMOTHERAPY DELIVERY. Several strategies have been used in the attempt to improve local delivery of chemotherapeutic agents to the tumor tissue. These include intraarterial chemotherapy (102), hyperosmolar BBB opening (103), and high-dose chemotherapy (104). None of these yet have been shown to provide any clinical benefit and have significant associated toxicity. For example, a randomized study of patients with newly diagnosed high-grade glioma found no benefit to intracarotid versus intravenous carmustine, and intraarterial administration produced significant neurological toxicity (105). High-dose myeloablative chemotherapy with thiotepa followed by bone marrow rescue has been used in the treatment of recurrent aggressive oligodendroglioma, but is associated with 20% mortality (106).

NEWER THERAPIES. Advances in understanding of the molecular biology of gliomas have led to the development of novel forms of chemotherapy. One novel target is type I topoisomerase, an enzyme critical for DNA replication and transcription. Irinotecan (CPT-11), which inhibits topoisomerase I, has shown activity as a single agent (107). Other newer agents target tumor invasion, signal transduction, and angiogenesis. For example, marimastat, a matrix metalloproteinase inhibitor that inhibits enzymes known to be involved in tumor invasion, is in phase III trials for patients with newly diagnosed GBM (108). Leflunomide (SU-101), which inhibits the PDGF (platelet-derived growth factor) signaling pathway, known to be upregulated in a subpopulation of human gliomas, has shown activity in phase I and II trials (109). Tamoxifen, an inhibitor of protein kinase C at high concentrations, has demonstrated efficacy for a subset of patients with recurrent gliomas (110). The angiogenesis inhibitor thalidomide has shown activity in phase II trials (111).

Tumor immunotherapy is another area of development. Tumor vaccines using cells engineered to secrete cytokines aim to boost host immunity against tumor-specific antigens with minimal effect on surrounding tissue, and this has shown promise in animal models (112,113). In another approach, recombinant toxins target tumor-associated antigens via a tumor-specific binding protein (e.g., antibody or growth factor) linked to a toxic moiety to combine tumor selectivity with increased potency (114). For example, because transferrin receptors are expressed on rapidly dividing cells, one approach uses a conjugate of human transferrin fused to a diphtheria toxin (TF-CRM107) to potently kill glioblastoma cells, which has shown efficacy in some patients (115).

Gene therapy also has been considered as a potential adjunct treatment for malignant gliomas. One approach is to transfer an exogenous gene into tumors that confers susceptibility to a given agent. For example, transfer of the gene that encodes the herpes simplex virus enzyme thymidine kinase (HSV-TK) followed by administration of the antiviral drug ganciclovir should in theory destroy rapidly proliferating cells that take up the viral gene (116). The first clinical trial using vector-producing cells was reported in 1997 (117). Fifteen patients with progressive recurrent malignant brain tumors were studied and an antitumor response was detected in five of the smaller tumors; however, gene transfer to tumors was limited. A subsequent study using a similar approach resulted in transient tumor control with limited effect on survival (118). Using a protocol based on a more efficient new vector construct, two phase I/II clinical trials in adult patients, a European-Canadian study (119) and a United States study were initiated. In the former trial, clinical benefit was marginal, although the treatment method was found to be feasible and sufficiently safe (119). A third phase I study using the modified vector was conducted on pediatric patients with recurrent malignant supratentorial tumors and concluded that the method may be used with satisfactory safety in select patients (120). Although this approach is promising, improved gene delivery vectors are needed to affect a sufficient proportion of tumor cells.

Conclusion

Prognosis remains poor despite intensive basic and clinical study of malignant gliomas. Factors influencing the clinical course of malignant gliomas include histological grade, age, neurological status, extent of resection, and radiation therapy (121,122). It is hoped that advances in noninvasive diagnosis, surgical technology and adjuvant treatment together with novel therapies derived from cellular and molecular understanding of glial tumorigenesis will significantly improve the clinical outcome from these devastating lesions.

References

1. Salcman M. Glioblastoma and malignant astrocytoma. In: Kaye AH, Laws ER, eds. *Brain tumors: an encyclopedic approach*. New York: Churchill Livingstone, 1995:449–477.
2. Preston-Martin S. Epidemiology. In: Berger MS, Wilson CB, eds. *The gliomas*. Philadelphia: WB Saunders, 1999:2–11.
3. Gudmundsson KR. A survey of tumours of the central nervous system in Iceland during the 10-year period, 1954–1963. *Acta Neurol Scand* 1970;46:538–552.
4. Annegers JF, Schoenberg BS, Okazaki H, et al. Epidemiologic study of primary intracranial neoplasms. *Arch Neurol* 1981;38:217–219.
5. Walker AE, Robins M, Weinfeld FD. Epidemiology of brain tumors: the national survey of intracranial neoplasms. *Neurology* 1985;35:219–226.
6. Burger PC, Scheithauer BW, Vogel FS. *Surgical pathology of the nervous system and its coverings*. New York: Churchill Livingstone, 1991.
7. Mork SJ, Lindegaard KF, Halvorsen TB, et al. Oligodendroglioma: incidence and biological behavior in a defined population. *J Neurosurg* 1985;63:881–889.
8. Burger PC. The grading of astrocytomas and oligodendrogliomas. In: Fields WS, ed. *Primary brain tumours: a review of histological classification*. New York: Springer-Verlag, 1989:171.
9. Kros JM, Van Eden CG, Stefanko SZ, et al. Prognostic implications of glial fibrillary acidic protein containing cell types in oligodendrogliomas. *Cancer* 1990;66:1204–1212.
10. Coons SW, Johnson PC, Pearl DK, et al. Prognostic significance of flow cytometry deoxyribonucleic acid analysis of human oligodendrogliomas. *Neurosurgery* 1994;34:680–687.
11. Schiffer D, Chio A, Giordana MT, et al. Histological prognostic factors in ependymoma. *Childs Nerv Syst* 1991;7:177–182.
12. Burger PC. Classification, grading, and patterns of spread of malignant gliomas. In: Apuzzo MLJ, ed. *Malignant cerebral glioma*. Park Ridge, IL: American Association of Neurological Surgeons, 1990:3–17.

13. Schiffer D. Patterns of tumor growth. In: Salcman M, ed. *Neurobiology of brain tumors*. Baltimore: Williams & Wilkins, 1991: 229–249.

14. Burger PC. Pathological anatomy and CT correlations in the glioblastoma multiforme. *Appl Neurophysiol* 1983;46:180–187.

15. Liang BC, Thornton AF, Sandler HM, et al. Malignant astrocytomas: focal tumor recurrence after focal external beam radiation therapy. *J Neurosurg* 1991;75:559–563.

16. Burger PC, Heinz ER, Shibata T, et al. Topographic anatomy and CT correlations in the untreated glioblastoma multiforme. *J Neurosurg* 1988;68:698–704.

17. Klatzo I. Neuropathological aspects of brain edema. *J Neuropathol Exp Neurol* 1967;26:1–11.

18. Rushton JG, Rooke ED. Brain tumor headache. *Headache* 1962;2: 139–146.

19. Forsyth P, Posner JB. Headaches in patients with brain tumors: a study of 111 patients. *Neurology* 1993;43:678–683.

20. Rasmussen T. Surgery of epilepsy associated with brain tumors. *Adv Neurol* 1975;8:227–239.

21. Ettinger AB. Structural causes of epilepsy. *Neurol Clin* 1994;12: 41–56.

22. Daumas-Duport C, Monsaigneon V, Blond S, et al. Serial stereotactic biopsies and CT scan in gliomas: correlative study in 100 astrocytomas, oligo-astrocytomas and oligodendrocytomas. *J Neurooncol* 1987;4:317–328.

23. Wulff JD, Proffitt PQ, Panszi JG, et al. False-negative CTs in astrocytomas: the value of repeat scanning. *Neurology* 1982;32:766–769.

24. Bolender NF, Cromwell LD, Graves V, et al. Interval appearance of glioblastomas not evident in previous CT examinations. *J Comput Assist Tomogr* 1983;7:599–603.

25. Brant-Zawadzki M, Berry I, Osaki L, et al. Gd-DTPA in clinical MR of the brain: 1. Intraaxial lesions. *AJR* 1986;147:1223–1230.

26. DeStefano N, Caramanos Z, Preul MC, et al. In vivo differentiation of astrocytic brain tumors and isolated demyelinating lesions of the type seen in multiple sclerosis using ^{1}H magnetic resonance spectroscopic imaging. *Ann Neurol* 1998;44:273–278.

27. Vigneron DB, Nelson SJ. Magnetic resonance spectroscopy. In: Bernstein M, Berger MS, eds. *Neuro-oncology: the essentials*. New York: Thieme, 2000:99–113.

28. Belliveau JW, Kennedy DN, McKinstry RC, et al. Functional mapping of the human visual cortex by magnetic resonance imaging. *Science* 1991;254:1224–1228.

29. Schulder M, Maldjian JA, Liu WC, et al. Functional image-guided surgery of intracranial tumors located in or near the sensorimotor cortex. *J Neurosurg* 1998;89:412–418.

30. Orrison WW. Magnetic source imaging in stereotactic and functional neurosurgery. *Stereotact Funct Neurosurg* 1999;72:89–94.

31. Szymanski M, Rowley H, Roberts T. A hemispherically asymmetrical MEG response to vowels. *NeuroReport* 1999;10:2481–2486.

32. Galicich JH, French L, Melby JC. Use of dexamethasone in treatment of cerebral edema associated with brain tumors. *Lancet* 1961; 1:46–53.

33. Leiguarda R, Sierra J, Pardal C, et al. Effect of large doses of methylprednisolone on supratentorial intracranial tumors: a clinical and CAT scan evaluation. *Eur Neurol* 1985;24:23–32.

34. Boarini DJ, Beck DW, Van Gilder JC. Postoperative prophylactic anticonvulsant therapy in cerebral gliomas. *Neurosurgery* 1985;16: 290–292.

35. Foy PM, Chadwick DW, Rajgopalan N, et al. Do prophylactic anticonvulsant drugs alter the pattern of seizures after craniotomy? *J Neurol Neurosurg Psychiatry* 1992;55:753–757.

36. Bernstein M, Parrent AG. Complications of CT-guided stereotactic biopsy of intra-axial brain lesions. *J Neurosurg* 1994;81:165–168.

37. Soo TM, Bernstein M, Provias J, et al. Failed stereotactic biopsy in a series of 518 cases. *Stereotact Funct Neurosurg* 1995;64:183–196.

38. Kulkarni AV, Guha A, Lozano A, et al. Incidence of silent hemorrhage and delayed deterioration after stereotactic brain biopsy. *J Neurosurg* 1998;89:31–35.

39. Ostertag CB, Mennel HD, Kiessling M. Stereotactic biopsy of brain tumors. *Surg Neurol* 1980;14:275–283.

40. Apuzzo ML, Chandrasoma PT, Cohen D, et al. Computed imaging stereotaxy: experience and perspective related to 500 procedures applied to brain masses. *Neurosurgery* 1987;20:930–937.

41. Lunsford LD, Martinez AJ. Stereotactic exploration of the brain in the era of computed tomography. *Surg Neurol* 1984;22:222–230.

42. Cook RJ, Guthrie BL. Complications of stereotactic biopsy. *Perspect Neurosurg* 1993;4:131–139.

43. Zakhary R, Keles GE, Berger MS. Intraoperative imaging techniques in the treatment of brain tumors. *Curr Opin Oncol* 1999; 11:152–156.

44. Roberts DW, Hartov A, Kennedy FE, et al. Intraoperative brain shift and deformation: a quantitative analysis of cortical displacement in 28 cases. *Neurosurgery* 1998;43:749–760.

45. Butler WE, Piaggio CM, Constantinou C, et al. A mobile computed tomographic scanner with intraoperative and intensive care unit applications. *Neurosurgery* 1998;42:1304–1310.

46. Black PM, Moriarty T, Alexander E, et al. Development and implementation of intraoperative magnetic resonance imaging and its neurosurgical applications. *Neurosurgery* 1997;41:831–845.

47. Tronnier VM, Wirtz CR, Knauth M, et al. Intraoperative diagnostic and interventional magnetic resonance imaging in neurosurgery. *Neurosurgery* 1997;40:891–902.

48. Steinmeier R, Fahlbusch O, Ganslandt O, et al. Intraoperative magnetic resonance imaging with the Magnetom open scanner: concepts, neurosurgical indications, and procedures: a preliminary report. *Neurosurgery* 1998;43:739–748.

49. Hammoud MA, Ligon BL, elSouki R, et al. Use of intraoperative ultrasound for localizing tumors and determining the extent of resection: a comparative study with magnetic resonance imaging. *J Neurosurg* 1996;84:737–741.

50. Giorgi C, Casolino DS. Preliminary clinical experience with intraoperative stereotactic ultrasound imaging. *Stereotact Funct Neurosurg* 1997;68:54–58.

51. McDermott MW. Image-guided surgery. In: Bernstein M, Berger MS, eds. *Neuro-oncology: the essentials*. New York: Thieme, 2000: 135–147.

52. Berger MS, Ojemann GA. Techniques for functional brain mapping during glioma surgery. In: Berger MS, Wilson CB, eds. *The gliomas*. Philadelphia: WB Saunders, 1999:421–435.

53. Keles GE, Berger MS. Functional mapping. In: Bernstein M, Berger MS, eds. *Neuro-oncology: the essentials*. New York: Thieme, 2000: 130–134.

54. Ojemann GA, Ojemann J, Lettich E, et al. Cortical language localization in left, dominant hemisphere: an electrical stimulation mapping investigation in 117 patients. *J Neurosurg* 1989;71:316–326.

55. Sartorius CJ, Berger MS. Rapid termination of intraoperative stimulation-evoked seizures with application of cold Ringer's lactate to the cortex. *J Neurosurg* 1998;88:349–351.

56. Coffey RJ, Lunsford LD, Taylor FH. Survival after stereotactic biopsy of malignant gliomas. *Neurosurgery* 1988;22:465–473.

57. Winger MJ, Macdonald DR, Cairncross JG. Supratentorial anaplastic gliomas in adults: the prognostic importance of extent of resection and prior low grade glioma. *J Neurosurg* 1989;71:487–493.

58. Ciric I, Ammirati M, Vick N, et al. Supratentorial gliomas, surgical considerations and immediate post-operative results. *Neurosurgery* 1987;21:21–26.

59. Berger MS, Deliganis AV, Dobbins J, et al. The effect of extent of resection on recurrence in patients with low-grade cerebral hemisphere gliomas. *Cancer* 1994;74:1784–1791.

60. Berger MS, Rostomily RC. Low grade gliomas: functional mapping resection strategies, extent of resection, and outcome. *J Neurooncol* 1997;34:85–101.

61. Berger MS, Wilson CB. Extent of resection and outcome for cerebral hemispheric gliomas. In: Berger MS, Wilson CB, eds. *The gliomas*. Philadelphia: WB Saunders, 1999:660–679.

62. Keles GE, Anderson B, Berger MS. The effect of extent of resection on time to tumor progression and survival in patients with glioblastoma multiforme of the cerebral hemisphere. *Surg Neurol* 1999;52: 371–379.

63. Rostomily RC. Management of adult recurrent supratentorial gliomas. *Neurosurg Quart* 1993;3:219–252.

64. Young B, Oldfield EH, Markesbery WR, et al. Reoperation for glioblastoma. *J Neurosurg* 1981;55:917–921.

65. Harsh GR, Levin VA, Gutin PH, et al. Reoperation for recurrent glioblastoma and anaplastic astrocytoma. *Neurosurgery* 1987;21: 615–621.

66. Chandler KL, Prados MD, Malec M, et al. Long-term survival in patients with glioblastoma multiforme. *Neurosurgery* 1993;32: 716–720.

67. Walker MD, Green SB, Byar DP, et al. Randomized comparisons

of radiotherapy and nitrosoureas for the treatment of malignant glioma after surgery. *N Engl J Med* 1980;303:1323–1329.

68. Leibel SA, Scott CB, Loeffler JS. Contemporary approaches to the treatment of malignant gliomas with radiation therapy. *Semin Oncol* 1994;21:198–219.

69. Wang Y, Pantelias GE, Iliakis G. Mechanism of radiosensitization by halogenated pyrimidines: the contribution of excess DNA and chromosome damage in BrdU radiosensitization may be minimal in plateau-phase cells. *Int J Radiat Oncol Biol Phys* 1994;66:133–142.

70. Prados MD, Scott CB, Rotman M, et al. Influence of bromodeoxyuridine radiosensitization on malignant glioma patient survival: a retrospective comparison of survival data from the Northern California Oncology Group (NCOG) and Radiation Therapy Oncology Group trials (RTOG) for glioblastoma multiforme and anaplastic astrocytoma. *Int J Radiat Oncol Biol Phys* 1998;40:653–659.

71. Prados MD, Scott C, Sandler H, et al. A phase 3 randomized study of radiotherapy plus procarbazine, CCNU, and vincristine (PCV) with or without BUdR for the treatment of anaplastic astrocytoma: a preliminary report of RTOG 9404. *Int J Radiat Oncol Biol Phys* 1999;45:1109–1115.

72. Chang EL, Loeffler JS, Reese NE, et al. Survival results from a phase I study of etanidazole (SR2508) and radiotherapy in patients with malignant glioma. *Int J Radiat Oncol Biol Phys* 1998;40:65–70.

73. Del Rowe J, Scott C, Werner-Wasik M, et al. A single-arm open label phase II study of intravenously administered tirapazamine for glioblastoma multiforme—an RTOG study. *Int J Radiat Oncol Biol Phys* 1998;42(suppl 1):266.

74. McDermott MW, Sneed PK, Gutin PH. Interstitial brachytherapy for malignant brain tumors. *Semin Surg Oncol* 1998;14:79–87.

75. Sneed PK, Prados MD, McDermott MW, et al. Large effect of age on the survival of patients with glioblastoma treated with radiotherapy and brachytherapy boost. *Neurosurgery* 1995;36:898–903.

76. Wen PY, Alexander E, Black PM, et al. Long term results of stereotactic brachytherapy used in the initial treatment of patients with glioblastoma. *Cancer* 1994;73:3029–3036.

77. Sneed PK, Stauffer PR, McDermott MW, et al. Survival benefit of hyperthermia in a prospective, randomized trial of brachytherapy boost ± hyperthermia for glioblastoma multiforme. *Int J Radiat Oncol Biol Phys* 1998;40:287–295.

78. Leksell L. The stereotaxic method and radiosurgery of the brain. *Acta Chir Scand* 1951;102:316–319.

79. Kondziolka D, Flickinger JC, Bissonette DJ, et al. Survival benefit of stereotactic radiosurgery for patients with malignant glial neoplasms. *Neurosurgery* 1997;41:776–783.

80. Masciopinto JE, Levin AB, Mehta MP, et al. Stereotactic radiosurgery for glioblastoma: a final report of 31 patients. *J Neurosurg* 1995;82:530–535.

81. Shrieve DC, Alexander EA, Black PM, et al. Treatment of primary glioblastoma multiforme with standard radiotherapy and radiosurgical boost: prognostic factors and long-term outcome. *J Neurosurg* 1999;90:72–77.

82. Snelling L, Miyamoto CT, Bender H, et al. Epidermal growth factor receptor 425 monoclonal antibodies radiolabeled with iodine-125 in the adjuvant treatment of high-grade astrocytomas. *Hybridoma* 1995;14:111–114.

83. Bigner DD, Brown MT, Friedman AH, et al. Iodine-131-labeled antitenascin monoclonal antibody 81C6 treatment of patients with recurrent malignant gliomas: phase I trial results. *J Clin Oncol* 1998;16:2202–2212.

84. Prados MD, Chang S, Mack EE. Chemotherapy of brain tumors. In: Youmans JR, ed. *Neurological surgery*. Philadelphia: WB Saunders, 1996:2893–2907.

85. Salcman M. Survival in glioblastoma: historical perspective. *Neurosurgery* 1980;7:435–439.

86. Fine HA, Dear KB, Loeffler JS, et al. Metaanalysis of radiation therapy with and without adjuvant chemotherapy for malignant gliomas in adults. *Cancer* 1993;71:2585–2597.

87. Levin VA, Silver P, Hannigan J, et al. Superiority of post-radiotherapy adjuvant chemotherapy with CCNU, procarbazine and vincristine (PCV) over BCNU for anaplastic gliomas: NCOG 6G61 final report. *Int J Radiat Oncol Biol Phys* 1990;18:321–324.

88. Prados MD, Scott C, Curran WJ, et al. Procarbazine, lomustine, and vincristine (PCV) chemotherapy for anaplastic astrocytoma: a retrospective review of radiation therapy oncology group proto-

cols comparing survival with carmustine or PCV adjuvant chemotherapy. *J Clin Oncol* 1999;17:3389–3395.

89. Jeremic B, Jovanovic D, Djuric LJ, et al. Advantage of postradiotherapy chemotherapy with CCNU, procarbazine, and vincristine (mPCV) over chemotherapy with VM-26 and CCNU for malignant glioma. *J Chemother* 1992;4:123–126.

90. Glass J, Hochberg FH, Gruber ML, et al. The treatment of oligodendrogliomas and mixed oligodendroglioma-astrocytomas with PCV chemotherapy. *J Neurosurg* 1992;76:741–745.

91. Cairncross JG, Macdonald DR, Ramsay DA. Aggressive oligodendroglioma: a chemosensitive tumour. *Neurosurgery* 1992;31:78–82.

92. Cairncross JG, Ueki K, Zlatescu MC, et al. Specific genetic predictors of chemotherapeutic response and survival in patients with anaplastic oligodendrogliomas. *J Natl Cancer Inst* 1998;90:1473–1479.

93. Streffer J, Schabet M, Bamberg M, et al. A role for preirradiation PCV chemotherapy for oligodendroglial brain tumors. *J Neurol* 2000;247:297–302.

94. Paleologos NA, Macdonald DR, Vick NA, et al. Neoadjuvant procarbazine, CCNU, and vincristine for anaplastic and aggressive oligodendroglioma. *Neurology* 1999;53:1141–1143.

95. Gornet MK, Buckner JC, Marks RS, et al. Chemotherapy for advanced CNS ependymoma. *J Neurooncol* 1999;45:61–67.

96. Huncharek M, Muscat J. Treatment of recurrent high grade astrocytoma: results of a systematic review of 1,415 patients. *Anticancer Res* 1998;18:1303–1312.

97. Yung WK, Prados MD, Yaya-Tur R, et al. Multicenter phase II trial of temozolomide in patients with anaplastic astrocytoma or anaplastic oligoastrocytoma at first relapse. *J Clin Oncol* 1999;17:2762–2771.

98. Osoba D, Brada M, Yung WK, et al. Health-related quality of life in patients treated with temozolomide versus procarbazine for recurrent glioblastoma multiforme. *J Clin Oncol* 2000;18:1481–1491.

99. Friedman HS, McLendon RE, Kerby T, et al. DNA mismatch repair and O6-alkylguanine-DNA alkyl transferase analysis and response to Temodal in newly diagnosed malignant glioma. *J Clin Oncol* 1998;16:3851–3857.

100. Brem H, Piantadosi S, Burger PC, et al. Placebo-controlled trial of safety and efficacy of intraoperative controlled delivery by biodegradable polymers of chemotherapy for recurrent gliomas. *Lancet* 1995;345:1008–1012.

101. Valtonen S, Timonen U, Toivanen P, et al. Interstitial chemotherapy with carmustine-loaded polymers for high-grade gliomas: a randomized double-blind study. *Neurosurgery* 1997;41:44–48.

102. Dropcho EJ. Intra-arterial chemotherapy for malignant gliomas. In: Berger MS, Wilson CB, eds. *The gliomas*. Philadelphia: WB Saunders, 1999:537–547.

103. Stewart DJ. Hyperosmolar disruption of the blood-brain barrier as a chemotherapy potentiator in the treatment of brain tumors. In: Berger MS, Wilson CB, eds. *The gliomas*. Philadelphia: WB Saunders, 1999:570–578.

104. Dunkel IJ, Finlay JL. High-dose chemotherapy followed by autologous bone marrow rescue for high-grade gliomas. In: Berger MS, Wilson CB, eds. *The gliomas*. Philadelphia: WB Saunders, 1999:549–554.

105. Shapiro WR, Green SB, Burger PC, et al. A randomized comparison of intra-arterial versus intravenous BCNU, with or without intravenous 5-fluorouracil, for newly diagnosed patients with malignant glioma. *J Neurosurg* 1992;76:772–781.

106. Cairncross JG, Swinnen L, Bayer R, et al. Myeloablative chemotherapy for recurrent aggressive oligodendroglioma. *Neuro-oncology* 2000;2:114–119.

107. Friedman HS, Petros WP, Friedman AH, et al. Irinotecan therapy in adults with recurrent or progressive malignant glioma. *J Clin Oncol* 1999;17:1516–1525.

108. Burton E, Prados M. New chemotherapy options for the treatment of malignant gliomas. *Curr Opin Oncol* 1999;11:157–161.

109. Malkin M, Mason W, Leiberman F, et al. A phase I study of SU101, a novel signal transduction inhibitor, in recurrent malignant glioma. *Proc Am Soc Clin Oncol* 1997;16:1371.

110. Couldwell WT, Weiss MH, DeGiorgio CM, et al. Clinical and radiographic response in a minority of patients with recurrent malignant gliomas treated with high-dose tamoxifen. *Neurosurgery* 1993;32:485–489.

111. Fine H, Loeffler J, Kyritsis A, et al. A phase II trial of the anti-

angiogenic agent thalidomide in patients with recurrent high-grade gliomas. *Proc Am Soc Clin Oncol* 1997;16:1372.

112. Wallenfriedman MA, Conrad JA, DelaBarre L, et al. Effects of continuous localized infusion of granulocyte-macrophage colony-stimulating factor and inoculations of irradiated glioma cells on tumor regression. *J Neurosurg* 1999;90:1064–1071.

113. Glick RP, Lichtor T. Novel therapeutic strategies. In: Bernstein M, Berger MS, eds. *Neuro-oncology: the essentials*. New York: Thieme, 2000:289–300.

114. Pastan I, Fitzgerald D. Recombinant toxins for cancer treatment. *Science* 1991;254:1173–1177.

115. Laske DW, Youle RJ, Oldfield EH. Tumor regression with regional distribution of the targeted toxin TF-CRM107 in patients with malignant brain tumors. *Nat Med* 1997;3:1362–1368.

116. Culver KW, Ram Z, Wallbridge S, et al. In vivo gene transfer with retroviral vector-producer cells for treatment of experimental brain tumors. *Science* 1992;256:1550–1552.

117. Ram Z, Culver KW, Oshiro EM, et al. Therapy of malignant brain tumors by intratumoral implantation of retroviral vector-producing cells. *Nat Med* 1997;3:1354–1361.

118. Klatzmann D, Valery CA, Bensimon G, et al. A phase 1/2 study of herpes simplex virus type 1 thymidine kinase "suicide" gene therapy for recurrent glioblastoma. *Hum Gene Ther* 1998;9:2595–2604.

119. Shand N, Weber F, Mariani L, et al. A phase 1-2 clinical trial of gene therapy for recurrent glioblastoma multiforme by tumor transduction with the herpes simplex thymidine kinase gene followed by ganciclovir. *Hum Gene Ther* 1999;10:2325–2335.

120. Packer RJ, Raffel C, Villablanca JG, et al. Treatment of progressive or recurrent pediatric malignant supratentorial brain tumors with herpes simplex virus thymidine kinase gene vector-producer cells followed by intravenous ganciclovir administration. *J Neurosurg* 2000;92:249–254.

121. Barker FG, Huhn SL, Prados MD. Clinical characteristics of long-term glioma survivors. In: Berger MS, Wilson CB, eds. *The gliomas*. Philadelphia: WB Saunders, 1999:710–722.

122. Curran WJ Jr, Scott CB, Horton J, et al. Recursive partitioning analysis of prognostic factors in three Radiation Therapy Oncology Group malignant glioma trials. *J Natl Cancer Inst* 1993;85:704–710.

104. Surgery for Glial Neoplasms within the Brain

Randall R. Johnson and Joseph M. Piepmeier

Primary brain tumors represent one of the most devastating events that can befall any individual. Likewise, craniotomy for tumor removal, adjuvant chemotherapy, and radiation therapy all represent highly significant departures from everyday life and are also associated with significant morbidity. Glial neoplasms are by far the most common primary brain neoplasm, accounting for approximately 40% to 60% of all primary brain tumors and occurring in approximately 4.1 to 5.7 per 100,000 population per year (1,2). Gliomas come in two peaks according to age-incidence, one in childhood consisting mostly of brainstem gliomas and cerebellar astrocytomas and a second in the fifth and sixth decades, containing a much larger percentage of aggressive tumors including anaplastic astrocytoma and glioblastoma multiforme (GBM).

Surgery for glial neoplasms largely coincides with the earliest historical evidence for craniotomy (3). The first resection of a glioma reported in the literature, however, was performed by Rickman Godlee in 1884 on a patient with an oligodendroglioma in rolandic cortex and focal motor seizures (4). Interestingly, Cushing initially advocated external decompressive craniotomy for the treatment of all gliomas, but by his later years had converted to gross total resection as the primary therapy, believing that removal of tumor itself had a positive impact on patient survival (5). Even as the modern era of neurosurgery enters the 21st century—with the advent of improved tumor markers to produce more accurate histology and molecular understanding of gliomas, imaging-guided stereotactic biopsy to improve early diagnosis of gliomas, and the development of more refined techniques of intraoperative guidance and localization to improve resection of tumor versus normal brain—there remains little consensus regarding the overall management of patients harboring glial neoplasms (6,7).

Classification of Gliomas

Historically, this lack of consensus has arisen in large part from difficulty in classifying these lesions (8,9). Cushing and Bailey first classified tumors in the late 1920s based on the presumed embryonic cell type of origin. Several decades later, however, Kernohan concluded the opposite, that gliomas arise from adult glial phenotypes via dedifferentiation, and thus can be classified as astrocytomas, oligodendrogliomas, and ependymomas. He classified gliomas into four grades of anaplasia on the basis of *amount* of pleomorphism, *number* of mitoses, *degree* of necrosis, and *amount* of vascular proliferation, recognizing that histopathological criteria have prognostic significance (10).

This system was codified by the World Health Organization (11), with grade assigned according to the predominant cell type found within the tumor (i.e., grade 1 = "pilocytic" astrocytoma; grade 2 = "fibrillary" and "gemistocytic" astrocytoma; grade 3 = "anaplastic" astrocytoma, and grade 4 = "glioblastoma"). Oligodendroglial tumors were assigned to grade 2 (oligodendrogliomas and oligoastrocytomas) and grade 3 (anaplastic oligodendrogliomas). Many institutions, however, have adopted some modification of the Daumas-Duport ("Mayo-St. Anne") system, which is based on more objective presence or absence of relevant histopathological features (nuclear atypia, mitoses, necrosis, and endothelial hyperplasia). In this system, grade is assigned on a scale of 1 to 4 according to the number of relevant features present, rather than subjective *amount* and *degree* of such findings (12).

In addition to evaluating tumor cell morphology, gliomas can be typed according to the topography of tumor cells in the brain (13,14). Correlation of sequential stereotactic biopsy results

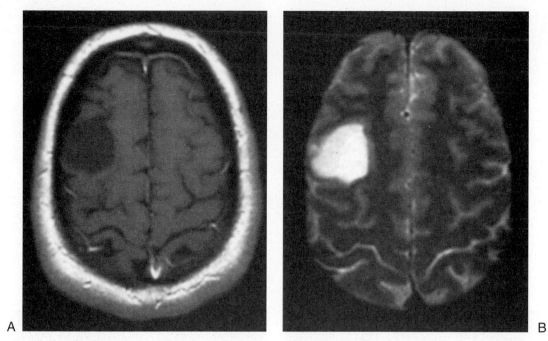

Fig. 1. Magnetic resonance scan of a type 1 glial neoplasm. The patient was an asymptomatic 48-year-old man who presented with this incidental mass noted on head computed tomography following a motor vehicle accident. **A:** The tumor was nonenhancing following gadolinium administration and had discrete border identifiable on T1 sequence. **B:** T2 sequence shows a lack of hyperintense signal surrounding the lesion, consistent with low probability of local invasion and lack of surrounding edema. Pathology returned as low-grade astrocytoma.

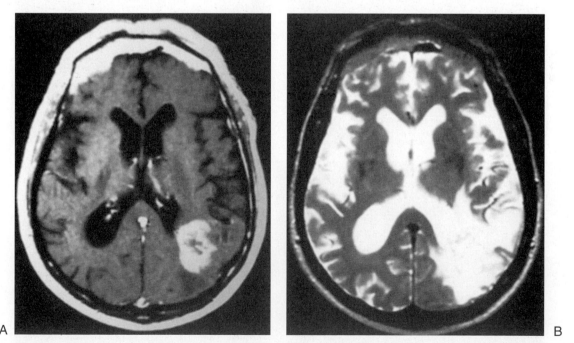

Fig. 2. Magnetic resonance imaging of a type 2 glial neoplasm in a 59-year-old woman who presented with headache and a single seizure. **A:** An irregular, hyperintense lesion T1 sequence which only mildly enhanced with gadolinium (not shown), suggestive of a tumor with central necrosis and hemorrhage. **B:** A high degree of surrounding hyperintensity on T2 sequence indicates high probability of local invasion and/or surrounding edema. Tissue obtained from surgical resection returned with the diagnosis of glioblastoma multiforme.

with imaging appearance demonstrates that hypodense areas on computed tomography (CT) and hyperintense regions on T2-weighted magnetic resonance imaging (MRI) contain isolated tumor cells that typically surround the central area of contrast enhancement. On this basis, three structural types are identified: type 1, composed of solid tumor tissue without intervening brain tissue and without surrounding isolated tumor cells (Fig. 1); type 2, composed of solid (commonly enhancing) tumor surrounded by infiltrative isolated tumor cells (Fig. 2); and type 3, composed only of isolated tumor cells without a central solid lesion (Fig. 3). Type 1 gliomas are most commonly pilocytic astrocytomas, whereas glioblastomas are the most common example of type 2 lesions. In contrast, type 3 lesions appear much more diffuse on imaging and virtually all are oligodendrogliomas. The surgical implications of tumor structural type are discussed later in this chapter.

Recently, a separate rating system for oligodendrogliomas has been proposed that is based on the presence of endothelial hyperproliferation and/or contrast enhancement (grade A = no endothelial hyperproliferation or contrast enhancement; grade B = hyperproliferation and/or contrast enhancement) (15,16). The current challenge in applying these criteria uniformly however is that tumors are often heterogeneous in terms of astrocytic and oligodendroglial features (mixed oligoastroglial histology), and the accuracy of sampling from the center versus surrounding tissue is often less than perfect. This is more than just an academic point however, because a subset of malignant oligodendrogliomas is responsive to chemotherapy, whereas malignant astrocytomas may show only a modest benefit (17).

The most significant contributions to accurate diagnosis of glial neoplasms, however, are now coming from work in molecular cytogenetics (18). It has been recognized recently that specific molecular markers can be used to predict chemotherapeutic response among subsets of anaplastic oligodendrogliomas. Interestingly, non–ring-enhancing tumors bearing deletions of 1p and 19q are uniquely sensitive to PCV (procarbazine, lomustine, and vincristine), whereas ring-enhancing tumors with

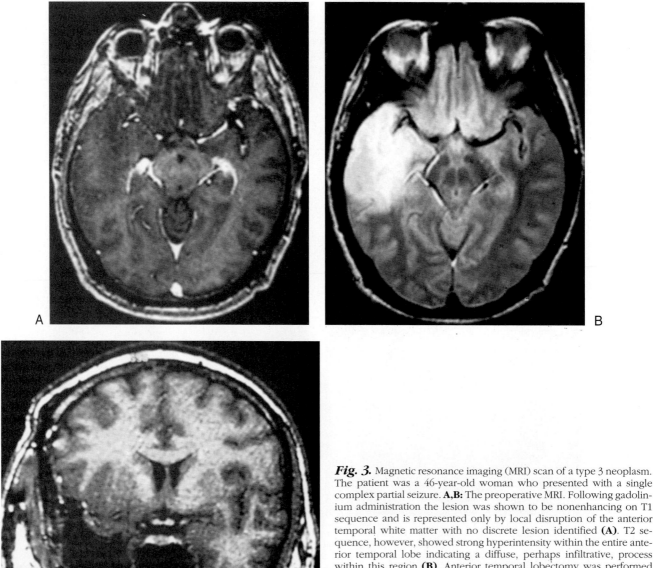

Fig. 3. Magnetic resonance imaging (MRI) scan of a type 3 neoplasm. The patient was a 46-year-old woman who presented with a single complex partial seizure. **A,B:** The preoperative MRI. Following gadolinium administration the lesion was shown to be nonenhancing on T1 sequence and is represented only by local disruption of the anterior temporal white matter with no discrete lesion identified **(A)**. T2 sequence, however, showed strong hyperintensity within the entire anterior temporal lobe indicating a diffuse, perhaps infiltrative, process within this region **(B)**. Anterior temporal lobectomy was performed with the postresection MRI **(C)**. Pathology provided abundant evidence for oligodendroglioma but a relative paucity of blood vessel hyperproliferation was noted, making this a type 3/grade A lesion.

deletions of CDKN2A are relatively insensitive to chemotherapy. These findings are likely to have an important function in shaping the role of operative intervention in the treatment of this subset of gliomas. Clearly, one of the primary roles of the neurosurgeon in the management of glial neoplasms is not only to obtain tissue for histology but for molecular analysis as well, resulting in a more accurate prognosis for patients.

Role of Surgery for Gliomas

To date no randomized, prospective study of surgery for gliomas has been performed, although several proposals for such a study are currently under consideration. Therefore, although cytoreductive surgery remains at the center of most current therapies for glioma, its benefit has not been formally proven. Retrospective series, however, have identified specific clinical parameters that correlate with better outcome for patients with gliomas, including age (under 40 years), functional status (Karnofsky performance score), presence of seizures, duration of symptoms, histological grade, tumor location, patient performance immediately postresection, and extent of resection (19–27). These series document a broad range of mean survival following open reduction of tumor: 2 to 12 years for low-grade astrocytoma, 12 to 39 months for anaplastic astrocytoma, and 30 weeks for GBM. Patients with oligodendroglioma on the whole tend to fare better than those harboring astrocytomas, with mean survivals of 5.5 to 13 years for low-grade lesions (with mixed oligoastrocytomas faring better than oligodendrogliomas) and 171 weeks for high-grade lesions.

In cases where tumor is located in "eloquent" brain, has non-diagnostic or ambiguous radiological characteristics, and is of sufficient size for stereotactic localization, stereotactic biopsy may provide a safe alternative to open resection in providing a diagnosis. This is important for patient management because the presence of aggressive histopathological features alters prognosis in major ways (6 to 10 years or more disease-free survival for a low-grade lesion versus 6 months or less for most stage 4 metastatic malignancies) (8). Patients with low-grade astrocytomas diagnosed by stereotactic biopsy and treated with radiation have a relatively favorable survival postsurgery (median survival = 9.8 years) (25). Interestingly, these data compare favorably to gross total resection for low-grade lesions. However, patients with anaplastic astrocytoma or glioblastoma diagnosed by stereotactic biopsy and treated with radiation (5,000 to 6,000 cGy total) do worse, as expected, and patients with deep-seated lesions do more poorly than those with hemispherical, lobar lesions (19.4 to 27 weeks for deep-seated lesions and 46.9 to 129 weeks for lobar lesions) (21).

The benefit of complete resection for low-grade gliomas is controversial. For tumors greater than 10 cm, more aggressive resection correlates with longer time to recurrence and with a lower histopathological grade at recurrence (28,29). The benefit from resection of lesions smaller than 10 cm^3 is less clear. Extent of resection of malignant lesions, likewise, has not consistently been shown to correlate with survival (30), and studies claiming a benefit for aggressive resection have only demonstrated modest improvement (28,29). Nonetheless, many surgeons have taken the approach that radical resection is the preferred approach for all gliomas if for no other reason than to decrease the amount of tumor that is left to undergo malignant transformation (31).

PATIENT PRESENTATION AND WORKUP. Patients harboring glial neoplasms present with complaint of seizures (38.3%), headache (35.2%), mental status change (16.5%), hemiparesis (10.3%), emesis (7.5%), dysphasia (6.9%), and/or visual change, hemianesthesia, or cranial nerve palsy (all less than 5%) (32). In our experience, the majority of gliomas are identified either in the course of a workup for seizures or following a workup for persistent headaches with or without a focal neurological deficit. Headaches associated with gliomas typically wax and wane over weeks or months and become refractory to over-the-counter analgesics, are worse in the morning after sleep and with recumbence, and improve as the day progresses and the patient walks about. Headaches typically become refractory to nonnarcotic analgesics, or the patient becomes increasingly drowsy, and a CT or MRI is obtained with subsequent referral to the neurosurgeon when a mass lesion is identified. Patients presenting with a more rapidly worsening focal deficit or mental status change in our experience tend to harbor a more aggressive lesion and have a poorer prognosis. On the other hand, patients with a more protracted time course of symptoms (greater than 3 to 4 months) tend to harbor a more benign lesion and have a more favorable outlook.

We have shown that gliomas found in chronic epilepsy patients represent a very different class of disease than those found in patients with no seizures (19). Gliomas associated with epilepsy are typically low grade, express tumor antigens representative of a distinct astrocytic lineage (type 1 astrocytes), and are most often located in the temporal lobe (26). In addition, patients who have had seizures for more than 3 months do better than those having their first seizure within the last 3 months. Interestingly, early surgery appears to have little benefit in patients with chronic epilepsy, since tumor-related outcome appears to be the same when surgery is deferred until the time of radiological progression of tumor (27). However, patients do appear to benefit from improved seizure control following surgery.

Physical Examination. Approximately one-half of patients with a glial neoplasm will present with a focal neurological finding at the time of initial diagnosis, and the frequency of finding any focal sign generally increases with grade of the lesion (32). Localizing signs at assessment include hemiparesis (45% to 70%), hemianesthesia (20% to 43%), hemianopia (19% to 39%), and dysphasia (22% to 36%). More generalized signs include mental status change (40% to 63%) and papilledema (47% to 60%). Other important but nonspecific signs of intracranial pathology include changes in deep tendon reflexes and release of frontal lobe reflexes including rooting, palmomental reflex, and glabellar reflex as well as Babinski reflex and Hoffman sign. In addition a complete cerebellar examination should be performed in all patients including assessment of finger-nose-finger, rapid alternating movements and heel-knee-shin maneuvers to rule out the presence of a cerebellar lesion, although these are much more common in children than adults. Also the skin of every patient with a suspected brain tumor should be thoroughly examined to rule out the presence of neurocutaneous syndromes and neurofibromatosis.

When considering surgical procedures that require neck flexion, it is advisable to assess range of motion in the neck to determine whether any limitations exist prior to intubation and positioning. Finally, a thorough general physical examination is performed including auscultation and percussion of the lung fields and abdomen, breast examination, stool guaiac, and digital rectal examination with the thought that final pathology may reveal an unexpected metastasis rather than glioma.

Preoperative Imaging and Operative Planning. Every patient with a suspected brain tumor should have, at the minimum, a CT scan of the brain with and without intravenous contrast. This is critical for both operative planning and prognostication.

In addition, MRI T1 sequence with and without gadolinium and T2 sequence is useful to differentiate peritumoral edema from local infiltration of tumor cells (8). One of the most important principles in planning surgery for gliomas is an understanding of the spatial relationship between the tumor and the brain (see earlier discussion regarding tumor types 1, 2, and 3). The surgical implications of structural typing are obvious. Solid tumor tissue that contains no intact parenchyma (type 1 tumors) theoretically can be removed without sacrificing functional brain tissue. In contrast, resection of many type 2 tumors is limited to the solid tumor tissue component. The isolated tumor cells that are found in type 2 tumors and compose the entirety of type 3 gliomas present a greater risk of resection because they require removal of the infiltrated, and presumably, functional brain tissue. The amount and severity of risk is dependent on the size and location of the tumor. Although most gliomas have characteristic imaging findings, there is sufficient variability among different gliomas that histopathological confirmation of a diagnosis remains essential for planning treatment (33,34).

In addition, it should be kept in mind that patients with suspected glioma may have a different primary central nervous system (CNS) neoplasm, or more commonly may harbor metastatic disease to the brain. Therefore, a chest radiograph should be obtained for all patients at risk for metastatic disease, as well as chest and abdominal/pelvic CT when history and physical examination are more suggestive of metastatic primary tumor than glioma of the brain. Finally, it must be recognized that patients presenting with history and findings of immune-compromised state are more likely to harbor other masses such as primary CNS lymphoma, abscess, or mycotic aneurysm as well as other infectious mass lesions. However, these patients often also require surgical biopsy or resection in order to make a firm diagnosis.

Practically speaking, the decision of which surgical procedure to undertake (open craniotomy versus stereotactic biopsy versus expectant management) is most often dictated by the aggressiveness of the lesion as determined clinically over time, as well as the location of the lesion, and its appearance on MRI (cystic and necrotic components as well as widespread enhancement and mass effect). Aggressive tumors may benefit from debulking and tissue for pathological diagnosis. However, isolated tumor cells are invariably present at the margins of resection, eventually giving rise to disease recurrence. On the other hand, less aggressive lesions, which appear well circumscribed and are located in surgically accessible areas, may benefit from complete resection. Theoretically by removing the greatest number of cells with malignant potential, the surgeon can minimize the rate of the tumor for malignant transformation.

INTRAOPERATIVE MANAGEMENT

Intraoperative Imaging Modalities. Imaging modalities to assist in tumor resection include visualization of regional blood flow using optical imaging (35) and visualization of blood–brain barrier preservation following systemic administration of florescent probes (36). One particularly intriguing technique uses preferential tumor uptake of fluorescein-conjugated porphyrins by malignant gliomas, enabling intraoperative identification of tumor with respect to normal tissue (37). This approach has the theoretical advantage of minimizing false-positive localization within peritumoral edema or surgically traumatized brain, both of which may disrupt the blood–brain barrier. On a more experimental basis other centers are using intraoperative CT or MRI as an adjunct to tumor localization (38–41). Although this modality has the theoretical advantage of maintaining lesion localization in the face of shifting intracranial contents secondary to resection and/or swelling, its use is cur-

rently prohibitively expensive for most medical centers, and its efficacy remains unproven.

The converse of the principle of maximal tumor resection is to provide the greatest protection to critical brain regions during a resection. In cases where tumor and/or associated edema encroach upon behaviorally critical areas of cortex including motor and speech areas, several adjunctive imaging studies are available both preoperatively and intraoperatively to the surgeon. These include functional MRI (42,43) for motor and sensory mapping and language localization, intraoperative electrophysiology in the awake patient for motor and language mapping, intraoperative electroencephalogram, and somatosensory evoked potentials. In addition, intraoperative localization of relatively small tumors can be greatly aided by the use of frameless stereotaxy (discussed later in this chapter). Finally, one particularly innovative approach involves *a priori* determination of tumor contours and location of eloquent brain regions using preoperative MRI and CT with projection of these contours into the operative microscope using "heads-up display" to guide the surgeon (44).

Patient Positioning and Tumor Exposure. Patient positioning is important to provide the most efficient access to the tumor while protecting the patient. Most hemispherical tumors can be accessed by placing the patient in the semi-Fowler position. This provides for head and leg elevation to facilitate venous drainage and to remove stress from the patient's spine and legs. Addition of mild neck extension can help with surgical access by using gravity to provide retraction. Lateral head exposure is facilitated by turning the patient to a partial or full lateral position to reduce the danger of neck injury. Posterior hemisphere access can be achieved either by full lateral positioning and neck flexion or by placing the patient prone. Care is needed, however, to prevent overflexion, which can result in cervical spine injury, jugular obstruction, or airway compromise.

Most craniotomies are performed with the patient's head fixed in a three-point (Mayfield) head-holder. This device is attached to the head of the operating table and provides for strict limitation of head movement without impeding access. Adequate padding of the axilla (lateral position), elbows, knees, and heels is needed to guard against pressure ischemia to the skin and to avoid compression injury to peripheral nerves. Once the final position is achieved, it is advisable for the anesthesiologist to recheck the airway and breath sounds to ensure that the endotracheal tube did not move during positioning.

We prefer to use linear scalp incisions with minimal to no hair shaving. Precise localization of the lesion is usually achieved with careful examination of the preoperative imaging. For example, if a tumor is located 13 cm from the nasion, as measured from the sagittal MRI, and 3 cm lateral to the midline on the coronal images, a relatively short linear area can be made at exactly this site, minimizing the need for extensive shaving. Alternatively, frameless stereotactic devices can provide precise localization of the tumor as well as the site for incision. These devices are particularly helpful when the location of the lesion precludes placing the incision and craniotomy directly over the tumor.

Tumor Resection. The operating microscope is indispensable for improving illumination and providing sufficient magnification to help define the tumor–brain interface. Gliomas are grossly identified by color, consistency, and vascularity. Although the differences between tumor and brain tissue can be subtle, typically small, but consistent differences in color and vascularity help to demarcate gross tumor from edematous brain. We prefer to avoid the use of mannitol unless the patient's intracranial pressure prevents opening the dura without further brain relaxation. Mannitol can decrease swelling and can reduce the need for retraction on edematous tissue; however, osmotic diuresis also can change the texture of the brain surrounding the tumor and obscure the subtle differences in tissue turgor.

At the time of diagnosis most gliomas are much larger than the size of the cortical incision used to access them. Consequently, tumors are removed in pieces by delivering the tumor to the region of exposure by a combination of suctioning and coagulation. The texture of the tissue assessed by suction and bipolar coagulation helps to identify the tumor. This technique requires careful attention to the tumor–brain interface to minimize the risk of unintended injury or unanticipated inadequate resection, and meticulous hemostasis is absolutely necessary to maintain clear definition of the tumor margin. Ultrasonic aspirators can be useful tools for resection of large gliomas, but in our opinion they do not provide the same tactile information found with simple bipolar coagulation and suction. Clearly, opinions vary on the usefulness of these techniques, however, and the optimal technique is ultimately dependent on the experience of each individual surgeon.

Intraoperative imaging (ultrasound, MRI, CT) also can provide a visual display of the resection region. All of these imaging techniques have been used successfully for the purposes of checking to determine whether the goals of surgery have been adequately achieved. The use of frameless stereotaxis also can help with glioma resection by comparing the intraoperative findings with an imaging study performed just prior to surgery. A number of commercially available devices exist and all appear to be accurate and reliable. The major limitation for frameless stereotaxis is that the images acquired prior to surgery do not reflect movement in the tumor and the brain that occurs during glioma surgery. Consequently, the surgeon must interpret the intraoperative findings and compare them with the imaging with an understanding of how this shift can generate false information.

Intraoperative Monitoring. Neurophysiological monitoring is very helpful for resection of gliomas that border the primary somatosensory or language cortex (45). In general, most surgeons are familiar with the technique of recording somatosensory evoked responses from the primary sensory cortex and the wave shift seen across the central sulcus to the primary motor cortex. These recordings are most often performed for the hand region because of the ease in generating a response, the relatively large cortical region that subserves hand function and the functional significance of maintaining use of the hand and arm. Most recordings are made with an electrode grid placed over the central sulcus that covers both primary motor and sensory regions. This recording can be completed successfully under light general anesthesia. Direct cortical stimulation for motor responses also can be achieved under general anesthesia without the use of muscle relaxation. However, these responses are easier to achieve with local anesthesia and neuroleptic anesthesia. Awake craniotomies are mandatory for mapping speech and language function. It is beyond the scope of this chapter to address the technical aspects of these techniques. However, direct cortical mapping can be completed in a relatively short period of time and in our experience, this is well tolerated by the patient who has received preoperative instruction on the tasks to be performed.

Stereotactic Biopsy. Some gliomas are not amenable to surgical resection based primarily on their location. When resection of a tumor poses an unacceptable risk, stereotactic biopsy can provide accurate tissue sampling for the purposes of diagnosis. The usefulness of stereotactic biopsy has been shown in the initial diagnosis of a glioma, as well as for evaluation of recurrent lesions in the setting of possible radiation necrosis versus tumor, or for evaluating potential anaplastic transformation in a low-grade glioma (21,25,46). Commercially available systems for MRI- or CT-guided biopsy are generally dependable and easy to use.

Stereotactic biopsies typically can be performed under local anesthesia. Sequential sampling that includes biopsies from areas with different imaging characteristics will improve the diagnostic reliability of the biopsy by reducing the chances of sampling error. For example, sampling the low-density center of a glioblastoma without obtaining tissue from the contrast-enhancing margin may reveal only necrosis that will prove to be inadequate to confirm the proper diagnosis. Conversely, a sample that does not include necrosis may be inadequate for some neuropathologists to confirm the presence of a glioblastoma. Gliomas are well recognized as heterogeneous lesions and sampling error can lead to inappropriate diagnoses. While the potential for sampling error cannot be eliminated, the risk of underdiagnosis can be minimized by including the imaging characteristics and neurological history along with the histopathological findings in determining a diagnosis.

The major risk of stereotactic biopsy is hemorrhage. This risk is reduced by careful technique, but the possibility of significant bleeding at the biopsy site is always present. One technique to moderate the risk of bleeding for deep lesions is to plan a biopsy trajectory so that the ventricular system is not entered. Ventricular puncture not only creates the possibility of venous bleeding, but also can create technical error by changing the position of the target with drainage of cerebrospinal fluid. Most image-guided biopsy systems permit the surgeon to follow the trajectory of the biopsy probe through axial, sagittal, and coronal planes to make sure the path does not enter the ventricles or cross major vascular areas. In addition, a general rule of stereotactic biopsy is to cross the arachnoid plane only once at the entry site. For example, biopsy of a temporal lobe lesion from a frontal entry carries the risk of vascular injury to the middle cerebral vessels and should be avoided if possible.

Surgically Implanted Interstitial Therapies. Surgical implantation of therapies for the treatment of gliomas have been attempted for several decades. The more commonly used interstitial treatments include brachytherapy with temporary or permanent iodine-125, chemotherapy impregnated biodegradable wafers, and catheters for convection delivery of chemotherapy and immunotherapy (47,48). Most of these treatments are potentially useful for relatively well-localized lesions and all (except for convection strategies) have limited effectiveness on infiltrative tumor cells. Convection delivery offers a potential mechanism for reaching infiltrative tumors cells by distributing relatively large volumes through slow infusion rates. The success of this treatment strategy awaits development of better agents for tumor-specific activity and better catheters for optimal agent distribution.

POSTOPERATIVE EVALUATION. Patients with a stable postoperative examination are assessed by elective, routine imaging. The optimal method for assessing the adequacy of resection is judged by routine postoperative MRI with and without gadolinium. This study should be obtained within the first 72 hours postoperatively to minimize the artifact of postoperative enhancement that can be falsely interpreted as residual tumor (33). This study is then used as a baseline against which all future scans will be compared. In general, repeat imaging is performed after each stage in therapy to assess the response. Specific criteria have been established to quantify the tumor's response which is particularly important in clinical trials to quantify the size of the tumor by objective criteria (49). Patients presenting with a new neurological deficit in the immediate postoperative period are taken for emergency head CT. The rare patient with a symptomatic clot is returned to the operating room for reexploration and clot evacuation. Symptomatic patients with a negative head CT are typically found to have seizures on subsequent workup and are loaded with anticonvulsants, usually phenytoin. Only patients on anticonvulsants preoperatively are routinely given anticonvulsants during and after surgery given conflicting data regarding the prophylactic use of anticonvulsants perioperatively (50,51).

One modality that may prove useful in predicting which low-grade astrocytomas are at risk for malignant transformation is preoperative positron emission tomography using 2-DG (52, 53). Interestingly, we have demonstrated increased uptake in 9 of 28 patients with tumors that were subsequently diagnosed as low-grade astrocytomas and were indistinguishable based on histology alone. Of these nine patients, all experienced tumor recurrence at later follow-up (52).

Reoperation is indicated for patients with tumor recurrence following initial low-grade glioma for the purpose of staging, and the same principles of maximal resection apply. Regarding reoperation for GBM, improvement in survival with reoperation appears to be 2 to 3 months at best compared with patients who are not operated on for recurrence (54,55). These results are likely to be biased by patient selection however, and actual improvements in survival may be even less. Therefore, reoperation is typically viewed less favorably for patients already harboring high-grade lesions.

References

1. Codd M, Kurland L. Descriptive epidemiology or primary intracranial neoplasms. *Prog Exp Tumor Res* 1985;29:1–11.
2. Walker A, Robins M, Weinfeld F. Epidemiology of brain tumors: the national survey of intracranial neoplasms. *Neurology* 1985;35:219–226.
3. Kaye AH, Laws ER. Historical perspective. In: Kaye AH, Laws ER, eds. *Brain tumors: an encyclopedic approach*. New York: Churchill Livingstone, 1995:3–8.
4. Bennett H, Godlee RJ. Excision of a tumour from the brain. *Lancet* 1884;2:1090–1091.
5. Cushing H. *Intracranial tumors: notes upon a series of two thousand verified cases with surgical-mortality percentages pertaining thereto*. Springfield, IL: Charles C Thomas Publisher, 1932.
6. Cairncross JG. Low-grade glioma: the case for delayed surgery. *Clin Neurosurg* 1995;42:391–398
7. Wilson CB, Prados MD. Surgery for low-grade glioma: rationale for early intervention. *Clin Neurosurg* 1995;42:383–390.
8. Daumas-Duport C. Histoprognosis of gliomas. *Adv Tech Stand Neurosurg* 1994;21:43–76.
9. Giles GG, Gonzales MF. Epidemiology of brain tumors and factors in prognosis. In: Kaye AH, Laws ER, eds. *Brain tumors: an encyclopedic approach*. New York: Churchill Livingstone, 1995:47–67.
10. Kernohan JW, Mabon RF, Svien HJ, et al. Symposium on a new and simplified concept of gliomas (a simplified classification of gliomas). *Mayo Clin Proc* 1949;24:71–75.
11. World Health Organization. *Histological classification of tumors of the central nervous system*. Geneva: World Health Organization, 1976.
12. Daumas-Duport C, Scheithauer B, O'Fallon J. Grading of astrocytomas: a simple and reproducible method. *Cancer* 1988;62:2152–2165.
13. Daumas-Duport C, Scheithauer B, Kelly P. A histologic and cytologic method for the spatial definition of gliomas. *Mayo Clinic Proc*, 1987;62:435–449.
14. Kelly P, Daumas-Duport C, Scheithauer B, et al. Stereotactic histologic correlations of computed tomography and magnetic resonance imaging defined abnormalities in patients with glial neoplasms. *Mayo Clin Proc* 1987;62:450–459.
15. Daumas-Duport C, Tucker M-L, Beuvon F, et al. Oligo-dendrogliomas. Part I: patterns of growth, histological diagnosis, clinical and imaging correlations: a study of 153 cases. *J Neuro-Oncol* 1997;34:37–59.
16. Daumas-Duport C, Tucker M-L, Kolles H, et al. Oligodendrogliomas. Part II: a new grading system based on morphological and imaging criteria. *J Neuro-Oncol* 1997;34:61–78.
17. Forsyth PAJ, Cairncross JG. Treatment of malignant glioma in adults. *Curr Opin Neurol* 1995;8:414–418.
18. Cairncross JG, Ueki K, Zlatescu MC, et al. Specific genetic predictors of chemotherapeutic response and survival in patients with anaplastic oligodendrogliomas. *J Natl Cancer Inst* 1998;90:1473–1479.
19. Bartolomei JC, Christopher SC, Vives K, et al Low-grade gliomas of chronic epilepsy: a distinct clinical and pathological entity. *J Neuro-Oncol* 1997;34:79–84.
20. Berger MS, Rostomily RC. Low grade gliomas: functional mapping, resection strategies, extent of resection, and outcome. *J Neuro-Oncol* 1997;34:85–101.
21. Coffey R, Lunsford D, Taylor F. Survival after stereotactic biopsy of malignant gliomas. *Neurosurg* 1988;22:465–473.
22. Devaux BC, O'Fallon JR, Kelly PJ. Resection, biopsy, and survival in malignant glial neoplasms. *J Neurosurg* 1993;78:767–775.
23. Janny P, Cure H, Mohr M, et al. Low grade supratentorial astrocytomas. *Cancer* 1994;73:1937–1945.
24. Laws ER, Taylor WF, Clifton MB, et al. Neurosurgical management of low-grade astrocytoma of the cerebral hemispheres. *J Neurosurg* 1984;61:665–673.
25. Lunsford D, Somaza S, Kondziolka D, et al. Survival after biopsy and irradiation of cerebral nonanaplastic astrocytoma. *J Neurosurg* 1995;82:523–529.
26. Piepmeier J, Christopher S, Spencer D, et al. Variations in the natural history and survival of patients with supratentorial low-grade astrocytomas. *Neurosurgery* 1996;38:872–879.
27. van Veelen ML, Avezaat CJ, Kros JM, et al. Supratentorial low grade astrocytoma: prognostic factors, de-differentiation, and the issue of early versus late surgery. *J Neurol Neurosurg Psychiatry* 1998;64:581–587.
28. Berger MS, Deliganis AV, Dobbins J, et al. The effect of extent of resection on recurrence in patients with low grade cerebral hemisphere gliomas. *Cancer* 1994;74:1784–1791.
29. Berger M. The impact of technical adjuncts in the surgical management of cerebral hemispheric low-grade gliomas of childhood. *J Neuro-Oncol* 1996;28:129–155.
30. Kowalczuk A, MacDonald RL, Amidei C, et al. Quantitative imaging study of extent of surgical resection and prognosis of malignant astrocytomas. *Neurosurgery* 1997;41:1028–1038.
31. Laws ER. Radical resection for the treatment of glioma. *Clin Neurosurg* 1995;42:480–487.
32. McKeran RO, Thomas GT. The clinical study of gliomas. In: Thomas DGT, Graham DI, eds. *Brain tumors: scientific basis, clinical investigation, and current therapy*. London: Butterworth, 1980;194–230.
33. Byrne T, Piepmeier J, Yoshida D. Imaging and clinical features of gliomas. In: Tindall G, Cooper P, Barrow D, eds. *The practice of neurosurgery*. Baltimore: Williams & Wilkins 1995;637–648.
34. Holt R, Maravilla K. Supratentorial gliomas: imaging. In: Wilkins R, Rengachary S, eds. *Neurosurgery*. New York: McGraw-Hill 1996;752–775.
35. Haglund MM, Berger MS. Enhanced optical imaging and tumor margins. *Neurosurgery* 1996;38:308–317.
36. Kabuto M, Kubota T, Kobayashi H, et al. Experimental and clinical study of detection of glioma at surgery using fluorescent imaging by a surgical microscope after fluorescein administration. *Neurol Res* 1997;19:9–16.
37. Stummer W, Stocker S, Wagner S, et al. Intraoperative detection of malignant gliomas by 5-aminolevulinic acid-induced porphyrin fluorescence. *Neurosurgery* 1998;42:518–526.
38. Hall W, Martin A, Liu H, et al. Brain biopsy using high-field strength interventional magnetic resonance imaging. *Neurosurgery* 1999;44:807–814.
39. Steinmeier R, Fahlbusch R, Ganslandt O, et al. Intraoperative magnetic resonance imaging with the magnetom open scanner: concepts, neurosurgical indications, and procedures: a preliminary report. *Neurosurgery* 1998;739–747.
40. Black PM, Moriarty T, Alexander E, et al. Development and imple-

mentation of intraoperative magnetic resonance imaging and its neurosurgical applications. *Neurosurgery* 1997;831–842.

41. Wirtz CT, Bonsanto MM, Knauth M, et al. Intraoperative magnetic resonance imaging to update interactive navigation in neurosurgery: method and preliminary experience. *Comput Aided Surg* 1997;2: 172–179.

42. Mueller WM, Yetkin FZ, Hammeke TA, et al. Functional magnetic resonance imaging mapping of the motor cortex in patients with cerebral tumors. *Neurosurgery* 1996;30:515–520.

43. Schulder M, Maldjian JA, Liu WC, et al. Functional MRI-guided surgery of intracranial tumors. *Stereotact Funct Neurosurg* 1997;68: 98–105.

44. Roessler K, Ungersboeck K, Czech T, et al. Contour-guided brain tumor surgery using a stereotactic navigating microscope. *Stereotact Funct Neurosurg* 1997;68:33–38.

45. Gunel M, Piepmeier J. Management of low-grade gliomas. *Contemp Neurosurg* 1997;19:1–6.

46. Muller W, Afra D, Schroder R. Supratentorial recurrences of gliomas. Morphological studies in relation to time intervals with astrocytomas. *Acta Neurochir* 1977;37:75–91.

47. Brem H, Piantadosi S, Burger P, et al. Placebo-controlled trial of safety and efficacy of intraoperative controlled delivery by biodegradable polymers of chemotherapy for recurrent gliomas. *Lancet* 1995;345:1008–1012.

48. Laske D, Ilercil O, Akbasak A, et al. Efficacy of direct intratumoral therapy with targeted protein toxins for solid human gliomas in nude mice. *J Neurosurg* 1994;80:520–526.

49. Macdonald D, Cascino T, Schold C. Response criteria for phase II studies of supratentorial malignant gliomas. *J Clin Oncol* 1990;8: 1277–1280.

50. North JB, Penhall RK, Hanieh A, et al. Phenytoin and postoperative epilepsy. *J Neurosurg* 1980;52:359–366.

51. Foy PM, Chadwick DW, Rajgopalan N, et al. Do prophylactic anticonvulsant drugs alter the pattern of seizures after craniotomy? *J Neurol Neurosurg Psychiatry* 1992;55:753–757.

52. Dewitte O, Levivier M, Violon P, et al. Prognostic value positron emission tomography with [18F]fluoro-2-deoxy-D-glucose in the low-grade glioma. *Neurosurgery* 1996;39:470–477.

53. Glantz MJ, Hoffman JM, Coleman RE, et al. Identification of early recurrence of primary central nervous system tumors by [18F] fluoro-deoxyglucose positron emission tomography. *Ann Neurol* 1991;29: 347–355.

54. Barker FG, Chang SM, Gutin PH, et al. Survival and functional status after resection of recurrent glioblastoma multiforme. *Neurosurgery* 1998;42:709–720.

55. Berger MS. Tucker A, Spence A, et al. Reoperation for glioma. *Clin Neurosurg* 1992;39:172–186.

105. *Radiotherapy for Glial Neoplasms*

Viviane Tabar and Philip H. Gutin

Glial neoplasms, particularly malignant gliomas, represent an enormous challenge in oncology. Therapeutic options remain suboptimal despite significant technological progress in diagnostic imaging and an improved knowledge of the molecular basis of neurocarcinogenesis. Radiation plays a significant role in tumor control and is currently the mainstay of adjuvant therapy. Eventual treatment failure, however, remains the rule, and in spite of the widely infiltrative nature of the disease, recurrence is often local. A better understanding of radiation biology, coupled with advances in the design of biological vectors and sophisticated radiation equipment, may finally rise to meet this formidable challenge. Precise three-dimensional (3D) planning or 3D-conformal radiation therapy (3D-CRT) is one of the major innovations of the last decade. This evolving technology aims at optimizing radiation delivery to the target tissue while minimizing exposure of surrounding normal tissue. This is achieved by directing multiple-shaped fields in various planes at the tumor, delivered in static or dynamic modes. It is estimated that 3D-CRT results in 30% less brain tissue exposure when compared to conventional radiation (1). Advances in computer technology and imaging, particularly the incorporation of high resolution magnetic resonance imaging (MRI) in 3D-CRT treatment planning and further refinement in the design and flexibility of beam-shaping devices, continue to widen the application and sophistication of this technology as well as improving its therapeutic index.

High-Grade Gliomas

Malignant gliomas constitute up to 45% of all primary adult gliomas, and are mostly supratentorial. They predominantly in-

clude glioblastoma multiforme (WHO grade IV) as well as high-grade oligodendrogliomas, anaplastic astrocytomas (WHO grade III), mixed oligoastrocytomas, and gliosarcomas. High proliferative rates, necrotic areas, and an array of genetic abnormalities causing activation of many oncogenes and inactivation of tumor suppressor genes characterize this group of tumors.

EXTERNAL BEAM RADIATION. The impact of radiation therapy on glioma control is substantial, and it represents the single most effective adjuvant treatment. This has been established by several trials presenting class I evidence in support of significantly improved survival following postoperative radiation therapy. The most classically cited studies include Brain Tumor Study Group 6901 (BTSG) (2) published in 1978. This study showed a median survival of 36 weeks following postoperative standard radiation treatment (RT) compared to 14 weeks in the control group receiving supportive care ($n = 222$, $p < .001$). In 1980, the BTSG published another prospective trial (7201) of 358 patients randomized to undergo surgery followed by lomustine (CCNU), standard RT, RT and CCNU, or RT and carmustine (BCNU) (3). The lowest median survival was 24 weeks in the CCNU group. Statistically significant survival was achieved in the other three groups at 36, 42, and 51 weeks, respectively. The Scandinavian Glioblastoma Study Group published yet another confirmatory trial in 1981 (4). These trials thus established unequivocally the role of radiation therapy in effective glioma treatment.

Radiation Dose. A review of three BTSG trials (66-01, 69-01, and 72-01) concluded that a real survival response exists at doses between 50 and 60 Gy. The Medical Research Council of Canada (5) published a randomized study involving 443 patients with malignant gliomas (MG) randomized between 60 and 45 Gy, which revealed a survival advantage for the first group (12 months versus 9 months). A joint study by the Radiation Therapy Oncology Group (RTOG) and the Eastern Cooperative Oncology Group (ECOG) determined that dose escalation up to 70 Gy does not provide an additional survival advantage (6). Based on these data, most centers have adopted 60 Gy as a standard dose for initial radiation of malignant gliomas.

Target Volume. The volume of brain irradiated varies among different studies. Initial series administered whole brain radiation based on the infiltrative nature of the tumor. There are histologic studies supporting the presence of infiltrating cells beyond the enhancing tumor margins seen on computed tomography (CT). However, a more targeted approach is now adopted with increasing awareness of the late side effects of radiation, mostly in the form of neurocognitive impairment among survivors (6). This is further supported by the widely documented patterns of recurrence of gliomas post radiation that do not appear to have changed with the switch from whole brain to partial RT and are mainly limited to the resection bed (7). Standards for defining the volume to be irradiated vary among groups and institutions, but partial brain RT has replaced whole brain radiation nearly universally. Many centers define their target as encompassing a 2- to 3-cm margin beyond the area of enhancement or low density on CT, or beyond the region of abnormal T2 signaling on MRI. Current recommendations for initial or postoperative "standard" external beam radiation for malignant gliomas involve 30 to 33 daily fractions of 1.8 to 2.0 Gy for a total of 60 Gy.

HYPERFRACTIONATION AND ACCELERATED FRACTIONATION.
Altered fractionation approaches are designed to circumvent the limitation on radiation dose imposed by normal tissue tolerance. Hyperfractionation (HRT) involves the administration of two or more daily treatments in a smaller fraction than standard RT, often in 1 to 1.2 Gy. A higher dose of radiation thus could be administered in the same amount of time required for conventional fractionation (6 weeks). Maintaining a lower dose per fraction carries the theoretical advantage of reduction of late normal tissue complications (8). Accelerated hyperfractionation (AHT) involves the delivery of multiple daily fractions of standard doses (1.6 to 2.0 Gy), thus providing the total treatment over a shortened period of time. The theoretical advantage is in limiting the time interval during which tumor cells attempt to repair radiation damage and repopulation, and by maintaining small doses per fraction, avoiding additional normal tissue toxicity. It has been shown that injury to the central nervous system or radionecrosis is related directly to fraction size and inversely to the number of fractions (9).

Clinical Trials. Several clinical trials of unconventional fractionation have been published, some in conjunction with chemotherapy. The studies are difficult to compare because of the variation of individual fraction doses and total dose or the concomitant administration of sensitizing or chemotherapeutic agents. Many of these studies were nonrandomized or uncontrolled; however, the overall results do not indicate a substantial survival advantage associated with altered fractionation.

In a prospective randomized study of 157 patients with malignant gliomas, Payne and associates (10) reported no significant difference in survival or neurotoxicity between conventional and accelerated fractionation. In addition to chemotherapy, the patients received 5,000 rads in 25 daily fractions over 5 weeks, or 3,600 to 4,000 rads in 36 to 40 fractions of 100 rads four times a day over 2 weeks. In another study (11), 69 patients were randomized to receive 5,000 rads in conventional daily frac-

tions, or in 50 fractions over 4 weeks. Median survival was 13 months versus 9 months in favor of the hyperfractionated group; however, this difference was not statistically significant. Moreover, the patient subgroups were too small in number and poorly controlled for performance status, age, and histology. A more favorable study was reported in a randomized trial by Fulton and colleagues (12), who compared a regimen of 89 rads three times a day for a total of 6,140 rads (over 4.5 weeks, with and without misonidazole) to 193 rads once a day for a total of 5,800 rads over 6 weeks. The difference in survival was statistically significant: 45 to 50 weeks in the hyperfractionation group versus 29 weeks in the group receiving conventional fractionation. The same investigators conducted a later trial with escalating doses of radiation using hyperfractionation. Patients received 6,141 rads, 7,120 rads, or 8,000 rads in three daily fractions. There was no significant impact on survival or time to progression (13). More recently, the RTOG conducted a phase III trial of 712 patients randomized to receive 72.0 Gy HRT or 60 Gy in conventional daily fractions. This trial (RTOG 90-06) has not identified a survival benefit to hyperfractionation on preliminary analysis (15). Thus, current clinical data for altered fractionation do not convincingly support the theoretical advantages foreseen by radiobiologists.

BRACHYTHERAPY. Brachytherapy or interstitial irradiation refers to radiation at very short range, such as by placement of a radiation source within or in the immediate vicinity of a tumor. The rationale is to allow delivery of high-dose radiation to tumor cells while minimizing exposure of normal tissue. Radiation source placement can be planned so as to generate isodose curves conforming to the 3D target volume (16,17). The surrounding normal tissue receives a much lower dose because of rapid falloff and tissue attenuation. The most commonly used sources of radiation are ^{125}I and ^{192}Ir isotopes. Another advantage of interstitial irradiation is its low dose rate of 0.3 to 1.0 Gy per hour, compared to about 3 Gy per minute for external RT. Low-dose rate radiation favors accumulation of the rapidly proliferating tumor cells in the G2 phase of the cell cycle, when cells are most vulnerable to radiation-mediated death. Variations in radiosensitivity at different phases of the cell cycle are not clearly understood, but cells are most radioresistant during the S phase and least so during G2 and M. This differential sensitivity may relate to the cell's ability to activate DNA repair mechanisms at specific cell cycle points. Moreover, continuous low-dose radiation inhibits cells from entering or proceeding through the M phase, thus affecting repopulation. Minimizing the radioresistance exhibited by hypoxic cells offers another theoretical advantage to this approach. This may result from the fact that radioresistant hypoxic cells tend to become "reoxygenated" during continuous low-dose rate radiation and thus are more vulnerable. Alternatively, they may be further impaired in their capacity to repair radiation damage (18).

Technique. Treatment is preplanned so as to achieve an isodose contour that conforms best to the tumor volume. Radiation rate is usually 0.4 to 0.8 Gy per hour. Radioisotope sources are placed within catheters alternating with spacers of variable length. The number of seeds per catheter and total catheter number vary per tumor and per planning method. Catheters can be placed variably or through a rigid template in parallel and 1 cm apart. Treatment planning also takes into consideration the type of radioisotope used: ^{192}Ir delivers a higher energy output and is less attenuated by tissue, compared to ^{125}I. It also carries a longer half-life (74.2 versus 59.6 days) (19). The catheters are subsequently implanted in the tumor bed using CT- or MRI-guided stereotactic procedures under local or general anesthesia. Technical details regarding radiation protection, shielding, and the use of after loaders vary significantly among different centers. Catheters are removed within 1 week of placement, at the bedside or in the operating room.

Patient Selection. Patient selection also varies among treating institutions. In North America, brachytherapy has been used mostly as adjuvant treatment in patients with recurrent malignant gliomas or, perhaps less frequently, as a boost to radiation therapy (XRT) for primary disease. Patients must have a Karnofsky score of 70 or better and tumor targets have to be relatively circumscribed and not exceed 5 to 6 cm in diameter (20). Most reported data of brachytherapy treatments are the results of uncontrolled or nonrandomized retrospective series, making it difficult to establish definite conclusions. This is compounded by the fact that patient numbers per study are usually low and patient eligibility is subject to biasing criteria (e.g., a good Karnofsky score and a smaller tumor size) and therefore not readily comparable to historic controls. However, the results of most of these studies were encouraging, demonstrating improved survival in patients receiving brachytherapy (21,22). There are two randomized controlled studies reported to date. A multiinstitutional study was reported in 1995 (BTCG-8701) in which patients with newly diagnosed malignant glioma were randomized to receive XRT with or without a preceding brachytherapy boost. The results showed a significant improvement in survival in the brachytherapy group ($p < .05$). To date, the data have been published in abstract form only (23). Conflicting data from another prospective randomized trial also emerged, however. In a study by the University of Toronto, a total of 140 patients with anaplastic astrocytomas were randomized to receive external beam with or without ^{125}I implants (0.7 Gy per hour, total dose of 60 Gy) (24). The authors did not find a statistically significant difference in survival between the two groups. Selection bias was fairly well accounted for, because the two groups were balanced for age, Karnofsky Performance Status (KPS), and reoperation rate. The authors of the study acknowledge the shortcomings of a small patient number and the lack of 3D planning for the brachytherapy array placement. Definite data as to the benefit of brachytherapy remain inconclusive; therefore, any advantages may be limited to selected patients.

Complications. The rate of significant complications following brachytherapy treatment is variable. In the Univeristy of California at San Francisco series of 307 patients (25), 8% experienced severe or life-threatening complications. In the Toronto series, 15 of 63 patients (24%) suffered significant complications. These complications include infection, bleeding at the catheter site, neurological deficits, and stroke (26). The rate of reoperation is consistently elevated in most series (56% at a median of 36 weeks in the UCSF series, 64% the Brigham and Women's group series) (27). The reasons for reoperation are an increase in mass effect commonly because of a combination of radionecrosis and tumor recurrence. Dexamethasone requirements for brachytherapy patients also are consistently elevated. Patterns of recurrence are local in most cases (28).

RADIOSURGERY. The use of radiosurgery in glioma treatment is based on the improvement in survival demonstrated by escalating doses of external beam radiation (5,29). Normal tissue tolerance and plateaus at 70 Gy limit this improvement (30). Radiosurgery allows the administration of significantly increased radiation dosage within the tumor volume with very rapid falloff at normal tissue margin. This theoretical advantage is further substantiated by the local patterns of failure demonstrated by recurrent tumors. The obvious major shortcoming is the infiltrative nature of the tumor, well beyond identifiable margins. Expanding the field exposed to high-dose radiation defeats the purpose of focal treatment. Nevertheless, several authors have attempted to establish radiosurgery protocols as upfront primary treatment in the form of a local boost following external beam radiation, or as a treatment option at recurrence.

Technique. Radiosurgery (RS) is performed using precisely targeted photon beams via a gamma knife, or the linear accelerator (LINAC). A few centers have the capacity to deliver charged particles or proton beams via a cyclotron. Relatively few patients with malignant gliomas have been treated with the latter technique. The gamma knife and LINAC differ in many technical aspects, but clinical outcomes in malignant gliomas have been similar with either device and are mostly dependent on accurate planning by an experienced team. In fact, strategies used in radiosurgery planning vary significantly among investigators. Some favor isodose curves that are tightly conformal to the tumor volume, thus diminishing risk to the surrounding (often previously irradiated) normal tissue. Others prefer to include a variable margin of normal tissue within the confines of the isodose prescription in order to target infiltrating cells. Current data do not allow separate evaluation of these strategies.

Clinical Trials. Results of clinical series of radiosurgical treatment of malignant gliomas vary considerably. This is because of small patient numbers and variation of selection criteria. Mehta and co-workers (31) conducted a prospective uncontrolled study of 31 patients with glioblastoma who underwent RS in addition to 54 Gy of external beam RT. Median patient age was 57, median KPS of 70, and median tumor volume was 17.4 cc. Tumor dose ranged between a median of 12 and 18.75 Gy. Median survival was 42 weeks, which does not represent a significant improvement over historic controls. However 2-year actuarial survival was 28%, which is significantly better than an expected value derived from a comparison to previous RTOG patients treated conventionally. The authors did not encounter significant acute toxicity, but 13% of patients developed necrosis. Kondziolka and associates (32) reported a series of 64 patients with GBM and 43 patients with anaplastic astrocytoma (AA) who underwent RS in addition to conventional treatment. RS was given as adjuvant at time of primary diagnosis or at recurrence. Overall median survival for GBM was 26 months with a 2-year survival rate of 51%. For AA, survivals were 32 months and 67%, respectively. These data show a significant survival benefit for RS, when compared to historic controls, but raise the issue of selection advantage. In fact, Curran and colleagues (33) compared radiosurgery-eligible and -ineligible patients who were enrolled in RTOG 83-02, a phase I/II hyperfractionated RT trial with BCNU. The criteria they used to evaluate eligibility for a stereotactic boost were: KPS greater than 60, tumor less than 4 cc, no subependymal spread, and a location not adjacent to brainstem or optic apparatus. SRS-eligible patients were shown to have a survival benefit compared to the ineligible group. Multivariate analysis proved age, KPS, and pathology to be strongly predictive of survival. The BWH group (34) also reported a median survival of 26 months from the time of diagnosis in their GBM patients treated with conventional RT and a 10- to 20-Gy stereotactic boost. Age under 40 was a statistically significant variable predictive of improved survival.

Complications. Acute complications have been reported in some studies. They typically consist of edema, mass effect, confusion, memory loss, focal neurological signs, or seizures (35, 36). Chronic complications are consistently reported when patients are followed for 12 months or more. They include headaches, numbness, weakness, ataxia, radionecrosis, cranial nerve damage, visual changes, focal neurological signs, and others. Late complication rates vary from 13% (31) to 27% (37).

Dexamethasone requirements and reoperation rates for radiation-induced necrosis also are more elevated.

Brachytherapy versus Radiosurgery. Radiosurgery and brachytherapy are often compared (38). Both techniques provide highly focal radiation with normal tissue sparing. Radiosurgery is less invasive and avoids catheter complications. Radiosurgical planning is probably more accurate and provides a more homogeneous distribution within the target volume. Brachytherapy, on the other hand, can target much larger volumes and might possess a biological advantage in its low-dose rate delivery. Advances in radiosurgery planning and the possibility of stereotactic fractionation will probably lead to the eventual replacement of brachytherapy, as is already the case in many institutions. Although there are no randomized trials comparing the two techniques, the BWH group conducted a retrospective study of their brachytherapy and RS patients and found similar median survival and 2-year survival rates (38).

Radiosurgery can be an effective tool in gaining local control in the management of malignant gliomas, but outcome is highly dependent on favorable selection criteria, such as smaller tumor volumes and better KPS. The EORTC has now proposed a randomized study of focal fractionated stereotactic boost following conventional treatment in patients with malignant gliomas (EORTC 22972) (39). This study should provide some guidelines as to the indications and effectiveness of radiosurgery.

RADIATION SENSITIZERS. A radiation sensitizer is a compound that modulates the response to radiation, leading to amplified tumor cell kill while minimizing injury to normal tissue. Tumor radioresistance is a wide topic that is beyond the scope of this chapter but is discussed in great detail in many publications. Briefly, radioresistance is the result of complex interactions among dynamic factors, such as the genetic makeup of the cell, which is a parameter subject to mutations, and many microenvironmental variables. One of the major and better-described contributing factors to radiation resistance is hypoxia. In fact, hypoxic cells are three to five times more radioresistant than normally oxygenated cells. Radiation sensitizers (e.g., nitroimidazole compounds) bind to large molecules in the cell under hypoxic conditions. They can act as electron donors on irradiation of the cell, leading to an increase in free radicals and DNA damage. Early experience with these compounds was discouraging. Newer generation nitroimidazole chemicals, such as etanidazole, are more promising owing to lower toxicity and higher tumor penetration. A phase I trial has already been conducted and maximal dose tolerance determined (40,41). Further RTOG trials have been proposed. Another approach to sensitization of hypoxic tumor cells consists of increasing the oxygen-carrying capacity of blood and subsequently of the tumor environment using perfluorocarbons (e.g., Fluosol). Evans and colleagues (42) conducted a pilot study using Fluosol along with external beam RT in patients with malignant gliomas but found no survival benefit.

Other classes of radiation sensitizers have also been investigated. These include halogenated pyrimidine analogues, such as BUdR and IUdR. These compounds act independently of oxygen and become incorporated in rapidly proliferating cells by substituting for thymidine during DNA synthesis. The mechanism of radiosensitization is unclear. Clinical studies have not shown a significant improvement in survival or time to progression in glioblastoma (43), but were more encouraging in anaplastic astrocytoma. In a NCOG/UCSF uncontrolled study of 148 patients with AA treated with BUdR during radiation, followed by chemotherapy, median survival was 5 years (44). However a recently published randomized phase III study (RTOG 9404) (45), comparing external beam RT and PCV chemotherapy with and without BUdR sensitization in 189 patients, had to curtail enrollment and close before full accrual. This was because of an interim analysis suggesting a lack of benefit to the addition of BUdR. There were early deaths in the BUdR arm apparently not related to toxicity. A final analysis of this data is pending. Other compounds under investigation as potentiators of radiation therapy include paclitaxel (46,47) (Taxol) and cisplatin/carboplatin, both of which have failed to demonstrate a significant impact in preliminary studies.

Although the clinical use of radiation sensitizers has not resulted in significant progress in glioma therapy so far, it has allowed a better understanding of mechanisms of radioresistance, particularly those involved in hypoxia.

Low-Grade Gliomas

Low-grade gliomas (LGG) are a group of heterogeneous slowly proliferating tumors. Histopathologically, they are classified as oligodendrogliomas, astrocytomas, or mixed oligoastrocytomas and graded as WHO grade I or II. Astrocytomas are further subdivided according to histologic characteristics: pilocytic (grade I), fibrillary, pleomorphic xanthoastrocytoma. They are characterized by an initially indolent clinical presentation and slow but progressive and infiltrating growth. The biology of these tumors is poorly understood, particularly their rate of progression into a more malignant phenotype. Management remains controversial and comprises a range of options, including observation with or without biopsy, surgery with or without radiation, and chemotherapy.

Earlier retrospective studies have demonstrated a beneficial role for postoperative radiation in patients older than 30 or 40 years of age. However, these studies did not distinguish between pilocytic tumors and other low-grade astrocytomas (LGA). Pilocytic astrocytomas have a distinctly better prognosis independently of RT and occur in younger individuals (48,49). Leibel and associates (50) reviewed the UCSF experience over 25 years, whereby patients with LGG underwent subtotal resection followed by observation or radiation. The 5-year survival rate differed significantly and reached 19% versus 46%, respectively. Patients with gemistocytic astrocytomas fared significantly worse. Shaw and colleagues (51) report a similar experience from the Mayo Clinic, whereby patients with astrocytomas or mixed oligoastrocytomas had an improved 5- and 10-year survival rate when surgery was followed by radiation when compared to surgery alone. Patients with pilocytic astrocytomas fared best and did not show evidence of improved survival after radiation. However, the preceding studies consist of class II or III data, as does most literature regarding LGG and radiation. An exception may be the EORTC/MRC phase III study, a randomized controlled trial (52) (EORTC 22845) that may provide class I data but is published in abstract form only. A total of 311 patients with grade II astrocytoma, oligodendroglioma, or mixed histology were randomized to receive 54 Gy immediately postoperatively (incomplete resection or biopsy) or at time of recurrence as documented by imaging and neurological evidence. The study concluded that immediate postoperative RT improves the progression-free survival (5-year, 47% versus 37%, $p = .02$) but not the overall survival (5-year, 63% versus 66%, $p = .49$). Another EORTC trial (22844) (53) had previously determined the absence of a radiotherapeutic dose-response for patients with LGG at least for two dose levels investigated (45 and 59.4 Gy), while recognizing tumor size as an important prognostic factor. Of note is a follow-up study investigating quality of life following high- or low-dose radiation among patients enrolled in EORTC 22844 (54). Higher radiation doses were associated with a greater incidence of fatigue, insomnia, and poor emotional functioning.

A major question in the management of LGG, for which current evidence is not decisive, concerns the timing of intervention. Some clinicians opt to defer therapy until patients are symptomatic or develop uncontrollable seizures. Others refer patients to surgery only if the tumor appears to be totally resectable. The majority of LGG in fact are not amenable to a true complete resection because of large infiltration or involvement of speech or other highly functional areas. A major modulating factor in assessing current data is patient selection. Clinicians use several prognostic variables to a variable extent in determining a treatment course. The presence of one or a combination of the following findings is often considered a basis for intervention. These include: presence of enhancement or mass effect, age more than 40 years, lobar versus diffuse tumor, or presence of a neurological deficit other than controllable seizures. Therefore, the interpretation of nonrandomized studies is significantly biased. The young patient (less than 40 years old) who is asymptomatic or presents with seizures but is otherwise intact and has no mass effect or enhancement on MRI presents the greatest dilemma. The EORTC randomized study answered some of these questions but only partially, leaving management of these difficult cases open to significant variation.

References

1. Thornton AF Jr, Hegarty TJ, Ten Haken RK, et al. Three-dimensional treatment planning of astrocytomas: a dosimetric study of cerebral irradiation. *Int J Radiat Oncol Biol Phys* 1991;20:1309–1315.
2. Walker MD, Alexander E Jr, Hunt WE, et al. Evaluation of BCNU and/or radiotherapy in the treatment of anaplastic gliomas. A cooperative clinical trial. *J Neurosurg* 1978;49:333–343.
3. Walker MD, Green SB, Byar DP, et al. Randomized comparisons of radiotherapy and nitrosoureas for the treatment of malignant glioma after surgery. *N Engl J Med* 1980;303:1323–1329.
4. Kristiansen K, Hagen S, Kollevold T, et al. Combined modality therapy of operated astrocytomas grade III and IV. Confirmation of the value of postoperative irradiation and lack of potentiation of bleomycin on survival time: a prospective multicenter trial of the Scandinavian Glioblastoma Study Group. *Cancer* 1981;47:649–652.
5. Bleehen NM, Stenning SP. A Medical Research Council trial of two radiotherapy doses in the treatment of grades 3 and 4 astrocytoma. The Medical Research Council Brain Tumour Working Party. *Br J Cancer* 1991;64:769–774.
6. Chang CH, Horton J, Schoenfeld D, et al. Comparison of postoperative radiotherapy and combined postoperative radiotherapy and chemotherapy in the multidisciplinary management of malignant gliomas. A joint Radiation Therapy Oncology Group and Eastern Cooperative Oncology Group study. *Cancer* 1983;52:997–1007.
7. Wallner KE, Galicich JH, Krol G, et al. Patterns of failure following treatment for glioblastoma multiforme and anaplastic astrocytoma. *Int J Radiat Oncol Biol Phys* 1989;16:1405–1409.
8. Withers HR. Biologic basis for altered fractionation schemes. *Cancer* 1985;55:2086–2095.
9. Sheline GE. Radiation therapy of brain tumors. *Cancer* 1977;39:873–881.
10. Payne DG, Simpson WJ, Keen C, et al. Malignant astrocytoma: hyperfractionated and standard radiotherapy with chemotherapy in a randomized prospective clinical trial. *Cancer* 1982;50:2301–2306.
11. Shin KH, Muller PJ, Geggie PH. Superfractionation radiation therapy in the treatment of malignant astrocytoma. *Cancer* 1983;52:2040–2043.
12. Fulton DS, Urtasun RC, Shin KH, et al. Misonidazole combined with hyperfractionation in the management of malignant glioma. *Int J Radiat Oncol Biol Phys* 1984;10:1709–1712.
13. Fulton DS, Urtasun RC, Scott-Brown I, et al. Increasing radiation dose intensity using hyperfractionation in patients with malignant glioma. Final report of a prospective phase I-II dose response study. *J Neurooncol* 1992;14:63–72.
14. Deleted in proof.
15. Scott CB, Scarantino C, Urtasun R, et al. Validation and predictive power of Radiation Therapy Oncology Group RTOG. Recursive partitioning analysis classes for malignant glioma patients: a report using RTOG 90-06. *Int J Radiat Oncol Biol Phys* 1998;40:51–55.
16. Weaver K, Smith V, Lewis JD, et al. A CT-based computerized treatment planning system for I-125 stereotactic brain implants. *Int J Radiat Oncol Biol Phys* 1990;18:445–454.
17. Anderson LL, Harrington PJ, Osian AD, et al. A versatile method for planning stereotactic brain implants. *Med Phys* 1993;20:1457–1464.
18. Hall EJ. *Radiobiology for the radiologist*. Philadelphia: JB Lippincott, 1994.
19. Weaver KA, Anderson LL, Meli JA. Source characteristics. In: Anderson LL, Nath R, Weaver KA, et al, eds. *Interstitial brachytherapy: physical, biological and clinical considerations*. New York: Raven, 2001:3–19.
20. Sneed PK, Gutin PH. Issues in the use of conventional and altered fractionation radiation therapy for pediatric and adult gliomas. In: Berger MS, Wilson CB, eds. *The gliomas*. Philadelphia: WB Saunders, 2001:480–488.
21. Wen P, Alexander III E, Black P, et al. Long term results of stereotactic brachytherapy used in the initial treatment of patients with glioblastomas. *Cancer* 1994;73:3029–3036.
22. Sneed PK, Prados MD, McDermott MW, et al. Large effect of age on the survival of patients with glioblastoma treated with radiotherapy and brachytherapy boost. *Neurosurgery* 1995;36:898–903.
23. Shapiro WR, Green S, Burger P, et al. A randomized trial of interstitial radiotherapy IRT boost for the treatment of newly-diagnosed malignant glioma glioblastoma-multiforme, anaplastic astrocytoma, anaplastic oligodendroglioma, malignant mixed glioma. BTCG study-8701. *Neurology* 1994;44:A263–A263.
24. Laperriere NJ, Leung PM, McKenzie S, et al. Randomized study of brachytherapy in the initial management of patients with malignant astrocytoma. *Int J Radiat Oncol Biol Phys* 1998;41:1005–1011.
25. Scharfen CO, Sneed PK, Wara WM, et al. High activity iodine-125 interstitial implant for gliomas. *Int J Radiat Oncol Biol Phys* 1992;24:583–591.
26. Bernstein M, Lumley M, Davidson G, et al. Intracranial arterial occlusion associated with high-activity iodine-125 brachytherapy for glioblastoma. *J Neurooncol* 1993;17:253–260.
27. Wen PY, Alexander E, III, Black PM, et al. Long term results of stereotactic brachytherapy used in the initial treatment of patients with glioblastomas. *Cancer* 1994;73:3029–3036.
28. Agbi CB, Bernstein M, Laperriere N, et al. Patterns of recurrence of malignant astrocytoma following stereotactic interstitial brachytherapy with iodine-125 implants. *Int J Radiat Oncol Biol Phys* 1992;23:321–326.
29. Walker MD, Strike TA, Sheline GE. An analysis of dose-effect relationship in the radiotherapy of malignant gliomas. *Int J Radiat Oncol Biol Phys* 1979;5:1725–1731.
30. Nelson DF, Diener-West M, Horton J, et al. Combined modality approach to treatment of malignant gliomas—re-evaluation of RTOG 7401/ECOG 1374 with long-term follow-up: a joint study of the Radiation Therapy Oncology Group and the Eastern Cooperative Oncology Group. *NCI Monogr* 1988;279–284.
31. Mehta MP, Masciopinto J, Rozental J, et al. Stereotactic radiosurgery for glioblastoma multiforme: report of a prospective study evaluating prognostic factors and analyzing long-term survival advantage [see comments]. *Int J Radiat Oncol Biol Phys* 1994;30:541–549.
32. Kondziolka D, Flickinger JC, Bissonette DJ, et al. Survival benefit of stereotactic radiosurgery for patients with malignant glial neoplasms. *Neurosurgery* 1997;41:776–783.
33. Curran WJ Jr, SCOTT CB, Weinstein AS, et al. Survival comparison of radiosurgery-eligible and -ineligible malignant glioma patients treated with hyperfractionated radiation therapy and carmustine: a report of Radiation Therapy Oncology Group 83-02. *J Clin Oncol* 1993;11:857–862.
34. Loeffler JS, Alexander E, III, Shea WM, et al. Radiosurgery as part

of the initial management of patients with malignant gliomas [see comments]. *J Clin Oncol* 1992;10:1379–1385.

35. Larson DA, Gutin P, McDermott MW, et al. Experience with gamma knife radiosurgery in the United States. *Proceedings of the US-Japan Radiation Oncology Conference*, San Francisco, 1995.

36. Shrieve DC, Alexander E III, Wen PY, et al. Comparison of stereotactic radiosurgery and brachytherapy in the treatment of recurrent glioblastoma multiforme. *Neurosurgery* 1995;36:275–282.

37. Buatti JM, Friedman WA, Bova FJ, et al. LINAC radiosurgery for high-grade gliomas: the University of Florida experience. *Int J Radiat Oncol Biol Phys* 1995;32:205–210.

38. Alexander E, Loeffler JS. The role of radiosurgery for glial neoplasms. *Neurosurg Clin N Am* 1999;10:351–358.

39. Brada M, Baumert B. Focal fractionated conformal stereotactic boost following conventional radiotherapy of high-grade gliomas: a randomized phase III study. A joint study of the EORTC 22972 and the MRC BR10. *Front Radiat Ther Oncol* 1999;33:241–243.

40. Wasserman TH, Lee DJ, Cosmatos D, et al. Clinical trials with etanidazole SR-2508 by the Radiation Therapy Oncology Group RTOG. *Radiother Oncol* 1991;20(suppl 1):129–135.

41. Reise N, Loeffler J, When P. Results of a Phase I trial using radiotherapy and etanidazole in malignant glioma patients. *Proceedings of the 8th International Conference of Chemical Modifiers of Cancer Treatment*, Kyoto, Japan, 1993:345.

42. Evans RG, Kimler BF, Morantz RA, et al. Lack of complications in long-term survivors after treatment with Fluosol and oxygen as an adjuvant to radiation therapy for high-grade brain tumors. *Int J Radiat Oncol Biol Phys* 1993;26:649–652.

43. Phillips TL, Levin VA, Ahn DK, et al. Evaluation of bromodeoxyuridine in glioblastoma multiforme: a Northern California Cancer Center Phase II study [see comments]. *Int J Radiat Oncol Biol Phys* 1991;21:709–714.

44. Levin VA, Prados MR, Wara WM, et al. Radiation therapy and bromodeoxyuridine chemotherapy followed by procarbazine, lomustine, and vincristine for the treatment of anaplastic gliomas. *Int J Radiat Oncol Biol Phys* 1995;32:75–83.

45. Prados MD, Scott C, Sandler H, et al. A phase 3 randomized study of radiotherapy plus procarbazine, CCNU, and vincristine PCV with or without BUdR for the treatment of anaplastic astrocytoma: a preliminary report of RTOG 9404 [see comments]. *Int J Radiat Oncol Biol Phys* 1999;45:1109–1115.

46. Prados MD, Schold SC, Spence AM, et al. Phase II study of paclitaxel in patients with recurrent malignant glioma. *J Clin Oncol* 1996;14:2316–2321.

47. Forsyth P, Cairncross G, Stewart D, et al. Phase II trial of docetaxel in patients with recurrent malignant glioma: a study of the National Cancer Institute of Canada Clinical Trials Group. *Invest New Drugs* 1996;14:203–206.

48. Garcia DM, Fulling KH, Marks JE. The value of radiation therapy in addition to surgery for astrocytomas of the adult cerebrum. *Cancer* 1985;55:919–927.

49. Laws ER Jr, Taylor WF, Clifton MB, et al. Neurosurgical management of low-grade astrocytoma of the cerebral hemispheres. *J Neurosurg* 1984;61:665–673.

50. Leibel SA, Sheline GE, Wara WM, et al. The role of radiation therapy in the treatment of astrocytomas. *Cancer* 1975;35:1551–1557.

51. Shaw EG, Daumas-Duport C, Scheithauer BW, et al. Radiation therapy in the management of low-grade supratentorial astrocytomas. *J Neurosurg* 1989;70:853–861.

52. Karim AB, Cornu P, Bleehen NM, et al. Immediate post-operative radiotherapy in low grade glioma improves progression free survival, but not overall survival: preliminary results of an EORTC/MRC randomized phase III study. *J Clin Oncol* 1998;17:400a.

53. Karim AB, Maat B, Hatlevoll R, et al. A randomized trial on dose-response in radiation therapy of low-grade cerebral glioma: European Organization for Research and Treatment of Cancer EORTC. Study 22844. *Int J Radiat Oncol Biol Phys* 1996;36:549–556.

54. Kiebert GM, Curran D, Aaronson NK, et al. Quality of life after radiation therapy of cerebral low-grade gliomas of the adult: results of a randomised phase III trial on dose response EORTC trial 22844. EORTC Radiotherapy Co-operative Group. *Eur J Cancer* 1998;34:1902–1909.

106. Innovative Treatments for Intracranial Gliomas

Wei Zhang, Chiedozie Nwagwu, and William T. Couldwell

Malignant gliomas present a formidable clinical challenge. In the United States, approximately 13,000 new cases of primary brain tumors are diagnosed yearly and brain tumors are the fourth leading cause of death in both genders in the age range between 15 and 34 years (1). About 80% of these new primary brain tumors are gliomas (2). According to the World Health Organization (WHO), diffuse cerebral gliomas have been classified based on histological characteristics: low-grade gliomas (astrocytoma and oligodendroglioma), anaplastic gliomas, and glioblastoma multiforme (WHO grade IV). Over 50% of newly diagnosed primary brain tumors are anaplastic gliomas or glioblastomas (3). The prognosis for patients with malignant gliomas has not significantly changed despite advances in surgery, radiation therapy, and cytotoxic chemotherapy. The median survival of patients diagnosed with high-grade gliomas remains estimated at 26 to 52 weeks (4). It is clear that new strategies aimed at novel therapeutic targets are needed to combat these devastating tumors. In this chapter, such therapeutic strategies as targeting glioma signal transduction pathways, glioma invasion and angiogenesis, gene therapy, and glioma immunotherapy are discussed.

Therapy Targeting Glioma Signal Transduction Pathways

Cellular proliferation, migration, differentiation, and eventual apoptosis (programmed cell death) normally are tightly regulated processes that depend on complex signaling mechanisms. Aberrations in a number of signal transduction pathways have been identified as playing a key role in the molecular pathogenesis of gliomas. These signaling mechanisms use small molecules—mostly polypeptides—that interact with their cognate

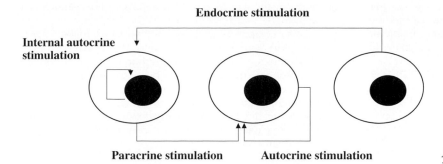

Fig. 1. Schematic representation of intercellular and internal signaling.

receptors. Potential approaches to more effective treatment of gliomas have developed from further understanding of the molecular basis of tumorigenesis. An increase in gene expression of growth factors and their receptors has been implicated in the genesis and progression of most human neoplasms. Growth factors have been shown to stimulate tumor proliferation, angiogenesis, and invasion by the formation of autocrine and paracrine stimulatory loops. Autocrine stimulation occurs when a tumor cell secretes both a particular growth factor and its corresponding receptor, whereas paracrine stimulation involves the production of a ligand adjacent to its site of action (Fig. 1). The major signal transduction pathways that play a role in the pathogenesis of malignant gliomas and some agents that have been developed to target these aberrant pathways in glioma cells are discussed in the following.

RECEPTOR PROTEIN TYROSINE KINASES AND THEIR INHIBITORS.

Malignant gliomas are characterized by overexpression or mutation of genes that encode a variety of growth factors and their receptors, particularly the receptors for epidermal growth factor (EGF), platelet-derived growth factor (PDGF), and vascular endothelial growth factor (VEGF). There are four major classes of receptors and ligands that activate these receptors on the basis of similar structural and functional characteristics (Fig. 2). Among them, the first three are receptors expressed at the cell surface that bind extracellular ligands. The first class of receptors is activated by a number of neurotransmitters and hormones. Their structure is similar in that they contain seven transmembranous domains, and they are functionally similar in that their activation results in the activation of heterotrimeric G-proteins. The second major class of receptors is the receptor protein tyrosine kinases (RPTKs). An extracellular domain that binds the polypeptide growth factors, hydrophobic membrane-spanning region, and cytoplasmic tyrosine kinase domain that transduces the extracellular signal to the cell characterize these receptors. Signal transduction occurs by ligand-induced stabilization of receptor homodimers or heterodimers, followed by receptor autophosphorylation and recruitment of specific intracellular signaling proteins, which initiates downstream signaling cascades. The third class of receptors is ligand-gated ion channels. The fourth major class of receptors differs

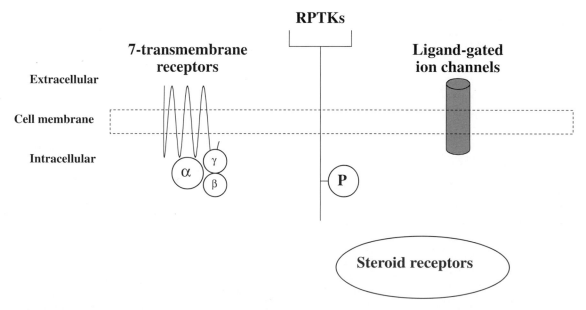

Fig. 2. Schematic representation of the four major receptor types in mammalian cells: *1,* 7-transmembrane receptors that are activated by a number of neurotransmitters (dopamine γ-aminobutyric acid A, serotonin) and hormones (glucagons, adrenocorticotropic hormone, luteinizing hormone, thyroid-stimulating hormone). *2,* Single transmembrane domain receptor protein tyrosine kinases. *3,* Ligand-gated ion channels that do not activate downstream signaling. *4,* Receptors of steroid hormones, which are lipophilic and located within the cytoplasm.

from the other three in that they are not surface-bound, but located within the cytoplasm. These receptors are activated by steroid hormones that are lipophilic, and thus are capable of crossing the plasma membrane, which most other polypeptide ligands cannot.

Among the four major receptor classes, the receptor protein tyrosine kinases have been clearly linked to the pathogenesis of gliomas. These receptors are so named because they are activated when specific tyrosine residues on the intracellular domain of the receptor are phosphorylated. Ligand binding occurs on the extracellular domain of RPTK, resulting in receptor dimerization. The kinase domain of one receptor phosphorylates specific tyrosine residues on the intracellular domain of the other receptor, and vice versa, through this dimerization. This is a process known as transautophosphorylation. The activated receptor's phosphotyrosine residues are then targets for signaling proteins, which recognize the phosphotyrosine residues in the context of specific adjacent amino acids. RPTKs are known to play an important role in cellular proliferation, migration, differentiation, and apoptosis, particularly during embryogenesis. To date, 14 subclasses of RPTKs have been described, largely on the basis of structural similarities. Because two major RPTKs—PDGFR and EGFR—are implicated in the pathogenesis of human gliomas, recent work has concentrated

on inhibiting the activation of these RPTKs for novel antiglioma therapy (5).

A variety of approaches have been taken to inhibit RPTKs, including: (a) disrupting the initial autophosphorylation of the receptor and the subsequent phosphorylation of its downstream substrates; (b) inhibiting the binding of the growth factor to its particular receptor; and (c) inhibiting the activity of one of the downstream signal transduction pathways (Fig. 3). The success of tyrosine kinase inhibitors depends on their selectivity, cell permeability, bioavailability, pharmacokinetic properties, and degree of toxicity.

Tyrosine kinase inhibitors can be divided into two classes: naturally occurring inhibitors and synthetic organic compounds (tyrphostins). Certain naturally occurring fungal-derived tyrosine kinase inhibitors have shown promise, including quercetin, genistein, erbstatin, herbimysin A, and lavendustin A. The major disadvantage of these agents is their nonspecific tyrosine kinase inhibitory spectrum, but they have served as useful models for the development of more selective kinase inhibitors. Genistein, which is found in soybean foods, is a potent competitive inhibitor of adenosine triphosphate (ATP) in kinase reactions and a noncompetitive inhibitor of the protein substrate. However, tyrphostins can more specifically inhibit protein tyrosine ki-

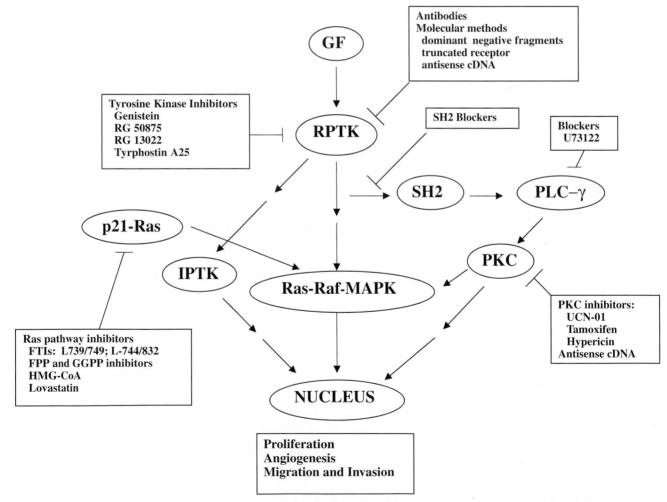

Fig. 3. Currently studied agents and methods targeting signal transduction pathways of malignant gliomas. *FTI,* farnesyl transferase inhibitor; *FPP,* farnesyl diphosphate; *GF,* growth factor; *GGPP,* geranylgeranyl diphosphate; *HMG-CoA,* 3-hydroxy-3-methylglutaryl-CoA; *IPTK,* intracellular protein tyrosine kinase; *MAPK,* mitogen-activated protein kinase; *PKC,* protein kinase C; *PLC,* phospholipase C; *RPTK,* receptor protein tyrosine kinase; *SH2,* Src homology 2.

nases compared with other kinases, because they act by competing for the substrate site and not the ATP binding site.

Most tyrosine kinase inhibitors have been studied in cell culture and in *in vivo* animal experiments. In one study with two human glioma cell lines, genistein was shown to inhibit both EGF- and PDGF-stimulated autophosphorylation of the receptors and induction of DNA synthesis. In this same study, two tyrphostins—RG13022 and RG50875—demonstrated a dose-dependent reduction in DNA synthesis, and RG13022 was able to completely inhibit it. The selective PDGFR-inhibitor, leflunomide (SU101) has been shown to inhibit PDGF-mediated signaling events, including receptor tyrosine phosphorylation, DNA synthesis, cell cycle progression, and cell proliferation in C6 rat glioma cells (6). Other strategies also have been used to block the activation of PDGF receptors. PDGF-neutralizing antibodies and a truncated receptor have been used successfully to antagonize PDGF-mediated effects on glioma cells. In fact, the truncated PDGF receptor was shown to impair the growth of glioma cells transplanted as a xenograft in nude mice.

Limited data are available on the clinical use of tyrosine kinase inhibitors in patients with gliomas. The selective PDGFR inhibitor SU101 has been shown to be safe in human phase I clinical trials; phase II trials recently were completed (7). Fifteen patients with recurrent malignant gliomas refractory to treatment were given a loading dose followed by a weekly maintenance dose. This administration schedule was shown to be optimal for SU101. Three patients showed minor responses with a duration of 18 to 56 weeks, and three had stable disease for 16 to 26 weeks. The remainder had no response to treatment (7).

RAS PATHWAY AND ITS INHIBITORS. Activation of PDGFR and EGFR results in receptor tyrosine phosphorylation and the recruitment of adapter signaling proteins, which initiate a cascade resulting in the activation of Ras. Ras is a 21-kDa protein that is now known to play a pivotal role in normal cell proliferation, differentiation, and apoptosis. Recent studies indicate that p21-Ras is significantly overactive in high-grade gliomas, although these tumors demonstrate an extremely low rate of mutations in Ras (8). Three genes encode four Ras proteins (H-Ras, N-Ras, K4A-Ras, K4B-Ras), and these proteins resemble the α-subunit of heterotrimeric G proteins in their function. It is becoming increasingly evident that Ras activation results in further signal transduction down multiple pathways, because a large number of Ras effector molecules have been discovered. The best-documented and -understood proliferative pathway downstream of Ras is the mitogen activated protein kinase (MAPK) pathway. This pathway is initiated with the activation of the 70- to 75-kDa serine/threonine kinase Raf, which then activates MAPK kinase (MAP/ERK kinase, MEK). MEK is a dual specificity (tyrosine and serine/threonine) kinase. Activated MEK phosphorylates the MAPK proteins ERK1 (p44) and ERK2 (p42) (extracellular-signal regulated kinase, ERK) at both a tyrosine and threonine residue. These proteins are able to phosphorylate a wide range of substrates, both within the cytosol and nucleus. It has been reported that EGF and PDGF stimulation of established human astrocytoma cells as well as operative glioblastoma multiforme specimens resulted in their cognate receptors being activated and complexing with upstream activators of p21-Ras, suggesting that growth factor-mediated proliferative signaling indeed utilized p21-Ras–mediated signal transduction in these cells. Therefore, there has been great interest in developing pharmacological agents that inhibit the Ras signaling pathway (Fig. 3).

p21-Ras requires posttranslational "lipid modification" for localization to the cell membrane, where it plays a pivotal role in growth signaling. Ras pathway inhibition has focused in particular on the generation of farnesyltransferase inhibitors (FTIs), which block this posttranslation modification of Ras. Various FTIs, including L-739,749, L-744,832, and BMS-191563 have been evaluated for their ability to inhibit the progression of a large number of human tumor cell lines. All these three FTIs showed growth inhibition, and L-744,832 produced a profound inhibitory effect (100% tumoricide) with an IC_{50} ranging between 2 and 17 μM.

Competitive inhibitors (peptidominetics) of farnesyl diphosphate (FPP) and geranylgeranyl diphosphate (GGPP), as well as tetrapeptide analogues of the C AAX (cysteine, aliphatic amino acid, aliphatic amino acid, other amino acid), can disturb the posttranslational modification process. Recent studies have demonstrated that three C AAX-peptidominetics p21-Ras inhibitors (FTase inhibitor FTI-27; GGTase I inhibitors GGTI-286 and GGTI-298) significantly antagonize glioma proliferation. Each of the tested mimics produced profound inhibition of proliferation in two established glioblastoma cell lines (U87 and LN-Z308) and a low-passage pediatric high-grade glioma cell line (SG-388) with median effective concentrations ranging between 3 and 12 μM, which was compatible with median inhibitory concentrations found in other tumor models. The efficacy of farnesyltransferase inhibition also has been examined in a series of preliminary animal glioma model studies. In a nude mouse subcutaneous model, administration of FTI-276 at a dose of 50 mg/kg per day using a continuous infusion osmotic minipump for 7 days produced a significant delay in the growth of U87 xenografts. Objective tumor regression was observed in three of four inhibitor-treated mice; two of these animals achieved durable (>90 days) complete remissions without further treatment. Comparable treatment in an intracranial xenograft model also produced a significant delay in tumor growth with a median survival of 80 ± 10 days in five FTI-276-treated animals versus 59 ± 7 days in six controls. None of the drug-treated animals exhibited weight loss or any other signs of overt toxicity from the inhibitor.

To date, clinical application of p21-Ras inhibition has been largely restricted to non-central nervous system (CNS) tumors. Because Ras and related G-proteins play important roles in normal cellular physiology, clinical use of Ras inhibitors raises concerns about the potential for undeserved side effects. At present, the inhibitors for Ras pathway, such as farnesyltransferase inhibitors, are not specific and face drug resistance of tumor cells, as well as inefficient cell penetration and metabolic instability owing to rapid degradation. The application of these agents to the treatment of patients with high-grade gliomas will necessitate further studies. In fact, a phase I/II clinical trial of lovastatin has been completed for a series of patients harboring malignant glioma (9), which showed that high doses of lovastatin are well tolerated with concurrent radiation. This suggests that CNS toxicity will not be significantly limiting as more selective farnesyltransferase inhibitors are brought to trial as radiation sensitizers.

PROTEIN KINASE C INHIBITORS. Protein kinase C (PKC) is a large family of phospholipid-dependent serine/threonine kinases with at least 11 defined members for mammalian cells, which are involved in a variety of signal transduction pathways. Three classes of PKC isoforms have been described based on their activation by calcium and diacylglycerol. The first group consists of four "conventional" PKC isoenzymes (cPKC)—α, β1, β2, and γ—which require calcium, diacylglycerol, and phosphatidylserine, or alternatively tumor-promoting phorbol ester, for their activation. The second group includes five "novel" PKC isoforms (nPKC)—δ, ε, η, θ, and μ—which lack the C2 region, a putative Ca^{2+}-binding domain, and thus do not require Ca^{2+} for activation. The last group comprises two "atypical" PKC isoenzymes (aPKC)—ξ and λ. aPKCs require neither calcium nor diacylglycerol or phorbol esters, but only phosphatidylserine for activation because they likewise lack the Ca^{2+}-binding C2 region and contain an atypical C1 region. The set of isoenzymes expressed in a cell varies during development, transformation, differentiation, and senescence. PKC is expressed at high levels in normal brain tissue and is important in normal development. Activation of PKC in fetal neonatal glial cells leads to marked proliferation and differentiation, a phenomenon not observed in adult glial cells. Numerous studies have demonstrated that PKC is dramatically overexpressed in neoplastic astrocytes in comparison with nonneoplastic adult glial cells, perhaps as a result of dedifferentiation. Certain isozymes appear to be particularly overexpressed, with some reports demonstrating marked overexpression of the α isoform (10). Transfection of astrocytomas with antisense constructs directed against the α isoform of PKC has resulted in reversion of the malignant phenotype in some experiments. Other PKC isozymes expressed in astrocytomas at high levels include the γ, ε, and ξ isoforms. The observations that PKC is overexpressed and overactive in malignant gliomas and represents a common downstream effector of growth factor signaling have fostered significant interest in targeting this enzyme as a means of inhibiting glioma growth.

To date, a variety of nonspecific and specific PKC inhibitors have been used to determine whether direct inhibition of PKC would effectively control glioma cell proliferation without causing unacceptable systemic toxicity (Fig. 3). Tamoxifen, a triphenylethylene antiestrogen, has been extensively studied. It produces modest inhibition of tyrosine kinases, PKC, cAMP-dependent protein kinase and calmodulin-dependent protein kinase. Multiple clinical trials have shown that tamoxifen is associated with a modest increase in duration of survival, clinical stabilization of disease, and tumor regression. In a study of chronic oral high-dose tamoxifen administration in 32 patients with malignant glioma, 25% of the patients (eight of 32) demonstrated a 50% decrease in the volume of lesion enhancement on magnetic resonance imaging, and an additional 19% (six of 32) exhibited stabilization of disease (11). However, a limitation in the clinical application of tamoxifen is its weak potency and poor specificity as a PKC inhibitor. Accordingly, current work has focused on more potent and selective inhibitors of PKC. One such compound is 7-hydroxy-staurosporine (UCN-01). UCN-01 produced inhibition of glioma growth *in vitro* with 100-fold greater potency than tamoxifen. The ED_{50} values for inhibition of proliferation of 20 to 100 nM correlated closely with the *in vitro* IC_{50} values for PKC inhibition of 20 to 60 nM. Animal studies in rat subcutaneous and intracranial glioma models showed reduced tumor size and increased survival (12). A phase I study of this agent in patients with progressive malignant gliomas is underway based on these results. Recently, a naturally occurring plant compound, hypericin, has been studied in patients with malignant gliomas (13). Hypericin is an aromatic polycyclic dine derived from plants of the *Hypericum* family (Saint John's wort, *Hypericum perforatum*). The molecular structure of hypericin is similar to calphostin C, a relatively potent inhibitor of protein kinases, especially PKC. *In vitro*, hypericin inhibits cell proliferation, induces apoptosis, enhances radiosensitivity, and inhibits cell invasion at concentrations in the low micromolar range in glioma cells. A clinical trial of hypericin has been undertaken in patients with recurrent malignant gliomas that had failed to respond to radiation therapy with or without standard chemotherapy.

Antisense-based PKC inhibition also is an avenue explored for experimental glioma therapy. As there is substantial evidence that an increase in PKCα expression might be a general finding in proliferating astrocytes that accounts for their elevated PKC activity, this isoform might comprise a favorable target for selective inhibition of glioma proliferation. Several groups have employed recombinant DNA technology to block

PKCα expression on translational levels. Yazaki and associates demonstrated that the growth of glioblastoma multiforme can be suppressed by an antisense S-oligodeoxynucleotide against the 3'-untranslated region PKCα mRNA in subcutaneous and intracranial mouse tumor models (14). However, it is not yet available for clinical use because of present difficulties with delivery of the antisense agents.

Gene Therapy for Gliomas

One of the most exciting areas of molecular biology is the potential for gene therapy, in which either modifying the expression of a mutant gene or introducing new genetic information into defective tissue *in vivo* would treat a given disease. Gene therapy refers to the transfer of genetic material into mammalian cells with the aim of eliciting a therapeutic response. Gene therapy is a technology with numerous applications, including anti-angiogenesis, immunotherapy, replacement of defective genes, and suppression of harmful genes (15).

Gene therapy offers significant advantages with the addition of specifically and uniquely engineered mechanisms of halting malignant proliferation through cytotoxicity or reproductive arrest. A favorable therapeutic ratio (the relative toxicity to tumor compared to normal tissue) must be achieved in order to confer a true benefit; thus, a vector or the transgene it carries must selectively affect or access tumor cells. Vectors can be targeted to tumors through a number of methods, including selective delivery, vector competence and toxicity for specific cell types or dividing cells, transgene or transgene product toxicity, cell entry (receptor targeting), and transcriptional activation (promoter targeting).

The majority of the molecular strategies for gliomas aim at three targets: (a) controlling cell cycle or inducing apoptosis; (b) use of suicide genes and enzyme–prodrug systems; and (c) enhancement of the immune system by immunogene therapy. In addition, gene therapy is used in other important fields including antiangiogenesis and oncolytic viruses.

Common vectors that have potential in the treatment of gliomas and in which significant work on targeting modifications has been done include: retrovirus (primarily Moloney murine leukemia virus or MMLV), adenovirus, adeno-associated virus (AAV), herpes simplex virus (HSV-1), HSV-1 amplicons, liposomes, and polylysine–DNA complexes. High-grade gliomas present an optimal disease for the development of such novel experimental therapies because they are usually confined to brain parenchyma where they are localizable as the only population of rapidly dividing cells, thus limiting the intrinsic cell cycle-dependent toxicity of many common transgene systems and vectors to tumor, as opposed to normal tissue.

CELL CYCLE CONTROL AND APOPTOSIS. Specific chromosomal abnormalities and associated genetic defects are found to be responsible for glioma development, as the glioma cell progresses from a low-grade astrocytoma cell to a glioblastoma multiforme cell. Sequential loss of the p53, Rb-1, p16, and amplification of epidermal growth factor receptor and other genes represent insights that will propel future molecular genetic and pharmacological intervention. As the pathways leading to tumorigenesis are being elucidated and shown to involve genes that control progression through the cell cycle and DNA repair, targeting their fundamental molecular defects can treat malignant gliomas. In general, the most successful therapeutic results have been achieved with adenovirus vectors injected into established tumors at a relatively high ratio of vector-to-tumor cell.

TUMOR SUPPRESSOR GENES. The concept for tumor suppressor gene therapy was sparked by two observations: (a) Somatic cell hybridization between neoplastic and normal cells yields hybrids that are nontumorigenic; and (b) the inactivation of specific genes leads to carcinogenesis. The p53, p16, Rb, and MMAC1/PTEN genes are implicated in the genesis of astrocytic neoplasms (Table 1), and the list of genes involved in glioma malignancy, lineage, and patterns of spread continues to grow. Much useful genetic information needed to fully conceptualize the genesis of primary gliomas has been discovered.

P53 Gene. The wild-type p53 is involved in several aspects of cell cycle control, and its protein suppresses transformation either by blocking cell cycle progression to allow for repair of DNA damage or inducing apoptosis of cells that are not able to achieve such repair functions. Loss of function mutations of the p53 gene are present in more than 30% of astrocytomas and constitute the earliest detectable genetic alteration in these tumors. The p53 protein directly induces the expression of the p21 gene, which in turn results in block of the cell cycle in the G1 phase, and it also transcriptionally activates the death gene BAX, an apoptosis-promoting member of the Bcl-2 family. In addition to the p53-direct effect, other molecules may enhance the p53-apoptosis ability. It is known that coexpression of p16 and p53 induces apoptosis in p53-resistant cells. Thus, the p53 gene is a critical target to develop gene therapy strategies for cancer, and the toxicity and anticancer effect of the transfer of p53 to gliomas is currently being tested in a clinical trial (Table 2). Replacement of defective p53 genes has been described in several tumor models, including medulloblastoma, lung cancer, head, and neck squamous cell carcinoma, and prostate tumors. However, because many gliomas already express wild-type p53, the value of this therapy in all gliomas has yet to be determined.

The Network p16/Rb/E2F. Several proteins modulate the cell cycle during cellular replication. Complexes of cyclins and cyclin-dependent kinases inactivate by phosphorylation key regulators of the cell cycle and promote cell proliferation. The p16 gene (CDKN2) encodes a cdk4/6 inhibitor protein, which inhibits the formation of cyclin D1–cdk4/6 complex, preventing the phosphorylation of Rb and the release of the E2F transcription factor, resulting in growth arrest. To complete the feedback regulation, Rb modulates p16 expression at the transcriptional level. In a variety of human cell lines, including 80% of glioma cell lines, p16 is mutated, methylated, or deleted. There is a high frequency of homozygous p16 gene deletion (>50%) in gliomas, and some gliomas lacking p16 expression exhibit in-

tact p16 gene, suggesting that p16 is downregulated at the transcriptional level. Restoration of p16 expression in p16-null glioma cells can be achieved by a gene transfer technique using a replication-defective adenovirus construct. The exogenous p16 inhibited the cell growth by blocking cell cycle progression in G1 phase, influenced the cell morphology, and modified several properties of the transformed cells, including colony formation (16). Moreover, overexpression of p16 gene considerably reduced the ability of glioma cells to invade normal brain (17).

PTEN/MMAC1 Pathway. Deletions of chromosome 10 are probably the most frequent cytogenetic alterations in glioblastoma multiforme, and the PTEN/MMAC1 is a tumor suppressor gene that has been found mutated in malignant gliomas. Restoration of the MMAC1 activity to glioma cells led to suppression of their neoplastic phenotype (18). The data from experiments with knockout mice indicate that MMAC1 can suppress tumorigenesis through its ability to regulate cellular differentiation and anchorage-independent growth, although its function is not yet completely understood. In addition, MMAC1 is inactivated in the latest stages of the glioma progression, and it may play a role in angiogenesis or invasiveness.

ACTIVATE PRODRUGS: SUICIDE GENE. Suicide gene therapy involves the conferring of drug sensitivity by transfecting tumor cells with a gene encoding an enzyme that can metabolize a nontoxic prodrug to its toxic form (suicide genes). Mool-

Table 2. Selected Clinical Gene Therapy for Malignant Gliomas

Target Genes	Vehicle
Tumor suppressor genes and antisense	
p53	Adenovirus
Insulin-like growth factor	Plasmid
Immunogene therapy	
Transforming growth factor/interleukin 2	Plasmid DNA
Interleukin 4	Retrovirus
Interleukin 2	Retrovirus
Interferon-β	Adenovirus
Interleukin 4/HSV-tk	Retrovirus
Drug-sensitivity genes	
Herpes simplex virus thymidine kinase (HSV-tk)	Adenovirus Retrovirus
Oncolytic virus	
Herpes simplex virus	

From Rosenberg SA, Blaese RM, Brenner MK, et al. Human gene marker/therapy clinical protocols. *Hum Gene Ther* 2000;11:919–979, with permission.

Table 1. Several Tumor Suppressor Genes in Gliomas

Tumor Suppressor	Chromosome	Function	Tumor Grade	Frequency (%)
p53	17	Cell-cycle control/apoptosis	A, AA GBM	30–50
p16	9	Cell-cycle control/senescence	AA, GBM	50–70
Rb	13	Cell-cycle control/senescence	AA, GBM	30
PTEN/MMAC1	10	Phosphatase	GBM	30
DMBT1	10	SRCR protein	GBM	25
H-neu	10	Unknown	GBM	Unknown

A, Astrocytoma; AA, anaplastic astrocytoma; DMBTI, deleted in malignant brain tumor; GBM, glioblastoma multiforme; H-neu, human homologue of the *Drosophila* neurolized gene; MMACI, mutated in malignant advanced cancers; PTEN, phosphatase and tensin homologue deleted from chromosome 10; SRCR, scavenger receptor cysteine-rich protein.

ten in 1986 described the first example of such a gene and it consists of the thymidine kinase (tk) gene from herpes simplex virus type 1 (HSV-1) (19). Its encoded enzyme converts nucleoside analogues, such as acyclovir and ganciclovir, into their phosphorylated metabolites. These then act as competitive inhibitors of endogenous nucleotides for incorporation into the DNA chains of proliferating cells, leading to their death. Tk-gene transfer can generate ganciclovir-mediated killing of tumor cells both in *in vitro* and animal models.

The thymidine kinase-ganciclovir approach has been recently or currently used in several clinical trials (Table 2) for malignant brain tumors. Recombinant retroviruses can target suicide gene delivery into rapidly multiplying tumor cells while sparing the background of nondividing neural tissue. In the initial phase I trial, 15 patients (12 with recurrent malignant glioma and three with metastatic tumors) received stereotactic inoculation of tk-retrovirus producer cells into their brain tumor. Fourteen days later, patients were treated with a 14-day course of ganciclovir (20). Adverse events included neurologic dysfunction in one patient and intratumoral hemorrhage in another. There were no complete tumor regressions by magnetic resonance imaging studies, although the authors did report evidence of partial regression in the early posttreatment period. In a few case, biopsies were obtained after inoculation of the producer cells. These revealed that the extent of tk-gene expression (assayed by the polymerase chain reaction) was less than 1% in the biopsied tumor sample. The lack of gene transfer led the authors to conclude that "bystander" mechanisms were primarily responsible for the observed partial tumor responses (21).

A subsequent phase II clinical trial was then conducted in multiple centers throughout the United States. The treatment scheme involved resection of the malignant brain tumor with injection of the tk-retrovirus producer cells into multiple sites within the wall of the cavity. This was then followed by placement of a catheter within the cavity connected to an Ommaya reservoir, to allow for reinjection of producer cells. Thirty patients were treated. Four patients died of causes unrelated to injection of the producer cells. The average survival time of 18 evaluated patients was 25 weeks from the initial injection of producer cells. Adverse events were related to inadvertent injection of producer cells into the ventricle, producing a severe aseptic meningeal reaction. MRI findings were consistent with a transient inflammatory response and evidence of partial antitumor responses. The authors concluded that this approach demonstrates safety and modest antitumor efficacy (22).

Based on these results, a prospective randomized trial was instituted involving 240 patients in three countries (United States, Germany, and Canada), comparing the standard treatment of a newly diagnosed glioblastoma (surgery plus radiation and chemotherapy) with surgical excision, followed by injection into the tumor margin with tk-retrovirus producer cells and subsequent treatment with ganciclovir and radiation therapy (and/or chemotherapy). Results from this trial are pending. These trials have been sponsored by Genetic Therapy Incorporated (Gaithersburg, MD); results are pending. Similar trials employing tk-retrovirus producer cells and ganciclovir as a treatment for malignant brain tumors have been performed in France (Genopoietic, Paris).

Two phase I clinical trials are currently being conducted in the United States, which employ a replication-defective adenovirus that bears the tk-gene to provide ganciclovir susceptibility to malignant brain tumors. In one trial, the tk-adenovirus is stereotactically inoculated into the tumor. Two days later, ganciclovir is administered. Seven days after injection of the adenovirus, the tumor is resected. The resected specimen then will be assayed for extent of gene transfer, immune responses, and tumor necrosis (23).

ACTIVATE IMMUNE RESPONSE: IMMUNOGENE THERAPY. Immunogene therapy is based on the use of recombinant DNA constructs to express cytokines and lymphokines, by which a systemic immune response against the tumor is generated. There are at least three different approaches for this strategy.

Antigen-Presenting Cells. Autologous antigen-presenting cells (APCs) can be harvested by mobilization from the blood of the patient or biopsy specimens of the brain tumor and then expanded *in vitro* with cytokines. To generate the antitumor immune response, antigen-presenting cells are transduced with the DNA or message RNA coding for the tumor antigen and then injected into the patient. Among these antigen-presenting cells, dendritic cells (DCs) have emerged as the most potent member of the class of APCs (24). Because of their immunostimulatory capacity, immunization with DCs presenting tumor antigens has been proposed as a treatment regimen for cancer.

Cytokine-Expressing Tumor Cells. This approach is based on the use of *ex vivo* vaccination with tumor cells expressing cytokines. Disadvantages of this approach include the unavailability of tumor cells from every patient (inaccessible tumors) and the failure of the transduced cells to express the cytokine gene.

Expression of Costimulatory Molecules on the Surface of Tumor Cells. The transfer of costimulatory molecules (e.g., HLA-type molecules) into tumor cells aims at generating T-cell responses against the tumor. The identification of tumor rejection antigens from brain tumors and the critical components of afferent and efferent arms of the immune response are necessary to increase the efficiency of these systems.

One of the first immunogene strategies employed an antisense insulin-like growth factor 1 (IGF-1) construct to provide rejection of C6 glioma cells grown in rats (25), which provided the basis for a clinical trial in patients with malignant gliomas. Other strategies have used transfer of the interleukin 4 gene, with evidence of tumor regression (26). Most recently, a phase I trial is ongoing with IL-4-HSV-tk gene therapy. The gene encoding for granulocyte/macrophage colony stimulating factor (GM-CSF), which probably involves facilitation of antigen presentation by antigen-presenting cells, also was studied. Transfer of this gene has been shown to produce rejection of tumor cells (27). On the other hand, some gliomas secrete TGF-β, which exerts potent immunosuppressive effects, including the inhibition of cytotoxic T lymphocytes. Antisense TGF-β gene therapy abolishes secretion of TGF-β and produces rejection of 9L gliosarcoma in animal models. It is likely that a combination of approaches or the discovery of new immune-enhancing molecules will provide further evidence of therapeutic benefits for these tumors.

MODULATE ANGIOGENESIS: ANTIANGIOGENIC GENE THERAPY. The process of neovascularization of expanding brain tumors offers one of the most suitable targets for an experimental gene therapy approach. Angiogenesis modulators are extraordinarily important in tumor growth, as shown by the fact that neovascularization must occur for solid tumors to grow beyond a diameter of 2 to 3 mm. Molecules and corresponding receptors involved in regulation of angiogenesis include basic FGF and its receptor, VEGF and its receptors (VEGFR-1 or flt-1, and VEGFR-2 or flk-1), TGF-α and -β, EGF receptor, and human platelet factor 4 (PF4) and its receptor. These molecules are especially important in gliomas because neovascularization is a major feature of these tumors. Indeed, the progression of an astrocytoma to anaplastic astrocytoma or glioblastoma multiforme is characterized by increased neovascularization. Several lines of evidence indicate that VEGF plays a major role in the growth of gliomas. The VEGF-messenger RNA is overexpressed in the highly vascularized glioblastoma multiforme. In addition, the transfection of VEGF complementary DNA to rat glioma cells results in hypervascularized tumors with abnormally large vessels, and the abrupt withdrawal of VEGF results in the regression of preformed tumor vessels. Selectivity in the angiogenesis strategies is provided by at least two factors: The molecules targeted are preferentially found in blood vessels within brain tumors and not in normal brain, and inhibition of these ligand–receptor interactions primarily affects rapidly dividing cells, which require continuous nourishment. Recent studies demonstrated that genetic methods can be used to disrupt angiogenesis in brain tumors, and the VEGF/flk receptor has provided the most fruitful target for therapeutic exploitation. When a dominant-negative version of the VEGFR-2 was introduced into C6 glioma cells by means of a retroviral vector, tumor involution was observed in a nude mouse model. Saleh and associates employed an antisense VEGF cDNA and found that the stable transfectants of C6 glioma cells produced markedly reduced quantities of VEGF (28). These tumor cells were significantly inhibited in their ability to form neoplasms in nude mice when compared to parental cells, and this correlated with a statistically significant decrease in blood vessel formation. In addition, expression of antisense bFGF cDNA correlated with reduced proliferation of glioma cells in culture.

ONCOLYTIC VIRUSES. Viruses have been tested in the past in an attempt to directly kill tumor cells by lysis. The first studies that described use of herpes viruses for destruction of cultured tumor cells were by Levaditi and Nicolau in 1922, but were not successful, presumably because of the poor infectivity of human herpes virus for rodent tumor cells. The perfect oncolytic virus must be able to distinguish between normal tissue and abnormal cancer cells, and should be able to efficiently eliminate the cancer cells and propagate the anticancer effect to surrounding tumor cells. In addition, it should be able to avoid the neutralizing immune response of the host. Finally, this kind of virus should be controllable pharmacologically. The current advances of genetic engineering allow the modifications of wild-type viruses to improve their safety and efficiency. At least two of the oncolytic viruses have been explored successfully for glioma treatment in animal models (29,30). Genetically engineered herpes simplex viruses have proved proficient in the elimination of glioma cells *in vitro* and *in vivo*. Martuza and associates employed a deletion mutant of the viral tk gene to show selective killing of human glioma cells both *in vitro* and in animal models (31). The mammalian tk enzyme probably generated the observed selectivity, which is upregulated during the G1/S phase transition of the cell cycle. This enzyme could complement the function of the deleted viral thymidine kinase, thus allowing for viral growth in dividing cells but not in postmitotic cells. Another strategy has employed deletion of the viral ribonucleotide reductase gene, which can also selectively replicate and kill glioma cells in culture and *in vivo* (32). One advantage provided by this virus is that it retains the endogenous tk gene, allowing for ganciclovir sensitivity. However, these viruses are highly toxic and may induce encephalitis in human beings. Current research is focused on the generation of genetically altered viruses with low virulence for normal cells.

Another viral oncolysis approach is the use of replication-competent adenoviruses. Replication of the virus is directly tied to the ability of E1B 55 kDa protein to bind and inactivate wild-type p53 in cells, which allows the cell to enter into S phase and synthesize the viral proteins necessary for viral replication. Bischoff and colleagues designed and generated an E1B-mu-

tated adenovirus that was not able to replicate in wild-type TP53 cells but was able to replicate and kill mutant TP53 cancer cells. Injection of gliomas growing in mice with the mutant adenovirus led to complete regression of the tumors. The disadvantages include the high heterogeneity of gliomas that express wild-type and mutant TP53 cells inside the same tumor. In addition, the neutralizing immune response of the host against this adenovirus is the principal barrier to a successful therapy in humans.

Therapy Targeting Invasion and Angiogenesis

Invasion and angiogenesis are critical components of malignant gliomas and undoubtedly contribute to their poor clinical outcomes. Diffuse gliomas are invasive in normal surrounding white matter from the moment they are detected, which ultimately limits local attempts at tumor control. The basic scientific studies of malignant glioma cell invasion and angiogenesis are leading to therapeutic strategies.

BIOLOGICAL AND MOLECULAR MECHANISMS OF TUMOR INVASION AND ANGIOGENESIS. Invasion of glioma cells involves three major interrelated steps: adhesion, proteolysis, and migration. Cellular adhesion, which includes cell–matrix and cell–cell adhesion, is the first step in the invasive process. Cell–matrix interactions include cellular binding to the extracellular matrix glycoproteins, such as type IV collagen, laminin, and fibronectin, through both high- and low-affinity receptors. Cell–cell interactions involve distinct classes of receptors present on the cell surface, including cell adhesion molecules and cadherins (33). The second crucial step in tumor invasion is the degradation of basement membrane extracellular matrix (ECM). Among the major components of the brain's ECM are the collagens (particularly type IV), chondroitin sulfate, laminin, elastin, fibronectin, entactin, vitronectin, tenascin, heparan sulfate proteoglycan, and hyaluronic acid. These components are considered to have an important role in the adhesive, ligand–receptor, and signal transduction messenger interactions that are prerequisites for tumor cell invasion. All the major proteinase classes are involved, including matrix metalloproteinases (MMPs), serine/threonine proteinase (SP), urokinase and tissue plasminogen activators (uPA and tPA), cysteine proteinases (cathepsin B and S), aspartic proteinases (cathepsin D), and glycosidases. Cellular migration is the third step for local brain tumor invasion, which is a dynamic process necessary for both local glioma invasion and neovascularization. Malignant glioma cells have been observed to migrate extensively along white matter, crossing hemispheres and extending along blood vessels without invading them (34). Multiple migration-stimulating factors have been identified and characterized. Tumor cells or host cells secrete autocrine or paracrine motility factors. Cytokines such as the insulin-like growth factors, hepatocyte growth factor/scatter factor, fibroblast growth factors, and tumor necrosis factor also have been shown to stimulate cell motility (35).

Angiogenesis is a necessary event for cellular proliferation and extensions of solid masses of tumor into the surrounding brain tissue. The development of a network of blood vessels is a prerequisite for the local expansion of tumor colonies beyond the region restricted by oxygen and nutrient diffusion. Tumor neovascularization begins with the sprouting of new capillary buds from an existing vessel in response to direct or

Table 3. Selected Agents Against Invasion and Angiogenesis in Glioma Clinical Trials

Drug	Effect	Mechanism	Clinical Status
AGM-1470 (TNP-470)	Antiangiogenic	Unknown, possible cell-cycle blocker	Phase II
BB-94	Inhibits proteolysis	Inhibits MMP-2 activity	Phase II/III
CAI (carboxyamido triazole)	Antiinvasive, antiangiogenic Antiproliferation	Inhibits nonvoltage gated calcium influx	Phase I/II
Marimastat	Inhibits proteolysis Antiinvasive, antiangiogenic	Inhibits MMP-2 activity	Phase II/III
Safingol	Antiinvasive	Inhibits protein kinase C	Phase I
SU5416	Antiangiogenic, invasive	Inhibits VEGF/FIK-1 pathway	Phase I/II
Suramin	Antiangiogenic	Inhibits angiogenic growth factors	Phase II
Thalidomide	Antiangiogenic	Unknown	Phase II
Tyrphostins	Inhibit cell growth and antiinvasive	Inhibits selected tyrosine kinases	Preclinical

From NCI clinical trials database. *http://cancernet.nci.nih.gov*

indirect angiogenic stimuli. The angiogenesis response occurs as a result of proteinase secretion and basement membrane remodeling, endothelial cell proliferation, and endothelial cell migration to form capillary sprouts and neovascular lumina (36). Tumors may produce multiple cytokines that are angiogenic. Angiogenesis in gliomas is stimulated by VEGF and, to a lesser extent, basic fibroblast growth factor (bFGF) and lesser cytokines.

INHIBITION OF GLIOMA INVASION AND ANGIOGENESIS.

Invasion and angiogenesis are the newest therapeutic targets to yield agents for clinical trials (Table 3). Three general strategies for anti-invasive and antiangiogenic intervention have arisen: (a) inhibition of the production of stimulatory factors by tumor cells; (b) blockade of invasive activity; and (c) interdiction of the signal directing the proliferative or invasive command.

Today, drugs to block tumor cell invasion are directed toward protease secretion by tumor cells. There is an association among the various grades of astrocytic tumors and a large number of proteases such that the level of protease increases with increasing tumor grade. Inhibitors directed against 72- and 92-kDa gelatinase, such as collagenase type IV, appear to block the movement of invasion of glioma cells into cellular invasion models and to produce antitumor activity in animal models. Clinical trials are now ongoing using Marimastat, an orally bioavailable analogue, in a number of tumor types, including a phase III trial in newly diagnosed malignant gliomas. Also, it appears that most of the anti-invasion drugs studied have antiangiogenic properties as well. Other trials using protease inhibitors are being conducted or planned.

To reduce angiogenesis, a variety of drugs have been evaluated in patients. They include interferon-α, -β, 13-cis-retinoic acid, all-trans-retinoic acid, and thalidomide. Newer agents include a fumagillin analogue (TNP-470), antibodies to compete with the VEGF receptor, and drugs to block the protein tyrosine kinase activity of the VEGF receptor and/or the FGF receptor. Thalidomide, a well-known teratogen, has been found to be a potent antiangiogenic factor (37). Using a rabbit cornea micropocket assay, orally administered thalidomide could inhibit corneal neovascularization induced by bFGF. Most recently, a phase II trial using thalidomide for patients with recurrent high-grade gliomas has been completed (38). A total of 39 patients (GBM 25, anaplastic astrocytomas and other anaplastic gliomas 14) were initially treated with thalidomide 800 mg per day with increase in dose by 200 mg per day every 2 weeks until a final daily dose of 1,200 mg was achieved. Thalidomide was well tolerated, with constipation and sedation being the major toxici-

ties. Two patients showed radiographic partial responses, two minor responses and 12 patients had stable disease. The data show that thalidomide is a generally well-tolerated drug that may have antitumor activity in a minority of patients with malignant gliomas.

Several agents that inhibit signaling events have been shown to have anti-invasive or antiangiogenic activity. Carboxyamidotriazole (CAI), an inhibitor of non-voltage–gated calcium influx, has been demonstrated to inhibit tumor cell migration and angiogenesis, and has been undertaken into phase I and II clinical trials for glioma therapy (39). Tyrphostins, the synthetic agents targeted against receptor protein tyrosine kinases, inhibit invasion and proliferation in a cytokine receptor-selective fashion (5). Signaling of several classes of molecules also modulates interaction of tumor and endothelial cells with the ECM. Recently described fragments of ECM components have direct angioregulatory effects, including endostatin and angiostatin (40, 41). In addition, antiangiogenic gene therapy is also under development as described elsewhere in this chapter.

It seems logical and experimentally feasible to combine other types of drugs to activate tumor cell apoptosis to maximize the antitumor activity of both antiangiogenic and anti-invasion drugs. Today, this can be achieved by the coadministration of DNA-damaging cytotoxic drugs. It is reasonable to assume that future drugs that effectively interfere with important signaling pathways also may work to effect apoptotic cell death with fewer systemic toxic effects.

Immunotherapy of Malignant Gliomas

The CNS represents a complex microenvironment in which immune responses are modulated. In general, cell-mediated immune responses are diminished while humoral responses are normal or increased (42). It is known that the blood–brain barrier breaks down in many pathological conditions, resulting in free lymphocyte traffic into the CNS. Much literature has attempted to address the importance of perivascular lymphocytic infiltration and the clinical behavior of the tumor (43).

GLIOMA IMMUNOLOGY AND IMMUNOTHERAPY.

Gliomas express tumor-specific antigens and have access to pathways for both Class I and II MHC-restricted antigen presentation, suggesting that gliomas may be sensitive to cell-mediated immune response. It is also demonstrated that glioma cells express Fas, and most appear sensitive to Fas-mediated apoptosis, the major pathway for cytotoxic T-cell–mediated killing. However, gliomas also express several immunosuppressive factors (e.g., TGF-β2, prostaglandin E2, and possibly Fas-L) that hinder lymphocyte activation.

Classically, there are four approaches for immunotherapy of malignant gliomas, administering: (a) nonspecific immune adjuvants (cytokines); (b) antitumor antibodies (serotherapy); (c) antitumor lymphocytes (adoptive immunotherapy); and (d) antitumor vaccines (active immunotherapy) (Table 4).

Nonspecific immune adjuvants (cytokines) have been studied for many different tumors by systemic administration to stimulate subtherapeutic antitumor immunity. Several cytokines, including IL-2, IL-4, IFN-α, and TNF-α, have been administered for clinical trials. Unfortunately, cytokine administration has produced limited clinical benefits for glioma patients to date, although preclinical animal studies have been promising. Furthermore, IL-2 requires high doses to achieve therapeutic activity, which has resulted in treatment-limiting cerebral edema (44).

Glioma serotherapy also has been extensively investigated in a number of clinical trials. Monoclonal antibodies that direct against several glioma antigens have been identified and administered to patients with malignant gliomas. In phase I/II clinical trials, it has been shown that ^{131}I-labeled monoclonal antibody directed against tenascin, a relatively glioma-specific ECM protein, induced response rates up to 51% and minimal toxicity (45,46). The phase I/II studies of intracranial ^{131}I-labeled anti-tenascin monoclonal antibody 81C6 in patients with malignant brain tumors are ongoing. In addition, monoclonal antibodies directed against other glioma antigens, such as EGFR, have undergone preclinical studies.

Adoptive transfer immunotherapy is administration of autologous lymphocytes that have been activated and expanded *in vitro*, specifically producing lymphokine-activated killer (LAK) cells. LAK cells can kill glioma cells *in vitro* and *in vivo*, but clinical trials using LAK cells have not shown clear benefits (44). A phase II study of intracavitary IL-2 and LAK therapy is ongoing

in patients with primary, recurrent, or refractory malignant gliomas (NCI-V97-1326). The other adoptive immunotherapy approach is stimulating lymphocytes with autologous tumor cells to generate Class I MHC-restricted cytotoxic T cells. Recently, a phase I clinical trial was performed of T-cell adoptive immunotherapy for patients with newly diagnosed malignant gliomas (47). Fresh tumor samples were minced and digested to produce a single-cell suspension. These tumor cells were irradiated and administered intradermally to each upper thigh. Inguinal lymph nodes were removed 8 to 10 days later and mechanically dissociated to obtain a single-cell suspension. The cells were stimulated with IL-2 for 6 to 8 days and then infused back to the patient through a peripheral vein. No long-term toxicity was observed in the 12 patients with malignant gliomas.

Antitumor vaccination is a cornerstone of standard immunotherapy. Tumor antigens or cells are administered to stimulate systemic antitumor immunity in this active immunotherapeutic approach. Several clinical trials were done in the 1970s and early 1980s, but the results were conflicting with no predominant efficacy demonstrated. In a randomized clinical trial, 65 patients with malignant gliomas were divided into four groups and received radiation, vaccination with autologous tumor cells and Freund's adjuvant, radiation plus vaccination with autologous tumor cells and Freund's adjuvant, or supportive care (48). Survival was prolonged for patients receiving radiation plus vaccination (10.1 months) compared with those receiving radiation alone (7.5 months); however, other studies have not shown a clear clinical advantage (49,50). Further studies are required.

NOVEL GLIOMA IMMUNOTHERAPY STRATEGIES. Rapid advances in molecular biology and immunology have produced some novel approaches for antitumor immunotherapy, although classical immunotherapy for malignant gliomas has been disappointing clinically. Such strategies for glioma immunotherapy include immunogene therapy and autologous antigen-presenting cells, specifically dendritic cells.

Immunogene therapy currently is revolutionizing cancer im-

Table 4. Immunotherapy of Malignant Gliomas

Immunotherapy Type	Method	Clinical Status
Nonspecific immune adjuvants (cytokines) IL-2, IL-4, IFN-α, -β, -γ, TFN-α	Administering cytokines to promote antitumor immunity	Phase I/II
Antitumor antibodies (serotherapy) Tenascin, gp 240, EGFRvIII	Administering toxin, drug, or radioisotope-conjugated antibodies directed against tumor-specific antigens	Phase I/II
Antitumor lymphocytes (adoptive immunotherapy) LAK and TIL cells, cytotoxic T cells	Administering autologous lymphocytes that have been activated and expanded *in vitro*	Phase I/II
Vaccines (active immunotherapy) Tumor antigens and tumor cells	Administering vaccines to stimulate systemic antitumor immunity	Phase I
Immunogene therapy Vaccination Genes encoding proinflammatory cytokines: IFN-γ, GM-CSF, IL-2 T-cell costimulatory molecules: B7-1, B7-2 MHC molecules Antisense: TGF-β2, IGF-1, or IGF-1 receptor Common glioma antigen: EGFRvIII Nontumor gene products carrier cells	Autologous tumor cells genetically modified to enhance their immunogenicity	Phase I
In situ gene transfer Local immunogene therapy	Intratumoral delivery of proinflammatory gene or gene-transduced carrier cells	Preclinical
Dendritic cell manipulation Tumor antigens and tumor cells	Vaccination with tumor antigen or mRNA-primed dendritic cells	Preclinical

EGFRvIII, epidermal growth factor receptor isoform; GM-CSF, granulocyte-macrophage colony-stimulating factor; IFN, interferon; IGF, insulin-like growth factor; IL, interleukin; LAK, lymphokine-activated killer cells; MHC, major histocompatibility complexes; TGF, transforming growth factor; TIL, tumor-infiltrating lymphocytes; TNF, tumor necrosis factor.

munotherapy, in which immunostimulatory genes are transferred to human cells to stimulate antitumor immune responses. Gene transfer can be performed either *in situ* or *in vitro* and both viral and nonviral vectors are available. Immunogene therapy vaccines are the major aim. Tumor cells from a given patient are cultured *in vitro* and genetically modified with genes encoding proinflammatory cytokines or antisense molecules targeting growth factors to increase their immunogenicity. The genetically modified tumor cells are irradiated to prevent further cell division and readministered subcutaneously to the same patient. Successful brain tumor immunogene therapy has been reported in several animal models, and clinical trials are ongoing. However, it is not always possible to successfully establish cultures from human gliomas and many early-passage human glioma cultures grow too slowly. To solve this problem, efforts have been made to develop vaccines using universal tumor antigens, such as EGFRvIII (51) or use a nontumor carrier cell to deliver immunotherapeutic gene products (e.g., IL-2 and IFN-γ) (52). In addition, several studies have examined the effect of local cytokine production on intracranial glioma growth. Local immunogene therapy in rodent glioma models using IL-2, IL-3, IL-4, TNF-α, GM-CSF, IFN-γ, and T-cell costimulatory molecule (B7) show potentially stimulated effective antiglioma responses (53,54). Clinical trials for immunogene therapy strategy are under development as described elsewhere in this chapter.

Another new approach for glioma immunotherapy involves the use of dendritic cells, which are extremely potent antigen-presenting cells that are bone marrow–derived similar to monocyte/macrophages (55). Dendritic cells conditioned by CD40/CD40–ligand interactions can provide "help" directly to Tk cells without need for Th cells (56). Dendritic cells exposed to tumor cells, isolated tumor antigens, or even tumor mRNAs are capable of stimulating potent antitumor cytotoxic T lymphocytes (55). It has been reported recently that immunization with tumor cells mixed with autologous dendritic cells resulted in cure for rats harboring established intracranial gliomas (57). In another *in vivo* study using an intracranial 9L gliosarcoma rat model, vaccination with syngeneic dendritic cells pulsed with 9L-derived protein prolonged the survival of these animals (58). These dramatic preclinical results are prompting clinical trials.

Conclusion

Malignant gliomas continue to be a devastating clinical problem. These tumors demonstrate phenotypic heterogeneity after treatment by surgery, radiation, and/or cytotoxic chemotherapy. Local multifocal targeting of various tumor cell types and their numerous molecular pathways, therefore, has been considered as a possible therapeutic strategy. The advances in glioma cell biology, molecular biology, immunology, and biotechnology offer us powerful therapeutic methods to fight these challenging tumors. The explosion in knowledge about normal cellular function and their aberrations in cancer are likely to lead to improved therapeutic options. A large number of focused therapeutic agents and their delivery systems have been developed. Numerous *in vitro* and *in vivo* studies using therapies targeting glioma cell signaling pathways, glioma invasion and angiogenesis, oncogenes, and immunity have demonstrated encouraging results. These new therapeutic strategies will lead to effective therapies in the future.

References

1. Boring CC, Squires TS, Tong T. Cancer statistics, 1993. *CA Cancer J Clin* 1993;43:7–26.

2. Mikkelsen TEK. Tumor invasiveness. In: Black PLJ, ed. *Cancer of the nervous system.* Cambridge, UK: Blackwell Scientific, 1997:834–857.

3. Walker AE, Robins M, Weinfeld FD. Epidemiology of brain tumors: the national survey of intracranial neoplasms. *Neurology* 1985;35: 219–226.

4. Davis FG, Freels S, Grutsch J, et al. Survival rates in patients with primary malignant brain tumors stratified by patient age and tumor histological type: an analysis based on Surveillance, Epidemiology, and End Results (SEER) data, 1973–1991. *J Neurosurg* 1998;88:1–10.

5. Levitzki A, Gazit A. Tyrosine kinase inhibition: an approach to drug development. *Science* 1995;267:1782–1788.

6. Shawver LK, Schwartz DP, Mann E, et al. Inhibition of platelet-derived growth factor-mediated signal transduction and tumor growth by N-[4-(trifluoromethyl)-phenyl]5-methylisoxazole-4-carboxamide. *Clin Cancer Res* 1997;3:1167–1177.

7. Malkin MGRL, Lopez AM, et al. Phase II study of SU101, a PDGF-R signal transduction inhibitor, in recurrent malignant glioma. *34th Annual Meeting of the American Society of Clinical Oncology.* Los Angeles, 1998:390.

8. Bredel M, Pollack IF. The p21-Ras signal transduction pathway and growth regulation in human high-grade gliomas. *Brain Res Brain Res Rev* 1999;29:232–249.

9. Larner J, Jane J, Laws E, et al. A phase I-II trial of lovastatin for anaplastic astrocytoma and glioblastoma multiforme. *Am J Clin Oncol* 1998;21:579–583.

10. Misra-Press A, Fields AP, Samols D, et al. Protein kinase C isoforms in human glioblastoma cells. *Glia* 1992;6:188–197.

11. Couldwell WT, Hinton DR, Surnock AA, et al. Treatment of recurrent malignant gliomas with chronic oral high-dose tamoxifen. *Clin Cancer Res* 1996;2:619–622.

12. Pollack IF, Kawecki S, Lazo JS. Blocking of glioma proliferation *in vitro* and *in vivo* and potentiating the effects of BCNU and cisplatin: UCN-01, a selective protein kinase C inhibitor. *J Neurosurg* 1996; 84:1024–1032.

13. Couldwell WT, Gopalakrishna R, Hinton DR, et al. Hypericin: a potential antiglioma therapy. *Neurosurgery* 1994;35:705–709; discussion 709–710.

14. Yazaki T, Ahmad S, Chahlavi A, et al. Treatment of glioblastoma U-87 by systemic administration of an antisense protein kinase C-alpha phosphorothioate oligodeoxynucleotides. *Mol Pharmacol* 1996;50: 236–242.

15. Alavi JB, Eck SL. Gene therapy for malignant gliomas. *Hematol Oncol Clin North Am* 1998;12:617–629.

16. Arap W, Nishikawa R, Furnari FB, et al. Replacement of the p16/CDKN2 gene suppresses human glioma cell growth. *Cancer Res* 1995;55:1351–1354.

17. Chintala SK, Fueyo J, Gomez-Manzano C, et al. Adenovirus-mediated p16/CDKN2 gene transfer suppresses glioma invasion *in vitro. Oncogene* 1997;15:2049–2057.

18. Cheney IW, Johnson DE, Vaillancourt MT, et al. Suppression of tumorigenicity of glioblastoma cells by adenovirus-mediated MMAC1/PTEN gene transfer. *Cancer Res* 1998;58:2331–234.

19. Moolten FL. Tumor chemosensitivity conferred by inserted herpes thymidine kinase genes: paradigm for a prospective cancer control strategy. *Cancer Res* 1986;46:5276–5281.

20. Ram Z, Culver KW, Oshiro EM, et al. Therapy of malignant brain tumors by intratumoral implantation of retroviral vector-producing cells. *Nat Med* 1997;3:1354–1361.

21. Oldfield EH, Ram Z, Chiang Y, et al. Intrathecal gene therapy for the treatment of leptomeningeal carcinomatosis. GTI 0108. A phase I/II study. *Hum Gene Ther* 1995;6:55–85.

22. Deliganis AV, Baxter AB, Berger MS, et al. Serial MR in gene therapy for recurrent glioblastoma: initial experience and work in progress. *AJNR Am J Neuroradiol* 1997;18:1401–1406.

23. Eck SL, Alavi JB, Alavi A, et al. Treatment of advanced CNS malignancies with the recombinant adenovirus H5.010RSVTK: a phase I trial. *Hum Gene Ther* 1996;7:1465–1482.

24. Banchereau J, Steinman RM. Dendritic cells and the control of immunity. *Nature* 1998;392:245–252.

25. Trojan J, Johnson TR, Rudin SD, et al. Treatment and prevention of rat glioblastoma by immunogenic C6 cells expressing antisense insulin-like growth factor I RNA. *Science* 1993;259:94–97.

26. Yu JS, Wei MX, Chiocca EA, et al. Treatment of glioma by engineered interleukin 4-secreting cells. *Cancer Res* 1993;53:3125–3128.

27. Dranoff G, Jaffee E, Lazenby A, et al. Vaccination with irradiated tumor cells engineered to secrete murine granulocyte-macrophage

colony-stimulating factor stimulates potent, specific, and long-lasting anti-tumor immunity. *Proc Natl Acad Sci USA* 1993;90: 3539–3543.

28. Saleh M, Stacker SA, Wilks AF. Inhibition of growth of C6 glioma cells *in vivo* by expression of antisense vascular endothelial growth factor sequence. *Cancer Res* 1996;56:393–401.

29. Bischoff JR, Kirn DH, Williams A, et al. An adenovirus mutant that replicates selectively in p53-deficient human tumor cells. *Science* 1996;274:373–376.

30. Mineta T, Rabkin SD, Yazaki T, et al. Attenuated multi-mutated herpes simplex virus-1 for the treatment of malignant gliomas. *Nat Med* 1995;1:938–943.

31. Martuza RL, Malick A, Markert JM, et al. Experimental therapy of human glioma by means of a genetically engineered virus mutant. *Science* 1991;252:854–856.

32. Mineta T, Rabkin SD, Martuza RL. Treatment of malignant gliomas using ganciclovir-hypersensitive, ribonucleotide reductase-deficient herpes simplex viral mutant. *Cancer Res* 1994;54:3963–3966.

33. Edvardsen K, Chen W, Rucklidge G, et al. Transmembrane neural cell-adhesion molecule (NCAM), but not glycosyl-phosphatidylinositol-anchored NCAM, down-regulates secretion of matrix metalloproteinases. *Proc Natl Acad Sci USA* 1993;90:11463–11467.

34. Pedersen PH, Marienhagen K, Mork S, et al. Migratory pattern of fetal rat brain cells and human glioma cells in the adult rat brain. *Cancer Res* 1993;53:5158–5165.

35. Kohn EC, Liotta LA. Molecular insights into cancer invasion: strategies for prevention and intervention. *Cancer Res* 1995;55: 1856–1862.

36. Folkman J, Klagsbrun M. Vascular physiology. A family of angiogenic peptides. *Nature* 1987;329:671–672.

37. D'Amato RJ, Loughnan MS, Flynn E, et al. Thalidomide is an inhibitor of angiogenesis. *Proc Natl Acad Sci USA* 1994;91:4082–4085.

38. Fine HA, Figg WD, Jaeckle K, et al. Phase II trial of the antiangiogenic agent thalidomide in patients with recurrent high-grade gliomas. *J Clin Oncol* 2000;18:708–715.

39. Kohn EC, Reed E, Sarosy G, et al. Clinical investigation of a cytostatic calcium influx inhibitor in patients with refractory cancers. *Cancer Res* 1996;56:569–573.

40. O'Reilly MS, Boehm T, Shing Y, et al. Endostatin: an endogenous inhibitor of angiogenesis and tumor growth. *Cell* 1997;88:277–285.

41. O'Reilly MS, Holmgren L, Shing Y, et al. Angiostatin: a novel angiogenesis inhibitor that mediates the suppression of metastases by a Lewis lung carcinoma. *Cell* 1994;79:315–328.

42. Cserr HF, Knopf PM. Cervical lymphatics, the blood-brain barrier and the immunoreactivity of the brain: a new view. *Immunol Today* 1992;13:507–512.

43. Brooks WH, Markesbery WR, Gupta GD, et al. Relationship of lymphocyte invasion and survival of brain tumor patients. *Ann Neurol* 1978;4:219–224.

44. Rosenberg SA, Lotze MT, Muul LM, et al. A progress report on the treatment of 157 patients with advanced cancer using lymphokine-activated killer cells and interleukin-2 or high-dose interleukin-2 alone. *N Engl J Med* 1987;316:889–897.

45. Bigner DD, Brown MT, Friedman AH, et al. Iodine-131-labeled anti-tenascin monoclonal antibody 81C6 treatment of patients with recurrent malignant gliomas: phase I trial results. *J Clin Oncol* 1998; 16:2202–2212.

46. Riva P, Franceschi G, Arista A, et al. Local application of radiolabeled monoclonal antibodies in the treatment of high grade malignant gliomas: a six-year clinical experience. *Cancer* 1997;80:2733–2742.

47. Plautz GE, Miller DW, Barnett GH, et al. T cell adoptive immunotherapy of newly diagnosed gliomas. *Clin Cancer Res* 2000;6: 2209–2218.

48. Trouillas P. Immunology and immunotherapy of cerebral tumors. Current status. *Rev Neurol (Paris)* 1973;128:23–38.

49. Bloom HJ, Peckham MJ, Richardson AE, et al. Glioblastoma multiforme: a controlled trial to assess the value of specific active immunotherapy in patients treated by radical surgery and radiotherapy. *Br J Cancer* 1973;27:253–267.

50. Mahaley MS, Bigner DD, Dudka LF, et al. Immunobiology of primary intracranial tumors. Part 7: active immunization of patients with anaplastic human glioma cells: a pilot study. *J Neurosurg* 1983;59: 201–207.

51. Ashley DM, Sampson JH, Archer GE, et al. A genetically modified allogeneic cellular vaccine generates MHC class I-restricted cytotoxic responses against tumor-associated antigens and protects against CNS tumors *in vivo. J Neuroimmunol* 1997;78:34–46.

52. Griffitt W, Glick RP, Lichtor T, et al. Survival and toxicity of an allogeneic cytokine-secreting fibroblast vaccine in the central nervous system. *Neurosurgery* 1998;42:335–340.

53. Sampson JH, Ashley DM, Archer GE, et al. Characterization of a spontaneous murine astrocytoma and abrogation of its tumorigenicity by cytokine secretion. *Neurosurgery* 1997;41:1365–1372; discussion 1372–1373.

54. Tseng SH, Hwang LH, Lin SM. Induction of antitumor immunity by intracerebrally implanted rat C6 glioma cells genetically engineered to secrete cytokines. *J Immunother* 1997;20:334–342.

55. Grabbe S, Beissert S, Schwarz T, et al. Dendritic cells as initiators of tumor immune responses: a possible strategy for tumor immunotherapy? *Immunol Today* 1995;16:117–121.

56. Bennett SR, Carbone FR, Karamalis F, et al. Help for cytotoxic-T-cell responses is mediated by CD40 signalling. *Nature* 1998;393: 478–480.

57. Siesjo P, Visse E, Sjogren HO. Cure of established, intracerebral rat gliomas induced by therapeutic immunizations with tumor cells and purified APC or adjuvant IFN-gamma treatment. *J Immunother Emphasis Tumor Immunol* 1996;19:334–345.

58. Liau LM, Black KL, Prins RM, et al. Treatment of intracranial gliomas with bone marrow-derived dendritic cells pulsed with tumor antigens. *J Neurosurg* 1999;90:1115–1124.

107. *Intracranial Meningiomas*

Saleem I. Abdulrauf and Ossama Al-Mefty

Harvey Cushing, in 1922, coined the term "meningioma" to describe a benign tumor arising from or in proximity of the meninges (1). Subsequently, meningiomas were recognized as originating from arachnoidal cap cells commonly found within arachnoid villi at the dural venous sinuses and their tributaries, at the cranial nerve foramina, at the cribriform plate, and at the medial middle fossa (2). Intraventricular, pineal region, and spinal meningiomas are thought to originate from meningothelial cells found in the choroid plexus, the tela choroidea, and arachnoid villi at the spinal nerve exit zones (2).

Epidemiology

The incidence of meningiomas has been based on a number of different types of studies: hospital-based studies, community-based studies, and autopsy observations. Cushing and Eisenhardt's review of meningiomas in 1938 found that meningiomas constituted 13.4% of all intracranial tumors (1). In the population-based clinical study performed in Manitoba from 1980 through 1985, 22% of primary intracranial tumors were meningiomas, and the overall incidence was 2.3 per 100,000 (3). A number of large studies have shown a higher incidence of meningiomas in women, with a ratio of female to male ranging from 1.4:1 to 2.8:1 (4–6). These differences are less evident among those of African descent, who seem to have equal preponderance between the sexes (7). Moreover, in a Los Angeles County population-based study, the incidence for blacks was found to be higher (average 3.1 per 100,000) than for whites (average 2.3 per 100,000) (5).

The incidence of intracranial meningiomas increases with age (5–7). In the study by Rohinger and colleagues, the incidence of meningioma in the male population peaked in the eighth decade at 6.0 per 100,000, while in the female population it peaked at 9.5 per 100,000 in the 70 to 79 age group (3). The decline in the incidence of meningiomas observed in these studies following the eighth decade may be due to less aggressive diagnostic testing in this age group.

Etiology

Historically, meningiomas have been linked to a number of environmental factors. Genetic factors will be discussed separately.

TRAUMA. Although in the 1930s Cushing suggested that head trauma may be a significant etiological factor for meningiomas, little subsequent evidence has supported this theory. In Cushing's series of 313 patients with meningiomas, 101 had a history of trauma (8). Preston-Martin and colleagues, in a large case control study of 189 women with meningioma and a control group, found significantly more recall of prior trauma requiring medical attention in the meningioma group than in the control group (5). Other studies, however, including the study by Annegers and associates, a prospective study of 2,953 patients with head injury over 29,859 person-years, found no significant increase in the number of intracranial tumors (including meningiomas), a finding that is far more objective than the earlier smaller case control studies which relied on "recall" (9).

VIRUSES. Strong evidence currently exists associating deoxyribonucleic acid (DNA) tumor viruses with human meningiomas; however, the role of the virus in tumor development in humans remains largely unknown. Some viruses, when inoculated into laboratory animals, will produce central nervous system tumors (10). All polyomaviruses (Polyoma, SV-40), which form a subgroup of papovaviruses (human, simian, and avian), have this ability. Papovaviruses are ubiquitous in humans, and most adults have circulating antibodies against them. Antibodies against the papovavirus tumor antigen (TAg), however, have been difficult to identify in humans. Immunohistochemical techniques have demonstrated the presence of the papovavirus large TAg in meningiomas (11). The significance of this finding for tumor genesis remains unclear.

RADIATION. It is well established that radiation is capable of producing both single-stranded nicks and double-stranded breaks in DNA, which may result in deletions or translocations (10). In the early 1900s, the treatment of scalp tinea capitis (ringworm) included radiation of the head. Between 1949 and 1960, approximately 17,000 children immigrating to Israel underwent radiation therapy for tinea captis. Modan and co-work-

ers retrospectively reviewed the incidence of head and neck tumors in 11,000 of these children (12). Meningiomas occurred four times more often in the irradiated group (4 per 10,000) than in the control group (1 per 10,000). The latent period between the irradiation and the appearance of tumor ranged from 16 to 21 years.

Subsequent work in evaluating radiation-induced meningiomas revealed certain distinguishing features. Radiation-induced meningiomas are more likely to occur on the convexity, be multiple, have a greater chance to recur after surgery, and are more often malignant (13,14). A number of authors have reported the occurrence of meningiomas following cranial irradiation for a variety of tumors including pituitary adenoma, medulloblastoma, glioma, and craniopharyngioma (12–20).

HORMONAL FACTORS. In 1979 Donnell and colleagues were the first to demonstrate that meningiomas possessed estrogen receptor binding protein (21). Since then numerous reports have described the presence of estrogen receptors in meningiomas based on using *in situ* hybridization and Western or Northern blot analysis (22–28).

More recent studies indicate the minimal presence or absence of estrogen receptor and confirm generally high levels of progesterone receptors in meningioma tissue using competitive binding assay techniques. In 1997 Hsu and co-workers correlated receptor status with patient outcome in 70 patients with meningiomas. They found a statistically significant benefit in longer disease-free survival in patients whose tumors had progesterone receptors (29).

In 1986 Reubi and associates identified a high incidence of somatostatin receptors in meningioma tissue (30). *In vivo* studies using radioactive labeling of somatostatin analogues have allowed imaging of somatostatin receptors in meningiomas (31). The function of these receptors is unknown.

GENETICS AND MOLECULAR BIOLOGY. Familial cases of meningiomas as well as the higher incidence of meningiomas in neurofibromatosis prompted researchers in the past two decades to study meningiomas using cytogenetic and molecular techniques.

The most common cytogenetic finding has been the loss of one copy of chromosome 22 (32–34). In addition to this monosomy, restriction fragment length polymorphism (RFLP) mapping techniques have shown deletions within the long arm of an otherwise karyotypically normal chromosome 22 (35,36). The finding of monosomies and deletions in chromosome 22 supports the theory that loss of a tumor suppressor gene leads to the formation of meningiomas (37). According to this hypothesis, the formation of a sporadic meningioma would require both a recessive oncogene on chromosome 22 and loss of the function of a tumor suppressor gene on chromosome 22 (10). In neurofibromatosis type 2 (NF2), the recessive oncogene is thought to be inherited dominantly, therefore only a single mutation is needed, namely the deletion of the tumor suppressor gene (38). In addition to aberrations found in chromosome 22, in atypical or malignant meningiomas structural aberrations or loss of chromosomes 1p, 10q, or 14q as well as chromosome instability including rings and dicentric and telemetric associations have been demonstrated (39–43). Simon and others examined benign, atypical, and malignant meningiomas for loss of heterozygosity (LOH) on chromosomes 1p, 6p, 9q, 10q, and 14q. They found LOH of loci on chromosomes 1p and 10q in tumors of all grades and observed an increased frequency of LOH in these three subregions with increasing tumor grade (44).

Ozaki and colleagues have demonstrated that genetic alterations are more common in malignant and atypical meningiomas when compared to benign meningiomas (45). These authors, using comparative genomic hybridization analysis, showed that losses of 1p, 2p, 6p, and chromosomes 10 and 14q and gain of 20q are all genetic alterations associated with malignant transformation in meningiomas. Other studies confirm the findings of the Ozaki group and showed that alterations on chromosomes 1, 10, and 14 are especially important in the malignant progression of meningiomas (46–48).

Pathology

Macroscopically, meningiomas are generally well-circumscribed, smooth, lobulated tumors with focal attachment to the dura. Although, most meningiomas are globular in shape, some may be diffuse (i.e., *en plaque*). In general, meningiomas can easily be separated from the pia, and the senior author (O. Al-Mefty) has advocated separating the double-layered arachnoid around meningiomas to achieve a more favorable microsurgical resection. Typical histological features of meningiomas are discussed subsequently.

FIBROBLASTIC MENINGIOMA. This tumor has multi-laminated sheets or fascicles formed from elongated meningothelial cells (49).

MENINGOTHELIAL MENINGIOMA. Also known as "syncytial" meningioma, this tumor is formed from cells that are densely packed, arranged in sheets with no discernible cytoplasmic borders (49).

TRANSITIONAL MENINGIOMA. This represents a combination of both fibroblastic and meningothelial meningioma. This tumor characteristically contains cellular whorls. Psammoma bodies or hyaline cores may also be prominent in some of the whorls (49).

ANGIOMATOUS MENINGIOMA. This type of meningioma is characterized by a large number of vascular channels of varying size with intervening rests of meningothelial, fibroblastic, and transitional zones (49).

ATYPICAL MENINGIOMA. Most meningiomas exhibit benign histological features and tend to follow a benign clinical course following resection. Certain meningiomas, however, tend to recur even with lack of frank malignant histological features. The de le Monte group reviewed 82 meningiomas and identified seven histological features that correlated with recurrence: (a) hypervascularity, (b) hemosiderin deposition, (c) loss of architectural pattern, (d) increased mitotic figures, (e) necrosis, (f) prominent nucleoli, and (g) moderate or marked nuclear pleomorphism (50).

MALIGNANT MENINGIOMA. The definition of "malignant" meningiomas has been somewhat controversial. It is, however, generally accepted that this diagnosis should require evidence of brain invasion or distant metastasis. Local invasion (dura, muscle, bone, sinus) is often seen in otherwise clinically and histologically benign meningiomas and cannot be used as a criterion for malignancy in meningiomas. Hence, brain parenchymal invasion by tumor becomes the central feature of malignant meningiomas, although, in some cases of previously operated tumors with distortion of local barriers, this feature may be difficult to discern. Invasion of brain parenchyma is usually accompanied by other anaplasia, mitotic activity, and necrosis (50,51). Distant metastasis is unequivocal evidence of malignancy. The most common sites of metastasis are the lung, liver, pleura, and lymph nodes (49).

Hyperostosis associated with intracranial meningiomas has been well described, but the cause of this phenomenon has been well understood. Pieper and colleagues performed histological examination on 26 hyperstolic bones and found tumor invasion in 25 (52). Bony invasion alone, however, does not reflect malignancy in meningiomas. Dural invasion surrounding the tumor similarly does not reflect malignancy.

HEMANGIOPERICYTOMA. Hemangiopericytoma is classified as an angioblastic meningioma by some pathologists, but is given a separate identity outside the family of meningiomas by others. This tumor is virtually indistinguishable from the hemangiopericytoma arising in other parts of the body (49). The neoplasm is highly cellular and vascular, and may behave aggressively at its site of origin or may metastasize. It tends to have less crisply defined borders than true meningiomas.

The various anatomical locations of meningiomas with their presentation, natural history, surgical approaches, and outcome are discussed in the following section.

Convexity Meningiomas

Convexity meningiomas are characterized by their site of dural attachment, which lies on the hemispheres without extension to the dura mater of the skull base. In general they do not invade the dura of the venous sinus.

Cushing and Eisenhardt subclassified convexity meningiomas into precoronal, coronal, postcoronal, paracentral, parietal, occipital, and temporal (1). The clinical presentation is related to the specific location of the meningioma on the convexity. However, it is not uncommon for these lesions to attain a significant size before the development of symptoms. Seizures and incidental findings on imaging remain the most common form of presentation.

The aim of surgery for convexity meningiomas is gross total resection of the tumor, its dural attachments, and any abnormal associated bone. The extent of resection of meningiomas was graded by Simpson in 1957 in an attempt to form a correlation with the risk of recurrence (53). For convexity meningiomas, the senior author (O. Al-Mefty) has advocated that an additional 2-cm margin of dura be removed, and this resection is termed "grade zero" removal. Using this strategy, Kinjo demonstrated zero recurrence in 37 meningiomas (54).

Removal of convexity meningiomas uses the following principles of technique.

1. A series of burr holes, each placed so as to circumscribe the tumor completely, are made far from the margin of the tumor to obtain healthy dura around the tumor.
2. The dura is opened circumferentially around the tumor 2 cm from the margin of the lesion.
3. Under the operating microscope, the tumor capsule is dissected from the cerebral cortex. Maintaining dissection within the arachnoid plane is crucial to preserve the cortical layer.

4. Cortical vessels underneath the tumor should be preserved completely.
5. The tumor is then removed en bloc.
6. In some larger, more adherent tumors, central enucleation under the microscope is needed followed by the above steps.

Parasagittal Meningiomas

Cushing and Eisenhardt defined parasagittal meningiomas as those that fill the parasagittal angle with no brain tissue between the tumor and the superior sagittal sinus (1). They defined falcine tumors separately, whereas other authors, such as Olivecrona, Elsberg, and Merrem have grouped all parasagittal meningiomas with falcine meningiomas (55–60).

Cushing indicated in 1922 that meningiomas comprised 11.3% of his 751 intracranial tumors, and among these, 32% were parasagittal meningiomas. Subsequent large series have shown that parasagittal meningiomas account for 17% to 32% of all meningiomas (56,60–65).

In reviewing 154 parasagittal meningiomas, Gautier-Smith found that 62% at presentation had seizures, 54% had headaches, 49% had unilateral weakness, and 43% had mental symptoms (66). The technique of parasagittal meningioma resection is based on the following principle:

1. We prefer a bicoronal incision as it allows maximal preservation of vascularity to the skin especially if subsequent craniotomies are performed.
2. A pericranial flap is reflected separately.
3. Multiple burr holes are made at the periphery of the tumor.
4. Burr holes straddle the superior sagittal sinus to allow safe separation of the dura from the bone.
5. Microsurgical separation of the tumor capsule from surrounding cortex is done while preserving the vessels overlying the normal cortex. If the tumor has grown into the lateral aspect of the superior sagittal sinus, but the sinus is not occluded, then there are three choices:
   a. Ligate the sinus. This option has the risk of venous infarction, especially if done posterior to the anterior third of the sinus (67).
   b. Leave the portion of the tumor attached to the sinus in place with the understanding that this most likely will grow in the future, and possibly cause slow occlusion of the sinus with formation of collateral venous channels, thus allowing easier resection in the future.
   c. Resect the portion of the sinus that is involved and then repair the sinus primarily or use a patch.

Falcine Meningiomas

Falcine meningiomas, as defined by Cushing, arise from the falx, are completely concealed by overlying cortex, and typically do not involve the superior sagittal sinus (1).

Falcine meningiomas can be divided into anterior, middle, and posterior, depending on their origin on the falx. The anterior third extends from the crista galli to the coronal suture, the middle third from the coronal suture to the lambdoid suture, and the posterior third from the lambdoid suture to the torcula (68). Yaşargil and colleagues have classified falcine meningiomas into outer and inner types (69). Outer falcine meningiomas arise from the main body of the falx in the frontal (anterior or posterior), central parietal, or occipital regions. Inner falcine meningiomas arise in conjunction with the inferior sagittal sinus.

Surgical principles in the resection of falcine meningiomas are as follows:

1. Microsurgical interhemispherical exposure is achieved.
2. For unilateral tumor, early devascularization along the falx is preferred.
3. For larger tumors, central enucleation allows subsequent microsurgical separation of tumor capsule from surrounding arachnoidal areas.
4. Liberal use of cotton pledgets along the dissection plane helps prevent injury to surrounding cerebral cortex and protects the pericallosal arteries in the inferior margin of the dissection.

Tentorial Meningiomas

Yaşargil and colleagues have classified tentorial meningiomas as follows: (a) those that arise from the inner aspect of the tentorium or the free edge; (b) those that arise from the outer ring or along the transverse sinus; (c) those that arise from the central leaflet of the tentorium; and (d) those that arise at the falcotentorial junction (69).

Surgical excision of tumors involving the tentorium can be challenging, mainly due to difficulties of access, especially for medially located lesions, as well as their relationship to the brainstem, cranial nerves, temporal lobe, blood vessels, and venous sinuses. The downward sloping of the tentorium, from its apex anteriorly to the petrous bones laterally, and to the occipital bones posteriorly adds an extra geometric complicating factor to the surgical exposure of these lesions. More recent advances in microsurgical techniques and skull base approaches have made access and resection of the larger and medially located tumors less formidable.

Although medial tentorial ring meningiomas may appear very similar to petroclival and sphenopetroclival meningiomas on radiographic examination, they differ significantly in their local anatomical relationships and ultimately this is reflected in the operative difficulty and outcome (70). Petroclival meningiomas originate medial to cranial nerve V, and based on the senior author's observations, usually only have one layer of arachnoid separating them from the brainstem to which they are usually adherent, thus making total resection technically difficult. Tentorial meningiomas on the other hand, arise from the tentorial edge, where there is convergence of the interpeduncular, crural, and ambient cisterns, and as they grow, they push multiple layers of arachnoid ahead of them. This provides a clear demarcation between the tumor, brainstem, and cranial nerves, thus making total resection relatively less risky.

Delineation of the vascular anatomy, especially that of the venous system, is crucial for planning surgery. This should include bilateral demonstration of the transverse and sigmoid sinuses and their connection at the torcular herophili for lateral and posterior approaches. Venous drainage of the temporal lobe must be thoroughly studied. This system includes the vein of Labbé and basal temporal veins, and it is important to identify their relationship to the superior petrosal sinus, tentorium, and sigmoid sinus. The jugular bulb and its location must also be delineated. These structures are best seen during the venous stage of angiography; however, magnetic resonance venography may be sufficient to obtain this information (71).

The surgical resection of tentorial meningiomas is based on

their specific location. Tumors involving anterior to midmedial incisural ring and petrous apex with extension into the perimesencephalic area can be resected using the zygomatic extended middle fossa approach. We prefer this approach to the standard subtemporal approach, since it allows a far more inferior window and thus less temporal lobe retraction. This approach can be combined with an anterior petrosectomy for lesions extending posteriorly into the lateral pontine area. Lesions involving the middle to posterior part of the inner ring of the tentorium with involvement of the petroclival area and extension into perimesencephalic cistern can be approached using the petrosal method. Falcotentorial lesions can be accessed using a posterior interhemispherical transtentorial approach. Tumors at the falcotentorial junction that are mainly infratentorial can be accessed via a supracerebellar infratentorial approach. Larger tentorial leaf tumors with superior extension into the occipital lobe and inferior extension into the cerebellum can be approached using the combined supra-infratentorial method.

Olfactory Groove Meningiomas

The anatomy, pathology, and the surgical principles of the management of olfactory groove meningiomas were eloquently described by Cushing in 1938 (1). In this monograph, based on his management of 29 patients with olfactory groove meningiomas, Cushing emphasized the importance of tumor decompression prior to tumor capsule dissection and the importance of preserving the anterior cerebral arteries and their branches, which may be adherent to the tumor capsule.

These tumors tend to grow slowly and gradually compress the frontal lobes. Due to lack of focal functional areas in the inferomesial frontal lobes, these meningiomas may attain a large size before presenting clinically.

Smaller olfactory groove meningiomas can be approached through a unilateral frontal or pterional approach. Larger olfactory groove meningiomas are best addressed using a standard bifrontal approach or a bilateral frontal cranio-orbital approach, which allows early devascularization of the tumor, minimal or no brain retraction, resection of the dural base, and repair of the anterior cranial base.

Sphenoidal Wing and Clinoidal Meningiomas

These meningiomas are classified based on their point of origin along the sphenoidal wing, as clinoidal, middle sphenoidal, or lateral sphenoidal wing tumors.

Meningiomas *en plaque* also occur in the area of the sphenoidal wing. These are characterized by marked hyperostosis of the sphenoidal bone and diffuse tumor invasion leading to proptosis or cranial neuropathies resulting from foraminal encroachment. The surgical approach to this type of meningioma is the complete removal of the greater wing of the sphenoidal wing, and the anterior clinoid, as well as the removal of the superior and lateral orbital walls. This is followed by generous removal of the affected dura. Careful dural repair with autologous fat, temporalis muscle, and/or fascia is undertaken (72).

Lateral sphenoidal wing meningiomas can be resected following extradural drilling of the sphenoidal ridge, which also aids in the devascularization of the tumors. Those meningiomas that arise from the middle third of the sphenoidal wing are also

resected following extradural drilling of the sphenoidal wing, and for tumors that involve the orbital margins, the superior orbital fissure, and grow toward the cavernous sinus, a cranio-orbitozygomatic craniotomy may be the optimal approach.

The more medially located clinoidal meningiomas represent a distinct clinical-anatomical entity, and historically the resection of these lesions has been associated with significant morbidity and mortality. Recent advances in cranial base surgery have allowed for more complete resection with lower risks of morbidity and mortality. Al-Mefty has classified clinoidal meningiomas into three categories based on the anatomical site of origin and degree of surgical difficulty (73).

After emerging from the cavernous sinus inferior and medial to the anterior clinoid process, the carotid artery enters the subdural space, where it lacks an arachnoidal covering over a distance of 1 to 2 mm. The carotid artery then enters the carotid cistern and is invested in arachnoid. Thus, if the origin of the meningioma is proximal to the carotid cistern (group I), as is the case in a meningioma originating at the inferior aspect of the anterior clinoid process, the tumor will enwrap the carotid artery, directly adhering to the adventitia without an interfacing arachnoidal membrane. As the tumor grows, this direct attachment to the vessel wall advances to the carotid bifurcation and along the middle cerebral artery, pushing the arachnoid membrane ahead of it. This anatomical arrangement accounts for the inability of the surgeon to dissect the tumor from the carotid artery and the middle cerebral branches.

Group II clinoidal meningiomas originate from the superior or lateral aspect of the anterior clinoid process above the segment of the carotid artery, which has already been invested by the arachnoid of the carotid cistern. As this tumor grows, the arachnoidal membrane of the carotid cistern and, more distally, of the sylvian cistern, separates the tumor from the arterial adventitia. This plane allows dissection of the tumor from the vessels even though they may be entirely engulfed. In group I and II tumors, the optic chiasm and nerves are wrapped in the arachnoidal membrane of the chiasmatic cistern, allowing microsurgical dissection of the tumor from these structures.

Group III clinoidal meningiomas originate at the optic foramen and extend into the optic canal and at the tip of the anterior clinoid process. These tumors are generally small, appearing early with optic nerve compression and decreased visual acuity. The arachnoidal membrane investing the carotid artery is present. Because this tumor arises proximal to the chiasmatic cistern, however, there may be no arachnoidal investment between the optic nerve and the tumor (74).

We recommend the cranio-orbitozygomatic approach for the resection of clinoidal meningiomas. This provides the surgeon a low-based approach with multiple avenues of dissection, requires minimal brain retraction, and offers the ability to enter the cavernous sinus if needed.

Tuberculum Sellae Meningiomas

Tuberculum sellae meningiomas account for 5% to 10% of intracranial meningiomas (75–79). The mean age of their occurrence is the fourth decade with a predominance of women in a ratio of 3:1 (80–82). The "chiasmal syndrome," a primary optic atrophy with bitemporal field defect in adult patients showing an essentially normal sellae, has been the classic presentation of this tumor since its recognition in 1927 by Holmes and Sargent (83). This was subsequently documented further by Cushing (84).

In most patients, visual loss is insidious in onset and progressive in course. It may, however, be acute or fluctuating (77,80, 82). Approximately two-thirds of patients complain of failing vision in one eye as the first symptom, and monocular blindness may be present in half of cases prior to surgery (85). Schlezinger and associates (86) emphasize that uniform visual fields in these lesions are not possible for anatomical reasons and stress the early occurrence of scotomatous field defects. Incongruity and asymmetry of the field defect is the common finding.

The classic and most common funduscopic finding is primary optic atrophy, which is asymmetrical in both eyes and different in degree (87). This may be accompanied by an incongruous bitemporal hemianopsia, and unilateral optic atrophy is usually associated with a suprasellar meningioma (88).

Anosmia rarely presents in patients with suprasellar meningioma (87). Poppen (89) emphasizes that olfactory groove meningiomas present with anosmia early on, while visual symptoms are a late finding. He notes, however, that suprasellar meningiomas present with a history of visual deficit, while anosmia is a late finding. Mental changes (memory impairment, personality changes, depression, anxiety) are present in 10% of cases (79, 90). Motor deficits are rare findings. Other clinical findings include seizures and dizziness.

The surgical resection of tuberculum sellae meningiomas is best done using a unilateral supraorbital, subfrontal approach. Tuberculum sellae meningiomas typically displace both optic nerves outward and backward, often to the extent that the optic nerve lies above and lateral to the internal carotid artery, with the chiasm stretched far back from the tuberculum sellae.

Identifying the optic nerve can be quite difficult when it has been completely engulfed by the tumor or when it has been distorted to an almost unrecognizable thin band in the tumor capsule. Extreme caution and piecemeal removal of the tumor, using fine-tipped bipolar forceps and microdissectors, are necessary. The tumor is slowly stripped from the flattened and engulfed nerve. Despite apparent encasement or severe adherence, a plane of dissection can be obtained under high magnification (88).

Diaphragma sellae meningiomas are a separate clinical-anatomical entity, although in the literature they are largely grouped with the tuberculum sellae tumors. Kinjo and associates have classified these lesions into three categories (91):

- type A, originating from the upper leaf of the diaphragma sellae anterior to the pituitary stalk
- type B, originating from the upper leaf of the diaphragma sellae posterior to the pituitary stalk
- type C, originating from the inferior leaf of the diaphragma sellae

For types A and B, surgery is technically more difficult due to the deep location and the difficulty of dissecting these tumors from the pituitary stalk.

Cavernous Sinus Meningiomas

In 1965 Parkinson (92) was the first to systematically address the cavernous sinus and its anatomy specifically for vascular and neoplastic lesions. Advances in skull base and microvascular surgery over the past two decades have made it possible to safely resect lesions within the cavernous sinus.

Meningiomas involving the cavernous the sinus may start primarily within it, or the cavernous sinus may be involved secondary to extension from clinoidal, sphenoidal wing, tuberculum sellae, or sphenopetroclival meningioma.

Detailed study of the internal carotid artery and its collateral systems is of paramount importance prior to surgical excision of a cavernous sinus meningioma. Magnetic resonance angiography, conventional angiography, and balloon test occlusion in association with cerebral blood flow studies, such as xenon computed tomography or radioisotope spectroscopy, are available to study cerebral blood flow dynamics in this setting.

The surgical approach to the cavernous sinus most often uses the cranio-orbitozygomatic approach. Proximal and distal control of the internal carotid artery is needed prior to dissection within the cavernous sinus. Proximal control may be achieved by exposing the internal carotid artery within the petrous bone in the middle fossa or by exposing the cervical internal carotid artery.

Entry into the cavernous sinus may be either through the medial triangles or the lateral triangles. Dissection of the tumor progresses in a stepwise fashion, beginning by opening the dura propria of the optic nerve sheath longitudinally along the length of the optic canal (74). The distal dural ring is opened next, with the opening extending posteriorly to the oculomotor trigone, and thereby also opening the proximal dural ring and allowing a wide entry into the anterior and superior cavernous sinus space. The carotid artery can be mobilized laterally by releasing it from its proximal and distal dural rings, which then allows dissection in the medial cavernous sinus space. Lateral entry into the cavernous sinus begins by an incision beneath the projected course of the third nerve, allowing elevation of the outer dural layer of the lateral wall of the cavernous sinus, which is peeled away. The internal carotid artery can be located by dissection between the third and fourth nerves and the first division of the trigeminal nerve (Parkinson triangle). The course of the sixth nerve, which runs lateral to the internal carotid artery and is usually in direct apposition to it, is usually parallel but deep to the first division of the trigeminal nerve. The tumor is removed from within the cavernous sinus space by suction, bipolar coagulation, and microdissection. A plane of cleavage along the carotid artery can usually be developed. Venous bleeding, typically not a problem when the tumor fills the sinus, may occur as the venous plexus is decompressed by tumor removal. In that event, homeostasis can be obtained by packing the cavernous sinus space with oxidized cellulose or another similar hemostatic agent.

In the senior author's series, gross total removal of cavernous sinus meningioma has been possible in 76% of patients. The major surgical morbidity and mortality rates were 4.8% and 2.4%, respectively. Preoperative cranial nerve deficits improved in 14%, remained unchanged in 80%, and permanently worsened in 6%. Seven patients experienced 10 new cranial nerve deficits (93). However, gross total removal does not imply care and regrowth from microscopic remnants of tumor may occur.

Petroclival Meningiomas

Cushing and Eisenhardt recognized early on that petroclival meningiomas were a formidable entity as they involved both the supratentorial and infratentorial compartments, and they included five patients in their "gasserpetrosal" group (1). The differentiation between clival, petroclival, and sphenopetroclival meningiomas is based on the surgical anatomy of the lesion. Those tumors that arise from the superior two-thirds of the clivus and displace the brainstem posteriorly are considered clival meningiomas. Petroclival meningiomas also involve the superior two-thirds of the clivus and are located medial to the fifth cranial nerve with the bulk of the tumor being more lateral along the spheno-occipital synchondrosis. In the latter group the brainstem and basilar artery are typically displaced to the contralateral side. Sphenopetroclival meningiomas have similar characteristics to petroclival meningiomas but also invade the lateral wall of the cavernous sinus along the medial sphenoidal wing.

Headache and ataxia from cerebellar compression are the most often identified clinical findings. Other findings including long tract signs, spastic paresis, and cranial neuropathies are also common. The natural history of these tumors almost uniformly leads to a fatal outcome in the absence of treatment. However, surgical treatment of these lesions prior to the 1980s was associated with very poor outcomes and an operative mortality exceeding 50% (94–96).

With advancements in microsurgical technique, neuroanesthesia, intensive care unit management, and improved knowledge of skull base anatomy, surgical resection of these lesions is now feasible with acceptable risk of morbidity and mortality. The principles of petroclival meningioma resection involve using a lateral skull base approach while avoiding brain retraction, avoidance of venous injury especially the vein of Labbé, and connecting the middle and posterior fossa by drilling the petrous ridge and splitting the tentorium. Two main approaches should be considered for these lesions: the petrosal approach and the middle fossa approach.

PETROSAL APPROACH. The petrosal approach offers a number of advantages:

1. The surgeon's operative distance to these regions is shorter than in the retrosigmoid approaches.
2. There is minimal retraction of the cerebellum and temporal lobe.
3. The neural structures (seventh and eighth nerves) are preserved.
4. The otological structures (cochlea, labyrinth, semicircular canals) are preserved.
5. The major venous sinuses (transverse and sigmoid), along with the vein of Labbé and other temporal and basal veins, are preserved (88).

MIDDLE FOSSA APPROACH. This approach is best suited for those tumors that primarily involve the supratentorial compartment with minimal extension into the posterior fossa. The exposure provides access to the cavernous sinus and Meckel cave. Lesions extending below the porus acusticus should not be approached through this exposure.

The extended petrosal approach is a combination of the middle fossa approach and the posterior petrosal approach, and can be used in cases where a single lateral window is not enough to allow resection of the lesion. Total petrosectomy affords the widest exposure of the petroclival region as well as the cavernous sinus and the parasellar areas. By definition this approach sacrifices hearing and therefore we use this technique mainly with patients with large tumors who lack hearing in the ipsilateral ear. The exposure also requires mobilization of the seventh cranial nerve and the majority of the patients suffer from temporary facial paresis.

Using such approaches, recent reports have indicated total tumor removal in 25% to 85% of patients (97–100).

Foramen Magnum Meningiomas

Foramen magnum meningiomas are divided into two main types (1,101):

1. Ventral foramen magnum meningiomas, which originate from the basal groove at the lower third of the clivus anterior to the medulla and project inferiorly toward the foramen magnum.
2. Spinocranial meningiomas, which originate from the upper cervical area, usually posterior or posterolateral to the spinal cord, and project superiorly into the cerebellomedullary cistern.

Patients with lesions in this location may present with unusual symptoms and can often be misdiagnosed. Cervical pain, usually unilateral, and motor and sensory deficits, especially involving the upper extremities and in later stages progressing to spastic quadriplegia, are well-documented clinical findings in foramen magnum meningiomas.

Lateral or posterior foramen magnum meningiomas can be resected using a standard inferior suboccipital approach. Ventral foramen magnum meningiomas, however, can be challenging and clearly pose a formidable challenge due to the involvement of the lower cranial nerves and vertebrobasilar artery complex and significant brainstem compression. The latter type, in the opinion of the authors, is best resected using the transcondylar approach (102–106).

Historically, surgical results of foramen magnum meningioma resection have been poor overall, especially for ventrally situated tumors. Recent advances in microsurgical techniques, neuroanesthetic management, and skull base approaches have led to improved results. In the experience of the senior author in the surgical management of 18 patients with ventral foramen magnum meningiomas using the transcondylar approach, statistically significant improvement in Karnofsky performance scores was documented overall. Ninth and tenth cranial nerve deficits were the most common complications, and there was no perioperative mortality (101).

References

1. Cushing H, Eisenhardt L. Meningiomas: Their classification, regional behavior, life history, and surgical end results. Springfield, IL: Hafner Publishing Co., 1938.
2. DeMonte F, Marmor R, Al-Mefty O. Meningiomas. In: Kaye AH, Laws ER, eds. *Brain tumors: an encyclopedic approach*, 2nd ed. London: Churchill Livingstone, 2001:719–750.
3. Rohinger M, Sutherland GR, Louw DF. Incidence of clinicopathological features of meningiomas. *J Neurosurg* 1989; 71: 665–692.
4. Kurland LT, Schoenberg BS, Annegers JF, et al. The incidence of primary intracranial neoplasms in Rochester, Minnesota. *Ann N Y Acad Sci* 1982;381: 6–16.
5. Preston-Martin S, Paganini-Hill A, Henderson BE, et al. Case control study of intracranial meningiomas in women in Los Angeles County. *J Natl Cancer Inst* 1980;65:67–73.
6. Sutherland GR, Florell R, Louw D, et al. Epidemiology of primary intracranial neoplasms in Manitoba, Canada. *Can J Neurolog Sci* 1987;15:586–592.
7. Fan K, Pezeshkpour GH. Ethnic distribution of primary central nervous system tumors in Washington, D.C., 1971 to 1985. *J Natl Med Assoc* 1992;84:858–863 .
8. Cushing H, Weed LH. Studies on the cerebrospinal fluid and its pathways. No. IX. Calcaseous and osseous deposits in the arachnoidea. *Johns Hopkins Hosp Bull* 1915;26:367–372.
9. Annegers J, Laws E, Kurland L, et al. Head trauma and subsequent brain tumors. *Neurosurgery* 1979;4:203–206.
10. Rachlin J, Rosenblum M. Etiology and biology of meningiomas. In: Al-Mefty O, ed. *Meningiomas*. New York: Raven Press, 1991.
11. Tabuchi K, Kirsch W, Low M, et al. Screening of human brain tumors for SV-40 related T antigen. *Int J Cancer* 1978;21:12–17.
12. Modan B, Baidatz D, Mart H, et al. Radiation-induced head and neck tumours. *Lancet* 1974;1:277–279.
13. Rubinstein AB, Shalit MN, Cohen ML, et al. Radiation-induced cerebral meningiomas: a recognizable entity. *J Neurosurg* 1984;61: 966–971.

14. Soffer D, Pittaluga S, Feiner M, et al. Intracranial meningiomas following low dose irradiation to the head. *J Neurosurg* 1983;59: 1048–1053.

15. Bogdanowicz WM, Saches E Jr. The possible role of radiation in oncogenesis of meningioma. *Surg Neurol* 1974;2:379–383.

16. Iancono RP, Apuzzo MLJ, Davis RL, et al. Multiple meningiomas following radiation therapy for medulloblastoma. Case report. *J Neurosurg* 1981;55:282–286.

17. Norwood CW, Kelly DL Jr, Davis CH, et al. Irradiation induced mesodermal tumors of the central nervous system: report of 2 meningiomas following x-ray treatment for gliomas. *Surg Neurol* 1974; 2:161–164.

18. Robinson RG. A second brain tumour and irradiation. *J Neurol Neurosurg Psychiatry* 1978;41:1005–1012.

19. Spallone A, Gagliordi FM, Vagnozzi R. Intracranial meningiomas related to external cranial irradiation. *Surg Neurol* 1979;12: 153–159.

20. Waga S, Handa H. Radiation-induced meningiomas with review of the literature. *Surg Neurol* 1976;5:215–219.

21. Donnell MS, Meyer GA, Donegan WL. Estrogen-receptor protein in intracranial meningiomas. *J Neurosurg* 1979;50:499–502.

22. Blaauw G, Blankenstein MA, Lamberts SWJ. Sex steroid receptors in human meningiomas. *Acta Neurochir* 1986;79:42–47.

23. Cahill DW, Bashirelahi N, Solomon LW, et al. Estrogen and progesterone receptors in meningiomas. *J Neurosurg* 1984;60:985–993.

24. Lesch KP, Fahlbusch R. Simultaneous estradiol and progesterone receptor analysis in meningiomas. *Surg Neurol* 1986;26:257–263.

25. Markwalder T-M, Zava DT, Goldhirsch A, et al. Estrogen and progesterone receptors in meningiomas in relation to clinical and pathologic features. *Surg Neurol* 1983;20:42–47.

26. Martuza RL, MacLaughlin DT, Ojemann RG. Specific estradiol binding in schwannomas, meningiomas, and neurofibromas. *Neurosurgery* 1981;9:665–671.

27. Poisson M, Pertuiset BF, Hauw J-J, et al. Steroid hormone receptors in human meningiomas, gliomas and brain tumors. *J Neuro-Oncol* 1983;1:179–189.

28. Schnegg J-F, Gomez F, LeMarchand-Beraud T, et al. Presence of sex hormone receptors in meningioma tissue. *Surg Neurol* 1981; 15:415–418.

29. Hsu DW, Efird JT, Hedley-Whyte ET. Progesterone and estrogen receptors in meningiomas: prognostic considerations. *J Neurosurg* 1997;86 (1):113–20.

30. Reubi JC, Maurer R, Klijn JGM, et al. High incidence of somatostatin receptors in human meningiomas: biochemical characterization. *J Clin Endocrinol Metab* 1986;63:433–438.

31. Lamberts SWJ, Reubi JC, Krenning EP. Somatostatin receptor imaging in the diagnosis and treatment of neuroendocrine tumors. *J Steroid Biochem Molec Biol* 1992a;43:185–188.

32. Casalone R, Gronata P, Simi E, et al. Recessive cancer genes in meningiomas? An analysis of 31 cases. *Cancer Genet Cytogenet* 1987;27:145–159.

33. Katsuyama J, Papenhausen PR, Herz F, et al. Chromosome abnormalities in meningiomas. *Cancer Genet Cytogenet* 1986;22:63–68.

34. Zang KD. Cytological and cytogenetical studies on human meningioma. *Cancer Genet Cytogenet* 1982;6:249–274.

35. Seizinger BR, Martuza RL, Gusella JF. Loss of genes on chromosome 22 in tumorigenesis of human acoustic neuroma. *Nature* 1986;322:644–647.

36. Seizinger BR, Rouleau GA, Ozelius GJ, et al. Common pathogenetic mechanism for three tumor types in bilateral acoustic neurofibromatosis. *Science* 1987;336:317–319.

37. Rouleau GA, Wertelecki W, Haines JL, et al. Genetic linkage of bilateral acoustic neurofibromatosis to a DNA marker on chromosome 22. *Nature* 1987;329:246–248.

38. Collins VP, Nordenskjold M, Dumanski JP. The molecular genetics of meningiomas. *Brain Pathol* 1990;1:19–24.

39. Al-Saadi A, Latimer F, Madercic M, et al. Cytogenetic studies of human brain tumors and their clinical significance: II. Meningioma. *Cancer Genet Cytogenet* 1987;26:127–141.

40. Bello JM, et al. Allelic loss at 1p is associated with tumor progression of meningiomas. *Genes Chrom Cancer* 1994;9:296–298.

41. Perry A, Jenkins RB, Dahl RJ, et al. Cytogenetic analysis of aggressive meningiomas. *Cancer* 1996;77:2567–2573.

42. Rey JA, Bello MJ, de Campos JM, et al. Chromosomal involvement secondary to -22 in human meningiomas. *Cancer Genet Cytogenet* 1988;33:275–290.

43. Vagner-Capodano AM, Grisoli F, Gamgarelli D, et al. Correlation between cytogenetic and histopathological findings in 75 human meningiomas. *Neurosurgery* 1993;32:892–900.

44. Simon M, von Deimling A, Larson JJ, et al. Allelic losses on chromosomes 14, 10, and 1 in atypical and malignant meningiomas: a genetic model of meningioma progression. *Cancer Res* 1995;55: 4696–4701.

45. Ozaki S, Nishizaki T, Ito H, et al. Comparative genomic hybridization analysis of genetic alterations associated with malignant progression of meningioma. *J Neuro-Oncol* 1999;41 (2):167–174.

46. Lamszus K, Kluwe L, Matschke J, et al. Allelic losses at 1p, 9q, 10q, 14q and 22q in the progression of aggressive meningiomas and undifferentiated meningeal sarcomas. *Cancer Genet Cytogenet* 1999;110 (2):103–110.

47. Leone PE, Bello MJ, de Campos JM, et al. NF2 gene mutations and allelic status of 1p, 14q and 22q in sporadic meningiomas. *Oncogenet* 1999;18 (13):2231–2239.

48. Weber RG, Bostrom J, Wolter M, et al. Analysis of genomic alterations in benign, atypical, and anaplastic meningiomas: toward a genetic model of meningioma progression. *Proc Natl Acad Sci USA* 1997;94 (26):14719–14724.

49. Chou SM, Miles JM. The pathology of meningiomas. In: Al-Mefty O, ed. *Meningiomoas*. New York: Raven Press, 1991.

50. de la Monte SM, Flickeringer J, Linggood RM. Histopathologic features predicting recurrence of meningiomas following sub-total resection. *Am J Surg Pathol* 1986;10:836–843.

51. Jaaskelainen J, Haltia M, Laasonen E, et al. The growth of intracranial meningiomas and its relation to histology: an analysis of 43 patients. *Surg Neurol* 1985;24:165–172.

52. Pieper DR, Al-Mefty O, Hanada Y, et al. Hyperostosis associated with meningioma of the cranial base: secondary changes or tumor invasion. *Neurosurgery* 1999;44 (4):742–746;discussion 746–747.

53. Simpson D. The recurrence of intracranial meningiomas after surgical treatment. *J Neurol Neurosurg Psychiatry* 1957;20:22–39.

54. Kinjo T. Grade zero removal of supratentorial convexity meningiomas. *Neurosurgery* 1993;33:394–399.

55. Elsberg CA. The parasagittal meningeal fibroblastomas. *Bull Neurol Inst NY* 1931;1:389–418.

56. Merrem G. Die parasagittalen meningiome. Fedor Krause-Gedachtnisvorlesung. *Acta Neurochir (Vienna)* 1970;23:203–216.

57. Olivecrona H. Die parasagittalen meningeome. *Zentralbl Chir* 1932;59:2954–2958.

58. Olivecrona H. Die parasagittalen meningeome. Leipzig: Georg Thieme, 1934.

59. Olivecrona H. The parasagittal meningiomas. *J Neurosurg* 1947;4: 327–341.

60. Olivecrona H. The surgical treatment of intracranial tumors. In: Olivecrona H, Tonnis W, eds. *Handbook of clinical neurosurgery*, vol. 4, part 4. Berlin: Springer-Verlag, 1967:1–191.

61. Giombini S, Solero CL, Lasio G, et al. Immediate and late outcome of operations for parasagittal and falx meningiomas: report of 342 cases. *Surg Neurol* 1984;21:427–435.

62. Hoessly GF, Olivecrona H. Report on 280 cases of verified parasagittal meningioma. *J Neurosurg* 1955;12:614–626.

63. Janisch W, Guthert H, Schrieber D. Pathologie der tumoren des zentralnervensystems. Jena: Fischer, 1976.

64. Mahaley MS Jr, Mettlin C, Natarajan N, et al. National survey of patterns of care for brain-tumor patients. *J Neurosurg* 1989;71: 826–836.

65. Zulch KJ. *Brain tumors: their biology and pathology*, 3rd ed. Berlin: Springer-Verlag, 1986.

66. Gautier-Smith PC. *Parasagittal and falx meningiomas*. London: Butterworth, 1970.

67. Jaeger R. Observations on resection of the superior longitudinal sinus at and posterior to the rolandic venous inflow. *J Neurosurg* 1951;8:103–109.

68. Lanman TH, Becker DP. Falcine meningiomas. In Al-Mefty O, ed. *Meningiomas*. New York: Raven Press, 1991.

69. Yaşargil MG. *Microneurosurgery of CNS tumors, IV-B*. Stuttgart/New York: Georg Thieme-Verlag, 1996:134–165.

70. Harrison MJ, Al-Mefty O. *Tentorial meningiomas*. Montreal: Williams & Wilkins, 1996:451–466.

71. Al-Mefty O. *Operative atlas of meningiomas.* New York: Lippin-cott-Raven, 1998:209–286.
72. DeMonte F, Al-Mefty O. Meningiomas. In: Kaye AH, Laws ER Jr, eds. *Brain tumors: an encyclopedic approach.* New York: Church-ill Livingstone, 1995:675–704.
73. Al-Mefty O. Clinoidal meningiomas. In: Al Mefty O, ed. *Meningiomas.* New York: Raven Press, 1991:427–443.
74. DeMonte F, Al-Mefty O. Anterior clinoidal meningiomas. In: Rengachary SS, Wilking RH, eds. *Neurosurgery: operative atlas,* Vol 3, No. 1. Baltimore: Williams & Wilkins, 1993:49–61.
75. Earle KM, Richany SF. Meningiomas: a case study of the histology, incidence, and biologic behavior of 243 cases from the Frazier-Grant collection of brain tumors. *Med Ann DC* 1969;38:353–356.
76. Kadis GN, Mount LA, Granti SR. The importance of early diagnosis and treatment of the meningiomas of the planum sphenoidale and tuberculum sellae: a retrospective study of 105 cases. *Surg Neurol* 1979;12:367–371.
77. Kunicki A, Uhl A. The clinical picture and results of surgical treatment of meningioma of the tuberculum sellae. *Cesk Neurolie* 1968; 31:80–91.
78. MacCarty CS, Taylor WF. Intracranial meningiomas: experiences at the Mayo Clinic. *Neurol Med Chir (Tokyo)* 1979;19:569–574.
79. Solero CL, Giombini S, Morello G. Suprasellar and olfactory meningiomas: report on a series of 153 personal cases. *Acta Neurochir (Vienna)* 1983:181–194.
80. Finn JE, Mount LA. Meningiomas of tuberculum sellae and planum sphenoidale: a review of 83 cases. *Arch Ophthalmol* 1974;92: 23–27.
81. Krenkel W, Frowein RA. Suprasellar meningiomas. *Acta Neurochir (Vienna)* 1975;31:280.
82. Symon L, Jakubowski J III. Meningiomas. Clinical features, technical problems, and results of treatment of anterior parasellar meningiomas. *Acta Neurochir (Vienna)* 1979;28(suppl):367–370.
83. Holmes G, Sargent P. Suprasellar endotheliomata. *Brain* 1927;50: 518–537.
84. Cushing H, Eisenhardt L. Meningiomas arising from the tuberculum sellae with the syndrome of primary optic atrophy and bitemporal field defects combined with a normal sellae turcica in a middle-aged person. *Arch Ophthalmol* 1929;1:1–41;168–206.
85. Krenkel W, Frowein RA. The suprasellar meningiomas. *Adv Neurosurg* 1975;2:55–58.
86. Schlezinger NS, Alpers BJ, Weiss BP. Suprasellar meningiomas associated with scotomatous field defects. *Arch Ophthalmol* 1946; 35:624–642.
87. Ehlers N, Malmros R. The suprasellar meningiomas: a review of the literature and presentation of a series of 31 cases. *Acta Ophthalmol (Copenh)* 1973;121(suppl):1–74.
88. Al-Mefty O, Smith RR. Tuberculum sellae meningiomas. In: Al-Mefty O, ed. *Meningiomas.* New York: Raven Press, 1991:395–411.
89. Poppen JL. Operative techniques for removal of olfactory groove and suprasellar meningiomas. *Clin Neurosurg* 1963;11:1–7.
90. Symon L, Rosenstein J. Surgical management of suprasellar meningioma, part I: the influence of tumor size, duration of symptoms, and microsurgery on surgical outcome in 101 consecutive cases. *J Neurosurg* 1984;61:633–641.
91. Kinjo T, Al-Mefty O, Ciric I. Diaphragma sellae meningiomas. *Neurosurgery* 1995;36:1082–1092.
92. Parkinson D. A surgical approach to the cavernous portion of the carotid artery: anatomical studies and case report. *J Neurosurg* 1965;23:474–483.
93. DeMonte F, Al-Mefty O. Neoplasms and the cranial nerves of the posterior fossa. In: Barrow DL, ed. *Surgery of the cranial nerves of the posterior fossa.* Park Ridge, IL: American Association of Neurological Surgeons, 1993:253–274.
94. Campbell E, Whitefield RD. Posterior fossa meningiomas. *J Neurosurg* 1948;5:131–153.
95. Dany A, Delcour J, Laine E. Les meningiomes du clivus. *Neurochirurgie* 1963;9:249–277.
96. Harsh GR, Sekhar LN. The subtemporal transcavernous, anterior transpetrosal approach to the upper brain stem and clivus. *J Neurosurg* 1992;77:709–717.
97. Al-Mefty O, Fox JL, Smith RR. Petrosal approach for petroclival meningiomas. *Neurosurgery* 1988;22:510–517.
98. Samii M, Ammirati M, Mahran A, et al. Surgery of the petroclival meningiomas: report of 24 cases. *Neurosurgery* 1989;24:12–17.
99. Symon L. Surgical approaches to the tentorial hiatus. In: Krayenbuhl H, ed. *Advances and technical standards in neurosurgery.* Vol 9. Vienna: Springer-Verlag, 1982:69–112.
100. Yaşargil MG, Mortara RW, Curcic M. Meningiomas of basal posterior fossa. In: Krayenbuhl H, ed. *Advances and technical standards in neurosurgery.* Vol 7. Vienna: Springer-Verlag, 1980:1–115.
101. Arnautovic KI, Al-Mefty O, Husain M. Ventral foramen magnum meningiomas. *J Neurosurg* 2000;92(1 suppl):71–80.
102. Al-Mefty O, Borba LAB, Aoki N. The transcondylar approach to extradural non-neoplastic lesions of the craniovertebral junction. *J Neurosurg* 1996;84:1–6.
103. George B, Lot G. Anterolateral and posterolateral approaches to the foramen magnum: technical description and experience from 97 cases. *Skull Base Surg* 1995;5:9–19.
104. Baldwin HZ, Miller CG, van Loveren HR, et al. The far lateral/combined supra- and infratentorial approach. A human cadaveric prosection model for routes of access to the petroclival region and ventral brain stem. *J Neurosurg* 1994;81:60–68.
105. Sen CN, Sekhar LN. An extreme lateral approach to intradural lesions of the cervical spine and foramen magnum. *Neurosurgery* 1990;27:197–204.
106. Wellington B, Al-Mefty O. Foramen magnum tumors. In: Cohen AR, ed. *Surgical disorders of the fourth ventricle.* Cambridge: Blackwell Science, 1996:251–261.

108. Intraventricular Tumors: Lateral Ventricles

Albert L. Rhoton, Jr.

The lateral ventricles, in addition to being the site of deeply situated lesions, also provide deep cavities through which the third ventricle and basal cisterns may be approached. The neural and vascular relationships that provide the basis for optimizing the results obtained with intraventricular operations are reviewed before describing the individual operative approaches.

Neural Relationships

Each lateral ventricle is a C-shaped cavity situated deep within the cerebrum. The walls of each ventricle are formed predominantly by the thalamus, septum pellucidum, corpus callosum, caudate nucleus, and fornix (Figs. 1 to 3) (1–3). The thalamus

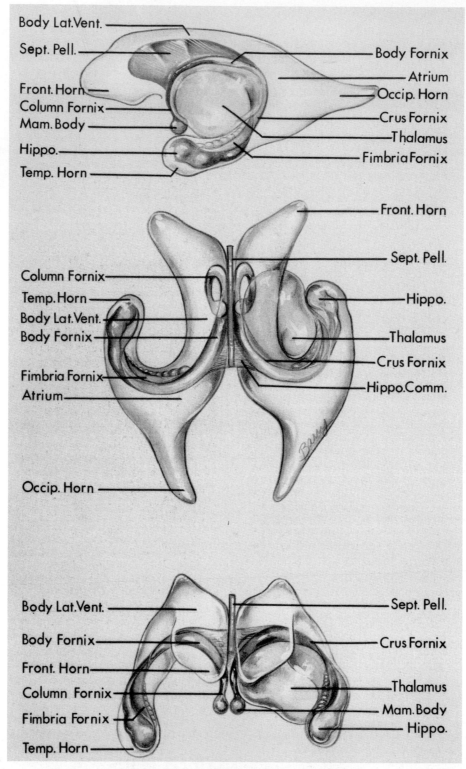

Fig. 1. Neural relationships of the lateral ventricles. **A:** Relationship of the septum pellucidum, thalamus, hippocampal formation, and fornix to the lateral ventricles. *Top,* lateral view. *Middle,* superior view. *Bottom,* anterior view. Each lateral ventricle wraps around the thalamus. The frontal horn *(Front. Horn)* is anterior to the thalamus; the body *(Body Lat. Vent.)* is above the thalamus; the atrium and occipital horn *(Occip. Horn)* are behind the thalamus; and the temporal horn *(Temp. Horn)* is below and lateral to the thalamus. The septum pellucidum *(Sept. Pell.)* is in the medial wall of the frontal horn and body. The hippocampal formation *(Hippo.)* is in the floor of the temporal horn. The fornix, which arises in the hippocampal formation and wraps around the thalamus, is in the medial part of the temporal horn, atrium, and body. The fimbria of the fornix arises on the surface of the hippocampal formation in the temporal horn. The crus of the fornix are posterior to the thalamus in the wall of the atrium. The body of the fornix passes above the thalamus in the lower part of the medial wall of the body. The columns of the fornix are formed at the level of the foramen of Monro and passed inferiorly to the mamillary bodies *(Mam. Body).* The crura of the fornix are connected across the midline in the roof of the third ventricle by the hippocampal commissure *(Hippo. Comm.). (Figure continues.)*

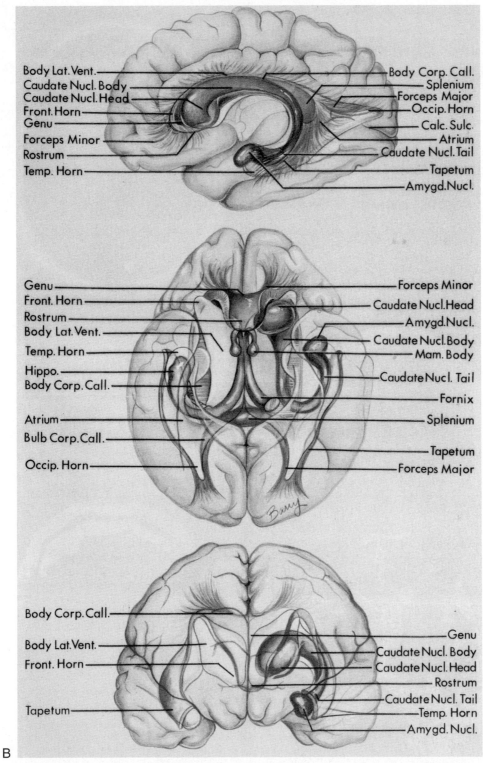

Fig. 1. *Continued.* **B:** Relationship of the corpus callosum *(Corp. Call.)*, caudate nucleus *(Caudate Nucl.)*, and hippo-campal formation to the lateral ventricles. *Top,* View through medial surface of the hemisphere; middle, view through the inferior surface the hemisphere. *Bottom,* View through the anterior surface of the hemisphere. The head and body of the caudate nucleus form the lateral wall of the frontal horn and body of the lateral ventricle. The tail of the caudate nucleus extends into the anterior part of the lateral wall of the atrium and into the medial part of the roof of the temporal horn to the level of the amygdaloid nucleus *(Amygd. Nucl.).* The corpus callosum is made up of the rostrum, which is in the floor of the frontal horn, the genu, which forms the anterior wall, and roof of the frontal horn, the body, which forms the roof of the body of the lateral ventricle and the splenium, which carries the fibers that forms a prominence in the medial wall of the atrium called the bulb of the corpus callosum. The splenium also gives rise to a fiber bundle, called the tapetum, which sweeps downward to form the roof and lateral wall of the atrium and temporal horn. A prominence in the medial wall of the atrium, called the calcar avis, overlies the calcarine sulcus *(Calc. Sulc.).* (From Timurkaynak E, Rhoton AL Jr, Barry M. Microsurgical anatomy of the lateral ventricles. *Neurosurgery* 1986;19:685–723, with permission.)

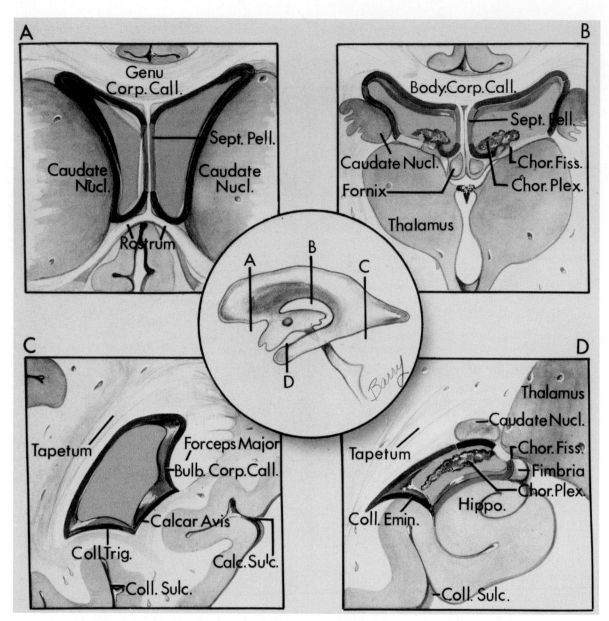

Fig. 2. Structures in the walls of the lateral ventricles. The central diagram shows the level of the cross sections through the frontal horn *(A)*, body *(B)*, atrium *(C)*, and temporal horn *(D)*. **A:** Frontal horn. The genu of the corpus callosum *(Corp. Call.)* is in the roof, the caudate nucleus *(Caudate Nucl.)* is in the lateral wall, the rostrum of the corpus callosum is in the floor, and the septum pellucidum *(Sept. Pell.)* is in the medial wall. **B:** Body of the lateral ventricle. The body of the corpus callosum is in the roof, the caudate nucleus is in the lateral wall, the thalamus is in the floor, and the septum pellucidum and fornix are in the medial wall. The choroidal fissure *(Chor. Fiss.)*, the site of the attachment of the choroid plexus *(Chor. Plex.)* in the lateral ventricle, is situated between the fornix and the thalamus. **C:** Atrium. The lateral wall and roof are formed by the tapetum of the corpus callosum, and the floor is formed by the collateral trigone *(Coll. Trig.)*, which overlies the collateral sulcus *(Coll. Sulc.)*. The inferior part of the medial wall is formed by the calcar avis, the prominence that overlies the deep end of the calcarine sulcus *(Calc. Sulc.)*, and the superior part of the medial wall is formed by the bulb of the corpus callosum, the prominence that overlies the forceps major. **D:** Temporal horn. The medial part of the floor of the temporal horn is formed by the prominence overlying the hippocampal formation *(Hippo.)*, and the lateral part of the floor is formed by the prominence called the collateral eminence *(Coll. Emin.)*, which overlies the deep end of the collateral sulcus. The roof is formed by the caudate nucleus and the tapetum of the corpus callosum. The lateral wall is formed by the tapetum of the corpus callosum. The medial wall is little more than the cleft between the fimbria of the fornix and the inferolateral aspect of the thalamus. (From Timurkaynak E., Rhoton AL Jr, Barry M. Microsurgical anatomy of the lateral ventricles. *Neurosurgery* 1986;14:685–723, with permission.)

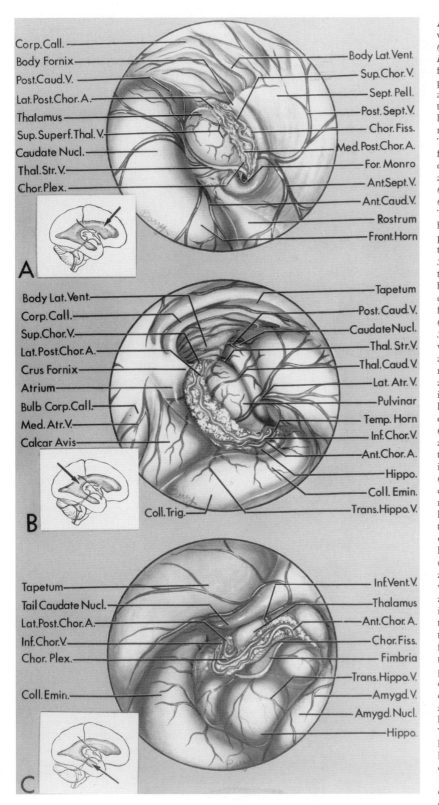

Corp. Call.
Body Fornix
Post. Caud. V.
Lat. Post. Chor. A.
Thalamus
Sup. Superf. Thal. V.
Caudate Nucl.
Thal. Str. V.
Chor. Plex.

Body Lat. Vent.
Sup. Chor. V.
Sept. Pell.
Post. Sept. V.
Chor. Fiss.
Med. Post. Chor. A.
For. Monro
Ant. Sept. V.
Ant. Caud. V.
Rostrum
Front. Horn

A

Body Lat. Vent.
Corp. Call.
Sup. Chor. V.
Lat. Post. Chor. A.
Crus Fornix
Atrium
Bulb Corp. Call.
Med. Atr. V.
Calcar Avis

Tapetum
Post. Caud. V.
Caudate Nucl.
Thal. Str. V.
Thal. Caud. V.
Lat. Atr. V.
Pulvinar
Temp. Horn
Inf. Chor. V.
Ant. Chor. A.
Hippo.
Coll. Emin.
Trans. Hippo. V.

Coll. Trig.

B

Tapetum
Tail Caudate Nucl.
Lat. Post. Chor. A.
Inf. Chor. V.
Chor. Plex.

Coll. Emin.

Inf. Vent. V.
Thalamus
Ant. Chor. A.
Chor. Fiss.
Fimbria
Trans. Hippo. V.
Amygd. V.
Amygd. Nucl.
Hippo.

C

Fig. 3. Views into the lateral ventricles. **A:** Anterior view, along the arrow in the insert, into the frontal horn (*Front. Horn*) and body of the lateral ventricle (*Body Lat. Vent.*). The frontal horn is located anterior to the foramen of Monro (*For. Monro*), and has the septum pellucidum (*Sept. Pell.*) in the medial wall, the genu and the body of the corpus callosum (*Corp. Call.*) in the roof, the caudate nucleus (*Caudate Nucl.*) in the lateral wall, the genu of the corpus callosum in the anterior wall, and the rostrum of the callosum in the floor. The body of the lateral ventricle has the thalamus in its floor, the caudate nucleus in the lateral wall, the body of the fornix and septum pellucidum in the medial wall, and the corpus callosum in the roof. The choroid plexus (*Chor. Plex.*) is attached along the choroidal fissure (*Chor. Fiss.*), the cleft between the fornix and thalamus. The superior choroidal vein (*Sup. Chor. V.*) and branches of the lateral (*Lat. Post. Chor. A.*) and medial posterior choroidal arteries (*Med. Post. A.*) course on the surface of the choroidal plexus. The anterior (*Ant. Sept. V.*) and posterior septal veins (*Post. Sept. V.*) cross the roof and the medial wall of the frontal horn and body. The anterior (*Ant. Caud. V.*) and posterior caudate veins (*Post. Caud. V.*) cross the lateral wall of the frontal horn and body and join the thalamostriate vein (*Thal. Str. V.*). A superior superficial thalamic vein (*Sup. Superf. Thal. V.*) courses on the thalamus. **B:** Posterior view, along the arrow in the insert, into the atrium. The atrium has the tapetum of the corpus callosum in the roof, the bulb of the corpus callosum, and the calcar avis in its medial wall, the collateral trigone (*Coll. Trig.*) in the floor, the caudate nucleus and tapetum in the lateral wall, and the crus of the fornix, pulvinar and choroid plexus in the anterior wall. The temporal horn (*Temp. Horn*) has the hippocampal formation (*Hippo.*) and collateral eminence (*Coll. Emin.*) in the floor and the thalamus, tail of the caudate nucleus, and tapetum in the roof and the lateral wall. Branches of the anterior (*Ant. Chor. A.*) and lateral posterior choroidal arteries course on the surface of the choroid plexus. The thalamocaudate vein (*Thal. Caud. V.*) drains the part of the lateral wall of the body behind the area drained by the thalamostriate vein. The inferior choroidal vein (*Inf. Chor. V.*) courses on the choroid plexus in the temporal horn. The lateral (*Lat. Atr. V.*) and medial atrial veins (*Med. Atr. V.*) cross the medial and lateral walls of the atrium and temporal horn. Transverse hippocampal veins (*Trans. Hippo. V.*) cross the floor of the atrium and temporal horn. **C:** Anterior view along the arrow in the insert, into the temporal horn. The floor of the temporal horn is formed by the collateral eminence and the hippocampal formation. The roof and lateral wall, from medial to lateral, are formed by the thalamus, the tail of the caudate nucleus, and the tapetum of the corpus callosum. The medial wall is little more than the cleft between the thalamus and the fimbria, called the choroidal fissure, along which the choroid plexus is attached. The amygdaloid nucleus (*Amygd. Nucl.*) bulges into the anteromedial part of the temporal horn. The fimbria of the fornix arises on the surface of the hippocampal formation. Branches of the anterior and lateral posterior choroidal arteries course on the surface of the choroid plexus. The inferior ventricular vein (*Inf. Vent. V.*) drains the roof of the temporal horn and receives the amygdalar vein (*Amygd. V.*). The inferior choroidal vein joins the inferior ventricular vein. The transverse hippocampal veins drain the floor of the temporal horn. (From Timurkaynak E, Rhoton AL Jr, Barry M. Microsurgical anatomy of the lateral ventricles. *Neurosurgery* 1986;19:685–723, with permission.)

is located in the center of each lateral ventricle. The body of the lateral ventricle is above the thalamus; the atrium and occipital horn are posterior to the thalamus; and the temporal horn is inferolateral to the thalamus. The caudate nucleus is an arched, C-shaped, cellular mass that wraps around the thalamus and constitutes an important part of the wall of each lateral ventricle. Its head bulges into the lateral wall of the frontal horn and body of the lateral ventricle. Its body forms part of the lateral wall of the atrium, and its tail extends from the atrium into the roof of the temporal horn.

The fornix is another C-shaped structure that wraps around the thalamus in the wall of the ventricle. In the body of the lateral ventricle, the body of the fornix is in the lower part of the medial wall; in the atrium, the crus of the fornix is in the medial part of the anterior wall; and, in the temporal horn, the fimbria of the fornix is in the medial part of the floor. The body of the fornix crosses the thalamus approximately halfway between the medial and lateral edge of the superior surface of the thalamus: The part of the thalamus lateral to the body of the fornix forms the floor of the body of the lateral ventricle and the part medial to the fornix forms part of the wall of the velum interpositum and third ventricle. The crux of the fornix crosses the pulvinar approximately midway between the medial and lateral edge of the pulvinar: The part of the pulvinar lateral to the crus of the fornix forms part of the anterior wall of the atrium and the part medial to the fornix forms part of the anterior wall of the quadrigeminal cistern. The fimbriae of the fornix pass below the inferolateral part of the thalamus just lateral to the medial and lateral geniculate bodies. The part of the thalamus medial to the fimbria forms the roof of the ambient cistern. The body of the fornix separates into two columns that arch along the superior and anterior margins of the foramen of Monro.

The corpus callosum, which forms the largest part of the ventricular walls, contributes to the wall of each of the five parts of the lateral ventricle. The rostrum of the corpus callosum is situated below and forms the floor of the frontal horn. The bundle of fibers in the genu called the forceps minor, forms the anterior wall of the frontal horn. The genu and the body of the corpus callosum form the roof of both the frontal horn and the body of the lateral ventricle. The splenium contains a large fiber bundle, the forceps major, which forms a prominence, called the bulb, in the upper part of the medial wall of the atrium. Another fiber tract, the tapetum, which arises in the posterior part of the body and selenium of the corpus callosum, sweeps laterally and inferiorly to form the roof and lateral wall of the atrium and temporal horns. The tapetum separates the fibers of the optic radiations from the temporal horn.

The septum pellucidum, which is composed of paired laminae, separates the frontal horns and bodies of the lateral ventricles in the midline. There may be a cavity, the cavum septum pellucidum, in the midline between the laminae of the septum pellucidum.

The close relationship of the internal capsule to the lateral wall of the frontal horn and body of the lateral ventricle is often forgotten in planning operative approaches to the ventricles. The anterior limb of the internal capsule, which is located between the caudate and lentiform nucleus, is separated from the frontal horn by the head of the caudate nucleus, and the posterior limb, which is situated between the thalamus and lentiform nucleus, is separated from the body of the lateral ventricle by the thalamus and body of the caudate nucleus. However, the genu of the internal capsule comes directly to the ventricular surface and touches the wall of the lateral ventricle immediately lateral to the foramen of Monro in the interval between the caudate nucleus and thalamus (Fig. 4).

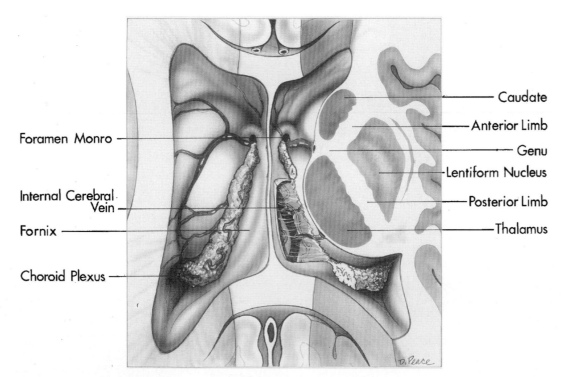

Fig. 4. Relationship of the internal capsule to the right lateral ventricle. The anterior limb of the internal capsule is separated from the lateral ventricle by the caudate nucleus and the posterior limb is separated from the ventricle by the thalamus. The genu comes directly to the ventricular surface in the area lateral to the foramen of Monro in the interval between the caudate nucleus and thalamus. The right half of the body of the fornix has been removed to expose the internal cerebral veins in the roof of the third ventricle.

Ventricular Walls

FRONTAL HORN. The frontal horn, the part of the lateral ventricle located anterior to the foramen of Monro, has a medial wall formed by the septum pellucidum, an anterior wall formed by the genu of the corpus callosum, a lateral wall composed of the head of the caudate nucleus, and a narrow floor formed by the rostrum of the corpus callosum (Figs. 2 and 3). The columns of the fornix, as they pass anterior and superior to the foramen of Monro, are in the posteroinferior part of the medial wall.

BODY. The body of the lateral ventricle extends from the posterior edge of the foramen of Monro to the point where the septum pellucidum disappears and the corpus callosum and fornix meet (Figs. 2 and 3). The roof is formed by the body of the corpus callosum, the medial wall by the septum pellucidum above and the body of the fornix below; the lateral wall by the body of the caudate nucleus; and the floor by the thalamus. The caudate nucleus and thalamus are separated by the striothalamic sulcus, the groove in which the stria terminalis and thalamostriate vein course.

ATRIUM AND OCCIPITAL HORN. The atrium and occipital horn together form a roughly triangular cavity, with the apex posteriorly in the occipital lobe and the base anteriorly on the pulvinar (Figs. 2 and 3). The roof of the atrium is formed by the body, splenium, and tapetum of the corpus callosum. The medial wall is formed by two roughly horizontal prominences that are located one above the other. The upper prominence, called the bulb of the corpus callosum, overlies and is formed by the large bundle of fibers called the forceps major, and the lower prominence, called the calcar avis, overlies the deepest part of the calcarine sulcus. The lateral wall has an anterior part, formed by the caudate nucleus; and a posterior part, formed by the fibers of the tapetum. The anterior wall has a medial part composed of the crus of the fornix and a lateral part, formed by the pulvinar of the thalamus. The floor is formed by the collateral trigone, a triangular area that bulges upward over the collateral sulcus.

The occipital horn extends posteriorly into the occipital lobe from the atrium. It varies in size from being absent to extending far posteriorly in the occipital lobe and it may vary in size from side to side. Its medial wall is formed by the bulb of the corpus callosum and the calcar avis, the roof and lateral wall are formed by the tapetum, and the floor is formed by the collateral trigone.

TEMPORAL HORN. The temporal horn extends forward from the atrium below the pulvinar into the medial part of the temporal lobe and ends blindly in an anterior wall that is situated immediately behind the amygdaloid nucleus (Figs. 2 and 3). The floor of the temporal horn is formed medially by the hippocampus, the smooth prominence overlying the hippocampal formation, and laterally by the collateral eminence, the prominence overlying the collateral sulcus that separates the parahippocampal and occipitotemporal gyri on the inferior surface of the temporal lobe. The roof is formed medially by the inferior surface of the thalamus and the tail of the caudate nucleus, and laterally by the tapetum of the corpus callosum. The medial wall is little more than a narrow cleft, the choroidal fissure, situated between the inferolateral part of the thalamus and the fimbria of the fornix.

Choroid Plexus and Choroidal Fissure

The choroid plexus in the lateral ventricle has a C-shaped configuration that parallels the fornix (Figs. 1 to 3) (1,4). It is attached along the choroidal fissure, the narrow C-shaped cleft that is situated between the fornix and thalamus. The edges of the thalamus and fornix bordering the choroidal fissure have small ridges, called the teniae, that anchor the choroid plexus to the fornix and thalamus. The tenia on the thalamic side is called the tenia choroidea. The tenia on the fornical side of the fissure is called the tenia fornicis except in the temporal horn where it is referred to as the tenia fimbriae.

Opening through the choroidal fissure from the body of the ventricle exposes the velum interpositum and the roof of the third ventricle. Opening through the fissure from the atrium exposes the quadrigeminal cistern, the pineal region, and the posterior portion of the ambient cistern. Opening through the choroidal fissure from the temporal horn exposes the structures in the ambient and posterior part of the crural cisterns.

Velum Interpositum

The velum interpositum is located in the roof of the third ventricle below the body of the fornix and between the superomedial surfaces of the thalami (3). The upper and lower walls of the velum interpositum are formed by the two membranous layers of tela choroidea in the roof of the third ventricle. The layer that is attached to the lower surface of the fornix and the hippocampal commissure forms the upper wall. The lower wall is attached to the small ridges on the free edge of the striae medullaris thalami. The posterior part of the lower wall is attached to the superior surface of the pineal body. The internal cerebral veins arise in the anterior part of the velum interpositum just behind the foramen of Monro and they exit the velum interpositum above the pineal body to enter the quadrigeminal cistern, where they join the great vein. The medial posterior choroidal arteries also course in the velum interpositum.

Tentorial and Cisternal Relationships

The lateral ventricles are situated above the tentorial incisura, the triangular space situated between the free edges of the tentorium and the dorsum sellae (5). The midbrain is situated in the center of the incisura. The area between the midbrain and the free edges is divided into: (a) an anterior incisural space located in front of the brainstem; (b) paired middle incisural spaces situated lateral to the midbrain; and (c) a posterior incisural space located behind the midbrain. The frontal horns are located above the anterior incisural space; the bodies of the lateral ventricles are located directly above the central part of the incisura, where they sit on and are separated from the central part of the incisura by the thalamus; the atria are located above the posterior incisural space; and the temporal horns are situated superolateral to the middle incisural space.

Arterial Relationships

Each part of the lateral ventricle has surgically important arterial relationships: All of the arterial components of the circle of Willis are located in the anterior incisural space below the frontal horns and bodies of the lateral ventricles; the internal carotid arteries bifurcate into the anterior and middle cerebral arteries in the area below the frontal horns and give rise to the anterior choroidal arteries, which send branches through the choroidal fissures to the choroid plexus; the posterior part of the circle of Willis and the apex of the basilar artery are situated below the thalami and bodies of the lateral ventricles; the anterior cerebral arteries pass around the floor and anterior wall of the frontal horns to reach the roof of the frontal horns and bodies; and the posterior cerebral arteries pass medial to the temporal horns and atria in the ambient and quadrigeminal cisterns and give rise to the posterior choroidal arteries, which supply the choroid plexus in the temporal horns, atria, and bodies (Fig. 3) (1,4,5).

The arteries most intimately related to the lateral ventricles and choroidal fissures are the choroidal arteries, which supply the choroid plexus in the lateral and third ventricles. They arise from the internal carotid and posterior cerebral arteries in the basal cisterns and reach the choroid plexus by passing through the choroidal fissures. The most common pattern is for the anterior choroidal artery to supply a portion of the choroid plexus in the temporal horn and atrium; the lateral posterior choroidal arteries to supply a portion of the choroid plexus in the atrium, body, and posterior part of the temporal horn; and the medial posterior choroidal arteries to supply the choroid plexus in the roof of the third ventricle and part of that in the body of the lateral ventricle.

The anterior choroidal artery arises from the internal carotid artery and passes around the uncus and through the choroidal fissure to enter the temporal horn at the posterior margin of the uncus. The lateral posterior choroidal arteries arise in the ambient and quadrigeminal cisterns from the posterior cerebral artery and pass laterally through the choroidal fissure to reach the choroid plexus in the temporal horn and atrium. The medial posterior choroidal arteries arise from the proximal part of the posterior cerebral artery in front of the midbrain, encircle the midbrain medial to the main trunk of the posterior cerebral artery, turn forward at the side of the pineal gland, course in the velum interpositum adjacent to the internal cerebral veins, and pass through the choroidal fissure to reach the choroid plexus in the body.

Venous Relationships

During operations on the lateral ventricles, the veins provide orienting landmarks more commonly than do the arteries because the arteries in the ventricular walls are small and poorly seen, but the veins are larger and are easily visible through the ependyma (Fig. 3). These venous landmarks are especially helpful in the presence of hydrocephalus, when the normal angles between the neural structures disappear.

The deep venous system of the brain collects into channels that course in a subependymal location through the walls of the lateral ventricles and pass through the margins of the choroidal fissure to reach the internal cerebral, basal, and great veins (1, 3,6). In general, the veins draining the frontal horn and body of the lateral ventricle drain into the internal cerebral vein as it courses through the velum interpositum; those draining the temporal horn drain into the segment of the basal vein coursing through the ambient cistern; and the veins from the atrium drain into the segments of the basal, internal cerebral, and great veins coursing through the quadrigeminal cistern.

The ventricular veins are divided into medial and lateral groups based on whether they course through the thalamic or forniceal side of the choroidal fissure: The lateral group passes through the thalamic or inner side of the fissure, and the medial group passes through the outer or fornical circumference of the fissure.

The anterior and posterior septal veins form the medial group of veins in the frontal horn and body; and the lateral group consists of the thalamostriate, thalamocaudate, and anterior and posterior caudate veins. The veins of the lateral group are larger than those of the medial group. The veins in the lateral group penetrate the thalamic side of the choroidal fissure to reach the velum interpositum. The thalamostriate vein passes forward in the sulcus between the caudate nucleus and thalamus toward the foramen of Monro, where it turns sharply posterior through the posterior margin of the foramen of Monro and enters the velum interpositum to join the internal cerebral vein. In some cases, the thalamostriate vein does not approximate the site of the foramen of Monro because it passes through the choroidal fissure well behind the foramen of Monro, in which case it is called the thalamostriate vein.

The medial group of veins in the atrium and occipital horn consists of the medial atrial veins, and the lateral group is composed of the lateral atrial veins. The inferior ventricular and amygdalar veins form the lateral group in the temporal horn and the transverse hippocampal veins form the medial group. The inferior ventricular vein, which courses along the roof, is the largest in the temporal horn. The superior and inferior choroidal veins are the largest veins on the choroid plexus.

Operative Approaches

The selection of the best operative approach to a lesion in the lateral ventricles is determined by the site of the lesion, the size of the lateral ventricles, and the relationship of the lesion to the third ventricle and basal cisterns (Fig. 5) (7). The routes to the lateral ventricles are divided into anterior, posterior, and inferior approaches (Fig. 5). The anterior approaches are directed to the frontal horn and body of the lateral ventricle. The posterior approaches are directed to the atrium and the inferior approaches are directed to the temporal horn. In all of the approaches to be described, image guidance, in selected cases, increases the accuracy of the approach and minimizes the required neural incision.

ANTERIOR APPROACHES. Lesions within the frontal horn and anterior portion of the body of the lateral ventricle are most commonly reached by the anterior transcallosal or anterior transcortical approaches (Figs. 6 and 7). The transcallosal approach is easier to perform than the transcortical approach if the ventricles are of a normal size or are minimally enlarged. On occasion an anterior frontal approach may be combined with an approach along the adjacent part of the interhemispheric fissure to reach the anterior wall and floor of the frontal horn (Fig. 8).

ANTERIOR TRANSCALLOSAL APPROACH. This approach is suitable for reaching lesions located within the frontal horn

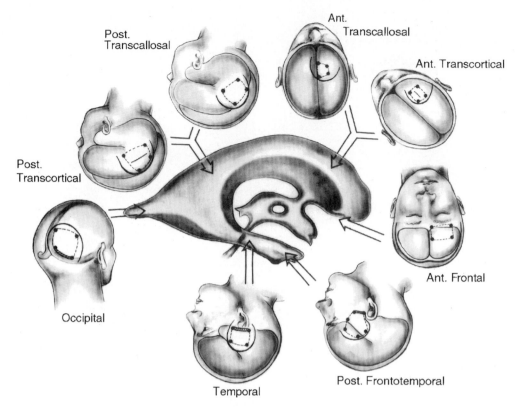

Fig. 5. Surgical approaches to the lateral ventricles. The site of the skin incision *(solid line)* and the bone flap *(interrupted line)* are shown for each approach. The anterior part of the lateral ventricle may be reached by the anterior transcallosal, anterior transcortical, and frontal approaches. The posterior routes to the lateral ventricle are the posterior transcallosal, posterior transcortical, and occipital approaches. The inferior part of the lateral ventricle is reached using the frontotemporal and temporal approaches. (From Timurkaynak E, Rhoton AL Jr, Barry M. Microsurgical anatomy of the lateral ventricles. *Neurosurgery* 1986;19:685–723, with permission.)

and body of the lateral ventricle, and for exposing the anterior–superior part of the third ventricle through the lateral ventricle (Fig. 6) (8,9). The patient is positioned supine with the head elevated 20 to 30 degrees and facing straight upward. Occasionally, the side of the approach, which is almost always the right side, is positioned downward in order to allow the medial surface of the right hemisphere to fall away from the falx, especially if the lesion is in the left lateral ventricle. A Souttar or a right frontal horseshoe scalp incision is positioned behind the hairline and posterior edge of the planned bone flap. The right frontal bone flap extending to the lateral edge of, or across the sagittal sinus is centered one-third behind and two-thirds in front of the coronal suture. The dura is opened with the base on the sagittal sinus. The cortical veins entering the superior sagittal sinus are protected: Some, usually no more than one, may have to be divided in order to retract the medial surface of the right frontal lobe away from the falx when the bone flap is centered as described. The arachnoid membrane, encountered deep to the free edge of the falx, is opened. The right and left cingulate gyri, which face each other, are separated to expose the corpus callosum and anterior cerebral arteries. The approach is directed between the pericallosal arteries, although some of their branches may cross the midline above the corpus callosum.

The part of the corpus callosum above the foramen of Monro is split in the midline. An incision approximately 2 cm in length provides satisfactory access to both lateral ventricles. On opening the ventricle by either the transcallosal or transventricular approaches, the foramen of Monro is found by following the attachment of the choroid plexus and the thalamostriate vein

anteriorly because both converge on this foramen. The opening into the lateral ventricle may expose the frontal horn and body on the same or opposite side of the cranial exposure, but the anatomy makes this obvious. A simple rule for determining whether the left or right lateral ventricle has been exposed is to determine whether the thalamostriate vein is to the left or right side of the choroid plexus: The left lateral ventricle has been opened if the thalamostriate vein is further to the patient's left side than the choroid plexus, and the right lateral ventricle has been entered if the thalamostriate vein is further to the patient's right side than the choroid plexus. Opening the septum pellucidum provides access to the opposite lateral ventricle and the opening of the foramen of Monro into both lateral ventricles. Entry into a cavum between the leaves of the septum pellucidum may be confusing until one realizes that no intraventricular structures are present.

The close relationship of the genu of the internal capsule to the foramen of Monro should be kept in mind when retracting the walls of the lateral ventricle. The genu of the internal capsule touches the wall of the ventricle in the area lateral to the foramen of Monro near the anterior pole of the thalamus.

Routes through the lateral ventricles to the anterior part of the third ventricle include working through the foramen of Monro, especially if enlarged by tumor or by enlarging the foramen by incising the ipsilateral column of the fornix. Other alternatives include the interforniceal approach, in which the body of the fornix is split longitudinally in the midline in the direction of its fibers, or the transchoroidal approach, in which the choroidal fissure is opened, thus allowing the fornix to be pushed to the opposite side in order to expose the structures in the roof of

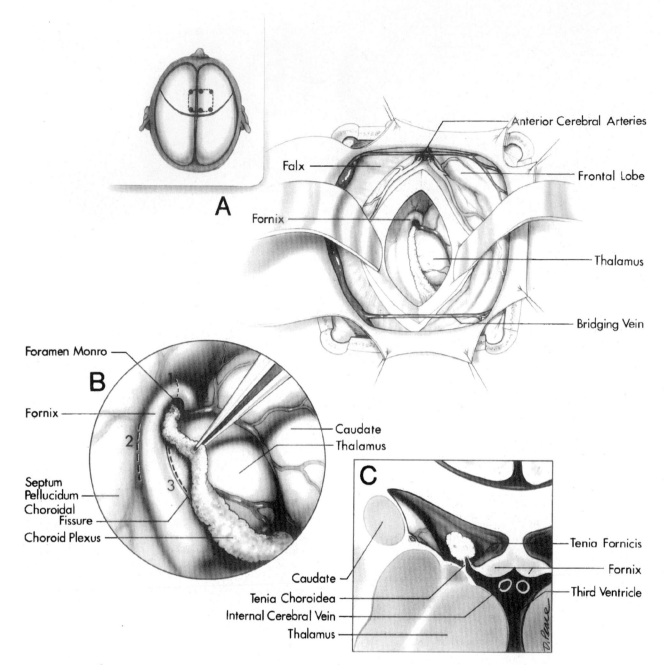

Fig. 6. Transcallosal approach to the lateral and third ventricles. **A–C:** Normal ventricular anatomy. **A:** The body and frontal horn of the right lateral ventricle have been exposed through an incision in the anterior part of the corpus callosum. The insert on the upper left shows the head position, scalp incision behind the hairline *(solid line)* and bone flap *(interrupted line)*. The bone flap extends across the superior sagittal sinus. An alternative would be to use a Souttar incision and to have the bone flap extend only to the lateral edge of the superior sagittal sinus. **B:** Sites of neural incisions used to reach lesions in the third ventricle. *1,* The foramen of Monro may be enlarged by incising the ipsilateral column of the fornix, at the anterior superior margin of the foramen of Monro. *2,* The interforniceal approach is completed using an incision along the body of the fornix in the midline. *3,* The transchoroidal approach is completed by opening the choroidal fissure by incising along the tenia fornicis. **C:** The transchoroidal approach is completed by incision along the tenia fornicis rather than the tenia choroidea because more veins and arteries pass through the tenia choroidea than the tenia fornicis. The internal cerebral veins course in the roof of the third ventricle. *(Figure continues.)*

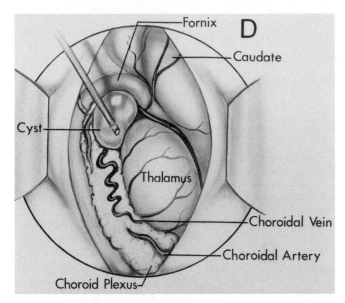

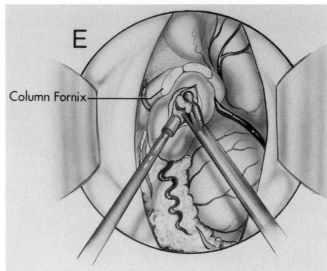

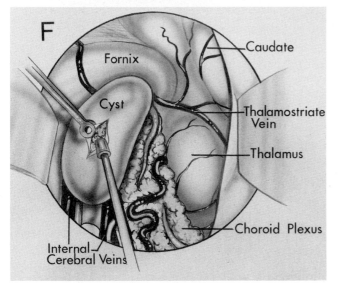

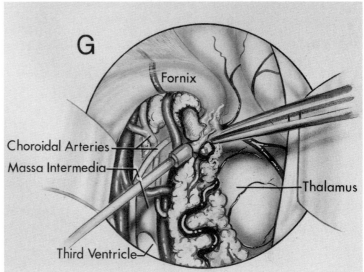

Fig. 6. *Continued.* **D,E:** Removal of a colloid cyst using an incision in the ipsilateral column of the fornix. **D:** A colloid cyst that obstructs the foramen of Monro is being aspirated with a needle. **E:** The column of the fornix has been divided to enlarge the foramen of Monro and the semigelatinous material within the cyst is being removed using a suction and cup forceps. A preferable method for enlarging the opening into the third ventricle is to open the choroidal fissure behind the foramen of Monro. **F,G:** Large colloid cyst being removed using an approach through the choroidal fissure. **F:** A colloid cyst that obstructs the foramen of Monro has been exposed by opening the choroidal fissure along the attachment of the choroid plexus to the fornix. This exposes the internal cerebral veins and medial posterior choroidal arteries behind the foramen of Monro. **G:** The final remnant of the attachment of the cyst to the choroid plexus is being coagulated. *(Figure continues.)*

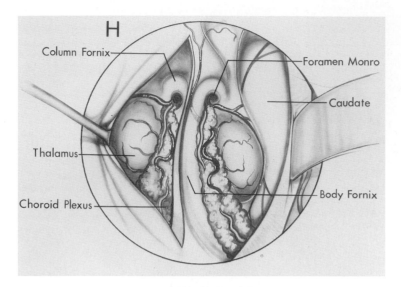

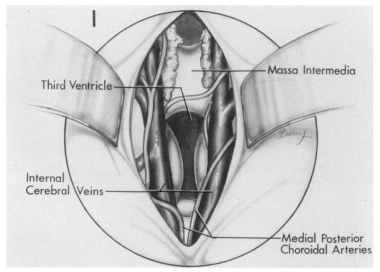

Fig. 6. *Continued.* **H:** The septum pellucidum has been opened to expose the frontal horns and bodies of both lateral ventricles. The columns of the fornix arch anterior and superior to the openings of the foramen of Monro into both lateral ventricles. The body of the fornix forms part of the roof of the third ventricle. **I:** The body of the fornix has been split in the midline to expose the third ventricle. The internal cerebral veins and medial posterior choroidal arteries course in the roof of the third ventricle. This interforniceal approach may be suitable for exposing lesions located in the third ventricle behind the foramen of Monro, although the author prefers the transchoroidal approach.

the third ventricle (3,10–14). The transchoroidal approach has the advantage of giving access to the central portion of the third ventricle behind the foramen of Monro by displacing, rather than incising, the fornix. The transchoroidal approach is preferred over incising the ipsilateral half of the fornix or the longitudinal interforniceal incision when there is a need to enlarge the opening into the third ventricle. With the transcortical approach through the middle frontal gyrus, the transchoroidal approach provides a better view into the third ventricle than the interforniceal route. It is both easier and safer to direct the transchoroidal approach through the tenia fornicis than the tenia choroidea because the large veins draining the central part of the cerebrum pass through the tenia choroidea rather than the tenia fornicis. The transchoroidal approach is especially well suited to lesions that are fed by the terminal branches of the choroidal arteries because these arteries pass through the choroidal fissure.

In the transchoroidal approach, the third ventricle is exposed by opening the choroidal fissure along the tenia fornices and displacing the fornix to the opposite side, after which the roof of the third ventricle is entered by opening the layers of tela choroidea. Opening through the velum interpositum in the interval between the internal cerebral veins allows a more extensive exposure of the third ventricle than if the third ventricle

is exposed between the ipsilateral internal cerebral vein and thalamus. It is often necessary to sacrifice some of the branches of the internal cerebral vein if the third ventricle is entered on the lateral side of the internal cerebral vein; however, the roof of the third ventricle commonly can be entered without sacrificing any branches of the internal cerebral veins if the approach is directed between these veins.

An incision is made anteriorly through one column of the fornix at the anterosuperior edge of the foramen of Monro only if needed to explore a deeper portion of the anterior part of the third ventricle. To prevent the complications associated with sectioning the fornix, Hirsch and associates sectioned the thalamostriate vein at the posterior margin of the foramen of Monro to enlarge the opening into the third ventricle; however, this may cause drowsiness, hemiplegia, and mutism, because of hemorrhagic infarction of the basal ganglia (15,16).

ANTERIOR TRANSCORTICAL APPROACH. This approach is suitable for lesions in the anterior part of the lateral ventricle and the anterosuperior part of the third ventricle, especially if the tumor is situated predominantly in the lateral ventricle on the side of the approach (Fig. 7). It is more difficult to expose the anterior part of the lateral ventricle on the side opposite

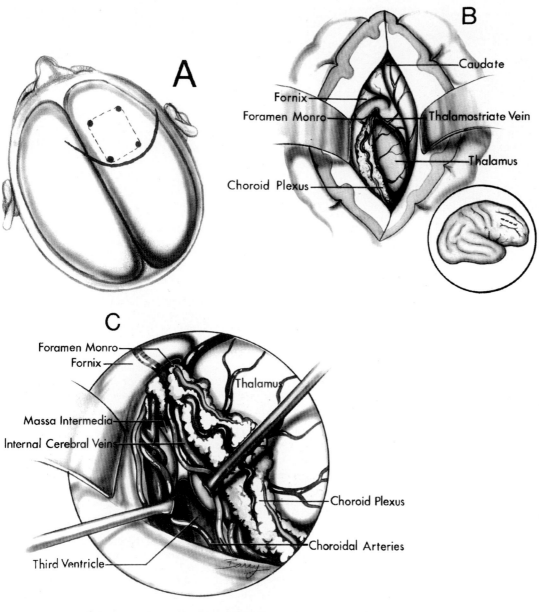

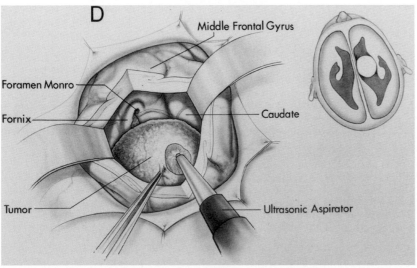

***Fig.* 7.** Transcortical approach to the lateral and third ventricles. **A:** The scalp incision positioned behind the hairline *(solid line)* and bone flap *(dotted line)* are centered over the middle frontal gyrus. **B,C:** Normal ventricular anatomy. **B:** The cortical opening exposes the right lateral ventricle. The insert on the lower right shows the site of the cortical incision. The opening into the right lateral ventricle exposes the caudate nucleus, fornix, foramen of Monro, thalamus, and thalamostriate vein. **C:** The third ventricle has been exposed by opening the choroidal fissure along the site of the attachment of the choroid plexus to the fornix. This exposes the internal cerebral veins and medial posterior choroidal arteries in the roof of the third ventricle. **D:** A choroid plexus papilloma has been exposed using the transcortical approach. The insert on the upper right shows the site of the tumor and the position of the head for the operation. The tumor is being removed using the ultrasonic aspirator. *(Figure continues.)*

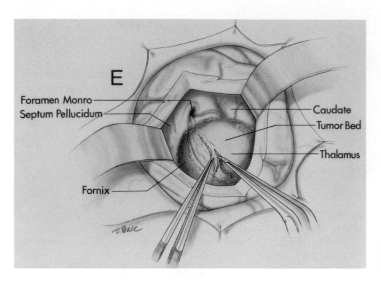

Fig. 7. *Continued.* **E:** The last remnant of tumor is being removed from its attachment to the choroid plexus. The tumor has compressed the structures in the floor at frontal horn.

the approach through the transcortical than the transcallosal approach. The transcortical approach is facilitated if the lateral ventricles are enlarged.

With the patient in the supine position, the head is rotated slightly to the side opposite the frontal lobe through which the ventricle is to be approached. The scalp and bone flaps are positioned over the central part of the middle frontal gyrus. If the approach is through the dominant hemisphere, then are is taken to place the cortical incision above and anterior to the expressive speech centers on the inferior frontal gyrus and anterior to the precentral motor strip. The dilated frontal horn is reached through a small cortical incision located in the long axis of the middle frontal gyrus or in an adjacent sulcus having its depths near the wall of the ventricle. Image guidance may assist in minimizing the length of the cortical incision needed to reach the target in the ventricle. Once inside the ventricle, the landmarks and approaches to the third ventricle are the same as those described far the transcallosal approach.

ANTERIOR FRONTAL APPROACH. The anterior frontal approach may be considered for a lesion involving the floor and lower part of the anterior wall of the frontal horn that extends

into the third ventricle behind the lamina terminalis (Fig. 8) (1, 17). This approach is not suitable for reaching a lesion in the body of the lateral ventricle or in the third ventricle behind the foramen of Monro.

The patient is positioned supine with the face looking directly upward. A Souttar scalp incision is used. A unilateral bone flap extending to the edge of the superior sagittal sinus is elevated. The lower margin of the flap is positioned just above the supraorbital ridge if the lesion is in the rostrum and adjacent part of the lamina terminalis, but is placed higher if the lesion is located in the lower part of the genu of the corpus callosum. The dura is opened with the base on the superior sagittal sinus. The orbital surface of the frontal lobe is elevated and the arachnoid is opened to expose the optic nerves and chiasm, lamina terminalis, and anterior cerebral and anterior communicating arteries. The olfactory nerve usually can be separated from the arachnoid and left resting on the anterior fossa floor. The medial surface of the frontal lobe is retracted away from the falx to expose the rostrum and genu of the corpus callosum. One or two small bridging veins entering the superior and inferior sagittal sinuses may need to be sacrificed in order to retract the frontal pole away from the falx. The arachnoid in the depths of the interhemispheric fissure is opened to expose the anterior

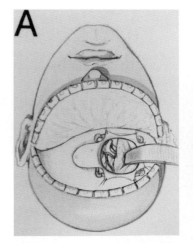

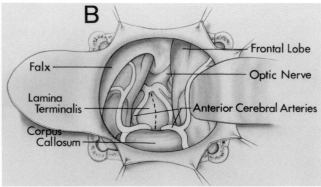

Fig. 8. Anterior frontal approach to the anterior part of the lateral and third ventricles. **A:** Site of scalp and bone flaps. **B:** The right frontal lobe has been retracted away from the falx to expose the optic nerves, lamina terminalis, rostrum of the corpus callosum and the anterior cerebral arteries. *(Figure continues.)*

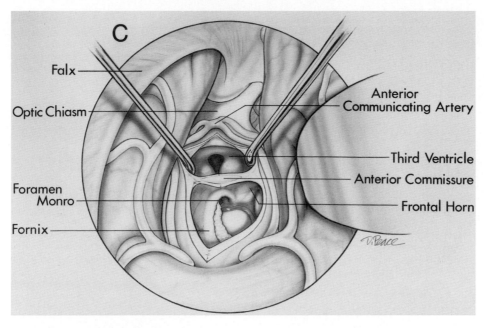

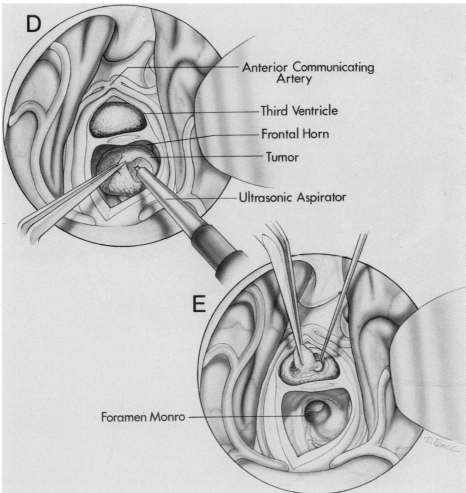

Fig. 8. *Continued.* **C:** Normal ventricular anatomy. The lamina terminalis and rostrum of the corpus callosum have been opened to expose the third ventricle and the frontal horn. The anterior commissure and column of the fornix have been preserved although the ipsilateral column of the fornix may be divided to increase the size of the opening into the third ventricle. **D:** A tumor that straddles the foramen of Monro and extends into both the frontal horn and third ventricle has been exposed. The portion of the tumor within the frontal horn is being removed using the ultrasonic aspirator. **E:** The part of the tumor within the third ventricle is being removed using a fine dissector.

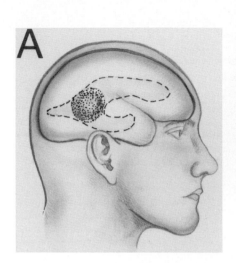

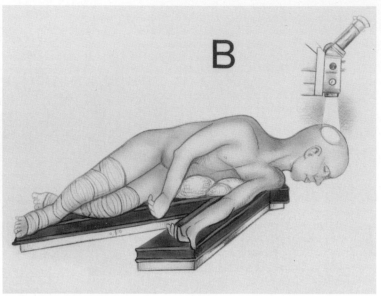

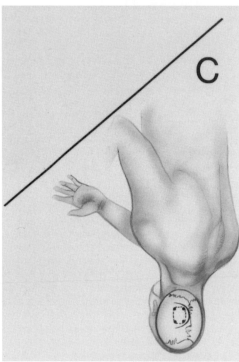

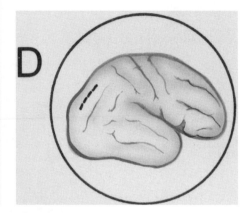

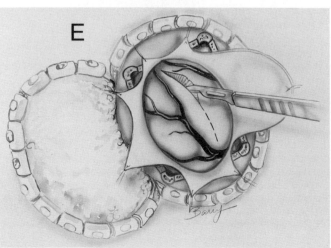

Fig. 9. Transcortical approach to a tumor in the atrium of the right lateral ventricle. **A:** Site of tumor within the right atrium. **B:** Park bench (three-quarter prone) position. **C:** Site of scalp incision *(solid line)* and bone flap *(dotted line)*. **D:** Site of the cortical incision in the superior parietal lobule. **E:** The dura is opened with the pedicle toward the superior sagittal sinus and the cortical incision is directed along the superior parietal lobule. The cortical veins pass forward at this level to reach the superior sagittal sinus. *(Figure continues.)*

cerebral arteries and their bifurcation into the pericallosal and callosomarginal arteries. The corpus callosum is exposed between the anterior cerebral arteries. Care should be taken to avoid occluding the perforating branches of the anterior communicating artery that extend into the walls of the third ventricle to supply columns of the fornix. A vertical incision beginning in the lamina terminalis and extending upward into the rostrum will expose a lesion in the floor of the frontal horn or straddling the lateral and third ventricular sides of the foramen of Monro. The landmarks within the ventricle have already been described.

POSTERIOR APPROACHES. Lesions situated within the posterior part of the body and atrium are most commonly exposed using a posterior transcortical approach. Selected lesions may be exposed by the posterior transcallosal or occipital approaches. The transcallosal approach may be considered if the

lesion involves the splenium of the corpus callosum and extends into the ventricle from the roof or the upper part of the medial wall of the atrium. The approach directed along medial side of the occipital pole is selected if the lesion arises in the medial wall of the atrium and extends into the ventricle and quadrigeminal cistern from the medial wall. Pineal tumors have been removed by a posterior transventricular approach directed through the medial wall of the atrium; however, the narrowness and heavy vascularization of the pineal area make it difficult to approach pineal tumors by this route (18). The occipital-transtentorial and infratentorial-supracerebellar approaches are most commonly used for exposing pineal tumors.

POSTERIOR TRANSCORTICAL APPROACH. This is the preferred approach to a lesion situated entirely within the atrium or arising in the region of the glomus of the choroid plexus (Fig. 9). Opening through the choroidal fissure from the

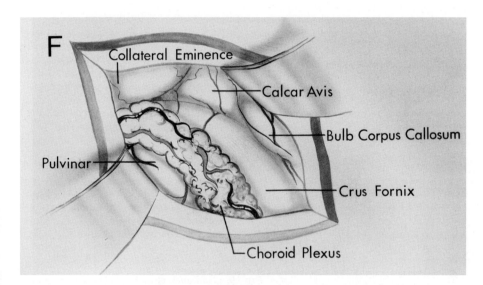

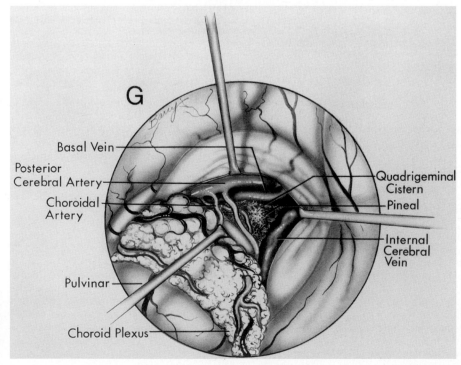

Fig. 9. Continued. **F,G:** Normal ventricular anatomy. **F:** The atrium of the right lateral ventricle has been opened to expose the fornix, collateral eminence, pulvinar, bulb of the corpus callosum, calcar avis, and choroid plexus. **G:** The choroidal fissure has been opened by incising along the attachment of the choroid plexus to the crus of the fornix. The choroid plexus has been retracted forward to expose the structures in the quadrigeminal cistern, which include the pineal body, posterior cerebral, and choroidal arteries, and the internal cerebral and basal veins. *(Figure continues.)*

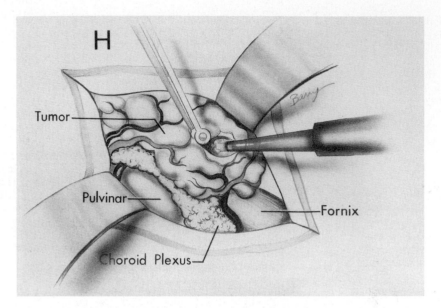

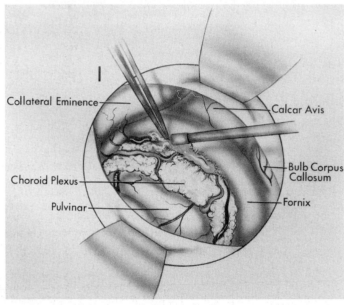

Fig. 9. *Continued.* **H:** A meningioma that arises in the atrium is being debulked using an ultrasonic aspirator. **I:** The last remnant of tumor has been removed and its attachment to the choroid plexus is being coagulated.

atrium exposes the quadrigeminal cistern and pineal region. The transchoroidal approach to the quadrigeminal cistern is most commonly used for arteriovenous malformations or vascular tumors that are located behind the pulvinar in the region of the choroidal fissure.

The patient is positioned in the three-quarter prone position with the face turned toward the floor and the parietal area to be operated uppermost. A high posterior parietal bone flap, centered behind the postcentral gyrus over the superior parietal lobule, is elevated. The cortex is incised in the long axis of the superior parietal lobule, preferably in a sulcus crossing the lobule. Image guidance may aid in minimizing the length of the incision. The atrium also has been approached through cortical incisions in the superior and middle temporal gyri, and the temporoparietal junction; however, exposing the atrium through the temporoparietal area may cause a homonymous visual field deficit because of the interruption of the optic radiations in either hemisphere, disturbances of visuospatial function in the nondominant hemisphere, and aphasia and agnostic disorders in the dominant hemisphere (5,19). Opening through the middle temporal gyrus might be considered for a lesion in the dominant hemisphere; however, cortical mapping during surgery has revealed an occasional extension of the speech representative into the middle temporal gyrus (20). In the approach through the superior parietal lobule, the ventricle is entered above the junction of the body and crus of the fornix. This approach exposes the glomus of the choroid plexus. The medial and lateral atrial veins are seen converging on the choroidal fissure. The arterial supply of lesions in this area is predominantly from the lateral posterior choroidal arteries. To reach the quadrigeminal cistern the choroidal fissure is opened by retracting the glomus of the choroid plexus laterally and opening along the tenia fornicis. Care is taken to avoid damaging branches of the posterior cerebral arteries on the medial side of the choroidal fissure from which the lateral posterior choroidal arteries arise. Retracting the crus medially and posteriorly exposes the quadrigeminal cistern and the caudal portion of the ambient cistern. The retraction should be carefully applied because it may damage the calcar avis and underlying visual cortex. Retraction of the pulvinar should be minimized in order to prevent language and speech disturbances in the dominant hemisphere. If the pulvinar bulges too far posteriorly, a supplemental horizontal incision in the medial wall of the atrium behind the crus may be needed in order to avoid retraction of the pulvinar; however, extending this incision posteriorly into the calcar avis will cause a visual field deficit. The opening into the quadrigeminal cisterns also may be obtained by making an arcuate incision along the direction of the fibers in the crus of the fornix. This incision should spare the contralateral half of the fornix; however, avoiding the contralateral half of the fornix is easier in this area than in the body of the ventricle because the crura have separated at the level of the atrium.

POSTERIOR TRANSCALLOSAL APPROACH. This approach is best suited to lesions that arise in the splenium and extend into the atrium rather than those situated entirely within the atrium (Fig. 10) (21). The patient is positioned in the three-quarter prone position with the face toward the floor and the parietal region to be operated uppermost. Occasionally, the side to be operated is positioned downward in order to allow the medial surface of the hemisphere on the side of the approach to fall away from the falx The parieto-occipital scalp flap and the craniotomy extend up to or across the superior sagittal sinus and have their anterior margin behind the postcentral gyrus. The dura is opened with the pedicle reflected toward the sagittal sinus. A bridging vein entering the superior sagittal sinus posterior to the Rolandic vein may need to be divided so that the hemisphere may be retracted away from the falx. Opening the arachnoid below the falx will expose the distal branches of the anterior cerebral arteries and occasionally the splenial branches of the posterior cerebral arteries. Opening the posterior part of the corpus callosum in the midline will expose the pineal region and the posterior part of the third ventricle. For the approach to the atrium an incision is made in the cingulate gyrus behind the posterior-superior part of the corpus callosum. This cortical incision is directed obliquely forward through the lateral part of the splenium to enter the atrium

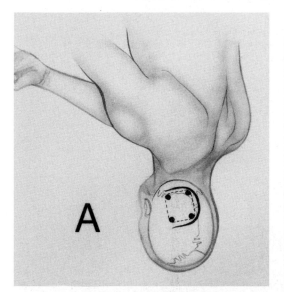

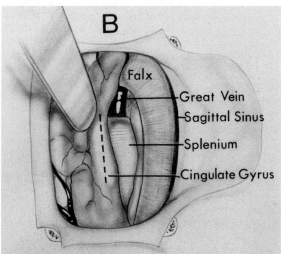

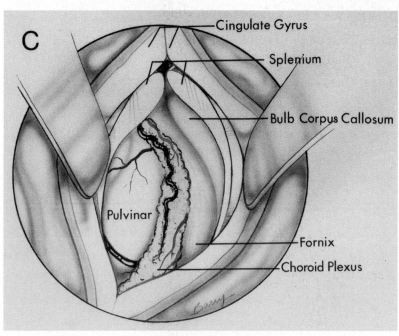

Fig. 10. Posterior transcallosal approach to the atrium of the right lateral ventricle. **A:** Three-quarter prone position. The scalp incision *(solid line)* and the bone flap *(interrupted line)* extends up to or across the midline. **B:** The dura is open with the pedicle toward the superior sagittal sinus. The medial surface of the right parietal lobe has been elevated away from the falx. The cortical incision extends through the posterior part of the cingulate gyrus. The corpus callosum is opened to the right of the midline to expose the right atrium. **C:** Normal ventricular anatomy. The opening through the cingulate gyrus encounters the lateral part of the splenium. Opening through the splenium in the midline would expose the roof of the third ventricle. The opening through the lateral part of the splenium into the atrium exposes the crus of fornix, bulb of the corpus callosum, and pulvinar and choroid plexus. *(Figure continues.)*

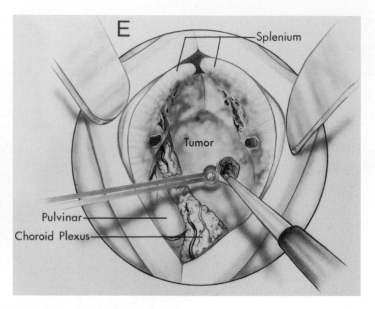

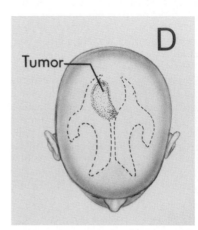

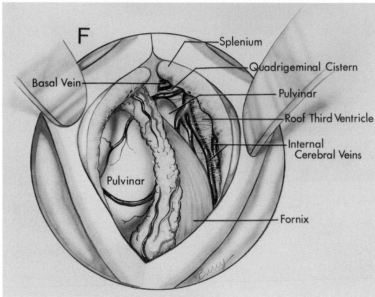

Fig. 10. *Continued.* **D:** The glial tumor is situated in the forceps major and the bulb of the corpus callosum. **E:** The tumor is being removed with the ultrasonic aspirator. The choroid plexus and pulvinar are pushed forward by the tumor. **F:** The tumor has been removed. Removing the bulb of the corpus callosum exposes the internal cerebral veins in the roof of the third ventricle and the quadrigeminal cistern.

just above the bulb of the corpus callosum. It should be remembered that the ventricles have started to deviate laterally at this point. The landmarks within the ventricle are described in the section on the posterior transcortical approach. The approach is directed lateral to the junction of the internal cerebral veins with the great vein. Dandy in some cases resected the great and internal cerebral veins, and the straight sinus in this region without neurological dysfunction; however, every effort should be made to spare these venous structures because their obliteration may cause major deficits (22,23).

OCCIPITAL APPROACH. This approach is suitable for approaching tumors that arise in the medial wall of the atrium and extend in the atrium or quadrigeminal cistern from the medial wall (Fig. 11) (24). These lesions are situated in the region of the atrial part of the choroidal fissure, in the posteromedial part of the pulvinar or in the region of the calcar avis and bulb of the corpus callosum. In order to use this approach, the lesion should come through the medial wall of the atrium

to the cisternal surface. It might also be considered for a lesion such as an arteriovenous malformation, in which it is desirable to expose the feeding choroidal arteries in the quadrigeminal cistern prior to exposing the lesion in the ventricle.

The patient is positioned in the three-quarter prone position with the occipital area to be operated uppermost and the face turned toward the floor. Occasionally, the side to be operated is positioned on the down side. The occipital scalp flap and craniotomy are placed so that they extend to the edge of or across the transverse and sagittal sinuses and the torcular. The dura is opened using two flaps, one based on the superior sagittal sinus and the other on the transverse sinus. The inferomedial aspect of the occipital pole is retracted superiorly and laterally. The occipital lobe usually can be retracted superolaterally without sacrificing any bridging veins because there are infrequently bridging veins between the medial occipital pole and the transverse, straight, and superior sagittal sinuses. The arachnoid over the ambient and quadrigeminal cisterns is opened. The internal occipital vein, which usually crosses from the anteromedial surface of the occipital lobe to the quadrigeminal cistern, is transected if necessary to expose the tumor. The ventricle is exposed by opening through the isthmus of the cingulate gyrus in front of the calcarine sulcus. The opening enters the medial wall of the atrium behind the choroidal fissure.

The tumor should extend into the cortical area near the junction of the vein of Galen and straight sinus for this approach to be successful. The branches of the posterior cerebral artery and its bifurcation into the calcarine and parieto-occipital branches course medial to the tumor. The lateral posterior choroidal arteries pass through the choroidal fissure in this area and the medial posterior choroidal arteries and basal vein is seen beside the pineal body. The lower portion of the splenium is divided, if necessary, to reach a lesion in the medial wall of the atrium near the crus of the fornix. The quadrigeminal plate,

trochlear nerve, superior cerebellar artery, and precentral cerebellar vein may be seen in the depths of the exposure.

INFERIOR APPROACHES. The inferior approaches are the posterior frontotemporal, transtemporal, and subtemporal approaches. The posterior frontotemporal approach exposes as much as the anterior two thirds of the temporal lobe and permits the anterior part of the temporal horn to be exposed through a small cortical incision or a temporal lobectomy. The transtemporal and subtemporal exposures done through a temporal craniotomy centered above the ear permit the full length of the temporal horn to be opened through cortical incisions on the lateral or inferior surfaces of the temporal lobe.

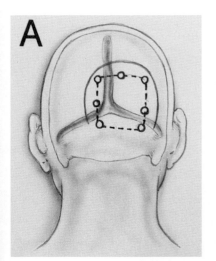
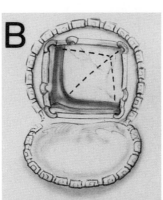
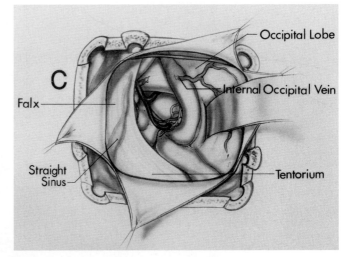
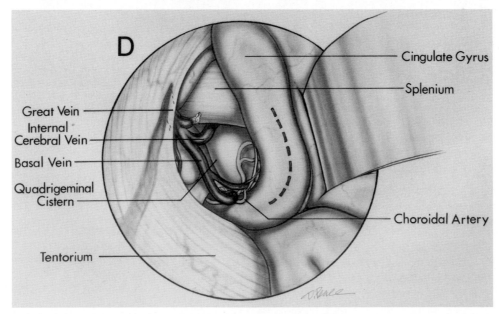

Fig. 11. Occipital-transcingulate approach to an arteriovenous malformation of the right atrium. **A:** Right occipital scalp *(solid line)* and bone flaps *(interrupted line)* are elevated. The bone flap extends up to or across the margin of the transverse and sagittal sinuses. **B:** The dura is opened with pedicles on the transverse and sagittal sinuses. **C:** The right occipital lobe is elevated away from the falx to expose the isthmus of the cingulate gyrus. An internal occipital vein is often sacrificed to reach this area. **D:** Enlarged view. The interrupted line shows the site of the: cortical incision through the isthmus of the cingulate gyrus. The internal cerebral, basal and great veins are exposed in the quadrigeminal cistern. *(Figure continues.)*

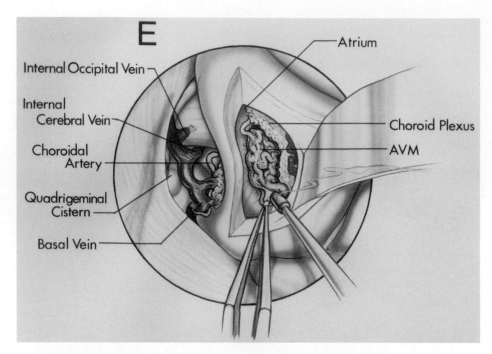

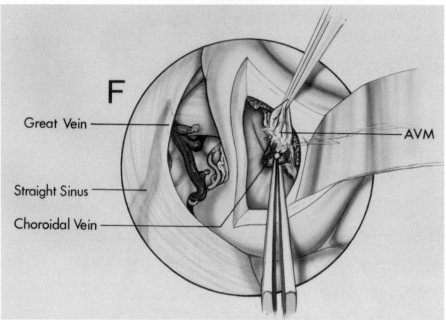

Fig. 11. *Continued.* **E:** The malformation is situated in the choroid plexus. The arteries entering and the veins exiting the malformation pass through the choroidal fissure to reach the quadrigeminal cistern. **F:** The choroidal arteries that feed the malformation have been coagulated and divided and the last draining vein from the malformation is being obliterated with bipolar coagulation.

POSTERIOR FRONTOTEMPORAL APPROACH. The posterior frontotemporal approach should be used for a lesion involving the anterior portion of the temporal horn that could be exposed through a temporal lobectomy or a small cortical incision in the anterior part of the temporal lobe (Fig. 12). The patient is placed in the supine position with a sandbag under the shoulder on the side to be operated. The head is tilted a bit backward and turned 45 degrees away from the side of the operation. The scalp incision begins in the frontal area and extends in a "question mark" configuration back to the area above the ear and then downward to the zygoma in front of the ear. The scalp, temporalis muscle and fascia, and pericranium are reflected as a single layer. A free frontotemporal bone flap that exposes the anterior half of the lateral surface of the temporal lobe is elevated and the lateral aspect of the sphenoid ridge is removed with a rongeur or drill. The dura is opened with the main flap pulled anterior–inferior along the region of the pterion. After opening the dura a decision is made as to whether to enter the temporal horn through a cortical incision or temporal lobectomy. The cortical incision should be selected if the lesion is strictly localized to the region of the tip of the temporal horn. The temporal lobectomy should be considered

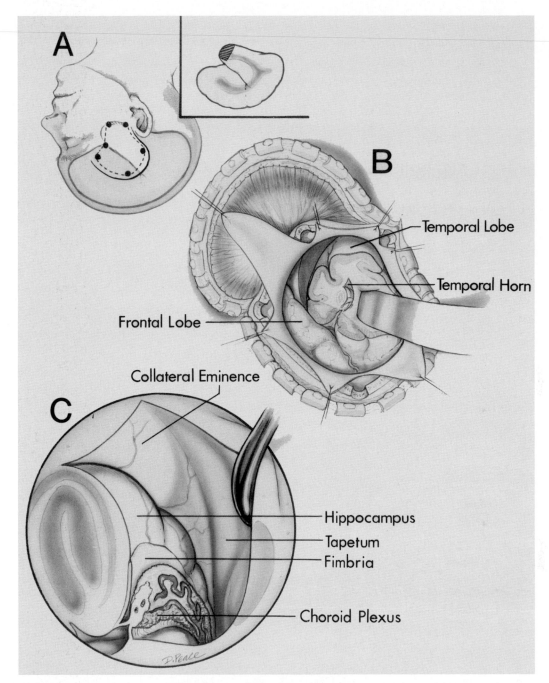

Fig. 12. Frontotemporal craniotomy and approach to temporal horn through a temporal lobectomy. **A:** Right frontotemporal scalp *(solid line)* and bone flaps *(interrupted line)* are elevated. The insert shows the extent of the temporal lobectomy. **B,C:** Normal ventricular anatomy. **B:** The lobectomy extends across the anterior part of the temporal horn. **C:** Structures exposed in the wall of temporal horn include the hippocampal formation, fimbria, choroid plexus, collateral eminence, and the tapetum of the corpus callosum.

if the lesion involves not only the tip of the temporal horn, but also extends into the temporal lobe around the temporal horn. For the transcortical approach, the lower part of the middle temporal gyrus or the upper part of the inferior temporal gyrus is opened in the long axis of the gyrus and the incision is directed backward through the temporal lobe to the anterior part of the temporal horn.

For the approach using a temporal lobectomy, the vertical incision through the temporal lobe should be situated no more than 4.5 cm from the temporal tip in order to avoid the optic radiations, and the horizontal incision paralleling the Sylvian fissure should be directed medially through the lower part of the superior temporal gyros or the upper part of the middle temporal gyros. Medially, an incision through the superior temporal gyrus encounters the pia arachnoid and the medial surface of the lower lip of the Sylvian fissure that covers the lower branches of the middle cerebral artery as they course over the insults. This incision paralleling the Sylvian fissure is extended anteriorly and medially into tuhe anterior pole of the temporal lobe just below the Sylvian fissure and sphenoid ridge. The

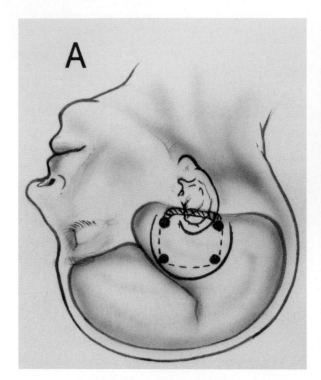

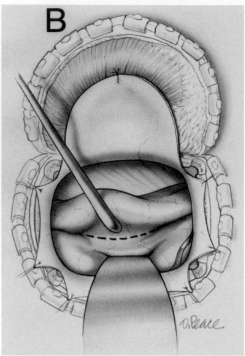

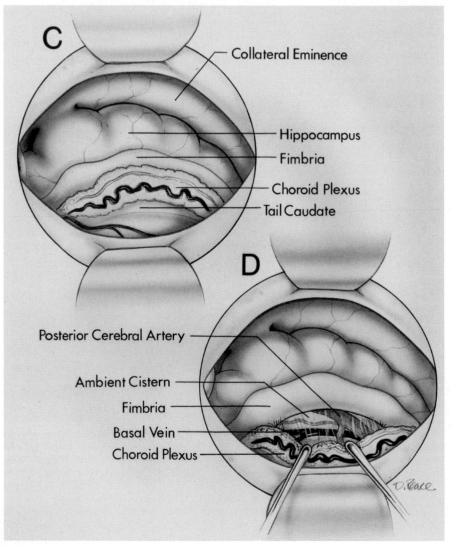

Collateral Eminence

Hippocampus
Fimbria
Choroid Plexus
Tail Caudate

Posterior Cerebral Artery

Ambient Cistern

Fimbria

Basal Vein

Choroid Plexus

Fig. 13. Subtemporal approach to the temporal horn and basal cisterns. **A:** Right temporal scalp *(solid line)* and bone flaps *(interrupted line)* are elevated. A small craniectomy *(cross-hatched area)* at the lower margin of the exposure gives access to the floor of the middle fossa. **B:** The dura has been opened with the pedicle inferiorly. The temporal horn is approached through a cortical incision *(interrupted line)* in the sulcus between the inferior temporal and occipitotemporal gyri. **C,D:** Normal anatomy of the temporal horn and ambient cistern. **C:** The temporal horn has been opened to expose the collateral eminence, hippocampus, fimbria, choroid plexus, and the tail of the caudate nucleus. *(Figure continues.)*

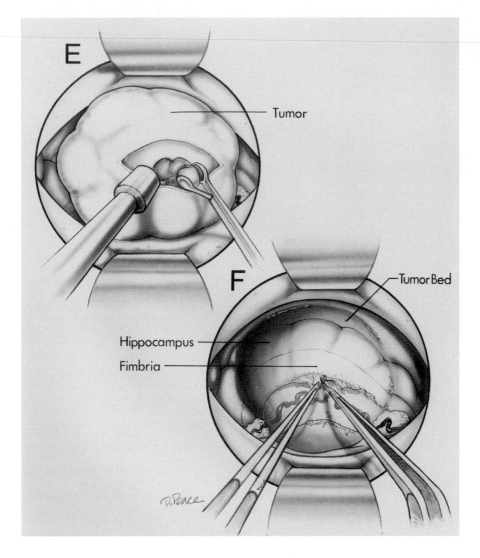

Fig. 13. *Continued.* **D:** The choroidal fissure has been opened by incising the attachment of the choroid plexus to the fimbria in order to expose the posterior cerebral artery and basal veins in the ambient cistern. **E:** An epidermoid tumor in the temporal horn has been opened and the intracapsular contents are being removed using a suction and cup forceps. **F:** A remnant of tumor capsule attached to the choroid plexus and adjacent part of the fimbria is being excised.

depths of the cortical incision encounter the uncus and parahippocampal gyrus, which are removed using subpial dissection with a fine suction in order to avoid injury to the perforating branches of the middle cerebral and anterior choroidal arteries that pass through the anterior perforated substance to supply the internal capsule. The cortical incision extending around the temporal tip often can be completed without sacrificing the major Sylvian veins that enter the sphenoparietal sinus just below the edge of the sphenoid ridge. These approaches expose the anterior part of the temporal horn as far back as the head of the hippocampus and where the anterior choroidal artery passes through the choroidal fissure. The prominence over the hippocampus and collateral eminence may be seen in the floor of the temporal horn and the inferior ventricular vein may be seen in the roof. The amygdaloid nucleus lies directly anterior and slightly above the tip of the temporal barn and is directly lateral to the cisternal surface of the anterior half of the uncus. Opening through the amygdaloid nucleus and uncus exposes the structures in the crural cistern. Opening the choroidal fissure at the posterior edge of the approach exposes the ambient cistern.

TRANSTEMPORAL AND SUBTEMPORAL APPROACHES.
A temporal craniotomy and transtemporal or subtemporal cortical incision should be used for a lesion in the middle or poste-

rior one third of the temporal horn and for selected lesions in the ambient and crural cisterns (Fig. 13).

For the temporal craniotomy centered above the ear, the patient is positioned in the supine position with the shoulder on the side of the lesion elevated, and the head tilted 60 to 80 degrees away from the side of the operation. The scalp incision extends from above the zygoma anterior to the ear to the area above the ear, and then posteriorly and downward to the region of the asterion posterior to the ear. The scalp, temporalis muscle and fascia, and pericranium are reflected as a single layer. The temporal horn may be exposed using a cortical incision in the middle temporal gyrus anterior to the optic radiations in the nondominant hemisphere and the inferior temporal gyrus in the dominant hemisphere. An alternative, and often preferable route, that minimizes the possibility of damage to the optic radiations and speech centers is the subtemporal route, in which an incision is directed medial to the inferior temporal or occipitotemporal gyrus on the inferior surface of the temporal lobe or through the collateral sulcus on the lateral margin of the parahippocampal gyrus. The risk of hemorrhage, venous infarction, and edema of the temporal lobe is reduced by avoiding occlusion of the bridging veins, especially the vein of Labbé. The opening into the temporal horn exposes the choroidal fissure and branches of the anterior and lateral posterior choroidal arteries as they enter the choroid plexus. The choroidal fissure is opened by incising along the tenia fimbriae, thus avoiding damage to the vessels that pass through the tenia choroidea. Opening the choroidal fissure between the tenia fimbriae and choroid plexus permits the arteries and veins that pass through the tenia choroidea to be retracted upward with the choroid plexus. This exposes the posterior cerebral and anterior and posterior choroidal arteries, and the basal vein without extensive retraction of the temporal lobe. The approach is especially useful for exposing arteriovenous malformations of the temporal horn, hippocampus, and medial part of the temporal lobe that are fed by the arteries entering and drained by the veins exiting the choroidal fissure (25). The transchoroidal approach to the basal cisterns reduces the risks of injury to the vein of Labbé and the swelling and hematoma of the temporal lobe that may result from the extensive retraction required to reach the posterior cerebral artery in the ambient cistern by the subtemporal extracerebral approach.

SELECTION OF OPERATIVE APPROACHES. Lesions within the anterior portion of the lateral ventricle are most commonly reached by the anterior transcallosal and anterior transcortical approaches. This anterior transcallosal approach is suitable for lesions in the frontal horn and body of the lateral ventricle, and for reaching the anterosuperior part of the third ventricle through the lateral ventricle. The transcallosal approach is easier to perform than the transcortical approach if the ventricles are of a normal size or are minimally enlarged. This anterior transcortical approach is suitable for reaching tumors in the anterior part of the lateral ventricle and the anterosuperior part of the third ventricle, especially if the tumor is situated predominantly in the lateral ventricle on the side of the approach. It is more difficult to expose the lateral ventricle on the opposite side through the transcortical than through the transcallosal approach. The transcortical approach is facilitated if the lateral ventricles are enlarged. Routes through the lateral ventricles to the anterior part of the third ventricle, other than by incising the ipsilateral column of the fornix, are by the transchoroidal approach in which the choroidal fissure is opened, and by the interforniceal approach in which the body of the fornix is split longitudinally in the midline. The transchoroidal and interforniceal approaches have the advantage of giving access to the central portion of the third ventricle behind the foramen of Monro by displacing, rather than transecting, the fibers in the fornix. The transchoroidal approach is preferred because there is no incision in the neural tissue. The interforniceal and transchoroidal routes provide a satisfactory view into the third ventricle when the ventricle is exposed through the corpus callosum. On the other hand, the transchoroidal opening provides a better view into the third ventricle than the interforniceal approach when the ventricle is exposed through the middle frontal gyrus. An anterior frontal approach may be considered for a lesion that involves the region of the rostrum and lower half of the genu of the corpus callosum or that extends from the rostrum into the third ventricle behind the lamina terminalis.

The posterior transcortical approach is the preferred route for exposing lesions situated entirely within the atrium, or arising in the glomus of the choroid plexus. Selected lesions may be exposed by the posterior transcallosal or medial occipital approaches. The transcallosal approach should be considered for a lesion that arises in the splenium and extends into the ventricle from the roof or the upper part of the medial wall of the atrium. The occipital approach directed along the falacotentorial junction should be used if the lesion arises in the medial wall of the atrium or extends from the atrium to the cisternal surface of the medial wall.

The temporal horn may be approached by the posterior frontotemporal, temporal, or subtemporal approach. The posterior frontotemporal approach should be used for a lesion involving the anterior portion of the temporal horn, which could be exposed through a small cortical incision in the anterior part of the temporal lobe or through a temporal lobectomy. The temporal and subtemporal routes to the temporal horn should be used for a lesion in the middle or posterior one-third of the temporal horn or for selected lesions in the cisterns medial to the temporal horn. The subtemporal route using a cortical incision is in the collateral sulcus or occipitotemporal gyrus and the inferior surface of the temporal lobe is preferred. The opening into the temporal horn exposes the choroidal fissure. Opening through the choroidal fissure in the temporal horn provides a transventricular view of the posterior cerebral artery and basal vein in the ambient cistern. In all of the approaches described, image guidance, in selected cases, will increase the accuracy of the approach and minimize the required neural incision.

References

1. Nagata S, Rhoton AL Jr, Barry M. Microsurgical anatomy of the choroidal fissure. *Surg Neurol* 1988;30:3–59.
2. Rhoton AL Jr. Microsurgical anatomy of the lateral ventricles. In: Wilkins RH, Rengachary SS, eds. *Neurosurgery,* 2nd ed. New York: McGraw-Hill, 1996:1419–1434.
3. Rhoton AL Jr. Microsurgical anatomy of the region of the third ventricle. In: Apuzzo MLF, ed. *Surgery of the third ventricle,* 2nd ed. Baltimore: Williams & Wilkins, 1998:89–157.
4. Fujii K, Lenkey C, Rhoton AL Jr. Microsurgical anatomy of the choroidal arteries: lateral and third ventricles. *J Neurosurg* 1980;52:165–188.
5. Timurkaynak E, Rhoton AL Jr, Barry M. Microsurgery anatomy of the lateral ventricles. *Neurosurgery* 1986;19:685–723.
6. Ono M, Rhoton AL Jr, Peace D, Rodriquez RJ. Microsurgical anatomy of the deep venous system of the brain. *Neurosurgery* 1984;15:621–655.
7. Rhoton AL Jr. Operative approaches to the lateral ventricles (supratentorial intraventricular tumours). In: Dudley H, Carter D, Russell RCG, eds. *Rob & Smith's operative surgery.* 4th ed. 1989:288–326.
8. Shucart WA, Stein BM. Transcallosal approach to the anterior ventricular system. *Neurosurgery* 1978;3:339–343.
9. Stein BM. Transcallosal approach to third ventricular tumors. In: Schmidek HH, Sweet WH, eds. *Operative neurosurgical techniques. Indications, methods and results.* New York: Grune & Stratton, 1982:575–584.
10. Apuzzo MLJ, Chikovani OD, Gott PS, et al. Transcallosal, interforniceal approaches for lesions affecting the ventricle: surgical consideration and consequences. *Neurosurgery* 1982;10:547–554.
11. Apuzzo MLJ, Giannotta SL. Transcallosal interforniceal approach. In: Apuzzo MLJ, ed. *Surgery of the third ventricle.* Baltimore: Williams & Wilkins, 1987:354–379.
12. Lavyne MH, Patterson RH Jr. Subchoroidal trans-velum interpositum approach. In: Apuzzo MLJ, ed. *Surgery of the third ventricle.* Baltimore: Williams & Wilkins, 1987:381–397.
13. Viale GL, Turtas S. The subchoroidal approach to the third ventricle. *Surg Neurol* 1980;14:71–76.
14. Wen HT, Rhoton AL Jr, de Oliveira E. Transchoroidal approach to the third ventricle: an anatomic study of the choroidal fissure and its clinical application. *Neurosurgery* 1998;42:1205–1219.
15. Hirsch JF, Zouaoui A, Renier D, et al. A new surgical approach to the third ventricle with interruption of the striothalamic vein. *Acta Neurochir (Wein)* 1979;47:135–147.
16. McKissock W. The surgical treatment of the colloid cyst of the third ventricle: a report based upon twenty-one personal cases. *Brain* 1951;74:1–9.
17. Rhoton AL Jr, Yamamoto I, Peace D. Microsurgery of the third ventricle: Part 2. Operative approaches. *Neurosurgery* 1981;8:357–373.
18. Van Wagenen WP. A surgical approach for the removal of certain

pineal tumors: report of a case. *Surg Gynecol Obstet* 1931;53: 216–220.
19. Brodal A. *Neurological anatomy in relation to clinical medicine,* 3rd ed. New York: Oxford University Press, 1981:832–841.
20. Ojemann GA. Individual variability in cortical localization of language. *J Neurosurg* 1979;50:164–169.
21. Horrax G. Extirpation of a huge pinealoma from a patient with pubertas praecox: a new operative approach. *Arch Neurol Psychiatry* 1937;37:385–397.
22. Dandy WE. An operation for the removal of pineal tumors. *Surg Gynecol Obstet* 1921;33:113–119.
23. Dandy WE. Operative experience in cases of pineal tumor. *Arch Surg* 1936;33:19–46.
24. Poppen JL. The right occipital approach to a pinealoma. *J Neurosurg* 1966;25:706–710.
25. Heros RC. Arteriovenous malformations of the medial temporal lobe: surgical approach and neuroradiological characterization. *J Neurosurg* 1982;56:44–52.

109. Intraventricular Tumors: Third Ventricle

Arun Paul Amar and Michael L.J. Apuzzo

Despite the highly refined nature of contemporary microneurosurgery, operations in and around the third ventricle continue to pose significant technical challenges. Optimal outcomes from such surgeries require careful preoperative evaluation and planning, fastidious intraoperative technique, and vigilant postoperative management. The intricacies of such treatment constitute the subject matter of entire volumes (1).

The goals of this chapter are to survey the relevant surgical anatomy, pathological conditions, and operative strategies that apply to lesions of the anterior third ventricle, with special emphasis on transcallosal approaches. The details of specific techniques, however, can be found elsewhere (2–8). The anatomical and functional considerations that pertain to lesions of the pineal region and the surgical approaches that are applied to access them are described in Chapter 112.

Pathology of Third Ventricular Lesions

Pathological lesions affecting the anterior third ventricle encompass a wide range of neoplastic and inflammatory processes (4, 9). Usually, such lesions deform the third ventricle by encroachment from the surrounding parenchyma, but rarely, masses arising from the ventricle itself prove to be the source of clinical disease.

Colloid cysts are the most common lesions intrinsic to the third ventricle. Typically, they originate from the anterior roof of the ventricle and project inferiorly. They possess an inner epithelium composed of cuboidal cells, which secrete a mucinous substance that accumulates under pressure. Symptoms may result from persistent or intermittent obstruction of the foramen of Monro; often, however, they may remain asymptomatic.

Choroidal plexus papillomas are benign neoplasms that usually present within the first 2 years of life. Although only 10% to 30% of these arise from the third ventricle, mobile tumors that arise within the lateral ventricle may slip through the foramen of Monro, where they become trapped, and thus present as a third ventricular mass (9).

Neurocytomas are intraventricular tumors of young adults that arise near the foramen of Monro and thus may involve the lateral or third ventricular regions. Although they account for only 0.5% of brain tumors in some series (9), their true incidence may be higher because, prior to their first description in 1982 and even subsequently, these tumors have often been misdiagnosed as either oligodendroglioma or ependymoma by light microscopy.

Intraventricular meningiomas are rare tumors with a disproportionate incidence in children, in whom they comprise 15% to 17% of meningiomas, compared with only 1.6% in adults (9). The majority of such tumors occur in the lateral ventricles, and a recent review of the literature found fewer than 50 reported cases of meningioma arising within the third ventricle (9). More commonly, intraventricular meningiomas occur as basal tumors that may extend up into the floor of the third ventricle.

Most other lesions encroach upon the third ventricle from the surrounding parenchyma. Many of these are neoplastic, with glial tumors representing the most common third ventricular neuroepithelial tumors. Astrocytomas include the fibrillary astrocytoma and the juvenile pilocytic astrocytoma. The latter occurs more commonly in the region of the hypothalamus. Subependymal giant cell astrocytomas may also occur adjacent to the ventricles, especially in younger patients with tuberous sclerosis.

Although the ependymal surface of the third ventricle is greater than that of the fourth, ependymomas arising from the former are rare, accounting for fewer than 8% of all ependymomas (9). Nonetheless, they often enter into the differential diagnosis of third ventricular neoplasms.

The subependymoma, first described in 1945, is a common tumor of the ventricular system in adults. Usually, it constitutes an incidental autopsy finding but may occasionally come to clinical attention. The majority of tumors occur in the fourth or lateral ventricles, and third ventricular tumors are rare.

Craniopharyngiomas are frequent diagnostic considerations in this region. Most of these tumors arise from the suprasellar region and subsequently expand into the third ventricle, where they may produce hydrocephalus or visual loss. However, 24 cases of purely intraventricular tumors have also been reported (9). These latter tumors occur almost exclusively in adults and are almost always of the papillary variant, unlike the adamantinomatous type that constitutes the majority of craniopharyngiomas in children. The prognostic implications of these differences, however, remain unclear.

Like subependymomas, xanthogranulomas and xanthomas are common incidental findings at autopsy, with a frequency ranging from 2% to 7% (9), but symptomatic lesions are rare. They arise from the choroidal plexus of the glomus of the lateral ventricle or the third ventricle and are speculated to result from cellular degeneration, tissue reaction to hemorrhage, or general disturbances of lipid metabolism. Lesions in these two locations differ in their clinical and histopathological findings, the latter being far more lethal.

Primary lymphomas of the brain may occur in the region of the third ventricle. They have been more frequently encountered since the onset of the current epidemic of acquired immune deficiency syndrome (AIDS). Depending on geography, infectious processes such as neurocysticercosis or tuberculomas may also involve the third ventricular region. Cavernous vascular malformations of the third ventricle are infrequent lesions, with fewer than 20 reported cases in the literature (9). Other, uncommon lesions include teratomas, dermoid and epidermoid cysts, germ cell tumors, histiocytosis X, sarcoidosis, arachnoid cysts, and expansive pituitary adenomas.

Clinical Presentation

The anterior third ventricle is delimited by a number of densely packed, vital anatomical structures subserving functions that range from basic preservation of consciousness and homeostasis to the more refined agencies of memory, emotion, and personality (Fig. 1). As a result, damage to any of these vascular or neural elements from direct compression, ischemia, or invasion can result in a multitude of signs and symptoms. These include cranial nerve deficits (e.g., diplopia), features of elevated intracranial pressure from hydrocephalus (e.g., lethargy,

visual obscuration, headache, nausea, or vomiting), changes in higher cognitive function (e.g., memory deficits, apathy, abulia, dementia), or even autonomic dysregulation (e.g., diabetes insipidus). In some cases, such as colloid cysts or neurocysticercosis, the symptoms may be episodic due to intermittent obstruction of the foramen of Monro. However, recent reports suggest that the risk of sudden death from this mechanism in incidentally discovered colloid cysts is probably lower than was once feared (10).

Relevant Anatomical Principles

The major topographic elements of the midline corridor that require identification and consideration during transcallosal approaches include the coronal suture, the sagittal sinus, the parasagittal veins, the falx cerebri, the cingulate gyrus, the pericallosal arteries, the corpus callosum, the fornix and its components, the tela choroidea, the medial posterior choroidal arteries, and the internal cerebral veins (2). Consideration of the consequences of injury to each neural or vascular component is essential as a stepwise progression evolves through the corridor of exposure. Discussions of the physiological cost of manipulating these critical brain structures are beyond the scope of this chapter, but have been reviewed in detail elsewhere (2,3).

Although a number of complications may result from dissection of lesions within the third ventricle itself (e.g., alteration of consciousness, gastrointestinal hemorrhage, endocrinopathy, visual loss, mutism, and other signs of diencephalic injury), the major hazards in establishing the transcallosal corridor are the development of hemiparesis and memory loss. Moreover, transcortical-transventricular approaches carry the additional risks of injury to the cerebral cortex, caudate nucleus, and centrum semiovale. Other possible untoward events include aseptic or infectious meningitis, seizures, hydrocephalus, intraventricular hemorrhage, and nonspecific postoperative complications.

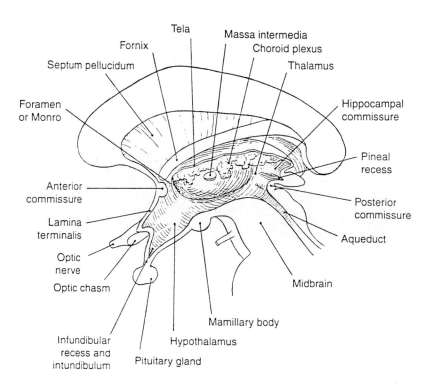

Fig. 1. Surgical anatomy of the third ventricle, viewed in midsagittal section. Damage to the neural or vascular elements that delimit this chamber may result from direct compression, ischemia, or invasion by the offending lesion. (From Amar AP, Albuquerque FC, Apuzzo MLJ: Anterior third ventricle lesions (including colloid cysts). In: Black P, Kaye A, eds. *Operative neurosurgery*. New York: Churchill Livingstone, 2000, with permission.)

Dissection of the interhemispherical corridor may result in injury to the bridging veins. Although we have sacrificed tributaries anterior to the coronal suture without adverse effects, we always attempt to preserve them whenever possible because of the risks of proximal or remote cortical injury. Experimental evidence suggests that venous infarction is much more likely to occur with a combination of brain retraction and sacrifice of a bridging vein than with either manipulation alone (2,3). With care during midline entry in relation to cortical venous anatomy and minimization of midline retraction, the incidence of permanent paresis will approach zero and that of transient paresis will be less than 10% (2).

Section of the corpus callosum (with sparing of the splenium) generally does not result in appreciable neurological sequelae (1–3). An acute syndrome following division of the anterior portion of the corpus callosum is characterized by a decrease in the spontaneity of speech, ranging from a mild slowness in initiating speech to frank mutism. This syndrome typically occurs in the hours and days following surgery but may persist for several months. Its reported incidence, as well as the segment of the corpus callosum that is implicated in the genesis of mutism consequent to sectioning, ranges widely. The protean manifestations of this acute syndrome, which may include paresis of the leg, incontinence, emotional disturbances, Babinski responses, focal motor seizures, and a disinhibited grasping reflex in the hand, suggest that other neural structures are likely to be involved. In addition to the effects of dividing the corpus callosum, mutism following transcallosal surgery may result from either direct retraction of the anterior cingulate gyrus, septum pellucidum, and fornix, or from circulatory disturbances in the supplementary motor area, thalamus, and basal ganglia (1–3).

Major callosal incision and limited but strategically placed interruption of posterior callosal pathways have been shown to result in disorders of interhemispherical transfer of information such as visual spatial transfer, tactile informational transfer, and bimanual motor learning, but these functions are usually preserved as long as the splenium remains intact. We studied six patients with 2.5-cm incisions in the callosal trunk (2). These results indicated no measurable deficits in interhemispherical transfer of somatesthetic information or complex perceptual motor learning tasks requiring continual sensory motor integration. Therefore, the majority of data support the concept that limited incision of the callosal trunk effects a minimal physiological alteration.

Once lateral ventricular entry has been effected, third ventricular lesions may be approached by a number of surgical maneuvers that involve an element of manipulation of the fornix. These maneuvers have been undertaken with trepidation because of the considered risk of amnesia during the postoperative period. Review of the literature related to the role of the fornix and memory processes provides contradictory opinions. There are clear instances of destruction of the fornix with absence of detectable amnesia and also those in which forniceal damage has been implicated in amnesia.

Approximately one-third of patients undergoing transcallosal-transforniceal surgery experience transient short-term memory difficulties manifesting as amnesia for recent events, typically occurring 24 to 72 hours after surgery. We believe that this effect is related more to the texture of the offending lesion than to its size, with firm masses creating a greater need for local manipulation. In our series, about 75% of cases resolved in less than 1 week, and all patients returned to their preoperative baseline status by 3 months postoperatively. Thus, in our experience, incision of the forniceal raphe and retraction of the body has not resulted in persistent amnestic syndromes, with mentation evaluated not only by standard bedside examination but also by formal psychometric assessment (2). Additional compli-

cations of forniceal manipulation may include confabulation, aphasia, and astereognosis (2,3).

Principles of Preoperative Evaluation

Before operative management of lesions within the third ventricle is undertaken, extensive planning and workup must precede (2,3). This preparation provides the surgeon with necessary information about the pathological nature of the third ventricular mass, as well as definition of the anatomical substrate peculiar to that given patient and identification of the major structures at risk from surgery. In addition, thorough neuropsychological assessment establishes baseline functional data for each patient, allowing for selection of the best management strategy in individualized circumstances.

Preoperative radiographic assessment is directed toward establishing clear perspectives of the individual's anatomy along the operative corridor and of all aspects of distortion and redisposition of anatomical elements by the lesion. Magnetic resonance imaging (MRI) in axial, coronal, and particularly midline sagittal planes will usually accomplish this objective. Furthermore, cerebral angiography may provide important information relevant to surgical planning, including cortical venous anatomy, parasagittal venous detail, tumor vascularity, and displacement of the internal cerebral veins, pericallosal arteries, and other deep vessels that may be altered by third ventricular lesions. Computed tomography angiography and magnetic resonance venography are noninvasive techniques that may supplant the need for catheter angiography in the preoperative definition of vascular anatomy.

Strict definition of surgical strategy and economy of tissue manipulation can be enhanced by careful consideration of the precise midpoint of bone flap placement, the angulation of retractor placement relative to the midpole of the lesion, and the distance of the corridor to the corpus callosum, fornix, and lesion. The size and extent of callosal and forniceal incisions may be estimated preoperatively in relation to the apparent type, size, and disposition of the lesion within the ventricle. The relation of the fornix to the corpus callosum and the area of the septum pellucidum may be determined. There is considerable variability regarding not only the relationship of all normal anatomical elements, but also the structural substrate deformed by the pathological process; absolute definition of the entire complex will permit maximal economy of manipulation and thus provide for ultimate safety and satisfactory management of the pathological process.

Planning of bone flap placement in the pericoronal area and the extent and mode of brain retraction or deformation should take into account the parasagittal venous anatomy as an important guiding factor. It has been our experience that appropriate placement of an economically sized craniotomy flap may be suitably devised in relation to venous anatomy as defined by preoperative cerebral angiography rather than strictly by bony landmarks (2,3).

Operative Strategies: Overview

Although the neural and vascular structures delimiting the anterior third ventricle constrain the possible approaches to this region, several methodologies have been developed (1) (Fig.

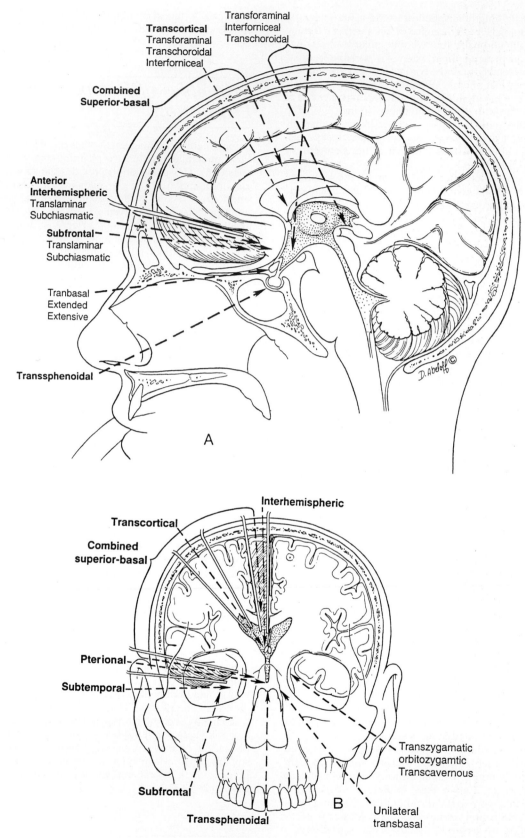

Fig. 2. Sagittal (**A**) and coronal (**B**) representations of various corridors of access to the anterior third ventricular region. Stereotactic and endoscopic approaches (not depicted) may be the most appropriate methodologies in certain circumstances. (From Apuzzo MLJ, Zee CS, Breeze RB, et al: Anterior and mid-third ventricular lesions: a surgical overview. In: Apuzzo MLJ, ed. *Surgery of the third ventricle*, 2nd ed. Baltimore: Williams & Wilkins, 1998, with permission.)

2). Selection of the optimum technique depends upon the goals of surgery in individual cases (e.g., biopsy to establish tumor histology for chemotherapy or radiotherapy, aspiration and decompression of a cystic lesion, or complete surgical extirpation). These aims, in turn, depend on the preoperative estimation of the lesion's excisability, based upon knowledge of its exact location, size, extension, encapsulation, and differential diagnosis as characterized by preoperative imaging studies, tumor markers, patient demographics, and other information.

Establishment of a tissue diagnosis and reconstitution of cerebrospinal fluid (CSF) pathways are the primary objectives in all cases. Depending on the pathological nature of the lesion (e.g., colloid cyst, cysticercosis), surgical excision may also be a reasonable goal; otherwise, cytoreduction is a realistic objective.

In addition to mass management, CSF diversion may be necessary to treat hydrocephalus. If cytoreductive surgery is likely to restore aqueductal or foraminal flow of CSF, temporary placement of a ventriculostomy may obviate the need for a permanent shunt and thus prevent the peritoneal spread of a dyscohesive tumor, although the likelihood of such a complication is probably lower than the frequency of its mention would indicate (11). For patients who undergo a biopsy followed by prolonged radiotherapy or chemotherapy, however, insertion of a ventriculoperitoneal shunt may be obligatory. The size of the lateral ventricles is also an important consideration in selecting between transcortical or transcallosal approaches to the third ventricle.

For patients whose lesions do not manifest the classic features of a benign tumor, stereotactic biopsy is often the first phase of treatment. Stereotactic biopsy of third ventricular masses introduces a number of potential hazards, including the risks of catastrophic hemorrhage, venous compromise, and implantation of tumor cells along the course of the biopsy instrument. Furthermore, since some of these lesions comprise admixtures of different histology, a theoretical possibility of sampling error also exists. In spite of these pitfalls, the safety, feasibility, and diagnostic yield of stereotactic biopsies of third ventricular lesions have been confirmed by many centers (9). Stereotactic aspiration of cystic lesions is also a well-established methodology but is associated with the possibility of recurrence or incomplete evacuation if the contents are viscous (12).

Endoscopy is a useful diagnostic and therapeutic tool in the management of various third ventricular lesions, especially those with cystic contents. Aspiration of both colloid and cysticercal cysts have been successfully performed through this modality (3,12), and endoscopic biopsy under direct visualization has also been described. The use of stereotactic guidance eliminates the requirement of ventricular dilation, and passage through the foramen of Monro is generally not problematic, especially when flexible endoscopes are used (12).

For patients with noncystic, benign-appearing lesions of the third ventricle, craniotomy is often the most appropriate primary strategy. Based on the works of Dandy, exposure of the third ventricle has historically been achieved via the transcortical route (Fig. 2). This approach permits access to the lateral ventricle and is well suited to lesions that arise from or extend into this chamber, especially when accompanied by lateral ventricular dilation. More recently, the studies of Sperry and Bogen confirmed the relative safety of callosal sectioning when the splenium is spared (1). As a result, an increased interest in interhemispherical (transcallosal) approaches to the third ventricle has been witnessed over the past 20 years (2). These latter routes have been applied to access both the anterior third ventricle as well as the region of the pineal body (11).

Generally, if there is no associated hydrocephalus, a transcallosal approach to the lateral ventricle should be used. The surgeon can then gain passage into the third ventricular chamber by a number of secondary maneuvers that involve some manipulation of forniceal structure, either by traversing the foramen of Monro (which may be expanded by the lesion or by the operative procedure), by the transchoroidal transvelum interpositum approach, or by the interforniceal corridor.

If the lesion is confined to the third ventricle, the transcallosal approach provides superior visualization of the entire ventricle. If, however, an extraaxial lesion arises inferiorly and extends upward into the caudal third ventricle, cranial base approaches may be more appropriate since the greatest volume of the mass may be accessed in this manner. Such approaches include the pterional, subfrontal, subtemporal, and transnasal-transsphenoidal routes (Fig. 2). The orbitozygomatic craniotomy has been popularized as an approach to skull base lesions that secondarily invade the floor of the third ventricle. Originally developed to gain improved access to basilar territory aneurysms (8), this technique combines previously described zygomatic and temporopolar modifications of the classic pterional and subtemporal craniotomies. Removal of the zygomatic process allows the microscope to be maneuvered into a basal-to-vertex trajectory, thus enhancing exposure to areas of extension above the dorsum sellae. Likewise, removal of the orbital rim permits retraction of the globe and exposure of the interpeduncular fossa along the anteroposterior axis. The enhanced operative corridor afforded by this approach may permit a greater extent of resection than is possible with conventional routes.

Compared with transcortical routes, the major advantages afforded by the transcallosal approach include the following:

- a short trajectory to the third ventricle
- flexibility to explore the entire third ventricular chamber, including the basal and posterior components
- the absence of cortical transgression and, hence, diminished probability of subsequent seizures
- bilateral exposure of the foramen of Monro
- no requirement of ventriculomegaly (2–4).

Transcallosal Approach: Operative Technique

The operative technique for the transcallosal approach (2–4) begins with the administration of high potency glucocorticoids, anticonvulsants, and perioperative antibiotic prophylaxis. After the induction of general anesthesia, the patient is positioned supine. The head is then placed in neutral pin fixation and flexed to 15 degrees. Other options such as the lateral decubitus position offer some potential advantages but may distort the midline structures due to the effects of gravity, risking loss of orientation for the inexperienced surgeon. Various scalp flaps may be used, although we generally employ a two-limbed curvilinear incision that affords visualization of the coronal suture and at least 1 cm of the sagittal suture.

For anterior third ventricular lesions, we prefer to use a 6×4×3-cm trapezoidal bone flap with complete sagittal sinus exposure, principally based on the right (Fig. 3). In order to reduce the potential for venous infarction, placement of the bone flap in the anteroposterior dimension should be based on assessment of the venous anatomy as determined by preoperative imaging. Review of 100 angiograms with particular attention to the distribution of the parasagittal venous complex disclosed that 42 studies had evidence of significant venous tributaries draining within 2 cm of the coronal suture, with the majority (70%) entering the sagittal sinus behind the suture and the remainder (30%) entering in front of it (2). Thus, whenever

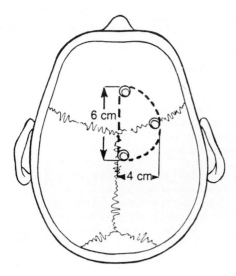

Fig. 3. Typical bone flap for transcallosal (interhemispherical) approaches to the third ventricle. Exposure of the superior sagittal sinus is critical. Commonly, the flap is placed two-thirds anterior and one-third posterior to the coronal suture, but placement in the anteroposterior dimension should be based on assessment of the venous anatomy as determined by preoperative imaging. (From Apuzzo MLJ, Amar AP: Transcallosal interforniceal approach. In: Apuzzo MLJ, ed. *Surgery of the third ventricle*, 2nd ed. Baltimore: Williams & Wilkins, 1998, with permission.)

possible, the flap should be placed two-thirds anterior and one-third posterior to the coronal suture. Placement of the bone flap as far anteriorly as possible also provides an optimum angle of view to the foramen of Monro. Although some authors suggest making the bony opening large enough so that the surgical strategy could be converted to a transcortical approach if a large parasagittal vein was encountered that required sacrifice in order to proceed with the transcallosal route, this maneuver should not be necessary if adequate definition of venous tributaries and paramedian venous anatomy has been undertaken preoperatively. Recently, we have relied on magnetic resonance venography or computed tomographic venography for such planning, with both modalities revealing an average of 4.3 cortical veins draining into either side of the superior sagittal sinus (2,3).

After the application of dural tenting stitches, the Budde halo self-retraining retractor system is secured in place. We then make a trapezoidal dural incision, with the broad base placed medially toward the sinus. This flap may be secured to the halo by several sutures, providing absolute midline exposure of the falx. As this flap is reflected, the bridging veins must be identified and preserved. Although we have sacrificed bridging veins that reside anterior to the coronal suture without untoward effects, every effort should be made to preserve them.

The falx-cortical interface is then identified, and the plane is then developed by placement of a large cotton patty into the space, followed by application of a 19-mm retractor blade from the right side of the field. This process is repeated in a serial fashion as the exposure is deepened. The surgeon should pause for 2 to 3 minutes between each advancement of the retractor blade to allow the brain to relax in the face of the pressure exerted by the retractor. This interhemispherical corridor should not exceed 5 cm in length and 1.5 cm in width, so as to minimize retraction injury. After identification of the inferior sagittal sinus, further dissection is accomplished with the aid of the operating microscope using either a 275-mm or 300-mm lens. Separation of the cingulate gyri often requires blunt

dissection with microinstrumentation. Inexperienced surgeons commonly mistake the cingulate gyrus for the corpus callosum, but these structures can be distinguished by the fact that the former has the typical tan-gray color of the cortical-pial surface, whereas the latter is strikingly white.

Eventually, the white callosal carpet is identified, with its associated pericallosal arteries. Once the corpus callosum is exposed, cotton balls or patties may be placed into the depths of the exposure at the anterior and posterior poles to aid in the maintenance of hemispherical retraction. The size of the callosal exposure should be 1×3 cm. The falx is maintained as the midline reference point, with the original position of the pericallosal arteries serving as a secondary landmark.

After the corpus callosum and the pericallosal arteries are identified, ventricular entry is undertaken. The site of the callosal incision depends on the position of the pericallosal arteries and may be either between the arteries or lateral to them. This entry is generally oval-shaped and 2 to 2.5 cm in length, depending on variables related to the angle of entry and the size of the lesion. Although some authors recommend sectioning the thinnest part of the trunk in order to minimize postoperative neuropsychological deficits, others argue that it is more important to plan the incision according to the most appropriate trajectory, which is usually anterior to the midportion of the corpus callosum. This region of the trunk may be approximated by the intersection of the corpus callosum with an imaginary line defined by the coronal suture in the midsagittal plane and the external auditory meatus; if continued inferiorly, this line would pass through the foramen of Monro (3). With No. 5 French catheter suction and bipolar coagulation, the corpus callosum is incised (Fig. 4). The thickness of the trunk varies greatly and can range from a thin layer in the presence of hydrocephalus to over 1 cm. Absolute control of ependymal bleeding must be obtained before proceeding, since failure to do so may result in postoperative intraventricular hemorrhage. Once the ventricles are entered, the blade is advanced to retract the corpus callosum and the ipsilateral hemisphere, being careful not to overadvance the blade to the basal ganglia (Fig. 4).

Depending on the location of the callosal incision and its relation to the anterior-to-posterior and medial-to-lateral planes, either the right or left lateral ventricle, forniceal body, or a cavum septum pellucidum, may be entered. Establishing proper orientation is critical before proceeding. If a cavum has been entered, the septum should be widely fenestrated. Otherwise, this maneuver should be performed after identification of ventricular landmarks, such as the choroidal fissure and foramen of Monro. Fenestration or excision of the septum provides potential bilateral midline exposure and alternate pathways for CSF flow. Fenestration should be no less than 1 cm².

Once the foramen and choroidal plexus are identified, one of the following three routes may be used for entry into the third ventricular chamber: (a) transforaminal, (b) transchoroidal transvelum interpositum, or (c) interforniceal (Fig. 5). Lesion character (size, vascularity, texture, location), foramen caliber, view lines, and personal skills and experience all guide the surgeon in selecting the most appropriate route. All strategies should be directed toward avoiding midline manipulation and minimizing the transmission of pressure gradients to paraventricular structures.

TRANSFORAMINAL CORRIDOR. Inspection of the foramen of Monro often reveals the presence of the lesion. Initially, an attempt to decompress the mass should be made via a transforaminal corridor, especially if it is distended by presence of the mass itself or by attendant hydrocephalus. Cystic, soft, or easily resectable lesions may usually be removed via the foramen of Monro. Obviously, these lesions must be located far

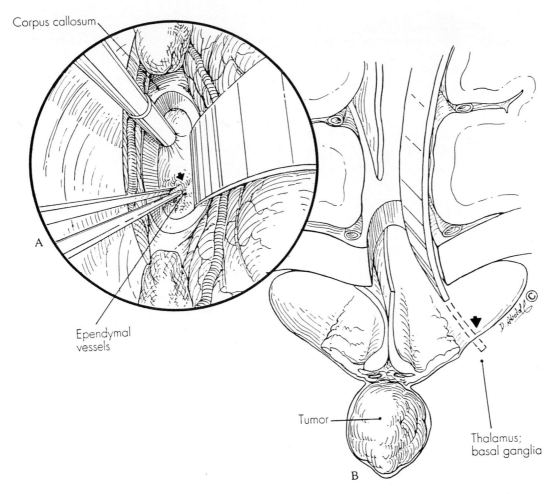

Fig. 4. An oval callosotomy measuring 2 to 2.5 cm in length is performed using bipolar forceps and a 5 French catheter suction (**A**). A retractor blade is then advanced in order to displace the callosal trunk and enhance exposure (**B**). In general, only unilateral retraction is employed, since bilateral cingulate gyrus retraction risks mutism. Care is taken not to overadvance the blade to the basal ganglia. (From Apuzzo MLJ, Litofsky NS: Surgery in and around the anterior third ventricle. In: Apuzzo MLJ, ed. *Brain surgery: complication avoidance and management*. New York: Churchill Livingstone, 1993, with permission.)

enough anteriorly within the ventricle to allow transforaminal visualization.

When attempting to remove lesions through the foramen, the surgeon should never try to deliver the mass if it exceeds the size of the foramen because this action may injure the paraforniceal region. Moreover, all attachments to the third ventricular roof must be freed to avoid bleeding from the tela choroidea and injury to the fornix. Some surgeons have advocated partial resection of the anterior nucleus of the thalamus or section of the forniceal column to enlarge the foramen, but we do not endorse these maneuvers, since the former risks uncontrollable bleeding from the internal cerebral vein while the latter may cause severe neuropsychological impairment, especially if the contralateral fornix has already been compromised by the third ventricular lesion (5).

In the management of colloid cysts, the cyst may be aspirated through the foramen, and subsequently, its wall may be coagulated with bipolar forceps. This may be a definitive treatment if the cyst remnant does not appear to present a significant residual mass or obstruct CSF flow.

TRANSCHOROIDAL CORRIDOR. If transforaminal dissection fails to provide a safe route for access to the lesion, a transchoroidal transvelum interpositum approach may be used to enter the third ventricle. Like the interforniceal approach, it is especially well suited for lesions occupying the superior half of the third ventricle posterior to the foramen of Monro. It may be technically more feasible than the interforniceal approach, however, when the two internal cerebral veins are not clearly separate structures.

Wen and colleagues (7) clarified two possible routes through the choroidal fissure that separates the thalamus inferiorly from the body of the fornix superiorly. In the classic "subchoroidal" approach, an incision is made along the taenia choroidea, the ependymal reflection between the dorsal surface of the thalamus and the inferolateral surface of the choroidal plexus in the body of the lateral ventricle. Alternatively, access to the velum interpositum in the roof of the third ventricle can be gained along the taenia fornicis, the reflection of ependyma off the forniceal body onto the superomedial aspect of the choroidal plexus. Although either taenia may be incised, Wen contends that the "suprachoroidal" approach between the dorsal aspect of the choroidal plexus and the fornix is safer, since superficial thalamic and caudate veins risk injury when the taenia choroidea is manipulated. In the subchoroidal approach, for instance, sacrifice of one thalamostriate vein is often necessary in lieu of

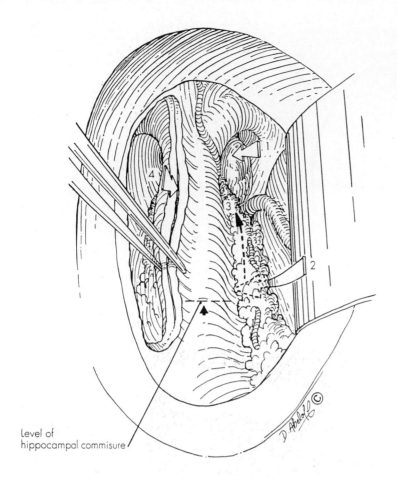

Level of
hippocampal commisure

Fig. 5. Once lateral ventricular entry has been effected, third ventricular lesions may be approached by a number of secondary maneuvers that involve some element of manipulation of the fornix. *1*, The transforaminal corridor may be attempted initially, especially if the foramen is already distended by the lesion. *2*, The transchoroidal transvelum interpositum corridor may be developed in order to gain wider exposure of the ventricle. *3*, The thalamostriate vein may be sectioned during this approach. *4*, The interforniceal plane is useful for lesions that bulge upward, distending the fornices. (From Apuzzo MLJ, Litofsky NS: Surgery in and around the anterior third ventricle. In: Apuzzo MLJ, ed. *Brain surgery: complication avoidance and management.* New York: Churchill Livingstone, 1993, with permission.)

sectioning or excessive local manipulation of the fornix. Although this maneuver may generally be accomplished without neurological sequelae, complications such as hemiplegia, mutism, and drowsiness have been reported.

Once lateral ventricular entry is accomplished, the choroidal fissure is readily appreciated by the presence of the overlying choroidal plexus. This structure serves as a guide to the foramen of Monro. In the subchoroidal route, the choroidal plexus is elevated or coagulated, thereby exposing the thalamus. As the choroidal plexus is mobilized medially, the attachments of the velum interpositum must be divided. Subsequently, the third ventricular roof is dissected medially, thus opening the ventricle. Eventually the thalamostriate vein is encountered at the foramen. This vein may then be divided, completing the opening into the third ventricle.

INTERFORNICEAL CORRIDOR. Busch initially described the interforniceal approach to a third ventricular lesion in 1944 (2). Using this route, he was able to decompress a malignant glioma. This method is best suited for large lesions that distend the roof of the third ventricle and cannot be removed via the foramen of Monro. The method results in a wide exposure of the entire third ventricle, and it allows for simultaneous bilateral transforaminal and interforniceal manipulation of the mass, thereby increasing the technical maneuvers available for tumor resection.

Once the septum pellucidum is fenestrated, the midline forniceal raphe in the roof of the third ventricle may be identified. This natural cleavage plane is developed with the use of a Sheehy canal knife, commencing at the foramen of Monro and extending posteriorly for 1 to 2 cm. The posterior dissection is

limited by the presence of the hippocampal commissure, which, along with the internal cerebral veins and medial posterior choroidal arteries, must be preserved. Secondary retraction at the level of the fornix is often not necessary; however, a 5-mm retractor blade tapered to 2-mm at the tip may be used to maintain exposure.

Large lesions tend to present themselves under pressure, thereby facilitating their dissection. Once exposure is accomplished, the lesion is internally decompressed and then dissected from the surrounding structures.

Summary

Transcallosal approaches to the third ventricle provide avenues for the establishment of tissue diagnoses, reconstitution of CSF pathways, and, occasionally, surgical cure of selected lesions. Proper understanding of the spectrum of third ventricular pathology and appropriate anatomical substrate will optimize patient selection and surgical outcomes.

References

1. Apuzzo MLJ, ed: *Surgery of the third ventricle*, 2nd ed. Baltimore: Williams & Wilkins, 1998.
2. Apuzzo MLJ, Amar AP: Transcallosal interforniceal approach. In:

Apuzzo MLJ, ed. *Surgery of the third ventricle*, 2nd ed. Baltimore: Williams & Wilkins, 1998; 421–452.

3. Amar AP, Albuquerque FC, Apuzzo MLJ: Anterior third ventricle lesions (including colloid cysts). In: Black P, Kaye A, eds. *Operative neurosurgery*. New York: Churchill Livingstone, 2000; 753–768.
4. Amar AP, Apuzzo MLJ: Transcallosal approach to the third ventricle. In: Schmidek HH, Sweet WH, eds. *Schmidek and Sweet's operative neurosurgical techniques: indications, methods, and results, 4th ed.* Philadelphia: WB Saunders, 2000.
5. Apuzzo MLJ, Litofsky NS: Surgery in and around the anterior third ventricle. In: Apuzzo MLJ, ed. *Brain surgery: complication avoidance and management.* New York: Churchill Livingstone, 1993; 541–579.
6. Apuzzo MLJ, Zee CS, Breeze RB, et al: Anterior and mid-third ventricular lesions: a surgical overview. In: Apuzzo MLJ, ed. *Surgery of the third ventricle*, 2nd ed. Baltimore: Williams & Wilkins, 1998; 635–680.

7. Wen HT, Rhoton AL, de Oliveira E: Transchoroidal approach to the third ventricle: an anatomic study of the choroidal fissure and its clinical application. *Neurosurgery* 1998;42:1205–1217.
8. Zabramski JM, Kiris T, Sankhla SK, et al: Orbitozygomatic craniotomy: technical note. *J Neurosurg* 1998;89:336–341.
9. Chen TC, Lavine S, Amar AP, et al: Stereotactic applications in third ventricular lesions. In: Apuzzo MLJ, ed. *Surgery of the third ventricle*, 2nd ed. Baltimore: Williams & Wilkins, 1998; 847–884.
10. Pollock BE, Huston J: The natural history of asymptomatic, untreated colloid cysts. *J Neurosurg* 1999;90:418A(abst).
11. Albuquerque F, Amar AP, Apuzzo MLJ: Pineal region tumors. In: Bernstein M, Berger MS, eds. *Neuro-oncology: the essentials.* New York: Thieme, 2000.
12. King WA, Ullman JS, Frazee JG, et al: Endoscopic resection of colloid cysts: surgical considerations using the rigid endoscope. *Neurosurgery* 1999;44:1103–1111.

110. Intraventricular Tumors: Fourth Ventricle

Tina Lin, Carl B. Heilman, and William A. Shucart

Surgery for mass lesions in the fourth ventricle presents unique surgical challenges because of the delicate neighboring anatomy and unique position of the fourth ventricle in the outflow of cerebrospinal fluid (CSF). Victor Horsley was the first to document surgical exploration of the posterior fossa in 1886 (1). William Macewen performed the first successful posterior fossa surgery in 1889 when he removed multiple tuberculous abscesses from the cerebellum (1). The surgery was performed in two stages: first the exposure, then the resection 1 week later. Since that time, the surgical treatment of posterior fossa and fourth ventricular tumors has advanced considerably because of improvements in surgical technique, anesthesia, and modern neuroimaging. Successful surgery of fourth ventricular tumors requires a thorough understanding of the anatomical and physiological considerations of this region.

Anatomy

The fourth ventricle serves as a conduit for the passage of CSF from the lateral and third ventricles to the craniospinal subarachnoid space. The tent-shaped roof of the fourth ventricle marks its dorsal boundary and consists of the cerebellum and its peduncles. The floor consists of the pons and medulla. Both lateral recess of the fourth ventricle have a foramen (Luschka) through which CSF flows to the cerebellopontine angle cisterns. The caudal-most extent of the fourth ventricle is marked by the foramen of Magendie, which opens into the cisterna magna. Detailed anatomy of the fourth ventricle has been studied and published by Matsushima and Rhoton, and is outside the scope of this chapter (2).

Most tumors within the fourth ventricle can be resected using a posterior midline approach, which will be discussed elsewhere in this chapter. Opening the suboccipital area exposes the two cerebellar hemispheres that are separated by the midline posterior cerebellar incisura (Fig. 1). Within the posterior cerebellar incisura lies the cerebellar vermis, which is divided into eight named lobules. Most prominent from the suboccipital surface are the two most inferior lobules: the pyramid and uvula, both named for their shapes. The uvula is partially obstructed by the overlying cerebellar tonsils, which are the inferior–medial extensions of the cerebellar hemispheres. Lateral retraction of the cerebellar tonsils uncovers the uvula and reveals the cisterna magna and foramen of Magendie, which lie below. Fourth ventricular tumors occasionally protrude through the foramen of Magendie. Large tumors often displace the cerebellar tonsils laterally.

Access to the fourth ventricle is best achieved by elevation or dissection of the inferior roof. The inferior roof is formed by the nodule, uvula, inferior medullary velum, and tela choroidea. The tela extends from the inferior medullary velum to the cerebellomedullary fissure, where it attaches to the dorsal medulla along narrow white ridges called the taenia ventricularis (Fig. 2). Sharp dissection of the tela at the telovelar junction toward the lateral recess can allow wide exposure to the fourth ventricle without violating important neural structures.

The fourth ventricular floor is just dorsal to many cranial nerve nuclei located in the dorsal pons and medulla (Fig. 3). The transition between pons and medulla is marked by the transversely oriented striae medullaris that extend to the lateral recesses of the ventricle. The cerebral aqueduct of Sylvius and the obex are the superior and inferior apices of the ventricle. The longitudinally oriented median sulcus divides the floor into symmetric halves. The sulcus limitans further divides each half into the median eminence and lateral vestibular area. The median eminence in the pontine region houses the facial colliculus with the underlying abducent nucleus and facial nerve fibers. The median eminence in the medullary region contains three

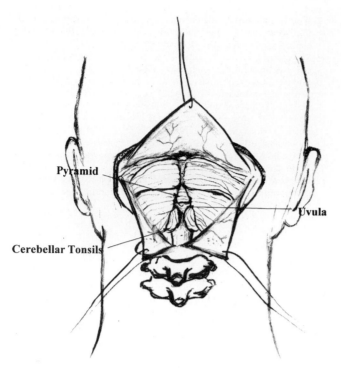

Fig. 1. The suboccipital surface. Most fourth ventricular tumors can be reached by this exposure. The posterior arch of C1 is removed in this illustration.

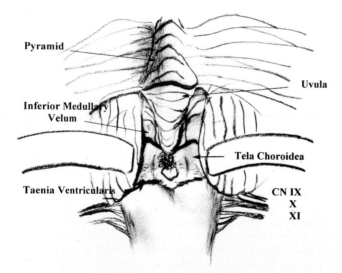

Fig. 2. Inferior roof of the fourth ventricle. Lateral retraction of the cerebellar tonsils reveals the roof of the fourth ventricle. Dissection of the thin tela gains access to the fourth ventricle without violating neural structures.

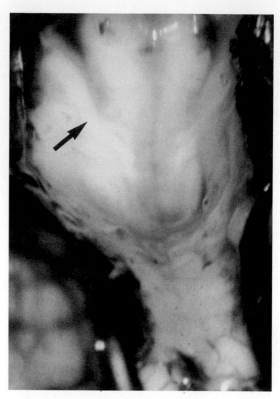

Fig. 3. Operative view of the fourth ventricular floor. Note the striae medullaris *(arrow),* which are the transversely oriented bands, separating the superior and inferior floor of the fourth ventricle. The facial colliculi are seen above the striae. Less distinct are the prominences below the striae: the hypoglossal trigone, vagal trigone, and area postrema.

trigones: hypoglossal, vagal, and area postrema, stacked superior to inferior. The lateral vestibular area houses the vestibular nuclei and auditory tubercle, which contains the dorsal cochlear nucleus and cochlear portion of cranial nerve VIII.

Clinical Presentation and Differential Diagnosis

Various lesions arise from the floor and walls of the fourth ventricle or extend into the ventricular system from the cerebellum or brainstem (Table 1). Lesions that obstruct the flow of CSF can cause hydrocephalus and increased intracranial pressure. Lesions that compress or invade the cerebellum can produce truncal, appendicular, or gait ataxia, dysarthric scanning speech, and nystagmus, depending on the area involved. Lesions on the floor of the fourth ventricle as well as those in the brainstem can cause various cranial nerve palsies. Long tract signs can be seen from pressure or tumor invasion of the brainstem.

MEDULLOBLASTOMAS. Medulloblastomas are the most common central nervous system (CNS) malignancy in childhood and account for 25% of all brain tumors in children. Seventy percent of medulloblastomas occur in patients younger than 8 years of age, with a slight male predominance. Medullo-

Table 1. Differential Diagnosis of Fourth Ventricular Tumors

Tumors and Cysts	Vascular Lesions	Infections
Medulloblastoma	Arteriovenous	Cysticercosis
Astrocytic tumors	malformations	Tuberculous
Ependymoma	Cavernous	Bacterial
Hemangioblastoma	angiomas	Fungal
Choroid plexus papilloma	Aneurysm	Other
Dermoid	(PICA)	
Epidermoid		
Subependymomas		
Meningioma		
Metastasis		
Teratoma		
Ganglioglioma		
Lymphoma		
Leukemia (chloroma)		
Myxofibroxanthoma		
Lhermitte-Duclos disease		
Hemangioma calcificans		
Arachnoid cyst		
Neuroepithelial/colloid cyst		
Choroidal epithelial cyst		

blastomas are classified as primitive neuroectodermal tumors (PNET), given their embryonal or primitive cell origin. Most medulloblastomas consist of dense sheets of undifferentiated cells with intensely basophilic nuclei and scant cytoplasm, sometimes referred to as "small blue cell tumors." In 30% of cases, pathognomonic neuroblastic Homer Wright rosettes (cells with fibrillary processes forming a false central lumen) are seen. A less common histological variant is the desmoplastic type, which has a rich reticulin background with cells lined up "Indian File." The desmoplastic variant is more likely to be found in patients over the age of 15, located laterally in the cerebellar hemisphere close to the dura; these carry a better prognosis.

Medulloblastomas usually originate from the inferior medullary velum and extend into the fourth ventricle (Fig. 4); however, 15% of all medulloblastomas arise as lateral hemispheric cerebellar tumors (3). As noted, lateral lesions are more typically the desmoplastic variant and often abut the dura. Medulloblastomas can spread through the subarachnoid space producing a characteristic "sugar-coated" appearance of the cerebellum. Distant metastases throughout the CNS are seen in 20% to 30% of cases (4). Most patients present with a 1- to 2-month history of symptoms owing to obstructive hydrocephalus; most commonly headache, vomiting, and irritability. Lateral hemispheric medulloblastomas more commonly cause limb ataxia.

Medulloblastomas have a hyperdense appearance on computed tomographic (CT) imaging because of their hypercellularity and usually brightly enhance with contrast (5). The presence of calcium, blood products, or microcysts is common. Medulloblastomas are hypointense to isointense on T1-weighted MR images and isointense to hyperintense on T2 and proton density techniques. Bright enhancement with gadolinium is typical. Enhancement may be minimal on rare occasions.

Total resection is the goal in medulloblastoma surgery as residual tumor less than 1.5 cc is associated with a better 5-year disease-free survival (6,7). Some treatment for hydrocephalus or increased intracranial pressure may need to be done prior to definitive surgery. Placement of a temporary ventriculostomy drain rather than a shunt usually is favored because permanent shunts are required in only 55% to 60% of cases (8). In the past, concern over extraneural spread led to use of shunts with Millipore filters, but these often became occluded. Subsequent

data have shown no difference in the incidence of extraneural spread in patients with or without shunts (9).

Evaluation of metastasis requires entire neuraxis imaging. Cerebrospinal fluid cytology is best studied 2 weeks after surgery to avoid false-positive results from tumor shedding associated with surgery.

Total craniospinal radiation has been considered standard therapy, given the high likelihood of metastases. Recurrence has been reported in the gaps of radiation fields. There is a trend toward the use of adjuvant chemotherapy and reduced-dose radiation because of the side effects of radiation (10). Chemotherapy is the preferred adjuvant treatment in very young children (under the age of 3 years).

ASTROCYTOMAS. Posterior fossa astrocytomas occur more frequently in children than adults. Cerebellar astrocytomas comprise 10% to 20% of all childhood brain tumors; brainstem astrocytomas account for another 10% to 20%. A host of histological subtypes with different biological behaviors are encountered, including juvenile pilocytic, well-differentiated, anaplastic astrocytomas and glioblastoma multiforme.

Most cerebellar astrocytomas in children are juvenile pilocytic (Fig. 5). Many of these extend into the cerebellar hemispheres, but most arise from the cerebellar vermis (11). Vermian astrocytomas usually are solid, whereas purely hemispheric cerebellar astrocytomas are more often cystic with a mural nodule. Cerebellar astrocytomas can compress the fourth ventricle and produce obstructive hydrocephalus, although this is usually late in the course and occurs only in about one third of cases.

The solid component of cerebellar astrocytomas is usually hypodense to isodense on CT and enhance brightly with contrast. Cyst walls usually do not enhance. Calcifications are infrequently seen. On MRI, the solid nodule is hypointense on T1-weighted images, and hyperintense on T2-weighted images.

Removal of all solid tumor is the goal in resection of cerebellar astrocytomas. It is preferable to remove the cyst wall if it enhances, because this suggests tumor involvement. Given the benign nature and excellent prognosis of most cerebellar astrocytomas, even incomplete resection is associated with a good prognosis. Aggressive extirpation of the tumor is not warranted on the occasion where there is tumor extension to a cerebellar peduncle or brainstem. Incomplete tumor resection should be followed with serial scans. Tumor recurrence can be treated with reoperation, radiation, or chemotherapy.

The diffuse pontine glioma is the most common brainstem astrocytoma. This is an infiltrative tumor that expands the entire pons and can penetrate the pial envelope into the floor of the fourth ventricle. Distortion or obstruction of the fourth ventricle causes hydrocephalus late in the course of this malignancy. Symptoms at presentation usually include extraocular muscle palsies, facial weakness and other cranial nerve deficits, ataxia, and motor weakness. The tumors are typically hypodense on CT scan, hypointense on T1-weighted MRI, and hyperintense on T2-weighted images. Enhancement is uncommon. These tumors are associated with a very poor prognosis, with greater than 90% mortality within 18 months of diagnosis (12). Diagnosis of diffuse pontine glioma may be made based on imaging characteristics, history, and examination, obviating the need for biopsy (13). There is no role for surgery, as intervention has not improved the dismal outcome.

Diffuse pontine gliomas must be differentiated from the more rare, focally occurring astrocytomas of the brainstem, which also may obstruct the fourth ventricle (14). Long-term stable disease is seen in the some of these patients after subtotal excision (15). These lesions tend to be low grade and remain histologically benign, even with regrowth.

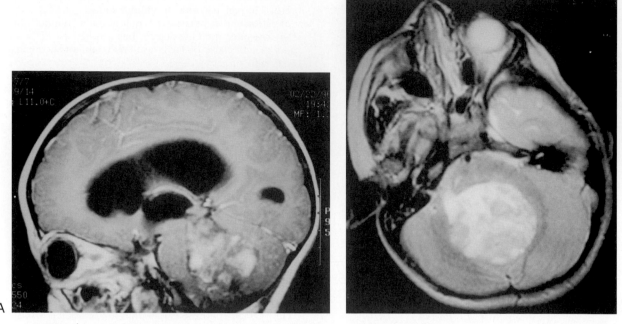

Fig. 4. Medulloblastoma in a 4-year-old girl. **A:** Enhancing mass is seen filling the fourth ventricle. Note the hydrocephalus. **B:** Mixed areas of isointensity and hyperintensity are seen in this T2-weighted image.

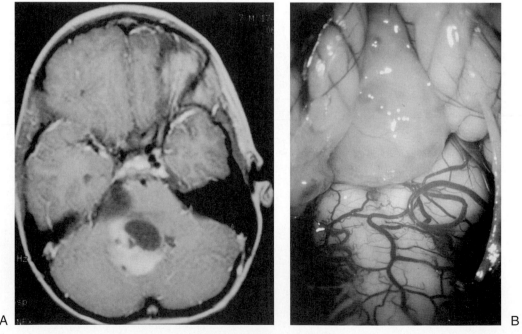

Fig. 5. Juvenile pilocytic astrocytoma in a 7-year-old boy. **A:** Brightly enhancing fourth ventricular mass with multiple cystic components. **B:** Intraoperative view of same patient. The tumor extends from the fourth ventricle through the foramen of Magendie.

EPENDYMOMAS. Ependymomas constitute 10% of all posterior fossa tumors in childhood. They are of neuroectodermal origin, arising from the cells lining the ventricles and central canal. Histologically, they can express characteristics of both glial and epithelial origin. The most common type consists of unpatterned proliferation of ovoid cells with dense chromatin among lucent areas of cytoplasmic processes reaching toward vessels, forming perivascular pseudorosettes. Epithelial properties are less commonly identified, but the ependymal rosette consisting of columnar cells forming a true lumen is characteristic.

The most common intracranial site for ependymomas in childhood is the floor of the fourth ventricle, particularly in the region of the obex, hypoglossal, or vagal trigone. These tumors usually grow into the fourth ventricle and can expand into the lateral recesses and foramina of Luschka. Often a tongue of tumor extends below the foramen magnum (16). Ependymo-mas can infiltrate the pontine/medullary tegmentum. Obstructive hydrocephalus can be seen at the time of diagnosis but there is usually a history of vomiting preceding the onset of headaches because of area postrema involvement. Patients also can present with posterior cervical pain, nuchal rigidity, or head tilt. Presence of cranial nerve palsies has been associated with worse prognosis (17).

Ependymomas tend to be solid (Fig. 6). On CT, the lesion is typically isodense with moderate enhancement with contrast. Focal calcifications are seen in 50% of cases, and areas of hemorrhage and cyst formation are common. On MRI, ependymomas are isointense to hypointense on T1-weighted images and isointense to hyperintense on T2 and proton density images. Heterogeneity on MRI is the rule, owing to areas of calcification, cysts, blood products, and necrosis. Intense enhancement usually is seen with gadolinium administration.

The goal of ependymoma surgery is complete resection be-

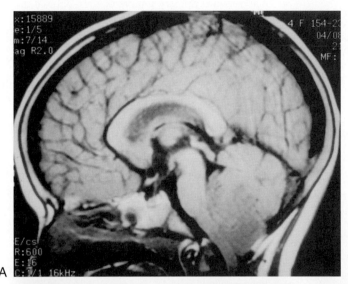

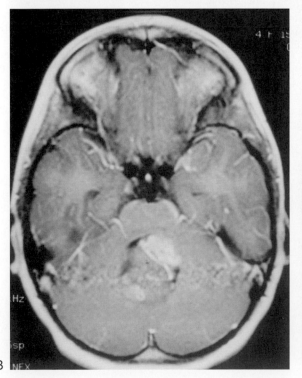

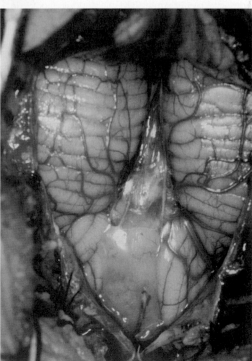

Fig. 6. Ependymoma in a 4-year-old girl. **A:** This solid mass is hypointense to isointense on T1-weighted MRI. **B:** Heterogenous enhancement is seen after Gd-DTPA administration. **C:** Intraoperative view shows the tumor splaying the cerebellar tonsils.

cause recent studies have shown better survival when complete resection is achieved by radiographic standards (17). Repeat operation by a lateral posterior approach may be indicated in cases where tumor extends into the lateral recesses or radiographic evidence of residual tumor is present (18). In one series, a 75% 5-year progression-free survival was documented in patients of all ages after total resection, compared to a 5-year survival rate of 14% to 50% in children and 76% in adults (19, 20). Unfortunately, complete resection can be achieved in only 20% to 40% of cases, as ependymomas are often adherent to normal subependymal parenchyma. In a recent multicenter retrospective study, a higher event-free survival rate was associated with gross-total resection, age greater than 3 years and low histological grades (21). Given the tendency for tumor extension down the cervical canal, posterior fossa craniotomy may need to be combined with C1-2 laminectomy. If done, follow-up plain films are used to assess cervical stability in young children.

Ependymomas may disseminate in the CSF. This has been seen in up to 30% in autopsy series, whereas only 3% were clinically apparent (16). CSF seeding is usually seen in the context of failed tumor control at the primary site; therefore, initial adjuvant radiation therapy for histologically benign ependymomas is targeted focally. This has been shown to improve overall survival (22).

The efficacy of chemotherapeutic agents has not yet been demonstrated for the treatment of ependymomas; however, several protocols are currently in progress.

HEMANGIOBLASTOMA. Hemangioblastomas are rare tumors accounting for 1% to 2.5% of all intracranial and 7% to 12% of posterior fossa tumors in adults (23). They occur sporadically as isolated tumors of the central nervous system or as part of the von Hippel–Lindau (VHL) syndrome. This syndrome is characterized by multiple hemangioblastomas of the cerebellum, spinal cord, or brainstem, as well as retinal angiomatosis, pheochromocytoma, and visceral cysts. Approximately 20% of patients with cerebellar hemangioblastomas have VHL syndrome, which is inherited in an autosomal dominant pattern with highly variable penetrance. The VHL gene has been located on the short arm of chromosome 3 (24). Hemangioblastomas are commonly tumors of young adulthood, typically occurring in the fourth decade, with a slightly earlier presentation in VHL.

Hemangioblastomas are uniformly benign vascular tumors of the CNS. The cell lineage is uncertain, but histologically the tumor consists of three cell types: endothelial cells, pericytes, and stromal cells. The key histological feature is numerous capillary channels lined by a single layer of plump endothelial cells that form an anastomosing plexiform pattern. Hemangioblastomas are often cystic lesions with a mural nodule.

The most common location for hemangioblastomas is in the cerebellar hemisphere or vermis. On rare occasions they arise within the fourth ventricle at the obex, where the lesions tend to be solid. Headache caused by hydrocephalus occurs in up to 95% of cases. Vomiting, ataxia, and vertigo are also frequent symptoms.

Characteristically CT scan shows a cystic lesion with an isodense to hyperdense mural nodule with intense contrast enhancement. The cyst wall does not contain tumor cells, but may enhance on rare occasion. On MRI, the tumor nodule is hypointense to isointense on T1-weighted images and hyperintense on T2-weighted images. Evidence of hemorrhage is seen in up to 20% of cases. Serpentine flow voids representing large draining veins are often seen.

The primary goal of surgery is removal of the tumor nodule.

The solid mass often is located adjacent to the pial surface. There is no true capsule, although the solid tumor appears well circumscribed. After drainage of the cyst fluid, the nodule must be dissected away from the surrounding glial cells and compressed cerebellar tissue. Piecemeal removal of the tumor leads to troublesome blood loss. Preoperative arteriography is helpful in identifying the mural nodule as well as arterial feeders. Embolization of feeding arteries occasionally is helpful.

Hemangioblastomas can extend locally into the subarachnoid space, but distant metastasis has never been documented. Surgical resection is considered curative for solitary hemangioblastomas. Patients with VHL often have multiple tumors; therefore, complete neuraxis imaging should be performed. Recurrence rate is 3% to 10% in patients with VHL. More recently, the use of stereotactic radiosurgery has been used in the management of patients with multiple lesions (25).

CHOROID PLEXUS PAPILLOMAS. Choroid plexus papillomas are rare primary tumors of the CNS that arise from cells of the choroid plexus. They account for 0.42% to 1.0% of all intracranial tumors. Choroid plexus papillomas occur most in the lateral ventricles during the first decade of life. The fourth ventricle and cerebellopontine angle are the most common locations in older children and adults.

Choroid plexus papillomas are lobulated masses that are continuous with and engulf the normal choroid plexus. They are histologically benign, and composed of a single layer of cuboidal epithelium. Rarely, they spread through the subarachnoid space and involve the leptomeninges but maintain a benign course (26). Choroid plexus carcinomas comprise 1% of choroid plexus tumors. Patients usually present with symptoms of obstructive hydrocephalus. Hydrocephalus out of proportion to the degree of ventricular obstruction caused by the tumor can be seen owing to either repeated small hemorrhages into the CSF, or less likely, oversecretion of CSF.

CT scans of choroid plexus papillomas show an isodense mass, often with calcifications. On MRI the tumor is hypointense to isointense on T1-weighted images, depending on the degree of calcification, and isointense to hyperintense on T2-weighted images (Fig. 7).

Choroid plexus papillomas of the fourth ventricle can be highly vascular. The blood supply, usually from branches of the posterior inferior cerebellar artery (PICA), should be eliminated early in the surgery. Branches of the anterior inferior cerebellar artery (AICA) usually feed tumors in the cerebellopontine angle. Complete surgical resection is curative. In contrast, choroid plexus carcinomas have a high recurrence rate, with the 5-year disease-free survival being only 50% (27). Although adjuvant radiation and chemotherapy have been tried, they are of unproved benefit (28).

EPIDERMOIDS AND DERMOIDS. Epidermoids and dermoids are cysts of cutaneous origin, thought to result from misplaced epithelial tissue during closure of the neural groove in embryogenesis. They may be found throughout the CNS, and constitute 0.5% to 1.0% of all intracranial tumors. Epidermoid cysts are lined with stratified squamous epithelium and connective tissue, although dermoid cysts also contain sweat glands, sebaceous glands, and hair follicles.

Most intracranial epidermoid and dermoid cysts arise in the basal cisterns but can occur in the fourth ventricle (29). Presenting symptoms vary depending on the location of the tumor. Epidermoids are ten times as common as dermoids. Dermoids are more common in the fourth ventricle, and can be associated with congenital dermal sinus tracts (30). Patients with dermoid

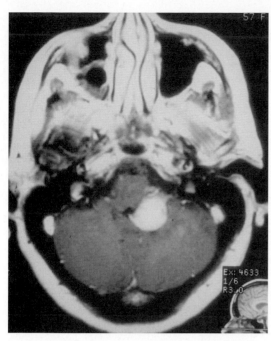

Fig. 7. Choroid plexus papilloma in a 57-year-old woman. This highly vascularized tumor enhances brightly after gadolinium administration. The tumor extends to the left lateral recess and through the foramen of Lushka.

cysts typically present in the first two decades of life as the cyst grows slowly from desquamation of epithelial cells and glandular secretions. When associated with an occipital dermal sinus, the overlying scalp may become inflamed or infected. Patients with epidermoid cysts typically present later in life, between the ages of 20 to 50 years, as epidermoid cysts tend to enlarge at a slower rate. Despite an epidermoid completely filling of the ventricle, hydrocephalus may not develop, presumably because of slow growth of the cyst, which conforms to the CSF space (31).

On CT epidermoids are hypodense and the cyst wall typically does not enhance. On MRI epidermoids are hypointense to brain tissue but hyperintense to isointense to CSF on T1-weighted images. T2-weighted images show a more heterogeneous signal that is hyperintense compared to brain. Dermoids tend to be more heterogenous, even on CT. The cyst contents are typically isodense to CSF. Enhancement of the cyst capsule and calcification are common. On MRI, dermoids have mixed signal intensity, likely produced by the lipid content.

Complete resection of both cyst wall and content is the goal of surgery, as recurrence rate is high with subtotal resection. In a recently published series recurrence-free survival was 95% at 13 years in patients who had complete resection of posterior fossa epidermoids, and 65% with those who had subtotal resection (32). These histologically benign tumors can adhere to vascular and neural structures that can limit resection. Spillage of cyst contents into the CSF space can cause aseptic meningitis (33).

UNUSUAL LESIONS OF THE FOURTH VENTRICLE. Subependymomas are rare lesions that arise in the ventricular system (Fig. 8). Approximately 70% are infratentorial, with equal numbers arising from the floor and roof of the fourth ventricle (34). In Scheithauer's review of 90 patients with subependymoma, 80% were male. The cell origin of subependymomas remains controversial, but is thought to be from the subependymal glia.

Subependymomas are lobulated intraventricular masses with attachments to the ependyma. Histologically, subependymomas consist of nests of astrocytic nuclei separated by broad bands of neuroglial fibers. Calcification often is present. Subependymomas must be differentiated from ependymomas because of the former's significantly better prognosis. Subependymomas often are found incidentally at autopsy, although some patients present with neurological symptoms. In a recent retrospective review from a single center, no tumor recurrence was found in the 12 patients who underwent either total or subtotal resection (35).

Fourth ventricular meningiomas are extremely uncommon. They have been found to arise from the inferior tela choroidea, choroid plexus, or within the cisterna magna without dural attachments. Meningiomas of the fourth ventricle usually produce symptoms of obstructive hydrocephalus, and are typically greater than 3 cm in diameter at the time of presentation (36).

Several vascular lesions may involve the fourth ventricle. These include cavernous angiomas, arteriovenous malformations, and berry aneurysms. Aneurysms within the fourth ventricle are extremely rare, and arise from distal branches of the posterior inferior cerebellar artery. In a recent case report, MRI was needed to demonstrate the intraventricular location of a PICA aneurysm, which was previously diagnosed by conventional angiography (37).

Cysticercosis is the most common CNS parasite in the world. *Taenia solium* is the parasite whose larval cyst can migrate to brain parenchyma, meninges, or ventricles. The fourth ventricle is the most commonly affected intraventricular location. The cyst can lodge in the fourth ventricle, producing obstructive hydrocephalus and inducing an inflammatory reaction. A ventriculoperitoneal shunt usually is needed in addition to surgical removal of the cyst.

Other CNS parasites include *Schistosoma japonicum* and less frequently *Schistosoma mansoni*. Bacterial, mycobacterial, and fungal abscesses also can occur in the posterior fossa and involve the fourth ventricle.

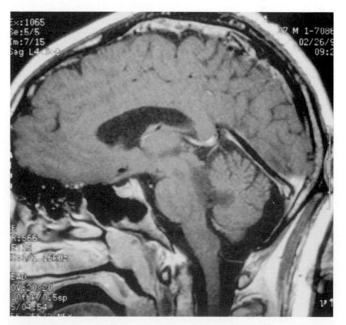

Fig. 8. Subependymoma in a 27-year-old man. Characteristic T1 hypointensity is demonstrated in this sagittal view; however, these rare tumors more typically are found in elderly men.

Surgical Considerations

CEREBROSPINAL FLUID DIVERSION. Hydrocephalus is common in patients with fourth ventricular tumors. When patients present with acute hydrocephalus and altered mental status, CSF diversion may need to be performed prior to tumor resection. Although a ventriculo-peritoneal shunt may be placed, many surgeons prefer an external ventriculostomy, because various patients do not require permanent CSF diversion (8). An external drain provides the additional benefit of being easily regulated, as well as the availability of CSF for further studies. Postoperatively, the drain may be set at 5 cm above the tragus to allow more rapid clearing of cellular debris and blood products. The drain pressure can be raised slowly over the period of 1 week. The external drain is removed when the pressure normalizes.

If CSF diversion is not necessary prior to tumor resection, it is still helpful to place a parietal burr hole at the time of surgery to provide ventricular access if needed. In adults, a small vertical incision is placed 7 cm rostral to the inion and 3 cm lateral to the midline, and a burr hole is made. A straight ventricular catheter can then be passed into the lateral ventricle if intracranial pressure reduction is needed.

INTRAOPERATIVE MONITORING. Some centers routinely employ electrophysiological monitoring for resection of fourth ventricular tumors. Brainstem auditory evoked responses (BAERs) monitor pathways that are laterally placed but have not been reliable indicators of brainstem function during surgery involving the fourth ventricular floor (38). Monitoring of blood pressure and pulse can be used to gauge brainstem function because reflex cardiovascular control centers (e.g., the nucleus of the tractus solitarius and dorsal motor nucleus of the vagus nerve) are near the floor of the fourth ventricle. Alterations in blood pressure and pulse can indicate brainstem compromise. Others have suggested the use of direct intraoperative stimulation of the facial colliculus and hypoglossal trigone to aid in the removal of tumors infiltrating the floor of the fourth ventricle (39).

POSITIONING. Access to most fourth ventricular tumors is achieved using either the prone or sitting positions. There are advantages and disadvantages to each position, and ultimately surgeon preference prevails. For the prone position the intubated patient is placed in a three-pin fixation head frame such as the Mayfield. Care is taken to prevent placing the pins into venous sinuses, the thin temporal squamous bone, or shunt tubing if the patient has had a previously placed shunt. In children younger than 2 years of age, a padded horseshoe head holder may be used instead. The patient is carefully turned prone onto a padded frame or chest roles. The operative field should be parallel to the floor. The head is slightly elevated above the heart. All pressure points should be generously padded. The prone position is advantageous because it allows both the surgeon and the assistant easy access to the operative field. Reaching rostrally positioned fourth ventricular tumors can sometimes be difficult in this position. Prolonged surgery in the prone position causes oropharyngeal, tongue, and facial edema, so nasotracheal intubation should be used.

For the sitting position, the patient is also placed in a Mayfield frame, which is attached to a crosstable support bar. The neck is in a military attitude with the chin tucked and neck straight. The foramen magnum should be at the surgeon's eye level. The patient's knees are gently flexed to prevent sciatic nerve compression. An armrest is helpful for the surgeon.

Those who favor the sitting position cite the advantages of a clearer operative view and gravitational drainage of CSF and blood from the operative field. Additionally, access to the airway is improved. The disadvantages associated with the sitting position include the potential for venous air embolism, which necessitates the use of precordial Doppler to monitor and placement of a central venous catheter to potentially aspirate air emboli. The sitting position also can cause hemodynamic instability such as hypotension. Subdural hematomas and tension pneumocephalus can occur in this position, especially in patients who have ventricular shunts. If there is an external ventricular catheter, it is important to drain CSF only as needed.

SURGICAL APPROACH. Complicated skin incisions such as Cushing's crossbow and Dandy's upward curving mastoid-to-mastoid incision has been replaced by the more simplified midline vertical incision. A linear incision is made 1 cm above the inion to approximately C3, superficial to the deep fascia. This plane is widely developed by dissection and retracted with self-retaining retractors.

A Y-shaped incision through the fascia-muscle layer is made, leaving a cuff attached to the bone (Fig. 9). The superior flap is reflected rostrally and held on tension sutures. The inferior limb of the incision is carried down to the ligamentum nuchae of C2. Care should be taken when clearing soft tissues off the superior-lateral arch of C1. Venous bleeding from the plexus surrounding the vertebral arteries at this level warns of the vertebral artery's proximity.

A craniectomy may be performed, but a craniotomy offers the advantage of better closure and protection of the posterior

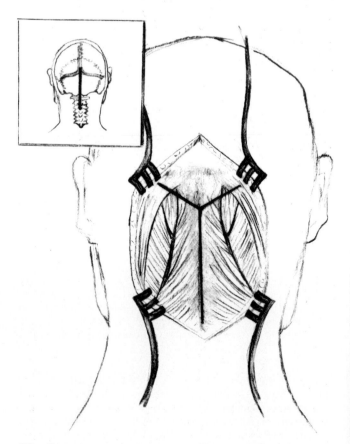

Fig. 9. Surgical approach. After a midline vertical skin incision, a Y-shaped fascia-muscle incision is made to optimize a watertight closure.

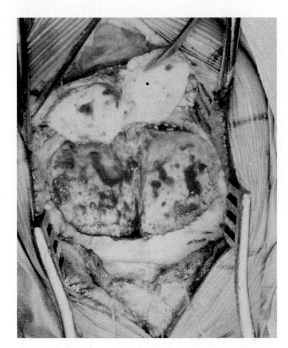

Fig. 10. The suboccipital bone flap is removed.

fossa (Fig. 10). Burr holes are placed below the torcula on either side of the midline. The dura is stripped off the bone. A drill or Kerrison rongeur may be used to connect the burr holes across the midline. Clearing the dura at the foramen magnum is performed to avoid bleeding from the annular sinus. A craniotome is used to connect the burr holes and create the bone flap. The bone edge is thoroughly waxed because this provides an entry for venous air embolism. The arch of C1 may need to be removed depending on the inferior extent of the tumor.

The dural opening is made with a Y-shaped incision. The occipital sinus can be a source of bleeding, especially in young children. Hemostatic clips can be used to occlude the occipital sinus. The dura is tented and reflected out of the field. It should be kept moist to prevent desiccation and facilitate closure.

Access to the fourth ventricle is achieved by lateral retraction of the cerebellar tonsils. Most fourth ventricular tumors can be seen protruding through the foramen of Magendie. Dissection of the inferior tela in the cerebellomedullary fissure often can gain adequate exposure without splitting the cerebellar vermis (40). A third retractor can be used to elevate the inferior vermis. Lesion removal is facilitated by the use of an ultrasonic aspirator. As the technology advances, the use of endoscopy may become useful for achieving total resection (41).

A dural graft may be needed to achieve a watertight dural closure. The bone flap is replaced using screws and plates. The fascia and scalp are closed in layers.

Complications

Manipulation of the floor of the fourth ventricle can cause cranial nerve palsies resulting in eye movement disorders or facial weakness. Hypoglossal or vagal nerve dysfunction is less common, but may necessitate placement of tracheostomy and gastrostomy feeding tube. Injury to the inferior vermis and flocculonodular lobe can cause gait ataxia. Limb dysmetria occurs with injury to the dentate nucleus, red nucleus, or superior cerebellar peduncle.

Aseptic meningitis with persistent fevers, headache, neck pain, and malaise can occur. Corticosteroids are effective treatment. Pseudomeningoceles and CSF leaks are potential complications in any posterior fossa surgery. Watertight closure and replacement of the bone flap reduce the risk of these complications. If they do occur, placement of a lumbar drain can relieve pressure enough to allow healing.

A well-described but poorly understood complication of posterior fossa surgery is a syndrome usually seen in children in which the patient is confused, combative, paranoid, and may have visual hallucinations. The patient can also develop "cerebellar mutism," but be otherwise awake, alert, and following commands. Patients also can develop scanning speech with orofacial apraxia, otherwise called the posterior fossa pseudobulbar palsy. These symptoms usually occur several days after surgery and reverse within weeks to months. The mechanism of injury leading to these deficits is unclear. Monoaminergic pathways have been implicated; several patients with akinetic mutism following posterior fossa surgery have been successfully treated with bromocriptine (42).

References

1. Cohen AR. The history of fourth ventricular surgery. In: Cohen AR, ed. *Surgical disorders of the fourth ventricle.* Cambridge, UK: Blackwell Scientific, 1996:3–19.
2. Matsushima T, Rhoton AL Jr, Lenkey C. Microsurgery of the fourth ventricle: Part 1. Microsurgical anatomy. *Neurosurgery* 1982;11: 631–667.
3. Zimmerman RA, Bilaniuk LT, Pahlajani H. Spectrum of medulloblastomas demonstrated by computed tomography. *Radiology* 1978; 126:137–141.
4. Packer RJ, Siegel KR, Sutton LN, et al. Leptomeningeal dissemination of primary central nervous system tumors of childhood. *Ann Neurol* 1985;18:217–221.
5. Tortori-Donati P, Fondelli MP, Rossi A, et al. Medulloblastoma in children: CT and MRI findings. *Neuroradiology* 1996;38:352–359.
6. Park TS, Hoffman HJ, Hendrick EB, et al. Medulloblastoma: clinical presentation and management. Experience at the hospital for sick children, Toronto, 1950–1980. *J Neurosurg* 1983;58:543–552.
7. Norris DG, Bruce DA, Byrd RL, et al. Improved relapse-free survival in medulloblastoma utilizing modern techniques. *Neurosurgery* 1981;9:661–664.
8. Culley DJ, Berger MS, Shaw D, et al. An analysis of factors determining the need for ventriculoperitoneal shunts after posterior fossa tumor surgery in children. *Neurosurgery* 1994;34:402–407; discussion 407–408.
9. Berger MS, Baumeister B, Geyer JR, et al. The risks of metastases from shunting in children with primary central nervous system tumors. *J Neurosurg* 1991;74:872–877.
10. Packer RJ. Childhood medulloblastoma: progress and future challenges. *Brain Dev* 1999;21:75–81.
11. Gusnard DA. Cerebellar neoplasms in children. *Semin Roentgenol* 1990;25:263–278.
12. Packer RJ. Brain tumors in children. *Arch Neurol* 1999;56: 421–425.13 Albright AL, Roger JP, Zimmerman R, et al. Magnetic resonance scans should replace biopsies for the diagnosis of diffuse brain stem gliomas: a report from the Children's Cancer Group. *Neurosurgery* 1993;33:1026–1029.
14. Hoffman HJ, Becker L, Craven MA. A clinically and pathologically distinct group of benign brain stem gliomas. *Neurosurgery* 1980;7: 243–248.
15. Pollack IF, Hoffman HJ, Humphreys RP, et al. The long-term outcome after surgical treatment of dorsally exophytic brain-stem gliomas. *J Neurosurg* 1993;78:859–863.
16. Kun LE, Kovnar EH, Sanford RA. Ependymomas in children. *Pediatr Neurosci* 1988;14:57–63.

17. Nazar GB, Hoffman HJ, Becker LE, et al. Infratentorial ependymomas in childhood: prognostic factors and treatment. *J Neurosurg* 1990;72:408–417.
18. Foreman NK, Love S, Gill SS, Coakham HB. Second-look surgery for incompletely resected fourth ventricle ependymomas: technical case report. *Neurosurgery* 1997;40:856–860; discussion 860.
19. Healey EA, Barnes PD, Kupsky WJ, et al. The prognostic significance of postoperative residual tumor in ependymoma. *Neurosurgery* 1991;28:666–671; discussion 671–672.
20. Berger MS, Geyer JR. Ependymomas of the fourth ventricle. In: Cohen AR, ed. *Surgical disorders of the fourth ventricle*. Cambridge, UK: Blackwell Scientific, 1996:209–221.
21. Horn B, Heideman R, Geyer R, et al. A multi-institutional retrospective study of intracranial ependymoma in children: identification of risk factors. *J Pediatr Hematol Oncol* 1999;21:203–211.
22. Ernestus RI, Schroder R, Stutzer H, et al. The clinical and prognostic relevance of grading in intracranial ependymomas. *Br J Neurosurg* 1997;11:421–428.
23. Neumann HP, Eggert HR, Weigel K, et al. Hemangioblastomas of the central nervous system. A 10-year study with special reference to von Hippel-Lindau syndrome. *J Neurosurg* 1989;70:24–30.
24. Seizinger BR, Rouleau GA, Ozelius LJ, et al. Von Hippel-Lindau disease maps to the region of chromosome 3 associated with renal cell carcinoma. *Nature* 1988;332:268–269.
25. Niemela M, Lim YJ, Soderman M, et al. Gamma knife radiosurgery in 11 hemangioblastomas. *J Neurosurg* 1996;85:591–596.
26. Leblanc R, Bekhor S, Melanson D, et al. Diffuse craniospinal seeding from a benign fourth ventricle choroid plexus papilloma. Case report. *J Neurosurg* 1998;88:757–760.
27. Ellenbogen RG, Winston KR, Kupsky WJ. Tumors of the choroid plexus in children. *Neurosurgery* 1989;25:327–335.
28. Packer RJ, Perilongo G, Johnson D, et al. Choroid plexus carcinoma of childhood. *Cancer* 1992;69:580–585.
29. Wagle WA, Jaufmann B, Mincy JE. Magnetic resonance imaging of fourth ventricular epidermoid tumors. *Arch Neurol* 1991;48:438–440.
30. Goffin J, Plets C, Van Calenbergh F, et al. Posterior fossa dermoid cyst associated with dermal fistula: report of 2 cases and review of the literature. *Childs Nerv Syst* 1993;9:179–181.
31. Rosario M, Becker DH, Conley FK. Epidermoid tumors involving the fourth ventricle. *Neurosurgery* 1981;9:9–13.
32. Talacchi A, Sala F, Alessandrini F, et al. Assessment and surgical management of posterior fossa epidermoid tumors: report of 28 cases. *Neurosurgery* 1998;42:242–251; discussion 251–252.
33. Yasargil MG, Abernathey CD, Sarioglu AC. Microneurosurgical treatment of intracranial dermoid and epidermoid tumors. *Neurosurgery* 1989;24:561–567.
34. Scheithauer BW. Symptomatic subependymoma. Report of 21 cases with review of the literature. *J Neurosurg* 1978;49:689–696.
35. Prayson RA, Suh JH. Subependymomas: clinicopathologic study of 14 tumors, including comparative MIB-1 immunohistochemical analysis with other ependymal neoplasms. *Arch Pathol Lab Med* 1999;123:306–309.
36. Matsumura M, Takahashi S, Kurachi H, et al. Primary intraventricular meningioma of the fourth ventricle—case report. *Neurol Med Chir (Tokyo)* 1988;28:996–1000.
37. Schelhaas HJ, Brouwers PJ, van der AHE, et al. MRI locates a posterior fossa aneurysm in the fourth ventricle. *Clin Neurol Neurosurg* 1998;100:216–218.
38. Piatt JH Jr, Radtke RA, Erwin CW. Limitations of brain stem auditory evoked potentials for intraoperative monitoring during a posterior fossa operation: case report and technical note. *Neurosurgery* 1985;16:818–821.
39. Strauss C, Romstock J, Nimsky C, et al. Intraoperative identification of motor areas of the rhomboid fossa using direct stimulation [see comments]. *J Neurosurg* 1993;79:393–399.
40. Kellogg JX, Piatt JH Jr. Resection of fourth ventricle tumors without splitting the vermis: the cerebellomedullary fissure approach [see comments]. *Pediatr Neurosurg* 1997;27:28–33.
41. Matula C, Reinprecht A, Roessler K, et al. Endoscopic exploration of the IVth ventricle. *Minim Invasive Neurosurg* 1996;39:86–92.
42. Caner H, Altinors N, Benli S, et al. Akinetic mutism after fourth ventricle choroid plexus papilloma: treatment with a dopamine agonist. *Surg Neurol* 1999;51:181–184.

111. Intrinsic Tumors of the Brainstem

Ian F. Pollack

Intrinsic neoplasms of the brainstem are uncommon lesions that most typically are detected during childhood and early adulthood (1,2). These tumors were once considered to have a uniformly poor prognosis. However, with improvements in neuroimaging, it has become clear that this broad category of lesions actually encompasses a number of distinct subgroups that differ significantly in terms of their growth characteristics, histology, and response to therapy (3–8). Refinements in surgical and intraoperative monitoring techniques during the last two decades have facilitated extensive surgical resection of histologically benign brainstem lesions that in the past would have been considered unresectable.

Magnetic resonance imaging (MRI) is an essential adjunct for the classification of brainstem gliomas, providing the surgeon with a fairly reliable assessment of the histopathology as well as the growth pattern of a given lesion. Coupled with a thorough history and neurological examination, it is generally possible to accurately distinguish lesions that are appropriate for extensive resection from those that are not. In general, lesions that exhibit a focal growth pattern, with relatively crisp borders on both gadolinium-enhanced T1-weighted and T2-weighted images, are histologically benign and, in some instances, may be amenable to extensive removal. Such lesions exhibit several anatomically distinct patterns of growth, and can be subclassified as (a) focal intrinsic tumors; (b) dorsally and laterally exophytic tumors; (c) cervicomedullary tumors; and (d) tectal tumors. In contrast to these lesions, so-called diffuse intrinsic brainstem tumors exhibit poorly defined borders with minimal or irregular enhancement and widespread infiltration of the entire transverse diameter of the brainstem (typically the pons). Such lesions are histologically and biologically malignant and are not amenable to resection (9).

MRI is also useful for distinguishing nonneoplastic brainstem lesions, such as cavernous malformations, vascular malformations, and infectious processes, from true neoplasms. Although this chapter will focus predominantly on the clinical presentation, management, and expected outcomes for brainstem neoplasms, many of the same surgical principles and anatomical considerations also apply to the treatment of nonneoplastic brainstem lesions.

Clinical Presentation

DIFFUSE TUMORS. These biologically aggressive, highly invasive lesions typically manifest with rapidly progressive ataxia, weakness, and multiple, often bilateral, cranial nerve deficits. The inexorable progression of these lesions fostered a sense of therapeutic nihilism regarding brainstem tumors in general. However, high-resolution imaging has helped to distinguish these lesions from other, less common, prognostically favorable, categories of brainstem gliomas (6,8,9–13). The appearance of a diffuse brainstem glioma on computed tomography (CT) often underestimates the extent of the tumor, typically showing an enlarged pons with variable enhancement that often appears focal. This pattern of enhancement belies the true infiltrative nature of these tumors, which may lead the surgeon to mistakenly expect that this is a focal, rather than a diffuse

tumor. MRI provides a much more reliable assessment of the extent of the tumor. T1-weighted images generally show a diffusely enlarged pons with no clear borders around the lesion (Fig. 1A). Although, MRI with gadolinium administration occasionally shows focal enhancement (Fig. 1B), the irregular nature of the enhancement usually helps to distinguish these lesions from true focal tumors. Moreover, these lesions exhibit a characteristic appearance on T2-weighted images, with diffuse high signal intensity that extends through the entire transverse diameter of the pons and often into the midbrain and medulla (Fig. 1C). Because this appearance is so strongly indicative of a malignant glioma in the pediatric age group, biopsy is rarely warranted if the clinical syndrome is consistent with that of a diffuse brainstem glioma; this procedure subjects the patient to risk without providing any clear benefit (9,10). In such patients, therapy is instituted based strictly on the history and MRI findings.

This empirical approach to treatment is less applicable in

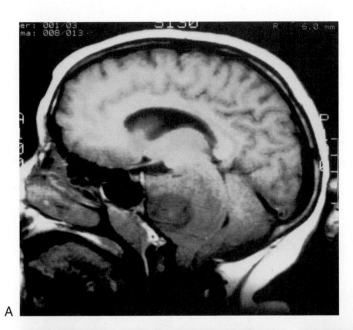

A

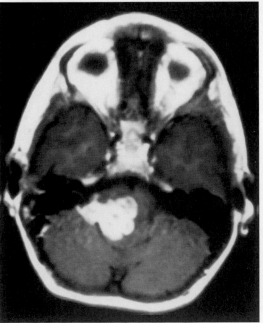

B

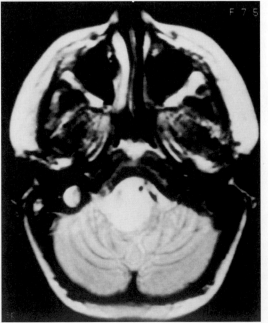

C

Fig. 1. **A:** Sagittal T1-weighted MRI of a diffuse intrinsic glioma, showing diffuse expansion of the brainstem. **B:** Such lesions can sometimes exhibit focal enhancement. **C:** T2-weighted image from the same patient as in **B**, showing diffuse signal abnormality that extends throughout the transverse diameter of the pons.

adults, in whom the possibility of brainstem encephalitis, demyelinating disease, metabolic disorders (e.g., central pontine myelinolysis), or inflammatory etiologies must also be considered in the differential diagnosis. Accordingly, additional workup, and in some cases biopsy, may be warranted in such patients before instituting therapy for a presumed diffuse brainstem glioma.

In addition, empirical institution of therapy is not warranted in children and adults with neurofibromatosis 1 (NF1) who have imaging evidence of a diffuse brainstem tumor because the natural history of such lesions often differs considerably from that of a typical diffuse intrinsic brainstem glioma (14–19). Affected patients often exhibit long-standing cranial nerve or long tract dysfunction at the time of presentation and have MRI evidence of diffuse brainstem enlargement in association with increased signal on T2-weighted images. Those lesions that have been biopsied have been found to be low-grade gliomas (16, 19), in contrast to the typically high-grade histological findings in diffuse brainstem gliomas in non-NF1 patients. However, in many cases, the behavior of these lesions is even more indolent than would be expected for typical low-grade gliomas because they may remain stable for years without specific therapy. Therapeutic intervention should therefore be limited to those tumors that do progress, and the remainder should be followed expectantly.

FOCAL INTRINSIC TUMORS. Focal intrinsic tumors may arise in the midbrain, pons, or medulla, and are characterized by a long natural history. These lesions commonly manifest with isolated cranial nerve impairments or with mild cerebellar or long-tract signs. Midbrain lesions commonly present with impairments in extraocular motility (20,21), pontine lesions with facial paresis (22), and medullary lesions with swallowing dysfunction (23,24). On imaging evaluation, these lesions are typically hypodense on CT, hypointense on T1-weighted MRI, and either uniformly enhancing, nonenhancing, or cystic with an enhancing mural nodule. On T2-weighted images, the pattern of signal abnormality often overlaps completely with that observed on T1-weighted images, which helps to distinguish even large focal tumors (generally benign) from diffuse tumors. In addition, because these lesions mainly grow by displacing rather than invading normal tissues, a surrounding cuff of normal brainstem tissue can be observed on both T1- and T2-weighted images, even with large lesions.

The clinical presentation and imaging appearance of benign brainstem gliomas can sometimes resemble that observed with cavernous malformations. However, cavernomas characteristically manifest with a stuttering course of symptom progression indicative of multiple bleeding episodes. These lesions often exhibit an inhomogenous appearance on CT and T1-weighted MRI, because they incorporate blood products of various ages. Cavernous malformations also have a characteristic appearance on T2-weighted MRI, with a surrounding dark rim indicative of hemosiderin staining.

DORSALLY AND LATERALLY EXOPHYTIC TUMORS. Because dorsally exophytic brainstem gliomas grow by expansion into the fourth ventricle, these tumors typically manifest with symptoms of obstructive hydrocephalus, such as headache, nausea, vomiting, and ataxia. The benign nature of the majority of these lesions is signaled by their long natural history, which may involve months of gradually progressive symptoms (3,5, 25–27). Because these lesions arise from the subependymal region of the fourth ventricle and show little invasion of the underlying brainstem tissue, cranial nerve dysfunction and long-tract signs, if present, are usually mild. Rarely, exophytic tumors can originate from the lateral brainstem surface and present as a cerebellopontine angle mass with focal cranial nerve deficits.

On imaging evaluation, these lesions are typically hypodense on CT, hypointense on T1-weighted MRI, and enhance uniformly (Figs. 2A,B). These features help to distinguish these

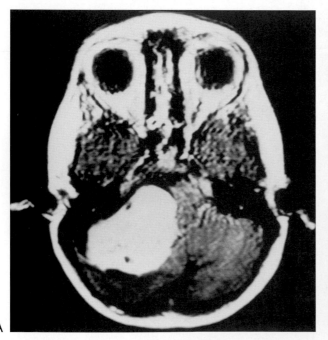
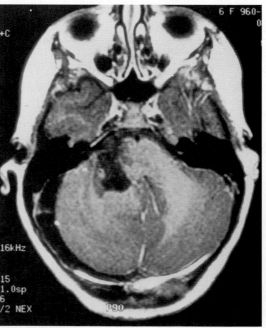

Fig. 2. A: This axial T1-weighted MRI, obtained following gadolinium administration, demonstrates a laterally exophytic brainstem tumor. The lesion was found to be a pilocytic astrocytoma. **B:** Postoperative MRI, demonstrating an apparent gross total resection. The patient remains progression-free 5 years postoperatively.

lesions from other common posterior fossa tumors, such as medulloblastoma or ependymoma, but are identical to those seen with cerebellar astrocytomas. In small lesions, the origin of the tumor from the brainstem can be determined preoperatively, but in larger lesions, it is sometimes impossible to determine preoperatively that the tumor has arisen from the brainstem, rather than merely compressed it.

CERVICOMEDULLARY TUMORS. Because cervicomedullary tumors generally represent cervical cord astrocytomas that extend rostrally into the medulla (rather than the converse) (7, 28), the majority of patients exhibit symptoms referable to the spinal cord rather than the brainstem, specifically neck pain, paresthesias, and gradually progressive weakness. On MRI, the epicenter of growth is usually within the cervical cord, with the rostral pole of the tumor appearing to push the medulla upward (Fig. 3A), presumably blocked from further rostral extension by the decussating white matter tracts of the medulla (28). The dome of the tumor often extends into the cisterna magna in the region of the obex, occasionally occluding the fourth ventricular outlets and leading to obstructive hydrocephalus. As with the other low-grade gliomas, most of these lesions are hypointense on T1-weighted images and uniformly enhancing, or cystic with an enhancing rim or mural nodule.

TECTAL TUMORS. Tectal tumors comprise a group of particularly benign focal midbrain astrocytomas that often produce symptoms of obstructive hydrocephalus, specifically headache, nausea, and vomiting, which can progress insidiously during a long interval (21,29–32). In contrast to other pineal region tumors, these lesions rarely manifest with Parinaud syndrome. The most common extraocular movement abnormality in such patients is simply a sixth nerve palsy referable to increased intracranial pressure. Because these tumors are often difficult to visualize on CT, children and adults with tectal gliomas were often assumed to have "idiopathic late-onset aqueductal stenosis" in the pre-MRI era, and were treated solely with cerebrospinal fluid (CSF) diversion. In some patients, the existence of a tectal tumor was revealed on MRI as many as 10 to 20 years after the initial detection of their hydrocephalus, attesting to the benign natural history of these lesions (31,32). Those tumors that have been biopsied have almost uniformly been found to be low-grade gliomas (21,29–32). More recent natural history studies that have monitored lesion size with serial MRI scans have confirmed that the majority of these tumors show little if any radiological progression during prolonged intervals (29, 30). This contrasts with the behavior of other focal intrinsic brainstem gliomas, which tend to progress, albeit insidiously, over time. Tectal lesions also differ from other focal brainstem gliomas in that they are commonly isointense to brain on T1-weighted MRI and are usually nonenhancing or at most show focal enhancement that sometimes fades over time (Fig. 4A). These lesions are usually visualized most clearly on T2-weighted or proton-density images as a hyperintense region in comparison to the surrounding brain that is centered on the tectum (Fig. 4B). Occasionally, signal abnormality may extend into the tegmentum and caudal diencephalon, but if the bulk of the signal abnormality is in these regions, then the diagnosis of a "tectal tumor" should probably not be made because the natural history of these more extensive lesions may be less indolent than that of a typical tectal tumor (21). In particular, large enhancing tegmental masses (Fig. 4C) are more appropriately

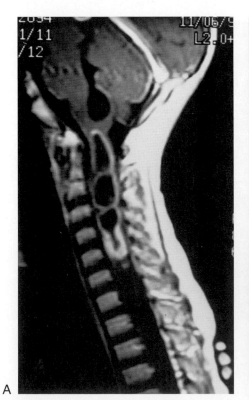
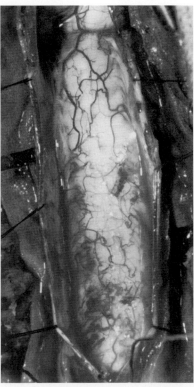

A   B

Fig. 3. **A:** Sagittal T1-weighted MRI demonstrating a partially cystic cervicomedullary lesion with irregular enhancement. **B:** Intraoperative view after dural opening, showing marked enlargement of the cervicomedullary region. *Figure continues.*

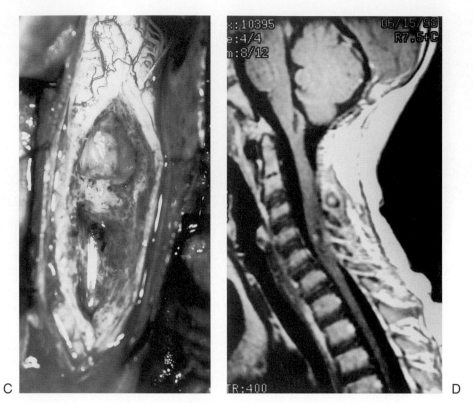

C   D

Fig. 3. *Continued.* **C:** A myelotomy has been performed and the majority of the tumor has been removed from within the cervical cord up to the cervicomedullary junction. Histopathological examination demonstrated the lesion to be a pilocytic astrocytoma. **D:** Postoperative MRI, demonstrating a nearly total resection.

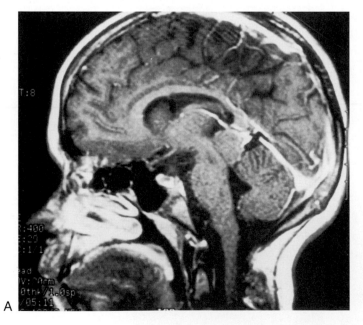

A

Fig. 4. **A:** Sagittal T1-weighted MRI after gadolinium administration demonstrates a nonenhancing globular tectal mass that manifested with obstructive hydrocephalus. *Figure continues.*

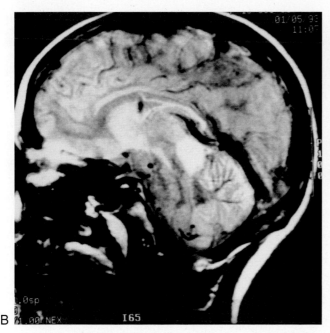
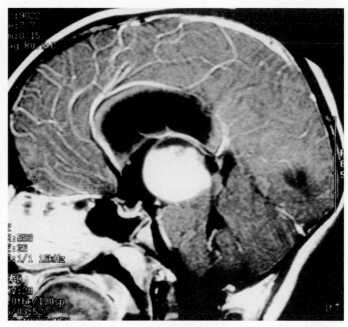

Fig. 4. *Continued.* **B:** Proton-density image shows hyperintensity within the lesion relative to normal brain. **C:** Large, densely enhancing tegmental lesion, which is distinguished from the more indolent tectal tumors shown in (**A**) and (**B**). The lesion was resected and found to be a pilocytic astrocytoma.

classified both in terms of prognosis and management with other focal intrinsic brainstem tumors.

Relevant Anatomical Principles

Because the brainstem is densely packed with critical anatomical structures, surgical intervention for a brainstem tumor is justified only if it is likely that the information gained from a diagnostic biopsy will influence the treatment plan or that the prognosis of a given lesion can be improved by extensive resection. For diffuse intrinsic gliomas, neither of these indications usually applies: an extensive resection is precluded by the infiltrative growth characteristics of the tumor and, because the histopathology is generally established by the characteristic MRI findings, a biopsy is rarely warranted to confirm the diagnosis (9,10). If the diagnosis of infection or inflammation is being entertained or the natural history is more suggestive of a benign rather than a malignant tumor, a stereotactic biopsy may provide a safer alternative than open exploration for obtaining a tissue diagnosis (33). Similarly, for benign intrinsic tectal gliomas, which typically infiltrate the entire tectum and exhibit an extremely indolent course, there is little to be gained from an attempted resection, and biopsy confirmation of the histological diagnosis is rarely required. The optimal treatment approach usually consists simply of CSF diversion with expectant management of the tumor, reserving biopsy for the rare lesion that progresses.

Lesions that are appropriate for resection are those that exhibit a well-circumscribed growth pattern, with displacement rather than invasion of the surrounding brainstem, and that produce progressive symptoms over time. Such lesions include cervicomedullary and dorsally exophytic gliomas and some focal intrinsic tumors. Although these lesions appear to be well circumscribed radiologically, they are not encapsulated, and all

are at least somewhat invasive along their borders. Thus, a truly complete resection is not safely feasible because of the risk of damage to the surrounding cranial nerve nuclei and long tracts. With midbrain tumors, the extraocular motor nuclei and the white matter pathways coordinating conjugate gaze are the structures at most risk during an extensive tumor removal, whereas with dorsally exophytic and focal intrinsic pontine tumors, the facial and abducens nuclei are most vulnerable to injury. Medullary tumors are the most treacherous, in view of their proximity to lower cranial nerve nuclei and respiratory centers.

Although the sensorimotor pathways are vulnerable to injury during resection of all brainstem gliomas, medullary and cervicomedullary junction lesions pose the greatest risk of profound sensorimotor loss because these pathways are immediately adjacent to the tumor. The corticospinal tracts are often severely flattened and distorted by these tumors, and catastrophic functional deterioration can follow attempts at extensive tumor resection. Similarly, the dorsal columns and dorsal column nuclei can be injured by either inadvertent transection (if a myelotomy is placed off the midline) or excessive traction.

In view of the high risks involved in resecting brainstem tumors, some surgeons use functional neurophysiological monitoring to help localize relevant structures and to warn of early signs of injury so that the operative approach can be modified accordingly. However, the usefulness of these approaches has not been confirmed in a prospective, randomized study, and the rationale for their application is strictly based on the favorable results of single-institution studies, such as our own (34–37). Cranial nerve electromyography (EMG) can be elicited by stimulation to identify the location of cranial nerve nuclei that may overlie a focal tumor or lie adjacent to an exophytic tumor, allowing modification of the operative trajectory (34–36). During the course of a resection, the EMG recordings also alert the surgeon that the relevant nerves or nuclei are being manipulated or if injury has occurred. Somatosensory evoked potentials (SSEPs) and brainstem auditory evoked responses (BSERs) provide feedback on the status of white matter tracts coursing within the brainstem and can be helpful in warning of impending injury during tumor resection. This theoretically can allow a surgeon to modify the operative approach before an irreversible deficit has occurred.

Surgical Approach

OPERATIVE PREPARATION. Patients are given corticosteroids (e.g., dexamethasone 0.1 mg per kg q6h) preoperatively,

which is continued intraoperatively and tapered postoperatively. Prophylactic antibiotics are also administered during the skin preparation and every 6 to 8 hours during the procedure. Because of the potential for hemodynamic changes during the course of the tumor resection, a central line, an arterial line, and a urinary drainage catheter are inserted before beginning the operation. Electrodes for evoked potential monitoring and EMG are also placed. Depending on the location and growth properties of the tumor, motor function from cranial nerves 3, 4, 5, 6, 7, 9, 10, and 12, evoked potentials from cranial nerves 5 and 8, and upper and lower extremity SSEPs can be monitored, either unilaterally or bilaterally. Achieving reliable monitoring while keeping the patient appropriately anesthetized requires

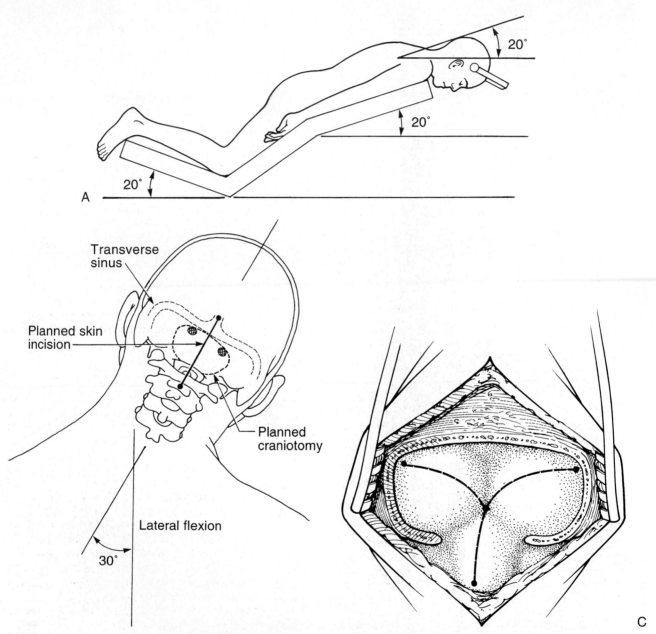

Fig. 5. **A:** A side view of the modified prone position used for resection of dorsal brainstem gliomas. **B:** A dorsal view of the planned approach. **C:** After the bone has been removed, the dura is opened in a V-shaped fashion over the cerebellar hemispheres. The occipital sinus is then controlled, and the apex of the incision is extended inferiorly toward the top of C1. For cervicomedullary tumors, a laminotomy is performed from the rostral surface of C1 to the inferior margin of the tumor and the dural opening is extended in the midline to the caudal extent of the tumor (as illustrated in Fig. 3C).

that the anesthesiologist be made aware of the surgeon's plans preoperatively; often, the anesthetic technique must be adjusted several times during the operation to achieve these goals.

If the patient presents with obstructive hydrocephalus or is at high risk for developing hydrocephalus during the perioperative period, CSF diversion forms an important early step in the operative plan. If the surgery is likely to open the CSF pathways, then an external ventricular drain is inserted in preference to a shunt or a third ventriculostomy. We generally place this via a coronal trajectory, although others prefer an occipital approach. In most cases, the drain can be "weaned" by progressive elevation of the drip chamber during the first postoperative week; otherwise a shunt or third ventriculostomy is subsequently performed.

PATIENT POSITIONING AND INITIAL EXPOSURE. Most brainstem tumors are exposed via a midline infratentorial approach, the trajectory of which can be varied depending on the growth characteristics of the tumor. For dorsally exophytic and dorsally located focal medullary and pontine tumors, a modified prone (concorde) position allows exposure of most lesions (Figs. 5A & B). With this approach, the neck is flexed forward and laterally away from the surgeon by approximately 30 degrees and the back is elevated by the same amount, which keeps the operative field relatively flat. Care must be taken to pad pressure points and to avoid excessive flexion of the neck, which can compromise jugular venous return. Pin fixation of the head is employed in adults and children older than 2 years and a horseshoe headrest is used in younger children. A midline skin incision is then made extending from the inion to the spinous process of C2 and a suboccipital craniectomy or craniotomy (my preference) is performed. The bone removal extends to the foramen magnum caudally and to the inferior margin of the transverse sinus rostrally.

If the dura is tense, the surgeon can ask the anesthesiologist to release 10 to 20 mL of CSF from the ventriculostomy before beginning the dural opening. The dura is then opened in a Y-shaped fashion beginning over the cerebellar hemispheres and extending toward the midline at the occipitocervical junction (Fig. 5C). Large venous sinuses at the foramen magnum region should be anticipated and occluded either using clips, sutures, or hemostats to avoid major bleeding. The incision is then extended inferiorly in the midline to the top of C1.

The approach is modified if the tumor arises more rostrally within the midbrain or caudally within the cervicomedullary junction. For dorsal midbrain tumors, the bony exposure must be carried upward to clearly visualize the transverse sinuses. Some surgeons prefer to approach such tumors using a sitting position; because of the higher risk of air embolism and the more tedious nature of the operation in this position, the modified prone position is preferred, with the back elevated a bit more than for a standard infratentorial exposure. Alternatively, a suboccipital transtentorial approach can be employed, although achieving the anatomical orientation needed for resecting brainstem lesions may be more difficult.

For cervicomedullary tumors, a standard midline cervico-occipital approach is used. Although the neck is flexed 30 degrees, no rotation is employed, and the back is kept in a neutral position. The suboccipital craniotomy is combined with a cervical laminectomy or laminotomy that extends from the rostral surface of C1 down to the inferior margin of the tumor. The use of a laminotomy rather than a laminectomy may reduce the likelihood of postoperative kyphosis, although this remains to confirmed. The extent of the suboccipital craniotomy and the rostral component of the dural opening is less than for a standard infratentorial approach because these lesions rarely extend significantly above the cisterna magna.

For tumors that extend laterally or ventrally within the brainstem, dorsal midline approaches will usually not provide the safest and most direct route to the tumor, and alternate approaches are preferred. For lesions within the lateral medulla or pons, a retromastoid craniectomy or craniotomy extending laterally to expose the sigmoid sinus provides optimal exposure. A subtemporal approach is required for the occasional tumor that extends into the cerebral peduncle through the anterolateral midbrain. Rarely, a transcallosal approach is required for midbrain tumors that expand anteromedially and fill the third ventricle.

Tumor Resection

FOCAL TUMORS. In general, the route that provides the shortest trajectory to the tumor is employed for initial exposure. Tumors that present laterally are best approached using a retromastoid exposure, whereas those that are close to the dorsal surface of the brainstem are best reached using a suboccipital exposure. The former lesions are exposed between the cranial nerve nuclei within the cerebellopontine and cerebellomedullary cisterns. The latter lesions, which are more common, are exposed by gentle separation of the cerebellar tonsils within the cisterna magna and, if necessary, division of the caudal vermis. An important element in the approach to these lesions is to have a clear idea of the relationship of the tumor to the surrounding bulbar structures. Stimulation of the fourth ventricular floor provides localization of the cranial nerve nuclei and, combined with visual inspection (which may reveal discoloration of the brainstem surface over the apex of the tumor) and in some cases ultrasound (to delineate the borders of the lesion), an appropriate trajectory to the tumor can be selected. Clearly, the approach must avoid traversing lower cranial nerve nuclei and the abducens/facial nerve complex, and must be situated off the midline to avoid inadvertent bilateral injury.

Once the location of the lesion and its relationship to the surrounding brainstem structures have been established, the brainstem surface is incised and the tumor is exposed. For cystic lesions with a well-defined mural nodule, the cyst is usually entered first and the solid tumor component is resected from within the wall of the cyst without violating the surrounding brain parenchyma. For solid tumors, the lesion is entered and then debulked from the inside using gentle suction. Because these lesions are bordered by functionally critical tissue, great care must be taken to avoid entering the surrounding brainstem to minimize the risk of irreversible injury. The resection must be performed meticulously, using the ultrasonic aspirator at a low setting or a small suction tip to gently remove tumor from within the cavity. Because these lesions are benign and potentially amenable to treatment with adjuvant chemotherapy or even stereotactic radiotherapy or radiosurgery in the event of subsequent progression, overly aggressive attempts at achieving a gross total resection are not advisable. Instead, the surgeon should strive for an extensive subtotal resection, which often achieves long-term disease control, even without further therapy.

DORSALLY EXOPHYTIC TUMORS. These tumors are approached in the same manner as other fourth ventricular tumors. The cisterna magna is opened and the cerebellar tonsils are gently separated using self-retaining retractors. In many cases, the tumor is apparent within the cisterna magna, but if not, is readily exposed by elevating, or coagulating and incising, the inferior vermis. The rostral and caudal margins of the tumor are then delineated within the cavity of the fourth ventricle. The dorsal wall of the tumor is incised and the inside of the lesion is debulked using the ultrasonic aspirator. The goal of the resection is to remove the tumor flush with the surrounding brainstem surface, and to avoid violating the adjacent brainstem structures to minimize the risk of cranial nerve morbidity. This goal is facilitated by clearly defining the borders of the tumor with the surrounding brainstem before embarking on an aggressive resection. Because dorsolaterally exophytic tumors often push the underlying brainstem ventromedially, the surgeon is able to remain within the tumor while the resection proceeds well beneath the plane of the adjacent brainstem; however, the key technical caveat is that the surgeon must avoid violating the tumor/brainstem interface. EMG and SSEP monitoring are useful for indicating early signs of cranial nerve and long tract manipulation during the course of the tumor resection.

Because the majority of these lesions are histologically benign, extended periods of disease control are usually possible after an extensive subtotal tumor resection. In several cases we have encountered, the surgeon was convinced that tumor was left behind, but no evidence of tumor growth was apparent on subsequent imaging, presumably because the residual tumor remained quiescent or actually regressed over time.

CERVICOMEDULLARY TUMORS. These lesions are initially approached in the same manner as spinal cord astrocytomas, beginning with a midline myelotomy over the region of maximum tumor diameter to expose the lesion (Fig. 3B). An essential step in this approach is to ensure that the cord is indeed being opened in the midline to avoid injury to the posterior columns. Identification of the dorsal root entry sites often helps to guide orientation if the location of the midline is unclear. A myelotomy is then performed using either a no. 11 blade or the surgical laser. The tumor or an associated cyst is usually apparent immediately beneath the cord surface and pial traction sutures (e.g., 7-0 Prolene) are secured to the dural margins. The lesion is then debulked from the inside. Cystic areas, if present, are helpful for identifying transition zones between tumor and normal cord parenchyma. In addition, ultrasound is useful for delineating the margins of the lesion and assuring an adequate resection. It is usually not necessary or advisable to extend the myelotomy to the caudal tip of the tumor (because this would involve incising a significant thickness of normal cord). Instead, the inferior pole of the lesion is resected from within the myelotomy cavity.

The resection is then extended rostrally toward the inferior medullary region. As noted earlier, the medulla is often displaced upward by the lesion; in such cases, the rostral portion of the tumor can usually be removed from within the cervical myelotomy cavity without necessitating a direct incision within the medulla (Fig. 3C). Care is taken to avoid overly aggressive tumor resection in this region to minimize the risk of permanent respiratory impairment and swallowing dysfunction, and also to avoid inadvertent injury to the posterior inferior cerebellar arteries. After the bulk of the tumor has been removed with the ultrasonic aspirator, a small suction is used to gently remove small residual fragments of tumor. Despite the fact that the spinal cord is often severely flattened by the tumor and that only a thin cuff of normal tissue is apparent at the conclusion of the resection (Fig. 3D), patients commonly awaken with minimal neurological deficits, provided that the surrounding parenchyma has not been violated. Although we generally use SSEPs as an indicator of early compromise to the spinal cord and dorsal column nuclei during the resection, these studies are sometimes so abnormal preoperatively that reproducible responses are difficult to elicit, limiting their use. Motor evoked potentials have also been reported to have some efficacy in

warning of impending injury to the corticospinal tracts (37), although as with SSEPs, these responses may be difficult to elicit reproducibly in some patients. Recognizing the limitations of current monitoring techniques, some surgeons avoid monitoring entirely in these patients, although we prefer to obtain as much neurophysiological information as possible during the resection to guide operative decision making. In addition to SSEPs, we usually incorporate EMGs of cranial nerves 10 and 12 to warn of inadvertent injury during resection of the rostral pole of the tumor.

CLOSURE. Upon completion of the tumor resection, meticulous hemostasis is confirmed. Hemostatic agents are usually not required and, because they can complicate interpretation of postoperative imaging studies, are best avoided. The dura is closed in a watertight fashion, incorporating a dural graft if needed. If a craniotomy or laminotomy has been performed, the bone is replaced and secured to the surrounding bone edges with 2-0 sutures or microplates. The wound is then closed in layers with absorbable sutures.

Complications and Their Management

Because lesions within the brainstem carry a high risk of neurological deterioration, patients are monitored closely in an intensive care unit setting for at least 48 hours postoperatively. Patients generally undergo a postoperative MRI study during this interval both to confirm the extent of the tumor resection and to rule out hemorrhage or injury to the brain around the resection cavity. Lesions involving the medulla may pose particularly serious problems, because the initial symptoms of neurological deterioration may be respiratory depression and airway compromise. If there is any question about the integrity of the patient's airway protective reflexes, a prolonged interval of ventilation may be warranted. A formal swallowing evaluation, consisting at a minimum of a "barium swallow" using various consistencies of feedings is also advisable in many instances. Some patients may require a temporary gastrostomy to ensure adequate nutrition without the risk of aspiration. For patients with more rostral brainstem lesions, facial and extraocular muscle palsies are common sequelae. In such patients, we typically defer operative reconstruction or strabismus surgery for at least 3 months, because substantial recovery often occurs during this interval.

Outcome and Therapeutic Alternatives

As noted earlier, surgical resection has limited use for diffuse intrinsic brainstem gliomas. These tumors are best treated with radiotherapy, which unfortunately is largely palliative, but often provides patients with a several-month period of disease stability. Attempts to enhance the effectiveness of radiotherapy by using high-dose hyperfractionated techniques have been disappointing, as have efforts to improve disease control by using adjuvant or intensive neoadjuvant chemotherapy in conjunction with irradiation (12,13,38). In most large studies, median progression-free survival is less than 1 year and fewer than 5% of patients survive for longer than 5 years (10,12,13,38). Although single-institution reports have suggested that diffuse brainstem gliomas in adults may have a somewhat less aggressive course than in children, with 5-year survivals in the range of 20% to 40% (39–41), such series have generally not excluded patients with tectal tumors and focal brainstem gliomas, which biases the results toward a more favorable overall outcome. Ongoing protocols are evaluating the role of various radiosensitizing techniques for improving disease control in these tumors.

Another group of brainstem tumors for which surgical resection has a limited role are the tectal gliomas, in this case because of the generally benign natural history of these lesions. These tumors are best managed strictly with CSF diversion, using a shunt or, preferably, a third ventriculostomy to treat the presenting symptoms of obstructive hydrocephalus. Biopsy and adjuvant therapy are reserved for the small percentage of lesions that progress. In our institutional series of more than 20 such tumors, less than 25% have ultimately required adjuvant therapy (29). The others have remained progression-free during periods of expectant management that exceed 10 years. Those lesions that have progressed have generally been found to be low-grade astrocytomas, which have been well controlled subsequently after focal irradiation. This largely mirrors the experience of other authors regarding the generally indolent nature of these lesions (30–32).

Most low-grade dorsally exophytic and cervicomedullary gliomas and some focal intrinsic tumors are best managed strictly as surgical lesions and, after an extensive resection, are monitored with serial imaging studies. Several institutional studies with median follow-up intervals ranging from 3 to 10 years have noted that only about 20% to 30% of patients require additional treatment for progressive disease, despite the fact that a complete tumor resection has not been achieved (5,20,25,42), and the majority of patients improve symptomatically following tumor resection. The small percentage of tumors that progress after an initial resection are usually amenable to a second attempt at radical resection (25). In young children, progressive lesions that are not believed to be resectable or that recur after a second resection can potentially be controlled with adjuvant chemotherapy. We have had favorable results with the combination of carboplatin and vincristine (43) in a handful of cases. In addition, a variety of other regimens have been successfully employed in the treatment of low-grade gliomas in young children (e.g., vincristine-actinomycin D and 6-thioguanine-procarbazine-dibromodulcitol-CCNU-vincristine) with response rates of 20% to 80% and response or stabilization rates of 75% to 100% (44,45), although reports of their application for brainstem gliomas are limited. In older patients, focused radiotherapy or stereotactic radiosurgery are alternate options, and favorable results in terms of long-term disease control have been reported (46,47).

Because focal tumors within the pons and medulla carry significant risks of neurological impairment after surgical resection, evidence supporting the role of surgery versus alternative treatment approaches is less well established for these tumors than for the above groups of low-grade gliomas. Although Abbott and colleagues (23) have reported favorable results in terms of disease control in a small series of focal medullary gliomas, the potential morbidity is high, with four of seven patients exhibiting persistent deterioration in lower brainstem function. Although surgery is an appropriate option for such tumors, it remains to be confirmed that the long-term results are better than those achieved with biopsy followed by focused radiotherapy, radiosurgery, or chemotherapy (22,46,47).

Finally, because the natural history of brainstem tumors in patients with NF1 is often much more indolent than that of seemingly identical lesions in patients without this disorder (14–19), the management of these lesions in NF1 patients must

be modified accordingly (14). The fact that patients with NF1 are at risk for developing multiple neoplasms within the neuraxis during their lifetimes mandates that for any given lesion, particularly careful consideration be given to the potential consequences of intervention. For example, the decision to treat a brainstem tumor with radiation may not only subject the patient to the potential morbidity associated with this modality, but may also limit the therapeutic options available for a lesion that may develop several years later in another intracranial location. Thus, in a patient with NF1 who is found to have a diffuse intrinsic brainstem tumor, it is important to confirm that the lesion is indeed enlarging or causing progressive symptoms before embarking on a course of therapeutic irradiation. Similarly, the finding on a screening MRI in a patient with NF1 of a small, focal enhancing brainstem tumor should not immediately signal the need for surgical resection or focused radiotherapy in the absence of objective evidence of disease progression. Although some such lesions clearly progress and warrant treatment, others remain stable in size or, rarely, regress spontaneously without intervention (14). In view of the variability in the natural history of these lesions, we have undertaken treatment only in those patients with progressive tumor enlargement in association with local mass effect or with the development of progressive clinical symptoms. Since the natural history of any given lesion remains uncertain, we advocate routine follow-up imaging in patients who are managed conservatively.

Summary

Brainstem tumors are a diverse group of lesions that differ significantly in terms of their growth properties and biological behavior. Although several large groups of brainstem tumors, specifically the diffuse intrinsic and benign tectal tumors, are best managed nonsurgically or with simple CSF diversion, other tumors are clearly amenable to extensive resection. For dorsally exophytic, cervicomedullary, and focal midbrain tumors, the postoperative results are often gratifying and appear to be far better than those achieved with nonsurgical approaches. For focal pontine and medullary tumors, the high risks of surgery mandate that careful consideration also be given to alternative treatment approaches (e.g., biopsy followed by stereotactic radiotherapy or radiosurgery) and that the patient and family be well informed of the potential risks and involved in the therapeutic decision-making process. In view of the more indolent natural history of many brainstem lesions in patients with NF1, it is important to consider this diagnosis when evaluating a patient with a brainstem glioma, because a correspondingly more conservative approach to intervention may be warranted.

Acknowledgment

The work was supported in part by a grant from the National Institutes of Health (NS01810).

References

1. Pollack IF. Brain tumors in children. *N Engl J Med* 1994;331: 1500–1507.

2. Young JL. Cancer incidence, survival, and mortality for children younger than 15 years. *Cancer* 1986;58:561–568.
3. Hoffman HJ, Becker L, Craven MA. A clinically and pathologically distinct group of benign brain stem gliomas. *Neurosurgery* 1980;7:243–248.
4. Stroink AR, Hoffman HJ, Hendrick EB, et al. Diagnosis and management of pediatric brain stem gliomas. *J Neurosurg* 1986;65:745–750.
5. Stroink AR, Hoffman HJ, Hendrick EB, et al. Transependymal benign dorsally exophytic brain stem gliomas of childhood: diagnosis and treatment recommendations. *Neurosurgery* 1987;20:439–444.
6. Epstein F, McCleary EL. Intrinsic brain-stem tumors of childhood: surgical indications. *J Neurosurg* 1986;64:11–15.
7. Epstein FJ, Wisoff JH. Intra-axial tumors of the cervicomedullary junction. *J Neurosurg* 1987:67:483–487.
8. Epstein FJ, Wisoff JH. Brainstem tumors in childhood: surgical indications. In: McLaurin RL, Schut L, Venes JL, et al, eds. *Pediatric neurosurgery. Surgery of the developing nervous system,* 2nd ed. Philadelphia: WB Saunders, 1989;357–365.
9. Albright AL, Packer RJ, Zimmerman R, et al. Magnetic resonance scans should replace biopsies for the diagnosis of diffuse brain stem gliomas: a report from the Children's Cancer Group. *Neurosurgery* 1993;33:1026–1030.
10. Sanford RA, Freeman CR, Burger P, et al. Prognostic criteria for experimental protocols in pediatric brain stem gliomas. *Surg Neurol* 1988;30:276–280.
11. Albright AL, Guthkelch AN, Packer RJ, et al. Prognostic factors in pediatric brain-stem gliomas. *J Neurosurg* 1986;65:751–755.
12. Packer RJ, Boyett JM, Zimmerman RA, et al. Hyperfractionated radiation therapy (7200 cGy) for children with brain stem gliomas: a Children's Cancer Group phase I/II trial. *Cancer* 1993;72:1414–1421.
13. Kaplan AM, Albright AL, Zimmerman RA, et al. Brainstem gliomas in children: a Children's Cancer Group review of 119 cases. *Pediatr Neurosurg* 1996;24:185–192.
14. Pollack IF, Shultz B, Mulvihill JJ. The management of brainstem gliomas in patients with neurofibromatosis 1. *Neurology* 1996;46:1652–1660.
15. Sevick RJ, Barkovich AJ, Edwards MSB, et al. Evolution of white matter lesions in neurofibromatosis type 1: MR findings. *AJR* 1992;159:171–175.
16. Raffel C, McComb JG, Bodner S, et al. Benign brain stem lesions in pediatric patients with neurofibromatosis: case reports. *Neurosurgery* 1989;25:959–964.
17. Molloy PT, Bilaniuk L, Needle M, et al. Brain-stem mass lesions in neurofibromatosis type-1. A distinct clinical entity. *Ann Neurol* 1994;36:549.
18. Itoh T, Magnaldi S, White RM, et al. Neurofibromatosis type-1—the evolution of deep gray and white-matter MR abnormalities. *Am J Neurorad* 1994;15:1513–1519.
19. Cohen ME, Duffner PK, Heffner RR, et al. Prognostic factors in brain stem gliomas. *Neurology* 1986;36:602–605.
20. Vandertop WP, Hoffman, HJ, Drake JM, et al. Focal midbrain tumors in children. *Neurosurgery* 1992;31:186–194.
21. Robertson PL, Muraszko KM, Brunberg JA, et al. Pediatric midbrain tumors: a benign subgroup of brainstem gliomas. *Pediatr Neurosurg* 1995;22:65–73.
22. Edwards MSB, Wara WM, Ciricillo SF, et al. Focal brain-stem astrocytomas causing symptoms of involvement of the facial nerve nucleus: long-term survival in six pediatric patients. *J Neurosurg* 1994;80:20–25.
23. Abbott R, Shiminski-Maher T, Wisoff JH, et al. Intrinsic tumors of the medulla: surgical complications. *Pediatr Neurosurg* 1992;17:239–244.
24. Constantini S, Epstein F. Surgical indication and technical considerations in the management of benign brain stem gliomas. *J Neuro-oncol* 1996;28:193–205.
25. Pollack IF, Hoffman HJ, Humphreys RP, et al. The long-term outcome after surgical treatment of dorsally exophytic brainstem gliomas. *J Neurosurg* 1993;78:859–863.
26. Hoffman HJ. Dorsally exophytic brain stem tumors and midbrain tumors. *Pediatr Neurosurg* 1996;24:256–262.
27. Pierre-Kahn A, Hirsch JF, Vinchon M, et al. Surgical management of brain-stem tumors in children: results and statistical analysis of 75 cases. *J Neurosurg* 1993;79:845–852.
28. Epstein FJ, Farmer J-P. Brain-stem glioma growth patterns. *J Neurosurg* 1993;78:408–412.
29. Pollack IF, Pang D, Albright AL. The long-term outcome in children with late-onset aqueductal stenosis resulting from benign intrinsic tectal tumors. *J Neurosurg* 1994;80:681–688.
30. Boydston WR, Sanford RA, Muhlbauer MS, et al. Gliomas of the tectum and periaqueductal region of the mesencephalon. *Pediatr Neurosurg* 1991–1992;17:234–238.
31. Chapman PH. Indolent gliomas of the midbrain tectum. In: Marlin AE, ed. *Concepts of pediatric neurosurgery.* Vol 10. Basel: Karger, 1990;97–107.
32. May PL, Blaser SI, Hoffman HJ, et al. Benign intrinsic tectal "tumors" in children. *J Neurosurg* 1991;74:867–871.
33. Kondziolka D, Lunsford LD. Results and expectations with image-integrated brainstem stereotactic biopsy. *Surg Neurol* 1995;43:558–562.
34. Moroto N, Deletis V, Lee M, et al. Functional anatomic relationship between brain stem tumors and cranial motor nuclei. *Neurosurgery* 1996;39:787–794.
35. Strauss C, Lutjen-Drecoll E, Fahlbusch R. Pericollicular surgical approaches to the rhomboid fossa. Part I. Anatomical basis. *J Neurosurg* 1997;87:893–899.
36. Grabb PA, Albright AL, Pollack IF, et al. Continuous intraoperative electromyography of cranial nerves during resection of fourth ventricular tumors in children. *J Neurosurg* 1997;86:1–4.
37. Morota N, Deletis V, Constantini S, et al. The role of motor evoked potentials during surgery for intramedullary spinal cord tumors. *Neurosurgery* 1997;41:1327–1336.
38. Jennings MT, Freeman ML, Murray MJ. Strategies in the treatment of diffuse pontine gliomas: the therapeutic role of hyperfractionated radiotherapy and chemotherapy. *J Neuro-oncol* 1996;28:207–222.
39. Landolfi JC, Thaler HT, DeAngelis LM. Adult brainstem gliomas. *Neurology* 1998;51:1136–1139.
40. Grigsby PW, Garcia DM, Simpson JR, et al. Prognostic factors and results of therapy for adult thalamic and brainstem tumors. *Cancer* 1989;63:2124–2129.
41. Guiney MJ, Smith JG, Hughes P, et al. Contemporary management of adult and pediatric brain stem gliomas. *Int J Radiat Oncol Biol Phys* 1993;25:235–241.
42. Konovalov AN, Gorelyshev SK, Khuhlaeva EA. Surgery of diencephalic and brainstem tumors. In: Schmidek HH, Sweet WH, eds. *Operative neurosurgical techniques,* 3rd ed. Philadelphia: WB Saunders, 1995;765–782.
43. Packer RJ, Lange B, Ater J, et al. Carboplatin and vincristine for recurrent and newly diagnosed low-grade gliomas of childhood. *J Clin Oncol* 1993;11:850–856.
44. Packer RJ, Sutton LN, Bilaniuk LT, et al. Treatment of chiasmatic/hypothalamic gliomas of childhood with chemotherapy: an update. *Ann Neurol* 1988;23:79–85.
45. Petronio J, Edwards MSB, Prados M, et al. Management of chiasmal and hypothalamic gliomas of infancy and childhood with chemotherapy. *J Neurosurg* 1991;74:701–708.
46. Somaza SC, Kondziolka D, Lunsford LD, et al. Early outcomes after stereotactic radiosurgery for growing pilocytic astrocytomas in children. *Pediatr Neurosurg* 1996;25:109–115.
47. Mundinger F, Braus DF, Krauss JK, et al. Long-term outcome of 89 low-grade brain-stem gliomas after interstitial radiation therapy. *J Neurosurg* 1991;75:740–746.

112. Tumors of the Pineal Region

Jeffrey N. Bruce

Strategies for surgical management of pineal region tumors are heavily influenced by the wide variety of histologically diverse pathologies that can occur in this anatomical location. It is imperative to establish an accurate diagnosis because the specific tumor histology influences subsequent management decisions. The ability to safely accomplish this has been facilitated by the advances in microsurgical technique, neuroanesthesia, stereotactic technology, and postoperative care that have reduced surgical morbidity and improved the attainment of surgical goals.

Pathology

Tumors of the pineal region can be grouped into four different tumor categories: (a) germ cell tumors; (b) pineal cell tumors; (c) glial cell tumors; and (d) miscellaneous tumors. A continuum of diverse cellular subtypes exists within each category ranging from benign to highly malignant, with many of an intermediate grade (1–4). Additionally, tumors within a given category can be of a mixed tumor variety, composed of more than one cell type.

Tumors in the miscellaneous category can include a wide variety of pathologies from metastatic tumors, meningiomas, lymphoma, hemangioblastoma, choroid plexus papilloma, chemodectoma, and adenocarcinoma (1). The histological profile is complicated by a variety of vascular lesions that also can occur in the pineal region, including arteriovenous malformations, cavernous malformations, and vein of Galen malformations.

Pineal cysts are being discovered with increasing frequency as people undergo magnetic resonance imaging (MRI) scans for routine neurological complaints. Pineal cysts are actually anatomical variants of the normal pineal gland that are rarely symptomatic and therefore rarely require treatment (5,6). Surgeons should resist coercion to remove these cysts from patients who have incidental and unrelated neurological symptoms. Progression of the cyst or development of symptoms clearly referable to it should raise the possibility that it is actually a low-grade cystic neoplasm such as a pilocytic astrocytoma and therefore may require surgical removal.

Preoperative Evaluation

MRI with and without gadolinium is the preferred modality for evaluating pineal region tumors (Fig. 1) (7,8). In addition to visualizing the size and geometric configuration of the tumor, MRI depicts the tumor's relationship to important surrounding structures such as the deep venous system and brainstem. Contrast enhancement provides some degree of information about tumor vascularity. High-resolution MRI allows the margins of the tumor to be visualized to estimate its invasiveness, although such findings are not always a reliable indicator of whether a tumor can be completely removed. Additionally, the presence of hydrocephalus and aqueductal compromise can be evaluated. Computed tomography (CT) scans are optional but can be complementary to MRI scanning by providing information

regarding calcification. Angiography generally is not needed unless a vascular anomaly is suspected or if questions exist regarding the patency or involvement of the deep venous system.

The preoperative evaluation should include the measurement of markers for malignant germ cells, including α-fetoprotein and human chorionic gonadotropin (2,9–11). These levels can be measured in the blood; however, cerebrospinal fluid (CSF) levels are slightly more sensitive and should be obtained when possible. Elevation of germ cell markers is pathognomonic for the presence of a malignant germ cell tumor. Surgery is not necessary for either debulking or establishing a diagnosis because these tumors are best treated with chemotherapy and radiation. After treatment with radiation and chemotherapy, if the tumor is still present, a surgical exploration can be considered to remove what are likely to be residual benign tumor elements that are resistant to adjuvant treatment (12).

Management of Hydrocephalus

The majority of patients with pineal region tumors present with hydrocephalus, which must be addressed as an initial step in the clinical management. Patients with only mild degrees of hydrocephalus who are neurologically stable often can be managed without any shunting procedure if it appears that the tumor is likely to be completely removed at surgery. In those instances, a ventricular drain may be necessary prior to surgery and then removed afterward. Conversely, patients who are symptomatic and progressive often benefit from a reduction of their increased intracranial pressure prior to undergoing their craniotomy. The procedure of choice is a stereotactically guided endoscopic third ventriculostomy, which is desirable because it avoids shunt-related complications such as infection, overshunting, and peritoneal seeding by malignant cells (13).

Surgical Indications

Except in unusual extenuating clinical circumstances, nearly all patients require some type of surgical procedure to, at minimum, establish a histological diagnosis (1,14,15). Despite advances in radiographic imaging, alternative methods have been insufficient to reliably obtain a histological diagnosis without a biopsy specimen. (Patients with elevated germ cell markers are the exception.) The initial management decision is whether to perform an open operative approach or stereotactic biopsy. Each approach has its risks and benefits. Stereotactic biopsy of pineal region tumors has many advocates because of its technical ease and reduced morbidity compared to open procedures (1,15–17). Surgeons who are relatively inexperienced with complex neurosurgical procedures such as pineal region surgery often prefer it. However, this strategy must be balanced against the potential for misdiagnosis from the limited sampling that can be achieved (14,18). Tissue sampling is particularly problematic in the pineal region because tumors often are heterogeneous, and neuropathologists often have difficulty distinguishing between the diverse tumor possibilities in the small

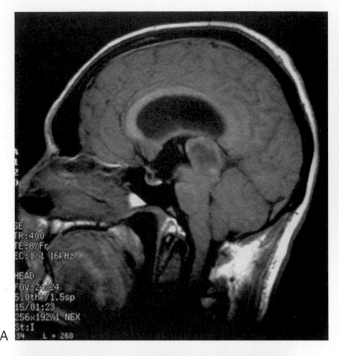

A

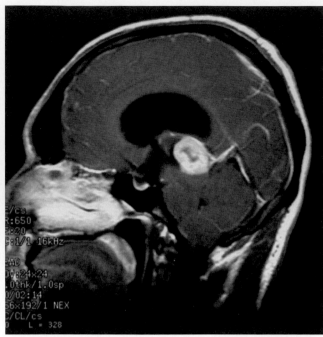

B

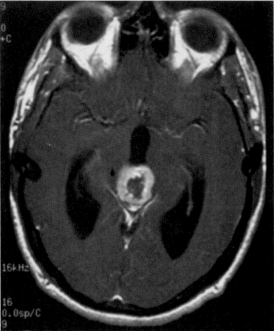

C

Fig. 1. Magnetic resonance image of a patient with a mixed pineal parenchymal tumor. **A:** T1-weighted sagittal. **B:** T1-weighted sagittal with gadolinium. **C:** T1-weighted axial.

samples provided. Additionally, stereotactic biopsy is not without hazard (19,20). These tumors often are highly vascular and adjacent to critical vascular structures in the third ventricle and quadrigeminal cistern. The potential for bleeding into the ventricle is significant because pressure from tissue turgor is not available to tamponade the minor bleeding that can occur. Stereotactic biopsy also ignores the benefit that open procedures can achieve in terms of tumor removal. In many instances, the ability to remove tumors can be curative or can improve the response to adjuvant therapy (21–23). Furthermore, surgical resection can avoid shunting procedures by directly relieving obstructive hydrocephalus. However, the ability to perform a stereotactic biopsy is a useful procedure and is critical to the surgeon's choice of the best approach for each patient. Patients

with multicentric or disseminated tumors or who have medical contraindications to surgery are excellent candidates for stereotactic biopsy. Certain patients with highly invasive tumors of the brainstem or thalamus also may be best served by a stereotactic biopsy.

Surgical Techniques

STEREOTACTIC BIOPSY. Stereotactic biopsies of pineal tumors are more complicated and have reduced margin of error compared to tumors in other locations. Advances in radiographic imaging and software planning provide several alternatives for safely planning biopsy trajectories. CT-guided procedures are acceptable because of their high degree of accuracy and common availability. Although nearly any stereotactic frame system is sufficient, target-centered stereotactic frame systems such as the CRW (Cosman-Roberts-Wells) have the versatility to facilitate even complex biopsies. Local anesthesia with mild sedation is safe and usually sufficient to perform biopsies.

The most common surgical trajectory to the pineal region is via an anterolaterosuperior approach anterior to the coronal suture and lateral to the midpupillary line (24). This trajectory passes through the frontal lobe and the internal capsule. The ependyma of the lateral ventricle and the internal cerebral vein should be avoided. An alternative approach is a posterolaterosuperior approach through the parietal–occipital junction, which is best suited for large tumors that have a lateral extension.

Multiple serial biopsy specimens should be obtained whenever possible. Obviously, the risks of bleeding for each additional specimen must be considered, taking into account the size of the mass. A frozen section intraoperatively may be useful in verifying pathological tissue; however, the wide diversity of tissue types reduces the accuracy of a frozen tissue diagnosis.

Advances in endoscopic technique have led to investigations of biopsies via this method (25–27). Endoscopy is sometimes performed in conjunction with an endoscopic third ventriculostomy to relieve hydrocephalus. Performing a ventriculostomy and biopsy simultaneously requires the use of a flexible endoscope because of the limited trajectory to the tumor through the foramen of Munro. A rigid endoscope can be used but would necessitate a second burr hole and trajectory with a more inferior entry point on the forehead. The risks of an endoscopic biopsy are considerable owing to the limited tissue sampling and difficulty achieving hemostasis within the ventricle. Even minor bleeding can obscure the operative field making it difficult to identify the target. In general, given these limitations, a stereotactic biopsy is preferable to endoscopic biopsy in situations where diagnostic tissue is desired.

OPEN OPERATIVE APPROACHES

Anesthesia Considerations. Standard general anesthesia techniques are used. Problems related to hydrocephalus or increased intracranial pressure should be addressed prior to surgery. If the sitting position is used, precordial Doppler monitoring is desirable to detect air emboli. Additionally, a central venous catheter should be placed to remove air that may become entrapped.

Operative Approaches. There are variations on the surgical approaches to the pineal region but basically they are categorized as either supratentorial or infratentorial approaches. The most common supratentorial approaches are the occipital-transtentorial and the transcallosal-interhemispheric approaches with the transcortical–transventricular approach rarely used (1,28–32). The infratentorial approach is through a corridor between the tentorium and cerebellum and is therefore known as the infratentorial-supracerebellar approach. Any of these approaches can be adequate for the majority of pineal region tumors; the ultimate choice is based on the surgeon's comfort and experience with a given technique. Our personal preference is for the infratentorial-supracerebellar approach because it provides a relatively bloodless midline approach that allows gravity to facilitate tumor removal when the patient is in the sitting position (1,23). Although the positioning is somewhat awkward because of the deep working depth, it allows the cerebellum to naturally drop downward and the tumor to be

encountered ventral and inferior to the deep venous system, where it can be more easily dissected off these structures.

Supratentorial approaches have the advantage of providing greater exposure and working room, but have the disadvantage of encountering the tumors deep to the deep venous system, which interferes with tumor removal. Generally, tumors that have a large extension either laterally or superiorly benefit from one of the supratentorial approaches.

Patient Positioning. A variety of patient positions have been described for these approaches, each having advantages and disadvantages (Fig. 2) (33–39). Some of the positions can be used interchangeably with the different approaches.

SITTING POSITION. The sitting position is the most commonly preferred position for the infratentorial-supracerebellar approach (1). Gravity works in the surgeon's favor by allowing the cerebellum to drop down with minimal retraction facilitating dissection of the tumor off of the deep venous system. Precautions can be taken to anticipate and minimize the risks from air emboli, pneumocephalus, or subdural hematoma associated with cortical collapse (35). Doppler monitoring and constant monitoring of end tidal Pco_2 can detect small amounts of air before it becomes problematic.

An operative table capable of being lowered close to the floor is desirable. The table is used in the reverse position to allow the surgeon to sit behind the patient. The patient's head is placed in a three-point vise type of head holder and is stabilized by the assistant as the patient is brought into the sitting position (Fig. 2A). The table is manipulated into a degree of Trendelenburg that allows the trunk and pelvis to be stabilized on the operative table so the patient does not shift if the table is moved. The head should be flexed until the tentorium is nearly parallel to the floor. Precautions should be taken to make sure that there is at least a two-finger breadth of space between the chin and sternum to avoid airway compromise.

LATERAL POSITION. Several variations of the lateral approach exist. In the lateral decubitus position, the nondominant right hemisphere is placed in a dependent position (Fig. 2B) (33). If the occipital-transtentorial approach is used, the head should be positioned with the patient's nose rotated 30 degrees toward the floor.

The three-quarter prone position is an extension of the lateral position, where the head is at an oblique 45 degree angle with the nondominant hemisphere dependent (Fig. 2C) (37,39). This is most commonly used for the occipital-transtentorial approach. It has the advantage of allowing the nondominant hemisphere to be easily retracted with the aid of gravity. Many surgeons find this approach more comfortable because the surgeon's hands are in a horizontal plane and do not need to be extended as in the sitting position. Although this is a very suitable position, it can be cumbersome to set up. A padded axillary roll is placed under the left thorax and the three-point head pin vise holder is fixed with the head slightly extended and rotated to the left at a 45-degree oblique angle.

PRONE POSITION. The prone position is simple, safe, and particularly suitable for the supratentorial approaches (Fig. 2D) (34). The drawbacks include the fact that the operative field is considerably raised making it difficult for the surgeon to be seated and also, unlike the sitting position, venous drainage is not facilitated and the brain has a tendency to collapse into the tumor bed. This approach can be useful, particularly in the pediatric population. The steep angle of the tentorium makes it impractical for the infratentorial-supracerebellar approach. A variation of this approach known as the Concorde position is useful and involves positioning of the head rotated 15 degrees away from the side of the craniotomy (38).

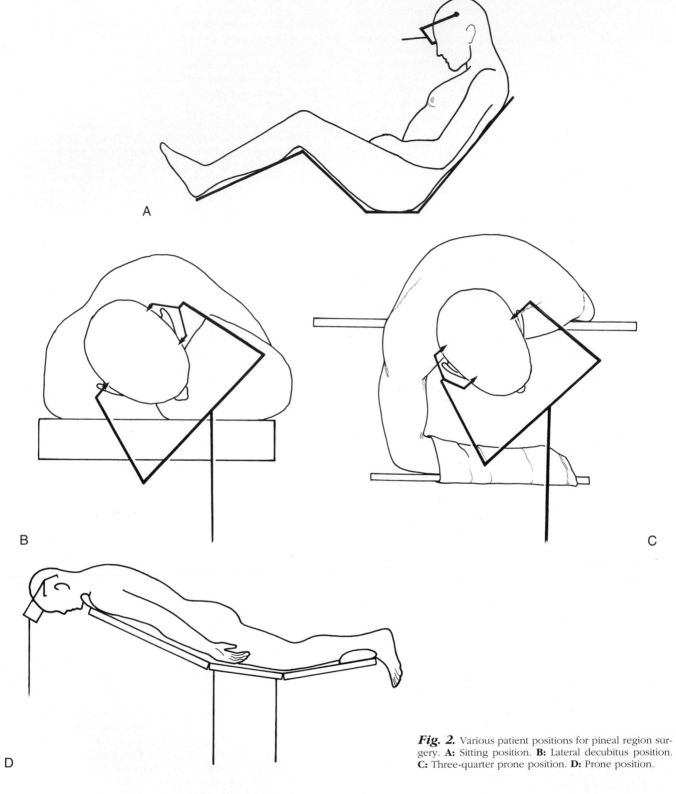

Fig. 2. Various patient positions for pineal region surgery. **A:** Sitting position. **B:** Lateral decubitus position. **C:** Three-quarter prone position. **D:** Prone position.

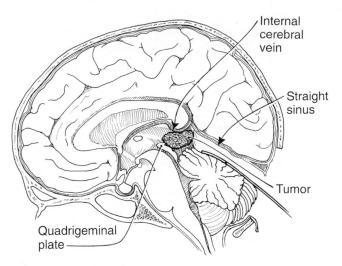

Fig. 3. Sagittal view of infratentorial-supracerebellar approach to the pineal region.

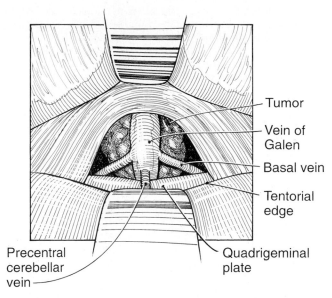

Fig. 4. Operative view of exposure with the infratentorial-supracerebellar approach with the precentral cerebellar vein overlying the tumor.

Infratentorial-Supracerebellar Approach. The sitting position is generally preferred for the infratentorial-supracerebellar approach (Fig. 3) (40). If a ventricular drain is needed, it can be placed through a burr hole at the lambdoid suture in the midpupillary line. A midline incision is made through the nuchal ligament of the suboccipital musculature extending from just above the external occipital protuberance down to approximately the level of C4 spinous process. A low profile self-retaining retractor is used to expose the suboccipital region. It is not necessary to open the foramen magnum or detach the muscles from the spinous process of C1 and C2. The craniotomy is centered just below the torcular and is facilitated by drilling burr hole slots over the transverse sinus on both sides as well as over the sagittal sinus just above the torcular. A midline burr hole just above the foramen magnum facilitates the use of the craniotome to turn the craniotomy. A sufficient extension above the transverse sinus is necessary to allow for the instruments and microscope to be utilized and for sufficient light to fill the operative field. A craniotomy is generally desirable over a craniectomy, as it appears to reduce postoperative discomfort and fluid collections. Attention should be given to avoiding sources of air emboli by waxing bone edges and cauterizing any venous bleeding.

The dura is opened in a gentle curve extending to the lateral exposure of the transverse sinus bilaterally. The dura is reflected upward with a gentle retraction, avoiding over-retraction that might occlude the sinus. The inferior dura acts as a "sling" support for the cerebellum. If the posterior fossa is tight, CSF can be removed from either the cisterna magna or the ventricular drain.

Cauterizing and dividing the bridging veins and freeing up the arachnoidal adhesions between the cerebellum and the tentorium open the infratentorial corridor. The cerebellum will drop down from the natural force of gravity because these are detached. The dorsal surface of the cerebellum is covered with protective padding such as Telfa, and a Greenberg retractor system (or similar system) is used to retract the cerebellum posteriorly and inferiorly. At this point the thickened arachnoid over the quadrigeminal cistern will begin to be visible.

An operating microscope with a variable objective is useful to accommodate the different depths encountered along the operative approach. Extralong instruments are necessary and a freestanding armrest is needed to avoid the surgeon's arm fatigue. With the microscope in place, the arachnoid is opened and the precentral cerebellar vein is cauterized and divided (Fig. 4). Great care should be taken to avoid any damage or compromise of the deep venous system into which the precentral cerebellar vein flows.

The trajectory of the microscope has been aimed at the vein of Galen at this point. The trajectory should now be aimed several degrees downward so that it is more in line with the geometric center of the tumor. It is usually possible with sufficient retraction to see the interface between the tumor and quadrigeminal plate (Fig. 5).

The posterior central surface of the tumor can be cauterized and sharply opened. This allows the tumor to be internally debulked, using a variety of instruments such as suction, tumor forceps, cautery, or a Cavitron if necessary. Specimens should be sent for frozen section analysis; however, the potential inac-

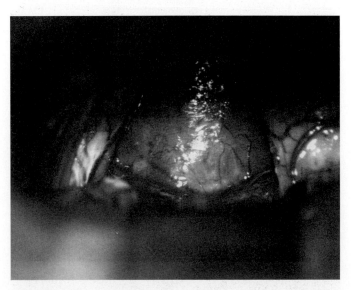

Fig. 5. Operative photo showing exposure of the tumor after the precentral cerebellar vein has been sacrificed.

curacy of these results must be taken into consideration when making surgical decisions. Most tumors are very soft and can be easily decompressed. It is gradually dissected from the surrounding brainstem, thalamus, and deep venous system after the tumor is decompressed. Maintaining the tumor capsule will facilitate this dissection. The surgeon's judgment and experience are critical at this point to determine the resectability of an individual tumor. Tumors that are invasive may not be conducive to complete removal; however, any residual tumor left behind increases the risk of postoperative bleeding.

The surgeon has an excellent view into the third ventricle once the tumor is removed (Fig. 6). Mirrors can be used to view the inferior portion of the tumor bed to make sure that removal is complete and hemostasis has been achieved. Careful attention must be paid to hemostasis because any bleeding can have devastating effects on ventricular flow, causing acute obstructive hydrocephalus. Hemostatic agents are used sparingly because they can float into the ventricle and cause obstruction.

The dura is closed as water tightly as possible when hemostasis is achieved. The bone flap is then plated into place using a miniplate system and the muscle and fascia are closed in layers. It is desirable to extubate the patient in the sitting position to avoid excessive shifting of the decompressed brain within the cranial vault.

Transcallosal-Interhemispheric Approach. Any of the previously described patient positions can be used for the transcallosal-interhemispheric approach, although the prone or sitting position are preferred because of the midline trajectory that they use. The operative corridor is between the falx and nondominant hemisphere at around the level of the parietal-occipital junction (Fig. 7) (41–43).

The bone flap is centered at the vertex, but the exact location depends on where the tumor is positioned within the third ventricle. The craniotomy must extend across the sagittal sinus to facilitate subsequent retractor placement. Bleeding from the sagittal sinus can be controlled with hemostatic agents. The advantage of this approach is that it is generally centered over the parietal lobe, avoiding retraction of the occipital lobe and possible visual deficits. A larger craniotomy is desirable so that it allows for more flexibility in choosing an approach that avoids the bridging veins. The dura is opened in a U-shaped fashion

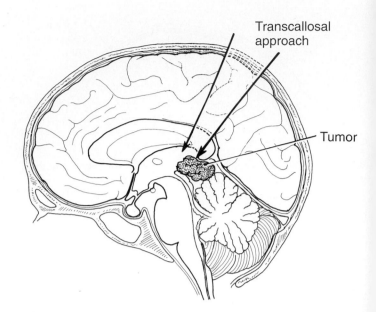

Fig. 7. Sagittal diagram demonstrating the transcallosal-interhemispheric approach.

and reflected toward the sagittal sinus. The interhemispheric fissure is inspected and bridging veins are evaluated. It is rarely possible to achieve the exposure necessary without sacrificing at least one bridging vein; however, it is undesirable to sacrifice more than one. Even a small exposure provides a wide angle because the tumors are deeply seated. The hemisphere is covered with protective padding, such as Telfa, and a retractor is placed in the interhemispheric fissure to gently retract the hemisphere laterally. If necessary, a retractor can be placed on the falx to provide additional exposure. The falx can be divided inferiorly if necessary to facilitate retraction of the left hemisphere.

The operating microscope is brought in at this point and the corpus callosum is easily identified by its white appearance. The pericallosal arteries are identified and are carefully retracted to avoid injury. An opening of approximately 2 cm is made in the midline of the corpus callosum. The opening is made anterior to the splenium, although we have had patients with large tumors in whom the splenium was opened without any neurological deficit. The corpus callosum is generally thinned out and callosotomy should not result in any measurable neurological deficit.

The tumor is usually readily identified by its vascular appearance following the opening in the corpus callosum. The internal cerebral veins are identified just below the corpus callosum and over the dorsal surface of the tumor. Every effort must be made to avoid injuring these vascular structures. At this point the tumor is internally debulked and subsequent tumor removal is as previously described for the infratentorial supracerebellar approach.

Occipital-Transtentorial Approach. The occipital-transtentorial approach is simply a more posterior approach than the transcallosal approach with several important caveats (29,42). A three-quarter prone position is generally preferred providing an oblique trajectory, which must be kept in mind to avoid disorienting the surgeon. It is usually not necessary to divide any part of the corpus callosum with this approach. By dividing the tentorium, however, an excellent exposure is provided to

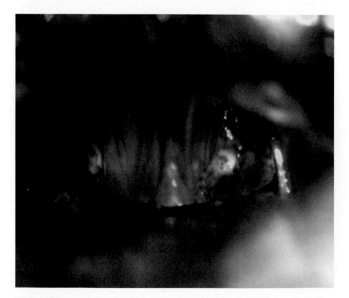

Fig. 6. Operative photo showing view into the third ventricle after the tumor has been resected.

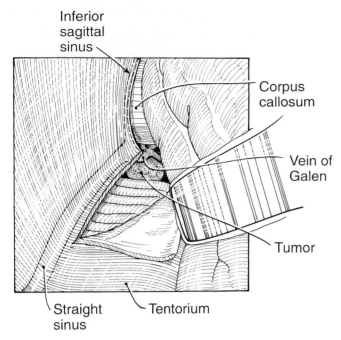

Fig. 8. Diagram demonstrating surgical view via the occipital-trans-tentorial approach.

the pineal region and quadrigeminal plate (Fig. 8). A linear or U-shaped incision can be used to facilitate placement of a craniotomy centered just above the torcular. A burr hole is made in the sagittal sinus just above the torcular with another placed over the sagittal sinus 6 to 10 cm above this. Bringing the craniotomy across the sagittal sinus makes it easier to retract the occipital lobe. The occipital lobe is covered with padding such as Telfa, and a retractor is used to gently retract the occipital pole from the falx and tentorium along the line of the straight sinus. The operating microscope is brought into place and the tentorium is divided adjacent to the straight sinus, extending to the incisura. At this point there is an excellent view of the tumor, quadrigeminal plate, and vein of Galen extending from the deep venous system. The tumor is visualized similar to the infra-tentorial-supracerebellar approach, although the angle is slightly more oblique and there is a better view of the quadrigeminal plate and its interface with the tumor. The tumor removal proceeds as previously described.

Postoperative Care

The most significant immediate postoperative problems include bleeding within the tumor bed and hydrocephalus (23,35). It is critical to be vigilant in the immediate postoperative period to aggressively treat these potentially reversible problems. It is necessary to obtain a CT scan at the earliest sign of an impending problem. Careful monitoring of the neurological examination is essential but can be difficult because air within the third ventricle or subdural space may result in blunting of mental status. Patients with incompletely removed tumors are at risk for problems related to obstructive hydrocephalus. Patients previously shunted or with third ventriculostomy can be compromised by operative debris. Prompt diagnostic scanning and placement of a ventricular drain is essential to avoid complications from this treatable condition. Patients should remain on

high doses of steroids until their clinical condition is stable. Early ambulation and mobilization are encouraged.

Complications

The majority of patients have some degree of impairment of extraocular movements, notably limited upgaze and convergence (23,35). Impaired pupillary response can cause difficulty with focusing. These problems are generally transient and resolve within several days to weeks. Permanent compromise is rare although many patients have some impaired upgaze, which is of limited clinical consequence. Extraocular movement problems tend to be more common in patients who already had significant impairment preoperatively.

Ataxia sometimes is seen and is likely related to cerebellar retraction. This problem also tends to resolve within a couple of days and most patients are fully ambulatory by the time they are discharged.

Complications related to brainstem trauma should be avoided but often are associated with invasive tumors. This can lead to cognitive impairment, which in extreme forms can result in akinetic mutism. Such brainstem problems also can be the result of cerebellar swelling and increased posterior fossa pressure. This problem is more common in patients with previous surgery or radiation therapy in addition to higher frequency with invasive tumors.

Complications related to brain retraction can occur when the supratentorial approach has been used (42,44). In the parietal region, this can cause contralateral sensory or stereognostic deficits and occasionally, hemiparesis. Seizure prophylaxis is desirable for a short time after surgery, although long-term use is not necessary. These complications can be the result of brain retraction or sacrifice of bridging veins. Fortunately, most deficits that occur are temporary. Similarly, occipital lobe retraction can result in visual field deficits (29,45). Disconnection syndromes can occur if the splenium has been divided; however, it is rare that this complication is related to simply opening the corpus callosum (42).

Complications relating to positioning can include subdural hematomas, hygromas, or ventricular collapse (35,44). These conditions generally are self-limiting.

Surgical Outcome

Advances in surgical technique have improved results for patients undergoing surgery by experienced surgeons (23,46). The surgeon's degree of experience correlates with improved outcome. The use of modern microsurgical technique should result in an operative mortality ranging from 0% to 8%, with permanent morbidity from 0% to 12%. Patients with benign encapsulated tumors such as teratomas, pineocytomas, pilocytic astrocytomas, and dermoid tumors can expect a complete removal with minimal complications. Although the degree of encapsulation may be less in a patient with a malignant tumor, many times these tumors can be aggressively removed, thereby avoiding the risk of postoperative bleeding, improving the likelihood that hydrocephalus will resolve, and improving the response to adjuvant therapy.

Postoperative Workup

Patients should have an MRI scan with gadolinium within 72 hours after surgery so that a baseline can be established to determine the completeness of resection (10,46). If tumor markers are elevated preoperatively, they should be evaluated in the postoperative period. Patients with malignant tumors, particularly of pineal cell, germ cell, or ependymoma origin, should have a spinal MRI to look for spinal seeding. Overall, the incidence of spinal seeding is relatively low, but if present it represents a poor prognostic sign and suggests the need for spinal radiation.

Adjuvant Therapy

Benign tumors that have been completely removed require no additional treatment but should be monitored closely with yearly MRI scans. Patients with malignant tumors require radiation therapy (10,46–49). Generally this consists of 5,500 cGy given in 180-cGy daily fractions with 4,000 cGy to the ventricular system and an additional 1,500 cGy to the tumor bed. Malignant germ cell tumors may benefit from chemotherapy as well (10). Tumors such as germinomas are highly sensitive to radiation, and radiation can be curative in many instances. A careful evaluation of the histology should be determined and the adjuvant therapy plan individualized for each patient. Radiosurgery sometimes can be beneficial; however, the indications from limited long-term follow-up are not known with certainty (15, 50).

Conclusions

Recent advances have improved the outcome for patients with pineal region tumors. Surgery is a mainstay of management because it allows establishment of an accurate diagnosis as well as facilitating tumor removal. A variety of surgical options have been developed carefully and offer many possibilities for the safe removal of these tumors. An advanced degree of comfort and experience with microsurgical technique is essential to avoid potential pitfalls and complications of this surgery.

References

1. Bruce JN. Management of pineal region tumors. *Neurosurg Quart* 1993;3:103–119.
2. Bruce J, Connolly E, Stein B. Pineal and germ cell tumors. In: Kaye A, Laws E, eds. *Brain tumors: an encyclopedic approach,* 2nd ed. London: Churchill Livingstone, 2001.
3. Sano K. Pineal region tumors: problems in pathology and treatment. *Clin Neurosurg* 1984;30:59–89.
4. Horowitz MB, Hall WA. Central nervous system germinomas. *Arch Neurol* 1991;48:652–657.
5. Lee DH, Norman D, Newton TH. MR imaging of pineal cysts. *J Comput Assist Tomogr* 1987;II:586–590.
6. Fetell MR, Bruce JN, Burke AM, et al. Non-neoplastic pineal cysts. *Neurology* 1991;41:1034–1040.
7. Müller-Forell W, Schroth G, Egan PJ. MR imaging in tumors of the pineal region. *Neuroradiology* 1988;30:224–231.
8. Tien RD, Barkovich AJ, Edwards MSB. M.R. imaging of pineal tumors. *AJNR* 1990;11:557–565.
9. Allen JC, Nisselbaum J, Epstein F, et al. Alpha-fetoprotein and human chorionic gonadotropin determination in cerebrospinal fluid. An aid to the diagnosis and management of intracranial germ-cell tumors. *J Neurosurg* 1979;51:368–374.
10. Allen JC, Bruce JN, Kun LE, et al. Pineal region tumors. In: Levin VA, ed. *Cancer in the nervous system.* New York: Churchill Livingstone, 1996:171–186.
11. Bjornsson J, Scheithauer B, Okazaki H, et al. Intracranial germ cell tumors: pathobiological and immunohistochemical aspects of 70 cases. *J Neuropathol Exp Neurol* 1985;44:32–46.
12. Herrmann H-D, Westphal M, Winkler K, et al. Treatment of non-germinomatous germ-cell tumors of the pineal region. *Neurosurgery* 1994;34:524–529.
13. Goodman R. Magnetic resonance imaging-directed stereotactic endoscopic third ventriculostomy. *Neurosurgery* 1993;32:1043–1047.
14. Edwards MSB, Hudgins RJ, Wilson CB, et al. Pineal region tumors in children. *J Neurosurg* 1988;66:689–697.
15. Dempsey PK, Kondziolka D, Lunsford LD. Stereotactic diagnosis and treatment of pineal region tumours and vascular malformations. *Acta Neurochir (Wien)* 1992;116:14–22.
16. Kreth F, Schatz C, Pagenstecher A, et al. Stereotactic management of lesions of the pineal region. *Neurosurgery* 1996;39:280–291.
17. Regis J, Bouillot P, Rouby-Volot F, et al. Pineal region tumors and the role of stereotactic biopsy: review of the mortality, morbidity, and diagnostic rates in 370 cases. *Neurosurgery* 1996;39:907–914.
18. Chandrasoma PT, Smith MM, Apuzzo MLJ. Stereotactic biopsy in the diagnosis of brain masses: comparison of results of biopsy and resected surgical specimen. *Neurosurgery* 1989;24:160–165.
19. Peragut JC, Dupard T, Graziani N, et al. De la prévention des risques de la biopsie stéréotaxique de certaines tumeurs de la région pinéale: a propos de 3 observations. *Neurochirurgie* 1987;33:23–27.
20. Pecker J, Scarabin J-M, Vallee B, et al. Treatment in tumours of the pineal region: value of stereotaxic biopsy. *Surg Neurol* 1979;12:341–348.
21. Sano K. Diagnosis and treatment of tumours in the pineal region. *Acta Neurochir* 1976;34:153–157.
22. Lapras C, Patet JD. Controversies, techniques and strategies for pineal tumor surgery. In: Apuzzo MLJ, ed. *Surgery of the third ventricle.* Baltimore: Williams & Wilkins, 1987:649–662.
23. Bruce JN, Stein BM. Surgical management pineal region tumors. *Acta Neurochirurgica (Wien)* 1995;134:130–135.
24. Maciunas R. Stereotactic biopsy of pineal region lesions. In: Kaye A, Black P, eds. *Operative neurosurgery.* London: Churchill Livingstone, 2000:841–848.
25. Oka K, Kin Y, Go Y, et al. Neuroendoscopic approach to tectal tumors: a consecutive series. *J Neurosurgery* 1999;91:964–970.
26. Gaab MR, Schroeder HW. Neuroendoscopic approach to intraventricular lesions. *J Neurosurg* 1998;88:496–505.
27. Ferrer E, Santamarta D, Garcia-Fructuoso G, et al. Neuroendoscopic management of pineal region tumours. *Acta Neurochir* 1997;139:12–20.
28. Stein BM. The infratentorial supracerebellar approach to pineal lesions. *J Neurosurg* 1971;35:197–202.
29. Lapras C, Patet JD, Mottolese C, et al. Direct surgery of pineal tumors: occipital-transtentorial approach. *Prog Exp Tumor Res* 1987;30:268–280.
30. Dandy WE. An operation for the removal of pineal tumors. *Surg Gynecol Obstet* 1921;XXXIII:113119.
31. Dandy WE. Operative experience in cases of pineal tumor. *Arch Surg* 1936;33:19–46.
32. Van Wagenen WP. A surgical approach for the removal of certain pineal tumors. *Surg Gynecol Obstet* 1931;53:216–220.
33. McComb JG, Apuzzo MLJ. The lateral decubitus position for the surgical approach to pineal location tumors. *Concepts Pediat Neurosurg* 1988;8:186–199.
34. Bruce JN, Fetell MR, Stein BM. Surgical approaches to pineal tumors. In: Wilkins RH, Rengachary SS, eds. *Neurosurgery.* New York: McGraw-Hill, 1996:1023–1033.
35. Bruce J, Stein B. Supracerebellar approaches in the pineal region. In: Apuzzo M, ed. Brain surgery: complication avoidance and management. New York: Churchill-Livingstone, 1993:511–536.
36. Reid WS, Clark WK. Comparison of the infratentorial and transtentorial approaches to the pineal region. *Neurosurgery* 1978;3:1–8.

37. McComb J, Apuzzo M. Posterior intrahemispheric retrocallosal and transcallosal approaches. In: Apuzzo M, ed. *Surgery of the third ventricle.* Baltimore: Williams & Wilkins, 1987:611–641.

38. Kobayashi S, Sugita K, Tanaka Y, et al. Infratentorial approach to the pineal region in the prone position: Concorde position. *J Neurosurg* 1983;58:141–143.

39. Ausman JI, Malik GM, Dujovny M, et al. Three-quarter prone approach to the pineal-tentorial region. *Surg Neurol* 1988;29:298–306.

40. Bruce JN, Stein BM. Infratentorial supracerebellar approach. In: Apuzzo MLJ, ed. *Surgery of the third ventricle,* 2nd ed. Baltimore: Williams & Wilkins, 1998:697–719.

41. Bruce J. Posterior third ventricular tumors. In: Kaye A, Black P, eds. *Operative neurosurgery.* London: Churchill Livingstone, 2000: 769–775.

42. Apuzzo M, Tung H. Supratentorial approaches to the pineal region. In: Apuzzo M, ed. *Brain surgery: complication avoidance and management.* New York: Churchill-Livingstone, 1993:486–511.

43. McComb J, Levy M, Apuzzo M. The posterior intrahemispheric retrocallosal and transcallosal approaches to the third ventricle region. In: Apuzzo M, ed. *Surgery of the third ventricle,* 2nd ed. Baltimore: Williams & Wilkins, 1998:743–777.

44. Bruce JN, Stein BM. Complications of surgery for pineal region tumors. In: Post KD, Friedman ED, McCormick PC, eds. *Postoperative complications in intracranial neurosurgery.* New York: Thieme, 1993:74–86.

45. Nazzaro JM, Shults WT, Neuwelt EA. Neuro-ophthalmological function of patients with pineal region tumors approached transtentorially in the semisitting position. *J Neurosurg* 1992;76:746–751.

46. Bruce J. Pineal tumors. In: Winn H, ed. *Youman's neurological surgery,* 5th ed. Philadelphia: WB Saunders, in press.

47. Sung DI, Harisiadis L, Chang CH. Midline pineal tumors and suprasellar germinomas: highly curable by irradiation. *Radiology* 1978; 128:745–751.

48. Linstadt D, Wara WM, Edwards MSB, et al. Radiotherapy of primary intracranial germinomas: the case against routine craniospinal irradiation. *Int J Radiat Oncol Biol Phys* 1988;15:291–297.

49. Matsutani M, Sano K, Takakura K, et al. Primary intracranial germ cell tumors: a clinical analysis of 153 histologically verified cases. *J Neurosurg* 1997;86:446–455.

50. Casentini L, Colombo F, Pozza F, et al. Combined radiosurgery and external radiotherapy of intracranial germinomas. *Surg Neurol* 1990; 34:79–86.

113. Brain Metastasis

**Yashail Y. Vora and
Raymond Sawaya**

Metastasis refers to the spread of malignant tumor cells from a primary neoplasm to distant tissues to form new growths (1). Intracranial metastases can deposit tumor in the extraaxial compartment (e.g., involving the skull and dura or the leptomeninges and subarachnoid space, which is addressed in a separate chapter), or more commonly in the intraaxial compartment leading to intraparenchymal brain metastasis. Rarely intracranial oncotic aneurysms may arise (2). A *single* brain metastasis refers to a single cerebral lesion that has arisen outside the central nervous system, without any reference to the systemic status, whereas *solitary* brain metastasis describes a single brain lesion without evidence of metastatic spread elsewhere in the body. *Multiple* brain metastases imply the presence of more than one brain metastasis, also without alluding to the presence or absence of any extracranial disease. The purpose of this chapter is to provide a concise yet current evidence-based review of intraparenchymal brain metastasis, using previously published guidelines for evaluating medical literature (3).

Epidemiology

Interpretation of incidence studies of brain tumors is undermined by variation in the diagnostic modalities employed, a low percentage of histological confirmation of diagnosis, and selection bias (4–6). Some of the most recent population-based studies suggest that brain metastases are the most common *adult* intracranial neoplasms, comprising slightly more than half and outnumbering primary tumors; however, this statistic is contested by some (7–10). Nevertheless, the diagnosis of metastasis has undoubtedly risen over the past 20 years, partly from advances in diagnostic technology, namely magnetic resonance imaging (MRI), and partly owing to longer survival (11,12). About 20% to 40% of patients with systemic malignancies suffer brain metastasis with the peak incidence occurring between the ages 50 to 60 years and without predisposition by gender (13–20). The former figure varies markedly, depending on the histology. For example, less than 1% to 2% of ovarian and prostate cancers spread to the brain in contrast to 50% or more of bronchial carcinomas and melanomas (21–24). Approximately 75% to 85% of lesions are located supratentorially and 15% to 25% infratentorially. About two-thirds of the lesions are multiple, based on MR imaging (18,21,25–27). The most common primary source is the lung (40% to 60%) followed by breast (15% to 20%) and melanoma (10% to 20%), depending on whether it is a clinical or autopsy series. Colorectal and renal cell carcinomas account for 5% to 10% each. The preceding five sources are responsible for 85% to 90% of cerebral metastases (13,15, 16,18,26). Melanoma has the highest propensity to metastasize to the brain. Among lung tumors, adenocarcinoma, followed by squamous cell carcinoma, are the most common culprits, accounting for 50% to 75% of lung primaries with small-cell lung carcinoma (SCLC) comprising 10% to 20% (13,28,29). Prostate carcinoma has a particular propensity to form dural based metastases (Fig. 1). Intracerebral metastases are rare among children and occur in less than 5% of pediatric malignancies (30–33). The most common sources are neuroblastoma, Wilms tumor, sarcoma (especially, rhabdomyosarcoma), and melanoma.

Pathophysiology

The mode of spread to the brain is almost always hematogenous through the arterial circulation; however, venous spread via the

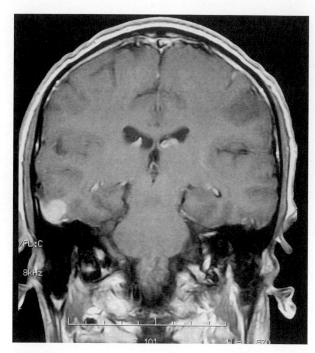

Fig. 1. Gadolinium-enhanced, T1-weighted coronal MRI. Dural-based right inferior temporal metastasis from prostate carcinoma in a 44-year-old man.

spinal epidural Batson's plexus also has been proposed as a possible mechanism (33,34). Metastases themselves can be a source of tumor emboli resulting in a "cascade" of metastases elsewhere (13,35,36). Primary tumors are biologically heterogenous. The metastatic process is highly selective for preexisting subpopulations of cells that possess the biological prerequisites for favorable interactions with host microenvironment and homeostatic mechanisms that allow these cells to segregate from the parent tumor and migrate to distant sites where they can evolve into new growths. Paget's "seed and soil" theory is the generally accepted explanation for the observation that metastatic spread of specific tumors occurs in specific patterns and is not a random process (32,37,38). The essential steps in the formation of a metastatic lesion include tumor cell adhesion to the local extracellular matrix, cell locomotion, and proteolysis, allowing invasion into lymphatics, venules, and capillaries followed by hematogenous embolism to a distant site, whereas the tumor cells interact with various blood components such as platelets in order to survive the hostile environment of the circulation. Once again, adhesion and extravasation must take place in the new host vascular bed followed by tissue invasion. If the new host environment ("soil") is conducive to proliferation of these cells ("seed"), then metastasis is established. Angiogenesis is a critical step without which the tumor mass cannot exceed about 2 mm in diameter. Evasion of host immune mechanisms also must occur. None of the preceding processes is novel or unique to tumor cells; instead, they represent an alteration of normal homeostatic processes that are routinely active during growth of the human embryo, tissue renewal, and injury repair. Fidler demonstrated that fewer than 0.1% of tumor cells survive to potentially evolve into a metastatic lesion 24 hours after entry into the circulation because failure to complete any one of the preceding steps eliminates the neoplastic cells (1,39–41).

Clinical Features

At least two thirds of patients with cerebral metastases experience neurological symptoms. The three most common symptoms are headaches, focal deficits (e.g., weakness or dysphasia), and higher cognitive dysfunction. The latter is found in the majority of patients with detailed testing and may not be obvious by history alone (27,42,43). The symptoms largely reflect intracranial hypertension or neurological dysfunction, depending on the location of the lesion(s). For example, patients may present with behavioral changes with frontal lobe involvement or gait ataxia and poor coordination resulting from a cerebellar lesion. Frontal and parietal lobes are the most common locations, whereas the brainstem and pituitary gland only rarely are invaded. Usually the presentation is subacute and progressive with the symptoms dating back over days to several weeks. However, the patient may present acutely as a result of a seizure or a vascular event. Partial or generalized seizures occur in 10% to 20% of patients and are more common with multiple metastases and melanoma (19,42–47). Vascular events include hemorrhage into the tumor or ischemic stroke from vessel compression or nonbacterial thrombotic endocarditis. Overt hemorrhage into the tumor may complicate 5% to 15% of patients, and even though it may occur with any neoplasm, three primaries are particularly prone to bleeding: melanoma (40%), renal cell (70%), and choriocarcinoma (virtually 100%). However, for an intracerebral hemorrhage caused by a possible secondary lesion, the cause is most likely bronchial or breast carcinoma simply because they are the most prevalent overall (16, 24,42,48–50). Hence, the differential diagnosis of multiple intracerebral hematomas bilaterally includes hemorrhagic metastases (e.g., choriocarcinoma or melanoma), bleeding disorder, venous sinus thrombosis, which itself may result from an underlying malignancy (Fig. 2). On imaging, substantial vasogenic edema surrounding a *recent* hematoma not more than a few hours old may serve as a clue to a malignancy underlying the hematoma. Cerebral ischemia rarely can occur from embolization of cardiac vegetations or vessel thrombosis from an associated hypercoagulopathy (42). Weight loss and cachexia may be evident in patients with disseminated cancer.

Investigations

Neuroimaging of the brain in the form of plain and enhanced computed tomography (CT) scan or preferably MRI scan is the initial diagnostic modality of choice. Gadolinium-enhanced MRI is the most sensitive test available for detecting cerebral metastasis, even when compared to double-dose delayed contrast CT, which in turn is more sensitive than standard contrast CT. This is especially true for disclosing small and multiple lesions (36,48,49).

COMPUTED TOMOGRAPHY. On plain CT most metastases are isodense with abundant surrounding hypodense vasogenic edema that is often strikingly disproportionate to their size. A homogenous hyperdense appearance in a lesion without any evidence of hemorrhage usually signifies the presence of melanin (*melanotic* melanoma), mucin-secreting tumors (e.g., colorectal and bronchial adenocarcinoma), or a high nucleus-to-cytoplasmic ratio in a hypercellular tumor (e.g., SCLC). A hypodense cystic component may be present (51–55).

MRI. On non-enhanced T1-weighted MR image most metastases are slightly hypointense to isointense compared to gray matter and they are surrounded by hypointense edema. The lesions are usually hyperintense on T2. Cysts and edema are markedly hyperintense. Differentiating hemorrhagic metastases from nonneoplastic causes often is difficult. Nonhemorrhagic enhancing areas, an incomplete T2 hypointense hemosiderin ring, and persistent edema are suggestive of the former. Almost all metastases enhance on CT and MRI, but the pattern may be variable, ranging from densely homogenous to heterogenous or a ring pattern, and on MRI it must be distinguished from the heterogenous signal characteristics caused by hemorrhage. Rarely small lesions may not enhance, signifying the relative preservation of the blood–brain barrier. On MRI *melanotic* melanoma (unlike *amelanotic* melanoma) and adenocarcinoma usually are relatively hyperintense on T1 and isointense or hypointense on T2 even in the absence of hemorrhage (Fig. 3) (52–54). Mucinous secretions have been shown to be unrelated to the MRI appearance of adenocarcinomas, which may originate from diverse primaries such as lung, breast, or the gastrointestinal tract (56).

CT and MRI characteristics that favor the diagnosis of metastasis include multiple well-circumscribed lesions that enhance and are located at the gray–white matter junction, often in watershed territories such as the parieto-occipital junction, with abundant surrounding vasogenic edema (Fig. 4). Their predilection for the preceding locations is felt to be the result of tumor emboli precipitation in end arterioles and capillaries (43,57). Metastases from melanoma, choriocarcinoma, and SCLC are most likely to be multiple, whereas single metastases are most likely to arise from breast, thyroid, renal cell, and colon carcinoma as well as adenocarcinoma of the lung. The rim of the ring-enhancing lesion is typically thick and irregular unlike in abscesses, resolving hematomas, or demyelinating lesions. Metastases on occasion may be calcified; this may portend a more benign course (58). Despite all the preceding guidelines, the only reliable rule is that exceptions are possible and false-negatives as well as -positives are common. In one study, the diagnosis of a single brain metastasis using MR imaging was shown to be erroneous following resection or stereotactic biopsy in 11% of patients with systemic cancer (59). In another study, only 15% of patients with multiple brain lesions evaluated with CT or MRI and without evidence of neoplasms outside the nervous system had metastasis based on stereotactic biopsy (60). Differential diagnoses that can mimic metastases include glioma, abscess, encephalitis, demyelinating lesion, ischemic in-

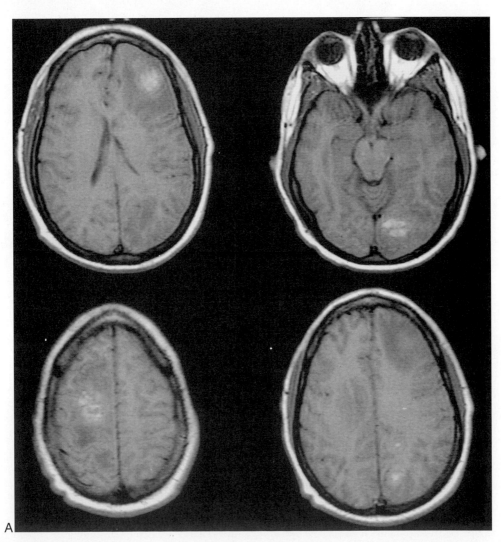

Fig. 2. Multiple hemorrhagic brain metastases from choriocarcinoma in a 31-year-old man. **A:** Nonenhanced axial T1-weighted MRI. *Figure continues.*

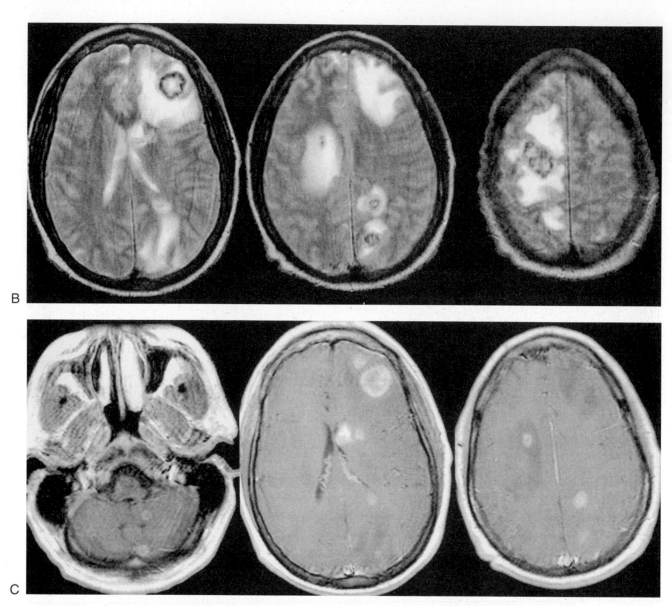

Fig. 2. *Continued.* **B:** T2-weighted axial MRI. **C:** Gadolinium-enhanced T1-weighted axial MRI.

farct, resolving hematoma, and radiation necrosis (36,53, 61–64). Multifocal demyelinating lesions resembling metastases in reaction to a regimen of levamisole and 5-FU (administered to patients with stage III colon adenocarcinoma) have been reported (65). Other diagnostic strategies may aid in establishing the pathology because of diagnostic dilemmas arising from these possibilities.

Increasing the gadolinium dose from 0.1 to 0.3 mmol/kg increases the MRI sensitivity for the number and size of lesions. The resolution of the study also is enhanced. Delayed imaging following a second gadolinium dose after 30 minutes also aids detection of small lesions less than 5 mm (54). However, the role of these additional maneuvers in clinical practice is unclear because increased detection of minute subclinical lesions has not been shown to improve outcome (66,67). Moreover, the threshold of detection requiring a change in management also remains to be established because patients with a single radiologically evident metastasis may harbor additional microscopic disease that remains invisible even with triple-dose, delayed gadolinium-enhanced MR imaging. Single-photon emission CT,

positron emission tomography, diffusion MRI, and magnetic resonance spectroscopy may help distinguish metastasis from its mimics (54,65,68). Cerebrospinal fluid (CSF) and serum carcinoembryonic antigen (CEA) and beta-human chorionic gonadotropin (HCG) have been shown to be of diagnostic utility in some cases (13,69,70). In one study CSF CEA had a sensitivity of 31% but a specificity of 90% (70). However, the routine use of CSF CEA levels is not useful. Beta-HCG serves as a useful marker of germ cell tumors.

UNKNOWN PRIMARY. Approximately 20% to 40% of patients with symptomatic cerebral metastasis present with previously undiagnosed primaries in the modern era (44,46,59,71, 72). Investigations should be tailored to the most statistically probable primaries, namely lung, breast, melanoma, colorectal, and renal cell carcinoma. They also should be geared to the clinical findings. An anteroposterior and lateral chest x-ray (CXR) is the single most useful and accessible study and up to 97% of patients with bronchial carcinoma demonstrate an

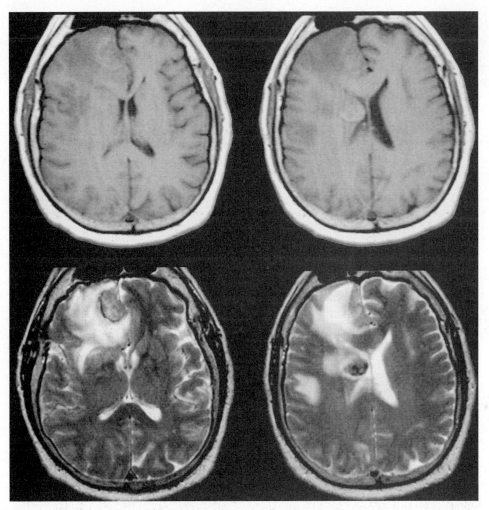

Fig. 3. Melanotic melanoma brain metastases in a 56-year-old man. The lesions exhibit hyperintensity on T1-weighted *(top)* and hypointensity on T2-weighted *(bottom)* axial MRIs.

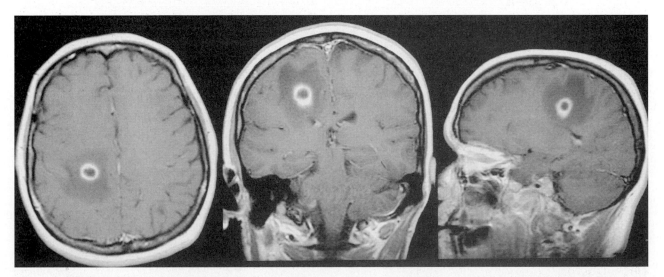

Fig. 4. Gadolinium-enhanced T1-weighted MRI. A single brain metastasis is located in the deep white matter underlying the right motor cortex. This metastatic breast carcinoma lesion presented with left hemiparesis in a 36-year-old woman and was treated with radiosurgery.

abnormality on the CXR (71). Although breast is one of the most common primary sources of brain metastases overall, it is conspicuously uncommon among this patient group and more than 80% of patients with previously unknown primaries subsequently are found to harbor bronchial (65% to 70%), gastrointestinal, or renal carcinoma, or melanoma. Melanoma lesions are most commonly found on the trunk or lower limbs. In general a CXR, mammogram (in women), urinalysis, complete blood count, and routine blood chemistry should be obtained. If these tests are fruitless, then a CT scan of the chest, abdomen, and pelvis should be undertaken. It can suggest the diagnosis or provide additional helpful clues in 25% to 30% of patients; moreover, it can be useful for ruling out systemic disease because false negatives are uncommon (46,55,71). Unexplained anemia may warrant colonoscopy. Bone scan reveals metastatic lesions to the skeletal system. It has a low yield if the preceding studies are negative but in the few positive cases it may offer alternative sites for biopsy in the hunt for the primary. In the absence of any accessible extracranial tumor, stereotactic biopsy or resection of the cerebral tumor should be undertaken to confirm the diagnosis prior to definitive treatment because other lesions imitating metastasis are common (47,59,60). Histological examination of cerebral lesions most commonly reveals adenocarcinoma but rarely points to the specific organ of origin (73). Even after all above investigations the primary tumor may remain undiagnosed until new signs arise on prolonged follow-up in about 15% of patients. Autopsy may be required to determine the primary tumor type in another about 15% of patients. Even an autopsy may be unrevealing in 2% to 3% of patients (19,46,71).

Treatment

Two decades ago the mainstays of management included steroids and fractionated external beam whole brain radiation treatment (RT) (74). The management of this entity has become complex and controversial in the current era of burgeoning medical literature and advances. The current principal options for the treatment of cerebral metastasis include RT, surgery, and radiosurgery (RS). It is more imperative than ever to critically apprise the growing number of studies for the weight and quality of scientific evidence they present in order to make sound clinical decisions. To this end the American Association of Neurological Surgeons (AANS) has adopted a classification scheme for the levels of evidence for various therapeutic options in the literature (3,75). The following overview, guided by the preceding system, attempts to provide a current evidence-based outline of the various treatment alternatives.

MEDICAL MANAGEMENT. Steroids have been used since the 1950s to treat brain tumor patients (74,76–81). Dexamethasone is most commonly employed because of its high glucocorticoid potency and minimal mineralocorticoid activity. The usual dose of 16 mg per day (4 mg q.i.d.) following a bolus of 10 mg finds its roots in the largely arbitrary doses thought to be beneficial during early studies of the drug. There is ample evidence that the dose required for a satisfactory response varies considerably among patients, ranging from about 3 to 96 mg per day, and once benefit is achieved its magnitude varies little by increasing the dose, unlike the adverse effects, which are amplified (74,77–83). One randomized study showed that the improvement at 1 week was comparable between daily doses of 4, 8, and 16 mg (82). Clinical improvement is noted in 60% to 80% of patients, often within 8 to 12 hours of starting steroids but the peak effects may not be realized for 5 to 7 days.

The mechanism of action has not yet been entirely elucidated, but it appears to be mediated mainly through stabilization of the leaky blood–brain barrier and reduction in the extravasated sodium, water, and protein constituting vasogenic edema surrounding metastatic lesions. However, this may take several days; hence, the more immediate benefits may be mediated through a separate mechanism. Other postulated mechanisms include improvement of local blood flow, local vasoconstriction, direct oncolytic effects on the tumor, and diminution of CSF production (47,80,83,84). Glucocorticoids in two to four times daily divided doses should be considered standard treatment beginning at the time of diagnosis (Class I evidence). Most patients can be tapered off this medication over several weeks following definitive treatment.

Seizures should be treated with anticonvulsants such as phenytoin. There is no evidence that prophylactic anticonvulsants reduce the incidence of seizures or improve outcome in this patient population. One case-control study showed the absence of any benefit (44). In the absence of any demonstrable advantage and given its potential side effects, limited Class II evidence suggests as a guideline that anticonvulsants be withheld until the time of first seizure or the availability of Class I evidence to the contrary (43–45). A randomized controlled trial (RCT) investigating this issue is currently underway at The University of Texas M.D. Anderson Cancer Center (M.D. Anderson). Dexamethasone and anticonvulsants such as phenytoin or phenobarbital reduce each other's levels by inducing hepatic microsomal enzymes that hasten the metabolism of the drugs; therefore, anticonvulsant levels should be monitored and the doses for all such drugs may need to be increased (27,81,85).

SINGLE BRAIN METASTASIS. Patients with brain metastasis assume a steady downhill course without any treatment, with a median survival of about 1 month. The addition of steroids improves the median survival to about 2 months. Historically, RT alone has been the preferred treatment for most patients, resulting in temporary symptomatic amelioration in 60% to 80% of patients and improving median survival to 3 to 6 months (35, 59,74,86–91). Prior to the first RCT in 1990 addressing surgery, several retrospective case series suggested a survival benefit for patients with single metastasis undergoing resection followed by RT (19,74,92,93). Table 1 summarizes the three RCTs to date comparing surgery plus RT with RT alone (59,72,94). The results by Patchell and associates and Vecht and associates are quite similar and confirm a significant benefit of surgery on overall survival as well as the quality of life. Improvement in the functional quality of life lasts up to 1 to 3 months short of the total survival (46,47,59,94). Local recurrence and death from neurological dysfunction also was significantly diminished according to the first study. Obviously brain surgery does not impact systemic progression of cancer, which is the cause of death in majority of patients and the single most important prognostic factor in these patients (19,27,74,76,95–100). In Vecht's study, the survival advantage of patients in the surgery group vanished with progressive systemic cancer. With systemically controlled cancer, death from progressive neurological disease becomes important and this is where surgery has a major role to play. Only in those with controlled systemic disease is local cure likely to translate into a longer and more functional survival. Herein lies the likely explanation for the lack of positive results in the study by Mintz and colleagues, in which almost half the patients had disseminated disease. Also, patients with lower Karnofsky Performance Scale (KPS) score of 50 to 69 were included, reflecting a generally more advanced status of the cancer in this study population. Moreover, they reported protocol violations, including failure to receive the allocated treatment, in a quarter of the enrollees. Although the two study groups were comparable in all three trials, the higher extracranial bur-

Table 1. Comparison of the Three Randomized Clinical Trials Evaluating the Role of Surgery

	Patchell, 1990 (59)	Vecht, 1993 (94)	Mintz, 1996 (72)
Number	48	63	84
Inclusion criteria	≥18 years old, single lesion, Karnofsky ≥70, lesion accessible, no LMD or highly radiosensitive tumors[a]	≥18 years old, single lesion, function level[b] ≥2, life expectancy >6 months, no LMD/SCLC/lymphoma	<80 years old, single lesion, Karnofsy ≥50, no deep lesion/LMD/SCLC/lymphoma/leukemia/nonmelanoma skin cancer
Median time to diagnosis	4 weeks (RT group) 8 weeks (surgery group)	Not specified	89.4 weeks (RT group) 62.3 weeks (surgery group)
Disseminated cancer	37.5% of patients (18/48)	31.7% of patients (20/63)	45.2% of patients (38/84)
Imaging modality	MRI	CT	CT
Histological verification in RT group	Yes, stereotactic biopsy	No	Not routinely, biopsy only if diagnosis uncertain on CT
Protocol violations	None	Two Patients lost to follow-up; one patient in RT group had glioma	10 (surgery group) + 11 (RT group) = 21
Time before treatment	Surgery within 3 d, RT within 2 wk (postop) or 2 d (if primary treatment)	RT within 3 wk postop, otherwise not specified	Surgery within mean 5.3 days/SD 3.1 d, RT within 4 wk (postop) or mean 10.5 d/SD 6.4 d (primary treatment)
RT regimen	36 Gy, 12 fractions	40 Gy, 2 Gy per fraction twice a day	30 Gy, 10 fractions
Follow-up	CT 2–5 days postop, clinical + CT or MRI q 3 mo	Clinical only q 1 mo	Clinical + CT q 1 mo
Outcome	With surgery, survival longer (40 vs. 15 wk), longer FIS (38 vs. 8 wk), lower local recurrence (20% vs. 52%)	With surgery, survival longer (10 vs. 6 mo), longer FIS (7.5 vs. 3.5 mo)	No significant difference in survival (about 6 mo) or quality of life scores between the two groups

[a] SCLC, germ cell tumors, lymphoma, leukemia, multiple myeloma.
[b] Based on five-point World Health Organization scale and a four-point neurological scale.
LMD, leptomeningeal disease; SCLC, small-cell lung carcinoma; SD, standard deviation; FIS, functionally independent survival; RT whole-brain radiation treatment.

den of disease among the patients in the last study tended to curtail the lifespan in both groups, as indicated by a shorter median survival of about 6 months in both groups, thereby obviating the potential benefits of surgery from being realized in that group of patients. This is partly evidenced by the premature death or deterioration of eight patients, even before their allocated treatment could be completed. Thus, the results of this study concur with the conclusions of the previous two trials that proper patient selection is key to avoiding an unnecessary operation. Class I evidence suggests that three variables should be considered when selecting patients with a single metastasis for resection: (a) the patient's clinical status, (b) the surgical accessibility of the tumor, and (c) its radiosensitivity. The extent of the primary cancer and the patient's functional status are the two most important prognostic variables. Only patients with absent or controlled systemic disease and no leptomeningeal disease (LMD) stand to derive a significant benefit from resection of cerebral metastatic lesions. Although the distinction between the absence and presence of systemic cancer is straightforward, the definition of "controlled" or "limited" systemic disease is more nebulous because of the absence of any formal criteria. A practical approach is to estimate the life expectancy notwithstanding the cerebral metastasis, with an expected survival greater than about 3 to 4 months qualifying the patient for surgery (100). Significant functional debilitation, which is another important indicator of the disease status, advanced age, medical instability, and KPS less than 70 argue against surgery. In such patients the risk-to-benefit ratio rarely justifies an invasive approach (46,101). Neurological dysfunction itself does not necessarily preclude surgery because significant improvement may be expected following the removal of a large lesion. Im-

provement with steroids predicts an increased likelihood of postoperative recovery. Surgical accessibility can be defined on the basis of the risk and amount of neurological deficit the patient is prepared to accept. A nonsurgical approach also may be preferred for deep tumor locations such as the white matter of eloquent brain, the basal ganglia, thalamus, or brainstem, where the morbidity associated with surgical manipulation may offset the benefits (Figs. 4 and 5) (85). Nonsurgical alternatives to be considered in such cases include RS, RT, and chemotherapy; these are discussed in the following. Highly radiosensitive or chemosensitive tumors indicated in Table 1 were excluded from the three trials and initially should be treated with a combination of radiation and chemotherapy. Yet another level of complexity in decision making is introduced when considering the definition of "*single* lesion." Lesions previously invisible on contrast CT may become evident on MRI as it becomes increasingly ubiquitous. Theoretically, patients with a single lesion may harbor microscopic metastases invisible to even triple-dose contrast MRI, metastases that may one day fall within the resolution limits of a more sophisticated diagnostic instrument. As mentioned, no study has defined the threshold of detection when the treatment algorithm should switch from the one for single metastasis to the one for multiple metastases. Given that the results using contrast CT in the study by Vecht are similar to those using MRI in the study by Patchell, if a single lesion on contrast CT is deemed to be operable, then discovery of additional lesions on MRI should not necessarily deter the clinician from offering surgery.

Radiosurgery and surgical resection are both considered forms of local therapy, whereas RT also addresses microscopic metastases in the remainder of the brain but is not as effective

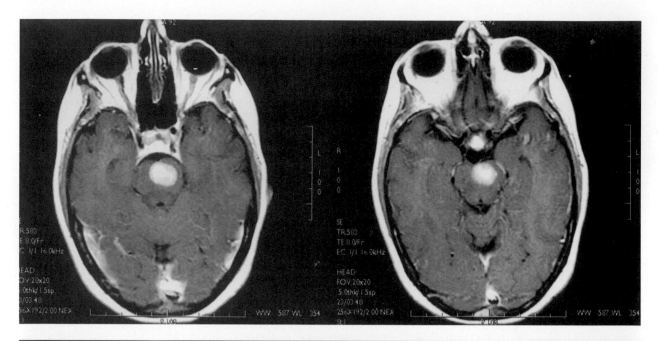

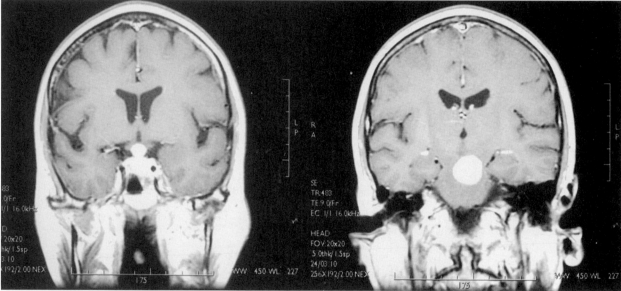

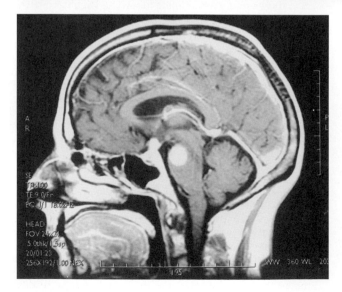

Fig. 5. Gadolinium-enhanced T1-weighted axial *(top)*, coronal *(middle)*, and sagittal *(bottom)* MRIs. Presumed metastatic breast carcinoma in the upper pons/midbrain and infundibulum. This 46-year-old woman was offered radiosurgery to the brainstem lesion and whole brain radiation for the infundibular lesion.

as RS for individual lesions because the radiation fraction dose per lesion must be reduced to minimize harm to normal tissue. The current controversy revolves around two issues: (a) the choice of local therapy (i.e., surgical resection versus RS) (76, 100,102–106), and (b) the role of RT as an adjunct to local treatment of a single lesion (45,97,101,107–118). The former issue is discussed first.

Since Lars Leksell introduced RS in the 1950s, it has emerged as a useful option in the management of brain metastases in selected cases. It can be delivered using either a linear accelerator (LINAC) or the gamma knife. Radiosurgery may be administered as primary treatment, as part of a multimodal approach involving surgery and RT for multiple metastases, as a local boost following RT, to treat a recurrence following surgery or RT, or for an incompletely excised tumor. Its advantages include noninvasiveness, ability to treat surgically inaccessible lesions or patients who are unfit for surgery, the short duration of hospital stay, and reduced cost. Even the traditionally "radioresistant" tumors (e.g., melanoma, renal cell carcinoma, and soft-tissue sarcomas) respond to RS just as well as the more radiosensitive tumors. The selection criteria for this form of local therapy are similar to those for surgery. Its principal disadvantage is its limited effectiveness on lesions larger than 3 to 3.5 cm (106,119). Also, it does not usually completely eradicate the tumor as the vast majority of surgical resections do. Rather, its goal is to provide "local control" by reducing the size of the tumor or arresting progressive growth. These effects are not immediate and patients may be steroid dependent for edema for a longer period of time. Resolution of symptoms and edema may require 1 to 3 months. In fact, about 10% of tumors may first transiently enlarge by more than 25% in the first 5 months (not after 6 months) before stabilizing or receding (106,120). Also, it does not allow a tissue diagnosis. Finally, there is currently no Class I or II evidence comparing RS to open resection, which is the current gold standard treatment that has been proven to improve outcome (102,103,107). Over the past decade numerous case series comprising over 2,000 patients have documented comparable outcomes between surgery and RS when survival, functional improvement, and adverse events are considered (76,119,121–128). Evidence to the contrary exists also (104). It has been demonstrated amply in the past that retrospective uncontrolled studies have a high propensity to magnify treatment effects regardless of the number of patients used in the analysis, in large part because of selection bias (129–131). Another pitfall of the various reports on RS is their common use of "local control" as the outcome variable, but there has been inconsistent definition of this parameter. The description of local control has ranged from "no growth or shrinkage," to growth less than 25% (106,116,119–121,123,127). Nevertheless, such studies serve a useful purpose by proposing alternative therapies, generating new hypotheses, and most important, setting the stage for the more conclusive RCTs. Two recent studies, albeit retrospective, have shown that even after accounting for the major prognostic factors to minimize selection bias, the overall survival and functionally independent survival were similar to the results of the preceding two RCTs by Patchell and Vecht involving surgery (132,133). The selection criteria for RS are not unlike those for surgery, the two most important being the absence of uncontrolled, disseminated systemic cancer or poorly controlled primary tumor, and a relatively independent functional status despite the presence of deficits (KPS 70). The median survival of patients treated with RS is 8 to 13 months, with or without RT, with the higher end of the range applying to patients in the better prognostic categories (76,102,119–128, 132,133). The 1-year local control rate is between 70% and 95%, with about half of these lesions shrinking and the other half remaining stable. The rate drops by about 20% at 2 years. The survival figures based on most studies are similar to those for

surgery; that is, 40% 1-year and 20% 2-year survivals (59,94, 134). The local recurrence rate after surgery plus RT is about 15% to 20%; therefore, similar to the local failure rate for RS (100% − 70% to 95%). Recurrence is usually seen a median of 5 to 7 months after initial treatment. The following complications may each result in a probability of 4% to 10% after RS: exacerbation of cerebral edema requiring prolonged steroid dependency, radiation necrosis requiring reoperation for mass effect, acute seizure or focal neurological deterioration, hemorrhage, and alopecia (76,104,106,117–119,121,123,124,126,127). In contrast to RS, worsening of cerebral edema is unusual after resecting a metastasis and the majority of patients improve substantially allowing the discontinuation of steroids within 1 to 2 weeks. Thirty-day operative mortality is about 2% to 5% and morbidity is about 10% to 15% (16,46,59,94,99,119,135–138). Infectious, thromboembolic, and pulmonary complications predominate among systemic causes of postoperative morbidity.

In summary, local therapy for a single metastasis in a patient selected according to the described criteria is considered *standard* treatment based on Class I evidence. Surgery should be considered in individual patients not conforming to these criteria but presenting with marked mass effect and impending herniation. The choice of local treatment between surgical resection and RS is controversial. Currently Class I evidence proving the benefit of local therapy exists only for surgery; however, a preponderance of Class III evidence suggests that there is at least an equivalent outcome using RS instead for small lesions, thereby justifying an RCT. An ongoing RCT at M.D. Anderson comparing the two forms of local treatment should help resolve this dilemma; however, until then the use of RS in patients with single metastases must be considered a treatment *option*. RS should be regarded as a complementary rather than competitive form of treatment. Radiosurgery is the preferred local treatment for lesions smaller than 3 cm in the following situations: patients unfit for surgery because of their age or medical comorbidities, deep lesion location, and informed patient preference. Local treatment is not warranted in debilitated patients with advanced cancer and life expectancy of less than 3 to 4 months because there is no benefit in addition to the palliation afforded by RT and steroids alone. The role of adjuvant RT in conjunction with local therapy and as primary treatment is controversial; it is discussed in the following.

All three RCTs involving surgery administered RT postoperatively (59,72,94). Numerous retrospective studies as well as the results of the only RCT on this topic raise questions about the indications for RT following surgery or RS (45,97,100,101,107, 108,110–118,123,124,133). This question becomes especially relevant given the long-term neurotoxicity that may be observed, because more patients survive longer with multimodal approaches using improved microsurgical techniques in combination with RS. The current conventional dose of RT is 3,000 cGy in 10 fractions because larger fraction sizes are associated with an increased risk of neurotoxicity (90,91). The optimal dose of RT has not been established firmly (45). A dose of 4,000 cGy with smaller fractions of 180 to 200 cGy may be used in patients with a longer life expectancy (more than 1 year) to minimize delayed adverse effects. Studies conducted by the Radiation Therapy Oncology Group (RTOG) and others have shown that various dose schedules, including different total doses with local boosts and hypofractionation and hyperfractionation regimes do not confer any additional benefit (87–91, 139–141). Patchell and associates recently reported the results of a well-conducted RCT evaluating postoperative RT (112). Previous retrospective surgical series generally had suggested a reduced recurrence rate in brain and a possible survival advantage, but the results were inconclusive (101,108,110,113, 114). Patchell's study included 95 patients more than 18 years old with a Karnofsky score of 70 or more who had a single metastasis that was resected completely. The postoperative observation group and RT group were well balanced in terms of the main prognostic factors. RT consisted of 50.4 Gy in 28 fractions. The follow-up was complete with only three protocol violations. Postoperative RT was found to significantly lower the local recurrence (10% versus 46%) and new distant brain metastases (14% versus 37%). Multivariate analysis revealed that only postoperative RT influenced this change. The time to recurrence was longer and death from neurological causes was reduced. Most important, the marginal differences in overall survival (48 versus 43 weeks) and functionally independent survival (37 versus 35 weeks) were not statistically significant. The two groups were not compared for late toxic effects of RT. Two caveats apply: Approximately one fourth of the patients (24/95) had disseminated disease, and the treatment policy for patients with recurrence was not specified. The former may have diluted a greater survival benefit despite well-balanced groups, especially because death from neurological causes was reduced. In addition, the power calculation for the number of patients required was based on recurrence of metastasis and not survival. As Haines and Walters have pointed out, a lack of statistical significance does not necessarily imply the absence of difference between groups (142). A larger number of patients may have demonstrated a statistically significant survival benefit, albeit slight. The second caveat is relevant because it may have influenced the overall survival and cause of death, both of which were secondary end points.

Retrospective series evaluating RT following local therapy with RS reported a lower recurrence rate and possibly an improved survival among patients with favorable prognostic features (117,118,123,124,133). These results generally parallel the conclusions of their counterpart surgical studies. Hence, the key question that remains to be answered is whether up-front adjuvant RT is superior to delayed administration in case of recurrence or LMD, because effective options such as repeat surgery or RS exist for salvage of a failed initial treatment.

The issue of adjuvant RT remains unresolved based on conflicting Class III evidence and limited Class I evidence for surgical patients showing no improvement in clinical outcome but only decreases in radiological recurrences and death specifically from neurological causes. Administering whole-brain radiation for single lesions after surgical extirpation or RS is considered a treatment *option,* as is withholding RT and monitoring the patient regularly for recurrences (at which point local therapy may or may not be repeated), followed by RT or close observation again. The decision to administer RT must be individualized based on the number of cerebral lesions and their size and radiosensitivity. RT is favored with multiple lesions (especially more than 3), smaller size (tumors greater than 2 cm are poorly responsive to RT), and radiosensitivity. Radioresistant tumors (e.g., renal cell carcinoma, melanoma, and sarcomas) do not respond to RT as they do to RS where radiosensitivity is less of an issue (116). Only large RCTs can further clarify treatment options for this patient population. The European Organization for the Research and Treatment of Cancer is currently conducting a Phase III study comparing initial observation with immediate RT following either resection or RS for single metastases (143). At least one other similar trial is planned (123).

Multiple Metastases

Traditionally, multiple brain metastases have been considered a contraindication for local therapy such as surgery; treatment has been confined to RT in most cases (19,35,102,144–146).

MRI often is performed after identifying only a single lesion on contrast CT with a view to avoid surgery should other metastases be identified. As mentioned, no evidence in support of this logic exists. Several retrospective case series and case control studies have advocated local therapy in the form of multiple surgical resections via one or more craniotomies, or RS, targeting up to four lesions in selected patients (99,114,147–150). One case control study showed that despite multiplicity of lesions being associated with a worse prognosis, the survival of patients undergoing *complete* resection of up to three metastases via up to three craniotomies concurrently was significantly better than those who had one or more lesions left unresected, and was similar to those with a single metastasis, without an increase in the morbidity or mortality (147). Others have corroborated these findings (18,99,114). However, no guidance from Class I data is available for this patient population. Recently an attempt at a RCT was made comparing RS plus RT to RT alone (150). However, the study was closed prematurely after the accrual of only 27 patients because of a marked improvement in local control in the RS plus RT arm. The subjects were highly selected and highly functioning (median KPS of 100) with two to four brain metastases, all smaller than 2.5 cm. The groups were well matched and similarly treated with a complete follow-up. The 1-year local failure rate was 100% after RT alone but only 8% in those who received boost RS as well. There was "no neurological or systemic morbidity" associated with RS. Such extraordinarily divergent findings and extreme results should be interpreted cautiously because they may be partly ascribed to unintentional and unidentifiable selection bias inadequately addressed by the randomization process. The lack of any statistical significance of the improvement in survival observed with RS is not surprising because of the small numbers (142). Validation of these findings is required in a larger RCT. Currently RT alone as well as local therapy followed by RT or observation are all considered treatment options for patients with multiple metastases based on Class III evidence. Surgery should be strongly considered if there is a single dominant surgically accessible lesion causing mass effect and neurological compromise (Fig. 6), a need for a histological diagnosis or the possibility of resecting all lesions through a single craniotomy. In many of the larger centers, including this one, local therapy followed by RT is offered for multiple metastases after the consideration of four factors: the extent of systemic disease, the patient's functional status, the number of brain lesions on contrast MRI, and the radiosensitivity of the tumor type (26,85,107, 147,151). Local therapy is reserved for patients with absent or controlled systemic cancer, a KPS score of at least 70, no more than four lesions, and life expectancy greater than 3 months. Radioresistant tumors such as renal cell carcinoma and melanoma are also favored for local therapy because RT alone provides suboptimal control. As detailed, the choice of local therapy is debatable and must take into account the guidelines set forth previously for single metastasis. Surgery may be preferred in patients with diabetes mellitus as steroids can be weaned off sooner and more readily than following RS, thereby minimizing glucose intolerance. In a typical scenario, lesions greater than 3 cm are resected with the remainder, especially those surgically inaccessible, being subjected to RS. For lesions less than 3 cm all the lesions must be resectable before embarking on surgery, because resection of only some lesions is not beneficial. Generally, but not routinely, RT is administered after local therapy for multiple metastases. Future RCTs will help further elucidate the indications for the various treatment options. RTOG 9508 is a phase III study comparing RT alone versus RT plus RS boost for one to three metastases and 172 out of a projected 262 patients had enrolled as of March 2000 (152).

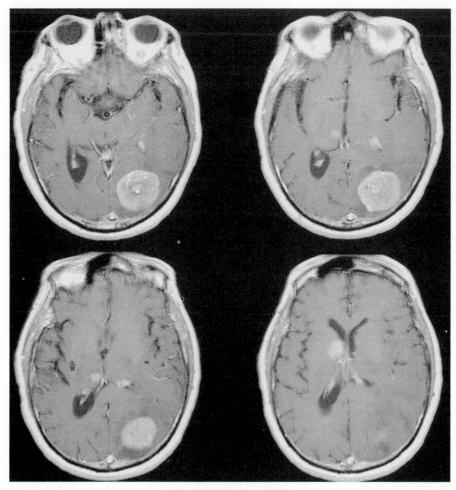

Fig. 6. Gadolinium-enhanced T1-weighted MRI. Multiple non–small-cell lung carcinoma metastases to the brain in a 62-year-old man presenting with confusion, ataxia, and right homonymous hemianopsia. The large symptomatic left occipital lesion was resected and radiosurgery was offered for the other two lesions in the right thalamus and internal capsule.

Recurrence of Brain Metastases

The probability of local or distant recurrence in the brain after local therapy plus RT for single metastasis is 10% to 20% each (26,59,94,105,116,134). The rate of distant brain metastasis in the absence of RT is higher at 30% to 40% (112,116). The probability rises with multiple metastases as most of these patients will experience recurrences. Local recurrences represent the growth of residual tumor cells not eradicated at first surgery, whereas distant recurrences arise from new tumor deposits. The median time to recurrence is 5 to 7 months (147,153,154). In these patients death is ascribed to neurological progression more commonly than to systemic disease, in contrast to patients without recurrences (154–156). The treatment decisions facing the clinician are not unlike those at the time of initial presentation. Similar treatment options and selection criteria for each option apply at the time of recurrence. In addition, the time to recurrence also should be taken into account because an interval of less than 4 months before recurrence bodes poorly for the patient (154). The majority of patients with recurrent brain metastases also harbor progressive extracranial disease; hence, only supportive measures are undertaken. Re-irradiation with RT has produced mixed results in offering symptomatic relief to patients with advanced cancer and a limited life span of less than 4 to 5 months. Clinical response rates range from 42% to 75% (97,155). This approach is discouraged in patients with limited extracranial disease and nondebilitated patients so that the brain tolerance dose of RT may not be exceeded and unacceptable neurological disability during the patient's remaining lifetime may be avoided. In the healthier subset of patients fulfilling the previously listed selection criteria for local therapy, RS or reoperation represent the options of choice. RT also is offered if not previously administered. Three retrospective case series have documented experiences with reoperation for recurrent metastases (153,154,156). Reoperation led to a median survival of 9 to 11.5 months in these selected patients. Neurological improvement occurred in 62% to 75% and 25% to 33% remained stable. Surgical morbidity occurred in 10% to 31%. In an attempt to better predict which patients stand to benefit most from reoperation, Bindal and colleagues proposed a grading system based on five prognostic factors: (a) systemic disease absent versus present (0 versus 1 point), (b) Karnofsky score greater than 70 versus less than 70 (0 versus 1 point), (c) time to recurrence 4 months versus less than 4 months (0 versus 1 point), (d) age less than 40 versus greater than 40 (0 versus 1 point), and (e) primary tumor nonmelanoma/breast versus melanoma or breast (0 versus 1 point) (150). Patients are scored by adding the points. The points are converted to the corresponding grade from 0 to IV. The grade was found to correlate with the median survival: grade I, median survival not reached; II, 13.4 months; III, 6.8 months; IV, 3.4 months. This scale was based on retrospective data and grades I and IV contained fewer than 10 patients. Hence, validation in a larger prospective study is necessary; nonetheless, it serves as a useful paradigm for deciding which patients may be reasonable candidates for reoperation. The authors caution against re-operating on grade IV patients. This grading system "is not valid for patients with advanced systemic disease who are expected to die within 4 months" and for those with multiple lesions if they are not all resectable.

There is a single study investigating the role of RS for recurrent metastases (152). This phase I/II study recently published its final report on 156 patients with recurrent primary tumors (36%) and brain metastases (64%) entered from 17 institutions between August 1990 and December 1994. Patients with a Karnofsky score greater than or equal to 60, single tumor less than or equal to 4 cm requiring further treatment after RT 3 months or more previously, and a life expectancy of 3 or more months were included. The RS dose was escalated to determine adverse effects and the maximum tolerable dose. This was found to range from 15 to 24 Gy, the dose being inversely proportional to tumor size. Unacceptable neurological toxicity developed in 22%, the likelihood being proportional to the tumor size. The incidence of radiation necrosis was 5% to 11% arising between 6 and 24 months following RS. Resumption of previously discontinued steroids was required in 27%, and continued use in those already on them was necessary in 68%. Local tumor progression rate was not specified for metastases, but based on the data it appears to be about 35% to 40% over 1 to 2 years. Median survival for patients with brain metastases was 7.5 months. One and two-year survivals were 26% and 8%, respectively. Functional status improved in 13%, remained stable in 41%, and deteriorated in 45% of the combined primary tumor/metastases patient group. It is difficult to directly compare these results, which include both primary and secondary tumors (although mostly the latter) to those from the aforementioned surgical series; however, the relatively high incidence of untoward side effects is concerning. Only a randomized study comparing the two treatments in patients selected based on predetermined criteria can provide the much-needed answers. In the meantime, based on Class III evidence, both RS and surgical resection are considered treatment options for patients with a high functional status (e.g., Karnofsky greater than or equal to 70) and absent or controlled systemic disease, with recurrent cerebral metastasis. For the remaining patients RT (repeat treatment or for the first time), interstitial brachytherapy or chemotherapy may be considered. The latter two options are discussed in the following.

Interstitial Brachytherapy and Chemotherapy

The role of these therapies for brain metastasis remains undefined. Anecdotal reports and retrospective case series suggest a potential role for brachytherapy when surgical resection or RS are unsuitable, to salvage highly selected patients with recurrent metastases and occasionally as adjuvant therapy to RT (36,85, 157–160). Brachytherapy consists of stereotactic implantation of ^{125}I or ^{192}Ir into the tumor. In general, results for *de novo* tumors have been disappointing compared to the other standard treatments. Median survivals range from 6 to 15 months. Significant morbidity in the form of neurological worsening, increased edema, seizures, major arterial occlusion, radiation necrosis requiring surgery, and infection may occur in 20% to

25% of patients (36,159). Given the relatively high risk-to-benefit ratio, the role of brachytherapy is limited with the advent of radiosurgery and microneurosurgery.

Chemotherapy generally has not had a major impact in the treatment of cerebral metastasis (19,90,95). The long-espoused belief that the brain represented a pharmacological sanctuary for metastatic lesions has been challenged as responses by chemosensitive solid tumors such as breast carcinoma, SCLC, and germ cell tumors have been demonstrated (29,109,144,161, 162). Similar responses also have been shown in a minority of patients with non-SCLC as part of phase II studies (163,164). As stated, SCLC and germ cell tumors initially are treated with RT and chemotherapy. The advantage of chemotherapy lies in its ability to simultaneously treat extracranial disease. Encouraging data were obtained in a RCT comparing RT with RT plus two different chemotherapeutic combinations in 100 patients (29). However, more than half the patients were excluded from analysis because of prior complete surgical resection of the tumor and there was no volumetric comparison of the amount of tumor subjected to nonsurgical treatment in the above three arms. Furthermore, patients with single and multiple metastases were both included. It is difficult to draw valid conclusions from the data because of these shortcomings. Based on CT imaging, higher rates of resolution were observed in the chemotherapy arms of the study compared to the RT alone arm, but there was no difference in survival. Common to the preceding studies is the lack of a survival advantage despite transient and variable responses to the drug regimen; the principal drawback is systemic toxicity from chemotherapy such as myelosuppression. Another randomized phase III study conducted by the RTOG failed to show any efficacy of misonidazole (a radiation sensitizer) in the treatment of brain metastasis (28). Hence, current Class III evidence and limited Class I evidence suggest a role for chemotherapy as an option in patients with recurrent non–germ cell and non–SCLC metastases who cannot be treated with surgery or RS, and in the context of clinical trials. Chemotherapy effects little change in survival or quality of life in most patients and usually represents a last resort after other failed treatments.

Prophylactic Cranial Radiation Treatment for Small-Cell Lung Carcinoma

This issue has been contentious since the 1970s and 1980s when RCTs were performed evaluating prophylactic RT for this highly radiosensitive tumor (165–167). More recent RCTs and non-RCT studies generally have agreed with the findings of the earlier studies that prophylactic brain RT reduces the incidence of brain metastases. However, a significant overall survival difference could not be demonstrated in any single study despite including only patients in complete remission, although trends toward a survival benefit were observed in some studies (168–171). The enthusiasm for routine prophylactic whole brain radiation initially was tempered by concerns regarding potential detrimental neurological sequelae from RT in those who survived more than 1 year (169,171,172). Acute side effects may include headaches, nausea, vomiting, and hair loss. A "somnolence syndrome" of increased fatigue may be noted subacutely 1 to 4 months later. Radiation necrosis can occur beyond 6 months. Previous studies reporting neurological toxicity were retrospective and employed dose fractions of more than 2 Gy, with chemotherapy being administered concurrent to the RT. The first RCT to clarify this issue found no significant difference in cognitive changes with careful neuropsychological testing when compared to the controls (168). Each fraction was 1.8 Gy and concurrent chemotherapy was disallowed. These findings later were confirmed (170). For unclear reasons patients with SCLC without radiologically evident brain metastasis perform worse on neuropsychological testing when compared to age-matched controls without SCLC. One of the most recent reports analyzed individual data pooled from seven RCTs, which included patients in complete remission, making it the largest study to date on this topic (173). A small but statistically significant survival benefit of 5.4% (20.7% in controls versus 15.3% in prophylactic group) at 3 years was demonstrated after the data on 987 patients were analyzed. The small magnitude of this difference explains why previous trials lacked the power to reveal a significant advantage with prophylactic RT. This metaanalysis confirmed a significant decrease in the incidence of brain metastasis from 58.6% to 33.3% (relative risk 0.46); however, it did not address functional or neuropsychological changes. According to the authors, "prophylactic cranial irradiation should now be considered part of the standard treatment of patients with SCLC in complete remission." Based on Class I evidence showing a survival advantage of about 5% at 3 years and a reduction in the incidence of brain metastases by about 25%, prophylactic whole brain radiation is considered standard treatment for patients with SCLC *who are in complete remission* following initial treatment. There is no support for this approach in patients who are not in complete remission. The magnitude of survival benefit is small and the applicability of these results of population-based studies to individual patients must be individualized, taking into account factors such as systemic status and patient performance and preferences. Fraction doses should not exceed 2 Gy and should be administered sequentially and not concurrently to chemotherapy in order to minimize the risk of neurotoxicity.

Prognosis

Immeasurable advances in diagnostic technology have taken place since the days of radioisotope brain scans and pneumoencephalography, as well as progress in therapeutic measures such as microneurosurgery and RS. Yet the overall prognosis of patients with cerebral metastasis remains bleak. The median survival has only risen from 3 to 6 months with RT and steroids, to 9 to 12 months currently. The 1- and 2-year survivals for single brain metastasis are about 40% and 20%, respectively. Only about 10% to 30% of patients with multiple metastases survive 2 years. Death is ascribed to neurological progression in 30% to 40% of cases, with systemic disease being the more common culprit in the remainder. This figure is reversed among patients with recurrence of brain metastasis. Despite these discouraging statistics, hope and encouragement should be instilled in patients because the prognosis is not invariably dismal. Exceptionally long survivals of more than 5 to 10 years have been documented and personally witnessed (174,175). Study after study has confirmed systemic status, the patient's functional status, and age to be the three most important prognostic variables (59,72,94–96,98,133,134,140,176). These factors must guide treatment decisions because older patients with advanced disease and poor functional status not only benefit less from surgery but also tend to get more treatment-related complications (137). Other relevant but sometimes debated negative prognostic indicators include shorter time interval (less than 1 year) between diagnosis of primary tumor and brain metastasis, and incomplete surgical excision (16,26,93,100,101). Survival of patients with more than 2 metastases is worse, about 10% at 2 years (18,19,26,73,91). Tumor histology also may be a determinant of survival; however, this is controversial (16,45,55,76, 95,124,154). Melanomas often portend a shorter survival, whereas breast carcinoma is associated with a longer survival (120,154). Infratentorial versus supratentorial location of a brain metastasis may augur an inferior outcome (93,95).

There have been only two attempts at systematically classifying the preceding myriad prognostic parameters in order to interpret the numerous outcome studies on brain metastasis more meaningfully. The first attempt by Bindal and colleagues has already been described and applies to reoperation for recurrences of brain metastases (154). More recently, the RTOG developed the recursive partitioning analysis (RPA) model of prognostic factors based on a database of 1,200 patients who had undergone RT as part of one of three previous RTOG trials (98). The three most significant prognostic factors were the Karnofsky performance score, systemic status of the cancer, and age. There are 3 RPA classes. Class 1 includes patients with KPS greater than 70, controlled primary tumor with solitary brain metastasis (i.e., no extracerebral site), and age less than 65; class 2 includes patients with KPS greater than 70 but either uncontrolled primary tumor, age more than 65 or extracerebral metastasis; and class 3 includes those with KPS less than 70. The median survivals for the three classes of patients were 7.1, 4.2, and 2.3 months, respectively. This grading scheme has been validated in three retrospective studies with patients who underwent surgery plus RT (median survival times of 14.8, 9.9, and 6.0 months for the three classes), RS plus RT (median survival times of 11.2 for class 1 and 6.9 months for classes 2 and 3), and RT alone (median survival times of 6.2 and 3.8 months for classes 1 and 2, no patients in class 3) (133,134,176). It is expected that future prospective studies will employ this scale and confirm its validity so that the results of outcome studies can be standardized. This will enable clinicians to supply their patients with more concrete recommendations, which are currently scarce because of a paucity of Class I evidence for many clinical situations. In the palliative care of patients with metastatic cancer where treatments are increasingly toxic, inconvenient to the patient and provide diminishing returns, quality of life, and functional status assume an even greater prominence as end points. The biggest gains in outcome for these patients in the future are likely to be realized in targeted immunotherapy and biotherapy using molecular and genetic techniques.

References

1. Radinsky R, Aukerman SL. The pathogenesis of cancer metastasis: relevance to biotherapy. In: Oldham RK, ed. *Principles of cancer biotherapy*, 3rd ed. Dordrecht: Kluwer, 1998:16–38.
2. Hove B, Andersen BB, Christiansen TM. Intracranial oncotic aneurysms from choriocarcinoma. Case report and review of the literature. *Neuroradiology* 1990;32:526–528.
3. Walters BC. Clinical practice parameter development in neurosurgery. In: Bean JR, ed. *Concepts in neurosurgery. Neurosurgery in transition. The socioeconomic transformation of neurological surgery*, vol. 9. Baltimore: Williams & Wilkins, 1998:99–111.
4. Counsell CE, Collie DA, Grant R. Incidence of intracranial tumours in the Lothian region of Scotland, 1989–90. *J Neurol Neurosurg Psychiatry* 1996;61:143–150.
5. Torres LF, Almeida R, Avila S, et al. Brain tumours in south Brazil: a retrospective study of 438 cases. *Arq Neuropsiquiatr* 1990;48:279–285.
6. Walker AE, Robins M, Weinfeld FD. Epidemiology of brain tumors: the national survey of intracranial neoplasms. *Neurology* 1985;35:219–226.
7. Grant R, Whittle JR, Collie DA, et al. Referral pattern and management of patients with malignant brain tumours in south east Scotland. *Health Bull* 1996;54:212–222.

8. Helseth E, Cappelen J, Kvinnsland S, et al. [Intracranial tumors in adults (over 15 years)]. *Tidssk Nor Laegeforen* 1993;113:1347–1350.
9. Crowley MJ, O'Brien DF. Epidemiology of tumours of the central nervous system in Ireland. *Ir Med J* 1993;86:87–88.
10. Lassouw GM, Twijnstra A, Schouten LJ, et al. The neuro-oncology register. *Neuroepidemiology* 1992;11:261–266.
11. Mao Y, Desmeules M, Semenciw RM, et al. Increasing brain cancer rates in Canada. *CMAJ* 1991;145:1583–1591.
12. Muir CS, Storm HH, Polednak A. Brain and other nervous system tumours. *Cancer Surv* 1994;19–20:369–392.
13. Karrer K, Fleischmann E, Hochpochler F. Site of the primary in intracranial metastases. *Adv Neurosurg* 1984;12:10–14.
14. Johnson JD, Young B. Demographics of brain metastasis. *Neurosurg Clin N Am* 1996;7:337–344.
15. Kehrli P. Epidmiologie des metastases cerebrales. *Neurochirurgie* 1999;45:357–363.
16. Nataf F, Emery E, Kherli P, et al. Etude multicentrique neurochirurgicale de metastases cerebrales. *Neurochirurgie* 1999;45:369–374.
17. Sorensen JB, Hansen HH, Hansen M, et al. Brain metastases in adenocarcinoma of the lung: frequency, risk groups, and prognosis. *J Clin Oncol* 1988;6:1474–1480.
18. Arbit E, Wronski M, Galicich J. Surgical resection of brain metastasis in 670 patients: the Memorial Sloan-Kettering Cancer Center experience, 1972–1992. *J Neurosurg* 1994;80:386A.
19. Pladdet I, Boven E, Nauta J, et al. Palliative care for brain metastases of solid tumour types. *Netherlands J Med* 1989;34:10–21.
20. Takakura K, Sano K, Hojo S, et al. *Metastatic tumors of the central nervous system*. New York: Igaku-Shoin, 1982.
21. Cormio G, Maneo A, Parma G, et al. Central nervous system metastases in patients with ovarian carcinoma. A report of 23 cases and a literature review. *Ann Oncol* 1995;6:571–574.
22. Cox JD, Yesner RA. Causes of treatment failure and death in carcinoma of the lung. *Yale J Biol Med* 1981;54:201–207.
23. Fervenza FC, Wolanskyj AP, Eklund HE, et al. Brain metastasis: an unusual complication from prostatic adenocarcinoma. *Mayo Clin Proc* 2000;75:79–82.
24. Reider-Groswasser I, Merimsky O, Karminsky N, et al. Computed tomography features of cerebral spread of malignant melanoma. *Am J Clin Oncol* 1996;19:49–53.
25. Pickren JW, Lopez G, Tsukada Y, et al. Brain metastases: an autopsy study. *Cancer Treat Symp* 1983;2:295–313.
26. Pollock BE. Management of patients with multiple brain metastases. *Contemp Neurosurg* 1999;21:1–6.
27. Oneschuk D, Bruera E. Palliative management of brain metastases. *Support Care Cancer* 1998;6:365–372.
28. Komarnicky LT, Phillips TL, Martz K, et al. A randomized phase III protocol for the evaluation of misonidazole combined with radiation in the treatment of patients with brain metastases (RTOG-7916). *Int J Radiat Oncol Biol Phys* 1991;20:53–58.
29. Ushio Y, Arita N, Hayakawa T, et al. Chemotherapy of brain metastases from lung carcinoma: a controlled randomized study. *Neurosurgery* 1991;28:201–205.
30. Farinotti M, Ferrarini M, Solari A, et al. Incidence and survival of childhood CNS tumours in the Region of Lombardy, Italy. *Brain* 1998;121:1429–1436.
31. McKinney PA, Parslow RC, Lane SA, et al. Epidemiology of childhood brain tumours in Yorkshire, UK, 1974–1995: geographical distribution and changing patterns of occurrence. *Br J Cancer* 1998;78:974–979.
32. Tasdemiroglu E, Patchell RA. Cerebral metastases in childhood malignancies. *Acta Neurochir (Wien)* 1997;139:182–187.
33. Shah SH, Soomro IN, Hussainy AS, et al. Clinico-morphological pattern of intracranial tumors in children. *J Pak Med Assoc* 1999;49:63–65.
34. Batson O. The role of the vertebral veins in metastatic processes. *Ann Intern Med* 1941;16:38–45.
35. Black P. Brain metastasis: current status and recommended guidelines for management. *Neurosurgery* 1979;5:617–631.
36. Greenberg HS, Chandler WF, Sandler HM. *Brain tumors*. New York: Oxford University Press, 1999.
37. Fidler IJ. Modulation of the organ microenvironment for treatment of cancer metastasis. *J Natl Cancer Inst* 1995;87:1588–1595.
38. Akslen LA, Heuch I, Hartveit F. Metastatic patterns in autopsy cases of cutaneous melanoma. *Invasion Metastasis* 1988;8:193–204.
39. Aznavoorian S, Murphy AN, Stetler-Stevenson WG, et al. Molecular aspects of tumor cell invasion and metastasis. *Cancer* 1993;71:1368–1383.
40. Fidler IJ, Hart IR. Biological diversity in metastatic neoplasms: origins and implications. *Science* 1982;217:998–1003.
41. Paget S. The distribution of secondary growths in cancer of the breast. 1889 [classical article]. *Cancer Metastasis Rev* 1989;8:98–101.
42. Das A, Hochberg FH. Clinical presentation of intracranial metastases. *Neurosurg Clin N Am* 1996;7:377–391.
43. Chidel MA, Suh JH, Barnett GH. Brain metastases: presentation, evaluation, and management. *Cleveland Clin J Med* 2000;67:120–127.
44. Cohen N, Strauss G, Lew R, et al. Should prophylactic anticonvulsants be administered to patients with newly-diagnosed cerebral metastases? A retrospective analysis. *J Clin Oncol* 1988;6:1621–1624.
45. Coia LR, Aaronson N, Linggood R, et al. A report of the consensus workshop panel on the treatment of brain metastases. *Int J Radiat Oncol Biol Phys* 1992;23:223–227.
46. Salvati M, Cervoni L, Raco A. Single brain metastases from unknown primary malignancies in CT-era. *J Neurooncol* 1995;23:75–80.
47. Vecht CJ. Clinical management of brain metastasis. *J Neurol* 1998;245:127–131.
48. Davis PC, Hudgins PA, Peterman SB, et al. Diagnosis of cerebral metastases: double-dose delayed CT vs contrast-enhanced MR imaging. *AJNR Am J Neuroradiol* 1991;12:293–300.
49. Mastonardi L, Lunardi P, Puzzilli F, et al. The role of MRI in the surgical selection of cerebral metastases. *Zentralbl Neurochir* 1999;60:141–145.
50. Schiff D, DeAngelis LM. Therapy of venous thromboembolism in patients with brain metastases. *Cancer* 1994;73:493–498.
51. Cooper JS, Ransohoff J, Rush S, et al. CT detection of cerebral metastases inapparent on magnetic resonance imaging scan. *J Comput Tomogr* 1988;12:182–186.
52. Dewulf P, Demaerel P, Wilms G, et al. Cerebral metastatic malignant melanoma: CT and MR findings with pathological correlation. *J Belge Radiol* 1993;76:318–319.
53. Osborne AG. *Diagnostic neuroradiology*. St. Louis: Mosby, 1994.
54. Schaefer PW, Budzik RF Jr, Gonzalez RG. Imaging of cerebral metastases. *Neurosurg Clin N Am* 1996;7:393–423.
55. Pechova-Peterova V, Kalvach P. CT findings in cerebral metastases. *Neuroradiology* 1986;28:254–258.
56. Carrier DA, Mawad ME, Kirkpatrick JB, et al. Metastatic adenocarcinoma to the brain: MR with pathologic correlation. *AJNR Am J Neuroradiol* 1994;15:155–159.
57. Hwang TL, Close TP, Grego JM, et al. Predilection of brain metastasis in gray and white matter junction and vascular border zones. *Cancer* 1996;77:1551–1555.
58. Hwang TL, Valdivieso JG, Yang CH, et al. Calcified brain metastasis. *Neurosurgery* 1993;32:451–454; discussion 454.
59. Patchell RA, Tibbs PA, Walsh JW, et al. A randomized trial of surgery in the treatment of single metastases to the brain. *N Engl J Med* 1990;322:494–500.
60. Franzini A, Leocata F, Giorgi C, et al. Role of stereotactic biopsy in multifocal brain lesions: considerations in 100 consecutive cases. *J Neurol Neurosurg Psychiatry* 1994;57:957–960.
61. Lecky BRF, Jeyagopal N, Smith ETS, et al. Cerebral CT lesions in multiple sclerosis mimicking multiple metastases. *J Neurol Neurosurg Psychiatry* 1991;54:92.
62. Okamoto K, Ito J, Furusawa T, et al. Small cortical infarcts mimicking metastatic tumors. *Clin Imaging* 1998;22:333–338.
63. Roberts WS, Sell JJ, Orrison WW Jr. Multiple ischemic infarcts versus metastatic disease. *Acad Radiology* 1994;1:75–77.
64. Schnittker JB, Thomas HG, Johns RD, et al. Late appearance of a radiodense lesion at the site of an irradiated metastasis: neuropathological findings. *Neurosurgery* 1988;23:785–788.
65. Savarese DM, Gordon J, Smith TW, et al. Cerebral demyelination syndrome in a patient treated with 5-fluorouracil and levamisole. The use of thallium SPECT imaging to assist in noninvasive diagnosis: a case report. *Cancer* 1996;77:387–394.
66. Sze G, Johnson C, Kawamura Y, et al. Comparison of single- and triple-dose contrast material in the MR screening of brain metastases. *AJNR Am J Neuroradiol* 1998;19:821–828.
67. Ginsberg LE, Lang FF. Neuroradiological screening for brain metas-

tases—can quadruple dose gadolinium be far behind? *AJNR Am J Neuroradiol* 1998;19:829–830.

68. Desprechins B, Stadnik T, Koerts G, et al. Use of diffusion-weighted MR imaging in differential diagnosis between intracerebral necrotic tumors and cerebral abscesses. *Am J Neuroradiol* 1999;20: 1252–1257.

69. Eden EA, Muggia JM, Hiesiger EM, et al. Plasma carcinoembryonic antigen as an indicator of cerebral metastases. *J Neurooncol* 1990; 8:281–287.

70. Twijnstra A, Nooyen WJ, van Zanten AP, et al. Cerebrospinal fluid carcinoembryonic antigen in patients with metastatic and nonmetastatic neurological diseases. *Arch Neurol* 1986;43:269–272.

71. Merchut MP. Brain metastases from undiagnosed systemic neoplasms. *Arch Intern Med* 1989;149:1076–1080.

72. Mintz AH, Kestle J, Rathbone MP, et al. A randomized trial to assess the efficacy of surgery in addition to radiotherapy in patients with a single cerebral metastasis. *Cancer* 1996;78:1470–1476.

73. Eapen L, Vachet M, Catton G, et al. Brain metastases with an unknown primary: a clinical perspective. *J Neurooncol* 1988;6:31–35.

74. Posner JB. Management of central nervous system metastases. *Semin Oncol* 1977;4:81–91.

75. Low-Grade Glioma Guidelines Team in Association with the Guidelines and Outcomes Committee of the American Association of Neurological Surgeons. Practice parameters in adults with suspected or known supratentorial nonoptic pathway low-grade glioma. *Neurosurg Focus* 1998;4:Article 10, 11 pp.

76. Boyd TS, Mehta MP. Radiosurgery for brain metastases. *Neurosurg Clin N Am* 1999;10:337–350.

77. French LA, Galicich JH. The use of steroids for control of cerebral edema. *Clin Neurosurg* 1962;10:212–223.

78. French LA. The use of steroids in the treatment of cerebral edema. *Bull NY Acad Med* 1966;42:301–311.

79. Galicich JH, French LA. Use of Dexamethasone in the treatment of cerebral edema resulting from brain tumors and brain surgery. *Am Pract* 1961;12:169–174.

80. Gutin PH. Corticosteroid therapy in patients with brain tumors. *Natl Cancer Inst Monogr* 1977;46:151–156.

81. Renaudin J, Fewer D, Wilson CB, et al. Dose dependency of Decadron in patients with partially excised brain tumors. *J Neurosurg* 1973;39:302–305.

82. Vecht CJ, Hovestadt A, Verbiest HB, et al. Dose-effect relationship of dexamethasone on Karnofsky performance in metastatic brain tumors: a randomized study of doses of 4, 8, and 16 mg per day. *Neurology* 1994;44:675–680.

83. Koehler PJ. Use of corticosteroids in neuro-oncology. *Anti-Cancer Drugs* 1995;6:19–33.

84. Bodsch W, Rommel T, Ophoff BG, et al. Factors responsible for the retention of fluid in human tumor edema and the effect of dexamethasone. *J Neurosurg* 1987;67:250–257.

85. Davey P. Brain metastases. *Curr Probl Cancer* 1999;23:59–98.

86. Reddy S, Hendrickson FR, Hoeksema J, et al. The role of radiation therapy in the palliation of metastatic genitourinary tract carcinomas. A study of the Radiation Therapy Oncology Group. *Cancer* 1983;52:25–29.

87. D' Elia F, Bonucci I, Biti GP, et al. Different fractionation schedules in radiation treatment of cerebral metastases. *Acta Radiol Oncol* 1986;25:181–184.

88. Epstein BE, Scott CB, Sause WT, et al. Improved survival duration in patients with unresected solitary brain metastasis using accelerated hyperfractionated radiation therapy at total doses of 54.4 gray and greater. Results of Radiation Therapy Oncology Group 85-28. *Cancer* 1993;71:1362–1367.

89. Harwood AR, Simson WJ. Radiation therapy of cerebral metastases: a randomized prospective clinical trial. *Int J Radiat Oncol Biol Phys* 1977;2:1091–1094.

90. Priestman TJ, Dunn J, Brada M, et al. Final results of the Royal College of Radiologists' trial comparing two different radiotherapy schedules in the treatment of cerebral metastases. *Clin Oncol (R Coll Radiol)* 1996;8:308–315.

91. Ziegler JC, Cooper JS. Brain metastases from malignant melanoma: conventional versus high-dose-per-fraction radiotherapy. *Int J Radiat Oncol Biol Phys* 1986;12:1839–1842.

92. Sause WT, Crowley JJ, Morantz R, et al. Solitary brain metastasis: results of an RTOG/SWOG protocol evaluation surgery + RT versus RT alone. *Am J Clin Oncol* 1990;13:427–432.

93. Yardeni D, Reichenthal E, Zucker G, et al. Neurosurgical management of single brain metastasis. *Surg Neurol* 1984;21:377–384.

94. Vecht CJ, Haaxma-Reiche H, Noordijk EM, et al. Treatment of single brain metastasis: radiotherapy alone or combined with neurosurgery? *Ann Neurol* 1993;33:583–590.

95. Bindal RK, Bindal AK, Sawaya R. Outcome of surgical therapy for metastatic cancer to the brain. *Adv Surg* 1998;31:351–373.

96. Noordijk EM, Vecht CJ, Haaxma-Reiche H, et al. The choice of treatment of single brain metastasis should be based on extracranial tumor activity and age. *Int J Radiat Oncol Biol Phys* 1994;29: 711–717.

97. Vermeulen SS. Whole brain radiotherapy in the treatment of metastatic brain tumors. *Semin Surg Oncol* 1998;14:64–69.

98. Gaspar L, Scott C, Rotman M, et al. Recursive partitioning analysis (RPA) of prognostic factors in three Radiation Therapy Oncology Group (RTOG) brain metastases trials. *Int J Radiat Oncol Biol Phys* 1997;37:745–751.

99. Meyer B, Stangl A, Neuloh G, et al. Prospective study on neurosurgical treatment of cerebral metastases. In: Wiegel T, Hinkelbein W, Brock M, et al., eds. *Controversies in neuro-oncology,* vol. 33. Basel: Karger, 1999:332–342.

100. Lang FF, Sawaya R. Craniotomy for single and multiple cerebral metastases. In: Maciunas RJ, ed. *Advanced techniques in central nervous system metastases.* Park Ridge, IL: The American Association of Neurological Surgeons, 1998:35–56.

101. Smalley SR, Laws ER Jr, O'Fallon JR, et al. Resection for solitary brain metastasis. Role of adjuvant radiation and prognostic variables in 229 patients. *J Neurosurg* 1992;77:531–540.

102. Alexander E 3rd, Loeffler JS. Intracranial metastatic tumor management. The case for radiosurgery. *Clin Neurosurg* 1999;45:32–40.

103. Haines SJ. Intracranial metastatic tumor management. Surgical or radiosurgical treatment for brain metastases? Opportunity lost, responsibility shirked. *Clin Neurosurg* 1999;45:30–31.

104. Bindal AK, Bindal RK, Hess KR, et al. Surgery versus radiosurgery in the treatment of brain metastasis. *J Neurosurg* 1996;84:748–754.

105. Sawaya R. Intracranial metastatic tumor management. Surgical treatment of brain metastases. *Clin Neurosurg* 1999;45:41–47.

106. Young RF. Radiosurgery for the treatment of brain metastases. *Semin Surg Oncol* 1998;14:70–78.

107. Lang FF, Sawaya R. Surgical treatment of metastatic brain tumors. *Semin Surg Oncol* 1998;14:53–63.

108. Armstrong JG, Wronski M, Galicich J, et al. Postoperative radiation for lung cancer metastatic to the brain. *J Clin Oncol* 1994;12: 2340–2344.

109. Buckner J. Surgery, radiation therapy, and chemotherapy for metastatic tumors to the brain. *Curr Opin Oncol* 1992;4:518–524.

110. DeAngelis LM, Mandell LR, Thaler HT, et al. The role of postoperative radiotherapy after resection of single brain metastases. *Neurosurgery* 1989;24:798–806.

111. Mintz AP, Cairncross JG. Treatment of a single brain metastasis. The role of radiation following surgical resection. *JAMA* 1998;280: 1527–1529.

112. Patchell RA, Tibbs PA, Regine WF, et al. Postoperative radiotherapy in the treatment of single metastases to the brain: a randomized trial. *JAMA* 1998;280:1485–1489.

113. Smalley SR, Schray MF, Laws ER Jr, et al. Adjuvant radiation therapy after surgical resection of solitary brain metastasis: association with pattern of failure and survival. *Int J Radiat Oncol Biol Phys* 1987; 13:1611–1616.

114. Weber F, Riedel A, Koning W, et al. The role of adjuvant radiation and multiple resection within the surgical management of brain metastases. *Neurosurg Rev* 1996;19:23–32.

115. Cho KH, Hall WA, Gerbi BJ, et al. Patient selection criteria for the treatment of brain metastases with stereotactic radiosurgery. *J Neurooncol* 1998;40:73–86.

116. Goyal LK, Suh JH, Reddy CA, et al. The role of whole brain radiotherapy and stereotactic radiosurgery on brain metastases from renal cell carcinoma. *Int J Radiat Oncol Biol Phys* 2000;47: 1007–1012.

117. Pirzkall A, Debus J, Lohr F, et al. Radiosurgery alone or in combination with whole-brain radiotherapy for brain metastases. *J Clin Oncol* 1998;16:3563–3569.

118. Sneed PK, Lamborn KR, Forstner JM, et al. Radiosurgery for brain metastases: is whole brain radiotherapy necessary? *Int J Radiat Oncol Biol Phys* 1999;43:549–558.

119. Muacevic A, Kreth FW, Horstmann GA, et al. Surgery and radiotherapy compared with gamma knife radiosurgery in the treatment of solitary cerebral metastases of small diameter. *J Neurosurg* 1999; 91:35–43.

120. Peterson AM, Meltzer CC, Evanson EJ, et al. MR imaging response of brain metastases after gamma knife stereotactic radiosurgery. *Radiology* 1999;211:807–814.

121. Adler JR, Cox RS, Kaplan I, et al. Stereotactic radiosurgical treatment of brain metastases. *J Neurosurg* 1992;76:444–449.

122. Kornblith PL, Walker MD, eds. *Advances in neuro-oncology II.* Armonk, NY: Futura, 1997.

123. Flickinger JC, Kondziolka D, Lunsford LD, et al. A multi-institutional experience with stereotactic radiosurgery for solitary brain metastasis. *Int J Radiat Oncol Biol Phys* 1994;28:797–802.

124. Chen JCT, Petrovich Z, O'Day S, et al. Stereotactic radiosurgery in the treatment of metastatic disease to the brain. *Neurosurgery* 2000; 47:268–281.

125. Kihlstrom L, Karlsson B, Lindquist C, et al. Gamma knife surgery for cerebral metastasis. *Acta Neurochir Suppl (Wien)* 1991;52:87–89.

126. Kihlstrom L, Karlsson B, Lindquist C. Gamma knife surgery for cerebral metastases. Implications for survival based on 16 years experience. *Stereotact Funct Neurosurg* 1993;61:45–50.

127. Nataf F. Place de la radiochirurgie dans le traitement des metastases cerebrales. *Neuro-Chirurgie* 1999;45:393–397.

128. Somaza S, Kondziolka D, Lunsford LD, et al. Stereotactic radiosurgery for cerebral metastatic melanoma. *J Neurosurg* 1993;79: 661–666.

129. Irish WD, Macdonald DR, Cairncross JG. Measuring bias in uncontrolled brain tumor trials: to randomize or not to randomize. *Can J Neurol Sci* 1997;24:307–312.

130. Shapiro WR. Bias in uncontrolled brain tumor trials. *Can J Neurol Sci* 1997;24:269–270.

131. Hu X, Wright JG, McLeod RS, et al. Observational studies as alternatives to randomized clinical trials in surgical clinical research. *Surgery* 1996;119:473–475.

132. Auchter RM, Lamond JP, Alexander E, et al. A multi-institutional outcome and prognostic factor analysis of radiosurgery for resectable single brain metastasis. *Int J Radiat Oncol Biol Phys* 1996;35: 27–35.

133. Chidel MA, Suh JH, Reddy CA, et al. Application of recursive partitioning analysis and evaluation of the use of whole brain radiation among patients treated with stereotactic radiosurgery for newly diagnosed brain metastases. *Int J Radiat Oncol Biol Phys* 2000;42: 155–159.

134. Agboola O, Benoit B, Cross P, et al. Prognostic factors derived from recursive partition analysis (RPA) of Radiation Therapy Oncology Group (RTOG) brain metastases trials applied to surgically resected and irradiated brain metastatic cases. *Int J Radiat Oncol Biol Phys* 1998;42:155–159.

135. Wronski M, Arbit E, Burt M, et al. Survival after surgical treatment of brain metastases from lung cancer: a follow-up study of 231 patients treated between 1976 and 1991. *J Neurosurg* 1995;83: 605–616.

136. Wronski M, Arbit E, Russo P, et al. Surgical resection of brain metastases from renal cell carcinoma in 50 patients. *Urology* 1996;47: 187–193.

137. Sawaya R, Hammoud M, Schoppa D, et al. Neurosurgical outcomes in a modern series of 400 craniotomies for treatment of parenchymal tumors. *Neurosurgery* 1998;42:1044–1056.

138. Cabantog AM, Bernstein M. Complications of first craniotomy for intra-axial brain tumour. *Can J Neurol Sci* 1994;21:213–218.

139. De Santis M, Balducci M, Basilico L, et al. Radiotherapy, local control and survival in brain tumors. *Rays* 1998;23:543–548.

140. Murray KJ, Scott C, Greenberg HM, et al. A randomized phase III study of accelerated hyperfractionation versus standard in patients with unresected brain metastases: a report of the Radiation Therapy Oncology Group (RTOG) 9104. *Int J Radiat Oncol Biol Phys* 1997; 39:571–574.

141. Sause WT, Scott C, Krisch R, et al. Phase I/II trial of accelerated fractionation in brain metastases RTOG 85-28. *Int J Radiat Oncol Biol Phys* 1993;26:653–657.

142. Haines SJ, Walters BC. Proof of equivalence. The inference of statistical significance. "Caveat emptor." *Neurosurgery* 1993;33: 432–433.

143. Shaw EG. Radiotherapeutic management of multiple brain metastases: "3000 in 10" whole brain radiation is no longer a "no brainer." *Int J Radiat Oncol Biol Phys* 1999;45:253–254.

144. Ellis R, Gregor A. The treatment of brain metastases from lung cancer. *Lung Cancer* 1998;20:81–84.

145. Miller JD. Surgical excision for single cerebral metastasis? *Lancet* 1993;341:1566.

146. Hazuka MB, Burleson WD, Stroud DN, et al. Multiple brain metastases are associated with poor survival in patients treated with surgery and radiotherapy. *J Clin Oncol* 1993;11:369–373.

147. Bindal RK, Sawaya R, Leavens ME, et al. Surgical treatment of multiple brain metastases. *J Neurosurg* 1993;79:210–216.

148. Chang SD, Lee E, Sakamoto GT, et al. Stereotactic radiosurgery in patients with multiple brain metastases. *Neurosurg Focus* 2000;9: Article 3, 5 pp.

149. Cho KH, Walter AH, Gerbi BJ, et al. The role of radiosurgery for multiple brain metastases. *Neurosurg Focus* 2000;9:Article 2, 7 pp.

150. Kondziolka D, Patel A, Lunsford LD, et al. Stereotactic radiosurgery plus whole brain radiotherapy versus radiotherapy alone for patients with multiple brain metastases. *Int J Radiat Oncol Biol Phys* 1999;45:427–434.

151. Chang SD, Adler JR, Jr. Current treatment of patients with multiple brain metastases. *Neurosurg Focus* 2000;9:Article 5, 5 pp.

152. Shaw E, Scott C, Souhami L, et al. Single dose radiosurgical treatment of recurrent previously irradiated primary brain tumors and brain metastases: final report of RTOG protocol 90-05. *Int J Radiat Oncol Biol Phys* 2000;47:291–298.

153. Arbit E, Wronski M, Burt M, et al. The treatment of patients with recurrent brain metastases. A retrospective analysis of 109 patients with nonsmall cell lung cancer. *Cancer* 1995;76:765–773.

154. Bindal RK, Sawaya R, Leavens ME, et al. Reoperation for recurrent metastatic brain tumors. *J Neurosurg* 1995;83:600–604.

155. Alexander E 3rd, Loeffler JS. Recurrent brain metastases. *Neurosurg Clin N Am* 1996;7:517–526.

156. Sundaresan N, Sachdev VP, DiGiacinto GV, et al. Reoperation for brain metastases. *J Clin Oncol* 1988;6:1625–1629.

157. Heros DO, Kasdon DL, Chun M. Brachytherapy in the treatment of recurrent solitary brain metastases. *Neurosurgery* 1988;23:733–737.

158. McDermott MW, Cosgrove GR, Larson DA, et al. Interstitial brachytherapy for intracranial metastases. *Neurosurg Clin N Am* 1996;7: 485–495.

159. Bernstein M, Laperriere N, Leung P, et al. Interstitial brachytherapy for malignant brain tumors: preliminary results. *Neurosurgery* 1990; 26:371–379; discussion 379–380.

160. Kreth FW, Warnke PC, Ostertag CB. Interstitial implant radiosurgery for cerebral metastases. *Acta Neurochir Suppl (Wien)* 1993; 58:112–114.

161. Korfel A, Thiel E. Chemotherapy of brain metastases. In: Wiegel T, Hinkelbein W, Brock M, et al, eds. *Controversies in neuro-oncology,* vol. 33. Basel: Karger, 1999:343–348.

162. Twelves CJ, Souhami RL, Harper PG, et al. The response of cerebral metastases in small cell lung cancer to systemic chemotherapy. *Br J Cancer* 1990;61:147–150.

163. Kelly K, Bunn PA Jr. Is it time to reevaluate our approach to the treatment of brain metastases in patients with non-small cell lung cancer? *Lung Cancer* 1998;20:85–91.

164. Minotti V, Crino L, Meacci ML, et al. Chemotherapy with cisplatin and teniposide for cerebral metastases in non-small cell lung cancer. *Lung Cancer* 1998;20:93–98.

165. Cox JD, Stanley K, Petrovich Z, et al. Cranial irradiation in cancer of the lung of all cell types. *JAMA* 1981;245:469–472.

166. Hansen HH, Dombernowsky P, Hirsch FR, et al. Prophylactic irradiation in bronchogenic small cell anaplastic carcinoma. A comparative trial of localized versus extensive radiotherapy including prophylactic brain irradiation in patients receiving combination chemotherapy. *Cancer* 1980;46:279–284.

167. Jackson DV Jr, Richards FD, Cooper MR, et al. Prophylactic cranial irradiation in small cell carcinoma of the lung. A randomized study. *JAMA* 1977;237:2730–2733.

168. Arriagada R, Le Chevalier T, Borie F, et al. Prophylactic cranial irradiation for patients with small-cell lung cancer in complete remission. *J Natl Cancer Inst* 1995;87:183–190.

169. Einhorn LH. The case against prophylactic cranial irradiation in limited small cell lung cancer. *Semin Radiat Oncol* 1995;5:57–60.

170. Gregor A, Cull A, Stephens RJ, et al. Prophylactic cranial irradiation

is indicated following complete response to induction therapy in small cell lung cancer: results of a multicentre randomised trial. United Kingdom Coordinating Committee for Cancer Research (UKCCCR) and the European Organization for Research and Treatment of Cancer (EORTC). *Eur J Cancer* 1997;33:1752–1758.

171. Russell AH, Pajak TE, Selim HM, et al. Prophylactic cranial irradiation for lung cancer patients at high risk for development of cerebral metastasis: results of a prospective randomized trial conducted by the Radiation Therapy Oncology Group. *Int J Radiat Oncol Biol Phys* 1991;21:637–643.

172. Ball DL, Matthews JP. Prophylactic cranial irradiation: more questions than answers. *Semin Radiat Oncol* 1995;5:61–68.

173. Auperin A, Arriagada R, Pignon JP, et al. Prophylactic cranial irradiation for patients with small-cell lung cancer in complete remission. Prophylactic Cranial Irradiation Overview Collaborative Group. *N Engl J Med* 1999;341:476–484.

174. Kocher M, Muller RP, Staar S, et al. Long-term survival after brain metastases in breast cancer. *Strahlenther Onkol* 1995;171:290–295.

175. Salvati M, Artico M, Carloia S, et al. Solitary cerebral metastasis from lung cancer with very long survival: report of two cases and review of the literature. *Surg Neurol* 1991;36:458–461.

176. Gaspar LE, Scott C, Murray K, et al. Validation of the RTOG recursive partitioning analysis (RPA) classification for brain metastases. *Int J Radiat Oncol Biol Phys* 2000;47:1001–1006.

114. Primary Central Nervous System Lymphoma

**Alejandro Torres-Trejo and
Lisa Marie DeAngelis**

Cerebral Lymphoma

HISTORY AND NOMENCLATURE. Primary central nervous system lymphoma (PCNSL) was first described by Bailey in 1929 (1). He called it "perithelial or perivascular sarcoma of leptomeningeal origin." Cerebral lymphoma was described under a variety of names over the following two to three decades, including reticulum cell sarcoma, microglioma, histiocytic sarcoma, adventitial sarcoma, reticuloendothelial sarcoma, malignant lymphoma, malignant reticulohistiocytic encephalitis, atypical granulomatous encephalitis, and lymphoproliferative disorder, highlighting the debate regarding the malignant cell of origin (2,3). However, in 1974, Henry and colleagues (2) demonstrated that the pathologic features seen in this central nervous system tumor were histologically similar to other tumors arising in the reticuloendothelial system. Modern immunohistochemical studies definitively established the lymphocytic nature of this tumor (4).

EPIDEMIOLOGY. PCNSL affects immunocompetent and immunodeficient individuals of all ages and gender. Acquired immunodeficiency syndrome (AIDS) patients are at highest risk among the immunocompromised (5). Congenital immunodeficiency states such ataxia-telangiectasia, X-linked immunodeficiency, severe combined immunodeficiency, and Wiskott-Aldrich syndrome also confer an increased risk for PCNSL (5). Patients who undergo kidney transplantation have a 350 times higher risk of developing lymphoma than the general population, with 2.2 cases per 1,000 transplants; 50% of these were cranial lymphomas and most occurred in the first year after transplantation (4,6). The risk is higher in heart-transplanted individuals, with three cases in 182 organ recipients (4,7,8).

PCNSL was considered an extremely rare neoplasm for decades. It accounted for only about 1% of all primary brain tumors, less than 1% of all malignant lymphomas, and about 2% of extranodal lymphomas. However, the incidence of PCNSL has risen dramatically in the past 15 to 20 years, both in the immuno-

competent and immunocompromised population (4,9–11). A recent study showed that there has been a threefold increased incidence from 2.5 cases per ten million from 1973 to 1975 to 7.5 cases per ten million from 1982 to 1984 in the United States. Never-married men, a relatively high-risk group for AIDS, were excluded from this study. This increase in incidence appears to be real; it antedates the AIDS epidemic and is not related to organ transplantation, better ascertainment, or time trends in nosology (12). Devesa and Fears reanalyzed this increased incidence and found the threefold increase was sustained through 1988 (11). It is estimated that in the year 2000, the projected incidence rate of brain lymphoma reached 51.1 per 10 million population and 118.2 per 10 million population, with never-married men excluded and included, respectively. Furthermore, the incidence of primary ocular lymphoma, a variant of PCNSL, has increased 1.5-fold during the same interval. The overall incidence of systemic non-Hodgkin's lymphoma has not risen significantly (13); however, the increase in PCNSL and ocular lymphoma is part of an overall trend of increasing extranodal lymphomas. This increased incidence of PCNSL also has been reported in Western Europe but not in Alberta, Canada (14). These geographic variations are unexplained.

In immunocompetent patients, PCNSL most often is diagnosed in the sixth decade or later and is more common in men than women in a ratio of 2 to 1 (15). The demographics of AIDS-related PCNSL are different from those seen in immunocompetent individuals. The usual age of onset is in the fourth or fifth decade and is much more common in men, as is HIV-1 infection.

Early in the AIDS epidemic, PCNSL was thought to occur in 1.9% of patients with AIDS (16), but we now recognize that it occurs between 5% and 10% during life (17,18). It is the second most common cause of an intracranial mass in adults and the most common in children (19–21). At autopsy 10% to 20% of patients who died of AIDS have PCNSL (22), and 20% to 25% of all lymphomas diagnosed in individuals with AIDS are PCNSL, which far exceeds the proportion of brain lymphomas in the immunocompetent population. AIDS patients are now living longer with the improvement of treatment for AIDS and opportunistic infections. Long survival has been associated with an increased incidence of lymphoma, including cerebral lymphoma (23,24). The risk of developing lymphoma in the AIDS population is 1,000 times that of the general population, with an estimate of 600 new cases per year (4,25); however, there is a clinical impression that the incidence of PCNSL is falling among those AIDS patients using highly active antiretroviral therapy (HAART). PCNSL is associated with severe depression of T-4 lymphocyte counts; HAART can partially reconstitute the immune response, which likely accounts for the decreasing incidence of PCNSL.

PATHOGENESIS. The etiology of PCNSL in immunocompetent patients is unknown, but the Epstein-Barr virus (EBV) has been implicated in the pathogenesis of PCNSL in immunocompromised patients, particularly AIDS patients. The EBV genome has been detected by *in situ* hybridization and polymerase chain reaction (PCR) in 50% to 100% of AIDS-associated PCNSL (17,26–31). This is not true for immunocompetent patients with PCNSL (32,33). EBV DNA can be detected by PCR in the CSF of individuals with HIV-associated PCNSL with a sensitivity of 100% and a specificity of 98% (34,35). This has become a critical test for any AIDS patient with an intracranial mass, and it has facilitated early, noninvasive diagnosis of PCNSL.

Most adults have had acute EBV infection at a young age, and after the initial infection, a population of B-lymphocytes becomes immortalized by the virus. T lymphocytes control the proliferation of this latently infected B-cell population in immunocompetent individuals, but T cells are incapable of suppressing uncontrolled growth of these latently infected lymphocytes in immunocompromised patients, which in turn leads to tumor formation (3,4). EBV-related lymphomas probably tend to develop in the nervous system because the brain, an immunologically privileged site, offers further protection from immune surveillance (36).

The mechanisms that cause B-cell proliferation in the immunocompetent population are unknown; there are three hypotheses: (a) lymphocytes trafficking through the CNS become transformed; (b) B cells are attracted into the CNS by an antigenic stimulus; and (c) lymphocytes are transformed systemically and home into the CNS.

PATHOLOGY. The appearance of PCNSL tumors on gross examination is variable: They can be well defined, homogeneous, gray, granular masses. Other lesions are more diffuse and infiltrate normal brain. Hemorrhage or necrosis rarely is seen. PCNSL does not have cysts, which are a common feature of malignant astrocytomas. Most commonly, PCNSL arises in the hemispheric white matter or in the deep gray structures of brain (2,9,37). The lesions are solitary in 60% of cases, and 40% are multiple. Most lesions are periventricular, which predisposes to subependymal and CSF extension (4,9). Multifocality is seen in almost all patients with AIDS-related PCNSL; these tumors more often are hemorrhagic and necrotic than non-AIDS PCNSL and often are found to coexist with CNS infections (36).

In 68 immunocompetent patients with 109 lesions, 70 were located in the cerebrum, 21 in the brainstem, 14 in the cerebellum, and four in the spinal cord (2). The eye represents another site of involvement, affecting 20% of patients, and may be the initial site of presentation (10,38).

Leptomeningeal involvement can be documented in 42% of patients at diagnosis, and is always present at autopsy. Isolated meningeal lymphoma in the absence of parenchymal disease is distinctly unusual (39). Extraneural involvement of organs occurs in less than 4% of patients at the time of presentation (40). Systemic metastasis may occur in 6% to 7% of patients

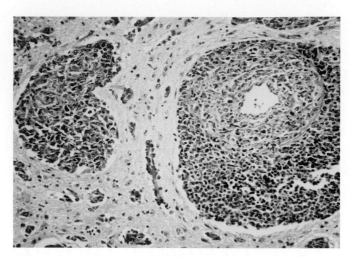

Fig. 1. Photomicrograph of primary central nervous system lymphoma demonstrating perivascular aggregation of tumor.

with very late-stage disease, usually in association with CNS relapse (2,10,41).

Microscopically the lymphomatous infiltrates are dense, patchy, poorly demarcated, and strikingly angiocentric. The last is a key histological feature of PCNSL (Fig. 1) (2,37). Angiocentricity and angioinvasion, although most apparent at the edges of the lesion, also are present in densely cellular portions of the tumor (42). PCNSL cells freely infiltrate the brain parenchyma, but they involve much wider regions of brain than malignant glial cells. Furthermore, PCNSL is frequently multifocal at the microscopic level, often with discontinuous areas of involvement (10,37,42). The vasculature of all lymphomas has a characteristic increase in perivascular reticulin (9,43), from which the name reticulum cell sarcoma was derived. Associated reactive astrocytosis, particularly at the tumor margins, can produce positive staining for glial fibrillary acidic protein (GFAP), which may obscure the diagnosis (37); this may be a problem when a biopsy is obtained from the periphery of the tumor. Prior corticosteroid therapy may cause a marked cytolytic effect on the tumor, seriously affecting the histological diagnosis (44).

The vast majority of PCNSLs are non-Hodgkin's lymphomas composed of B cells, although T-cell lymphomas have been identified (9,10). Some authors have noted an unfavorable prognosis for patients with T-cell lymphoma (45); however, others have found that this type of lymphoma has the tendency to develop in younger people and has an improved prognosis (46). The majority of PCNSLs can be classified histologically according to the International Working Formulation of Lymphoma (4,47). Most are large-cell or large-cell immunoblastic tumors. Rarely they may be composed of small noncleaved cells or mixed cells (10,37). The histological differentiation between B-cell lymphoma versus the rare T-cell lymphoma is made by immunotyping with a panel of monoclonal antibodies in a small sample obtained by stereotactic biopsy (33). Sometimes reactive T-cells infiltrate B-cell lymphomas, which may cause diagnostic confusion (48). Genotypic analysis establishes the monoclonal nature of B- or T-cell lymphomas by identifying gene rearrangements of the Ig heavy- and light-chain genes or the T-cell receptor gene (9). PCNSL has not been associated with arrangements of the *c-myc* oncogene, as in AIDS-associated systemic lymphomas (49).

CLINICAL PRESENTATION. The majority of patients present with altered level of alertness and cognitive impairment (36%), because of the frequency of bilateral and deep frontal lobe involvement (4). More than two thirds of patients develop cognitive dysfunction during the course of PCNSL (3,4). Twenty-two percent of patients have headache as a presenting symptom, and more than 50% develop headache during their illness (3,4). Cerebellar signs are seen in 31%, seizures in 20%, motor dysfunction in 17%, and visual changes in 12% (4). The majority of patients present in a subacute fashion with an average duration of symptoms from 2 weeks to 2.5 months prior to diagnosis (2,3). Neurologic dysfunction often progresses quickly because these tumors grow rapidly and have a high labeling index.

Ocular lymphoma usually involves the vitreous, uvea, or retina (38,50). It is different from orbital lymphoma, an extranodal site of systemic lymphoma, which affects the lacrimal gland, eyelid, and conjunctiva (51). The ocular involvement can be bilateral in 67% to 81%, but is usually asymmetric (38,50,52). The symptoms of ocular lymphoma often are subtle and consist of floaters, blurry vision, or rarely, eye pain. These symptoms are nonspecific and often are misdiagnosed as uveitis or vitreitis of unknown etiology (38,51). Slit-lamp examination usually reveals inflammatory cells in the vitreous, which can cause visual loss, although this is rare in the early stages. The diagnosis of ocular lymphoma should be considered in the absence of a durable clinical response to standard corticosteroid therapy for "uveitis" or "vitreitis" (3).

Primary leptomeningeal lymphoma is rare, accounting for at most 7% of all cases of PCNSL. It usually presents with lumbosacral polyradiculopathy that may be painful, followed by cranial neuropathies, confusion, and symptoms of increased intracranial pressure with headache, nausea, and vomiting, or a combination of these symptoms (53). Spinal lymphoma presents as an intramedullary expansile spinal cord mass with painless myelopathy producing bilateral leg weakness, and sensory and sphincter dysfunction (54).

RADIOGRAPHIC FEATURES. Typically, PCNSL is located in the deep gray matter or around the ventricles. The precontrast images usually are isodense or hyperdense on CT scans and isointense or hypointense on T1 technique on MR scans (15, 55,56). There is a variable degree of surrounding edema; after administration of contrast, there is usually homogeneous enhancement (Fig. 2) (57). The tumor occasionally enhances in a heterogeneous fashion or ring-enhancing pattern (56,58); the tumor is rarely nonenhancing (59). In the immunocompromised patient, the lesions on precontrast T1 MRI appear hypointense and enhance in a ringlike pattern in 19% to 59% of patients (60). The lesions are usually hypodense on a precontrast CT scan and enhance in a patchy or ringlike fashion after contrast administration (61). The preceding features make AIDS-related PCNSL indistinguishable radiographically from other CNS neoplasms or infections, particularly toxoplasmosis, which may even coexist in the same patient (62,63). Positron emission tomography (PET) and single photon emission tomography (SPECT) imaging may differentiate PCNSL from toxoplasmosis (18,64).

DIFFERENTIAL DIAGNOSIS. PCNSL can be confused with malignant primary brain tumors in immunocompetent patients with a single lesion. Multiple PCNSL lesions may be mistaken for metastases. Approximately 15% of patients with PCNSL have a past history of a prior malignancy. This may encourage the physician's assumption that the new brain lesions are metastases, leading to empirical palliative whole brain radiotherapy, which may compromise the patient's outcome (65).

Corticosteroid treatment often is given immediately to patients with a mass lesion identified on cranial imaging, to decrease swelling and improve the patient's neurological status. This approach may be effective for most intracranial masses; however, corticosteroids function as a cytotoxic agent in PCNSL producing cell lysis of malignant lymphocytes. This can destroy the opportunity to establish the diagnosis of lymphoma by giving a false negative brain biopsy, vitrectomy, or CSF examination (44). Furthermore, if there is a prominent T-cell infiltrate in the PCNSL, the malignant cells may be lysed, leaving behind the reactive lymphocytes and misleading the pathologist into a diagnosis of an inflammatory condition. When a mass lesion

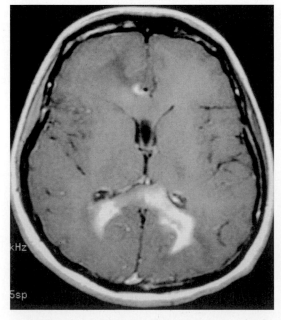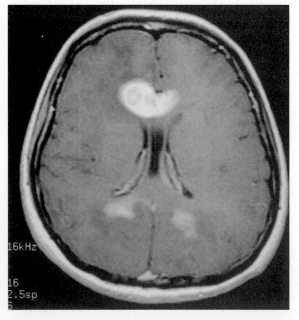

Fig. 2. Gadolinium-enhanced MRI demonstrating multifocal periventricular diffusely enhancing primary central nervous system lymphoma. Note the absence of central necrosis and the relative lack of edema.

resolves with corticosteroids, lymphoma often is presumed. However, other entities such as sarcoid or multiple sclerosis also may resolve after the administration of steroids (66); therefore, when PCNSL is considered, steroids should be deferred until after tissue has been obtained unless there is imminent danger of cerebral herniation.

As mentioned, AIDS-related PCNSL cannot be distinguished, clinically or radiographically, from other brain lesions seen in the AIDS patient. Diagnosis is even more difficult because some opportunistic infections may coexist with PCNSL (67). The use of PET or SPECT and EBV PCR on CSF usually establishes the diagnosis of PCNSL when the patient presents with neurological symptoms and a mass is identified on imaging. These tests have largely replaced empiric diagnosis after failure of 2 weeks of antitoxoplasma therapy (17,18,26–31,57,64).

DIAGNOSTIC WORKUP. Enhanced MR scan of the brain is the single most important diagnostic procedure used to evaluate a patient with PCNSL (3,41). It identifies the parenchymal brain involvement and occasionally defines leptomeningeal involvement. Patients with spinal or radicular symptoms should undergo spinal MRI with gadolinium. All patients should have a lumbar puncture to evaluate for leptomeningeal extension, particularly because most patients with positive cytology do not have symptoms of leptomeningeal disease. The documentation of positive CSF cytology is important prognostically and therapeutically (3). All patients should have an ophthalmological examination, including slit-lamp to identify ocular involvement (38,50). The need for systemic staging in immunocompetent patients is controversial. The yield is less than 4% and systemic sites of disease were identified on abdominal and pelvic CT or bone marrow biopsy in all; thus, systemic testing can be limited to these tests (40). Lymphoma can be more extensive in the immunocompromised patient; therefore, a chest CT should be added to the evaluation (41). HIV testing should be done in all patients (3).

TREATMENT. PCNSL is not a surgical disease. Resection has no therapeutic role in the treatment of PCNSL and may cause unnecessary neurologic deficits, because of the deep-seated location of many lesions (68,69). Stereotactic biopsy is the best surgical modality for deep lesions. A frozen section should be obtained for cortically based lesions, and no further resection is necessary if it confirms lymphoma. Occasionally patients may require emergency debulking for cerebral herniation; most improve dramatically with resection. The focus of PCNSL treatment has been medical. Glucocorticoids have a cytolytic effect on PCNSL; however, this is not lasting. Radiotherapy (RT) can cause tumor regression, but the response is not durable and most patients relapse in the first year (68). Combined multiagent chemotherapy is used increasingly because it significantly prolongs life and disease-free survival.

Radiotherapy has been used in both immunocompetent and immunocompromised patients with PCNSL with clinical and radiographic improvement. Due to the multifocal nature of this disease, whole brain radiation is used, usually to a total dose of 45 Gy (70). When RT is used alone, median survival is 12 to 18 months in non-AIDS PCNSL (71,72), whereas the median survival is 2 to 5 months in the AIDS population. However, most patients with AIDS die of opportunistic infections rather than PCNSL progression (16,60–62,73). Ocular lymphoma should be treated with 36 Gy RT. Both eyes should be included because the disease is bilateral in more than 80% of patients (38,50). Craniospinal irradiation is not used even for patients with a positive CSF cytology. It does not improve survival and can compromise bone marrow reserve. These patients are treated with high-dose systemic chemotherapy supplemented with intrathecal methotrexate. Patients with parenchymal spinal cord lymphoma receive focal RT. When primary leptomeningeal lymphoma is documented, craniospinal radiation occasionally is used with intrathecal (IT) methotrexate (MTX) (53), but high-dose systemic chemotherapy may be an alternative.

Chemotherapy now is being used as adjuvant or neoadjuvant therapy with or without RT (Table 1). The goal is to use an agent that crosses the blood–brain barrier (BBB). The types of chemotherapeutic agents used to treat PCNSL are different from those used to treat systemic lymphoma, typically doxorubicin and cyclophosphamide. Standard systemic lymphoma regimens have been added to WBRT but have not proven effective, likely because these agents do not penetrate the BBB (74,75). In addition, these drugs add considerable systemic toxicity.

One approach used by Dahlborg and colleagues (76) has been to use BBB disruption with intraarterial (IA) mannitol followed by IA methotrexate, cyclophosphamide, procarbazine, and dexamethasone monthly for 12 months. Radiation was given only for tumor progression or recurrence. The median survival was 44.5 months. The procedure is associated with significant acute toxicity, but the authors claim there is no long-term neurotoxicity despite exposing the brain to high concentrations of methotrexate, a known neurotoxin.

DeAngelis and colleagues (70) treated 31 immunocompetent patients with preradiation systemic MTX and six doses of intra-Ommaya MTX, followed by a full course of RT. Two cycles of high-dose cytarabine were given post-RT. This approach gave a median survival of 42.5 months. Recent follow-up demonstrated a stable median survival with seven patients still alive. However, there was a high incidence of late neurotoxicity particularly in patients over age 60. Prolonged survival revealed that chemotherapy combined with radiotherapy had a synergistic toxic effect on normal brain; therefore, many began to explore the use of chemotherapy alone. Freilich and colleagues (77) treated 13 patients over age 50 (mean age 74 years) with MTX and procarbazine; in addition, five received thiotepa, four vincristine, and four vincristine and cytarabine. Ten patients had a complete response (CR) and two had a partial response (PR). The median survival was 30.5 months. Others have reported good responses to high-dose MTX alone.

High-dose cytarabine can be used in ocular lymphoma, since this agent is one of the few that penetrates into the vitreous humor (78). Ocular lymphoma responds to high-dose MTX (3), and refractory ocular disease has been successfully treated with intraocular injections of MTX. For patients who received WBRT as initial therapy, adjuvant chemotherapy can be beneficial. Chamberlain and Levin (79) treated 16 immunocompetent patients with adjuvant chemotherapy using procarbazine, CCNU, and vincristine (PCV), with a median survival of 41 months. This therapeutic approach is an alternative for patients who cannot receive chemotherapy prior to RT. PCV given after RT does not seem to potentiate radiation toxicity; however, MTX

Table 1. Treatment of Primary Central Nervous System Lymphoma and Median Survival

Therapy	Median Survival (mo)	5-Year Survival (%)
BBBD + intraarterial MTX	44.5	30
HD-MTX + WBRT	42.5	30
WBRT	12–18	4

BBBD, blood–brain barrier disruption; HD-MTX, high-dose methotrexate; WBRT, whole brain radiotherapy.

post-RT should be avoided because of the enhanced potential for leukoencephalopathy.

AIDS-related PCNSL presents a challenge regarding treatment. Most patients are too sick to receive more than palliative WBRT; however, some benefit from chemotherapy (80). New approaches include antiviral therapy and new antiretroviral treatments.

PROGNOSIS. Age and performance status are important prognostic factors regardless of treatment; however, even older patients can benefit from a vigorous approach with multiagent chemotherapy. PCNSL behaves much more aggressively than a comparable systemic stage IE lymphoma, despite the fact that both are histologically similar. If patients with PCNSL are given supportive care only, the expected survival is 1 to 2 months. Surgery alone does not prolong survival, radiotherapy alone gives a median survival of 12 to 18 months, and WBRT plus chemotherapy gives a median survival of about 40 months. The future challenge is to improve survival while minimizing the potential for neurotoxic damage. The primary focus has been to maximize chemotherapy and defer RT. In AIDS-related PCNSL novel therapeutic approaches may focus on better antiviral therapies.

References

1. Bailey P. Intracranial sarcomatous tumors of leptomeningeal origin. *Arch Surg* 1929;18:1359–1402.
2. Henry JM, Heffner RR Jr, Dillard SH, et al. Primary malignant lymphomas of the central nervous system. *Cancer* 1974;34:1293–1302.
3. DeAngelis LM. Primary central nervous system lymphoma. In: Gilman S, Goldstein G, Waxman S, eds. *Neurobase.* San Diego: Arbor, 1998.
4. Hochberg FH, Miller DC. Primary central nervous system lymphoma. *J Neurosurg* 1988;68:835–853.
5. Kersey JH, Shapiro RS, Filipovich AH. Relationship of immunodeficiency to lymphoid malignancy. *Pediatr Infect Dis J* 1988;7:S10–12.
6. Hoover R, Fraumeni JF Jr. Risk of cancer in renal-transplant recipients. *Lancet* 1973;2:55–57.
7. Weintraub J, Warnke RA. Lymphoma in cardiac allotransplant recipients: clinical and histological features and immunological phenotypes. *Transplantation* 1982;33:347–351.
8. Velasquez WS. Primary central nervous system lymphoma. *J Neurooncol* 1994;20:177–185.
9. Grant JW, Isaacson PG. Primary central nervous system lymphoma. *Brain Pathol* 1992;2:97–109.
10. Miller DC, Hochberg F, Harris N, et al. Pathology with clinical correlations of primary central nervous system non-Hodgkin's lymphoma. The Massachusetts General Hospital Experience 1958-1989. *Cancer* 1994;74:1383–1397.
11. Devesa SS, Fears T. Non-Hodgkin's lymphoma time trends: United States and international data. *Cancer Res* 1992;52:S5432–5440.
12. Eby NL, Grufferman S, Flannelly CM, et al. Increasing incidence of primary brain lymphoma in the US. *Cancer* 1988;62:2461–2465.
13. Corn BW, Marcus SM, Topham A, et al. Will primary central nervous system lymphoma be the most frequent brain tumor diagnosed in the year 2000? *Cancer* 1997;79:2409–2413.
14. Hao D, DiFrancesco LM, Brasher PM, et al. Is primary CNS lymphoma really becoming more common? A population-based study of incidence, clinicopathological features and outcomes in Alberta from 1975-1996. *Ann Oncol* 1999;10:65–70.
15. O'Neill BP, Illig JJ. Primary central nervous system lymphoma. *Mayo Clin Proc* 1989;64:1005–1020.
16. Rosenblum ML, Levy RM, Bredesen DE, et al. Primary central nervous system lymphomas in patients with AIDS. *Ann Neurol* 1988;23:S13–16.
17. Auperin I, Mikol J, Oksenhendler E, et al. Primary central nervous system malignant non-Hodgkin's lymphomas from HIV-infected and non-infected patients: expression of cellular surface proteins and Epstein-Barr viral markers. *Neuropathol Appl Neurobiol* 1994;20:243–252.
18. Ruiz A, Ganz WI, Post MJD, et al. Use of Thallium-201 brain SPECT to differentiate cerebral lymphoma from toxoplasma encephalitis in AIDS patients. *AJNR Am J Neuroradiol* 1994;15:1885–1894.
19. Goldstein J, Dickson DW, Rubenstein A, et al. Primary central nervous system lymphoma in a pediatric patient with acquired immune deficiency syndrome. Treatment with radiation therapy. *Cancer* 1990;66:2503–2508.
20. Del Mistro A, Laverda A, Calabrese F, et al. Primary lymphoma of the central nervous system in two children with acquired immune deficiency syndrome. *Am J Clin Pathol* 1990;94:722–728.
21. Schulman H, Hertzanu Y, Maor E, et al. Primary lymphoma of brain in childhood. *Pediatr Radiol* 1991;21:434–435.
22. Ling SM, Roach M 3rd, Larson DA, et al. Radiotherapy of primary central nervous system lymphoma in patients with and without human immunodeficiency syndrome virus. Ten years of treatment experience at the University of California San Francisco. *Cancer* 1994;73:2570–2582.
23. Gail MH, Pluda JM, Rabkin CS, et al. Projections of the incidence of non-Hodgkin's lymphoma related to acquired immunodeficiency syndrome. *J Natl Cancer Inst* 1991;83:695–701.
24. Pluda JM, Yarchoan R, Jaffe ES, et al. Development of non-Hodgkin lymphoma in a cohort of patients with severe human immunodeficiency virus (HIV) infection on long-term antiretroviral therapy. *Ann Intern Med* 1990;113:276–282.
25. Beral V, Peterman T, Berkelman R, et al. AIDS-associated non-Hodgkin lymphoma. *Lancet* 1991;337:805–809.
26. Morgello S. Epstein-Barr and human immunodeficiency viruses in acquired immunodeficiency syndrome-related primary central nervous system lymphoma. *Am J Pathol* 1992;141:441–449.
27. DeAngelis LM, Wong E, Rosenblum M, et al. Epstein-Barr virus in acquired immune deficiency syndrome (AIDS) and non-AIDS primary central nervous system lymphoma. *Cancer* 1992;70:1607–1611.
28. Bignon YJ, Clavelou P, Ramos F, et al. Detection of Epstein-Barr virus sequences in primary brain lymphoma without immunodeficiency. *Neurology* 1991;41:1152–1153.
29. Rouah E, Rogers BB, Wilson DR, et al. Demonstration of Epstein-Barr virus in primary central nervous system lymphomas by the polymerase chain reaction and in situ hybridization. *Hum Pathol* 1990;21:545–550.
30. List AF, Greer JP, Cousar JP, et al. Primary brain lymphoma in the immunocompetent host: relation to Epstein-Barr virus. *Mod Pathol* 1990;3:609–612.
31. MacMahon EM, Glass JD, Hayward SD, et al. Epstein-Barr virus in AIDS-related primary central nervous system lymphoma. *Lancet* 1991;338:969–973.
32. Rosenberg NL, Hochberg FH, Miller G, et al. Primary central nervous system lymphoma related to Epstein-Barr virus in a patient with acquired immune deficiency syndrome. *Ann Neurol* 1986;20:98–102.
33. Bashir R, Luka J, Cheloha K, et al. Expression of Epstein-Barr virus proteins in primary CNS lymphoma in AIDS patients. *Neurology* 1993;43:2358–2362.
34. Cinque P, Brytting M, Vago L, et al. Epstein-Barr virus DNA in cerebrospinal fluid from patients with AIDS-related primary lymphoma of the central nervous system. *Lancet* 1993;342:398–401.
35. De Luca A, Antinori A, Cingolani A, et al. Evaluation of cerebrospinal fluid EBV-DNA and IL-10 as markers for in vivo diagnosis of AIDS-related primary central nervous system lymphoma. *Br J Haematol* 1995;90:844–849.
36. Greenberg HS, Chandler WF, Sandler HM. *Brain tumors.* New York: Oxford University Press, 1999.
37. Russell DS, Rubinstein LJ. Primary cerebral lymphoma. In: Russell DS, Rubinstein LJ, eds. *Pathology of tumours of the nervous system,* 5th ed. Baltimore: Williams & Wilkins, 1989:592–608.
38. Peterson K, Gordon KB, Heinemann MH, et al. The clinical spectrum of ocular lymphoma. *Cancer* 1993;72:843–849.
39. Balmaceda C, Gaynor JJ, Sun M, et al. Leptomeningeal tumor in primary central nervous system lymphoma: recognition, significance and implications. *Ann Neurol* 1995;38:202–209.
40. O'Neill BP, Dinapoli RP, Curtin PJ, et al. Occult systemic non-Hodgkin's lymphoma (NHL) in patients initially diagnosed as primary

central nervous system lymphoma (PCNSL): how much staging is enough? *J Neurooncol* 1995;25:67–71.

41. DeAngelis LM. Current management of primary central nervous system lymphoma. *Oncology (Huntingt)* 1995;9:63–71.

42. Burger PC, Scheithauer BW. Primary tumors of hematopoietic tissue. In: *Atlas of tumor pathology. Tumors of the central nervous system.* Washington, DC: Armed Forces Institute of Pathology, 1994: 321–331.

43. Kleihues P, Burger PC, Scheithauer BW. *Histological typing of tumours of the central nervous system,* 2nd ed. Berlin: World Health Organization, Springer-Verlag, 1993.

44. Geppert M, Ostertag CB, Seitz G, et al. Glucocorticoid therapy obscures the diagnosis of cerebral lymphoma. *Acta Neuropathol (Berl)* 1990;80;629–634.

45. Mineura K, Sawataishi J, Sasajima T, et al. Primary central nervous system involvement of the so called "peripheral T-cell lymphoma." Report of a case and review of the literature. *J Neurooncol* 1993;16: 235–242.

46. Ferracini R, Bergmann M, Pileri S, et al. Primary T-cell lymphoma of the central nervous system. *Clin Neuropathol* 1995;14:125–129.

47. The non-Hodgkin's lymphoma pathologic classification project: The National Cancer Institute sponsored study of classifications of non-Hodgkin's lymphomas: summary and description of a working formulation for clinical usage. *Cancer* 1982;49:2112–2135.

48. Morgello S, Petito CK, Mouradian JA. Central nervous system lymphoma in the acquired immunodeficiency syndrome. *Clin Neuropathol* 1990;9:204–215.

49. Meeker TC, Shiramizu L, Kaplan B, et al. Evidence for molecular subtypes of HIV-associated lymphoma: division into peripheral monoclonal, polyclonal and central nervous system lymphoma. *AIDS* 1991;5:669–674.

50. Char DH, Ljung BM, Miller T, et al. Primary intraocular lymphoma (ocular reticulum cell sarcoma) diagnosis and management. *Ophthalmology* 1988;95:625–630.

51. Trudeau M, Shepherd FA, Blackstein ME, et al. Intraocular lymphoma: report of three cases and review of the literature. *Am J Clin Oncol* 1988;11:126–130.

52. Whitcup SM, deSmet MD, Rubin BI, et al. Intraocular lymphoma clinical and histopathologic diagnosis. *Ophthalmology* 1993;100: 1399–1406.

53. Lachance DH, O'Neill PB, Macdonald DR, et al. Primary leptomeningeal lymphoma: report of 9 cases, diagnosis with immunocytochemical analysis, and review of the literature. *Neurology* 1991;41:95–100.

54. Hautzer NW, Aiyesimoju A, Robitaille Y. "Primary" spinal intramedullary lymphomas: a review. *Ann Neurol* 1983;14:62–66.

55. Amadori M, Maltoni M, Ravaioli A, et al. Primary lymphoma of the central nervous system. *Tumori* 1991;77:32–35.

56. Zimmerman RA. Central nervous system lymphoma. *Radiol Clin North Am* 1990;28:697–721.

57. Mendenhall NP, Thar TL, Agee OF, et al. Primary lymphoma of the central nervous system. Computerized tomography scan characteristics and treatment results for 12 cases. *Cancer* 1983;52:1993–2000.

58. DeAngelis LM, Yahalom J, Rosenblum M, et al. Primary CNS lymphoma: managing patients with spontaneous and AIDS-related disease. *Oncology (Huntingt)* 1987;1:52–62.

59. DeAngelis LM. Cerebral lymphoma presenting as a nonenhancing lesion on computer tomographic/magnetic resonance scan. *Ann Neurol* 1993;33:308–311.

60. Forsyth PA, Yahalom J, DeAngelis LM. Combined modality therapy in the treatment of primary central nervous system lymphoma in AIDS. *Neurology* 1994;44:1473–1479.

61. Baumgartner JE, Rachlin JR, Beckstead JH, et al. Primary central nervous system lymphomas: natural history and response to radiation therapy in 55 patients with acquired immunodeficiency syndrome. *J Neurosurg* 1990;73:206–211.

62. Goldstein JD, Zeifer B, Chao C, et al. CT appearance of primary CNS lymphoma in patients with acquired immunodeficiency syndrome. *J Comp Assist Tomogr* 1991;15:39–44.

63. Dina TS. Primary central nervous system lymphoma versus toxoplasmosis in AIDS. *Radiology* 1991;179:823–828.

64. Hoffman JM, Waskin HA, Schifter T, et al. FDG-PET in differentiating lymphoma from nonmalignant central nervous system lesions in patients with AIDS. *J Nucl Med* 1993;34:567–575.

65. DeAngelis LM. Primary central nervous system lymphoma as a secondary malignancy. *Cancer* 1991;67:1431–1435.

66. DeAngelis LM. Primary central nervous system lymphoma imitates multiple sclerosis. *J Neurooncol* 1990;9:177–181.

67. Loureiro C, Gill PS, Meyer PR, et al. Autopsy findings in AIDS-related lymphoma. *Cancer* 1988;62:735–739.

68. DeAngelis LM, Yahalom J, Heinemann MH, et al. Primary CNS lymphoma: combined treatment with chemotherapy and radiotherapy. *Neurology* 1990;40:80–86.

69. Michalski JM, Garcia DM, Kase E, et al. Primary central nervous system lymphoma: analysis of prognostic variables and patterns of treatment failure. *Radiology* 1990;176:855–860.

70. DeAngelis LM, Yahalom J, Thaler HT, et al. Combined modality therapy for primary CNS lymphoma. *J Clin Oncol* 1992;10:635–643.

71. Leibel SA, Sheline GE. Radiation therapy for neoplasms of the brain. *J Neurosurg* 1987;66:1–22.

72. Nelson DF, Martz KL, Bonner H, et al. Non-Hodgkin's lymphoma of the brain: can high dose, large volume radiation therapy improve survival? Report on a prospective trial by the Radiation Therapy Oncology Group (RTOG): RTOG 8315. *Int J Radiat Oncol Biol Phys* 1992;23:9–17.

73. Formenti SC, Gill PS, Lean E, et al. Primary central nervous system lymphoma in AIDS. Results of radiation therapy. *Cancer* 1989;63: 1101–1107.

74. O'Neill BP, O'Fallon JR, Earle JD, et al. Primary central nervous system non-Hodgkin's lymphoma: survival advantages with combined initial therapy? *Int J Radiat Oncol Biol Phys* 1995;33:663–673.

75. Lachance DH, Brizel DM, Gockerman JP, et al. Cyclophosphamide, doxorubicin, vincristine, and prednisone for primary central nervous system lymphoma: short-duration response and multifocal intracerebral recurrence preceding radiotherapy. *Neurology* 1994;44: 1721–1727.

76. Neuwelt EA, Goldman DL, Dahlborg SA, et al. Primary CNS lymphoma treated with osmotic blood-brain barrier disruption: prolonged survival and preservation of cognitive function. *J Clin Oncol* 1991;9:1580–1590.

77. Freilich RJ, Delattre J-Y, Monjour A, et al. Chemotherapy without radiation therapy as initial treatment for primary CNS lymphoma in older patients. *Neurology* 1996;46:435–439.

78. Strauchen JA, Dalton J, Friedman AH. Chemotherapy in the management of intraocular lymphoma. *Cancer* 1989;63:1918–1921.

79. Chamberlain MC, Levin VA. Primary central nervous system lymphoma: a role for adjuvant chemotherapy. *J Neurooncol* 1992;14: 271–275.

80. Chamberlain MC. Long survival in patients with acquired immune deficiency syndrome-related primary central nervous system lymphoma. *Cancer* 1994;73:1728.

115. Diagnosis and Treatment of Pituitary Adenomas

Ivan Ciric, Sami Rosenblatt, and Jin Cheng Zhao

The twentieth century witnessed a remarkable progress in the understanding of the nature of pituitary tumors, their diagnosis, and treatment. It was not until the 1920s that Cushing realized that acromegaly, first described by Pierre Marie in the late nineteenth century, is the result of a pituitary adenoma. Cushing also first described the disease that today bears his name. The pituitary-dependent syndrome of amenorrhea, galactorrhea, and hyperprolactinemia was not known as such until the latter part of the twentieth century. The diagnosis of pituitary adenomas was, until relatively recently, based principally on clinical grounds and skull radiographs showing evidence of an enlarged sella. Tomography of the sella universally employed by endocrinologists and neurosurgeons in the late 1960s and 1970s enabled them to discover microadenomas that eroded only one side of the sella. Angiography and pneumoencephalography were the mainstays of diagnosis of large pituitary adenomas until computed tomography (CT) became available approximately 30 years ago and magnetic resonance imaging (MRI) less than 20 years ago. Sophisticated laboratory testing of many hypothalamic-pituitary-adrenal axis hormones was not available until recently. A burgeoning expansion of molecular biological research and understanding of the pathogenesis of pituitary adenomas taking place today will certainly bear heavily on the treatment of pituitary adenomas in the twenty-first century.

Diagnosis of Pituitary Adenomas

PROLACTINOMAS. The clinical syndrome of amenorrhea and galactorrhea in women and impotence and gynecomastia in men, associated with a serum prolactin level of greater than 300 to 400 ng per mL, is diagnostic of a prolactin-secreting adenoma. Prolactin levels of less than 200 ng per mL are not diagnostic of, but they are consistent with, a prolactin-secreting pituitary adenoma, especially in patients with a microadenoma. Conversely, they are also consistent with the presence of the so-called stalk effect secondary to an interference with the free passage of the prolactin-inhibiting factor from the hypothalamus via the stalk circulation to the anterior pituitary, as well as with a variety of physiological and pathophysiological conditions other than an adenoma. However, there are also patients who present with the classical clinical syndrome of a prolactinoma and an MRI that demonstrates a pituitary adenoma, often an invasive one, but whose serum prolactin level may be in the normal range and yet, the immunocytochemical examination of the removed tumor tissue will show indisputable evidence for a lactotrophic adenoma. This discrepancy can be explained by the so-called high-dose hook effect of the chemiluminometric assay used (1). As for the imaging of prolactin-secreting pituitary adenomas, the majority of macroprolactinomas tend to be invasive and indeed, giant invasive pituitary adenomas are almost invariably prolactinomas in nature.

GROWTH HORMONE-SECRETING TUMORS. The endocrine diagnosis of acromegaly rests on the clinical presentation and on the laboratory evidence of an elevated insulin growth-like factor-1 (IGF-1) and the lack of suppressibility of the growth hormone (GH) to below the 1 ng per mL level by the glucose load [oral glucose tolerance test (OGTT)]. A preoperatively elevated GH level is not necessarily a *conditio sine qua non* in the diagnosis of acromegaly. Indeed, the diagnosis of acromegaly is possible with GH levels under 5 ng per mL (2,3). Hourly GH determinations conducted over 24 hours in these patients will show, however, a lack of pulsatility in GH secretion compared to healthy individuals who exhibit a pulsatile pattern of secretion, with the GH usually reaching its peak in the mid-afternoon hours (4). Preoperatively elevated GH levels, on the other hand, are an excellent marker for postoperative follow-up.

ACTH-SECRETING TUMORS. The endocrine diagnosis of Cushing disease rests on a sequential series of laboratory tests, beginning with the determination of hypercortisolism and proceeding to the evidence that the pituitary-adrenal feedback loop is set at a higher level, the evidence of a brisk responsiveness of adrenocorticotropin hormone (ACTH) secretion to the ACTH-releasing hormone (CRH) stimulation and, if indicated, on the presence of a ACTH gradient greater than 100% between the petrosal and the peripheral venous blood. Hypercortisolism can be established when the urinary free cortisols are elevated and when, during the 24-hour half hourly plasma cortisol determination, the plasma cortisol is greater than 5 to 10 μg per dL in the early morning hours, usually around 2:00 a.m. Under physiological circumstances this level is always less than 5 μg per dL. A normal or intermediately elevated serum ACTH, concordance of ACTH and plasma cortisol secretion, and a suppression of ACTH and plasma cortisol levels with high dexamethasone doses over a 48-hour period are all evidence that the pituitary-adrenal feedback loop is intact, though set at a higher level. Perhaps most importantly, a brisk stimulation of ACTH secretion by CRH infusion is very much diagnostic of a pituitary-dependent Cushing disease. Given that there is evidence of a pituitary-dependent hypercortisolism, a positive MRI study for a pituitary adenoma (most commonly a microadenoma) is sufficient for diagnosis. In this regard, a difficult-to-detect microadenoma can be shown with increased resolution if the MRI is performed either immediately or after a 20-minute delay following a double-dose contrast infusion. In the absence of a positive MRI, the petrosal sinus sampling test in search of a ACTH gradient of more than 100% between the petrosal and peripheral venous blood should be carried out. If such gradient is found following CRH infusion, the petrosal sinus sampling test can be considered as 100% specific and 100% sensitive. However, this test is only 75% accurate in predicting the laterality of the adenoma. The reason for this is that venous drainage from the sella is not always ipsilateral.

Current Concepts in the Treatment of Pituitary Adenomas

PROLACTINOMAS. Dopamine agonists remain the mainstay in the treatment of prolactin-secreting pituitary adenomas. In addition to bromocriptine (Parlodel), the availability of cabergoline (Dostinex) has greatly enhanced our ability to treat these tumors. Cabergoline efficacy is reported to be equal to or greater than that of bromocriptine and just as importantly, its side effects may be less than those of bromocriptine (5–7). Indeed, the number of endocrinologists using cabergoline as a start-up medication is growing daily.

It is generally accepted that microprolactinomas are the prime indication for treatment with dopamine agonists. On the other hand, we believe that patients should be made aware of the possibility that approximately 10% of microprolactinomas can grow and that some will become invasive into the surrounding structures, especially if the treatment is stopped at some time in the future. Patients should also be made aware that invasiveness very often means incurability. Finally, patients with microprolactinomas should also be informed of the excellent prognosis for cure following transsphenoidal microadenomectomy and of the minimum morbidity associated with this procedure in the hands of an experienced pituitary surgeon.

Our indications for surgical treatment of microprolactinomas are thus as follows:

- the endocrine syndrome must be supported by an unequivocally positive MRI
- dopamine agonists are ineffective, be it in terms of containing the tumor size or in terms of achieving euprolactinemia.
- the patient is intolerant to dopamine-agonist therapy due to side effects
- infertility persists in spite of dopamine-agonist therapy
- side effects of hyperprolactinemia (galactorrhea, dyspareunia, etc.) and other symptoms of a pituitary adenoma (headaches) are not relieved by dopamine agonist-therapy
- patient preference after a thorough discussion regarding all treatment options and their implications

Evidence of a surgical cure with a small or no chance for recurrence rests on a postoperative prolactin (PRL) level of 5 ng per mL or less (8). The incidence of recurrences in our experience increases to approximately 10% to 20% when the postoperative PRL level is between 5 and 10 ng per mL, with the frequency of recurrences rising even higher when the postoperative PRL level is between 10 and 20 ng per mL. As for macroprolactinomas, including invasive prolactinomas, it is usually assumed that surgical decompression is not only an acceptable form of treatment (usually after pretreatment with a dopamine agonist), but also under certain circumstances the necessary initial form of treatment. It is our experience, however, that pharmacotherapy of large, and certainly of invasive, macroprolactinomas is far superior to the surgical therapy in palliating the mass effect and the endocrine abnormality. Giant invasive prolactinomas are usually rather fibrous and tough tumors that are very difficult to remove because a surgical palliation of the mass effect is not only difficult to achieve, but often hazardous. Similarly, an attempt to achieve endocrine palliation in such tumors with surgical means is nearly impossible. In contrast, dopamine agonists are overwhelmingly and rapidly effective in decompressing large invasive prolactinomas and in palliating the endocrine abnormality, even when the patient presents with an advanced neurological deficit (9).

ACROMEGALY. Surgery remains the primary treatment modality for acromegaly. The incidence of surgical cures following transsphenoidal surgery in patients with microadenomas is in the 90th percentile range (10–13). There are a few series, however, that base their data regarding the surgical cure rates on the strict critera of a postoperative GH level of ≤ 2.5 ng per mL and normalization of the OGTT and of the IGF-1 level (11,

14). There is ample evidence in the literature indicating that a GH level of ≤ 5 ng per mL is consistent with biologically active acromegaly (15). Even more important, a comparison of the survival curves in patients with a postoperative or a last follow-up GH level of ≤ 2 ng per mL and those with a GH level of higher than 2 ng per mL shows a statistically significant longer survival in the former group (16). Consequently, reported cure rates in some series that are based on the postoperative basal GH level of ≤ 5 ng per mL should not be considered as representative of the true value of transsphenoidal surgery in the cure of acromegaly (17). Surgical results in the treatment of enclosed, noninvasive GH-secreting adenomas are also quite good, although the results do not approximate those in microadenomas. The surgical results are significantly better and the procedure much safer in experienced hands (18–20). Invasive pituitary adenomas are largely incurable with surgical means alone unless there is a limited invasion of the medial wall of the cavernous sinus when they can be occasionally extracted and removed completely.

Medical management of GH-secreting pituitary adenomas has made considerable progress in the last decade. The advent of the somatostatin analogue octreotide (21) and the long-acting somatostatin analogue Sandostatin LAR (22,23), injectable on a once every 28-day basis, has given us a new treatment modality for acromegaly. It is the conventional wisdom that somatostatin analogues can lower and eventually normalize GH in approximately 65% of all patients and reduce the size of the tumor to about 50% or less of its baseline size in approximately 40% to 50% of patients (24). The preoperative use of somatostatin analogues does not appear to influence the resectability of the tumor, while it does seem to be associated with improved results in both enclosed and invasive adenomas (25–27). The dopamine agonists bromocriptine and cabergoline, alone or in combination with somatostatin analogues, are also reported as being effective in the treatment of acromegaly (28). GH-receptor antagonists have been tested for efficacy in the treatment of acromegaly. One study reports normalization of IGF-1 in 92% of 38 patients treated with the investigational drug Trovert (29).

Radiation therapy has also become one of the important pillars in the treatment of acromegaly (29). Conventional radiation therapy, however, while capable of lowering the GH to about 20% of its pretreatment baseline values over a period of 10 to 20 years, is rarely, if ever associated with normalization of the postoperative GH levels or the IGF-1 levels. Consequently, conventional radiation therapy does not prevent the biological ravages of acromegaly in the long run (30). In contrast, radiosurgery, especially with the "gamma knife," has proven effective in normalizing the postoperative GH level in about 50% to 60% of patients (31). The main indication for radiosurgery is failed surgical therapy with residual acromegaly secondary to unremoved tumor tissue, usually in the region of the cavernous sinus (31–33).

Various guidelines in the treatment of acromegaly have been proposed (34). In our practice, patients with large and invasive GH-secreting adenomas are usually pretreated with somatostatin analogues for a period of about 6 to 8 weeks before undergoing transsphenoidal microsurgery. In addition, older patients and those incapable of undergoing surgery are treated with the long-acting somatostatin analogue. Transsphenoidal microsurgery is the first treatment choice for all other patients. If cure is achieved, patients are followed for the remainder of their life. If cure is not achieved, imaging studies are obtained and treatment with a somatostatin analogue is instituted. A reoperation can be very effective in patients in whom another surgeon may have missed a portion of the tumor for whatever reason (experience, exposure, etc.). Also, patients with recurrent enclosed adenomas can be amenable to surgical cure (35). On the other hand, if the initial surgery was performed adequately, and the residual or recurrent tumor tissue is not readily accessible because of its location and invasiveness, a reoperation tends to be unsuccessful (36). If reoperation is deemed contraindicated, radiosurgery is recommended for the residual/recurrent tumor.

CUSHING DISEASE. Surgical removal of a ACTH-secreting pituitary adenoma, usually a microadenoma, is by far the single most effective treatment of this disease. The pivotal factor in achieving a surgical cure is localizing the microadenoma on the preoperative imaging studies and finding it at the time of surgery. Clearly, these efforts require the involvement of a sophisticated endocrinologist and neuroradiologist and the availability of an experienced pituitary surgeon. In the process of removal of the ACTH-secreting pituitary microadenoma, it is important to remove a thin layer of the surrounding compressed normal anterior pituitary tissue in order to assure cure.

The pharmacotherapy of Cushing disease tends to be ineffective. Focused radiosurgery in the treatment of ACTH-secreting microadenoma is not being used often for the simple reason that a microadenoma can usually be removed successfully in the hands of an experienced pituitary surgeon. Additionally, in contrast to GH-secreting adenomas, ACTH-secreting microadenomas do not tend to be invasive. The cure is defined when the postoperative basal plasma cortisol levels are ≤ 2.5 μg per dL. It is our practice not to start steroid replacement therapy for the first 24 hours after surgery and to obtain 6-, 18-, and 24-hour postoperative plasma cortisol levels. Normalization is usually achieved at the 18-hour drawing with symptoms of hypocortisolism beginning to emerge between 18 and 24 hours postoperatively when replacement therapy is started and continued for several months until the pituitary-adrenal axis function is reestablished.

NONSECRETING TUMORS. Nonsecreting tumors diagnosed incidentally, if perceived nonthreatening, can be followed with repeat visual examinations and MRI studies, especially in older adults. If symptomatic, transsphenoidal surgery is performed always with the goal of attempting a gross total removal. This is possible more often than not, especially in patients with tumors that have symmetrical suprasellar extension. Consequently, postoperative radiation therapy is rarely necessary immediately after surgery and is usually reserved for when there is evidence of a recurrence. Even then, if this is deemed appropriate, a reoperation is preferred to radiation therapy.

Prognosis

If diagnosed early and appropriately treated, the prognosis for high-quality, long-term survival in patients with pituitary tumors is excellent. This is especially true for hypersecreting microadenomas. While the percentage of cures diminishes as the tumor size increases, surgical results in the treatment of enclosed macroadenomas, both nonfunctioning and hypersecreting are also very good. On the other hand, our ability to eradicate and achieve endocrine cure in patients with invasive tumors is nearly impossible. Decompression of the optic chiasm, following removal of a macroadenoma, is associated with a visual improvement that usually occurs within the first 24 hours after surgery. The incidence of recurrences ranges from 1% to 2% to approximately 10% in long-term follow-up studies. We do not advocate immediate postoperative radiation therapy in patients

who had a gross total removal of a macroadenoma and we are deliberate in our recommendation for such therapy in patients with subtotally removed tumors.

Various studies have been proposed to determine future biological behavior of incompletely removed pituitary adenomas (37,38). Among these, immunohistochemistry using antibodies to the KI-67 and proliferating cell nuclear antigen (PCNA), which are expressed in cells that have entered mitosis, can be used to assess the proportion of the cells in a tumor that is proliferating. The percentage of such cells, the so-called labeling index (LI), has been shown to be proportionate with invasiveness and a tendency toward recurrences. However, the LI has not proven a reliable predictor of future biological behavior of a pituitary adenoma, in that there are aggressively growing pituitary adenomas with a low LI and conversely, there are slow-growing tumors with a relatively high LI. On molecular biological grounds, and, thus, on a less practical side, it has been variously shown that, in addition to a loss of the p53 suppressor gene expression (39), invasive behavior of a pituitary adenoma can also be associated with an increased expression of the human pituitary transforming gene (40) of the epidermal growth factor (41) and of fibroblast growth factors 2 and 4 (42). Finally, measurement of deoxyribonucleic acid ploidy has not been found useful in patients with pituitary adenomas. For example, aneuploidy, usually associated with tumor aggressiveness, was reported in one study as being associated with biologically indolent pituitary adenomas (43).

Surgical Technique

Transsphenoidal microsurgery is the surgical technique of choice among pituitary surgeons. Recent technological advances with the frameless stereotaxis and interactive image-guided transsphenoidal microsurgery have further increased the safety of this procedure (44). On the other hand, the use of an intraoperative MRI, while advocated by some (45), has not been widely accepted as a singular advantage.

Concerning the endoscopic transsphenoidal surgical technique, we should be very careful to encourage those who have shown facility with this procedure to continue their work and demonstrate its safety and usefulness, especially in achieving endocrine cures (46). At the same time, our enthusiasm with this procedure should be tempered with our concern for misuse of the technique in the hands of the less initiated and improperly trained. Neurosurgeons have struggled over the years to operate with two eyes and two hands. Definitely, the operating microscope has provided a breakthrough in allowing neurosurgeons the luxury, beauty, and elegance of a three-dimensional view, enlarged at will, in a sunlit field of otherwise, under direct vision, barely perceptible deep-seated structures, including pituitary adenomas. In contrast, endoscopic surgery is monocular and largely one-handed—counterintuitive to everything neurosurgeons have strived for to date. If endoscopic surgery is to challenge microscopic surgery to the extent of replacing it, it will have to do so by achieving binocularity (i.e., three-dimensionality) and by allowing the surgeon to use both hands in a field that is free of the still rather bulky and cumbersome endoscopic shafts. While there are centers where various holders are being applied to the endoscope in order to allow the surgeon the freedom of using both hands during surgery, to the best of our knowledge, this has not been duplicated in other centers to the same extent. In short, endoscopic surgery is still in its infancy, but it is hoped that it will rise to its challenges in the years to come.

It is of concern to us that there are still neurosurgeons who advocate craniotomy for any pituitary adenoma extending into the suprasellar space, each neurosurgeon setting the standard as to where the cutoff point is with the transsphenoidal approach in terms of the degree of the suprasellar extension. The reason for this may be actually quite appropriate. Lack of training and subsequent lack of exposure in a center where this procedure is not often being done may result in a trepidation toward engaging in a surgical endeavor in an unfamiliar territory and using unfamiliar techniques, simply doing an operation that can be associated with significant complications. A change in this attitude toward transsphenoidal microsurgery can only be achieved if neurosurgeons were to specialize in this field by acquiring additional training and devoting their career toward becoming an accomplished pituitary surgeon. Clearly, this would require support from the neurosurgical community at large in terms of other neurosurgeons avoiding performing transsphenoidal surgery on a sporadic basis.

Molecular Biology of Pituitary Adenomas

It has been suggested that pituitary adenomas can arise as a consequence of abnormal regulatory influences exerted by the hypothalamus or due to intrinsic abnormalities within the pituitary itself. Recent molecular biological research has demonstrated that the majority of pituitary adenomas arise as a result of a somatic mutation in a progenitor cell with subsequent monoclonal expansion of the mutated cell into an adenoma. Conversely, normal pituitary and hyperplastic pituitary tissue are polyclonal in nature (47–49).

The proliferation of a mutated pituicyte into an adenoma occurs as a consequence of a variety of extrinsic and intrinsic factors within the pituitary itself. Genetic alterations that have been implicated in the origin of a variety of other benign and malignant tumors include loss of tumor suppressor genes or the activation of cellular proto-oncogenes. Published data have shown that a loss of expression of p53 suppressor gene in pituitary adenomas correlates directly with aggressive growth and invasiveness (39). In addition, the loss of chromosome 11q13 sequence, which contains the MEN-1 gene locus, has been found in a certain subset of GH-secreting adenomas suggesting that the inactivation of a tumor suppressor gene in this region may play a role in pituitary tumorigenesis (50). On the oncogene side, activating mutations have been found in the α-subunit gene (*gsp*) of the stimulatory guanine nucleotide-binding protein (G protein), in the H-*ras* gene, and in protein kinase Cα. The stimulatory G-protein is involved in the activation of adenylyl cyclase that, under physiological circumstances, mediates the regulatory action of GH-releasing hormone in the stimulation of GH synthesis and secretion. This stimulatory effect of the G-protein is, under physiological circumstances, tempered by the α-subunit of this protein that inactivates adenylyl cyclase. Mutation in the α-subunit gene will thus result in a persistent activation of the adenylyl cyclase and, consequently, in a continuous autonomous GH secretion by the adenoma. Indeed, this is the most commonly described genetic defect associated with pituitary tumors (50,51).

A novel pituitary tumor transforming gene (*pttg*) has been discovered. Human *pttg* is demonstrated to be more abundant in pituitary tumors compared to normal controls, and the *pttg* expression is even more elevated in invasive tumors when compared with enclosed tumors. Thus, it is suggested that human *pttg* expression level may be a marker for invasiveness in hyperfunctioning pituitary tumors (40). Furthermore, extrahypotha-

lamic GH-releasing hormone gene expression has been demonstrated in GH-producing adenomas suggesting that GH-releasing hormone may act to stimulate GH adenoma growth and hypersecretion. Overexpression of GH-releasing hormone gene in these tumors correlates directly with the adenoma invasiveness (52,53).

The recent molecular biological research on prolactin-secreting tumors has shown that a loss of D_2-receptor gene expression is associated with aggressive growth, invasiveness, and resistance to dopamine-agonist therapy (54,55). Furthermore, tissue specimens from such tumors showed a paucity of nerve growth factor (NGF) gene expression. Addition of NGF to such tumor tissue *in vitro* and *in vivo* resulted in an increase in the D_2-receptor gene expression and in a phenotypic change from an aggressively growing, invasive, dopamine-agonist resistant tumor to a less aggressively growing, noninvasive, dopamine-agonist–sensitive adenoma (56). It is anticipated that such phenotypic changes toward less aggressivity and greater responsiveness to pharmacotherapy, under the influence of genetic manipulation, will become an important arm in the management of various pituitary tumors in this century.

Summary

Significant advances have been made in the molecular biological understanding of pituitary tumorigenesis. These advances will have an impact on the gene therapy of pituitary tumors in the twenty-first century. Transsphenoidal surgery remains the mainstay of treatment for the majority of pituitary adenomas, with endoscopic surgery being used at some centers in select patients. Pharmacotherapy of pituitary adenomas has made great strides in the management of prolactinomas and GH-secreting pituitary adenomas. Finally, radiosurgery has become a very important adjuvant therapy in the treatment of hypersecreting pituitary adenomas.

References

1. Barkan AL, Chandler WF. Giant pituitary prolactinoma with falsely low serum prolactin: the pitfall of the "high-dose hook effect." Case report. *Neurosurgery* 1998;42:913–915.
2. Brockmeier SJ, Buchfelder M, Adams EF, et al. Acromegaly with 'normal' serum growth hormone levels. Clinical features, diagnosis and results of transsphenoidal microsurgery. *Hormone Metab Res* 1992;24:392–400.
3. Mohr G, Chen ZP, Schweitzer M. Acromegaly with normal basal growth hormone levels. *Can J Neurol Sci* 1997;24:250–253.
4. Barkan AL. Acromegaly: diagnosis and therapy. *Endocrinol Metab Clin North Am* 1989;18:277–310.
5. Colao A, Di Sarno A, Sarnacchiaro F, et al. Prolactinomas resistant to standard dopamine agonists respond to chronic cabergoline treatment. *J Clin Endocrinol Metab* 1997;82:876–883.
6. Ferrari CI, Abs R, Bevan JS, et al. Treatment of macroprolactinoma with cabergoline. A study of 85 patients. *Clin Endocrinol* 1997;46:409–413.
7. Biller BM, Molitch ME, Vance ML, et al. Treatment of prolactin-secreting macroadenomas with the once-weekly dopamine agonist cabergoline. *J Clin Endocrinol Metab* 1996;81:2338–2343.
8. Feigenbaum SL, Downey DE, Wilson CB, et al. Transsphenoidal pituitary resection for preoperative diagnosis of prolactin-secreting pituitary adenoma in women: long term follow up. *J Clin Endocrinol Metab* 1996;81:1711–1719.
9. Ciric I. Giant and invasive prolactin-secreting pituitary adenoma. In:

Winchester DP, Brennan MF, Dodd GD Jr, et al, eds. *Tumor board case management*. Philadelphia: Lippincott-Raven, 1997;631–634.

10. Davis DH, Laws ER Jr, Ilstrup DM, et al. Results of surgical treatment for growth hormone-secreting pituitary adenomas *J Neurosurg* 1993; 79:70–75.
11. Swearingen B, Barker FG II, Katnelson L, et al. Long-term mortality after transsphenoidal surgery and adjunctive therapy for acromegaly [Comment]. *J Clin Endocrinol Metab* 1998;83:3419–3426.
12. Tindall GT, Oyesiku NM, Watts NB, et al. Transsphenoidal adenomectomy for growth hormone-secreting pituitary adenomas in acromegaly: outcome analysis and determinants of failure. *J Neurosurg* 1993;78:205–215.
13. Fahlbusch R, Honegger J, Buchfelder M. Evidence supporting surgery as treatment of choice for acromegaly. *J Endocrinol* 1997; 155(suppl):S53–S55.
14. Sheaves R, Jenkins P, Blackburn P, et al. Outcome of transsphenoidal surgery for acromegaly using strict criteria for surgical cure. *Clin Endocrinol* 1996;45:407–413.
15. Holdaway IM, Rajasoorya C. Epidemiology of acromegaly. *Pituitary* 1999;2:29–41.
16. Rajasoorya C, Holdaway IM, Wrightson P, et al. Determinants of clinical outcome and survival in acromegaly. *Clin Endocrinol* 1994; 41:95–102.
17. Clayton RN. New developments in the management of acromegaly. Should we achieve absolute biochemical cure? *J Endocrinol* 1997; 155(suppl 1):S23–S29.
18. Ciric I, Ragin A, Baumgartner C, et al. Complications of transsphenoidal surgery: results of a national survey, review of the literature and personal experience. *Neurosurgery* 1997;40:225–237.
19. Lissett CA, Peacey SR, Laing I, et al. The outcome of surgery for acromegaly: the need for a specialist pituitary surgeon for all types of growth hormone (GH) secreting adenoma [Review]. *Clin Endocrinol* 1998;49:653–657.
20. Ross DA, Wilson CB. Results of transsphenoidal microsurgery for growth hormone-secreting pituitary adenoma in a series of 214 patients. *J Neurosurg* 1988;68:854–867.
21. Farooqi S, Bevan JS, Shepperd MC, et al. The therapeutic value of somatostatin and its analogues. *Pituitary* 1999;2:79–88.
22. Gisslis JC, Noble S, Goa KL. Octreotide long-acting release (LAR). *Drugs* 1997;53:681–699.
23. Lancranjan I, Atkinson AB. Sandostatin LAR® in acromegalic patients. Results of a European multicare study with Sandostatin LAR® in acromegalic patients. *Pituitary* 1999;1:105–114.
24. Newman CB. Medical therapy for acromegaly [Review]. *Endocrinol Metab Clin North Am* 1999;28:171–190.
25. Colao A, Ferone D, Cappabianca P, et al. Effect of octreotide pretreatment on surgical outcome in acromegaly. *J Clin Endocrinol Metab* 1997;82:3308–3314.
26. Lucas-Morante T, Garcia-Uria J, Estrada J, et al. Treatment of invasive growth hormone pituitary adenomas with long-acting somatostatin analog SMS 201-995 before transsphenoidal surgery. *J Neurosurg* 1994;81:10–14.
27. Stevenaert A, Beckers A. Presurgical octreotide treatment in acromegaly. *Acta Endocrinol* 1993;129(suppl 1):18–20.
28. Colao A, Ferone D, Marzullo P, et al. Effect of different dopaminergic agents in the treatment of acromegaly. *J Clin Endocrinol Metab* 1997;82:518–523.
29. Van der Lely AJ, de Herder WW, Lamberts SW. New medical treatment for acromegaly. *Pituitary* 1999;2:89–92.
30. Jaffe CA. Reevaluation of conventional pituitary irradiation in the therapy of acromegaly. *Pituitary* 1999;2:55–62.
31. Jackson IMD, Norene G. Role of gamma knife radiosurgery in acromegaly. *Pituitary* 1999;2:71–78.
32. Landolt AM, Haller D, Lomax N, et al. Stereotactic radiosurgery for recurrent surgically treated acromegaly: comparison with fractionate radiotherapy. *J Neurosurg* 1998;88:1002–1008.

33. Morange-Ramos I, Regis J, Defour H, et al. Gamma-knife surgery for secreting pituitary adenomas. *Acta Neurochir* 1998;140:437–443.
34. Melmed S, Jacons I, Kleinberg D, et al. Current treatment guidelines for acromegaly. *J Clin Endocrinol Metab* 1998;83:2646–2652.
35. Abe R, Ludecke DK. Recent results of secondary transnasal surgery for residual or recurring acromegaly. *Neurosurgery* 1998; 42: 1013–1021.
36. Long H, Beauregard H, Somma M, et al. Surgical outcome after repeated transsphenoidal surgery in acromegaly. *J Neurosurg* 1996; 85:239–247.
37. Amar AP, Hinton DR, Krieger MD, et al. Invasive pituitary adenomas: significance of proliferation parameters. *Pituitary* 1999;2:117–122.
38. Zhang X, Horwitz GA, Heaney A, et al. Pituitary adenomas: marker for functional tumor invasiveness. *J Clin Endocrinol Metab* 1999; 84:761–767.
39. Thepar K, Scheithauer BW, Kovacs K, et al. p53 expression in pituitary adenomas and carcinomas: correlations with invasiveness and tumor growth fractions. *Neurosurgery* 1996;38:763–770.
40. Zhang X, Horwitz GA, Prezant TR, et al. Structure, expression, and function of human pituitary tumors transforming gene (PTTG). *Mol Endocrinol* 1999;13:156–166.
41. LeRiche VK, Asa SL, Ezzat S. Epidermal growth factor and its receptor (EGFR) in human pituitary adenomas: EFG-R correlates with tumor aggressiveness. *J Clin Endocrinol Metab* 1995;81:656–662.
42. Ezzat S, Smyth HS, Raymar L, et al. Heterogeneous in vivo and in vitro expression of basic fibroblast growth factor by human pituitary adenomas. *J Clin Endocrinol Metab* 1995;80:878–884.
43. Anniko M, Wersall J. DNA studies for prediction of prognosis of pituitary adenomas. *Adv Biosci* 1988;69:45–52.
44. Sandeman D, Moufid A. Interactive image-guided pituitary surgery. An experience of 101 procedures. *Neurochirurgie* 1998;44:331–338.
45. Martin CH, Schwartz R, Jolesz F, et al. Transsphenoidal resection of pituitary adenomas in an intraoperative MRI unit. *Pituitary* 1999;2: 155–162.
46. Jho HD, Carrau RL. Endoscopic endonasal transsphenoidal surgery: experience with 50 patients. *J Neurosurg* 1997;87:44–51.
47. Herman V, Fagin J, Gonsky R, et al. Clonal origin of pituitary adenomas. *J Clin Endocrinol Metab* 1990;71:1427–1433.
48. Shimon I, Melmed S. Genetic basis of endocrine disease: pituitary tumor pathogenesis. *J Clin Endocrinol Metab* 1997;82:1675–1681.
49. Biller BMK, Alexander JM, Zervas NT, et al. Clonal origins of adrenocorticotropin-secreting pituitary tissue in Cushing's disease. *J Clin Endocrinol Metab* 1992;75:1303–1309.
50. Jameson JL. Molecular pathogenesis of pituitary tumors: an overview. In: Melmed S, ed. *Molecular and clinical advances in pituitary disorders*. Marina del Ray, CA: Third International Pituitary Congress, 1993;15–19.
51. Drange MR, Melmed S. Molecular pathogenesis of acromegaly. *Pituitary* 1999;2:43–50.
52. Wakahayayashi I, Inokuchi K, Hasegawa O, et al. Expression of growth hormone (GH)-releasing factor gene in GH-producing pituitary adenoma. *J Clin Endocrinol Metab* 1992;74:357–361.
53. Thapar K, Kovacs K, Stefaneanu L, et al. Overexpression of the growth hormone-releasing hormone gene in acromegaly-associated pituitary tumors. An event associated with neoplastic progression and aggressive behaviour. *Am J Pathol* 1997;151:769–784.
54. Pellegrini-Boullier I, Morange-Ramos I, Barlier A, et al. Pituitary-1 gene expression in human lactotroph and somatotroph pituitary adenomas is correlated to D2 receptor gene expression. *J Clin Endocrinol Metab* 1996;81:3390–3396.
55. Caccavelli L, Feron F, Morange I, et al. Decreased expression of the two D2 dopamine receptor isoforms in bromocriptine resistant prolactinomas. *Neuroendocrinology* 1994;60:314–322.
56. Missale C, Sigala S, Fiorentini C, et al. Nerve growth factor suppresses the tumoral phenotype of human prolactinomas [Review]. *Hormone Res* 1997;47:240–244.

116. Craniopharyngiomas in Children and Adults

Edward R. Laws and Kamal Thapar

As early as 1900, Babinski described a patient with sexual infantilism and dystrophic obesity who had a cystic sellar-suprasellar lesion, almost certainly a craniopharyngioma (1). The profound effects on growth and development produced by craniopharyngiomas make these lesions among the most dramatic and challenging abnormalities encountered in medical practice.

Clinical Presentation

The clinical presentation of craniopharyngiomas is determined by the age of the patient and size and location of the tumor (2–11). In general, symptoms can be categorized as endocrine, visual, cognitive, and those deriving from increased ICP (Table 1).

Virtually all children with craniopharyngiomas have an abnormal growth curve and impairment in development of secondary sexual characteristics. In young adults, endocrine symptoms are often subtle, particularly those related to partial hypopituitarism. The effects of moderate hyperprolactinemia from infundibular or hypothalamic compression generally are more obvious, especially in young women, in whom prolactin elevations manifest as amenorrhea and galactorrhea. Diabetes insipidus may occur as part of the presenting symptom complex in both age groups.

Relevant Anatomical Principles

Craniopharyngiomas are generally believed to be developmental lesions, thought to arise from remnants of Rathke's pouch. These embryonic remnants occur as epithelial "rests," deposited between the tuber cinereum and pituitary gland itself, along the tract of an incompletely involuted hypophyseal-pharyngeal duct; craniopharyngiomas can arise anywhere along this pathway. It also has been postulated that craniopharyngiomas might arise from squamous metaplasia of normal cells of the pars intermedia situated along the pituitary stalk (12). Craniopharyngiomas encompass a broad biological spectrum from the standpoints of size, location, contents, pathological appearance, and overall clinical behavior. At the one extreme are tumors of microscopic proportions situated wholly within a normal pituitary gland. At the other and more common extreme are larger tumors whose progressive growth enables them to compress the pituitary gland and stalk, optic apparatus, and hypothalamic structures. These larger lesions may extend into the third ventricle, causing hydrocephalus. Craniopharyngiomas can be solid or cystic, and the overwhelming majority exhibit both features. The cyst contents, although classically described as "machinery oil" in appearance and consistency, can range from a shimmering cholesterol-laden fluid to a brown-black purulent sludge admixed with desquamated debris. Calcification is a common feature of craniopharyngiomas, ranging from microscopic specks to large and even bonelike concretions of considerable size. Histopathologically, the epi-

thelial elements comprising these tumors range from cuboidal to columnar to squamous in appearance.

Topologically, approximately 60% to 80% of craniopharyngiomas arise in the suprasellar region. Approximately 30% to 40% of craniopharyngiomas originate within the sella, resulting in its enlargement in a fashion similar to that seen with pituitary adenomas (8). Rare examples have been reported of craniopharyngiomas wholly situated within the third ventricle, optic chiasm, or sphenoid bone.

Principles of Preoperative Evaluation

ENDOCRINE DIAGNOSIS. The endocrine diagnosis of craniopharyngioma rests on physical signs and laboratory studies. Laboratory measurements include basal and provoked tests of pituitary-hypothalamic function as clinically indicated. These include basal determinations of growth hormone (GH), insulin-like growth factor, type I (IGF-1), prolactin (PRL), cortisol, thyroid function (TSH and T4), gonadotrophs (FSH, LH), testosterone, and estradiol. Determination of alpha subunit levels and ACTH occasionally can be helpful.

An insulin tolerance test with measurement of cortisol and growth hormone offers a helpful dynamic evaluation of the pituitary-hypothalamic axis. Urine and serum osmolality determinations or a water-deprivation test may be helpful if diabetes insipidus is suspected.

IMAGING DIAGNOSIS. Magnetic resonance imaging (MRI) is the diagnostic procedure of choice for craniopharyngioma. (Figs. 1 and 2). Both solid and cystic components are identified, along with important anatomical relationships and various extensions of tumor and cyst outside of the immediate suprasellar region. Cerebral angiography generally is not required with

Table 1. Clinical Characteristics of Craniopharyngioma

Age Range	Clinical Features
Infants and children	Increased intracranial pressure Growth and sexual retardation Headache, nausea, and vomiting Visual loss Diabetes insipidus
Adolescents and young adults	Sexual retardation Infertility Pseudoprolactinoma Headache
Adults and elderly persons	Headache Hypopituitarism Mental changes

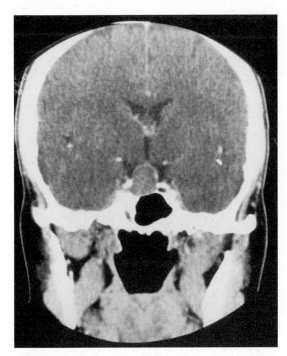

Fig. 1. Coronal computed tomography scan of intrasellar craniopharyngioma. This young woman presented with amenorrhea-galactorrhea—a "pseudoprolactinoma."

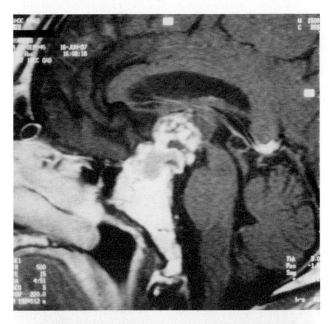

high resolution MRI, and is reserved for cases of presumed vascular tumors or those that have a particularly difficult relationship to blood vessels in the region. Computed tomography (CT) still plays some role in the anatomical diagnosis of craniopharyngiomas and has the advantage of showing calcifications and some aspects of bony distortion associated with the tumor more effectively than does MRI (Figs. 3 and 4). Radiological evaluation may identify a suprasellar or intrasellar lesion, but the differential diagnosis of such lesions is broad and surgery may be needed to establish diagnosis (Table 2).

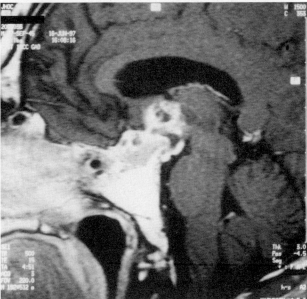

Fig. 3. Sagittal MRI: suprasellar craniopharyngioma.

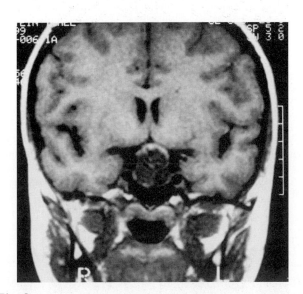

Fig. 2. Coronal MRI of intrasellar craniopharyngioma. Note deformed optic chiasm draped over the dorsal aspect of the tumor.

Table 2. Differential Diagnosis of Craniopharyngioma

Rathke's cleft cyst
Dermoid
Epidermoid
Pituitary adenoma
Germinoma
Hamartoma
Suprasellar aneurysm
Arachnoid cyst
Suprasellar abscess, Inflammatory disease
Langhans cell histocytosis
Sarcoid, tuberculosis
Glioma of optic chiasm

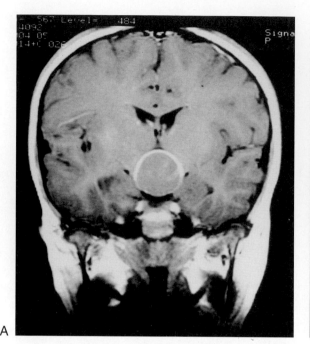
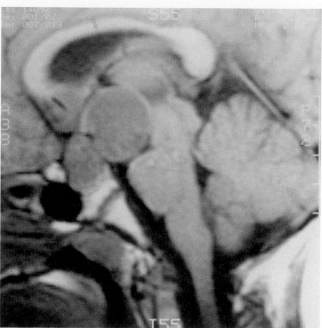

Fig. 4. Coronal (**A**) and sagittal (**B**) MRI studies of an 8-year-old patient with a sellar and suprasellar craniopharyngioma.

Principles of Management

Maximum *safe* tumor resection is often a reasonable initial goal in newly diagnosed patients (Table 3). This can be achieved via craniotomy in many instances (13–24), although transsphenoidal resection provides safer access in selected cases (17, 25–32), whereas complete excision requires a combination of both approaches in others (33). Tumors unassociated with sellar enlargement generally arise and remain suprasellar; therefore, a transcranial (pterional or subfrontal) route manages them best. It usually becomes evident during the course of tumor resection whether or not complete removal is a safe and feasible strategy (21). Aggressive attempts to remove tumor fragments, which are tenaciously adherent to neural and vascular structures, are accompanied by an unacceptable functional cost (11, 19,34). Alternatively, other tumors are less adherent and complete excision can be achieved safely.

As a rule, craniopharyngiomas associated with sellar enlargement can be regarded as subdiaphragmatic in origin. Even though such tumors may exhibit significant intracranial extension, they invariably maintain an "extra-pial" and "extra-arachnoid" disposition. Accordingly, they remain amenable to complete excision via a transsphenoidal route.

Completeness of surgical removal usually can be confirmed by postoperative imaging studies. Some form of postoperative radiation therapy generally is recommended when complete removal is not feasible, except in very young children (35–38).

The management of the recurrent craniopharyngioma is considerably more complex, because therapeutic goals must be especially well defined. In some cases, and despite the technical demands of reoperation, total resection still can be achieved. For many recurrent tumors, however, palliative surgery is often the most realistic goal. Recurrent lesions with a significant cystic component often can be treated by repetitive aspiration. This can be achieved by inserting a silastic tube attached to an Ommaya reservoir into the cyst cavity. Alternatively, the transsphenoidal insertion of a silastic tube from the tumor cavity into the posterior nasal space can provide prolonged drainage, or Bleomycin may be instilled to shrink and toughen the cyst wall.

Stereotactic needle aspiration of fluid contents may be remarkably effective in reversing symptoms and signs. In some cases a radioactive isotope (colloidal ^{32}P, yttrium, or gold) may be instilled into the cyst cavity to provide local B particle-mediated radiotherapy (39). Radiosurgery delivered by gamma knife or a stereotactic linear accelerator also may provide dramatic results in patients who are not suitable surgical candidates (40).

Table 3. Management Options for Craniopharyngioma

Clinical observation (monitoring MRI, visual fields, replacement therapy)
Cerebrospinal fluid shunt (when hydrocephalus is present)
Stereotactic procedures
    Puncture and aspiration
    Catheter/Ommaya reservoir drainage
    Instillation of bleomycin
    Instillation of radioisotope (P^{32}, yttrium)
Surgical removal (complete or partial)
    Craniotomy
    Transsphenoidal
Radiotherapy (initial versus adjunctive)
Stereotactic radiotherapy
Radiosurgery

Surgical Techniques (Table 4)

TRANSSPHENOIDAL REMOVAL OF CRANIOPHARYNGIOMA. The rationale for the transsphenoidal approach in the microsurgical removal of craniopharyngioma lies in the patho-

Table 4. Surgical Approaches for Resection of Craniopharyngioma

Craniotomy
    Unilateral subfrontal
    Bilateral subfrontal and interhemispheric
    Subfrontal translamina terminalis
    Subfrontal transsphenoidal
    Frontotemporal (pterional)
    Temporal and petrosal (for retroclinoidal tumors)
    Orbitofrontal and zygomatic
Transsphenoidal
    Transseptal
    Lateral rhinotomy
    Transethmoidal
    Extended anterior skull base approaches

logical anatomy of those lesions, which take origin below the diaphragma sellae. Craniopharyngiomas arise from epithelial cell rests or areas of squamous metaplasia that are related to the embryogenesis of the pituitary. These cell rests can occur anywhere along the path of the craniopharyngeal duct, and are found from the tuber cinereum rostrally to the sphenoid bone caudally. They frequently are related to the infundibulum, pars intermedia, or pars tuberalis of the hypophysis. When craniopharyngiomas arise above the diaphragm, the sella and its contents usually appear normal in size and configuration in imaging studies. When these tumors arise below the diaphragm, they produce progressive enlargement of the sella, a radiographic feature of 30% to 60% of previously reported series. When a craniopharyngioma arises below the diaphragm, this membrane tends to remain an effective barrier, even though it may stretch dramatically as a tumor extends into the suprasellar compartment. For this reason, craniopharyngiomas associated with sellar enlargement rarely, if ever, have intimate attachments to the optic chiasm, hypothalamus, or other intracranial structures. The dorsal capsule of the craniopharyngioma fuses with the diaphragm of the sella, but ordinarily cannot transgress this anatomical barrier. This feature of the pathological anatomy of infradiaphragmatic craniopharyngiomas theoretically permits "total" removal of the lesion so long as the surgeon is willing to resect the diaphragm and create the potential for a large cerebrospinal fluid (CSF) leak. It must be acknowledged that the lateral capsule of the intrasellar craniopharyngioma may be intimately attached to the medial dural wall of the cavernous sinus. Stripping away of the capsule may be difficult and risk bleeding from the sinus, damage to the cavernous carotid artery, or trauma to the cranial nerves in the cavernous sinus.

The transsphenoidal approach also may be useful in the management of craniopharyngiomas, which are predominantly suprasellar. In these cases, and in patients who have been operated on previously by craniotomy, a "total" removal usually cannot be accomplished safely, but the goal of palliation may be achieved by drainage of the cystic component of such tumors or by subtotal removal of tumor contents, decompressing the optic apparatus, and other intracranial structures.

Surgical techniques are similar to those used for the transsphenoidal management of pituitary adenomas. Patients with large tumors and suprasellar extension have a lumbar catheter inserted so that air can be injected or CSF withdrawn during the operative procedure. The sella is carefully and widely exposed. It is usually possible to create a sellar floor by removing first the cortical bone and then the medullary bone of the sphenoid in children with poorly pneumatized sphenoid sinuses. The posterior cortical surface then becomes the floor of the

sella. This procedure can be done with a drill or combination of fine chisel and curette.

The floor of the sella is removed as widely as possible to create the greatest possible working area. Lateral exposure should extend from one cavernous sinus to the other. Vertical exposure should extend from the floor of the sella to the junction of the face of the sella with the anterior fossa. The dura should be opened with caution. If pituitary gland tissue is present, it is usually just behind the dura. It should be displaced laterally and preserved. Once a plane of cleavage has been established, the cystic component of the tumor may be aspirated. Further vigorous dissection may be necessary to detach the capsule of the craniopharyngioma from the walls of the sella. When the intrasellar portion of the tumor has been fully mobilized, the diaphragm must be incised, usually at the anterolateral margin. This creates a sizable CSF leak. Further dissection mobilizes the anterior attachment of the tumor capsule that is fused with the diaphragm. The pituitary stalk usually is visualized as the tumor is depressed into the sella. Careful bipolar cauterization and sharp dissection allow detachment of the tumor from the stalk with minimal trauma. Further intracranial dissection is performed under direct microscopic, endoscopic, and fluoroscopic control, often with image-guided methods. The majority of tumors associated with enlarged sellas can be removed completely.

The resection of the diaphragm makes effective closure a major challenge of this operative approach. Occlusive packing of the sella with muscle or fat is almost always necessary. This is done under fluoroscopic control. Once packed, the sella is carefully reconstructed. The floor is replaced with a plate of bone or nasal cartilage designed to apply broad pressure to the graft. Epidural placement of the bone is preferred when feasible. If septal bone and cartilage are not available, bank bone or methacrylate fashioned to form a plate can be used. In most cases, the sphenoid sinus also is packed with muscle or fat. The use of biologic glue or postoperative spinal drainage has not been mandatory, but often is useful.

Steroid support is given before and after surgery until accurate baseline blood corticosteroid determinations can be made. Diabetes insipidus is controlled with parenteral DDAVP (desmopressin) until the nasal formulation can be used (ordinarily the fourth postoperative day).

Transsphenoidal and craniotomy approaches have been used in the same patient in a number of cases. This has occurred in urgent situations where transsphenoidal decompression was followed by definitive transcranial surgery. It is employed also when a solid tumor has intracranial and intrasellar components.

The transsphenoidal route has been used for palliative resections and attempted prolonged drainage of cystic lesions. It is possible to insert a silastic drain from the tumor cavity into the posterior nasal space if the subarachnoid space is not entered. Although such drainage tubes tend to become obstructed and are eventually extruded, they have functioned well for up to 5 years in some patients.

CRANIOTOMY. A large number of craniotomy approaches for craniopharyngiomas have been developed and used. Historically, the unilateral subfrontal approach has been the most common. Most surgeons recommend fashioning the bone flap on the side of worse vision. Bifrontal craniotomy with subfrontal or interhemispheric approach also has been advocated. Heuer and Dandy advocated a unilateral approach along the sphenoid wing for tumors of the hypophyseal region. This approach has matured into the pterional craniotomy, which has become favored by many surgeons using microsurgical techniques. Poppen suggested a temporal approach; this has been sophisticated and adapted to microtechniques by Symon (23).

Transventricular and transcallosal approaches have been advocated for tumors lying primarily within the third ventricle (16).

Patterson proposed a variant of trans-frontal craniotomy: a transcranial, transsphenoidal approach where in the tuberculum sellae is drilled away and the sphenoid sinus is entered, giving access to the anterior wall of the sella (18).

The choice of craniotomy approach depends on the nature and anatomy of the tumor. Several routes may obtain access to the tumor once the brain is exposed. Some lesions may be removed from between the optic nerves. In many patients, particularly children, the optic chiasm is prefixed, limiting access between the nerves. Further dissection along the dorsal surface of the optic chiasm allows an approach through the lamina terminalis. This has the advantage of midline exposure, but may limit visualization of the lateral extents of the tumor. An approach between the optic nerve and carotid artery allows good exposure of the lateral aspect of the tumor, but may be limited by the optic tract posteriorly and other aspects of the anatomy of the supraclinoid carotid and optic apparatus. The temporal approach requires either surgical removal or extensive mobilization and retraction of the anterior temporal lobe. This provides good access to the lateral and posterior aspects of the tumor, but is limited again by the anatomical relationships of the optic nerve and tract, the carotid artery and its branches, and the third cranial nerve. Combinations of these approaches, along with the transcranial, transsphenoidal exposure mentioned in the preceding, may be required to removed particularly difficult tumors.

Controversies in Management

Some investigators have advocated various forms of subtotal removal of craniopharyngiomas or their contents, followed by radiation therapy (21,41). Most forms of radiation therapy currently given for craniopharyngioma produce hypothalamic and pituitary damage, although radiation therapy is of proven benefit in delaying recurrence and controlling tumor growth (34,35, 38). There is also a small but constant risk of radiation-induced optic neuropathy leading to blindness, diffuse brain damage leading to dementia, focal brain necrosis affecting the hypothalamus or septal region, vascular pathology leading to occlusion, and a moyamoya-type vasculopathy, and the late induction of secondary tumors, many of which are malignant. New forms of radiation therapy are being evaluated, and should represent a major advance in the avoidance of such complications. Hopefully they will be more effective in destroying the tumor and its potential for recurrence.

Data from the University of Virginia are now available for some 30 patients treated by cyst aspiration and gamma knife radiosurgery, with encouraging results (40). Cyst aspiration and instillation of colloidal radioactive isotopes also has been used in a small number of appropriate cases.

One must recognize the selection bias that affects previously reported retrospective studies. Rapidly growing large tumors that cause progressive visual loss and hydrocephalus demand surgical management, and the outcome of many of those patients reflects the aggressiveness of the tumor. Those patients with small, indolent, relatively asymptomatic tumors are over represented in the group of patients treated by less radical surgery and radiation. Naturally, their end results reflect the less aggressive nature of their tumors.

It is important to individualize the plan of management to the patient and to what is known about the anatomy and biology of the tumor because each craniopharyngioma is different. Several issues should be addressed in previously untreated patients. Total removal remains a reasonable goal for many tumors, especially those with enlargement of the sella and no major involvement of or attachment to the hypothalamus or optic apparatus. It is occasionally prudent to delay therapy until growth is complete in infants and children who are growing normally.

Conclusion

The goal of treatment, a neurologically intact patient living as normal a life as possible, is accomplished by using a judicious combination of careful surgery, meticulous medical and endocrine management, and appropriate radiation therapy. Improvements in diagnosis and the technical and conceptual aspects of medical, surgical, and radiotherapeutic management should lead to continuing improvement in the outlook for patients with craniopharyngioma.

Acknowledgment

The authors are grateful to Pamela Leake for her expert assistance in the preparation of the manuscript.

References

1. Babinski MJ. Tumeur du corps pituitare sans acromegalie et avec arret de development des organes genitaux. *Rev Neurol (Paris)* 1900;8:531–533.
2. Banna M, Hoare RD, Stanley P, et al. Craniopharyngioma in children. *J Pediatr* 1973;83:781–785.
3. Carmel PW. Craniopharyngiomas. In: Wilkins RH, Rengachary SS, eds. *Neurosurgery*. New York, McGraw-Hill, 1985:905–915.
4. Carmel PW, Antunes JL, Chang CH. Craniopharyngiomas in children. *Neurosurgery* 1982;11:382–389.
5. Choux M, Lena G, Genitori L. Le craniopharyngiome de l'enfant. *Neurochirurgie* 1991;37:12–165.
6. Hoff JT, Patterson RH. Craniopharyngiomas in children and adults. *J Neurosurg* 1972;36:299–302.
7. Laws ER Jr. Craniopharyngioma: diagnosis and treatment. *Endocrinologist* 1992;2:184–188.
8. Laws ER Jr. Craniopharyngiomas: diagnosis and treatment. In: Sekhar LN, Schramm VL Jr, eds. *Tumors of the cranial base: diagnosis and treatment*. Armonk, NY: Futura, 1987:347–371.
9. Laws ER Jr. Diagnosis and management of craniopharyngioma in children and adolescents. *Curr Opin Endocrinol Diabetes* 1996;3:110–114.
10. Randall RV, Laws ER Jr, Abboud CF. Clinical presentation of craniopharyngioma: a brief review of 300 cases. In: Givens JR, ed. *The hypothalamus*. Chicago: Year Book Medical Publishers, 1984:335–347.
11. Till K. Craniopharyngiomas. *Child Brain* 1982;9:179–187.
12. Carmichael H. Squamous epithelial rests in the hypophysis cerebri. *Arch Neurol Psychol* 1931;26:966–975.
13. Cushing H. The craniopharyngiomas. In: *Intracranial tumors. Notes upon a series of two thousand verified cases with surgical mortality percentages pertaining thereto*. Springfield, IL: Charles C Thomas, 1932:93–98.
14. Hoffman HJ. Surgical management of craniopharyngioma. *Pediatr Neurosurg* 1994;21:44–49.

15. Hoffman HJ, De Silva M, Humphreys RP, et al. Aggressive surgical management of craniopharyngiomas in children. *J Neurosurg* 1992;76:47–542.
16. Konovalov AN. Operative management of craniopharyngiomas. In: Krayenbuhl H, ed. *Advances and technical standards in neurosurgery.* Vienna: Springer-Verlag, 1981:281–318.
17. Maira G, Anile C, Rossi GF, et al. Surgical treatment of craniopharyngiomas: an evaluation of the transsphenoidal and pterional approaches. *Neurosurgery* 1995;36:715–724.
18. Patterson RH, Danyelevich A. Surgical removal of craniopharyngiomas by transcranial approach through the lamina terminalis and sphenoid sinus. *Neurosurgery* 1980;7:111–117.
19. Rougerie J. What can be expected from the surgical treatment of craniopharyngiomas in children. Report of 92 cases. *Child Brain* 1979;5:433–449.
20. Samii M, Tatagiba M. Craniopharyngioma. In: Laws ER Jr, Kaye AH, eds. *Encyclopedia of brain tumors.* New York: Churchill Livingstone, 1995:873–894.
21. Shillito J Jr. Craniopharyngiomas: the subfrontal approach, or none at all? *Clin Neurosurg* 1980;27:188–205.
22. Sweet WH. Radical surgical treatment of craniopharyngioma. *Clin Neurosurg* 1976;23:52–79.
23. Symon L, Sprich W. Radical excision of craniopharyngioma. *J Neurosurg* 1985;62:174–181.
24. Yasargil MG, Curcic M, Kis M, et al. Total removal of craniopharyngiomas. Approaches and long-term results in 144 patients. *J Neurosurg* 1990;73:3–11.
25. Baskin DS, Wilson CB. Surgical management of craniopharyngiomas: a review of 74 cases. *J Neurosurg* 1986;65:22–27.
26. Bouche J, Rougerie J, Freche CH, et al. L'abord des craniopharyngiomes part la voie transsphenoidale basse. *Ann Otolaryngol (Paris)* 1967;84:655–658.
27. Ciric IS, Cozzens JW. Craniopharyngiomas: transsphenoidal method of approach—for the virtuoso only? *Clin Neurosurg* 1980;27:169–187.
28. Hamberger CA, Hammer G, Norlen G, et al. Surgical treatment of craniopharyngioma: radical removal by transsphenoidal approach. *Acta Otolaryngol* 1960;52:285–292.
29. Landolt AM, Zachmann M. Results of transsphenoidal extirpation of craniopharyngiomas and Rathke's cysts. *Neurosurg* 1991;28:410–415.
30. Laws ER Jr. Transsphenoidal approach to lesions in and about the sella turcica. In: Schmidek HH, Sweet WH, eds. *Operative neurosurgical techniques.* New York: Grune and Stratton, 1982:327–341.
31. Laws ER Jr. Transsphenoidal microsurgery in the management of craniopharyngioma. *J Neurosurg* 1980;52:661–666.
32. Laws ER Jr, Randall RV, Kern EB, et al. Craniopharyngioma—the transsphenoidal microsurgical approach. In: Givens JR, ed. *The hypothalamus.* Chicago: Year Book Medical Publishers, 1984:335–347.
33. Kobayashi T, Nakane T, Kageyama N. Combined transsphenoidal and intracranial surgery for craniopharyngioma. *Prog Exp Tumor Res* 1987;30:341–349.
34. Cavazutti V, Fischer EG, Welch K, et al. Neurological and psychophysiological sequelae following different treatments of craniopharyngioma in children. *J Neurosurg* 1983;59:409–417.
35. Constine LS, Woolf PD, Cann D, et al. Hypothalamic-pituitary dysfunction after radiation for brain tumors. *N Engl J Med* 1993;328:87–94.
36. Lichter AS, Wara WM, Sheline GE, et al. The treatment of craniopharyngiomas. *Int J Radiat Oncol Biol Phys* 1977;2:675–683.
37. Richmond IL, Wara WM, Wilson CB. Role of radiation therapy in the management of craniopharyngiomas in children. *Neurosurgery* 1980;6:513–517.
38. Samaan NA, Bakdash MM, Cadero JB, et al. Hypopituitarism after external irradiation: evidence for both hypothalamic and pituitary origin. *Ann Intern Med* 1975;83:771–777.
39. Backlund EO, Axelsson B, Bergstrand CG, et al. Treatment of craniopharyngiomas: the stereotactic approach in a ten to twenty-three years' perspective. I. Surgical, radiological and ophthalmological aspects. *Acta Neurochir* 1989;99:11–19.
40. Prasad D, Steiner M, Steiner L. Gamma knife surgery for craniopharyngioma. *Acta Neurochir* 1995;134:167–176.
41. Fischer EG, Welch K, Shillito J Jr, et al. Craniopharyngiomas in children: long-term effects of conservative surgical procedures combined with radiation therapy. *J Neurosurg* 1990;73:534–540.

117. Craniofacial Surgery for Tumors of the Anterior Skull Base

Andrew H. Kaye

Most intracranial anterior skull-base tumors can be resected using standard neurosurgical techniques. Carcinomas of the paranasal sinuses extending to the floor of the anterior cranial fossa and esthesioneuroblastoma are by far the most common tumors presenting that require a craniofacial resection involving the anterior skull base. These tumors, and the resection techniques, will be described in detail in this chapter. Less common tumors requiring craniofacial resection include sarcomas of the skull base and meningiomas that invade through the anterior fossa floor into the paranasal sinuses. The principles of resection of these tumors are similar to that which will be described for the paranasal sinus carcinomas (PSCs). Rarely, craniofacial resection techniques may be necessary for fi-

brous dysplasia when functional or esthetic deformity requires surgery.

Epidemiology: Paranasal Sinus Carcinoma

PSC is a relatively rare group of tumors with an incidence of 0.3 to 1 cases per 100,000 people per year in most Western countries (1–5). PSC is responsible for less than 1% of cancer deaths in the United States and comprises 3% of all head and neck carcinomas in Western series (2). The lifetime risk of developing PSC for men is 1 in 1,000 and for women, 1 in 3,000 (5). PSC is exceedingly rare in childhood, with an incidence of about 0.1 per 100,000 per year. The incidence increases significantly with age after the fourth decade to 5 to 6 per 100,000 per year in the eighth decade (1,5). The peak age at presentation is 55 to 65 years for men and 60 to 80 years for women with a median age at diagnosis of 62 and 72 years, respectively. There is an apparent decline in incidence after 85 years of age, which may be due to underreporting in this age group. Our series of 86 patients with PSC suitable for craniofacial resection from the Royal Melbourne Hospital (RMH) ranged in age from 58 to 75 years with a median age of 66 years. There is a male preponderance, and the male-to-female ratio varies between 1.5 to 3.1 in all age groups over 35 years of age (1,5). The male predominance is related to the histology of the tumors; in cases of adenocarcinoma, the overall male-to-female ratio is 4:1 while in squamous cell carcinoma (SCC) it is 1.5:1. The explanation for this male preponderance relates to occupational factors discussed later in this chapter. In the RMH series 79 of 86 patients (92%) were men, giving a male-to-female ratio of nearly 13:1. No familial or genetic tendency has been described with PSC.

The incidence of PSC varies about threefold worldwide. Asia, Africa, and South America are three regions of relatively high incidence. In Japan and Colombia the reported incidence has been between 2 to 396 per 100,000 people per year (3). The age-standardized rate in these countries is estimated to be four times that of the white population in the United States. In Uganda the rate is also similarly high but this is largely due to cases of Burkitt lymphoma (2).

Anatomical Distribution

A large English registry-based series reports the site of predilection for PSC to be the maxillary sinus where 60% of these cancers originate. Other paranasal sinuses, principally the ethmoid sinus, comprised 16% of the total, while 20% of cases arose in the nasal cavity and 4% in the nasal vestibule (1); these figures are similar to hospital-based series from the United States (2). In the RMH series of 86 patients who underwent craniofacial resection for PSC, the paranasal sinus of origin was the ethmoid sinus in 54%, maxillary sinus in 19%, nasal cavity in 10%, and frontal sinus in 8%, the distribution reflecting the bias for treatment by craniofacial resection.

The different histological types of tumors have various sites of predilection (1,6). SCC tends to arise mostly in the maxillary sinus where it comprises 60% of tumors. Adenocarcinoma is principally located in the ethmoid sinuses and upper nasal cavity. Transitional cell and anaplastic carcinomas are more evenly distributed among the sinuses, however, in many cases it can be difficult to determine the exact site of origin because the tumor has invaded far beyond the confines of the sinus of origin.

PSC is rare in the general population, however, local clusters of cases have been recognized and careful epidemiological studies have been performed to pinpoint various causes. The relative risks of those exposed to the occupational hazards described have been as high as 30 to 1,000 times that of the normal population. Alterations of the working environment to reduce exposure to hazardous carcinogens have been followed in many situations by a reduction in the incidence of PSC (7,8). The occupational hazard where the association was first demonstrated was nickel refining (9); nickel workers in Canada,

Table 1. Environmental Correlations of PNC

Squamous cell carcinoma	Nickel refining
	Mustard gas manufacturing
	Isopropyl alcohol manufacturing
	Watch face painting
	Thorium dioxide contrast medium
	Snuff and tobacco smoking
Adenocarcinoma	Hardwood dusts in woodworking
	Footware soles machining
	Flour milling
	Polyaromatic hydrocarbon exposure
	Asbestos inhalation

From Kaye AH, Danks RA. *Brain tumors — an encyclopedic approach,* New York: Churchill Livingstone, 1995: Chap 42, with permission.

Norway, the former Soviet Union, and Wales suffered a relative risk of over 100 times that of the rest of the population. The typical histology of the tumors was anaplastic or SCC; there was also an associated large increase in the risk of lung cancer. With correct management of the workplace environment a zero incidence was achieved at one Canadian plant over a 30-year period (8). The carcinogenicity of nickel has been confirmed in multiple animal and *in vitro* studies (2). Other hazardous materials include radium (encountered by watch face painters), mustard gas, isopropyl alcohol, and hydrocarbon (2) (Table 1). Recreational snuff inhalation has been suggested as a risk factor in several studies, but the association was clear in African studies (2). While tobacco smoking has been correlated with a threefold increase in the risk of SCC (10,11), other studies report no association with cigarette smoking (4,12). An iatrogenic cause of SCC is the radioactive contrast medium thorium dioxide, retained in the maxillary sinus after radiological investigations; tumors have developed after a latent period of decades postexposure. The high incidence of PSC in Japan is principally due to an elevated incidence of SCC of the maxilla. Despite epidemiological studies demonstrating very modest associations with chronic sinusitis, nasal polyposis, cigarette smoking, and woodworking, this incidence has not been adequately explained (3, 12–14), although it has become less common (3,10,15).

Adenocarcinoma of the ethmoid sinus is a rare tumor in the general population; there is a very strong association, however, between the incidence of this tumor and inhalation of hardwood dusts, particularly from high-speed machining. The occupational association of hardwoods was first convincingly demonstrated in the Buckinghamshire furniture industry (16). The relative risk to workers in this industry was 1,000 times that of the general population, making it as common as carcinoma of the lung in this group. By taking detailed occupational histories the authors were able to pinpoint that the risk was to those workers who were exposed to hardwood dust during the machining and sanding of furniture, rather than to those exposed to varnishes and lacquers during the stage of French polishing. Insecticides and other chemical treatments of the wood were not employed prior to woodworking during the period of risk studied in this report. The mean latency period from first exposure to tumor diagnosis was 43 years and there was a strong correlation between the length of exposure and the risk of tumor formation (7). The shortest period of exposure to development of tumor was only 5 years in a patient who developed the tumor 33 years after leaving the industry. The association between adenocarcinoma of the ethmoid sinus and exposure to hardwood dusts has been confirmed by reports from Germany, the United States, Canada, Denmark, Finland, Sweden, the Netherlands (17), France (18), and Australia

(19–21); there is also an association with carpentry in the building trade in those countries. In the Australian reports and in one from United States concerning the state of Georgia (22), there is a strong association between adenocarcinoma and the processes of timber cutting and machining. In England, where softwoods are the material used by workers in such industries, no cases of adenocarcinoma have been observed (23).

In our region of the state of Victoria, Australia, there is a substantial timber industry and adenocarcinoma comprises 35% of the cases of PSC in registry statistics (5). In the RMH series of 86 cases of PSC suitable for craniofacial resection, there were 32 cases of adenocarcinoma and 31 (97%) patients gave a history of prolonged hardwood exposure. Interestingly, 19 (50%) of 38 patients with SCC also gave such a history, indicating the possibility of a weaker association with this histological type (24). Of our 10 patients with adenoid cystic carcinoma, 9 had been occupationally exposed to hardwoods, while none of the 6 patients with esthesioneuroblastoma gave such an occupational history. Other case series and formal epidemiological studies have demonstrated a two- to fourfold increase in paranasal sinus SCC in woodworkers, but no clear dose-response relation was evident (14,17,25).

It would suggest that a crucial factor in the risk of PSC is the type of wood dust to which the workers are exposed. At least 48 types of wood are known to have been used in workshops in which workers have developed these tumors; these woods are derived from both deciduous and evergreen trees and from trees native to both the Northern and Southern hemispheres. Hardwood species tend to be the wood types most associated with PSC. Hardwoods, by definition, come from deciduous trees, in contrast to softwoods that derive from conifer trees. Generally the terms "hard" or "soft" connote the density of the wood but there are notable exceptions (e.g., the well-known light balsa wood is actually from a deciduous tree and is therefore a hardwood).

Clinical Features

The common presenting symptoms of PSC are nasal obstruction (often unilateral), epistaxis, and nasal discharge. There is often a preceding history of chronic rhinitis causing similar symptoms which contributes to the common delay in diagnosis. Less often, patients present with facial pain, facial sensory disturbance, swelling of the cheek, proptosis, diplopia, or visual disturbance (26). Presentation with symptoms referable to intracranial involvement is rare. Likewise, lymph node involvement or metastatic disease at presentation is rare. Anosmia, usually unilateral, is a common presenting sign in patients with ethmoid sinus or nasal involvement.

In one U.S. series, the diagnosis of PSC was delayed between 3 and 14 months (27). The authors recommend vigorous examination in all adults presenting with sinonasal complaints of greater than 6 weeks' duration, including telescopic endonasal examination and biopsy of all suspicious areas. If the symptoms do not resolve within 2 weeks of vigorous medical therapy, a limited computed tomography (CT) of the sinuses is recommended. Using this regimen, the authors were able to reduce the mean diagnostic delay in their patients from 8 to 4 months, with 33% of the tumors in their series being diagnosed at a relatively early stage (T1 or T2). This is much earlier than in other series and the authors suggest that this reflects their more vigorous investigation of suspicious presenting complaints.

Cancers of the nasal cavity tend to present earlier due to more pronounced early symptoms and easier diagnosis, and this is reflected in the better prognosis of these lesions (6).

Imaging Diagnosis

CT scanning and magnetic resonance imaging (MRI) are the investigations of choice for assessment of PSC. Typical CT findings include a soft-tissue density tumor mass with erosion of the bony walls around the sinus of origin and invasion into adjacent anatomical structures. The tumor enhances nonuniformly with contrast. Multiple fine cuts using window settings for bone and soft tissue are required for detailed presurgical assessment, allowing assessment of tumor extent and bony erosion (Figs. 1 and 2). Direct coronal scans are useful and are particularly valuable in assessment of orbital roof, cribriform plate, olfactory groove, and intracranial involvement (Fig. 3). CT assessment of sinus involvement may be misleading as inspissated mucus in an obstructed sinus may mimic the appearance of tumor; this is particularly crucial when assessing the sphenoid sinus as tumor involvement there may dictate whether the tumor is resectable in its entirety. MRI can usually differentiate between tumor and inspissated mucus (28) (Figs. 4 and 5) and may demonstrate invasion of tumor along the perineural space (29). MRI may show orbital apex or small intracranial deposits better than CT. Inspissated mucus is variable in its MRI-signal intensity but is often different from tumor on T1- or T2-weighted images. Most commonly, entrapped mucus is seen as a high signal on T2-weighted images (Fig. 4). MRI appears to be the most useful imaging modality for postoperative surveillance (30).

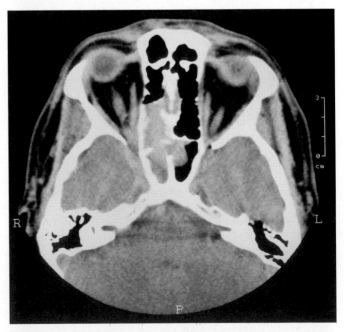

Fig. 1. Axial CT scan of patient with adenocarcinoma of the ethmoid, displayed on soft-tissue window settings. There is soft-tissue mass in the sphenoid sinus, but one cannot be sure if this is a tumor or only trapped mucus. (From Kaye AH, Danks RA, Kleid S, et al. Cranio-facial resection in the management of cancer of the paranasal sinuses. *J Clin Neurosci* 1994;1:111–117, with permission.)

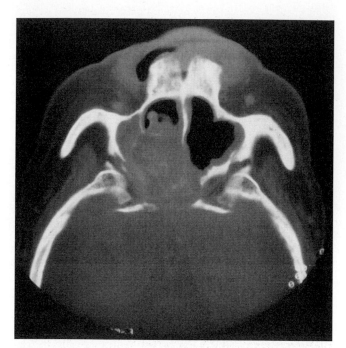

Fig. 2. CT scan of patient with extensive adenocarcinoma using bone windows to display bony erosion.

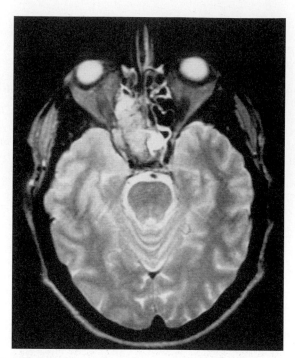

Fig. 4. Axial MRI of patient showing tumor involvement of the right side of the sphenoid sinus, but accumulation of mucus on the left, as shown by the high signal. (From Kaye AH, Danks RA, Kleid S, et al. Cranio-facial resection in the management of cancer of the paranasal sinuses. *J Clin Neurosci* 1994 1:111–117, with permission.)

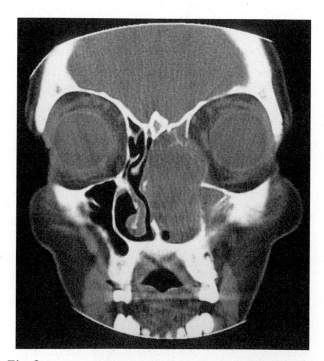

Fig. 3. Coronal CT using bone windows. This displays tumor involvement of the maxilla and ethmoid sinuses, erosion of the orbital wall, and tumor extending right up to the olfactory groove but with no erosion evident. Nevertheless, microscopic dural involvement was present.

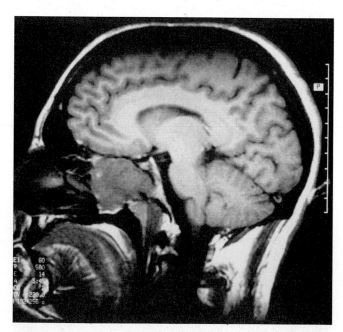

Fig. 5. Parasagittal MRI slightly to the right of the midline in a patient with adenocarcinoma of ethmoid showing the tumor involvement of the sphenoid sinus. The bony floor of the anterior cranial fossa appears intact as a black line in this section. (From Kaye AH, Danks RA, Kleid S, et al. Cranio-facial resection in the management of cancer of the paranasal sinuses. *J Clin Neurosci* 1994 1:111–117, with permission.)

Laboratory Diagnosis

Endoscopic or open examination of the nasal cavity and nasal sinuses, with biopsy of suspicious areas, is the key method of confirming the diagnosis, which is essential before major surgery is undertaken. Cytological diagnosis of maxillary sinus disease has been suggested by examination of washings of the sinus. While malignancy may be diagnosed by this method, there were two false-negative cytology reports among the seven cases of malignant tumor in one Japanese series (31). Systemic investigations will be required to assess the general condition of the patient. No other specific investigations are required except that we find it useful to perform preoperative nasal swabs to guide antibiotic prophylaxis during craniofacial resection.

Gross Morphological Features

PSC commences in one cavity but then invades the bony walls to involve adjacent structures. Often tumors grow extraperiosteally before invading further into the invaded cavity, particularly with respect to the orbit where some surgeons have selectively resected periosteum in an attempt to avoid orbital exenteration (32). When the tumor arises in or involves the ethmoid sinus, early spread to the dura of the olfactory groove is the rule rather than the exception (24); gross intradural disease is less common, reflecting the barrier provided by the dura.

The majority of the tumors are gray to pink or red, friable fungating growths that are susceptible to contact bleeding (6). Some tumors may have a papillomatous appearance or be found in a papilloma after removal. Papillomas are benign but may be bulky and even cause bony erosion by pressure on occasion, and tend to be firm or rubbery in texture (33).

Maxillary cancers typically invade into the hard palate, facial skin, and nose as well as into the ethmoid and sphenoid sinuses, the intracranial cavity, the orbit, and posteriorly into the pterygopalatine fossa.

Adenoid cystic carcinomas are notorious for their diffuse infiltration, which is difficult to demarcate, as well as their tendency to spread along neural pathways. These features contribute to the very high recurrence rate of this tumor type (6).

Salivary carcinoma (principally adenoid cystic), lymphoma, melanoma, sarcoma, and esthesioneuroblastoma are less common (1); these are more common in the Armed Forces Institute of Pathology series, but this may reflect a secondary referral bias (6). The distribution of histologies in our surgical experience is shown in Table 2. Adenocarcinoma is very strongly represented, reflecting both its high incidence in our region and also a referral bias in patients referred for craniofacial resection. Meningioma, hemangiopericytoma, and basal cell carcinoma are rare as primary paranasal sinus tumors but may invade the sinuses by direct spread from adjacent sites and present similar management problems. There is a large number of other rare tumor types that may involve the paranasal sinus region (6).

Table 2. Histological Distribution of Carcinoma of Paranasal Sinuses in the Royal Melbourne Hospital Series of 86 Patients Treated by Craniofacial Resection

Squamous cell carcinoma	38 (44%)
Adenocarcinoma	32 (37%)
Adenoid cystic carcinoma	10 (12%)
Esthesioneuroblastoma	6 (7%)

Esthesioneuroblastoma, or olfactory neuroblastoma, is a variant of neuroblastoma arising from the olfactory apparatus, tending to occur in the upper nasal cavity and ethmoid sinuses. Derivation from nerve cells in the olfactory mucosa (pattern I of Mendelhoff) or supporting epithelial cells (pattern II of Mendelhoff) has been described but does not appear to correlate with patient outcome (34). This tumor occurs throughout life with bimodal peaks in the second and sixth decades. Grading and staging systems have been proposed and correlate with prognosis (6). Lymphomas in this region tend to be high grade, both histologically and in their clinical behavior. They can be typed histochemically for B- and T-cell markers (35).

Management

Patients with PSC often present to the neurosurgeon at an advanced stage when radical resection is difficult or impossible. The results of treatment are highly dependent on the stage of the disease at presentation. In most series the 5-year survival for T1 or T2 disease is 3 to 5 times better than that for T4 disease. Unfortunately the vast majority of patients present with stage T3 or T4 disease. Esthetic considerations weigh heavily in the planning of treatment options as well as the consequences of untreated disease. Distal spread to regional lymph nodes or other organs is uncommon but may occur in the more malignant tumors.

There are at least six classification systems currently in use to stage maxillary sinus tumors. The use of different systems in the various series confuses the interpretation of results and makes it difficult to compare different treatment strategies. All systems are based on the TNM system. The T stage is of paramount importance because nodal and distal spread are relatively uncommon and occur late in the disease. A review of 205 patients revealed Harrison's classification to be the most valid of the six classification systems (36). This system allowed a balanced distribution of cases with good correlation with treatment and survival in the different stages. Another similar review (37) of 70 patients found that Harrison's classification and also that of the Japanese Joint Committee were the most practical and appropriate for staging PSC. Harrison's classification and those of the American and Japanese Joint Committees are shown in Table 3.

There are no widely accepted staging systems of ethmoid carcinoma although a three-stage system has been proposed by Parsons and colleagues (38). Stage 1 tumor is limited to the sinus of origin. Stage 2 includes extension to adjacent areas such as the upper nasal cavity, the orbit, or the sphenoid sinus. Stage 3 includes destruction of the skull base, pterygoid plates, or intracranial extension. On the basis of our experience with patients treated by craniofacial resection and radiotherapy we consider that sphenoid sinus or orbital apex involvement are the worst prognostic indicators, while dural involvement by itself correlates less strongly with a worse outcome (39). Thus we do not entirely concur with the classification of Parsons and colleagues, however, others have found dural involvement to be a significant prognostic factor for survival (40).

The ideal management of PSC incorporates early diagnosis by vigorous investigation of presenting complaints, however, most cases are generally far advanced at the time of presentation. The emphasis in this chapter is on the treatment of advanced PSC as it is these tumors that usually involve the neurosurgeon.

The results of conventional local removal by transnasal or lateral rhinotomy have proven to be very disappointing, conventional radiotherapy alone has also led to poor results. The

Table 3. Staging of Carcinoma of the Maxillary Sinus

	American Joint Committee	Japanese Joint Committee	Harrison's
T1	Tumor confined to antral mucosa of infrastructure with no bone erosion or destruction	Tumor confined to the maxillary sinus with no evidence of bony involvement	Tumor confined to maxillary sinus with no evidence of bony involvement
T2	Tumor confined to suprastructure without bony destruction or to infrastructure with destruction of medial or inferior walls only	Tumor causing destruction of bony wall with external periosteum remaining intact as the capsule and surrounding tissue not invaded but only compressed. Minimal invasion into the ethmoid cells and the exophytic tumor in the middle nasal meatus included.	Bony erosion without evidence of involvement of facial skin, orbit, pterygopalatine fossa, or ethmoid labyrinth
T3	More extensive tumor invading skin of cheek, orbit, anterior ethmoid sinuses, or pterygoid muscles	Tumor infiltrated deeply into the surrounding tissue by penetration of external periosteum	Involvement of orbit, ethmoid labyrinth, or facial skin
T4	Massive tumor with invasion of cribriform plate, posterior ethmoids, sphenoid, nasopharynx, pterygoid plates, or base of skull	Tumor extending to the base of skull, nasopharynx, maxilla of opposite side, and/or facial skin with ulceration. This includes deep infiltration into the orbit with limited eye movement or visual impairment or extension into the temporal fossa or invasion of the pterygoid muscles.	Tumor extension to nasopharynx, sphenoidal sinus, cribriform plate, or pterygopalatine fossa

From Kaye AH, Danks RA. *Brain tumors — an encyclopedic approach,* New York: Churchill Livingstone, 1995: chap 42, with permission.

5-year survival rate with either modality alone did not exceed 25% and was often less (41). Subsequently, management has used different combinations of radiotherapy and surgery, generally using radiotherapy doses above 50 Gy. Ten large, mixed series from 1968 to 1983 were reviewed (42). The mean 5-year survival with these treatments was a disappointing 35%, only a modest improvement on either radiotherapy or surgery alone.

Other authors (41,43,44) have developed craniofacial resection to adequately excise the tumors with some apparent improvement in long-term results. Japanese groups developed different approaches using multimodal therapy. They combined chemotherapy and radiotherapy with surgery but the surgery was often less radical than in other series, and chemotherapy was often intraarterial and also applied topically inside the tumor cavity. More interesting advances include the concurrent use of intravenous infusions of *cis*-platinum and 5-fluorouracil (5-FU) during radiotherapy and the use of three-dimensional computer planning and semi-stereotactic methods of delivering high-dose radiotherapy. These modalities will be discussed in detail later in this chapter.

Unfortunately, meaningful comparison between the different published series is extremely difficult for several reasons. Most series are small or extend over many years because PSCs are uncommon. Several series span the period before and after the introduction of CT and MRI. Many series are retrospective and draw conclusions between treatment groups that were selected on various criteria and thus cannot be easily compared. The series all include different mixtures of tumors, histologies, site, and stage and also differ considerably in the ratio of recurrent to previously untreated cases. Finally results are reported in different ways in the series. The length of follow-up in many of these series is relatively short for most of the cases in the understandable effort to maximize analysis, and the patient numbers to calculate 5-year results are often only a modest proportion of the series. In 6 of the 7 series where 5-year follow-up was assessable, one-third to one-fourth of the total 5-year recurrences occurred between 2 and 5 years after treatment. Therefore, series that quote follow-up for only 2 to 3 years do

not adequately describe the results of treatment. Recurrences may occur after 5 years; of the patients in one large series who died, 8% did so more than 5 years after treatment (26). This delayed recurrence is especially marked with adenoid cystic carcinoma where the 10-year cure rate may be as low as 7% (6); to a lesser degree this also applies to adenocarcinoma. Any patient who survives 5 years cannot be regarded as cured. Finally, many series do not adequately discuss morbidity and mortality.

Despite a detailed and exhaustive review of the literature, conclusions as to the relative merits of different modalities of treatment can only be inferential. Many authors appropriately conclude their reports by recommending a properly constructed prospective multicenter trial of the different treatment modalities available but, unfortunately, no such studies have been performed to date.

Surgical Management

The goal of surgery is to achieve a radical tumor resection with a margin of normal tissue; this margin is necessarily limited by the close confines and important relationships of PSC. Orbital resection is required where tumor invasion has occurred although this is controversial and will be discussed subsequently. When a tumor involves the ethmoid sinuses, the resection will usually be inadequate unless craniofacial resection is employed to fully resect the roof of the ethmoid sinuses (45). Posterior extension into the pterygopalatine fossa or nasopharynx may make radical resection difficult or impossible. In our experience, extensive posterior sphenoid or cavernous sinus involvement has precluded radical curative resection; this may often be suspected on preoperative imaging, but it is often only at surgery that direct inspection and frozen section biopsies can definitively establish resectability. Some authors report radical resection involving the cavernous sinus, but detailed results

propriate in cases of esthesioneuroblastoma because of its known sensitivity to radiotherapy and chemotherapy.

Craniofacial resection incorporating the anterior cranial fossa floor has, in the past, been associated with significant morbidity and mortality due to cerebrospinal fluid (CSF) fistula and resultant intracranial infection. However, in our RMH series of 86 patients (24) there have been no cases of CSF fistula requiring repair or mortality but we have had one case of infection (a superficial facial cellulitis). There has also been one case of postoperative tension pneumocephalus, requiring reoperation and temporary tracheostomy. Certain technical points are emphasized in the following paragraphs that have been crucial in achieving our results.

All patients are under the care of the neurosurgical department. Preoperative nasal swabs are taken to guide perioperative antibiotics, which are vigorously employed, including 24 hours of preoperative intranasal Soframycin (in the initial 42 patients), intraoperative and postoperative intravenous prophylaxis with flucloxacillin, amoxicillin, and metronidazole, and intraoperative topical antibiotic irrigation using flucloxacillin and amoxicillin. In the last 3 years of the series, cephalothin has replaced the combination of flucloxacillin and amoxicillin.

An intraoperative lumbar drain and neurosurgical anesthetic techniques are employed to ensure adequate brain relaxation. The head is positioned in slight extension in a three-pin headrest to allow gravity to assist with brain retraction and exposure of the anterior cranial fossa floor. A bicoronal scalp flap is positioned well posteriorly to allow a large pericranial flap based upon the supraorbital and supratrochlear vessels of both sides to be reflected inferiorly. A low, free bifrontal bone flap is cut just above the supraorbital ridges. We do not employ the approach via a shell-shaped craniotomy through the frontal sinus (49) nor do we incorporate the superior orbital margin in our craniotomies (50) as we have not encountered complications from brain retraction, which only needs to be light due to the CSF drainage.

The dura is dissected from the anterior cranial fossa floor using magnification and head light for adequate visualization. Involved dura is resected and then grafted with temporalis fascia or fascia lata. All dural tears are meticulously closed with 5-0 polypropylene, the integrity of the dural closure is the key to preventing CSF leaks. En-bloc tumor dissection is then performed in conjunction with a lateral nasal approach performed by the ear, nose, and throat (ENT) surgeon and the tumor is passed out inferiorly via that incision. Frozen-section examination of the surgical margins or any suspicious-looking areas is very useful in guiding the resection and assessing resectability.

After the resection, liberal antibiotic irrigation is used before and after suturing the pericranial flap to the margin of the bony defect to hold it firmly to the skull base (Fig. 8). No graft is used on the nasal side of this vascularized pericranial flap as the nasal epithelium covers this gradually over a 3- to 4-week period.

The pericranial flap technique (24,51,52) is crucial in achieving satisfactory results with low morbidity. This is confirmed by an analysis of the published series of craniofacial resection with and without this technique. There was a four- to tenfold reduction in the rate of CSF fistula, intracranial infection, and operative mortality in those series employing this technique over those other techniques for cranial base reconstruction (Table 4).

Craniotomy without employing resection from below, via a facial excision, has been reported by a group who also had performed craniofacial resection for PSC (53). These patients tended to have a greater number of local complications including frontal lobe retraction injuries and postoperative hematomas thought to be due to the more limited exposure.

In cases where orbital exenteration is required, the dura of

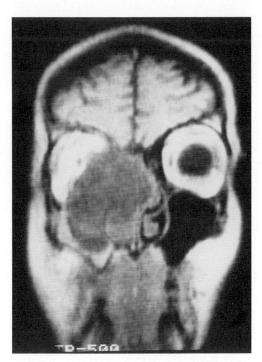

Fig. 6. Coronal magnetic resonance imaging showing extensive squamous cell carcinoma invading through the floor of anterior cranial fossa.

have not been reported (32). On the other hand, a large mass of intracranial disease extending superiorly from the olfactory groove has not precluded successful radical resection; these tumors can be resected by conventional neurosurgical techniques, along with the cranial base which is then grafted (24, 46). However, in some cases multiple intradural nodules of tumor spreading over the anterior cranial fossa floor may prevent curative resection. (Fig. 6.)

In the RMH series of 86 cases of PSC treated by craniofacial resection, sphenoid sinus involvement was the major predictor of later tumor recurrence. Dural or orbital involvement, however, correlated more weakly with the risk of later recurrence, indicating adequate treatment of these sites by this operative strategy (24,39). (Fig. 7.)

The decision to undertake orbital resection is controversial and this should certainly not be undertaken unless all other disease can be adequately resected. The conventional wisdom is that if there is invasion of the bony walls of the orbit, then orbital exenteration is required. However in a detailed retrospective analysis of a series of 41 patients where there was a strong commitment to preserving the eye (32), local recurrence did not occur in the orbit; yet, 10 of these 14 tumors were esthesioneuroblastomas, an otherwise uncommon tumor. Ketcham and van Buren's experience in a series dominated by advanced SCC was that there was a 30% survival rate in those who had preservation of the orbit, compared with a 50% survival rate in those who had orbital resection (47). In a large series of 209 patients followed for over 10 years, Lund and colleagues adopted a policy of orbital sacrifice only if the periosteum was breached by tumor; their figures showed no survival difference for orbital involvement with or without periosteal invasion (48). Our policy is to preserve the orbit where there is extensive bilateral orbital invasion or other involvement that precludes radical resection. We prefer to exenterate the orbit if there is breach of the bony orbital walls by tumor in cases where a radical and complete tumor clearance can be achieved. Perhaps the more conservative option would be ap-

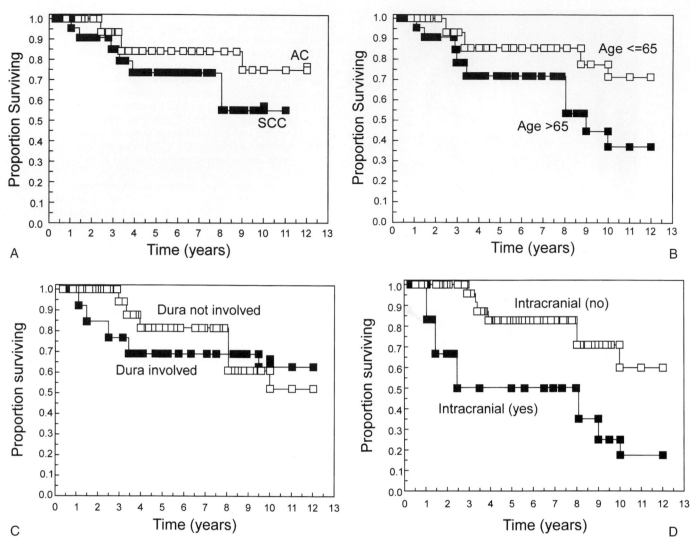

Fig. 7. Actuarial survival curves from the Royal Melbourne Hospital series of 86 patients showing the survival for patients with adenocarcinoma (*ac*) and squamous cell carcinoma (*SCC*) **(A)**, by age **(B)**, dural involvement **(C)**, and intracranial extension of tumor **(D)**.

Table 4. Pericranial Flaps in Craniofacial Resection

	Pericranial flap not used[a]	Pericranial flap used[b]	Current Royal Melbourne Hospital series (86 patients)
No series	3	5	1
Cerebrospinal fluid fistula	16%	2%	0%[c]
Intracranial infection	13%	5%	0%
Mortality	6%	2%	0%

[a] Data from Terz et al., 1980 (41); Ketcham and van Buren, 1985 (47); Cheeseman et al., 1986 (49)
[b] Data from Sundaresan and Shah, 1988 (46); Blacklock et al., 1989; Snyderman et al., 1990 (40), Kaye et al., 1994 (24); Sekhar et al., 1992 (50).
[c] No case required surgical repair of cerebrospinal fluid fistula.

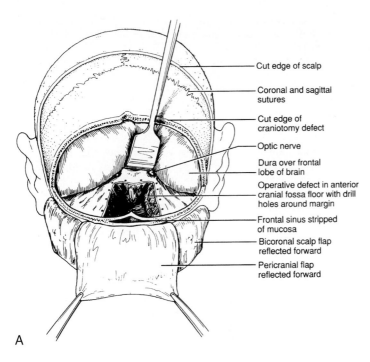

A

Cut edge of scalp

Coronal and sagittal sutures

Cut edge of craniotomy defect

Optic nerve

Dura over frontal lobe of brain

Operative defect in anterior cranial fossa floor with drill holes around margin

Frontal sinus stripped of mucosa

Bicoronal scalp flap reflected forward

Pericranial flap reflected forward

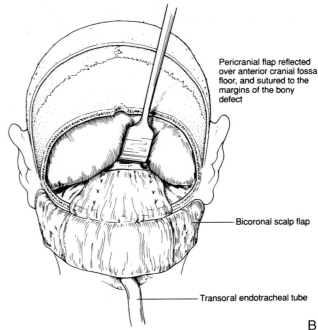

B

Pericranial flap reflected over anterior cranial fossa floor, and sutured to the margins of the bony defect

Bicoronal scalp flap

Transoral endotracheal tube

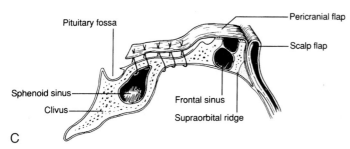

C

Pituitary fossa

Pericranial flap

Scalp flap

Sphenoid sinus

Clivus

Frontal sinus

Supraorbital ridge

Fig. 8. The pericranial flap is designed and positioned to close the defect in the anterior cranial fossa floor. **A:** The defect in the anterior cranial fossa floor following the en-bloc removal of the tumor. Fine holes are drilled around the margins of this defect for suturing down the pericranial flap. **B:** Midsagittal section of the operative field showing the pericranial flap being sutured into position around the bony defect. **C:** The pericranial flap in position sutured to the margins of the operative defect, and covering a wide area of the anterior cranial fossa floor beyond that. Fibrin glue is used to seal the edges of the flap. (From Kaye AH, Danks RA, Kleid S, et al. Cranio-facial resection in the management of cancer of the paranasal sinuses. *J Clin Neurosci* 1994;1:111–117, with permission.)

the optic nerve is closed to prevent CSF leak. The eyelids are sutured together and the orbital cavity is filled by transposition of the temporalis muscle. This local flap is more convenient than a microvascular free flap, however, a free flap is required if substantial facial skin needs to be sacrificed due to tumor involvement.

In our series of 86 patients there have been no significant complications other than one case of tension pneumocephalus requiring reexploration, five cases of nonfatal venous thromboembolism (three deep vein thromboses and two cases of pulmonary embolism), and one case of postoperative facial cellulitis. Reported complications of craniofacial resection include CSF fistula and infections such as meningitis, intracranial abscess, or bone flap infection (53–57). Other complications may occur due to brain retraction causing frontal lobe edema, hemorrhage, or epilepsy, but correct positioning of the head, minimization of brain retraction, and careful technique can eliminate these problems. Intracranial aerocele may occur due to excessive lumbar drainage late in the operation and postoperatively. The eye may be damaged due to exposure to the air or alcoholic skin preparation or by pressure, we use ointment and then suture the eyelids closed before skin preparation and are vigilant to prevent pressure on the orbital structures throughout the operation. Damage to the optic nerve may occur due to dissection at the orbital apex, damaging that structure. This may lead to the dreaded complication of bilateral blindness if the other orbit is exenterated.

There are four published series assessing the 5-year results

of craniofacial resection and radiotherapy in advanced (T4) SCC (41,46,47,58). The 5-year survival was in the range of 50% to 70%. In our series the 5-year survival was 74%. A similar number of series employing conventional noncraniofacial surgery and radiotherapy for such tumors gave a 5-year survival of 7% to 25% (27,59–62). For adenocarcinoma of the ethmoid sinus, two series employing craniofacial surgery and radiotherapy had 5-year survival rates of 78% and 83%, respectively (24,39,58), compared with 25% to 46% for transnasofacial surgery and radiotherapy (27,38,63). In both of these comparisons there was a much higher ratio of recurrent to untreated tumors in the craniofacial series, thus the therapeutic advantage from a craniofacial approach is possibly even greater than these figures suggest. Our updated RMH series had a 60% incidence of recurrent PSC proceeding to craniofacial resection (52 recurrent cases in 86 patients).

For esthesioneuroblastoma, good results are achieved by radical surgical resection and radiotherapy with 86% to 100% 5-year control (64,65). This is clearly better than the results with single-modality treatment.

Radiotherapy

Several studies have compared patient groups treated with surgery alone against similar groups given additional postoperative radiotherapy (48,61,66–68). All but the series of Wustrow and others found that adjuvant radiotherapy gave significant improvement in outcome. A recent large series compared the effect on survival of administering radiotherapy before or after craniofacial resection and no statistically significant difference was found (48). It appears widely accepted in the literature that postoperative radiotherapy offers additional benefit to the patient after radical tumor resection.

Several series have suggested that many PSCs can be cured by radical high-dose radiotherapy combined with subradical surgery or even surgical biopsy only (38,60,63,69–71). There are no series that have compared different radiotherapy dosages in a controlled manner, but comparison between series suggests that doses of 60 to 80 Gy produce an improved outcome compared to lower doses. In the three series employing the higher dose there was a 5-year survival averaging 56% compared with those series where 45 to 55 Gy was given where the 5-year survival averaged 37%. One series employing high-dose radiotherapy used vigorous orbital shielding to try to limit ocular toxicity but this group suffered a high rate of orbital relapse leading to a 5-year survival of only 37% (69).

The literature indicates that radical radiotherapy can give results similar to those achieved by simple transnasal surgery and radiotherapy combined, but the results are still marginally inferior to those series that have employed radical craniofacial surgery to achieve as complete a tumor resection as possible. Furthermore, comparison of two similar groups of patients treated in Toronto by either radiotherapy alone or radiotherapy and surgery revealed better results in the combined therapy group (51% versus 40% 5-year survival) (72). Unfortunately many patients suffer significant morbidity following radical radiotherapy, particularly dry eyes, but the most serious morbidity is damage to the visual apparatus. Optic nerve or retinal damage to the ipsilateral eye occurs in 25% to 100% of cases (73) while frank blindness occurs in 7% to 22%. Several authors claim that blindness is inevitable if the orbit is radically treated, although this may be delayed for up to 5 years. Such morbidity is defended by the argument that orbital exenteration would otherwise be necessary to control tumor, the dreaded complication of bilateral blindness has occurred in 2% to 8% of cases (38,62, 69). Osteoradionecrosis occurred in a similar number in these series but was up to 17% in one series (69). Transient central nervous system disturbances occurred in up to 10% of cases but no long-term sequelae were detected.

Two series attest that reduction in morbidity can be achieved by the use of immobilizing shells and three-dimensional CT-guided computerized treatment planning systems to deliver precise differential dosimetry to the tumor and surrounding important structures (60,70). Both of these series also claim a modest improvement in disease control attributable to this technique.

A number of reports have favored preoperative radiotherapy (21,49) but the results do not differ clearly from those in similar series. However, the authors of these reports believe this technique allowed them to better preserve the orbital contents in some cases. The morbidity of craniofacial resection subsequent to radiotherapy did not appear worse than in other series using similar techniques (49). Pre- and postoperative radiotherapy were compared at one center and no difference in outcome or morbidity was evident (27). Preoperative radiotherapy does allow observation of changes in tumor histology to document the effectiveness of the treatment (e.g., in 6 of 19 patients with adenocarcinoma treated with preoperative radiotherapy, no tumor could be found at operation 6 weeks later) (21); none of these patients developed recurrence on prolonged follow-up. A substantial number of other tumors in this series exhibited large areas of tumor necrosis, emphasizing that this tumor type is significantly radiosensitive. Among cases of SCC, combined preoperative radiotherapy and chemotherapy produced elimination of all viable tumor in 34 of 86 cases on the basis of histopathology (74).

Esthesioneuroblastoma appears to be more sensitive than other PSCs to both radiotherapy and chemotherapy (75,76). A recent small series has shown that even bulky disease can be well controlled with chemotherapy using cis-platinum and etoposide followed by proton beam radiation for good responders, or surgery and conventional radiotherapy for poor responders (77).

There are two relatively recent advances that have found application in the treatment of PSC. The use of chemotherapeutic agents as radiosensitizers and hyperfractionated radiotherapy may improve the therapeutic ration in treating these tumors. These therapies rely on normal tissue being better able to repair itself after sublethal damage from each treatment while tumor cells typically have defects in their DNA repair mechanisms that render this repair less likely. Tissue culture and experiments performed in animal models have demonstrated that concomitant intravenous infusions of cis-platinum may act as a radiosensitizer (78). Infusions of cis-platinum were given in conjunction with hyperfractionated radiotherapy (60 to 70 Gy in 60 fractions over 8 weeks). Eleven of twelve (92%) patients with T4 tumors achieved a complete response with this treatment and 7 of 12 (58%) were alive 3 to 6 years after treatment (79); 4 of 12 (33%) patients suffered local recurrence. Ophthalmic complications occurred in only 1 patient. These results appear clearly better than in similar patients treated with radiation alone and are supported by other studies in these and other tumor types in one review (78).

In summary, it is certainly widely accepted that radiotherapy is of major benefit in the treatment of PSC. The most widely accepted view is that radiotherapy should be given after radical surgical resection of the tumor. To achieve maximal effect the radiotherapy needs to be given in high doses, of the order of 60 to 80 Gy. CT-guided, computer-assisted, three-dimensional treatment planning appears to offer benefits in terms of reduced morbidity and possibly increased effectiveness.

Chemotherapy

Chemotherapy has not been widely used in the primary treatment of PSC in the English-speaking world. However, regimens containing cis-platinum and 5-FU have a beneficial effect; such treatments have been pioneered in Japan where intraarterial and topical routes have been combined with intravenous therapy. Treatment regimens have evolved over many years prompted by two factors: the relatively high incidence of PSC in Japan; and the realization that the mean 5-year survival treated by surgery and radiotherapy was only 35% (42). Maximal combination therapy using preoperative radiotherapy, intraarterial 5-FU, and intravenous bromodeoxyuridine combined with surgery achieved a 5-year survival rate of 50% (74,80). Subsequently, the intraarterial 5-FU therapy was replaced by repeated applications of topical 5-FU with maintenance of these good results (42,81,82). In another Japanese series the use of preoperative intraarterial cis-platinum and pepleomycin was believed to be the major factor in improving the 5-year survival rate of 22% to 55% despite a reduction in the rate of radical maxillectomy from 50% to 18% (82). Another series found no improvement in patients treated with intraarterial 5-FU although the patients who received 5-FU received lower doses of radiotherapy than the control group, severely confounding the results of this study (60). A prospective study was performed in Rotterdam based on this Japanese work (42). A vigorous surgical internal decompression of the PSC was performed via an anterior maxillectomy but without removing orbital periosteum or dura, even if involved. The cavity was then packed, internally debrided thrice weekly, and topical 5-FU applied to the walls of the cavity before repacking; this was continued over several weeks depending on the progress and appearance of the cavity. 4 Gy radiotherapy was administered preoperatively followed by 10 Gy over 1 week postoperatively. The 5-year survival in cases of SCC and undifferentiated maxillary sinus carcinoma was 52%. In 20 cases of ethmoid adenocarcinoma, a 100% 5-year disease-free survival was achieved even though dura and/or periorbita were involved, although not penetrated, in many cases. The treatment mortality was 1% due to one case of postoperative pulmonary embolism but there were no cases of major morbidity. The conclusions of Knegt and colleagues are appropriately cautious but they suggest that their less aggressive treatment, which did not disturb the patient's appearance, could achieve results equal to or better than conventional combined radical surgery and high-dose radiotherapy (42).

A randomized clinical trial of methotrexate with folinic acid rescue or placebo given synchronously with radiotherapy showed clear improvement in a mixed group of SCCs of the head and neck (83).

Three U.S. series investigating the use of chemotherapy have concentrated on salvage treatment of massive recurrent SCCs (84–86); 90% of the cases demonstrated significant response to treatment and 45% of tumors resolved completely on radiological criteria producing a mean survival of over 21 months. These authors all employed several courses of chemotherapy based on *cis*-platinum and 5-FU, and all patients had radiotherapy but did not have additional surgery. One study tested different protocols and found that a 5-day infusion of *cis*-platinum and 5-FU gave significantly better results than other regimens tested (84). In the rare esthesioneuroblastoma, combination radiotherapy and chemotherapy with cyclophosphamide and vincristine rendered several advanced tumors operable and appeared to produce improved disease control (64). Esthesioneuroblastoma appears to be particularly chemosensitive; a recent series reported an 89% response rate to two courses of *cis*-platinum and etoposide (VP-16) (77).

In conclusion, there is evidence to suggest that regimens based on *cis*-platinum and 5-FU improve the results in the treatment of PSC. These therapies deserve closer examination than they have thus far received in the English literature.

Other Adjuvant Therapies

Techniques based on molecular biology promise improved results in the treatment of many tumor types, one interesting example of this is a case report that described adoptive immunotherapy in combination with radiotherapy causing cellular differentiation of an adenoid cystic carcinoma into normal-appearing bone (80). The immunotherapy involved intraarterial injection of lymphokine-activated killer cells and intravenous recombinant interleukin-2. Gene therapy trials using many different strategies have also been conducted in diverse tumor types (87).

Patterns of Failure

Prevention of local recurrence is the major challenge facing those who treat patients with PSC. Traditional limits to resection

have been the common sites of recurrence in earlier series, these sites include the floor of the anterior cranial fossa, particularly the olfactory groove, the orbit, and the pterygopalatine fossa. More distant recurrence may occur due to extension of tumor along nerves such as the trigeminal or vidian nerves, particularly well documented with adenoid cystic carcinoma (29).

Spread to local lymph nodes is uncommon at presentation (8%) and occurs in a further 5% to 10% of cases in long-term follow-up. Generally this form of recurrence is adequately treated by radical neck dissection and radiotherapy (74). Distant metastases to bone, lung, and liver occur in a similar proportion of patients (5% to 10%); however, in the subgroup with anaplastic carcinoma distal metastases occur in up to 50% of cases within 1 year (26,74). Local radiotherapy to symptomatic metastases and systemic chemotherapy have a role in the management of these problems. Intracranial metastases are rare although we noted two cases of cerebellar metastasis in our initial experience of 45 cases (88); these were treated by local excision and neuraxis radiotherapy.

Treatment of Recurrent Disease

Recurrent disease can be effectively treated in many cases. Many of the series discussing advanced disease include a high proportion of recurrent cancers.

The patient should be assessed fully by clinical examination, CT and MRI, chest radiograph, and other tests as appropriate. Interpretation of postoperative scans can be difficult as the healing tissues used in reconstruction may exhibit contrast enhancement that may simulate tumor recurrence (89). Radical or palliative surgical resection may be appropriate; craniofacial resection has a major role in cases where there is involvement of the anterior cranial fossa floor. In the large craniofacial series, including our own, over half of the patients treated with a craniofacial resection had recurrent disease. Despite that, a high proportion (50% to 70%) have enjoyed long-term disease control and probable cure. If previous craniofacial resection has been performed the pericranium may not be available for reconstruction. Frontal galeal flaps (90) or a microvascularized free flap of omentum (91) or other donor material (50) can be used for reconstruction.

Many patients will already have received radiotherapy and may only be able to receive limited further therapy. Chemotherapy with *cis*-platinum and 5-FU–based regimens has a demonstrable effect on these tumors, as already discussed. Palliative subtotal surgical resections can be of value in the slower growing tumor types such as adenocarcinoma, adenoid cystic carcinoma, and transitional cell carcinoma, and may provide surprisingly long periods of tumor control.

Management Outcome

The management outcomes differ widely between series but, as previously discussed, it is often difficult to compare series due to the many differences in the groups of patients. Nonetheless, on review of many series, several broad patterns emerge.

Treatment by conventional noncraniofacial surgery and radiotherapy gives a 5-year survival of approximately 35% in series including all grades of tumor (42); such treatment yields only a 7% to 25% 5-year survival in patients with T4 disease

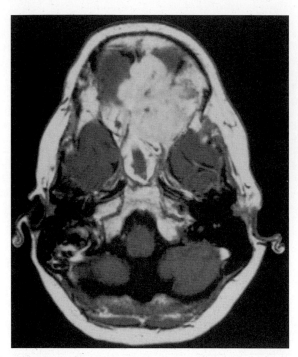

Fig. 9. MRI showing adenocarcinoma invading both frontal lobes.

- CT and MRI are essential and complementary investigations in the assessment of PSC.
- Involvement of the upper nasal cavity by PSC, and particularly the cribriform plate and fovea ethmoidalis (i.e., floor of anterior cranial fossa), mandates craniofacial resection rather than a purely endonasal/endosinus approach.
- Involvement of sphenoid sinus or intracranial extension by PSC are adverse predictors for survival.
- We reserve orbital exenteration when a bony orbital wall is breached by PSC and when complete tumor resection is believed to be achievable.
- The key to avoidance of postoperative CSF leak after craniofacial resection is obvious—the dura must be fastidiously repaired and closed watertight; the pericranial flap over the anterior cranial fossa floor is a physical, not watertight, support.
- Radiotherapy is recognized as a valuable adjuvant to craniofacial resection, probably in higher doses (e.g., 60 to 80 Gy) but the optimal timing (pre- or postoperative) and dose are yet to be adequately determined.
- Other adjunctive therapies need to be studied and considered as there have been reports of the benefits of chemotherapy, particularly based on *cis*-platinum and 5-FU.
- Better treatment of PSC will come with improved understanding of its molecular biology.

(27,59–62). In series employing craniofacial resection, about 50% to 70% of patients with T4 SCC were alive and free of disease at 5 years (24,41,46,47,58). Of 38 patients with SCC in the current RMH series, there was a 74% 5-year survival; the figures are somewhat better (84% 5-year survival) for 32 patients with adenocarcinoma (Fig. 9). In earlier series there has been a 25% to 46% 5-year survival for conventional therapy and 78% to 83% 5-year survival for craniofacial series (24,58); there is a greater tendency for delayed recurrence in this tumor type resulting in more late recurrences after the 5-year period.

Multimodality therapy employing chemotherapy by various routes, preoperative radiotherapy, and noncraniofacial surgery has produced an approximately 70% 5-year survival for the overall group (74,80), a treatment that also enjoys the advantage of a lower rate of disfiguring surgery. One group achieved the spectacular result of 100% 5-year, disease-free survival employing multimodality therapy based on topical 5-FU in adenocarcinoma.

Despite the serious nature of PSC and the restrictions placed on treatment by the important surrounding structures, at least temporary disease control can be achieved in a majority of patients and many patients have a long period of relief from the tumor. There remain many challenges in developing more effective therapies and refining their application to improve the results of present therapies.

Summary of Key Points

- Almost all paranasal sinus adenocarcinomas and approximately half of all SCC relate to prolonged exposure to hard wood.
- Late presentation of PSC can be diminished by vigorous examination of all adult patients with sinonasal complaints of more than 6 weeks, including biopsy of suspicious areas.

References

1. Robin PE, Powell DJ, Stansbie JM. Carcinoma of the nasal cavity and paranasal sinuses: incidence and presentation of different histological types. *Clin Otolaryngol* 1979;4:431.
2. *Roush GC. Epidemiology of cancer of the nose and paranasal sinuses: current concepts. *Head Neck Surg* 1979;2:3.
3. Muir C, Waterhouse J, Mack T, et al. *Cancer incidence in the five continents*, 5th ed. Lyon: IARC, 1987.
4. Olsen JH. Epidemiology of sinonasal cancer in Denmark 1943–1982. *Acta Pathol Microbiol Immunol Scand* 1987;95:171.
5. *Giles G, Farrugia H, Silver B, et al. *Cancer in Victoria 1982–1987*. Melbourne, Australia: Anti-Cancer Council of Victoria, 1992.
6. Hyams VJ, Batsakis JG, Michaels L. *Tumors of the upper respiratory tract and ear*, 2nd ed. Washington, DC: Armed Forces Institute of Pathology, 1988.
7. Acheson ED, Winter PD, Hadfield E, et al. Is nasal adenocarcinoma in the Buckinghamshire furniture industry declining? *Nature* 1982; 299:263.
8. Egedahl RD, Coppock E, Homit K. Mortality experience at a hydrometallurgical nickel refinery in Fort Saskatchewan, Alberta between 1954 and 1984. *J Soc Occupation Med* 1991;41:29.
9. Doll R, Morgan LG, Speizer FE. Cancer of the lung and nasal sinuses in nickel workers. *Br J Cancer* 1970;24:623.
10. Fukuda K, Shibata A. Demographic correlation between occupation and maxillary cancer mortality in Japan. *Kurume Med J* 1985;32:151.
11. Hayes RB, Kardaun JW, de Bruyn A. Tobacco use and sinonasal cancer: a case-control study. *Br J Cancer* 1987;56:843.
12. Shimizu H, Hozawa J, Saito H. Chronic sinusitis and woodworking as risk factors for cancer of the maxillary sinus in northeast Japan. *Laryngoscope* 1989;99:58–63.
13. Muir CS, Nectoux J. Descriptive epidemiology of malignant neoplasms of nose, nasal cavities, middle ear and accessory sinuses. *Clin Otolaryngol* 1980;5:195–211.
14. Fukuda K, Shibata A, Harada K. Squamous cell cancer of the maxillary sinus in Hokkaido, Japan: a case control study. *Br J Industr Med* 1987;44:263.
15. Waterhouse J, Muir C, Correa P, et al. *Cancer incidence in five continents*, 3rd ed. Lyon: IARC, 1976.
16. Acheson ED, Cowdel RH, Jolles B. Nasal cancer in the Northamptonshire boot and shoe industry. *Br Med J* 1970;1:385.
17. Hayes RB, Gerin M, Raatgever JW, et al. Wood-related occupations,

wood dust exposure and sinonasal cancer. *Am J Epidemiol* 1986; 124:569.

18. Luce D, Leclerc A, Marne MJ, et al. Sinonasal cancer and occupation: a multicenter case-control study. *Rev Epidemiol Sante-Publique* 1991;39:7.

19. Ironside P, Matthews J. Adenocarcinoma of the nose and paranasal sinuses in woodworkers in the State of Victoria. *Cancer* 1975;36: 1115.

20. Franklin CIV. Adenocarcinoma of the paranasal sinuses in Tasmania. *Australasian Radiol* 1982;26:49.

21. Klintenberg C, Olofsson J, Hellquist H, et al. Adenocarcinoma of the ethmoid sinuses. A review of 28 cases with special reference to wood dust exposure. *Cancer* 1984;54:482.

22. Wills JH. Nasal carcinoma in woodworkers: a review. *J Occupation Med* 1982;24:526–535.

23. *Acheson ED, Cowdel RH, Hadfield E, et al. Nasal cancer in woodworkers in the furniture industry. *Br Med J* 1968;2:587.

24. *Kaye AH, Danks RA, Kleid S, et al. Cranio-facial resection in the management of cancer of the paranasal sinuses. *J Clin Neurosci* 1994;1:111–117.

25. Mohrashampiur E, Norpoth K, Luhmann F. Cancer epidemiology of wood working. *J Cancer Res Clin Oncol* 1989;115:503–522.

26. Lund VJ. Malignant tumours of the nasal cavity and paranasal sinuses. *Otolaryngology* 1983;45:1.

27. Sisson OS, Toriumi DM, Aniyah RA. Paranasal sinus malignancy: a comprehensive update. *Laryngoscope* 1989;99:143.

28. Maroldi R, Farina D, Battaglia G, et al. MR of malignant nasosinusal neoplasms: frequently asked questions. *Eur J Radiol* 1997;24: 181–190.

29. Pandolfo I, Gaeta M, Blandino A, et al. MR imaging of perineural metastasis along the vidian nerve. *J Comput Assist Tomogr* 1989;13: 498.

30. Lund VJ, Lloyd GAS, Howard DJ, et al. Enhanced magnetic resonance imaging and subtraction techniques in the postoperative evaluation of craniofacial resection for sinonasal malignancy. *Laryngoscope* 1996;106:553–558.

31. Nishioka K, Masuda Y, Yanagi E, et al. Cytologic diagnosis of the maxillary sinus re-evaluated. *Laryngoscope* 1989;99:842.

32. *Perry C, Levine PA, Williamson BR, et al. Preservation of the eye in paranasal sinus cancer surgery. *Arch Otolaryngol Head Neck Surg* 1988;114:632.

33. *Orvidas LJ, Lewis JE, Olsen KD, et al. Intranasal verrucous carcinoma: relationship to inverting papilloma and human papillomavirus. *Laryngoscope* 1999;109:371–375.

34. Mills S, Freison H. Olfactory neuroblastoma: a clinicopathologic study of 21 cases. *Am J Surg Pathol* 1985;9:317–327.

35. Ratech H, Burke JS, Blayney DW, et al. A clinicopathologic study of malignant lymphomas of the nose, paranasal sinuses, and hard palate, including cases of lethal midline granuloma. *Cancer* 1989; 64:2525–2530.

36. Willatt DJ, Morton RP, McCormick MS, et al. Staging of maxillary cancer. Which classification? *Ann Otol Rhinol Laryngol* 1987;96: 137–141.

37. Har-El G, Hadar T, Krespi YP, et al. An analysis of staging systems for carcinoma of the maxillary sinus. *Ear Nose Throat J* 1988;67:511.

38. Parsons JT, Mendenhall WM, Mancuso AA, et al. Malignant tumours of the nasal cavity and ethmoid and sphenoid sinuses. *Intl J Radiat Oncol Biol Phys* 1988;14:11.

39. Kaye AH, Popovic EA. Craniofacial resection for paranasal sinus tumours. *Neurosurg Q* 1998;8(1):55–69.

40. Bilsky MH, Kraus DH, Strong EW, et al. Extended anterior craniofacial resection for intracranial extension of malignant tumors. *Am J Surg* 1997;174:565–568.

41. Terz JJ, Young HF, Lawrence W. Combined craniofacial resection for locally advanced carcinoma of the head and neck: carcinoma of the paranasal sinuses. *Am J Surg* 1980;140:618.

42. Knegt PP, de Jong P, van Anfri JG, et al. Carcinoma of the paranasal sinuses. Results of a prospective pilot study. *Cancer* 1985;56:57.

43. Ketcham AS, Chretion PB, van Buren JM, et al. The ethmoid sinuses: a re-evaluation of surgical resection. *Am J Surg* 1973;126:469.

44. Millar HS, Petty PG, Hueston JT. A combined intracranial and facial approach for excision and repair of cancer of the ethmoid sinuses. *Aust NZ J Surg* 1973;43:179.

45. Cantu G, Solero CL, Marlani L, et al. Anterior craniofacial resection

for malignant ethmoid tumors—a series of 91 patients. *Head Neck Surg* 1999;21:185–191.

46. Sundaresan N, Shah JP. Craniofacial resection for anterior skull base tumours. *Head Neck Surg* 1988;10:219.

47. Ketcham AS, van Buren J. Tumors of the paranasal sinuses: a therapeutic challenge. *Am J Surg* 1985;150:406–413.

48. *Lund VJ, Howard DJ, Wei WI, et al. Craniofacial resection of tumors of the nasal cavity and paranasal sinuses: a 17 year experience. *Head Neck Surg* 1998;20:98–107.

49. Cheeseman AD, Lund VJ, Howard DJ. Craniofacial resection for tumours of the nasal cavity and paranasal sinuses. *Head Neck Surg* 1986;8:429.

50. Sekhar LN, Nanda A, Seri CN, et al. The extended frontal approach to tumours of the anterior, middle and posterior skull base. *J Neurosurg* 1992;76:198.

51. Johns ME, Winn HR, McLean WC, et al. Pericranial flap for the closure of defects of craniofacial resections. *Laryngoscope* 1981;91:952.

52. Horowitz JD, Persing JA, Nichter LS, et al. Galeal-pericranial flaps in head and neck reconstruction. *Am J Surg* 1984;148:489.

53. *McCutcheon IE, Blacklock JB, Weber RS, et al. Anterior transcranial (craniofacial) resection of tumors of the paranasal sinuses: surgical technique and results. *Neurosurgery* 1996;38:471–480.

54. Bebear JP, Darrouzet V, Stoll D. Surgery of the anterior skull base: total ethmoidectomy for malignant ethmoidal tumors. *Isr J Med Sci*1992;28:169.

55. Kraus DH, Shah JP, Arbit E. Complications of craniofacial resection for tumors involving the anterior skull base. *Head Neck Surg* 1994; 16:307–312.

56. *McCaffrey TV, Olsen KD, Yohanan JM, et al. Factors affecting survival of patients with tumors of the anterior skull base. *Laryngoscope* 1994;104:940–945.

57. Catalano PJ, Hech CS, Biller JF, et al. Craniofacial resection: an analysis of 73 cases. *Arch Otolaryngol Head Neck Surg* 1994;120: 1203–1208.

58. Bridger GP, Mendelsohn MS, Baldwin M, et al. Paranasal sinus cancer. *Aust NZ J Surg* 1991;61:290.

59. Lavertu P, Roberts JK, Kraus DH, et al. Squamous cell carcinoma of the paranasal sinuses. The Cleveland Clinic Experience 1977–1986. *Laryngoscope* 1989;99:1130.

60. Tsuji H, Kamada T, Matsuoka Y, et al. The value of treatment planning using CT and an immobilising shell in radiotherapy for paranasal sinus carcinomas. *Intl J Radiat Oncol Biol Phys* 1989;16:243.

61. Anniko M, Franzen L, Lofroth PO. Long-term survival of patients with paranasal sinus carcinoma. *Otorhinolaryngology* 1990;52:187.

62. *Logue JP, Slevin NJ. Carcinoma of the nasal cavity and paranasal sinuses: an analysis of radical radiotherapy. *Clin Oncol* 1991;3:84.

63. Ellingwood KE, Million RR. Cancer of the nasal cavity and ethmoid/sphenoid sinuses. *Cancer* 1979;43:1517.

64. O'Connor TA, McLean P, Juillard GJ, et al. Olfactory neuroblastoma. *Cancer* 1989;63:2426.

65. Beitler JJ, Fass DE, Brenner HA. Esthesioneuroblastoma: is there a role for elective neck treatment? *Head Neck Surg* 1991;13:321.

66. Gabriele P, Besozzi MC, Pisano P, et al. Carcinoma of the paranasal sinuses. Results with radiotherapy alone or with a radiosurgical combination. *Radiologica Med (Torino)* 1986;72:210.

67. Kenady DE. Cancer of the paranasal sinuses. *Surg Clin North Am* 1986;66:119.

68. Wustrow J, Rudert H, Diercks M, et al. Squamous epithelial carcinoma and undifferentiated carcinoma of the inner nose and paranasal sinuses. *Strahlenther Onkol* 1989;165:468.

69. Bush SE, Bagshaw MA. Carcinoma of the paranasal sinuses. *Cancer* 1982;50:154.

70. Karim ABMF, Kratendonk JH, Njo KH, et al. Ethmoid and upper nasal cavity carcinoma: treatment, results and complications. *Radiother Oncol* 1990;19:109–130.

71. Haylock BJ, John DG, Paterson IC. The treatment of squamous cell carcinoma of the paranasal sinuses. *Clin Oncol (Royal Coll Radiol)* 1991;148:489–501.

72. Beale FA, Garrett PG. Cancer of the paranasal sinuses with particular reference to maxillary sinus cancer. *J Otolaryngol* 1983;12:377.

73. Midena E, Segato T, Piermarocchi S, et al. Retinopathy following radiation therapy of paranasal sinus and nasopharyngeal carcinoma. *Retina* 1987;7:142–145.

74. Konno A, Togawa K, Inoue S. Analysis of the results of our com-

bined therapy for maxillary cancer. *Acta Otolaryngol* 1980; 372(suppl):2.

75. *Morita A, Ebersold MJ, Olsen KD, et al. Esthesioneuroblastoma: prognosis and management. *Neurosurgery* 1993;32:706–715.

76. Irish J, Dasgupta R, Freeman J, et al. Outcome and analysis of the surgical management of esthesioneuroblastoma. *J Otolaryngol* 1997; 26:1–7.

77. Bhattacharyya N, Thornton AF, Joseph MP, et al. Successful treatment of esthesioneuroblastoma and neuroendocrine carcinoma with combined chemotherapy and proton radiation. Results of 9 cases. *Arch Otolaryngol Head Neck Surg* 1997;123:34.

78. Roman M, Aziz H. Concomitant continuous infusion chemotherapy and radiation. *Cancer* 1990;65:823–829.

79. Choi KN, Roman M, Aziz H, et al. Locally advanced paranasal sinus and nasopharynx tumours treated with hyperfractionated radiation and concomitant infusion of cisplatin. *Cancer* 1991;67:2748.

80. Sato Y, Morita M, Takahashi H, et al. Combined surgery, radiotherapy and regional chemotherapy in carcinoma of the paranasal sinuses. *Cancer* 1970;25:571.

81. Sakai S, Ebinhara T, Ono I, et al. A comparison of AJC and JJC proposals on TNM classification of maxillary sinus carcinoma. *Arch Otorhinolaryngol* 1983;237:139.

82. Inuyama Y, Kavaurs M, Toji M, et al. Intra-arterial chemotherapy of maxillary sinus carcinoma. *Gan To Kagaku Ryoho* 1989;16:2688.

83. Gupta NK, Pointon RC, Wilkinson PM. A randomised clinical trial to contrast radiotherapy with radiotherapy and methotrexate given synchronously in head and neck cancer. *Clin Radiol* 1987;38: 575–581.

84. *Rooney M, Kish J, Jacobs J, et al. Improved complete response rate and survival in advanced head and neck cancer after three course induction therapy with 120 hour 5FU infusion and cisplatinum. *Cancer* 1985;55:1123.

85. LoRusso P, Tapazoglou E, Kish JA, et al. Chemotherapy for paranasal sinus carcinoma. A 10-year experience at Wayne State University. *Cancer* 1988;62:1.

86. Lee YY, Dimery IW, van Tassell P, et al. Super-selective intra-arterial chemotherapy of advanced paranasal sinus tumors. *Arch Otolaryngol Head Neck Surg* 1989;115:503–508.

87. Culver KW, Ram Z, Wallbridge S, et al. In vivo gene transfer with retroviral vector-producer cells for treatment of experimental brain tumors. *Science* 1992;256:1550.

88. Murphy MA, Kaye AH, Hayes IP. Intracranial metastasis from carcinoma of the paranasal sinus. *Neurosurgery* 1991;28:890.

89. Som PM, Lawson W, Biller HF, et al. Ethmoid sinus disease: CT evaluation in 400 cases. *Radiology* 1986;159:605–630.

90. *Snyderman CH, Janecka IP, Sekhar LN, et al. Anterior skull base reconstruction: role of galeal and pericranial flaps. *Laryngoscope* 1990;100:607.

91. Yanaki T, Uede T, Tano-oka A, et al. Vascularized omentum graft for the reconstruction of the skull base after removal of a nasoethmoidal tumor with intracranial extension: case report. *Neurosurgery* 1991; 28:877–879.

* Key references.

118. Current Management of Tumors of the Cavernous Sinus

Gail L. Rosseau

Anatomy of the Cavernous Sinus

The cavernous sinus is a paired structure located on either side of the sella turcica. It is trapezoidal in shape and filled with venous plexuses and sinusoids. Running through these venous structures is the entrance of the carotid artery into the intracranial space. Cranial nerves III, IV, V, and VI pass through the cavernous sinus en route to their exits from the skull through the orbit or the floor of the middle cranial fossa (Fig. 1).

The cavernous sinus is a site of important venous communication among the orbit, the brain, and the extracranial venous system. Two layers of dura mater are involved in the cavernous sinus. Three of the dural walls, the lateral, superior, and medial, are formed by the meningeal layer of dura mater, while the inferior wall is made of the periosteal dura which lines the sphenoid bone. The lateral dural wall is the largest and is located in the middle cranial fossa inferomedial to the temporal lobe. This lateral wall becomes the superior wall of the cavernous sinus at the anterior petroclinoid fold. The bony anterior clinoid process overhangs the anterior half the cavernous sinus. This process is covered by the meningeal dura which splits, thereby encircling the process. The medial wall of the cavernous sinus dura separates the pituitary gland from the sinus contents and is the inferior continuation of the diaphragma sella. In coronal section, each cavernous sinus is larger posteriorly, narrowing anteriorly to form the superior orbital fissure where it joins the orbital apex.

The most critical structure traversing the cavernous sinus is the internal carotid artery (ICA). It enters the petrous temporal bone, traveling vertically, then over the foramen lacerum. The ICA enters the cavernous sinus through the posterior periosteal dura of the inferior wall. The ICA travels anteriorly and exits the cavernous sinus medially to the anterior clinoid process through the meningeal dura of the superior wall.

It is important to note that two layers of dura make up the lateral wall of the cavernous sinus. The outer layer facing the temporal lobe is thick and well developed. The inner layer is much thinner and incomplete in places. It invests the cranial nerves located in the lateral cavernous sinus. These nerves pierce the meningeal dura on entry to the cavernous sinus and carry dural epineurial sheaths with them, thus forming the incomplete inner layer of the lateral wall. Cranial nerves III, IV, and V_1 are located in the lateral wall. Cranial nerve VI is more medial in location, traveling within the body of the cavernous sinus inferolaterally to the ICA.

A number of critical structures are located around the cavernous sinus. The orbital apex is located anteriorly and is where cranial nerves III, IV, and VI and the ophthalmic artery continue into the orbit. The pituitary gland and sphenoid sinus are medial to each cavernous sinus. Posteriorly, the posterior fossa is separated from the cavernous sinus by the clival dura and the ten-

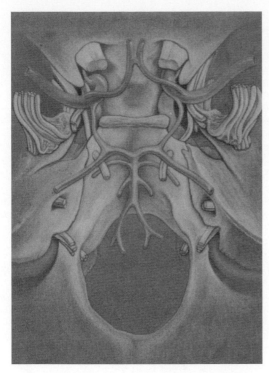

Fig. 1. Anatomy of the cavernous sinus in relation to other neurovascular structures of the skull base.

torium. The trigeminal ganglion and its cistern are located posterolaterally. Inferior to the middle fossa are the pterygopalatine, parapharyngeal, and infratemporal spaces (1–4).

Histology of Tumors of the Cavernous Sinus

BENIGN TUMORS. Benign tumors involving the cavernous sinus include meningiomas, neurilemmomas, cavernous he-

Table 1. Classification of Intracavernous Neoplasms

Grade	CS involvement	Intracavernous ICA
I	One area only (A, P, L, or M)	Not involved
II	More than one area	Displaced, not totally encased
III	Entire CS	Totally encased, at least a short length
IV	Entire CS	Encased, with narrowing, pseudoaneurysm or occlusion
V	Bilateral CS	Encased

CS, cavernous sinus; ICA, internal carotid artery; A, anterior; P, posterior; L, lateral; M, medial.
From Spetzler RF, et al. Petrous carotid to intradural carotid saphenous vein graft for intracavernous giant aneurysm, tumor, and occlusive cerebrovascular disease. *J Neurosurg* 1990; 73: 496–501, with permission.

mangiomas, juvenile angiofibromas, craniopharyngiomas, and pituitary adenomas.

SLOW-GROWING MALIGNANCIES. Slow-growing malignancies that may encountered within the cavernous sinus include chordomas and chondrosarcomas.

MALIGNANT LESIONS. These lesions generally begin within the paranasal sinuses and include adenoid cystic carcinoma and squamous cell carcinoma, among others.

A classification system has been proposed for tumors involving the cavernous sinus. Adoption of such a classification system would allow assessment of the risks of microsurgery, as well as comparison among various means of microsurgical and radiosurgical treatment. This classification system is outlined in Table 1.

Preoperative Evaluation of the Cavernous Sinus Tumors

CT. Computed tomography (CT) and magnetic resonance imaging (MRI) are complementary in the evaluation of cavernous sinus lesions. CT is superior in defining bony anatomy. Axial and coronal CT with bone windows are obtained to evaluate for bony hyperostosis, as is the case when meningioma is suspected. CT is also useful when a malignancy is suspected, as the pattern of bone destruction typical of high-grade malignancies may be best elucidated on CT.

MRI. MRI is the best screening procedure for suspected cavernous sinus involvement. It is performed with and without gadolinium enhancement. MRI is the study of choice for distinguishing vascular from neoplastic lesions and is the single best study for demonstrating the relationship of the lesion to the carotid artery.

Particularly in the region of the cavernous sinus, it is often difficult to distinguish on MRI residual tumor versus postoperative changes. Often, periodic follow-up, with surveillance images over time, is needed to make this distinction. Serial MRI is the most accurate and noninvasive way of following a lesion presumed to be benign. Often, slow-growing benign lesions, such as meningiomas, are followed in this way before any decision to intervene is undertaken.

MAGNETIC RESONANCE ANGIOGRAPHY. Spherical or oval lesions in the sellar or parasellar area may represent an aneurysm. Even the post-enhanced MRI may not readily distinguish a partially thrombosed giant aneurysm from a neoplasm. With this in mind, a magnetic resonance angiography (MRA) may be a useful noninvasive adjunct to MRI in the preoperative evaluation of patients with suspicious lesions or those who harbor other known aneurysms.

ANGIOGRAPHY. Despite its invasive nature, angiography remains an important part of preoperative evaluation of patients with cavernous sinus lesions. A carotid angiogram is the "gold standard" for defining the exact nature and origin of vascular lesions within the cavernous sinus. In the evaluation of neoplastic processes, the carotid angiogram is the single best test for defining details of the degree and location of involvement of the carotid artery by the neoplasm. The angiogram reveals the source of vascularity of a neoplasm, allowing for potential pre-operative embolization of tumor blood supply. Finally, carotid angiography may be critically important in defining the contra-lateral or collateral blood supply in the region. It also allows for the performance of balloon test occlusion of the ipsilateral ICA.

BALLOON TEST OCCLUSION. It has been estimated that 80% of patients will tolerate occlusion of one ICA without neu-rological deficit. Twenty percent of patients, however, remain at risk for infarction if the ICA ipsilateral to a lesion is sacrificed. Clinical and radiographic data alone are not completely specific in revealing which group of patients may be at risk for delayed cerebral ischemia.

For this reason, balloon test occlusion of the ICA, with neuro-logical examination and stable xenon CT blood flow determina-tion has been advocated as one means of allowing the risk of stroke with carotid occlusion to be more precisely quantified (5). Using this methodology, patients with no change in clinical examination or cerebral blood flow (CBF) during occlusion (CBF greater than 35 cc per 100 g per minute) are considered to be at low risk; patients with no change in examination but diminished blood flow (CBF 10 to 35 m per 100 g per minute) may be considered at intermediate risk; and patients with neu-rological deficits during test occlusion are considered to be at high risk. It has been estimated that 75% of patients are low risk, 15% are intermediate risk, and 10% are high risk. Using these quantifications of risk, some surgeons have stressed the need for graft reconstruction of the ICA in patients at high or intermediate risk (1). The recommendation that reconstruction of the ICA is preferred, especially in younger patients with be-nign or low-grade malignant tumors, is controversial (5–10).

Summary of Surgical Approaches to the Cavernous Sinus

The surgical approach to the cavernous sinus is dictated by the changes in normal anatomy that have occurred in the areas involved by the tumor. The lateral wall, with the largest surface area, offers the most extensive access to the region. Occasion-ally, the tumor will have enlarged the spaces between cranial nerves, allowing advantageous surgical access. The use of "sur-gical triangles," which are routes of access between the neuro-vascular structures of the cavernous sinus, has been advocated (2).

The evolution of the subspecialty of cranial base surgery has led to several general principles that may be considered practice guidelines and are useful in determining the microsurgical treat-ment of these lesions:

1. Wherever possible, bone removal is preferred in order to avoid brain retraction. This has led to the frequent use of zygomatic or orbitozygomatic osteotomies, bone removal from the roof and lateral walls of the orbit, and extensive bone removal in the sphenoid wing to expand the pterional approach.
2. Large craniotomies are preferred because the target area of the cavernous sinus is deep. The wide exposure provided by large craniotomy allows inspection of the cavernous sinus region from several directions, thereby allowing the surgeon the potential choice of several surgical triangles.

3. Proximal control of the ICA is an essential step and can be obtained in the neck or the petrous bone.
4. Intracavernous dissection should only be performed when one has a thorough understanding of the complex anatomical relationships of the neurovascular structures involved. A foundation in cadaveric dissection is a prerequisite to surgery in this area.
5. The cavernous sinus portion of the nerves to the extraocular muscles (III, IV, and VI) are highly susceptible to paresis from traction or ischemic injury following cavernous sinus dissection (2).

Although details of the surgical approach depend on the ac-cess required to the specific region of the cavernous sinus, there are some general steps common to all craniotomies performed for exploration of the cavernous sinus. The patient is generally placed in the supine position, with the neck extended so that the frontal and temporal lobes will fall away by gravity, requir-ing only limited retraction. Head elevation to reduce venous bleeding is useful. A scalp incision is selected to allow for gener-ous bony opening. We have not found it necessary to shave the hair. The inferior limb of the incision extends to the zygoma and is just anterior to the tragus of the ear, thereby minimizing any risk of injury to the facial nerve or its branches. The subfas-cial dissection on the temporalis muscle is done with care to preserve the frontalis branch of the facial nerve. The orbit and the zygomatic arch are exposed. The temporalis muscle is ele-vated from the temporal fossa and freed from the undersurface of the zygoma. A frontotemporal craniotomy is created to ex-tend medially to the supraorbital notch and posteriorly and infe-riorly to the external auditory canal.

Zygomatic or orbitozygomatic osteotomy is then performed with the reciprocating saw. A zygomatic osteotomy may be sufficient when access is needed only to the lateral and posterior portions of the cavernous sinus. Additional extradural bone re-moval may then be carried out at the orbital roof to the superior orbital fissure and the greater wing of the sphenoid, depending on the region of the cavernous sinus to be explored.

If proximal control of the ICA is planned for the petrous segment, the foramina ovale and spinosum are exposed, allow-ing identification of the horizontal portion of the petrous ICA. The arcuate eminence of the temporal bone is identified in the floor of the middle fossa. The greater superficial petrosal nerve (GSPN) is identified anteromedial to the arcuate emmi-nence and is sharply divided in order to avoid traction on the geniculate ganglion of the facial nerve with its potential for postoperative cranial nerve VII paresis. The GSPN travels paral-lel to the horizontal segment of the petrous ICA, which is visible if its bony canal is dehiscent. If the carotid canal is covered by bone, a diamond drill is used to uncover it. The artery is fol-lowed anteriorly until it disappears from the middle fossa medi-ally to V_3. The eustachian tube is identified lateral to the carotid artery and medial to the middle meningeal artery. The tube is divided in its cartilaginous portion and its bony segment oc-cluded with bone wax.

If proximal control of the ICA is planned at the cervical carotid segment, this is generally performed prior to the craniotomy. The surgeon's preference dictates whether the anterior clinoid process is removed extradurally or intradurally (2).

ANGLES OF APPROACH TO THE CAVERNOUS SINUS (1,2,5,11)

Superior Approach. This approach is used for lesions in the anterior portion of the cavernous sinus involving the clinoidal segment to anterior genu and the horizontal segment back to the posterior genu of the carotid artery. This approach requires removal of the anterior clinoid process and transsylvian dissection.

The approach begins with a wide opening from lateral to medial along the sylvian fissure, exposing the anterior petroclival ligament and the tentorial edge. The supraclinoid ICA and optic nerves come into view. A flap of dura mater is elevated from the orbital roof and the lesser wing of the sphenoid bone is then drilled using a high-speed drill. The distal dural ring and optic nerve sheath are opened laterally and cranial nerve III is identified at the proximal ring. The dural incision continues posteriorly into the superior wall of the cavernous sinus, medial to cranial nerve III and lateral to the intracavernous ICA. Mobilization of the anterior genu of the ICA is limited because it is tethered to the ophthalmic artery in the region of the "carotid cave." Superior exposure gives access to the horizontal segment of the ICA, the sella, and the pituitary gland.

Lateral Approach. This approach is ideally suited for tumors such as schwannomas, which involve the trigeminal ganglion and its branches, as well as tumors that involve the precavernous and posterior vertical portion of the cavernous ICA.

The patient's head is rotated further to the contralateral side than with the superior approach, generally about 45 degrees. The craniotomy generally does not extend as far anteriorly unless a combination of this superior approach with the lateral approach is being performed. A zygomatic osteotomy is generally sufficient.

The temporal lobe is gently elevated extradurally. The greater wing of the sphenoid is removed to the foramen spinosum and ovale. The middle meningeal artery is coagulated and divided. When V_2 and V_3 have been unroofed, the outermost layer of dura is incised just lateral to V_2 and V_3. The trigeminal ganglion is exposed extradurally by creation of an incision between V_2 and V_3. With further posterior dissection, the dura of the floor of the Meckel cave is exposed. With retraction of V_3 laterally and V_2 superiorly, the ICA may be followed into the cavernous sinus. This extradural lateral approach allows exposure of the lower portion of the cavernous sinus.

Intradural exposure via the lateral approach allows more superior access to the cavernous sinus. This includes exposure of the III, IV, V_1, and VI cranial nerves. In this approach, the anterior clinoid process is removed intradurally.

Care is taken to locate the IV cranial nerve prior to reflecting the dura of the lateral wall. The tentorium may be incised vertically, posterior to the entry of the IV nerve. The outer layer of the lateral wall may also be incised inferior and parallel to the IV nerve, leaving a strip of tentorial edge intact to protect the IV nerve.

Tumor removal proceeds by working within involved triangles. The Parkinson triangle is the space between V_1 and cranial nerve IV. Another surgical triangle may be used to advantage by working between V_1 and V_2, and so forth.

Medial Approach. The medial approach is used for tumors situated medially to the cavernous ICA. These would include pituitary tumors, chordomas, and some meningiomas. These approaches include the transsphenoidal, transmaxillary, and bicoronal approaches. The bicoronal approach with or without orbitozygomatic osteotomy offers the attractive feature of providing a vascularized pericranial flap which may be used to repair a defect in the midline of the anterior cranial base once the tumor and bone in this region have been removed. Further details and surgical approaches to the cavernous sinus region may be found in other chapters in this text.

Decision Making for Lesions of the Cavernous Sinus

SYMPTOMATIC OR ASYMPTOMATIC. Many tumors of the cavernous sinus are serendipitously discovered when studies are performed for other reasons such as trauma. The first question to be asked, therefore, is, "Is the patient symptomatic or asymptomatic?" The asymptomatic patient with a benign-appearing lesion may be reasonably followed with serial imaging studies, as meningiomas and pituitary adenomas are common in this region and may grow slowly or not at all.

If the patient is symptomatic, however, diagnosis and possible intervention should be considered.

HISTOLOGY: BENIGN OR MALIGNANT. While benign lesions are common in this area, lesions that appear to have destroyed bone, particularly if the epicenter appears to be in the paranasal sinuses, may be malignant. Such a lesion could represent a highly aggressive malignancy; therefore, biopsy and a definitive treatment should occur promptly. In some cases, it may be possible to perform a transoral or transnasal biopsy, perhaps even in the outpatient setting. This allows establishment of diagnosis prior to complete surgical planning. Also, if a benign histology is established, the surgical approach can be tailored to the pathology.

Illustrative Cases

CASE 1

Intracavernous Meningioma. A 37-year-old woman presented with transient right eye pain and mild ptosis. Imaging studies (Fig. 2) revealed the presence of a completely intracavernous lesion, consistent with meningioma. Because of the history of progressive symptoms, the patient was treated with stereotactic radiosurgery, without biopsy.

CASE 2

Extracavernous Meningioma. A 47-year-old man presented with headache and left retro-orbital pain and intermittent ptosis. Imaging studies (Fig. 3) revealed the presence of an enhancing lesion involving the lateral wall of the cavernous sinus, consistent with meningioma. The patient was taken to surgery, where the tumor was completely resected via a lateral approach to the cavernous sinus. The entire lateral wall of the cavernous sinus was removed, with a complete tumor resection. Ptosis completely resolved postoperatively. There is no evidence of residual recurrent disease 5 years postoperatively.

CASE 3

Adenoid Cystic Carcinoma. A 62-year-old man presented with nasal congestion and diplopia. Imaging studies (Fig. 4) revealed the presence of an enhancing lesion involving the paranasal sinuses, cavernous sinus, and skull base extending into the right temporal lobe. Transnasal biopsy in the outpatient setting revealed adenoid cystic carcinoma.

Using a subtemporal/infratemporal fossa approach, which included orbital exenteration, the tumor was completely removed and the cavernous ICA was skeletonized. Reconstruction was with a microvascular anastomosis of a rectus abdominous graft.

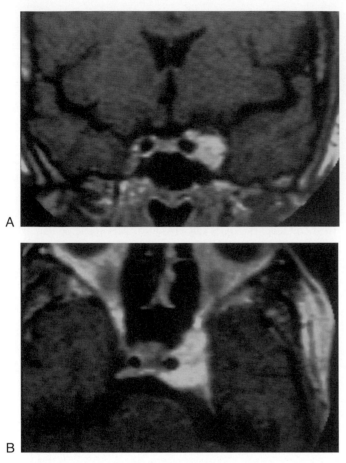

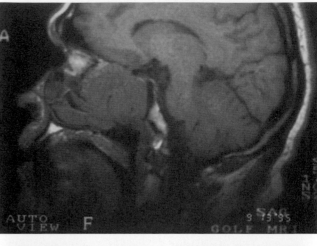

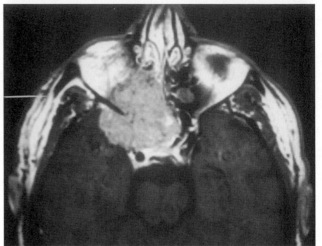

Fig. 2. A: Gadolinium-enhanced T1-weighted coronal MRI depicting totally intracavernous meningioma. **B:** Axial post-enhanced MRI of the same patient.

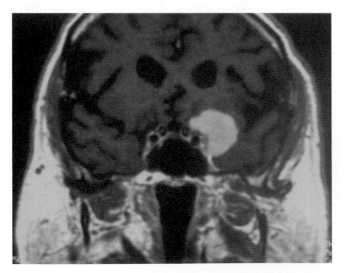

Fig. 3. Gadolinium-enhanced coronal image of primarily extracavernous meningioma.

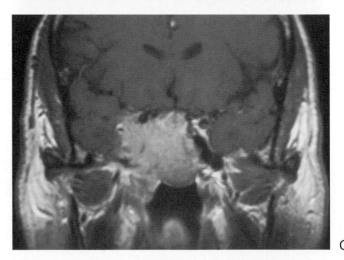

Fig. 4. Sagittal **(A)** and post-gadolinium enhanced T1-weighted MRIs in the axial **(B)** and coronal **(C)** planes, demonstrating adenoid cystic carcinoma invading the skull base, including the cavernous sinus.

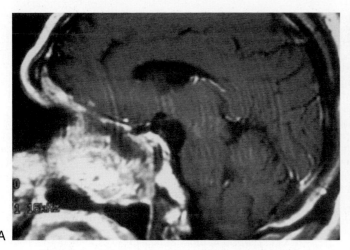
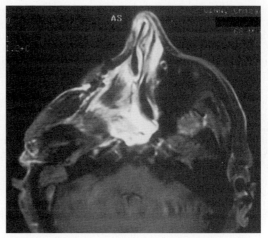

A   B

Fig. 5. Gadolinium-enhanced sagittal **(A)** and axial **(B)** MRIs demonstrating complete tumor resection, and reconstruction using practice abdominous microvascular free flap. The patient is alive and well with no evidence of disease at 7 years postsurgery.

At 7 years postsurgery (Fig. 5) the patient is alive and well with no evidence of recurrent or residual disease. Surgery was followed by adjunctive chemotherapy and radiotherapy.

References

1. Sekhar LN, Ross DA, Sen C. Cavernous sinus and sphenocavernous neoplasms. In: Sekhar LN, Janecka IP, eds. *Surgery of the cranial base tumors.* New York: Raven Press, 1993;37:521–564.
2. Sen C, Chen S, Post KD, eds. *Microsurgical anatomy of the skull base and approaches to the cavernous sinus.* New York: Thieme Medical Publishers, 1997;11:190–266.
3. Spetzler RF, Fukushima T, Martin N, et al. Petrous carotid to intradural carotid saphenous vein graft for intracavernous giant aneurysm, tumor, and occlusive cerebrovascular disease. *J Neurosurg* 1990;73:496–501.
4. Taptas JN. The so-called cavernous sinus: a review of the controversy and its implications for neurosurgeons. *Neurosurgery* 1982; 2(5):712–717.
5. Sekhar LN, Buchanan RI, Wright DC, et al. The case for aggressive resection. *Clin Neurosurg* 1997;45:263–278.
6. Friedlander RM, Ojemann RG, Thornton AF. Management of meningiomas of the cavernous sinus: conservative surgery and adjuvant therapy. *Clin Neurosurg* 1997;45:279–282.
7. Rosseau GL. Benign tumors of the cavernous sinus. *Clin Neurosurg* 1997;45:260–262.
8. Rosseau GL, Cerullo LJ. Current challenges in management of cranial base meningiomas. *Am J Otology* 1995;16(1):1–3.
9. Rosseau GL, Sekhar L. Surgery of cranial base tumors. In: Moranty RA, Walsh KW, eds. *Brain tumors: a comprehensive text.* New York: Marcel Dekker, New York, 1994;451–491.
10. Sanson M, Cornu P. Biology of meningiomas. *Acta Neurochir* (Wien) 2000;142:493–505.
11. Inoue T, Rhoton AL, Theele D, et al. Surgical approaches to the cavernous sinus: a microsurgical study. *Neurosurgery* 1990;26(6): 903–932.

119. Approaches to the Posterior Skull Base

Aymara Triana, Chandranath Sen, Naresh P. Patel, and Caleb Lippman

The posterior skull-base region is comprised of all of the intra- and extradural structures related to the petrous temporal bone, the clivus, and the foramen magnum. A variety of malignant and benign tumors occur in this area. Substantial progress has been made in the diagnosis and surgical treatment of these tumors over the last two decades. This can be traced to several factors, namely exquisite imaging, detailed knowledge of the applied anatomy, and several innovative operative techniques.

Despite the high quality of modern imaging, many of these tumors attain a large size by the time they are diagnosed because of their slow growth. Their location in relation to the brainstem, the cranial nerves, and internal carotid and vertebrobasilar arteries makes them a surgical challenge.

Many surgical approaches to this region have been described and can be broadly divided into anterior, anterolateral, posterolateral, and posterior. Each of these strategies has its benefits and shortcomings and should be carefully analyzed. A thorough firsthand knowledge of the surgical anatomy of this region, which is obtained by careful dissections, is invaluable in defining the extent of exposure and limitations of each of these approaches. For large lesions involving midline and lateral extensions, or those with intra- and extradural extensions, a single approach may be insufficient. Multiple simultaneous approaches or staged procedures may be considered. The surgical team for the transtemporal approaches usually consists of a neurosurgeon and a neuro-otologist. For the anterior approaches, namely the transoral, transfacial and their modifications, and the extended subfrontal, the neurosurgeon usually works with an otolaryngologist or an oral surgeon. The approaches for intradural tumors of the posterior skull base are discussed in Chapter 121.

Anatomy of the Posterior Skull Base

The body of the sphenoid and basiocciput form the clivus, which occupies the central region of the posterior cranial fossa and extends from the dorsum sella down to the foramen magnum. On either side of the clivus the petrous portion of the temporal bones extends out laterally and backward. The petroclival synchondrosis separates the clivus from the petrous bones. The tentorium attaches to the posterior superior edge of the petrous bone, enclosing the superior petrosal sinus, one on each side. The dura covering the clivus has two distinct layers—the periosteal and the meningeal layers—which enclose a rich venous plexus. The cavernous sinus occupies the area immediately lateral to the upper clivus extending laterally and anteriorly from the free edge of the tentorium. The inferior petrosal sinus courses along the petroclival synchondrosis. The superior petrosal sinus thus connects the cavernous sinus to the sigmoid sinus while the inferior petrosal sinus connects the clival venous plexus and posterior cavernous sinus to the jugular bulb (1). The midbrain, pons, and the medulla are in direct relation to the clivus and the middle cerebellar peduncle rests on the posterior face of the petrous bones. The basilar artery and its branches lie between the brainstem and the clivus. The cranial nerves III through XII traverse the area between the brainstem and the posterior skull base and are always related to the tumors or aneurysms in this area, depending on their rostrocaudal extension.

The petrous temporal bones transmit the internal carotid arteries, the VII and VIII cranial nerves, and the jugular bulb and occupy the lateral portions of the posterior skull base. The entire auditory and vestibular apparatus including the external, middle, and inner ear structures occupies the petrous bone.

Preoperative Evaluation

The patient's baseline preoperative neurological status is important in establishing surgical goals in terms of preserving function. Preoperative cranial nerve deficits are seldom reversible, although there are exceptions, and often tumor resection is undertaken to halt their progression rather than to improve them. In addition, the surgical goals, whether a conservative or a radical excision, can be modified depending on the cranial nerve deficits that may already be present (i.e., certain cranial

nerve deficits may allow the surgeon to be more aggressive with the resection).

A detailed radiological evaluation of the lesion and surrounding structures is crucial to developing a successful surgical treatment plan. High-resolution computed tomography (CT) with soft tissue and bone algorithms, before and after contrast administration, gives invaluable information regarding areas of bone involvement and destruction as well as the relation to the bony structures, useful in planning the surgical approach. Direct imaging in the axial and coronal planes in 1.5-mm slices allows precise localization of tumor involvement at the bony foramina of the skull base and in the temporal bone. Characteristics of the bone destruction and calcification are useful to narrow the differential diagnosis.

Magnetic resonance imaging (MRI) with T1- and T2-triplanar views, before and after contrast administration, provides key information about tumor location, brain, soft tissue, and tumor relationships. CT and MRI provide complementary information regarding skull-base bone involvement because bone marrow is better seen on MRI. Especially useful is the tumor–brainstem interface in the T2-weighted image, which is an extremely useful determinant for surgery.

Involvement of the arterial and venous structures can be performed, in most instances with an MR arteriogram (MRA) and venogram (MRV). For a more detailed view of the vessels a conventional angiogram is preferred. The caliber of involved vessels and perforators as well as the adequacy of collateral circulation are best seen on conventional angiography. Conventional angiography is important to detect the presence of significant tumor blood supply and its source in order to plan the surgery and/or embolization. Embolization of feeding vessels may be accomplished at the same time in order to reduce intraoperative blood loss during tumor resection. In the event of internal carotid artery (ICA) involvement, a balloon test occlusion (BTO) of the ICA may be undertaken depending on the type of lesion and how much manipulation of the artery is anticipated. Although not an absolute predictor of stroke, the BTO can help guide the surgical approach, aggressiveness of tumor resection, and need for constructing a bypass. The venous phase of the angiogram is studied carefully as well, with particular attention paid to temporal lobe draining veins, and specifically, the transverse and sigmoid sinuses. The jugular bulb and cross-communication at the torcula are evaluated as well.

General Considerations

All patients receive anticonvulsants and high-dose steroids preoperatively. Antibiotic prophylaxis begins during the induction of anesthesia, and is continued for a few days postoperatively if a patient has a lumbar drain or a ventricular catheter.

Neurophysiological Monitoring/ Anesthesia

Intraoperative monitoring of cranial nerve responses and neural pathways is a useful adjunct for patients with posterior skull-base tumors. Facial electromyography, motor evoked potentials, brainstem auditory evoked responses, and somatosensory evoked potentials all alert the surgeon to possible neurological compromise. The positioning of the patient, prolonged brain

Table 1. Transoral Approach

	Structures Exposed	Main Steps of Access
Basic	Lower clivus Anterior arch of the atlas Odontoid process Body of C2	Midline incision of the posterior pharyngeal wall Retraction of the mucosa and muscle as a single layer Subperiosteal dissection
Variants Transpalatal Labiomandibular or labioglossomandibular	Additional cephalad exposure Additional longitudinal exposure	Opening of the soft palate, or the soft and hard palate Incision of the lip, chin, mandible, and possibly the tongue and the floor of the mouth (labioglossomandibular variant)

Table 2. Transsphenoidal Approach

Structures Exposed	Main Steps of Access
Upper third of the clivus and medial portion of cavernous sinus	Sublabial incision Resection of the vomer Entry into the sphenoid sinus Resection of the floor of the sella turcica

retraction and manipulation, or temporary vascular occlusion may all jeopardize function, and having intraoperative awareness of such potential dangers may help avoid permanent deficits.

Communication between the surgeon, the anesthesiologist, and the neurophysiologist is vital. Other standard monitoring devices include arterial and central venous lines, pneumatic compression stockings over the lower extremities, and an indwelling Foley catheter.

Brain relaxation may be obtained via the proper use of hyperventilation, osmotic diuretics, or cerebrospinal fluid (CSF) drainage. In the absence of a significant intradural mass or brain distortion, CSF drainage through a spinal subarachnoid drain may be safely employed.

An overview of the various approaches is provided in Tables 1–6. Some selected approaches are discussed in this chapter.

Anterior Approaches

Anterior approaches are most suitable for extradural midline lesions. These include the transoral, transmaxillary, transcervi-

cal, transsphenoidal, and the extended subfrontal approaches (2,3). If any of these approaches are to be used for tumors with lateral extensions, an additional approach may be necessary. The extended subfrontal approach is discussed here with emphasis on indications and technique. The other approaches are discussed in other chapters.

THE EXTENDED SUBFRONTAL APPROACH. The extended subfrontal approach is a modification of the transbasal approach described by Derome (4), with the addition of an orbito-fronto-ethmoidal osteotomy (2). The removal of both orbital rims allows better access to deep-seated lesions while simultaneously allowing for less retraction. This approach is most useful for extradural midline tumors involving the clivus and sphenoid sinus, extending from the base of the dorsum sellae to the foramen magnum. The limits of the approach laterally are the optic nerves, the cavernous and petrous internal carotid arteries, and the hypoglossal nerves. The inferior extent of this exposure is the rim of the foramen magnum, while the superior extent is the base of the sella turcica.

Position and Scalp Incision. The patient is positioned supine on a horseshoe rest or in head pins. A bicoronal incision is made beginning at the level of the ear, and carried vertically up and over to the other side (Fig. 1).

Scalp Flap/Bone Flap. The scalp and the pericranium are elevated together, down to the nasion. The supraorbital nerves and vessels are carefully freed from their foramen by converting it into a notch by the help of an osteotome. The periorbita is then stripped from the roofs and lateral orbital walls. A bifrontal craniotomy is performed with the craniotome, following which the supraorbital rims and the anterior orbital roofs are removed (Fig. 2).

Table 3. Bifrontal Transbasal Approach

	Structures Exposed	Main Steps of Access
Basic	Ethmoid bone Sphenoid bone Clivus	Bifrontal free bone flap Elevation of subfrontal dura Division of olfactory nerves at the cribriform plate Resection of the sphenoid lesser wing, tuberculum sella, and the base of the anterior clinoid To reach the clivus: Resection of the posterior part of the anterior cranial fossae, upper walls of ethmoid and sphenoid sinuses, and the floor of the sella turcica
Variant Extended subfrontal	Frontal sinus Orbit Medial wall of cavernous sinus	Orbitofrontoethmoidal osteotomy (supraorbital ridges, part of the orbital roofs, upper nasion, roof of the ethmoid sinuses, and cribriform plate are removed in a single block)

Table 4. Middle Fossa Approach

	Structures Exposed	Main Steps of Access
Basic	Internal acoustic meatus Intrapetrous course of the seventh cranial nerve	Temporal craniotomy (above ear and zygoma) Elevation of middle fossae floor dura (with identification of the eminence arcuatae and greater petrosal nerve) Exposure of middle meningeal artery and third trigeminal division Exposure of geniculate ganglion and greater petrosal nerve junction Unroofing of the internal auditory canal Identifying the vertical crest toward the meatal fundus
Variant Extended middle cranial fossa approach	Additional exposure with a wider opening of the posterior part of the petrous pyramid Whole intrapetrosal course of the facial nerve Horizontal petrous ICA	Extension of the resection to the posterior part of the petrous bone Drilling of the petrous apex medial to the petrous ICA Exposure of superior petrosal sinus and dura in front of the upper brainstem

ICA, internal carotid artery.

Table 5. Subtemporal Preauricular Infratemporal Approach

	Structures Exposed	Main Steps of Access
Basic	Middle cranial fossae Anterior part of the petrous bone located medial to the cochlea, jugular foramen, and petroclival region Petrous ICA Infratemporal fossae Cervical carotid artery, internal jugular vein, the vagus, accessory and hypoglossal nerves	Frontopreauricular curvilinear incision Division of the zygoma Frontotemporal craniotomy Separation of the dura from the middle fossa floor Exposure of meningeal artery, eminence arcuatae, third division of the trigeminal and greater petrosal nerves Removal of the middle fossa floor (including part of the superior orbital fissure and foramen ovale)
Variant Extended subtemporal preauricular infratemporal approach	Additional exposure: Clival region to the level of the foramen magnum Dura of the anterior and lateral aspects of the posterior fossa Meckel cave (superiorly) Cochlea and ICA (laterally) Abducens nerve (medially) Hypoglossal canal (inferiorly) Inferolateral portion of the cavernous sinus	Removal of zygomatic arch with the condylar fossa Resection of the bone medial to the mandibular fossa Exposure of the ascending portion of the petrous ICA Mobilization and displacement of the entire petrous ICA Continue the bone drilling toward the clivus Division of the third trigeminal branch above the foramen ovale

ICA, internal carotid artery.

Table 6. Extreme or Far Lateral Transcondylar Approach

	Structures Exposed	Main Steps of Access
Basic	Muscle, joint, bone, and neurovascular structures of the lateral posterior cranial fossa and cervico-occipital region	Posterolaterally placed skin incision Muscular dissection, including occipital triangle, early identification of the VA and venous plexuses, exposure of transverse process of the atlas, and upper cervical nerves Extradural dissection, including suboccipital craniectomy or craniotomy with removal of at least half of the posterior arch of the atlas. Does not include removal of the posterior part of the occipital condyle Intradural exposure, including neurovascular structures and dentate ligament
Variant		
Supracondylar	Median region of the hypoglossal canal and jugular tubercle	
Paracondylar	Posterior part of the jugular foramen and posterior aspect of the facial nerve and mastoid on the lateral side of the jugular foramen	Extent of the bony resection to the occipital condyle according to the variants
Transcondylar	Allows more lateral exposure and provides access to the lower clivus and the paramedullary area	
Transcondylar extension		
Atlanto-occipital transarticular	Additional exposure of the dura surrounding the VA	Removal of the adjacent posterior part of the occipital condyle and superior articular facet of C1
Occipital transcondylar	Lower clivus and the area in front of the medulla	Above part of AO joint, through the occipital condyle mass and below the hypoglossal canal
Transtubercular	Area in front of the brainstem and origin of the PICA	Extradural removal of the prominence of the jugular tubercle

VA, vertebral artery; AO, atlanto-occipital; PICA, petrous internal carotid artery.

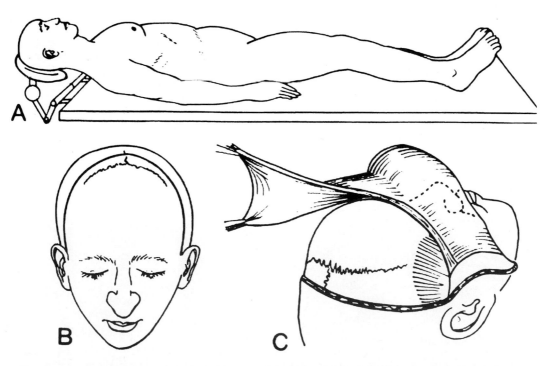

Fig. 1. Extended subfrontal approach. **A:** Surgical position. **B:** Bicoronal incision. **C:** Scalp and pericranial flap.

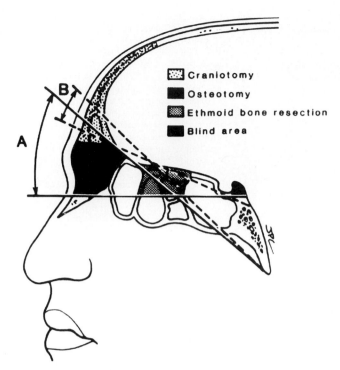

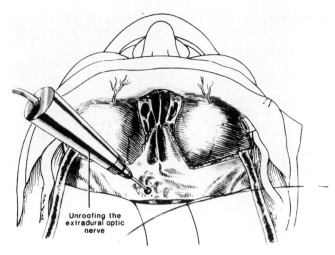

Fig. 2. Improved angle of view (*A*) with the fronto-orbito-ethmoidal osteotomy. Lateral view.

Fig. 4. Drilling of the planum after the fronto-orbito-ethmoidal osteotomy. Axial view.

The orbito-frontal osteotomy, which is made with a reciprocating saw, provides an additional 2 cm of room under the frontal lobes and thus reduces the amount of brain retraction needed (Fig. 3).

Elevation of the frontal lobes extradurally usually involves sacrificing the olfactory nerves at the cribriform plate (2,4). For posterior skull-base tumors one can attempt to preserve smell by making osteotomies around the cribriform plate and the roof of the nasal vault, leaving the whole olfactory apparatus attached to the dura and elevating the entire complex with the frontal lobes. Gentle frontal retraction is then used to gain access to both optic nerves, which are unroofed extradurally using a high-speed diamond drill and plenty of irrigation. It is not necessary to drill the anterior clinoid processes unless a lateral

approach is also being combined. The optic nerves are unroofed toward the orbits for about 2 cm and the planum sphenoidale is drilled between the nerves (Fig. 4).

The posterior ethmoid air cells are also drilled away. The bone underneath the optic nerve is carefully drilled away to expose the medial surface of the intracavernous ICA in its anterior portion (2). The dura of the medial surface of the cavernous sinuses is exposed by carefully drilling away from anterior to posterior, leading toward the petrous apex. Thus, a wide exposure of the sphenoid sinus is accomplished, medial to the cavernous sinuses. The floor of the sphenoid sinus is drilled down, exposing the clivus (Fig. 5). Visualization of the petrous apex is carried out by angling the microscope from over the opposite orbit. A wide angle of visualization is thus required at the surface in order to see the entire extent of the clivus.

Tumor Resection. The extradural tumor is usually encountered while drilling into the sphenoid sinus and the clivus. Tumor removal is accomplished with the help of curets and rongeurs. If there is extension of the tumor through the dura,

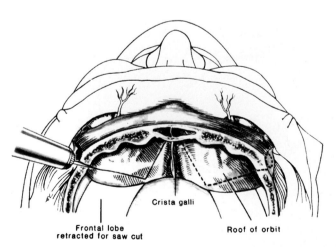

Fig. 3. After removal of the frontal free bone flap and before the fronto-orbito-ethmoidal osteotomy. Axial view.

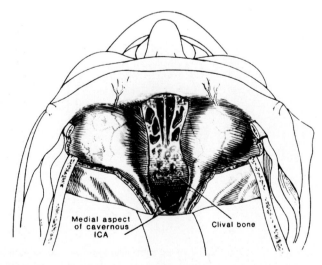

Fig. 5. Exposure of the clivus after drilling down the floor of the sphenoid sinus and the medial walls of the cavernous sinus. Axial view.

it can also be removed by this route. However, the exposure is not wide enough to remove a primarily intradural tumor. Tumor extensions into the cavernous sinuses can also be removed from this exposure. A straight and angled rigid endoscope is a useful adjunct to the surgical microscope in looking around the corners at a depth, especially in the posterior cavernous sinus and clivus. After removal of the soft tumor, the surrounding bone is drilled away until healthy bone is seen.

Closure. A pericranial flap and autologous free fat graft are used to reconstruct the floor following tumor removal. The flap is based on both supraorbital vessels and passed between both optic nerves to cover the clivus. It is placed before replacing the supraorbital rims so that sufficient length is available to cover the clivus (Fig. 6).

If the olfactory preservation technique has been used, the pericranial flap is split down the middle to accommodate the cribriform plate, but a watertight closure will not be achieved. The bone flap and the supraorbital rims are carefully replaced, avoiding pressure and ischemia on the pericranial flap. The scalp is closed in multiple layers. Lumbar CSF drainage is continued in the postoperative period for 3 to 4 days, carefully regulated by volume in order to avoid overdrainage.

Advantages and Disadvantages. The extradural nature of this approach makes it well suited for lesions, which are primarily extradural. Approaching from the midline makes the surgical anatomy easier to comprehend, and provides direct access to midline tumors. Intracranial approaches (in contrast to transsphenoidal or transoral) allow one to easily reconstruct the skull base, especially when there is a substantial communication with the CSF.

The major disadvantage of the procedure is the complete loss of olfaction with resultant loss of taste due to elevation of the frontal lobes (2,4). Olfaction can be preserved in certain instances where there has been no communication with the CSF. In addition, for tumors involving the medial cavernous sinus it will be necessary to remove the posterior ethmoidal cells and widely unroof the optic nerves superiorly and medially, placing these structures at risk. Furthermore, carotid artery injury cannot be safely dealt with because of the lack of proximal control. Lastly, the presence of the sellar contents prevents access to the dorsum sellae and posterior clinoids, which are hidden from the surgeon's view.

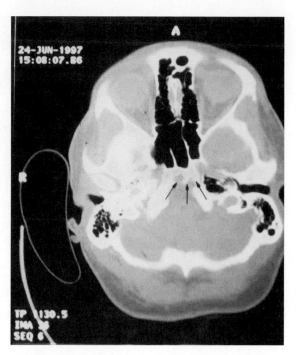

Fig. 7. Preoperative CT scan (Illustrative Case 1).

ILLUSTRATIVE CASE 1

Extended Subfrontal Approach. A 25-year-old man experienced two episodes of severe headache with nausea and vomiting, lasting for 1 day and resolving spontaneously, within a 6-month interval. The day after the second episode he woke up with diplopia at the left gaze and noted a convergent strabismus on his left eye, lasting for 2 days and also resolving spontaneously. Physical examination at the consultation showed no particular sign.

CT and MRI revealed a lesion located at the clivus and left petrous apex with bone destruction and indentation of the brainstem extending into the sphenoid sinus. The tumor was also apposed to the left ICA in its intracavernous segment as well as in close proximity to the VI cranial nerve (Figs. 7 and 8).

A bifrontal craniotomy, supraorbital osteotomy, exenteration of the frontal, ethmoid and sphenoid sinuses, resection of the clival tumor, repair of the dura mater with pericranial patch graft and abdominal fat, repair of the anterior fossa defect with pericranial rotation flap, and the placement of a right frontal ventriculostomy were performed. Postoperatively, a left VI cranial nerve palsy (that subsequently recovered) and some difficulties with the left temporomandibular joint were noted.

The histopathology analysis reported a chordoma (Figs. 9 and 10).

Lateral Approaches

Lateral approaches may be used for both intra- and extradural lesions of the posterior skull base. These include the anterolateral approaches: extended middle cranial fossa (anterior transpetrosal) approach and the subtemporal preauricular infratemporal approach. The posterolateral approaches include the subtemporal and presigmoid retrolabyrinthine, translabyrinthine, and transcochlear approaches. The area of the foramen

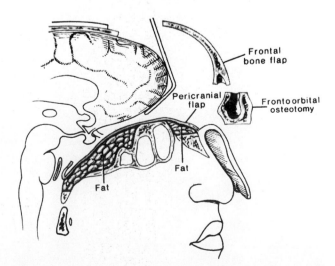

Fig. 6. Lateral view of the approach, before closure, showing the placement of the pericranial flap and the replacement of the osteotomy.

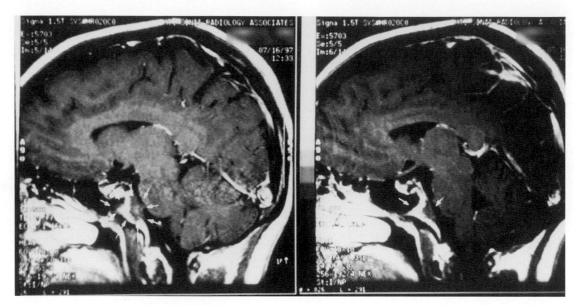

Fig. 8. Preoperative MRI (Illustrative Case 1).

magnum is accessed by the extreme lateral transcondylar approach. A combination of these approaches may be employed in the case of large tumors. These approaches are useful for predominantly ventral and ventrolateral tumors that involve the cavernous sinus and the temporal bone. They afford excellent control of the ICA and unilateral cranial nerves and allow many options for reconstruction to prevent or repair a CSF fistula.

THE SUBTEMPORAL PREAURICULAR INFRATEMPORAL APPROACH. Tumors of the posterior skull base that are eccentric in location and involve the petrous temporal bone are better approached through an anterolateral approach (5). This ap-

proach is suitable for intra- and extradural tumors anterior and anterolateral to the brainstem. A major benefit in using an anterolateral approach is that the surgeon avoids working in between multiple cranial nerves in order to get in front of the brainstem. The subtemporal preauricular infratemporal approach is predominantly an extradural approach that allows access to the area in front of the brainstem (6). By opening the dura of the temporal lobe and in front of the brainstem and dividing the tentorium, the approach allows access from the posterior clinoids down to the hypoglossal canals (7). Lesions treated with this approach include meningiomas, chordomas, chondrosarcomas, neurilemmomas, and cholesteatomas.

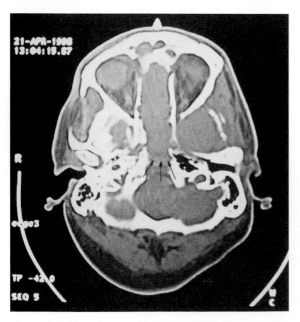

Fig. 9. Postoperative CT scan showing the area of clival bone removal (Illustrative Case 1).

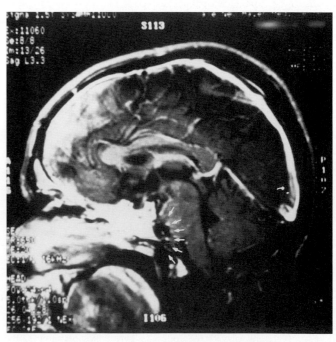

Fig. 10. Postoperative MRI (Illustrative Case 1).

Patient Position and Incision. The patient is placed supine with the head and neck turned to the side opposite to the surgical approach. The head is fixed in a three-point fixation or placed on a horseshoe headrest. The incision is a unilateral "?" fashion starting at the hairline and then brought down very close to and in front of the ear, to just below the tragus. A temporoparietal fascial flap is raised during the opening (Fig. 11).

This corresponds to the galeal layer based on the superficial temporal artery and is a versatile flap for reconstruction of the surgical bed and prevention of a CSF leak. A subfascial dissection is used to elevate the scalp from the temporalis muscle preserving the frontal branch of the facial nerve (8–10). The zygomatic arch, lateral rim of the orbit, and the mandibular condyle, including a short portion of its neck, are exposed. The caudal exposure is carefully done so as not to injure the superficial temporal artery or the facial nerve. The temporalis muscle is elevated and also freed from the zygomatic arch.

Craniotomy and Osteotomies. A frontotemporal craniotomy is carried out in the standard fashion and the sphenoid wing is rongeured down to the floor of the middle fossa. Drainage of CSF from the lumbar drain relaxes the brain and allows the temporal lobe to be elevated extradurally. The temporomandibular joint is opened and the condyle is dislocated down. A reciprocating saw is used to remove the zygomatic arch. The anterior cut is made at the junction with the lateral rim of the orbit. The posterior cut includes the condylar fossa. This is accomplished by making a "V"-shaped osteotomy in front of and behind the condylar fossa. The posterior cut of this "V" should not violate the middle ear cavity (Fig. 12).

The entire zygomatic arch is removed along with the mandibular fossa. Both are replaced at the end of the operation. Depending on the extent of the caudal exposure that is needed, the mandibular condyle may be resected or only dislocated downward and out of the way. If its resection is needed, a saw cut is made at the neck of the mandible. The condyle is discarded and does not create any significant impairment. It should be noted that resection of the mandibular head produces less trismus than dislocating and retracting it down for an extended period of time.

Extradural Dissection. The temporal lobe is elevated extradurally, exposing the foramen rotundum, ovale, and spinosum.

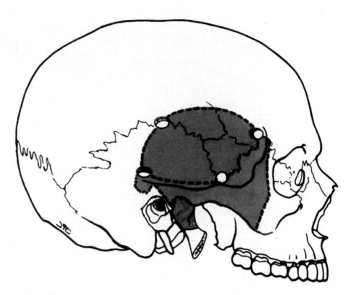

Fig. 12. Extent of the temporal craniotomy, zygomatic osteotomy after dislocation of the temporomandibular joint. Lateral view.

The sphenoid wing is drilled away to unroof these foramina. The middle meningeal artery is coagulated and divided. The horizontal segment of the petrous ICA is exposed posteromedial to the foramen ovale and underneath the course of the greater petrosal nerve after it emerges from the facial hiatus anterior to the arcuate eminence. The horizontal and vertical intrapetrous portion of the ICA is completely exposed down to its entry into the skull base. Bone in front of the third division of the trigeminal nerve (V3) and between the ICA and V3 is removed, and the ICA is gently lifted and mobilized laterally by establishing a subperiosteal plane (Fig. 13).

The eustachian tube is divided during exposure of the vertical portion of the artery. The fibrocartilaginous ring at the entrance of the ICA into the carotid canal is incised so that the entire artery can be freely mobilized out of the bony canal and rotated out laterally (9,10). Bone removal must be avoided posterior to the genu of the petrous ICA due to its proximity with the cochlea and geniculate ganglion of the facial nerve. The petrous temporal bone and clivus are thus exposed medial to the displaced ICA (Fig. 14).

The clivus may now be drilled to expose the clival dura. Drilling in this location requires familiarity with the relationship between the jugular bulb, pars nervosa of the jugular foramen, and the hypoglossal canal. The jugular vein lies immediately posterolateral to the artery at the skull base, while the nerves are located between the two and just medial to the vein. The styloid process, which can be palpated, is located adjacent and lateral to the jugular bulb.

Clival and Petrous Apex Exposure. The soft, cancellous bone of the petrous apex and clivus can be drilled away with a diamond burr. The major foramina (hypoglossal canal, jugular foramen, and foramen magnum) consist of bone that is hard and cortical. The field of exposure narrows considerably as the surgeon approaches the hypoglossal foramen because the jugular bulb and foramen partially obstruct the caudal view. The clival dura has two layers: an outer periosteal layer and an inner meningeal layer. Between the two layers lies a prominent venous plexus including the inferior petrosal sinus. The dural window exposed extends superiorly to the Meckel cave, inferiorly to the hypoglossal foramen, medially to the Dorello canal, and laterally to the internal auditory meatus. The extradural

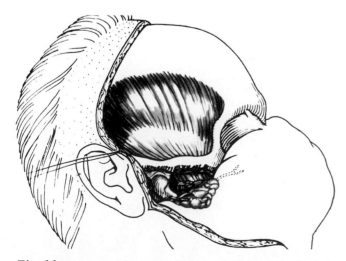

Fig. 11. Subtemporal preauricular infratemporal approach. Skin incision, scalp flap reflected forward, muscular and bony exposure. Lateral view.

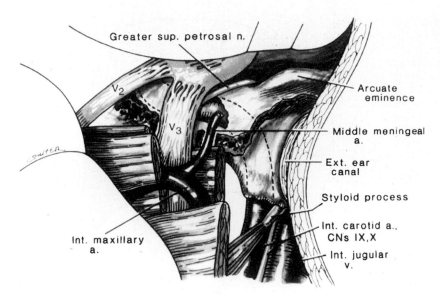

Fig. 13. Lateral anatomical view of the subtemporal and infratemporal regions exposed during the approach emphasizing the course of the petrous carotid artery. Lateral view.

tumor is usually visualized in the bone during clival bone work and is removed using curets and suction.

Intradural Exposure. Intradural tumor extension is followed by opening the clival dura inferior to the Meckel cave in a cruciate manner and the edges are coagulated. The VI cranial nerve travels through the dura in the anterior edge of the bony opening and should not be injured. The pons and pontomedullary junction are exposed. The bone drilling can be carried posteriorly to the anterior surface of the internal auditory canal. The basilar artery and the ipsilateral vertebral artery are exposed through this exposure. If cephalad intradural exposure is needed, the temporal dura can be opened and the tentorium incised to view the upper clivus.

Reconstruction. After the completion of tumor resection a piece of autologous fat is used to fill the clival bony defect (Fig. 15). The temporoparietal fascial flap is rotated to cover the defect and separate the middle ear from the CSF around the brainstem. The zygomatic arch is fixed in position with

titanium plates and screws. The bone flap and temporalis muscle are secured in position. If the mandibular head has been removed, the ramus is left floating.

Advantages and Disadvantages. The main advantage of the subtemporal preauricular infratemporal approach is its ability to provide direct access to the ventral brainstem, clivus, and petrous temporal bone without much brain retraction. In addition, this approach preserves the hearing apparatus, minimizes the manipulation of the facial nerve, and avoids traversing septic spaces. Furthermore, full exposure and control of the petrous ICA is achieved, making this useful for tumors encasing this segment of the ICA. Extradural, intradural, and transdural tumors can all be approached by this route.

The major disadvantages include trismus or malocclusion in the contralateral temporomandibular joint, mostly as a result from the ipsilateral mandibular condyle resection. Also, division of the eustachian tube leads to a temporary conductive hearing loss, which is reversible with a tympanostomy. The approach provides a unilateral exposure of the clivus and petrous region

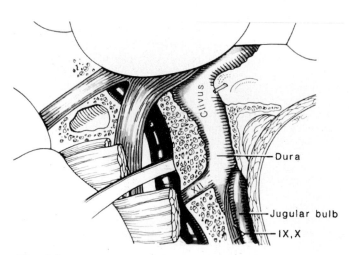

Fig. 14. Exposure of the clivus after displacement of the petrous carotid artery. Lateral view.

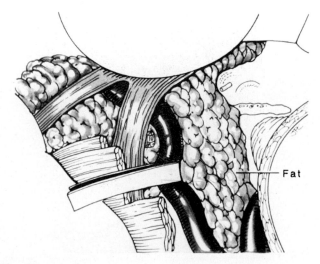

Fig. 15. Reconstruction with fat graft, after clivus drilling and resection, before closure. Lateral view.

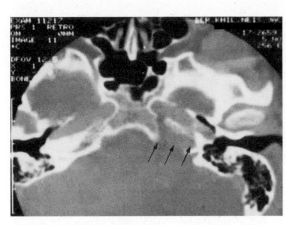

Fig. 16. Preoperative CT scan (Illustrative Case 2).

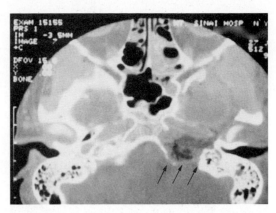

Fig. 18. Postoperative CT scan showing the area of bone resection (Illustrative Case 2).

and must be carefully selected for tumors that are entirely intradural in this location.

ILLUSTRATIVE CASE 2

Subtemporal Preauricular Infratemporal Approach. An 18-year-old boy complained of vague visual difficulty that subsided spontaneously. Physical examination at the consultation showed no particular sign.

CT and MRI showed a destructive lesion in the left petrous apex extending down into the petroclival region with a bulging at the posterior fossa dura mater. The lesion was immediately medial to the petrous carotid artery. An arteriogram with BTO appeared well tolerated (Figs. 16 and 17).

A left temporal craniotomy, zygomatic osteotomy and osteotomy of the mandibular condyle, exposure and displacement of the petrous carotid artery, removal of tumor, and reconstruction of the mandibular condyle and zygomatic arch with titanium miniplates were performed. Postoperatively, cranial nerve palsy of the left VI and VII cranial nerves (that recovered completely) as well as an autonomic dysfunction (diaphoresis, sialorrhea, and discoloration of the face) due to section of the greater petrosal nerve were noted.

The histopathology analysis reported a low-grade chondrosarcoma (Figs. 18 and 19).

ILLUSTRATIVE CASE 3

Extended Middle Fossa Approach. A 22-year-old woman complained of right progressive decreased hearing and tinnitus, as well as paresthesias in the right side of the face. Physical examination confirmed the right hypacusia without any other particular sign.

CT and MRI revealed a lesion located on the right clivus, indenting the pons and the midbrain, extending into the Meckel cave, anterior to the VII and VIII cranial nerves, and surrounding completely the trigeminal nerve (Fig. 20).

A right frontotemporal craniotomy, zygomatic osteotomy, anterior petrosal temporal bone resection, combined supra- and infratentorial approach with total removal of the tumor, and an intraoperative endoscopy (to confirm total tumor resection and viewing around the corners) were performed (Figs. 21 and 22). Postoperatively. a right VI cranial nerve palsy, diplopia, and hypoesthesia of the right V2 and V3 territories were noted (all recovered progressively).

The histopathology analysis reported an epidermoid tumor (Figs. 23 and 24).

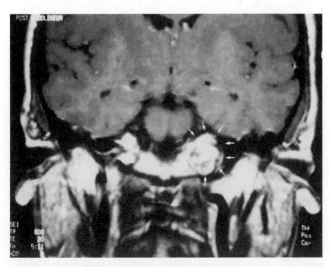

Fig. 17. Preoperative MRI (Illustrative Case 2).

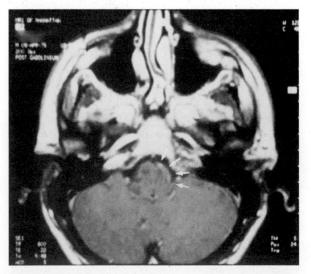

Fig. 19. Postoperative MRI (Illustrative Case 2). *Arrows* indicate area of tumor resection.

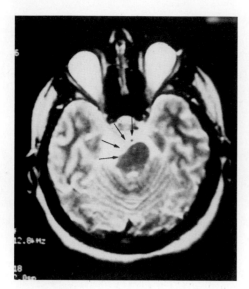

Fig. 20. Extended middle fossa approach. Preoperative magnetic resonance image showing the brainstem indentation by the epidermoid tumor (*arrows*) (Illustrative Case 3).

THE EXTREME LATERAL TRANSCONDYLAR APPROACH. The extreme lateral transcondylar approach is used for ventrally situated tumors of the lower clivus and foramen magnum with extension into the upper cervical spine. It may be employed for lesions involving the vertebral artery and lower cranial nerves. It is suitable for both intra- and extradural lesions, allows control over the aforementioned structures, permits dissection of the brainstem–tumor interface tangentially along this plane, and avoids approaches that traverse contaminated spaces like the oral and nasal cavities. Large glomus tumors of the temporal bone may also be managed by this approach.

Position and Skin Incision. The patient is positioned in the lateral decubitus position with the head in a neutral position in three-point fixation (11–13). For the resection of extradural tumors that involve the occipital condyle, the resection may be

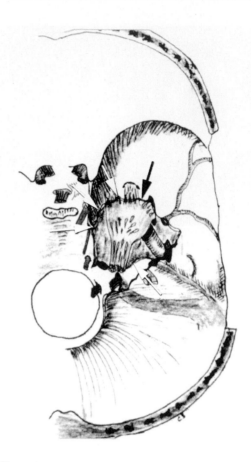

Fig. 22. Axial view of the final exposure obtained with this approach. After the bone drilling and opening the dura the area in front of the upper brainstem is exposed.

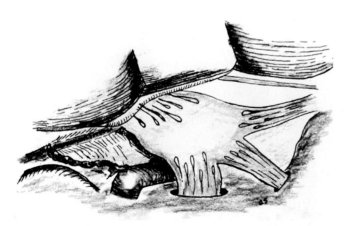

Fig. 21. Subtemporal view showing the drilling of the petrous apex medial to the petrous internal carotid artery. The clival dura and the superior petrosal sinus have been exposed. On opening the dura and sectioning the superior petrosal sinus and the tentorium, an anterior approach to the upper petroclival region is achieved.

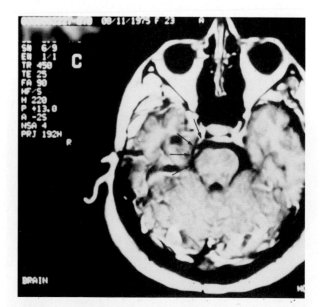

Fig. 23. Postoperative magnetic resonance image showing the normal brainstem contour after removal of the tumor (*arrows*) (Illustrative Case 3).

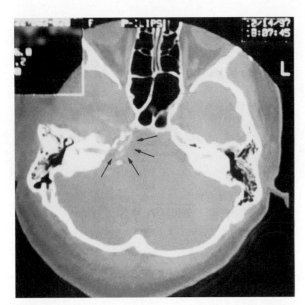

Fig. 24. Postoperative computed tomography scan showing the bone defect in the petrous apex which was reconstructed with hydroxyapatite cement to prevent cerebrospinal fluid leakage (Illustrative Case 3).

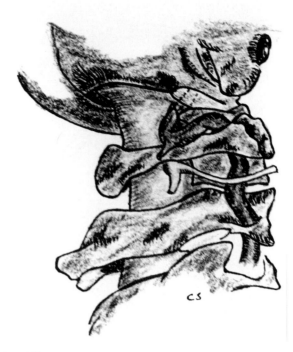

Fig. 26. Exposure of the vertebral artery in its third segment (V3) and the second cervical nerve root (C2) with its ganglion and main branches. Posterolateral view from below.

accompanied by an occipitocervical fusion. In this instance an inverted "U"-shaped incision is made by starting in the midline curving on to the back of the head and then down behind the ear. If a considerable temporal bone involvement is present, a "C"-shaped retroauricular incision is used. For purely intradural tumors at the foramen magnum an inverted "L"-shaped incision is used with the horizontal arm at the level of the top of the ear and the vertical arm along the posterior border of the sterno-cleidomastoid muscle (14) (Fig. 25).

Soft-Tissue Dissection and Identification of the Vertebral Artery. The sternocleidomastoid muscle is reflected downward and the spinal accessory nerve and internal jugular vein are identified. The splenius capitus, recti, and oblique muscles must then be removed from the occipital bone, mastoid process, and transverse process of C1. The oblique muscles are dissected carefully since the vertebral artery and the surrounding venous plexus are underneath the muscles. The transverse process of C1 is an excellent guide (15). The artery can be identified below C1 or above C1 depending on the level of the lesion and the proximal control that would be needed (Fig. 26).

Bone Removal. A retrosigmoid craniectomy is performed first. The vertebral artery is followed toward the foramen magnum where it enters the dura (Fig. 27). It is isolated from the venous plexus by incising the sheath longitudinally along the vessel and circumferentially coagulating it around the artery. The condylar emissary vein is controlled by packing with Surgicel. Further bone removal is dictated by the type and extent of the lesion. If it is an extradural tumor involving a portion of the temporal bone, a mastoidectomy and temporal bone removal is carried out, preserving the facial nerve and rerouting it. If the tumor is extradural and is only in the lower clivus and foramen magnum region, the occipital condyle is drilled away. Depending on the cephalad extension of the tumor, the resection can be carried up to the labyrinth also including the jugular foramen. During drilling of the occipital condyle, the course of the hypoglossal nerve is carefully noted and protected. Bone is drilled away until healthy bone is seen. For intradural tumors, only a small portion of the posterior part of the occipital condyle is drilled away. The jugular tubercle between the occipital condyle and the jugular bulb is also drilled away to provide a clear access to the anterior surface of the lower clivus and the foramen magnum (Figs. 28–30).

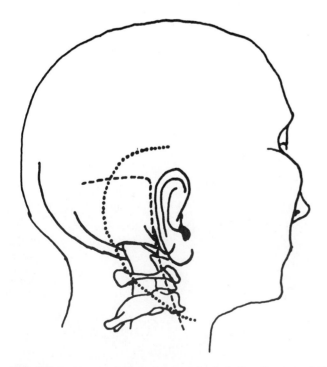

Fig. 25. Extreme or far lateral approach. A choice of two surgical scalp and skin incisions: C-shape and inverted L-shape. Posterolateral view.

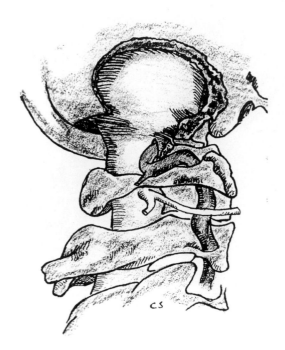

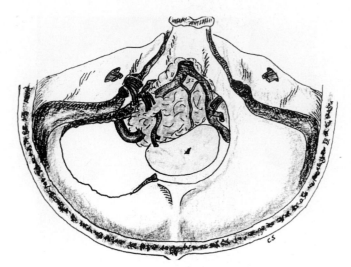

Fig. 29. Axial view of the exposure with the tumoral mass encasing the left vertebral artery and compressing the brainstem. It also shows the occipital craniotomy, the jugular tubercle resection, the partial resection of the occipital condyle, and its relationship with the artery.

Fig. 27. Occipital craniotomy with resection of the posterior part of the occipital condyle and the jugular tubercle. Posterolateral view from below.

Dural Opening and Tumor Removal. For intradural tumors, the dura is opened posterior to the sigmoid sinus and the vertebral artery in a vertical linear manner. The dural incision is carried circumferentially around the vertebral artery entry area and the artery is gently displaced posteriorly, allowing an unobstructed view of the anterior aspect of the foramen magnum (Fig. 31).

In the case of extradural tumors the bone drilling is much more extensive and the overlying dura may also be excised. If the tumor involves the anterior aspect of the C1 and C2 bones, the vertebral artery may be displaced from the foramen transversarium of C1 after opening the bony foramen and dissecting the artery in a subperiosteal plane. The artery is then reflected laterally, allowing access to the anterior structures. If the tumor reaches up into the jugular foramen, the sigmoid sinus is ligated as well as the internal jugular vein. The jugular bulb is opened and the cranial nerves are followed from the brainstem to the area of tumor involvement and carefully freed from the tumor, if possible. Tumor removal is carried out in a piecemeal manner with full control of the vertebral artery and the cranial nerves.

Closure. In order to achieve as tight a closure as possible, a dural graft may be needed. In addition, fibrin glue supplemented with an autologous fat graft is recommended. In some instances, a lumbar spinal drain may be left for up to 4 days' postoperatively.

If one or both surfaces of the occiput-C1 joint are entirely removed, or if more than two-thirds of the occipital condyle is removed, the patient may suffer from mechanical instability.

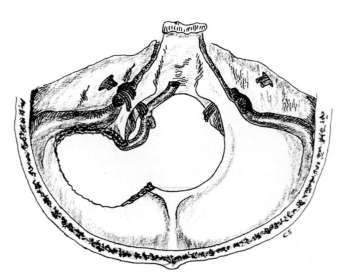

Fig. 28. Axial view of the routine retrosigmoid craniectomy before the resection of the occipital condyle and the jugular tubercle.

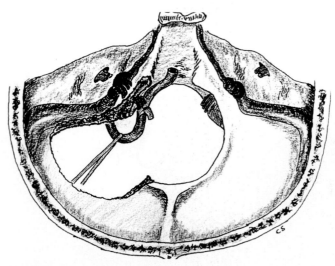

Fig. 30. Axial view of the exposure with resection of the left occipital condyle and the jugular tubercle allowing the space anterior to the vertebral artery and the anterior portion of the foramen magnum.

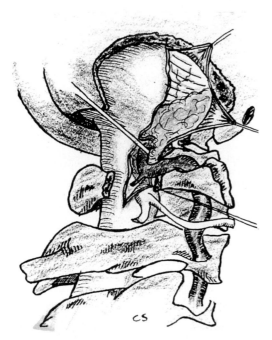

Fig. 31. Intradural view, posterolateral from below, showing the dural entry of the vertebral artery as well as the entry into the tumor at the V1 segment level. The artery has been released at its dural entry to facilitate its separation from the tumor.

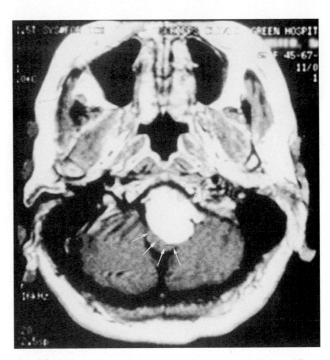

Fig. 32. Preoperative magnetic resonance image, axial plane (Illustrative Case 4). *Arrows* indicate brain stem compression.

This could lead to a painful torticollis. In these cases, stabilization is indicated and may be performed at the same sitting or in a subsequent procedure. Options available for occiput-C1 fusion include plates and screws, contoured titanium loops and sublaminar wires, and contoured Steinmann pins. An autologous bone graft is essential for achieving an adequate fusion.

Advantages and Disadvantages. This approach is advantageous because it directly exposes the tumor and its interface with the brainstem and cervicomedullary junction, reducing manipulation and retraction of these structures (16,17). The surgeon has complete control of the vertebral artery and the lower cranial nerves. The access is completely extrapharyngeal and can be used with equal ease in intra- and extradural tumors. Aggressive bone removal can be accomplished and a fusion operation, if needed, can be performed at the same sitting. The approach does not provide good access to structures across the midline in case of tumor extension. Since a watertight dural closure cannot be achieved, good soft tissue closure is necessary in order to avoid a CSF fistula.

ILLUSTRATIVE CASE 4

Extreme Lateral Transcondylar Approach. A 60-year-old woman complained of left occipitocervical headaches for 5 years as well as a progressive sensitivity loss in both upper extremities that descended to the trunk and the left lower extremity 1 month before being admitted to the hospital.

Physical examination showed impaired dexterity and grasp in both hands as well as hyperreflexia, without clonus, in the four extremities.

CT and MRI revealed a large lesion located in the region of the lower clivus, foramen magnum, and C1, a lateral displacement of both vertebral arteries with encasement of the left one, and a severe compression of the cervicomedullary junction and brainstem (Figs. 32 and 33).

A left suboccipital craniectomy, C1 hemilaminectomy, partial excision of the occipital condyle, decompression and mobilization of the vertebral artery, and resection of the tumor were performed. Postoperatively, bilateral cranial nerve palsies of the VI, IX, and left XII cranial nerves as well as a slight sensorimotor loss in the upper extremities were noted. All regressed completely within 6 months. The histopathology analysis reported a meningioma (Figs. 34 and 35).

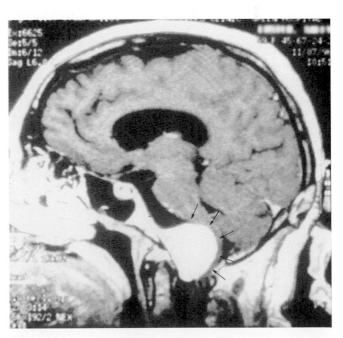

Fig. 33. Preoperative magnetic resonance image, sagittal plane (Illustrative Case 4). *Arrows* indicate brain stem compression.

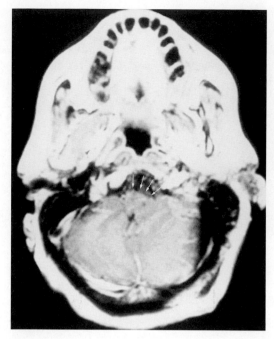

Fig. 34. Postoperative magnetic resonance image, axial plane (Illustrative Case 4). *Arrows* indicate area of tumor resection.

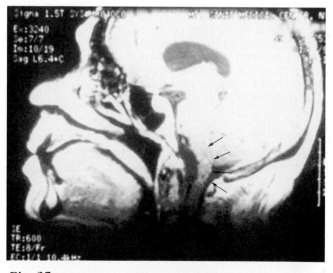

Fig. 35. Postoperative magnetic resonance image, sagittal plane (Illustrative Case 4). *Arrows* indicate area of tumor resection.

References

1. Rhoton AL Jr: Anatomical basis of surgical approaches to the region of the foramen magnum. In: Dickman CA, Spetzler RF, Sonntag VKH, eds. *Surgery of the craniovertebral junction.* New York: Thieme Medical Publishers, 1998:13–57.
2. Sekhar LN, Nanda A, Sen CN, et al: The extended frontal approach to tumors of the anterior, middle and posterior skull base. *J Neurosurg* 76:198–206, 1992.
3. Hitotsumatsu T, Matsushima T, Rhoton AL Jr: Surgical anatomy of the midface and the midline skull base. In: Spetzler RF, ed. *Operative techniques in neurosurgery.* Vol 2. Philadelphia: WB Saunders, 1999:160–180.
4. Derome P: The transbasal approach to tumors invading the base of the skull. In: Schmidek HH, Sweet WH, eds. *Current techniques in operative neurosurgery.*New York: Grune & Stratton, 1977:223–245.
5. House WF: Middle cranial fossa approach to the petrous pyramid. *Arch Otolaryngol* 78: 460–469, 1963.
6. Fisch U, Fagan P, Valavanis A: The infratemporal fossa approach for the lateral skull base. *Otolaryngol Clin North Am* 7: 513–552, 1984.
7. Kawase T, Shiobara R, Toya S: Anterior transpetrosal transtentorial approach for sphenopetroclival meningiomas: surgical method and results in 10 patients. *Neurosurgery* 28: 869–876, 1991.
8. Sekhar LN, Schramm VL Jr, Jones NF: Operative management of large neoplasms of the lateral and posterior cranial base. In: Sekhar LN, Schramm VL Jr, eds. *Tumors of the cranial base. Diagnosis and treatment.* Mount Kisco, NY: Futura Publishing Co, 1987:655–682.
9. Sekhar LN, Schramm VL Jr, Jones NF: Subtemporal preauricular infratemporal fossa approach to large lateral and posterior cranial base neoplasms. *J Neurosurg* 67: 488–499, 1987.
10. Sen CN, Sekhar LN: The subtemporal and preauricular infratemporal approach to intradural structures ventral to the brain stem. *J Neurosurg* 73: 345–354, 1990.
11. Babu RP, Sekhar LN, Wright DC: Extreme lateral transcondylar approach: technical improvements and lessons learned. *J Neurosurg* 81: 49–59, 1994.
12. Baldwin HZ, Miller CG, Van Loveren HR, et al: The far lateral/combined supra and infratentorial approach: a human cadaveric prosection model for routes of access to the petroclival region and ventral brainstem. *J Neurosurg* 81:60–68, 1994.
13. Lang DA, Neil-Dwyer G, Iannotti F: The suboccipital transcondylar approach to the clivus and cranio-cervical junction for ventrally placed pathology at and above the foramen magnum. *Acta Neurochir* (Wien) 125: 132–137, 1993.
14. Wen H, Rhoton AL Jr, Katsuta T, et al: Microsurgical anatomy of the transcondylar, supracondylar, and paracondylar extensions of the far-lateral approach. *J Neurosurg* 87: 555–585, 1997.
15. Sen CN, Sekhar LN: Extreme lateral transcondylar and transjugular approaches. In: Sekhar LN, Janecka IP, eds: *Surgery of cranial base tumors.* New York: Raven Press, 1993: 389–341.
16. Sen CN, Sekhar LN: Surgical management of anteriorly placed lesions at the craniocervical junction: an alternative approach. *Acta Neurochir* (Wien) 108: 70–77, 1991.
17. Sen CN, Sekhar LN: An extreme lateral approach to intradural lesions of the cervical spine and foramen magnum. *Neurosurgery* 27: 197–204, 1990.

120. Tumors of the Cerebellopontine Angle

John G. Golfinos, Stephen M. Russell, and J. Thomas Roland, Jr.

The first cerebellopontine angle tumor successfully removed was likely a meningioma by Ballance in 1892 (1). Three years later, Annandale, in what Cushing described as "a brilliant surgical result, the first recorded," successfully removed an acoustic neuroma using the "enucleating finger" technique. Over the ensuing years, many surgeons finger enucleated acoustic neuromas, only attempting the procedure once the tumors became large and symptomatic. The mortality for this procedure was shockingly high, with surgeons reporting a 72% to 84% fatality rate (2). This poor result was attributed to avulsion of the anterior inferior cerebellar artery, causing horrendous bleeding and brainstem infarction. Cushing compared this complication with the infamous fence corner at the battle of Gettysburg, suggesting that the cerebellopontine angle should be called 'the bloody angle' (1).

The prognosis and quality of life following acoustic neuroma surgery improved dramatically following the widespread application of new operative adjuncts, including the operating microscope, skull base techniques, bipolar cautery, magnetic resonance imaging (MRI), stereotactic radiosurgery, and even antibiotics. Recently, a large clinical series boasted a greater than 90% complete resection rate and a 1% mortality rate, a far cry from surgical results a century ago (3–5).

This chapter begins with a brief overview of the cerebellopontine angle's anatomical relationships, with special emphasis on relevant surgical anatomy. The core of this chapter describes the clinical presentation, radiographic evaluation, and treatment of the most common cerebellopontine angle tumors: acoustic neuromas, meningiomas, epidermoids, and arachnoid cysts. The final third discusses the three surgical approaches used to resect tumors in this anatomical region.

Microsurgical Anatomy

The microsurgical anatomy of the cerebellopontine angle has been exhaustively described and catalogued by Rhoton; any surgeon hoping for success in this region should read the original landmark contributions by Rhoton and colleagues (6–8). The relevant anatomical relationships are summarized here.

OSSEOUS STRUCTURES AND VENOUS SINUSES. The posterior petrosal surface of the temporal bone defines the anterior-lateral margin of the cerebellopontine angle with its surface topography relevant to all surgical approaches to this region. The internal auditory meatus is located in the center of the posterior petrosal surface and receives the VII–VIII nerve complex, labyrinthine artery, and occasionally a loop of the anterior inferior cerebellar artery (AICA). The internal auditory canal is usually 1 cm long.

Approximately 1 cm inferior and slightly posterior to the internal auditory meatus is the jugular foramen housing the jugular bulb, which receives venous drainage anteriorly from the inferior petrosal sinus and posteriorly from the sigmoid sinus. The sigmoid sinus runs in a prominent groove along the poste-

rior margin of the petrous temporal bone, from the asterion to the jugular foramen. The inferior petrosal sinus runs in the inferior petrosal sulcus from the petrous apex along the inferior margin of the posterior petrosal surface to the jugular foramen. The superior petrosal sinus runs in the superior petrosal sulcus located along the petrosal ridge, and empties into the sigmoid-transverse junction. The operculum, where the endolymphatic sac communicates with the vestibular aqueduct, is located approximately 1 cm posterior and slightly inferior to the internal auditory meatus.

NEURAL STRUCTURES. The VII–VIII nerve complex is the major nervous structure in the cerebellopontine angle. These two cranial nerves originate from the lateral pontomedullary junction and travel anterolateral to the internal auditory meatus. The cerebellar flocculus lies just lateral to their origin at the brainstem and serves as a useful surgical landmark. Throughout its intracranial course, the VIIth cranial nerve is closely associated with the nervus intermedius, which contains the facial nerve's parasympathetic and sensory fibers. The VIIIth cranial nerve has three components, the cochlear, superior vestibular, and inferior vestibular nerves. The spatial organization of the VII–VIII nerve complex is constant at its origin (at the brainstem) and terminus (at the internal auditory canal fundus). In between these points, the organization of the VII–VIII complex is often unpredictable. At the brainstem, the VIIth cranial nerve (including the nervus intermedius) originates inferior and medial to the VIIIth nerve. The components of the VIIIth nerve originate from the brainstem with the cochlear nerve inferior, the superior vestibular nerve superior and medial, and the inferior vestibular nerve superior and lateral.

The fundus of the internal auditory canal is divided into four quadrants by a vertical bony crest (Bill's bar, named for William House who described it) and a horizontal ridge called the falciform crest. At the fundus of the canal, the VIIth nerve runs in the superior-anterior quadrant, the cochlear nerve in the inferior-anterior quadrant, the superior vestibular nerve in the superior-posterior quadrant, and the inferior vestibular nerve in the inferior-posterior quadrant.

The trigeminal nerve originates from the pons and runs laterally through the subarachnoid space of the superior cerebellopontine angle above the VII–VIII nerve complex en route to the porus trigeminus and Meckel's cave at the petrous bone apex. The petrosal vein (of Dandy) is associated with the trigeminal nerve.

Below, in the inferior portion of the cerebellopontine angle, the IXth and Xth cranial nerves originate in the postolivary sulcus and travel to the jugular foramen. Located just lateral to the IXth and Xth cranial nerves, at their origin from the brainstem, is the foramen of Luschka containing a tuft of choroid plexus protruding into the cerebellopontine angle.

ARTERIES. The AICA is the major arterial vessel in the cerebellopontine angle and the first major branch of the basilar artery. It originates at the midpontine level and travels laterally toward the cerebellopontine angle. AICA can be divided into premeatal, meatal, and postmeatal segments based on the vessel's relationship with the internal auditory meatus.

The premeatal segment passes from the origin of AICA off the basilar artery to the internal auditory meatus. The premeatal segment gives off small perforating branches to the pons. The meatal segment is the portion of the artery adjacent to the internal auditory meatus. A loop of AICA enters the internal auditory canal for a variable distance in approximately 50% of patients. AICA may be injured when the internal auditory canal is unroofed during surgery for acoustic neuromas in these cases. In the majority of patients, AICA passes inferior to the VII–VIII nerve complex *en route* to the petrosal surface of the cerebellum; therefore, it is usually displaced inferiorly by acoustic neuromas. Occasionally AICA passes superior to, or between, the VIIth and VIIIth cranial nerves. If AICA is superior, an acoustic neuroma displaces the artery superiorly, and if AICA passes between the VIIth and VIIIth nerves, an acoustic neuroma displaces AICA anteriorly. The meatal segment has three inconstant branches, the subarcuate artery, labyrinthine artery, and a recurrent brainstem perforator. The subarcuate artery enters the petrous bone at the subarcuate fossa and irrigates a portion of the bony labyrinth. The labyrinthine artery enters the internal auditory meatus and provides blood to the intracanalicular nerves and the majority of the bony labyrinth. This artery, therefore, must be preserved if hearing preservation is attempted in order to prevent ischemia of the cochlea or cochlear nerve. The third branch of the meatal segment is a recurrent perforator to the pons. This last often is found nestled just between the VIIIth nerve and facial nerve at the brainstem and can serve as a useful surgical landmark for the facial nerve (as discussed in the following in the retrosigmoid approach). The postmeatal segment heads laterally from the internal auditory meatus to irrigate the petrosal surface of the cerebellum. An exaggerated rostral loop of the posterior inferior cerebellar artery may reach the VII–VIII nerve complex in the cerebellopontine angle in some patients.

VEINS. The petrosal vein (the vein of Dandy) and its tributaries is the dominant venous structure in the cerebellopontine. The petrosal vein receives venous drainage from the pons, medulla, and petrosal surface of the cerebellum. The major, named tributaries of the petrosal vein include the medial anterior pontomedullary vein, vein of the middle cerebellar peduncle, medial anterior medullary vein, vein of the cerebellopontine fissure, and transverse pontine vein. Usually the petrosal vein is located in the upper cerebellopontine angle, lateral to the trigeminal nerve, and may appear as a complex of several small veins instead of one large vein. The petrosal vein deposits the venous drainage of the cerebellopontine angle into the superior petrosal sinus. The sacrifice of small veins draining this region usually is tolerated without neurological consequence, yet every effort is made to maintain the integrity of small bridging petrosal veins during the resection of cerebellopontine angle tumors.

Cerebellopontine Angle Tumors

Tumors of almost every type and description have been found in the cerebellopontine angle, but the surgical pathology of this region is dominated by acoustic neuromas and meningiomas. Epidermoid tumors are found here as well, although in far smaller numbers. Of course, acoustic neuroma is a misnomer, because these tumors are schwannomas of the vestibular nerves in almost all cases. The term acoustic neuroma has been so ingrained in the neurosurgical vernacular, though, that too much history is sacrificed by using the more anatomically correct term. Schwannomas of the facial nerve and even the cochlear nerve are rarely found in the cerebellopontine angle as well.

ACOUSTIC NEUROMAS. Acoustic neuromas are benign tumors arising from one of the two vestibular nerves, usually the superior one. They are the most common mass lesions in the cerebellopontine angle, representing 80% to 90% of all tumors in this area. The true incidence of acoustic neuromas is not known. In a review of 1,400 temporal bones, one postmortem investigation found the incidence of occult acoustic neuromas to be 570 per 100,000 (9). The 1991 NIH consensus statement estimated that there are 2,000 to 3,000 new cases of acoustic neuroma diagnosed in the United States each year (an incidence of 1 per 100,000) (10). Considering some may remain asymptomatic or even spontaneously regress, thus never coming to medical attention, the actual acoustic neuroma incidence is probably somewhere between these two numbers. Histologically, acoustic neuromas (schwannomas) arise from the perineural Schwann cells. Although they are predominantly sporadic tumors, those associated with neurofibromatosis type 2, an autosomal dominant syndrome characterized by bilateral acoustic neuromas, form one relatively common exception to this rule (11,12).

These tumors originate in the internal auditory canal and extend along an intracranial trajectory, compressing nearby neurovascular structures as they grow (13–15). Because of their slow growth, unilateral loss of vestibular function is readily compensated for, and the patient remains asymptomatic in that regard. The most common presentation of acoustic neuromas is unilateral hearing loss and tinnitus, with speech discrimination being affected out of proportion to pure tone loss. The facial nerve is infrequently affected, even by large tumors. The next cranial nerve that is sometimes involved is the trigeminal nerve, with patients experiencing anesthesia of the cornea. In the modern era of MRI, most tumors are diagnosed before they reach sizes sufficient to cause trigeminal neuropathy. Brainstem compression causing obstructive hydrocephalus or hemiparesis may also occur; however, the tumor is usually diagnosed and treated prior to causing these problems as well.

Acoustic neuromas are best evaluated using gadolinium-enhanced MR images (16–19). They appear hypointense on T1-weighted sequences and display robust gadolinium enhancement, with one third of cases appearing inhomogeneous (Fig. 1). Ten percent of acoustic neuromas have intratumoral cysts and/or necrosis, and occasionally these lesions hemorrhage within the tumor capsule. Acoustic neuromas are globular in shape, based within, or directly over, the internal auditory meatus. Because of their shape, they make an acute angle with the adjacent dura, unlike meningiomas, which are sessile and make an obtuse angle with the petrous pyramid dura. Acoustic neuromas usually cause a marked widening of the internal auditory meatus, whereas meningiomas generally do not, as is evident on temporal bone computed tomography (CT) scans.

There is a considerable amount of controversy surrounding the treatment of acoustic neuromas. Points of contention include: (a) microsurgery versus stereotactic radiosurgery for definitive treatment of small acoustic neuromas less than 2 to 3 cm in diameter; (b) the best approach if hearing preservation is the goal of surgery; (c) the optimal approach for larger tumors in patients with poor preoperative hearing; (d) whether mildly symptomatic intracanalicular acoustic neuromas should be observed or resected; and (e) the respective roles neuro-otologists and neurosurgeons play in the treatment of this disease. Despite these uncertainties, the current treatments for acoustic neuromas are both efficacious and safe (Table 1). Acoustic neuromas have gone from being a death sentence at the turn of the century, to being safely treated with multiple therapeutic options that concentrate on hearing preservation, sophisticated cranial base exposures with minimal brain retraction, and cranial nerve preservation and reconstruction. Optimally, an otologist and neurosurgeon should jointly manage patients, both as outpatients and during the surgical procedure. The combined expertise with skull base approaches, microsurgery, cerebrospinal fluid (CSF) leak management, and stereotactic radiosurgery allows such teams to provide comprehensive, unbiased treatment.

The goal of microsurgical treatment is complete tumor resection, including any intracanalicular component, with anatomical preservation of the facial and cochlear nerves. Total resection is not possible in rare cases, as determined by the consistency of the tumor and its adherence to the facial nerve. The surgeon may find that discretion is the better part of valor in some patients, and leaving a minimal remnant of tumor on the facial nerve is preferable to risking complete facial paralysis. It is the rare patient who escapes reoperation or radiosurgery and presents with a massive recurrence in the modern era of MR imaging with excellent visualization of any residual contrast-enhancing tumor.

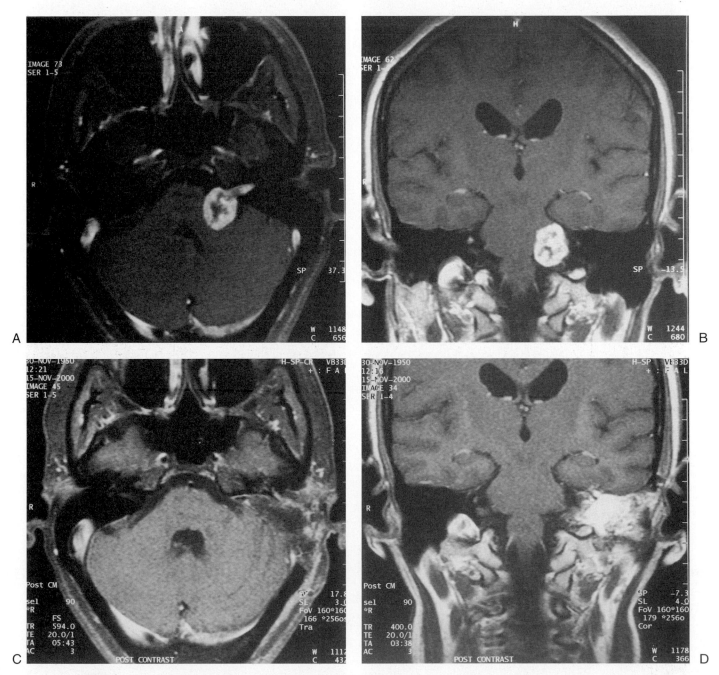

Fig. 1. The typical MRI appearance of an acoustic neuroma. This patient had no hearing remaining, and the tumor was removed using the translabyrinthine approach. Preoperative axial (**A**) and coronal (**B**) T1-weighted images postcontrast. Postoperative axial (**C**) and coronal (**D**) T1-weighted MR images postcontrast confirming complete tumor resection. *Figure continues.*

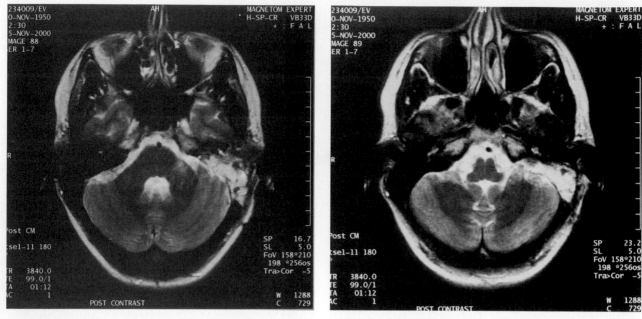

Fig. 1. *Continued.* **E,F:** Postoperative axial T2-weighted images demonstrating the extent of temporal bone removal for the translabyrinthine approach.

There are three surgical approaches used to access this region: the retrosigmoid, translabyrinthine, and middle fossa approach. The retrosigmoid and middle fossa approaches preserve hearing, and therefore are used for patients with useful hearing preoperatively. The middle fossa approach is optimal for small acoustic neuromas mostly contained within the internal auditory canal (20,21). The retrosigmoid approach is more versatile and may be used to resect most acoustic neuromas (4). The translabyrinthine approach is another surgical option for resecting acoustic neuromas (22,23). The use of this transmastoid approach is limited to patients with poor preoperative hearing because traversing the bony labyrinth causes deafness. These approaches are discussed in detail in the following.

In 1997, Madjid Samii in Hannover, Germany described his extensive experience with removing 1,000 acoustic neuromas using the retrosigmoid approach (3–5). Tumor removal was complete in 98% of cases. Anatomical cochlear nerve preservation was achieved in 68% of cases, with functional hearing preserved in 47% of patients. The facial nerve was anatomically preserved in 93% of cases, with 51% of these patients having normal facial nerve function postoperatively. In all cases, 79% had good eye closure postoperatively. He attributes this high rate of facial nerve preservation to the use of intraoperative facial nerve neurophysiological monitoring (24,25). An immedi-

ate nerve reconstruction was recommended in cases of facial nerve transection. The mortality rate for this series was 1.1%. This large, well-documented series of tumor resections provides an excellent measure of the results achievable with resection.

The neurosurgeon who is able to intelligently discuss both microsurgical resection and radiosurgery based on personal experience with both techniques presents an unbiased façade to the acoustic neuroma patient seeking guidance. Not all patients are good surgical candidates and not all patients are reasonable radiosurgery candidates. The best outcomes result from matching the proper treatment to the individual patient. Stereotactic radiosurgery should be used to treat acoustic neuromas in patients with medical conditions or advanced age precluding safe surgical extirpation. It must be understood that complete surgical resection is almost always curative, whereas radiosurgery fails to control tumor growth in 6% to 8% of cases (26,27). Prasad and associates retrospectively reviewed 153 acoustic neuromas that received stereotactic radiosurgery (27). In this series, 37% of tumors were subtotally resected. Overall, 75% of tumors mildly decreased in size, 17% remained stable, and 8% grew. The treatment morbidity included facial numbness (3%), facial weakness (2%), and progressive hearing loss (60%). Kondziolka and colleagues reported similar results in 162 consecutive patients, 25% of whom had previous surgery (26). In this series, 62% of tumors

Table 1. Treatment Outcome for Acoustic Neuromas

Study	Year	No. Patients	Mean Age (Years)	Previous Surgery (%)	Treatment Modality	Mean Diameter (mm)	Complete Removal	Tumor Control[a] (%)	Hearing Preservation (%)	Facial Weakness (%)	Mortality (%)
Samii (4)	1997	1,000	46	5.6	Surgery	29.5	97.9	99.3	39.5	49	1
Kondziolka (26)	1998	162	60	26	Gamma knife	22	0	94	51	21	0
Prasad (27)	2000	153	65	37	Gamma knife	NA[b]	0	94	60	2	0

[a] Failed tumor control is defined as posttreatment tumor growth documented with magnetic resonance imaging.
[b] Mean tumor diameter was not reported. Tumor volumes ranged from 0.02 to 18.3 cm³.

became smaller, 53% remained unchanged, and 6% grew. The morbidity rates were higher than in the previous study, with 21% of patients having facial weakness, 27% facial numbness, and 49% further hearing loss. The exact cause of morbidity following radiosurgery is not known. Post-radiosurgery cranial nerve dysfunction can be from radiation damage, progressive tumor growth, or radiation-induced tumor swelling. The long-term rate of cranial neuropathy beyond 5 years owing to radiosurgery also is unknown. An unsettled question is whether hearing remains stable in radiosurgical cases of attempted hearing preservation or whether it continues to deteriorate with time. In the series of Prasad and co-workers (27), almost all hearing changes began more than 2 years after radiosurgery and continued into the eighth postoperative year. Finally, the debate continues to rage in the literature on the risk of malignant tumor induction from the low radiation doses found in the penumbra of the radiosurgically treated target. This is a question that will be definitively settled by the passage of time. Until the answer is known, surgeons should very judiciously recommend radiation to patients who lack contraindications to surgery—a curative procedure for a histologically benign disease.

MENINGIOMAS. Meningiomas are the second most common tumor found in the cerebellopontine angle and account for approximately 5% to 15% of lesions in this region (28–32). Overall, the cerebellopontine angle is the eighth most common location for intracranial meningiomas. Meningiomas are benign, slow-growing tumors that arise from the epithelial lining of the arachnoid villae, which are sinus-based structures responsible for CSF absorption. Meningiomas of the cerebellopontine angle often grow from these arachnoid villae lining the sigmoid sinus, jugular bulb, superior petrosal sinus, and inferior petrosal sinus. A small percentage of meningiomas follow a more aggressive course, as predicted by high mitotic indices found on histopathological analysis.

In general, meningiomas of the cerebellopontine angle present with a similar clinical presentation to other mass lesions compressing neurovascular structures in this area (33). Meningiomas present with facial weakness, facial numbness, vertigo, unsteadiness, hearing loss, tinnitus, and headache. In contrast to acoustic neuromas, which frequently present with hearing loss and tinnitus, meningiomas of the cerebellopontine angle rarely cause hearing loss until the tumors become very large. Alternatively, meningiomas more commonly present with facial numbness secondary to trigeminal nerve compression. All other clinical signs and symptoms occur with equal frequency for both acoustic neuromas and meningiomas.

Preoperative MR imaging reliably differentiates acoustic neuromas from meningiomas by observing subtle radiographic findings (34,35). On T1-weighted sequences both tumors are hypointense, on T2-weighted sequences both have variable intensity, and following gadolinium administration both enhance vigorously. Acoustic neuromas are present in the internal auditory canal, are symmetrically based on the internal auditory meatus, globular in shape, and do not have a dural tail. On the other hand, meningiomas do not involve the internal auditory canal, are either anterior or posterior to the internal auditory meatus, are sessile, dural based, and have a pathognomonic dural tail (the meningeal sign). Furthermore, acoustic neuromas widen the internal auditory meatus demonstrated with temporal bone CT scans. Meningiomas do not widen the internal auditory meatus.

Meningiomas of the cerebellopontine angle are resected using either the retrosigmoid or translabyrinthine approach (31, 32,36,37). The middle fossa approach is infrequently used because meningiomas in this region are commonly large and not localized in and near the internal auditory meatus. One excep-

tion would be small petrous apex meningiomas near the trigeminal nerve, which may be resected via a middle fossa approach supplemented with an anterior petrosectomy. The retrosigmoid approach is the most common trajectory used to remove cerebellopontine angle tumors, considering useful hearing is most often present preoperatively, thus making a translabyrinthine approach contraindicated. For patients with large meningiomas and poor preoperative hearing, the translabyrinthine approach may be an option (36). Meningiomas in the cerebellopontine angle are located either anterior (premeatal) or posterior (retromeatal) to the VII–VIII complex (38). Retromeatal meningiomas are usually removed via a retrosigmoid approach, while premeatal meningiomas are optimally removed with a presigmoid transpetrosal transtentorial approach with or without sacrifice of the labyrinth depending on hearing status. When possible, 5 to 10 mm of bone beneath the meningioma is also resected to help prevent recurrence.

Voss and co-workers reported the surgical results for 40 patients with cerebellopontine angle meningiomas (32). Total tumor resection was achieved in 82% of cases. The most common morbidity was facial nerve palsies in 30% of patients following resection. Sekhar and associates removed 22 cerebellopontine angle meningiomas, with 14 patients enjoying a complete resection (37). Five patients suffered from new cranial nerve palsies postoperatively. These and other smaller clinical studies demonstrate that cerebellopontine angle meningiomas may be completely resected with acceptable morbidity.

EPIDERMOID CYSTS. Epidermoids are nonneoplastic, extraparenchymal cysts that slowly spread along normal subarachnoid cleavage planes and extend into, and occupy, multiple intracranial compartments over time (29,39). They arise from ectopic dorsal midline ectodermal cell rests from aberrant closure of the dorsal neural tube. The most common location for intracranial epidermoids is the cerebellopontine angle (40%), followed by the parasellar region. Epidermoids are the third most common tumor of the cerebellopontine angle, accounting for 5% to 9% of space-occupying lesions in this region.

Epidermoids are characterized by a protracted clinical course with a slow progression of symptoms. In the cerebellopontine angle, epidermoids usually present with a long history of hearing loss and tinnitus. Less commonly, they present with headaches, hemifacial spasm, or trigeminal neuralgia. Aseptic meningitis suddenly may occur secondary to epidermoid rupture spilling toxic keratinaceous debris into the subarachnoid space, which causes an intense inflammatory reaction. Epidermoids tend to envelop and densely adhere to cranial nerves, vascular structures, and the brainstem over time, making surgical resection hazardous.

Epidermoids are characteristically well demarcated on CT scan with irregular, scalloped margins, and frequent displacement of the brainstem and cerebellum. Epidermoids are homogeneous, hypodense, and appear similar to CSF on CT scan. Rarely epidermoids may be hyperdense or have calcified margins. On MRI, epidermoids also appear like CSF, being hypointense on T1-weighted sequences and hyperintense on T2-weighted images (40). They do not enhance with gadolinium or have a vascular blush on cerebral angiography. Considering that epidermoids have similar signal characteristics to CSF, they can be difficult to distinguish from arachnoid cysts. Heterogeneity within the lesion on MRI is more common for epidermoid than arachnoid cysts. Diffusion-weighted MR sequences establish the diagnosis, with epidermoids having a high signal intensity, easily distinguishing them from low intensity arachnoid cysts (Fig. 2).

Epidermoids of the cerebellopontine angle are best treated

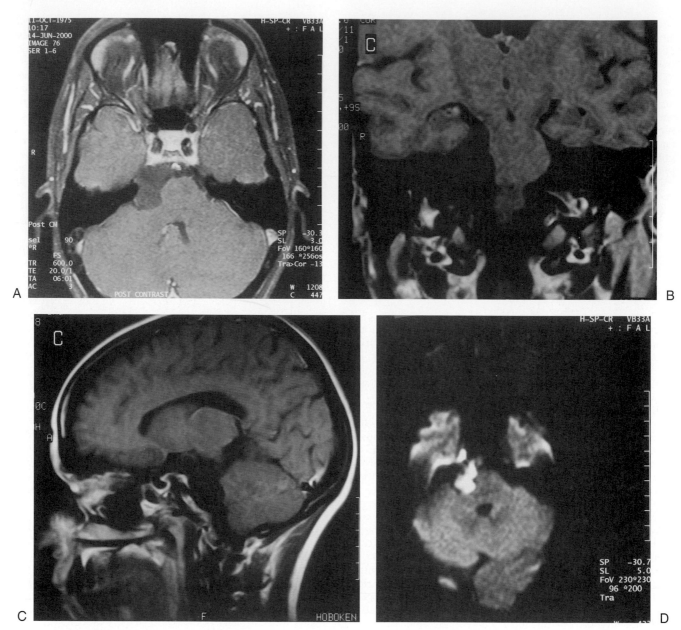

Fig. 2. A 25-year-old patient with right-sided facial numbness. The MRI is consistent with an epidermoid tumor. Because of its extent, this tumor was resected via a retrolabyrinthine transpetrosal transtentorial approach. Preoperative axial **(A)**, coronal **(B)**, and sagittal **(C)** T1-weighted MR-images postcontrast. **D:** High signal intensity on an axial diffusion-weighted MR image clinches the diagnosis of epidermoid. *Figure continues.*

with complete surgical resection of the cyst capsule with meticulous removal of all keratinaceous debris. Complete resection is not possible in up to 50% of cases because epidermoids encase vital neurovascular structures, and in some instances provoke a granulomatous reaction causing adhesions. Considering epidermoids accumulate debris slowly, partial resection may be therapeutic for more than a decade. Sacrificing cranial nerves to achieve a complete resection, therefore, is not warranted. Patients should be placed on prophylactic high-dose steroids following epidermoid resection to prevent aseptic meningitis from intraoperative spillage of keratinaceous debris.

Mohanty and colleagues reported the clinical outcome of 25 epidermoids of the cerebellopontine angle that were surgically resected (41). The lesions were completely resected in 12, nearly resected in eight, and partially resected in five patients.

They aggressively dissected the adherent capsule from the involved neurovascular structures. Eleven patients experienced significant cranial nerve dysfunction postoperatively, with some improvement over time. They concluded that a more conservative approach is indicated for patients in whom the epidermoid capsule is adherent to the brainstem and cranial nerves. Samii and co-workers reported their surgical results for 40 consecutive cerebellopontine angle epidermoid cysts (39). Thirty epidermoids (75%) were completely resected. Only 40% of patients were in excellent condition on discharge, with this postoperative result improving to 93% at 6-month follow-up.

ARACHNOID CYSTS. Arachnoid cysts are abnormal CSF collections in the subarachnoid space thought to be developmental

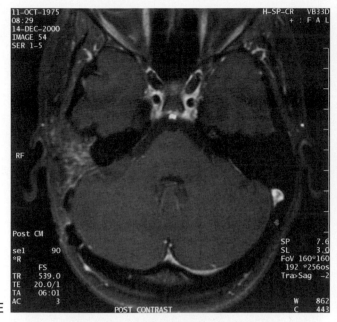
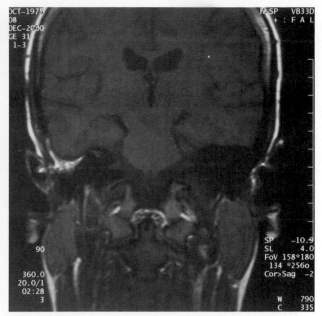

Fig. 2. *Continued.* Postoperative axial (**E**) and coronal (**F**) T1-weighted images confirm complete tumor resection and demonstrate the intact labyrinth.

in origin (29,42). Other etiologies have been proposed, including trauma, arachnoiditis, subarachnoid hemorrhage, and meningitis. Although some arachnoid cysts communicate with their adjacent subarachnoid cisterns, others become disconnected and grow, causing progressive, symptomatic compression of surrounding neural structures. The cerebellopontine angle is the second most common location for an arachnoid cyst, second only to the Sylvian fissure. Most arachnoid cysts are asymptomatic, and when they become symptomatic they often present in early childhood.

Cerebellopontine angle arachnoid cysts have a similar clinical presentation to other mass lesions in this region, including hearing loss, tinnitus, vertigo, and unsteadiness. Rarely arachnoid cysts cause raised intracranial pressure secondary to obstructive hydrocephalus. Arachnoid cysts can produce vague, intermittent neurological symptoms, causing a delay between symptom onset and diagnosis. With a fluctuating clinical course, patients with arachnoid cysts are often misdiagnosed with multiple sclerosis.

Arachnoid cysts have the same imaging qualities as CSF on CT scan and MRI. They do not enhance and are often indistinguishable from epidermoids on conventional T1- and T2-weighted sequences. The diagnosis of arachnoid cyst is made using diffusion-weighted MR images, because unlike epidermoids, arachnoid cysts have low signal intensity on these sequences, as pointed out in the preceding.

The vast majority of arachnoid cysts are asymptomatic and do not require surgical treatment. Arachnoid cysts should be decompressed or resected when symptoms become severe, progressive, or if increased intracranial pressure is present. Surgical options include complete cyst resection, a wide fenestration communicating the cyst cavity with the basal cisterns, and cyst-to-peritoneum shunt placement. Corticosteroids and diuretics may provide a temporary relief of symptoms in some patients. Jallo and co-workers reported the clinical outcome of five patients who received wide fenestration of their cerebellopontine angle arachnoid cysts through a retrosigmoid approach (42). Although one patient underwent two procedures, all five patients had symptom resolution following fenestration. They

reported no clinical or radiographic recurrence, with a mean follow-up of 5 years.

OTHER TUMORS. Although acoustic neuromas, meningiomas, epidermoids, and arachnoid cysts represent most tumors in the cerebellopontine angle, a laundry list of more obscure pathologic processes also occur in this region (43). These rare lesions may be incorrectly diagnosed and treated as acoustic neuromas. They include: lipomas (44), metastatic tumors (45–47), choroid plexus papillomas (48), basilar artery ectasia (49), arachnoiditis (50), hamartomas (51), plasmacytomas (52), angiomas (53), aneurysms (54), salivary gland heterotopias (55), craniopharyngiomas (56), granulomatous abscesses (57), pneumocephalus (58), amyloidomas (59), mixed gliomas (60), exophytic glioblastomas (61), teratomas (62), triton tumors (63), sarcomas (64), lymphoma (65), hemangioblastomas (66), cavernomas (67), paragangliomas (68), chordomas (69), neuroblastomas (70), primitive neuroectodermal tumors (71), fibromatosis (72), medulloblastomas (73), Ramsey-Hunt syndrome (74), thrombosed vertebral arteries (75), rhabdomyoma (76), disseminated pituitary adenoma (77), papillary adenomas of the endolymphatic duct (78), ependymomas (79), sarcoidosis (80), germinomas (81), ceruminomas(82), and Hodgkin's disease (83). Radiologists with poor experience in neuro-oncology may incorrectly identify any mass lesion near the cerebellopontine angle as an acoustic neuroma (Fig. 3).

Surgical Approaches

The surgical approaches for cerebellopontine angle tumors are virtually the same regardless of the tumor pathology. Approach selection is governed by the factors discussed in the preceding, primarily hearing status, tumor size, and medial extent of the tumor. Creatures of habit that they are, surgeons always have

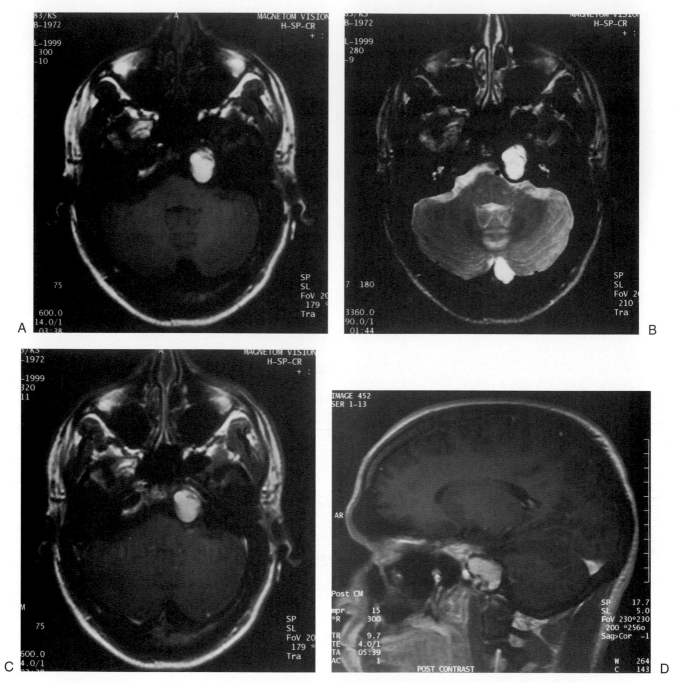

Fig. 3. This MRI scan was interpreted by a radiologist as showing an acoustic neuroma despite the fact that the lesion is entirely contained within the petrous apex. Careful examination of the MRI shows the lesion is hyperintense on both T1- and T2-weighted images. The lesion was a symptomatic petrous apex cholesterol cyst that was resected via a middle fossa approach. Preoperative axial T1-weighted **(A)** and T2-weighted **(B)** MR images revealed a high intensity lesion in the left petrous apex prior to contrast administration. Preoperative axial **(C)** and sagittal **(D)** T1-weighted MR images postcontrast. *Figure continues.*

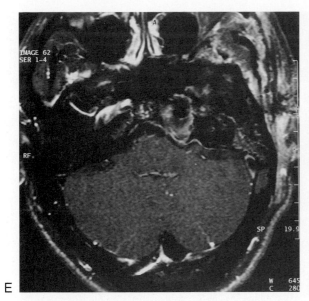
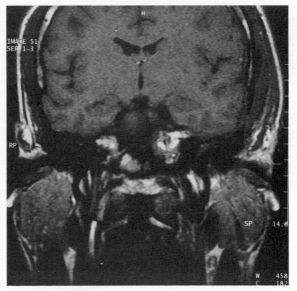

Fig. 3. *Continued.* No contrast enhancement was present. Postoperative axial (**E**) and coronal (**F**) T1-weighted MR images postcontrast. Postoperative blood products were present in the resection cavity.

their personal preferences and should use the approach with which they personally achieve the best results (21,84,85).

RETROSIGMOID APPROACH. The retrosigmoid craniotomy is by far the workhorse of surgical approaches to the posterior fossa (4). Its popularity results from two main advantages: hearing preservation and a direct view along the posterior face of the petrous pyramid all the way to the midline. The retrosigmoid craniotomy is an extension of the classic suboccipital craniectomy, and as such, is the oldest approach to the cerebellopontine angle (1). By moving the craniotomy flush against the sigmoid sinus, the surgeon obtains the greatest access to the cerebellopontine angle with a direct view of the choroid plexus in the foramen of Luschka. This approach has been in use long enough that most surgeons have their own technical idiosyncrasies. A unifying characteristic of all these operative nuances is emphasis on exposing the dura right up to the sigmoid sinus.

Nowhere is it truer that there are many ways to skin a cat than in the variations of the retrosigmoid approach. Patient positioning is the first point of departure and bone of contention. Some surgeons with vast experience swear by the sitting position, whereas others condemn it for its torturous effects on the surgeon's shoulders and neck (4,86–88). Potentially disastrous complications of the sitting position, such as air embolism and compartment syndrome, are well described (89,90). For these reasons, we have favored the supine position with the patient's head turned at our institution (87). For larger patients, especially obese patients with short, bull-like necks, in whom we suspect jugular venous outflow may be compromised with head rotation, we use a lateral recumbent position with minimal rotation of the neck. For acoustic neuroma removal, we rarely use three-point head fixation. For particularly large tumors, and for transpetrosal-transtentorial approaches, we use three-point head fixation with the patient supine and head turned. A bolster placed under the ipsilateral shoulder reduces neck rotation, relieving compression of the contralateral jugular vein.

Skin incisions show the same variability as does patient positioning. Some surgeons prefer the classic lazy S incision behind the ear, and many surgeons continue to use a straight incision. We have had good success with an inferiorly based horseshoe

incision behind the ear. The anterior limb is along the posterior border of the pinna down to the mastoid tip. The posterior limb is placed 4 cm posteriorly, with the superior edge of the flap reaching the top of the pinna. A separate periosteal flap is raised, and reapproximated at the end of the procedure to hold the fat graft in place.

Exposing the sigmoid sinus and sigmoid transverse junction completely with a partial mastoidectomy provides several benefits (86,87). First, no burr hole is necessary because the footplate of the drill can be placed directly under the bone at the transverse sigmoid junction. A 2.5-cm circular craniotomy that extends to the transverse and sigmoid sinuses can be turned with replacement of the bone flap at the end of the procedure with no need for a cranioplasty. Second, all large mastoid air cells are exposed and can be more easily obliterated with a fat graft and fibrin glue to reduce the incidence of spinal fluid leak. Third, the dural opening can extend exactly to the edge of the transverse and sigmoid sinuses providing maximal anterior exposure (Fig. 4). Last, the sigmoid sinus itself can be gently retracted anteriorly with the dural flap to augment this anterior exposure. We have used a single, triangular dural flap based against the sigmoid sinus. A small 2-mm hole drilled through the wall of the external auditory canal provides excellent anchorage for a tack-up suture that gently displaces the dural flap and sigmoid sinus anteriorly.

The cerebellum is almost always full on opening the dura, except in particularly thin individuals. Hyperventilation and reverse Trendelenburg positioning relieves any cerebellar fullness and allow for a small dural opening. Mannitol can be administered if necessary for further relaxation. The microscope is brought into the operative field and Telfa strips are placed over the cerebellum for protection. Using the bipolar and a gentle 7F suction, the cerebellum can be lifted superiorly and slightly posteriorly to expose the cistern over the lower cranial nerves and lateral-most extension of the cisterna magna. Puncture of the arachnoid with either the microbipolar or small arachnoid knife results in immediate and gratifying release of spinal fluid and complete relaxation of the cerebellar hemisphere. No further retraction is necessary on the cerebellum for the remainder of the procedure and no retractor blades are used at any time. Occasionally, in large and particularly bloody

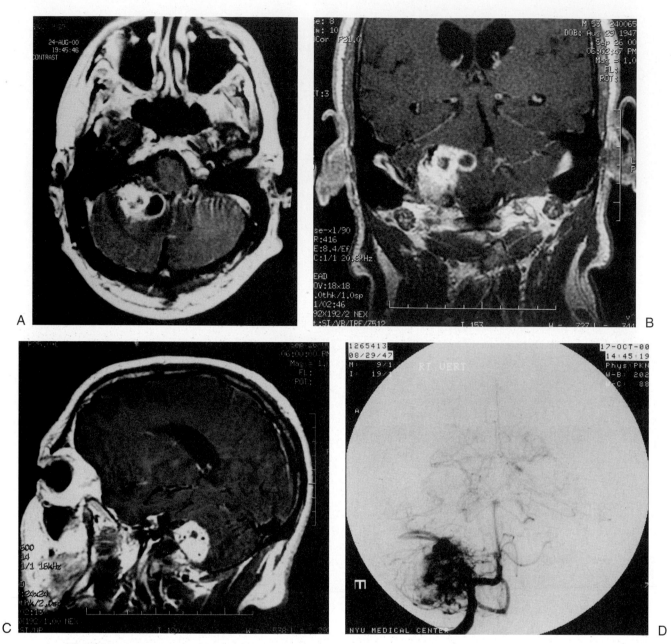

Fig. 4. This 53-year-old patient presented with gait instability, dysphagia, and headaches. Radiographic workup demonstrated a right-sided hemangioblastoma in the cerebellopontine angle. It was resected via a retrosigmoid approach following preoperative polyvinyl alcohol embolization. Preoperative axial **(A)**, coronal **(B)**, and sagittal **(C)** T1-weighted MR images postcontrast. **D–F:** Preoperative cerebral angiography. *Figure continues.*

tumors, the surgeon may find that the cerebellum appears once again full, protruding sufficiently to obscure the previously wide exposure. A quick examination usually reveals the culprit to be coagulated blood obstructing the CSF pathways. Removal of this blood results in a second release of CSF and further relaxation of the cerebellum.

In order to effect a complete resection of an acoustic neuroma or meningioma that has entered the internal auditory canal, it is mandatory to drill the posterior petrous ridge over the posterior lip of the internal auditory canal. This exposes the lateral canal and any contained tumor. Whether this step is performed before or after dissection of the tumor from the brainstem is a matter of personal choice, although completing the drilling first has advantages. Drilling the posterior canal wall first provides

a complete view of the tumor and allows access to both the medial and lateral ends of the facial nerve from the start (88). To achieve this exposure, the dura on the posterior face of the petrous ridge lateral to the porus acusticus is incised in a fashion to create two flaps resembling "saloon doors," which can be reapproximated at the end of the procedure. These dural flaps are further retracted with a microcurette. The exposed bone is the drilled away using successively smaller burrs to expose the dura of the internal auditory canal.

Much has been written about individual microsurgical techniques in dissection of acoustic neuromas and other cerebellopontine angle tumors (7,91–93). The unifying characteristic of successful dissection in this region is a thorough knowledge of the complex anatomy and spatial relationship of the cranial

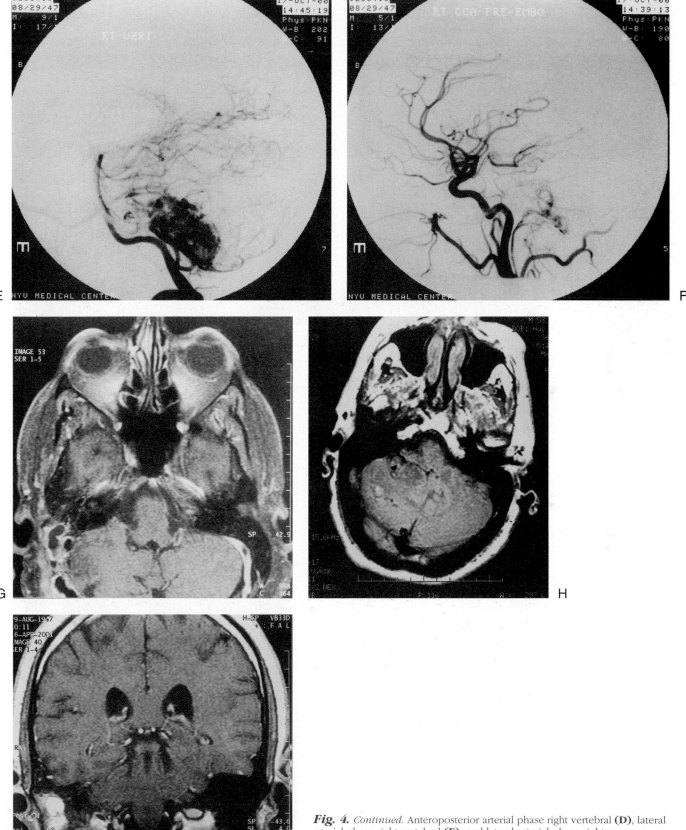

Fig. 4. *Continued.* Anteroposterior arterial phase right vertebral **(D)**, lateral arterial phase right vertebral **(E)**, and lateral arterial phase right common carotid **(F)** injections revealed extensive tumor vascularity and blood supply from the external carotid artery via the ascending pharyngeal artery. Postoperative axial **(G,H)** and coronal **(I)** T1-weighted MR images postcontrast confirming complete tumor resection.

nerves to the tumor (6). Sampath and associates (92) studied over 1,000 acoustic neuroma resections, striving to identify reliable landmarks for the position of the facial and cochlear nerves in the presence of acoustic neuromas. The facial nerve was displaced anteriorly in almost 80% of cases with a true posterior location of the nerve occurring rarely (92). This should not be surprising because these tumors originate from the vestibular nerves, which lie posterior to the facial nerve in the canal. Fortunately, less than 2% of tumors have the facial nerve lying on their posterior surface, creating a difficult problem in dissection. The surgeon should be attuned to the fact that the facial nerve must travel from its brainstem origin inferior to the eighth nerve root entry zone to end in a superior position in the internal auditory canal. This means that the facial nerve occasionally loops around the inferior or superior poles of the tumor where it is vulnerable to injury early in the dissection process. In the series of Sampath and colleagues, the facial nerve was encountered at the superior pole in 14% of cases, regardless of tumor size. Rhoton points out a useful anatomical detail (8): the facial nerve at the brainstem can be found by following the ninth cranial nerve back to its medullary junction. The facial nerve exits the brainstem at a point 2 to 3 mm superior to the entry of the glossopharyngeal nerve along an imaginary line that connects the lower cranial nerve rootlets at their junction with the pontomedullary sulcus (8). The eighth nerve root entry zone is a prominent landmark when it is identified. The facial nerve lays a few millimeters medial to the eighth nerve entry zone separated by a small, unnamed branch of the anterior inferior cerebellar artery that is a recurrent perforator from the meatal segment. When this small artery is recognized, the facial nerve entry zone is found just on its medial side. Once the facial nerve is identified at the brainstem, its lateral end can be found in the internal auditory canal by rolling the tumor medially. With both ends of the facial nerve identified, the dissection proceeds with the projected course of the nerve in mind.

Preservation of the facial nerve requires patience and persistence. Most surgeons agree that the first step in preserving the cranial nerves is converting a large tumor to a small one by debulking the interior of the tumor with a dissector or ultrasonic aspirator (4,5,7,88). The tumor capsule can then be folded in on itself and used as a handle to free the tumor from the brainstem and cranial nerves. The newest ultrasonic aspirators feature multiple vibration/power settings and small tips useful even for intracanalicular tumors. Occasionally in small tumors it is possible to roll the tumor off the nerve en bloc without causing undue tension on the nerve. Some surgeons have even promoted this technique for tumors up to 25 mm in diameter (94). The most difficult dissection always occurs at the level of the porus acusticus, where the nerves are most attenuated and in greatest danger of inadvertent transection (5,88,95). Intraoperative monitoring and stimulation of the facial nerve are tools that have radically improved facial nerve preservation rates (96, 97). The stimulating probe can readily identify the thinned out fibers of the facial nerve and differentiate them from adjacent vestibular nerve fibers. The stimulating probe at times can be used as a fine dissector along the facial nerve, although care must be taken to avoid overstimulation of the nerve. At the end of the resection, comparing the response amplitudes of the facial nerve at its lateral and then medial ends is predictive of postoperative facial nerve function (98,99). The threshold for stimulation of the nerve at the brainstem seems to have predictive value in patients with good immediate postoperative facial function (100,101).

Preservation of the cochlear nerve provides an even greater challenge (87,102–106). The cochlear nerve is particularly intolerant of stretch or distortion of any kind. Monitoring of the cochlear nerve is more difficult and less reliable than facial nerve monitoring (25,107–112). Direct monitoring of compound action potentials from the nerve itself, via a small electrode, can be rewarding at times and quite frustrating at other times (113). The electrode may move and electrical noise in the operating room may confound the recordings. On occasion the small electrode may record a contralateral far field response when there is no compound action potential in the cochlear nerve of interest. Moreover, there are few corrective measures to take when there is a change in either the far field or direct nerve action potential recording. Some surgeons administer papaverine topically on the nerve in hopes of reversing ischemia, although it is not clear if this is beneficial (114). Generally, stopping the dissection and gentle warm irrigation helps the auditory potentials recover. Most surgeons eschew bipolar cautery as much as possible in hearing preservation cases in hopes that blood supply to the cochlear nerve and cochlea itself will be maintained (3,4). The best hope for hearing preservation lies in identifying the cochlear nerve on the anteroinferior surface of the tumor early in the dissection. Larger tumors generally distort the cochlear nerve to such a degree that achieving reasonable rates of hearing preservation is not possible, although it is possible occasionally to preserve hearing in tumors up to 2.5 cm. Fahlbusch, on the other hand, reported hearing preservation rates of 23.5% in patients with tumors greater than 3 cm (including the canalicular portion) and recordable ipsilateral brainstem auditory evoked responses (BAERs) (115). These excellent results not withstanding, most authors agree that tumor size is a significant predictor of hearing preservation (116–118).

The surgeon must perform a meticulous closure after tumor resection. The risk of CSF leak is underappreciated following the retrosigmoid approach (119–122). A thorough and complete exposure of the internal auditory canal will often expose perimeatal air cells that may be difficult to occlude. Surgeons who do not routinely perform a partial mastoidectomy must take special pains to insure a watertight dural closure to prevent leakage into mastoid air cells near the sigmoid sinus. A fat graft placed in the IAC will help obliterate any exposed air cells. The dural flaps, or "saloon doors," are closed and sutured with one or two interrupted sutures. Fibrin glue, autologous or otherwise, helps secure the fat graft in place. The dura is sutured in a watertight fashion using a graft of temporalis fascia as necessary to bridge gaps in the suture line. Fibrin glue is deposited over the suture line and the bone is replaced with titanium miniplates for a rigid fixation. Fat is placed into the partial mastoidectomy cavity and the periosteal flap is reapproximated to hold the fat in place. Patients are awakened in the operating room so that a neurological examination can be performed.

TRANSLABYRINTHINE AND RETROLABYRINTHINE APPROACHES. William House stunned the neurosurgical world and encountered stiff resistance in 1964 when he presented a series of acoustic neuromas resected via transtemporal approaches, including the translabyrinthine approach (123). The translabyrinthine approach, however, has stood the test of time and remains an important part of the cerebellopontine angle surgeon's arsenal (22,23,36,124,125). The translabyrinthine approach, as the name indicates, obliterates the labyrinth en route to exposing the tumor, and of necessity destroys whatever residual hearing the patient may have. For this reason, and because of a perceived small exposure, many neurosurgeons have only utilized a translabyrinthine approach for patients with poor hearing and a small tumor. Properly executed, however, the translabyrinthine approach is the archetype of a "keyhole surgery." This surgical technique relies on the close cooperation of a neurosurgeon and a neuro-otologist. Proper drilling of the petrous bone by the neuro-otologist provides the neurosurgeon with more than enough room to remove even the largest tumors (23,125). This approach has the advantage of exposing the facial nerve laterally in the internal auditory canal at the beginning of the procedure. Additionally, the more anterior exposure, compared with the retrosigmoid approach, obviates the need for cerebellar retraction and provides a better view of the brainstem posteriorly, to the point where the foramen of Luschka can be visualized and used for insertion of brainstem auditory implants. The main disadvantage of the translabyrinthine approach is the higher incidence of CSF leak (23,126–128). In experienced hands, the translabyrinthine approach probably affords a higher chance of facial nerve preservation owing to the improved visualization of the lateral end of the nerve, although no study has proven this. The technical details of petrous bone drilling are extensively covered in several sources (22). Once the drilling is complete, the dura is opened from the lateral internal auditory canal out to the sigmoid sinus with a

perpendicular T incision. The technique of intradural dissection then becomes virtually identical to the retrosigmoid approach, except for more movement of the patient and microscope in order to take advantage of the keyhole exposure. Prevention of CSF leak involves reapproximation of the two dural flaps and a fat graft to obliterate any rents in the dura or open-air cells (121,129).

The translabyrinthine approach can be extended to a transcochlear approach that allows direct vision to the basilar artery at the midline in cases of particularly large tumors with extension to the midline. In our institution, we modify this approach so that the facial nerve is not translocated, the dissection occurring posterior and if necessary anterior to the intact nerve (Fig. 5). On the other hand, small tumors, including meningiomas of the posterior petrous face, can be approached through a

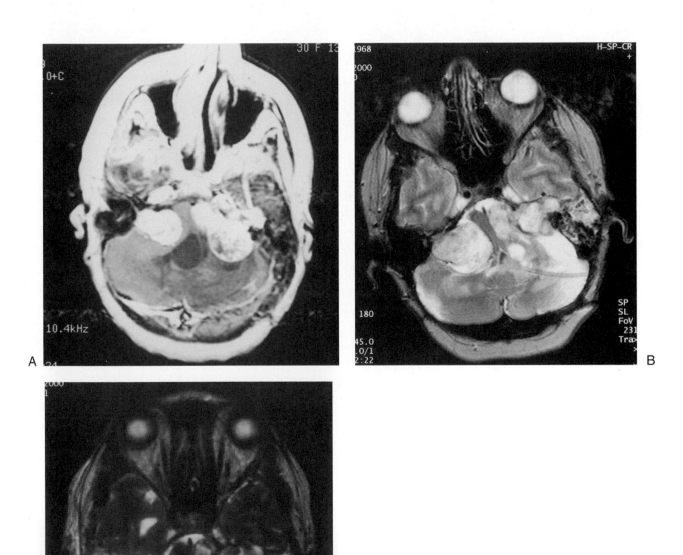

Fig. 5. The classic bilateral acoustic neuromas of neurofibromatosis type 2 in a 32-year-old patient. The right-sided acoustic neuroma was resected via a transcochlear approach. Preoperative axial postcontrast T1-weighted **(A)** and T2-weighted **(B)** MR images. **C:** Postoperative axial T2-weighted MR image demonstrating the amount of temporal bone removed during a transcochlear approach. The left-sided tumor was removed at a later date.

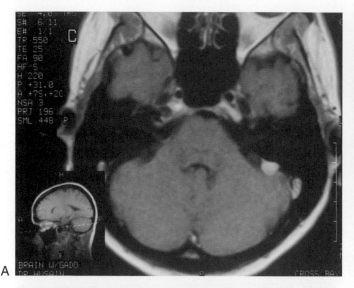

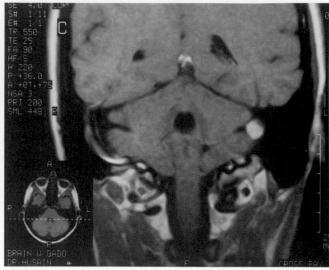

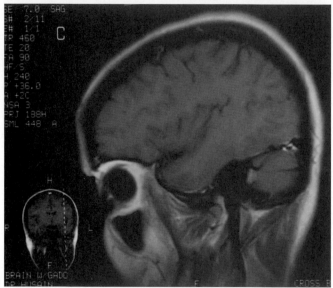

Fig. 6. This 35-year-old patient presented with intermittent vertigo. Radiographic evaluation revealed a left-sided meningioma near the endolymphatic sac. This tumor was resected through a retrolabyrinthine approach. Preoperative axial **(A)**, coronal **(B)**, and sagittal **(C)** T1-weighted MR images postcontrast.

retrolabyrinthine approach (Fig. 6). This is a presigmoid approach in which the labyrinth is left intact. The exposure is limited, but this is a relatively noninvasive avenue to resect small tumors (130). The poor exposure of the lateral end of the internal auditory canal makes this an infrequently utilized exposure in acoustic neuroma surgery (131). It is well suited for small lesions that are easily resected, such as arachnoid cysts or small epidermoid tumors. The surgeon who is comfortable with both presigmoid and retrosigmoid approaches is able to use them in a complementary fashion for reoperation or recurrences. If the initial approach was retrosigmoid, then a translabyrinthine approach for reoperation avoids scarring and obscuration of key anatomical landmarks (132).

MIDDLE FOSSA. Evolving imaging techniques have allowed early diagnosis of acoustic neuromas smaller than 5 mm. This has greatly expanded the range of candidates for hearing preservation operations to include those with small, wholly intracanalicular tumors. William House also introduced an approach through the middle fossa to the superior aspect of the internal auditory canal for acoustic neuroma resection in addition to

setting the neurosurgical world on its ear with the translabyrinthine approach (123) (Fig. 7). The middle fossa approach has steadily gained favor because it is associated with superior rates of hearing preservation (20,21,85,84,133,134). Unfortunately, all direct comparisons to date of the retrosigmoid and middle fossa approaches have been retrospective in nature and therefore complicated by learning effects and surgeons' bias. Nonetheless, investigators have shown higher hearing preservation rates for the middle fossa approach, especially for wholly intracanalicular tumors. Some have promoted the middle fossa approach as providing a greater exposure of the internal auditory canal fundus, but studies have not clearly supported this contention (20,135). Many surgeons remain married to a retrosigmoid approach, even for intracanalicular tumors (3,136), and hints of increased rates of facial nerve injury owing to the extensive drilling in and around the facial nerve during the middle fossa approach support this viewpoint (21,134).

We use the middle fossa approach at our institution for wholly intracanalicular tumors where hearing preservation is the goal. The patient is placed supine on the operating table with the head turned toward the contralateral side, almost completely lateral. A small pillow under the ipsilateral shoulder pre-

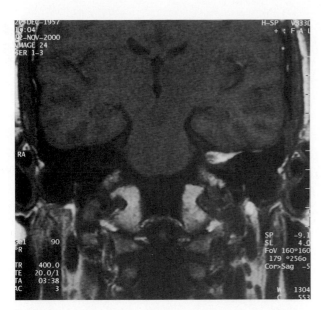

Fig. 7. This 43-year-old patient had a small left-sided intracanalicular acoustic neuroma resected via the middle fossa approach. The postoperative coronal T1-weighted MR image demonstrates the amount of temporal bone removed superior to the internal auditory canal via this approach. This is evidenced by the amount of fat graft located on the medial left petrous ridge above the unroofed internal auditory canal.

vents excessive torsion of the neck and obstruction of venous outflow. We have not used three-point head fixation except for large tumors that require an extended middle fossa approach. A small question mark incision is made beginning just in front of and above the tragus, extending posteriorly over the pinna and then 5 cm superiorly, where it turns anteriorly and ends well short of the hairline. The skin flap is dissected free of the temporalis muscle, which is brought down as a separate flap. The bone flap is centered two thirds in front of the external auditory meatus and one third behind. The craniotome is used to turn a rectangular bone flap 4.5 cm wide and 5.5 cm tall. Tack-up sutures are placed at the periphery of the bone flap superiorly, leaving the inferior dura without tack-up sutures until the closure. The brain is relaxed with the intravenous administration of moderate doses of mannitol and furosemide. The dura is dissected off the middle fossa floor with the facial nerve monitor functional to prevent injury to the geniculate ganglion. We prefer to transect the middle meningeal artery at the foramen spinosum in almost all cases to allow greater mobilization of the dura. The arcuate eminence and greater superficial petrosal nerve provide relatively constant landmarks pointing toward the more medial meatal plane, a triangular, flat area of bone over the medial internal auditory canal. The Sterkers middle fossa retractor is fixed in position and the retractor blade placed on the temporal lobe extradurally. The tip of the retractor blade is gently wedged into position at the tip of the petrous ridge in the superior petrosal sulcus where the superior petrosal sinus reaches its medial extent. This provides excellent exposure of the bone covering the internal auditory canal. As much bone as possible is removed to fully expose the internal auditory canal without damage to the cochlea or semicircular canals. The dura then is opened on the posterior portion of the canal to avoid damaging the facial nerve.

Dissection techniques are the same as for the other approaches except that it is often possible to use an en bloc technique with very small tumors. Surgeons accustomed to the retrosigmoid approach have to reorient their view of the nerves

in the canal, realizing that the facial nerve now lies directly anterior to, or almost on top of, the tumor. The stimulating probe aids in identifying the cleavage plane between the facial nerve and superior vestibular nerve. If the tumor is of superior vestibular nerve origin, this plane is often obvious, with only wisps of the remaining superior vestibular nerve being present. If the tumor is of inferior vestibular nerve origin, then the superior vestibular nerve first must be transected to give access to the tumor. The tumor is gently dissected free from the undersurface of the facial nerve and rolled out of the canal from anterior to posterior. The cochlear nerve is then usually found displaced anteriorly in the canal and preserved. Some authors have promoted medial to lateral dissection rather than lateral to medial dissection to prevent traction on cochlear nerve fibers (8,21). Often it seems that the tumor determines the best avenue of dissection. Monitoring of the brainstem auditory evoked responses and direct recording of compound action potentials from the cochlear nerve are always used in these cases. Closure involves replacing the dural flap gently over the facial nerve. A small fat graft is placed over the internal auditory canal. The retractor is removed and the brain allowed to settle into place. The remaining dural tack-up sutures are placed and the bone flap replaced with titanium miniplates. The temporalis muscle is reapproximated and the skin closed in layers. We do not use lumbar drains or subgaleal wound drainage.

Familiarity with the three major approaches for cerebellopontine angle tumor resection affords the surgeon with the greatest range of options. We have developed the following treatment paradigm in our institution using these approaches. For nonacoustic tumors where hearing is usually intact, the retrosigmoid approach is used. For acoustic tumors where hearing preservation is attempted, the middle fossa approach is used, unless the cisternal portion of the tumor is greater than 9 mm in diameter or the patient is elderly. In all other hearing preservation cases, the retrosigmoid approach is used. For patients without useful hearing, the translabyrinthine approach is used almost without regard to tumor size. For particularly large tumors, a transcochlear approach or even a transpetrosal-transtentorial approach is used.

In the final analysis, the surgical approach used is not so important as the close working relationship between the neurosurgeon and the neuro-otologist. The existence of a tightly knit acoustic neuroma team benefits all patients with cerebellopontine angle pathology (137–139).

References

1. Ramsden RT. The bloody angle: 100 years of acoustic neuroma surgery. *J Roy Soc Med* 1995;88:464P–468P.
2. Krause F. Zur freilegung der hinteren felsenbeinflache und des kleinhorns. *Beitr Klin Chir* 903;37:728–764.
3. Samii M, Matthies C. Management of 1000 vestibular schwannomas (acoustic neuromas): hearing function in 1000 tumor resection. *Neurosurgery* 1997;40:248–260; discussion 260–262.
4. Samii M, Matthies C. Management of 1000 vestibular schwannomas (acoustic neuromas): surgical management and results with an emphasis on complications and how to avoid them. *Neurosurgery* 1997;40:11–21; discussion 21–23.
5. Samii M, Matthies C. Management of 1000 vestibular schwannomas (acoustic neuromas): the facial nerve—preservation and restitution of function. *Neurosurgery* 1997;40:684–694; discussion 694–695.
6. Rhoton AL Jr. Microsurgical anatomy of the posterior fossa cranial nerves. *Clin Neurosurg* 1979;26:398–462.
7. Rhoton AL Jr, Tedeschi H. Lateral approaches to the cerebellopontine angle and petroclival region (honored guest lecture). *Clin Neurosurg* 1994;41:517–545.

8. Rhoton AL Jr, Tedeschi H. Microsurgical anatomy of acoustic neuromas. *Otolaryngol Clin North Am* 1992;25:257–294.

9. Schuknecht H. Pathology of vestibular schwannoma (acoustic neuroma). In: Silverstein H, Norell H, eds. *Neurological surgery of the ear.* Birmingham, UK: Aesculapius, 1977:193–197.

10. NIH consensus statement. 1991;9:1–24.

11. Baldwin D, King TT, Chevretton E, et al. Bilateral cerebellopontine angle tumors in neurofibromatosis type 2. *J Neurosurg* 1991;74: 910–915.

12. Bikhazi NB, Slattery WH 3rd, Lalwani AK, et al. Familial occurrence of unilateral vestibular schwannoma. *Laryngoscope* 1997;107: 1176–1180.

13. Matthies C, Samii M. Management of 1000 vestibular schwannomas (acoustic neuromas): clinical presentation. *Neurosurgery* 1997;40: 1–9; discussion 9–10.

14. Rosenberg SI. Natural history of acoustic neuromas. *Laryngoscope* 2000;110:497–508.

15. van Leeuwen JP, Cremers CW, Thewissen NP, et al. Acoustic neuroma: correlation among tumor size, symptoms, and patient age. *Laryngoscope* 1995;105:701–707.

16. Curati WL, Graif M, Kingsley DP, et al. Acoustic neuromas: Gd-DTPA enhancement in MR imaging. *Radiology* 1986;158:447–451.

17. Held P, Fellner C, Seitz J, et al. The value of T2(*)-weighted MR images for the diagnosis of acoustic neuromas. *Eur J Radiol* 1999; 30:237–244.

18. Mawhinney RR, Buckley JH, Worthington BS. Magnetic resonance imaging of the cerebello-pontine angle. *Br J Radiol* 1986;59: 961–969.

19. Sheppard IJ, Milford CA, Anslow P. MRI in the detection of acoustic neuromas—a suggested protocol for screening. *Clin Otolaryngol Allied Sci* 1996;21:301–304.

20. Haberkamp TJ, Meyer GA, Fox M. Surgical exposure of the fundus of the internal auditory canal: anatomical limits of the middle fossa versus the retrosigmoid transcanal approach. *Laryngoscope* 1998; 108:1190–1194.

21. Slattery WH 3rd, Brackmann DE, Hitselberger W. Middle fossa approach for hearing preservation with acoustic neuromas. *Am J Otol* 1997;18:596–601. [Published erratum appears in *Am J Otol* 1997; 18:796.]

22. Glasscock ME, Hays JW. The translabyrinthine removal of acoustic and other cerebellopontine angle tumors. *Ann Otol Rhinol Laryngol* 1973;82:415–427.

23. Lanman TH, Brackmann DE, Hitselberger WE, et al. Report of 190 consecutive cases of large acoustic tumors (vestibular schwannoma) removed via the translabyrinthine approach. *J Neurosurg* 1999;90:617–623.

24. Matthies C, Samii M. Management of vestibular schwannomas (acoustic neuromas): the value of neurophysiology for evaluation and prediction of auditory function in 420 cases. *Neurosurgery* 1997;40:919–929; discussion 929–930.

25. Matthies C, Samii M. Management of vestibular schwannomas (acoustic neuromas): the value of neurophysiology for intraoperative monitoring of auditory function in 200 cases. *Neurosurgery* 1997;40:459–466; discussion 466–468.

26. Kondziolka D, Lunsford LD, McLaughlin MR, et al. Long-term outcomes after radiosurgery for acoustic neuromas [see comments]. *N Engl J Med* 1998;339:1426–1433.

27. Prasad D, Steiner M, Steiner L. Gamma surgery for vestibular schwannoma [see comments]. *J Neurosurg* 2000;92:745–759.

28. Laird FJ, Harner SG, Laws ER Jr, et al. Meningiomas of the cerebellopontine angle. *Otolaryngol Head Neck Surg* 1985;93:163–167.

29. Lalwani AK. Meningiomas, epidermoids, and other nonacoustic tumors of the cerebellopontine angle. *Otolaryngol Clin North Am* 1992;25:707–728.

30. Rhoton AL Jr. Meningiomas of the cerebellopontine angle and foramen magnum. *Neurosurg Clin North Am* 1994;5:349–377.

31. Thomas NW, King TT. Meningiomas of the cerebellopontine angle. A report of 41 cases. *Br J Neurosurg* 1996;10:59–68.

32. Voss NF, Vrionis FD, Heilman CB, et al. Meningiomas of the cerebellopontine angle. *Surg Neurol* 2000;53:439–446; discussion 446–477.

33. Granick MS, Martuza RL, Parker SW, et al. Cerebellopontine angle meningiomas: clinical manifestations and diagnosis. *Ann Otol Rhinol Laryngol* 1985;94:34–38.

34. Lalwani AK, Jackler RK. Preoperative differentiation between men-

ingioma of the cerebellopontine angle and acoustic neuroma using MRI. *Otolaryngol Head Neck Surg* 1993;109:88–95.

35. Mikhael MA, Ciric IS, Wolff AP. Differentiation of cerebellopontine angle neuromas and meningiomas with MR imaging. *J Comput Assist Tomogr* 1985;9:852–856.

36. Giannotta SL, Pulec JL, Goodkin R. Translabyrinthine removal of cerebellopontine angle meningiomas. *Neurosurgery* 1985;17: 620–625.

37. Sekhar LN, Jannetta PJ. Cerebellopontine angle meningiomas. Microsurgical excision and follow-up results. *J Neurosurg* 1984;60: 500–505.

38. Schaller B, Merlo A, Gratzl O, et al. Premeatal and retromeatal cerebellopontine angle meningioma. Two distinct clinical entities. *Acta Neurochirur* 1999;141:465–471.

39. Samii M, Tatagiba M, Piquer J, et al. Surgical treatment of epidermoid cysts of the cerebellopontine angle. *J Neurosurg* 1996;84: 14–19.

40. Savader SJ, Murtagh FR, Savader BL, et al. Magnetic resonance imaging of intracranial epidermoid tumours [see comments]. *Clin Radiol* 1989;40:282–285.

41. Mohanty A, Venkatrauma S, Rao B, et al. Experience with cerebellopontine angle epidermoids. *Neurosurgery* 1997;40:24–30.

42. Jallo G, Woo H, Meshki C, et al. Arachnoid cysts of the cerebellopontine angle: diagnosis and surgery. *Neurosurgery* 1997;40: 31–38.

43. Kohan D, Downey LL, Lim J, et al. Uncommon lesions presenting as tumors of the internal auditory canal and cerebellopontine angle. *Am J Otol* 1997;18:386–392.

44. Jallo JI, Palumbo SJ, Buchheit WA. Cerebellopontine angle lipoma: case report. *Neurosurgery* 1994;34:912–914; discussion 914.

45. Kingdom TT, Lalwani AK, Pitts LH. Isolated metastatic melanoma of the cerebellopontine angle: case report. *Neurosurgery* 1993;33: 142–144.

46. Knorr JR, Ragland RL, Smith TW, et al. Squamous carcinoma arising in a cerebellopontine angle epidermoid: CT and MR findings. *AJNR Am J Neuroradiol* 1991;12:1182–1184.

47. Nelson DR, Dolan KD. Cerebellopontine angle metastatic lung carcinoma resembling an acoustic neuroma. *Ann Otol Rhinol Laryngol* 1991;100:685–686.

48. Martin N, Pierot L, Sterkers O, et al. Primary choroid plexus papilloma of the cerebellopontine angle: MR imaging. *Neuroradiology* 1990;31:541–543.

49. Gibson WP, Wallace D. Basilar artery ectasia. (An unusual cause of a cerebello-pontine lesion and hemifacial spasm.) *Am J Laryngol Otol* 1975;89:721–731.

50. Adeloye A, Ogan O, Olumide AA. Arachnoiditis presenting as a cerebello-pontine angle tumour. *Am J Laryngol Otol* 1978;92: 911–913.

51. Babin RW, Fratkin JD, Cancilla PA. Hamartomas of the cerebellopontine angle and internal auditory canal: report of two cases. *Arch Otolaryngol* 1980;106:500–502.

52. Fujiwara S, Matsushima T, Kitamura K, et al. Solitary plasmacytoma in the cerebellopontine angle. *Surg Neurol* 1980;13:211–214.

53. Viale GL, Pau A, Viale ES, et al. Angiomas of the cerebellopontine angle. *J Neurol* 1981;225:259–267.

54. Cantore GP, Ciappetta P, Vagnozzi R, et al. Giant aneurysm of the anterior inferior cerebellar artery simulating a cerebellopontine angle tumor. *Surg Neurol* 1982;18:76–78.

55. Curry B, Taylor CW, Fisher AW. Salivary gland heterotopia: a unique cerebellopontine angle tumor. *Arch Pathol Lab Med* 1982; 106:35–38.

56. Altinors N, Senveli E, Erdogan A, et al. Craniopharyngioma of the cerebellopontine angle. Case report. *J Neurosurg* 1984;60:842–844.

57. Cholankeril JV, Lieberman H. Chronic granulomatous abscess simulating cerebellopontine angle tumor. *AJNR Am J Neuroradiol* 1984;5:637–638.

58. Ganapathy K, Govindan R. Cerebellopontine pneumocephalus acting as a space-occupying lesion: CT demonstration. *J Comput Assist Tomogr* 1985;9:407.

59. Matsumoto T, Tani E, Maeda Y, et al. Amyloidomas in the cerebellopontine angle and jugular foramen. Case report. *J Neurosurg* 1985;62:592–596.

60. Millen SJ, Campbell BH, Meyer GA, et al. Mixed glioma of the cerebellopontine angle. *Am J Otol* 1985;6:503–507.

61. Ahn MS, Jackler RK. Exophytic brain tumors mimicking primary

lesions of the cerebellopontine angle. *Laryngoscope* 1997;107: 466–471.

62. Waters DC, Venes JL, Zis K. Childhood cerebellopontine angle teratoma associated with congenital hydrocephalus. *Neurosurgery* 1986;18:784–786.

63. Best PV. Malignant triton tumour in the cerebellopontine angle. Report of a case. *Acta Neuropathol* 1987;74:92–96.

64. Kao SC, Yuh WT, Sato Y, et al. Intracranial granulocytic sarcoma (chloroma): MR findings. *J Comput Assist Tomogr* 1987;11:938–941.

65. Yang PJ, Seeger JF, Carmody RF, et al. Cerebellopontine angle lymphoma. *AJNR Am J Neuroradiol* 1987;8:368–369.

66. Young S, Richardson AE. Solid haemangioblastomas of the posterior fossa: radiological features and results of surgery. *J Neurol Neurosurg Psychiatry* 1987;50:155–158.

67. Bordi L, Pires M, Symon L, et al. Cavernous angioma of the cerebello-pontine angle: a case report [see comments]. *Br J Neurosurg* 1991;5:83–86.

68. Jamjoom ZA, Sadiq S, Naim Ur R, et al. Cerebello-pontine angle paraganglioma simulating an acoustic neurinoma. *Br J Neurosurg* 1991;5:307–312.

69. Hardie RC. Magnetic resonance appearance of a rare intradural chordoma. *Wisconsin Med J* 1992;91:627–628.

70. Sohma T, Tuchita H, Kitami K, et al. Cerebellopontine angle ganglioneuroblastoma. *Neuroradiology* 1992;34:334–336.

71. Papaefthymiou G, Tritthart H, Kleinert R, et al. Primitive neuroectodermal tumor (PNET) extending into the cerebellopontine angle: case report. *Wiener Klinische Wochenschrift* 1993;105:614–617.

72. Pulec JL. Aggressive fibromatosis (fibrosarcoma) of the facial nerve. *Ear, Nose, Throat J* 1993;72:460–467, 470–472.

73. Yamada S, Aiba T, Hara M. Cerebellopontine angle medulloblastoma: case report and literature review. *Br J Neurosurg* 1993;7: 91–94.

74. Goldsmith P, Zammit-Maempel I, Meikle D. Ramsay Hunt syndrome mimicking acoustic neuroma on MRI. *Am J Laryngol Otol* 1995;109:1013–1015.

75. Morris DP, Ballagh RH, Hong A, et al. Thrombosed posterior-inferior cerebellar artery aneurysm: a rare cerebellopontine angle tumour. *Am J Laryngol Otol* 1995;109:429–430.

76. van Leeuwen JP, Pruszczynski M, Marres HA, et al. Unilateral hearing loss due to a rhabdomyoma in a six-year-old child. *Am J Laryngol Otol* 1995;109:1186–1189.

77. Depper MH, Carlow TJ, Crooks LA, et al. Intracranial dissemination of a pituitary adenoma: presentation as an unusual mass in the cerebellopontine angle [letter]. *AJR Am J Roentgenol* 1996;166: 1500–1501.

78. Folker RJ, Meyerhoff WL, Rushing EJ. Aggressive papillary adenoma of the cerebellopontine angle: case report of an endolymphatic sac tumor. *Am J Otolaryngol* 1997;18:135–139.

79. Sanford RA, Kun LE, Heideman RL, et al. Cerebellar pontine angle ependymoma in infants. *Pediatr Neurosurg* 1997;27:84–91.

80. Lipper MH, Goldstein JM. Neurosarcoidosis mimicking a cerebellopontine angle meningioma. *AJR Am J Roentgenol* 1998;171: 275–276.

81. Nagendran K, Rice-Edwards M, Kendall B, et al. Germinoma in the cerebellopontine angle [letter]. *J Neurol Neurosurg Psychiatry* 1985; 48:955–956.

82. Rossato RG, Timperley WR. Posterior fossa ceruminoma. *Acta Neurochirur* 1973;28:315–322.

83. Antonio G, Dahlstrom J, Chandran KN, et al. Cerebellopontine angle Hodgkin's disease. *Australas Radiol* 2000;44:115–117.

84. Sanna M, Zini C, Mazzoni A, et al. Hearing preservation in acoustic neuroma surgery. Middle fossa versus suboccipital approach. *Am J Otol* 1987;8:500–506.

85. Staecker H, Nadol JB Jr, Ojeman R, et al. Hearing preservation in acoustic neuroma surgery: middle fossa versus retrosigmoid approach. *Am J Otol* 2000;21:399–404.

86. Shelton C, Alavi S, Li JC, et al. Modified retrosigmoid approach: use for selected acoustic tumor removal. *Am J Otol* 1995;16:664–668.

87. Cohen NL, Lewis WS, Ransohoff J. Hearing preservation in cerebellopontine angle tumor surgery: the NYU experience 1974–1991. *Am J Otol* 1993;14:423–433.

88. Samii M, Turel KE, Penkert G. Management of seventh and eighth nerve involvement by cerebellopontine angle tumors. *Clin Neurosurg* 1985;32:242–272.

89. Poppi M, Giuliani G, Gambari P, et al. A hazard of craniotomy in the sitting position: the posterior compartment syndrome of the thigh. Case report. *J Neurosurg* 1989;71:618–619.

90. Young ML, Smith DS, Murtagh FR, et al. Comparison of surgical and anesthetic complications in neurosurgical patients experiencing venous air embolism in the sitting position. *Neurosurgery* 1986;18. 157–161.

91. Sampath P, Holliday MJ, Brem H, et al. Facial nerve injury in acoustic neuroma (vestibular schwannoma) surgery: etiology and prevention [see comments]. *J Neurosurg* 1997;87:60–66.

92. Sampath P, Rini D, Long DM. Microanatomical variations in the cerebellopontine angle associated with vestibular schwannomas (acoustic neuromas): a retrospective study of 1006 consecutive cases. *J Neurosurg* 2000;92:70–78.

93. Matula C, Diaz Day J, Czech T, et al. The retrosigmoid approach to acoustic neurinomas: technical, strategic, and future concepts. *Acta Neurochirur* 1995;134:139–147.

94. Colletti V, Fiorino FG. Retrosigmoid-transmeatal en bloc removal of small to medium-sized acoustic neuromas. *Otolaryngol Head Neck Surg* 1999;120:122–128.

95. Tos M, Youssef M, Thomsen J, et al. Causes of facial nerve paresis after translabyrinthine surgery for acoustic neuroma. *Ann Otol Rhinol Laryngol* 1992;101:821–826.

96. Nissen AJ, Sikand A, Welsh JE, et al. A multifactorial analysis of facial nerve results in surgery for cerebellopontine angle tumors [see comments]. *Ear Nose Throat J* 1997;76:37–40.

97. Grey PL, Moffat DA, Palmer CR, et al. Factors which influence the facial nerve outcome in vestibular schwannoma surgery. *Clin Otolaryngol Allied Sci* 1996;21:409–413.

98. Goldbrunner RH, Schlake HP, Milewski C, et al. Quantitative parameters of intraoperative electromyography predict facial nerve outcomes for vestibular schwannoma surgery. *Neurosurgery* 2000; 46:1140–1146; discussion 1146–1148.

99. Fenton JE, Chin RY, Shirazi A, et al. Prediction of postoperative facial nerve function in acoustic neuroma surgery. *Clin Otolaryngol Allied Sci* 1999;24:483–486.

100. Axon PR, Ramsden RT. Intraoperative electromyography for predicting facial function in vestibular schwannoma surgery. *Laryngoscope* 1999;109:922–926.

101. Mandpe AH, Mikulec A, Jackler RK, et al. Comparison of response amplitude versus stimulation threshold in predicting early postoperative facial nerve function after acoustic neuroma resection. *Am J Otol* 1998;19:112–117.

102. Cohen NL. Retrosigmoid approach for acoustic tumor removal. *Otolaryngol Clin North Am* 1992;25:295–310.

103. Cohen NL. Acoustic neuroma surgery with emphasis on preservation of hearing. *Laryngoscope* 1979;89:886–896.

104. Cohen NL, Hammerschlag PE, Berg H, et al. Acoustic neuroma surgery: an eclectic approach with emphasis on preservation of hearing. *Ann Otol Rhinol Laryngol* 1986;95:21–27.

105. Cohen NL, Ransohoff J. Hearing preservation: posterior fossa approach. *Otolaryngol Head Neck Surg* 1984;92:176–183.

106. Rosenberg RA, Cohen NL, Ransohoff J. Long-term hearing preservation after acoustic neuroma surgery. *Otolaryngol Head Neck Surg* 1987;97:270–274.

107. Battista RA, Wiet RJ, Paauwe L. Evaluation of three intraoperative auditory monitoring techniques in acoustic neuroma surgery. *Am J Otol* 2000;21:244–248.

108. Jackson LE, Roberson JB Jr. Acoustic neuroma surgery: use of cochlear nerve action potential monitoring for hearing preservation. *Am J Otol* 2000;21:249–259.

109. Harner SG, Harper CM, Beatty CW, et al. Far-field auditory brainstem response in neurotologic surgery [see comments]. *Am J Otol* 1996;17:150–153.

110. Moller AR. Monitoring auditory function during operations to remove acoustic tumors. *Am J Otol* 1996;17:452–460.

111. Roberson J, Senne A, Brackmann D, et al. Direct cochlear nerve action potentials as an aid to hearing preservation in middle fossa acoustic neuroma resection. *Am J Otol* 1996;17:653–657.

112. Zappia J, Wiet RJ, O'Connor CA, et al. Intraoperative auditory monitoring in acoustic neuroma surgery. *Otolaryngol Head Neck Surg* 1996;115:98–106.

113. Butler S, Coakham H, Maw R, et al. Physiological identification of the auditory nerve during surgery for acoustic neuroma. *Clin Otolaryngol Allied Sci* 1995;20:312–317.

114. Eisenman DJ, Digoy GP, Victor JD, et al. Topical papaverine and

facial nerve dysfunction in cerebellopontine angle surgery. *Am J Otol* 1999;20:77–80.

115. Fahlbusch R, Neu M, Strauss C. Preservation of hearing in large acoustic neurinomas following removal via suboccipito-lateral approach. *Acta Neurochirur* 1998;140:771–777; discussion 778.

116. Robinette MS, Bauch CD, Olsen WO, et al. Nonsurgical factors predictive of postoperative hearing for patients with vestibular schwannoma. *Am J Otol* 1997;18:738–745.

117. Dornhoffer JL, Helms J, Hoehmann DH. Hearing preservation in acoustic tumor surgery: results and prognostic factors. *Laryngoscope* 1995;105:184–187.

118. Hecht CS, Honrubia VF, Wiet RJ, et al. Hearing preservation after acoustic neuroma resection with tumor size used as a clinical prognosticator. *Laryngoscope* 1997;107:1122–1126.

119. Nutik SL, Korol HW. Cerebrospinal fluid leak after acoustic neuroma surgery. *Surg Neurol* 1995;43:553–556; discussion 556–557.

120. Millen SJ, Meyer G. Surgical management of CSF otorhinorrhea following retrosigmoid removal of cerebellopontine angle tumors. *Am J Otol* 1993;14:585–589.

121. Fishman AJ, Hoffman RA, Roland JT Jr, et al. Cerebrospinal fluid drainage in the management of CSF leak following acoustic neuroma surgery. *Laryngoscope* 996;106:1002–1004.

122. Kabuto M, Kubota T, Kobayashi H, et al. MR imaging of cerebrospinal fluid rhinorrhea following the suboccipital approach to the cerebellopontine angle and the internal auditory canal: report of the two cases [see comments]. *Surg Neurol* 1996;45:336–340.

123. House WF. Evolution of transtemporal bone removal of acoustic tumours. *Arch Otolaryngol* 1964;80:731–741.

124. Hardy DG, Macfarlane R, Baguley D. Surgery for acoustic neurinoma: an analysis of 100 translabyrinthine operations. *J Neurosurg* 1989;71:799–804.

125. Leonetti JP, Reichman OH, Smith PG. Additional exposure during translabyrinthine surgery. *Laryngoscope* 1992;102:213–216.

126. Lebowitz RA, Hoffman RA, Roland JT Jr, et al. Autologous fibrin glue in the prevention of cerebrospinal fluid leak following acoustic neuroma surgery. *Am J Otol* 1995;16:172–174.

127. Mass SC, Wiet RJ, Dinces E. Complications of the translabyrinthine

approach for the removal of acoustic neuromas. *Arch Otolaryngol Head Neck Surg* 1999;125:801–804.

128. Celikkanat SM, Saleh E, Khashaba A, et al. Cerebrospinal fluid leak after translabyrinthine acoustic neuroma surgery. *Otolaryngol Head Neck Surg* 1995;112:654–658.

129. Ekvall L, Bynke O. Prevention of cerebrospinal fluid rhinorrhea in translabyrinthine surgery. *Acta Oto-Laryngol* 1988;449(suppl): 15–16.

130. Brackmann DE, Hitselberger WE. Retrolabyrinthine approach: technique and newer indications. *Laryngoscope* 978;88:286–297.

131. Molony TB, Kwartler JA, House WF, et al. Extended middle fossa and retrolabyrinthine approaches in acoustic neuroma surgery: case reports. *Am J Otol* 1992;13:360–363.

132. Roberson JB Jr, Brackmann DE, Hitselberger WE. Acoustic neuroma recurrence after suboccipital resection: management with translabyrinthine resection. *Am J Otol* 1996;17:307–311.

133. Brackmann DE, Owens RM, Friedman RA, et al. Prognostic factors for hearing preservation in vestibular schwannoma surgery. *Am J Otol* 2000;21:417–424.

134. Irving RM, Jackler RK, Pitts LH. Hearing preservation in patients undergoing vestibular schwannoma surgery: comparison of middle fossa and retrosigmoid approaches [see comments]. *J Neurosurg* 1998;88:840–845.

135. Driscoll CL, Jackler RK, Pitts LH, et al. Is the entire fundus of the internal auditory canal visible during the middle fossa approach for acoustic neuroma? *Am J Otol* 2000;21:382–388.

136. Rowed DW, Nedzelski JM. Hearing preservation in the removal of intracanalicular acoustic neuromas via the retrosigmoid approach. *J Neurosurg* 1997;86:456–461.

137. Kelly DL Jr, Britton BH, Branch CL Jr. Cooperative neuro-otologic management of acoustic neuromas and other cerebellopontine angle tumors. *South Med J* 1988;81:557–561.

138. Hardy DG. Acoustic neuroma surgery as an interdisciplinary approach [comment] [editorial]. *J Neurol Neurosurg Psychiatry* 2000; 69:147–148.

139. Tonn JC, Schlake HP, Goldbrunner R, et al. Acoustic neuroma surgery as an interdisciplinary approach: a neurosurgical series of 508 patients [see comments]. *J Neurol Neurosurg Psychiatry* 2000;69: 161–166.

121. Petroclival Meningiomas

Caleb Lippman and Chandranath Sen

Clival and petroclival meningiomas, by definition, encompass the upper two-thirds of the clivus and the area medial to the trigeminal nerve at the petroclival junction. Tumors of the lower one-third of the clivus, along with the foramen magnum tumors, and those originating lateral to the trigeminal nerve are considered to be tumors of the cerebellopontine angle (1,2). The strategic location of this region and the numerous vital structures it is related to, including the basilar artery, the brainstem, and multiple cranial nerves, makes tumors of this region particularly challenging to the neurosurgeon.

Before the development of modern microsurgical techniques, patients with these tumors fared poorly. The natural history is one of a relentless progression to an ultimately fatal outcome, and surgery was, and still is, seen as the primary treatment of choice. The early literature shows a cumulative surgical mortality that is greater than 50% (1). With these modern techniques, which include the use of the operative microscope, high-resolution preoperative imaging studies, intraoperative monitoring, and innovative surgical approaches, there has

been progressive improvement in morbidity and mortality, increased frequency of complete tumor removal, and overall improved clinical outcome.

Classification

Posterior fossa meningiomas account for approximately 10% of all meningiomas (3). Castellano and Ruggiero classify posterior fossa meningiomas by the site of dural attachment. Based on postmortem studies, they classify meningiomas as posterior petrous (42%), tentorium (30%), clivus (11%), cerebellar convexity (10%), or foramen magnum (4%), and further note tumors that extend from the Meckel cave into the posterior fossa (4). Yasargil classifies these tumors based on intraoperative findings into those with primary attachment to dura as clival, petroclival, sphenopetroclival, foramen magnum, or cerebellopontine angle tumors (5). However, several authors (2,6,7) believe that these classifications do not differentiate the distinct and clinically recognized petroclival location from other posterior fossa locations. For this reason, the strict definition of petroclival meningiomas stated at the beginning of this chapter is suggested.

Clinical Presentation

Patients present from 5 months to 69 years old—the average age of presentation is in the mid-40s (1). Some series report a higher incidence in females (2,3,7–11), while in other series there is an equal sex distribution (4,12). Symptoms present insidiously, with an average range of 3 to 5 years, although duration prior to diagnosis has ranged from as short as 1 month to as long as 17 years (2,3,7–11). The most common presenting symptoms are headache or slowly progressive gait disturbance (2,7–11). The most common signs on physical examination are usually cranial nerve palsies (most commonly V, VII, and VIII, and less often III and VI) (2,7–10), followed by brainstem compression, and cerebellar compression (1). Rarely, these tumors may present as basilar artery insufficiency (13).

Preoperative Evaluation

The patient's preoperative neurological status should first be considered. All cranial nerve deficits must be noted, as some are not reversible. A preexisting deficit may be considered an opportunity to widen the exposure, furthering tumor resection. For example, a translabyrinthine approach may be considered in a patient who is already deaf, or a more aggressive resection may be attempted in a patient with existing cranial nerve deficits.

A detailed preoperative radiological evaluation is essential for proper planning and execution of the surgical procedure. High-resolution computed tomography (CT) scanning in the axial and coronal planes with and without contrast provides a good detail of the bony anatomy of the region of interest, including bone destruction, the relation of the lesion to the basal foramina, and the anatomy of the temporal bone structures.

Magnetic resonance imaging (MRI) provides information absolutely invaluable for predicting the nature of the lesion and pretreatment planning, and is complementary to the information provided by CT. MRI is superior to CT for evaluation of the tumor and its relationship to nearby neurovascular structures. Although CT is superior to MRI when evaluating bony anatomy, MRI demonstrates marrow invasion better. Lastly, MRI is used to examine the relationships of the tumor to brain, particularly the displacement and invasion of brain and pia, amount of cerebral edema, and presence of an arachnoid plane. Magnetic resonance angiography has been refined extensively, and may be used to evaluate cerebral vascular anatomy

Conventional angiography permits visualization of the small vessels, changes in vessel caliber caused by tumor encasement, adequacy of collateral circulation, and vascular supply to the tumor. Most of these tumors obtain their vascular supply from the external carotid arteries (ECAs) or the meningohypophyseal branch of the internal carotid artery (ICA), although about 20% will have some blood supply coming from the basilar artery and its branches (11).

Angiography allows for the evaluation of the tumor's blood supply, and for the preoperative embolization of tumor vessels. The venous side should be evaluated for major draining veins. The size and configuration of temporal draining veins, size and dominance of the sigmoid sinus, and competence and drainage of the torcula are noted. The temporal draining veins must be carefully preserved and transection of the sigmoid sinus is considered only if adequate collateralization of the venous drainage is present.

Treatment

The natural history of these lesions is that of relentless progression, with ultimate neurological decline and death. Management options include observation alone, microsurgical resection, and radiation therapy (external beam fractionated radiotherapy or stereotactic radiosurgery), either alone or in combination with surgery (14). It is generally believed that microsurgical resection is the treatment of choice for these lesions (9). Radiosurgery may be considered an alternative if a patient is a very poor surgical candidate, or if there is residual tumor (14).

Preoperative Preparation

High-dose steroids are administered for a day or two before surgery (if a patient is not receiving them), with the intention of tapering them off rapidly a few days after surgery. Anticonvulsants are usually started when the surgery begins when supratentorial approaches are used. Antibiotic prophylaxis begins during the induction of anesthesia, and is continued for a few days postoperatively if a patient has a lumbar drain or a ventricular catheter.

Intraoperative Monitoring

Integrity of the brainstem pathways is assessed in real time by monitoring the brainstem auditory evoked potentials, somatosensory evoked potentials, and motor evoked potentials. Cranial nerve monitoring may also be performed, mainly of VII nerve. Intraoperative monitoring requires the help of an experienced neurophysiologist and an active dialogue with the anesthesiologist.

Anesthesia

General inhalation anesthesia is used. Use of intraoperative neurophysiological monitoring places certain special constraints on the anesthetic techniques. Arterial lines and central venous catheters are placed for hemodynamic monitoring. Sequential pneumatic compression stockings are used to reduce the risk of deep venous thrombosis and pulmonary embolism. An indwelling urinary catheter is used to measure fluid output accurately. If temporary arterial occlusion is necessary, barbiturates, mild hypothermia, and induced hypertension may be used for neuroprotection.

Cerebrospinal Fluid Drainage

Brain relaxation is one of the most important prerequisites for a successful operative procedure. Although dehydrating agents can afford some amount of relaxation, cerebrospinal fluid (CSF) drainage is far superior because of its controllability. A frontal or a temporal ventriculostomy accomplishes this well. If the tumor is small, a lumbar spinal subarachnoid drain can also serve the purpose. The drainage can also be continued in the postoperative period as a preventive against a CSF leak.

Approaches

Approaches to this region are difficult—few are straightforward and direct—and traditional approaches are usually inadequate for pathological processes of this area. The target area is far from the surface, and exposure is often limited by normal vascular and neuronal elements nearby. Brain retraction can be extensive, and is one of the major causes of morbidity and mortality associated in these cases. Several approaches have been developed to overcome the difficulties associated with the traditional approaches.

The best approaches provide a combination of wide exposure, decreased distance to the target, and minimize brain retraction; the approaches to the clivus all emphasize these basic principles. Thus, excess bone removal, ventricular and cisternal drains, and the use of osmotic agents all serve to reduce the degree of brain retraction necessary, widen the area of exposure, and increase the safety and efficacy of the surgery.

Numerous surgical approaches and combinations of approaches have been used to remove petroclival meningiomas. In the following sections we will review our three preferred approaches: the transsylvian and subtemporal approach (along with anterior transpetrosal bone removal), the petrosal (subtemporal/presigmoid) approach, and the retrosigmoid (suboccipital) approach.

Transsylvian and Subtemporal Approach

Although the entire range of the approach is described, the specific steps are tailored to the individual patient and lesion.

POSITION AND SCALP INCISION. The patient is placed supine with the head fixed in a three-point pin headrest, which is turned 45 degrees to the side opposite the approach and extended so that the malar eminence is higher than the cranium. The incision runs from level of the tragus, below the zygomatic arch and just in front of the ear so that the scar will be in the normal skin crease. The incision is brought to just approach the forehead. (Fig. 1)

SCALP FLAP/SOFT TISSUE FLAP/BONE FLAP (CRANIOTOMY, ORBITOZYGOMATIC OSTEOTOMY). The scalp flap is elevated, exposing the superior and lateral rim of the ipsilateral orbit and zygomatic arch. A subfascial dissection is performed on the temporalis muscle to protect the frontal branch of the facial nerve.

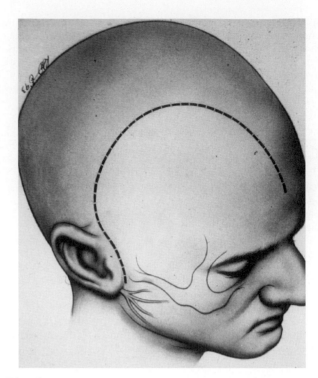

Fig. 1. Artist's illustration. The skin incision for the subtemporal/transsylvian approach is shown.

The temporalis muscle is elevated from the temporal fossa and zygomatic arch, exposing the temporal region and temporomandibular joint (TMJ) capsule. The periorbita is further stripped from the roof and lateral wall of the orbit.

The frontotemporal craniotomy is made such that the anterior extent is over the roof of the orbit and the posterior limit is the external ear canal. An orbitozygomatic osteotomy is completed and the piece of bone is removed in one piece (Fig. 2).

The greater sphenoid wing is drilled away to provide a flat approach along the middle fossa floor and sylvian fissure.

EXTRADURAL DISSECTION FOR EXPOSURE OF THE PETROUS INTERNAL CAROTID ARTERY AND REMOVAL OF THE PETROUS APEX. To expose the foramen spinosum and ovale, the temporal lobe is elevated extradurally. The middle meningeal artery is coagulated and divided, and the arcuate eminence of the petrous bone is identified. The greater superficial petrosal nerve (GSPN) is identified as it emerges from the facial hiatus of the temporal bone. The GSPN can be preserved by leaving a small portion of the periosteal dura attached to it while elevating the temporal lobe dura.

The horizontal portion of the petrous ICA is found medial to V3 and anteromedial to the arcuate eminence along the course of the GSPN. It may be partially devoid of a bony covering. The artery is unroofed in its entire horizontal segment using the diamond burr up to its genu posteriorly. Of note, the eustachian tube is lateral to the ICA; these two structures are separated by a layer of bone less than 1-mm. The bone medial to the artery is drilled away, exposing clival dura (Fig. 3). The bone drilling can be taken posteriorly to include unroofing the internal auditory meatus. This bone work will serve to improve the exposure of the area in front of the upper brainstem from the intradural subtemporal route.

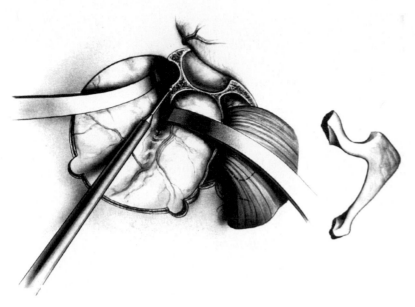

Fig. 2. Artist's illustration. An orbitozygomatic osteotomy is shown. It is performed after completing the craniotomy.

DURAL OPENING AND DIVISION OF THE TENTORIUM.
At this point, the frontal and temporal dura is opened and the sylvian fissure split widely, starting over the lateral convexity and following the middle cerebral artery branches into the fissure (Fig. 4). To increase temporal lobe mobilization, draining veins at the temporal tip are sacrificed and the tentorial incisura and upper clival area are exposed. The temporal lobe is now elevated to visualize the medial edge of the tentorium (Fig. 5A).

The edge of the tentorium is everted with a small hook, revealing cranial nerve IV. The tentorium is divided laterally, posterior to cranial nerve IV, over and lateral to the trigeminal ganglion (Fig. 5B). Venous bleeding is controlled by coagulating the dural edges or packing with Surgicel. The dura is also opened inferior to the root of cranial nerve V, and anterior to the brainstem. Thus, the clivus is exposed from the level of the

posterior clinoid process to the level of the horizontal petrous ICA, below the root of cranial nerve V. The premesencephalic and prepontine area above and below cranial nerve V is visualized, including the origin of cranial nerve III. The basilar artery is exposed from its summit to the origin of the anterior ICA. The petrous apex, which was drilled extradurally in this case, can also be drilled intradurally if desired.

TUMOR REMOVAL. Access to the upper clivus is provided by working both transsylvian and subtemporally (Fig. 6). Tumor removal is performed by working between cranial nerves and blood vessels, taking care to preserve the arachnoid planes. The tumor is thoroughly debulked while working between the supraclinoid ICA and cranial nerve III, cranial nerve III and IV,

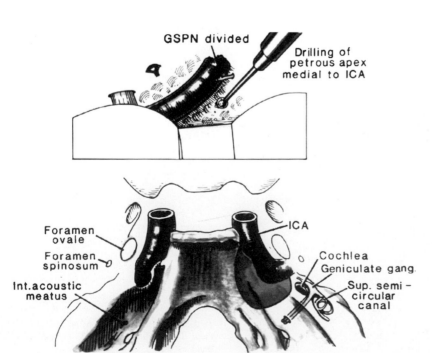

Fig. 3. Artist's illustration. The shaded area indicates the drilling of the petrous apex in relation to the petrous internal carotid artery and the geniculate ganglion.

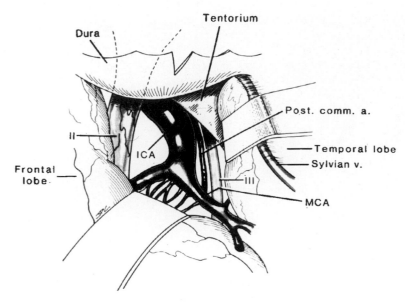

Fig. 4. Artist's illustration. The sylvian fissure is split, exposing the internal carotid artery *(ICA)* and its bifurcation, the tentorial edge, and the optic (cranial nerve II) and oculomotor (cranial nerve III) nerves. *MCA*, middle cerebral artery.

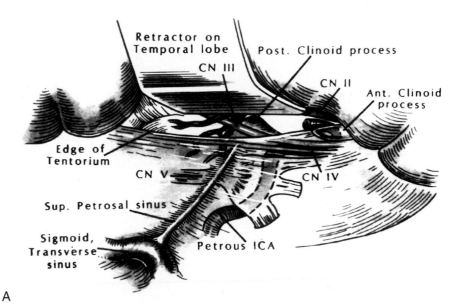

A

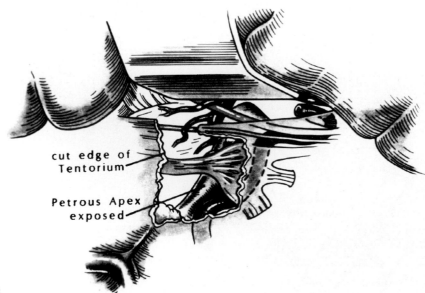

B

Fig. 5. Artist's illustration. **A:** Subtemporal view of the tentorial edge. **B:** Tentorium has been incised.

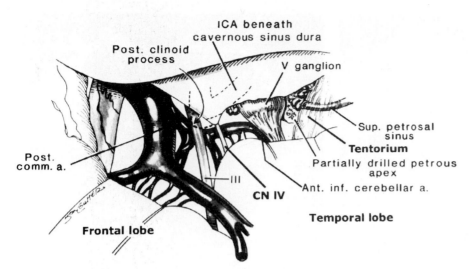

Fig. 6. Artist's illustration. The final preparation showing the combined use of the transsylvian and subtemporal routes. *ICA,* internal carotid artery.

or between cranial nerve IV and V. Drilling of the posterior clinoid process and dorsum sella can improve visualization across the midline (6). In removing the tumor capsule from the brainstem, the dissection must be kept in the arachnoid plane at all times, and care taken not to lose it. If the plane cannot be found because of pial invasion by the tumor, it is better to leave tumor than to risk injuring normal neurovascular structures.

CLOSURE. The temporal lobe is inspected for contusions, and hemostasis is achieved. Petrous air cells are waxed, and the eustachian tube inspected for any breaches. A piece of autologous fat is left over the petrous ICA to plug the hole in the petrous apex. The convexity dura is closed and the craniotomy flap, zygoma, and orbital rim replaced and secured with titanium plating.

EXTENT OF EXPOSURE. The clivus is seen from the level of the posterior clinoid processes rostrally to the horizontal por-

tion of the ICA caudally. The basilar artery is exposed from its summit to the origin of the anterior-inferior cerebellar artery. The anterolateral surface of the midbrain and superior pons are seen, including the origin of the oculomotor and trigeminal nerves.

EXAMPLE 1. A 55-year-old woman presented with a history of progressive right cranial nerve VI palsy, which had been complete for several months. MRI and CT revealed a small right petrous apex tumor in the vicinity of cranial nerve VI (Fig. 7). A right frontotemporal craniotomy, zygomatic osteotomy with exploration of the posterior cavernous sinus was performed. After complete removal of the tumor, cranial nerve VI was seen to be atrophic distally, and a sural nerve graft was sutured in continuity. Postoperatively, the patient had numbness on the right side of her face. She developed right nasal ulceration as a result of the new cranial nerve V palsy, but this resolved with conservative management. The cranial nerve VI palsy did not

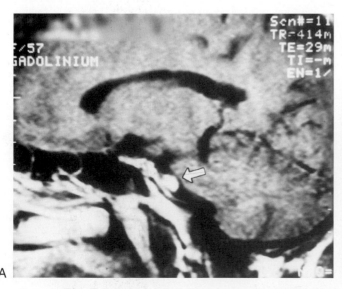

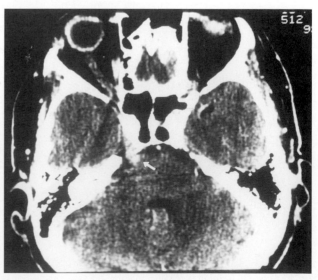

Fig. 7. **A:** Preoperative sagittal contrast-enhanced, T1-weighted MRI reveals a homogenously enhancing lesion (*arrow*) anterior to the brainstem. **B:** Preoperative contrast-enhanced CT shows the tumor at the petrous apex.

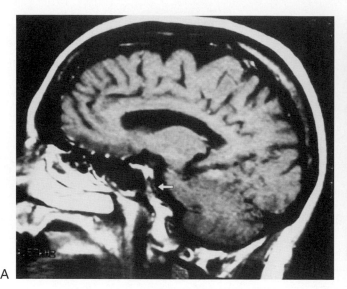
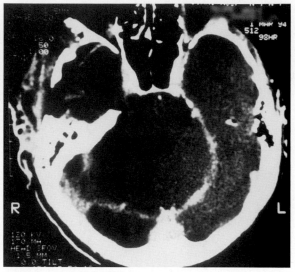

Fig. 8. A: Postoperative sagittal contrast-enhanced, T1-weighted MRI shows good tumor resection, with only a small amount of residual lesion (*arrow*). **B:** Postoperative contrast-enhanced CT shows the drilled petrous apex.

improve. No recurrence has been observed in 5 years of follow-up (Fig. 8).

Petrosal Approach

The petrosal approach described in this section is a combination of the subtemporal and presigmoid approaches (Fig. 9) and is indicated for meningiomas of the upper and middle clivus, cerebellopontine angle, and the tentorial incisura. This combined supra- and infratentorial approach is a modification of an approach first described by Malis (15), in which the sigmoid-transverse sinus junction was divided to achieve exposure.

POSITION AND SCALP INCISION. The patient is placed supine with the head fixed in a three-point Mayfield head clamp and turned 60 degrees away from the side of the tumor and tilted, so that the vertex is inferior to the ear. The incision starts horizontally 2.5 cm above the ear and is then curved down in the occipital region 2.5 cm medial (posterior) to the mastoid (Fig. 10).

SCALP FLAP/SOFT TISSUE FLAP/BONE FLAP/MASTOID-ECTOMY. The scalp flap is elevated up to the external ear canal. A horizontal incision is made into the musculature extending posteriorly from the zygomatic root. The temporalis flap is raised anteriorly while the nuchal muscles are reflected

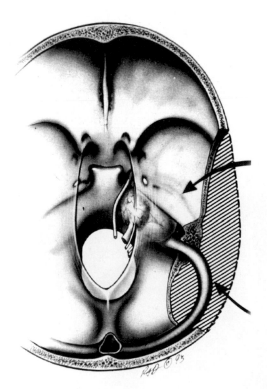

Fig. 9. Artist's illustration. The petrosal approach is a combination of the subtemporal approach (*anterior arrow*) and the presigmoid posterior fossa approach (*posterior arrow*).

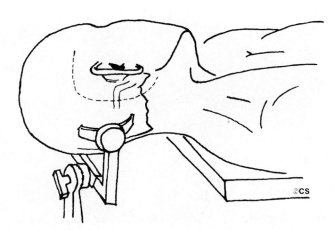

Fig. 10. Artist's illustration. The patient position and scalp incision is depicted for a right-sided approach.

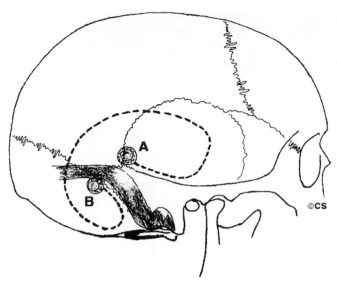

Fig. 11. Artist's illustration. After the skull is exposed, two burr holes are made which straddle the transverse sinus. The outline of the bone flap is shown.

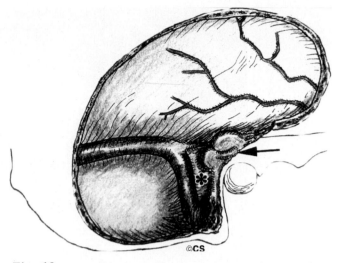

Fig. 13. Artist's illustration. After mastoidectomy, the semicircular canals are identified (*arrow*), and the presigmoid dura is visible (*asterisk*).

inferiorly. The squamous temporal, mastoid, and suboccipital regions are thus exposed.

The craniotomy is made, straddling the transverse sinus, which lies in a line joining the root of the zygoma to the inion. Two burr holes are made which straddle the transverse-sigmoid sinus junction (Fig. 11). One is made at the asterion, which will open into the posterior fossa below the transverse-sigmoid junction. The other, which opens into the supratentorial compartment, is made at the squamous and mastoid junction of the temporal bone, along the superior temporal line. A bony trough is drilled joining the two burr holes to unroof the sinus. A single bone flap is raised over the temporal lobe and the posterior fossa starting from the two burr holes (Fig. 12). In older patients where the dura is adherent, additional burr holes may be made or the temporal and posterior fossa craniotomies may be made separately.

The mastoid and petrous bones are drilled away, unroofing the sigmoid sinus down to the jugular bulb. The semicircular

canals and facial nerve are left intact. The temporal floor dura, presigmoid dura, and superior petrosal sinus are exposed (Fig. 13). If the patient is deaf, the labyrinth itself may be drilled away, increasing the bony opening and increasing tumor exposure, essentially converting the procedure into a subtemporal-translabyrinthine approach (Fig. 14).

DURAL OPENING/MANAGEMENT OF VENOUS STRUCTURES. As mentioned before, a relaxed brain is essential before opening the dura. The dura is opened on both sides of the superior petrosal sinus anterior to the sigmoid sinus. The temporal incision is horizontal, making a "T" with the vertical presigmoid incision (Fig. 15). For better exposure below cranial nerve VII and VIII, when the jugular bulb is high, the sigmoid sinus may be divided. This can be done safely if both transverse sinuses are (a) patent, (b) connected to and drain the torcula, and (c) if there is no increase of intrasinus pressure when the sinus is temporarily clamped. After division the dural incision is extended downward. If the sinus cannot be divided, the presigmoid approach can be combined with a retrosigmoid approach to provide a lower exposure and the surgeon can work both in front of and behind the sigmoid sinus. The posterior temporal lobe is gently elevated to inspect the floor for temporal lobe draining veins, all of which should be preserved by incising the dura and tentorium in front of these veins (Fig. 16).

The superior petrosal sinus is clipped or coagulated and divided. The tentorial cut is carried all the way to the incisura, taking care to stay posterior to the entry of cranial nerve IV.

TUMOR RESECTION. The tumor is progressively devascularized by coagulating and dividing its base at the tentorium and petrous ridge. The tumor is debulked, with the surgeon working between the cranial nerves. Caution must be exercised in looking for cranial nerves and vessels encased within the tumor. The tumor capsule is carefully dissected from the brainstem and cerebellum, maintaining the dissection in the arachnoid planes and preserving the neurovascular structures. Tumor in the Meckel cave is removed by opening the overlying dura. During the entire operation, temporal lobe and cerebellar retraction is used judiciously.

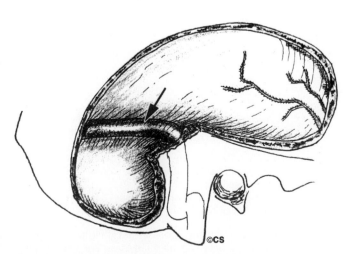

Fig. 12. Artist's illustration. After craniotomy, the transverse sinus (*arrow*) is exposed.

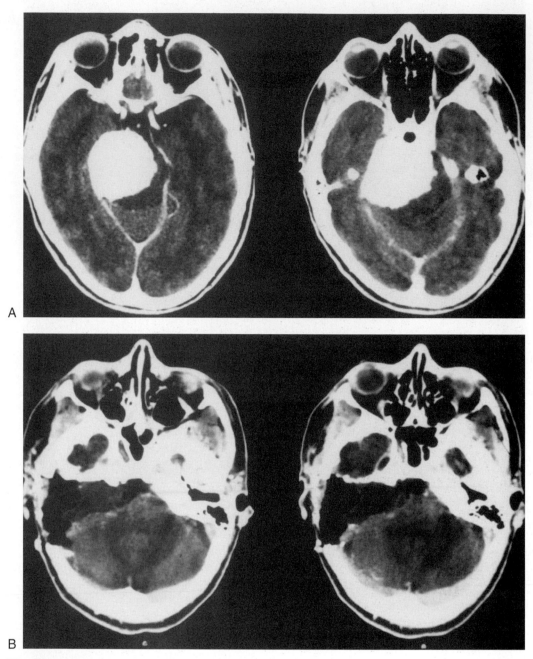

Fig. 14. **A:** Axial contrast-enhanced CT scan. Preoperative imaging reveals a large clival/cerebellopontine angle tumor with brainstem and cerebellar compression. The patient presented with right-sided deafness. A subtemporal-translabyrinthine approach was used with complete drilling of the temporal bone structures. **B:** Postoperative axial CT scan shows removal of the tumor and the extent of the temporal bone drilling.

CLOSURE. Dura is closed in a watertight fashion with a dural graft. The mastoid antrum is closed with a small piece of bone followed by bone wax, which is used to coat the entire surface of the bone. The soft tissues are closed in multiple layers after the bone flap is replaced.

ADVANTAGES AND DISADVANTAGES. There are several important advantages with this approach. These include:

• minimized brain retraction
• shortened operative distance to the clivus

• an exposure that puts the surgeon's line of sight in a direct line with the lesion and with the anterior and lateral aspects of the brainstem
• preservation of all neural, vascular, and otological structures (including the transverse and sigmoid sinuses, the cochlea, and the facial canal)
• provision of multiple axes for dissection
• early interruption of the tumor's vascular supply (3)

The disadvantages of this approach are that it still requires the surgeon to work between cranial nerves. The risk of injury is less if the cranial nerves have been chronically stretched. This leaves more room between the cranial nerve for the surgeon

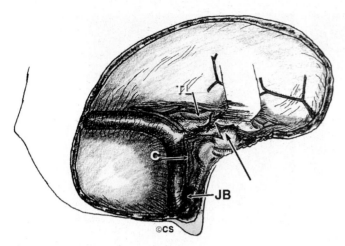

Fig. 15. Artist's illustration. The dural opening is shown over the temporal lobe and the posterior fossa. *C,* cerebellum; *JB,* jugular bulb; *TL,* temporal lobe.

to operate (as in the case of laterally extending petroclival meningiomas) than in the case of more centrally situated tumors (i.e., purely clival tumors) where the cranial nerves are shorter. Further, the sigmoid sinus is exposed and at risk of thrombosis or injury, the posterior temporal lobe tolerates retraction poorly, and a high jugular bulb can restrict the presigmoid dural opening (6).

EXAMPLE 2. A 44-year-old woman presented with poor vision in the left eye, partial III and VI cranial nerve palsies, left-sided hemiparesis, and recent urinary incontinence. MRI revealed a large petroclival meningioma compressing the brainstem and displacing the basilar artery (Fig. 17). The patient underwent left temporal and posterior fossa craniotomies, mastoidectomy, and tumor resection (Fig. 18). Postoperatively, she had a complete ophthalmoplegia of the left eye and anesthesia in the left V1 and V2 distribution. At follow-up, 3 months later, there was partial recovery of III and V cranial nerve function.

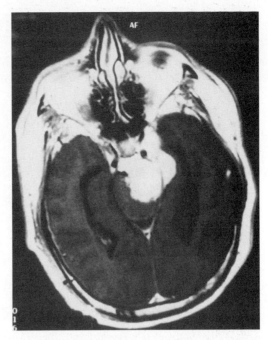

Fig. 17. Axial contrast-enhanced, T1-weighted MRI. This preoperative film reveals a large petroclival meningioma with significant brainstem compression, displacing the basilar artery.

EXAMPLE 3. A 41-year-old man presented with trouble swallowing, gait difficulty, and emotional lability. MRI revealed a large meningioma involving the clivus, tentorium, and left middle cranial fossa with brainstem compression (Fig. 19). In his first operation, a left temporal craniotomy, posterior fossa craniotomy, and mastoidectomy were performed to resect the tumor within the posterior fossa. The second stage involved a temporal craniotomy (which was in continuity with the first bone flap), and resection of the tumor from the middle fossa (Figs. 20 A–C). Postoperatively he had left cranial nerve VI paralysis and left facial hypesthesia, from which he recovered.

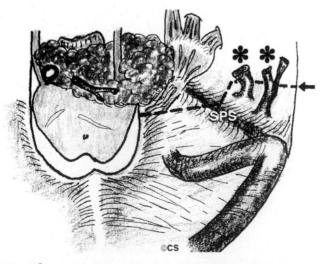

Fig. 16. Artist's illustration. Division of the tentorium. The tentorium is divided (*dotted line*) anterior to the temporal draining veins (*asterisks*), carried across the superior petrosal sinus (*SPS*), posterior to the trigeminal ganglion, and carried to the incisura.

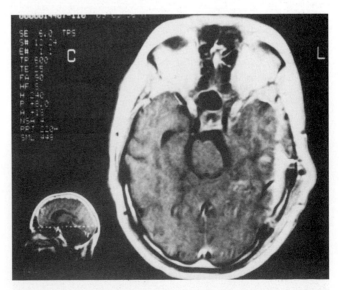

Fig. 18. Postoperative axial contrast-enhanced, T1-weighted MRI reveals the tumor resection.

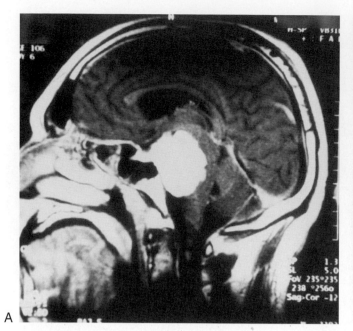
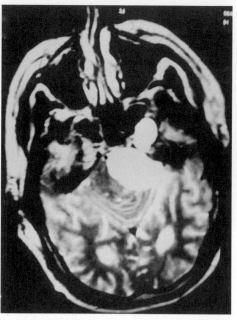

A   B

Fig. 19. Preoperative sagittal contrast-enhanced, T1-weighted MRI **(A)** and axial contrast-enhanced, T2-weighted MRI **(B)** reveal a large tumor anterior to the brainstem with significant brainstem compression.

Retrosigmoid Approach

The retrosigmoid approach (also known as the suboccipital approach) is primarily indicated for tumors involving the cerebellopontine angle, although it was commonly used for meningiomas of the mid- or upper clivus before the more extensive exposures were developed. Some authors believe that this approach is the preferred approach for tumors of the upper clivus (2), although others believe that it is best suited for tumors of the cerebellopontine angle, rather than tumors of the clivus and petrous apex (16). When used for clival tumors, this approach is best suited for small or medium-sized tumors located at the mid- or upper clivus, and with limited dural attachment (7), which are centrolaterally (rather than purely centrally) located (2).

POSITION AND SCALP INCISION. Numerous patient positions have been used, including the supine position with shoulder roll, sitting position, prone, concorde, and lateral oblique (park bench). We prefer the full lateral position, as this position is associated with a reduced risk of air embolism and decreased operator hand fatigue. The head is positioned so that its long axis is parallel to the floor. A vertical incision 6- to 8-cm long is made 3-cm medial to the mastoid tip.

SCALP FLAP/MUSCLE FLAP/BONE FLAP. The underlying muscles are incised in line with the skin incision, and retracted medially and laterally. A craniectomy is made, which extends superiorly to the transverse sinus, laterally to the sigmoid sinus, and inferiorly down to the flat part of the posterior fossa but not including the foramen magnum.

DURAL OPENING. The dural opening is made so that the base is medially located, and the edges parallel to the transverse

sinus and foramen magnum. Dura is drawn upward and sideways so that the lateral and sigmoid sinuses are drawn away. Thus, a very lateral access to the cerebellopontine angle is created, parallel to the posterior petrous ridge and insertion of the tentorium on the petrous bone. This angle allows for less cerebellar retraction.

The cerebellum is retracted medially, exposing the basal cisterns and tumor. Arachnoid is opened, allowing CSF to drain, and providing brain relaxation.

TUMOR EXCISION. The tumor is the debulked, working through the spaces created by cranial nerves V, VII, and VIII and cranial nerves IX, X, and XI. After debulking, the capsule is removed in succession from cranial nerves and brainstem, again taking care to work within arachnoid planes. Lastly, the tumor's insertions on the petrous apex, tentorium, and clivus are coagulated or excised.

According to Bricolo and colleagues, although this is predominantly an infratentorial approach, it is possible at this stage in the operation to access the supratentorial portion of tumor. When the cerebellopontine tumor component is removed, a space between the brainstem and free margin of tentorium exists. Through this space the supratentorial tumor may be accessed and removed. The tentorium may be incised to provide more room (2).

CLOSURE. Once tumor is removed the dura is closed primarily. Any openings in mastoid air cells are rechecked to ensure that they were sealed properly with bone wax. The soft tissues are closed in multiple, watertight layers.

ADVANTAGES AND DISADVANTAGES. The advantages to this approach are that it is a classical approach and familiar to most neurosurgeons. It affords the simplest access to the cerebellopontine angle and lateral clivus. Furthermore, the surgeon begins tumor removal earlier in the procedure than for

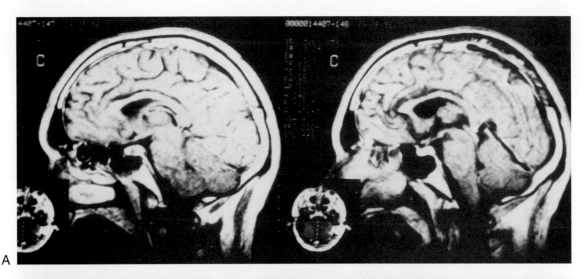

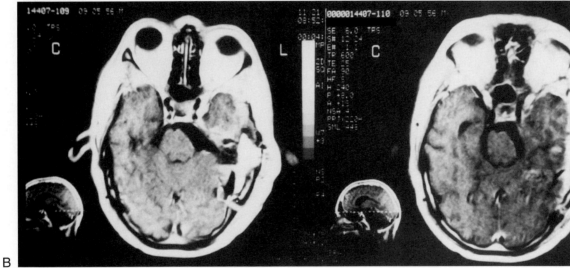

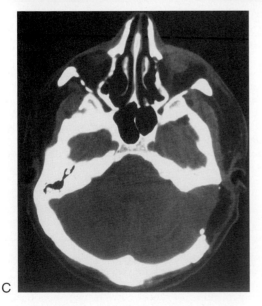

Fig. 20. Postoperative sagittal **(A)** and axial **(B)** contrast-enhanced, T1-weighted MRIs reveal total resection of the lesion and that the brainstem has shifted to a normal position. **C:** Postoperative axial CT shows the extent of the temporal bone removed.

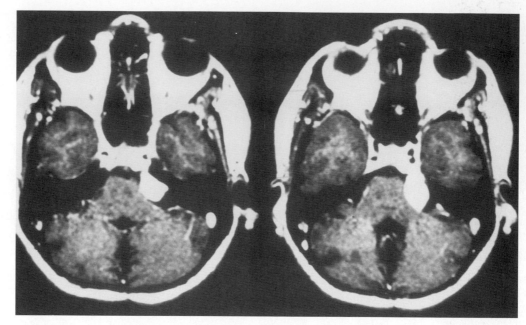

Fig. 21. Axial contrast-enhanced CT. Preoperative films show an enhancing cerebellopontine angle mass with a small amount of brainstem compression.

other approaches, and the mild to moderate cerebellar retraction is well tolerated (6).

Disadvantages are found in that the tumor is at a considerable depth from the surface, and that the resection is carried on through fissures made by cranial nerves V, VII, and VIII and cranial nerves IX, X, and XI, placing those nerves at risk of injury (2). The brainstem is poorly visualized when indented by the tumor, making tumor excision difficult and, at times, dangerous (6).

EXAMPLE 4. A 32-year-old woman presented with a grand mal seizure. Imaging showed multiple supratentorial and sev-

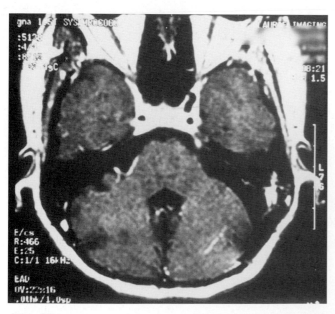

Fig. 22. Axial contrast-enhanced CT. Postoperative MRI shows no residual tumor after retrosigmoid removal.

eral small brainstem cavernous angiomas, as well as a small left cerebellopontine angle meningioma of the medial incisura with brainstem compression (Fig. 21). The patient underwent a left suboccipital craniectomy and drilling of the internal auditory canal for tumor resection (Fig. 22). She remained neurologically intact postoperatively, and has been free of tumor recurrence for 3 years.

Postoperative Management

Postoperative care is extremely important in ensuring a good outcome. Because patients can deteriorate rapidly from a variety of problems, vigilance is essential. Patients must be kept in an intensive care unit, preferably one dedicated to the care of neurosurgical patients. Ventilation status, neurological status, blood pressure, and electrolyte levels are closely followed, and adjustments made accordingly. In the event of a poor postoperative mental status, a patient is kept intubated and a CT scan is obtained emergently. The blood pressure should be well controlled, and the judicious use of antihypertensive agents or pressors as indicated is essential. Ventricular or spinal fluid drainage is continued postoperatively for 4 to 5 days.

Complications

Many of the postoperative complications may be predicted from the surgical approach, type of lesion, and patient history (i.e., primary surgery or reoperation, or a history of irradiation). Meticulous planning of preoperative management (i.e., embolization), surgical execution, and postoperative care is essential for successful treatment.

We have broadly divided the postoperative complications into wound-related, brain-related, and cranial nerve-related problems.

WOUND-RELATED. The scalp flap must be planned so that the blood supply is maintained, promoting wound healing and preventing infection and CSF leak. This is especially true in the case of reoperations or after irradiation. The dura should be closed as watertight as possible, using dural grafts as needed, and be reinforced by multiple layers of muscle and soft-tissue closure.

BRAIN-RELATED. Brain-related problems are further divided into mass lesions, CSF fistulae, vascular problems, and infections.

Cerebral edema and contusions are the most serious postoperative complications. Other mass lesions include subdural and epidural collections. The best treatment is prevention. Paying particular attention to posterior temporal draining veins lessens risk of contusion and edema; they should be preserved at all costs and their manipulation minimized. Venous infarction can be caused by excessive or extensive retraction on the brain. For long operations, it is worthwhile to intermittently release the retraction on the brain for several minutes. If the brain appears full during closure, an ultrasound can be used to determine the presence of an intracerebral hematoma, which can be promptly evacuated. Fluid status, hydration, and anticonvulsant levels are all followed closely. Surgical decompression of the temporal lobe should be performed if there is any clinical indication to do so, such as poor mental status or hemiparesis. We have a low threshold for intervention; deterioration can be rapid, and once that has started it is difficult to regain that lost ground

CSF fistulae are a serious complication that, if not addressed promptly, can result in meningitis. We often put in a ventricular catheter or lumbar drain at the time of surgery and leave it in for up to a week thereafter, giving the wound time to heal. Subgaleal and subcutaneous collections of CSF are often encountered and resolve spontaneously. However, a leak from the incision or the mastoid may require surgical reexploration.

Vascular-related problems include all those related to venous and arterial structures, and include venous infarction (discussed previously) and arterial infarction. Infarctions usually result from loss of basilar artery perforators. Injury to larger vessels should be immediately repaired. Tumor removal should be meticulous with good judgment to leave some tumor on the small vessels rather than risk their irreversible loss.

CRANIAL NERVE-RELATED. Cranial nerves III through XII are at risk during surgeries of the petroclival region. Many patients will experience some level of postoperative neurapraxia after surgery, usually diplopia related to injury of the nerves controlling extraocular movements. Most of these are transient by nature.

The most serious problems are those related to the lower cranial nerves—IX, X, and XI. Airway protection and swallowing function are impaired, increasing the risk for aspiration pneumonia and malnutrition. If there is any concern about the functioning of these nerves, the patient's swallowing function should be evaluated and the diet slowly advanced so that aspiration pneumonia does not occur. Unilateral paralysis can be easily compensated in the younger patient, but older patients can rarely compensate adequately. In these patients, a feeding gastrostomy and a tracheostomy can, by preventing pneumonia and malnutrition, be lifesaving, and also hasten recovery. Once the patient has compensated for the deficit, these tubes can be removed.

Permanent loss of cranial nerve X function may require vocal cord augmentation and cricopharyngeal myotomy. After an injury to the facial nerve, the cornea should be protected immediately with the use of an eye bubble, artificial tears, and lubricant. A gold weight should be placed in the eyelid for further protection. If the nerve is severed, it can be reconstructed intraoperatively with an end-to-end anastomosis or cable graft (using the greater auricular or sural nerves). In these situations, the best outcome possible is a House-Brackman grade III (17). If such measures are not possible, or if facial nerve in continuity has not recovered after 12 months, an extracranial VII to XII anastomosis can be performed (18). Passive reanimation with facial slings can be considered in long-standing situations. These latter two options, while not providing facial function, will at least provide some cosmetic relief.

Trigeminal nerve impairment can give rise to corneal anesthesia and predispose to corneal ulcers. The eye must be carefully protected. If corneal problems develop, tarsorrhaphy may be needed. Deafferentation type of facial pain syndrome can also occur and is treated medically.

RESULTS. The mortality of modern surgical series ranges from 0% (3,8,9) to 17% (2,5–7,10). Most deaths are caused by complications from a worsened neurological status (such as pulmonary embolus, sepsis, and aspiration pneumonia) (6,7,10). Intraoperative deaths are relatively rare—Couldwell and colleagues reported 4 in their series of 109 patients (7). Gross total resection has been achieved in 69% to 91% of cases (2,3,6–9). Of all patients, 0 to 15% of petroclival meningiomas recurred or regrew (2,6,7,10).

Morbidity remains high. Cranial nerve deficits remain the most common neurological deficit after surgery, with an incidence of 33% to 76% of patients having new postoperative deficits (2,3,7,9,10). While approximately 50% of these deficits are permanent (3,6), they are often well tolerated, have little effect on patient independence, and do not prevent a meaningful existence (2,10). The cranial nerves most often involved are V, VII, and VIII, with cranial nerves III, IV, and VI being involved less often (10).

Motor weakness is another significant cause of morbidity, occurring in 12% to 46% of patients (2,3,7,9,10). These deficits have been shown to be transient in 7% to 50% of cases (3,6). A transient change in mental status postoperatively has been observed in 12% to 31% of patients (6,10).

Several authors believe that morbidity and mortality are more significant for the patients they treat at the earlier stages of their surgical series, and decrease with increasing experience (2,6,10). It has also been stated that patients with smaller tumors did better than those with larger tumors (6,10). Sekhar and associates also believe that complications are more likely in patients who have undergone prior radiation therapy or are undergoing a second operation (6).

Sekhar and co-workers published a retrospective study of 75 patients who had undergone surgery for clival meningiomas (upper, middle, and lower clival), and found that 45 patients (60%) had early postoperative deterioration (11). Tumor size was the most significant variable predicting this deterioration—patients with large and giant tumors were 6.7 and 13 times more likely to have early postoperative deterioration than those harboring smaller meningiomas. Other factors found to be significant included blood supply from the basilar artery (as demonstrated on angiography), the presence of brainstem edema on MRI (Fig. 23), encasement of vertebrobasilar arteries, preoperative Karnofsky score, male gender, and lack of arachnoid plane between tumor and brainstem on MRI (Fig. 24). Of these 45 patients, 12 (27%) had permanent postoperative dysfunction, which was associated with blood supply from the basilar artery, difficult surgical dissection, subtotal resection, and the presence of early postoperative dysfunction (11).

Some petroclival meningiomas are invasive, and due to the

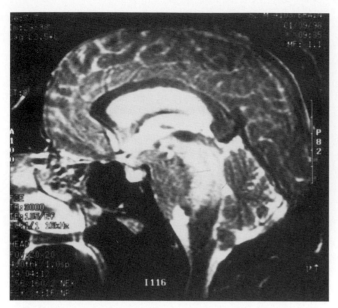

Fig. 23. Sagittal contrast-enhanced, T2-weighted MRI reveals a large petroclival meningioma, notable for the high degree of brainstem edema, which is a poor prognostic indicator.

high degree of brainstem indentation (2), lack of arachnoid plane (8), tumor encasement of important arteries and cranial nerves (2,7), or bony invasion (2), gross total resection is either not possible or will result in unacceptable morbidity for the patient (2,7,8). These tumors can be well tolerated for a long time after a successful subtotal resection. In Mayberg and Symon's series, 26 of 35 patients (74%) underwent subtotal tumor resection. Of these, 4 ultimately died of recurrent disease (at 9,

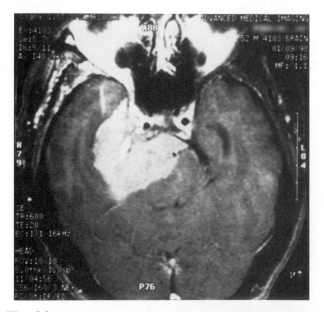

Fig. 24. Axial contrast-enhanced, T1-weighted MRI shows a large petroclival meningioma with significant brainstem compression, which is encasing, narrowing, and displacing the basilar artery. There is no arachnoid plane between the tumor and the brain. Both characteristics are poor prognostic indicators.

10, 15, and 32 months after surgery), while 3 showed radiographic evidence of recurrence but were asymptomatic (10).

Conclusion

The treatment of petroclival meningiomas has improved significantly. The powerful combination of detailed preoperative radiological imaging, intraoperative monitoring, modern microneurosurgical techniques, and critical care management have made total excisions of these tumors common, with a better patient outcome than could be expected two decades ago. As experience with these tumors grows, current questions regarding the use of adjunctive therapy will be answered, and we will further know how to treat these difficult lesions and offer the best chance for a long and productive life for our patients.

References

1. Al-Mefty O, Smith RR. Clival and petroclival meningiomas. In: Al-Mefty O, ed. *Meningiomas.* New York: Raven Press, 1991:517–538.
2. Bricolo AP, Turazzi S, Talacchi A, et al. Microsurgical removal of petroclival meningiomas. *Neurosurgery* 1992;31:813–828.
3. Al-Mefty O, Fox JL, Smith RR. Petrosal approach for petroclival meningiomas. *Neurosurgery* 1988;22:510–517.
4. Castellano F, Ruggerio G. Meningiomas of the posterior fossa. *Acta Radiol Suppl* 1953;104:1–157.
5. Yasargil MG, Mortara RW, Curcic M. Meningiomas of basal posterior cranial fossa. *Adv Tech Stand Neurosurg* 1980;7:3–115.
6. Sekhar LN, Jannetta PJ, Burkhart LE, et al. Meningiomas involving the clivus: a six-year experience with 41 patients. *Neurosurgery* 1990;27:764–781.
7. Couldwell WT, Fukushima T, Giannotta SL, et al. Petroclival meningiomas: surgical experience in109 cases. *J Neurosurg* 1996;84:20–28.
8. Spetzler RF, Daspit CP, Pappas CTE. The combined supra- and infratentorial approach for lesions of the petrous and clival regions: experience with 46 cases. *J Neurosurg* 1992;76:588–599.
9. Samii M, Ammirati M, Mahran A, et al. Surgery of petroclival meningiomas: report of 24 cases. *Neurosurgery* 1989;24:12–17.
10. Mayberg MR, Symon L. Meningiomas of the clivus and apical petrous bone. *J Neurosurg* 1986;65:160–167.
11. Sekhar LN, Swamy NKS, Jaiswal V, et al. Surgical excision of meningiomas involving the clivus: preoperative and intraoperative features as predictors of postoperative functional deterioration. *J Neurosurg* 1994;81:860–868.
12. Hakuba A, Nishimura S, Jang BJ. A combined retroauricular and preauricular transpetrosal-transtentorial approach to clivus meningiomas. *Surg Neurol* 1988;30:108–116.
13. Haddad GF, Al-Mefty O. Infratentorial and foramen magnum meningiomas. In: Wilkins RH, Rengachary SS, eds. *Neurosurgery.* New York: McGraw-Hill, 1996:951–958.
14. Subach BR, Lunsford LD, Kondziolka D, et al. Management of petroclival meningiomas by stereotactic radiosurgery. *Neurosurgery* 1998;42:437–445.
15. Malis LI. Surgical resection of tumors of the skull base. In: Wilkins RH, Rengachary, eds. *Neurosurgery.* New York: McGraw-Hill, 1985:1011–1021.
16. Haddad GF, Al-Mefty O. Approaches to petroclival tumors. In: Wilkins RH, Rengachary SS, eds. *Neurosurgery.* New York: McGraw-Hill, 1996:1695–1706.
17. Stephanian E, Sekhar LN, Janecka IP, Hirsch B. Facial nerve repair by interposition nerve graft: results in 22 patients. *Neurosurgery* 1992;31:73–77.
18. Pitty LF, Tator CH. Hypoglossal-facial nerve anastomosis for facial nerve palsy following surgery for cerebellopontine angle tumors. *J Neurosurg* 1992;77:764–781.

122. Clival Chordomas

Franco DeMonte

Chordomas are rare neoplasms, accounting for 0.1% to 0.2% of all primary intracranial tumors. They are believed to originate from remnants of the primitive notochord and occur along the craniospinal axis. About 35% of chordomas involve the cranium and two-thirds of these lie in the clivus. The peak incidence occurs between 35 and 50 years of age (1). Only 5% occur in those younger than 20 years of age (2–4). Chordomas in children younger than 5 years of age tend to have a heightened biological aggressiveness (3).

Tumors arising from the rostral clivus have been classified as basi-sphenoidal chordomas, whereas those arising caudal to the spheno-occipital synchondrosis have been classified as basi-occipital. These tumors usually grow extradurally but may penetrate the dura as they become large or recur (5,6). The majority of clival chordomas are large at diagnosis and extend to the anterior cranial fossa or parasellar region, whereas a third extend ventrally into the nasal cavities, paranasal sinuses or nasopharynx, or middle fossa (1). Cavernous sinus invasion is present in 50% to 75% of patients at diagnosis (7–9). Basisphenoidal chordomas tend to cause dysfunction of the upper cranial nerves (i.e., visual loss and cavernous sinus syndrome) and pituitary endocrinopathy by virtue of their relation to the upper brainstem and sella. Basi-occipital chordomas are more likely to result in palsy of the lower cranial nerves and long tract signs (Table 1). Lateral extensions of tumor give rise to unilateral symptoms. In 1945, Givner reviewed the 100 cases of spheno-occipital chordomas reported at that time and found that paresis of the abducens nerve was the most frequent symptom, occurring in 34 patients (10). This paresis tended to precede the onset of paralysis of other ocular nerves. The paresis initially was unilateral, but became bilateral in the later stages of the disease. He also noted that in every instance of facial nerve dysfunction, the abducens nerve was also affected. Diplopia was the most common and usually the first symptom reported in the patient series described by Raffel and associates (11). An abducens palsy was the cause of the diplopia in approximately 70% of patients. Oculomotor palsy affected the remainder. Similarly, more recent papers by Sen and colleagues (6) and Forsyth and co-workers (1) report abducens palsy in nine of 17 and 29 of 51 patients, respectively. This represents the most frequent clinical abnormality in both series. Spontaneously remitting abducens palsy has been documented to occur, emphasizing the need for the radiological evaluation of all patients with a new onset of diplopia (12,13). Review of the preceding series of patients reinforces the significance of the classical presentation of clival chordoma: unilateral abducens nerve paresis, followed by bilateral cranial nerve signs, followed by bulbar signs.

Chordomas are locally invasive and must be considered malignant, although most commonly they are histologically benign and slow growing. These tumors often involve and infiltrate surrounding bone, even though they appear well localized. Recurrence has been the rule for this reason. Pathologically these tumors often are lobulated and contain compact masses or elongated cords of clear cells with intracytoplasmic vacuoles that appear bubblelike (physaliphorous) and usually are intersected by thick fibrous connective tissue strands (Fig. 1). Immunocytochemically, a mixed epithelial–mesenchymal phenotype is identified. Vimentin, cytokeratin, and epithelial membrane antigen reactivity is present. S-100 Reactivity also may be seen. Dedifferentiated tumors and distant metastases occur, although they are uncommon. Of the 63 patients with recurrence identified by Fagundes, 13 had evidence of distant metastasis, most commonly to the lung and bone (14).

The average length of survival for untreated patients after the onset of symptoms is about 1 year. Heffelfinger and associates in 1973, reported median survival times of 0.9 years without therapy, 1.5 years after surgery alone, 4.8 years after radiation therapy alone, and 5.2 years after surgery and radiation therapy (15). Twenty years later, Forsyth and co-workers reported overall 5- and 10-year survivals of 51% and 35% and disease-free survival rates of 33% at 5 years and 24% at 10 years (1). Treatment consisted of biopsy or subtotal resection followed by external beam radiotherapy. This form of management occasionally has resulted in long-term survival and even cure, but the mean survival of treated patients has remained at 50 to 60 months, with 5-year survival rates near 50%, and 10-year survival rates around 30% (1,16,17). Factors correlating with improved survival were a greater extent of resection, younger age, and absence of mitoses. Conventional postoperative radiation therapy did not improve survival time but had a significant effect on prolonged disease-free survival (1), suggesting the benefit of attempts at gross total resection. Series advocating radical resection have reported similar survival rates of 65% at 5 years (8) and disease-free incidence rates of 70% at 2 years (2). Menezes and colleagues reported an 86% survival in their 36 patients followed for a mean of 5 years (18).

Conventional external beam radiation therapy has resulted in generally poor progression-free and overall survival (19), with recurrence rates of 50% to 100% following treatment (20). Charged particle irradiation has shown increased effectiveness when compared to conventional external beam radiotherapy. Austin-Seymour and colleagues using mean proton-beam treatment doses of 69.4 cGyE (cGy Equivalents), reported actuarial survival rates of 76% at 5 years (21). Similarly, Berson and associates achieved 5-year disease free survivals of 62%. This increased to 80% for smaller tumor sizes. The overall 2-year local control rate was 78% for initial disease, but decreased to 33% for recurrent disease (22). Hug and associates reported on 33 patients with chordoma treated with proton irradiation to mean doses of 70.7 cGyE. A 76% tumor control rate by the end of the follow-up period (mean of 33 months) was observed. The actuarial 5-year survival rate was determined to be 79% (20). Treatment failures following charged particle irradiation are usually seen with large tumors and in regions receiving less than 67 to 72 cGyE (23). Deliberate reductions in radiation dose typically are made adjacent to the optic nerve and chiasm, spinal cord, and brainstem.

Table 1. Symptoms of Clival Chordoma Based on Site of Origin

Site of Origin	Symptoms
Upper clivus	Pituitary endocrinopathy, visual loss, chiasmal syndrome, cavernous sinus syndrome
Mid clivus	Nasopharyngeal mass, abducens nerve palsy, multiple cranial neuropathies, brainstem syndrome, hydrocephalus, cerebellopontine angle syndrome
Lower clivus	Hypoglossal nerve palsy, foramen magnum syndrome

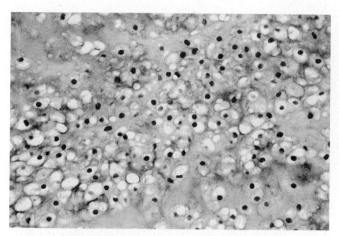

Fig. 1. Photomicrograph of a typical chordoma. The tumor cells contain bubblelike intracytoplasmic vacuoles (physaliphorous cells).

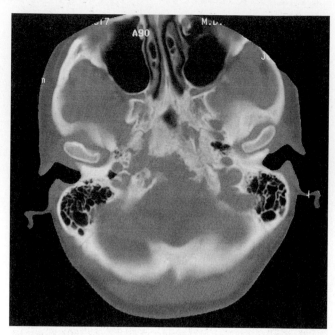

Fig. 2. Axial CT scan at bone window settings. Extensive destruction of the skull base is present.

The efficacy of radiosurgical treatment of clival chordomas is being evaluated. Muthukumar and colleagues treated nine patients with clival chordomas with stereotactic radiosurgery for marginal doses of 12 to 20 Gy. The average tumor diameter was 2.1 cm. A number of patients improved during the median clinical follow-up of 40 months. Mean radiosurgical follow-up was not mentioned and patient outcome was not discussed (24).

Principles of Preoperative Evaluation

All patients have a complete history and physical examination as well as a careful neuro-ophthalmologic evaluation, which assesses visual acuity and fields, pupillary function, and ocular motility. Less than one third of these patients have a normal neuro-ophthalmological examination. Patients with upper clival chordomas undergo a complete endocrinological assessment to identify evidence of pituitary or hypothalamic dysfunction. Patients with mid to lower clival chordomas are assessed by an otolaryngologist with specific attention to hearing and lower cranial nerve function. An audiogram and direct laryngoscopy usually are performed. High-resolution computed tomographic (CT) scanning allows the accurate assessment of bony destruction by the tumor, which is present universally (Fig. 2). Integrity of the optic and carotid canals can be best assessed in this way. Tumoral calcification, usually consisting of a few scattered punctate densities, is well seen if present. Typically the tumor is of increased density relative to brain and enhances brightly with contrast administration (25). If there is a question of occipitocervical instability, plain x-ray films of the cervical spine are performed, both in flexion and extension.

Multiplanar magnetic resonance imaging (MRI), with and without contrast enhancement, best demonstrates the extent of the tumor and best identifies important adjacent neurovascular structures such as the brainstem, optic nerves and chiasm, and internal carotid and basilar arteries (Fig. 3). Chordomas generally have low to intermediate signal intensity on T1-weighted images and moderately high to very high signal intensity on T2-weighted images. Scattered foci of variable intensity also can be seen and generally represent small sites of hemorrhage or

mucinous collections. The signal intensity on T2-weighted studies is heterogeneous in about 80% of tumors. The tumors all evidence contrast enhancement. This enhancement usually is heterogeneous in nature (25,26). The differential diagnosis of an invasive clival mass includes chordoma, chondrosarcoma (although these tumors are usually found in a paramedian location), pituitary adenoma, metastasis, meningioma, nasopharyngeal carcinoma (especially in patients of Chinese descent), and primary sphenoid sinus malignancy.

Cerebral angiography is typically not necessary for the diagnosis of clival chordomas. It is used when felt necessary by the surgeon to obtain a detailed view of the head and neck and intracranial vasculature, which at times is significantly distorted, encased, or narrowed by the tumor. Important anatomical variations are noted, such as the pattern of venous drainage, especially if the planned surgical approach places these structures at risk. Preoperative temporary balloon occlusion testing of the ICA is performed if ICA occlusion or sacrifice is planned, or if risk of arterial injury is deemed high. In most centers one or more complimentary investigations of cerebrovascular reserve—such as transcranial doppler (TCD), cerebral blood flow (CBF), or single photon emission computed tomography (SPECT)—are used in conjunction with the temporary balloon occlusion test.

General Surgical Principles

Clival chordomas are primarily extradural tumors, and only transgress the dura in advanced cases or when they recur (6). They rarely affect only one anatomical region, thus complicating the choice of operative approach, and decreasing the likeli-

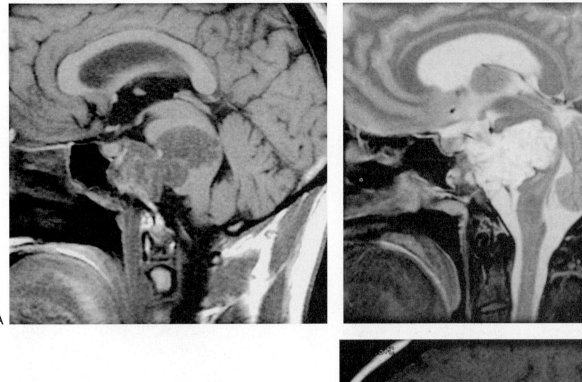

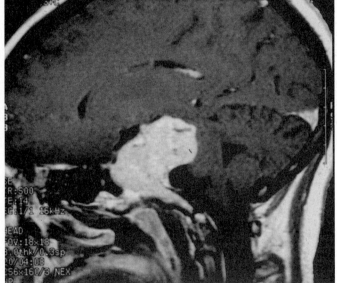

Fig. 3. T1-weighted **(A)**, T2-weighted **(B)**, and T1-weighted postcontrast **(C)** MRIs all in the sagittal plane depicting the imaging characteristics of chordoma. **A:** On T1-weighted scans the tumor is hypointense to brain, although areas of increased signal intensity are also seen. **B:** The tumor is of increased intensity on T2-weighted studies. **C:** The pattern of enhancement in this particular instance is fairly homogenous. A more heterogenous pattern of enhancement is common.

hood of complete resection. Most often these tumors are soft and gelatinous in consistency; however, they may be fibrous and tenacious, making removal difficult and dangerous, especially through limited approaches. A wide surgical field also allows more extensive bone removal with greater safety, and facilitates dural repair should it be necessary.

There have been numerous surgical approaches used to access the clivus. The choice of one approach over another needs to factor in the parameters of tumor location, size, extension, unique patient anatomy and functional requirements, and experience, expertise, and preference of the surgical team. Small, midline upper clival chordomas without lateral extension, for example, are probably best removed through a transsphenoidal approach, whereas large tumors with lateral and intradural extensions may require both a transfacial and intracranial approach for adequate tumor removal. Table 2 lists the various surgical approaches that are useful for clival chordoma resection. The transbasal and transmandibular approaches are dealt with in detail, although each is discussed briefly.

Extended Transbasal Approach

Developed by Tessier and Derome, the transbasal approach to the clivus subsequently was modified to incorporate orbital osteotomies in an effort to reduce frontal lobe retraction and allow exposure of more laterally related structures, such as the medial walls of the cavernous sinus and the hypoglossal canals (8,27–30). The approach consists of a bifrontal craniotomy, bilateral orbital osteotomy (removal of supraorbital bar), eth-

Table 2. Surgical Approaches to the Clivus

Transsphenoidal
Transsphenoethmoidal
Transoral–transpalatal
Transmaxillary
Transmandibular circumglossal retropharyngeal
Extended transbasal
Transtemporal
   Anterior
   Posterior
   Combined
Transcondylar

moidectomy, sphenoidectomy, and extradural resection of the clivus. The limits of exposure are the foramen magnum inferiorly and the hypoglossal canals inferolaterally, whereas the intracavernous carotid arteries form the superolateral limits. The posterior clinoids, dorsum sellae, and region behind and above the pituitary gland are obscured by the gland, rendering this a blind area via the extended transbasal approach (Fig. 4) (8,29, 30).

Following a bicoronal scalp incision, the scalp is elevated sharply from the periosteum and loose connective tissue layers (collectively named the pericranium) immediately deep to the galea in order to maintain the maximal thickness and vascularity of the pericranium medial to the superior temporal lines bilaterally. Separation of these layers should only be taken to a level 1 cm above the supraorbital bar to preserve the rich vascular supply to the pericranium. Both superficial and deep layers of

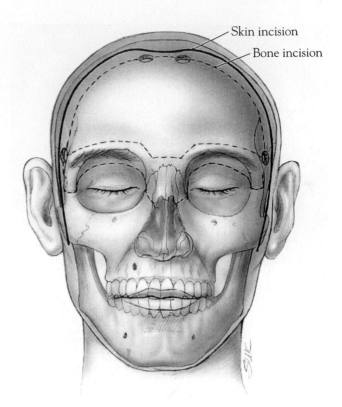

Fig. 5. The skin incision used for the extended transbasal approach *(solid line)*. The osteotomies used to elevate the bifrontal craniotomy and biorbital osteotomy *(broken lines)*. (Used with the permission of the Department of Neurosurgery, University of Texas, MD Anderson Cancer Center.)

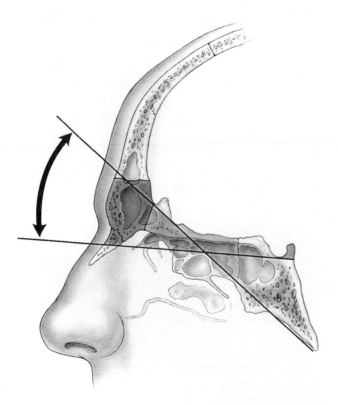

Fig. 4. Artist's depiction of the improved arch of visualization of the clivus when an orbital osteotomy is added to a standard frontal craniotomy. However, the view to the dorsum sellae remains obscured by the pituitary gland. (Used with the permission of the Department of Neurosurgery, University of Texas, MD Anderson Cancer Center.)

the temporalis fascia are incised. Dissection deep to the fascial layer minimizes the risk of injury to the frontalis branches of the facial nerve. Lateral subperiosteal dissection exposes the zygomatic process of the frontal bones, frontozygomatic sutures, and upper lateral orbital rims. Medially, the subperiosteal dissection exposes the glabella, frontonasal suture, and superior orbital rims (Fig. 5).

The dura is dissected from the posterior wall of the frontal sinuses following a bifrontal craniotomy. The frontal sinuses then are cranialized and demucosalized with the high-speed drill and rongeurs. Careful dissection of the dura from the orbital surface of the frontal bones allows access to the orbital osteotomies. The orbital periosteum is dissected down from the roof and walls of the orbit. It has not been necessary in our experience to free the medial canthal ligaments. With protection of the orbital contents and dura, osteotomies are placed in the lateral wall, roof, and upper medial walls of the orbits and across the nasal bones to just in front of the crista galli. This bifronto-orbital osteotomy piece is freed with an osteotome and removed (Fig. 6).

The dura is dissected along the side of the cribriform plate bilaterally to the level of the posterior ethmoidal artery if an attempt at olfactory sparing is to be made. Under the microscope, a reciprocating saw is used to cut across the anterior planum sphenoidale at the level of the frontosphenoid suture (Fig. 6). A generous cuff of nasal mucosa is preserved with the cribriform plate (31). Attempts at olfactory preservation generally are successful in less than one third of patients. Olfactory sparing is contraindicated for nasopharyngeal malignancies because of the neurotropism that many of these neoplasms exhibit.

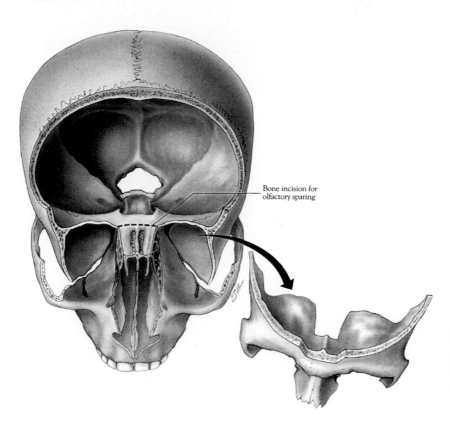

Bone incision for
olfactory sparing

Fig. 6. The biorbital free osteotomy is removed and a bifrontal craniotomy has been performed. The osteotomy line for a olfactory sparing procedure is illustrated. (From the Department of Neurosurgery, University of Texas, MD Anderson Cancer Center, with permission.)

If olfactory preservation is not an issue, as is most often the case, then the crista galli is removed and the dural sleeves of the olfactory groove are cut on either side and closed primarily. The planum sphenoidale then is opened and a wide sphenoidotomy is performed with a high-speed drill. The medial wall of the orbit is removed anteromedially to the optic nerves (Fig. 7). One or both of the optic nerves may require decompression. All but the lateral wall of the optic canal can be removed from this approach. The walls of the sphenoid are progressively removed from anterior to posterior. The sella then is unroofed. Access to the dorsum sellae is blocked by the pituitary gland and tumor in this area is not well seen. The cavernous sinuses and intracavernous internal carotid artery (ICA) are completed unroofed on the medial aspect (Fig. 7). Although covered by a thin periosteal layer, bleeding from the cavernous plexus may occur and is controlled by tamponade. Similarly, bleeding from the clival basilar venous plexus can be considerable but controlled with surgical packs. The cavernous ICA can be exposed from its anterior vertical segment to its entry into the cavernous sinus posterolaterally. The clival tumor and bone are progressively removed in a superior to inferior direction, with the foramen magnum being the lower limit of resection. At the level of the foramen magnum the resection can be carried laterally up to the hypoglossal canals. Clival bone removal continues to include a margin of normal-appearing bone if possible.

Reconstruction begins by closure of any dural defects. Temporalis fascia or fascia lata are used as dural patches as necessary if primary closure is not possible. Typically it is difficult if not impossible to get a watertight closure of the clival dura. In this case, a fascial cover is tacked down with sutures and reinforced with fibrin glue and autologous fat.

The open ethmoid sinuses are packed with fat and then the pericranial flap is turned down to cover and reinforce the exposed dura and separate it from the paranasal sinuses. The bifrontal orbital osteotomy is replaced in its anatomical position and rigidly fixated with titanium plates. Care is taken not to compress the pericranial graft as it passes over the orbital soft tissues and nasal bones. The remainder of the closure follows standard techniques. Graduated, intermittent lumbar spinal drainage is continued for 48 to 72 hours postoperatively if the dural closure is tenuous.

Transmandibular, Circumglossal, Retropharyngeal, and Transpalatal Approaches to Clivus and Upper Cervical Spine

Initially described by Biller and colleagues (32) and popularized by Krespi (33–35) and later Ammirati (36,37), the transmandibular approach to the skull base provides simultaneous exposure of the middle and lateral compartments of the skull base, allows excellent vascular control and access to cranial nerves 9 to 12, and by straightforward expansion allows an exposure that extends from the ipsilateral infratemporal fossa (ITF) to the contralateral medial pterygoid plate, from the anterior cranial fossa to the lower clivus, and the anterior cervical spine down to C7. The main indications for this approach are large tumors involving both the middle and lateral compartments and tumors of the craniocervical junction and upper cervical spine (38). Tumors of the parapharyngeal space and complicated decompressions of the craniocervical junction also can be approached in this manner. The wide exposure allows for anterior reconstruction and internal fixation. Intradural extensions

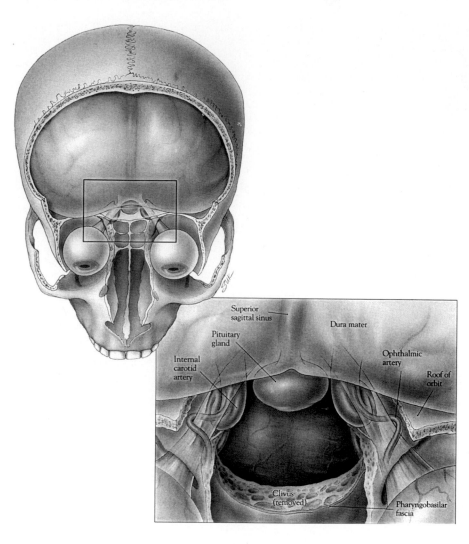

Fig. 7. Progressing from anterior to posterior, the medial orbital walls are resected and an ethmoidectomy is performed. The sphenoid sinus is entered and its bony walls removed as needed. The optic nerves may be decompressed as needed. Tumor removal and partial clivectomy is performed exposing the clival dura. (From the Department of Neurosurgery, University of Texas, MD Anderson Cancer Center, with permission.)

certainly can be removed by this approach, although it is ideally suited for extradural pathology and the risk of meningitis increases. The elevation and subsequent replacement of the laterally based pharyngeal flap helps buttress any needed dural repairs, even though dural repair is rarely watertight in this region. This minimizes the incidence of cerebrospinal fluid (CSF) leakage along with the judicious use of subcutaneous fat and facial grafts, fibrin glue, and lumbar spinal drainage.

A good deal of anatomical dissection is required for this approach, which results in predictable morbidity. A temporary tracheostomy is required. Conductive hearing loss and serous otitis media result from section of the eustachian tube. Temporary swallowing difficulties induced by the circumglossal and palatal incisions, extensive retropharyngeal dissection, and section of the tensor and levator palatini muscles occasionally necessitate the insertion of a gastrostomy. Preoperative consultation with dentistry should be obtained to fashion a palatal stent to be used for support of the palatal mucosa after closure. This stent allows for improved apposition of the mucosa against the residual hard palate, which helps prevent acute mucosal loss. Careful consideration should be given to the use of this approach because of this inherent morbidity. It should be reserved for instances where surgical cure or significant palliation are likely.

Following a tracheostomy, a curvilinear incision is begun just below the mastoid and extended inferiorly and medially along a skin crease to the mentum and through the lip split (Fig. 8). Subplatysmal flaps are elevated to expose the upper neck, submandibular gland, and surrounding tissues (Level I). A selective neck dissection removes the contents of Level I, allowing for the clear identification and preservation of the lingual and hypoglossal nerves. The internal carotid artery (ICA) and internal jugular vein (IJV) are identified and vessel loops are placed. Continued elevation of the flap exposes the mandible. The mandibulotomy site is carefully marked and an internal fixation plate is placed. The plate position is carefully marked, and the plate removed and saved for closure. A stairstep mandibulotomy is performed between the lower medial-two incisors (tooth numbers 24 and 25). Dissection follows the floor of the mouth posteriorly toward the glossopharyngeal sulcus. This allows the mandible to swing laterally and the tongue medially. The styloid process is palpated and the muscular attachments are separated. The ICA, IJV, and CNs IX through XII are traced superiorly to the skull base (Fig. 9). As the incision approaches the anterior tonsillar pillar, it splits into two limbs. The upper limb extends to the soft palate, which is separated from its lateral attachments. This incision then is carried onto the hard palate approximately 1 cm medial to the alveolar ridge. It then passes anteriorly around to the contralateral hard palate. The

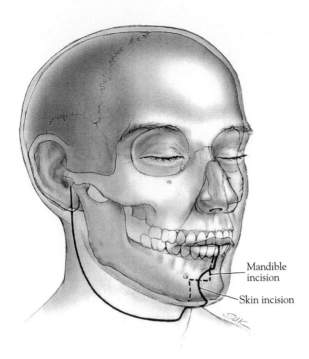

Fig. 8. The *solid line* depicts the skin incision, and the *broken line* depicts the stair-step mandibulotomy necessary for the transmandibular approach to the clivus. (From the Department of Neurosurgery, University of Texas, MD Anderson Cancer Center, with permission.)

base of the hard palate is resected as needed for visualization into the sphenoid sinus. The lower limb of the incision extends into the hypopharynx passing lateral to the tonsil and the orifice of the eustachian tube. The eustachian tube is transected and retropharyngeal dissection follows the subperiosteal plane to expose the clivus and upper cervical spine. This pharyngeal flap is elevated and rotated medially. The clivus and upper cervical spine are covered by the longus capiti muscles and the prevertebral fascia. Removal of the posterior hard palate reveals the posterior bony nasal septum (vomer) and anterior inferior face of the sphenoid sinus. Removal of this bone allows wide exposure of the sphenoid sinus, sella turcica, and upper clivus (Fig. 10).

At this point clivectomy may be performed, and may extend from the sella turcica to the foramen magnum (Fig. 11). Repair with fascial and subcutaneous fat grafts and fibrin glue may be necessary if the dura is deficient.

Closure begins by reattaching the superior constrictor muscle to the muscles at the base of the skull. The palatal flap is reapproximated and the soft palate and hard palate mucosa is sutured. The preoperatively fashioned palatal stent is placed to support the palatal mucosa. The floor of the mouth is closed in a double layer. The pharyngeal flap is allowed to return to its normal position and closure is by careful reapproximation of the posterolateral mucosal edges. The mandible is reapproximated and the reconstruction plate secured. Drains are placed in the neck and a nasogastric tube is inserted. Precise alignment of the vermilion border is assured during lip closure and the platysma and skin are closed in a standard fashion. As for the extended transbasal approach, graduated, intermittent lumbar spinal drainage is continued for 48 to 72 hours postoperatively if the dural closure is tenuous.

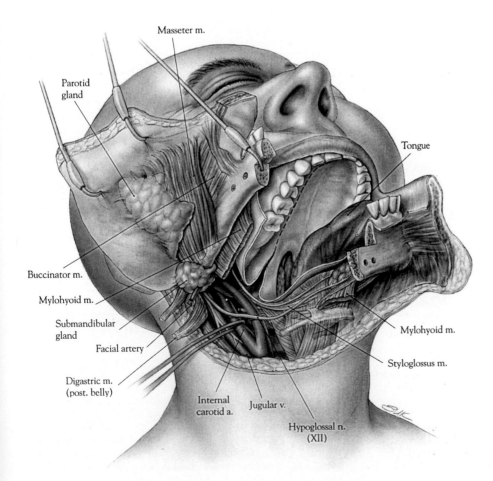

Fig. 9. An upper neck dissection is performed exposing and controlling the internal and external carotid arteries and internal jugular vein. The lower cranial nerves are dissected and preserved. The beginning of the palatal incision is shown. The inferior limb of this incision extends into the hypopharynx and allows for retropharyngeal dissection. (From the Department of Neurosurgery, University of Texas, MD Anderson Cancer Center, with permission.)

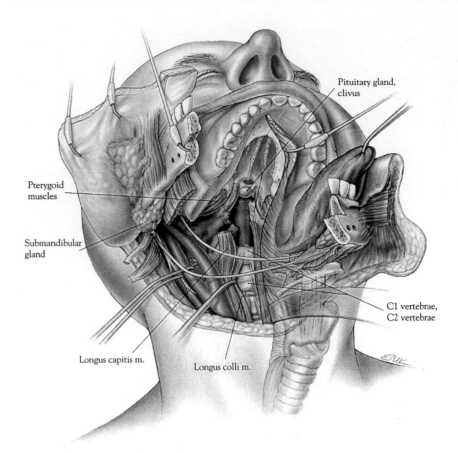

Pituitary gland, clivus

Pterygoid muscles

Submandibular gland

Longus capitis m.

Longus colli m.

C1 vertebrae, C2 vertebrae

Fig. 10. The palatal flap and pharynx have been retracted to the left. A portion of the hard palate has been removed and a clivectomy performed. (From the Department of Neurosurgery, University of Texas, MD Anderson Cancer Center, with permission.)

Transsphenoidal Approach

The transsphenoidal approach works well for smaller tumors located in the upper and middle clivus (11). Excellent exposure of the sphenoid sinus, sella turcica, and upper and middle clivus is possible (5). It has the disadvantages of limited inferior and lateral exposure, although the lateral exposure can be improved by entry into the medial maxillary sinus (2,7). The surgical field is typically deep and narrow and thus there is little room to allow aggressive bone resection. The transsphenoidal approach is quite satisfactory if the goals of surgery are confirmation of diagnosis, decompression of the tumor and palliation of neurologic symptoms and signs (39).

Transsphenoethmoidal Approach

An external ethmoidectomy with or without a medial maxillectomy can be employed in order to expand the exposure offered by the transsphenoidal approach. Lalwani and associates (40) found this approach to be "adequate for the majority of tumors and disease processes present in the sphenoid sinus and clivus." The addition of the medial maxillectomy in instances of a narrow ethmoid sinus or inferiorly extending tumor allows improved access. Disadvantages include the necessity of a facial incision and relatively limited exposure. The inferior limits can be extended by a medial maxillectomy as described in the preceding, but lateral reach is limited to approximately 2 cm from the midline.

Transoral-Transpalatal

Following the placement of an appropriate oral retractor system, the posterior pharyngeal wall and soft palate are divided to expose the clivus and upper cervical spine. Most commonly employed for odontoidectomy, the exposure obtained with this approach is relatively quite limited. It is adequate for tumor biopsy or in the case of small lower clival tumors. Repair of intraoperative cerebrospinal fluid leakage is problematic. Although fat and/or fascial tissue can be placed posterior to the pharyngeal wall, the pharyngeal wall rarely approximates well and gaps are common, thus increasing the risk of CSF leakage. The transoral-transpalatal approach should not be the primary approach to intraarachnoidal lesions at the foramen magnum unless other approaches prove ineffective (41).

Transmaxillary Approaches

The transmaxillary approaches have proven useful for clival chordomas that extend into the nasopharynx or craniocervical junction with minimal lateral extension (2,42,43). Numerous variations of this approach have been described; the most basic consisting of a simple Le Fort I osteotomy with or without midline splitting of the hard and soft palates (2,7,31,43). Alternatively, a unilateral maxillotomy with median or paramedian splitting of the hard and soft palates can be used (44,45). Access to the maxilla is best obtained via a facial degloving approach, although a classic lateral rhinotomy with lip split can be used

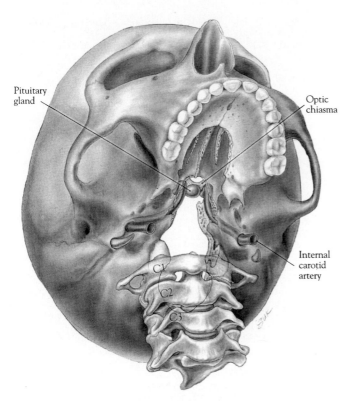

Pituitary gland

Optic chiasma

Internal carotid artery

Fig. 11. Artistic representation of the extent of clivectomy that may be performed. Note that the internal carotid artery is vulnerable both at the cavernous sinus and medial end of the foramen lacerum. (From the Department of Neurosurgery, University of Texas, MD Anderson Cancer Center, with permission.)

the tumor. Anterior, posterior, or rarely, total petrosectomy may be necessary.

An anterior petrosectomy accesses tumor extensions in and around the petroclival synchondrosis, the posterior cavernous sinus, and prepontine and cerebellopontine cisterns. The limits of bone removal include the ICA laterally, superior petrosal sinus medially, inferior petrosal sinus inferiorly, and internal auditory canal posteriorly (2). Sacrifice of the mandibular nerve and anterolateral displacement of the ICA allows for further inferior exposure of the clivus (46,47). Although a few appropriately located small chordomas can be resected through this surgical corridor, an anteriorly based approach is typically required as a second stage.

Of the posterior transpetrous approaches the petrosal or subtemporal—retrolabyrinthine approach is best suited for large posterolateral intradural tumor extensions (48,49), whereas the ITF approach can be used for both extradural and intradural tumor extensions (50). In the later approach the structures of the jugular foramen can be identified and skeletonized with the high-speed drill. The extradural removal of chordoma from around the exiting lower cranial nerves can result in neurological improvement. The approach can be extended inferiorly by the posterior mobilization of the vertebral artery from the foramina transversaria of C1 and C2. In this way, the region of the odontoid process and arch of C1 can be exposed. Craniospinal fixation may be necessary.

Total petrosectomy allows access from the sphenoid sinus to the foramen magnum and from the upper cervical spine to the intradural structures of the middle and posterior fossae. Destruction of the inner ear and complete mobilization of the facial nerve, with their attendant morbidities, are consequences of this approach. The problem of limited midline access remains.

(42). The use of maxillary osteotomies unifies and enlarges the surgical field in a rostrocaudal direction. Access extends from the anterior cranial fossa to the upper cervical spine (C2-3 disc space). Lateral exposure is limited by the pterygoid plates, ICA at the level of the foramen lacerum and cavernous sinus, hypoglossal canal, and jugular foramen. Removal of the pterygoid plates allows for some degree of access to the ITF.

Disadvantages of the transmaxillary approaches include the risk of ischemic osteonecrosis with multisegment osteotomies. This risk can be minimized by subtotally splitting the soft palate if palatal osteotomies are necessary and leaving wide soft-tissue attachments to freed maxillary compartments during swing procedures (44,45). The principal disadvantage of the transmaxillary approach, however, is the inability to reliably stop CSF leakage. This is particularly problematic during the midline maxillary approaches as direct repair rarely is possible and the whole area must be packed with fat, fascia, and fibrin glue without the availability of firm tissue support to hold the repair in place. The maxillary swing procedures allow greater options for repair, including temporalis muscle transfer and septally based mucoperichondrial flaps (44,45).

Transtemporal Approaches

Adequate access for tumor resection may necessitate the use of a variety of transtemporal approaches in the presence of clival chordomas with lateral or posterolateral extensions. The amount of petrous bone resection is tailored to the location of

Transcondylar Approach

Chordomas of the lower clivus with lateral extension to the atlanto-occipital joint, jugular foramen, or upper cervical spine are well addressed via this approach (7,51–53). Important advantages of the transcondylar approach include a short, wide, and uncontaminated surgical field, and vascular control of the vertebral artery (52). The direct lateral exposure of the craniocervical junction afforded by this approach allows for a direct line of sight to the structures ventral to the cervicomedullary junction and upper cervical cord (52,54). This is an excellent approach for large lower clival chordomas. Neural decompression can be confirmed directly and craniocervical fixation performed should it be necessary. Typically this removes the patient from immediate danger and allows time for a staged anterior approach, which is required for maximal tumor removal in most cases.

References

1. Forsyth PA, Cascino TL, Shaw EG, et al. Intracranial chordomas: a clinicopathological and prognostic study of 51 cases. *J Neurosurg* 1993;78:741–747.
2. Al-Mefty O, Borba LA. Skull base chordomas: a management challenge. *J Neurosurg* 1997;86:182–189.
3. Borba LA, Al-Mefty O, Mrak RE, et al. Cranial chordomas in children and adolescents. *J Neurosurg* 1996;84:584–591.

4. Wold LE, Laws ER, Jr. Cranial chordomas in children and young adults. *J Neurosurg* 1983;59:1043–1047.

5. Maira G, Pallini R, Anile C, et al. Surgical treatment of clival chordomas: the transsphenoidal approach revisited. *J Neurosurg* 1996;85:784–792.

6. Sen CN, Sekhar LN, Schramm VL, et al. Chordoma and chondrosarcoma of the cranial base: an 8-year experience. *Neurosurgery* 1989;25:931–940.

7. Borba LA, Al-Mefty O. Skull-base chordomas. *Contemp Neurosurg* 1998;20:1–6.

8. Gay E, Sekhar LN, Rubinstein E, et al. Chordomas and chondrosarcomas of the cranial base: results and follow-up of 60 patients. *Neurosurgery* 1995;36:887–896.

9. Lanzino G, Sekhar LN, Hirsch WL, et al. Chordomas and chondrosarcomas involving the cavernous sinus: review of surgical treatment and outcome in 31 patients. *Surg Neurol* 1993;40:359–371.

10. Givner I. Ophthalmologic features of intracranial chordoma and allied tumors of the clivus. *Arch Ophthalmol* 1945;33:397–403.

11. Raffel C, Wright DC, Gutin PH, et al. Cranial chordomas: clinical presentation and results of operative and radiation therapy in twenty-six patients. *Neurosurgery* 1985;17:703–710.

12. Volpe NJ, Lessell S. Remitting sixth nerve palsy in skull base tumors. *Arch Ophthalmol* 1993;111:1391–1395.

13. Volpe NJ, Liebsch NJ, Munzenrider JE, et al. Neuro-ophthalmologic findings in chordoma and chondrosarcoma of the skull base. *Am J Ophthalmol* 1993;115:97–104.

14. Fagundes MA, Hug EB, Liebsch NJ, et al. Radiation therapy for chordomas of the base of skull and cervical spine: patterns of failure and outcome after relapse. *Int J Radiat Oncol Biol Physiol* 1995;33:579–584.

15. Heffelfinger MJ, Dahlin DC, MacCarty CS, et al. Chordomas and cartilaginous tumors at the skull base. *Cancer* 1973;32:410–420.

16. Magrini SM, Papi MG, Marletta F, et al. Chordoma: natural history, treatment and prognosis. *Acta Oncol* 1992;31:847–851.

17. Watkins L, Khudados ES, Kaleoglu M, et al. Skull base chordomas: a review of 38 patients, 1958–88. *Br J Neurosurg* 1993;7:241–248.

18. Menezes AH, Gantz BJ, Traynelis VC, et al. Cranial base chordomas. *Clin Neurosurg* 1996;44:491–509.

19. Catton C, O'Sullivan B, Bell R, et al. Chordoma: long-term follow-up after radical photon irradiation. *Radiother Oncol* 1996;41:67–70.

20. Hug EB, Loredo LN, Slater JD, et al. Proton radiation therapy for chordomas and chondrosarcomas of the skull base. *J Neurosurg* 1999;91:432–439.

21. Austin-Seymour M, Munzenrider J, Goitein M, et al. Fractionated proton radiation therapy of chordoma and low-grade chondrosarcoma of the base of the skull. *J Neurosurg* 1989;70:13–17.

22. Berson AM, Castro JR, Petti P, et al. Charged particle irradiation of chordoma and chondrosarcoma of the base of skull and cervical spine: the Lawrence Berkeley Laboratory experience. *Int J Radiat Oncol Biol Physiol* 1988;15:559–565.

23. Austin JP, Urie MM, Cardenosa G. Probable causes of recurrence in patients with chordoma and chondrosarcoma of the base of skull and cervical spine. *Int J Radiat Oncol Biol Physiol* 1993;25:439–444.

24. Muthukumar N, Kondziolka D, Lunsford LD, et al. Stereotactic radiosurgery for chordoma and chondrosarcoma: further experiences. *Int J Radiat Oncol Biol Physiol* 1998;41:387–392.

25. Oot RF, Melville GE, New PF, et al. The role of MR and CT in evaluating clival chordomas and chondrosarcomas. *Am J Roentgenol* 1988;151:567–575.

26. Meyers SP, Hirsch WL Jr, Curtin HD, et al. Chordomas of the skull base: MR features. *Am J Neuroradiol* 1992;13:1627–1636.

27. Fujitsu K, Saijoh M, Aoki F, et al. Telecanthal approach for meningiomas in the ethmoid and sphenoid sinuses. *Neurosurgery* 1991;28:714–719.

28. Kawakami K, Yamanouchi Y, Kawamura Y, et al. Operative approach to the frontal skull base: extensive transbasal approach. *Neurosurgery* 1991;28:720–724.

29. Sekhar LN, Nanda A, Sen CN, et al. The extended frontal approach to tumors of the anterior, middle, and posterior skull base. *J Neurosurg* 1992;76:198–206.

30. Terasaka S, Day JD, Fukushima T. Extended transbasal approach: anatomy, technique, and indications. *Skull Base Surg* 1999;9:177–184.

31. Beals SP, Joganic EF, Hamilton MG, et al. Posterior skull base transfacial approaches. *Clin Plast Surg* 1995;22:491–511.

32. Biller HF, Shugar JM, Krespi YP. A new technique for wide-field exposure of the base of the skull. *Arch Otolaryngol* 1981;107:698–702.

33. Krespi YP, Har-El G. Surgery of the clivus and anterior cervical spine. *Arch Otolaryngol Head Neck Surg* 1988;114:73–78.

34. Krespi YP, Sisson GA. Skull base surgery in composite resection. *Arch Otolaryngol* 1982;108:681–684.

35. Krespi YP, Sisson GA. Transmandibular exposure of the skull base. *Am J Surg* 1984;148:534–538.

36. Ammirati M, Bernardo A. Analytical evaluation of complex anterior approaches to the cranial base: an anatomical study. *Neurosurgery* 1998;43:1398–1407.

37. Ammirati M, Ma J, Cheatham ML, et al. The mandibular swing-transcervical approach to the skull base: anatomical study. [technical note] *J Neurosurg* 1993;78:673–681.

38. DeMonte F, Diaz E, Callender D, et al. The transmandibular, circumglossal, retropharyngeal approach for chordomas of the clivus and upper cervical spine. *Neurosurg Focus* 2001;10:1–5.

39. Laws ER Jr. Transsphenoidal surgery for tumors of the clivus. *Otolaryngol Head Neck Surg* 1984;92:100–101.

40. Lalwani AK, Kaplan MJ, Gutin PH. The transsphenoethmoid approach to the sphenoid sinus and clivus. *Neurosurgery* 1992;31:1008–1014.

41. Menezes AH, VanGilder JC. Transoral-transpharyngeal approach to the anterior craniocervical junction. Ten-year experience with 72 patients. *J Neurosurg* 1988;69:895–903.

42. Harbour JW, Lawton MT, Criscuolo GR, et al. Clivus chordoma: a report of 12 recent cases and review of the literature. *Skull Base Surg* 1991;1:200–206.

43. Uttley D, Moore A, Archer DJ. Surgical management of midline skull-base tumors: a new approach. *J Neurosurg* 1989;71:705–710.

44. Catalano PJ, Biller HF. Extended osteoplastic maxillotomy. A versatile new procedure for wide access to the central skull base and infratemporal fossa. *Arch Otolaryngol Head Neck Surg* 1993;119:394–400.

45. Wei WI, Lam KH, Sham JS. New approach to the nasopharynx: the maxillary swing approach. *Head Neck* 1991;13:200–207.

46. Harsh GR, IV, Sekhar LN. The subtemporal, transcavernous, anterior transpetrosal approach to the upper brain stem and clivus. *J Neurosurg* 1992;77:709–717.

47. Sen CN, Sekhar LN. The subtemporal and preauricular infratemporal approach to intradural structures ventral to the brain stem. *J Neurosurg* 1990;73:345–354.

48. Blevins NH, Jackler RK, Kaplan MJ, et al. Combined transpetrosal-subtemporal craniotomy for clival tumors with extension into the posterior fossa. *Laryngoscope* 1995;105:975–982.

49. Megerian CA, Chiocca EA, McKenna MJ, et al. The subtemporal-transpetrous approach for excision of petroclival tumors. *Am J Otol* 1996;17:773–779.

50. Leonetti JP, Reichman OH, al-Mefty O, et al. Neurotologic considerations in the treatment of advanced clival tumors. *Otolaryngol Head Neck Surg* 1992;107:49–56.

51. Canalis RF, Martin N, Black K, et al. Lateral approach to tumors of the craniovertebral junction. *Laryngoscope* 1993;103:343–349.

52. Sen CN, Sekhar LN. An extreme lateral approach to intradural lesions of the cervical spine and foramen magnum. *Neurosurgery* 1990;27:197–204.

53. Sen CN, Sekhar LN. Surgical management of anteriorly placed lesions at the craniocervical junction—an alternative approach. *Acta Neurochir* 1991;108:70–77.

54. George B, Dematons C, Cophignon J. Lateral approach to the anterior portion of the foramen magnum. Application to surgical removal of 14 benign tumors: technical note. *Surg Neurol* 1988;29:484–490.

123. Principles of Radiotherapy for Tumors of the Craniospinal Axis

Shiao Y. Woo and Bin S. Teh

Radiotherapy plays a central role in the management of tumors of the craniospinal axis in both children and adults. Improved imaging modalities such as magnetic resonance imaging (MRI), computed tomography (CT), and positron emission tomography (PET) imply more accurate tumor and normal tissue localization. Advances in computers have aided in very complex conformal treatment planning and delivery such as intensity-modulated radiation therapy (IMRT) using inverse planning. A better understanding of radiobiology and tumor biology has given rise to new fractionation schedules, use of radiosensitizers, and to more innovative approaches, which offer a hope of improving the therapeutic index.

Radiation Tolerance of the Central Nervous System

RADIATION TOLERANCE OF THE BRAIN. The development of the brain is most rapid during the first 3 years of life. It slows down after age 6. Axonal growth and synaptogenesis are most active during the growth phase (1). The maturation of the brain, judged by degree of myelinization, is not complete until puberty (2). Thus, radiation-induced brain injury is most pronounced during the early years of childhood. Radiation injury to the brain is generally regarded as one of the most serious complications of radiotherapy for brain tumors and thus constitutes the major limitation in delivering high-dose radiation. As a rule, radiotherapy for brain tumors is more likely to produce side effects in infants than in older children and adults. Dose modification, especially lower fraction size, is often employed in younger children.

OTHER CRITICAL STRUCTURES IN THE CRANIOSPINAL AXIS

Brainstem. The brainstem has traditionally been regarded as more radiosensitive than the cerebrum, especially in the era of orthovoltage. However, in the modern era of high-energy radiotherapy, brainstem necrosis is rare. In view of the high concentration of white matter, a reduction of 10% from brain tolerance dose is usually recommended (3). Fraction size is also very important. Other factors influencing the development of radionecrosis include chemotherapy and preexisting vascular pathology.

Spinal Cord. In view of its critical function, the tolerance of the spinal cord to radiation is a major dose-limiting factor in delivering high-dose radiation not only to tumors involving the cord (e.g., astrocytoma) but also to extramedullary tumors in the vicinity. In pediatric radiation oncology, craniospinal irradiation is common especially in the treatment of medulloblastoma, in both standard and high-risk groups. Also, when certain head and neck tumors in childhood (e.g., rhabdomyosarcoma and nasopharyngeal angiofibroma) are irradiated, the spinal cord will usually receive some radiation. If the spinal cord is overdosed, devastating neurological deficits may ensue. Radia-tion myelopathy can occur from one year to several years after delivery of the irradiation (4). Tumor cure rather than quality of life then becomes a very important issue. The traditional dogma in the pathogenesis of radiation myelopathy is postmitotic cell death in the endothelial cells and/or oligodendrocytes. Current concepts view radiation as producing cell death which in turn induces a complex pathophysiological reaction in which the response of surviving cells may contribute to determining the impact of radiation on tissue integrity and functions. Cytokines such as tumor necrosis factor and interleukin-6 also play important roles (4). There is also some suggestion that the tolerance of the spinal cord is 5% to 10% lower in children (4). In view of low α/β ratio, the radiation tolerance depends strongly on fraction size.

Interfractional interval also plays an important role in radiation myelopathy. It has been generally accepted that the dose to the spinal cord should be reduced when the volume irradiated is large. A primate study indicates that an increase in the treatment volume reduces the threshold and steepens the slope of the sigmoid dose-response curve for myelopathy. The effect, however, is less pronounced at a low-incidence level (e.g., 1% to 2 % incidence) than at a high-incidence level (4).

Cranial Nerves. Most cranial nerves are relatively resistant to radiation-induced damage. Two cranial nerves are worth mentioning in the radiation treatment of pediatric cancers.

1. Optic nerve (cranial nerve II) and visual pathway can be damaged when delivering therapeutic radiation to periorbital tumors (e.g., orbital rhabdomyosarcoma, optic glioma, paranasal, and nasopharyngeal tumors) and suprasellar tumors (e.g., craniopharyngioma, pituitary adenoma, germ cell tumor, hypothalamic-chiasmatic glioma). A linear-quadratic model has yielded an α/β estimate of 1.6 Gy for optic neuropathy (5). The risk of radiation-induced optic neuropathy is related to total radiation dose, fraction size, and the irradiated volume (6). It has been shown that no injuries were observed in 106 optical nerves that received a total dose (TD) of less than 59 Gy. The 15-year actuarial risk of optic neuropathy after dose greater than 60 Gy was 11% when treatment was administered in fraction sizes of less than 1.9 Gy, as compared to 47% when given in fraction sizes of greater than 1.9 Gy (7).

2. Vestibulocochlear nerve (cranial nerve VIII) and auditory apparatus should be considered in the delivery of high-dose radiation to tumors in the posterior fossa (e.g., medulloblastoma, ependymoma, and astrocytoma). It is most important in the case of medulloblastoma, as *cis*-platinum–based chemotherapy is given after completion of radiotherapy and will increase the ototoxicity.

Retina. The retina, a specialized neural end organ supplied by an end-arterial system, is very sensitive to vascular injury and has a small probability of repair (7). It is very sensitive to radiation. Deterioration of vision resulting from radiation-induced progressive obliteration of small retinal vessels can occur from 1.5 to 6 years after irradiation. The dose response curve is very steep between 50 and 60 Gy, and 45 Gy for a TD 5/5 (the probability of 5% complication within 5 years of treatment) for visual loss is realistic (3). Again as the fraction size increases (up to 2.5 Gy or more), the frequency of injury increases (8).

Lens. The lens is one of the most radiosensitive organs. Even very low-dose radiation (i.e., 1 Gy) can lead to cataract formation. From total body irradiation data, the risk of developing a cataract requiring surgery was 20% for fractionated doses of 12 to 16 Gy (9). Currently, the TD 5/5 is 10 Gy.

Hypothalamus and Pituitary Areas. Irradiation of the hypothalamus and pituitary areas can result in significant neuroendocrine abnormality and long-term sequelae. This is especially important in children. The hormones affected include growth hormone (GH), thyroid-stimulating hormone (TSH), adrenocorticotropic hormone (ACTH), follicle-stimulating hormone (FSH), and luteinizing hormone (LH). Data are most readily available on the effect of cranial irradiation on GH production and release. The irradiated anatomical site responsible for GH deficiency has been shown to be the hypothalamus (10). Between 60% and 80% of pediatric brain tumor patients will ultimately have impaired serum GH response to provocative stimulation (10). There is a dose-response relationship with a threshold of 18 to 25 Gy. The higher the radiation dose, the earlier the GH deficiency will occur. Deficiencies of other hypothalamic-pituitary hormones have also been described (11). The responsible irradiated site can be either hypothalamus or pituitary or both.

Reactions of Brain to Radiation

The responses of brain tissues to radiation are classified into three groups: (a) acute reactions that occur during or shortly after treatment; (b) early delayed (subacute) reactions that occur a few weeks to 2 to 3 months after treatment; and (c) late delayed reactions that occur several months to years after treatment (12).

ACUTE REACTIONS. The pathogenesis is thought to be radiation-induced edema. The reactions are manifested as headache, nausea, vomiting, or worsening of preexisting neurological symptoms. These symptoms are generally mild when conventional daily 180 to 200 cGy is used. The acute symptoms can be more common and severe when a larger fraction size or a larger volume of brain is irradiated. Corticosteroids are useful for management of symptoms as they occur, or as a prophylaxis.

EARLY DELAYED (SUBACUTE) REACTIONS. Damage to oligodendroglial cells leading to inhibition of myelin synthesis and damage to the vascular endothelium leading to white mat-

ter necrosis are two possible mechanisms of the early delayed reactions. Common symptoms include somnolence, lethargy, and transient deterioration of neurological symptoms. The symptoms usually improve with or without corticosteroids. Early delayed reactions should be considered as one of the differential diagnoses in interpreting follow-up MRI changes.

LATE DELAYED REACTIONS. These make up the most serious sequelae of brain irradiation. The reactions range from asymptomatic focal white matter change to progressive radionecrosis. Various mechanisms have been proposed for the pathogenesis including injury of oligodendroglial cells and vascular endothelial damage. The clinical manifestations depend on the involved volume and location. Late neuropsychological effects include intellectual impairment, memory deficits, and inability to acquire new knowledge. Impairment in cognition is most pronounced in young children. Deterioration in IQ could occur in children following whole brain or supratentorial irradiation for primary brain tumors.

Treatment-Related Sequelae

The important late sequelae of brain irradiation are summarized in Table 1. The presence and severity of radiation reactions depend on (a) radiation treatment factor, which includes TD, fraction size, interfractional interval, and treatment volume; (b) patient factor, which includes age, presence of preexisting brain injury by tumor, hydrocephalus or surgery, infection, and vascular diseases; and (c) other treatment modality (i.e., surgery and/or chemotherapy). The new conformal radiation therapy technologies are aimed at decreasing the volume of normal brain irradiated with the hope of minimizing toxicity.

When is Radiotherapy Indicated?

Management of tumors of the craniospinal axis depends on histopathological diagnosis. A needle biopsy may be performed on virtually all tumors when stereotactically guided by MRI or CT. There are some exceptions such as brainstem glioma and optic glioma, in which a diagnosis can be made with high certainty on imaging. Gross total resection is a desirable goal if it can be done safely. Radiotherapy is generally required for

Table 1. Late Sequelae of Radiation Therapy and Its Clinical Significance

Late Sequelae	Clinical Significance	Comments
1. Neurocognitive	Adverse effect on intelligence, learning, and social emotional adjustment. Memory deficits if large volume of temporal lobe is involved.	Complicated by the effects from tumor itself, surgery, and chemotherapy
2. Neuroendocrine	Development delay and multitude of problems from hormonal deficiencies	Growth hormones, thyroid, gonadal, prolactin, and/or adrenal abnormality
3. Vision	Optic neuropathy, retinopathy, lacrimal atrophy, cataract, corneal scarring, and glaucoma	Worsened with additional effects from tumor and surgery
4. Hearing	Hearing loss leading to difficulty in communication, speech, and language which has an adverse effect on learning	Combined radiotherapy and cisplatinum have increased the risk of ototoxicity more than either treatment alone
5. Second malignancy	The incidence of second malignancy increases with higher radiation dose.	Genetic predisposition and chemotherapy (alkylators) both further increase the risk

malignant invasive tumors even after gross total resection [e.g., high-grade glioma (12), medulloblastoma (13), ependymoma (14), and germ cell tumor (15)]. It is also indicated for low-grade tumors that are either incompletely or not resected. This group of tumors includes low-grade gliomas, meningiomas, craniopharyngiomas, chordomas, neurilemmomas, oligodendrogliomas, pituitary adenomas, optic gliomas, and pineal tumors, among others. The role of radiotherapy in brain metastases is well established (16).

Radiation Dose

The dose of therapeutic radiation depends on the histopathology types, radioresponsiveness, treatment intent, anatomical sites, and critical tissue tolerance. In general, total tumor dose ranges from 4,500 to 6,000 cGy over 5 to 7 weeks with daily fractions of 150 to 200 cGy. For more radioresponsive tumors such as germinoma and nongerminoma, a TD of 3,000 to 5,000 cGy is used.

Brain Tumor Cooperative Group (BTCG) randomized trials have shown a survival benefit for patients with high-grade glioma receiving postoperative radiotherapy (50 to 60 Gy in single daily fractions of 1.7 to 2.0 Gy, 5 days a week), either alone or with chemotherapy as compared to those treated with either resection and supportive care only or with chemotherapy alone (17,18). A dose of 60 Gy has been shown to result in significantly prolonged survival as compared to 50 Gy (19).

Radiation Treatment Volume

Radiation treatment volume is determined by the anatomical extent of the tumor and the potential areas of spread as well as the patterns of failure. Advances in MRI and CT have made tumor localization more accurate. In general, the treatment volume is more generous for a high-grade glioma, which has a tendency to infiltrate beyond the identifiable tumor on imaging. The majority of recurrences in patients with glioblastoma multiforme occur within 2 to 3 cm of the initial tumor (20). The treatment volume therefore usually includes the contrast-enhancing tumor with 2 to 3 cm margins (Fig 1). For more benign and noninfiltrative tumors, such as meningioma, craniopharyngioma, acoustic neuroma, and pituitary adenoma, a more limited radiation field is employed (i.e., gross tumor is covered with a margin) (Fig. 2).

Whole brain irradiation is reserved for multifocal lesions and lesions with significant leptomeningeal involvement. Whole brain irradiation is also used for brain metastases, especially when they are multiple. In solitary brain metastasis, whole brain irradiation usually follows surgical resection (21). A radiosurgical boost has been shown to produce a comparable outcome (22).

Craniospinal irradiation is usually delivered to patients who have tumors with a high propensity to seed the subarachnoid space (i.e., when both the brain and spinal cord are at high risk for tumor recurrence). These tumors include medulloblastoma, other primary neuroectodermal tumors, germ cell tumors, and high-grade tumors with positive cerebrospinal fluid cytology or gross spinal metastases.

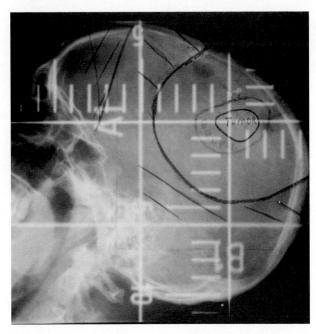

Fig. 1. Radiation treatment volume for glioblastoma usually includes the contrast-enhancing tumor with 2 to 3 cm margins.

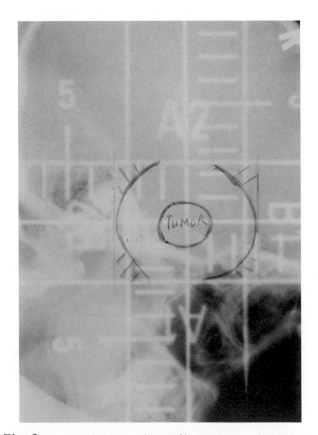

Fig. 2. For more benign and noninfiltrative tumors (e.g., pituitary adenomas), a more limited field is employed.

Radiobiological Considerations

The biology of fractionation in radiotherapy is based on four "R's"—*re*oxygenation, *re*distribution of cells within the cell cycle, *re*pair of sublethal damage, and *re*population.

Between 10% to 40% of cells in tumors are hypoxic and it is the hypoxic cell survival curve that determines the overall survival curve. Radiation tends to kill a greater proportion of oxygenated than hypoxic cells because the former are more radiosensitive. Reoxygenation is the process by which cells that are hypoxic at the time of irradiation become oxygenated after or during the next fraction. This is due to the fact that when enough cells are killed, cells that were once far from a vessel are now close to the vessel. Reoxygenation appears to be a fairly quick dynamic process. Thus, dose fractionation is aimed at overcoming hypoxia and increasing tumor cell kill.

The cell cycle can be divided into four phases: mitosis (M), G1, DNA synthetic phase (S), and G2. Cells are most radiosensitive in the M and G2 phases and most resistant in the late S phase. In theory, variations in sensitivity through the cell cycle are important in radiotherapy; therefore a fractionated regimen will lead to sensitization of cells due to redistribution or reassortment within the cell cycle.

Repair of sublethal damage describes the increase in survival when a dose of radiation is split into two fractions separated in time. It is slower in most late-responding tissues than in rapidly responding tissues. Thus, at least a 6- to 8-hour interfractional interval is generally needed between dose fractions for critical normal tissues (e.g., spinal cord) with a slow rate of repair.

Acute responding normal tissues but not late responding tissues can repopulate better than tumor. Tumors have the capacity to repopulate during an extended course of radiation therapy as well as after a lag period. Rapid repopulation of tumor clonogens during a radiotherapy course is usually not evident because the surviving cells form a small proportion of the shrinking tumor mass. This effect is especially evident in head and neck cancer.

In short, dividing radiotherapy dose into a number of fractions spares normal tissues because of repopulation of cell clones and repair of sublethal damage, and also increases tumor cell kill because of reoxygenation and redistribution of cells into radiosensitive phases of the cell cycle.

The effect of radiation on the brain is generally characterized by delayed reactions as the normal brain parenchymal cells are either slowly dividing or nondividing. As a late-responding tissue the normal central nervous system (CNS) is very sensitive to radiation dose fraction size. Small radiation fraction sizes tend to produce a lesser effect on the CNS than on tumor cells. One can take advantage of this phenomenon by decreasing the fraction size from the conventional fraction size and delivering more than one fraction each day. This is called hyperfractionation.

Hyperfractionated radiotherapy has the following theoretical benefits: (a) it gives dose escalation without increasing damage to late-responding tissues; (b) it overcomes tumor hypoxia which contributes to radioresistance, and (c) it increases tumor cell kill by the dose escalation. Generally, a sufficient interfractional interval (6 to 8 hours is commonly used) is necessary to allow normal tissue repair of radiation-induced damage between the radiation fractions. This approach has been used in the treatment of supratentorial and brainstem high-grade glioma. However, to date there are no convincing data to suggest any survival benefits with the use of a hyperfractionated radiotherapy approach, probably because the total radiation dose is still insufficient to show a significant increase in tumor cell kill. In a Pediatric Oncology Group phase III randomized trial comparing conventional versus hyperfractionated radiotherapy in children with newly diagnosed diffuse intrinsic brainstem tumors, hyperfractionated radiotherapy did not improve event-free or overall survival (23).

Accelerated fractionation radiotherapy is another approach to fractionation with the aim of delivering the total radiotherapy dose over a shortened period of time. It involves multiple daily radiotherapy fractions in conventional radiotherapy fraction size (1.6 to 2.0 Gy). The total radiotherapy dose may be equivalent or less than that delivered with conventional fractionation. Shortening of overall treatment time has the theoretical benefit of overcoming the accelerated repopulation of tumor clonogens between radiation fractions (24). Again, there are no convincing data to suggest survival advantage with the use of the accelerated fractionation scheme over conventional radiotherapy in the treatment of glioblastoma.

Techniques in Radiotherapy

CONVENTIONAL EXTERNAL-BEAM RADIOTHERAPY TECHNIQUES. Conventional radiotherapy techniques remain the most common techniques used today. These techniques use simple geometrical radiation field arrangements with a small number of treatment fields. Head immobilization is important so that the treatment target is not missed during radiotherapy. A customized head-fixation device (e.g., Aquaplast mask) is often used (Fig. 3). Other immobilization devices such as a body cast or alpha-cradle are used when appropriate (Fig 4).

The advantages of conventional techniques are their relative simplicity and the general familiarity with such techniques by radiation oncologists and technologists. The major disadvantage is the usual inclusion of more normal brain tissue than necessary in the high-radiation dose regimen because of the limited field arrangements.

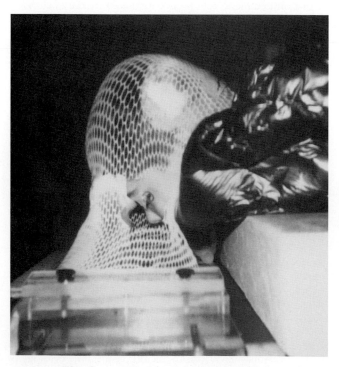

Fig. 3. Head fixation device (Aquaplast mask).

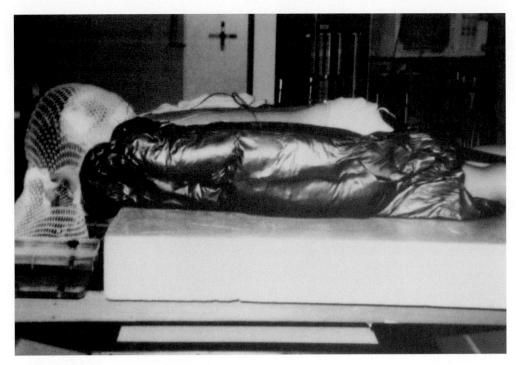

Fig. 4. Immobilization device (body cast).

CLASSIC THREE-DIMENSIONAL CONFORMAL RADIO-THERAPY. Advances in neuroimaging and computers have made it possible to deliver high-dose radiation more precisely to the tumor while significantly sparing the surrounding normal tissues when using classic three-dimensional conformal radiotherapy (3D-CRT). 3D-CRT may involve multiple-shaped fields directed at the tumor arranged in coplanar, nonaxial, and non-coplanar orientation and delivered in either static or dynamic modes (12). It has been shown that approximately 30% less normal brain tissue receives high-dose radiation using a 3D-CRT technique when compared to conventional radiotherapy (25,26). This reduction could lead to fewer side effects, especially in young children.

INTENSITY-MODULATED RADIOTHERAPY. Intensity-modulated radiotherapy (IMRT), an advanced form of 3D-CRT, combines two advanced concepts to deliver 3D-CRT: (a) inverse treatment planning with optimization by computer and (b) computer-controlled intensity modulation of the radiation beam during treatment (27). IMRT allows a high degree of flexibility in reducing the dose to the surrounding normal tissues by the creation of so-called avoidance areas during the treatment plan process (Color Plate 32). The initial experience with IMRT in the treatment of brain tumors has been encouraging (27).

STEREOTACTIC RADIOSURGERY. Radiosurgery can be administered by a gamma-knife unit using 201 cobalt sources, or by a modified linear accelerator unit. It is designed to deliver a very high-radiation dose to a small intracranial target in one sitting by focusing multiple small radiation beams on the target from different directions. Usually the application of radiosurgery is limited to tumors measuring 3.5 cm or less in maximum diameter in order to achieve a steep-dose gradient at the treatment field edge. Radiosurgery is commonly used for the man-

agement of brain metastases, acoustic neuromas, and meningiomas, and is being investigated as a boost treatment for small high-grade gliomas (28).

BRACHYTHERAPY. Brachytherapy or interstitial irradiation involves the implantation of radioactive sources directly into brain tumors. Iodine-125, iridium-192, and gold-198 have all been used as either permanent or temporary implants. Brachytherapy has been used in patients with glioblastoma as an additional boost after external-beam radiotherapy and in selected patients with recurrent high-grade glioma. Patient selection criteria are important. These are based on a good Karnofsky Performance Scale (KPS greater than 70) and the presence of a well-defined unifocal supratentorial lesion (without subependymal spread) measuring less than 5 cm and away from eloquent areas of the brain.

The University of California at San Francisco reported their experience in a cohort of patients with glioblastoma treated with brachytherapy to 50 Gy after conventional external-beam radiation therapy (29). The median age was 52 years and the median KPS was 90. The median survival was 19 months, with 1-year, 2-year, and 3-year survival probabilities of 85%, 36%, and 20%, respectively. A prospective randomized trial of the BTCG assigned patients with high-grade glioma to brachytherapy (60 Gy), external-beam radiotherapy, and carmustine versus external-beam radiotherapy and carmustine. Median survival for the patients undergoing brachytherapy was 16 months as compared to 13 months for the patients not receiving brachytherapy (30). Brachytherapy appears to have a small beneficial role in the treatment of some patients with newly diagnosed glioblastoma or with recurrent glioblastoma.

Conclusion

Radiotherapy is an important treatment modality for both benign and malignant tumors of the craniospinal axis. Advances in neuroimaging and radiotherapeutic technology have made possible a more precise delivery of high-radiation dose while sparing critical normal tissues. This will have a significant impact on tumor control with the ability to escalate radiation dose, and in addition, may decrease treatment-related toxicity with increased sparing of normal tissues. More innovative approaches including combining radiotherapy and biological therapy, as well as new radiosensitizers, cytotoxins, and antiangiogenesis agents are all currently in progress and hold promise for the future.

References

1. Packer RJ, Meadows AT, Rocke RB, et al. Long-term sequelae of cancer treatment of the central nervous system in childhood. *Med Pediatr Oncol* 1987;15:241–253.
2. Dobbing J, Sands J. The quantitative growth and development of the human brain. *Arch Dis Child* 1963;48:757–767.
3. Emami B, Lyman J, Brown A, et al. Tolerance of normal tissue to therapeutic irradiation. *Int J Radiat Oncol Biol Phys* 1991;21:109–122.
4. Ang KK, Stephens LC. Prevention and management of radiation myelopathy. *Oncology (Huntingt)* 1994;8:71–76.
5. Jiang GL, Tucker SL, Guttenberger L, et al. Radiation-induced injury to the visual pathway. *Radiother Oncol* 1994;30:17–25.
6. Parsons JT, Bova FJ, Fitzgerald CR, et al. Radiation optic neuropathy after megavoltage external beam irradiation: analysis of time-dose factors. *Int J Radiat Oncol Biol Phys* 1994;30:755–763.
7. Leibel SA, Sheline GE. Tolerance of the central and peripheral nervous system to therapeutic irradiation. *Adv Radiat Biol* 1987;12:257–288.
8. Wara WM, Irvine A, Neger R, et al. Radiation retinopathy. *Int J Radiat Oncol Biol Phys* 1979;5:81–83.
9. Deeg H, Flournoy N, Sullivan K. Cataracts after total body irradiation and marrow transplantation. *Int J Radiat Oncol Biol Phys* 1984;10:957–964.
10. Halperin EC, Constine LS, Tarbell NJ, et al. Late effects of cancer treatment. In: Halperin EC, Constine LS, Tarbell NJ, eds. *Pediatric radiation oncology*, 3rd ed. Philadelphia: Lippincott Williams & Wilkins, 1999:457–537.
11. Constine L, Woolf P, Cann D, et al. Hypothalamic-pituitary dysfunction after radiation for brain tumors. *N Engl J Med* 1993;328:87–94.
12. Leibel SA, Scott SB, Loeffler JS. Contemporary approaches to the treatment of malignant glioma with radiotherapy. *Semin Oncol* 1994;21:198–219.
13. Kun LE, Constine LS. Medulloblastoma: caution regarding new treatment approaches. *Int J Radiat Oncol Biol Phys* 1991;20:897–899.
14. Shaw EG, Evans RG, Scheithauer BW, et al. Postoperative radiotherapy of intracranial ependymoma in pediatric and adult patients. *Int J Radiat Oncol Biol Phys* 1987;13:1457–1462.
15. Rich TA, Cassady JR, Strand RD. Radiation therapy for pineal and suprasellar germ cell tumors. *Cancer* 1985;55:932–940.
16. Coia LR. The role of radiation therapy in the treatment of brain metastases. *Int J Radiat Oncol Biol Phys* 1992;23:229–238.
17. Walker MD, Alexander E, Hunt WE, et al. Evaluation of BCNU and/or radiotherapy in the treatment of anaplastic glioma. *J Neurosurg* 1978;49:333–343.
18. Walker MD, Green SB, Byar DP, et al. Randomized comparisons of radiotherapy and nitrosoureas for the treatment of malignant glioma after surgery. *N Engl J Med* 1980;303:1323–1329.
19. Walker MD, Strike TA, Sheline GE. An analysis of dose-effect relationship in the radiotherapy of malignant glioma. *Int J Radiat Oncol Biol Phys* 1979;5:1725–1731.
20. Wallner KE, Galicich JH, Krol G, et al. Patterns of failure following treatment for glioblastoma multiforme and anaplastic astrocytoma. *Int J Radiat Oncol Biol Phys* 1989;16:1405–1409.
21. Patchell RA, Tibbs PA, Walsh JW, et al. A randomized trial of surgery in the treatment of single metastasis to the brain. *N Engl J Med* 1990;322:494–500.
22. Alexander E III, Moriarty TM, Davis RB, et al. Stereotactic radiosurgery for the definitive, noninvasive treatment of brain metastases. *J Natl Cancer Inst* 1994;87:34–40.
23. Mandell LR, Kadota R, Freeman C, et al. There is no role for hyperfractionated radiotherapy in the management of children with newly diagnosed diffuse intrinsic brainstem tumors: results of a Pediatric Oncology Group phase III trial comparing conventional vs. hyperfractionated radiotherapy. *Int J Radiat Oncol Biol Phys* 1999;43:959–964.
24. Thames HD, Peters LJ, Withers HR, et al. Accelerated fractionation vs. hyperfractionation: rationales for several treatments per day. *Int J Radiat Oncol Biol Phys* 1983;9:127–138.
25. Cooley G, Gillin MT, Murray JF, et al. Improved dose localization with dual energy photon irradiation in treatment of lateralized intracranial malignancies. *Int J Radiat Oncol Biol Phys* 1991;20:815–821.
26. Thornton AF Jr, Hegarty TJ, Ten Haken RK, et al. Three-dimensional treatment planning of astrocytoma: a dosimetry study of cerebral irradiation. *Int J Radiat Oncol Biol Phys* 1991;20:1309–1315.
27. Teh BS, Woo SY, Butler EB. Intensity-modulated radiation therapy (IMRT): a new promising technology in radiation oncology. *Oncologist* 1999;4:433–442.
28. Garden AS, Maor MH, Yung WKA, et al. Outcome and patterns of failure following limited-volume irradiation for malignant astrocytoma. *Radiother Oncol* 1991;20:99–110.
29. Sneed PK, Prado MD, McDermott MW, et al. Large effect of age on the survival of patients with glioblastoma treated with radiotherapy and brachytherapy boost. *Neurosurgery* 1995;36:898–903.
30. Green SB, Shapiro WR, Burger PC, et al. A randomized trial of interstitial radiotherapy (RT) boost for newly diagnosed malignant glioma: Brain Tumor Cooperative Group (BTCG) trial 8701. *Proc Am Soc Clin Oncol* 1994;13:174(abst).

124. Stereotactic Radiosurgery for Intracranial Tumors

Walter A. Hall and Kwan H. Cho

Worldwide, more than 20,000 patients have been treated with stereotactic radiosurgery for a variety of benign and malignant conditions since 1951 (1). With stereotactic radiosurgery, a single high dose of ionizing radiation, a gamma ray or a charged-particle beam, is delivered precisely to a radiographically well-defined intracranial volume of normal or pathological tissue without including a significant amount of adjacent brain parenchyma in the treatment field (1). The radiation is administered using multiple narrow collimated beams, non-coplanar converging arcs, or a single beam that passes through a common point (1). The margin of the lesion is usually encompassed within the 40% to 90% isodose lines and an insignificant dose of radiation is delivered to the surrounding normal brain (2). Radiosurgery delivers an ablative dose to the target margin with a higher dose delivered centrally (2). An inhomogeneous dose distribution can develop within the treatment volume because of the rapid radiation fall off. Dose inhomogeneity is a foreign concept in radiation oncology where the goal is to administer a uniform dose of radiation throughout the entire treatment field since radiotherapy relies on the susceptibility difference between tumor tissue and normal brain.

Indications for using stereotactic radiosurgery instead of conventional neurosurgery include advanced age, the presence of severe medical disease precluding general anesthesia, lesion location within eloquent cerebral tissue, surgical inaccessibility of the target, radioresistant tumor histology, the presence of recurrent or residual tumor, and patient preference (1,2). Commonly treated benign tumors include skull base meningiomas, acoustic schwannomas, and pituitary adenomas, with brain metastases and astrocytomas comprising those malignant tumors usually considered for radiosurgery.

Technical Considerations

When evaluating a patient with an intracranial tumor for stereotactic radiosurgery, the computed tomography (CT) and magnetic resonance imaging (MRI) scans, tumor histology, and prior surgical and radiation treatments need to be taken into consideration. On the day of treatment, the stereotactic head frame is applied using local anesthesia. For children under the age of 14 years, general anesthesia is often necessary. Neuroradiological tests performed prior to treatment planning are a high-resolution CT scan or MRI. Previously, MRI with standard T1- and T2-weighted spin-echo images had inherent localization inaccuracies of 3 to 4 mm due to the magnetic field. Correction of these errors and the use of magnetization prepared-rapid gradient echo (MP-RAGE) sequencing allows for the generation of 1-mm thick contrast-enhanced axial, coronal, and sagittal projections through the target with resolution comparable to that obtained with CT (1,2). During treatment, the patient is positioned on the couch and the stereotactic head frame is attached to either a couch mount or to a floor stand for the linear accelerator (LINAC) or particle beam generator. Isocenter coordinates, collimator size, arc-start angle, arc-end angle, couch angle, gantry arc rotation interval, and collimator field size are set on the LINAC and particle beam generator (1). The radiation delivered usually requires less than 1 hour per isocenter and the patient is usually discharged home thereafter.

The shape of a single radiosurgical treatment field is usually spherical or oval. Although beam shaping is possible with the LINAC or charged-particle beam generators, multiple overlapping isocenters provide more conformal radiation coverage for irregular lesions. Charged-particle beam generators and LINACs generally require 2 to 3 isocenters to treat an irregular lesion in contrast to the gamma knife where multiple isocenters can be used for a single treatment plan. The least standardized aspect of stereotactic radiosurgery is dose prescription (1). Before prescribing the radiation dose to be administered, lesion histology, volume, anatomical location, and dose to adjacent eloquent structures should be considered.

Normal tissue tolerance for ionizing radiation depends on the treatment volume, the size of the fraction delivered over time, and the total dose delivered (1). With stereotactic radiosurgery, the ability to limit the amount of normal brain tissue within the treatment field decreases with an increase in the target volume (1,3). As the target volume increases in size, the number of required isocenters, the diameter of the treatment beams, the overlap between treatment beams, and the amount of normal tissue included in the entrance and exit paths will also increase (1,3). An integrated logistical formula has been derived for all stereotactic radiosurgery techniques that applies standard radiotherapy equations to small radiation fields and allows clinicians to predict the minimum dose of radiation that is associated with a 3% risk of causing central nervous system (CNS) injury (4). These 3% isoeffect lines are similar to the 1% dose-diameter line for brain necrosis determined for the cyclotron (3). The integrated logistical formula estimates the probability of brain necrosis over the entire radiation dose distribution (3,4).

GAMMA KNIFE RADIOSURGERY. The current gamma knife has 201 radioactive cobalt-60 sources arranged hemispherically within an 18,000-kg shielding vessel. Each cobalt source has an activity of 30 Ci, a radiosurgical dose rate of 3 to 4 Gy per minute, and a half-life of 5.7 years. The radiation beams intersect 403 mm from the sources with the central source fixed at a 55-degree angle relative to the horizontal and the remaining sources arranged ± 48 degrees from the central source and ± 80 degrees relative to the transverse axis (5). The inner collimator helmet has four variable sizes of 4 mm, 8 mm, 14 mm, and 18 mm, allowing variation in the size of the radiation-dose distribution. Multiple overlapping exposures using the different size collimator helmets are necessary to treat large lesions. The position of the radiation sources allows production of a spherical isodose distribution in the coronal and axial planes and an elliptical configuration in the sagittal projection. Beam channel blocking some of the radiation sources allows additional shaping of the isodose configuration.

A modified Leksell stereotactic head frame is fixed to the skull before obtaining the radiological localization data to determine the rectilinear coordinates (X, Y, Z) of the target necessary for treatment planning. Axis bars that extend from the collimator helmet attach to the stereotactic frame and position the target at a central location in the collimator helmet where the cobalt sources intersect at a single point. The patient and treatment couch move into the gamma unit and align the inner collimator with the collimator helmet. After the appropriate radiation dose has been delivered over time, the couch is withdrawn from the unit and the head frame removed. Variables that are determined during treatment planning include isocenter coordinates, collimator size, and relative weighting of each isocenter. Most targets are treated with the 50% or higher isodose shell.

The accuracy of the gamma knife is assured by the absence of any moving parts, which obviates the need for treatment verification films and reduces the need for medical physics support. Advantages of the gamma knife are its high degree of accuracy, reliable beam delivery, effective dose distributions, rapid treatment time, uncomplicated treatment planning, and ease and speed of field shaping with multiple isocenters (6). Disadvantages associated with the gamma knife are the high acquisition cost, recommended source replacement every 5 to 10 years, limited field sizes, inability to perform fractionation, and the lack of potential for individually shaped isocenter fields (6).

PARTICLE-BEAM GENERATOR RADIOSURGERY. Synchrocyclotron, cyclotron, and bevatron particle-beam generator radiosurgery are uncommon because of their cost and the need to affiliate with a nuclear physics research center (2). The unit in Boston generates a 10-mm Bragg peak with a 160-million electron volt (MeV) proton beam through 12 portals in 1 fraction. The Berkley unit uses 165 MeV helium ions to deliver 25 to 45 Gy of radiation through 3 to 5 entry ports in 1 to 3 fractions (1).

Protons, deuterons, or helium ions of one energy are accelerated to a high-energy state and propelled as a beam to destroy tissue. Proton beam characteristics that are advantageous for radiosurgery are their narrow size, a specific depth of tissue penetration, and a high degree of collimation with very little scatter (2). The treatment uses a fully energized beam to pass through the lesion (plateau ionization region) or the greatly enhanced energy emitted at the point of most rapid deceleration known as the Bragg peak, beyond which point there is no tissue damage (2,5). Several modifications are necessary to adapt a charged-particle beam generator for radiosurgery. These include adjusting the range of the beam, spreading out the Bragg peak, and shaping the beam in the lateral direction to define the cross-sectional shape (1,6). Each beam requires a customized range-modifying absorber, a variable-thickness rotating absorber, and a beam-shaping aperture in order to conform to the lesion geometry (6). Some centers have used custom-formed collimator apertures to further refine the beam shape to conform more accurately to the target.

Advantages of charged-particle radiosurgery are the ability to produce excellent dose distributions and the potential for fractionation. Disadvantages of charged-particle generators are their substantial cost, time-consuming treatment planning, the need for beam modification devices, and the uncertainty between dose and biological effectiveness (6).

LINAC RADIOSURGERY. LINAC-based stereotactic radiosurgery uses single plane rotations, multiple non-coplanar converging arcs, and dynamic radiosurgery where the couch and gantry rotate simultaneously to create dose distributions (1). Multiple non-coplanar converging arcs and dynamic radiosurgery generate dose distributions similar to those obtained with the gamma unit (1). Photon beams of 4 to 18 MeV produced by the LINAC have equivalent energies to the gamma radiation produced by the gamma knife. The LINAC generates radiographs, produced after a stream of electrons strikes a metal target, which are then focused toward the lesion by two collima-

tion systems. To modify a LINAC for stereotactic radiosurgery, a third collimator is necessary to more accurately focus the increased dose of radiation on the target. Maintaining the accuracy of this instrument to 0.2 mm ± 0.1 mm requires additional time and medical physics personnel to recalibrate the LINAC using photographic quality control procedures before each radiosurgical treatment.

Stereotactic head frames used for LINAC radiosurgery include the Brown-Roberts-Wells, Talaraich, and Leksell frames (1). Treatment planning involves adjusting the isocenter location, couch angle, gantry arc rotation interval, collimator field size, arc-start angle, arc-end angle, the number of treatment arcs, and the relative dose distribution (1). Commonly, three to seven arcs are necessary to deliver the radiation dose through 250 to 500 degrees of arc rotation with the total dose administered being the sum of all individual arcs.

Advantages of LINAC-based radiosurgery are the low acquisition cost, dose distributions similar to those of the gamma unit, no field size limitation, flexibility in altering the pattern of beam delivery, fractionation, and ease of field shaping (6). Disadvantages of LINAC radiosurgery are the extensive quality assurance necessary to assure safety, reliability, and accuracy, time-consuming machine preparation, and longer treatment times required per isocenter (6).

Benign Intracranial Tumors

ACOUSTIC TUMORS. The first acoustic tumor was treated in Stockholm in 1969 with the gamma unit. Patients with acoustic tumors who have been treated with stereotactic radiosurgery (Fig. 1) are usually older, have medical problems that increase the risk of surgery, have type 2 neurofibromatosis and bilateral lesions, have a tumor in the only ear with preserved hearing, or refuse conventional neurosurgery (1,7,8). Acoustic tumors that have been treated with stereotactic radiosurgery are acellu-

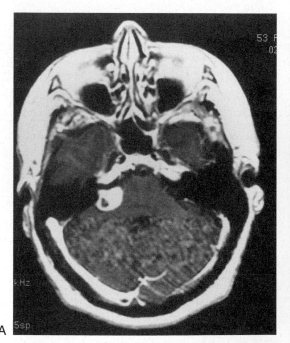
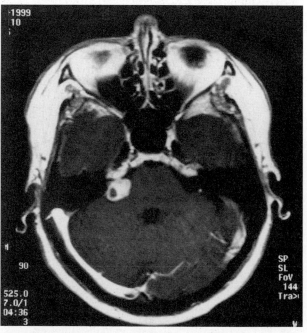

Fig. 1. Acoustic tumor. **A:** Left acoustic tumor prior to stereotactic radiosurgery on enhanced magnetic resonance imaging. **B:** Tumor appearance 1 year after treatment.

lar and have few blood vessels, abundant collagen, and central necrosis on histological examination (1,8).

The largest number of acoustic tumors have been treated in Sweden with the gamma knife, where the minimum dose to the tumor periphery was 18 to 25 Gy and the maximum central dose was 22 to 25 Gy (7). Patients with unilateral tumors who were followed after treatment from 12 to 206 months (mean, 54 months) demonstrated that 44% to 56% of tumors decreased in size, 32% to 42% were stable, and 9% to 15% enlarged (1,2, 7,8). The overall tumor growth control rate was 86%. In patients with neurofibromatosis and bilateral acoustic tumors who were treated with the gamma knife, 25% to 32% of tumors decreased in size, 43% were stable, and 25% to 33% progressed (1,2,8). Facial weakness developed at 4 to 15 months after treatment in 15% of patients and usually resolved within 6 to 12 months (1,2,8). Hearing was preserved in 56% at 1 year, 54% at 2 years, and 28% at 6 years (8). By decreasing the radiation dose to the tumor periphery from 25 to 35 Gy to 10 to 15 Gy, transient facial numbness or weakness decreased to 5% or less, without an increase in the rate of tumor growth (8).

When 20 Gy was administered to the periphery of the acoustic tumor, 60% decreased in size and 40% were stable in size at a follow-up of more than 20 months (7,9). The volumes of the treated tumors ranged from 0.12 to 17 cm^3 (median, 2.75 cm^3) and the 4-year actuarial tumor growth control rate defined as reduced tumor size or absence of growth was 89.2% ± 6% for 136 tumors (9). Central contrast enhancement was absent in 78% of tumors at a median of 6 months after treatment (9). At a median duration of 5 months after radiosurgery, hearing deteriorated in 60% of patients and 24% had transient facial weakness (7). In 92 patients who received 16 to 18 Gy to the tumor margin, 21 (23%) tumors decreased in size, 68 (74%) were stable in size, and 3 (3%) enlarged after an average period of 12 months (10). The 4-year actuarial incidence of post-radiosurgical facial and trigeminal neuropathies were 29% ± 4.4% and 32.9% ± 4.5%, respectively (9).

In 402 patients with acoustic tumors treated with stereotactic radiosurgery, 30% showed a decrease in size, 63% stabilized, and 7% increased at a mean follow-up of 36 months (8). Using MRI-based treatment planning, facial nerve function was maintained in 92%, trigeminal nerve function in 92%, and auditory nerve function in 68%. A cranial nerve deficit was most likely to occur within 2 years of treatment. When microsurgery was compared to stereotactic radiosurgery for the treatment of acoustic tumors less than 3 cm in diameter, radiosurgery was more effective in preserving normal facial function ($p < .05$) and hearing ($p < .03$) with less treatment-related morbidity ($p < .01$) (11). The total management charges were lower and the length of hospital stay was shorter in the radiosurgical group ($p < .001$). In patients who had stereotactic radiosurgery after a previous microsurgical resection of their acoustic tumor, the growth control rate was 94% at a median follow-up of 43 months (12). The incidence of delayed microsurgery after previous stereotactic radiosurgery was approximately 3% in 452 patients at a median follow-up of 27 months (13). Another series reported comparable morbidity, mortality, and cranial nerve function preservation rates for stereotactic radiosurgery compared to microsurgery for tumors 3 cm or less in diameter with a 6.6-year median follow-up in 27 patients with 29 tumors (14).

Fractionated stereotactic radiotherapy has been used for large acoustic tumors with excellent results. In 33 patients with tumors having a mean volume of 7.8 cm^3, 25 tumors (74%) decreased in size and 9 (26%) remained stable at a median MRI follow-up of 18 months (15). Patients with tumors smaller than 3 cm in diameter received 500 cGy in four daily fractions and larger tumors were treated with 400 cGy in five daily fractions. Of the 28 patients with evaluable hearing, 4 (15%) improved, 21 (75%) had stable hearing, and 3 (10%) worsened. After treat-ment, two patients with facial weakness improved and no patient developed a new trigeminal or facial nerve neuropathy (15). In another series of 26 patients with 27 acoustic tumors who were treated with fractionated stereotactic radiotherapy, no patient developed a treatment-related facial neuropathy, although 13% experienced a trigeminal neuropathy (16).

Nonacoustic schwannomas have been successfully treated with stereotactic radiosurgery (17). At a mean follow-up of 21 months after radiosurgery, all six trigeminal nerve tumors were stable in size, whereas one of seven jugular foramen tumors had enlarged by 7 months. No patient experienced injury to the cranial nerves or brainstem after treatment.

MENINGIOMAS. Radiosurgery has been used to treat recurrent or inoperable intracranial meningiomas. Small meningiomas have been treated with radiosurgery alone, whereas large tumors have required a combination of surgical resection followed by radiosurgery. Radiation doses administered to the tumor periphery have ranged from 12 to 25 Gy. After treatment most lesions remain stable in size and central hypodensity, suggesting necrosis can develop at 6 to 12 months.

An early study with long-term follow-up in 30 patients showed a decrease in tumor size in approximately half, 12 stabilized, and 4 continued to grow (2,8). Seven of 20 patients (35%) had improved cranial nerve function and 5 (25%) had partial improvement. Eighteen (60%) patients had no improvement after treatment and none had complications (2,8). Of the 59 tumors followed for 1 to 3 years, 31 (53%) decreased in size, 23 were stable (39%), and 5 enlarged (8%) (2,18). Clinical improvement was seen in 9 patients (15%), 44 (75%) were stable, and 6 (10%) worsened (1,2). A decrease in contrast enhancement within the center of the tumor, suggestive of necrosis, was seen in 22 (37%) patients (2,8). The actuarial 2-year tumor control rate was 96% (8,18).

Of 28 meningiomas treated with LINAC radiosurgery that were followed for 2 to 86 months (mean, 27 months), 4 (14%) decreased in size, 19 (68%) did not change, and 2 (7%) enlarged (2). Six (21%) patients improved clinically, 17 (61%) were stable, and 2 (7%) worsened (2). In another LINAC-based series of 55 patients with meningiomas, tumor stabilization was seen in 38 (69%), 16 (29%) decreased in size, and 1 (2%) enlarged (19). The duration of follow-up in this series was 48.4 months. Central contrast enhancement decreased on MRI in 20% of patients after treatment. Fifteen patients (27%) improved neurologically and 34 were unchanged (63%). The actuarial 2-year growth control rate was 98% (19).

Stereotactic radiosurgery has been advocated as an alternative treatment to microsurgery for meningiomas, particularly for tumors less than 3 cm in diameter (20,21). Meningiomas are ideal for radiosurgery because they are well circumscribed, rarely invasive, easily visualized by current imaging techniques, can be encompassed within the radiosurgical field even when irregular in shape, are identified when small, and their dural blood supply can be included in the treatment field (1,8). The 4-year actuarial growth control rate was 92% in 94 tumors treated with radiosurgery (20). In 34 patients with recurrent cavernous sinus meningiomas treated with stereotactic radiosurgery and followed for a median of 26 months, the tumor control rate was 100% and permanent cranial nerve palsies developed in only 2 patients (8). In 72 middle fossa meningiomas treated with radiosurgery, 50 (69%) tumors decreased in size, 18 (25%) stabilized, 2 (3%) progressed, and 2 (3%) initially decreased and then progressed (8). The treatment of petroclival meningiomas with radiosurgery was associated with a low rate of complications despite their location near critical neural structures (22). Tumor volumes decreased in 14 patients (23%), remained stable in 42 (68%), and increased in 5 (8%) of 62 petroclival tumors after treatment (22). Only 5 patients (8%) developed cranial nerve deficits within 24 months of radiosurgery which resolved completely within 6 months of onset in 2 patients.

PITUITARY TUMORS AND CRANIOPHARYNGIOMAS. Pituitary adenomas were among the first tumors to be treated with stereotactic radiosurgery. Nearly 3,000 adenomas have been treated with charged-particle beam generators of which 1,149 were growth-hormone–secreting tumors, 535 were adrenocorticotropic hormone (ACTH)-secreting tumors, 264 were prolactin-secreting tumors, and 220 were nonsecreting tumors (23). Bragg peak proton radiosurgery has been used to treat acromegaly, Cushing disease, Nelson syndrome, prolactinoma, and nonsecreting adenoma. Panhypopituitarism following radiosurgery for acromegaly and Cushing disease occurred in 10% to 15% of patients and 2% had temporary oculomotor disturbances (7). Visual field deficits and loss of vision can occur after radiosurgery because of the proximity of the pituitary gland to the optic chiasm and nerves.

Patients with acromegaly who were treated with 30 to 50 Gy of helium ion radiosurgery in 4 fractions over 5 days had clinical improvement and decreased hormone levels within 3 to 6 months (8). Mean growth hormone levels decreased by 70% within 1 year and some patients had normal levels for more than 10 years (8). Clinical improvement was seen in 90% of patients with acromegaly within 2 years of Bragg peak proton irradiation and growth-hormone levels decreased to less than 10 ng per mL in 60% (2,8). More than 50% of patients with Cushing disease treated with 50 to 150 Gy in 3 or 4 fractions had normal cortisol levels within 1 year which remained normal for 10 years (2,8). Complete clinical and endocrinological remission was seen in 65% of 175 patients, 20% improved, and 15% did not respond after Bragg peak radiosurgery for Cushing disease (2,8).

In 21 patients with acromegaly, up to 3 treatments were necessary with the gamma knife using either 40 to 70 Gy for each treatment or 30 to 50 Gy if prior radiation therapy had been administered (23). Two patients (10%) had near normal hormone levels with complete clinical remission, 8 (38%) improved clinically or endocrinologically, and 11 (52%) had little or no improvement at 1- to 21-year follow-up (23). Two patients who had prior radiotherapy developed pituitary insufficiency after stereotactic radiosurgery (23).

Gamma knife radiosurgery was used to create 1 to 4 small lesions within the pituitary gland at intervals ranging from 5 to 55 months in 35 adults and 8 children with ACTH-producing microadenomas (7,8). If improvement was not seen after the first lesion was placed in the center of the adenohypophysis, anterior and lateral lesions were generated using 70 to 100 Gy in adults or 50 to 70 Gy in children (7,8). Fourteen patients had normal urinary free-cortisol levels with 1 treatment and 8 patients had clinical remission with near normal urinary cortisol levels after 2 to 3 treatments at 3- to 9-year follow-up. Five patients failed to respond to radiosurgery and 12 of 22 patients (55%) in remission later developed panhypopituitarism (8). Complete clinical remission and normal urinary cortisol levels were reported in 7 of 8 children (88%); the child who did not respond was retreated, required bilateral adrenalectomy, and later lost pituitary function (2).

Four patients with acromegaly, 6 with Cushing disease, and 8 with nonsecreting pituitary tumors were treated with the gamma unit and followed for up to 32 months (8,24). Nine (50%) patients had macroadenomas and 9 had microadenomas. Visual acuity and the visual fields were normal in 12 (67%) patients and 6 (33%) had impaired vision (24). Eleven tumors were recurrent and 5 patients had received prior irradiation (8).

Eight (44%) tumors decreased in size, 9 (50%) were unchanged, and 1 (6%) macroadenoma in the cavernous sinus progressed after treatment with 28 to 60 Gy. Normal hormone levels were achieved in 3 of 10 patients and 3 had improved hormone levels within 3 to 5 months after treatment. Patients with normal vision remained stable and 2 of 6 patients with impaired vision improved. One patient who had received prior radiotherapy experienced severe, sudden visual loss (24).

Treatment of craniopharyngiomas consists of combination of stereotactic radiosurgery for the solid portion and intracavitary radionuclide for the cyst wall. Craniopharyngiomas that recur after microsurgery or are located within the sella turcica and are at least 3 to 5 mm away from the optic chiasm or optic nerves can be treated safely with stereotactic radiosurgery. Nearly 80 craniopharyngiomas have been treated with 20 to 50 Gy using the gamma knife (2,8). Tumor growth was arrested in all patients, two experienced visual impairment, and none lost pituitary function.

Malignant Intracranial Tumors

METASTATIC TUMORS. Stereotactic radiosurgery is an excellent treatment option for some patients with brain metastases (Fig. 2). Radiosurgery has been used to treat brain metastases located in deep, inoperable areas or those that recur or persist after whole-brain radiation therapy. Although some metastases are considered resistant to fractionated radiation therapy based on their histology, these tumor types can respond dramatically to stereotactic radiosurgery. Brain metastases are considered ideal targets for radiosurgery because most are less than 3 cm in diameter, are spherical in shape, and are radiographically distinct from surrounding brain parenchyma on CT and MRI. They are also not locally invasive, and most displace normal brain tissue away from the radiosurgery treatment volume diminishing the potential for radiation injury (25–27). Metastases treated with radiosurgery that infiltrate outside the enhancing tumor margin will ultimately recur at the edge of the treatment field (28).

In a review of more than 20 independent reports where brain metastases were treated with stereotactic radiosurgery, the results were analyzed in more than 1,250 patients with more than 2,100 lesions (25). The composite data demonstrated an average local control rate of 83% and a median survival time of 9.6 months. This length of survival is comparable to that reported for patients with a solitary brain metastasis who have surgical excision and whole-brain radiation therapy (27,29). Prognostic factors associated with prolonged survival are the presence of fewer than three tumors, Karnofsky performance scale $\geq$ 70, and absent or controlled systemic disease (25,30). A dose-response relationship appears to exist when $\geq$ 18 Gy is used as the treatment dose. Whole-brain radiation therapy may enhance local tumor control rate but does not seem to prolong survival. Most patients can be withdrawn from their corticosteroids within 1 to 3 months after radiosurgery and will have improvement in their quality of life (28).

Whether stereotactic radiosurgery alone without whole-brain radiation therapy is satisfactory treatment for brain metastases is unknown. In a series of 236 patients with 311 metastatic lesions, 158 patients received radiosurgery alone and 78 patients had radiosurgery and whole-brain radiation therapy (31). The overall median survival was 5.5 months and control of the CNS disease was achieved in 92%. The results were not significantly different between the two treatment groups (31). In patients with metastatic melanoma who were treated with stereotactic radiosurgery alone, neurological progression was halted in 35

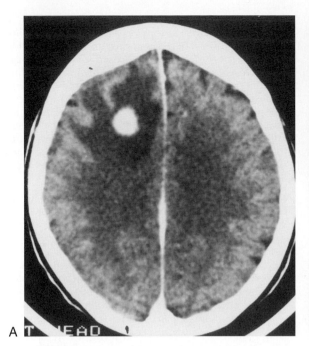
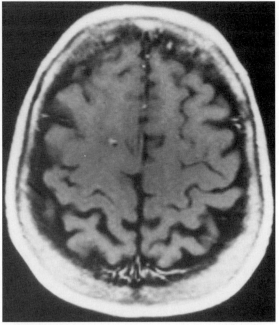

Fig. 2. Brain metastasis. **A:** Single brain metastasis from uterine carcinoma before stereotactic radiosurgery on enhanced computed tomography. **B:** Tumor 3 months after treatment on enhanced magnetic resonance imaging.

of 45 (77.8%) patients and only 7.7% of patients died as a result of their neurological disease (32).

ASTROCYTOMAS. The infiltrative nature of astrocytomas as confirmed by stereotactic biopsy suggests that radiosurgery should not be beneficial for these tumors. For this reason, stereotactic radiosurgery has primarily been used to "boost" an area either suspected of or confirmed to be recurrent tumor in patients who have already received external-beam radiation therapy. For the treatment of recurrent glioblastoma multiforme, stereotactic radiosurgery has been compared to brachytherapy using high-activity iodine-125 sources (33). For patients having radiosurgery, the actuarial median survival was 10.2 months with 12- and 24-month survivals of 45% and 19%, respectively (33). The actuarial median survival for those treated with brachytherapy was 11.5 months with 12- and 24-month survivals of 44% and 17%, respectively (33). The reoperation rate after radiosurgery was 22% compared to 44% for those receiving brachytherapy (33).

Whether radiosurgery should be given before conventional radiation therapy (up-front) or at the time of tumor recurrence for gliomas is not known. The median actuarial survival was 26 months for 23 patients with glioblastoma multiforme and has not been reached for anaplastic astrocytoma in 37 patients who received an up-front radiosurgical dose of 13 Gy to the enhancing tumor margin (8,34). In 30 patients with malignant gliomas who received a radiosurgical boost immediately after the completion of external-beam radiation therapy, the median survival was 13.9 months and the 1- and 2-year disease-specific survivals from diagnosis were 57% and 25%, respectively (35).

For 58 patients treated with radiosurgery at the time of tumor recurrence and then followed for a median of 12 months, the median survival rate was 10 months for patients with glioblastoma multiforme and the median survival has not been reached for anaplastic astrocytoma. In the 27 patients who have died, 4 had local failure at a median interval of 6 months, 12 had marginal failure at a median of 9 months, and 9 developed

distant disease in the CNS at a median of 6 months (34). Twelve (21%) patients required reoperation at a median interval of 7 months after radiosurgery for increasing mass effect and neurological deterioration (8). In 35 patients with recurrent malignant gliomas who were treated with stereotactic radiosurgery, the actuarial survival from treatment to death was 8 months (8,36). Seven patients required reoperation for increasing mass effect at a mean of 4 months after radiosurgery for an actuarial reoperation rate of 31% (8,36).

Seventy-one patients with recurrent malignant gliomas were treated with either stereotactic radiosurgery or fractionated stereotactic radiotherapy (37). The 46 patients treated with stereotactic radiosurgery received a median radiosurgical dose of 17 Gy delivered to the median isodose surface of 50% encompassing the target (37). A median dose of 37.5 Gy in 15 fractions was delivered to the median isodose surface of 85% in 25 patients who received fractionated stereotactic radiotherapy (37). The actuarial median survival for the radiosurgery group was 11 months compared to 12 months for those receiving the fractionated stereotactic treatment. Late complications developed in 14 patients in the radiosurgery group compared to 2 patients in the fractionated stereotactic radiotherapy group (37).

OTHER TUMOR TYPES. Recurrent chordomas and chondrosarcomas have been treated with gamma knife radiosurgery. Local tumor control was achieved with a dose of 20 Gy delivered to the tumor periphery (38). Half of the patients improved neurologically after treatment and the other half remained clinically stable.

LINAC radiosurgery has been used to treat recurrent head and neck tumors that were previously treated with external-beam radiation therapy. Three patients with squamous cell carcinoma, 1 with mucoepidermoid carcinoma, and 1 with adenoid cystic carcinoma received 17.5 to 35 Gy to the tumor periphery (2). All patients improved clinically within 5.5 to 7 months; 3 tumors were smaller in size and 2 were stable (2).

Pineal region tumors such as germinomas, pineocytomas, pineoblastomas, metastases, gliomas, ependymomas, craniopharyngiomas, and meningiomas have been treated with stereotactic radiosurgery. In 9 patients with pineal region tumors (4 meningiomas, 1 ependymoma, 1 craniopharyngioma, 1 pineocytoma, and 2 anaplastic astrocytomas) who had gamma knife radiosurgery and were followed for up to 32 months, 6 tumors decreased in size and 3 remained stable (8). Seven patients with small germinomas treated with LINAC radiosurgery (10 to 12 Gy) and external-beam radiation therapy (25 to 30 Gy) had tumor shrinkage at a follow-up of 26 to 86 months (8).

Hemangioblastomas, glomus jugulare tumors, and ocular melanomas have been treated with stereotactic radiosurgery (8). A case report demonstrates no tumor growth at 2 years for patients with cerebellar hemangioblastomas who received 14 to 16 Gy (39). A multi-institutional series of 38 hemangioblastomas treated with stereotactic radiosurgery found an actuarial absence rate of 86% ± 12% for tumor progression (40). Tumor control rates were better for smaller treatment volumes and for higher radiation doses.

In a report evaluating the efficacy of stereotactic radiosurgery in children, 11 recurrent brain tumors and one arteriovenous malformation were treated (8,41). Three of four children with malignant brain tumors died within 6 to 9 months after treatment. Six of eight (75%) children with low-grade tumors had radiographic reduction in the size of their tumors. A relationship was seen between lesion size and/or location and therapeutic response.

RADIATION INJURY. The development of radiation necrosis after stereotactic radiosurgery is related to the treatment volume and the dose of radiation administered. Increased intracranial pressure, increasing seizure frequency, and focal neurological deficits such as motor weakness have resulted from radiation necrosis. Symptoms of radiation injury can develop within 3 to 18 months after radiosurgery and usually resolve within 6 to 12 months in 50% of patients (8).

Symptomatic radiation necrosis after radiosurgery can develop in approximately 5% to 10% of patients with brain metastases who are followed for up to 18 months (8,25,28). Clinically apparent complications occurred in 14 of 40 (35%) patients with primary brain tumors after stereotactic radiosurgery (42). Five complications were considered moderate and nine were severe (3,42). These complications were significantly related to tumor-dose inhomogeneity, maximum tumor dose, number of isocenters, maximum normal tissue dose, and tumor volume, but not to the administration of prior radiotherapy (1,3,8).

The single-fraction radiation tolerance of the optic nerves and chiasm is 8 to 10 Gy with a 3- to 5-mm clearance being necessary to treat lesions near these structures. Other cranial nerves have a higher radiation tolerance but can be more vulnerable if they have received prior irradiation. Prescribing the radiation dose to a higher percentage isodose line was not found to decrease the incidence of trigeminal or facial nerve complications (3). The risk of trigeminal neuropathy was associated with radiation doses of more than 19 Gy for patients with skull-base meningiomas who were treated with stereotactic radiosurgery (43).

Future Considerations

TECHNICAL ISSUES. The Brown-Roberts-Wells stereotactic head frame has been adapted for noninvasive relocation to the head as the Gill Thomas locator. This frame is temporarily fixed to the maxillary teeth with a bite block and its accuracy has been confirmed by performing stereotactic brain biopsies of intracranial lesions (44). Conformal and dynamic field shaping are being developed for LINAC-based stereotactic radiosurgery to decrease the radiation dose to normal tissue and to reduce dose inhomogeneity within the treatment field. Stereotactic radiosurgery is being applied to other parts of the body such as the spine and liver (45). In 100 patients with primarily metastatic lesions in the liver and lungs who were treated with stereotactic radiosurgery to the body, 29% had tumor growth arrest, 39% had shrinkage, and 32% had complete disappearance of their tumors by a mean duration of 11 months (45).

CLINICAL ISSUES. A combination of cytoreductive surgery, conventional partial brain radiotherapy, and stereotactic radiosurgery may provide the best long-term control for skull-base meningiomas. Recurrent malignant glial tumors that have received conventional external-beam radiotherapy may be best treated at the time of recurrence with fractionated stereotactic radiotherapy to avoid the development of radiation necrosis. The beneficial effect of stereotactic radiosurgery for patients with three or more brain metastases is currently under investigation. As stereotactic radiosurgery becomes more accessible for patients, it is estimated that two-thirds of patients with acoustic tumors will be treated with this modality by the year 2020 (46).

OTHER ISSUES. Radiosurgical treatment of meningiomas has decreased the length of hospitalization, reduced the medical cost to patients, and allows patients to rapidly return to their preoperative functional status (1,8). When stereotactic radiosurgery was evaluated for acoustic tumors, arteriovenous malformations, and meningiomas, the average length of hospitalization was 2.24 days for radiosurgery compared to 11.44 days for craniotomy, and the hospital costs were reduced by 30% to 70% for patients treated with radiosurgery instead of microsurgery (1,8,47).

As the practice of medicine evolves, there is pressure for physicians to develop and recommend treatment options for patients that are effective and have a lower economical cost to society. In a cost-effectiveness analysis comparing stereotactic radiosurgery to surgical resection for the treatment of solitary brain metastases, radiosurgery has a lower total cost per procedure ($22,742 versus $30,461), a lower uncomplicated procedure cost, and a lower average complication cost per case (8, 48). By this analysis, radiosurgery is determined to be more cost-effective and has a better incremental cost-effectiveness than surgical resection. Another study suggests that stereotactic radiosurgery and whole-brain radiation therapy has a local control rate equal to or better than surgical resection and whole-brain radiation therapy and is 38% less expensive, based on average Medicare reimbursement rates (49).

References

1. Hall WA. Stereotactic radiosurgery in perspective. In: Cohen AR, Haines SJ, eds. *Concepts in neurosurgery: minimally invasive techniques in neurosurgery.* Baltimore: Williams & Wilkins, 1995; 104–117.
2. Walsh JW. Stereotactic radiosurgery. In: Morantz RA, Walsh JW, eds. *Brain tumors. A comprehensive text.* New York: Marcel Dekker, 1994;693–716.
3. Flickinger JC. Dosimetry and dose-volume relationships in radiosur-

gery. In: Alexander E III, Loeffler JS, Lunsford LD, eds. *Stereotactic radiosurgery.* New York: McGraw-Hill, 1993;31–42.

4. Flickinger JC. An integrated logistic formula for prediction of complications from radiosurgery. *Int J Radiat Biol Phys* 1989;17: 879–885.

5. Luxton G, Petrovich Z, Jozsef G, et al. Stereotactic radiosurgery: principles and comparison of treatment methods. *Neurosurgery* 1993;32:241–259.

6. Lutz W. Radiation physics for radiosurgery. In: Alexander E III, Loeffler JS, Lunsford LD, eds. *Stereotactic radiosurgery.* New York: McGraw-Hill, 1993;7–16.

7. Loeffler JS, Alexander E III. The role of stereotactic radiosurgery in the management of intracranial tumors. *Oncology* 1990;4:21–31.

8. Cho KH, Gerbi BJ, Hall WA. Stereotactic radiosurgery and radiotherapy. In: Levitt SH, Khan FM, Potish RA, et al, eds. *Levitt and Tapley's technological basis of radiation therapy. Clinical applications,* 3rd ed. Philadelphia: Lippincott Williams & Wilkins, 1999;147–172.

9. Kondziolka D, Lunsford LD, Linskey ME, et al. Skull base radiosurgery. In Alexander E III, Loeffler JS, Lunsford LD, eds. *Stereotactic radiosurgery.* New York: McGraw-Hill, 1993;175–188.

10. Flickinger JC, Lunsford LD, Coffey RJ, et al. Radiosurgery of acoustic neurinomas. *Cancer* 1991;67:345–353.

11. Pollock BE, Lunsford LD, Kondziolka D, et al. Outcome analysis of acoustic neuroma management: a comparison of microsurgery and stereotactic radiosurgery. *Neurosurgery* 1995;36:215–229.

12. Pollock BE, Lunsford LD, Flickinger JC, et al. Vestibular schwannoma management. Part I. Failed microsurgery and the role of delayed stereotactic radiosurgery. *J Neurosurg* 1998;89:944–948.

13. Pollock BE, Lunsford LD, Kondziolka D, et al. Vestibular schwannoma management. Part II. Failed radiosurgery and the role of delayed microsurgery. *J Neurosurg* 1998;89:949–955.

14. Forster DMC, Kemeny AA, Pathak A, et al. Radiosurgery: a minimally interventional alternative to microsurgery in the management of acoustic neuroma. *Br J Neurosurg* 1996;10:169–174.

15. Lederman GS, Wertheim S, Lowry J, et al. Acoustic neuromas treated by fractionated stereotactic radiotherapy. In: Alexander E III, Kondziolka D, Lindquist C, et al, eds. *Radiosurgery 1997.* Basel: Karger, 1998;25–30.

16. Andrews DW, Silverman CL, Glass J, et al. Preservation of cranial nerve function after treatment of acoustic neurinomas with fractionated stereotactic radiotherapy. Preliminary observations in 26 patients. *Stereotact Funct Neurosurg* 1995;64:165–182.

17. Pollack BE, Kondziolka D, Flickinger JC, et al. Preservation of cranial nerve function after radiosurgery for nonacoustic schwannomas. *Neurosurgery* 1993;33:597–601.

18. Kondziolka D, Lunsford LD, Coffey RD, et al. Stereotactic radiosurgery of meningiomas. *J Neurosurg* 1991;74:552–559.

19. Chang SD, Adler JR Jr. Treatment of cranial base meningiomas with linear accelerator radiosurgery. *Neurosurgery* 1997;41:1019–1027.

20. Lunsford LD. Contemporary management of meningiomas: radiation therapy as an adjuvant and radiosurgery as an alternative to surgical removal? *J Neurosurg* 1994;80:187–190.

21. Kondziolka D, Flickinger JC, Perez B, et al. Judicious resection and/ or radiosurgery for parasagittal meningiomas: outcomes from a multicenter review. *Neurosurgery* 1998;43:405–414.

22. Subach BR, Lunsford LD, Kondziolka D, et al. Management of petroclival meningiomas by stereotactic radiosurgery. *Neurosurgery* 1998;42:437–445.

23. Thorén M, Rähn T, Guo W-Y, et al. Stereotactic radiosurgery with the cobalt-60 gamma unit in the treatment of growth hormone-producing pituitary tumors. *Neurosurgery* 1991;29:663–668.

24. Stephanian E, Lunsford LD, Coffey RJ, et al. Gamma knife surgery for sellar and suprasellar tumors. *Neurosurg Clin North Am* 1992; 3:207–218.

25. Mehta MP, Boyd TS, Sinha P. The status of stereotactic radiosurgery for cerebral metastases in 1998. *J Radiosurg* 1998;1:17–30.

26. Hall WA. Stereotactic radiosurgery for brain metastases. *Crit Rev Neurosurg* 1996;6:257–262.

27. Hall WA. Solitary brain metastasis: surgery, stereotactic radiosurgery, and/or radiation therapy? In: Fischer III WS, ed. *Perspectives in neurological surgery.* Vol 9, No 1. New York: Thieme Medical Publishers, 1998;83–94.

28. Loeffler JS, Kooy HM, Wen PY, et al. The treatment of recurrent brain metastases with stereotactic radiosurgery. *J Clin Oncol* 1990; 8:576–582.

29. Cho KH, Hall WA, Lee AK, et al. Stereotactic radiosurgery for patients with single brain metastasis. *J Radiosurg* 1998;1:79–85.

30. Cho KH, Hall WA, Gerbi BJ, et al. Patient selection criteria for the treatment of brain metastases with stereotactic radiosurgery. *J Neuro-Oncol* 1998;40:73–86.

31. Pirzkall A, Debus J, Lohr F, et al. Radiosurgery alone or in combination with whole-brain radiotherapy for brain metastases. *J Clin Oncol* 1998;16:3563–3569.

32. Lavine SD, Petrovich Z, Cohen-Gadol AA, et al. Gamma knife radiosurgery for metastatic melanoma: an analysis of survival, outcome, and complications. *Neurosurgery* 1999;44:59–66.

33. Shrieve DC, Alexander E III, Wen PY, et al. Comparison of stereotactic radiosurgery and brachytherapy in the treatment of recurrent glioblastoma multiforme. *Neurosurgery* 1995;36:275–284.

34. Loeffler JS, Alexander E III, Shea WM, et al. Radiosurgery as part of the initial management of patients with malignant gliomas. *J Clin Oncol* 1992;10:1379–1385.

35. Gannett D, Stea B, Lulu B, et al. Stereotactic radiosurgery as an adjunct to surgery and external beam radiotherapy in the treatment of patients with malignant gliomas. *Int J Radiat Oncol Biol Phys* 1995;33:461–468.

36. Hall WA, Djalilian HR, Sperduto PW, et al. Stereotactic radiosurgery for recurrent malignant gliomas. *J Clin Oncol* 1995;13:1642–1648.

37. Cho KH, Hall WA, Gerbi BJ, et al. Single dose versus fractionated stereotactic radiotherapy for recurrent high-grade gliomas. *Int J Radiat Oncol Biol Phys* 1999;45:1133–1141.

38. Kondziolka D, Lunsford LD, Flickinger JC. The role of radiosurgery in the management of chordoma and chondrosarcoma of the cranial base. *Neurosurgery* 1991;29:38–46.

39. Chandler HC Jr, Friedmen WA. Radiosurgical treatment of a hemangioblastoma: case report. *Neurosurgery* 1994;34:353–355.

40. Patrice SJ, Sneed PK, Flickinger JC, et al. Radiosurgery for hemangioblastoma: results of a multiinstitutional experience. *Int J Radiat Oncol Biol Phys* 1996;35:493–499.

41. Weprin BE, Hall WA, Cho KH, et al. Stereotactic radiosurgery in children. *Pediatr Neurol* 1996;15:193–199.

42. Nedzi LA, Kooy LI, Alexander E III, et al. Variables associated with the development of complications from radiosurgery of intracranial tumors. *Int J Radiat Oncol Biol Phys* 1991;21:591–599.

43. Morita A, Coffey RJ, Foote RL, et al. Risk of injury to cranial nerves after gamma knife radiosurgery for skull base meningiomas: experience in 88 patients. *J Neurosurg* 1999;90:42–49.

44. Sofat A, Kratimenos G, Thomas DGT. Early experience with the Gill Thomas locator for computed tomography-directed stereotactic biopsy of intracranial lesions. *Neurosurgery* 1992;31:972–974.

45. Blomgren H, Lax I, Göranson H, Kræpelien T, et al. Radiosurgery for tumors in the body: clinical experience using a new method. *J Radiosurg* 1998;1:63–74.

46. Pollock BE, Lunsford LD, Norén G. Vestibular schwannoma management in the next century: a radiosurgical perspective. *Neurosurgery* 1998;43:475–483.

47. Lunsford LD, Flickinger J, Coffey RJ. Stereotactic gamma knife radiosurgery: initial North American experience in 207 patients. *Arch Neurol* 1990;47:169–175.

48. Rutigliano MJ, Lunsford LD, Kondziolka D, et al. The cost effectiveness of stereotactic radiosurgery versus surgical resection in the treatment of solitary metastatic brain tumors. *Neurosurgery* 1995;37: 445–455.

49. Sperduto PW, Hall WA. The cost-effectiveness for alternative treatments for single brain metastases. In: Kondziolka D, ed. *Radiosurgery 1995.* Basel: Karger 1996;180–187.

125. Preoperative Embolization of Intracranial Tumors

Herbert H. Engelhard III

Preoperative embolization of intracranial tumors, in selected cases, can be a valuable adjunct to their surgical removal. The goal of embolization is to devascularize the tumor, making it smaller, softer, less bloody, and therefore easier to resect (1,2). Types of intracranial tumors that have been treated by preoperative embolization are given in Table 1. Glomus jugulare and other "head and neck tumors" may invade the skull base and extend intracranially, and are also often embolized. Skull-base tumors are listed in Table 2. Meningioma, the most common benign brain tumor in adults, is also the type of brain tumor most often embolized (Fig. 1). Meningiomas typically have a rich blood supply from the dura adjacent to them, which originates from the external carotid artery. Because of this, embolization at the time of cerebral angiography has been used for many years to reduce the blood supply to meningiomas, as well as other vascular tumors.

Years ago, angiography was the primary diagnostic procedure for intracranial tumors. With the advent of computed tomography (CT), then magnetic resonance imaging (MRI), use of cerebral angiography for tumor diagnosis was sharply curtailed. Because of this, the option of preoperative embolization became more restricted. Use of the cerebral *micro*catheter, which ushered in the modern era of interventional neuroradiology, was pioneered by Serbinenko and colleagues almost 30 years ago (G. Debrun, personal communication). "Endovascular surgical neuroradiology" is now recognized as a subspecialty by the Accreditation Council for Graduate Medical Education. Neurosurgeons may be more aware of the benefits of endovascular approaches for aneurysms and cerebral arteriovenous malformations than for tumors. Those who have never operated on a meningioma treated by preoperative embolization may be unaware of the benefits of the procedure (1,3). Currently, intraarterial digital subtraction angiography continues to give the most precise information regarding the vascular anatomy of intracranial tumors, and is the most useful test for assessing the feasibility of preoperative embolization (1,4).

Cerebral Angiography and Imaging of the Neurovascular Anatomy of Brain Tumors

MRI currently dominates the diagnosis of intracranial disorders including tumors, providing superior information as to their anatomical location, size, and relationship to the dura and other structures (1,5). Yet, intraarterial digital subtraction cerebral angiography remains the best imaging technique for patients in whom there are potential neurovascular issues (1). Recent technical improvements have increased the speed, quality, and safety of diagnostic cerebral angiography (6). For a meningioma, angiography will demonstrate its arterial supply from meningeal vessels, and show the typical finding of a "delayed blush" (i.e., contrast persisting into the late venous phase) (7–9). The arterial pedicle usually enters the tumor at its meningeal attachment and supplies a radially arrayed vascular pattern resulting in a "spoke-wheel" or "sunburst" appearance (8,10),

as is demonstrated in Fig. 1B. Tumors in specific locations have characteristic arterial feeders, which are summarized in Table 3 (3,4,10,11).

The primary purpose in performing angiography on a patient with an intracranial tumor is to precisely define the relevant vascular anatomy including: (a) the location of feeding vessels; (b) any displacement or encasement of normal vascular structures; (c) identification of "vessels of passage" supplying normal brain, which should not be sacrificed; (d) the position of cortical draining veins; and (e) the degree of dural sinus invasion or occlusion (1,8). The nature of this information can have a significant impact upon surgical planning (11–13). As examples, conclusively establishing the lack of patency of a venous sinus simplifies the planning of its surgical resection along with the tumor. Also, knowing precisely where the major feeding vessels to the tumor are located facilitates their early identification and control. Lastly, being aware of the precise location of the cortical draining veins—and their collaterals—can help in planning the operative trajectory to the tumor, potentially improving the chance of a total resection while avoiding the possibility of venous infarction.

Angiography can be used to characterize the precise degree of tumor vascularity and the nature of the arterial blood supply of the tumor—dural, pial, or mixed (1). Angiography can be used to perform a trial temporary occlusion (i.e., with a deflatable balloon) of a potentially functional artery, which may need to be sacrificed to completely resect a tumor such as a medial sphenoid wing meningioma (3,10,14–16). Before the occlusion is done, the angiogram gives the most accurate information about the collateral circulation of the brain. Competing studies that might potentially be used to provide such information include MRI, conventional cerebral angiography, magnetic resonance angiography (MRA), and magnetic resonance venography (MRV).

Detection of vessels with a diameter less than 1 mm has remained elusive for MRA, and MRA may overestimate the degree of vessel stenosis (17). With MRA, it is also difficult to determine whether lack of visualization of an artery is the result of severe stenosis or complete occlusion (17). MRA (at 1.5 T) has not been reliable in revealing the characteristic vascular findings of a meningioma (13). The vascular supply of skull-base tumors cannot currently be adequately evaluated by MRA (16). MRV has the ability to noninvasively detect the patency of the dural venous sinuses (13,17). Yet nonvisualization of a sinus by MRV may not be sufficient to prove total occlusion. Vessels are more clearly shown with the new 3-T MRI units, however, and the availability of this test may impact upon the preoperative evaluation of patients in the near future (1).

Preoperative Embolization: Indications and Risks

How does one decide whether or not to recommend preoperative embolization? This topic continues to be an area of controversy in neurosurgery (18,19,20). At our institution, each patient's preoperative studies are reviewed with the interventional

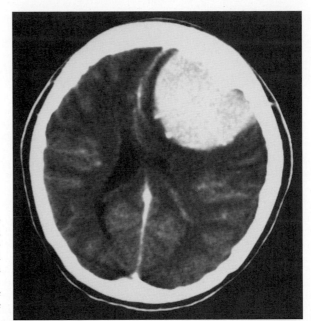

Fig. 1. A: Head CT scan with contrast, showing a large convexity meningioma that occurred in a 34-year-old woman. **B:** Preembolization digital subtraction angiogram. The feeding vessel from the middle meningeal artery is clearly seen. **C:** Postembolization angiogram showing that the feeding vessel is completely occluded. This tumor was soft, necrotic, and very easy to remove at the time of surgery, which was performed on the following day.

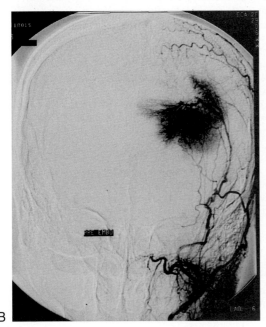

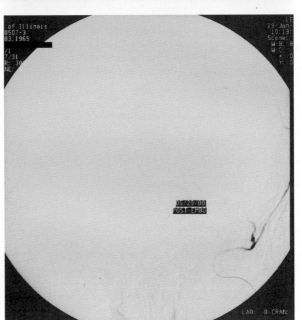

Table 1. Types of Intracranial Tumors Treated by Preoperative Embolization

Meningioma
Hemangioblastoma
Choroid plexus papilloma/carcinoma
Hemangioendothelioma
Hemangiopericytoma
Brain/skull metastases
Skull base tumors
Other rare tumors

Table 2. Representative Skull Base Tumors (Primary or Secondary)

Meningioma	Nasopharyngeal carcinoma
Paraganglioma (i.e., glomus tumor, chemodectoma)	Juvenile nasopharyngeal angiofibroma
Schwannoma	Rhabdomyosarcoma
Chordoma	Endolymphatic sac tumor
Chondroma	Skull metastases
Chondrosarcoma	Other rare tumors

Table 3. Characteristic Arterial Feeders, According to Tumor Location

Location	Parent Artery(ies)
Cerebral convexity	Middle meningeal, superficial temporal, cortical
Parasagittal	Middle meningeal, superficial temporal, anterior falx, cortical
Middle sphenoid wing	Middle meningeal
Medial sphenoid wing	Ophthalmic, intracavernous internal carotid
Olfactory groove	Ophthalmic, ethmoidal, sphenoid branches of middle meningeal, frontal branch of anterior cerebral
Falx	Ophthalmic, middle meningeal, superficial temporal, anterior falx, cortical
Tuberculum sellae	Internal carotid, ethmoidal, sphenoid branches of middle meningeal and meningohypophyseal trunk
Middle fossa	Internal carotid, middle meningeal, ophthalmic
Optic sheath	Ophthalmic
Tentorium	Meningohypophyseal trunk (tentorial branch), middle meningeal, occipital, vertebral
Cavernous sinus	Intracavernous internal carotid, ophthalmic, middle meningeal
Lateral ventricle	Anterior or lateral posterior choroidal
Pineal	Medial posterior choroidal
Cerebellopontine angle	Vertebral, ascending pharyngeal, occipital, middle meningeal, anterior inferior cerebellar
Cerebellar convexity	Occipital, posterior meningeal
Foramen magnum	Occipital, ascending pharyngeal, vertebral
Petroclival	Meningohypophyseal trunk (clival branch), ascending pharyngeal, occipital, middle meningeal

neuroradiologist in order to ascertain the feasibility of embolizing a particular tumor, and the potential risks involved. Certainly, most meningiomas do not need to be embolized—a proximal vascular occlusion can be performed intraoperatively, or is not needed. For a given patient, the benefit of devascularizing the tumor preoperatively has to be weighed against possible complications of embolization. It is advantageous to perform preoperative embolization on highly vascular tumors, especially those in which the feeding vessels are going to be encountered late in the procedure.

Many studies illustrate the benefits of preoperative embolization of meningiomas and other tumors (1–25). Softer, devascularized tumors should theoretically be easier to manipulate and remove, thus shortening operative time, and reducing blood loss and the potential for brain injury from dissection and retraction (4,10,11,14,15,26). Tumor firmness can often be determined from the preoperative MRI. Suzuki and colleagues studied 73 intracranial meningiomas, and concluded that the lower intensity portions of the tumor on T2-weighted images were harder and more fibrous in character, whereas the higher intensity portions were softer (26). Other authors have reported similar findings on both T2-weighted images and proton-density images (27–29).

While the experience with embolizing meningiomas is fairly extensive and the indications for doing so fairly clear, less information is available for other types of tumors. Hemangioblastomas are vascular tumors, but they often occur in the posterior fossa, and their blood supply is usually received through the pia mater. Nonetheless, some of these tumors are fed through branches of the external carotid artery (e.g., occipital artery) or branches of the internal carotid artery amenable to embolization (e.g., artery of Bernasconi and Cassinari) (30). Accordingly, there have been reports of embolizing these tumors (30–32). Choroid plexus papillomas (or carcinomas) are also usually quite vascular, and embolization of these tumors—by a variety of methods—has been reported to be valuable (33). Hemangiopericytomas, given their aggressive biological nature, have also been embolized more aggressively (5).

Skull-base tumors encompass a wide variety of pathological types, some of which are given in Table 2. Preoperative embolization may be of benefit for many types of skull-base tumors (15,16,34,35). Blood loss from such tumors can be a major contributor to postoperative morbidity. Some authors believe embolization is of benefit for treating convexity *and* skull-base lesions (1,7). Others believe it should be reserved only for surgically difficult tumors, such as those involving the skull base (10, 19). This is provided embolization can be accomplished without undue risk of infarcting normal brain and/or cranial nerves (i.e., the blood supply is predominantly from the external carotid artery). Whether or not to attempt a complete resection of meningiomas that invade the cavernous sinus at the base of the skull is another controversial topic. Permanent occlusion of the internal carotid artery before surgery (after a negative balloon occlusion test) has been used when the carotid is encased with tumor, in order to facilitate a complete resection. However, many neurosurgeons believe that the risk of cranial nerve damage is prohibitively high, especially considering results achieved with radiosurgery (36). Oka and co-workers studied 20 patients with skull-base meningiomas and demonstrated that for tumors less than 6 cm in diameter, the blood lost during subsequent surgery was significantly less in the embolized group. The embolized group also had a better clinical outcome (37). Embolization of a glomus jugulare tumor invading the skull base is demonstrated in Fig. 2.

Even in the major centers, cerebral angiography is not without risks. Embolization procedures, by their very nature, carry more risk than angiography alone. Complications from angiography can be divided into three categories: local (i.e., groin hematoma, leg numbness, or local infection), systemic (i.e., renal failure or allergic reaction to the contrast agent), and neurological (i.e., transient neurological deficits or infarction) (6). Headache often follows cerebral angiography (6). In a study of 1,000 consecutive patients undergoing cerebral angiography, Heiserman and associates found a 1% incidence of neurological deficits related to the procedure, with about half of these being persistent. All the complications occurred in patients presenting with a history of stroke, transient ischemic attack, and/or carotid bruit (38). A recent metaanalysis of cerebral angiography performed in neurovascular patients put the risk of permanent neurological complication at only 0.07%, and serious nonneurologic complications at 0.6%—much lower than expected (39). Factors that correlated with adverse events included age, volume of contrast used, length of the procedure, use of multiple catheters, and the presence of systolic hypertension (39).

While the *overall* incidence of complications of contemporary cerebral angiography has been reported, most of the angiograms in such series were not performed specifically in patients with brain tumors (1). In the 1970s, Mani and Eisenberg analyzed 5,000 catheter cerebral arteriograms, and found that the complication rate was lower for patients with tumors than for those with cerebrovascular occlusive disease and subarachnoid hemorrhage (40). It would seem that the risk of a significant complication from angiography in a patient with a tumor—in trained hands—is extremely low, but not nonexistent (1).

With embolization, neurological deficit can occur if the embolic material gets into vessels feeding either the cranial nerves

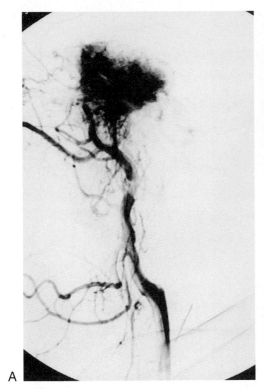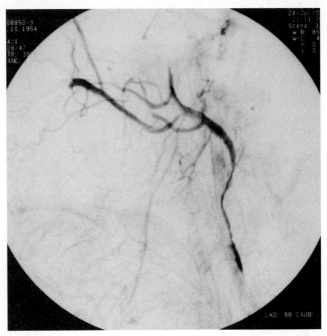

Fig. 2. Digital subtraction angiograms from the embolization of a glomus jugulare tumor invading the skull base found in a 38-year-old woman. **A:** Preembolization angiogram showing a highly vascular tumor. **B:** The tumor is completely devascularized, which made it much easier to resect.

or the brain itself. The use of provocative testing with amobarbital sodium and lidocaine, in order to reveal the presence of dangerous anastomoses to the internal carotid artery distribution and the blood supply to cranial nerves, has been described (41). Embolization of scalp vessels may cause ischemic necrosis of the scalp (and/or scalp flap, if a craniotomy was performed after the embolization) (11,42). This may even require reconstruction with a free flap. Microcatheters can become caught, or break during the procedure, especially if acrylic glue is used (43). Other reported complications include facial pain, trismus, and various types of hemorrhage (subarachnoid, peritumoral, intratumoral) (4,10,44–47). In a study published by Probst and colleagues, two out of 80 patients (2.5%) had neurological deficits after tumor embolization with fibrin glue. Both involved cranial nerves; one resolved within one year of the procedure and one persisted (20).

Considering all of this, at our institution embolization is likely to be recommended for a meningioma if it is highly vascular and most of the vascular supply comes from meningeal vessels safely accessible with superselective catheterization. Embolization is especially useful for larger tumors, or if it is anticipated that the blood supply will be reached only at the end of the operation (20). Others have attempted embolization alone, without subsequent surgery, to attempt to slow tumor growth as a palliative procedure in cases in which surgical treatment is contraindicated (3,4,14,16,18,46,48,49).

Tumor Embolization: Technical Considerations

Currently, preoperative tumor embolization is usually performed by neurosurgeons or radiologists who have completed

a fellowship in interventional neuroradiology. Ideally, the interventionalists work as a part of a team, which includes neurosurgeons, neurologists, and neuroradiologists. The interventional neuroradiologist must have a thorough knowledge of the vascular supply to the meninges, anatomy of potentially dangerous anastomoses between the external and internal carotid artery vascular territories, and functional neuroanatomy in relation to the vascular supply of the brain (1). Hazardous anastomoses may especially be present around the skull base (15). As mentioned previously, interventional neuroangiography techniques allow superselective catheterization of tumor vessels (8,11) which ideally originate from the external carotid artery. Internal carotid artery branches supplying the tumor are usually not embolized, due to the risk of stroke (14). Although there are reports to the contrary, optic nerve meningiomas, which are usually supplied by branches of the ophthalmic artery, are usually not embolized due to the risk of damage to the optic nerves (4). To avoid complications, the microcatheter must be advanced far past any anastomoses, and the risk of reflux of the embolic material carefully analyzed.

A typical room setup for performing intracranial tumor embolization is shown in Fig. 3. Such a room has the capability for real-time biplane digital subtraction angiography. Several different types of flow-directed microcatheters and guidewires are available. Using the transfemoral Seldinger technique, they can be navigated into selected branches of the intracranial or extracranial vasculature. Several excellent nonionic contrast agents are now available for visualization of the vessels during the procedure. Feeding vessels have been occluded with a variety of agents and devices including Gelfoam powder, polyvinyl alcohol (PVA) foam (with particles of various diameters), lyophilized dura, Silastic microspheres, trisacryl gelatin microspheres, N-butyl cyanoacrylate ("acrylic glue"), fibrin glue, dehydrated ethanol, latex or Silastic detachable balloons, and/or

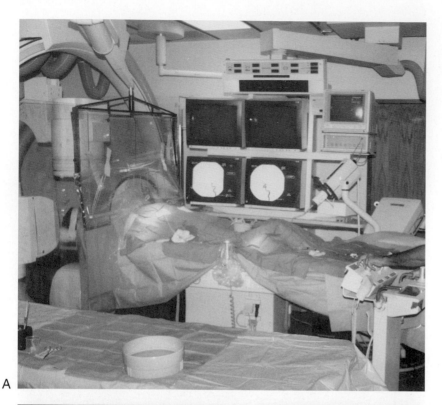

A

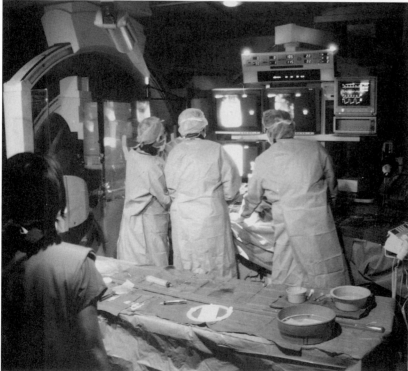

B

Fig. 3. Setup of room used for interventional neu-roradiology. **A:** Arrangement of sterile field, with the table used for arranging the catheters and other equipment in the foreground, patient (sterilely draped) in the center, and biplane digital subtrac-tion angiography display (with injector, right) in the background. Catheters as small as 2F can be used to provide access to the feeding vessels of tumors, as well as aneurysms and arteriovenous malforma-tions. **B:** The neurointerventional team at work.

detachable coils (2,3,5,10,11,20,46,48,50–52). While PVA microparticles are currently the most popular material for embolizing tumors, interventionalists disagree as to which of the materials is best. The choice of material is dictated by the location of the lesion and the anticipated end point of the procedure (2). The material used for embolization plays an important role in generating complications. Acrylic glue and ethanol seem to be more risky than PVA particles, and therefore should be used with great caution (G. Debrun, personal communication).

Brain tumors and especially meningiomas occur in characteristic locations, and have specific arterial "feeders," which have been carefully described and tabulated, as is summarized in Table 2 (3,11). It may not be possible, or safe, to embolize all of these vessels. The specific strategies for embolizing meningiomas according to their location has been described in detail

(4,10). The goal of the interventionalist is to reach the tumor's capillary bed and obliterate the arterial and arteriolar feeders, while preserving the integrity of normal brain, cranial nerves, and scalp vessels (1,10). If the vessel feeding the tumor cannot be selectively catheterized, embolization is usually not attempted. Blood supply from the pia can limit the effectiveness of embolization (10).

At our institution the embolization is done the day before surgery, using PVA particles in the 50- to 150-μm range. For tumors, we believe that solid particles are safer than acrylic glue, despite the fact that a liquid agent might provide deeper penetration into the tumor (2). The embolization procedure is done with the patient under general anesthesia and paralyzed so that there is no movement. Before the procedure, the patient must be optimized in terms of their hydration status, and ste-

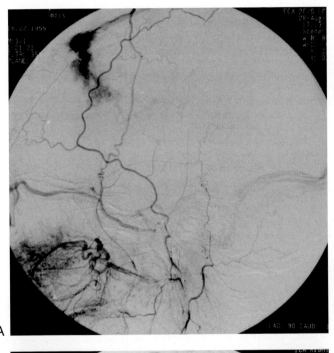

A

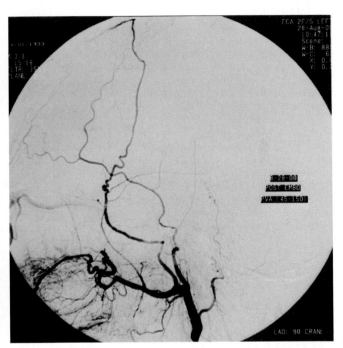

B

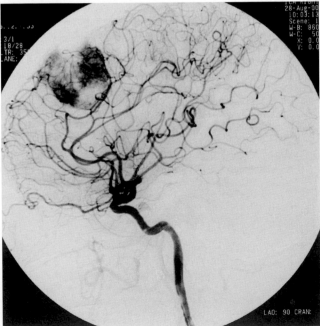

C

Fig. 4. Digital subtraction angiograms from the embolization of a recurrent parasagittal meningioma in a 45-year-old man. **A:** Preembolization angiogram clearly showing the feeding vessel from the middle meningeal artery. **B:** Postembolization angiogram demonstrating vessel occlusion. **C:** Internal carotid angiogram, showing multiple additional feeding vessels from the internal carotid circulation. This tumor remained vascular, and was only partially embolized.

roids are administered (10,52). Before injecting particles, superselective angiography through the microcatheter, under biplane digital subtraction angiography, must clearly show that there are no anastomoses with the ophthalmic artery or intracranial vessels. The margin of safety must be clearly determined so that it is known exactly how much reflux can be tolerated (G. Debrun, personal communication). The particles are injected slowly to avoid reflux. The most effective embolization occurs with the most distal loading of the vascular bed (20). The tip of the microcatheter only rarely reaches the tumor itself. Wedging of the catheter into the tumor vessels is to be avoided because it can cause the tumor to rupture and/or hemorrhage (4). Recurrent and malignant meningiomas are usually more difficult to embolize (10). This is illustrated in Fig, 4, which shows angiograms from the embolization of a recurrent parasagittal meningioma in a 45-year-old man. After the embolization procedure, observation in the neurosurgical intensive care unit is recommended.

There are several situations in which only a partial embolization of the tumor may be possible, or the attempt at embolization should be aborted. Attempts at embolization are stopped if (a) feeding branches to the tumor are found to be inaccessible, (b) catheter positions allowing for safe embolization cannot be achieved, and/or (c) the remaining feeders after partial embolization would be surgically accessible at an early stage of the tumor dissection (23). The case in Fig. 4 illustrates a situation in which only a partial tumor embolization could be achieved from the external carotid circulation. If embolization is not used, or is unsuccessful, it is beneficial to interrupt the tumor's blood supply as an initial step in its surgical removal.

Authors differ as to when embolization should be done prior to surgery (4,20,48). At our institution, surgery is usually performed the day after the embolization procedure. Others have recommended waiting 3 to 5 days (4,10,15) or even 1 to 2 weeks (48). These recommendations might depend on the type of material used for the embolization (15). If too long a time elapses before surgery, embolized vessels may recannulate. If a permanent balloon occlusion is performed before surgery (after the patient "passes" a temporary balloon occlusion test), surgery should be avoided for 8 weeks to allow organization of the thrombus, reducing the possibility of embolization of a clot during manipulation of the distal carotid artery (16). One must be particularly cautious when embolizing very large meningiomas associated with edema and/or shift of the intracranial contents. The embolization procedure could cause additional swelling and subsequent neurological deficit. It may be preferable to perform the surgery for these large meningiomas with mass effect *immediately* after embolization.

Following embolization, the success of the procedure can be assessed by several methods. First among these is the postembolization angiogram, which demonstrates the disappearance of the tumor blush. One must be aware, however, that the tumor could still have a partial blood supply from other routes, such as branches of the internal carotid artery (as demonstrated in Fig. 4). CT and MRI (and analysis of pathology specimens) have also been used, but may underestimate the effect of the procedure (1,46,52). CT can demonstrate low-density areas within a previously homogeneous tumor. An MRI done with gadolinium may show less intense enhancement, more heterogeneity, or increased signal on T2-weighted images. If more precise information is needed, mapping the relative regional cerebral blood volume seems to be an effective technique (21). Magnetic resonance spectroscopy (MRS) has been performed on patients with meningiomas after embolization (18,52,53). In embolized tumors, infarction is indicated by increased levels of lactate and aliphatic lipids (52,53). In patients who did not have surgery, long-term follow-up with MRS indicated the occurrence of fatty degeneration of the tumor (18).

Conclusions

While the possibility of embolizing intracranial and skull-base tumors has existed for many years, recent advances in the design of superselective microcatheters, improved embolic agents, and subspecialty-trained interventional neuroradiologists have made the procedure safer and more effective. Angiography performed alone is still useful for precisely defining the vascular anatomy of brain tumors, and assessing the collateral circulation and feasibility of embolization. At present, medical centers vary widely in their use of cerebral angiography, and in many locations embolization might not be available at all (1).

Patients for preoperative embolization are selected on a case-by-case basis. The goal of the procedure is to reduce a tumor's blood supply, making it softer, less vascular, and easier to resect. Embolization is usually not needed if the tumor's blood supply can be easily interrupted during the approach to the tumor. On the other hand, tumors expected to be very vascular, large, firm, or to have major feeding vessels that cannot be accessed early in the procedure are considered for embolization. While the complication rate of interventional neuroradiology in intracranial tumors is not known precisely, in trained hands it should be very low (less than 1%) (1,48). In the future, tumor embolization—perhaps combined with chemotherapy and/or medications that inhibit angiogenesis—might develop into a primary treatment modality (1,21,48).

Acknowledgments

The author wishes to thank Dr. Gerard M. Debrun for his careful review of the manuscript, suggestions about its content, and for supplying cases used in the figures. The assistance of Ms. Jacqueline Debrun and Ms. Clary Olichwier is also greatly appreciated.

References

1. Engelhard HH: Progress in the diagnosis and treatment of patients with meningiomas. Part I: diagnostic imaging, preoperative embolization. *Surg Neurol* 2001;55:89–101.
2. Bauza JA: Interventional neuroradiology. In Allen MB, Miller RH, eds. *Essentials of neurosurgery: a guide to clinical practice.* New York: McGraw-Hill, 1995:333–340.
3. Connors III JJ, Wojack JC: Meningiomas. In: Connors III JJ, Wojack JC, eds. *Interventional neuroradiology: strategies and practical techniques.* Philadelphia: WB Saunders, 1999:100–121.
4. Rodesch G, Lasjaunias P: Embolization and meningiomas. In: Al-Mefty O, ed. *Meningiomas.* New York: Raven Press, 1991:285–297.
5. Choi IS, Tantivatana J: Neurovascular management of intracranial and spinal tumors. *Neurosurg Clin North Am* 2000;11:167–185.
6. Pryor JC, Setton A, Nelson PK, et al: Complications of diagnostic cerebral angiography and tips on avoidance. *Neuroimag Clin North Am* 1996;6:751–758.
7. Black PM: Meningiomas. *Neurosurgery* 1993;32:643–657.
8. Jacobs JM, Harnsberger HR: Diagnostic angiography and meningiomas. In: Al-Mefty O, ed. *Meningiomas.* New York: Raven Press, 1991:225–240.
9. Zimmerman RD: MRI of intracranial meningiomas. In Al-Mefty O, ed. *Meningiomas,* New York: Raven Press, 1991:209–223.
10. Nelson PK, Setton A, Choi IS, et al: Current status of interventional neuroradiology in the management of meningiomas. *Neurosurg Clin N Am* 1994;5:235–259.

11. McDermott MW, Wilson CB: *Meningiomas.* In: Youmans JR, ed. *Neurological surgery,* 4th ed. Philadelphia: WB Saunders, 1996: 2782–2825.
12. Ojeman R: Meningiomas. *Neurosurg Clin North Am* 1990;1:181–197.
13. Murtagh R, Linden C: Neuroimaging of intracranial meningiomas. *Neurosurg Clin North Am* 1994;5:217–233.
14. Akeyson EW, McCutcheon IE: Management of benign and aggressive intracranial meningiomas. *Oncology* 1996;10:747–756.
15. Desai R, Bruce J: Meningiomas of the cranial base. *J Neuro-Oncol* 1994;20:255–279.
16. Thornton J, Bashi Q, Aletich VA, et al: Role of magnetic resonance imaging and diagnostic and interventional angiography in vascular and neoplastic diseases of the skull base associated with vestibulocochlear symptoms. *Top Magn Reson Imaging* 2000;11:123–137.
17. Van Hemert RL: MRA of cranial tumors and vascular compressive lesions. *Clin Neurosci* 1997;4:146–152.
18. Bendszus M, Martin-Schrader I, Warmuth-Metz M, et al: MR imaging and MR spectroscopy-revealed changes in meningiomas for which embolization was performed without subsequent surgery. *Am J Neuroradiol* 2000;21:666–669.
19. Latchaw RE: Preoperative intracranial meningioma embolization: technical considerations affecting risk-to-benefit ratio. *Am J Neuroradiol* 1993;14:583–586.
20. Probst EN, Grzyska U, Westphal M, et al: Preoperative embolization of intracranial meningiomas with a fibrin glue preparation. *Am J Neuroradiol* 1999;20:1695–702.
21. Bruening R, Wu RH, Yousry TA, et al: Regional relative blood volume MR maps of meningiomas before and after partial embolization. *J Comput Assist Tomogr* 1998;22:104–110.
22. Dean BL, Flom RA, Wallace RC, et al: Efficacy of endovascular treatment of meningiomas: evaluation with matched samples. *Am J Neuroradiol* 1994;15:1675–1680.
23. Gruber A, Killer M, Mazal P, et al: Preoperative embolization of intracranial meningiomas: a 17-year single center experience. *Minim Invasive Neurosurg* 2000;43:18–29.
24. Macpherson P: The value of pre-operative embolisation of meningioma estimated subjectively and objectively. *Neuroradiology* 1991; 33:334–337.
25. Morimura T, Takeuchi J, Maeda Y, et al: Preoperative embolization of meningiomas: its efficacy and histopathological findings. *Noshuyo Byori* 1994; 11:123–129.
26. Suzuki Y, Sugimoto T, Shibuya M, et al: Meningiomas: correlation between MRI characteristics and operative findings including consistency. *Acta Neurochir* 1994;129:39–46.
27. Chen TC, Zee C-S, Miller CA, et al: Magnetic resonance imaging and pathological correlates of meningiomas. *Neurosurgery* 1992;31: 1015–1022.
28. Maiuri F, Ianconetta G, de Divitiis O, et al: Intracranial meningiomas: correlations between MR imaging and histology. *Eur J Radiol* 1999; 31:69–75.
29. Yamaguchi N, Kawase T, Sagoh M, et al: Prediction of consistency of meningiomas with preoperative magnetic resonance imaging. *Surg Neurol* 1997;48:579–583.
30. Yamada SM, Ikeda Y, Takahashi H, et al: Hemangioblastomas with blood supply from the dural arteries—two case reports. *Neurol Med Chir* (Tokyo) 2000;40:69–73.
31. Standard SC, Ahuja A, Livingston K, et al: Endovascular embolization and surgical excision for the treatment of cerebellar and brain stem hemangioblastomas. *Surg Neurol* 1994;41:405–410.
32. Tampieri D, Leblanc R, TerBrugge K: Preoperative embolization of brain and spinal hemangioblastomas. *Neurosurgery* 199;33: 502–505.
33. Pencalet P, Sainte-Rose C, Lellouch-Tubiana A, et al: Papillomas and carcinomas of the choroid plexus in children. *J Neurosurg* 1998;88: 521–528.
34. Bingaman KD, Alleyne CH, Olson JJ: Intracranial extraskeletal mesenchymal chondrosarcoma: case report. *Neurosurgery* 2000;46: 207–211.
35. Davis KR, Debrun GM: Embolization of juvenile nasopharyngeal angiofibromas. *Semin Intervent Radiol* 1987;4:309–319.
36. Engelhard HH: Current role of radiation therapy and radiosurgery in the management of meningiomas. *Neurosurg Focus* 1997;2(4): 1–4.
37. Oka H, Kurata A, Kawano N et al: Preoperative superselective embolization of skull-base meningiomas: indications and limitations. *J Neuro-Oncol* 1998:40:67–71.
38. Heiserman JE, Dean BL, Hodak JA, et al: Neurologic complications of cerebral angiography. *Am J Neuroradiol* 1994; 15:1401–1407.
39. Cloft HJ, Joseph GJ, Dion JE: Risk of cerebral angiography in patients with subarachnoid hemorrhage, cerebral aneurysm, and arteriovenous malformation: a meta-analysis. *Stroke* 1999;30:317–320.
40. Mani RL, Eisenberg RL: Complications of catheter cerebral angiography: analysis of 5,000 procedures. II. Relation of complication rates to clinical and arteriographic diagnoses. *Am J Neuroradiol* 1978; 131:867–869.
41. Deveikis JP: Sequential injections of amobarbital sodium and lidocaine for provocative neurologic testing in the external carotid circulation. *Am J Neuroradiol* 1996;17:1143–1147.
42. Adler JR, Upton J, Wallman J, et al: Management and prevention of necrosis of the scalp after embolization and surgery for meningioma. *Surg Neurol* 1986;25:357–360.
43. Inci S, Ozcan OE, Benli K, et al. Microsurgical removal of a free segment of microcatheter in the anterior circulation as a complication of embolization. *Surg Neurol* 1996; 46:562–566.
44. Hayashi T, Shojima K, Utsunomiya H, et al: Subarachnoid hemorrhage after preoperative embolization of a cystic meningioma. *Surg Neurol* 1987;27:295–300.
45. Kallmes DF, Evans AJ, Kaptain GJ, et al: Hemorrhagic complications in embolization of a meningioma: case report and review of the literature. *Neuroradiology* 1997;39:877–880.
46. Richter H-P, Schachenmayr W: Preoperative embolization of intracranial meningiomas. *Neurosurgery* 1983;13:261–268.
47. Suyama T, Tamaki N, Fujiwara K, et al: Peritumoral and intratumoral hemorrhage after gelatin sponge embolization of meningioma: case report. *Neurosurgery* 1987;21:944–946.
48. Ahuja A, Gibbons KJ, Hopkins LN: Endovascular techniques to treat brain tumors. In Youmans JR, ed. *Neurological surgery.* Philadelphia: WB Saunders, 1996:2826–2840.
49. Koike T, Sasaki O, Tanaka R, et al: Long-term results in a case of meningioma treated by embolization alone—case report. *Neurol Med Chir* (Tokyo) 1990;30:173–177.
50. Bendszus M, Klein R, Burger R, et al: Efficacy of trisacryl gelatin microspheres versus polyvinyl alcohol particles in the preoperative embolization of meningiomas. *Am J Neuroradiol* 2000;21:255–261.
51. Guglielmi G: Use of the GDC crescent for embolization of tumors fed by cavernous and petrous branches of the internal carotid artery. Technical note. *J Neurosurg* 1998;89:857–860.
52. Wakhloo AK, Juengling FD, Van Velthoven V, et al: Extended preoperative polyvinyl alcohol microembolization of intracranial meningiomas: assessment of two embolization techniques. *Am J Neuroradiol* 1993;14:571–582.
53. Houkin K, Kamada K, Sawamura Y, et al: Proton magnetic resonance spectroscopy (1H-MRS) for the evaluation of treatment of brain tumors. *Neuroradiology* 1995;37:99–103.

126. The Neurosurgical Implications of Neurofibromatosis

Gelareh Zadeh and Abhijit Guha

Neurofibromatosis (NF) is a common germline disorder with a myriad of neural and extraneural manifestations. NF consists of at least two separate genetic diseases, termed NF1 and NF2, with loss of two separate tumor suppressor genes, although they may demonstrate some clinical overlap. Both NF1 and NF2 are considered to be part of the phakomatosis syndromes, with cutaneous and neural manifestations involving neuroectodermal derived structures. Other members of the phakomatosis family include tuberous sclerosis (Bourneville-Pringle disease), von Hippel-Lindau (retino-cerebellar angiomatosis), and neurocutaneous angiomatosis, among which is the ataxia-telangiectasia, Sturge-Weber, Rendu-Osler-Weber, and Fabry's disease. Among these syndromes, NF1 is the most prevalent and has the highest propensity to form tumors, making it the most common tumor-predisposing syndrome known in humans. The most common NF1-associated neoplasms arise from the nervous system, although there is an increased incidence of benign and malignant cancers in other organ systems. In addition to tumors, structural and developmental defects affecting the neural, skeletal, hematological, and cutaneous systems also are associated with NF1. This makes NF1 a systemic disorder requiring the attention of many medical and surgical disciplines, plus family counseling and patient advocacy groups.

Historical Background

Neurofibromatosis was long described as a single disease entity, with clinical subtypes under many different names. The first clinical reports of patients suggestive of having NF date back to as early as the sixteenth century, with some of these reports leading to erroneous diagnoses. The most famous of these is the "elephant man" popularized in a 1970s movie. In retrospect the "elephant man" did not have NF at all but rather suffered from the genetically distinct Proteus syndrome, although his vivid disfigured picture is still associated with and wrongly stereotypes NF (1). Friedrich von Recklinghausen first correctly identified the pathology of NF-associated cutaneous tumors as being composed of "skin and nerve tumors representing mingling of both neural and connective tissue" and coined the term neurofibroma (2,3). Thereby, since 1882 NF has become synonymous with "von Recklinghausen disease." Thompson described the hereditary nature and autosomal dominant mendelian transmission pattern of NF in the early 1900s (2,4).

The molecular biological explosion starting in the 1980s enabled diseases to be classified as per their genetic defects, and led to the realization that there are at least two forms of NF. Although both forms have some clinical overlap, they are two distinct diseases mapped to genetic defects on two different chromosomes (2,4). This led to subsequent refinement of the nomenclature so that today von Recklinghausen disease, peripheral neurofibromatosis, and NF1 refer to the same syndrome with its genetic defect on chromosome 17, as discussed in the following (5). In contrast, bilateral acoustic neurofibromatosis (BANF), central neurofibromatosis, or NF2 refer to a separate syndrome, which is a distinct disease with its genetic defect on chromosome 22 although sharing some clinical manifestations with NF1 (6). To distinguish these two forms of NF clinically,

the National Institute of Health (NIH) Consensus Conference on NF recommended a numerical classification of clinical criteria required to diagnose NF1 or NF2 in 1987 (Table 1) (7). These more rigid clinical criteria helped to define more homogenous patients and families with either forms of NF. Chromosomal linkage studies localized these two distinct diseases by the late 1980s to chromosome 17 and 22 for NF1 and NF2, respectively, with actual cloning of the two genes requiring further molecular analysis in the early 1990s (5,6). Current studies are focused on the function of the encoded proteins by the NF1 and NF2 genes, how they regulate cellular function normally, and how their loss leads to the clinical manifestations including tumorigenesis associated with the respective diseases.

Genetics and Molecular Biology

NF1 and NF2 are autosomal dominant transmitted disorders at a population genetic level. Half of the patients inherit the mutated gene from one of the parents, whereas the other half result from de novo mutations of the genes in the germline, especially the sperm (4,8). An incidence of approximately one in 4,000 live births being born with NF1 implies an extremely high spontaneous mutational rate of the NF1 gene (8,9). The exact reason for this is yet unresolved but may have to do with the extremely large size of the NF1 gene. Although a patient with either of the NF syndromes has a 50% chance of passing the gene to the next generation with a 100% penetrance, the clinical sequelae or expression is extremely variable, even among siblings who inherit the same mutated gene (8). The modifying factors are not known, in addition to the mutated NF1 gene that leads to this variable expression, which makes it extremely hard for genetic counseling to predict the long-term clinical course of a patient with NF1. Therefore, patients require ongoing vigilance. Variable gene expression, large NF1 gene size, lack of any mutational "hot spots," lack of a tight genotype-phenotype correlation, and ability to diagnose NF1 based on clinical manifestations very early in the majority of patients, make routine prenatal screening for NF1 mutations impractical. Specialized studies with protein truncation assays are utilized sometimes, with their sensitivity and specificity remaining uncertain. Hence, NF1 remains a clinical diagnosis as per the NIH criteria (Table 1), for which we are increasing our understanding of its molecular and genetic basis.

Both NF syndromes are caused by tumor suppressor genes at a genetic level, with mutation or loss of one allele in the germline and a somatic loss or mutation. This is based on the "two-hit" concept pioneered by Knudson in retinoblastomas (10). The NF1 gene was mapped by linkage studies to the centromeric region of the long arm of chromosome 17, with subsequent cloning of the gene revealing the protein product neurofibromin (10–12). Neurofibromin is a ubiquitously expressed large cytoplasmic protein with a molecular weight of 220 kd, that shares a domain with a family of proteins termed p21ras-guanosine triphosphatase (GTPase) activating proteins or ras-GAPs (13–16). These ras-GAPs play a pivotal role in regulation of cell proliferation and differentiation via modulation of a key intracellular signal transduction pathway mediated by activation

Table 1. Diagnostic Criteria for Neurofibromatosis (NF) 1 and 2 based on National Institute of Health Consensus Statement (1988)

Neurofibromatosis Type 1	Neurofibromatosis Type 2

Two or more of the following
  Six or more café-au-lait macules of over 5 mm in greatest diameter in prepubertal individuals and over 15 mm in postpubertal individuals
  Two or more neurofibromas of any type or one plexiform neurofibroma
  Freckling in the axillary or inguinal region
  Optic glioma
  Two or more Lisch nodules (iris hamartomas)
	Any of the following
	  Bilateral vestibular Schwannoma (VS), seen on computed tomography or magnetic resonance imaging
	  A family history of NF2 (first-degree relative) and either:
	    unilateral VS diagnosed <30 old
	    or
	    two of the following: meningioma, glioma, Schwannoma, juvenile posterior subcapsular lenticular opacities/juvenile cortical cataracts

A distinct osseous lesion such as a sphenoid dysplasia or thinning of the long bone cortex with or without pseudoarthrosis
 	
A first-degree relative (parent, sibling, or offspring) with NF1 by the preceding criteria.
	Individuals with following clinical features should be evaluated for NF2:
	  Unilateral VS <30 old plus one of: meningioma, glioma, Schwannoma, juvenile posterior subcapsular lenticular opacities/juvenile cortical cataracts
	  Multiple meningiomas plus unilateral VS diagnosed <30 old or one of meningioma, glioma, Schwannoma, juvenile posterior subcapsular lenticular opacities/juvenile cortical cataracts

of a G-protein called p21ras. The ras-GAPs serve to catalyze the inactivation of p21ras from its GTP-bound state to its inactive guanosine diphosphatase (GDP)-bound form (13,17,18). Simplistically, loss of both copies of neurofibromin causes elevated levels of activated ras-GTP, resulting in uncontrolled proliferation signals to the nucleus, facilitating tumorigenesis (13,17–19) (Fig. 1). This simple paradigm has been shown in some NF1-associated tumors such as neurofibromas by our laboratory and others (13), in NF1-associated sporadic childhood leukemias (20), and recently by us in NF1-associated astrocytomas (21). However, the role of neurofibromin as a ras-GAP does not fully explain tumorigenesis in several other NF1-associated tumors, benign NF1-associated clinical symptoms, or in certain preferentially affected tissues. The large size of neurofibromin suggests that it has other domains that function other than as a ras-GAP, whose loss also adversely alters cellular regulation.

NF2 is also a typical tumor suppressor gene that is transmitted in an autosomal dominant manner, with 50% of cases representing *de novo* mutations (22,23). Two varieties of the NF2 syndrome are recognized. The Wishart subtype is characterized by multiple central nervous system (CNS) tumors with an early and aggressive onset, whereas the Gardner subtype presents later with mainly bilateral acoustic neurofibromas (BANF). These two subtypes can be found in the same NF2 family, with additional genetic aberrations leading to other subtypes that remain unknown. The *NF-2* gene was identified on the long arm of chromosome 22 (20,24), with the gene product a 595–amino acid-encoded protein called Schwannomin or Merlin (moesin-ezrin-radixin–like protein) (24,25). Merlin derives its name from its homology with other members of the protein 4.1 family,

such as *ezrin*, *radixin*, and *moesin* (ERM), which are implicated as linkers between integral membrane glycoproteins and the cytoskeleton (26). Although Merlin is similar in function to the ERMs, it has notable differences and affects distinct critical signaling pathways. Typical of tumor suppressor genes, NF2 predisposes to a variety of other tumors in addition to the BANF, including astrocytomas, meningiomas, and ependymomas. Loss of Merlin has been demonstrated not only in these NF2-associated nervous system tumors, but also in their much more common sporadic counterparts (27). This suggests that Merlin also plays an important role in cellular regulation, perhaps through regulating the cytoskeleton, although much less is known about it compared to neurofibromin.

Clinical Presentation and Management

The management of NF requires lifelong careful follow-up because it is a germline disorder with a plethora of clinical and subclinical abnormalities affecting almost all organ systems. Judicious medical and/or surgical intervention should be used for symptomatic relief of a specific problem. With this underlying philosophy, fewer than 50% of NF1 patients require medical or surgical intervention, and the vast majority lead normal and productive lives (4). Sometimes, an NF1 patient goes undetected throughout his or her lifetime because of varying expression with few symptoms other than some cutaneous lesions. Monitoring and preservation of hearing for as long as possible is of paramount importance in the management of patients with BANF. Balance the natural progression of these bilateral benign but growing lesions against the risks of hearing loss with either microsurgical removal or focused radiotherapy. Screen for other intracranial and spinal lesions associated with NF2. Intervention depends on their clinical significance and/or radiological growth.

The team approach is important in the management of a pleiotropic genetic syndrome such as NF. NF clinics that provide education and psychological support to patients and their families as well as medical expertise are preferred. The medical team should consist of a primary physician—often a neurologist or neurogeneticist—and subspecialists, including dermatologists, ophthalmologists, orthopedic surgeons, plastic surgeons, psychiatrists, neuro-otologists, and neurosurgeons. Active participation in NF foundations is an excellent strategy for patients, family, and medical caregivers. In the following sections we discuss the main clinical issues related to NF1 and NF2 that may require neurosurgical attention and intervention.

Neurofibromatosis Type 1

CUTANEOUS LESIONS. The clinical manifestations of neurofibromatosis type 1 (NF1), especially the cutaneous ones, appear quite early. For example the characteristic café-au-lait spots (CLS) often are observed at birth, with an increase during childhood, and subsequent plateauing and sometimes a reduction in number and size in adulthood (Fig. 2A) (28). Greater than six CLS, especially those greater than 1.5 cm, are observed in more than 95% of NF1 patients, with this being the only visible manifestation in about 10% of all NF1 patients (8). The other characteristic NF1 cutaneous pigmentation is freckling (Fig. 2B), especially those in intertriginous areas such as the axilla, inguinal regions, upper eyelids, and base of neck; plus

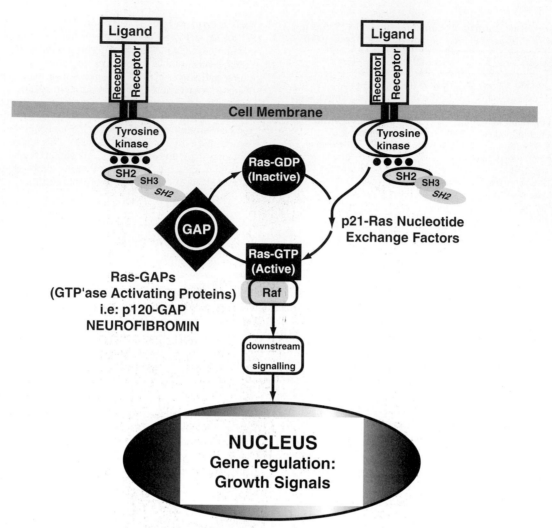

Fig. 1. Neurofibromin inactivates a key intracellular signaling protein called p21ras, which is inactive bound to guanosine diphosphatase (GDP) and active bound to guanosine triphosphatase (GTP). Inactivation of GTP to GDP bound p21ras is accelerated by p21ras-guanosine activating protein (GAP) proteins, among which neurofibromin is a major member. Therefore, loss of neurofibromin expression leads to an increase in p21ras-GAP activity and abnormal proliferative nuclear signals, as demonstrated in several NF1-associated tumors. In addition, the large neurofibromin protein also interacts with other intracellular signaling and cytoskeletal proteins, with loss of these functions probably also contributing to tumor formation.

areas of skin apposition such as submammary regions in women and skinfolds of obese people. CLS and freckling are histopathologically similar (4); both contain melanin macroglobules (giant melanosomes), which are organelles for synthesizing the skin's pigment, as described by Benedict in 1986 (29). Lisch nodules (Fig. 2C), as reported by the Austrian ophthalmologist Lisch in 1937, are melanin hamartomas of the iris that are prevalent in almost all NF1 patients by late childhood (4). Because of their prevalence, a slit-lamp examination for Lisch nodules is useful for diagnostic purposes in NF1, as they are rare in the general population and not associated with NF2 in which subcapsular cataracts are found more commonly. NF1 patients also have a significantly higher number of cutaneous angiomas termed Campbell de Morganii spots, and cutaneous xanthogranulomas (i.e., yellowish papules or nodules). In some families these may represent the salient feature of the disease, which are highly suggestive of NF1 if seen together with CLS (30). Malignant transformation of these cutaneous lesions does not occur; hence, they require no surgical intervention. Plastic and reconstructive surgery may be indicated if lesions create irritation or cosmetic defects.

PERIPHERAL NERVE LESIONS. The majority of neurofibromas and schwannomas, the two most common types of peripheral nerve sheath tumors, arise sporadically in the non-NF population with only the minority associated with NF1 or NF2 patients, respectively. Neurofibromas (Fig. 2D), the hallmark of NF1, are the most common reason for medical referral, with increasing numbers of lesions seen until middle or late adulthood (2). Histopathologically, neurofibromas demonstrate elongated, wavy, interlacing hyperchromatic cells with spindle-shaped nuclei on a disorderly mucoid background (Fig. 3A). Some tumor cells stain positive for S-100 and Leu-7 but not to the same extent found in schwannomas. Perineural cells, fibroblasts, lymphocytes, and mast cells are all present as an integral component of neurofibromas, with some debate as to the actual cell(s) of origin. The presence of axons within a neurofibroma, representing intraneural growth of the tumor, is the cardinal feature differentiating a neurofibroma from a schwannoma. As a general rule, NF1 patients with peripheral nerve tumors harbor neurofibromas and not schwannomas, whereas schwannomas are more prevalent in NF2 patients.

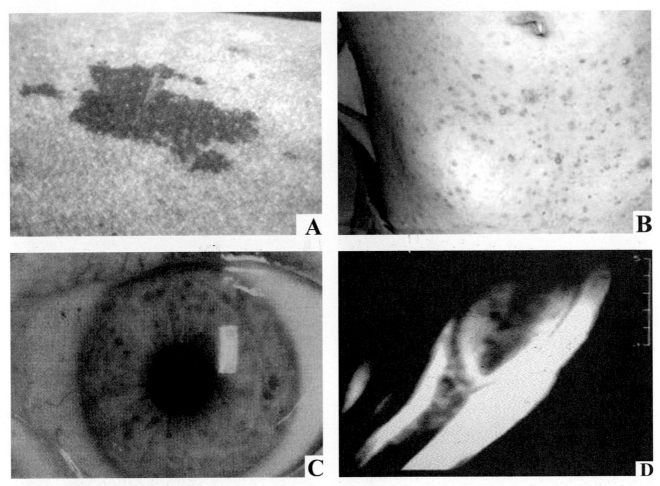

Fig. 2. NF1 remains a clinical diagnosis as per the National Institute of Health criteria (see Table 1). Clinical signs associated with NF1 include café-au-lait spots **(A)**, freckling in covered regions **(B)**, Lisch nodules **(C)**, and plexiform neurofibromas **(D)**.

However, some of the NF2-associated schwannomas may have more of an intraneural growth pattern, although the cells are S-100 positive Schwann cells, compared to the pure extraneural growth of sporadic schwannomas in the general population. Neurofibromas in the sporadic and NF1 population can be broadly classified into dermal and plexiform varieties, with the latter being closely associated with NF1 (28). Dermal neurofibromas are discrete, soft, and mobile, and may grow to become pedunculated. These lesions are readily palpable or visible with a purplish hue, often involving the trunk with relative sparing of the extremities. They can vary from a few to hundreds in number, and can occur anywhere from the dorsal spinal root to the spinal ganglia, including the cranial nerves. Dermal neurofibromas do not become malignant, although they can be cosmetically and psychologically disabling. Indications for removal by a plastic surgeon or neurosurgeon are rare, and should only be reserved for those lesions causing major cosmetic deformity or those that are subjected to repeated macerations from clothing.

Plexiform neurofibromas (Fig. 2D) are diffuse growths along more proximal nerves and spanning multiple branches. They have a predominant intrafascicular growth with convoluted mass formation referred to as "string of onions." They are characterized by redundant loops of nerve fascicles in random orientation with characteristic intervening spindle cells, collagen bundles, and mucinous substance. Solitary plexiform neurofibromas do occur in sporadic patients, but when multiple they

are highly suggestive of underlying NF1. Plexiform neurofibromas also can present as large subcutaneous swelling with the overlying skin being abnormal either because of hypertrophy, hyperpigmentation, or hypertrichosis. Most frequently these occur on the trunk, limbs, head, and neck. "Elephantitis" is a term often used to describe these very large plexiform neurofibromatosis. Most plexiform neurofibromas are asymptomatic and only require clinical or radiological follow-up, with the MRI being the modality of choice. Extent of tumor growth and invasion should be assessed, because they tend to grow further internally and erode through structures of the retroperitoneum, mediastinum, skull, and gastrointestinal and paraspinal regions (Fig. 3B). When symptomatic, neurological symptoms may include local and radiating pain, progressive weakness, and paralysis caused by invasion of the spinal canal, plus paresthesia/hypesthesia/anesthesia and autonomic dysfunction. In addition, their growth may impede the function of normal adjacent structures to cause secondary skeletal abnormalities, scoliosis, vascular occlusion, and airway and digestive system obstruction. Unfortunately, this unpredictable and relentless growth of a benign tumor can have grave consequences, creating significant morbidity and sometimes leading to death.

The indications and goals of surgical intervention for plexiform neurofibromas must be clearly defined and the risks discussed with the patient preoperatively. Total removal is rarely attempted if the origin is from a nerve of clinical significance, because it usually leads to significant deficits caused by the

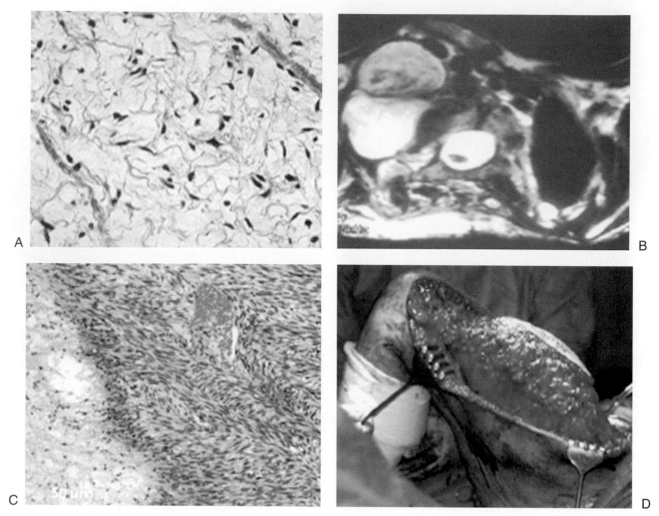

Fig. 3. The most common NF1-associated tumors are in the peripheral nervous system. **A:** Hematoxylin and eosin: Plexiform neurofibroma with intraneural growth arising from the sympathetic chain, with entrapped ganglion cells. **B:** MRI of a large intrathoracic plexiform neurofibroma arising from the sympathetic chain that was excised to improve pulmonary function, highlighting the need to carefully define the preoperative goals in managing these systemic tumors. **C:** Malignant peripheral nerve sheath tumor (MPNST) *(right)* arising from a previous plexiform neurofibroma *(left).* **D:** Compartmental resection of MPNST, supplemented by pathological examination for tumor-free margins, is as effective as full limb amputation for local control of these highly malignant tumors.

intraneural growth of neurofibromas, in contrast to schwannomas. Indications for surgical intervention comprising biopsy and/or debulking may include: (a) A new recognized lesion or progression of neurological symptoms in a prior tumor. Neuropathic pain often can be the most debilitating symptom from a plexiform neurofibroma, although surgical intervention is rarely efficacious for long term relief; (b) compression of adjacent vital neural and nonneural structures; and (c) rapid radiological growth. The usual main goals of surgery are amelioration of symptoms caused by compression of adjacent structures and assessment of potential malignant transformation resulting in new neurological symptoms or radiological growth. Microsurgical techniques with the use of intraoperative electrophysiological monitoring may allow removal of the bulk of the tumor while preserving function. If functional fascicles cannot be preserved, be conservative in resection and undertake just what is required to achieve the discussed preoperative goals. Nerve grafting usually is neither indicated nor practical because of the longitudinal and extensive involvement of neurofibromas in NF1 patients.

The risk of malignant transformation must be considered in a clinically symptomatic or radiologically growing plexiform neurofibroma in an NF1 patient. This risk, once thought to be much higher, is actually only 3% to 5% (31,32); nevertheless, it remains a source of major concern to the patient and physician. The malignant peripheral nerve sheath tumor (MPNST), also termed neurogenic sarcoma or neurofibrosarcoma, is lethal; 50% of these rare tumors occur in NF1 patients (33). Increasing pain, growth of a previously indolent tumor, and progressive focal deficits are warning signs of malignant transformation within a plexiform neurofibroma. The management of MPNST, as guided by our experience at the University of Toronto, has been published and involves a multidisciplinary approach (34). In brief we recommend that the initial surgery should comprise of open multiple quadrant biopsies if a MPNST is suspected, based on aggressive clinical and/or radiological growth. It is vital that evaluation of the neurofibroma be performed by an experienced neuropathologist, using both light and electron microscopy to assess degree of cellular pleomorphism, nuclear atypia, and mitotic figures, in order to exclude the small chance of malignant transformation to MPNST (Fig. 3C). After pathological confirmation of an MPNST, a metastatic screen comprising chest x-ray and CT scan of the chest and abdomen is undertaken to determine gross extent of the disease. For localized disease, after consultation with the patient and full knowledge of expected morbidity and disfigurement, a second compartmental resection comprised of the MPNST, adjacent fascia, and muscles should be undertaken with intraoperative pathological sampling to ensure negative tumor margins (Fig. 3D). This second oncological surgery is followed with external beam radiotherapy to the tumor bed site with adequate margins, and subsequent rehabilitation. Careful follow-up for both regional and distant pulmonary recurrence is undertaken, and any recurrence is managed by systemic chemotherapy protocols utilized for other soft-tissue sarcomas. The 5-year prognosis remains less than 50% for these generally young patients. The strongest prognosticators are localized or systemic disease at presentation, grade of the MPNST (grading schemes for the much more common soft-tissue sarcomas generally are used), and ability to obtain tumor-free margins at the primary site. Whether the

grade 505 of MPNST arising in NF1 patients have a different prognosis than those in the sporadic population is not clearly known, because of the small incidence of these tumors. There are anecdotal cases; a small series of patients suggests the NF1 population with MPNST do worse.

CENTRAL NERVOUS SYSTEM LESIONS: INTRACRANIAL

Gliomas. MRI brain imaging of NF1 patients often shows multiple abnormalities, although the significance of these unidentified bright objects (UBOs) remains unclear, because they also may represent hamartomas and/or developmental abnormalities (Fig. 4A). The number and types of CNS neoplasms in NF1 patients are much more limited compared to NF2. The most common are gliomas that involve the optic pathway, brainstem, and cerebellum. Optic gliomas (Fig. 4B), which account for 2% to 5% of all pediatric brain tumors, are indolent pilocytic

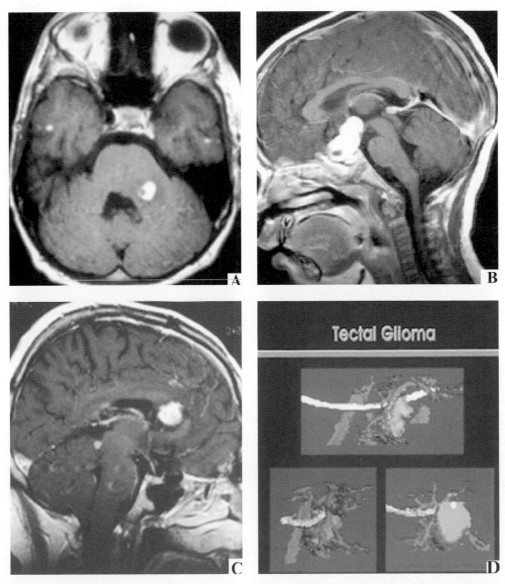

Fig. 4. Central nervous system lesions associated with neurofibromatosis type 1 include the following. **A:** Unidentified bright objects. **B:** Optic nerve glioma: whole mount hematoxylin and eosin cross section. **C:** Periventricular enhancing low-grade astrocytoma. **D:** Low-grade tectal glioma causing aqueductal stenosis treated with MRI–guided biopsy, shunt placement, and external beam radiation.

astrocytomas within the optic pathway that have little propensity for malignant transformation. They diffusely infiltrate and expand the optic nerve and often follow the nerve fibers of the optic radiation. At times they involve the hypothalamus, cause obstructive hydrocephalus, and occasionally infiltrate into the subarachnoid space (35). Depending on the method of radiological examination used, between 1.5% and 15% of patients with NF1 harbor optic gliomas, with 15% to 52% of these patients reported as ultimately becoming symptomatic (35–37). The majority of symptomatic NF1 patients with optic nerve gliomas present before 5 years of age and clinical consequences are rare if radiological diagnosis of tumor is made after 10 years of age (35). Signs and symptoms of optic nerve gliomas vary. In children, complaints of visual deterioration often are supported by decreased color vision, optic atrophy, strabismus, and pupillary abnormalities on neuro-ophthalmological examination. Other signs and symptoms may include precocious puberty, which is suggestive of hypothalamic involvement.

The natural history and optimal management of optic nerve gliomas remain controversial because of their relative nonresectability and indolent growth. A 1995 task force provided guidelines and recommendations for screening, follow-up, and treatment of these tumors (37). The recommended guidelines for screening of optic nerve gliomas include the following:

1. Screening of all NF1 children under 6 years of age without a known optic glioma with a yearly full neuro-ophthalmological examination. This includes visual acuity, color vision, visual fields, funduscopy, and slit-lamp examination. Visual evoked potentials (VEPs) have been advocated as a useful screening method, with one study citing a 100% sensitivity and 60% specificity for detection of optic nerve gliomas (37); however, the task force failed to demonstrate that VEPs, as a screening tool, add value to a thorough neuro-ophthalmological examination (37).
2. NF1 children older than 6 years of age are advised to undergo a full neuro-ophthalmological examination every 4 years.
3. Annual neuro-ophthalmological examination of NF1 patients with a known but asymptomatic optic nerve glioma is not required, as it has not been shown to improve the clinical outcome.
4. An NF1 child without a known optic nerve glioma who has an abnormal neuro-ophthalmological examination should be followed up with a gadolinium enhanced MRI. Whether T2-weighted MRI signal changes of the optic nerve pathway give a true indication of tumor involvement remains unclear, although gadolinium enhancement is confirmatory.

Surgical intervention for optic nerve gliomas is rarely needed and depends on the location of the tumor. In chiasmatic gliomas, surgery has a very limited role, because the tumor also may involve posterior visual pathways and the optic nerve itself. Lesions with mass effect or cystic components can be debulked, but the risk of increased visual and neurological morbidity is high. For optic nerve gliomas that are radiologically growing and clinically symptomatic, external beam radiotherapy with 150 to 180 cGy daily for a total of 4,500 to 5,500 cGy is a valid option. There is a small risk of radiation-induced visual deterioration; however, 80% stabilize or decrease in tumor size. The long-term efficacy of radiation therapy in controlling disease progression is questionable, however, with a small risk of inducing more aggressive malignant behavior (36). Chemotherapy also can be used for growing tumors, although its effectiveness is questionable, as is true for other astrocytomas.

NF1-associated gliomas also have an indolent course, with the majority being pilocytic astrocytomas requiring minimal intervention (38). They exhibit radiological growth rarely (Fig.

4C), with associated increased focal neurological deficits, obstruction of the CSF pathways, or an increase in seizure frequency, and require surgical removal. Brainstem gliomas also are relatively common, with the majority only managed by serial imaging and clinical follow-up. Better prognosis is observed in those brainstem gliomas that do not enhance after contrast, and in those that are dorsally exophytic into the fourth ventricle or localized to the cervicomedullary junction. Poor prognosis is seen with hypodense lesions with large areas of brainstem involvement and early signs and symptoms of cranial nerve dysfunction (37). Tumors around the periaqueductal region may cause CSF outflow obstruction secondary to aqueductal stenosis. Such patients are usually managed by biopsy combined with a CSF diversion procedure, and primary debulking is rarely indicated because of the associated morbidity (Fig. 4D). Meningiomas, medulloblastomas, ependymomas, and subependymal nodules or subependymomas occur with slightly higher frequency in NF1 patients, but the actual incidence is not known.

Hydrocephalus. Obstructive hydrocephalus, resulting from aqueductal stenosis caused by a space-occupying lesion of the tectum, may require CSF diversion sometimes combined with image-guided assisted biopsy of the causative lesion, as described in the preceding (Fig. 4D). Endoscopy with third ventriculostomy and biopsy may be an excellent approach in certain situations. Communicating hydrocephalus with generalized ventriculomegaly, which for the most part is asymptomatic, is also seen with higher frequency in NF1 patients. It should be noted that macrocephaly is slightly more prevalent in NF1 patients, with the head circumference being above the 95th percentile (2).

Epilepsy. Generalized epilepsy is seen with increased frequency in 5% of the NF1 population (4,38). No recognized pathology causing the seizure focus can be identified on radiological examination in the majority of cases (38). However, microscopic abnormalities of the cerebral cortex owing to developmental abnormalities have been hypothesized to be the underlying pathogenesis for seizure activity in NF1 patients (38). In general, neurosurgical management of NF1 patients suffering from intractable seizures without a structural identifiable abnormality is similar to that of the general public.

Cerebrovascular Pathology. The most common cerebrovascular pathology seen in NF1 is stenosis or occlusion of cerebral arteries. As a result, moyamoya disease is slightly more prevalent in NF1 patients, especially in those who have received cranial radiation for neoplasms. Intracranial aneurysms are rare, and mainly occur on the internal carotid artery circulation (39). Patients become symptomatic mainly because of ischemia or hemorrhage, and occasionally are identified incidentally.

SPINAL LESIONS

Tumors. Numerous spinal abnormalities are present in NF1 patients, although the vast majority are not of clinical significance, such as dural ectasia and T2 intramedullary MRI abnormalities. Compression of the spinal cord can occur anywhere along its course, from C1 to the conus, because of the growth of a neurofibroma arising from exiting spinal nerve root(s). These lesions can be dumbbell-shaped tumors with significant extradural extension into the thoracic or retroperitoneal cavity, combined with intradural extramedullary compression of the spinal cord, and sometimes intramedullary invasion (Fig. 5). Intramedullary extension may represent invasion of actual tumor cells or proliferation of benign Schwann's cells in the CNS, a process termed schwannosis. Like other paraspinal lesions, neuro-

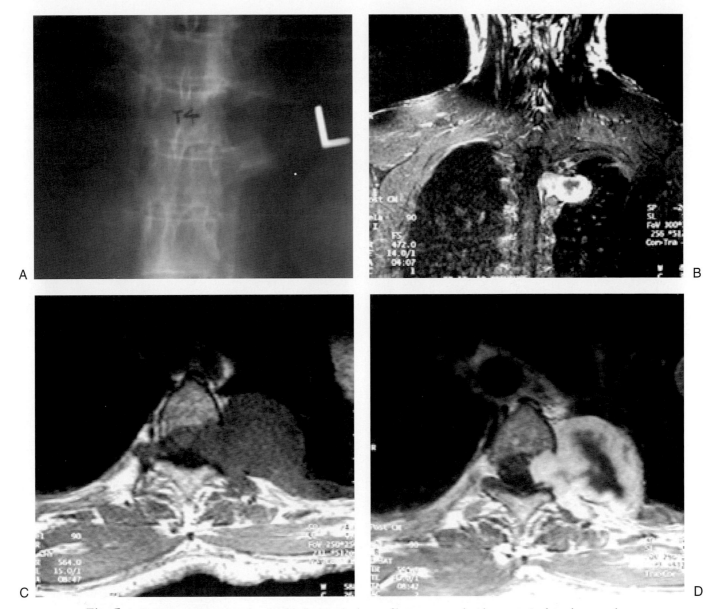

Fig. 5. **A–D:** MRI contrast enhancing dumbbell paraspinal neurofibroma resected with a posterior-lateral approach.

surgical intervention with the primary goals of spinal cord decompression, spinal column stabilization, and decompression of the extradural compressed visceral structures should be planned in that order. Often, all these objectives can be undertaken with a single posterior, posterolateral, or anterior approach in conjunction with stabilization. However, a staged approach can be the best choice if there is a large and clinically significant extradural component. Preoperative planning for spinal stabilization and use of MRI compatible hardware intraoperatively to allow subsequent follow-up imaging, needs to be emphasized. Bony and ligamentous instability may arise because of destruction from the primary tumor, or as a result of surgical manipulations, often requiring spinal stabilization because these patients are relatively young and have many years of active future life.

Intramedullary abnormalities, as visualized on T2-weighted MRI, are quite common in NF1 patients. The vast majority are

nonenhancing UBOs, probably representing hamartomas or other developmental abnormalities such as schwannosis. These are not clinically significant and do not require any active management other than follow-up imaging to document their benign nature. Spinal cord astrocytomas, which may involve large segments of the spinal cord, are more common in NF1 patients compared to the general population, although the prevalence of intramedullary spinal cord tumors is much lower than in NF2 patients. In addition, the vast majority of intramedullary spinal cord lesions in NF2 patients are surgically resectable ependymomas (Fig. 6A), compared to the infiltrative and surgically nonresectable astrocytomas that are more common in NF1 patients. The majority of the spinal astrocytomas in NF1 are pilocytic indolent tumors, requiring no intervention. Malignant transformation to spinal glioblastomas does occur, manifested by clinical and/or radiological progression, requiring surgery for diagnosis and sometimes debulking (40). In these cases, a

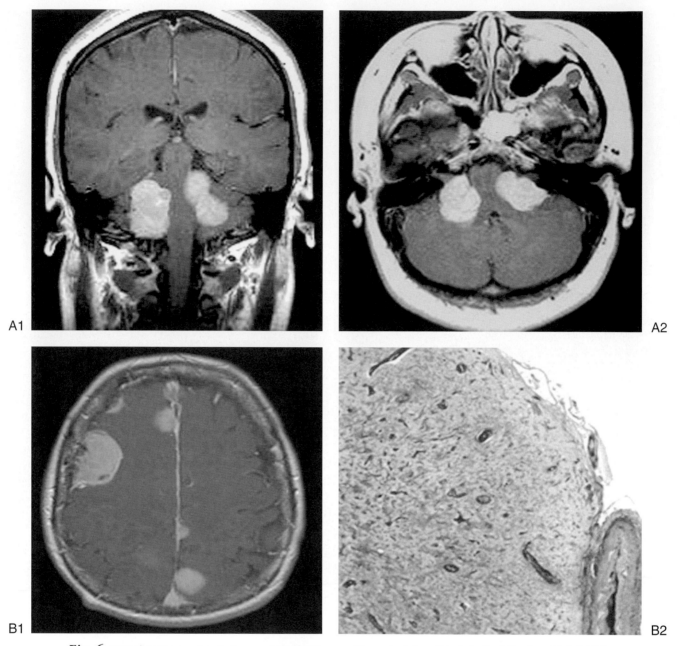

Fig. 6. Central nervous system lesions associated with neurofibromatosis type 2 include the following. **A1,2:** BANF, bilateral acoustic neurofibromas. Multiple meningiomas **(B1)** and meningiomatosis **(B2)**. *Figure continues.*

conservative resection or biopsy followed by external beam radiation therapy is the therapy of choice, although prognosis is extremely poor.

Scoliosis. The incidence of scoliosis in the NF1 population is high; it is estimated to be 10% to 20% (2,41). The vast majority of NF1-related scoliosis is idiopathic and asymptomatic, similar to the general population. The second most common group are the dystrophic scolioses, which are caused by vertebral dysplasia resulting from an underlying neurofibroma (28). They typically involve six to eight segments and cause distortion of vertebral bodies and ribs. They have a rapidly progressive course, requiring surgical intervention and early instrumentation. Additionally, scoliosis can be a consequence of unequal leg length caused by extremity hypertrophy in

cases of patients with segmental NF1. Further detailed discussion of the management of these axial and nonaxial skeletal abnormalities in NF1 patients is beyond the scope of this chapter and can be obtained in the orthopedic or spinal literature.

OTHER NEUROLOGICAL AND MEDICAL ISSUES OF NEUROFIBROMATOSIS TYPE 1. Contrary to the general perception, the average intelligence of NF1 patients is not vastly different from the general population, with NF1 patients undertaking the same types of occupations as those not afflicted by the disease. Although the majority of NF1 patients fall within the range of global intelligence quotients of the general population, some specific learning difficulties are more common with NF1.

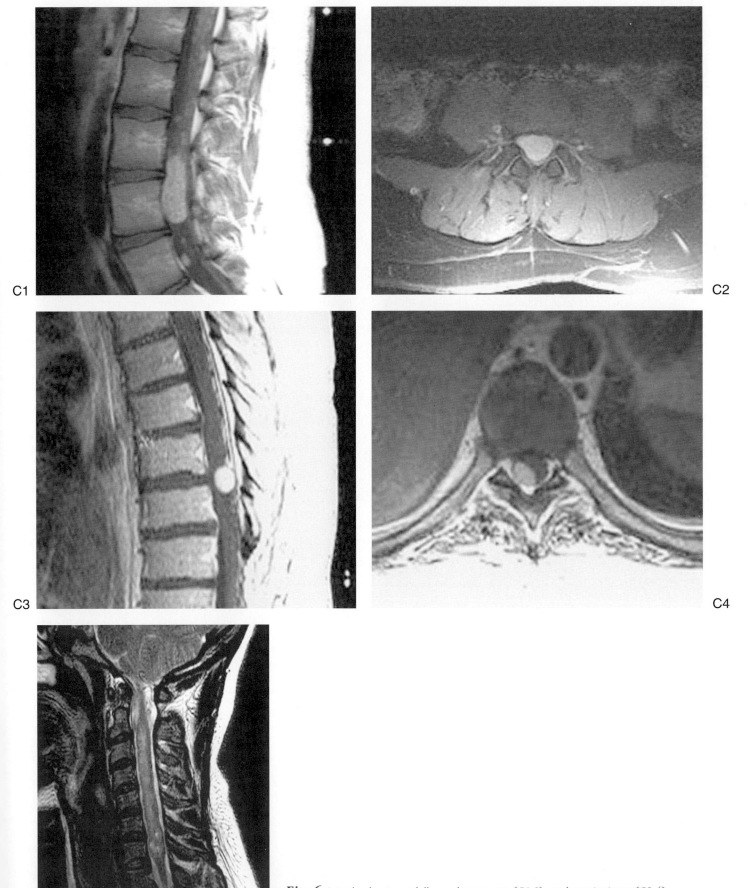

Fig. 6. Intradural extramedullary schwannoma **(C1,2)** and meningioma **(C3,4)**.
D: Intramedullary gliomas, which are mainly ependymomas.

Associations of learning deficits with intracranial pathologies, including the number of UBOs on MRI, have been postulated, but the data remain unclear. Unjustified stereotyping of lower intelligence in the NF1 population is undoubtedly caused to some degree by the systemic manifestations, such as the higher proportion of NF1 patients who harbor visible skeletal abnormalities such as short stature and macrocephaly. Forty-five percent of NF1 children have a head circumference greater than the 95th percentile, but this is not usually related to hydrocephalus or other intracranial pathology. The short stature involves the axial skeleton, with abnormalities in the vertebral bodies with scoliosis, but also affects limb development, with 30% of patients falling below the third percentile (2,4,38).

NF1 is the most common cancer predisposing syndrome in humans, with a 10^3 to 10^5 times higher risk of developing a tumor compared to the general population (4). Understandably, for most NF1 patients, this increased risk affects their ability to deal psychologically with their systemic cancer predisposition. A large proportion of NF1-associated tumors have neurological manifestations, as discussed, whereas several nonneural NF1-related cancers do have significant implications. For example, NF1 children may develop juvenile cell myelogenous leukemia (JCML). Overactivity of the p21ras-mediated signaling pathway has been implicated in both NF1 and sporadic JCML (20). In NF1-related JCML, the increased p21ras activity is owing to loss of neurofibromin, a major inactivator of p21ras or p21ras-GAP, as discussed. In contrast, oncogenic p21ras mutations, where p21ras is locked in its activated GTP bound state, are the etiology in sporadic JCML patients. Such laboratory findings have led to clinical trials with inhibitors of this key signaling pathway mediated by p21ras in both sporadic and NF1 JCML patients. Carcinoid tumors arising from enterochromaffin cells of the small intestine, thyroid, stomach, and pancreas are noted in 2% of patients with NF1 (8,9). Patients present with general symptoms of gastrointestinal distress, such as abdominal pain, dyspepsia, hematemesis, melena, and bowel obstruction. Multiple endocrine neoplasias (MEN) are three distinct autosomal dominant conditions that have similar features to NF1, specifically with respect to pheochromocytoma. These tumors are of neural crest origin; however, a genetic link between NF1 and MEN has not been identified (38).

Hypertension is another nonneural but significant medical issue with surgical implications; it is prevalent in about 6% of NF1 patients (32). NF1 patients presenting with hypertension should have a thorough biochemical and radiological investigation to exclude causes of secondary hypertension, of which renal artery stenosis and pheochromocytomas are the most common (32). Renal function should be studied (including renal angiogram) and biochemical investigations for pheochromocytoma performed in such patients; these should include measurement of 24-hour urinary catecholamines, vanillylmandelic acid, and other metabolites. Pheochromocytoma can present with unexpected paroxysmal hypertension during anesthesia; but with prior knowledge allowing prophylactic coverage with β- and α-adrenergic blockers.

Neurofibromatosis Type 2

With an incidence of one per 40,000 live births, neurofibromatosis type 2 (NF2) is less than one-tenth as frequent as NF1, but has a higher associated morbidity and mortality rate owing to the increased prevalence of CNS neoplasms, the most characteristic of which are the bilateral acoustic neuromas (BANF) (Fig. 6A). NF2 patients have multiple other CNS tumors in addition to schwannomas of multiple cranial and peripheral nerves.

These include multiple meningiomas or meningiomatosis of the entire dura (60%) (Fig. 6B), spinal schwannomas, gliomas, and ependymomas (90%) (Fig. 6C,D). Although there can be clinical similarities between NF1 and NF2, especially in the cutaneous lesions such as café-au-lait spots and peripheral nerve tumors found in both syndromes, these are two distinct diseases caused by loss of tumor suppressor genes on two different chromosomes, as discussed in the preceding. Perhaps the overlap reflects modifying genes that are altered in addition to the main NF mutation or undiscovered distinct genetic syndromes in the NF family. In addition to the prevalence of CNS tumors and BANF in NF2 patients, additional clinical–pathological differences help distinguish these two syndromes. For example, in NF2 patients the peripheral nerve tumors usually are schwannomas with extraneural growth allowing resection and preservation of passerby fascicles versus neurofibromas in NF1 patients with intraneural growth and associated surgical risks, as discussed. Some degree of overlap also is present, as exemplified by the entity of plexiform schwannoma seen more commonly in NF2 patients. The Schwann's cells grow more in an intraneural pattern, which is similar to plexiform neurofibromas in NF1. Another distinct clinical characteristic of NF2 patients is the ophthalmological examination, where a high proportion of NF2 patients develop subcapsular cataracts, which are usually asymptomatic, in contrast to NF1 patients with Lisch nodules.

BILATERAL ACOUSTIC NEUROMAS OR VESTIBULAR SCHWANNOMAS. The pathognomonic features of NF2, as described by the NIH classification (Table 1), are bilateral vestibular schwannomas, which are historically referred to as bilateral acoustic neuromas (BANF) (Fig. 6A). They are present in 95% of NF2 patients and account for 5% of total number of vestibular schwannomas (42,43). Differences and similarities exist between NF2 and sporadic patients with vestibular schwannomas, aside from the bilaterality and presence of other CNS neoplasms. Similarities include their clinical presentation, with early signs being gradual sensorineural hearing loss, high-pitched tinnitus, and vertigo. Seventh cranial nerve symptoms are usually a rare, late manifestation of large tumors in both NF2 and sporadic cases. Additional similarities are at the microscopic and molecular level, with loss of the NF2 gene product (Schwannomin or Merlin) also found in a large number of sporadic vestibular schwannomas (27,42). Differences between the two groups include age of presentation: 50% of NF2 patients become symptomatic by age 30, which is one to two decades earlier than the age of onset in the sporadic population (43). The prevalence among males and females is equal in NF2 patients, in keeping with its autosomal dominant pattern of familial transmission or germline *de novo* occurrence, whereas there is a slight female predilection for vestibular schwannomas in the general population. Additionally, unlike the unilateral sporadic vestibular schwannomas that tend to displace the auditory portion of the eighth cranial nerve, tumors associated with NF2 originate from the superior vestibular division of the eighth cranial nerve at the porus acusticus, and often infiltrate and engulf the cochlear and facial nerve (44). This has relevance to the ability of the surgeon to preserve hearing and facial nerve function, which is often harder to accomplish in NF2 vestibular schwannomas, if microsurgical removal is indicated. Presence of schwannomas in other cranial nerves in combination with unilateral vestibular schwannomas should raise the possibility of NF2, even though they do not have BANF. Multiple schwannomas in NF2 patients can occur on all cranial nerves other than the olfactory nerve, with the trigeminal nerve being the second most common site in both NF2 and sporadic populations (43–45).

Vestibular schwannomas in sporadic and NF2 patients grow through four stages (46).

1. Intracanalicular lesions where the tumor is present only within the internal auditory meatus 2. Cisternal or cerebellopontine angle (CPA) tumors, with continued progression of sensorineural hearing loss
3. Brainstem compression and associated cranial nerve palsies such a facial numbness, facial and lower cranial nerve weakness, in addition to progressive spasticity and unsteadiness of gait
4. Hydrocephalus, with headaches and change in level of consciousness and ultimately death.

Currently there are three management options for both sporadic and NF2 vestibular schwannomas:

1. Conservative management with close follow-up and serial imaging
2. Microsurgical resection of the tumor
3. Radiosurgery

In cases of brainstem compression and hydrocephalus the treatment of choice is relatively straightforward involving microsurgical decompression and relieving CSF outflow obstruction.

The management options need to be individualized to each patient and tumor in BANF, with high priority given to hearing preservation for as long as possible. The main factors determining whether to actively intervene in BANF or to watch include: (a) age, coexisting medical conditions, and hence life expectancy; (b) knowledge-based decision of the patient; (c) presence or absence of clinical brainstem compression; (d) functional and audiometric evaluation and follow-up of hearing status; (e) tumor size and either documented or expected growth rate; and (f) acute and long-term risks of any intervention, with an emphasis on hearing preservation. The definitive answers to many of the preceding factors, on which we might base our management recommendations, is not available because of the rarity of the condition and absence of any large experience from a single institution. Therefore, the management of BANF is guided largely by the neurosurgeon's experience and patient preference. It is highly recommended that these patients be managed by an NF clinic or experienced neurosurgeons and other caregivers, to whom all potential modalities of therapy are available for this complex clinical problem.

Early detection of BANF in NF2 patients is important for determining the frequency and mode of follow-up plus management options. A patient with a positive family history of NF2 can be screened genetically to determine whether he or she carries the mutated NF2 gene, a somewhat easier task than for *NF1* because of the smaller size of the *NF2* gene. If this test is not available, then yearly audiometric screening and a baseline MRI should be undertaken, with frequency of follow-ups individualized as per the clinical and radiological progression. Such screening tests usually detect the BANF in NF2 patients when the tumor is relatively small, and hearing is still functional, although compromised. Audiometric and MRI follow-up is recommended for these smaller tumors in patients with functional hearing, because hearing preservation with microsurgical tumor removal is not optimal. The suboccipital or middle fossa route allows for hearing preservation theoretically, with rates reported from 13% to 82%, depending on tumor size (45,47–49). The validity of these rates is subject to debate because of the ambiguity in definition of functional hearing preservation and variability between centers. In addition, the application of these preservation rates to BANF is suspect because the pattern of growth and involvement of the cochlear fibers by these tumors is different

from the pattern in sporadic vestibular schwannomas. Radiosurgery, although not posing an acute risk to hearing, does have a long-term risk owing to radiation induced neuritis of the cochlear and facial nerve complex, along with other issues, as discussed in the following. Another reason not to intervene in these small tumors is that most vestibular schwannomas grow extremely slowly, in the range of 0 to 3.7 mm per year (50,51), although erratic growth over time has been noted. Long-term follow-up has suggested that 38% of all vestibular schwannomas increase in size, 59% remain dormant and 5% actually decrease (51). Whether these statistics are also applicable to NF2-associated BANF is not known. This conservative approach requires lifelong follow-up and serial imaging because tumors have been documented to grow after many years of indolent behavior (50,52). Although the decline in hearing is slow and progressive mirroring the indolent growth, it may also occur in a fluctuating manner in the absence of any radiological growth, perhaps owing to vascular insufficiency in the vulnerable cochlear nerve from the compressive effects of the tumor. These fluctuating events require close follow-up by a team comprising both neuro-otologists and neurosurgeons, with occasional reevaluation of the management options with the patient and often courses of short-term steroids in an attempt to stabilize hearing.

Intervention with either microsurgery or radiosurgery may be used for those BANF tumors in which hearing preservation is not an issue, especially in moderate or enlarging lesions. The microsurgical approach of choice depends on tumor size and the preference of the surgical team, but the overall mortality rate is less than 1% (45). The middle fossa approach is restricted to extremely small tumors with less than 0.5 to 1 cm extension into the CPA; hence, it is usually not used in BANF, where tumors of this size are usually watched. The two main routes used in both sporadic and BANF tumors are the suboccipital and translabyrinthine approaches. The translabyrinthine route gives a more anterior-lateral view of the tumor, and may be combined with a transcochlear approach to widen the exposure for more medially and anteriorly extending lesions. The main advantage of the translabyrinthine approach is the ability to identify the normal facial nerve early in the temporal bone, leading to what we believe is a better facial nerve preservation rate. In addition, we believe that postoperative recovery is smoother because little to no cerebellar retraction is involved. Although a high jugular bulb and an extremely shallow posterior fossa are relative contraindications, these obstacles often can be managed and large tumors removed with experience. Lack of familiarity by neurosurgeons working without a neuro-otologist is probably the main reason this approach is less commonly used than the suboccipital route.

Facial nerve preservation and tumor debulking are the two main goals of microsurgery. The two main determinants of facial nerve preservation are the size of the tumor and the surgeon's experience. In specialized centers normal or near normal (Grade 1 or 2) postoperative facial nerve function in sporadic vestibular schwannomas is reported to be 90% in tumors less than 2 cm, and 67% in tumors 2 to 4 cm in diameter (53). A more representative rate of 44% for facial nerve palsy is reported on average (54). Whether these rates are similar for BANF is not known, but in our experience the success rate is lower because the more engulfing and sometimes infiltrating growth of the tumor in relation to the adjacent cranial nerves. Subtotal resection in cases where facial nerve integrity is in jeopardy is a viable option and radiographically significant tumor recurrence in these cases is reported at a rate of approximately 17% to 31% (55).

Focused radiosurgery, whereby smaller doses of radiation are delivered in a convergent fashion to achieve exposure of a tumor to extremely high radiation was pioneered by Lars Leksell, who coined the term "stereotactic radiosurgery" (SR). Vestibular schwannomas are good candidates for SR because they are usually spherical, well circumscribed, have essentially pathognomonic imaging characteristics, and occur in an area that carries significant potential risks of surgery. SR can be fractionated or delivered in one session (gamma knife), with high-resolution CT or MRI studies used to obtain appropriate isodose configuration and computer assisted radiation planning. The advantages and disadvantages of the various modalities and technical aspects to deliver stereotactic radiosurgery is an ongoing debate. The goal of SR is not tumor eradication, but rather prevention of tumor growth. In general, SR is usually restricted to vestibular schwannomas less than 3 cm in their largest diameter, which have no significant mass effect on the brainstem. In Pittsburgh, only 2% of patients required surgery 5 to 10 years after gamma knife treatment (56), whereas the Swedish group reported that 5% showed tumor progression (57). These results are with 18 to 20 Gy of radiation, rather than the more recently advocated 14 to 16 Gy (50% isodose) margins for which tumor control rates are yet to be determined (56).

The side effects of radiosurgery have decreased since its inception in 1969 with refinements in planning, delivery, and dosing. Facial and trigeminal numbness occurs in less than 10% (56,57). Hearing preservation is approximately achieved in 50% to 70% (56,57), which is superior to the surgical results, although there is a progressive decline with time attributed mainly to radiation injury to the blood supply of the cochlear nerve (51). Complications that are higher with radiosurgery than microsurgery include hydrocephalus because of acute radiation-induced intratumoral and peritumoral edema (seen in 1% to 4%) and trigeminal neuralgia (51,57). Specific experience with the gamma knife in NF2 patients is limited, with a recent series of 40 patients with 45 vestibular schwannomas reported from Pittsburgh, of which 29% had undergone prior microsurgical attempts (58). Over a median follow-up of 36 months, 36% of the tumors regressed, 62% were unchanged, and 2% showed progression (58). Although the minimal acute risk to the cochlear and facial nerve, and the documented ability of SR to effectively stagnate tumor growth, makes it appealing for the treatment of BANF, the long-term risks of radiation must be acknowledged, including radiation-induced neuritis and malignancy. The latter includes conversion of a benign tumor to a malignant one, or induction of a *de novo* primary within the radiation field, as recently reported from our group (59). These radiation-related complications in the setting of a germline cancer predisposition syndrome such as NF2 are not well understood. In our opinion the multidisciplinary team approach to BANF should allow use of all available modalities, including microsurgery and SR when required, individualized to the patient and his or her tumors.

MULTIPLE MENINGIOMAS. Meningiomas are the second most common neoplasms in NF2 patients, with most being multiple (Fig. 6B). They may be intracranial or intraspinal, and show a younger age at presentation and equal sex distribution, compared to the middle or older age group and female preponderance in the general population of sporadic meningiomas. Most NF2-associated meningiomas are benign, perhaps with an over-representation of the fibroblastic subtype. Meningiomatosis, whereby meningothelial cells surround vessels in multiple regions of the brain and spinal cord, is also found in NF2 patients, although this is usually asymptomatic and found incidentally on autopsy. A small number of patients have only multiple meningiomas, without any vestibular schwannomas or other NF2-associated lesions. Analysis of the *NF2* gene does not reveal any mutations and suggests that these small cohorts of patients represent a distinct population with a multiple meningi-

oma predisposition syndrome. The responsible gene is thought to be on the long arm of chromosome 22 near the *NF2* gene, though its exact location and identity remains unknown. It should be noted that loss of the NF2 protein, Schwannomin or Merlin is found in a large proportion of sporadic meningiomas than is true for those associated with NF2 (27).

The management of NF2-associated meningiomas is for the most part similar for those in the general population, with the location being the major determinant of the approach and the attendant morbidity. The main clinical difference in the management of NF2-associated meningiomas is their multiplicity and younger age of presentation. Thus, they require careful judgment and consultation with the patient similar to the management of BANF, as discussed in the preceding. Careful clinical and radiological follow-up is the main management modality for the multiple meningiomas in NF2, with active intervention indicated for those with significant clinical or radiological progression. The team approach is equally applicable in these tumors as in BANF, with judicious use of microsurgery and radiation when indicated. Occasionally there is accelerated growth in one or several of the meningiomas after a long period of dormancy that emphasizes the need for long-term follow-up.

SPINAL TUMORS. Spinal lesions are found in over 90% of NF2 patients, although most are intradural-extramedullary and/or extradural, with the vast majority asymptomatic (43). Most of these spinal lesions are slow-growing schwannomas or meningiomas (Fig. 6C), with the benign pathology and indolent growth rate found in the general population of such tumors. Schwannosis, which often presents as multiple nodules seen on MRI involving the dorsal roots, is usually asymptomatic in the setting of NF2. Younger age, equal male to female incidence, and multiplicity are the main features of the NF2 patients bearing these spinal tumors. Follow-up and intervention in clinically significant tumors is indicated as is true for other germline cancer predisposition tumors. The surgical approaches are no different than those used for these extramedullary tumors in the general population, with emphasis on stabilization of the spine because of the multiplicity of levels involved and relative youth and activity of these patients.

The vast majority of gliomas seen in NF2 patients occur in the spine although asymptomatic glial hamartomas are commonly seen as UBOs. Intramedullary spinal tumors are mainly ependymomas, with a small number being pilocytic astrocytomas (Fig. 6D). The ependymomas can be multiple, and occasionally are holocord in extent. Many of these intramedullary tumors are simply followed, but if they become symptomatic because of growth of the tumor or associated syrinx, early intervention is recommended. The preoperative neurological status of the patient is the main determinant of postoperative neurological deficits after excision of the spinal ependymoma. Therefore, if a spinal intramedullary tumor is starting to cause neurological decline, we suggest surgery to optimize long-term function. If a tumor such as an astrocytoma without a clear tumor-cord border is encountered at surgery, it is best not to attempt total excision but rather to follow the patient or give external beam radiation. A standard posterior laminectomy approach is used, although consideration should be given to a laminotomy or posterior stabilization to prevent delayed swan neck deformity of the cervical spine for multiple levels and in the younger NF2 age group.

Conclusion

Germ-line cancer syndromes such as NF1 and NF2 provide unique challenges as well as opportunities to learn about the more common but similar sporadic tumors. Because of the multiplicity of tumors in young patients with these syndromes, a team approach with the availability of not only all the active interventions (surgery, radiation, chemotherapy), but also genetic and psychological support is ideal. Most of the tumors are benign and do not require intervention, allowing these patients to lead a full and near-normal life. However, close follow-up with reevaluation and discussion with the patient is required on a lifelong basis. The *NF* genes have been identified, and now research is directed at increasing our knowledge of the role of the encoded proteins in normal cellular growth regulation that is lost in NF. NF directed research will be extremely useful in our understanding of the much larger group of sporadic patients afflicted with these tumors because NF and sporadic neurofibromas, schwannomas, meningiomas, astrocytomas, and so on share many similar molecular pathogenic mechanisms. In the future, it will be ideal to treat systemic diseases such as NF with biologically targeted therapies, or even by correction of the genetic defects by use of gene therapy. However, currently these treatment modalities are not practical and the need for neurosurgical and other interventions by neurosurgeons and supplementary specialists is required.

References

1. Tibbles JAR, Cohen MM. The Proteus syndrome: the elephant man diagnosed. *Br Med J* 1986;293:683–685.
2. North K. *Neurofibromatosis* type 1 in childhood. London: MacKieth Press, 1997.
3. Lott IT, Richardson Jr EP. Neuropathological findings and the biology of neurofibromatosis. *Adv Neurol* 1981;29:23–32.
4. Riccardi VM. *Neurofibromatosis: phenotype, natural history and pathogenesis,* 2nd ed. Baltimore: The John Hopkins University Press, 1992.
5. Barker D, Wright E, Nguyen K, et al. Gene for von Recklinghausen neurofibromatosis is in the pericentromeric region of chromosome 17. *Science* 1987;236:1100–1102.
6. Rouleau GA, Seizinger BR, Ozelius LG, et al. Genetic linkage analysis of bilateral acoustic neurofibromatosis to a DNA marker on chromosome 22. *Nature* 1987;329:246–248.
7. Stumpf S, Alksne JF, Annegers JF, et al. Neurofibromatosis conference statement. National Institute of Health. Consensus Development Conference. *Arch Neurol* 1988;45:575–578.
8. Crowe FW, Schull WJ, Neel JV. *A clinical, pathological and genetic study of multiple neurofibromatosis.* Springfield, IL: Charles C Thomas, 1956.
9. Riccardi VM. Von Recklinghausen neurofibromatosis. *N Engl J Med* 1987;305:1617–1627.
10. Knudson AG Jr. Mutation and cancer: statistical study of retinoblastoma. *Proc Natl Acad Sci USA* 1997;68:820–823.
11. Marchuk DA, Saulino AM, Tavakkol R, et al. CDNA cloning of the type I neurofibromatosis gene: complete sequence of the NF1 gene product. *Genomics* 1991;11:931–940.
12. Gutmann DH, Wood DL, Collins FS. Identification of the neurofibromatosis type 1 gene is expressed at highest abundance in neurons, Schwann cells and oligodendrocytes. *Neuron* 1992;8:415–428.
13. Guha A, Lau N, Huvar I, et al. Ras-GTP levels are elevated in human NF1 peripheral nerve tumors. *Oncogene* 1996;12:507–513.
14. Trahey M. Molecular cloning of two types of GAP from complementary DNA for human placenta. *Science* 1988;242:1697–1700.
15. Trahey M, McCormick F. A cytoplasmic protein stimulates normal N-ras p21 GTPase, but does not affect oncogenic mutations. *Science* 1987;238:542–545.
16. Vogel U. Cloning of bovine GAP and its interaction with oncogenic ras p21. *Nature* 1988;335:90–93.
17. Bollag G, McCormick F. Differential regulation of rasGap and neurofibromatosis gene product activities. *Nature* 1991;351:576–579.
18. Martin GA, Viskochil D, Bollag G, et al. The GAP related domain of neurofibromatosis type 1 gene product interacts with ras p21. *Cell* 1990;63:843–849.
19. Xu G, O'Connell P, Viskochil D, et al. The neurofibromatosis type 1 gene encodes a protein related to GAP. *Cell* 1990;62:599–608.
20. Shannon KM, O'Connell P, Martin GA, et al. Loss of the normal NF1 allele from the bone marrow of children with type 1 neurofibromatosis and malignant myeloid disorders. *N Engl J Med* 1994;30: 597–601.
21. Lau N, Feldkamp MM, Roncari L, et al. Loss of neurofibromin is associated with activation of RAS/MAPK and PI3-K/AKT signaling in a neurofibromatosis 1 astrocytoma. *Neuropathol Exp Neurol* 2000; 59:759–767.
22. Rouleau GA, Wertelecki W, Haines JL, et al. Genetic linkage of bilateral acoustic neurofibromatosis to DNA marker on chromosome 22. *Nature* 1987;329:246–248.
23. Seizinger BR, Rouleau G, Ozelius LJ, et al. Common pathogenetic mechanism for three tumor types in bilateral acoustic neurofibromatosis. *Science* 1987;236:317–319.
24. Trofalter JA, MacCollin MM, Rutter JL, et al. A novel moesin-ezrin-radixin-like gene is a candidate for the neurofibromatosis 2 tumor suppressor. *Cell* 1993;75:826–829.
25. Rouleau GA, Merel P, Lutchman M, et al. Alteration in a new gene encoding a putative membrane organizing protein causes neurofibromatosis type 2. *Nature* 1993;363:515–521.
26. Gusella JF, Ramesh V, MacCollin M, et al. Merlin: the neurofibromatosis 2 tumor suppressor. *Biochim Biophys Acta* 1999;1423: 1429–1436.
27. Gutmann DH, Giordano MJ, Fishback AS, et al. Loss of merlin expression in sporadic meningiomas, ependymomas and schwannomas. *Neurology* 1997;49:267–270.
28. Huson SM, Hughes RAC, eds. *The neurofibromatoses: a pathogenetic and clinical overview.* London: Chapman and Hall, 1994.
29. Benedict PH, Szabo G, Fitzpatrick TB, et al. Melanotic macules in Albright's syndrome and in neurofibromatosis. *JAMA* 1986;205: 618–626.
30. Wertelecki W, Superneau DW, Forehand LW. Angiomas and von Recklinghausen neurofibromatosis. *Neurofibromatosis* 1988;1: 137–145.
31. Kline DG, Hudson AR. *Nerve injuries: operative results for major nerve injuries, entrapments, and tumors,* 1st ed. Philadelphia: WB Saunders 1995.
32. Sorensen SA, Mulvihill JJ, Nielsen A. A long-term follow-up of von Recklinghausen neurofibromatosis: survival and malignant neoplasms. *N Engl J Med* 1986;314:1010–1015.
33. Weiss S. *Histological typing of soft tissue tumors.* Berlin: Springer-Verlag, 1994.
34. Angelov L, Davis A, O'Sullivan B, et al. Neurogenic sarcomas: experience at the University of Toronto. *Neurosurgery* 1998;43:56–64; discussion 64–65.
35. North K, Cochineas C, Tang E, et al. Optic gliomas in neurofibromatosis type 1: role of visual evoked potentials. *Pediatr Neurol* 1994; 10:117–123.
36. Listernick R, Louis DN, Packer RJ, et al. Optic pathway glioma in children with NF1: consensus statement from the NF1 optic pathway glioma task force. *Ann Neurol* 1997;41:13–19.
37. Mapstone TB. Neurofibromatosis and central nervous system tumors in childhood. *Neurosurg Clin North Am* 1992;3:771–779.
38. Upadhyaya M, Cooper DN. *Neurofibromatosis type 1, from genotype to phenotype.* Oxford: BIOS Scientific Publishers, 1988.
39. Zhao JZ, Han XD. Cerebral aneurysm associated with von Recklinghausen's neurofibromatosis: a case report. *Surg Neurol* 1998;50: 592–596.
40. Ciappetta P, Salvati M, Capoccia G, et al. Spinal glioblastomas: report of seven cases and review of the literature. *Neurosurgery* 1991;28: 302–306.
41. Akbarnia BA, Gabriel KR, Beckman E, et al. Prevalence of scoliosis in neurofibromatosis. *Spine* 1992;17:S244–S2248.
42. Gutmann DH. Molecular insights into neurofibromatosis-2. *Neurobil Dis* 1997;3:247–261.
43. Evans DG, Huson SM, Donnai D, et al. A genetic study of type 2 neurofibromatosis in United Kingdom I. Prevalence, mutation rate, fitness and confirmation of maternal transmission effect on severity. *J Med Genet* 1992;29:841–846.
44. Martuza RL, Ojeman RG. Bilateral acoustic neuroma. Clinical aspects and treatment. *Neurosurgery* 1982;10:1–12.
45. Samii M, Mathies C. Management of 1000 vestibular schwannomas (acoustic neuromas): surgical management and results with an em-

phasis on complications and how to avoid them. *Neurosurgery* 1997; 40:11–23.

46. Mazzoni A, Calabrese V, Moschini L. Residual and recurrent acoustic neuroma in hearing preservation procedures: neuroradiologic and surgical findings. *Skull Base Surg* 1996;6: 105–112.

47. Bance M, Ramsden RT. Management of neurofibromatosis type 2. *Ear Nose Throat J* 199;78:91–99.

48. Ebersold MJ, Harner SG, Beatty CW, et al. Current results of the retrosigmoid approach to acoustic neuroma. *J Neurosurg* 1992;76: 901–909.

49. Fischer G, Fischer C, Redmond J. hearing preservation in acoustic neuroma surgery. *J Neurosurg* 1992;76:910–917.

50. Charabi S. Acoustic neuroma/vestibular Schwannoma in vivo and in vitro growth models. *Acta Otolaryngol (Stockh)* 1997;530(suppl): 1–9.

51. Lunsford LD, Linskey ME. Stereotactic radiosurgery in the treatment of patients with acoustic neuromas. *Otolaryngol Clin North Am* 1992;25:471–491.

52. Noren G, Grietz D. The Natural history of acoustic neuroma. In: Tos M, Thomson J, eds. *Proceedings of the first international conference on acoustic neuroma.* Amsterdam: Kugler, 1992:191–192.

53. Friedman RA, House JW. Facial nerve results. In: House WF, Luetje C, et al., eds. *Acoustic tumors: diagnosis and management.* San Diego: Singular Publishing Group, 1997:251–259.

54. Wiegand DA, Ojemann RG, Fickel V. Surgical treatment of acoustic neuroma (vestibular schwannoma) in the United States: report from the Acoustic Neuroma Registry. *Laryngoscope* 1996;106:58–66.

55. Samii M, Mathies C, Tatagiba M. Management of vestibular schwannoma (acoustic neuromas): auditory and facial nerve function after resection of 120 vestibular schwannomas in patients with neurofibromatosis 2. *Neurosurgery* 1997;40:696–702.

56. Kondziolka D, Lunsford LD, McLaughlin MR, et al. Long term outcomes after radiosurgery for acoustic neuroma. *N Engl J Med* 1998; 39:1426–1433.

57. Noren G. Long term complications following gamma knife radiosurgery of vestibular schwannomas. *Sterotact Funct Neurosurg* 1998; 70(suppl):65–73.

58. Subach BR, Kondziolka D, Lunsford LD, et al. Stereotactic radiosurgery in the management of acoustic neuromas associated with neurofibromatosis Type2. *J Neurosurg* 1999;90:815–822.

59. Shamisa A, Bance M, Nag S, et al. Glioblastoma multiforme occurring in a patient treated with gamma knife surgery: case report and review of the literature. *J Neurosurg* 2001;94:816–821.

127. The Neurosurgical Implications of von Hippel-Lindau Disease

**Tung T. Nguyen and
Edward H. Oldfield**

von Hippel-Lindau (VHL) syndrome is an inherited autosomal dominant disease produced by a germline mutation in the VHL gene located on chromosome 3. Patients with VHL are predisposed to developing tumors in multiple organs (Table 1). The central nervous system (CNS) manifestations include hemangioblastomas in the cerebellum, spinal cord, and, rarely, in the cerebrum, and tumors of the endolymphatic sac. The multifocal and metachronous nature of tumor development has distinct implications for diagnosis, treatment, and ultimate overall neurological outcome. Although surgery and high-dose focused radiation are accepted therapies for these lesions, the challenge to neurosurgeons treating VHL patients with lesions of the CNS

is to define optimally if, when, and how to treat these multiple lesions.

Historical Aspects

In 1894 Treacher Collins initially described what are now known as retinal hemangioblastomas in two patients whose hereditary condition produced lesions best described as capillary nevi (1). In 1904 and 1911 Eugen von Hippel published his descriptions of two patients with retinal hemangioblastomas (2), and Arvid Lindau subsequently recognized the association between cerebellar hemangioblastomas and retinal angiomas, as well as the presence of uncommon visceral lesions in 1926 (3). Because of Lindau's accurate description of the constellation of tumors now known to be associated with inheritance of an abnormal "VHL" gene, many authors argue that the disease is most appropriately named Lindau disease (4). The disease is inherited in an autosomal dominant fashion, has high penetrance but variable expressivity, and predisposes affected individuals to tumors in many organ systems (Table 1).

TABLE 1. Typical Lesions of von Hippel-Lindau Disease

Hemangioblastomas
  Cerebellum
  Spinal cord
  Medulla
  Cerebrum
Retinal angiomas
Renal lesions
  Cysts
  Adenoma/carcinoma
Pheochromocytoma
Pancreatic lesions
  Cysts
  Adenoma/carcinoma
Epididymal cystadenoma

Tumor Biology

GENETICS OF VON HIPPEL-LINDAU DISEASE. Pedigree studies and linkage analyses of large affected kindred have established the autosomal dominant inheritance pattern of von Hippel-Lindau disease (5–8). Seizinger and colleagues (6) performed genetic-linkage analysis with polymorphic DNA markers in nine families with VHL. The results, expressed as a lod score, clearly established a linkage with the human RAF1 oncogene locus on chromosome 3p25, and, thus, showed that the genetic defect causing VHL is located on chromosome 3p25. The significance of this genetic defect was revealed in the detection of loss of alleles from chromosome 3p in hereditary tumors (renal cell carcinomas, pheochromocytoma, and spinal and cerebellar hemangioblastomas) found in VHL patients (9) and sporadic renal cell carcinomas (10,11). Loss of heterozygosity studies (12) of tumors from VHL families showed that these four types of tumors shared a common mechanism of tumorigenesis—that the VHL gene is a recessive tumor suppressor gene and that loss of the second copy of the gene is the critical event in the pathogenesis of neoplasms, which is consistent with Knudson's "two-hit" tumor suppressor hypothesis (13). The location of the VHL gene was eventually localized to the region of 3p25-26 (8,14–17) and sequenced (18). Germline mutations were found in a high percentage (75%) of families with VHL (19,20). When separated by absence (Type 1) or presence (Type 2) of pheochromocytomas, microdeletions/insertions, missense and nonsense mutations accounted for 56% of mutations responsible for VHL Type 1, whereas missense mutations accounted for 96% of mutations responsible for VHL Type 2.

CELLULAR AND MOLECULAR BIOLOGY. The details of the function of the VHL gene and the molecular mechanisms involved in tumor suppression remain to be fully established. Structurally, the cDNA has 852 nucleotides in three exons, and encodes a 30 kd protein (pVHL) that is unrelated to any known gene. The VHL protein is part of a functional complex, which includes the proteins elongin B, elongin C, and cullin-2, all of which are associated with elongation and degradation of mRNA during transcription (21–23).

The most important role of pVHL seems to be its role in regulating expression of genes involved in the cellular response to hypoxia (24), of which the hypoxia-inducible factor (HIF) transcriptional system is the most important. HIF-1, a heterodimer consisting of α and B subunits, plays a key role in the cellular response to hypoxia by activating the transcription of genes involved in angiogenesis, apoptosis, and metabolism. Genes identified as having a hypoxia-responsive element (HRE) include those encoding vascular epithelial growth factor (VEGF), erythropoietin, and glucose transporter-1 (GLUT-1). HIF-1 activity is regulated by the availability of the α subunit, which is ubiquinated and rapidly degraded under nonhypoxic conditions. pVHL, as part of a larger elongin-ubiquitin ligase complex, binds HIF-α and allows for the degradation process to proceed. Under hypoxic conditions this binding is inhibited, leading to accumulation of HIF-α, its transportation to the nucleus, dimerization with the B-subunit, binding of coactivators and activation of target gene transcription (25). When pVHL function is lost, such as in VHL-defective cells, HIF-α is constitutively stabilized and leads to upregulated expression and overproduction of VEGF/VPF (24,26–28). Therefore, the level of pVHL generated by changes in oxygen tension underlies the vascular nature of hemangioblastomas.

When wild-type VHL gene is restored in VHL-deficient renal carcinoma cells, the ability of these cells to follow the normal cell–cycle checkpoints is restored (29), suggesting a role for VHL in regulation of the cell cycle exit. VHL protein also negatively regulates the expression of carbonic anhydrases 9 and 12 (30), which are transmembrane proteins implicated in the acidification of the extracellular milieu surrounding tumor cells. Deletion of VHL function results in overexpression of carbonic

anhydrases types 9 and 12, acidification of the extracellular milieu, and an acidic environment that may enhance tumor growth and spread (31). Thus, overexpression of these enzymes suggests a role for VHL loss in dysregulation of extracellular pH and in cancer cell growth and invasion.

Patient Evaluation and Treatment

CLINICAL DIAGNOSIS. Melmon and Rosen (4) argued persuasively that the minimal criteria for the diagnosis of the syndrome as an association between cerebellar hemangioblastomas and one or more of the following lesions: retinal hemangioblastomas, spinal cord hemangioblastomas, pancreatic cysts, and renal or epididymal lesions. Patients with a single lesion and with a family member who has a documented CNS hemangioblastomas are also considered to have VHL. Use of a VHL registry in England (32) determined that 60.2% of VHL patients develop a cerebellar hemangioblastoma and 14.5% develop a spinal hemangioblastoma. In addition, 14% of all CNS hemangioblastomas were found in patients with VHL.

The most common lesions requiring neurosurgical evaluation in VHL patients are hemangioblastomas. These are well-vascularized lesions of various sizes involving primarily the cerebellum, brainstem, and spinal cord, with rare presentations in the supratentorial compartment. Symptomatic lesions often have associated cyst in the cerebellum or syrinx formation in the spinal cord.

Endolymphatic sac tumors (ELSTs) are in general very rare, and can be sporadic or inherited in a tumor syndrome such as VHL. Because of an increased incidence of hearing loss in patients with VHL, Manski and associates (33) demonstrated convincingly that hearing loss and ELSTs are components of VHL. In patients with hearing loss, tinnitus, vertigo, or facial paresis, brain magnetic resonance images (MRIs) revealed evidence of 15 ELSTs in 13 (11%) of 121 patients with VHL, but in none of 253 patients without evidence of VHL (p < .001). Furthermore, the role of VHL disease in ELST was confirmed by identification of germline VHL gene mutation and wild-type VHL gene deletion in VHL-associated ELST (34) and homozygous loss of VHL gene function by the combination of somatic mutation and VHL gene deletion in sporadic ELSTs (35).

RADIOLOGICAL FINDINGS. Hemangioblastomas typically present as a cystic tumor with an enhancing mural nodule. The tumors uniformly and intensely enhance on CT or MR imaging, and, with the availability of more sensitive noninvasive imaging techniques, they are found much sooner than they previously could be detected and can now be detected while they are very small and without associated cysts when they are detected during screening evaluation (Fig. 1). Spinal cord hemangioblastomas are usually on the dorsal aspect of the spinal cord, posterior to the dentate ligament. A majority of lesions have both intramedullary and extramedullary components, but approximately 30% of the spinal lesions are entirely intramedullary. Most symptomatic spinal hemangioblastomas are associated with syrinx formation (Fig. 2) in the cervical, thoracic, and lumbar regions.

Hemangioblastomas exhibit robust vascularity with prominent afferent and efferent vessels on cerebral or spinal arteriograms (Fig. 3). In the spinal cord the most prominent vessels, the draining veins, can have an appearance similar to a vascular malformation (Fig. 4). Despite the impressive vascularity of these tumors on preoperative arteriograms, preoperative embo-

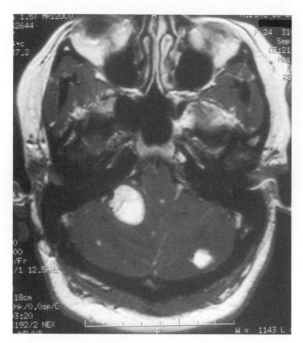

Fig. 1. Axial gadolinium-enhanced T1-weighted image showing several uniformly enhancing hemangioblastomas in the cerebellum. The largest ones are in the right cerebellopontine angle and left cerebellar hemisphere.

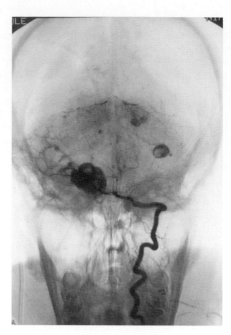

Fig. 3. Cerebral arteriogram. Left vertebral injection, anteroposterior projection. Multiple hemangioblastomas are noted, the largest of which is filled early after vertebral injection. No tumor vessels are present for selective embolization.

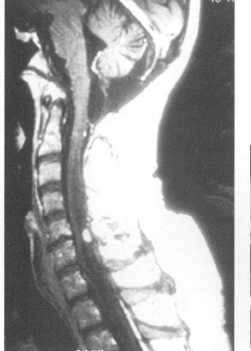

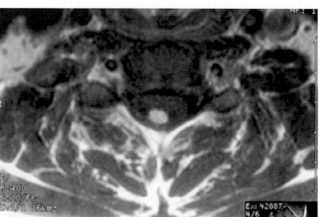

Fig. 2. Spinal hemangioblastoma. **A:** Sagittal gadolinium-enhanced MRI scan showing posteriorly located hemangioblastoma at C5-6 with associated spinal cord edema *(above)* and syrinx *(below the lesion)* and a smaller hemangioblastoma posteriorly at C2. **B:** Axial gadolinium-enhanced MRI scan at the level of the larger tumor showing dorsal location of the tumor.

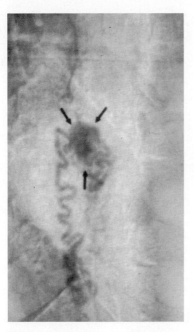

Fig. 4. Spinal arteriogram. Tumor *(arrows)* is associated with multiple serpiginous draining vessels that have an appearance that might be misinterpreted as a spinal arteriovenous malformation.

lization is not routinely used because it is rarely needed and because most hemangioblastomas do not have a predominant vessel selectively supplying the tumor.

ELSTs are seen on CT as an expansile, destructive lesion of the posterior petrous bone. On MRI, the tumor appears as a heterogeneously enhancing lesion, in some instances with expansion possible into the cerebellopontine angle and cerebellum posteriorly and medially, to the junction of the sigmoid sinus and jugular bulb inferiorly, or to the petrous apex superiorly (Fig. 5).

Histopathology

HEMANGIOBLASTOMAS

Macroscopic. Hemangioblastomas are well-circumscribed, red-orange tumors (Fig. 6) with large efferent and afferent vessels on the tumor surface, and multiple smaller feeders arising from the deeper portion of the tumors. Cerebellar lesions can present on the surface or lie deep within the hemisphere. There is always a sharp demarcation between the tumor capsule and the adjacent compressed gliotic tissue that can be exploited to facilitate microsurgical dissection. In the spinal cord the lesions are almost always posteriorly located, where they usually present to the surface laterally near the dorsal root entry zone.

Microscopic. The microscopic appearance of hemangioblastomas is similar from tumor to tumor and does not vary with the location of the lesions. The characteristic appearance of hemangioblastomas presents a mixture of background reticulin staining, multiple sinusoidal channels lined with normal-appearing endothelial cells, and stromal cells. The large, polygonal stromal cells are lipid-rich, and due to lipid removal during the fixation process, they have large cytoplasmic vacuoles. The reticulin staining of the vessels highlights the mass of arborizing vessels that are a prominent feature of hemangioblastomas. The walls of the cysts that are commonly associated with symptom-producing hemangioblastomas show dense gliosis with Rosenthal fibers, consistent with the nonneoplastic nature of these fluid-filled cavities.

The cell of origin of hemangioblastomas is unknown. VHL gene abnormalities were first detected in hemangioblastomas by RFLP analysis (9). Berkman and associates (36) subsequently demonstrated dense staining of the stromal cells for VEGF and proposed that the stromal cells were the cell of origin of the tumor, the vascular part comprising an epiphenomenon induced by the excess VEGF provided by the stromal cells. After isolation of the VHL gene, VHL gene abnormalities were detected in 10 of 20 CNS hemangioblastomas (37). Vortmeyer and colleagues (38) used microdissected tumor tissue to localize

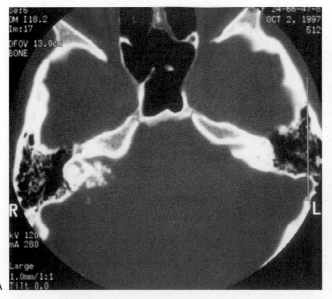
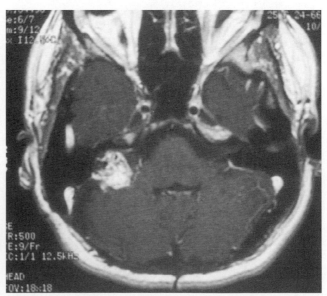

Fig. 5. Endolymphatic sac tumor. **A:** Axial CT scan shows bony erosion of the right internal auditory meatus. **B:** Axial gadolinium-enhanced MRI of the same area showing the heterogeneously enhancing tumor encroaching into the posterior fossa at the cerebellopontine angle on the right side.

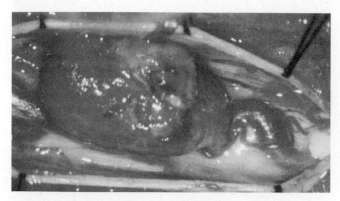

Fig. 6. Intraoperative exposure of spinal hemangioblastoma. The reddish-orange lesion is partially extramedullary, well encapsulated, and associated with large superficial draining veins.

the VHL mutations to stromal cells, confirming the neoplastic characteristic of these lipid-laden stromal cells. Stromal cells generally do not stain for glial fibrillary acidic protein, keratin or EMA, and although negative for neurofilaments, they do stain for neuron-specific enolase and other markers that suggest a neuroendocrine differentiation. The true origin of these cells, whether glial, neuronal, or endothelial, remains to be determined.

ENDOLYMPHATIC SAC TUMORS. Tumors that become large enough to encroach into the posterior fossa have cystic cavities filled with hemorrhagic fluid (Fig. 7). The adjacent dura often has proliferation of small vessels. The petrous bone may be completely replaced by the soft tumor, or have a porous appearance, due to tumor infiltration of the bone. Hematoxylin and eosin staining of endolymphatic sac tumors (ELSTs) shows areas of papillary proliferation that have a lining comprised of cuboidal epithelial cells. There also may be angiomatous cavities filled with recent or old hemorrhage.

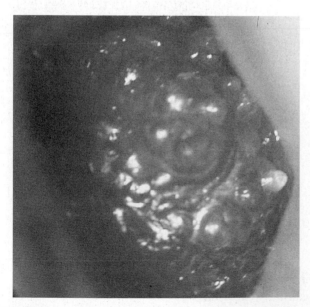

Fig. 7. Intraoperative exposure of endolymphatic sac tumor. This tumor expanded from the presigmoid dura to encroach on the cerebellum. Larger tumors typically have multiple cystic cavities filled with hemorrhagic fluid.

Neurosurgical Considerations

The development of hemangioblastomas in von Hippel-Lindau disease poses challenging questions for the neurosurgeon. The challenge is to define the patient who is at risk for neurological deterioration from one or more tumors, select the optimal treatment (surgery or focused radiation), and then execute the treatment safely and effectively.

PATIENT EVALUATION. Full evaluation of patients suspected of having the hereditary form of hemangioblastoma includes general physical, neurological, otological, and eye examinations; CT scans of the chest and abdomen; MRI of the head and spine; CBC (patients occasionally have polycythemia because of tumor production of erythropoietin); 24-hour urine catecholamines; ultrasound of the abdomen and testicles; chest x-ray; and a blood sample and/or cheek swab for genetic analysis for the VHL gene.

PATIENT COUNSELING. Patients with brainstem and cerebellar disease may manifest signs and symptoms of cerebellar and vestibular dysfunction. Brainstem lesions can produce posterior column disturbances, lower cranial nerve abnormalities, and motor deficits in the upper and lower extremities. Patients with spinal cord tumors can present with varying degrees of sensorimotor deficits in the limbs.

Recommendation of surgical resection is generally accepted with a diagnosis of a symptomatic hemangioblastoma in the neuraxis. Patients can be symptomatic from the mass effect of a large tumor or tumor-associated cerebellar or spinal cord cysts.

A challenge arises with management of patients who have multiple lesions of various sizes and different growth rates but who remain clinically asymptomatic. From a retrospective review of 160 patients with CNS and spinal hemangioblastomas followed at the National Institute of Health, preliminary data demonstrate that between 15% and 33% of patients had tumor progression over a 3-year period of observation (Wanabo and associates, personal communication). Of these, 47% of patients had continuous growth as demonstrated on serial MRI scans, whereas 53% had quiescent phases between growth phases. Cysts, once formed, enlarge or plateau but do not diminish in size. Cyst progression may occur in the absence of tumor growth; therefore, serial observation is an important part of patient evaluation.

Intervention

SURGICAL TECHNIQUES. The general surgical principles used for resection of hemangioblastomas in the cerebellum, spinal cord, and brainstem are similar to the general principles that pertain to tumor removal in general: adequate exposure, brain relaxation, careful exposure and definition of the tumor–neural interface, preservation of the tumor capsule, and complete resection of the tumor as a single mass if possible.

Hemangioblastoma of the Brainstem and Cerebellum. Patients are positioned prone with the head flexed, with rotation as necessary for lateral lesions. Exposure is provided by a wide suboccipital craniectomy. A C1 laminectomy is performed for exposure of lesions in the brainstem or cervicomedullary junction. An occipital or parietal bur hole should be considered if obstructive hydrocephalus is present. Intraoperative ultrasound with Doppler flow detection is used to localize the tumor and cyst before dural opening. The typical Y-shaped dural opening is used for midline lesions. A tumor cyst can be used to provide a convenient route to the tumor nodule for deep hemangioblastomas. The tumor capsule is identified and defined and the surrounding whitish-yellow gliotic layer is dissected from the tumor capsule with closed bipolar tips. This plane is developed circumferentially using microsurgical techniques, use of small cottonoid patties to maintain the plane, and gentle bipolar coagulation and sharp interruption of small vessels as they enter the tumor capsule. Rarely, a very large lesion requires piecemeal tumor removal. In this circumstance, portions of the tumor capsule and tumor interior are coagulated with broad-tipped bipolar forceps and removed with the Cavitron, after which complete hemostasis is achieved before repeating the cycle. Shunting or fenestration of cysts after tumor resection is unnecessary because the cyst collapses or disappears after tumor removal.

Hemangioblastoma of the Spinal Cord.

The radiologist marks the involved vertebral level the day before surgery. The patient is positioned prone on a chest roll or Wilson frame. Care is taken to pad all pressure points. We do not use intraoperative monitoring of somatosensory or motor-evoked potentials because we have found them to be unnecessary. A wide laminectomy overlying the level of the tumor is performed. Once the dura is exposed, intraoperative ultrasound (IOUS) with Doppler flow detection is used to locate the tumor and assess the relationship, if any, of a syrinx with the tumor.

The dura is incised with preservation of the arachnoid to avoid injury of the underlying vessels, and the dural leaves are reflected laterally with retention sutures to the paraspinous musculature. The arachnoid then is opened carefully under magnification. The arachnoid may be adherent to the superficial arterialized vessels of the coronal venous plexus. Sharp dissection is performed to remove the arachnoid overlying the tumor and its associated vessels and define the tumor margin.

The margin of a tumor that reaches the pial surface is exposed by gently coagulating the draining vessels at the margin of the tumor, where the capsule of the tumor reaches the pia of the spinal cord. The pia is incised precisely at its interface with the tumor capsule using a diamond-knife. This permits early identification of the tumor capsule, which is glossy and salmon-colored, in contrast to the whitish-yellow avascular gliotic tissue adjacent to the tumor capsule. Overzealous coagulation can discolor the surface of the tumor and obliterate easy visibility of the margin, making the dissection more difficult and producing more blood loss from entry into the capsule. Individual vessels should be managed discretely with bipolar coagulation at the tumor margin as the tumor capsule is exposed from sequential dissection through deeper layers. Large veins traversing the margin should be sharply divided after bipolar coagulation. Clips are never required. Draining veins are interrupted early without consequence. However, to minimize the risk of tumor engorgement, at least one major draining vein is preserved until the tumor margin has been completely dissected.

The tumor margin is dissected circumferentially, advancing each plane deeper in stages until the tumor has been shelled out entirely. We use small, custom-cut cottonoid patties without strings to protect the tumor capsule and neural tissue during dissection and to maintain a small space at the tumor margin, and expose the tumor–neural interface by applying the sucker tip to a cottonoid for tumor retraction.

By methodically interrupting the blood supply, blood loss and its consequent blood staining of the spinal cord can be minimized. This staining can make it more difficult to distinguish the spinal cord from tumor. Bipolar coagulation of the tumor capsule also can blur this distinction. However, the tumor capsule will regain its color and gloss if left undisturbed, and patience often helps to redefine the tumor–neural interface. In the event that the tumor is much too bulky to be resected in one piece, it may be necessary to resect part of it. This can be accomplished with little bleeding by progressively coagulating a small portion of the tumor capsule and tumor center, removing the coagulated tissue with microscissors (or the Cavitron for larger tumor fragments), obtaining complete hemostasis, and then resuming the piecemeal tumor resection.

Ventrally located hemangioblastomas in the cervical region are approached by an anterior exposure from a wide corpectomy. The advantages are that the anterior spinal artery can be identified and protected during tumor resection, and neural tissue is not traversed in order to expose the tumor. The microsurgical techniques are identical to those used for posteriorly located tumors. Following tumor resection, the dural opening is repaired with Gelfoam and fibrin glue. For anterior tumors, the cervical spine is reconstructed using MR-compatible cervical instrumentation.

Surgical Outcomes.

Results for VHL patients with hemangioblastomas are sparse as the patients form a subset of available published surgical outcome. Overall, with early diagnosis and improved microsurgical techniques, surgical outcomes are favorable. Conway and associates (39) reviewed outcomes for 40 patients with central nervous system hemangioblastomas, of whom 15 had VHL disease. Resolution or stabilization of symptoms was documented in 88% of patients at 12 months after surgery, with no difference in outcome between the sporadic or VHL groups. Serious complications were noted in 15% of patients. Neumann and colleagues (40) reported that 89% of patients with cerebellar lesions were in good condition without major residual symptoms 5 years after surgery, with a 7% morbidity rate.

Resection of spinal cord hemangioblastomas is also associated with good surgical outcome in most patients. Murota and co-workers (41) noted clinical improvement after complete excision in 72% of patients with spinal hemangioblastomas, similar to outcomes reported by others (42–44).

Tumor recurrence and multicentricity affect a high percentage of patients with VHL (39,45). The rate of new lesion formation (one lesion per 2.1 years) combined with other systemic manifestations of VHL disease contributed to increased morbidity over time for these patients (39). However, in that small series of VHL patients, repeat surgery was not associated with increased risks or poorer outcome.

Endolymphatic Sac Tumors.

Endolymphatic sac tumors (ELST) erode the mastoid bone and can grow posteriorly into the posterior fossa at the cerebellopontine angle, or inferiorly toward the jugular foramen. These tumors are removed using a combined retromastoid and transmastoid approach. The intracranial portion is undertaken first to protect the cerebellum, drain the CSF, and identify the VIIth and VIIIth nerves at the internal auditory canal, and then to define the IX–X–XIth nerve complex. The endolymphatic sac is identified using internal landmarks (46). A 1- to 2-mm dural cuff around the edge of the tumor is cut, with care taken to not enter the jugular bulb. Then the transmastoid exposure is performed to "blue-line" the posterior semicircular canal, expose the presigmoid dura, and find and complete the dural cut from intracranial exposure. Larger tumors can extend to the junction of the sigmoid sinus and jugular bulb, where exposure of the dura is difficult. Bony resection with a diamond drill is pursued until the margin of the more porous, tumor-infiltrated bone is no longer visible.

NONSURGICAL TREATMENT OPTIONS

Radiation. Stereotactic radiosurgery and whole brain irradiation have been used to treat sporadic and hereditary hemangioblastomas (47–57). The most common indications that have been used for treatment with irradiation of either type are: (a) inability to tolerate surgery, (b) residual tumor after surgery, (c) tumor recurrence, (d) multiple lesions, and (e) "unresectable" lesions. Several studies also used positive tumor margins as an indication to treat (50,51). Most authors have treated tumors between 5 and 30 mm in diameter with doses ranging from 40 to 55 Gy for conventional radiation and 10 to 15 Gy to the enhancing margin, or 20 to 25 Gy to the whole tumor, using stereotactic radiation. Solid and cystic tumors have been treated. Follow-up periods range from 4 months to more than 11 years. Clinical responses have been reported as actuarial and progression-free survival, or as rates of tumor disappearance, stability, or progression. In general, conventional external beam therapy resulted in 85% to 90% 5-year survival rates using high-dose (more than 40 Gy) radiotherapy (48,51). Stereotactic surgery is associated with 88% and 86% 2-year actuarial and progression-free survival, respectively (50). Tumor shrinkage was seen in 60% to 73% of lesions, and tumor control (no growth or shrinkage) was noted in 24% to 40% of hemangioblastomas treated with radiosurgery (52,58). Complications such as cerebellar edema, radiation necrosis, or hydrocephalus have occurred. Cyst enlargement requiring surgical drainage after radiation occurred frequently (37% to 100% of patients) (47,50–53). The indications for stereotactic radiosurgical and/or conventional radiation treatment of hemangioblastomas in VHL patients are evolving, and the appropriate use of this treatment choice should be clarified when data from longer follow-up review of patient outcome are available. Given the high rate of cyst enlargement requiring surgery, cystic hemangioblastomas should not now be considered candidates for irradiation treatment of any type. However, patients with surgically inaccessible tumors or for whom surgery is medically contraindicated may benefit from this less invasive technique. Relative indications for radiosurgery, such as size (small- to medium-sized tumors), whether or not lesions are enlarging or producing symptoms, and residual tumors after surgery, remain to be determined.

Future Treatments and Considerations

The pace of scientific discovery of the mechanism of the von Hippel-Lindau protein offers an exciting opportunity to seek new treatments to supplement or replace current therapy. Ideally, newer therapies would be targeted toward smaller, clinically silent hemangioblastomas that are likely to become symptomatic over a period of several years. There are several potential targets for future therapies. For example, blockade of the constitutive overexpression of hypoxia-inducible transcription factor (HIF) may prevent the downstream effects of target genes involved in angiogenesis. If CA isozyme expression is limited only to tumor cells, then the transmembrane protein may act as a tumor-specific antigen, which can then be targeted by antibodies in a highly selective manner.

Conclusion

Neurosurgical intervention in patients with VHL should be limited to selective resection of symptomatic hemangioblastomas.

Surgery, which can be performed safely, is the therapy of choice for most tumors, and radiation is beneficial in carefully selected tumors. With the elucidation of the mechanism of disease, treatments aimed at the biological factors in tumor development and progression are forthcoming and will help greatly in the care of patients with VHL.

References

1. Collins ET. Intra-ocular growths (two cases, brother and sister, with peculiar vascular new growth, probably primarily retinal, affecting both eyes). *Trans Ophthal Soc UK* 1894;14:141–149.
2. von Hippel E. Ueber eine sehr seltene Erkrankung der Netzhaut. Albrecht von Graefes. *Arch Ophthalmol* 1904;59:83–106.3.Lindau A. Zur Frage der Angiomatosis Retinae und Ihrer Hirncomplikation. *Acta Ophthalmol* 1927;4:193–226.
4. Melmon K, Rosen S. Lindau's disease: review of the literature and study of a large kindred. *Am J Med* 1964;36:595–617.
5. Atuk NO, et al. Familial pheochromocytoma, hypercalcemia, and von Hippel-Lindau disease. A ten year study of a large family. *Medicine (Balt)* 1979;58:209–218.
6. Seizinger BR, et al. Von Hippel-Lindau disease maps to the region of chromosome 3 associated with renal cell carcinoma. *Nature* 1988;332:268–269.
7. Seizinger BR, et al. Genetic flanking markers refine diagnostic criteria and provide insights into the genetics of Von Hippel Lindau disease. *Proc Natl Acad Sci USA* 1991;88:2864–2868.
8. Crossey PA, et al. Genetic linkage between von Hippel-Lindau disease and three microsatellite polymorphisms refines the localisation of the VHL locus. *Hum Mol Genet* 1993;2:279–282.
9. Tory K, et al. Specific genetic change in tumors associated with von Hippel-Lindau disease. *J Natl Cancer Inst* 1989;81:1097–1101.
10. Yamakawa K, et al. A detailed deletion mapping of the short arm of chromosome 3 in sporadic renal cell carcinoma. *Cancer Res* 1991;51:4707–4711.
11. Gnarra JR, et al. Molecular genetic studies of sporadic and familial renal cell carcinoma. *Urol Clin North Am* 1993;20:207–216.
12. Crossey PA, et al. Molecular genetic investigations of the mechanism of tumourigenesis in von Hippel-Lindau disease: analysis of allele loss in VHL tumours. *Hum Genet* 1994;93:53–58.
13. Knudson AG Jr. Mutation and cancer: statistical study of retinoblastoma. *Proc Natl Acad Sci USA* 1971;68:820–823.
14. Maher ER, et al. Mapping of von Hippel-Lindau disease to chromosome 3p confirmed by genetic linkage analysis. *J Neurol Sci* 1990;100:27–30.
15. Maher ER, et al. Mapping of the von Hippel-Lindau disease locus to a small region of chromosome 3p by genetic linkage analysis. *Genomics* 1991;10:957–960.
16. Richards FM, et al. Mapping the Von Hippel-Lindau disease tumour suppressor gene: identification of germline deletions by pulsed field gel electrophoresis. *Hum Mol Genet* 1993;2:879–882.
17. Richards FM, et al. Detailed genetic mapping of the von Hippel-Lindau disease tumour suppressor gene. *J Med Genet* 1993;30:104–107. [Published erratum appears in *J Med Genet* 1993;30:528.]
18. Latif F, et al. Identification of the von Hippel-Lindau disease tumor suppressor gene [see comments]. *Science* 1993;260:1317–1320.
19. Chen F, et al. Germline mutations in the von Hippel-Lindau disease tumor suppressor gene: correlations with phenotype. *Hum Mutat* 1995;5:66–75.
20. Zbar B, et al. Germline mutations in the Von Hippel-Lindau disease (VHL) gene in families from North America, Europe, and Japan. *Hum Mutat* 1996;8:348–357.
21. Duan DR, et al. Characterization of the VHL tumor suppressor gene product: localization, complex formation, and the effect of natural inactivating mutations. *Proc Natl Acad Sci USA* 1995;92:6459–6463.
22. Kibel A, Iliopoulos O, DeCaprio JA, et al. Binding of the von Hippel-Lindau tumor suppressor protein to Elongin B and C [see comments]. *Science* 1995;269:1444–1446.
23. Feldman DE, Thulasiraman V, Ferreyra RG, et al. Formation of the VHL-elongin BC tumor suppressor complex is mediated by the chaperonin TRiC. *Mol Cell* 1999;4:1051–1061.

24. Maxwell PH, et al. The tumour suppressor protein VHL targets hypoxia-inducible factors for oxygen-dependent proteolysis [see comments]. *Nature* 1999;399:271–275.

25. Semenza GL. HIF-1 and human disease: one highly involved factor. *Genes Dev* 2000;14:1983–1991.

26. Iliopoulos O, Levy AP, Jiang C, et al. Negative regulation of hypoxia-inducible genes by the von Hippel-Lindau protein. *Proc Natl Acad Sci USA* 1996;93:10595–10599.

27. Mukhopadhyay D, Tsiokas L, Sukhatme VP. High cell density induces vascular endothelial growth factor expression via protein tyrosine phosphorylation. *Gene Expr* 1998;7:53–60.

28. Mukhopadhyay D, Knebelmann B, Cohen HT, et al. The von Hippel-Lindau tumor suppressor gene product interacts with Sp1 to repress vascular endothelial growth factor promoter activity. *Mol Cell Biol* 1997;17:5629–5639.

29. Pause A, Lee S, Lonergan KM, et al. The von Hippel-Lindau tumor suppressor gene is required for cell cycle exit upon serum withdrawal. *Proc Natl Acad Sci USA* 1998;95:993–998.

30. Zbar B, Kaelin W, Maher E, et al. Third International Meeting on von Hippel-Lindau disease. *Cancer Res* 1999;59:2251–2253.

31. Ivanov SV, et al. Down-regulation of transmembrane carbonic anhydrases in renal cell carcinoma cell lines by wild-type von Hippel-Lindau transgenes. *Proc Natl Acad Sci USA* 1998;95:12596–12601.

32. Maddock IR, et al. A genetic register for von Hippel-Lindau disease. *J Med Genet* 1996;33:120–127.

33. Manski TJ, et al. Endolymphatic sac tumors. A source of morbid hearing loss in von Hippel-Lindau disease. *JAMA* 1997;277:1461–1466.

34. Vortmeyer AO, Choo D, Pack SD, et al. von Hippel-Lindau disease gene alterations associated with endolymphatic sac tumor [letter]. *J Natl Cancer Inst* 1997;89:970–972.

35. Vortmeyer AO, et al. Somatic von Hippel-Lindau gene mutations detected in sporadic endolymphatic sac tumors. *Cancer Res* 2000;60:5963–5965.

36. Berkman RA, et al. Expression of the vascular permeability factor/vascular endothelial growth factor gene in central nervous system neoplasms. *J Clin Invest* 1993;91:153–159.

37. Oberstrass J, Reifenberger G, Reifenberger J, et al. Mutation of the Von Hippel-Lindau tumour suppressor gene in capillary haemangioblastomas of the central nervous system. *J Pathol* 1996;179:151–156.

38. Vortmeyer AO, et al. von Hippel-Lindau gene deletion detected in the stromal cell component of a cerebellar hemangioblastoma associated with von Hippel-Lindau disease. *Hum Pathol* 1997;28:540–543.

39. Conway JE, et al. Hemangioblastomas of the central nervous system in von Hippel-Lindau syndrome and sporadic disease. *Neurosurgery* 2001;48:55–62; discussion 62–63.

40. Neumann HP, et al. Hemangioblastomas of the central nervous system. A 10-year study with special reference to von Hippel-Lindau syndrome. *J Neurosurg* 1989;70:24–30.

41. Murota T, Symon L. Surgical management of hemangioblastoma of the spinal cord: a report of 18 cases. *Neurosurgery* 1989;25:699–707; discussion 708.

42. Pietila TA, Stendel R, Schilling A, et al. Surgical treatment of spinal hemangioblastomas [in process citation]. *Acta Neurochir* 2000;142:879–886.

43. Xu Q, Bao W, Mao R. Magnetic resonance imaging and microsurgical treatment of intramedullary hemangioblastoma of the spinal cord. *Chin Med J (Engl)* 1995;108:117–122.

44. Yasargil MG, et al. The microsurgical removal of intramedullary spinal hemangioblastomas. Report of twelve cases and a review of the literature. *Surg Neurol* 1976; Sept (3):141–148.

45. de la Monte SM, Horowitz SA. Hemangioblastomas: clinical and histopathological factors correlated with recurrence. *Neurosurgery* 1989;25:695–698.

46. Ammirati M, et al. The endolymphatic sac: microsurgical topographic anatomy. *Neurosurgery* 1995;36:416–419.

47. Jeffreys R. Clinical and surgical aspects of posterior fossa haemangioblastomata. *J Neurol Neurosurg Psychiatry* 1975;38:105–111.

48. Sung DI, Chang CH, Harisiadis L. Cerebellar hemangioblastomas. *Cancer* 1982;49:553–555.

49. Page KA, Wayson K, Steinberg GK, et al. Stereotaxic radiosurgical ablation: an alternative treatment for recurrent and multifocal hemangioblastomas. A report of four cases. *Surg Neurol* 1993;40:424–428.

50. Patrice SJ, et al. Radiosurgery for hemangioblastoma: results of a multiinstitutional experience. *Int J Radiat Oncol Biol Phys* 1996;35:493–499.

51. Smalley SR, et al. Radiotherapeutic considerations in the treatment of hemangioblastomas of the central nervous system. *Int J Radiat Oncol Biol Phys* 1990;18:1165–1171.

52. Chang SD, et al. Treatment of hemangioblastomas in von Hippel-Lindau disease with linear accelerator-based radiosurgery. *Neurosurgery* 1998;43:28–34; discussion 34–35.

53. Niemela M, et al. Long-term prognosis of haemangioblastoma of the CNS: impact of von Hippel-Lindau disease. *Acta Neurochir* 1999;141:1147–1156.

54. Chakraborti PR, Chakrabarti KB, Doughty D, et al. Stereotactic multiple are radiotherapy. IV—Haemangioblastoma. *Br J Neurosurg* 1997;11:110–115.

55. Jawahar A, et al. Stereotactic radiosurgery for hemangioblastomas of the brain. *Acta Neurochir* 2000;142:641–644.

56. Pan L, et al. Gamma knife radiosurgery for hemangioblastomas. *Stereotact Funct Neurosurg* 1998;70:179–186.

57. Chandler HC, Friedman WA. Radiosurgical treatment of a hemangioblastoma: case report. *Neurosurgery* 1994;34:353–355; discussion 355.

58. Niemela M, Lim YJ, Soderman M, et al. Gamma knife radiosurgery in 11 hemangioblastomas. *J Neurosurg* 1996;85:591–596.

128. Preoperative and Intraoperative Mapping of Eloquent Cortex

Jayashree Srinivasan, Todd Parrish, and George A. Ojemann

Resection of lesions adjacent to eloquent areas of the brain poses a significant challenge for neurosurgeons. The ability to resect lesions such as tumors, arteriovenous malformations, and epileptic foci has improved as techniques for mapping the cerebral cortex have improved. Intraoperative cortical stimulation (ICS) remains the gold standard for identification of critical functional areas both on the cerebral cortex and in the subcortical tracts; however, in recent years, new technologies such as functional magnetic resonance imaging (fMRI) and $[^{15}O]H_2O$ positron emission tomography (PET) have been used for preoperative assessment and localization of functional cortex. Neurosurgeons who operate near eloquent cortex should familiarize themselves with the advantages and drawbacks of these various techniques.

Intraoperative Mapping

IDENTIFICATION OF ROLANDIC CORTEX. The location of the Rolandic cortex is relatively constant in human beings, although a lesion, particularly a congenital one, may displace it. For this reason, mapping of Rolandic cortex is the simplest mapping technique and may be performed under either local or general anesthesia. Direct cortical stimulation of the motor cortex may be done with a monopolar or bipolar stimulator. Most neurosurgeons use a bipolar cortical stimulator (Ojemann stimulator, Radionics, Burlington, MA) with a hand-held bipolar electrode that contains 5 mm of spacing between the tips. The advantage of bipolar stimulation is that the current is limited to the area between the tips with little spread out of this area. The stimulator is set to deliver a 60-Hz pulse with a 1-ms pulse width beginning at a setting of 2 mA for each phase of its biphasic wave form. The current level may be increased in 1-mA increments until a maximum level of 8 mA is reached or a response is obtained (1,2). If motor mapping is performed under general anesthesia, then paralytic agents obviously cannot be used. Instead, anesthesia is maintained with a combination of inhalation anesthetics, propofol, and fentanyl. The current requirement to generate a response is higher in the anesthetized patient than the awake patient (2,3). Currents up to 16 mA may be used for patients under general anesthesia and stimulation of subcortical fibers. This technique is very accurate (greater than 95%) for the identification of Rolandic cortex (4). However, one reason for failure is related to the depth of anesthesia and subsequent inability to elicit a motor response. Yingling and associates improved the efficiency of motor ICS by using multichannel electromyographic (EMG) recording in the face, arm, and leg contralateral to the Rolandic cortex being studied (2). They found that only EMG responses without visible motor activity were found in 9% of cases. The EMG also allowed early detection and therefore control of seizure activity. A significant source of error with motor mapping is found in patients with a neurological deficit (i.e., hemiparesis). A motor response may not be elicited with stimulation: EMG may potentially detect small responses, but this has yet to be studied. Rolandic cortex also may be identified by recording of somatosensory evoked potentials (SEP). In this method, a strip electrode is placed on the brain surface across the Rolandic cortex. SEPs then are recorded in a standard fashion and the location of the phase reversal noted. This corresponds to somatosensory cortex and identifies the central sulcus. Kombos and associates studied this technique in 68 patients and found it to be accurate in detection of the Rolandic cortex in 97% of patients (4). Failure of SEP recording may be related to shifting of the central sulcus by a mass, misplacement of the recording electrode, influence of general anesthesia, or presence of dural adhesions, which prevent correct placement of the electrode (4). The use of both direct motor stimulation and SEPs allows for a nearly 100% accuracy in identification of Rolandic cortex.

MAPPING OF LANGUAGE. Identification of eloquent language cortex in the brain is more difficult for several reasons. First, the location is extremely variable from patient to patient (5). Because the effect of cortical stimulation is to block function rather than evoke it (as in motor mapping), the currents required are larger and may provoke after-discharge potentials or even a seizure.

The craniotomy is performed under local anesthesia for language mapping. This technique is limited to children over the age of 12 years and most adolescents and adults because patient cooperation is necessary. The slides to be used intraoperatively for mapping are shown to the patient the day prior to surgery. This allows the patient to familiarize himself or herself with the test slides. Intraoperative mapping is inaccurate in patients with a naming error rate of greater than 25% because the random errors are difficult to distinguish from the evoked ones unless a large sample of stimulated responses is used (1).

The patient is placed in the lateral position and given intravenous (IV) propofol to induce anesthesia. Skeletal fixation is not used. Local anesthesia is given using 0.5% lidocaine and 0.2% bupivacaine with 1:200,000 epinephrine. This is combined with a sodium bicarbonate solution in a 9 to 1 ratio. Both the incision and areas around the major scalp nerves are infiltrated with anesthetic using a 30-gauge needle. A complete block is performed in this way. Small amounts of fentanyl may be given intravenously if the patient responds significantly to the injection of the local anesthetic.

The scalp incision and craniotomy then are performed in the usual fashion. Once the bone flap is removed, the propofol is discontinued; most patients are conversant within 7 to 12 minutes of stopping the propofol. Occasionally, a patient requires a longer period to awaken. The dura mater is opened in the standard fashion once the patient is awake. At this point, electrocorticography (ECoG) recording is performed. The after-discharge threshold is established with cortical stimulation during continuous ECoG recording. The current is increased in 1-mA increments until after-discharges are provoked or an upper limit of 10 mA is reached. The mapping is performed at the lowest threshold for after-discharge on any region of the brain surface.

The technique most commonly used for language mapping is visual object naming. This method, in addition to its simplicity, is preferred because all aphasic syndromes include naming deficits. Counting, which evaluates the function of Broca's area, and reading of short phrases, which assesses function in the posterior temporal region, may be performed in addition to object naming (3). Discrete cortical sites 1 to 2 cm^2 in size can be identified using bipolar stimulation. These language sites often are present in a mosaic pattern with noneloquent intervening brain tissue; most patients have at least two sites (5). For object naming, the slides with line drawings of objects are shown at four-second intervals. The surface is stimulated with the presentation of a new slide and contact maintained until the patient offers a correct response or until the next slide appears. A baseline response without stimulation is obtained following stimulation. Each site is stimulated at least three times but never in succession. A total of approximately 20 sites are stimulated (1,3). If seizure activity is noted on the ECoG, the cortex may be irrigated with cold saline solution, which inhibits the after-discharges. If the patient has a clinical seizure, it may be treated with IV methohexital (1 mm per kg) or an IV benzodiazepine.

Resection of Lesions

The resection may be carried out to the pial bank of the motor cortex for lesions located adjacent to hand motor cortex. Recovery of hand function following resection of hand motor cortex is poor. Face motor cortex may be safely resected in the nondominant hemisphere; however, in the dominant hemisphere, this resection carries a significant risk of dysarthria. Resection of leg motor cortex is possible; however, a prolonged period of weakness lasting months follows. Lesions invading primary somatosensory cortex may be resected somewhat more aggressively. The patient is left with a proprioceptive deficit postoperatively, and if this is in the dominant hemisphere, this deficit can be quite significant. The proximity of the sensory cortex to motor cortex mandates that motor stimulation be carried out during resection of these lesions at a current evoking responses with cortical stimulation (3).

Primary language sites are present essentially only on the surface cortex and not in buried cortex. Further, the fibers are organized in a vertical fashion with respect to the subcortical tracts (5). In resections for epilepsy, Ojemann and associates found that when anterior temporal resections came within 2 cm along the contiguous gyrus of a site where stimulation evoked repeated naming errors, testing with a sensitive aphasia battery 1 month after operation showed subtle language changes that were not present when the resection had not come within 2 cm (6). When Haglund and associates assessed postoperative deficits in tumors resected adjacent to eloquent cortex, they found that resection margins less than 1 cm away from a language site resulted in a permanent postoperative deficit in 40% of the patients. On the other hand, resections greater than 1.5 cm away from a language site led to no permanent deficits (7). Intraoperative mapping is essential for safe resection of all masses because of the variability of language sites between patients and because of some differences in language localization between patients with tumors and those without tumors (7). Black and colleagues found that resections close to sites of speech impairment seemed to produce less postoperative deficit than resections close to sites of speech arrest (8). The presence of an infiltrative lesion such as a glioma may result in functional tissue within the margins of the tumor. Skirboll and colleagues analyzed 28 patients who had motor or language function within the boundaries of a tumor, as determined by intraoperative mapping. This functional tissue limited the extent of resection in these patients. Their study population represented 7% of all patients who had undergone mapping for tumor resection during that time (9). Although functional tissue is present only in a minority of tumors, it is crucial that these areas be preserved.

Intraoperative mapping of eloquent cortex thus provides a measure of safety during resection of lesions in these regions. It is important to note that during mapping of language, different sites seem to be essential for naming in different languages (10), including sign and oral languages (11). Different sites are often essential for naming, reading, or verbal memory (12). Language mapping may need to be tailored to obtain an appropriate map in any given patient.

Preoperative Evaluation of Eloquent Cortex

Technological advances in imaging now allow preoperative evaluation of eloquent cortex. Although these methods are less accurate than intraoperative stimulation, they have the ability to visualize the entire brain and are not limited to the region of the craniotomy.

FUNCTIONAL MRI. The advent of fMRI introduces the possibility of identifying eloquent cortex preoperatively. fMRI is based on blood oxygenation level dependent (BOLD) imaging, usually using a 1.5 Tesla magnet. BOLD imaging takes advantage of susceptibility changes that occur locally because of the changing oxygenation levels in the blood in response to neuronal activation. Following cortical activation, there is an increase in cerebral blood flow approximately 4 to 8 seconds after activation. With the increase in perfusion, there is an increase in oxygenated blood and therefore a decrease in deoxyhemoglobin. The decrease in the deoxy Hb results in an increase in the susceptibility weighted magnetic resonance (MR) signal. When activity ceases, the perfusion falls and the MR signal returns to baseline; the actual percentage of MR signal change is in the 1% to 10% range (13). Because of this, a series of data points collected and processed with a statistical model is required to accurately localize functional cortex. A review of the physics of this technique is beyond the scope of this text; the reader is referred to an excellent review of the topic (13).

The use of fMRI to identify motor cortex has been studied extensively over the past few years. The largest study by Lehericy and associates assessed 60 patients harboring brain tumors close to Rolandic cortex. Motor deficit was either quite mild or absent in those patients. When the fMRI data were compared to intraoperative cortical stimulation, there was a 92% correlation between the two methods (14). The remaining sites were within 15 mm of the margins of the activated areas on fMRI. fMRI even identified functional cortex within the boundaries of a tumor. Of importance, the size of the activated sensorimotor cortex was frequently larger by fMRI than cortical stimulation (14). This finding obviously is significant with regard to extent of resection parameters. An interesting observation was made by Roux and co-workers when fMRI and intraoperative brain mapping were used to study patients with significant hemiparesis. They described five hemiparetic patients with a cerebral tumor who had significant ipsilateral activation on fMRI preoperatively. No hand movement could be elicited by the contralateral hemisphere with intraoperative stimulation. This activation pattern reversed to a normal pattern postoperatively, although it did not necessarily correlate with the extent of functional recovery (15). They hypothesized that this ipsilateral cortical activation was secondary to an unmasking of preexistent functional cortex owing to temporary disinhibition. For a neurosurgeon, the importance of this paper lies in the fact that the absence of contralateral Rolandic activity by fMRI or intraoperative cortical stimulation does not indicate irreversible damage to the motor cortex (Fig. 1).

The comparison between fMRI and intraoperative mapping of language areas has been more limited. In both fMRI and positron emission tomography (PET), visual object naming results in very diffuse activation of cerebral cortex, including the visual areas. Therefore, this has not been as useful a technique to identify discrete sites. Instead, other techniques have been used, including visual and auditory verb generation. Herholz and co-workers found a correlation of 81.9% between intraoperative object naming and verb generation using preoperative PET scanning (16). The concordance is not absolute. Few studies have compared functional MR imaging with intraoperative electrocortical stimulation. Fitzgerald and associates studied 11 patients with lesions by fMRI followed by intraoperative cortical stimulation. The intraoperative photograph was digitized and then compared to the fMRI image. For all language tests overall, they found a 48% sensitivity and a 44% specificity for fMRI if the areas identified by each technique were adjacent to one another. If a 1-cm separation was allowed between the areas identified by cortical stimulation versus functional MRI, an overall 63% sensitivity and 24% specificity was found. Using this criterion, verb generation had a sensitivity of 90% but persistently low specificity (17). Ruge and associates studied language

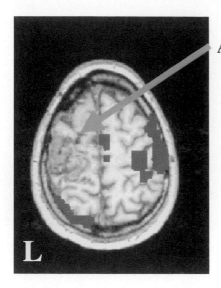
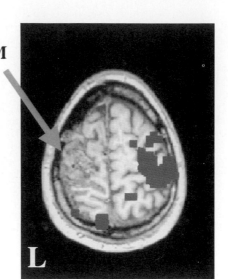

AVM

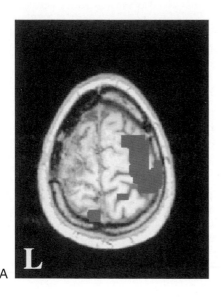
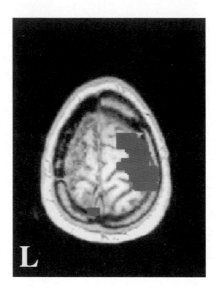

A

Fig. 1. A patient with a left frontal arteriovenous malformation (AVM) underwent functional MRI (fMRI) to evaluate the location of motor cortex. **A:** A left-hand motor task appropriately activates the right hemisphere Rolandic cortex. *Figure continues.*

function in five patients. They found a 100% correlation between fMRI and intraoperative physiology for both Broca's and Wernicke's areas, but they did not provide the specific criteria they used for this comparison, including the degree of overlap of the areas identified by the two techniques (18).

An error of 10 mm is not acceptable in operative decision making because the extent of resection is determined by the very specific localization of functional cortex. This is a significant disadvantage of fMRI when this information is transferred to the operating room. Another disadvantage is that although subcortical fibers may be identified by intraoperative stimulation, these cannot be identified by fMRI or PET. fMRI may become more precise for localization of eloquent cortex as the technology improves.

POSITRON EMISSION TOMOGRAPHY. PET using [^{15}O]H$_2$O has been used for functional mapping. Similar to fMRI,

PET measures the increase in regional cerebral blood flow with activation of functional cortex. Vinas and colleagues used PET in 12 patients and performed an MRI/PET coregistration. They then performed intraoperative mapping of motor or language cortex. They found good correlation in all patients but did not specify the size of the activated cortex by PET (19). They did note that during intraoperative stimulation, subcortical pathways were activated, which were not seen on the PET scan. Herholtz and associates studied language areas using PET and intraoperative stimulation. They found 73% sensitivity and 81% specificity for PET to predict aphasic disturbance during intraoperative stimulation (16). In addition, they found the overall resolution of PET to be approximately 10 mm. This level of specificity and sensitivity makes reliance on PET alone unacceptable. Bittar and colleagues compared fMRI and PET and found that the average distance between activation peaks was 7.9 ± 4.8 mm (20). The language cortex must be precisely mapped to obtain maximal resection of a lesion. At this point in time, such accuracy is not possible with PET scanning. In

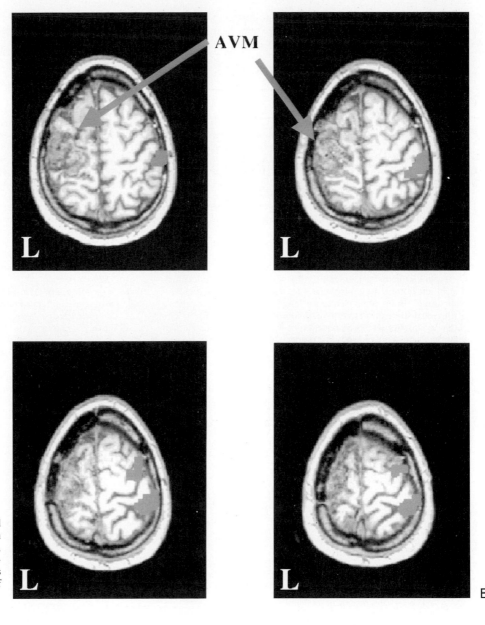

AVM

Fig. 1. *Continued.* **B:** A right-hand motor task results in cortical activation only in the ipsilateral right hemisphere, indicating rearrangement of motor function to this hemisphere. The fMRI allows detection of functional cortex outside of the boundaries of the craniotomy.

B

addition, a significant disadvantage of PET imaging is the high cost and limited availability of this technique.

Integration of Preoperative Mapping with Surgical Navigation Systems

Schulder and co-workers synthesized fMRI of sensorimotor cortex onto a frameless stereotactic surgical navigation device (STEALTH, Sofamor Danek, Memphis, TN). They were able to localize somatosensory cortex intraoperatively using this technique. However, they found an average error rate of 6.6 mm in the 12 patients, which results from a combination of the inherent error in the fMRI and the intrinsic error in the frameless

navigational system (21). At this time, such an error rate limits reliance on fMRI or PET as a substitute for intraoperative mapping. As these techniques become more refined in the future, they may allow neurosurgeons to transfer preoperative data with reasonable precision to the operating room.

Overview

Evaluation and identification of functional cortex allows safer resections of lesions located adjacent to eloquent cortex. Preoperative mapping techniques include PET and fMRI. However, they do not provide a degree of accuracy that can be used to guide surgical resection because of the inherent errors in these techniques and the transfer of the map to the operating theater. The intraoperative stimulation remains the gold standard for resection of lesions adjacent to functional cortex, particularly for identification of language areas. This may change in the future as imaging techniques improve.

References

1. Ojemann GA. Awake operations with mapping in epilepsy. In: Schmidek HH, Sweet WH, eds. *Operative neurosurgical techniques*, 3rd ed. Philadelphia: WB Saunders, 1995:1317–1322.
2. Yingling CD, Ojemann S, Dodson B, et al. Identification of motor pathways during tumor surgery facilitated by multichannel electromyographic recording. *J Neurosurg* 1999;91:922–927.
3. Matz PG, Cobb C, Berger MS. Intraoperative cortical mapping as a guide to the surgical resection of gliomas. *J Neuro-Oncol* 1999;42: 233–245.
4. Kombos T, Seuss O, Funk T, et al. Intra-operative mapping of the motor cortex during surgery in an around the motor cortex. *Acta Neurochir* 2000;142:263–268.
5. Ojemann G, Ojemann J, Lettich E, et al. Cortical language localization in left-dominant hemisphere. *J Neurosurg* 1989;71:316–326.
6. Ojemann G. Brain organization for language from the perspective of electrical stimulation mapping. *Behav Brain Sci* 1983;6:189–230.
7. Haglund MM, Berger MS, Shamseldin M, et al. Cortical localization of temporal lobe language sites in patients with gliomas. *Neurosurgery* 1994;34:567–576.
8. Black P, Ronner S. Cortical mapping for defining the limits of tumor resection. *Neurosurgery* 1987;20:914–919.
9. Skirboll SS, Ojemann GA, Berger MS. Functional cortex and subcortical white matter located within gliomas. *Neurosurgery* 1996;38: 678–685.
10. Ojemann GA, Whitaker HA. The bilingual brain. *Arch Neurol* 1978; 35:409–412.
11. Haglund MM, Ojemann G, Lettich E, et al. Dissociation of cortical and single unit activity in spoken and signed language. *Brain Lang* 1993;44:19–27.
12. Mateer CA, Polen SB, Ojemann GA, et al. Cortical localization of finger spelling and oral language: a case study. *Brain Lang* 1982; 17:46–57.
13. Parrish T. Functional MR imaging. *Magn Reson Imaging Clin N Am* 1999;7:765–782.
14. Lehericy S, Duffau H, Cornu P, et al. Correspondence between functional magnetic resonance imaging somatotopy and individual brain anatomy of the central region: comparison with intraoperative stimulation in patients with brain tumors. *J Neurosurg* 2000;92:589–598.
15. Roux FE, Boulanouar K, Ibarrola D, et al. Functional MRI and intraoperative brain mapping to evaluate brain plasticity in patients with brain tumours and hemiparesis. *J Neurol Neurosurg Psychiatry* 2000; 69:453–463.
16. Herholz K, Reulen H, von Stockhausen H, et al. Preoperative activation and intraoperative stimulation of language-related areas in patients with glioma. *Neurosurgery* 1997;41:1253–1262.
17. Fitzgerald DB, Cosgrove GR, Ronner S, et al. Location of language in the cortex: a comparison between functional MR imaging and eletrocortical stimulation. *AJNR Am J Neuroradiol* 1997;18: 1529–1539.
18. Ruge MI, Victor J, Hosain S, et al. Concordance between functional magnetic resonance imaging and intraoperative language mapping. *Stereotact Funct Neurosurg* 2000;72:95–102.
19. Vinas FC, Zamorano L, Mueller R, et al. [^{15}O]-water PET and intraoperative brain mapping: a comparison in the localization of eloquent cortex. *Neurol Res* 1997;19:601–608.
20. Bittar RG, Olivier A, Sadikoff AF, et al. Presurgical motor and somatosensory cortex mapping with functional magnetic resonance imaging and positron emission tomography. *J Neurosurg* 1999;91: 915–921.
21. Schulder M, Maldjian JA, Liu W, et al. Functional image-guided surgery of intracranial tumors located in or near the sensorimotor cortex. *J Neurosurg* 1998;89:412–418.

VI. Spinal Disorders

Section Editor
Stephen L. Ondra

129. Developmental Anatomy of the Spine

David G. McLone and Mark S. Dias

Vertebral column development begins during gastrulation, and continues through postnatal life. To properly understand this process, it is important to know how segmentation occurs in the developing organism.

In higher organisms segmental organization is necessary during development to allow the independent development of structurally and functionally different body regions. The antero-posterior and dorsoventral orientation of the embryo is determined by specific genes. The discovery of particular *homeobox* genes, which direct segmental development, provides proof of direct genomic control of segmentation; the development of single segments of the organism is under direct control of specific regions of the genome (1).

Normal Development of the Spine

GASTRULATION AND FORMATION OF SOMITES. Members of the subphylum Vertebrata, which is a division of the phylum Chordata, are characterized by the presence of a segmented bony or cartilaginous spinal column. In mammalian embryos, prospective mesodermal cells, which will form the vertebral column, are located in the epiblast; during gastrulation these cells ingress through the Hensen node and the cranial half of the primitive streak, and spread bilaterally to form the definitive mesodermal layer between the overlying ectoderm and underlying endoderm. Prospective mesodermal cells in the Hensen node will form the notochordal process, whereas prospective mesodermal cells of the primitive streak will form the remaining mesoderm. Mesodermal cells begin ingressing through the primitive streak during mid- to late gastrulation (during Hensen node regression) and do so in an orderly fashion. Prospective notochordal cells within the Hensen node are the first mesodermal cells to ingress and pass cranially in the midline between the ectoderm and the endoderm. Cells located within the primitive streak ingress in a craniocaudal sequence. Cells that will form more medial mesodermal structures (e.g., prospective somitic mesoderm) ingress first and are more cranially located within the primitive streak, whereas cells that will form more lateral mesodermal structures (e.g., prospective limb mesoderm) ingress later and are more caudally located (2).

The definitive mesoderm subsequently becomes organized, from medial to lateral, in paraxial (lying immediately lateral to the notochord) or somitic mesoderm, intermediate mesoderm, and lateral plate mesoderm. The paraxial mesoderm contributes to the formation of the somites, while the intermediate mesoderm contributes to the formation of the genitourinary system and the lateral plate mesoderm contributes to the musculoskeletal components of the limbs. The somitic mesoderm subsequently becomes segmented to form discrete blocks of tissue called somites (3,4). The somites are bilaterally paired structures which lie on either side of the midline notochord, and contribute to the formation of the axial skeleton (vertebrae and ribs),

as well as the muscles of the trunk and the dermis of the body wall. The fate of the cells that will form the vertebrae is already specified to a considerable extent at the time of somitic segmentation; however, as Bellairs and colleagues (5) have suggested, these cells must be supplemented by other cells from the primitive streak to fulfill their ultimate fate. The notochord involutes during later development; remnants of the notochord persist as the nucleus pulposus of the mature spine (6).

The formation of the neural tube both precedes and continues during somitic segmentation. The neural tube provides the principal stimulus for somitic segmentation (7). Prospective somitic cells within the paraxial mesoderm are located immediately subjacent to the neural plate during early neurulation, extending as far laterally as the lateral edges of the neural plate. As neurulation proceeds, these cells occupy a position immediately lateral to the developing neural tube (Fig. 1). Condensation of these paraxial mesodermal cells and cleavage of the cells into discrete masses produces the somites (Fig. 2). In chick embryos somitic cells surround a central lumen to form a complete rosette, whereas in mammalian embryos the lumen is incomplete inferomedially. Somitic cells are joined both apically and basally by junctional processes (8); the apical regions contain actin microfilaments similar to those found in neuroepithelial cells (9).

The somite is divided into a dorsal dermomyotome and a ventral sclerotome (10,11). The dermomyotomal portion gives rise to dermal elements and to the myocytes of the dorsal muscles. The cells of the sclerotomal portion surround the notochord and form the primordia of the developing axial skeleton (vertebrae and ribs).

The number of somites that develop appears to be species-specific and is relatively constant (12). If somitic mesoderm is removed prior to somitic segmentation, regulation occurs such that the number of somites that form is unchanged, but the size of the somites is somewhat reduced. During later development, even the sizes of the somites is reconstituted such that the fetus will appear to be normal (13,14).

The subsequent development of the somites into the vertebral elements can be divided into three overlapping phases (15). The initial, or *membranous* phase, begins at 5 weeks of gestation; the second, or *cartilaginous* phase, begins at 6 weeks of gestation; and the final, or *osseous* phase, begins at about 9 weeks of gestation.

MEMBRANOUS PHASE. During the membranous phase, sclerotomal cells move toward and surround the notochord (Fig. 3). The cells of the sclerotome are divided into a loosely packed rostral cell mass and a more dense caudal cell mass. The junction between the rostral and caudal portions of the sclerotome forms a cleft, called the fissure of von Ebner. Each vertebra has been thought to receive contributions from two adjacent somites in a process called *resegmentation* (16) (Fig. 4). Experiments in which chick vertebrae were excised and replaced with corresponding quail vertebrae (the fate of the transplanted quail tissue can be followed using a nucleolar marker) suggest that, during resegmentation, the centrum of

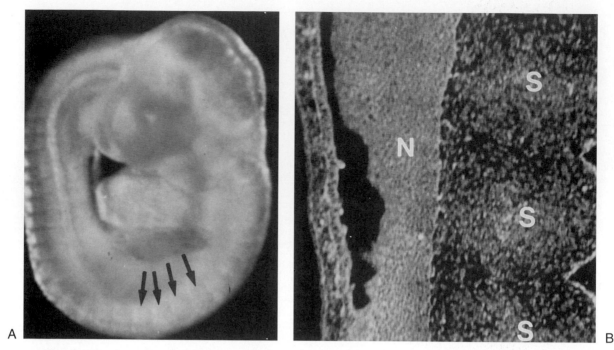

Fig. 1. A: Mouse embryo clearly shows the segmentation of spine with prominent somites *(arrows)*. **B:** A light micrograph shows the somites *(S)* separated next to the developing neural tube *(N)*.

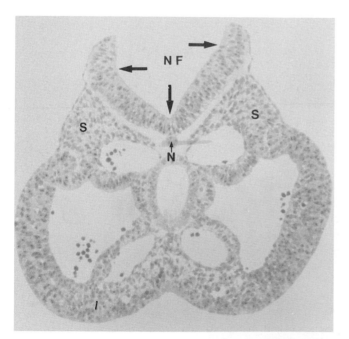

Fig. 2. A transverse section light micrograph of an embryo demonstrates the neural folds *(NF)* and bilateral somites *(S)*. The notochord *(N with arrow)* lies immediately ventral to the neural tube. (From McLone DG, Dias MS. Normal and abnormal development of the spine. In: Cheek WR, Marlin AE, McLone DG, et al., eds. *Pediatric neurosurgery: surgery of the developing nervous system.* Philadelphia: WB Saunders, 1994:40–50, with permission.)

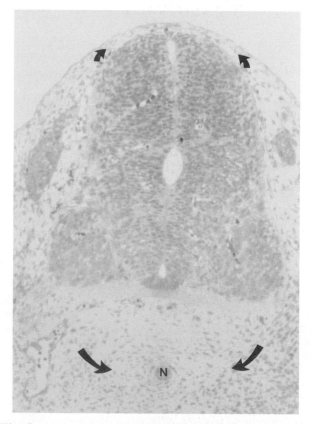

Fig. 3. A light micrograph of a mouse embryo at 11 days of gestation shows the notochord *(N))* has moved ventrally, away from the neural tube, and mesenchymal cells *(arrows))* are streaming from the adjacent somites to surround the notochord and dorsal neural tube. (From McLone DG, Dias MS. Normal and abnormal development of the spine. In: Cheek WR, Marlin AE, McLone DG, et al., eds. *Pediatric neurosurgery: surgery of the developing nervous system.* Philadelphia: WB Saunders, 1994:40–50, with permission.)

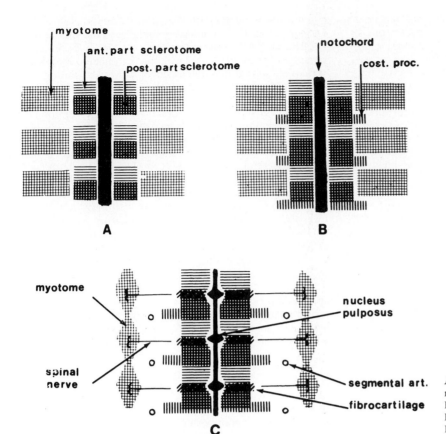

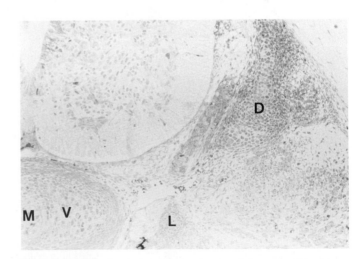

Fig. 4. Schematic illustration showing developmental changes in the sclerotome and notochord. **A:** Embryonic. **B:** Resegmentation. **C:** Mature. (From Park WW. Development of the spine. In: Rothman RH, Simeone FA, eds. *The spine.* Vol 1. Philadelphia: WB Saunders, 1975:1–17, with permission.)

each vertebral body is formed from the caudal region of the more rostral sclerotome and the rostral region of the more caudal sclerotome (17). However, the concept of resegmentation has been questioned by others (18), and equally plausible mechanisms have been proposed. The fate of the rostral and caudal portions of the sclerotome also differ in that only the caudal sclerotome participate in the formation of the neural arches and costal processes. The cells within the cleft of von Ebner proliferate and contribute to the intervening intervertebral disc.

The contributions of each of the somites to vertebrate development is unclear. Following unilateral removal of as much as 90% of the somites in the chick, the vertebrae are fully or very nearly reconstituted from the remaining somitic mesoderm such that normal or only minimally malformed vertebrae (i.e., those missing only a single process) result; hemivertebrae and other complex vertebral malformations of the type usually encountered in clinical practice are rare (14). Even following bilateral removal of somites at a single level, chick embryos are capable of establishing a normal pattern of vertebrae. This extraordinary ability for embryonic regulation may well explain the infrequent occurrence of vertebral anomalies in clinical practice.

CHONDRIFICATION PHASE. Chondrification centers appear during week 6 of embryogenesis. Initially, three paired centers of chondrification form (Fig. 5). The first pair surrounds the notochord and fuses ventral to the neural tube to form the centrum of the vertebral body. The second pair forms dorsolaterally and fuses dorsal to the neural tube to become the posterior neural arch and spinous process. The final pair develops between the ventral and dorsal pairs and forms the transverse

Fig. 5. A mammalian embryo during the chondrification phase shows the three paired centers of chondrification—ventral *(V)*, dorsal *(D)*, and intermediate or lateral *(L)*—surrounding the mucoid streak *(M)*. (From McLone DG. Development of the spine and spinal cord. In: Cockard A, Hayward R, Hoff J, eds. *Neurosurgery. The scientific basis of clinical practice,* Vol 1, 2nd ed. London: Blackwell Scientific, 1992: 84–91, with permission.)

process. Chondrification begins at the cervicothoracic junction and extends both cranial and caudal thereafter. The centrum is the first portion of the vertebra to chondrify; the dorsal neural arch chondrifies later. Chondrification is initiated in response to substances secreted by both the notochord and the ventral portion of the developing neural tube through a process known as "inductive tissue interaction" (19).

The anterior and posterior longitudinal ligaments form during the chondrification phase and are derived from the mesenchyme surrounding the cartilaginous vertebrae. The intervertebral disc develops from densely aggregated somitic mesoderm and receives contributions from both rostral and caudal halves of adjacent sclerotome. The vertebral cartilages are initially contiguous with the cartilage of the intervertebral discs so that the vertebral column exits as a continuous cartilaginous column. Later, as the vertebrae ossify, the discs become distinct from the adjacent vertebrae; the intervertebral cartilage differentiates to form the fibrocartilaginous component of the intervertebral disc (6). A ring of perinotochordal tissue forms the annulus fibrosus. Notochordal remnants contribute to the nucleus pulposus and mucoid streak within the vertebra centra.

OSSIFICATION PHASE. Ossification of the vertebral column begins in the second gestational month and continues into postnatal life (Fig. 6). Ossification is initiated within four *primary ossification centers,* two in the vertebral centrum and one in each side of the dorsal neural arch. The vertebral body becomes ossified from both dorsal and ventral ossification centers that fuse during weeks 20 to 24 of gestation to form a single ossification center. Cartilaginous zones develop rostral and caudal to the vertebral ossification centers and will form the cartilaginous end plates adjacent to the intervertebral discs. At the periphery of the cartilaginous end plates, a C-shaped ring of cartilaginous material, the *ring apophysis,* develops in intimate association with the lateral borders of the vertebral bodies and with the

annulus of the intervening discs at the centrum–disc interface and firmly attaches the intervertebral disc to the vertebral bodies. The ring apophysis is similar to the epiphysis of the long bones, and eventually fuses with the peripheral portions of the vertebrae during mid-adolescence. However, during childhood, the apophyseal ring may become fractured and dislocate posteriorly into the spinal canal; symptoms and signs of neural impingement simulate those of a herniated intervertebral disc.

Ossification of the paired dorsal neural arches proceeds medially within the laminae and ventrally within the pedicles; the junction of the dorsal and ventral ossification centers marks the neurocentral synchondrosis (20) (Fig. 7). The *neurocentral joint* lies within the developing vertebral body; therefore the terms centrum and vertebral body are not equivalent, since the vertebral body contains elements derived from both the centrum and dorsal ossification centers (Fig. 8).

Ossification of the vertebral bodies begins in the lower thoracic and upper lumbar spine and proceeds both cranially and caudally from this point. Ossification of the dorsal neural arch begins cranially in the cervical spine and proceeds caudally; however, the final union of the laminae begins in the lumbar spine and proceeds cranially (21,22).

Secondary ossification centers appear later during childhood, and are located in the transverse processes, spinous processes, and ring apophyses. These secondary centers fuse with the primary centers by 15 to 16 years of age.

An understanding of vertebral development allows some insight into how vertebral malformations might arise. For example, hemivertebrae may result from unilateral maldevelopment of a cartilaginous center and, secondarily, a vertebral centrum. In contrast, anterior or posterior anomalies of the vertebral bodies might arise from defects in ventral or dorsal vertebral body ossification centers (Fig. 9).

Dorsal laminar fusion usually occurs by 1 to 3 years of age. However, a localized failure of laminar fusion may occur at one or more segments as spina bifida occulta (23).

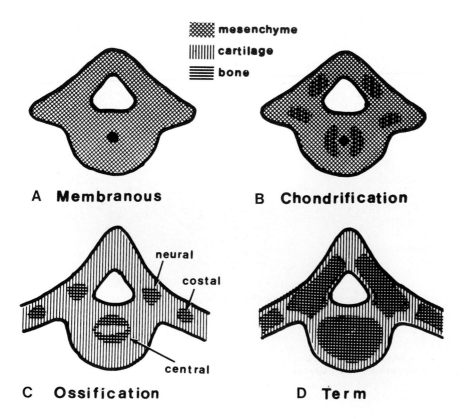

Fig. 6. Schematic illustration of the sequential development of vertebral components: membranous **(A)**, chondrification **(B)**, ossification **(C)**, term **(D)**. (From Parke WW. Development of the spine. In Rothman RH, Simeone FA, eds. *The spine.* Vol 1. Philadelphia: WB Saunders, 1975: 1–17, with permission.)

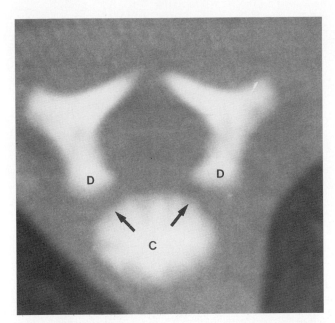

Fig. 7. CT scan through the vertebra of a term human infant shows the single ossification center in the centrum *(C)* and the paired dorsal ossification centers *(D)*. *Arrows* indicate the cartilaginous neurocentral synchondrosis. (From McLone DG, Dias MS. Normal and abnormal development of the spine. In: Cheek WR, Marlin AE, McLone DG, et al., eds. *Pediatric neurosurgery: surgery of the developing nervous system.* Philadelphia: WB Saunders, 1994:40–50, with permission.)

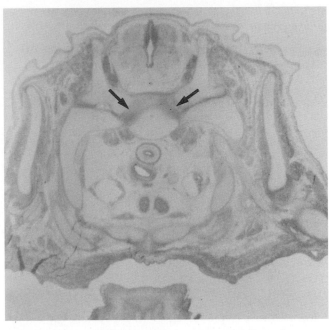

Fig. 8. Light micrograph of a human embryo at 35 days of gestation shows the contribution of the dorsal ossification center to the vertebral body *(arrows)*. (From McLone DG, Dias MS. Normal and abnormal development of the spine. In: Cheek WR, Marlin AE, McLone DG, et al., eds. *Pediatric neurosurgery: surgery of the developing nervous system.* Philadelphia: WB Saunders, 1994:40–50, with permission.)

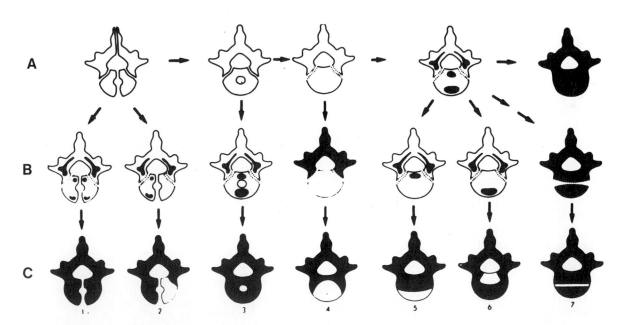

Fig. 9. Normal vertebral development and possible developmental malformations. Cartilaginous development is shown in *white,* ossification in *black.* **A:** Normal sequence. **B:** Intermediate stage of abnormal development. **C:** Final stage of abnormality. *1,* sagittal cleft of body (butterfly vertebrae) results from nonfusion of the bilaterally paired cartilaginous centers; *2,* hemivertebrae result from nonfusion of the cartilaginous centers and subsequent nondevelopment of the ossification centers on one side; *3,* notochordal remnants; *4,* absent vertebral body results from nondevelopment of ossification centers; *5,* hypoplastic vertebral body from nondevelopment of the anterior ossification center; *6,* hypoplastic vertebral body from nondevelopment of the posterior ossification center; *7,* failure of fusion of the anterior and posterior ossification centers. (From Harwood-Nash DC, Fitz CR. *Neuroradiology of infants and children.* St. Louis: CV Mosby, 1976, with permission.)

DEVELOPMENT OF THE CRANIOVERTEBRAL JUNC-
TION. While the general developmental plan previously discussed holds true for the majority of the spine, the two ends of
the spine (the craniovertebral junction and the sacrum) undergo
significant modifications. The development of the craniovertebral junction is particularly complex and embryologically unstable; malformations are therefore more frequent in this location. The development of this region is covered in greater detail
in Chapter 152; its development will be only briefly summarized
here.

The craniovertebral junction (encompassing the basicranium,
axis, and atlas) develops from the last four occipital somites
and the C-1 sclerotome (24). The basicranium is formed from
the first four somites and forms the clivus, occipital condyles,
and occipital squama. The C-1 vertebral ring develops from the
caudal portion of the first cervical sclerotome and the rostral
portion of the second cervical sclerotome. This vertebra does
not contain a centrum, but rather forms the C-1 vertebral ring.
The "body" of C-1 is actually incorporated into the axis as the
odontoid process. The odontoid also receives a contribution
form the fourth occipital sclerotome at its tip. The remainder
of the axis (the body and posterior neural arch) is derived from
the second cervical sclerotome.

The axis ossifies from two ossification centers, one in each
of the lateral masses. The axis ossifies from five separate ossification centers: one that gives rise to the tip of the dens (derived
from the fourth occipital sclerotome); two that form the dens
proper (derived from the first cervical sclerotome); and one
each for the body and posterior neural arch (both derived from
the second cervical sclerotome). The dens is formed from bilaterally paired ossification centers which are present by 10 to 24
weeks of gestation and which ultimately fuse to make a single
structure (Figs. 10 and 11). Fusion of the dens with the axis
body begins at about 4 years of age and is completed by about
8 years; fusion of the tip of the dens with the dens proper does
not occur until about 12 years.

A number of anomalies may arise through abnormal development of this complex region. The atlas may fail to completely
separate from the basiocciput and remain fused with the clivus,
a condition known as assimilation of the atlas. The anterior or
posterior atlas ossification centers may fail to develop or to fuse
properly, resulting in bifid or deficient C-1 laminae or anterior
arch. Failure of the odontoid to properly fuse with the axis body

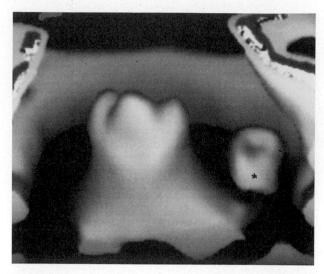

Fig. 11. Three-dimensional CT reconstruction of the atlas and axis
in a child demonstrates the three components of the odontoid. Note
also the presence of an accessory ossification center *(asterisk)*. (From
McLone DG, Dias MS. Normal and abnormal development of the spine.
In: Cheek WR, Marlin AE, McLone DG, et al., eds. *Pediatric neurosurgery: surgery of the developing nervous system*. Philadelphia: WB Saunders, 1994:40–50, with permission.)

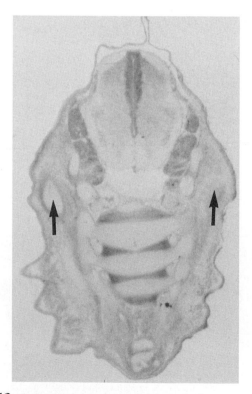

Fig. 12. Photomicrograph of the caudal vertebral segments of a 35-
day-old human embryo shows the segmental development of the sacrum with the two additional lateral centers *(arrows)*. (From McLone
DG, Dias MS. Normal and abnormal development of the spine. In:
Cheek WR, Marlin AE, McLone DG, et al., eds. *Pediatric neurosurgery:
surgery of the developing nervous system*. Philadelphia: WB Saunders,
1994:40–50, with permission.)

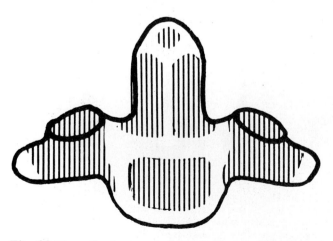

Fig. 10. The ossification centers of the axis. The paired lateral centers
and central ossification center are the same as for the remaining vertebrae; however, the odontoid shows two bilaterally paired primary centers and a single secondary apical center. (From Parke WW. Development of the spine. In: Rothman RH, Simeone FA, eds. *The spine*. Vol
1. Philadelphia: WB Saunders, 1975:1–7, with permission.)

results in an *os odontoideum;* failure of the odontoid tip to fuse with odontoid proper results in *ossiculum terminale* (or *os avis*). Failure of the odontoid to properly form from the second cervical sclerotome results in odontoid agenesis or hypoplasia. These malformations are discussed in greater detail in Chapter 152.

DEVELOPMENT OF THE SACRUM AND COCCYX. The sacral and coccygeal vertebrae are the last to develop at 31 days of gestation. In addition to the normal developmental sequence previously described, the first three sacral elements contain an extra pair of ossification centers (Fig. 12). Fusion of the sacral vertebrae begins during early puberty and is complete by the middle part of the third decade.

The coccyx is formed from rudimentary segments; ossification of the first segment begins between 1 and 4 years of age. The remaining coccygeal segments ossify in rostrocaudal order from 5 to 20 years of age. The coccyx is usually segmented, although fusion occasionally occurs.

POSTNATAL DEVELOPMENT OF THE SPINE. The developmental changes of the spine during childhood are readily evaluated by standard radiographs or with computed tomography (CT). Magnetic resonance imaging (MRI) techniques offer a new noninvasive means to study the developing spine (25). During the first two postnatal years, the spine demonstrates changes related to ossification of the cartilaginous end plates, conversion of red marrow to yellow marrow, responses to weight-bearing stresses, and changes in the water content of the disc. During the first six postnatal months, the spine is relatively straight due in part to the lack of weight-bearing forces. Red marrow occupies the vertebral body, and is hypointense on T1- and T2-weighted images. The cartilaginous end plates are hyperintense on T1-weighted images and hypointense on T2-weighted images.

By six postnatal months, the end plates have largely ossified, and become hypointense on both T1- and T2-weighted images. Between 6 and 12 months, the red marrow is replaced by yellow marrow; this gives a mixed signal that is slightly hyperintense on T1-weighted images and hypointense of T2-weighted images. The intervertebral disc at this age is isointense on T1-weighted images and hypointense on T2-weighted images (Figs. 13A–C).

The spine during gestation has a C-shaped profile. Postnatally, this curve begins to straighten and a lordotic curve devel-

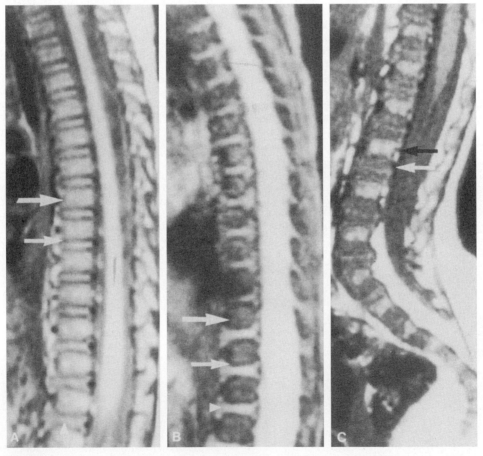

Fig. 13. MRIs of thoracic upper lumbar spine (sagittal view) in a 7-month-old infant. **A:** T1-weighted image shows slight hyperintensity of the bone marrow *(large arrow)*, hypointensity of the ossifying end plates *(small arrow)*, and isointensity of the intervertebral discs *(arrowhead)*. **B:** T2-weighted image shows hypointensity of the bone marrow *(large arrow)*, hypointensity of the cortical end plates *(small arrow)*, and hyperintensity of the intervertebral discs *(arrowhead)*. **C:** MRI of lower thoracic and lumbosacral spine (sagittal view) in a 7-month-old infant. T1-weighted image shows a striated appearance to the vertebral bodies with the upper half demonstrating hyperintensity *(black arrow)* and the lower half demonstrating hypointensity *(white arrow)*. (From Bryd SE, Wilczynski MA. Imaging modalities for the pediatric spine. *Curr Opin Radiol* 1991;6:906–918, with permission.)

ops in the lumbar region. The final configuration of spinal curvature develops during early childhood.

As the child begins to sit and then to stand, the normal spinal curvatures begin to appear. From 6 months to 2 years of age, the vertebral bodies undergo a normal but unusual change in imaging characteristics. The rostral half of each vertebral body becomes hyperintense on T1-weighted images, whereas the lower half becomes hypointense. This difference is not appreciated on T2-weighted images. By 2 years of age, these changes have disappeared, and the child has a more characteristic composition and a curvature reminiscent of the adult spine. The ossified cortex of the vertebrae at this age are hypointense on all sequences. The intervertebral disc, annulus fibrosus, and nucleus pulposus can all usually be differentiated by 5 years of age.

Congenital Anomalies of the Spine

As previously discussed, congenital anomalies of the spine are relatively rare and are perhaps related to the enormous capacity of the embryo to regulate and overcome developmental insults. The cause of many of these vertebral anomalies is obscure; however, extrapolating from what we know of normal spinal development allows some insight into the timing and pathogenesis of these insults.

Vertebral malformations may conveniently be divided into those that arise through a disorder of formation, and those that represent a disorder of segmentation. In many instances, disorders of both formation and segmentation will coexist.

Defects of vertebral formation may be partial or complete, and may be unilateral or bilateral. Examples of unilateral partial failures of formation include wedge or trapezoid vertebrae, whereas unilateral complete failure results in hemivertebrae (Fig. 14). Complete failure of the vertebral development usually

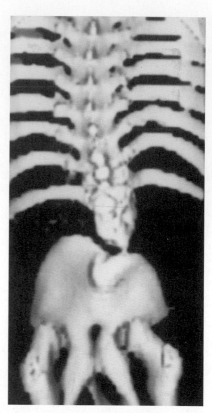

Fig. 15. A reformatted image of a spine CT in a child with caudal agenesis. Note the absence of most of the lumbar vertebrae and all of the sacral spine. (From McLone DG, Dias MS. Normal and abnormal development of the spine. In: Cheek WR, Marlin AE, McLone DG, et al., eds. *Pediatric neurosurgery: surgery of the developing nervous system.* Philadelphia: WB Saunders, 1994:40–50, with permission.)

involves the caudal spine and results in lumbar and/or sacral agenesis (Fig. 15).

Defects in segmentation result in failure of separation of the vertebrae and various degrees of vertebral fusion. Examples of defective segmentation include block vertebrae and unsegmented bars. The disorder may be limited to two adjacent vertebrae, or may extend over several vertebral segments. Anterior, posterior, or combined fusions may exist in isolation or combination. The Klippel-Feil syndrome represents a severe form of multifocal segmentation anomaly in which multiple adjacent vertebrae are fused in various combinations. Lateral segmentation anomalies are thought to arise during membranous and cartilaginous phases of vertebral development, whereas vertebral body segmentation anomalies are thought to arise through disordered ossification.

The outcome from vertebral anomalies is variable. Hemivertebrae or wedge-shaped vertebrae may contribute to asymmetrical growth of the spine and result in scoliosis; unilateral segmentation anomalies such as unsegmented bars have a similar fate, and carry the worst prognosis for progressive spinal deformity. Bilateral segmentation anomalies such as block vertebrae result in the least spinal deformity, but limit growth at that segment. Symmetrical anterior segmentation anomalies generally produce kyphosis, while posterior anomalies produce lordosis.

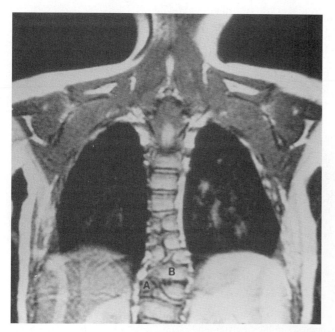

Fig. 14. MRI of the spine in a child shows multiple appropriate labeled segmentation anomalies. Both wedge **(A)** and hemivertebrae **(B)** are present. (From McLone DG, Dias MS. Normal and abnormal development of the spine. In: Cheek WR, Marlin AE, McLone DG, et al., eds. *Pediatric neurosurgery: surgery of the developing nervous system.* Philadelphia: WB Saunders, 1994:40–50, with permission.)

References

1. Keynes RJ, Stern CD. Mechanisms of vertebrate segmentation. *Development* 1988;103:413.

2. Schoenwolf GC, Garcia-Martinez V, Dias MS. Mesoderm movement and fate during avian gastrulation and neurulation. *Dev Dynamics* 1992;193:235.

3. Tam PPL, Meier S. The establishment of a somitomeric pattern in the mesoderm of the gastrulating mouse embryo. *Am J Anat* 1982; 164:209.

4. Lipton BH, Jacobson AG. Analysis of normal somite development. *Dev Biol* 1974;38:73.

5. Bellairs R, Veine M. Experimental analysis of control mechanisms in somite segmentation in avian embryos. II. Reduction of material in the gastrula stages of the chick. *J Embryol Exp Morph* 1984;79: 183.

6. Peacock A. Observations on the pre-natal development of the intervertebral disc in man. *J Anat* 1951;85:260.

7. Fraser RC. Somite genesis in the chick. III. The role of induction. *J Exp Zool* 1960;45:1 51.

8. Revel JP, Yip P, Chang LL. Cell junctions in the early chick embryo—a freeze etch study. *Dev Biol* 1973;35:302.

9. Ostrovsky K, Sanger JW, Lash JW. Light microscope observations on actin distribution during morphogenetic movements in the chick embryo. *J Embryol Exp Morph* 1983;78:23.

10. Christ B, Jacob HJ, Jacob M. On the formation of the myotomes in avian embryos. An experimental and scanning electron microscope study. *Experientia* 1978;34:514.

11. Christ B, Jacob M, Jacob HJ, et al. Myogenesis: a problem of cell distribution and cell interactions. In: Bellairs R, Ede DA, Lash JW, eds. *Somites in developing embryos.* New York: Plenum Press: 261–275.

12. Flint OP, Ede DA, Wilby OK, et al. Control of somite number in normal and amputated mutant mouse embryos: an experimental and a theoretical analysis. *J Embryol Exp Morph* 1978;45:189.

13. Tam PPL. The control of somitogenesis in mouse embryos. *J Embryol Exp Morph* 1981;65(suppl):103.

14. Bagnall KM, Sanders EJ, Higgins SJ, et al. The effects of somite removal on vertebral formation in the chick. *Anat Embryol* 1988; 178:183.

15. O'Rahilly R, Meyer DB. The timing and sequence of events in the development of the human vertebral column during the embryonic period proper. *Anat Embryol* 1979;157:167.

16. Remack R. *Untersuchungen uber die Entwicklung der Wirbelihiere.* Berlin: Reimer, 1855.

17. Bagnall KM, Higgins SJ, Saunders EJ. The contribution made by a single somite to the vertebral column: experimental evidence in support of resegmentation using the chick-quail chimaera model. *Development* 1988;103:69.

18. Verbout AJ. A critical review of the "Neugliederung" concept in relation to the development of the vertebral column. *Acta Biotheor* (Leiden) 1976;25:219.

19. Hall BK. *Developmental and cellular skeletal biology.* New York: Academic Press, 1978.

20. Sberk HH, Park WW. Developmental anatomy. In: Bailey RW, ed. *The cervical spine.* Philadelphia: JB Lippincott Co, 1983.

21. Noback CR, Robertson GG. Sequences of appearance of ossification centers in the human skeleton during the first five prenatal months. *Am J Anat* 1951;89:1.

22. O'Rahilly R, Meyer DB. Roentgenographic investigation of the human skeleton during early fetal life. *Am J Roentgenol* 1979;76: 455.

23. Schmori G, Junghanns H. *The human spine in health and disease,* 2nd ed. New York: Grune & Stratton, 1971.

24. Jenkins FA. The evolution and development of the dens of the mammalian axis. *Anat Rec* 1969;164:173.

25. Byrd S, Wilczynski MA. Imaging modalities for the pediatric spine. *Curr Opin Radiol* 1991;3:906.

130. Cervical Spine Biomechanics

William Mitchell, Gregory J. Przybylski, and Edward C. Benzel

The application of biomechanical principles to spinal anatomy and physiology over the past three decades has substantially enhanced our understanding of the spine and its supporting elements in both the normal and pathological states. However, the transition from a normal to a pathological state is indistinct and should be considered a continuum instead. The spine represents a multisegmented scaffolding that supports the body and head to allow the assumption of the upright posture and motion. Therefore, the evaluation of normal spine kinematics has led to an appreciation of the contributions of structures in the spine to the normal physiological range of motion. Similarly, the study of kinematics in pathological models has facilitated both a framework for describing the etiology of the pathology and as a guide for treatment. The application of biomechanics to the cervical spine has been extensively studied. The principles derived from these studies can be used to guide clinical decision-making process.

Terminology

The surgeon must understand basic biomechanical terminology and related anatomy to apply a biomechanical analysis to the spine. The motion of spinal components is described in terms of displacement. Its vector quantity (meters) defines both the magnitude and direction of migration from the original position. Velocity represents the displacement over time (m/sec), whereas acceleration represents the rate at which the velocity changes (m/sec^2). Force (or load) is determined by the product of an object's mass and its acceleration (kg-m/sec^2). A bending moment (or torque) is the product of an applied force at a given point and the distance from the axis of rotation (nm or kg-m^2/sec^2).

Forces and moments applied to an object can cause deformation and/or motion of the object. The direction of displacements (vector) within a three-dimensional space can be simplified and broken down into individual translational and/or rotational component vectors along or about three orthogonal (perpendicular) axes or planes.

This coordinate system has been applied to the human body and is helpful in understanding movements of the spine. The three orthogonal planes with three perpendicular axes consist of the sagittal, coronal, and transverse planes. There are a total of six degrees of freedom within this system because motion can occur either along or about an axis. For example, movement of the spine in the sagittal plane consists of rotation about the

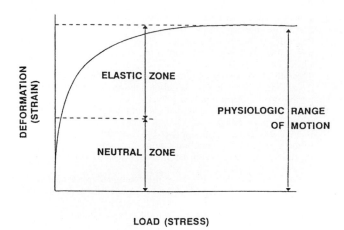

Fig. 1. A typical load deformation curve depicting the neutral and elastic zones (deformation or strain versus load or stress).

x-axis, which is perpendicular to this plane and results in flexion or extension. Likewise, rotation about the z-axis, which is perpendicular to the coronal plane, results in lateral bending, whereas rotation about the y-axis in the transverse plane results in axial rotation.

The structural and material properties of objects help define the predicted effects of forces applied to those objects. The structural properties of an object are easier to measure. They involve the determination of the relationship between force and displacement. Tension describes the application of forces away from an object, whereas compression describes the application of forces toward the object. Material testing machines typically apply a given force and measure the resultant displacement or provide a given displacement while measuring the required force. The rate of change along a measured load-displacement curve (Fig. 1) is termed "stiffness" (N/m). An elastic constant is identified for a linear relationship between force and displacement. For example, the force to stretch a simple spring is proportional to the displacement observed. Consequently, a structure with significant elasticity requires greater forces to achieve deformation.

Testing of many biological tissues (e.g., ligaments) reveals a nonlinear relationship between force and displacement, which is termed viscoelasticity. Creep, which is observed with such

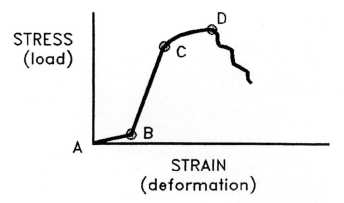

Fig. 2. A typical stress/strain curve for a biological tissue, such as a ligament. *AB*, the neutral zone; *BC*, the elastic zone. Permanent deformation can occur (permanent set) when the elastic limit is reached *(C)*; *CD*, the plastic zone, where a permanent set occurs. Past *D*, failure occurs and the load diminishes.

structures, is a phenomenon that describes smaller progressive displacements over time after a single force is applied and maintained. In contrast, stress relaxation describes the progressively smaller forces required to maintain a viscoelastic object at a given length. Both of these time-dependent properties demonstrate the importance of dynamic testing on human tissues.

An ultrastructural examination of an object allows the measurement of material properties, such as stress and strain. Stress describes the force applied to a given surface area (N/m^2), whereas strain measures the ratio of the change in length of a material and its original length. Elasticity allows an object to return to its original length after deformation. However, when the elastic limit is exceeded, plastic deformation occurs with only incomplete recovery of the original shape on removal of the force (Figs. 1 and 2). Failure occurs if the deformation exceeds the object's plastic limit (Figs. 1 and 2).

Structural Biomechanics and Kinematics

The application of biomechanical principles to the spine requires some understanding of its structural components. The simplest basic unit of the spine is termed the functional spinal unit. This consists of two adjacent vertebrae with their intervening discoligamentous structures. Bone is comprised predominantly of calcium salts, which imparts strength. Tensile forces are applied to the vertebrae by attached muscles, tendons, and ligaments. Although the tensile strength of bone is greatest along its predominant axis (which is associated with its muscular attachments) (1), most forces applied to the vertebra typically are applied in compression. Consequently, vertebrae are strongest in compression. Moreover, the stiffness of the vertebra is related to the rate of loading, with increased strength and energy absorption at higher rates of loading. This tissue behavior correlates with the increasing width, depth, and height of each caudal vertebral body (2–6). The cortical to cancellous ratio affects the axial load-bearing resistance of a vertebral body. This is also true for screw pullout resistance. A 50% reduction in bone density reduces the vertebral body strength by 25% (7).

The kinematics of the vertebrae are significantly influenced by the orientation of the facet joints, which can limit motion depending on their alignment. The coronal orientation of cervical facet joints facilitates axial rotation while allowing sagittal plane bending. Extension and compression are the major motions that are limited by the facet joints, although this coronal orientation resists ventral and dorsal translation. Furthermore, they help support the axial load when placed in extension. This alignment accounts for the significant mobility of the cervical spine (7). Finally, Zdeblick (8,9) found that more than 50% resection of the facet joints significantly affected the resistance conferred by the facets and their capsules.

The other major structural component of the functional spinal unit is the intervertebral disc. This joint is composed of circumferential layers of annular ligaments oriented at a 30-degree angle to the plane of the end plate and in opposite directions in alternating layers. The central viscoelastic nucleus pulposus, which is contained by the annulus fibrosis, helps distribute axial loads by causing compression of the cartilaginous end plates and tension within the annular ligaments. Aging reduces the water content of the nucleus pulposus, and thereby the ability of the nucleus to distribute axial forces (10).

The kinematic effects of the annular ligaments are observed in tension. In axial rotation, alternating annular layers are placed

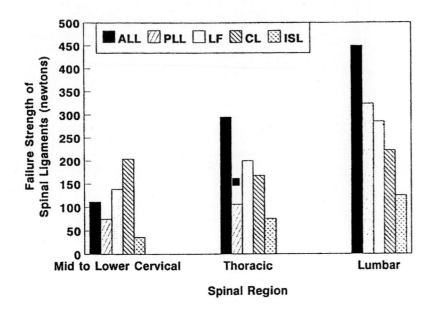

Fig. 3. Failure strength of spinal ligaments versus spinal region. *ALL*, anterior longitudinal ligament; *CL*, capsular ligament; *ISL*, interspinous ligament; *LF*, ligamentum flavum; *PLL*, posterior longitudinal ligament (7,10,15–19,21, 36,61,62).

in tension to resist excess rotation. In contrast, bending in either the sagittal or coronal planes places ligaments on the convex side of the bend in tension (11,12). Finally, some internal displacement of the nucleus pulposus is observed toward the convex side (13,14).

The other spinal ligaments are similarly composed of collagen, elastin, and reticulin fibers, although usually considered independently from the annular ligaments. Although these ligaments are designed to resist tensile forces, their behavior is dependent on the ratio of the component fiber types. For example, the flaval ligament is composed of the greatest proportion of elastin fibers of all the body ligaments, thereby permitting less resistance to tension. The strength of the ligament varies by the ligament type as well as the spinal segment of attachment (7,15–21).

The spinal ligaments stabilize joints when placed in tension. The distance between the ligament and the axis of rotation also contributes to the ability of a ligament to resist a given displacement because the lordosis of the cervical spine typically places the instantaneous axis of rotation in the dorsal third of the intervertebral disc (12). Moreover, tension lengthens the ligaments on the convex side of a bend and shorten or "buckle" ligaments on the opposite side of a bend. For example, the anterior longitudinal ligament and the ventral annulus fibrosis resist extension (7,22), whereas the dorsal annular, posterior longitudinal, capsular, flaval, and interspinous ligaments all resist flexion (7,23). In addition, capsular and annular ligaments resist lateral bending (24). Upper cervical spine stability (occiput-C2) relies on the integrity of the strong craniocervical ligaments (Fig. 3) to limit excessive motion. In particular, the tectorial membrane limits atlanto-occipital translation (less than 1 mm) and distraction (less than 5 mm) (25) as well as limiting atlantoaxial flexion-extension (26,27). The paired alar ligaments limit atlanto-occipital translation (28), lateral bending, and rotation (less than 8 degrees unilaterally) (29). The transverse ligament limits atlantoaxial translation. This ligament is attenuated when the displacement of the atlas in relation to the dens (ADI) is 3 to 5 mm, and it is ruptured when the displacement is more than 5 mm (30–32). However, some evidence suggests that certain ligaments may not be placed in tension within the physiological range of motion of the functional spinal unit (33,34).

One of the least understood components of the spine is the musculature. Although muscles provide both motion and stability to the spine, the complicated neurophysiological behavior of muscles has limited the understanding of their contribution to spinal stabilization. The location of the muscular attachments dictate the motion provided. The longus colli produce flexion, whereas the splenius muscles provide extension and rotation. In addition, muscle activity may provide spinal stability while reducing ligamentous tension within the physiological range of motion (35). The neutral zone of the upright spine is modulated by the continuous muscular influences that limit segmental movement and increase stability.

The alignment of the cervical spine is critical in assessing stability and the effects of injury. Normal sagittal plane cervical alignment has a lordosis that transmits axial loads symmetrically. This provides maximal support for axial loading, as evidenced by failure at lower forces when flexed or extended in comparison to neutral. Approximately 50% of the load required for axial compression failures resulted in flexion and extension injuries, but the direction of the force only partially correlated with the observed fracture (36). Variations from neutral significantly affect the fracture pattern and the net force that is "seen" by the spine (37). A feature of the cervical spine attributed to the uncovertebral joints is the coupling phenomenon (38). Coupling refers to the consistent association of translation or rotation about an axis that occurs with translation or rotation about another axis. For example, lateral bending in the cervical spine results in rotation of the spinous processes away from the concave side of the direction of the bend.

Determining Spinal Stability

A consensus agreement among spinal surgeons and scientists remains elusive, although describing spinal instability has been the topic of many publications. Displacement beyond the normal boundaries of motion may be sufficient to indicate instability in the acute phase, but the absence of such excess displacement on a static radiograph should not imply maintenance of stability. White and Panjabi (7) proposed that spinal instability represents the "loss of the ability of the spine under physiological loads to maintain relationships between vertebrae in such a way that there is neither damage nor subsequent irritation to the spinal cord or nerve roots, and, in addition, there is no development of incapacitating deformity or pain due to structural changes." Rather than suggesting an absolute limit, White and Panjabi describe a continuum of spinal stability in which accumulation of deficiencies within the normal properties of the spine leads to progressive instability. It should be noted that this definition could be applied to a broad spectrum of conditions. It may apply to a herniated cervical disc, spondylitic cervical myelopathy, tumor, vertebral body tumor, cervical discitis with or without osteomyelitis, inflammatory conditions, and trauma. A simpler definition describes an inability of the spine to resist displacement and resume its resting position (39).

The structure of the spine has been divided into components termed columns in order to understand the effects of partial injury to the spine on its stability. The two-column model separates the vertebral bodies and supporting ligaments from the elements dorsal to the posterior longitudinal ligament. Instability occurs after all of the elements of one column and any additional element of the second column are disrupted (40). In contrast, the three-column model separates the ventral column into an anterior and middle column based on the elements in the ventral two thirds of the vertebrae and dorsal third. Instability occurs after elements of two columns are disrupted (41). These theories provide a framework to assist the spine specialist in translating the radiographical findings to an estimation of spine instability.

A mechanistic classification of traumatic spinal injury was devised for the subaxial cervical spine (2). The scheme is based on compression or distraction occurring with the spinal segment in one of three positions (neutral, flexion, or extension). Compression with the cervical spinal segment in a neutral position results in application of forces along the axis of the spine. This may result in a "burst" fracture, with displacement of the body outward in the coronal plane. Compression with the cervical spinal segment in flexion applies forces ventral to the axis of rotation. This may result in a wedge-shaped fracture. Progressively greater forces additionally can cause dorsal retropulsion and/or dorsal ligamentous and facet joint damage. Compression with the cervical spinal segment in extension transmits forces dorsal to the axis of rotation and may result in dorsal fractures. Progressively greater forces can additionally cause ventral ligamentous injury. Distraction with the cervical spinal segment in flexion may result in a dorsal ligamentous rupture, causing various degrees of facet joint subluxation or dislocation. Distraction with the cervical spinal segment in extension may produce widening of the disc space ventrally, as the anterior longitudinal ligament and ventral annular ligaments fail. Progressively greater forces can cause dorsal ligamentous failure.

Although these methods analyze the bony structure of the spine, the assessment of the remaining spinal components is likewise essential in estimating stability. Neurological injury secondary to trauma implies instability. Bony displacements beyond the normal range imply ligamentous disruption. Modern imaging techniques can reveal ligamentous, muscular, and intervertebral disc injuries (42–44). Although there is no definitive algorithm for every spinal injury, one can synthesize an understanding of the normal anatomy, physiological range of motion, column theories, and mechanism of injury to estimate spinal stability as well as direct appropriate treatment.

Implants

Spinal instrumentation can be used to augment the stability of the spine. Regardless of the etiology (e.g., traumatic, iatro-

genic), the goals of instrumentation are restoration of alignment and supplementation of the deficient spinal elements; therefore, the mechanism causing the instability should determine the most desirable implant to restore stability. Load sharing and load bearing as well as the instantaneous axis of rotation are critical to devising a successful construct. Furthermore, segmental fixation is essential to counteract the inherent mobility of the cervical spine. Structural properties of the implants should be considered. The section modulus (pi × D3/32) is an indicator of strength, whereas the moment of inertia (pi × D4/16) is an indicator of stiffness. Therefore, the diameter of a rod and core diameter of a screw exponentially affect strength and stiffness.

Upper Cervical Spine Injuries

The upper cervical spine (occiput-C2), primarily allows rotation in the axial and sagittal planes. The normal axial rotations of the atlanto-occipital and atlantoaxial joints are 8 degrees and 56 degrees, respectively, whereas the normal flexion-extension range is 25 degrees for both joints (45,46). The tectorial membrane and alar ligaments provide the majority of the ligamentous stability of the craniovertebral junction (47–49). Atlanto-occipital dislocation is a hyperextension injury in which disruption of the craniovertebral ligaments, particularly the tectorial membrane and alar ligaments, results in atlanto-occipital instability. This injury typically occurs in children, perhaps related to the flatter articulation plane of the superior facets of the atlas with the immature occipital condyles (50). This ligamentous injury requires reduction and internal fixation because ligaments typically do not heal well. In contrast, occipital condyle fractures result from axial compression. These are typically stable injuries unless avulsion of the alar ligaments and tectorial membrane also occurs from off-axis loading. Although isolated fractures (types 1 and 2) can be managed with external immobilization, significant disruption of the supporting ligaments (some type 3) may require surgical stabilization (51).

The transverse ligament provides much of the resistance to sagittal translation of the atlas on the axis. Atlas fractures result from axial loading of the occipital condyles on the lateral masses of C1, displacing the lateral masses centripetally. This fracture is usually treated with external immobilization. However, lateral displacement of the lateral masses of C1 on C2 beyond 7 mm, as measured on an open-mouth anterior-posterior radiograph (32), or an atlantodental interval greater than 3 mm on a lateral radiograph (30), imply injury to the transverse ligament, which may require surgical stabilization. Odontoid fractures are classified into three types based on the scheme proposed in 1974 by Anderson and D'Alonzo (52). An avulsion of the tip of the dens (type 1) is uncommon and typically is treated with rigid collar immobilization. The more common fracture at the base of the dens (type 2) typically occurs from lateral bending (53). Advanced age and significant subluxation have been associated with frequent nonunion from external immobilization (54,55). Whereas some patients can be treated successfully with external immobilization, others at increased risk for nonunion may benefit from surgical fusion. In contrast, odontoid fractures extending into the vertebral body and facet (type 3) occur from flexion and usually achieve satisfactory union with external immobilization (53). Finally, traumatic C2 spondylolisthesis (hangman's fracture) typically occurs following hyperextension (56), resulting in bilateral axis fractures near the articular facets. These fractures are classified based on displacement and angulation (57). Unless substantial displacement from ligamentous injury occurs with facet dislocation (type 3), these bony injuries often can be treated with external immobilization.

Subaxial Cervical Spine Injuries

In the subaxial spine, the parameters measured on plain radiographs that suggest potential instability include sagittal plane angulation beyond 11 degrees on static and 20 degrees on dynamic lateral radiographs, or sagittal translation beyond 3.5 mm on lateral radiographs (28). Normal segmental ranges of motion include 5 to 10 degrees of axial rotation, 6 to 10 degrees of flexion-extension, and 6 to 10 degrees in lateral bending (24, 58). Several common patterns of injury appear whether one uses the scheme proposed by Allen and Ferguson (2), Holdsworth (59), Denis (41), or Benzel (60). Burst, wedge, and posterior fractures occur from axial loading in neutral, flexion, and extension, respectively. Distraction injuries usually result in ligamentous injury and when severe enough, bony fracture. The relation of the force to the instantaneous axis of rotation determines where the injury will occur. Many subaxial spine injuries require internal fixation to restore the spine to its physiological range of motion.

Conclusion

Application of biomechanics can assist the spinal surgeon in assessing the extent of bony and ligamentous injury. An analysis of the traumatized spine is essential for the guidance of appropriate treatment. Whether treating acute trauma, tumor, infection, degenerative diseases, or a herniated disc, basic biomechanical principles can and should be applied to facilitate optimum treatment in each individual clinical situation. The goal is often to restore the cervical spine to the physiological range of motion. Knowledge of the instantaneous axis of rotation, loads and bending moments, limitations of the range of motion that the spinal elements impose, and support that an implant imparts are some of the factors that the spine surgeon should consider as part of the decision-making process.

References

1. Cowin SC. The mechanical and stress adaptive properties of bone. *Ann Biomed Eng* 1983;11:263–295.
2. Allen BL Jr, Ferguson RL, Lehman TR, et al. A mechanistic classification of closed, indirect fractures and dislocations of the lower cervical spine. *Spine* 1982;7:1–27.
3. Pintar FA, Yoganandan N, Droese K, et al. Biomechanics of cervical spine column injury. *Proceedings of the fourth annual injury prevention through biomechanics symposium.* 1995;4:117–126.
4. Roaf R. A study of the mechanics of spinal injuries. *J Bone Joint Surg Br* 1960;42:810.
5. Yoganandan N, Pintar FA, Sances A, et al. Strength and kinematic response of dynamic cervical spine injuries. *Spine* 1991;16S: S511–S517.
6. Yoganandan N, Sances A, Pintar FA, et al. Injury biomechanics of the human cervical column. *Spine* 1990;15:1031–1039.
7. White AA, Panjabi M. *Clinical biomechanics of the spine,* 2nd ed. Philadelphia: JB Lippincott, 1990.
8. Zdeblick TA, Abitbol JJ, Kunz DN, et al. Cervical stability after sequential capsule resection. *Spine* 1993;18:2005–2008.
9. Zdeblick TA, Zou D, Warden KE, et al. Cervical stability following foraminotomy: a biomechanical in-vitro analysis. *J Bone Joint Surg Am* 1992;74:22–27.
10. White AA, Panjabi MM. The basic kinematics of the human spine: a review of past and current knowledge. *Spine* 1978;3:12–20.
11. Munro D. The factors that govern the stability of the spine. *Paraplegia* 1965;3:219–228.
12. Panjabi MM, Greenstein G, Duranceau J, et al. Three-dimensional quantitative morphology of lumbar spinal segments. *J Spinal Disord* 1991;4:54–72.
13. Broberg KB. On the mechanical behaviour of intervertebral discs. *Spine* 1983;8:151–165.
14. Krag MK, Seroussi RE, Wilder DG, et al. Internal displacement distribution from in vitro loading of human thoracic and lumbar spinal motion segments: experimental results and theoretical predictions. *Spine* 1987;12:1001–1007.
15. Chazal J, Tanguy A, Bourges M, et al. Biomechanical properties of spinal ligaments and a histological study of the supraspinal ligament in traction. *J Biomech* 1985;18:167–176.
16. Mykelbust JB, Pintar F, Yoganandan N, et al. Tensile strength of spinal ligaments. *Spine* 1988;13:526–531.
17. Nachemson A, Evans J. Some mechanical properties of the third lumbar inter-laminar ligament. *J Biomech* 1968;1:211–217.
18. Panjabi MM, Hausfield JN, White AA. A biomechanical study of the ligamentous stability of the thoracic spine. *Acta Orthop Scand* 1981; 52:315–326.
19. Posner I, White AA III, Edwards WT, et al. A biomechanical analysis of the clinical stability of the lumbar and lumbosacral spine. *Spine* 1982;7:374–389.
20. Przybylski GJ, Carlin GJ, Patel PR, et al. Human anterior and posterior cervical longitudinal ligaments possess similar tensile properties. *J Orthop Res* 1996;14:1005–1008.
21. Tkaczuk H. Tensile properties of human lumbar longitudinal ligaments. *Acta Orthop Scand* 1968;115(suppl):1–69.
22. Shea M, Wittenberg RH, Edwards WT, et al. In vitro hyperextension injuries in the human cadaveric cervical spine. *J Orthop Res* 1992; 10:911–916.
23. Bailey RW. Fractures and dislocations of the cervical spine. *Postgrad Med* 1964;588–599.
24. Lysell E. Motion in the cervical spine. *Acta Orthop Scand* 1969; 123(suppl):1–61.
25. Weisel SW, Rothman RH. Occipito-atlantal hypermobility. *Spine* 1979;4:187.
26. Dvorak J, Froelich D, Penning L, et al. Functional radiographical diagnosis of the cervical spine: flexion/extension. *Spine* 1988;13: 748.
27. Panjabi M, Dvorak J, Durnanceau J, et al. Three-dimensional movements of the upper cervical spine. *Spine* 1988;13:726.
28. White AA, Johnson RM, Panjabi MM. Biomechanical analysis of clinical stability in the cervical spine. *Clin Orthop Rel Res* 1975;109: 85–96.
29. Dvorak J, Panjabi MM. Functional anatomy of the alar ligaments. *Spine* 1987;12:183.
30. Fielding JW, Cochran GV, Lawsing JF. Tears of the transverse ligament of the atlas. *J Bone Joint Surg Am* 1974;56:1683–1691.
31. Fielding JW, Hawkins RJ, Ratzan SA. Spine fusion for atlanto-axial instability. *J Bone Joint Surg Am* 1976;58:400–407.
32. Spence KF, Decker S, Sell KW. Bursting atlantal fracture associated with rupture of the transverse ligament. *J Bone Joint Surg Am* 1970; 52:543–549.
33. Przybylski GJ, Patel PR, Carlin GJ, et al. Quantitative anthropometry of the subatlantal cervical longitudinal ligaments. *Spine* 1998;23: 893–898.
34. Schendel MJ, Wood KB, Butterman GR, et al. Experimental measurement of ligament force, facet force, and segment motion in the human lumbar spine. *J Biomech* 1993;26:427–438.
35. Wilke HJ, Wolf S, Claes LE, et al. Stability increase of the lumbar spine with different muscle groups: a biomechanical in vitro study. *Spine* 1995;20:192–198.
36. Maiman DJ, Sances A, Myklebust JB, et al. Compression injuries of the cervical spine: a biomechanical analysis. *Neurosurgery* 1983;13: 254–260.
37. Myers BS, McElhaney JH. *Cervical spine injury mechanisms: biomechanics and prevention.* New York: Springer-Verlag, 1993: 311–361.

38. Penning L, Wilmink JT. Rotation of the cervical spine: a CT study in normal subjects. *Spine* 1987;12:732–738.
39. Farfan HF, Gracovetsky S. The nature of instability. *Spine* 1984;9:714–719.
40. Hung TK, Chang GL, Chang JL, et al. Stress-strain relationship and neurological sequelae of uniaxial elongation of the spinal cord of cats. *Surg Neurol* 1981;15:471–476.
41. Denis F. The three-column spine and its significance in the classification of acute thoracolumbar spinal injuries. *Spine* 1983;8:817–831.
42. Dickman CA, Mamourian A, Sonntag VKH. Magnetic resonance imaging of the transverse atlantal ligament for the evaluation of atlantoaxial instability. *J Neurosurg* 1991;75:221–227.
43. Greene KA, Dickman CA, Marciano FF, et al. Transverse atlantal ligament disruption associated with odontoid fractures. *Spine* 1994;19:2307–2314.
44. Pathria MN, Petersilge CA. Spinal trauma. *Radiol Clin North Am* 1991;29:847–865.
45. Dvorak J, Hayek J, Zehnder R. CT-functional diagnostics of the rotatory instability of the upper cervical spine. *Spine* 1987;12:726–738.
46. White AA, Panjabi MM. The clinical biomechanics of the occipitoatlantoaxial complex. *Orthop Clin North Am* 1978;9:867–878.
47. Bucholz RW, Burkhead WZ. The pathological anatomy of fatal atlanto-occipital dislocations. *J Bone Joint Surg Am* 1979;61:248–250.
48. Dvorak J, Schneider E, Saldinger P, et al. Biomechanics of the craniocervical region: The alar and transverse ligaments. *J Orthop Res* 1988;6:452–461.
49. Werne S. Studies in spontaneous atlas dislocation. *Acta Scand* 1957;23(suppl):1–150.
50. Traynelis VC, Marano GD, Dunker RO, et al. Traumatic atlanto-occipital dislocation: case report. *J Neurosurg* 1986;65:863–870.
51. Anderson PA, Montesano PX. Morphology and treatment of occipital condyle fractures. *Spine* 1988;13:731–736.
52. Anderson LD, D'Alonzo RT. Fractures of the odontoid process of the axis. *J Bone Joint Surg Am* 1974;56:1663–1674.
53. Mouradian WH, Fietti VG Jr, Cochran GVB. Fractures of the odontoid: a laboratory and clinical study of mechanisms. *Orthop Clin North Am* 1978;9:985–1001.
54. Apuzzo MLF, Heiden JS, Weiss MH, et al. Acute fractures of the odontoid process. An analysis of 45 cases. *J Neurosurg* 1978;48:85–91.
55. Hadley MN, Browner C, Sonntag VKH. Axis fractures: a comprehensive review of management and treatment in 107 cases. *Neurosurgery* 1985;17:281–289.
56. Schneider RC, Livingston KE, Cave AJE, et al. "Hangman's fracture" of the cervical spine. *J Neurosurg* 1965;22:141–154.
57. Effendi B, Roy D, Cornish B. Fractures of the ring of the axis: a classification based o the analysis of 131 cases. *J Bone Joint Surg Br* 1981;63:313–318.
58. Holmes A, Wang C, Han ZH, et al. The range and nature of flexion-extension motion in the cervical spine. *Spine* 1994;19:2505–2510.
59. Holdsworth FW. Fractures, dislocations, and fracture-dislocations of the spine. *J Bone Joint Surg Am* 1970;52:1534–1551.
60. Benzel EC, Hart BL, Ball PA, et al. Fractures of the C2 vertical body. *J Neurosurg* 1994;81:206–212.
61. Goel VK, Njus GO. Stress-strain characteristics of spinal ligaments. *32nd Trans Orthop Res Soc* New Orleans, 1986:1–2.
62. Panjabi MM, Jorneus L, Greenstein G. Lumbar spine ligaments: an in vitro biomechanical study. *10th Meeting of the International Society for the Society of the Lumbar Spine* Montreal, 1984:1–3.

131. Thoracic Spine Anatomy and Biomechanics

Anthony K. Frempong-Boadu and Bernard H. Guiot

Appropriate management of thoracic spine lesions is based on a thorough understanding of the pertinent anatomy and biomechanics of the thoracic region. The thoracic spine is rigid compared to the hypermobile cervical and lumbar spines. This stiffness, which is a product of its complex osteoligamentous relationship with the rib cage, determines its biomechanics and reaction to various disease states.

The thoracic region is under different biomechanical loads and has different anatomical considerations in comparison to the other spinal regions. The thoracic spine is a transitional zone between the cervical and lumbar regions. It is naturally kyphotic, and the addition of the rib cage to the functional vertebral unit changes its stability and range of motion (1,2). Alterations of thoracic spine biomechanics result from degenerative changes, tumor, infection, trauma, and surgical decompression. The proper surgical management of these problems relates largely to the degree of biomechanical alterations that they cause (3,4); therefore, knowledge of the anatomy and biomechanics of the thoracic region is essential for the management of these processes.

Thoracic Spine Anatomy

The three-dimensional anatomy of the vertebral bodies, pedicles, transverse processes, rib heads, and rib articulations with the vertebral bodies and intervertebral discs is complex. Both the bony and ligamentous anatomy provide important clues for understanding the biomechanical characteristics of the thoracic spine.

The thoracic region can be divided into three distinct regions with unique morphological and biomechanical features (5). There are two transitional zones at the cervicothoracic and thoracolumbar junctions and a rigid middle zone. The transitional zones share their anatomy and biomechanical properties with those of the bordering cervical and lumbar regions (5). The remaining thoracic spine is unique both anatomically and biomechanically.

There are 12 thoracic vertebral bodies. The dorsal, ventral, and lateral diameters of the vertebral bodies increase from the cervicothoracic to thoracolumbar junction. The physiological kyphosis of the thoracic spine results from the wedge shape of the thoracic vertebral bodies. The dorsal thoracic vertebral wall has a greater rostral-caudal height than the ventral vertebral wall (6–8). The normal thoracic kyphosis ranges from 20 to 40 degrees and peaks at T7 (Fig. 1) (4,5).

The first thoracic vertebra is anatomically similar to its cervical cousins but has costal facets and no foramen transversarium. The spinal canal is larger at this level than in the caudal thoracic spine, in order to accommodate the distal portion of the cervical enlargement. It has an entire costal facet that articulates with

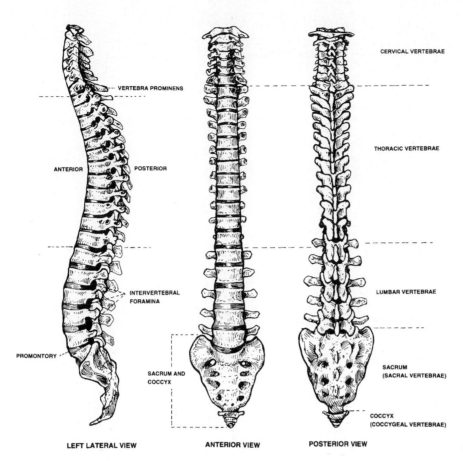

CERVICAL VERTEBRAE

VERTEBRA PROMINENS

THORACIC VERTEBRAE

ANTERIOR   POSTERIOR

INTERVERTEBRAL
FORAMINA

LUMBAR VERTEBRAE

PROMONTORY

SACRUM AND
COCCYX

SACRUM
(SACRAL VERTEBRAE)

COCCYX
(COCCYGEAL VERTEBRAE)

LEFT LATERAL VIEW   ANTERIOR VIEW   POSTERIOR VIEW

Fig. 1. Spinal column.

the first rib and a rostral demifacet that articulates with the second rib.

Between T1 and T11 the costovertebral articulation is made up of two semicircular halves known as demifacets (Fig. 2). The demifacets articulate with those from the neighboring vertebral bodies to form the articular facets for the rib heads. The T1 to T11 the thoracic vertebrae usually have rostral and caudal demifacets on their lateral surfaces, which together with the demifacets on the neighboring segments make complete articulations for the rib heads. The eleventh, twelfth, and occasionally the tenth thoracic vertebrae have complete costal facets for articulation with their rib heads (6–8).

The twelfth thoracic vertebra is similar to the lumbar vertebrae. The spinal canal is larger than in the midthoracic spine to accommodate the rostral portion of the lumbar enlargement, but unlike the lumbar vertebrae, it has costal facets (8).

PEDICLE ANATOMY. Thoracic pedicles are narrower and closer to the adjacent neural structures than those of the lumbar vertebra (9). They leave the vertebral bodies at their rostral ends. In the upper thoracic spine the pedicles are directed rostrally (Fig. 2) (10,11). The transverse pedicle angle decreases from 30 to 40 degrees at T1-2 to 10 degrees at T12 (10,11). The sagittal pedicle angle remains relatively constant throughout the thoracic region at about 15 degrees above the horizontal. The transverse diameter of the thoracic pedicles increases from 4.5 mm at T4 to 7.8 mm at T12 and the sagittal pedicle diameter increases in from 8 mm at T4 to greater that 15 mm at T12 (12–15).

TRANSVERSE PROCESS ANATOMY. From T1 to T10 the thoracic transverse processes provide support for the ribs via

their transverse costal articular facets (6,7). These transverse costal facets are ventrally located on the transverse processes from T1 to T7. They are located rostrally from T8 to T10 and are not present on the transverse processes of T11 and T12. The eleventh and twelfth ribs only articulate with the vertebral body (6,7). Tubercles on the thoracic transverse processes serve as muscular and ligamentous attachments (Fig. 2). The transverse process is located rostral to the pedicle above T6-7. The transverse process is found caudal to the pedicle below T6-T7 (11).

LAMINAR AND SPINOUS PROCESS ANATOMY. The midthoracic laminar and spinous processes are caudally oblique and overlap the body and intervertebral disc of the next caudal segment (6–8). The spinous processes of the upper and lower thoracic spine are less obliquely directed. The thoracic laminar are taller than they are wide. There are prominent tubercles on the thoracic spinous processes for the attachment of the muscles and ligaments (Fig. 1).

FACET ANATOMY. The thoracic facets are flat and project nearly vertically from the pedicle (16). Their orientation is intermediate between the relatively coronally oriented cervical and the sagittally oriented lumbar facet joints (Fig. 3). They provide stability during flexion and extension (17). Bony markings on the facets allow for the attachment of the radiate ligaments of the rib heads (7).

RIB ANATOMY. The paired ribs slope downward in their course from the vertebral bodies posteriorly to the sternum an-

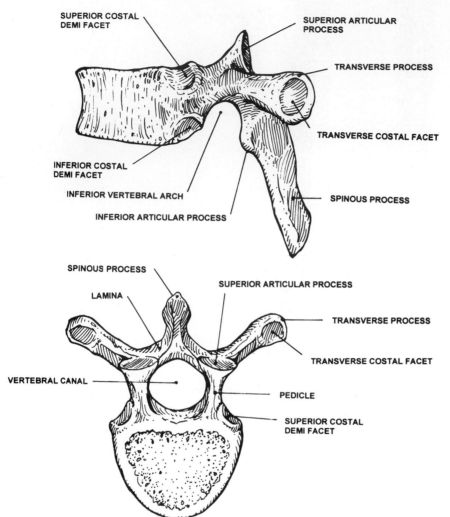

SUPERIOR COSTAL DEMI FACET

SUPERIOR ARTICULAR PROCESS

TRANSVERSE PROCESS

TRANSVERSE COSTAL FACET

INFERIOR COSTAL DEMI FACET

INFERIOR VERTEBRAL ARCH

INFERIOR ARTICULAR PROCESS

SPINOUS PROCESS

SPINOUS PROCESS

LAMINA

SUPERIOR ARTICULAR PROCESS

TRANSVERSE PROCESS

TRANSVERSE COSTAL FACET

VERTEBRAL CANAL

PEDICLE

SUPERIOR COSTAL DEMI FACET

Fig. 2. Bony relationships of the midthoracic vertebra. **A:** Lateral view. **B:** Superior view.

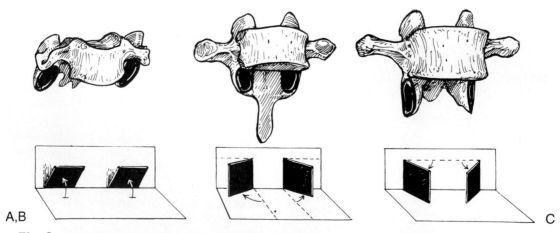

A,B

C

Fig. 3. Facet orientation. **A:** Cervical, coronal orientation. **B:** Thoracic, intermediate orientation. **C:** Lumbar, sagittal orientation.

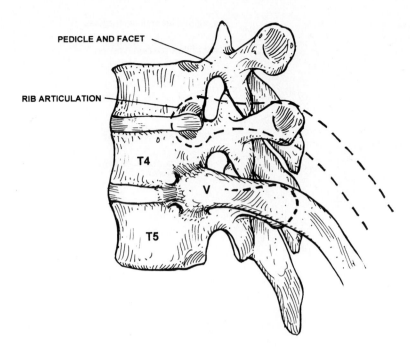

Fig. 4. Midthoracic rib articulation.

teriorly. This angle increases caudally to approximately 45 degrees (6). The ribs are divided into the sternal or true ribs (T1-7), which articulate directly with the sternum; and false ribs (T8-10), which do not. The eleventh and twelfth ribs are called floating ribs because they do not articulate with the costal cartilage anteriorly (6,7).

Each rib head except for the first, eleventh, twelfth, and often the tenth has two articular facets for articulation with the demifacets of the adjacent vertebra (Fig. 4) (7). The first, eleventh, and twelfth rib heads have a full facet for individual articulation with their numerically corresponding vertebral bodies, and they are named for the vertebral body that they articulate with (e.g., the eleventh rib articulates with the eleventh vertebral body). The second to ninth ribs articulate with two adjacent vertebral bod-

ies and the transverse process of the caudal of the two vertebral bodies. The second to ninth ribs are named after the caudal of the two vertebral bodies that they articulate (e.g., the fifth rib articulates with the fourth and fifth vertebral bodies). The eleventh and twelfth ribs do not articulate with the transverse processes of the eleventh and twelfth vertebral bodies (7).

LIGAMENTOUS ANATOMY. The anterior longitudinal ligament (ALL), the posterior longitudinal ligament (PLL), ligamentum flavum (LF), and the annulus surround the thoracic vertebral bodies and intervertebral disc spaces (7,18).

The ALL is a continuous band that attaches to the annulus and vertebral body end plates. It is thickest in the thoracic re-

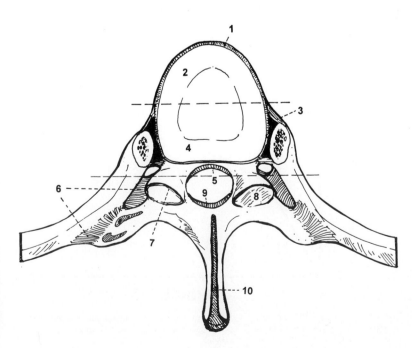

Fig. 5. Major thoracic ligamentous anatomy. *1*, anterior longitudinal ligament; *2*, anterior annulus; *3*, radiate and costovertebral ligaments; *4*, posterior annulus; *5*, posterior longitudinal ligament; *6*, costotransverse ligaments; *7*, capsular ligaments; *8*, facet joint; *9*, ligamentum flavum; *10*, interspinous ligament.

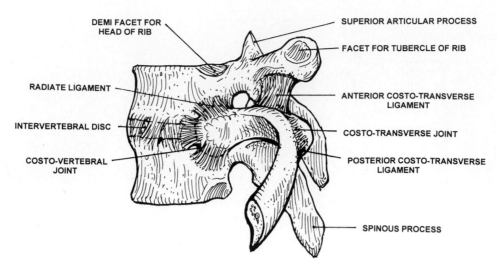

Fig. 6. Lateral thoracic ligamentous anatomy.

gion. The PLL also spans the entire spinal column and it is also thickest in the thoracic region. It attaches to the annulus and vertebral body endplates and is separated from the dura by loose connective tissue. The lateral vertebral ligaments attach to the annulus and endplates surrounding the disc space. They connect the ALL to the PLL and to the end plates at the level of the intervertebral discs. The ligamentum flavum connects the overlapping lamina at contiguous levels. Its fibers are perpendicularly oriented to the laminae. The interspinous ligaments connect the adjacent spinous processes. They attach at their base to the interlaminar ligament and above to the supraspinous ligament that attaches the spinous process tips to the aponeurosis of the thoracolumbar fascia (6,7). In addition, there are capsular ligaments that surround each facet joint and support the joint and attached ligaments (Fig. 5).

The costotransverse and costovertebral/radiate ligaments provide a strong, stable attachment of the thoracic vertebrae to the ribs. Each rib is attached to its adjacent intervertebral disc space and vertebral body by the radiate ligament ventrally and the costovertebral ligaments dorsolaterally. The costovertebral ligaments join the rostral portion of the rib neck to the caudal base of the transverse process. A costovertebral capsular ligament surrounds the costovertebral joint and attaches to the annulus of the intervening disc and radiate ligament (Figs. 5 and 6).

The costotransverse ligament attaches the rib neck at its tubercle to the transverse process of the corresponding vertebra. It runs from the transverse process of each vertebra to the rib and is divided into superior and lateral costotransverse ligaments. The superior costotransverse ligament attaches the rostral rib neck to the caudal portion of the transverse process above the rib. The lateral costotransverse ligament attaches the transverse process to the tubercle of the rib of its own vertebral body and the body below.

In addition, the capsular ligaments surround the attachment of the transverse process to the rib tubercle and secure the neck of the rib to the transverse process ventrally (Figs. 5 and 6) (6,7).

Thoracic Spine Biomechanics

The biomechanics of the thoracic spine contrasts with that of the cervical and lumbar spine because of its articulation with

the thoracic rib cage. It is this complex osteoligamentous relationship that determines its biomechanics and reaction to various pathological conditions (1–4).

Normal spinal motion is defined in terms of combinations of translations and rotations about a three-axis system. This gives a total of six degrees of freedom. A force on the spine generally results in movement in all six degrees of freedom (19,20); however, in the thoracic spine sagittal movement (flexion/extension) occurs in a single plane (3,19,20).

Load-deformation curves of the spine define three zones of movement that are altered by pathological processes. In the neutral zone the osteoligamentous system provides no resistance to movement. In the elastic zone the ligaments offer resistance to movement, and there is a linear relationship between movement and the force producing it. Together, the neutral and elastic zones constitute the functional range of motion (Fig. 7). The point at which the osteoligamentous system is stressed beyond its maximum tolerance is called the injury zone, and movement in this zone causes injury to the osteoligamentous structures of the spine. The properties of the tissues, including bony and ligamentous structures, determine the extent of resis-

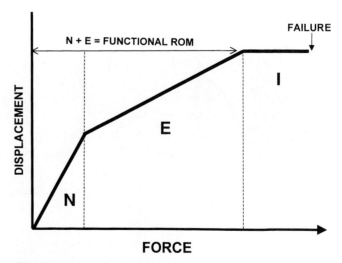

Fig. 7. Thoracic load-deformation curve. *E*, elastic zone; *I*, injury zone; *N*, neutral zone. N + E = FROM (functional range of motion).

tance and degree and direction of movement for any given load (19–21).

The naturally kyphotic rigid thoracic spine supports the axial load of the head, neck, and shoulders in flexion/kyphosis (Fig. 8). The vertebral bodies constitute the major load-bearing component in the thoracic spine. They can accommodate loads between approximately 350 pounds force and 1,800 pounds force from the first to the twelfth thoracic vertebrae (19,20). Along with the posterior ligamentous complex, the vertebral bodies represent the major anatomical structures necessary for spinal stability and the prevention of deformity in the thoracic spine. The posterior ligamentous complex (ligamentum flavum, supraspinous, intraspinous, and capsular ligaments) forms an effective dorsal tension band because it is positioned at a distance posterior to the instantaneous axis of rotation of the thoracic motion segment enabling it to act through a long lever

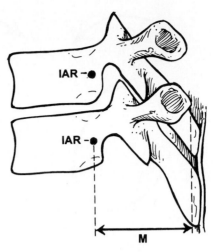

Fig. 9. The posterior ligamentous complex resists flexion because of its distance *(M)* from the instantaneous axis of rotation *(IAR)*.

arm (Fig. 9) (3,4,19,20). The posterior tension band acts to resist flexion forces, which constitutes the largest movement forces observed in the thoracic spine. Sectioning of the posterior ligamentous complex results in a 50% increase in range of motion (2,20).

Movement in the thoracic spine is limited by the anatomy and orientation of the facet joints and by the rib cage, which is firmly attached to the thoracic vertebrae by the costotransverse and costovertebral ligaments. The interaction of the sternum and rib cage with the posterior elements provides a significant degree of load sharing and limitation of movement in the thoracic spine (Fig. 10) (1,2). Oda and co-workers (2) demonstrated that the stabilizing effect of the thoracic cage is lost with bilateral division of the costovertebral joints and costosternal junctions, thereby disconnecting the thoracic spine and rib cage. The intact thoracic cage limits thoracic flexion/extension, lateral bending, and axial rotation by acting as a stabilizing lever arm that resists thoracic vertebral body movement. There were statistically significant increases in the range of motion of flexion/extension, lateral bending, and axial rotation ranging from 4 to 6 degrees under all loading conditions with destruction of the thoracic cage (2). Berg demonstrated similar findings, leading him to suggest that the rib cage complex should be considered a fourth column of stability in the thoracic spine (1).

The largest forces encountered by the thoracic spine are those involving flexion, and the vertebral bodies bear the vast majority of a flexion load (3,4). If vertebral body weight-bearing capacity is compromised by a pathological process, then progression of deformity is likely to produce further flexion and kyphotic angulation leading to instability (3,4,19,20).

Increase in the neutral zone of spinal movement is the essential feature of spinal instability. The neutral zone is associated with ligamentous laxity and is expanded by any pathological process that promotes or causes increased ligamentous laxity (19,20). If the osteoligamentous system develops an uncompensated expansion of the neutral zone, then instability and abnormal spinal movement will occur. White and Panjabi defined clinical instability as the loss of the ability of the spine under physiological loads to maintain its pattern of displacement so that there is no initial or additional neurological deficit, major deformity, and incapacitating pain (19,20).

Diseases that affect the thoracic spine tend to produce flexion or forward angulation of the spine and the naturally kyphotic posture of the thoracic region promotes progression of a flexion deformity (3,4,19,20).

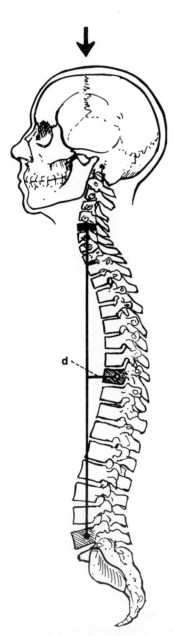

Fig. 8. The physiologically kyphotic thoracic segment counterbalances the lordotic cervical and lumbar segments, thus maintaining sagittal spine balance.

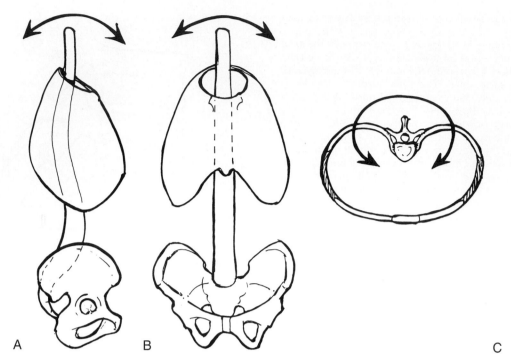

Fig. 10. Thoracic range of motion is limited in all plains of movement by an intact thoracic cage. **A:** Flexion/extension. **B:** Lateral bending. **C:** Axial rotation.

Biomechanics of Thoracic Spine Diseases

DEGENERATIVE DISEASE. Disc disease leads to osteophyte formation and facet hypertrophy secondary to abnormal movement (22,23). In addition, the facet gains an increasingly important role in axial load bearing as degenerative changes progress in the spine. The facet capsule thickens, as does the posterior ligamentous structures in an attempt to restore stability leading to eventual canal stenosis (24).

Aging also causes osteopenia that can lead to compression fractures and flexion deformity when the normal weight-bearing capacity of the osteopenic body is exceeded (4).

TRAUMA. Instability secondary to pure ligamentous injury in the thoracic spine is rare because of the osteoligamentous stabilization provided by the rib cage and supporting structures (1, 3,4). Unstable injuries of the thoracic spine usually involve vertebral body fractures. The extent of instability is determined using spinal stability models.

In 1983, Denis described the widely accepted three-column model of spinal stability. In this model the anterior column consists of the anterior longitudinal ligament and the anterior half of the vertebral body. The middle column consists of the posterior half of the vertebral body, and the posterior longitudinal ligament. The posterior column consists of the posterior elements, and the posterior ligamentous complex. Instability is defined as occurring with pathological involvement of two of the columns of support (25).

In general, pure loss of height (burst fractures) indicates pure axial column loading in excess of the load-bearing capacity of the vertebral body and failure of the anterior and middle columns. Anterior compression fractures indicate flexion injuries (pure anterior column failure) and coronal plane compression indicates lateral bending or rotation injuries in combination with anterior column failure (25).

The intervertebral disc is relatively resistant to axial loading, and the end plates fail first with loading in both normal and degenerated discs (26); however, with rotational and shear forces, the disc tears easily. Chance-type fractures secondary to shearing injuries of either the vertebral body or disc space are grossly unstable three-column injuries that require surgical stabilization (3,4,25).

INFECTION. Spinal infection may result in significant instability and biomechanical alterations, depending on the site and extent of involvement. With canal involvement by epidural abscess the bone and ligaments are generally not involved and biomechanics are not altered. Discitis usually leads to fusion of the adjoining vertebral bodies without any significant biomechanical alterations. However, disc space infections often are not discovered until the disc is destroyed and the vertebral bodies are involved. Vertebral body osteomyelitis can result in immediate instability if collapse results in acute catastrophic kyphotic deformity. Infection also can cause delayed instability, progressive kyphosis, chronic pain, and neurological deterioration; therefore, vigilant radiographic surveillance is necessary in all cases of vertebral body osteomyelitis (3,4).

INFLAMMATORY DISEASES. Chronic inflammatory diseases affect spinal biomechanics by altering the morphology and function of the synovial tissue, ligaments, and joints. They also can cause long segments of spontaneously fused vertebrae (e.g., ankylosing spondylitis, diffuse idiopathic skeletal hyperostosis [DISH]) that can transmit focused and magnified forces to the spinal cord resulting in catastrophic injuries with minor trauma (4,27).

NEOPLASTIC DISEASE. Tumors of the spinal column lead to altered biomechanics via the same mechanisms of traumatic instability. The vast majorities of thoracic spinal tumors are metastatic and cause disruption of the bony elements with relative preservation of the intervertebral disc and ligamentous structures.

SURGICAL DECOMPRESSION. Aggressive anterior and posterolateral surgical approaches can cause instability, especially if vertebral body resection is performed. The surgical approach and the extent of resection determine the degree of instability and need for reconstruction and stabilization. The goal of reconstruction and stabilization is to restore the load-bearing and biomechanical properties of the reconstructed spinal segment so that it performs adequately under physiological loads (4,25, 28).

References

1. Berg EE. The sternal-rib complex. A possible fourth column in thoracic spine fractures. *Spine* 1993;18:1916–1919.
2. Oda I, Abumi K, Lu D, et al. Biomechanical role of the posterior elements, costovertebral joints, and rib cage in the stability of the thoracic spine. *Spine* 1996;21:1423–1429.
3. Baldwin N. Biomechanics. In: Benzel E, Stillerman C, eds. *The thoracic spine.* St. Louis: Quality Medical Publishing, 1999:68–79.
4. Benzel E. *Biomechanics of spine stabilization: principles and clinical practice,* 1st ed. New York: McGraw-Hill, 1995.
5. Panjabi MM, Takata K, Goel V, et al. Thoracic human vertebrae. Quantitative three-dimensional anatomy. *Spine* 1991;16:888–901.
6. Clemente C. *Anatomy: a regional atlas of the human body,* 3rd ed. Baltimore: Urban & Schwarzenberg, 1987.
7. Goss C. *Gray's anatomy of the human body,* 29th ed. Philadelphia: Lea & Febiger, 1973.
8. Netter F. *Atlas of human anatomy.* Summit, NJ: Ciba-Geigy, 1989.
9. Ebraheim NA, Jabaly G, Xu R, et al. Anatomic relations of the thoracic pedicle to the adjacent neural structures. *Spine* 1997;22: 1553–1556; discussion 1557.
10. Ebraheim NA, Xu R, Ahmad M, et al. Projection of the thoracic pedicle and its morphometric analysis. *Spine* 1997;22:233–228.
11. McCormack BM, Benzel EC, Adams MS, et al. Anatomy of the thoracic pedicle. *Neurosurgery* 1995;37:303–308.
12. Kothe R, O'Holleran JD, Liu W, et al. Internal architecture of the thoracic pedicle. An anatomic study. *Spine* 1996;21:264–270.
13. Krag MH, Weaver DL, Beynnon BD, et al. Morphometry of the thoracic and lumbar spine related to transpedicular screw placement for surgical spinal fixation. *Spine* 1988;13:27–32.
14. Vaccaro AR, Rizzolo SJ, Balderston RA, et al. Placement of pedicle screws in the thoracic spine. Part II: An anatomical and radiographic assessment. *J Bone Joint Surg Am* 1995;77:1200–1206.
15. Vaccaro AR, Rizzolo SJ, Allardyce TJ, et al. Placement of pedicle screws in the thoracic spine. Part I: Morphometric analysis of the thoracic vertebrae. *J Bone Joint Surg Am* 1995;77:1193–1199.
16. Ebraheim NA, Xu R, Ahmad M, et al. The quantitative anatomy of the thoracic facet and the posterior projection of its inferior facet. *Spine* 1997;22:1811–1817; discussion 1818.
17. Panjabi MM, Oxland T, Takata K, et al. Articular facets of the human spine. Quantitative three-dimensional anatomy. *Spine* 1993;18: 1298–1310.
18. Jiang H, Raso JV, Moreau MJ, et al. Quantitative morphology of the lateral ligaments of the spine. Assessment of their importance in maintaining lateral stability. *Spine* 1994;19:2676–2682.
19. White A, Panjabi M. The basic kinematics of the human spine: a review of past and current knowledge. *Spine* 1978;3:12–20.
20. White A, Panjabi M. *Clinical biomechanics of the spine,* 2nd ed. Philadelphia: JB Lippincott, 1990.
21. Kumar S, Panjabi MM. In vivo axial rotations and neutral zones of the thoracolumbar spine. *J Spinal Disord* 1995;8:253–263.
22. Panjabi MM, Krag MH, Chung TQ. Effects of disc injury on mechanical behavior of the human spine. *Spine* 1984;9:707–713.
23. Markolf KL, Morris JM. The structural components of the intervertebral disc. A study of their contributions to the ability of the disc to withstand compressive forces. *J Bone Joint Surg Am* 1974;56: 675–687.
24. Shirazi-Adl A. Finite-element simulation of changes in the fluid content of human lumbar discs. Mechanical and clinical implications. *Spine* 1992;17:206–212.
25. Denis F. The three column spine and its significance in the classification of acute thoracolumbar spinal injuries. *Spine* 1983;8:817–831.
26. Brinckmann P, Frobin W, Hierholzer E, et al. Deformation of the vertebral end-plate under axial loading of the spine. *Spine* 1983;8: 851–856.
27. Boachie-Adjei O, Bullough PG. Incidence of ankylosing hyperostosis of the spine (Forestier's disease) at autopsy. *Spine* 1987;12: 739–743.
28. Ebraheim NA, Xu R, Ahmad M, et al. Anatomic considerations of anterior instrumentation of the thoracic spine. *Am J Orthop* 1997; 26:419–424.

132. Anatomy and Biomechanics of the Lumbar Spine

John J. Knightly

Knowledge of the anatomy of the thoracic and lumbar spine is crucial for understanding the normal function and mechanics of this region of the vertebral column. The purpose of this chapter is to review the anatomical relationships of the various osseous and ligamentous structures of the lumbar spinal junctions and the biomechanics of this segment in both normal physiological ranges and when placed under excessive stress. Only by a thorough understanding of these principles can abnormal thoracic and lumbar spinal segments be properly evaluated, and an appropriate treatment plan be initiated.

Anatomy

The human spine is a complex entity comprised of three basic elements: the osseous structures, their ligamentous attachments, and the neural structures they support and protect. The human spine also forms the main supporting structure of the trunk on which the head and extremities are attached. The thoracic and lumbar spine provide the majority of structural sup-

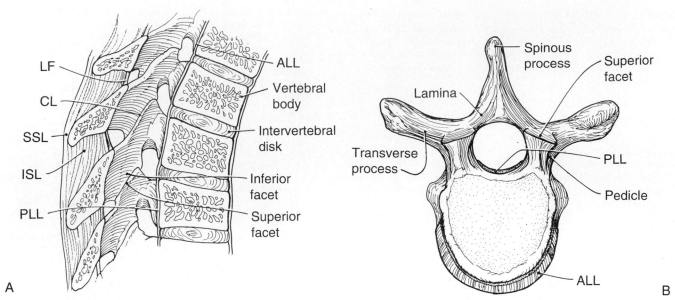

Fig. 1. Parasagittal **(A)** and axial **(B)** view of thoracic and lumbar spine. The osseous structures include the vertebral body, pedicle, superior and inferior facets, lamina, and spinous process. The ligamentous structures include the anterior longitudinal ligament *(ALL)*, posterior longitudinal ligament *(PLL)*, capsular ligaments *(CL)*, ligamentum flavum *(LF)*, interspinous ligament *(ISL)*, and supraspinous ligament *(SSL)*. (©2002, Thomas H. Weinzerl. Adapted from Knightly JJ, Sonntag VKH. Treatment of thoracolumbar fractures. In: Menezes AH, Sonntag VKH, eds. *Principles of spinal surgery.* New York: McGraw-Hill, 1996:919–950, with permission.)

port for the trunk as well as participate in movement of the trunk in relationship to the pelvis and lower extremities.

OSSEOUS STRUCTURES. The osseous structures in each segment of the lumbar spine are the vertebral bodies, pedicles, facets, lamina, spinous processes, and transverse processes. In addition, the thoracic cage is an integral part of the thoracic spine.

Vertebral Body. Each vertebral body is cylindrical in shape, formed by cortical bone at the end plate and supported by relatively thin cortical bone on the sides (Fig. 1). The vertebral body is filled with cancellous bone of varying density depending on the age and health of the individual. Both the end plates and walls are concave toward the cancellous core. Throughout the thoracic and lumbar segment, the vertebral bodies increase in size in both the anteroposterior (AP) and coronal plane (1–3). The height of the vertebral bodies also increases from T1 to L2, with the lower lumbar bodies decreased in height relative to L2 (1–4).

Pedicles. The pedicles connect the vertebral body to the remainder of the posterior elements (facets, transverse processes, lamina, and spinous processes). As depicted in Table 1, the size, shape, and angle of each paired pedicle change from each segment (thoracic or lumbar) and can vary at alternating levels. It is important to understand these differences, especially when using stabilization techniques such as pedicle screw fixation.

Descending caudally through the lumbar spine, there is a decrease in the height of the pedicle, with the shortest height being present at the L5 level, 14 mm (1,3–7). This loss of sagittal height in the lower lumbar spine is offset by the significant increase in pedicular width, with a maximum at L5 (18 mm) (3, 5–7). The angle of the pedicle in relationship to the vertebral body decreases over the thoracic segment to −4 degrees at

T12. From T12 there is a gradual increase in angulation to 30 degrees at L5 (1,3,5).

Facets. Each vertebral segment has matching superior and inferior facets extending from the area of the pedicle. In the lumbar spine (Fig. 2B), where the joint has a more curved surface than the thoracic spine, the facets are angulated approximately 90 degrees from the horizontal plane, and approximately 45 degrees from the sagittal plane (1,3). The angle from the sagittal plane also increases from L1 to L5, with the inferior facet of L5

Table 1. Mean Pedicle Dimensions in the Thoracic and Lumbar Spine[a]

Level	Width (mm)	Height (mm)	Angle with sagittal plane (degrees)	Angle with transverse plane (degrees)
T1	8 (5–10)	10 (7–15)	27 (16–34)	13 (4–25)
T5	5 (3–7)	12 (7–14)	9 (2–19)	15 (7–20)
T9	6 (4–9)	14 (11–16)	8 (0–11)	16 (9–14)
T12	7 (3–11)	16 (12–20)	−4 (−17–15)	12 (7–16)
L1	9 (5–13)	15 (11–21)	11 (7–15)	2 (−13–15)
L2	9 (4–13)	15 (10–18)	12 (5–18)	2 (−10–13)
L3	10 (5–16)	15 (8–18)	14 (8–24)	0 (−10–12)
L4	13 (9–17)	15 (9–19)	18 (6–28)	0 (−6–7)
L5	18 (9–29)	14 (10–19)	30 (19–44)	−2 (−8–6)

[a] Mean values (with range).
Adapted from White JI, Panjabi MM. *Clinical biomechanics of the spine,* 2nd ed. Philadelphia: JB Lippincott, 1990, with permission. Data from Zindrick MR, Wiltse LL, Doornik A, et al. Analysis of the morphometric characteristics of the thoracic and lumbar pedicles. *Spine* 1987;12:160–166; Berry JL, Moran JM, Berg WS, et al. A morphometric study of human lumbar and selected thoracic vertebral. *Spine* 1987;12:362–367; Krag MH, Weaver DL, Beynnon BD, et al. Morphometry of the thoracic and lumbar spine related to transpedicular screw placement for surgical spinal fixation. *Spine* 1988;13:27–32, with permission.

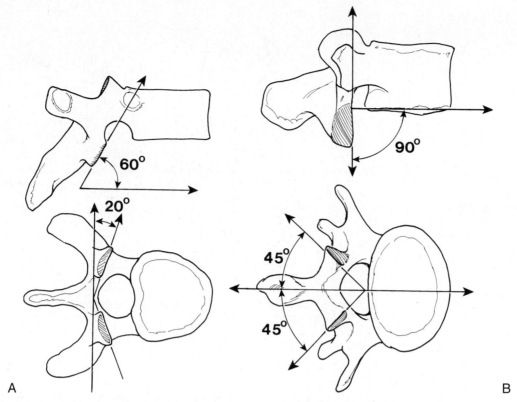

Fig. 2. Orientation of the facet joints. **A:** In the thoracic region, the face of the inferior facet is 60 degrees above the axial plane and 20 degrees off the coronal plane. **B:** In the lumbar spine, the facets take on a more sagittal alignment approximately 90 degrees from the axial plane and 45 degrees from the coronal plane. (©2002, Thomas H. Weinzerl. Adapted from White JI, Panjabi MM. *Clinical biomechanics of the spine,* 2nd ed. Philadelphia: JB Lippincott, 1990, with permission.)

being close to 50 degrees, giving a nearly vertical orientation of the L5-S1 joint, an orientation that tends to inhibit translational movement if the posterior elements remain intact (3,4).

Lamina. The lamina of the vertebral body forms the posterior margin of the vertebral canal. The shape and angle of the lamina in relationship to its origin at the pedicle dictate the diameter of the spinal canal and can have significant variation. The diameter of the canal is diminished in the upper thoracic segments and increases to its widest dimension at the thoracolumbar junction, where it remains fairly constant in the nondegenerated spine throughout the lumbar spine.

Spinous Process. The spinous processes arise from the midline at the junction of the lamina. In the thoracic spine, the spinous processes project in a more caudal direction than those processes in the lumbar spine, which project in a more straight dorsal direction without much angulation (4). The spinous processes serve with the dorsal surface of the lamina as an important site of attachment for the paraspinal musculature.

Transverse Process. There are significant differences between the transverse processes of the thoracic and lumbar spine. The transverse processes emerge from the junction of the pedicle and lamina, and, like the spinous processes, serve as an attachment site for the paraspinal musculature. In the lower thoracic spine, the transverse processes are small in size, with less rostral projection. In the lumbar spine, the transverse processes project in a more lateral-ventral direction.

LIGAMENTOUS STRUCTURES

Intervertebral Disc. The intervertebral disc may be the most complicated structure in the spinal column. It joins adjacent vertebral bodies throughout the thoracic and lumbar spine and contributes 20% to 33% of the height of the entire spinal column (3). The disc is made up of three structures: the annulus fibrosus, nucleus pulposus, and cartilaginous end plates.

Annulus Fibrosus. The annulus is comprised of layers of fibrous tissue formed into concentric bands, as shown in Fig. 3. In each layer, the fibers are orientated 30 degrees from the midline, but each adjacent band is oriented in the opposite direction, leading to a 120-degree difference in orientation (3, 4,8). The inner layers of the annulus attach directly to the cartilaginous end plates, whereas the outer layers attach directly to the vertebral body as Sharpey's fibers (3,4,9).

Nucleus Pulposus. The nucleus pulposus is a loose collection of fibrous tissue immersed in a gel containing various mucopolysaccharides occupying 30% to 50% of the cross-sectional area of the disc (3,4). The loose tissue gradually merges into the inner layers of the more organized annulus. The nucleus pulposus contains a high degree of water content that decreases with age. In the thoracic spine, the majority of the nucleus lies in the middle of the disc, whereas in the lumbar spine it is located in the more dorsal aspect of the disc (3).

Cartilaginous End Plate. The cartilaginous end plate separates the annulus and nucleus from the vertebral body at the cortical

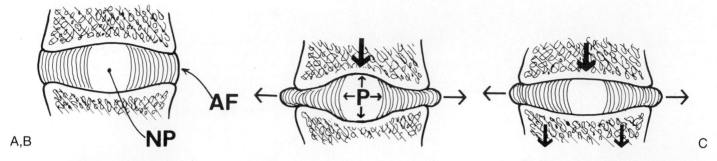

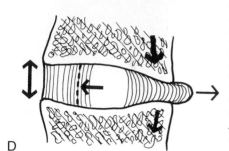

Fig. 3. Intervertebral disc under different loading conditions. **A:** The disc at rest comprised of the nucleus pulposus *(NP)* and annulus fibrosus *(AF)* with the annular fibers arranged in alternating strands 30 degrees from the end plate. **B:** A nondegenerated intervertebral disc subjected to axial loading. Pressure develops in the NP and is transmitted superiorly and inferiorly against the end plates, which deform; and circumferentially around the AF, which bulges out. **C:** A degenerated disc subjected to axial loading. Pressure does not build up within the NP and the axial forces are directed down through the AF around the periphery of the end plate. **D:** Axial load with lateral bending. On the side of the disc with compression forces, there is bulging of the disc outward, whereas on the contralateral side the AF is placed under tension and flattens. The NF shifts away from the side of compression. *P*, pressure; *arrows*, force vectors. (©2002, Thomas H. Weinzerl. Adapted from White JI, Panjabi MM. *Clinical biomechanics of the spine,* 2nd ed. Philadelphia: JB Lippincott, 1990; Benzel EC. *Biomechanics of spine stabilization: principles and clinical practice.* New York: McGraw-Hill, 1995, with permission.)

end plate. Comprised of hyaline cartilage, it is firmly attached to the cortical bone, from which it receives its blood supply (9).

Ligaments

ANTERIOR LONGITUDINAL LIGAMENT. The anterior longitudinal ligament (ALL) runs the entire length of the thoracic and lumbar spine. Although it attaches to both the vertebral body and annulus, the degree of attachment is less to the annulus (3). The fibers are thicker in the thoracic spine than the lumbar region.

POSTERIOR LONGITUDINAL LIGAMENT. The posterior longitudinal ligament (PLL), like the ALL, also runs posteriorly throughout the thoracic and lumbar segments. The PLL is interwoven with the fibers of the annulus and, as opposed to the ALL, is wider at the level of the intervertebral disc and narrows over the vertebral body (3).

LIGAMENTUM FLAVUM. The fibers of the ligamentum flavum run from the superior border of the lamina rostral to the anterior-inferior border of the superior segment and extend laterally to the undersurface of the facet complex. Although containing a high amount of elastic fibers, it has been shown to stiffen with age with a relative increase in the amount of fibrous tissue present (3,10).

INTERSPINOUS LIGAMENT. The interspinous ligaments extend from the superior surface of the spinous process to the inferior surface of the spinous process above, from the base up to the tip of the process. They are thicker in the lumbar segments than the thoracic region.

SUPRASPINAL LIGAMENT. The supraspinal ligament connects the tips of adjacent spines throughout both the thoracic and lumbar spine. Similar to the interspinous ligaments, it is thicker and broader in the lumbar spine than in the thoracic (3,4).

CAPSULAR LIGAMENT. The capsular ligaments surround the facet joint and attach to the bone outside of the synovial joint. The fibers run perpendicular to the plane of the joint (3,11).

NERVOUS STRUCTURES

Spinal Cord. The spinal cord is situated in the spinal canal surrounded by dura and suspended within cerebrospinal fluid of the subarachnoid space. The cord increases in size as travels caudally in the thoracic segment, especially between T11 and L1 where it forms the conus medullaris. Below L1, the cord terminates with the pia matter continuing on as the filum terminale. The nerve roots exiting from the lumbar and sacral levels continue to travel within the dura as the cauda equina.

Biomechanics

OSSEOUS STRUCTURES

Vertebral Body. The predominant biomechanical force affecting the vertebral body is axial loading. The overall increase in size of the vertebral bodies in the rostral-caudal direction of the thoracic and lumbar spine leads to an increase in strength and the ability to resist axial loading failure. Load to failure is highest at L4 and decreases progressively up the entire spinal column (3).

Although the facets can carry some of the axial load, the majority of the force is transferred from the superior end plate of the vertebra to the inferior end plate through the cortical shell and cancellous bone (3,11,12). Although cortical bone provides the majority of strength in most long bones, the cortical shell in the vertebral bodies is relatively small. Depending on the density and ash content (osseous tissue) of the body, the cortical shell provides from as little as 10% of the axial failure load to as much as 65% when there is a decrease in the load-sharing characteristics of the cancellous bone (3,13,14). A 25% loss of ash content leads to a 50% loss of vertebral strength (3, 15).

The load-to-failure characteristics of the cancellous bone depend on age and other pathological processes. Under the age of 40, trabecular bone accounts for 55% of the load share compared to 35% after age 40, leading to decreased vertebral strength (3,9,13). Lindahl has described three different qualities of cancellous bone when they fail. In Type I, there is decreased strength in the bone after failure; in Type II the strength of the bone is maintained after failure; and Type III there is an increase in the overall strength of the bone after the initial failure (3,16). Type III bone is more likely to be found in males under 40 (3, 16). Another factor influencing the failure rate of cancellous bone is the presence of bone marrow. Hays and Carter have shown that the collapse of trabecular bone constrains the movement of the bone marrow, which then acts as a hydraulic cushion (3,17).

Compression forces generated by various loading conditions affect the end plates of the vertebral bodies more than the cortical shell (3,9,18,19). End plate failure occurs centrally, peripherally, or in a combined fashion depending on the health of the disc (18). In a nondegenerated disc, force is directed through the nucleus, which absorbs a portion of the energy and transmits the remainder to the central portion of the adjoining end plate. The energy load may cause the center portion of the end plate to buckle, and if sufficient, and not enough support from the underlying cancellous bone is present, to fail. In the second scenario with a significantly degenerated disc, the force is transferred directly through the annulus, thus causing the peripheral portion of the end plate to fail. Combined failures occur when sufficient force is generated to cause the entire end plate to fail (3,18).

POSTERIOR ELEMENTS. Facets have fewer load-bearing characteristics than the vertebral body, but are still important in providing stability. Facets support 0% to 33% of axial loads, depending on the degree of flexion or extension involved (3,11,12). With the functional segment in extension, an increase in the amount of axial loading force is directed more posteriorly through the facet joints (3,4). In the lumbar spine, the facet joint absorb 45% and 33% of the torsional and shear forces, respectively, stabilizing against axial rotational forces (1,3,9,11). The facets also protect the intervertebral disc from being damaged by excessive rotation (3,20–22).

The pedicle is the only portion of the vertebral segment that has a high ratio of cortical to cancellous bone. This ratio is higher in the smaller pedicles of the thoracic and upper lumbar spine and somewhat decreased in the lower lumbar spine and sacrum. This increase in bone density affects screw pullout, with screw in smaller pedicles having more resistance than larger pedicles (4).

LIGAMENTOUS STRUCTURES

Disc. The intervertebral disc is the primary structure that transfers compressive forces between adjacent vertebral bodies (3, 9). Other tensile stresses are placed on the disc depending on the force moments being applied. Some degree of tension force is generated in the disc regardless of the direction of the stress (9). Figure 3 shows the intervertebral disc under different load conditions. The disc is stiffest under conditions of compression caused by buildup of pressure within the nucleus pulpous and weakest under tensile loading (3,9). How loads are transferred through the disc is dependent on the degree of degeneration (23). When a pure axial load is generated in a nondegenerative disc, pressure is developed within the nucleus pulposus and then directed against both vertebral end plates and the annular fibers (Fig. 3B) (19,24,25). This allows some of the energy to be absorbed by the annular fibers, and deformation of the vertebral end plate (3). With degenerative discs, the nucleus does not have the same load absorbing qualities; therefore, most of the load is transferred to peripheral portions of the end plate directly through the annulus (Fig. 3C) (3,9,19). When excessive loads are placed on the disc, there is predominant failure of the end plate rather than the disc (3,19).

Rarely is there an isolated pure axial loading of the disc. With lateral bending or asymmetric axial loading, the disc is put under conditions of both compression and tension (Fig. 3D). The portion of the disc under compression bulges while the side loaded under tension contracts. In addition to these changes in the annular fibers, the nucleus also shifts away from the side of compression toward the side under tension (3,4,26). Over time, and given that the disc is weaker under tension than compression, this phenomenon of the nucleus migrating toward the area of tension can explain prolapse of the nucleus through degenerating annular fibers. Radial fissuring and tissue fragmentation ("fissure and fragment") of the annulus has been found to contribute to this process (8,27). The disc is most loaded in flexion, and is exposed to large tension forces when placed under flexion and lateral bending (28).

The intervertebral disc also is subjected to loading in the form of torsion and shear forces. The strong attachment of the annular fibers to the vertebral body inhibits failure from these forces in most circumstances. Torque alone does not cause failure of the disc but enhances disruptive forces from other vectors, especially in flexion (29). Shear forces over time are thought to contribute to separation of the lamina within the annular ring and enhance degeneration (30). The posterior elements, specifically the facet joints, resist torsion and shear stresses; failure of the disc from these forces is unlikely if they are intact (3,20,21).

Spinal Ligaments. The spinal ligaments allow for varying degrees of movement in the vertebral column and help maintain structural support. Ligaments are most effective in resisting tensile loads directed along the course of their fibers. When subjected to a load, each ligament has a load-displacement curve, with variations dependent on the relative ratio of elastic to fibrous tissue within the ligament. Thus the ligamentum flavum, which has a high elastic content, has a different curve than the ALL, which is far more fibrous. As described by Panjabi, each load-displacement curve is broken into three sections: neutral, elastic, and plastic zone (Fig. 4) (31). The neutral zone is where the ligament is most flexible with deformation (lengthening) being produced with minimal load (stress). In the elastic zone, more load is needed to produce a deformation. The neutral and plastic zone together forms the physiological range of motion. With increasing loads above the plastic zone, deformation occurs only through microtrauma within the ligament until the load reaches a point where failure of the ligament results (31). Within the plastic zone, large amounts of energy can be absorbed before there is failure of the ligament (3,31). These characteristics of the spinal ligaments allow normal physiological motion and alignment within the spinal column to occur while eliminating extremes of motion under normal physiological loads, and prevention of failure of the ligament by resisting excessive loads.

As illustrated in Fig. 5, each ligament resists physiological loads differently because of its orientation and location in relationship to the instantaneous axis of rotation (IAR) of each vertebral segment (2,3,10,32–35). Paired ligaments also differ within an individual segment depending on the amount of lateral bending forces applied. The anterior longitudinal ligament is most important in resisting extension loads. The posterior longitudinal ligament is important in preventing flexion and lateral bending. The capsular ligaments inhibit lateral bending and axial rotation as well as some degree of flexion. The interspinous and supraspinous ligaments are both important in preventing flexion. Although these last two ligaments are individually not as strong as others (e.g., the anterior longitudinal ligament), their greater distance from the IAR gives them a longer lever arm to resist flexion (4). The capsular ligaments, with their fibers aligned perpendicular to the plane of the facet joint, are important in resisting rotation and contribute to control of both flexion and extension (3,11,20,35).

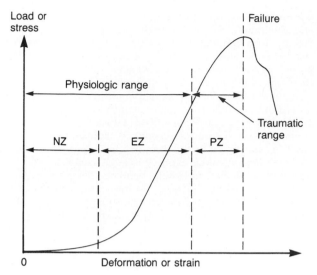

Fig. 4. Load-deformation curve for a typical ligament. The physiological range is made up of the neutral zone *(NZ)* and the elastic zone *(EZ)*. In the NZ, as the ligament is deformed (increased strain), there is little change in load (stress). As the ligament is further deformed, the EZ is entered where there is a significant increase in load on the ligament. As the ligament is stressed past its physiological range, the plastic zone *(PZ)* is entered where deformation occurs at the expense of microtrauma within the ligament until the load is increased to the point where there is failure of the entire ligament. The traumatic range is occurs with load and deformation past the physiological range. (Adapted from White JI, Panjabi MM. *Clinical biomechanics of the spine,* 2nd ed. Philadelphia: JB Lippincott, 1990, with permission.)

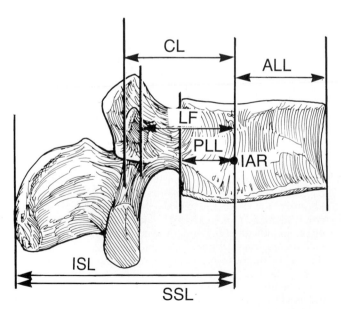

Fig. 5. The effective moment arms of the spinal ligaments. The longer the ligament is relative to the instantaneous axis of rotation (IAR), the longer the moment (or lever) arm. *Dot,* IAR; *ALL,* anterior longitudinal ligament; *CL,* capsular ligaments; *ISL,* interspinous ligament; *LF,* ligamentum flavum; *PLL,* posterior longitudinal ligament; *SSL,* supraspinous ligament. (©2002, Thomas H. Weinzerl. Adapted from Benzel EC. *Biomechanics of spine stabilization: principles and clinical practice.* New York: McGraw-Hill, 1995, with permission.)

The ligamentum flavum has special characteristics that are clinically important. Although this ligament has a high amount of elastic fibers, Evans and Nachemson found "resting" tension within the ligament (10). The ligamentum flavum is important in preventing lateral bending and flexion (3,35). When the ligament goes back into the neutral position, the "resting" tension is thought to contract the ligament to prevent buckling of the ligament into the canal, where it may compress the neural structures (3,10).

INSTABILITY. Clinical instability, as defined by White and Panjabi, "is the loss of the ability of the spine under physiologic loads to maintain its pattern of displacement so that there is no initial or additional neurological deficit, no major deformity, and no incapacitating pain" (3). Benzel to simplified this " . . . the inability to limit excessive or abnormal spinal displacement" (4). The thoracic and lumbar spinal segments are subjected to a high degree of physiological loads both during normal activities of daily living and in cases of trauma. Depending on the amount of load, vector of the force, and health of the involved vertebral segment, failure of the spine can develop leading to pain, deformity, and possible neurological compromise. The vertebral axis is divided anatomically in order to determine which structures are important in maintaining stability. As described by Holdsworth (Fig. 6), the osseous and ligamentous structures were divided into anterior and posterior elements with the posterior longitudinal ligament forming the posterior margin of the anterior elements (36). Holdsworth felt the posterior ligamentous complex was the predominant structure in stability. Denis devised a three-column system to help differentiate types of fractures leading to instability (Fig. 6): the anterior, middle, and posterior columns (37,38). The anterior column comprises the ALL and anterior half of the vertebral body and intervertebral disc. The middle column comprises the PLL and posterior half of the vertebral body and intervertebral disc. Finally, the posterior column comprises all osseous and ligamentous structures dorsal to the PLL.

Biomechanical studies indicate removal of the posterior column does not necessarily cause instability as long as integrity of the anterior and middle columns is maintained (3). However, as was noted in the preceding, loss of integrity of the posterior elements can lead to increased stress on the intervertebral disc and hasten degeneration. Clinically, the integrity of the posterior column is important in determining the stability of a lesion, especially burst fractures (39–41).

To better understand the concept of instability, White and Panjabi developed a point system that helps define what deformities are clinically unstable (3). Their point system helps quantify from a radiographical and clinical perspective whether instability is present at a particular vertebral motion segment. Table 2 shows the Benzel modification of this point system that can be used throughout the subaxial spine (4). With either system of point grading, a score of 5 or greater is indicative of overt spinal instability of the involved segment. Other factors certainly play a role in determining what the appropriate treatment is when diagnosing instability, because, as stated by Benzel, " . . . the spine surgeon must rely on common sense combined with clinical astuteness . . . . (t)here is no substitute for common sense" (4).

Instability of the spine can occur in several different pathological conditions ranging from severe trauma to progressive deformity secondary to degeneration of the vertebral segment. *Benzel categorized clinical instability as acute and chronic (4). Acute instability is subdivided into overt and limited instability.* Overt instability, usually seen in trauma but also found in destruction of the vertebral segment by neoplasm, infection, or severe degeneration, results in " . . . the inability of the spine

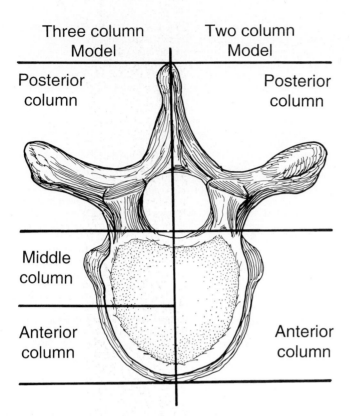

Fig. 6. The two-column versus three-column model of the spine. The two-column model, as described by Holdsworth (36), divides the spine in half with the anterior half containing all ventral structures up to and including the posterior longitudinal ligament (PLL). The posterior column contains all structures dorsal to the PLL. In the three-column model of Denis (37,38), the anterior column is comprised of the anterior longitudinal ligament (ALL) and the ventral half of the vertebral body and intervertebral disc. The middle column is comprised of the dorsal half of the vertebral body and intervertebral disc, and the PLL. The posterior column is all-osseous and ligamentous structures dorsal to the PLL. (©Thomas H. Weinzerl. Adapted from Knightly JJ, Sonntag VKH. Treatment of thoracolumbar fractures. In: Menezes AH, Sonntag VKH, eds. *Principles of spinal surgery.* New York: McGraw-Hill, 1996: 919–950.)

Table 2. Benzel Point System for Quantification of Acute Instability in the Subaxial Cervical, Thoracic, and Lumbar Spine[a]

Condition	Points
Loss of integrity of anterior (and middle) column[b]	2
Loss of integrity of posterior column (s)[b]	2
Acute resting translational deformity[c]	2
Acute resting angulation deformity[c]	2
Acute dynamic translational deformity exaggeration[d]	2
Acute dynamic angulation deformity exaggeration[d]	2
Neural element injury[e]	3
Acute disk narrowing at level of suspected pathology	1
Dangerous loading anticipated	1

[a] A score of 5 or greater points indicates overt instability, with 2 to 4 points implying the presence of limited instability, as discussed in text.
[b] From clinical or radiographic evaluation; one point if incomplete evidence exists.
[c] Based on static anteroposterior and lateral plain films using criteria of White and Panjabi.
[d] Based on standard flexion and extension views. To be done only if other assessments of instability have failed to confirm degree of instability and only by experienced clinician.
[e] Three points for cauda equina injuries, 2 points for cord injuries, and 1 for isolated root injuries.
Modified from Benzel EC. *Biomechanics of spine stabilization: principles and clinical practice.* New York: McGraw-Hill, 1995, with permission.
Original adaptation from White JI, Panjabi MM. *Clinical biomechanics of the spine,* 2nd ed. Philadelphia: JB Lippincott, 1990, with permission.

to support the torso during normal activity" (4). There must be failure of all three-columns for this to occur. In limited instability, there is " . . . loss of either ventral or dorsal spinal integrity, with preservation of the other—which is sufficient to support some normal activities" (4). Overt instability usually needs to be treated surgically, whereas cases of limited instability often can be managed conservatively.

Chronic instability is also subcategorized into *glacial instability and dysfunctional segmental motion* (4). As defined by Benzel, glacial instability is " . . . spinal instability that is not overt and that does not pose a significant chance of the rapid development or progression of kyphotic, scoliotic, or translational deformities; but in which, as in the motion of a glacier, the deformity progresses gradually, and substantial external forces do not cause immediate movement or progression of deformity" (4). An example of glacial instability is spondylolisthesis, but the etiology can include trauma, tumor, spondylosis, and infection. Whatever the etiology, a clinical situation develops where the involved segment is abnormal in some way and what may otherwise be normal physiological loads cause progressive failure. Treatment can range from observation to surgical correction of the deformity, depending on the degree of symptoms (usually pain) or the potential for neurological injury.

A dysfunctional segmental motion is " . . . a type of instability related to a disk interspace or vertebral body degenerative changes, tumor, or infection that results in the potential for pain of spinal origin" (4). Sometimes referred to as mechanical instability, there is neither evidence of significant deformity nor radiographical evidence of overt instability. The diagnosis of dysfunctional segmental motion is difficult to make either from a clinical or radiographical perspective, and thus has a potential for abuse as an indication for surgical fusion with possible poor clinical outcomes (4).

References

1. Panjabi MM, Takata K, Goel V, et al. Thoracic human vertebrae. Quantitative three-dimensional anatomy. *Spine* 1991;16:888–901.
2. Panjabi MM, White AA III. Basic biomechanics of the spine. *Neurosurgery* 1980;7:76–93.
3. White JI, Panjabi MM. *Clinical biomechanics of the spine,* 2nd ed. Philadelphia: JB Lippincott, 1990.
4. Benzel EC. *Biomechanics of spine stabilization: principles and clinical practice.* New York: McGraw-Hill, 1995.
5. Zindrick MR, Wiltse LL, Doornik A, et al. Analysis of the morphometric characteristics of the thoracic and lumbar pedicles. *Spine* 1987; 12:160–166.
6. Berry JL, Moran JM, Berg WS, et al. A morphometric study of human lumbar and selected thoracic vertebrae. *Spine* 1987;12:362–367.
7. Krag MH, Weaver DL, Beynnon BD, et al. Morphometry of the thoracic and lumbar spine related to transpedicular screw placement for surgical spinal fixation. *Spine* 1988;13:27–32.
8. Shirazi-Adl A. Strain in fibers of a lumbar disc. Analysis of the role of lifting in producing disc prolapse. *Spine* 1989;14:96–103.
9. Gertzbein SD. *Thoracolumbar fractures.* Baltimore: Williams & Wilkins, 1992.
10. Evans JH, Nachemson AL. Biomechanical study of human lumbar ligamentum flavum. *J Anat* 1969;105:188–189.
11. Shirazi-Adl A, Drouin G. Load-bearing role of facets in a lumbar segment under sagittal plane loadings. *J Biomech* 1987;20:601–613.
12. Nachemson A. The load on lumbar disks in different positions of the body. *Clin Orthop* 1966;45:107–122.

13. Rockoff SD, Sweet E, Bleustein J. The relative contribution of trabecular and cortical bone to the strength of human lumbar vertebrae. *Calcif Tissue Res* 1969;3:163–175.
14. McBroom RJ, Hayes WC, Edwards WT, et al. Prediction of vertebral body compressive fracture using quantitative computed tomography. *J Bone Joint Surg Am* 1985;67:1206–1214.
15. Bell GH, Dunbar O, Beck JS, et al. Variations in strength of vertebrae with age and their relation to osteoporosis. *Calcif Tissue Res* 1967;1:75–86.
16. Lindahl O. Mechanical properties of dried defatted spongy bone. *Acta Orthop Scand* 1976;47:11–19.
17. Carter DR, Hayes WC. The compressive behavior of bone as a two-phase porous structure. *J Bone Joint Surg Am* 1977;59:954–962.
18. Perry O. Fracture of the vertebral end plate in the lumbar spine. *Acta Orthop Scand* 1957;25(suppl).
19. Shirazi-Adl A. Finite-element simulation of changes in the fluid content of human lumbar discs. Mechanical and clinical implications. *Spine* 1992;17:206–212.
20. Shirazi-Adl A. Nonlinear stress analysis of the whole lumbar spine in torsion—mechanics of facet articulation. *J Biomech* 1994;27:289–299.
21. Oxland TR, Crisco JJ III, Panjabi MM, et al. The effect of injury on rotational coupling at the lumbosacral joint. A biomechanical investigation. *Spine* 1992;17:74–80.
22. Miller JA, Haderspeck, KA, Schultz, AB. Posterior element loads in lumbar motion segments. *Spine* 1983;8:331–337.
23. Horst M, Brinckmann P. 1980 Volvo award in biomechanics. Measurement of the distribution of axial stress on the end plate of the vertebral body. *Spine* 1981;6:217–232.
24. Brinckmann P, Frobin W, Hierholzer E, et al. Deformation of the vertebral end plate under axial loading of the spine. *Spine* 1983;8:851–856.
25. Reuber M, Schultz A, Denis F, et al. Bulging of lumbar intervertebral disks. *J Biomech Eng* 1982;104:187.
26. Krag MH, Seroussi RE, Wilder DG, et al. Internal displacement distribution from in vitro loading of human thoracic and lumbar spinal motion segments: experimental results and theoretical predictions. *Spine* 1987;12:1001–1007.
27. Brinckmann P, Porter RW. A laboratory model of lumbar disc protrusion. Fissure and fragment. *Spine* 1994;19:228–235.
28. Shirazi-Adl A. Biomechanics of the lumbar spine in sagittal/lateral moments. *Spine* 1994;19:2407–2414.
29. Shirazi-Adl A, Ahmed AM, Shrivastava SC. Mechanical response of a lumbar motion segment in axial torque alone and combined with compression. *Spine* 1986;11:914–927.
30. Goel VK, Monroe BT, Gilbertson LG, et al. Interlaminar shear stresses and laminae separation in a disc. Finite element analysis of the L3-L4 motion segment subjected to axial compressive loads. *Spine* 1995;20:689–698.
31. Panjabi MM. The stabilizing system of the spine. Part II. Neutral zone and instability hypothesis. *J Spinal Disord* 1992;5:390–396.
32. Panjabi MM, Greenstein G, Duranceau J, et al. Three-dimensional quantitative morphology of lumbar spinal ligaments. *J Spinal Disord* 1991;4:54–62.
33. Panjabi MM, Hausfeld JN, White AA III. A biomechanical study of the ligamentous stability of the thoracic spine in man. *Acta Orthop Scand* 1981;52:315–326.
34. Panjabi MM, Greenstein G, Duranceau J, et al. Three-dimensional quantitative morphology of lumbar spinal ligaments. *J Spinal Disord* 1991;4:54–62.
35. Panjabi MM, Goel VK, Takata K. Physiological strains in the lumbar spinal ligaments. An in vitro biomechanical study 1981 Volvo Award in Biomechanics. *Spine* 1982;7:192–203.
36. Holdsworth F. Fractures, dislocations and fracture-dislocations of the spine. *J Bone Joint Surg Am* 1970;53A:1534–1559.
37. Denis F. The three-column spine and its significance in the classification of acute thoracolumbar spinal injuries. *Spine* 1983;8:817–831.
38. Denis F. Spinal instability as defined by the three-column spine concept in acute spinal trauma. *Clin Orthop* 1984;189:65–76.
39. Cantor JB, Lebwohl NH, Garvey T, et al. Nonoperative management of stable thoracolumbar burst fractures with early ambulation and bracing. *Spine* 1993;18:971–976.
40. James KS, Wenger KH, Schlegel JD, et al. Biomechanical evaluation of the stability of thoracolumbar burst fractures. *Spine* 1994;19:1731–1740.
41. Knightly JJ, Sonntag VKH. Treatment of thoracolumbar fractures. In: Menezes AH, Sonntag VKH, eds. *Principles of spinal surgery*. New York: McGraw-Hill, 1996:919–950.

133. Anatomy and Biomechanics of Sacral Fractures

Jeffrey D. Gross and Seth M. Zeidman

The sacrum is a unique element of the spine which functions as a force transition unit, distributing the axial load of the spine to the pelvis and legs. Because of the relationship of the sacrum to the lumbar spine and pelvis, it has an impact on the development of degenerative changes at the lumbosacral junction. Acute injuries of the sacrum are not without neural and vascular sequelae. This chapter provides a review of the anatomy and biomechanics of the sacrum, and includes a discussion of sacral fractures.

Sacral Anatomy

OSSEOUS ANATOMY. The sacrum represents five fused vertebrae that articulate rostrally with the lumbar spine; the number of sacral vertebrae can vary from four to six. This lower portion of the spinal column forms the dorsal wall of the bony pelvis, situated between the paired iliac bones (Fig. 1). The wedge-shaped sacrum is concave ventrally, and narrows in two planes as it descends toward the caudal end of the bone. The coccygeal spine lies rostral to the sacrum (1–3).

The ventral sacral foramina are paired openings at each sacral level transmitting the ventral rami of the sacral nerves, which contribute to the lumbosacral plexuses (Fig. 2) (1–3). The ventral rami travel in grooves lateral to each ventral sacral foramen, while a transverse ridge runs horizontally between neighboring ventral sacral foramina (3). The portion of the sacrum lateral to the foramina is known as the lateral mass, which contains the venal grooves (4).

The sacral promontory refers to the most rostral and ventral

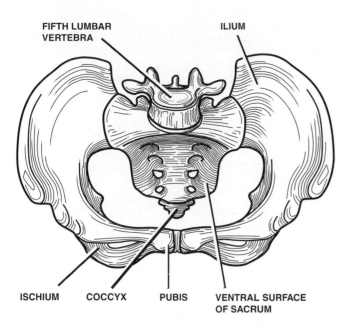

FIFTH LUMBAR VERTEBRA   **ILIUM**

ISCHIUM   COCCYX   PUBIS   VENTRAL SURFACE OF SACRUM

Fig. 1. A depiction of the sacrum and its relationship to the lumbar spine and pelvis.

edge of the ventral portion of the sacrum. The lateral borders of the sacrum, which are called the lateral sacral notches, articulate with the iliac bones; the lateral sacral notches are located opposite the second through fourth sacral segments (1). The lateral borders of the sacrum caudal to the lateral sacral notches are called the inferior lateral angles, which end caudally as the sacral apex.

The dorsal surface of the sacrum is convex and covers the sacral spinal canal with fused posterior sacral elements (1,2). The sacral hiatus is formed from the deficiency of these posterior elements near the caudal end of the canal (Fig. 2) (1,2). The sacral spinal canal tapers as it descends caudally. Sacral spinous processes are smaller than the processes of the lumbar vertebrae, and form the median sacral crest running the length of the midline of the dorsal surface of the sacrum. The paired sacral grooves lie lateral to the sacral crests, and represent the fused laminae medial to the fused facets. The sacral grooves end caudally at the sacral cornua, which articulate with the coccyx. Just lateral to these sacral grooves lie the four pairs of dorsal sacral foramina, which transmit the dorsal rami of the sacral nerves (1,2). The larger ventral sacral foramina lie in a horizontal plane from their corresponding dorsal sacral foramina. Lateral to the dorsal sacral foramina are the lateral sacral crests, which contain the sacral transverse tubercles. The sacral transverse tubercles represent transverse processes and costal elements at other spinal levels. The rostral sacral transverse tubercles comprise the sacral tuberosity (1–3).

The first sacral vertebra has enlarged lateral masses called the sacral ala (Fig. 2). These lateral prominences articulate with the pelvic iliac bones. The first sacral vertebral body articulates with the last lumbar vertebra via an intervertebral disc. This lumbosacral disc is often taller ventrally and thin dorsally. The dorsal portion of each ala contains an articular process known as the first sacral superior articular process, or facet joint. The superior facet of S-1 articulates with the inferior facets of L-5 in nearly the coronal plane (Fig. 3) (3,5,6). The rostral sacrum contains the superior sacral notches that transmit the fifth lumbar nerves.

The sacral pedicles are short and wide, while the first sacral pedicle is the largest in the entire spinal column (7). These

important landmarks of the sacrum may be angled 25 to 30 degrees from the midsagittal plane (Fig. 4) (2,7).

The lumbar spinal column forms an angle with the sacrum called the lumbosacral angle (Fig. 5); the average lumbosacral angle should be 210 to 220 degrees (1,3,6,8). Although the female sacrum is wider than the male sacrum, the sacroiliac articulations are longer in the male (1,9). Differences also include a more pronounced sacral curvature, and greater lumbosacral angle in the female (1,3). The inclusion of a coccygeal vertebra, a mobile (or lumbarized) first sacral vertebra, a rostrally located sacral hiatus, dorsal sacral canal deficiencies, and sacral agenesis in association with other musculoskeletal deformities are further variations in the sacrum (3).

The facet and disc of the sacrum articulate rostrally with the fifth lumbar vertebra, while caudally the sacrum articulates with the sacrococcygeal disc and the cornua. The sacrum articulates laterally with the paired ilium bones to form the sacroiliac joints (SIJs) (3). The sacroiliac articulations are composed of the interactions of the sacral ala and the iliac bones. The SIJs are synovial joints that are closely related to their strong ligamentous complexes (3). The SIJs may fuse with advancing age (3). The ventral portion of the articular surface of the ilium is significantly thicker than the dorsal portion (10). The sacrum articulates with the coccyx via the fibrocartilaginous and synovial sacrococcygeal disc (3). In humans, the coccyx is a rudimentary structure comprised of three to five vestigial vertebrae. The superior articular processes of the first coccygeal vertebra are called the coccygeal cornua, and articulate with the sacral cornua (1,11).

MUSCULOLIGAMENTOUS ANATOMY. The posterior longitudinal ligament (PLL) crosses the dorsal surface of the lumbosacral disc space and attaches to the ventral wall of the sacral spinal canal (Fig. 6). The ligamentum flavum extends caudally from the ventral surfaces of the lumbar laminae to the sacral laminae (3). The strong dorsal sacroiliac ligaments attach the dorsum of the sacrum to the iliac bones. The attachment of these ligaments occurs near the dorsolateral aspect of the lateral mass of the sacrum, opposite the first two sacral vertebrae, and helps to stabilize the dorsal sacroiliac joints (Fig. 6) (3). The dorsal sacroiliac ligaments can be divided into deep and superficial portions. The deep portion connects the sacral tuberosity to the iliac tuberosity, and the longer, superficial part bridges the posterior superior iliac spine to the lateral sacral crest (3). A stronger interosseous sacroiliac ligament blends with the deeper portion of the dorsal sacroiliac ligament to connect the sacral tuberosities with the iliac tuberosities.

The sacrotuberous ligaments blend, and extend over the dorsal sacroiliac ligaments. These sacrotuberous ligaments fasten the transverse tubercles of third (and sometimes fourth) sacral segment(s) to the posterior inferior spine of the ilium. Rostral fibers of the sacrotuberous ligament may be contiguous and indistinct from fibers of the oblique portion of the dorsal sacroiliac ligament. The remaining fibers of the sacrotuberous ligaments extend from the lower sacral transverse tubercles and coccyx, to the dorsal aspect of the ilium and ischial tuberosity (1,2). The gluteus maximus muscles follow the fibers of these ligaments from the ilium to the lower sacrum (Fig. 7).

The multifidus spinae muscle arises from the sacral groove that extends from the dorsal sacroiliac ligament. Superficial to the dorsal sacroiliac ligament lies the sacrospinalis muscles which attach the median sacral ridge to the ilium in a rostrocaudal direction (Fig. 7). The coccygeus muscles lie caudal to the multifidus. The coccygeus muscle fibers extend from the dorsocaudal sacrum to the coccyx, and are continuous rostrally with the sacrospinous ligament. This ligament extends from the lateral sacrum to the spine of the ischium, deep to the sacrotuberous ligament (1–3). The greater sciatic foramen is defined cau-

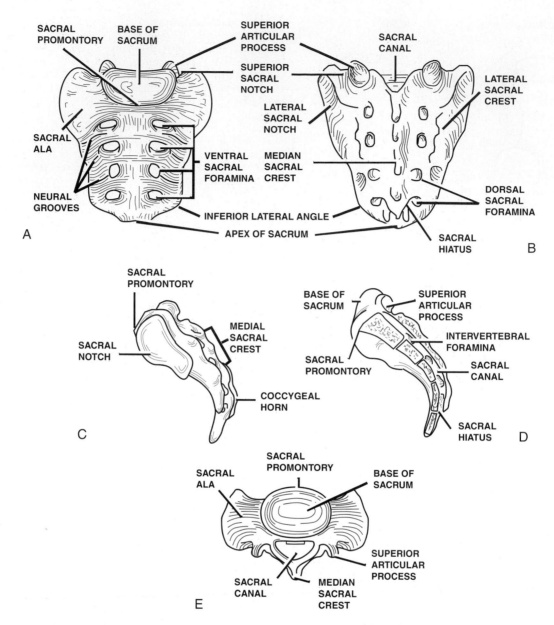

Fig. 2. Drawings of the sacrum. **A:** Ventral surface. **B:** Dorsal surface. **C:** A lateral sagittal view. **D:** A midline sagittal view. **E:** Axial view from the rostral vantage.

dally by the sacrospinous ligament (2,3). In addition, the interspinous and supraspinous ligaments extend from adjacent spinous processes of the sacrum, and are contiguous with lumbar spinous processes (1–3). The caudal continuation of these ligaments is known as the deep sacrococcygeal ligament.

The most caudal portion of the sacrospinous ligament extends beyond the sacral hiatus to the coccyx. These fibers become indistinct with fibers of the coccygeus muscle and other muscles that line the floor of the pelvis. The anococcygeal ligament extends from the coccyx to the anorectal musculature allowing for rectal sphincter muscular attachment points (1).

The latissimus dorsi, gluteus maximus muscles, and the erector spinae muscular group are part of the dorsal musculature involved in stabilizing the lumbosacral and iliosacral junctions. Both the latissimus dorsi and the gluteus maximus muscles insert onto the thoracolumbar fascia (1–3,9).

Ventrally, the anterior longitudinal ligament (ALL) continues caudally along the spinal column and attaches to the sacrum, medial to the ventral sacral foramina (Fig. 6) (3). The ventral sacroiliac ligaments extend from the sacral promontory to each ilium, near the insertions of the inferior iliolumbar ligaments. Caudal to those fibers, the sacrotuberous ligaments connect the caudolateral sacral tubercles near the lateral sacral notches to the ischial tuberosities. The sacrotuberous ligament continues to become part of the biceps femoris tendon (2). Further ventrocaudal ligamentous fibers bridge the sacral inferior lateral angles to the spines of the ischium to form the sacrospinous ligaments, which divide the greater and lesser sciatic foramina (2, 11). Additional superior and anterior iliolumbar ligaments, and the lumbosacral annulus fibrosus are also essential to the stability of the lumbosacral junction (6,11). Several texts refer to the caudal fibers of the iliolumbar ligaments as the lumbosacral

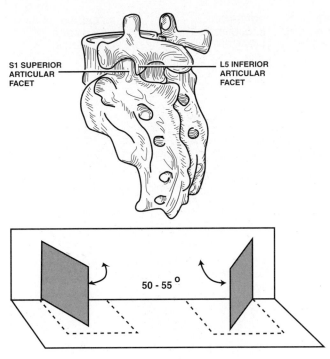

Fig. 3. The lumbosacral facet articulations.

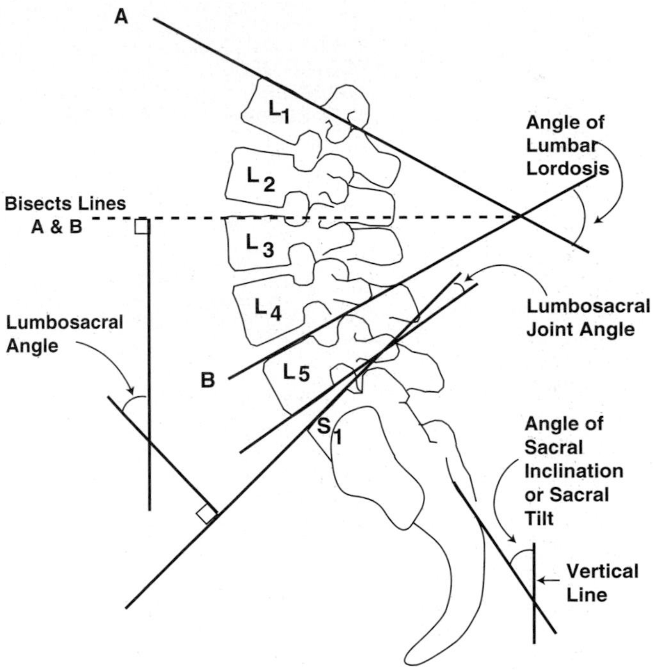

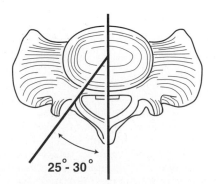

Fig. 4. An axial depiction of the first sacral vertebra to demonstrate the pedicular angles.

Fig. 5. Metrics of the lumbosacral junction.

ligament. The lumbosacral ligament joins the caudal portion of the transverse process of L-5 to the rostral portion of the ventral sacroiliac ligament (1,3,12). The lumbosacral ligament, ventral sacroiliac ligament, and sacrospinous and sacrotuberous ligaments all contribute to stabilizing the SIJs (3,11). The iliolumbar ligament has a role in stabilizing the lumbosacral junction (3, 6,11).

The piriformis muscle arises from bony ridges between the neural grooves on the dorsal portion of the sacrum and inserts onto the greater trochanter of the femur (3,9). The sacrotuberous ligament also sends a small number of fibers to attach to the fascia of the piriformis muscle (9). The more rostrally located iliacus muscle arises from the sacral ala (3).

The origin of the gluteus maximus is partially from the dorsal portion of the sacrotuberous ligament; this ligament serves to separate the gluteus maximus muscle from the piriformis muscle (3). In addition, forces from the latissimus dorsi muscles,

the erector spinae muscles, the thoracolumbar fascia, and the fascia of the serratus posteroinferior muscles are transferred to the sacrotuberous ligament (9).

The ventral sacrococcygeal ligaments are analogous to the ALL, securing the ventral coccygeal surface to the ventral sacrum, while the deep dorsal sacrococcygeal ligament is similarly analogous to the PLL (2,3). Although a superficial dorsal sacrococcygeal ligament extends further caudally, both dorsal sacrococcygeal ligaments cover the sacral hiatus. Laterally, the paired lateral sacrococcygeal ligaments, which resemble the intertransverse ligaments of more rostral spinal levels, connect the sacral transverse tubercles to the coccyx. The intercornual ligaments, which extend from the sacral cornua to the coccyx, are analogous to facet capsular ligaments (3).

NEURAL ANATOMY. The sacral spinal canal transmits the distal cauda equina and the filum terminale. The filum terminale attaches to the dorsal aspect of the first coccygeal segment to anchor the conus medullaris. Before attaching to the coccyx, the filum terminale combines with the dura mater of the sacral spinal canal. The dural sac of the sacral canal transmits the sacral and coccygeal nerve roots (Fig. 8) (2,3,11). The sacral nerve roots leave the cauda equina and branch into primary dorsal and ventral rami that exit the dorsal and ventral sacral foramina. The ventral rami are larger than their dorsal counterparts. The first three dorsal primary rami pass through their foramina and enter the substance of the multifidus muscle to divide into medial and lateral branches (1,3). Each sacral ramus carries a small dural sleeve through its foramina for a short distance, before fusing with the epineurium (3). The dorsal root ganglia lie within the sacral spinal canal, unlike other spinal levels (3,13).

The ventral sacral primary rami divide into dorsal and ventral divisions before entering the pelvis. The paired ventral sacral foramina transmit the ventral rami of the upper four sacral nerves; the fifth sacral nerve emerges near the caudal sacral

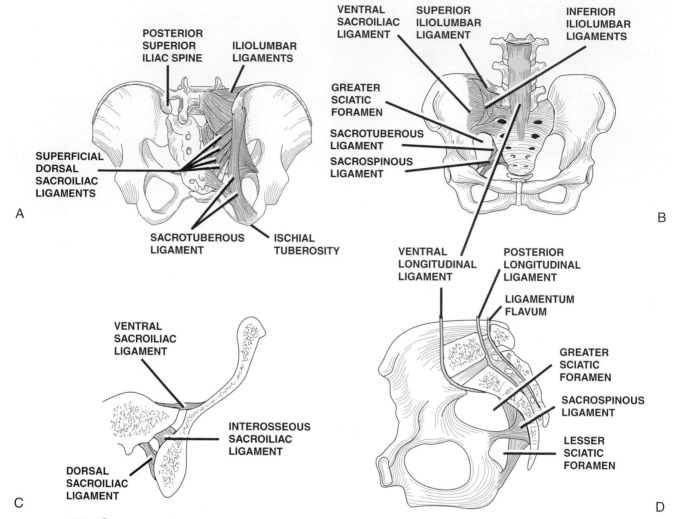

Fig. 6. Ligaments of the sacrum. **A:** Dorsal surface. **B:** Ventral surface. **C:** Axial view. **D:** Midsagittal view.

aperture and passes through the coccygeus muscle (1–3). The rostral three ventral sacral rami contribute to the sacral plexus, while the fourth and fifth ventral sacral rami contribute to the coccygeal plexus. Lumbar and sacral nerve roots combine to form the lumbosacral plexus. Distal branches of sacral nerve roots contribute nerve fibers that innervate pelvic and leg muscles, and also the pelvic viscera (Fig. 9).

Fibers from the ventral ramus of S-1 join the ventral rami of L-4 and L-5 to form the superior gluteal nerve, which courses dorsolaterally near the superior gluteal artery and leaves the pelvis through the greater sciatic foramen. The ventral rami of L-5, S-1, and S-2 contribute to the inferior gluteal nerve that runs in the sciatic notch near the sciatic nerve. The sciatic nerve receives fibers from the first three sacral roots. Branches from the lumbosacral plexus also innervate the short lateral rotator muscles of the leg, including the quadratus femoris, inferior gemellus, superior gemellus, and obturator internus. These nerves receive contributions from the first two sacral nerves. Contributions from the ventral and dorsal rami of the sacral plexus form the lateral femoral cutaneous nerve that leaves the pelvis lateral to the sacrotuberous ligament. Branches from the ventral rami of S-2, S-3, and S-4 contribute to the pudendal nerve; this nerve exits the pelvis through the greater sciatic

foramen and crosses the sacrospinous ligament close to its attachment to the ischial spine. The pudendal nerve accompanies the internal pudendal vessels, and reenters the pelvis through the lesser sciatic foramen to supply muscles of the pelvic floor and the sensory innervation to the skin of the perineum (2,3, 11). The dorsal rami of the second and third sacral nerves supply branches to the perforating cutaneous nerve to innervate the skin over the gluteus maximus muscle. The skin over the coccyx is supplied by the dorsal rami of S-4, S-5, and the coccygeal dorsal ramus.

Many autonomic nervous structures are found near the sacral region. The sympathetic trunk coalesces on the ventral surface of the sacrum (Fig. 9). Four or five sympathetic ganglia supply gray communicantes to two adjacent sacral roots. The sacral sympathetic plexus contributes fibers to the superior hypogastric plexus at the rostral end of the ventral sacrum. The superior hypogastric plexus contributes branches to the more laterally situated inferior hypogastric (or pelvic) plexuses (2,3). Parasympathetic fibers from S-2, S-3, and S-4 contribute branches to form the pelvic splanchnic nerves (Fig. 10). These nerves travel ventral to the sympathetic component en route to secondary parasympathetic ganglia to innervate the pelvic viscera (2,3).

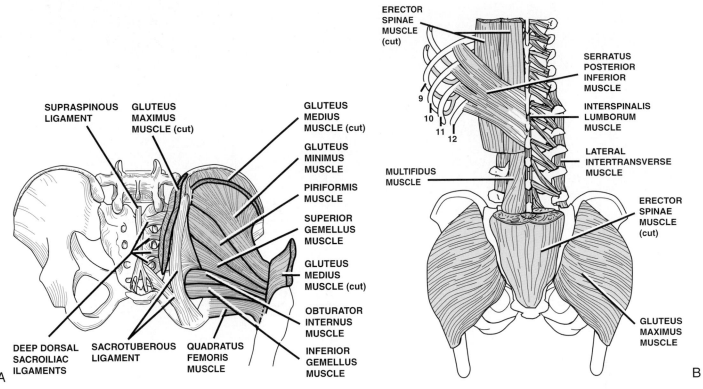

Fig. 7. Muscles of the sacrum. **A:** Dorsal surface. **B:** Ventral surface.

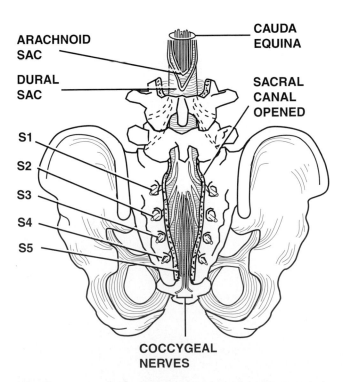

Fig. 8. A drawing of the sacral cauda equina and the filum terminale.

VASCULAR ANATOMY. The median sacral and the lateral sacral arteries provide the arterial supply to the sacrum. The median sacral artery is a branch of the aorta just above the bifurcation, and supplies the ventral surface of the sacrum and the coccyx (Fig. 11). The lateral sacral arteries come off the posterior trunks of the internal iliac arteries, and supply the sacral vertebrae and the sacral canal. The median and lateral sacral arteries anastomose anterior to the sacrum, and branches from the anastomosis enter the ventral sacral foramina. The middle rectal artery, a branch of the anterior trunk of the internal iliac, also contributes to this vascular anastomosis (2). Continuations of these arteries may exit the dorsal sacral foramina (2,3, 7). The iliolumbar artery, which comes off the posterior trunk of the internal iliac may supply the SIJs; the median sacral and iliolumbar arteries anastomose anterior to the L-5 vertebra. The superior gluteal artery is the largest branch of the internal iliac and usually runs between the first and second ventral sacral rami; it exits the pelvis through the greater sciatic foramen (3).

A venous network parallels the arterial vessels except that the vena cava is on the right side of the aorta; the arteries cross ventral to the veins. The median sacral vein or veins drain preferentially into the left common iliac vein, rather than directly into the vena cava because of the asymmetrical position of the venous drainage system. The iliolumbar veins also drain into the common iliac veins, instead of the internal iliac veins (3).

RELATIONAL ANATOMY. The peritoneal cavity lies directly ventral to the sacrum and its neurovascular elements (Fig. 12). The vascular and nervous elements that course along the ventral surface of the sacrum are retroperitoneal. The ascending and descending colon lie on the right and left sides of the pelvis, within the peritoneum (13). The ureters run in the retroperito-

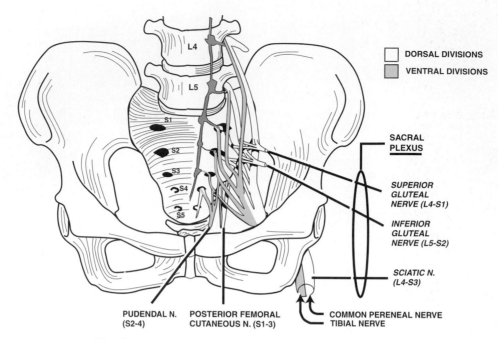

Fig. 9. A representation of the sacral plexus and its major branches.

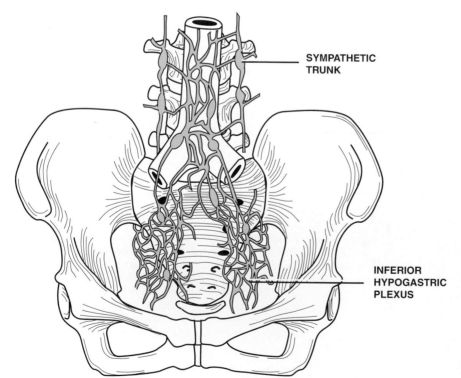

Fig. 10. A drawing of the lumbosacral sympathetic plexuses.

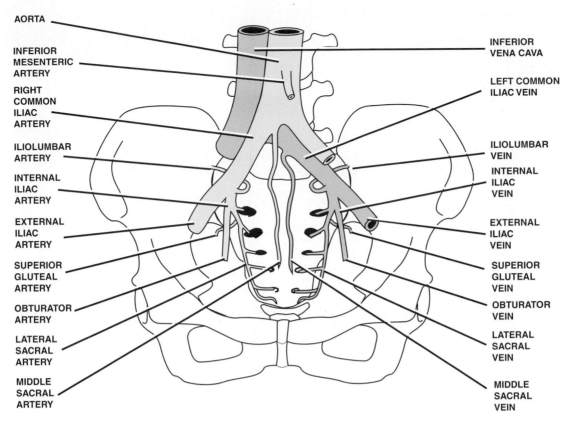

Fig. 11. A drawing of the arterial and venous anatomy of the sacrum.

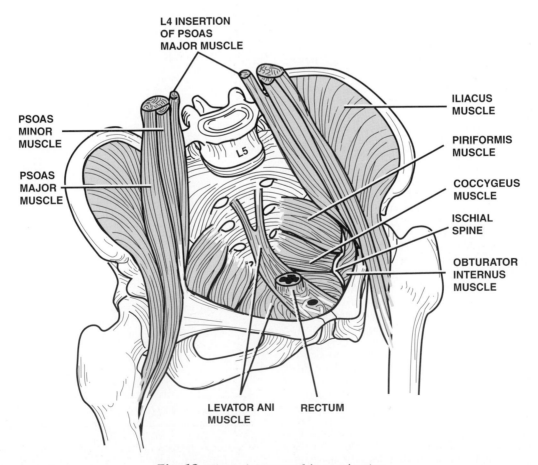

Fig. 12. Relational anatomy of the sacral region.

neal space near the sacral plexuses and the internal iliac veins (11).

Sacral Biomechanics

Because the sacrum is a relatively fixed structure, it has important interactions with the fifth lumbar vertebra and the iliac bones. The relationship of the sacrum to the coccyx has little importance for weight bearing and biomechanics. The sacrum serves as a force redirection unit allowing the axial loads of the spine to be dispersed to the pelvis, and ultimately the lower extremities (9). The angular relationship between the lumbar spine and the sacrum contributes to the significance of efficiently transferring the spinal load to the pelvis (3,6). Suboptimal lumbosacral relationships may accelerate degenerative changes and pathological conditions (6,13). Bony, ligamentous, and muscular elements all provide stability to the sacrum and its articulations, while the sacrum derives additional stability as part of the pelvic ring (13). Disruptions of the pelvic ring must occur in two distinct locations, requiring significant traumatic force. The sacrum therefore, is integral to the strong ring of the pelvis (14,15).

Normal motions of the sacrum are considered as part of pelvic tilting in relationship to the hip joints and the lumbar spine. These articulations allow maintenance of the vertical posture of the trunk during a wide range of load-bearing activities. Flexion and extension movements are possible at the lumbosacral juncture. Normal flexion may be considered to be up to 53 degrees with extension up to 30 degrees, but interaction of the lumbosacral facets limits extension (6,13). Although the sacral canal has fixed dimensions, lumbosacral flexion can cause widening of the lumbosacral foramina and elongation of the lumbar spinal canal. The end result of flexion is to provide additional room for the thecal sac, which is fixed to the sacrococcygeal junction by the filum terminale, and unloading of the lumbosacral facet joints (6,13).

The lumbosacral interaction is dominated by strong disc space with its supporting ligamentous stability, and the almost coronal orientation of the facet joints, which are designed to resist translational forces in the anteroposterior direction. A representational diagram of normal lumbosacral metrics is shown in Fig. 5. The sacrum experiences a shear force when axial forces of the spine reach the lumbosacral junction and cause spinal elements rostral to the sacrum to move ventrally. Shear force is directly resisted by the actions of the facet joints, the lumbosacral disc space, and musculoligamentous structures, particularly the iliolumbar ligament (3,6). The forces on the lumbosacral disc and facet joints are different when bending forward at the hips to lift a weight incorrectly, with the disc resisting most of the shear stress and the facet joints experiencing a compressive force (9,13). With this type of movement, flexion concentrates spinal load to the lumbosacral junction (6). Additional resistive forces that prevent dorsal and rostral rotatory motion of the sacrum caused by axial spinal loads are resisted by the sacrotuberous and sacrospinous ligaments (3). Conditions such as spondylolysis and spondylolisthesis, as well as decompressive and/or reconstructive surgery, can alter the biomechanical relationships of the lumbosacral junction (6,15, 16). Instability of the lumbosacral junction is implied when axial forces cannot be resisted and efficiently transferred to the pelvis and lower extremities without lumbosacral spondylolisthesis (15).

Normal sagittal spinal balance also plays a role in the biomechanics of the lumbosacral junction (Fig. 13). Deviation from this balance leads to perturbations both in local biomechanics

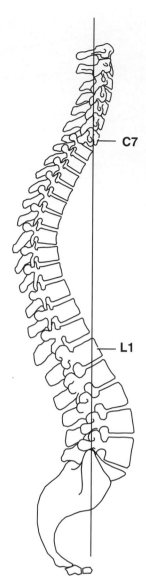

Fig. 13. A depiction of sagittal spinal balance.

and in responses to normal loading. Coupling also occurs at the lumbosacral joint, while axial rotation occurs with lateral bending in the same direction (16). This biomechanical relationship is accentuated in the extended position because additional engagement of the lumbosacral facet joints occurs (15).

The SIJs exhibit very little movement (16). It has been postulated that the strong sacroiliac ligaments provide most of the strength at the SIJs (16). The female SIJs relax somewhat during pregnancy to allow the fetus additional room for development and eventual delivery (3,9). Later in life the SIJs may fuse, a process that is more common in males (3,9).

Sacral Fractures

Fracture is the most significant clinical ailment and provides the best demonstration of the biomechanics of the sacrum. Sacral fractures may be associated with visceral, neural, and vascular injuries to the pelvis (17). Most sacral injuries are indirect, resulting from forces applied through the pelvis or spinal column (14,17). Indirect injuries are more often associated with sacral nerve root deficits. Mechanisms of injuries may result in one of two patterns: vertical or high transverse fractures (14,17).

Vertical sacral fractures occur more frequently and often are associated with pelvic fractures when the pelvic ring is fractured in two locations. Vertical sacral fractures can be subdivided anatomically to include the following subclassifications: lateral mass fractures, juxtaarticular fractures, cleaving fractures, and avulsion fractures (Fig. 14). Several texts indicate that vertical fractures are often associated with a lumbosacral radiculopathy (14,17,18).

Lumbosacral flexion injuries often cause high transverse sacral fractures that result in a traumatic high sacral spondylolisthesis. Such mechanisms are much less common than those causing vertical sacral fractures, and are also associated with neurological deficits (14,17). Although less commonly detected, direct injuries to the sacrum from falls or blunt or penetrating trauma may be classified anatomically. Falls or blunt trauma often result in a low transverse fracture of the sacrum, often through the S-4 foramina, the first sacral region caudal to the fixed SIJ (Fig. 15) (14,17).

Denis and colleagues (11,19) developed an anatomical classification to identify sacral fractures on the basis of sacral foramina and canal involvement. Fractures that occur in one of three zones define the likelihood for neurological injury in this classification scheme (Fig. 16). Fractures through zone I include the sacral ala, not involving the sacral foramina or canal, and are not often associated with neurological problems. Zone II injuries involve the sacral foramina but not the sacral canal, and

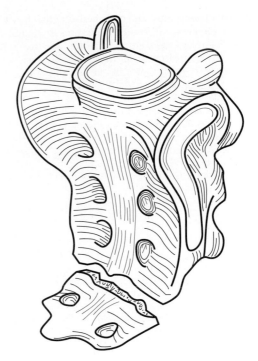

Fig. 15. Low transverse fracture of the sacrum.

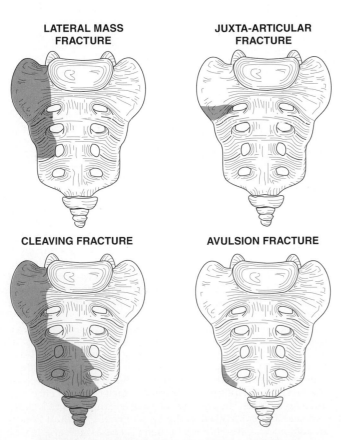

Fig. 14. The subclassification of vertical sacral fractures.

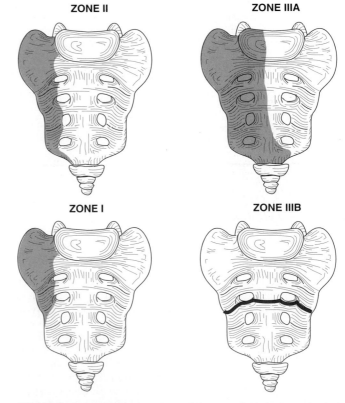

Fig. 16. The classification of sacral fractures based on anatomical zones. Zone I, the alar zone; zone II, the foraminal zone; zone IIIA, a transverse fracture through the central canal zone; zone IIIB, a horizontal fracture through the central canal zone.

are similar to a lateral mass fracture; neurological injury is also uncommon with a zone II fracture. Fractures involving the sacral canal are referred to as zone III fractures, and are commonly associated with neurological sequelae. Such zone III injuries include both transverse (zone IIIA) and horizontal (zone IIIB) fractures (11,15,17,19).

Gertzbein describes other classifications for spinal injuries that are extrapolated to the sacrum (20). Although the sacrum is derived and composed of spinal elements, the relationship between the sacrum and the pelvic ring changes the biomechanical nature of fracture mechanisms, and these schemes seem less applicable (15).

References

1. Breathnach AS, ed: *Frazer's anatomy of the human skeleton*, 5th ed. London: J & A Churchill, 1958.
2. Ronderos J, Sonntag VKH: Treatment of sacral fractures. In: Menezes AH, Sonntag VKH, eds. *Principles of spinal surgery*. Vol. 2. New York: McGraw-Hill, 1996.
3. Esses SI, Botsford DJ: Surgical anatomy and operative approaches to the sacrum. In: Frymoyer JW, ed. *The adult spine: principles and practice*. Vol. 2 New York: Raven Press, 1991.
4. Xu R, Ebraheim NA, Douglas K, et al: The projection of the lateral sacral mass on the outer table of the posterior ilium. *Spine* 21: 790–795, 1996.
5. Benzel EC: *Biomechanics of spine stabilization. Principles and clinical practice*. New York: McGraw-Hill, 1995.
6. Gross JD, Baldwin NG, Benzel EC: Lumbosacral junction biomechanics. *Perspectives Neurolog Surg* 10:75–99, 1999.
7. Zindrick MR, Hodges SD: Clinical anatomy of the lumbosacral junction and pelvis. In: Margulies JY, ed. *Lumbosacral and spinopelvic fixation*. Philadelphia: Lippincott–Raven Publishers, 1996.
8. Jackson RP, Peterson MD, McManus AC, et al: Compensatory spinopelvic balance over the hip axis and better reliability in measuring lordosis to the pelvic radius on standing lateral radiographs of adult volunteers and patients. *Spine* 23:1750–1767, 1998.
9. Vleeming A, Stoeckart R, Snijders CJ: A new perspective on the integrated function of spine, pelvis, and legs. In: Margulies JY, ed. *Lumbosacral and spinopelvic fixation*. Philadelphia: Lippincott–Raven Publishers, 1996.
10. Ebraheim NA, Lu J, Biyani A, et al: Anatomic considerations for posterior approach to the sacroiliac joint. *Spine* 21:2709–2712, 1996.
11. Kristiansen TK: Fractures of the sacrum and coccygodynia. In: Frymoyer JW, ed. The *adult spine: principles and practice*. Vol. 2. New York: Raven Press, 1991.
12. Gray H, Pickering PT, Howden R, eds: *Anatomy, descriptive and surgical*. Rev American ed. from the 15th British ed. New York: Portland House, 1977.
13. Louis RP: Anatomy, physiology, and biomechanics of the lumbopelvic junction. In: Margulies JY, ed. *Lumbosacral and spinopelvic fixation*. Philadelphia: Lippincott–Raven Publishers, 1996.
14. Schmidek HH, Smith DA, Kristiansen TK: Sacral fractures. *Neurosurgery* 15:735–746, 1984.
15. Benzel EC: Biomechanics of lumbar and lumbosacral spine fractures. In: Cooper P, ed. *Spinal trauma: current evaluation and management*. Park Ridge, IL: AANS Publications, 1996.
16. Laxer EB, Steffen T, Aebi M: Biomechanics of the lumbosacral junction and sacroiliac joints.
17. David CA, Green BA: Injuries to the sacrum and pelvis. In: Wilkins RH, Rengachary SS, eds. *Neurosurgery*, 2nd ed. New York: McGraw-Hill, 1996:3047–3053.
18. Bents RT, France JC, Glover JM, et al: Traumatic spondylopelvic dissociation. A case report and literature review. *Spine* 21: 1814–1819, 1996.
19. Denis F, Davis S, Comfort T: Sacral fractures: an important problem. Retrospective analysis of 236 cases. *Clin Ortho* 227:67–81, 1988.
20. Gertzbein SD: Disorders of the spinopelvic junction: indications for fixation and fusion in cases of trauma. In: Margulies JY, ed. *Lumbosacral and spinopelvic fixation*. Philadelphia: Lippincott–Raven Publishers, 1996.

134. Bone Biology

Alexander R. Vaccaro and Jonathan F. Rosenfeld

Bone Biology

BONE ANATOMY AND PHYSIOLOGY. Bone is composed of inorganic salts impregnating a collagenous mesh made of 95% type I collagen fibers with the remaining 5% consisting of ground substance, various proteins, and minerals. Calcium is the primary mineral of bone, making bone the body's reservoir for this and other ions. There are two main types of bone, cortical and cancellous. Cortical bone comprises 80% of the body's bone mass and contains less than 10% soft tissue. It is dense, solid, and contains only microscopic channels. Its main purpose is skeletal support and protection. Cancellous bone comprises the remaining 20% of the body's bone mass, consists of more than 75% soft tissue, and functions as the homeostatic regulator of bone metabolism. Cancellous bone is composed of trabeculae, which resemble plates and rods approximately 100- to 150-μm thick filled with hematopoietic or fatty marrow.

This trabecular system greatly increases the surface area to volume ratio of cancellous compared to cortical, explaining why cancellous bone accounts for two thirds of the bony surface area in the body. This large surface area allows for more rapid bone turnover, and therefore a susceptibility to bone loss in certain clinical settings such as osteoporosis (1). The trabecula of cancellous bone is continuous with the interior of cortical bone, with the transition from one type to another being gradual.

A long bone of the appendicular skeleton consists of three main anatomical regions: (a) The shaft portion or diaphysis, and the (b) proximal and (c) distal metaphyses where the bone widens prior to the articular surface. In the immature individual, a growth plate, referred to as the epiphyseal plate, is located between the metaphysis and epiphysis, the bone adjacent to the articular surface. The epiphyseal plate is composed of hyaline cartilage and is involved in the longitudinal growth of bones. In adulthood, when bone lengthening ceases, the epiphyseal plate transforms into cancellous bone, allowing the metaphysis and epiphysis to fuse, forming a solid synostosis. The diaphysis, or shaft, is mainly cortical bone, whereas the metaphysis and epiphysis are composed of a cancellous bone surrounded by a cortical shell; this allows for greater impact absorption at joint surfaces. The exact ratio of cortical to cancellous bone depends on the individual and its stress environment. Greater amounts of cancellous bone with a thinner cortical shell are found in flat bones (i.e., skull, pelvis) and short bones (i.e., tarsal, carpal, vertebrae).

The articular surface of a bone is covered by hyaline cartilage, whereas the rest of the bone, including its shaft, is covered by a periosteum made up of an outer fibrous connective tissue layer and an inner layer of undifferentiated cells called the cambium or osteogenic layer. The periosteum functions to create new bone during bone growth and fracture healing. The periosteum is deficient at the attachment sites of tendons, ligaments, and sesamoid bones, as well as along the femoral neck and subscapular surfaces (2). The inner surface or endosteal lining of bone consists of cells involved in bone remodeling, including osteoclasts, osteoblasts, and bone lining cells. The endosteum encloses all bony and soft-tissue structures (i.e., marrow) except for osteocytes.

Both cortical and cancellous bone may be of two microscopic types, woven or lamellar, depending on the level of maturity. Woven cancellous bone is found in the developing embryo and other sites of new bone formation such as fracture repair, ectopic ossification, and osteosarcoma. Cortical woven bone is formed at sites of injury or compression of diaphyseal bone. Composed of collagen fibers aligned in many directions interwoven with randomly placed osteocytes, woven bone is less organized than lamellar bone. Woven bone is eventually replaced by lamellar bone in approximately 2 to 3 years.

Lamellar bone is a layered structure with each layer measuring 3 to 7 μm. The fine collagen fibers that make up each layer all run in the same direction, alternating in direction between layers. The fibrils connect within and between lamellae, increasing bone strength. There are three types of lamellae in cortical lamellar bone: (a) concentric lamellae, consisting of circular rings surrounding a vascular channel (these concentric lamellae make up the osteon or haversian system); (b) circumferential lamellae, which are multiple layers of lamellae surrounding all or part of the shaft of the bone; and (c) interstitial lamellae, which are remnants of former concentric or circumferential lamellae. Cancellous lamellar bone is of two types, trabecular lamellae and interstitial lamellae.

The osteon, or haversian system of bony canals, makes up two thirds of cortical bone volume, with the remaining volume devoted to circumferential and interstitial lamellae. haversian canals are 200 to 250 μm in diameter and are made up of 20 to 30 concentric lamellae, usually oriented along the long axis of the bone. This orientation allows the bone to resist tensile and compressive forces but leads to less resistance against perpendicular forces. A cement line of mineralized matrix lacking collagen fibers surrounds the outer border of the osteon. This cement line marks where resorption stopped and new bone formation began. The central osteon canal is 40 to 50 μm in diameter and contains blood vessels, nerves, lymphatics, and connective tissue. The central haversian canals are connected to other central canals by a system of obliquely oriented Volkmann's canals. The contents of the canals continue through both the endosteum and periosteum (Fig. 1).

Cancellous bone has a system similar to the haversian system of cortical bone except the lamellae are parallel sheets at opposed to concentric circles. Cells of cancellous bone lie between lamellae on the trabecular surface; their increased metabolic activity versus cortical bone cells may result from greater blood–cell interaction.

Cortical and cancellous woven and lamellar bone have cavities known as lacunae that contain relatively inactive bone cells called osteocytes. These are connected to one another by canaliculi that contain the cytoplasmic processes of the osteocytes. Communication through cytoplasmic process contact or gap junctions provides important nutritional and metabolic support.

The vascular supply of bone may be divided into the periosteal-diaphyseal-metaphyseal system and the epiphyseal–physeal system. The former is comprised of nutrient arteries that penetrate the diaphysis, enter the marrow, and centrifugally distribute to the periosteum. In addition to nutrient arteries, epiphyseal and metaphyseal penetrating arteries as well as periosteal arterial plexuses that anastomose with muscular and cambium layer vessels are part of the periosteal-diaphyseal-metaphyseal system. The epiphyseal–physeal system supplies blood flow to the ends of long bones as well as the growth plates. Few vessels cross the physis during growth or after closure of the physis, leaving the epiphysis at risk for ischemic necrosis following damage to epiphyseal penetrating arteries. The elaborate blood supply of bone results in no bone cell being located more than 300 μm from a vessel.

THE CELLULARITY OF BONE. There are four types of bone cells: osteoclasts, osteoblasts, osteocytes, and bone lining cells. Greater than 90% of the volume of lamellar bone in made up of bone matrix (3). Matrix is a combination of organic (e.g., collagen) and inorganic (e.g., mineral) elements. The organic portion assists in resisting tension, whereas the inorganic portion resists compression.

Osteoclasts. Osteoclasts are multinucleated giant cells that function as bone resorbing cells. They possess tartrate-resistant acid phosphatase, dehydrogenases, carbonic anhydrase, and calcitonin receptors. Osteoclasts are located in Howship's lacunae, cavities located on the surface of cancellous or periosteal bone. The portion of the osteoclasts' plasma membrane closest to the bone surface is made up of an involuted portion, the ruffled border, which participates in bone resorption. Within cortical bone, small cavities or cutting cones are formed during bone resorption. Surrounding this structure is a organelle-free clear space that forms a sealed zone with the bone allowing for localized lysosomal activity within a closed resorbing area. Alendronate, a bisphosphonate drug currently prescribed for osteoporosis, interferes with this ruffled border to inhibit resorption.

Osteoclast activity is affected directly or indirectly by a variety of agents. Calcitonin and glucocorticoid act directly on osteoclasts to decrease bone resorption. Parathyroid hormone (PTH), activated vitamin D, and other factors activate osteoclastic bone resorption through osteoblast modification.

Osteoclasts are the only bone cell type to originate in hematopoietic tissue, arising from pluripotent stem cells of the marrow that are likely related to the monocyte-macrophage lineage (1, 2,4). Precursor cells from the stem cell colony forming unit (CFU-S) eventually transform into the granulocyte-macrophage line (CFU-GM) and become committed osteoclast progenitor cells, migrating from the blood to the bone. Further maturation takes place in the stromal mesenchyme of the bone, leading to preosteoclasts and then osteoclasts. It is possible that local factors influence this stem cell progression. The final maturation involves three steps: (a) the mitotic stage of proliferation and differentiation; (b) the postmitotic stage of acid phosphatase activity acquisition; and (c) the fusion stage in which multinucleated osteoclasts are formed.

The osteoclast has a 7-week life span, after which it moves into the bone marrow where hibernation or degeneration takes place. Hibernating osteoclasts, which do not have ruffled borders, are known as mobile osteoclasts.

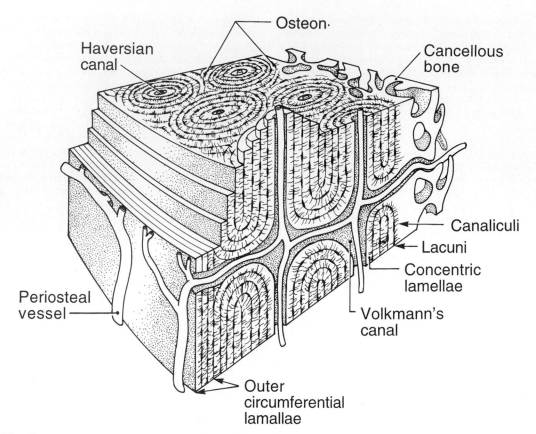

Fig. 1. A schematic depicting both cortical *(left)* and cancellous *(right)* bone in the proximal shaft of a long bone. Cortical lamellar bone contains three types of lamellae: concentric lamellae (circular rings surrounding a vascular channel), which make up the osteon or haversian system; circumferential lamellae (multiple layers of lamellae surrounding all or part of the shaft of the bone); and interstitial lamellae (remnants of former concentric or circumferential lamellae). The trabeculae of cancellous bone also are depicted. The haversian system makes up most cortical bone volume. Each osteon is oriented along the long axis of the bone and is composed of a central haversian canal (containing blood vessels, nerves, lymphatics, and connective tissue), concentric lamellae, a cement line, canaliculi, and lacunae. The central haversian canals are connected to other central canals by a system of obliquely oriented Volkmann's canals. (©2002, Thomas H. Weinzerl. Redrawn from Jee WSS. The skeletal tissues. In: Weiss L, ed. *Cell and tissue biology.* Baltimore: Urban and Schwarzenberg, 1988:221.)

Osteoblasts. Osteoblasts are the bone forming cells. They synthesize and secrete a large number of macromolecules and proteins, including type I collagen and osteoid, the unmineralized bone matrix. Osteoblasts are involved in extracellular mineralization of bone matrix, calcification of bone, resorption of bone (through osteoclastic activity), and regulation of calcium and phosphate transport. Osteoblasts are rich in alkaline phosphatase. Products of osteoblasts include type I collagen, bone matrix, various proteins (e.g., osteocalcin, bone sialoprotein, osteopontin, osteonectin, and phosphoproteins), various proteoglycans, growth factors, prostaglandins (E_1, E_2, and I_2), collagenase, and tissue plasminogen activator. The appearance of some of these products in the blood allows for the evaluation of bone formation.

After osteoid formation and calcification, the osteoblast subsequently functions in one of four paths. The cell may: (a) reenter the preosteoblastic pool; (b) become a bone lining cell; (c) become an osteocyte; or (d) die. Osteoblast-regulated mineralization activity differs between woven and lamellar bone. In woven bone, mineralization occurs away from the osteoblast plasma membrane in budding vesicles. In lamellar bone, mineralization begins in the interval between overlapping type I collagen fibers, and may be partly initiated by these fibers. Generally, matrix is deposited toward the bone surface; circumferential

patterns of deposition may lead to the surrounding of osteoblasts, resulting in the development of an osteocyte.

Osteoblasts arise from undifferentiated mesenchymal cells located in the periosteum, endosteum, and marrow. The exact nature of this progenitor cell in unknown, but current opinion favors its origin being nonhematopoietic marrow stroma that eventually differentiates into an osteoblast. A five-step histogenesis has been elucidated in the development of an osteoblast; the length of this process is thought to take a minimum of 60 hours.

Factors that stimulate osteoblast function include transforming growth factor (TGF)α and -β, platelet derived growth factor (PDGF), insulin-like growth factors (IGF) 1 and 2, interleukin 1 (IL-1), macrophage-derived growth factor (MDGF), prostaglandin E_2, and other systemic growth factors and hormones. Osteoblasts are also stimulated through treatment with autograft or allograft bone.

Osteocytes. Greater than 90% of bone cells in the mature human skeleton are osteocytes (3). Osteocytes are mature osteoblasts responsible for maintenance of the bony matrix and are involved with some synthetic and resorptive activity (5). As an osteoblast is surrounded by the product of its synthesis, it may become engulfed, transforming into an osteocyte. Single

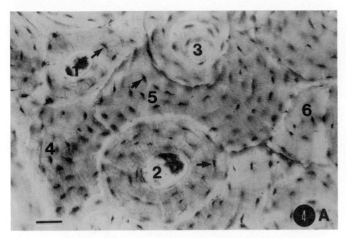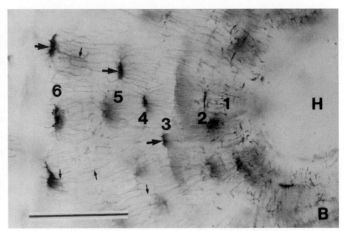

Fig. 2. **A:** A thin-ground cross-section of human cortical bone in which osteocyte lacunae *(arrows)* and canaliculi have been stained with India ink. Osteocytes, mature osteoblasts responsible for maintenance of the bony matrix, are located in lacunae and communicate with other osteocytes through gap junctions within canaliculi. This cross-section depicts active haversian systems *(1,2,3)* with concentric lamellae as well as older haversian systems *(4,5,6)* with their residual interstitial lamellae. (Original magnification: ×185. Bar, 50 μm.) **B:** Higher magnification demonstrating concentric lamellae with osteocytes *(large arrows)* in lacunae radiating from the central haversian canal *(H)*. The canaliculi are marked with small arrows. (Original magnification: ×718. Bar, 50 μm.) (From Marks SC Jr, Hermey DC. The structure and development of bone. In: Bilezikian JP, Raisz LG, Rodan GA, eds. *Principles of bone biology.* New York: Academic Press, 1996:6, with permission.)

osteocytes, located in lacunae, communicate with other osteocytes through gap junctions within canaliculi (Fig. 2). Osteocytes are involved in calcium storage and transport, and, in combination with bone-lining cells, the stabilization of the ionic state of bone. Osteocytes are also involved in the repair of microfractures. These cells are influenced by various stresses and strains placed on bone, and are instrumental in bone remodeling as a result of these forces.

Bone-Lining Cells. Bone-lining cells are flat, elongated cells directly apposed to quiescent bone. Gap junctions allow for communication with other bone-lining cells and with osteocytes. The quantity of bone-lining cells increase in hematopoietic portions of bone. The origin of bone-lining cells is unclear; they may originate from inactive osteoblasts or aborted osteoblast precursors. The development and decline of bone-lining cells is also unclear. Their eventual fate (i.e., return to a precursor pool or death) also is unclear. It has been hypothesized that bone-lining cells are actually osteoblast precursor cells (5).

In conjunction with osteoblasts and osteocytes, bone-lining cells participate in bone homeostasis and remodeling as determined by local stress and strain environments. The efflux of calcium may be regulated by the permeability of bone-lining cells as affected by various hormonal influences (e.g., PTH). Bone-lining cells also play a role in the hematopoietic function of bone marrow. Marrow stromal regeneration originates from cells localized to the bone-lining cells.

BONE FORMATION AND GROWTH. Bone formation begins during the fetal period as mesenchymal condensations that eventually ossify. Cell differentiation leads to the formation of osteoblasts which produce osteoid (unmineralized bone). This quickly mineralizes to form woven bone that eventually engulfs surrounding osteoblasts, leading to the creation of osteocytes. Woven bone will mature to lamellar bone in the postnatal period. Osteoclasts appear soon after formation of bone to begin the remodeling process (see the following). The process of formation is replayed during fracture repair, treatment with auto-

graft or allograft bone, growth factors, and in bone disease states.

Bone mineralization begins with the precipitation of calcium phosphate within the osteoid matrix. Bone is considered a hydroxyapatite crystal and is represented by the formula

$$Ca_{10x}H_x(PO_4)_6OH_{2x} \qquad [Eq.1]$$

where $x = 2$ as the crystal is first deposited. As bone ages, x approaches zero. The mineral portion of bone contains water as well as additional calcium salts.

Two types of ossification occur within humans: endochondral ossification and intramembranous ossification. The form of ossification depends on the specific bone in question. The shaft of most long bones participates in both processes. Endochondral, or indirect ossification begins through the development of a cartilage model involving the skull-base bones, vertebrae, and bones of the pelvis and extremities (weight-bearing bones). Cartilage cells proliferate within a mesenchymal condensation (blastema) and eventually calcify in the shape of a future bone. Vascular buds enter the cartilage, creating the marrow cavity and bringing osteoprogenitor cells to the bone. Osteoblasts then appose woven bone to unresorbed cartilage cores to form the primary spongiosa or native trabecular architecture of bone. Bone remodeling then results in mature lamellar trabecula.

Intramembranous or direct ossification describes bone formation involving most of the skull vault, face, clavicle, and mandible. Intramembranous ossification also participates in the formation of the outer cortical shell of most adult bones excluding the epiphysis. The process is "direct" because mesenchymal cells are transformed directly into osteoblasts without a cartilaginous precursor. Embryonic cellular condensations develop into primary centers of ossification containing blood vessels and osteoprogenitor cells. Osteoblasts form and appose bone to these centers, forming loose spicules that interconnect. This spongiosa continues to grow as the spicules increase in length and thickness through apposition. This bone is then remodeled through the development of primary and secondary osteons.

The formation of most long bones involves both direct and

indirect ossification. Within these bones, primary ossification centers develop from maturing chondrocyte columns that develop parallel to the long axis of the bone. As chondrocytic cells hypertrophy and release osteogenic factors, the surrounding intracolumnar cartilage matrix mineralizes, forming the scaffold for metaphyseal bone formation (6). Around the outside of long bones, beginning at the midshaft level, a collar of cartilage transforms into osteoblasts, forming a periosteal collar. This appositional formation of the periosteum continues with osteoblasts secreting osteoid on the outer surface of the bone, increasing the circumference in layers.

After its initial formation, bone grows and remodels through a process called apposition (i.e., laying down of new bone on existing surfaces). The resorbing (osteoclasts) and forming cells (osteoblasts) of bone participate in bone growth and remodeling. Both longitudinal and radial bone growth continues until the age of 16 in females and 18 in males (2,7).

Long bones grow in length through endochondral ossification of their secondary growth centers, or epiphyseal plates (growth plate cartilage) (Fig. 3). The cells of the growth plate are also arranged in a columnar manner as was seen in the formation of long bones. The top layer closest to the articular surface is composed of a series of chondrocyte columns. Deep to this layer, the chondrocyte cells hypertrophy leading to their mineralization in the intracolumnar matrix of the next layer. This results in formation of a scaffold for osteoblast deposition and mineralization. Osteoclasts assist in this overall process by removing about two thirds of cells to allow room for new bone and vascular growth. Vascular invasion of the hypertrophied chondrocyte level is considered a rate-limiting step in this process. The remaining step is the creation of the marrow cavity. The entire process of longitudinal growth is regulated by hormonal and local factors. These factors affect chondrocyte proliferation, cartilage matrix production, hypertrophy, and mineralization.

Growth of long bone width is accomplished by growth of the periosteum with concurrent resorption of the endosteum. This process is modified at the metaphysis where the periosteum is deficient and bone expansion at the extremes of the diaphysis is the result of endosteal bone growth.

As bone grows, external forces (e.g., strain) influence the remodeling process (6). The osteons of cortical bone and trabecula of cancellous bone are continuously replaced as the body responds to the biomechanical stresses and metabolic requirements of its environment. This remodeling continues throughout life even after longitudinal growth cessation. Aside from nutritional factors, bone requires mechanical forces to develop and adapt to its environment. This effect of mechanical forces on bone begins during fetal life with intrauterine muscle contractions. The combination of biological and mechano-biological factors was examined through computer modeling (6). Decreased bone loading beginning in fetal life resulted in decreased girth and periosteal development. Decreasing loading after age 20 results in extreme cortical thinning, whereas increasing loading above normal after age 20 results in greater girth and cortical thickness. The magnitude of loads applied to bone is directly related to its density. Further research is needed to elucidate the relationship between mechano-biological factors and bone cell biology.

BONE REMODELING UNIT. All of the cells described in the preceding combine to play a role in the bone remodeling unit, which controls the continuous degeneration and rebuilding of bone as well as shape modifications during growth. Bone exists in one of three states: formation, resorption, or quiescent. In the majority of time, bone is in a resting stage. On average, cortical bone is in the formation phase 3% of the time, resorp-

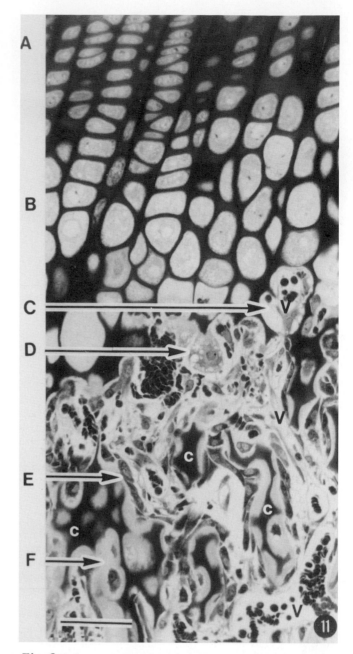

Fig. 3. Light micrograph of the proximal tibial epiphyseal plate and subjacent metaphyseal bone in a young rat. Long bones grow in length through endochondral ossification of their secondary growth centers, or epiphyseal. The cells of the growth plate are arranged in a columnar manner as was seen in the formation of long bones. The top layer closest to the articular surface is composed of a series of chondrocyte columns **(A)**. Deep to this layer, the chondrocyte cells hypertrophy **(B)**, leading to their mineralization in the intracolumnar matrix of the next layer. Vascular invasion *(V)* of the hypertrophied chondrocyte level **(C)** is considered a rate-limiting step in this process. Osteoclasts **(D)** remove cells to allow room for new bone and vascular growth. **E,F:** Osteoblast deposition and mineralization on the cartilage scaffold *(c)* leads to new bone formation. The remaining step is the creation of the marrow cavity. The process of longitudinal growth is regulated by hormonal and local factors affecting chondrocyte proliferation, cartilage matrix production, hypertrophy, and mineralization. (Original magnification: ×500. Bar, 50μm.) (From Marks SC Jr, Hermey DC. The structure and development of bone. In: Bilezikian JP, Raisz LG, Rodan GA, eds. *Principles of bone biology.* New York: Academic Press, 1996:10, with permission.)

tion phase .6% of the time, and quiescent phase 97% of the time. Cancellous bone is in the formation phase 6% of the time, resorption phase 1.2% of the time, and quiescent phase 93% of the time (2). The ratio of bone formation to resorption varies over one's life span. During the early years (birth through teens), bone is continuously remodeling with formation preceding and exceeding resorption. Over the next three decades, resorption precedes formation with the processes occurring in equal quantities with no net change in bone mass. During the sixth decade of life, bone resorption precedes and exceeds formation, resulting in decreased skeletal mass and strength and predisposing one to skeletal fractures (8).

Bone remodeling can be divided into six steps. The first step is the digestion at the endosteal membrane by bone lining cells resulting in the exposure of mineralized bone. This results in the recruitment of osteoclasts and osteoblasts into the local area. The second step is the resorption phase. During this phase, osteoclasts locate themselves in cavities known as Howship's lacunae within cancellous bone and resorption cavities (or cutting cones) in cortical bone. A low-pH environment is created by the release of lysosomal enzymes at the ruffled osteoclast membrane border. Bone minerals are solubilized and released with subsequent degradation of organic components, most of which are reused. In cortical bone, new cutting cones are developed through the haversian system resulting in new osteons of varying size and age. After the resorption phase is completed, a locally regulated 1- to 2-week coupling phase takes place (step three) in which removal of local waste products occurs. Osteoclasts are no longer present in the Howship's lacunae or resorption cavities during this time.

After the coupling phase, the building of new bone begins. Bone formation takes place in two phases. First (step four), bone matrix is formed at the osteoblast–osteoid interface. After about 10 days, mineralization of osteoid occurs along the mineralization front (step five). The osteoid seam is a layer of unmineralized matrix remaining. This seam is of decreased size in woven and embryonic bone owing to the decreased lag time between matrix formation and mineralization. When mineralization is completed, the seam disappears with remaining surface cells becoming bone-lining cells. As noted, osteoblasts trapped in the bone may become osteocytes or disappear.

Gain or loss of bone (both cortical and cancellous) through bone remodeling depends on many factors affecting a specific bone. The surface–volume ratio, mechanical stresses, proximity to joints and marrow, age, bone type, hormonal stimulation, mineral availability, and concurrent disease are all factors involved in bone turnover. The relationship between the mechanical stresses applied to bone and the microscopic and macroscopic appearance of bone is bidirectional. A bone undergoing increased mechanical usage (2,8) will increase its growth, remodeling, and mass conservation properties. Conversely, pathological osteopenia resulting in vertebral fractures is the result of bone that is no longer able to handle the mechanical stress applied to it. Vertebrae in the aged often show a decrease in short horizontal trabeculae and a retention of long vertical trabeculae that results in disconnection of the trabecular elements and increased fragility (2). In addition, osteocytes die as bone ages, which lead to the creation of brittle bones with canals filled with connective tissue.

REGULATION OF BONE GROWTH AND REMODELING.
Regulation of the bone remodeling unit includes systemic as well as local factors (1,2,4,8). Recall that the skeleton serves as the calcium reservoir for 99.5% of the body's calcium (7). Systemically, the major hormones affecting bone remodeling and calcium metabolism are the parathyroid hormone (PTH), activated vitamin D (1,25 OH_2D_3), and calcitonin. Calcitonin

increases the storage of calcium and inhibits the action of osteoclasts; no effect on osteoblasts is seen. PTH and vitamin D have an interesting method of increasing bone turnover: They affect only the osteoblast, even though the osteoclast cell is needed to increase overall bone resorption. Osteoblasts carry the receptors for the majority of proresorptive agents and influence the localization and stimulation of osteoclasts. PTH causes osteoblasts to become round through a cAMP-mediated change in the cell's cytoskeleton. Although this shape change decreases the activity of the osteoblast, it is not clear how osteoclast activity is increased. The surface previously covered by the osteoblast is now exposed because its cytoskeletal changes. Osteoclastic activity now begins with osteoblast collagenase-mediated removal of surface collagen (and demineralized collagen at the base of the lacunae) with release of plasminogen activators. Bone lining cells also retract through changes in their shape as osteoblasts secrete activating factors that lead to bone resorption by osteoclasts. No direct osteoclast activator has yet been discovered. Vitamin D also stimulates osteoblasts, with no receptors to date identified on osteoclast cells.

Locally, factors such as transforming growth factorβ (TGFβ), platelet derived growth factor (PDGF), insulin-like growth factors (IGF), interleukins (IL), prostaglandin E_2 and I_2, tumor necrosis factorsα and -β (TNFα and -β), and others influence bone resorption. TGFβ causes fibroblasts to form large colonies and has a mitogenic effect on osteoblasts. TGFβ is synthesized by bone cells and in addition serves to modulate collagen synthesis. TGFβ significantly stimulates bone turnover resulting in a high formation to resorption ratio (1). Bone morphogenetic protein is a member of the TGFβ superfamily and, as detailed in the next section, has been shown to stimulate ectopic bone formation in animal studies. PDGF stimulates DNA and protein synthesis as well as bone cell replication. IGF mediates the effect of growth hormone and is increased by PTH and prostaglandin E_2 secretion. It has been demonstrated to increase collagen synthesis. Prostaglandin E stimulates bone resorption, although less dramatically than PTH or vitamin D; it is produced locally by osteoblasts. Additionally, as discussed, the loading of bone (environmental effects) play a large part in the regulation and direction of bone growth.

Spinal Bone Grafting Alternatives

One of the most fascinating applications of our understanding of bone biology is our ability to extend the basic principle of bone healing to reconstructive surgical procedures that involve bony healing (i.e., bone fusion). Humans have attempted to influence the success of bone healing with the addition of internal fixation; however, long-term stability is gained only through bony healing. During a spinal arthrodesis procedure, bony healing may be assisted with various grafting materials in addition to the gold standard of autologous bone graft. Ideally, a bone graft should be osteogenic, osteoinductive, and osteoconductive (9). Osteogenesis is a cellularly derived feature dependent on osteoblasts and osteoprogenitor cells. Matrix proteins, such as bone morphogenetic protein, provide osteoinductive properties, allowing the transformation of osteoprogenitor cells into bone producing cells. Osteoconductive materials provide a framework (nonviable scaffolding) for new bone formation.

AUTOGRAFT. Autogenous bone theoretically has osteogenic, osteoinductive, and osteoconductive properties and is considered the gold standard grafting substance in spinal reconstructive surgery. Autogenous bone may be solely cancellous, cortical, or a combination of cortical and cancellous bone. The graft source may be harvested along with or without a vascular source (vascularized or nonvascularized). Cancellous bone has demonstrated improved graft incorporation as compared to cortical grafts, owing mainly to increased cell mass (osteoblasts and osteocytes) and availability of these cells to the graft host surface (9). Cortical bone provides greater initial strength compared to cancellous bone; however, cortical bone has less osteogenic and osteoinductive properties. Cancellous bone increases its strength over time because of osteointegration and accumulation of bone mass. Cortical bone initially provides optimum compressive strength when implanted. During remodeling nonviable bone is gradually replaced, a process that may take up to 18 months. Some nonviable bony islands may remain for the life of the individual. Vascularized cortical cancellous grafts retain their arterial and venous anastomoses and therefore undergo less cell necrosis. A vascularized graft has the potential to heal or repair a stress-related fracture better than a nonvascularized graft, and is a superior grafting choice in unsupported grafting segments greater than 12 cm. After 6 months there is no perceivable difference in biomechanical characteristics between a vascularized and a nonvascularized cortical autograft. The disadvantages of a vascularized graft include increased operating time and donor site morbidity.

Complications related to the use of autogenous bone include pain at the graft donor site (10), blood loss owing to graft harvesting, infection, increased operative time, lack of adequate autograft bone, and the potential for vascular injury. The advantages of autograft are foremost its lack of immunological reactivity and disease transmission, the potential for viable cell transfer, and improved arthrodesis potential.

ALLOGRAFT. As mentioned, the disadvantages of allogenic bone grafting material include disease transmission, immunological reactions (11), and decreased biological activity. The advantages include a lack of donor site pain (10,12), decreased operating time, decreased blood loss, and unlimited bone graft source, useful in revision surgery and procedures involving fixation to the pelvis or multilevel fusions.

Allograft may be processed as fresh, fresh-frozen, or freeze-dried. Fresh allografts require no preservation but require a quick transfer, resulting in decreased time for immunogenicity testing or sterilization of the graft. Often an intense immune reaction results from its use. Rarely is allograft used in this fashion in clinical situations due to these concerns. Fresh-frozen (below −60°C) processed allograft, technically easier to obtain, results in minimal alteration of graft properties and maintenance of many native osteoconductive properties. Although immunogenicity of frozen allograft is decreased compared to fresh processing, the potential adverse qualities of antigenicity continue to exist. Freeze-drying reduces this antigenicity further but decreases the structural and healing properties of the graft (loss of hoop and compressive strength). The process of freeze-drying removes all existing water. The specimen is then vacuum packed and stored at room temperature for up to 5 years. A review of the literature finds that the clinical pseudarthrosis rate for fresh-frozen and freeze-dried allograft is nearly identical (0% to 7.5% versus 0% to 5%) (13). Therefore, the concerns of viral transmission with fresh-frozen allograft may make freeze-dried allograft a better graft choice. So far, sterilization techniques such as ethylene oxide and radiation have altered the structural, biochemical, and biomechanical properties of the graft. The use of ethylene oxide gas-sterilized freeze-dried allograft in the posterior thoracolumbar spine has been shown to result in an increased pseudarthroses rate in multiple studies (10,14). As a

result, this type of allograft is not recommended for this application. Additionally, allograft bone has not been found useful in posterior cervical applications. Anteriorly, allograft bone has been used extensively in the cervical spine with varied results. A number of studies with allograft sources such as iliac crest, fibular, and femoral head bone have attested to its efficacy in single-level fusions (12,15,16). The similarities in fusion rate between allograft and autograft decrease markedly as the number of fused levels increases.

Structural allograft bone has proven useful in anterior column reconstructive procedures involving the thoracolumbar spine. Strut grafts consisting of allograft femoral shaft, femoral head, iliac crest, tibial shaft, and fibulas have provided adequate anterior column stability with radiographic evidence of incorporation in multiple clinical reviews (17). Allograft bone provides different levels of strength depending on its anatomical source and method of preservation. A biomechanical study (18) comparing cadaveric 24-hour freeze-dried partially demineralized microperforated femoral bone to fresh cadaveric fibular and iliac crest grafts found an increased load to failure and overall strength with the femoral bone allograft. *In vitro* testing of anterior structural allografts (19) revealed that femoral cortical ring allografts were stronger than tricortical ilium, fibular struts, or cancellous allograft cubes and dowels. In clinical applications, autograft is often morcellized and packed into the medullary canal of the femoral ring.

In clinical studies, Bridwell and colleagues (20) reviewed the results of 24 patients who underwent a combined anterior and posterior procedure with anterior fresh-frozen structural allograft and posterior instrumentation with autograft. Some patients also received anterior instrumentation. At follow-up, approximately 80% of patients were found to have radiographic remodeling of the bony trabeculae at the anterior fusion site.

In degenerative lumbar spine applications, results of fusion success with allograft alone or as an adjunct to autograft have been equivocal (21,22). However, densitometry studies have shown autograft fusions to be superior over allograft fusions.

Structural allograft bone also has shown usefulness in revision surgery for posterior lumbar pseudarthroses or flat back syndrome. In comparing anterior femoral ring to tricortical iliac autograft in anterior-posterior fusions with posterior instrumentation, Buttermann and co-workers (17) reported a lower pseudarthrosis rate in the allograft group (3% versus 7% for autograft) even in light of a greater number of segments fused in patients receiving allograft.

DEMINERALIZED BONE MATRIX. Demineralized bone matrix (DBM) is a composite of noncollagenous proteins, bone growth factors, and collagen formed by acid extraction of cortical or corticocancellous bone followed by freeze-drying. The preparation method reduces antigenicity and makes the bioactive proteins of the allograft more available to the host (23). One of the bone growth factors found in DBM is bone morphogenetic protein (BMP). BMP provides the bulk of the osteoinductive ability of DBM. The quantity of BMP in DBM is far less than in trials using recombinant BMP such as recombinant human BMP-2 (rhBMP-2). Although DBM does not provide strength to the graft site, it does facilitate bone growth. Its usefulness is now waning owing to our understanding of individual BMPs and their utility.

BONE MORPHOGENETIC PROTEIN. Perhaps the most exciting orthopedic biological discovery in recent decades is the role and application of bone morphogenetic protein (BMP) in bone growth and healing. BMP is an osteoinductive growth factor found in the bony matrix that induces endochondral bone formation and is proving viable as an alternative for autogenous bone grafting in long bones and spinal fusion. Recombinant DNA technology is providing the clinician with an unlimited supply of human BMP, avoiding the necessity of harvesting or the potential for disease transmission. Recombinant human bone morphogenetic protein (rhBMP) belongs within the superfamily of TGFβ (dimeric, disulfide cross-linked growth and differentiation factors found in many tissues). Through cloning, 12 related proteins have been identified. Each can induce cartilage and bone formation *in vivo* to varying degrees (24). Bone formation as induced by BMP is through a series of sequential steps including chemotaxis, proliferation, differentiation, calcification, angiogenesis, and bone differentiation and remodeling.

Long bone animal studies have demonstrated the usefulness of BMP. Yasko and co-workers (25) demonstrated union rates of 100% in a rat femoral bone defect model when BMP was combined with bone marrow. This value was three times greater than the cancellous autograft control.

The application of rhBMP-2 in spinal fusion has also been studied. Helm and colleagues (26) studied the efficacy of BMP in an adult beagle posterior spinal fusion model. A total of five groups were compared with each undergoing a unilateral decompression and contralateral autologous bone grafting. Group 1 underwent autologous bone grafting; group 2 the same but with the addition of demineralized bone matrix; group 3 underwent fusion with the addition of a type I collagen gel (an osteoconductive material); group 4 included both DBM and a type I collagen gel; and group 5 consisted of rhBMP-2 and autologous graft. At the conclusion of the study, the fusion masses were larger in group 5, the rhBMP-2 group, versus the control. rhBMP-2 was the only substance to significantly increase the number of solidly fused levels versus the control (3 versus 1.57). Additionally, only group 5 (BMP) showed significantly greater bone volume (average increase of 10.24 cm^3) at the fusion site versus the amount placed at surgery.

In a posterolateral lumbar intertransverse process fusion model in a rabbit, Schimandle and colleagues (22) demonstrated that fusions involving rhBMP-2 were stronger and stiffer than an autograft control. Seventeen rabbits underwent L5-6 single level posterolateral intertransverse arthrodeses with autogenous iliac crest on one side and one of four rhBMP-2 combinations on the other side (low- or high-dose rhBMP-2 with collagen carrier, combination autogenous graft, and high-dose rhBMP-2 with collagen carrier, or autogenous graft soaked with rhBMP-2). In the same study, a group of 39 rabbits underwent a similar fusion with autogenous iliac crest bone graft placed bilaterally, high-dose rhBMP-2 in a collagen carrier bilaterally, or the collagen carrier alone bilaterally. Although all rabbits in the first group were noted to have solid, localized fusions, the most radiographically and histologically mature fusions resulted in the high-dose rhBMP-2 group. In the bilateral group, the group containing rhBMP-2 with collagen carrier specimens all fused, whereas only 42% of the autograft group and none of the collagen carrier alone specimens were found to be healed. Radiographically, the rhBMP-2 fusion specimens revealed a homogeneous mass compared to the other groups. Histologically, the rhBMP-2 with collagen carrier fusions were mature with peripheral corticalization, remodeling, and marrow formation. Biomechanically, the rhBMP-2 fusions were significantly stronger and stiffer than the autograft-alone fusions.

David and associates (27) demonstrated a dose-dependent osteoinductive effect of rhBMP-2. They obtained 100% clinical and radiographic fusion in 12 canine spinal fusion specimens. The control group of iliac crest autograft demonstrated failed fusion by clinical and CT evaluation in two thirds of the cases. A third group consisting of collagen carrier alone demonstrated complete absence of fusion.

The application routes, dosages of rhBMP-2, and efficacy of decortication in obtaining a fusion have been extensively studied. In a single-level lumbar canine arthrodesis, Sandu and co-workers (28) demonstrated that a dose of 2,300 μg of rhBMP-2 in an open-pore polylactic acid polymer (OPLA) was superior to an autologous iliac crest control. The investigators went on to demonstrate (29) that varying the dose of rhBMP-2 between 58 and 2,300 μg did not result in mechanical, radiographic, or histological variations in the quality of intertransverse process fusions, with abundant bone formation in all samples by three months. Boden and co-workers (30) also studied various dosages of BMP. In a primate model of laparoscopic anterior lumbar interbody arthrodesis using an interbody-threaded titanium cage, the investigators soaked the cages in either 750 or 1,500 μg of rhBMP-2 prior to insertion. Bone formation and fusion were seen at both doses, but the higher dose of rhBMP-2 produced a more rapid fusion.

Collagen sponge carriers have been studied to evaluate their feasibility, efficacy, and safety in delivering BMP to the graft site. The goal of the carrier was to assist in performing minimally invasive intertransverse process fusions. Hecht and associates (31) investigated an absorbable collagen sponge carrier (Helistat) soaked with rhBMP-2 within a freeze-dried cortical dowel allograft in a rhesus macaque primate. When compared to cancellous iliac crest autograft and freeze-dried cortical dowel allograft controls, the BMP produced greater new bone formation and superior fusions.

CERAMICS. Ceramic materials provide a potential osteoconductive surface when used as a grafting source. Examples of ceramic grafting materials include hydroxyapatite (HA), tricalcium phosphate (TCP), or a combination of the two. The porosity of each material confers certain biochemical properties related to its ability to osetointegrate. TCP's greater porosity leads to faster degradation *in vivo,* better remodeling, but less mechanical strength. HA has the advantage of forming a strong bond between the graft and host bone; its greater strength makes it more useful in compression. Because ceramics are brittle until they have been incorporated and remodeled, they must be protected from loading forces until incorporation has occurred. One type of ceramic, replamineform ceramic, is derived from sea coral and results in a highly organized pore structure similar to human cancellous bone. A variety of genuses of sea coral result in differing coral graft pore sizes.

CORAL. Natural coral (97% calcium carbonate) is morphologically similar to cancellous bone and has been used experimentally as a carrier for autologous bone and even a bone graft substitute when used alone (32). It is biocompatible (i.e., rapidly resorbed and reossified), and has a very low immunogenicity. The calcium carbonate exoskeleton of sea coral in addition provides an excellent mold for a ceramic graft with the use of hydrothermal chemical conversion. Grafts similar to both cancellous and cortical bone can be formed depending on the genus of coral. The porosity of the coral allows quick and direct ingrowth of bone with direct connection to the host bone.

The testing of non-spinal coral implants in humans began in 1982 in the area of traumatic bone defects. Although mechanically weaker than cancellous bone, coral grafts have been associated with excellent fracture union in situations where they do not have to bear initial loads without additional stabilization.

XENOGRAFT. Although allografts and autografts are grafting materials derived from humans, a xenograft is a material derived from a different species. A xenograft provides the advantages of autograft and allograft. There is no donor site morbidity and lack of supply is of little concern, unlike the situation with autograft. Because the grafting material is from another species, the risk of immunological response is present. This necessitates appropriate processing to avoid graft resorption. Preparations have included frozen and freeze-dried calf bone, decalcified ox bone, deproteinized bone, anorganic bone, and Kiel Bone, a partly deproteinized bone of freshly killed calves (33). Most xenografts lack osteoinductive ability and therefore act as spacers to provide for appropriate healing; however, bovine xenograft has produced the most favorable osteoinductive results (34). Xenografts have been combined with autograft or bone marrow to increase its osteoinductive capabilities (33).

Conclusion

An understanding of bone biology is necessary to provide the optimum host–graft environment for successful bone healing. The growth, remodeling, and regulation of bone physiology is a complex interplay between patient specific internal biological factors and the external environment, including nutritional supplementation, grafting sources, and stresses from the physical environment. The resultant outcome of these interactions determines the success or failure of biological activities such as fracture repair and adaptation. A successful biological fusion is intended to impart localized mechanical stability and improve overall functionality. Grafting sources or alternatives should be compared to the gold standard of autologous iliac crest bone graft in determining its overall efficacy. Emerging allogeneic bone sources appear promising in that the critical biological functions of autologous bone, such as osteoinduction, are being simulated through recombinant technology (i.e., bone morphogenetic protein). Further research into the complex biology of bone physiology should substantially reduce the present morbidity related to autologous bone harvesting and hopefully improve overall fusion success rates.

References

1. Rodan GA. Introduction to bone biology. *Bone* 1992;13:3S–6S.
2. Jee WSS. Introduction to skeletal function: structural and metabolic aspects. In: Bronner F, Worrell RV, eds. *A basic science primer in orthopaedics*. Baltimore: Williams & Wilkins, 1991:3–34.
3. Buckwalter JA, Glimcher MJ, Cooper RR, et al. Bone biology, part I: structure, blood supply, cells, matrix, and mineralization. *JBJS* 1995;77A:1256–1275.
4. Bronner F. Bone formation and bone resorption. In: Bronner F, Worrell RV, eds. *A basic science primer in orthopaedics*. Baltimore: Williams & Wilkins, 1991:81–90.
5. Marks SC Jr, Hermey DC. The structure and development of bone. In: Bilezikian JP, Raisz LG, Rodan GA, eds. *Principles of bone biology*. New York: Academic Press, 1996:3–14.
6. Carter DR, Van Der Meulen MCH, Beaupre GS. Mechanical factors in bone growth and development. *Bone* 1996;18IS:5S–10S.
7. Marcus R. Endogenous and nutritional factors affecting bone. *Bone* 1996;18IS:11S–13S.
8. Buckwalter JA, Glimcher MJ, Cooper RR, et al. Bone biology, part II: formation, form, modeling, remodeling, and regulation of cell function. *JBJS* 1995;77A:1276–1289.
9. Lane JM, Muschler GF. Principles of bone fusion. In: Rothman RH, Simeone FA, eds. *The spine*. Philadelphia: WB Saunders, 1992: 1739–1752.
10. Jorgenson SS, Lowe TG, France J, et al. A prospective analysis of autograft versus allograft in posterolateral lumbar fusion in the same patient: a minimum of 1-year follow-up in 144 patients. *Spine* 1994; 19:2048–2053.
11. Gurr KR, Haddad BR, Mowbray RD. In vivo analysis of autograft versus allograft in posterior intertransverse fusions. *Orthop Trans* 1992;16:138.
12. Malinin TI, Brown MD. Bone allografts in spinal surgery. *Clin Orthop* 1981;154:668–673.
13. Yazici M, Asher MA. Freeze-dried allograft for posterior spinal fusion in patients with neuromuscular spinal deformities. *Spine* 1997;22: 1467–1471.
14. Herron LD, Newman MA. The failure of ethylene oxide gas-sterilized freeze-dried bone graft for thoracic and lumbar spine fusion. *Spine* 1989;14:496–500.
15. Grossman WC, Peppelman WC, Baum JA, et al. The use of freeze-dried fibular allograft in anterior cervical fusion. *Spine* 1992;17: 565–569.
16. Young WF, Rosenwasser RH. An early comparative analysis of the use of fibular allograft versus autologous iliac crest graft for interbody fusion after anterior cervical discectomy. *Spine* 1993;18: 1123–1124.
17. Buttermann GR, Glazer PA, Bradford DS. The use of bone allografts in the spine. *Clin Orthop* 1996;324:74–85.
18. Rao S, McKellop H, Chao D, et al. Biomechanical comparison of bone graft used in anterior spinal reconstruction. *Clin Orthop* 1993; 289:131–135.
19. Morales DO, Pettine KA, Salib RM. A biomechanical study of bone allografts. *Orthop Trans* 1993;17:12.
20. Bridwell KH, Lenke LG, McEnery KW, et al. Anterior fresh frozen structural allografts in the thoracic and lumbar spine: do they work if combined with posterior fusion and instrumentation in adult patients with kyphosis or anterior column defects? *Spine* 1995;20: 1410–1418.
21. Nasca RJ, Whelchel JD. Use of cryopreserved bone in spinal surgery. *Spine* 1987;12:222–227.
22. Schimandle JH, Boden SD, Hutton WC. Experimental spinal fusion with recombinant human bone morphogenetic protein-2. *Spine* 1995;20:1326–1337.
23. Morone MA, Boden SD. Experimental posterolateral lumbar spinal fusion with a demineralized bone matrix gel. *Spine* 1998;23: 159–167.
24. Sasano Y, Ohtani E, Narita K, et al. BMPs induce direct bone formation in ectopic sites independent of the endochondral ossification in vivo. *Anat Rec* 1993;236:373–380.
25. Yasko AW, Cole BJ, Lane JM, et al. Comparison of recombinant human BMP-2 versus cancellous bone to heal segmental bone defects. Transactions of the Orthopaedic Research Society 39th Annual Meeting. 1993;17:100.
26. Helm GA, Sheehan JM, Sheehan JP, et al. Utilization of type I collagen gel, demineralized bond matrix, and bone morphogenetic protein-2 to enhance autologous bone lumbar spinal fusion. *J Neurosurg* 1997;86:93–100.
27. David SM, Murakami T, Tabor OB, et al. Lumbar spinal fusion using recombinant human bone morphogenetic protein rhBMP-2: a randomized, blinded, and controlled study. International Society for the Study of the Lumbar Spine, Helsinki, Finland. 1995, June 18–22.
28. Sandu HS, Kanim LE, Kabo JM, et al. Evaluation of rhBMP-2 with an OPLA carrier in a canine posterolateral transverse process. Spinal fusion model. *Spine* 1995;20:2669–2682.
29. Sandu HS, Kanim LE, Kabo JM, et al. Effective doses of recombinant human bone morphogenetic protein-2 in experimental spinal fusion. *Spine* 1996;21:2115–2122.
30. Boden SD, Horton WC, Martin G, et al. Laparoscopic anterior spinal arthrodesis with rhBMP-2 in a titanium interbody threaded cage. Scoliosis Research Society 32nd Annual Meeting, St. Louis, MO. 1997, Sept. 25–27.
31. Hecht B, Fischgrund J, Herkowitz H, et al. The use of rhBMP-2 to promote spinal fusion in a non-human primate anterior interbody fusion model utilizing a freeze-dried allograft cylinder. NASS 12th Annual Meeting, New York. 1997, Oct. 22–25:280.
32. Guillemin G, Patat J, Fournie J, et al. The use of coral as a bone graft substitute. *J Biomed Mater Res* 1989;23:765–779.
33. Salama R. Xenogeneic bone grafting in humans. *Clin Orthop* 1983; 174:113–121.
34. Block JE, Poser J. Does xenograft demineralized bone matrix have clinical utility as a bone graft substitute? *Med Hypoth* 1995;45:27–32.

135. Clinical Syndromes of Spinal Cord Disease

Michael G. Fehlings,
Gordon D.C. Dandie,
and Wai Pui Ng

Despite advances in neuroimaging, accurate diagnosis of the segmental level and axial location of spinal cord pathology remains clinically challenging and intellectually stimulating. The level of the lesion usually can be deduced from the segmental distribution of impaired motor function, sensory changes, and altered reflexes. Knowledge of the functional anatomy of the spinal cord allows correlation of clinical examination findings for more accurate localization of the lesion within the cord. However, it should be borne in mind that spinal cord disease can present with false localizing signs that can lead to a variance between the clinically determined level and that ultimately disclosed by imaging. A difference as large as 11 segments has been reported (1), but the pathophysiological mechanism for this phenomenon has yet to be adequately explained.

Complete interruption of the spinal cord leads immediately to flaccid paralysis with loss of all sensation and reflex activity below the site of the lesion, and paralysis of the bladder and rectum. Incomplete spinal cord injuries result in characteristic patterns of motor, sensory, and reflex impairment depending on the location of the lesion within the cord. The degree of injury can be classified according to the standard published by the American Spinal Injury Association and International Medical Society of Paraplegia (ASIA/I MSOP) (2). The ASIA/I MSOP Classification of Spinal Cord Injury (SCI) consists of five grades of impairment (Table 1). Grade A is defined as complete SCI. Grades B to D represent varying degrees of incomplete injuries, and grade E denotes normal neurological function. This classification is based on a standardized system of examination as outlined in Fig. 1. Following this system requires the examination of 10 key muscle groups and 28 dermatomes bilaterally. The neurological level of an SCI then is defined by the sensory and motor levels on both sides of the body; hence, up to four levels may be identified. The "sensory level" is the most caudal segment with normal sensory function. The "motor level" is now defined as the most caudal key muscle group with at least grade 3 power (using the Medical Research Council [MRC] 0 to 5 scale). Determining whether a lesion is complete or incomplete requires testing of the S4 and S5 segments. An incomplete lesion is defined as any sensory or motor function preserved in these segments. A zone of partial preservation also may be identified if dermatomes or myotomes are found partially innervated below the identified "level." Patients with incomplete injuries have a more favorable prognosis for recovery. This chapter summarizes the various syndromes and patterns associated with spinal cord disease. Presentation of a particular "pure" syndrome, however, is relatively rare because most lesions of the spinal cord are irregular.

Root Syndromes

The dorsal roots can be affected by a wide variety of conditions as they enter the spinal cord, including herniated intervertebral disc, herpes zoster, and tabes dorsalis. Root syndrome also can be seen with neurofibroma, schwannoma, metastatic epidural tumor or an intradural extramedullary tumor (3). The syndrome is characterized by severe radicular pain, which may be constant or intermittent, and often is described as lancinating. The pain classically is aggravated by coughing, straining, and the Valsalva maneuver. This is thought to be related to the resultant fluid wave causing increased compression or irritation of the root. Some associated sensory impairment is usual, which may be either hyperesthesia or loss of superficial sensation in a dermatomal distribution.

Lower motor neuron weakness, with wasting and fasciculation, are only observed if the pathological process involves the anterior root.

Spinal Cord Syndromes

SPINAL CORD CONCUSSION. Spinal cord concussion refers to a syndrome of variable injury to the spinal cord, up to and including the clinical picture of a complete transverse myelopathy, which spontaneously resolves within 24 to 72 hours after the injury (4). There usually is a lack of radiological evidence of spinal stenosis or ligamentous instability, suggesting these concussive injuries are caused by the injuring force being transmitted to the cord without direct cord compression (5). It has been hypothesized that the immediate onset and rapid recovery of neurological deficit is related to functional disturbance of the axonal membrane, such as prolongation of the absolute refractory period, without disruption of its structural integrity (5).

SPINAL SHOCK. Spinal shock refers to the *initial* pattern of lost somatic motor, sensory, and autonomic function after acute

Table 1. American Spinal Injury Association and International Medical Society of Paraplegia Classification of Spinal Cord Injury

Grade	Impairment	Comments
A	Complete	No motor or sensory function is preserved in the sacral segments S4 and S5.
B	Incomplete	Sensory but not motor function is preserved below the neurological level and extends through the sacral segments S4 and S5.
C	Incomplete	Motor function is preserved below the neurological level, and the majority of key muscles below the neurological level have a muscle grade less than 3.
D	Incomplete	Motor function is preserved below the neurological level, and the majority of key muscles below the neurological level have a muscle grade greater than or equal to 3.
E	Normal	Motor and sensory function is normal.

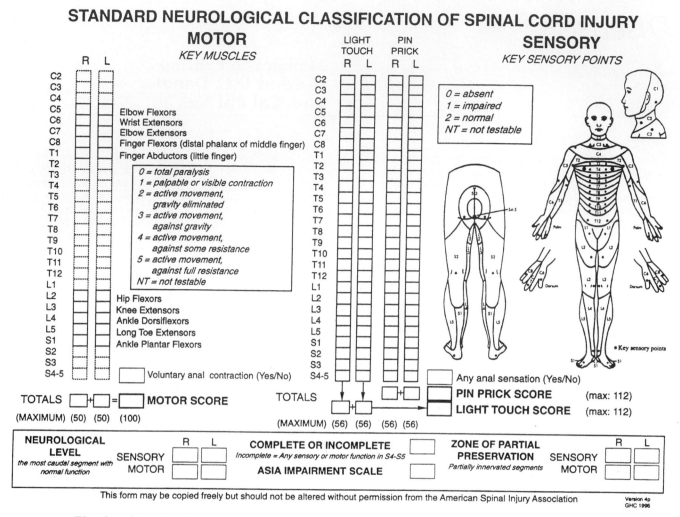

Fig. 1. American Spinal Injury Association, International Medical Society for Paraplegia classification of spinal cord injury. (Courtesy of American Spinal Injury Association, International Medical Society for Paraplegia. *International Standards for Neurological and Functional Classification of SCI.* Chicago: the Association and Society, 1996.)

SCI. The syndrome results from acute transection of, or severe injury to, the spinal cord with sudden loss of supraspinal innervation (6). It is characterized by flaccid paralysis and areflexia in all muscle groups below the level of injury. All sensory modalities distal to the level of injury are lost. The loss of autonomic function, predominantly sympathetic innervation, can manifest as hypotension, bradycardia, hyperemia, and skin warmth. In its most severe form, the loss of sympathetic tone to the heart and vasculature results in sustained hypotension and bradycardia leading to neurogenic shock.

The severity and duration of spinal shock varies, but it correlates with the severity and level of the injury. It is usually most severe in complete cervical and upper thoracic cord injuries, less severe in incomplete injuries and minimal in lumbar injuries. Complete spinal shock, though, rarely persists longer than 24 hours, but in some cases can last for weeks. The resolution of the spinal shock is usually followed by the development of radicular pain at the level of injury and gradual development of spastic paralysis below the level of injury with hyperreflexia (7). The autonomic effects of spinal shock tend to last longer than the motor and sensory manifestations. Urinary retention with overflow incontinence is observed initially, but irritability and spasticity with reflex emptying of the bladder subsequently develops after a few weeks (8).

The etiology of spinal shock is unknown, but suspected mechanisms include imbalances in transmembrane ionic concentrations and permeabilities secondary to local tissue trauma, causing inhibition of local neuronal excitability.

COMPLETE TRANSECTION OR TRANSVERSE MYELOPATHY. The most severe consequence of spinal cord trauma is complete transection or transverse myelopathy in which all sensory modalities and voluntary motor function below the level of injury is lost (9). Complete spinal cord injury can result from true anatomical disruption of the spinal cord, physiological disruption of neuronal function because of compression or ischemia, or a combination of both. This entity is frequently, if not always, associated with spinal shock in which there is impairment of sensation, flaccid paralysis, and absence of monosynaptic reflexes distal to the level of the lesion at the time of initial evaluation. This phase may mask the true extent of the SCI. As noted, complete spinal shock rarely persists longer than 24 hours after injury (6). If no recovery is noted within this period, there usually are permanent paralysis and sensory deficits below the lesion.

Following the initial phase of spinal shock, the motor deficit gradually conforms to that of upper motor neuron loss, with the development of hypertonia and hyperreflexia. The painless retention of urine with overflow incontinence in the acute phase is followed by bladder spasticity and irritability with reflex emptying in a few weeks (8). In the longer term, the chronic manifestations of SCI come to dominate the clinical presentation, such as decubitus ulcers, involuntary flexor withdrawal spasms, contractures, and chronic urinary tract problems.

INCOMPLETE SPINAL CORD TRANSECTION. Incomplete spinal cord injuries are those associated with preservation of some neurological functions below the level of injury (Table 2). The ASIA/IMSOP classification defines this as preserved sensation or motor function in the lowest sacral segments (S4 and S5). These injuries have a better prognosis for neurological recovery than do complete injuries (2). However, deterioration of partial injury to total neurological deficit can occur in the presence of spinal cord compression by bony fragments, extruded disc material, hematoma, or spinal instability, causing further cord damage.

Patients with incomplete SCI often follow specific patterns of neurological deficit. These syndromes generally are classified according to the anatomical location of the lesion within the spinal cord.

Cervicomedullary Syndrome. Cervicomedullary syndrome occurs in SCI involving the high cervical cord and lower brainstem. The lesion can extend caudally as low as C4, and rostrally to the pons. The syndrome is caused by direct injury (traction or compression) to the cord and medulla, or by concomitant disruption of the vertebral arteries during cervical spine trauma. In its most severe form, the syndrome consists of respiratory arrest, hypotension, quadriparesis or quadriplegia, and anesthesia, usually below C4 (10). Immediate resuscitation is required to prevent death shortly after the initial injury. Patients may also exhibit the Dejerine pattern of facial anesthesia (anesthesia of the periphery of the face with sparing of the midportion, including the nasal alae, to the vermilion border of the lips). This is caused by the topographic arrangement of the spinal trigeminal nucleus, which extends as low as C4, with the fibers from the periphery of the face synapsing in the more caudal portion at greatest risk of injury. In between the sensory impairment affecting the face and below C4, there can be sparing of the collar area supplied by C2-4. This may be related to the fact that sensation from this area is carried by two pathways, the lateral spinothalamic and spinal trigeminal tract, which cross higher in the brainstem. Varying degrees of bulbar dysfunction also may be present (10).

The cervicomedullary syndrome can also mimic the motor manifestations of the central cord syndrome (see the following) by producing greater weakness in the upper than lower extremities, in a pattern termed the cruciate paralysis of Bell (11). Originally it was thought to be caused by a lesion in the rostral portion of the pyramidal decussation selectively affecting the fibers to the arms, but recently this has been questioned because of the lack of evidence supporting topographic lamination of

Table 2. Summary of Incomplete Spinal Cord Syndromes

	Motor	Sensory	Sphincters	Other
Cervicomedullary syndrome	Quadriparesis, may be cruciate paralysis of Bell	Sensory loss below C4. May be Dejerine facial anesthesia	Usually involved	Respiratory arrest. Hypotension. May be bulbar dysfunction.
Brown-Séquard syndrome	Ipsilateral motor loss (upper motor neuron) below level of lesion	Ipsilateral loss of proprioception and vibration sense. Contralateral loss of pain and temperature sense below level of lesion.		
Syringomyelic syndrome	Bilateral weakness and wasting of upper limbs, especially intrinsic muscle of hands. Later develop upper motor neuron weakness in lower limbs.	Dissociate sensory loss (pain and temperature) in "cape" distribution		
Central cord syndrome	Bilateral motor loss, more prominent in upper limbs than lower limbs.	Variable sensory loss below the level of the lesion	Usually involved	
Anterior cord syndrome	Bilateral motor loss below the level of the lesion	Bilateral loss of pain and temperature sensation below the level of the lesion		
Posterior cord syndrome	Power intact. Patient has sensory ataxia and Rhomberg sign. Broad-based gait with slapping down of feet.	Bilateral loss of proprioception and vibration sensation below the level of the lesion		
Conus medullaris syndrome	Flaccid paralysis of lower limbs. Later develop signs of upper motor neuron loss.	Symmetrical bilateral anaesthesia in "saddle" distribution	Sphincter involvement early	Sexual function involved
Cauda equina syndrome	Variable motor changes (lower motor neuron loss)	Unilateral or asymmetrical bilateral anaesthesia in "saddle" distribution	Sphincter involvement late	Radicular pain early

the corticospinal tracts (12). It may be explained on the basis of the greater importance of the corticospinal tracts for hand function compared to lower limb functions.

Brown-Séquard Syndrome (Hemisection of the Spinal Cord). Brown-Séquard syndrome is characterized by loss of the lateral half of spinal cord functions. It is classically seen in penetrating injuries to the spinal cord (13), but also may result from lateral spinal cord compression by herniated cervical disc, tumor, or hematoma (14). Ipsilateral paralysis with increased muscle stretch reflexes and extensor plantar response owing to involvement of the corticospinal tract is observed. Loss of ipsilateral proprioceptive and vibration sensation occurs as a result of involvement of the posterior column, and contralateral loss of pain and temperature sensation occurs because of involvement of the spinothalamic tract, these fibers having already crossed before ascending. Occasionally, a thin band of lost pain and temperature sensation is detected on the ipsilateral side in the dermatome corresponding to the level of the lesion.

Brown-Séquard syndrome occurs more frequently in the cervical than thoracic cord and conus medullaris, and often occurs in combination with other incomplete syndromes. The prognosis for recovery varies widely.

Syringomyelic Syndrome. This syndrome usually is seen in patients with syringomyelia, but may result from trauma, infarction, hemorrhage, or tumor in the spinal cord (15). It is characterized by a bilateral, dissociate loss of pain and temperature sensation in a suspended, multisegmental pattern classically referred to as the "shawl" or "cape" distribution. It is caused by compression of the ventral commissure (containing the decussating spinothalamic fibers) secondary to expansion of the central canal or other centrally placed lesion. There is usually weakness and wasting of the hand and arm musculature. This is particularly evident in the intrinsic muscles of the hands and is thought to be related to anterior horn cell involvement. Impaired pain and temperature sensation can result in repetitive injuries, especially minor burns, and Charcot neuropathic arthropathy can develop if the condition becomes chronic (16). Although discriminative touch and proprioceptive and vibration sensation are preserved (hence the term dissociate sensory loss), the posterior columns can become involved with progression of the lesion (17).

Central Cord Syndrome. The central cord syndrome is typically observed in acute hyperextension injury to the cervical spine (18). This may be the result of a forward fall in an elderly patient or inadvertent hyperextension during endotracheal intubation or cervical manipulation. Spinal fracture is not a necessary feature of this syndrome (19), but it is usually associated with an anatomically narrow spinal canal in the anteroposterior plane. The stenotic spinal canal of cervical spondylosis increases the risk of simultaneous compression anteriorly by osteophytes and posteriorly by the bulging ligamentum flavum during hyperextension injury. The syndrome is characterized by a disproportionately greater loss of power in the upper limbs compared with the lower limbs. This pattern of deficit is sometimes referred to as "man in a barrel" syndrome. Paresis of both upper extremities with relative sparing of the lower extremities was hypothesized to result from hemorrhagic injury to the center of the cord affecting the medial laminations of the corticospinal tract, believed to carry the arm fibers. Fibers to the legs, traversing through the outer laminations, were thought less likely to be affected. However, evidence suggests that there is no somatotopic organization within the corticospinal tract. The disproportionate weakness of the upper versus lower extremities may be explained by the critical importance of the corticospinal tracts in hand functions but not locomotion (12). Further-

more, radiological and pathological observations indicated that the central cord syndrome is predominantly caused by diffuse axonal disruption of the corticospinal tracts in the lateral columns and that intramedullary hemorrhage in the cord is not a necessary feature (20). Varying degrees of sensory disturbance below the level of the lesion, as well as sphincter disturbances, may occur (21).

Central cord syndrome has a relatively good prognosis compared to other syndromes. There may be rapid, spontaneous recovery. The recovery of function usually follows a specific pattern, with power returning to the lower limbs first, followed by an improvement in bladder function, and finally movement in the upper limbs returns. Power in the hands and fingers is the very last to return, but may not recover completely. In contrast, any sensory recovery does not appear to follow a specific pattern.

Posterior Column Syndrome. The posterior columns can be affected selectively by a variety of pathological processes, including trauma, tumors, subacute combined degeneration, multiple sclerosis, and tabes dorsalis. The resulting syndrome is characterized by impairment of proprioceptive and vibration senses and discriminative tactile perception below the level of the lesion (22). Spinothalamic sensory function remains intact. The clinical manifestations remain basically the same regardless of where the lesion is along the posterior columns. Loss of proprioception causes a sensory ataxia with loss of smooth, coordinated movement and dysmetria. The ataxia is classically worse when the patient loses visual compensation, such as with eye closure or in a darkened environment, and this can be demonstrated with Romberg's test. The patient exhibits a characteristic gait, which is wide based and is marked by slapping down of the feet. The patient often watches his legs to help visually compensate for the proprioceptive loss.

Anterior Cord Syndrome. Anterior cord syndrome consists of bilateral paralysis and loss of pain and thermal sensation below the level of the lesion, with preservation of posterior column function (discriminative touch, proprioception, and vibration sense). Reflex activity below the level of the lesion usually is absent, and the degree of motor loss usually is equal in both the upper and lower extremities. The syndrome was initially described in cases of anterior compression of the spinal cord by either ruptured cervical disc, fracture-dislocation, or both. It was theorized that tissue injury resulted from compression and insufficiency of the anterior spinal artery. This artery, via the paramedian sulcal arteries, supplies the anterior two thirds of the spinal cord, including the corticospinal and anterolateral spinothalamic tract (23). However, in pathology studies evidence of occlusion in the anterior spinal artery was only demonstrated in a small number of patients (24). Thus, the pathophysiology of this syndrome has not been defined precisely. It may be related to injury because of direct trauma to the anterior and lateral aspect of the cord (25). Extension of the injury into the upper cervical cord can be associated with loss of sensation over the face because of involvement of the spinal trigeminal tract and Horner syndrome (26).

The chronic myelopathy form of this syndrome from gradual anterior cord compression secondary to calcified disc protrusion consists of hyperreflexia, hypertonia, spastic gait disturbance, weakness (more severe in the lower extremities), and subjective sensory disturbances. It has been proposed that this clinical presentation is caused by chronic traction on a cord fixed in position by the dentate ligaments, affecting the lateral corticospinal tracts.

The recovery from anterior cord syndrome varies considerably for both sensory and motor functions.

CONUS MEDULLARIS SYNDROME. The conus medullaris syndrome classically is characterized by a symmetrical anesthesia in the perineal or "saddle" region, loss of sphincter function with urinary retention, and flaccid paralysis of the lower extremities. Loss of sexual function with impotence also may occur. Pain usually is not a feature of this syndrome. In the chronic phase, the motor loss may revert to an upper motor neuron pattern including spasticity, hyperreflexia, and extensor Babinski responses (27).

The change in spinal anatomy from the stiff thoracic spine to the more mobile lumbar spine makes the thoracolumbar region prone to instability under stress. Burst fractures and fracture-dislocations, therefore, are most common in this part of the lower vertebral column, placing the conus at risk of direct injury.

The prognosis of conus medullaris syndrome is usually not very promising, possibly because of the destruction of the lower motor neuron cell bodies in the conus, which do not regenerate (28).

CAUDA EQUINA SYNDROME. Cauda equina syndrome tends to be grouped with the spinal syndromes, although it is caused by pathology below the L1-2 disc space (i.e., below the termination of the normal spinal cord), such as acute disc herniations, burst fractures, fracture-dislocations, or tumors. The syndrome is characterized by asymmetrical "saddle" sensory impairment, sphincter dysfunction, and radicular pain (29). Motor changes are variable, and may only affect an isolated myotome. It should be noted that central disc herniations predominantly may affect the centrally placed sacral roots; therefore, the patient may have normal leg strength and an absence of radicular pain (28).

Urgent surgical decompression usually is required for acute presentations of this syndrome, and generally the prognosis is better than for SCI because of the greater regenerative potential of the lower motor neuron axons and their relative resilience to trauma (28).

Chronic Posttraumatic Spinal Cord Syndromes

SYRINGOMYELIA. Approximately 3% of patients with SCI develop a clinically significant syrinx (a centrally placed, fluid-filled cavitation within the cord). The time of onset varies from months to years after the initial insult (30). The syndrome usually presents with some form of deafferentation pain, followed by progressive loss of sensory and motor function beyond that of the already existing deficit from the original injury. The motor deficit usually involves the lower motor neurons at the level of injury or above. Decompression of the syrinx may be required to preserve the patient's previous level of function.

A number of theories have been advanced to explain syrinx formation. Arachnoiditis and resultant adhesions at the site of original injury may be responsible for obstruction of normal intraspinal CSF flow. As a result, abnormal transmission of intraspinal CSF pressures during periods of increased pressure, such as during a Valsalva maneuver, may cause the fluid cavity to expand (31).

MICROCYSTIC MYELOMALACIA. Posttraumatic microcystic myelomalacia presents in a similar manner to posttraumatic syringomyelia, with a progression of the patient's original deficit. The cord shows microcystic degeneration without a continuous cavity. The cystic lesions can extend for several levels above and below the injury, and their continuity can be interposed by segments of normal cord. Occasionally, the lesions can be difficult to distinguish from syringomyelia, even on MRI, and surgical exploration may be required to elucidate which syndrome is responsible for clinical deterioration (32).

ARACHNOIDITIS. Arachnoiditis can occur after any form of SCI. It results in connective tissue adhesions between the spinal cord and its surrounding arachnoid, with or without involvement of the overlying theca. If the adhesions become clinically significant, there may be a stepwise or gradual neurological deterioration. Mechanisms proposed for the cause of the deterioration include tethering of the spinal cord, vascular congestion, ischemia as a result of fibrosis of arachnoid vessels, and obstruction of intraspinal CSF flow (33).

DEAFFERENTATION PAIN SYNDROMES. Unfortunately, up to 25% of patients with SCI can be affected by deafferentation pain syndromes in the chronic stage. They are believed to be the result of abnormal nociceptive impulses generated at various levels of the nervous system, including injured nerve roots, the spinal cord, and the brain after injury (34).

Spinal Cord Syndromes Not Associated with Trauma

DEMYELINATING DISEASES. The demyelinating diseases belong to a group of nervous system disorders characterized by pathological destruction of the myelin sheaths in the brain and spinal cord. Multiple sclerosis is the prototypical disease of the group and is associated with multiple or disseminated demyelinating lesions. A syndrome of transverse myelitis results when the demyelinating process is confined to the spinal cord. Transverse myelitis is associated with inflammatory demyelination of the spinal cord, often preceded by a viral infection or vaccine inoculation (35). In about half of the cases, it is the harbinger of multiple sclerosis (36). The onset is gradual and insidious over several days. Clinical manifestations can resemble those of acute spinal cord transection; however, recovery is rapid and often complete.

DEGENERATIVE DISEASES

Motor Neuron Diseases. The term "motor neuron disease" embraces a collection of inherited and acquired disorders characterized by progressive degeneration of motor neurons in the spinal cord with wasting and fasciculation of voluntary muscles. Similar lesions in the cranial nerve motor nuclei or motor cortex can accompany the loss of anterior horn cells in the spinal cord. In children, motor neuron diseases are likely to be inherited (mostly autosomal recessive) and usually are not accompanied by upper motor neuron involvement (37). In adults, amyotrophic lateral sclerosis (ALS) is the prototypical motor neuron disease with degeneration and loss of both upper and lower motor neurons. About 5% to 20% of the cases are familial with autosomal dominant inheritance (38).

ALS is defined by a pattern of both lower motor neuron disease (muscle weakness, wasting, and fasciculation) and upper motor neuron disease (spastic weakness and hyperreflexia).

The onset of the disease usually is in middle to late life. Clinical manifestations can vary; however, the combinations of hyperactive deep tendon reflexes; Babinski's sign; and clonus with weak, fasciculating, and wasted muscles are highly suggestive of ALS. Involvement of the cranial nerve motor nuclei results in dysphagia, dysarthria, and aspiration pneumonitis. The unrelenting course of the disease usually is terminated by respiratory failure, pneumonia, and the complications of prolonged immobility (38).

Subacute Combined Degeneration of the Cord. Extreme deficiency in intake (or use) of vitamin B12 (cyanocobalamin) may result in degeneration in the dorsal and lateral white matter columns (39). Loss of proprioception, tactile sensation, ataxic gait, spastic muscle weakness, hyperreflexia, and plantar extensor response are the characteristic features because of the involvement of the lateral corticospinal tract and posterior columns (39).

Inherited and Acquired Ataxias. Ataxias result from diseases in the cerebellum and its interconnection with many regions of the central nervous system. The main features of these diseases are slowly progressive ataxias that usually begin in the legs. However, posterior columns, pyramidal tracts, pontine nuclei, basal ganglia, and other regions of the brain also can be affected (40).

Classification of the ataxias remains problematic. Inherited ataxias can be subclassified according to the age of onset (< 20 years old = early; > 20 = late) or the biochemical defect causing the neurological dysfunction. An example of the latter is the abnormality in copper metabolism associated with Wilson disease that can result in ataxia (40). Friedreich ataxia is the prototypical ataxia of early onset without known biochemical defect.

The gene of Friedreich ataxia has been mapped to the long arm of chromosome 9 and is characterized by regions of multiple trinucleotide repeats (41). Symptoms usually begin between the ages of 8 and 15 years. The disease is defined by signs and symptoms of gait ataxia, posterior column sensory loss, loss of reflexes, dysarthria, corticospinal-type muscle weakness, and scoliosis. The corticospinal tract involvement results in plantar extensor response and spastic weakness in the legs, but there is a loss of deep tendon reflexes related to a peripheral neuropathy. Posterior column disease is seen in almost all patients. Impairment in proprioception and vibration sense occur in the legs first and later in the arms. Other clinical findings include nystagmus, insulin-dependent diabetes, optic atrophy, deafness, skeletal deformities, and cardiomyopathy. Most patients cannot walk within 15 years after onset of symptoms. Cardiac failure is a common cause of death (40).

Acquired ataxias can be caused by trauma, surgery, neoplasms, demyelination, toxins, and metabolic derangement.

INFECTION

Tabes Dorsalis. This syndrome is seen in tertiary neurosyphilis and is characterized by inflammatory demyelinating damage to the dorsal roots and posterior columns. Impairment of tactile sensation and proprioception, and loss of deep tendon reflexes are observed. Patients exhibit sensory ataxia and Romberg's sign is present because of the loss of proprioceptive input. Repeated injuries of insensitive joints can be present, resulting in Charcot arthropathy. Tabes dorsalis is now rare because of the availability of antibiotics (42).

Human Immunodeficiency Virus. Primary human immunodeficiency virus (HIV) infection of the spinal cord causes a condition called vacuolar myelopathy. Loss of myelin, predominantly in the lateral and posterior columns, leads to vacuolization of the cord substance, particularly affecting the thoracic region. The pathogenesis is unknown but is thought be related to abnormal transmethylation mechanisms induced by the HIV virus and cytokines (43). Although vacuolization of the spinal cord is present in more than one third of patients with acquired immunodeficiency syndrome (AIDS), it does not become clinically evident until there is significant loss of tissue.

The myelopathy is characterized by a slowly progressive spastic paraparesis, loss of proprioceptive and vibration sense, and bladder dysfunction. Sexual dysfunction also may occur, particularly in males.

Rarer manifestations of spinal cord disease caused by AIDS include viral myelitis and neoplastic and vascular myelopathies (43).

TUMORS

Extramedullary Tumors. The most common intradural extramedullary tumors of the spine are nerve sheath tumors and meningiomas. The clinical presentation is characterized by a slow progression of symptoms and signs that often precede diagnosis by 1 or 2 years. The major early symptom is pain, which is usually radicular and made worse on movement. The motor and sensory changes depend on the longitudinal position of the tumor and the direction in which the cord is being compressed; therefore, the patient may exhibit Brown-Séquard syndrome, anterior cord syndrome, posterior cord syndrome, or a combination of these. Frequently, however, there is very little clinical abnormality detected, in contrast to the sometimes severe distortion of the spinal cord revealed by imaging studies (44).

Intramedullary Tumors. Glial tumors, especially ependymomas and astrocytomas, are the most common intramedullary spinal tumors. The presentation is more likely to involve a poorly localized, burning pain. Motor and sensory changes may resemble the syringomyelia syndrome with a dissociate sensory loss and lower motor neuron-type weakness, later progressing to an upper motor neuron pattern (44).

VASCULAR LESIONS

Anterior Spinal Artery Thrombosis. Anterior spinal artery thrombosis causes ischemic necrosis and myelomalacia in the anterior two thirds of the spinal cord, particularly in the watershed region of the thoracic cord. This leads to the abrupt onset of anterior cord syndrome (see the preceding). Usually it is related to localized atherosclerosis, but may occur with dissection of an abdominal aortic aneurysm or procedures involving the aorta (45).

Spinal Vascular Malformations. Spinal vascular malformations include aneurysms, cavernomas, spinal dural arteriovenous fistulae (AVF), intramedullary arteriovenous malformations (AVM), and intradural AVFs. Differences in presentation can help the clinician delineate between spinal dural AVF (the most common malformation) and intradural AVM (46). Spinal dural AVFs tend to present in middle-aged males with a gradual onset of paraparesis. The weakness tends to be exacerbated by activity. In contrast, intradural spinal AVMs tend to present in younger males or females, frequently with sudden onset of neck or back pain, heralding a subarachnoid hemorrhage (46).

References

1. Jamieson DRS, Teasdale E, Willison HJ. Lesson of the week: false localizing signs in the spinal cord. *BMJ* 1996;312(7025):243–244.
2. Ditunno JF. American Spinal Injury Standards for Neurological and Functional Classification of Spinal Cord Injury: past, present, and future. *J Am Paraplegia Soc* 1993;17:7–11.
3. Ng WP, Fehlings MG. Intradural metastasis mimicking nerve sheath tumor. *Spine* 1995;20:2580–2583.
4. Del Bigio MR, Johnson GE. Clinical presentation of spinal cord concussion. *Spine* 1989;14:37–40.
5. Zwimpfer TJ, Bernstein M. Spinal cord concussion. *J Neurosurg* 1990;72:894–900.
6. Atkinson PP, Atkinson JL. Spinal shock. *Mayo Clin Proc* 1996;71:384–389.
7. Bach-y-Rita P, Illis LS. Spinal shock: possible role of receptor plasticity and non synaptic transmission. *Paraplegia* 1993;31:82–87.
8. Nygaard IE, Kreder KJ. Spine update. Urological management in patients with spinal cord injuries. *Spine* 1996;21:128–132.
9. Brazis PW, Masdeu JC, Biller J. *Localization in clinical neurology*, 3rd ed. Boston: Little, Brown, 1996.
10. Dickman CA, Hadley MN, Pappas CT, et al. Cruciate paralysis: a clinical and radiographic analysis of injuries to the cervicomedullary junction. *J Neurosurg* 1990;73(6):850–858.
11. Bell HS. Paralysis of both arms from injury of the upper portion of the pyramidal decussation: "cruciate paralysis." *J Neurosurg* 1970;33(4):376–380.
12. Levi AD, Tator CH, Bunge RP. Clinical syndromes associated with disproportionate weakness of the upper versus the lower extremities after cervical spinal cord injury. *Neurosurgery* 1996;38:179–183; discussion 183–185.
13. Roth EJ, Park T, Pang T, et al. Traumatic cervical Brown-Séquard and Brown-Séquard-plus syndromes: the spectrum of presentations and outcomes. *Paraplegia* 1991;29:582–589.
14. Rumana CS, Baskin DS. Brown-Séquard syndrome produced by cervical disc herniation: case report and literature review. *Surg Neurol* 1996;45:359–361.
15. Perrouin-Verbe B, Lenne-Aurier K, Robert R, et al. Post-traumatic syringomyelia and post-traumatic spinal canal stenosis: a direct relationship: review of 75 patients with a spinal cord injury. *Spinal Cord* 1998;36:137–143.
16. Williams B. Syringomyelia. *Neurosurg Clin North Am* 1990;1:653–685.
17. Kohli A, Gupta RK. Neurological picture. Gardner's hypothesis and magnetic resonance imaging. *J Neurol Neurosurg Psychiatry* 1997;63:143.
18. Maroon JC, Abla AA, Wilberger JI, et al. Central cord syndrome. *Clin Neurosurg* 1991;37:612–621.
19. Waters RL, Adkins RH, Sie IH, et al. Motor recovery following spinal cord injury associated with cervical spondylosis: a collaborative study. *Spinal Cord* 1996;34:711–715.
20. Quencer RM, Bunge RP, Egnor M, et al. Acute traumatic central cord syndrome: MRI-pathological correlations. *Neuroradiology* 1992;34:85–94.
21. Nath M, Wheeler JS Jr, Walter JS. Urologic aspects of traumatic central cord syndrome. *J Am Paraplegia Soc* 1993;16:160–164.
22. Ross RT. Dissociated loss of vibration, joint position and discriminatory tactile senses in disease of spinal cord and brain. *Can J Neurol Sci* 1991;18:312–320.
23. Suh DC, Kim SJ, Jung SM, et al. MRI in presumed cervical anterior spinal artery territory infarcts. *Neuroradiology* 1996;38:56–58.
24. Foo D, Rossier AB. Anterior spinal artery syndrome and its natural history. *Paraplegia* 1983;21:1–10.
25. Kowalske KJ, Herbison GJ, Ditunno JF, et al. Spinal cord injury syndrome with motor sparing in the absence of all sensation. *Arch Phys Med Rehabil* 1991;72:932–934.
26. Baumgartner RW, Waespe W. Anterior spinal artery syndrome of the cervical hemicord. *Eur Arch Psychiatry Clin Neurosci* 1992;241:205–209.
27. Anderson NE, Willoughby EW. Infarction of the conus medullaris. *Ann Neurol* 1987; 21(5):470–474.
28. Fehlings MG, Phan N. Spinal cord and related injuries. In: Brinker MR, ed. *Review of orthopaedic trauma*. Philadelphia: WB Saunders, 2001.
29. Bartleson JD, Cohen MD, Harrington TM, et al. Cauda equina syndrome secondary to longstanding ankylosing spondylitis. *Ann Neurol* 1983;14(6):662–669.
30. el Masry WS, Biyani A. Incidence, management, and outcome of post-traumatic syringomyelia. In memory of Mr Bernard Williams. *J Neurol Neurosurg Psychiatry* 1996;60(2):141–146.
31. Williams B. Post-traumatic syringomyelia: an update. *Paraplegia* 1990;28(5):296–313.
32. MacDonald RL, Findlay JM, Tator CH. Microcystic spinal cord degeneration causing posttraumatic myelopathy. Report of two cases. *J Neurosurg* 1988;68(3):466–471.
33. Park YK, Tator CH. Prevention of arachnoiditis and postoperative tethering of the spinal cord with Gore-Tex surgical membrane: an experimental study with rats. *Neurosurgery* 1998;42(4):813–823.
34. Siddall PJ, Taylor D, Cousins MJ. Pain associated with spinal cord injury. *Curr Opin Neurol* 1995;8(6):447–450.
35. al Deeb SM, Yaqub BA, Bruyn GW, et al. Acute transverse myelitis. A localized form of postinfectious encephalomyelitis. *Brain* 1997; 120:1115–1122.
36. Ungurean A, Palfi S, Dibo G, et al. Chronic recurrent transverse myelitis or multiple sclerosis. *Funct Neurol* 1996;11:209–214.
37. Ross MA. Acquired motor neuron disorders. *Neurol Clin* 1997;15:481–500.
38. Jackson CE, Bryan WW. Amyotrophic lateral sclerosis. *Semin Neurol* 1998;18:27–39.
39. Hemmer B, Glocker FX, Schumacher M, et al. Subacute combined degeneration: clinical, electrophysiological, and magnetic resonance imaging findings. *J Neurol Neurosurg Psychiatry* 1998;65:822–827.
40. Harding AE, Hewer RL. *Advances in neurology: inherited ataxias*. New York: Raven Press, 1993.
41. Moseley ML, Benzow KA, Schut LJ, et al. Incidence of dominant spinocerebellar and Friedreich triplet repeats among 361 ataxia families. *Neurology* 1998;51:1666–1671.
42. Rodgers CA, Murphy S. Diagnosis of neurosyphilis: appraisal of clinical caseload. *Genitourinary Med* 1997;73:528–532.
43. Di Rocco A. Diseases of the spinal cord in human immunodeficiency virus infection. *Semin Neurol* 1999;19(2):151–155.
44. Haerer AF. *Dejong's the neurologic examination,* 5th ed. Philadelphia: JB Lippincott, 1992.
45. Cheshire WP, Santos CC, Massey EW, et al. Spinal cord infarction: etiology and outcome. *Neurology* 1996;47(2):321–330.
46. Oldfield EH, Doppman JL. Spinal arteriovenous malformations. *Clin Neurosurg* 1988;34:161–183.

136. External Orthoses

Edward C. Benzel and William Mitchell

Frankel demonstrated that bed rest and immobilization are effective in achieving bony fusion (1). However, today's healthcare environment necessitates early mobilization of the patient in an effort to both minimize the medical complications of immobilization and maximize cost-effectiveness. External orthoses were developed to facilitate early mobilization while enabling fusion and/or protection of the spine and its neural elements. External orthoses are devices that are applied externally to minimize spine movement. These devices may be used alone or as a supplement to internal fixation.

It is critical to assess the dependence placed on an orthosis for immobilization. These devices have limitations conferred by their materials and obligatory biomechanical disadvantages. They are generally constructed from materials (e.g., plastic polymers) that permit some flexibility while maintaining support. One must understand some basic biomechanical principles as well as the normal motion of the spine to optimize the efficacy and safety of external immobilization techniques. All devices have limitations that must be balanced with their advantages. Each segment of the spine must be considered individually because of the variability of anatomy, mobility, and applicability of an orthosis.

Internal segmental fixation applies direct immobilization to spinal segments. However, most commonly employed spinal orthosis apply their forces at some distance from the spine. An inverse relationship between the thickness of the soft tissue separating the spine from the inner surface of the orthoses and the effectiveness of immobilization exists. Conformation of the brace to the body helps maintain the cylindrical body shell, thereby increasing the stability of the spine (2–5). Also, longer braces provide more stability than shorter ones; therefore, the length–width ratio of the orthotic significantly affects efficacy (Fig. 1).

A principal goal in long bone splinting is the immobilization of the fractured bone from one joint above to one joint below the site of injury. The axial skeleton is composed of five segments, each of which may be considered a long bone (cranial, cervical, thoracic, lumbar, and sacropelvic). One might then similarly consider the external splinting of an unstable spinal motion segment as being similar to long bone splinting (Figs. 1 and 2). Therefore, one segment above and one segment below the unstable motion segment would be included in the brace.

Direct points of fixation to the spine via an orthosis is uncommon (the Halo device is an exception). However, a brace can apply forces that are perpendicular to the long axis of the spinal column. This technique does not require conformation to the spine or body surface, but uses directed forces to maintain alignment. The Jewett brace uses the aforementioned biomechanical advantage of a three-point bending force application produced by applying dorsal forces at the sternum and pubis, in combination with a ventral force at the affected thoracic or lumbar vertebra (4,6). The long lever arms minimize the force required to produce sufficient bending moment.

The parallelogram effect and the "snaking" phenomenon describe segmental motion that occurs while the end points of the braced region remain relatively fixed along the spinal axis. The parallelogram effect refers to the situation when the rostral point of an immobilized region translates ventrally, whereas the caudal point of the immobilized region translates dorsally, or vice versa. The "snaking" phenomenon describes segmental motion that occurs while the end points of the immobilized region remain relatively fixed in the brace. Although there is no net movement, significant segmental (e.g., flexion and extension or lateral bending) motion can occur. Increasing the length and conformation of a brace minimizes the parallelogram deformation of the spine and the snaking phenomenon. This also maximizes the biomechanical effect of the brace. Close conformation to a large body surface area supports the intervening spinal segmental resistance to deformation. These basic principles must be individualized for each spinal region and clinical scenario.

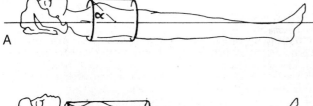

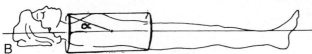

Fig. 1. The effectiveness of spinal bracing is inversely related to the axial distance between the spine and inner surface of the brace. This is *theoretically* defined by the following relationship: Efficacy of bracing is related to the cosine of *a* where *a* is the angle defined by the edge of the brace, the instantaneous axis of rotation (IAR) at the unstable segment, and the long axis of the spine. This angle is dictated by both the length of the brace and thickness of tissue between the spine and inner surface of the brace. **A:** A short brace (a = 15 degrees; cosine a = 0.966). **B:** A long brace (a = 45 degrees; cosine a = −0.707). Obviously, a significant reduction of efficacy comes with the use of a shorter, wider brace; that is, the length–width ratio of the brace is too small.

Cervical Spine

The cervical spine is the region of the spine that is most effectively stabilized by an external orthosis. It is also the region with the greatest intrinsic mobility. It has the least amount of surrounding soft tissue, thereby improving the orthoses' efficacy. There are also relatively solid points of fixation at each end of the cervical spine (i.e., the cranium and thoracic cage). However, rotation and bending in all directions is difficult to prevent by all techniques (7–13). Lateral bending and rotation have been assessed using a goniometer and anteroposterior radiographs (12,14); however, movement in the sagittal plane generally is emphasized with regard to clinical stability. Normal range of motion in the subaxial cervical spine generally is accepted as less than 3.5 mm of translation or less than 11 degrees of angulation on static lateral radiographs (15,16). Studies have compared the various orthoses and their segmental restriction of their motion (Tables 1 and 2).

Several problems arise with regard to immobilizing the cervical spine. These must be balanced with the limitation of motion that each device confers. The parallelogram effect is best dem-

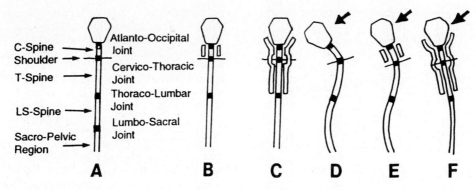

Fig. 2. The consideration of the axial skeleton as consisting of five segments. **A:** The segments are depicted and defined. **B:** A cervical collar. **C:** A brace embracing the mandible and thoracic regions. Responses to externally applied forces are depicted for the unbraced spine (**D**), the collar (**E**), and the extensively braced spine (**F**). Note the relative augmentation of protection provided by longer braces.

Table 1. Flexion and Extension Allowed at Each Segmental Level[a]

Test situation	Motion	0–C1	C1–2	C2–3	C3–4	C4–5	C5–6	C6–7	C7–T1
Normal unrestricted	Flexion	0.7 ± 0.5	7.7 ± 1.2	7.2 ± 0.9	9.8 ± 1.0	10.3 ± 1.0	11.4 ± 1.0	12.5 ± 1.0	9.0 ± 1.1
		18.1 ± 2.1	6.0 ± 1.2	4.8 ± 0.8	7.8 ± 1.1	9.8 ± 1.2	10.5 ± 1.3	8.2 ± 1.2	2.7 ± 0.7
Soft collar	Extension	1.3 ± 1.3	5.1 ± 1.9	4.5 ± 1.2	7.4 ± 1.5	8.4 ± 2.4	9.9 ± 1.7	9.7 ± 0.9	7.7 ± 2.5
	Flexion	13.7 ± 3.5	1.9 ± 1.4	3.9 ± 1.0	5.8 ± 1.7	6.8 ± 1.6	7.8 ± 1.2	7.4 ± 1.4	2.8 ± 1.9
	Extension								
Philadelphia collar	Flexion	0.9 ± 1.0	4.0 ± 1.8	1.6 ± 1.0	3.1 ± 1.1	4.6 ± 1.8	6.2 ± 1.9	6.2 ± 1.6	5.5 ± 1.8
	Extension	6.8 ± 2.2	4.5 ± 1.5	1.8 ± 0.9	3.4 ± 1.0	5.8 ± 1.2	5.9 ± 1.2	5.8 ± 2.0	1.3 ± 0.9
Somi brace	Flexion	3.6 ± 1.8	2.7 ± 1.8	0.9 ± 0.7	1.6 ± 1.1	1.9 ± 0.8	2.8 ± 1.2	2.9 ± 1.6	3.1 ± 1.8
	Extension	9.1 ± 2.6	5.4 ± 1.9	4.4 ± 1.1	6.3 ± 1.4	6.0 ± 1.8	6.0 ± 2.0	5.6 ± 1.8	2.1 ± 1.1
Four-poster brace	Flexion	2.9 ± 2.0	4.4 ± 2.1	1.6 ± 1.0	2.1 ± 1.1	1.8 ± 0.9	3.0 ± 1.2	3.9 ± 1.6	2.8 ± 1.4
	Extension	9.3 ± 2.2	3.2 ± 1.4	2.0 ± 0.7	3.2 ± 1.2	3.4 ± 1.3	2.9 ± 0.9	3.1 ± 1.5	1.6 ± 0.8
Cervicothoracic brace	Flexion	1.3 ± 0.9	5.0 ± 1.9	1.8 ± 0.8	2.9 ± 1.2	2.8 ± 0.7	1.6 ± 0.8	0.7 ± 0.6	2.4 ± 1.0
	Extension	8.4 ± 2.1	2.5 ± 0.8	2.1 ± 0.7	1.6 ± 0.7	2.2 ± 0.9	2.8 ± 0.9	3.4 ± 1.1	1.7 ± 0.8

[a] Data are expressed as mean degrees and 95% confidence limits of the mean.
From Panjabi MM, White AA, Johnson RM. Cervical spine mechanisms as a function of transection of components. *J Biomech* 1975; 8:327, with permission.

Table 2. Average Movement at Each Intervertebral Level from Maximum Flexion to Maximum Extension[a]

Stabilization device	0–C1	C1–2	C2–3	C3–4	C4–5	C5–6	C6–7	Sum of angles	Average movement at each level	Sum of angles 0 to C6 or C7	Measured movement
Halo jacket	4.5 ± 2.7	1.3 ± 1.1	4.1 ± 2.6	4.1 ± 3.2	3.1 ± 2.6	3.0 ± 1.9	6.3 ± 5.7	23.4 ± 13.7	3.7 ± 3.1	23.4 ± 13.7	5.2
Minerva jacket	3.5 ± 2.1	2.1 ± 1.1	1.7 ± 1.7	1.9 ± 1.2	2.0 ± 2.1	2.5 ± 1.6	2.3 ± 1.8	14.8 ± 4.4	2.3 ± 1.7	14.8 ± 4.4	5.2

[a] Data expressed in degrees as means ± standard deviations.
From Benzel EC, Hadden TA, Saulsbery CM. A comparison of the Minerva and Halo jackets for stabilization of the cervical spine. *J Neurosurg* 1989; 70:411–414, with permission.

onstrated in the cervical spine owing to its segmental mobility and lack of intermediate fixation points. Short braces that abut the mandible, occiput, and shoulder may increase this effect. Without intermediate points of fixation, the end points of fixation are subject to translational forces. A review of published data on the effectiveness of cervical orthoses illustrates this point (Tables 1 and 2) (12). Snaking becomes a significant issue when rigid fixation is applied (11,17,18). Flexion and extension movements at each vertebral level occur as a result of a simple movement, such as flexion or extension. The ends remain fixed, whereas the intermediate segments in between the end points move independently (8,12). Fixation to the upper thoracic spine appears to limit segmental movement at all cervical levels.

Assessing the efficacy of cervical orthoses is somewhat artificial and must be individualized. Most studies measure movement resulting from voluntary neck motion. There have been no consistent methods for assessing movement and thereby evaluating immobilization. The pros and cons of the available devices must be balanced during the decision-making process.

TRACTION. Traction generally is a preoperative and intraoperative immobilizing technique. It may be used to realign the cervical spine (e.g., facet dislocation, kyphosis, and so on) or simply maintain a specific alignment until internal fixation can be achieved. It is generally tolerated and safe, except with atlanto-occipital dislocations. Axial distraction applied via traction can be modified to also apply flexion or extension. Although 5 pounds per subaxial segment is a guide, extreme caution must be used in an unstable spine.

CERVICAL COLLAR. Cervical collars are commonly employed external cervical orthoses. "Soft" collars should not be used for immobilization purposes. They offer a mandibular point of fixation without a caudal point of fixation. They do not restrict motion because of their excessive flexibility; hence, they do not produce a parallelogram effect. They can be used as a support for patient comfort. When the brace is extended caudally to the shoulders and a more rigid material is used (e.g., the Philadelphia collar), movement is restricted. Flexion and extension are the motions most effectively limited by "rigid collars" (Table 1). However, this limitation of motion can produce a parallelogram effect. The ends remain fixed along the spinal axis, but motion can occur by the rostral segment translating ventrally and the caudal segment translating dorsally, or vice versa. Table 1 shows the limitation of motion provided by cervical collars (12,19). This type of orthosis does provide some restriction of movement, but the significance of the limitation of motion is difficult to ascertain; therefore, variable efficacy is provided by cervical collars (20–23).

Extending the orthotic further caudally to include the thorax adds a three-point bending moment that provides a significant biomechanical advantage. Such devices (e.g., SOMI, four-poster, and cervico-thoracic brace) substantially restrict motion in the mid to lower cervical spine (Table 1).

CRANIAL-THORACIC FIXATION. Cranial-thoracic fixation provides the greatest restriction of segmental cervical spine motion. The Halo device has been the gold standard of craniocervical and cervical immobilization for years (24,25). The rigid (Halo) and semirigid (Minerva) techniques limit mid to lower cervical motion, while minimizing the parallelogram effect. This is demonstrated by the decreased, allowed segmental movement in the upper cervical spine (Table 2).

Rigid cranial fixation, such as that achieved by the Halo, con-

siderably restricts capital flexion and extension movements. However, there is a significant difference between (a) the overall movement between the head and the thorax from flexion to extension and (b) the summation of segmental movements between these two regions (8,12). This difference can be quantitatively derived from radiographs (Fig. 3). This provides an objective measure of snaking (8). Snaking essentially is the intervening segmental motion that occurs while the end points of the immobilized region remain fixed. This segmental movement is more important than the overall movement between the head and thorax. Rigid cranial fixation exaggerates the snaking of the mid to lower cervical spine (Table 2). This correlates with clinical data demonstrating an unexpected deficiency of Halo efficacy in patients with unstable cervical spine injuries (26–29). The Minerva jacket similarly minimizes the parallelogram effect by providing a three-point bending biomechanical advantage (Fig. 4). This is provided in part by the chest fixation; however, it does not provide substantial control of capital flexion and extension and should not be used to provide these force applications. A significant advantage of the Minerva jacket is its minimal amplification of the snaking phenomenon (8,12,14,30).

If one compares Halo and Minerva data, it is apparent that the Minerva jacket controls subaxial sagittal plane segmental motion better than the Halo. On the other hand, the Halo is

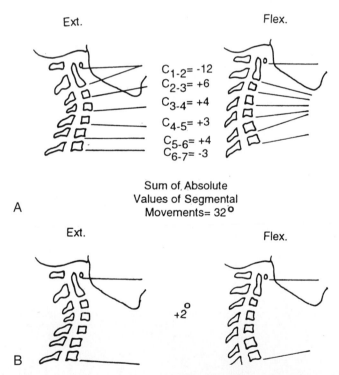

$C_{1-2} = -12$
$C_{2-3} = +6$
$C_{3-4} = +4$
$C_{4-5} = +3$
$C_{5-6} = +4$
$C_{6-7} = -3$

Sum of Absolute Values of Segmental Movements $= 32°$

$+2°$

Fig. 3. The assessment of segmental movement at each individual level (in degrees) can be measured and calculated from flexion and extension x-rays. The total movement is the sum of angles. The overall movement between the cranium and low cervical region (lowest segment assessed) is the measured movement. A: The difference is an objective assessment of snaking. The differences at segmental levels are depicted in this hypothetical example. The sum of angles is 32 degrees. *Ext*, the extension intersegmental angles; *Flex*, the flexion intersegmental angles. B: The overall movement between the cranium and the lowest segment assessed is 2 degrees. Therefore, in this case, the objective measure of snaking is 30 degrees. (From Benzel EC, Hadden TA, Saulsbery CM. A comparison of the Minerva and Halo jackets for stabilization of the cervical spine. *J Neurosurg* 1989;70:411–414, with permission.)

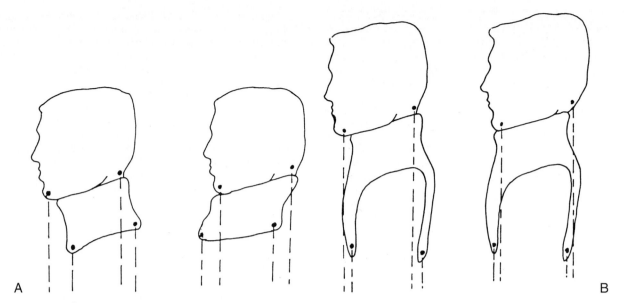

Fig. 4. A: The parallelogram-like bracing effort can be significantly diminished by the minimization of movement in the low cervical and cervicothoracic regions, via a three-point bending mechanism. **B:** This significantly restricts true neck flexion-extension.

obviously much better at controlling capital flexion and extension (8,12,14). The degree of control of capital flexion and extension (via manipulation of the degree of tilt of the Halo ring), combined with its additional ability to manipulate true neck flexion and extension (by movement of the ring ventrally or dorsally) makes the Halo unique as the only technique that provides the ability to manipulate cranio-cervical translational and flexion-extension movement. Orthosis selection should be based on the clinical, anatomical, and pathological scenario.

The different mechanisms by which the Minerva and Halo provide stability can be explained biomechanically. The former functions primarily as a three-point bending fixator and the latter primarily as a fixed moment arm cantilever beam fixator (Fig. 5). The Minerva is less rigid than the Halo, thereby explaining the observed differences in snaking (Table 2; Fig. 3) (8). However, the addition of a lower thoracic or lumbar attachment increases the lever arm available for a three-point bending force application. The length of the construct is proportionally related to its efficacy and the ability to resist bending moments at the unstable segment increases with the length of the construct.

Compression or distraction of the cervical spine is difficult to achieve with an external orthosis. However, Koch and Nickel

assessed distraction and compression forces with the Halo by inserting a transducer in the stabilizing bars of the Halo. A surprising variation of axial forces (22-lb) was observed during the assumption of several positions of normal daily activity (17). Lind and coworkers corroborated this data and concluded that: (a) significant flexion-extension motion occurs in each motion segment of the cervical spine; (b) the motion pattern is similar to a curling snake; (c) the motion decreases from rostral to caudal; (d) distraction is provided throughout the entire treatment interval; (e) the forces vary considerably depending on body position or movement (mean maximal variation: 175N); and (f) a tightly fitted vest exaggerates these variations (31).

All the aforementioned devices are associated with their own advantages, disadvantages, and complications. It is incumbent on the treating physician to understand these issues and balance them in an effort to achieve stability. There is no absolute answer regarding the definition of the "best cervical brace"; therefore, the normal range of motion of the affected segment of spine, limitations of a given brace, and dependence being placed on immobilization must be considered to determine the likelihood that this can be achieved. Finally, compliance and the patient's physical condition should be considered carefully.

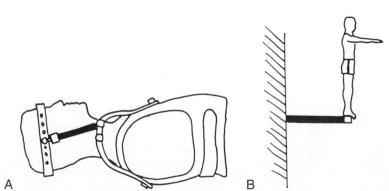

Fig. 5. A,B: The halo ring is rigidly attached to the calvarium. This provides a rigid cantilever (fixed moment arm cantilever beam) construct.

Thoracic Spine

The thoracic spine has two unique features that permit adequate immobilization via external orthoses. The two spinal regions above (cranial and cervical) and below (lumbar and sacral) the thoracic spine can be included in the brace. These additional points of fixation and the rib cage add truncal stability. Both factors minimize the effect of the soft-tissue thickness between the orthotic and spine. Data on the restriction of movement in the thoracic spine by external orthoses are lacking. However, it can be assumed that conventional methods are effective, as evidenced by the success of the nonoperative treatment of thoracolumbar fractures (32–34) and adolescent idiopathic scoliosis (35). Bracing for mild thoracolumbar fractures, however, has been legitimately questioned (36). This may be owing in part to the lack of support in the region. External orthoses that are commonly employed to immobilize the thoracic spine include: the body cast, "clam shell," Halo, Minerva with thoracic extension, and thoraco-lumbar-sacral orthoses (TLSO).

Lumbar Spine

The lumbar spine presents its own region-specific limitations to external immobilization. The lack of a caudal fixation segment limits the ability to obtain adequate fixation. Four levels proximal and distal to the target segment should be amenable to immobilization. The lack of caudal fixation in the lumbar spine is apparent. Hip flexion increases the motion in this region. Lengthening the brace and or adding a limb in the form of a hip spica helps minimize this motion. The hip-spica brace may function as a rigid cantilever-like construct, as well as apply or resist three-point bending forces. This may compensate for the excessive soft tissue between the brace and spine, as well as the lack of a caudal fixation point. This may explain the lack of correlation between length of brace and bracing efficacy observed by Triggs and co-workers (37). Sitting must be eliminated to effectively immobilize this segment. This generally is not well tolerated; therefore, compliance is suspect (38,39).

Sypert indicates that the discomfort the brace imparts is more effective than the forces transmitted (6). These devices use discomfort to remind the patient to restrict movement, support the abdomen, restrict upper lumbar spine motion, and maintain a straight or lordotic low back. The orthoses commonly employed for the lumbar spine include: the back belt; body cast; lumbosacral orthoses (LSO), with or without a hip spica; and Jewett brace (40,41). Efficacy has been demonstrated by higher fusion rates of uninstrumented lumbar fusions that were braced for 5 compared to 3 months (42). However, this does not necessarily imply biomechanical efficacy. Objective data on the efficacy of external lumbar orthoses are sparse (43). Back belts have not been shown to be effective in the workplace (44) and may contribute to weakening of the paraspinal musculature.

Junctions

The junctions of spinal segments (cervicothoracic and thoracolumbar) impart their own unique difficulties for the surgeon. They generally have characteristics that are a combination of the segments rostral and caudal to the junction. They are also located at a transition zone and, therefore, "see" the entire bending moment from above and below the junction. Finally, they are difficult to immobilize.

The cervicothoracic region can be effectively immobilized via an extension of a thoracic brace to include the cervical region or caudal extension of a cervical brace (e.g., Halo) to include the thoracolumbar region. Kock and Nickel have furnished interesting data demonstrating the progressive increased efficacy of Halo immobilization regarding the limitations of flexion and extension movement as one descends caudally in the cervical spine (Fig. 6) (17). Extrapolating this information into the upper thoracic spine with a caudally extended Halo technique, one might expect to achieve a substantial advantage with the Halo brace in this region. The thoracolumbar region can be immobilized by extending a thoracic brace caudally into the lumbar spine, and even to an extremity (e.g., hip spica). Alternatively, a lumbar brace can be extended into the thoracic spine.

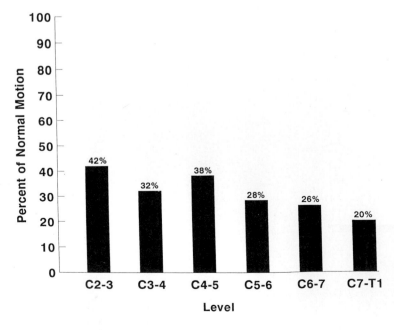

Fig. 6. Koch and Nickel determined the percentage of normal cervical spine motion allowed in a halo. The average was 31%; the range was from 42% in the upper cervical spine to 20% in the low cervical spine. The restriction of segmental motion increased as the spine was descended, as depicted. (From Koch RA, Nickel VL. The halo vest. An evaluation of motion and forces across the neck. *Spine* 1978;3:103–107, with permission.)

Conclusions

External immobilization is a complex tool in the spine surgeon's armamentarium. It must be employed judiciously and appropriately. Balancing the limitations and strengths of each device with the desired goal of immobilization and dependency on the device is critical to success. Ultimately, each situation must be individually approached with consideration of basic biomechanics, anatomy, and physiology.

References

1. Frankel HL, Hancock DO, Hyslop G, et al. The value of postural reduction in the initial management of closed injuries of the spine with paraplegia and tetraplegia. *Paraplegia* 1969;7:179–192.
2. Morris JM, Lucas DB, Bresler B. Role of the trunk in stability of the spine. *J Bone Joint Surg Am* 1961:43:327–351.
3. Morris JM. Spinal bracing. In: Wilkins RH, Rengachary SS, eds. *Neurosurgery.* New York: McGraw-Hill, 1985:2300–2305.
4. Norton PL, Brown T. The immobilizing efficiency of back braces. *J Bone Joint Surg Am* 1957;39:111–138.
5. Waters R, Morris J. Effects of spinal supports on the electrical activity of muscles of the trunk. *J Bone Joint Surg Am* 1970;52:51–60.
6. Sypert GW. External spinal orthotics. *Neurosurgery* 1987;20:642–649.
7. Askins V, Eismont FJ. Efficacy of five cervical orthoses in restricting cervical motion. *Spine* 1997;22:1193–1198.
8. Benzel EC, Hadden TA, Saulsbery CM. A comparison of the Minerva and Halo jackets for stabilization of the cervical spine. *J Neurosurg* 1989;70:411–414.
9. Hart DL, Johnson RM, Simmons EF, et al. Review of cervical orthoses. *Phys Ther* 1978;58:857–860.
10. Hartman JT, Palumbo F, Hill BJ. Cineradiography of the braced normal cervical spine. *Clin Orthop Rel Res* 1975;109:97–102.
11. Johnson RM, Hart DL, Owen JR, et al. The Yale cervical orthosis. *Spine* 1968;58:865–871.
12. Johnson RM, Hart DL, Simmons BF, et al. Cervical orthoses: a study comparing their effectiveness in restricting cervical motion in normal subjects. *J Bone Joint Surg Am* 1977;59:332–339.
13. Jones MD. Cineradiographic studies of the collar-immobilized cervical spine. *J Neurosurg* 1960;17:633–637.
14. Maiman D, Millington P, Novak S, et al. The effect of the thermoplastic Minerva body jacket on cervical spine motion. *Neurosurgery* 1989;25:363–368.
15. Panjabi MM, White AA, Johnson RM. Cervical spine mechanisms as a function of transection of components. *J Biomech* 1975;8:327.
16. White A, Panjabi M. *Spinal kinematics in the research status of spinal manipulative therapy.* Washington, DC: US Department of Health, Education, and Welfare, 1975.
17. Koch RA, Nickel VL. The halo vest. An evaluation of motion and forces across the neck. *Spine* 1978;3:103–107.
18. Mirza SK, Moquin RR, Anderson PA, et al. Stabilizing properties of the Halo apparatus. *Spine* 1997;22:727–733.
19. Kauppi M, Neva MH, Kautiainen H. Headmaster collar restricts rheumatoid atlantoaxial subiuxation. *Spine* 1999;24:526–528.
20. Coric D, Wilson JA, Kelly DL Jr. Treatment of traumatic spondylolisthesis of the axis with nonrigid immobilization: a review of 64 cases. *J Neurosurg* 1996;85:550–554.
21. Hughes SJ. How effective is the Newport/Aspen collar? A prospective radiographic evaluation in healthy adult volunteers. *J Trauma* 1998;45:374–378.
22. Murvis L. Biomechanics of cervical collars. *AANS Spine Section News* July 1994.
23. Sandler AJ, Dvorak J, Humke T, et al. The effectiveness of various cervical orthoses: an in vivo comparison of the mechanical stability provided by several widely used models. *Spine* 1996:21:1624–1629.
24. Bucholz RD, Cheung KC. Halo vest versus spinal fusion for cervical injury: evidence from an outcome study. *J Neurosurg* 1989;70:884–892.
25. Nickel VL, Perry J, Garrett A, et al. The halo. *J Bone Joint Surg Am* 1968;50:1400–1409.
26. Anderson PA, Budorick TE, Easton KB, et al. Failure of halo vest to prevent in vivo motion in patients with injured cervical spines. *Spine* 1991;16:S501–S505.
27. Kelly EG. Frequent lateral films key to control cervical displacement in halo cast. *Surg Pract News* 1981;10:21.
28. Tomonaga T, Krag MH, Novotny JE. Clinical, radiographic, and kinematic results from an adjustable four-pad Halovest. *Spine* 1997;22:1199–1208.
29. Whitehill R, Richman JA, Glaser JA. Failure of immobilization of the cervical spine by the halo vest. *J Bone Joint Surg Am* 1986;68:326–332.
30. Sharpe K, Rao S, Ziogas A. Evaluation of the effectiveness of the Minerva cervicothoracic orthosis. *Spine* 1995;20:1475–1479.
31. Lind B, Sihlbom H, Nordwall A. Forces and motions across the neck in patients treated with halo-vest. *Spine* 1988;13:162–167.
32. Cantor JB, Lebwohl NH, Garvey T, et al. Nonoperative management of stable thoracolumbar burst fractures with early ambulation and bracing. *Spine* 1993;18:971–976.
33. Chow GH, Nelson BJ, Gebhard JS, et al. Functional outcome of thoracolumbar burst fractures managed with hyperextension casting or bracing and early immobilization. *Spine* 1996;21:2170–2175.
34. Mumford J, Weinstein JN, Spratt KF, et al. Thoracolumbar burst fractures: the clinical efficacy and outcome of nonoperative management. *Spine* 1993;18:955–970.
35. Wiley JW, Thomson JD, Mitchell TM, et al. Effectiveness of the Boston brace in treatment of large curves in adolescent idiopathic scoliosis. *Spine* 2000;25:2326–2332.
36. Ohana N, Sheinis D, Rath E, et al. Is there a need for lumbar orthosis in mild compression fractures of the thoracolumbar spine? A retrospective study comparing the radiographic results between early ambulation with and without lumbar orthosis. *J Spinal Disord* 2000;13:305–308.
37. Triggs KJ, Ballock T, Byrne T, et al. Length dependence of a halo orthosis on cervical immobilization. *J Spinal Disord* 1993;6:34–37.
38. Axelsson P, Johnsson R, Stromqvist B. Effect of lumbar orthosis on intervertebral mobility. *Spine* 1992;17:678–681.
39. Axelsson P, Johnsson R, Stromqvist B. Lumbar orthosis with unilateral hip immobilization. *Spine* 1993;18:876–879.
40. van Poppel MNM, Koes BW, van der Ploeg T, et al. Lumbar supports and education for the prevention of low back pain in industry. *JAMA* 1998;279:1789–1794.
41. Willerns PC, Nienhuis B, Sietsma M, et al. The effect of a plaster cast on lumbosacral joint motion: an in vivo assessment with precision motion analysis system. *Spine* 1997;22:1229–1234.
42. Johnsson R, Stromqvist B, Axelsson P, et al. Influence of spinal immobilization on consolidation of posterolateral lumbosacral fusion: a roentgen stereophotogrammetric and radiographic analysis. *Spine* 1992;17:17–21.
43. van Poppel MNM, de Looze MP, Koes BW, et al. Mechanisms of action of lumbar supports. *Spine* 2000;25:2103–2113.
44. Wassell JT, Gardner LI, Landsittel DP, et al. A prospective study of back belts for prevention of back pain and injury. *JAMA* 2000;284:2727–2732.

137. Spinal Neuroendovascular Procedures

Richard D. Fessler,
Andrew J. Ringer, Lee R. Guterman,
and L. Nelson Hopkins

Cerebral angiography was first performed by Egas Moniz in 1927 (1). It was not until 1947 that the first spinal angiogram was performed by Tarlov (2). This study was performed intraoperatively and demonstrated a spinal extradural hemangioblastoma. Following this initial report, many years passed with case reports of cervical spinal intradural and extradural malformations and tumors identified serendipitously during vertebral artery angiography (3–7). Early case reports of complications ranging from renal failure to paraplegia led to perceptions of spinal angiography as a high-risk procedure (8–11). Improved access techniques, medical management, and catheter technology, along with the introduction of nonionic contrast media have resulted in significant reductions in procedure-related morbidity and mortality. Magnetic resonance imaging (MRI) has largely supplanted the role of diagnostic spinal angiography in the diagnosis of spinal pathology (12,13). However, a role for spinal angiography remains in cases of vascular malformations involving the spine, as well as in the evaluation and performance of neuroendovascular interventions for multiple spinal lesions. Newer catheters and superselective catheterization of segmental vessels supplying the spine now allow therapeutic infusions and interventions that were not possible in the past. This chapter details the technique of spinal angiography, provides a review of the pertinent anatomy, and discusses the current indications for spinal angiography with a particular emphasis on those neurosurgical diagnoses amenable to neuroendovascular interventions.

Anatomical Considerations

Proper interpretation of angiographic findings and planning for therapeutic intervention require an understanding of the vascular anatomy and supply of the spine and spinal cord. The vertebral column is supplied by 31 pairs of segmental arteries from which an equal number of posterior and anterior radicular arteries originate. Radicular arteries enter the vertebral column through the intervertebral foramina. Vessels supplying the spinal cord, termed medullary arteries, arise from the radicular arteries. During gestation, paired medullary vessels supply each segment of the spinal cord. Ultimately, the majority of these medullary vessels regress, and by the third trimester approximately six to 10 radiculomedullary vessels supply the spinal cord (14).

The spinal cord is supplied by three longitudinal arterial channels, the anterior spinal artery and paired posterior spinal arteries (Figs. 1–3). The anterior spinal artery lies within the anterior sulcus of the spinal cord, and the posterior spinal arteries lie over the posterolateral aspect of the spinal cord, medial to the dorsal root entry zone. The anterior spinal artery supplies approximately two thirds of the anterior spinal cord (15). From its location within the anterior sulcus, it supplies central branches to the anterior cord. Contributions to the anterior spinal artery may include its initial origin from the bilateral vertebral arteries, a variable number (typically one to five) of radi-

culomedullary contributions from the cervical vertebral arteries, and the ascending cervical, supreme intercostal, thoracic intercostal, and lumbar radicular arteries. Generally, one radiculomedullary vessel supplying the cervical spine at C5-6 is larger than the others and is called the artery of cervical enlargement. The upper thoracic spine is supplied by a contribution from an upper intercostal artery. Additionally, the mid to distal thoracic spinal cord and conus are supplied by a single large vessel arising from a lumbar radicular branch, the artery of Adamkiewicz, which arises from either an inferior intercostal or lumbar radicular artery (16,17). The artery of Adamkiewicz generally arises between T8 and L2 on the left and supplies the spinal cord from approximately T6 to the lumbar region (18). The posterior spinal arteries arise from multiple anastomoses of radiculomedullary vessels and supply the dorsal third of the spinal cord. At the caudal end of the spinal cord, the cruciate anastomosis consists of a "basket" formed by the terminal ends of the anterior spinal artery and paired posterior spinal arteries.

The spinal parenchyma drains into sulcal and radial veins. Sulcal veins in the anterior median fissure drain into the anterior median spinal vein, and radial veins drain the anterolateral and posterior spinal cord to the coronal venous plexus. Both sulcal and radial veins ultimately drain via radiculomedullary veins to the epidural venous plexus, also known as Batson's plexus (14, 19,20). Similar to the radiculomedullary arteries, radiculomedullary veins are not present at every level and exit the spinal canal adjacent to the nerve root.

The vertebral column is supplied by branches of radicular arteries as well as extrinsic contributions. The supply is conceptually easiest when divided into four regions: (a) an anterolateral supply to the anterior vertebral body originating from the ascending cervical or vertebral arteries in the cervical region and lumbar or intercostal radicular arteries in the thoracolumbar regions; (b) an anterior spinal canal supply composed of an arcade of vessels lying under the posterior longitudinal ligament, which is derived from the vertebral arteries in the cervical region and iliolumbar arteries in the lumbosacral region; (c) the posterior spinal canal, including the lamina and a portion of the spinous process, is supplied by vessels entering the spinal canal with the nerve root; (d) a posterior supply from a meshlike plexus over the spinous processes and a portion of the lamina formed by the dorsispinal artery (16,21,22).

Preprocedural Planning and Evaluation

It is of paramount importance to perform a complete neurological examination before the spinal neuroendovascular procedure. Not only does this familiarize the examiner with the patient, but also it allows for more rapid identification of neurological compromise in many cases. In addition, in those patients with preexisting neurological deficits, documentation before the procedure can result in confidence afterward that

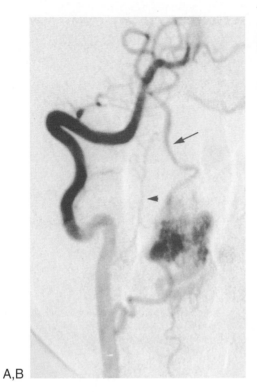

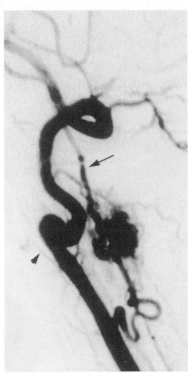

A,B

Fig. 1. Anteroposterior **(A)** and lateral **(B)** angiogram of a right vertebral artery injection in a patient with a cervical spinal cord arteriovenous malformation. The malformation has resulted in dilatation of the anterior spinal artery *(arrows)*. Spinal arteries to the anterolateral spinal column are also visible *(arrowheads)*.

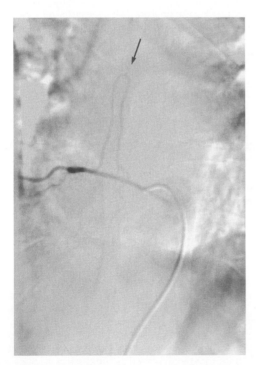

Fig. 2. Selective angiogram of a spinal intersegmental artery. The *arrow* indicates the medullary branch of the radicular artery. Note the typical hairpin curve of the artery as it enters the spinal canal.

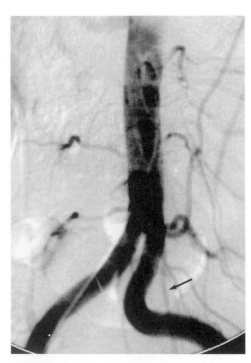

Fig. 3. Angiogram of the aortic bifurcation. The *arrow* indicates the lumbosacral artery to the spinal cord.

no additional deficit has accrued. Peripheral pulses should be noted, and if diminished, should be marked for easy identification during angiography. Review of any previous studies and an in-depth knowledge of the patient's history results in an appropriate plan and complete diagnostic study relative to each patient. Inappropriate review of available studies and inadequate review of the history of the patient's illness may lead to the performance of additional invasive procedures. A history of significant peripheral vascular occlusive disease or coronary artery disease should alert one to increased risk for an arterial access complication, periprocedural myocardial infarction, or stroke (23,24). Congestive heart failure requires judicious use of periprocedural fluid intake and contrast load. Necessary lab work includes at least the following: a baseline hemoglobin and hematocrit, platelet count, partial thromboplastin time, prothrombin time, blood urea nitrogen, serum creatinine, and blood glucose.

Numerous issues bear consideration before the performance of any endovascular procedure. The maximum potential contrast load for each patient should be calculated for patients with impaired renal function, and for all spinal angiography studies. For an assumed nonionic iodine (300 mg/mL) contrast preparation, the maximum contrast volume that can be used can be simply calculated as the patient's weight in kilograms (kg) multiplied by 5 and divided by the serum creatinine level. For example, a 90-kg patient with a 1.5 serum creatinine level would be able to receive 90(5)/1.5, or 300 mL of contrast. For longer procedures requiring large contrast loads, one can assume that a patient with adequate hydration and normal renal function has excreted approximately 50% of the administered contrast load and dosing can be recalculated. For those patients with a previous history of a reaction to contrast material, the administration of prednisone, diphenhydramine and acetaminophen before the procedure typically prevent unwanted contrast reactions and their sequelae (25). Generally, prednisone (10 mg, three times daily) is orally administered beginning 1 day before the procedure and as a single dose on the morning of the procedure. Diphenhydramine (25 to 50 mg, orally) and acetaminophen (10 mg, orally) are given approximately 1 to 2 hours before the procedure. Additionally, the mode of sedation or anesthesia should be addressed before the procedure. We generally perform all spinal angiography and interventional procedures using local anesthesia with sedative hypnotics and narcotic analgesics given intravenously before and throughout the procedure. However, the patient is maintained in a wakeful, cooperative state to allow serial neurological examinations that will alert the angiographer to changes in neurological function.

Indications for Spinal Angiography and Intervention

Vascular lesions of the vertebral column and spinal cord are listed in Table 1. Although MRI has supplanted spinal angiography for the diagnosis of most lesions, the role of spinal endovascular procedures likely increases as catheter technology allows improved access to the distal vasculature. Spinal angiography, although not indicated in the majority of cases imaged with MRI, should be seriously considered when MRI suggests a vascular lesion. Angiography is typically required to confirm the diagnosis and delineate or classify the lesion.

SPINAL VASCULAR MALFORMATIONS. The treatment of spinal vascular malformations has benefited tremendously from

Table 1. Vascular Lesions Most Commonly Found in the Spinal Cord and Vertebral Column

Vertebral column
  Tumors
    Aneurysmal bone cyst
    Giant cell
    Hemangioma
  Metastases
    Breast
    Thyroid
    Prostate
    Renal cell
Spinal cord
  Arteriovenous malformations
  Cavernous malformations
  Dural arteriovenous fistulae
  Hemangioblastoma

advances in spinal angiography and neuroendovascular techniques. A brief description of the common spinal vascular malformations and their neurangiographic diagnosis and current treatment options follows.

Spinal arteriovenous malformations (AVMs) must be described accurately and consistently to allow proper preoperative planning and operative intervention. Consistent nomenclature and diagnostic criteria are a necessity, and we adhere to the classification system categorizing AVMs as types I through IV as described by Anson and Spetzler (26). Type I AVMs are the most common spinal AVMs and predominantly affect males in their forties. Approximately 85% of lesions are below T6 and cause gradual onset of symptoms. Once the patient experiences symptoms, neurological impairment is generally progressive unless treatment is initiated (27). Type I lesions are dural arteriovenous fistulas (AVFs) arising from a dural radiculomedullary artery within the dural sleeve of a nerve root (28). The dural artery communicates directly with a radiculomedullary vein that carries the shunted blood in a retrograde fashion to the surface of the spinal cord. Owing to the limited auxiliary pathways of venous drainage from the spinal cord, the retrograde shunting of blood results in increased venous pressure within the coronal venous plexus and subsequently the radial veins, as well as venous hypertension and diminished spinal perfusion pressure. This sequence is the primary pathophysiological mechanism of myelopathy in patients with Type I AVMs. Type I A AVMs are characteristically supplied by a single fistula. Type I B lesions have two or more fistulas providing retrograde flow to the cord. It is of paramount importance that this be recognized on preoperative spinal angiography. Identification of a single feeding artery may not fully delineate the lesion. Therefore, selective catheterization must be performed in segmental arteries several levels above and below the lesion (Fig. 4). Current treatment options include open surgery for ligation of the fistula or endovascular embolization of the fistulous communication.

Type II AVMs are intramedullary, typically with a compact nidus. They are high-flow lesions with multiple feeding vessels from the anterior spinal as well as the posterior spinal arteries. Venous drainage is via the coronal venous plexus, which typically becomes enlarged and tortuous. Spinal AVMs tend to present equally in men and women in childhood or early adulthood. Symptoms may present in a stepwise fashion with periods of exacerbation and remission or acutely from intraspinal hemorrhage (29). On spinal angiography, these lesions are high flow with early venous drainage. Superselective catheterization of feeding vessels should be sought to fully delineate the extent

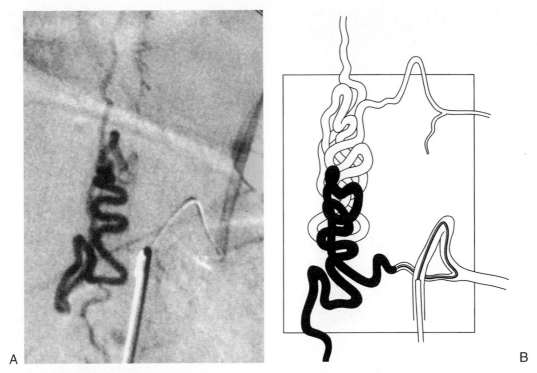

Fig. 4. Angiogram **(A)** and artist's rendering **(B)** of a spinal cord arteriovenous malformation. The injection of a single pedicle in the angiogram delineates only a fraction of the entire lesion, as depicted in **B**.

of the AVM. Neuroendovascular techniques are useful adjuncts to operative intervention or in certain cases as the sole therapy.

Type III AVMs are complex, large lesions that were formerly known as juvenile AVMs. They tend to occur in children and young adults and manifest symptoms such as progressive deficit, myelopathy, and pain. They are intramedullary but often have extensive extramedullary involvement, which may include the vertebral column or extraspinal tissues. The prognosis is generally poor. Spinal angiography reveals numerous feeding vessels from multiple spinal levels. Neuroendovascular embolization alone or in conjunction with surgery may be important as palliative treatment or for partial debulking.

Type IV spinal AVMs were described by Djindjian and coworkers in 1977 (30). Type IV AVMs are intradural extramedullary AVFs. The lesions are graded A through C. Type IV A lesions are typically located on the anterior surface of the spinal cord, although occasionally posterior malformations fed by the posterior spinal arteries occur. They are fed by a single arterial feeder, are low flow, and do not exhibit marked venous engorgement. The IV B subtype is characterized by engorged arterial feeders and dilated veins. The C subtype is a giant AVF with single or multiple pedicles.

Cavernous malformations of the spine are identical to those found in the brain. They represent up to 12% of spinal vascular lesions (31,32). MRI reveals evidence of hemosiderin consistent with multiple, repeated hemorrhages. Patients present with symptomology consistent with myelopathy owing to a number of factors, which include mass effect, hematomyelia, syrinx, and subarachnoid hemorrhage. Symptomatic lesions tend to have a progressive course, whereas other lesions are found incidentally on MRI (33). Those lesions that become symptomatic tend to do so from the third to sixth decade of life (33). They may present as either intramedullary or extramedullary in location. The MRI appearance is typically pathognomonic. Angiography reveals an avascular mass owing to the extremely slow flow. Occasionally, prolonged angiographic runs reveal a late blush.

There is no endovascular treatment. When necessary, surgery is the treatment of choice, but observation is reasonable in the absence of major hemorrhage.

Hemangioblastomas represent approximately 5% of spinal cord tumors (34). In the spine, hemangioblastomas frequently occur in association with von Hippel-Lindau disease (35). Patients typically present in the fourth decade with progressive myelopathy. The lesions are generally within the posterior portion of the spinal cord; 60% are intramedullary; and 80% are solitary. Approximately 50% are within the thoracic cord; 40% are within the cervical cord. It is not unusual for an associated syrinx to be present. Magnetic resonance imaging reveals vessel flow defects and an isointense lesion on T2-weighted imaging with enhancement after the administration of gadolinium (36). Angiographically, the lesions exhibit a well-circumscribed vascular blush that persists well into the venous phase (Fig. 5). There may be large engorged veins draining the tumor but the lack of evidence of arteriovenous shunting allows ready differentiation from spinal AVMs. Neuroendovascular embolization is frequently a useful adjunct before surgical removal to reduce intraoperative blood loss.

Metastatic tumors are the most common vascular lesions to involve the vertebral column and spine. The first symptom of compression is usually pain. However, many patients present with rapidly progressive neurological deterioration because of spinal cord compression. The most common metastatic spinal tumors in women are breast and thyroid cancer. In men, prostate and renal cell carcinoma are the most common sources of metastasis (37). Endovascular embolization can be of significant use for local control as well as an aid to controlling blood loss in patients who will undergo spinal reconstruction (38). For tumors such as metastatic renal cell or thyroid carcinoma, blood loss can be diminished as much as 50% by preoperative embolization (39). In patients with medical contraindications to surgery or in whom a lesion is not amenable to surgical resection, neuroendovascular embolization of metastatic lesions may pro-

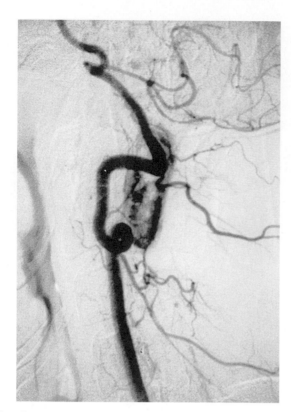

Fig. 5. Lateral angiogram of the left vertebral artery demonstrating a cervical spinal cord hemangioblastoma.

vide palliation of pain and temporize the progression of the lesion (40). One such patient in our practice with metastatic paravertebral renal cell carcinoma has undergone yearly embolization of a massive lesion with improvement and stabilization of his neurological status and control of pain (Fig. 6). Multiple investigators have reported improved surgical outcomes in case series in which preoperative embolization was performed as an adjunct to resection and stabilization. Diminished blood loss, greater margins of resection, and improved local tumor control are several of the benefits cited by surgical teams routinely utilizing preoperative embolization (38,39,41–44). Diagnostic studies, such as MRI, allow relative localization of metastatic lesions and can guide diagnostic angiography and embolization to minimize contrast load.

SPINAL TUMORS AND MASSES. Vertebral hemangiomas are typically benign lesions noted incidentally on MRI studies of the spine for back pain. Increased signal on T1- and T2-weighted images generally is confined to the vertebral body. Rarely, vertebral hemangiomas cause severe back pain, spinal cord compression, or nerve root compression. Aggressive, symptomatic vertebral hemangiomas are characterized by a constellation of signs that may include involvement of the entire vertebral body, extension to the neural arch, vertebral body collapse, increased soft-tissue mass, and/or an irregular honeycomb pattern on radiographs (45,46). Symptomatic vertebral hemangiomas are occasionally embolized through an endovascular approach before definitive resection or vertebroplasty (47). Currently, however, it is more common to perform percutaneous transpedicular injection of ethanol for sclerosis of the angioma followed by polymethylmethacrylate injection. In lesions with extensive epidural extension and spinal compression, sur-

gical decompression can be used adjunctively. In 50 patients treated in this fashion, Deramond and co-workers noted two episodes of intercostal neuralgia as the only periprocedural complications (46). Postprocedural irradiation with fractionated dosing (less than 4,000 centigray) has been used by some to treat residual lesions, but it is of questionable benefit and the risk of secondary radionecrosis argues against radiation therapy (48). Asymptomatic vertebral hemangiomas confined to the vertebral body can be managed conservatively.

Aneurysmal bone cysts have a slight female predilection, and 80% present in patients below the age of 20 years (49). They are cystic, blood-filled lesions lacking a normal endothelium. Approximately 30% to 50% of lesions are associated with preexisting bony abnormalities (50). Pain, mass effect, tenderness, and scoliosis are some of the presenting symptoms. Pathological compression fractures and spinal cord compression can also

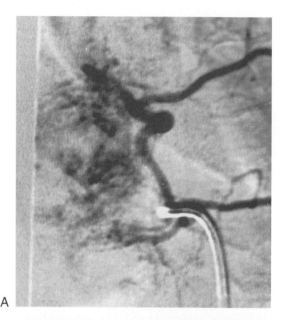

A

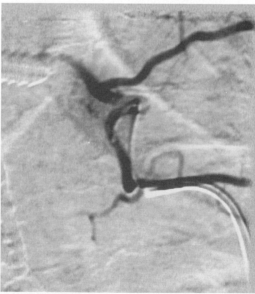

B

Fig. 6. Selective spinal angiogram of a spinal renal cell carcinoma metastasis before (**A**) and after (**B**) embolization. This patient underwent numerous staged embolizations for local tumor control and relief of pain.

occur. Plain films show cortical expansion and thinning in the affected area. Angiographic findings range from a faint blush to intense staining. Spinal angiography and embolization, either alone or as an adjunctive therapy prior to surgical resection, may be indicated in select cases.

Giant cell tumors occur in patients aged 20 to 50 years and represent approximately 5% of primary spinal column lesions. They are locally aggressive, containing sinusoidal vessels with a hypervascular stroma. However, they rarely cross the periosteum (49). Patients present with symptoms ranging from pain and radiculopathy to pathological compression fractures and spinal cord compression. Up to 10% of lesions may undergo malignant transformation with locally aggressive behavior or distant metastases. Spinal lesions most commonly occur in the sacrum, with the majority of nonsacral spine lesions occurring in females (51,52). Plain films depict a lytic, expansile lesion; MRI shows a heterogenous signal within a cystic lesion consistent with blood degradation products (36). Angiography reveals moderate to highly vascular lesions with evidence of arteriovenous shunting (53). Spinal angiography and preoperative embolization is typically a useful adjunct prior to surgical resection to diminish blood loss. Postprocedural radiation therapy may be warranted to diminish the risk of recurrence or metastasis. Recurrence rates as high as 50% have been reported.

Technique of Spinal Angiography

Patients are positioned supine on the neuroangiography table, with the knees slightly bent and supported if the patient has a history of lower back pain. Patients with a history of severe back pain or those in whom a lengthy procedure will be undertaken require intermittent position changes to alleviate pain and prevent pressure sores. Most of our procedures are performed using intravenous analgesics and sedative hypnotics, which allows serial neurological examinations and provocative testing during embolization procedures. We reserve general anesthesia for patients unable to tolerate recumbency for long periods. The maximum contrast load is calculated, and venous access is obtained well in advance of the procedure to permit intravenous hydration. A Foley catheter is placed for lengthy procedures expected to last 2 hours or more, such as spinal angiography. A radiopaque ruler may be placed lateral to the spine but within the field to allow localization of vertebral levels. In addition, the ruler allows accurate measurement of vessels and lesions as spinal angiography is typically performed in the anteroposterior (AP) plane, thus negating the calibrating and measuring functions of most biplane digital angiography units.

The inguinal regions are prepared and draped. The femoral pulse is palpated two to three finger breadths below the inguinal ligament. The inguinal ligament is approximated by a line drawn from the anterior superior iliac crest to the pubic tubercle. This site is chosen for ease of access and to allow compression of the femoral artery against the pubic bone following completion of the procedure. The common femoral artery is bordered by the femoral nerve lying deep to the lateral aspect of the artery and the femoral vein lying medial and slightly superficial to the artery. The neurovascular bundle overlies the medial aspect of the iliopsoas muscle and is just beneath the medial edge of the sartorius muscle. The skin is anesthetized and a small cut is made at the femoral access site. A percutaneous introducer needle is inserted at a 30- to 45-degree angle with the bevel up, and the needle oriented parallel to the direction of the femoral artery. The femoral artery should be palpated to determine its course prior to needle insertion. As many cases of spinal angiography involve heparinization for possible neu-

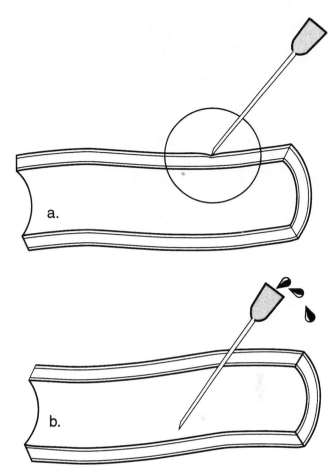

Fig. 7. Illustration of anterior wall puncture for femoral artery access. **a:** The needle is advanced slowly until the pulse is transmitted through the needle to the operator's hand. **b:** Gentle pressure at this point permits entry into the artery without posterior wall puncture.

roendovascular interventions, it is important to enter the artery on the first attempt and to avoid puncture of the posterior wall of the artery (Fig. 7). A J-wire is passed through the introducer needle, after which the needle is removed and an introducer sheath is placed. Introducer sheaths are used for cases in which catheter exchanges are anticipated and for patients in whom previous access or surgical bypass procedures have been performed. The introducer sheath should be large enough to accommodate the largest catheter that will be used.

Often, a limited angiogram can be performed because the relative site of the lesion is known from other diagnostic studies such as MRI. However, in some cases, a complete spinal angiogram is necessary and proper planning is imperative. Before insertion of a catheter, the region of interest must be aligned in the AP plane. The spinous processes should lie between the pedicles on AP view, without significant rotation. The type of catheter chosen depends on the level of interest. However, as a general rule, the orientation of the ostia of the segmental vessels changes from a steep upward orientation in the more rostral thoracic vessels to a more horizontal or slightly inferior plane in the caudal, lumbar segmental vessels. Additionally, lumbar segmental vessels are spaced more widely than are those of the thoracic aorta, and the aorta narrows as it passes from the descending aorta to the aortoiliac bifurcation. Thus, a catheter with a slight upward tip is most useful in the thoracic aorta and a catheter with a downward angled tip may be much more useful in the lumbar region. Several common catheter

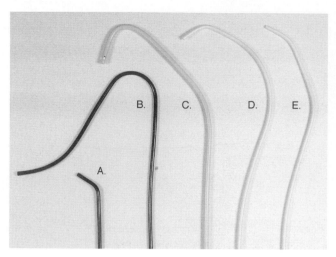

Fig. 8. Catheter tips used in selective spinal angiography and endovascular procedures. **A:** Angled taper (Meditech, Watertown, MA). **B:** Simmons curve (Meditech). **C:** Renal double curve (Cordis Neurovascular, Miami Lakes, FL). **D:** Cobra (Cordis). **E:** Headhunter (Cook, Bloomington, IN).

shapes that are useful in spinal angiography are shown in Fig. 8. In a capacious aorta, a catheter with a secondary curve may be used to increase the stability of the catheter while selectively catheterizing segmental arteries. It is important to document the level as each segmental artery is cannulated. One benefit of placing a ruler within the field is that, even if an angiographic run is labeled incorrectly, the correct level can be checked against a precontrast, unsubtracted scout film. In addition to the intercostal segmental vessels, the performance of a complete spinal angiogram involves imaging of all possible sources of pathology. A complete study includes the bilateral external carotid and vertebral arteries, costocervical trunk, thyrocervical trunk, and supreme intercostal arteries (T1-4). The segmental vessels span approximately from T5 to L3. In addition, the median sacral arteries arising from the aortic bifurcation and the lateral sacral arteries from the internal iliac vessels must be visualized. Bilateral access is necessary for visualization of the lateral sacral arteries. The vessels included in a complete spinal angiogram are listed in Table 2.

Spinal angiography is an exercise in patience and compulsion. In cases in which a complete spinal angiogram is warranted (i.e., multiple lesions or spinal subarachnoid hemorrhage with a negative MRI), the procedure should be approached in a systematic fashion, working from rostral to caudal. In some cases, the location of the lesion is known and angiography two levels above and two below generally suffices. Technically, the costocervical and thyrocervical trunks, supreme intercostals, vertebral arteries, and external carotid arteries are typically readily accessible; and one should take care to obtain appropriate views with minimal contrast use. All contrast

Table 2. Arteries Contributing to Spinal Cord
Vascular Supply and Included in Complete Spinal Angiography

Vertebral arteries (anterior spinal artery)
Costocervical trunk
Thyrocervical trunk
External carotid arteries
Segmental aortic branches (T3-L3)
Sacral artery

should be accounted for throughout the procedure. On occasion, it may be necessary to stop the procedure if the maximum contrast load has been administered.

Localization of spinal segmental arteries is accomplished by gently moving the catheter tip along the aorta from rostral to caudal and medial to lateral in the region of the inferior pedicle on AP views. The catheter tip will catch the ostia of the vessel and should be carefully advanced into the ostia by gently torquing a straight catheter or pulling back on a catheter with a secondary curve. Injections of contrast may be performed with a power injector or by hand. We inject 2 to 3 ccs of contrast by hand during a digital run at four to six frames per second. In cases of high flow AVFs or AVMs, frame rates as high as 30 frames per second may be used to delineate feeding vessels. The location of the first spinal vessel should be used as a guide to finding the contralateral vessel.

KEY POINTS: SPINAL ANGIOGRAPHY

- Position the patient supine in a comfortable position
- Maintain venous access
- Calculate contrast load, monitor contrast use
- Choose catheters
- Access femoral artery two finger breadths below inguinal ligament and place introducer sheath (minimum size: 5 French)
- Choose catheter, reconstitute over wire in aortic arch, and initiate angiography
- Work rostral to caudal and maintain record of levels in a consistent fashion

Interventional Spinal Neuroendovascular Procedures

If a lesion requiring endovascular embolization is identified, several additions to the technique of spinal angiography are necessary. Interventions require a coaxial system (i.e., a catheter within a catheter). One catheter serves as a guide or stabilizer, and an inner flow-directed catheter or catheter over a microguidewire is used to access the lesion. The introducer sheath must be of adequate diameter to accept the guide catheter. Given the relatively small size of many spinal vessels, a 6-French introducer and 5-French guide catheter generally suffices and allows the passage of a microcatheter as well as the injection of contrast around the microcatheter through the guide catheter for digital subtraction angiographic runs. All catheters used for intervention are continually flushed with heparinized saline (heparin 1 U/cc for routine diagnostic angiography; 4 U/cc for interventional procedures) through rotating hemostatic valves that allow for the passage of catheters in a watertight fashion. Additionally, patients are heparinized to maintain an activated coagulation time (ACT) of approximately 300 seconds (heparin, 50 to 70 U/kg body weight). The ACT is monitored on an hourly basis and heparin is readministered as necessary. Following catheterization of the pedicle selected for superselective catheterization with the guide catheter, the fluoroscopy unit (typically AP only) is placed to permit visualization of the microcatheter during manipulation. A road map is then produced, and the microcatheter is passed over a leading microguidewire and into the pedicle to the area of interest. After the feeding pedicle has been catheterized, provocative testing is performed with methohexital sodium, followed by an infusion of lidocaine to diminish the pain associated with embolization (54,55). Once superselective catheterization is verified by a microangiographic run through the microcatheter, provocative testing is performed by infusing methohexital sodium (1 cc, 10 mg/cc) into the pedicle; and a neurological examination is performed. If the patient is neurologically intact, embolization proceeds. Absorbable or nonabsorbable embolic agents or ethanol (see the following) are infused under constant fluoroscopy to verify that reflux of the agent into important anastomoses or proximal vessels does not occur. If necessary, adjacent normal arteries (e.g., intercostal vessels) may be occluded proximally with coils to prevent inadvertent delivery of ethanol to normal tissue. Distal collateral supply to the normal tissue compensates for the proximal vessel.

MATERIALS USED FOR SUPERSELECTIVE EMBOLIZATION. Embolic agents can be broadly classified into absorbable, nonabsorbable, and cytotoxic agents. Absorbable agents include autologous blood, Avitene (microfibrillar collagen; Medchem Products, Woburn, MA), and Gelfoam (absorbable gelatin; The Upjohn Company, Kalamazoo, MI). Autologous blood rarely is used today. Avitene and Gelfoam are often used preoperatively for the embolization of large vessels. They are generally mixed with 15 to 20 cc of contrast material under negative pressure and infused through the microcatheter. Nonabsorbable embolic agents include polyvinyl alcohol (packaged in vials with diameters ranging from 50 to 1,000 units), coils, and liquid embolic agents such as isobutylcyanoacrylate (IBCA) and n-butyl cyanoacrylate (NBCA) that polymerize on contact with ionic solutions (e.g., blood). The most commonly used cytotoxic embolization agent is alcohol, a potent denaturant that is cytotoxic to endothelium or cellular elements and thus promotes ischemia or anoxia. There is no immediate mechanical damage. Alcohol is available as a 95% to 100% solution. Up to 1 cc/kg body weight of alcohol may be administered. Ethanol generally provokes extensive necrosis secondary to severe intimal damage and subsequent vascular stasis but must be used with the utmost caution because reflux into a vessel supplying the spinal cord can result in irreversible damage (56).

Complications of Spinal Angiography

Spinal angiography has improved greatly since Tarlov performed the first spinal angiogram in 1947. Although complications were significant in the past, improvements in catheter technology and technique have lessened the risk of spinal angiography to approximately 3% for any type of neurological complication, the vast majority of which are transient (57,58). The use of nonionic contrast is mandatory, as ionic agents were associated with significantly greater complication rates. Of course, the most feared complication of spinal angiography is ischemic spinal cord damage. This can occur from iatrogenic dissection of any parent vessel supplying the cord as well as from dislodgement of atheroemboli within the aorta or from the introduction of air emboli. Neurological sequelae also may result from arterial obstruction induced by catheter wedging. In addition, as mentioned, embolic agents infused into vessels supplying the spinal cord or inadvertent reflux may be a source of severe ischemia. The importance of protective embolization should be emphasized: Many normal vessels may be temporarily occluded with Gelfoam or Avitene to allow selective flow of embolization material to the area of interest while sparing a normal territory. Peripheral complications include renal failure secondary to excessive contrast load and groin-related compli-

cations such as subcutaneous hematoma, retroperitoneal hematoma, infection, pseudoaneurysm, and distal emboli.

The management of spinal cord ischemia related to an interventional procedure should be predicated on the mechanism of the injury. The administration of high-dose steroids (e.g., methylprednisolone) and fluid hydration as well as further angiography (to determine the site of embolization if possible) are indicated. If an acute thrombus is present, lysis with urokinase or tissue plasminogen activator is possible. In cases in which it is not possible to determine the site of occlusion or the deficit is secondary to iatrogenic embolization with an embolic agent, the management is supportive. Consideration can be given to heparinization or antiplatelet agents to prevent possible secondary injury.

Conclusions

Advances in catheter-based technologies have resulted in the ability to access spinal lesions that previously were difficult or dangerous to manipulate from a neuroendovascular approach. In contrast to the risk years ago, the current risk associated with spinal angiography is similar to that of cerebral angiography. Spinal endovascular approaches can be used adjunctively to diminish intraoperative blood loss in patients with vascular tumors and, in some lesions, can be curative.

Acknowledgment

We thank Paul H. Dressel for preparation of the illustrations.

References

1. Antunes JL. Egas Moniz and cerebral angiography. *J Neurosurg* 1974; 40:427–432.
2. Tarlov IM. Spinal extradural hemangioblastoma roentgenographically visualized with Diodrast at operation and successfully removed. *Radiology* 1947;49:717–722.
3. DiChiro G. Combined retino-cerebellar angiomatosis and deep cervical angiomas: case report. *J Neurosurg* 1957;14:685–687.
4. Henson RA, Croft PB. Spontaneous spinal subarachnoid haemorrhage. *Q J Med* 1956;25:53–66.
5. Hook O, Lidvall H. Arteriovenous aneurysms of the spinal cord. A report of two cases investigated by vertebral angiography. *J Neurosurg* 1958;15:84–91.
6. Lindgren E. Another method of vertebral angiography. *Acta Radiol (Stockh)* 1956;46:257–261.
7. Morris L. Angioma of the cervical spinal cord: case report. *Radiology* 1960;75:785–787.
8. Antoni N, Lindgren E. Steno's experiment in man: as complication in lumbar aortography. *Acta Chir Scand* 1949;98:230–247.
9. McCormack JC. Paraplegia secondary to abdominal aortography. *JAMA* 1956;161:860–862.
10. Hol R, Skjerven O. Spinal cord damage in abdominal aortography. *Acta Radiol* 1954;42:276–284.
11. Boyarsky S. Paraplegia following translumbar aortography. *JAMA* 1954;166:1035–1037.
12. Dormont D, Gelbert F, Assouline E, et al. MR imaging of spinal cord arteriovenous malformations at 0.5 T: study of 34 cases. *AJNR Am J Neuroradiol* 1988;9:833–838.
13. Larsson E-M, Desai P, Hardin CW, et al. Venous infarction of the

spinal cord resulting from dural arteriovenous fistula: MR imaging findings. *AJNR Am J Neuroradiol* 1991;12:739–743.

14. Gillilan LA. The arterial blood supply to the human spinal cord. *J Comp Neurol* 1958;110:175.

15. Warwick R, Williams P. Spinal cord vasculature. *Gray's anatomy.* Philadelphia: WB Saunders, 1973:839–840.

16. Choi IS, Berenstein A. Surgical neuroangiography of the spine and spinal cord. *Radiol Clin North Am* 1988;26:1131–1141.

17. Djindjian R. Angiography of the spinal cord. *Surg Neurol* 1974;2:179–185.

18. Taveras J, Wood E. *Diagnostic neuroradiology,* 2nd ed. Baltimore: Williams & Wilkins, 1976.

19. Suh T, Alexander L. Vascular system of the human spinal cord. *Arch Neurol Psychiatry* 1939;41:659–663.

20. Batson OV. The function of the vertebral veins and their role in the spread of metastases. *Arch Surg* 1940;112:138–149.

21. Chiras J, Morvan G, Merland JJ. The angiographic appearance of the normal intercostal and lumbar arteries. Analysis of the anatomic correlation of the lateral branches. *J Neuroradiol* 1979;6:169–196.

22. Crock HV, Yoshizawa H. Origins of arteries supplying the vertebral column. In: Crock HV, Yoshizawa H, eds. *The blood supply of the vertebral column and spinal cord in man.* New York: Springer-Verlag, 1977:1–21.

23. Chimowitz MI, Kokkinos J, Strong J, et al. The Warfarin-Aspirin symptomatic intracranial disease study. *Neurology* 1995;45:1488–1493.

24. Marzewsky DJ, Furlan AJ, Louis P, et al. Intracranial internal carotid artery stenosis: longterm prognosis. *Stroke* 1982;13:821–824.

25. Westhoff-Bleck M, Bleck JS, Jost S. The adverse effects of angiographic radiocontrast media. *Drug Safety* 1991;6:28–36.

26. Anson JA, Spetzler RF. Interventional neuroradiology for spinal pathology. *Clin Neurosurg* 1992;39:388–417.

27. Aminoff MJ, Logue V. The prognosis of patients with spinal vascular malformations. *Brain* 1974;97:211–218.

28. Oldfield E, Di Chiro G, Quindlen EA, et al. Successful treatment of a group of spinal cord arteriovenous malformations by interruption of dural fistula. *J Neurosurg* 1983;59:1019–1030.

29. Thompson BG, Oldfield EH. Spinal vascular malformations. In: Carter LP, Spetzler RF, Hamilton MG, eds. *Neurovascular surgery.* New York: McGraw-Hill, 1994:1167–1195.

30. Djindjian M, Djindjian R, Rey A, et al. Intradural extramedullary spinal arterio-venous malformations fed by the anterior spinal artery. *Surg Neurol* 1977;8:85–93.

31. Cosgrove G, Bertrand G, Fontaine S, et al. Cavernous angiomas of the spinal cord. *J Neurosurg* 1988;68:31–36.

32. Simard JM, Garcia-Bengochea F, Ballinger W, et al. Cavernous angioma: a review of 126 collected and 12 new clinical cases. *Neurosurgery* 1986;18:162–172.

33. Ogilvy C, Louis D, Ojemann R. Intramedullary cavernous angiomas of the spinal cord: clinical presentation, pathological features, and surgical management. *Neurosurgery* 1992;31:219–229.

34. Jellinger K. Pathology of spinal vascular malformations and vascular tumors. In: Pia H, Djindjian R, eds. *Spinal angiomas: advances in diagnosis and therapy.* New York: Springer-Verlag, 1978:18–44.

35. Ho VB, Smirniotopoulos JG, Murphy FM, et al. Radiologic-pathological correlation: hemangioblastoma. *AJNR Am J Neuroradiol* 1992;13:1343–1352.

36. Osborn AG. Tumors, cysts, and tumorlike lesions of the spine and spinal cord. *Diagnostic neuroradiology.* St. Louis: Mosby-Year Book, 1994:876–918.

37. Fuller BG, Heiss J, Oldfield EH. Spinal cord compression. In: DeVita VT Jr, Hellman S, Rosenberg SA, eds. *Cancer: principles and practice of oncology,* 5th ed. Philadelphia: Lippincott-Raven, 1997:2476–2484.

38. Sundaresan N, Galicich JH, Lane JM, et al. Treatment of neoplastic epidural cord compression by vertebral body resection and stabilization. *J Neurosurg* 1985;63:676–684.

39. Gellad FE, Sadato N, Numaguchi Y, et al. Vascular metastatic lesions of the spine: preoperative embolization. *Radiology* 1990;176:683–686.

40. Soo CS, Wallace S, Chuang VP, et al. Lumbar artery embolization in cancer patients. *Radiology* 1982;145:655–659.

41. Ellman BA, Parkhill BJ, Curry TS 3rd, et al. Ablation of renal tumors with absolute ethanol: a new technique. *Radiology* 1981;141:619–626.

42. Hilal S, Michelsen JW. Therapeutic percutaneous embolization for extra-axial vascular lesions of the head, neck, and spine. *J Neurosurg* 1975;43:275–287.

43. Sundaresan N, Scher H, DiGiacinto GV, et al. Surgical treatment of spinal cord compression in kidney cancer. *J Clin Oncol* 1986;4:1851–1856.

44. King GJ, Kostuik JP, McBroom RJ, et al. Surgical management of metastatic renal carcinoma of the spine. *Spine* 1991;16:265–271.

45. Laredo JD, Reizine D, Bard M, et al. Vertebral hemangiomas: radiologic evaluation. *Radiology* 1986;180:161–163.

46. Deramond H, Depriester C, Galibert P, et al. Percutaneous vertebroplasty with polymethylmethacrylate: technique, indications, and results. *Radiol Clin North Am* 1998;36:533–546.

47. Merland JJ, Reizine D, Laurent A, et al. Embolization of spinal cord vascular lesions. In: Vinuela F, Halbach VV, Dion JE, eds. *Interventional neuroradiology: endovascular therapy of the central nervous system.* New York: Raven Press, 1992:153–165.

48. Yang ZY, Zhang LJ, Lhen ZX, et al. Hemangioma of the vertebral column: a report of 23 patients with special reference to functional recovery after radiation therapy. *Acta Radiol Oncol* 1985;24:129–132.

49. Dorwart RH, LaMasters DL, Watanabe TJ. Tumors. In: Newton TH, Potts DG, eds. *Computed tomography of the spine and spinal cord.* San Anselmo: Clavadel Press, 1983:115–147.

50. Manaster BJ. *Handbooks in radiology: skeletal radiology.* Chicago: Yearbook, 1989:1–106.

51. Goldenburg R, Campbell C, Bonfigliio M. Giant cell tumor of bone: an analysis of 218 cases. *J Bone Joint Surg* 1970;52:619–625.

52. Shikata J, Yamamuro T, Shimizu K, et al. Surgical treatment of giant-cell tumors of the spine. *Clin Orthop* 1992;278:29–36.

53. Djindjian R, Hurth M, Houdart R. *Angiography of the spinal cord.* Baltimore: University Park Press, 1970.

54. Rauch R, Vinuela F, Dion J, et al. Preembolization functional evaluation in brain arteriovenous malformations: the superselective Amytal test. *AJNR Am J Neuroradiol* 1992;13:303–308.

55. Touho H, Karasawa J, Ohnishi H, et al. Intravascular treatment of spinal arteriovenous malformations using a microcatheter—with special reference to serial Xylocaine tests and intravascular pressure monitoring. *Surg Neurol* 1994;42:148–156.

56. Ellman BA, Green CE, Eigenbrodt E, et al. Renal infarction with absolute ethanol. *Invest Radiol* 1980;15:318–322.

57. Forbes G, Nichols DA, Jack CR Jr, et al. Complications of spinal cord arteriography: prospective assessment of risk for diagnostic procedures. *Radiology* 1988;169:479–484.

58. Kendall B. Spinal angiography with iohexol. *Neuroradiology* 1986;28:72–73.

138. Electrophysiological Monitoring During Spinal Surgery: A Practical Approach

Lawrence P. Bernstein and Emmanuel K. Nenonene

Intraoperative electrophysiological monitoring of spinal cord and nerve root function has been widely used for the last 25 years. The techniques employed have included somatosensory evoked potentials (SSEPs), dermatomal evoked potentials, free-running electromyography (EMG), compound muscle action potentials (CMAPs), and motor evoked potentials (MEPs).

Three operational principles govern electrophysiological monitoring:

1. The modality being monitored is sensitive to the operative manipulation being employed.
2. Useful intervention can take place if a change is detected.
3. The monitoring procedure poses no or little risk to the patient.

Efficacy

Electrophysiological monitoring has become accepted as an effective means of reducing inadvertent injury during spinal surgery based on data from animal experimentation, case reports, and clinical series (1–3). Rigorous prospective studies in patients are not available. A particular problem is establishing the true positive rate (4), because not intervening following a major change in a monitored parameter would appear unethical, given available information. Formal evaluation of intraoperative electrophysiological monitoring, by means of receiver operating characteristic analysis (5), or other formal systems have not been carried out. Therefore, it is not appropriate to make quantitative statements about the advantages of monitoring, but rather to regard it as a likely helpful adjunct to surgery.

How Evoked Potentials Are Recorded

Successful recording of intraoperative evoked potentials depended on the development of the differential amplifier and digital computer. The former allows rejection of electrical noise common in phase and polarity and the latter allows increase in the signal to noise ratio of small signals by means of averaging a number of events time locked to a stimulus. The minimal sampling rate needed to define a wave is twice its frequency and is referred to as the Nyquist frequency (6). The ability of the amplifier to reject extraneous noise common in phase and amplitude to its input is termed common mode rejection. The signal to noise ratio of a displayed signal is increased by the square root of the number of stimulus presentations. For this reason evoked potentials are not real-time events and often take minutes to appear. Evoked potentials are categorized as near-field if electrode position has a large influence on their amplitude and polarity and far-field if this influence is small (7). Gold-plated cup, stainless steel subdermal needle, and stainless steel disc electrodes can all be employed for evoked potential recording. When potentials are recorded from the scalp, electrodes are placed according to the International 10-20 System (8), which is used to record the electroencephalogram. Potentials generated by peripheral nerves or the spinal cord, are acquired from electrodes placed in appropriate anatomical locations (9).

How Electromyographic Activity and Compound Muscle Action Potentials Are Recorded

Either surface disc electrode or subdermal needle electrodes produce satisfactory recordings. Pairs of electrodes are employed with one electrode placed centrally over the muscle, the other closer to its origin when possible. Higher impedance insulated monopolar or bipolar EMG needle electrodes can provide sharp definition of single motor unit potentials but will not necessarily record from more distant portions of a muscle when recording CMAPs. Recording of spontaneous activity should be continuous. In the case of CMAPs, activity is recorded following a shock delivered to a nerve, nerve root, or pedicle screw.

Electrical Safety

Most modern equipment provides adequate isolation to protect patients from electrical injury. Maintenance of an electrically safe patient environment is one of the prime responsibilities of the monitoring team. It is important to emphasize a few points. Patients with a low impedance path to the myocardium (pacemaker) may be at increased risk, particularly when upper extremity stimulation is employed. Small surface area electrodes (needle electrodes) can provide a dangerous path for current return in the event of an open cautery return lead. Ground connections must be isolated. Finally, equipment should be switched on before connecting it to a patient and the patient disconnected prior to turning equipment off, to avoid the effect of surges or possibly reveal a catastrophic fault in the equipment before a patient is connected. Clear review of this topic can be found in the literature (4,10,11).

Anesthetic Considerations

Inhalational agents, both halogenated agents and nitrous oxide, suppress SSEPs (12). However, it is relatively easy to record potentials in the presence of these agents provided doses are low. Other intravenous agents, with the exception of etomidate (which seems to enhance cortical potentials) and narcotics also have the ability to suppress evoked potentials. It is self-evident that EMG and CMAP recording cannot be carried out in the face of a high degree of neuromuscular blockade. All anesthetic regimens used in patients undergoing intraoperative monitoring represent a compromise between the need to maintain the patient safely anesthetized and the need to preserve evoked potential or EMG activity.

General Guidelines for Successful Monitoring

1. Always obtain a baseline prior to surgery. It is inefficient and frustrating to attempt to record SSEPs from patients in which they are absent secondary to underlying illness (peripheral neuropathy, lumbar stenosis, and so on) in the operating

---

EVANSTON HOSPITAL
CLINICAL NEUROPHYSIOLOGY LABORATORY

Patient Name _____ Age _34_ BD _12/2k/62_ Sex _F_

Height _5'3"_ Weight _145 LBS_ Date _1/21/97_ Preop. _Normal_ Date _1/7/97_

EP # _97-_ Room # _12_ Surgeon(s) _____

Anesthesiologist _____ Technologist _EKN/GV_

Surgery _L4-5 Discectomy_ Monitor _POST TIBIAL NERVE/DERMS_
        L5-S1 Decompression
Diagnosis _Herniated disk_

Time	B.P.	Forane %	COMMENTS
8:43	127/82	0.32%	Good Potentials / well defined - Exposure
9:24	99/54	0.29%	Derms Potentials / well defined. Decompression L4-L5 / Disk out.
11:01	112/68	.30%	
12:00	108/59	.33%	slight decrease of amplitude - Talked to Anesthesiologist / Broke disk out / Tapping.
12:53	99/58	.32%	Continous X-Ray on Start hardware -
13:50	105/63	.34%	Inserting Screws.
14:00	98/58	0.29%	Amplitude smaller / Anesthesiologist is aware.

SUMMARY _propofol_
        _N0 2_
        fentanol.

Fig. 1. Protocol sheet.

room. Identifying absent potentials preoperatively may allow alternative sites to be stimulated or (in the case of very small potentials) allow modification of anesthesia to enhance potentials.

2. Make sure the monitoring team knows what changes the surgeon wishes to be notified of and when.

3. Prior to making a manipulation, which may lead to a change in evoked potentials, check that no recent change in anesthesia has taken place, vital signs are stable, and the current set of averages is completed.

4. A protocol sheet for comments and data entry should be maintained (Fig. 1).

Lower or Upper Extremity Somatosensory Evoked Potentials

Posterior tibial or peroneal nerve
Median or ulnar nerve
Filters: 30 to 3,000 Hz

Analysis time: 50 ms for upper and 100 ms for lower extremity
Number of stimuli: 125 to 500
Stimulus duration: .2 to .3 ms
Stimulus amplitude: 10 to 40 mA
Stimulus rate: 4 to 7 Hz

Expected results are shown in Figures 2 and 3.

Interpretation of Lower Extremity Somatosensory Evoked Potentials

Because SSEPs vary to some extent during surgical procedures involving the spine (13), decision making depends in some degree on the experience of the monitoring personnel and specific intraoperative conditions. Amplitude as well as latency changes may be important indicators that intervention is needed (Fig. 4). Abrupt amplitude changes greater than 30% to 40% that are maintained for at least two averages are a cause to evaluate any manipulation that preceded them. This is particularly important in the case of bilateral simultaneous stimulation

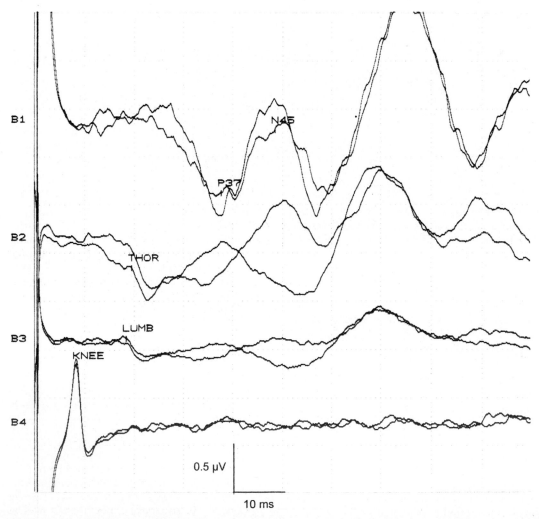

Fig. 2. Evoked responses for posterior tibial nerve stimulation. (*B1*, cortical; *B2*, thoracic; *B3*, lumbar; *B4*, popliteal fossa.)

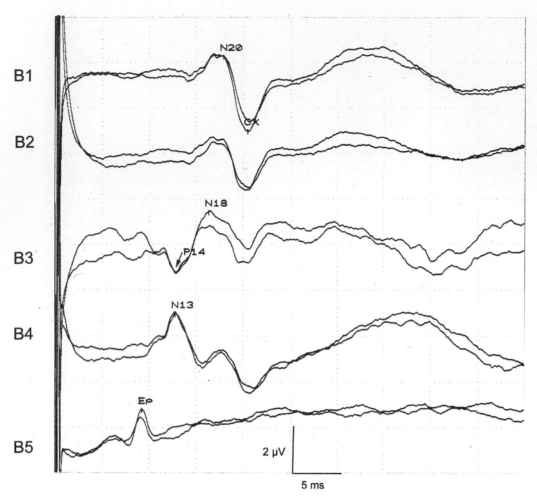

Fig. 3. Evoked responses from right median nerve stimulation at the wrist. (*B1*, cortical C3'-Fpz; *B2*, cortical C3'-C4'; *B3*, cortical C3'-Erb contra; *B4*, cervical C5S-Fpz; B5, Erb ipsi-Erb contra.)

where a unilateral deficit may be masked partially by maintained activity from the contralateral side. Slowly developing changes in amplitude and/or latency unrelated to a discrete manipulation frequently are related to factors other than spine injury, including decrease in body temperature, anesthetic effect, and changes in blood pressure. It is important to keep in mind that SSEPs are at best an indirect indicator of motor system integrity, so that their ability to detect motor system damage is uncertain. This is particularly true in the case of distraction during Harrington rod placement for scoliosis (2).

are absent preoperatively, monitoring upper extremity potentials is reasonable. If lower extremity potentials are obtainable, it has been our practice to monitor these during cervical procedures, although simultaneously monitoring upper extremity potentials is an option.

As is the case for lower extremity stimulation, intact SSEPs do not guarantee the integrity of the corticospinal tracts. Significant change in SSEP amplitude and latency is equivalent to those used for lower extremity stimulation.

Interpretation of Upper Extremity Evoked Potentials

Median nerve stimulation can be used with procedures at C-5 and above and ulnar stimulation at C-7 and above. It is probably best to use alternate rather than simultaneous stimulation of each side to make interpretation of waveform changes easier. Although it is possible to stimulate all four nerves, this type of paradigm makes interpretation of changes difficult (Fig. 3). Stimulation of upper extremity nerves does not yield direct information about the integrity of dorsal column pathways from the lower extremity. Despite this, if lower extremity potentials

Dermatomal Evoked Potentials

This subcategory of evoked potential is elicited by electrical stimulation of the skin of single dermatomes (Fig. 4). The methodology has been well described for both diagnostic studies and intraoperative use (14). These potentials have been used in monitoring pedicle screw placement and the integrity of dorsal roots. In our experience, they are of lower amplitude, more dispersed and less stable, and more difficult to record than SSEPs from mixed nerve stimulation. Typical stimulation and recording sites can be found in Toleikis and Sloan (14).

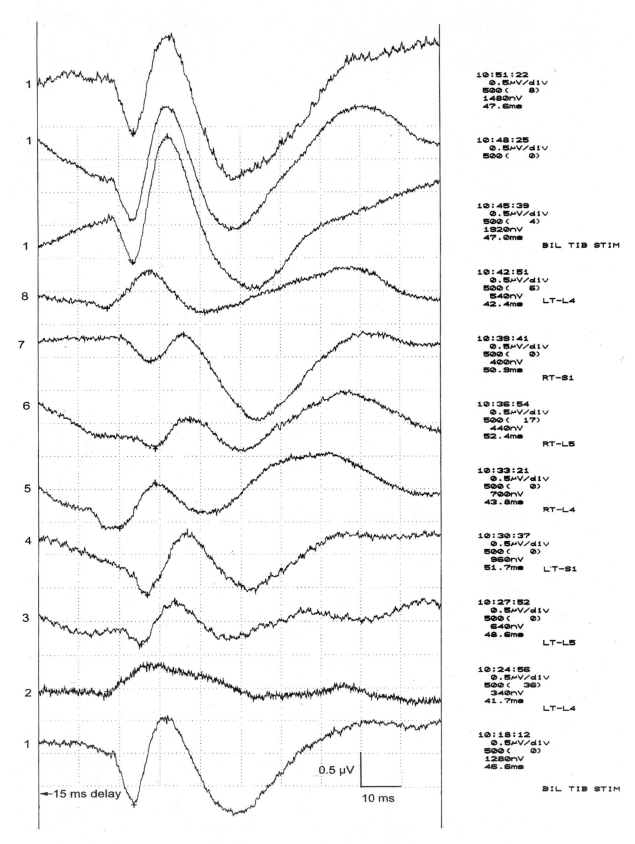

Fig. 4. Intraoperative cortical somatosensory evoked potentials. *1,* bilateral posterior tibial nerve response; *2* and *5,* left and right L4 dermatomal responses; *3* and *6,* left and right L5 dermatomal responses; *4* and *7,* left and right S1 dermatomal responses; *8,* left L4 dermatomal response.

Interpretation of Dermatomal Evoked Potentials

False positive or failed monitoring attempts are more frequent because these potentials are less stable than SSEPs. We have encountered a single false negative response using this technique during pedicle screw placement.

Pedicle Screw Stimulation

Pedicle screw stimulation is the electrophysiological measure for the evaluation of the integrity of the pedicle and pedicle screw placement. This technique for recording compound muscle action potentials (CMAPs) is used to monitor specific nerve roots that carry the risk of injury during pedicle screw placement

in lumbosacral surgery (1,15–17). The results to be expected are shown in Figure 5.

Interpretation of Free Running Electromyography and Pedicle Screw Stimulation

Free run EMG consists of monitoring of muscle activity during absence of electric stimulation of the pedicle or pedicle screw. Normally no spontaneous muscle activity is present. Partial neuromuscular blockade is used for muscle relaxation. We prefer a level low enough to be able to obtain three twitches in a train of four, stimulating the median nerve at the wrist. Bursts of motor unit potentials (MUPs) are associated with transient disturbance of the nerve root, whereas persistent trains of MUPs are associated with sustained traction or compression of the nerve root.

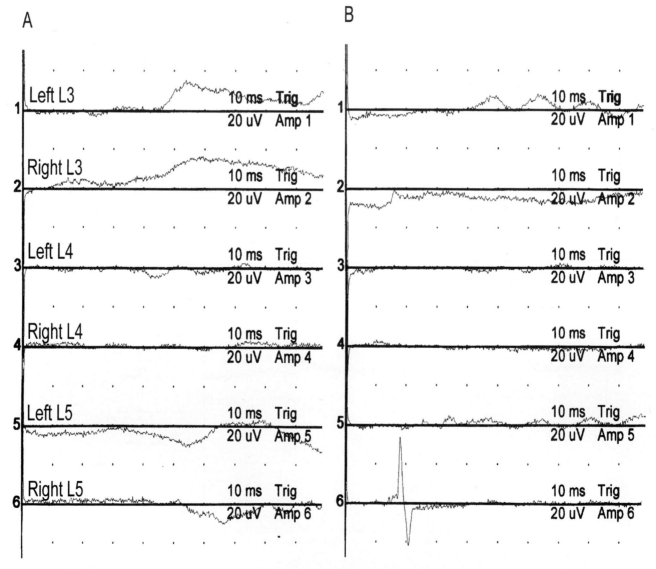

Fig. 5. Right L5 pedicle screw stimulation. **A:** 11 mA no compound muscle action potential (CMAP) present. **B:** 29 mA CMAP present. Note: thresholds greater than 11 mA correlate with proper screw placement and intact pedicle.

__4

Stimulation of the pedicle screw or of the hole drilled to accept the pedicle screw evokes activity of muscles connected to the ventral root contiguous with the pedicle (18). Our experience suggests that thresholds in excess of 11 mA correlate with successful screw placement in an intact pedicle. We estimate our false positive rate at 5% to 10% and have yet to encounter a false negative response in over 400 to 600 screw placements.

Spontaneous Electromyography and Compound Muscle Action Potentials

Virtually, any nerve or nerve root whose myotomal representation is accessible to surface or needle electrode placement can be studied. The most commonly studied nerves are cranial nerves, particularly the seventh nerve. Study of spinal nerves or roots is almost identical. Typical examples are given in Figure 6.

As is the case for pedicle screw stimulation, bursts of MUPs suggest irritation and sustained trains of MUPs or iteratively discharging single MUPs suggest injury. It may be necessary to adjust the time during CMAP recording depending on the distance between the point of stimulation and recording site. Monopolar stimulation is likely to give more reproducible thresholds and better localization than bipolar stimulation. A control stimulus to an inactive region is helpful when trying to identify a nerve or nerve root. If bipolar stimulation by means of forceps is used, constant voltage stimulation is essential because of shunting of current by conductive fluid surrounding the nerve or the nerve root. If monopolar stimulation is used (the cathode), we prefer to use constant current. Robust CMAPs

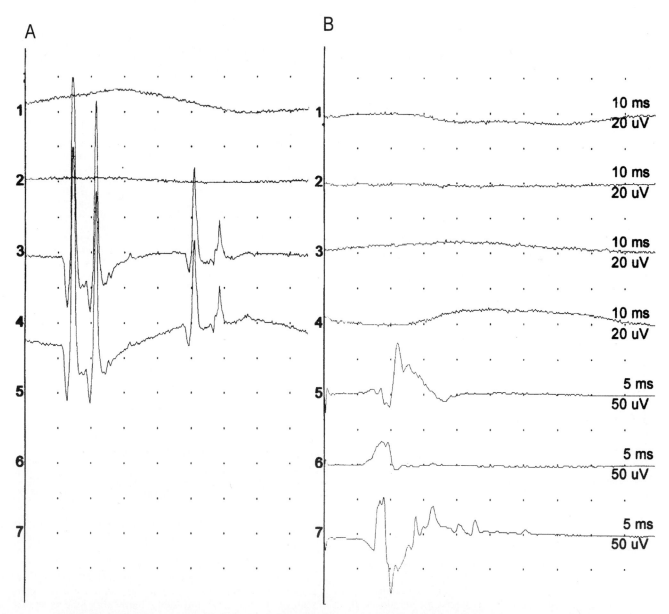

Fig. 6. Multichannel recording from facial muscles during acoustic neuroma surgery. **A:** Free running electromyography activity: manipulation of the seventh nerve gives rise to some injury discharges. **B:** Direct stimulation of the seventh nerve evokes a compound muscle action potential, confirming that the nerve remains intact distal to the point of stimulation.

are obtainable provided neuromuscular blockade is limited as in pedicle screw stimulation.

Motor Evoked Potentials Recording

Despite the fact that motor evoked potentials have been successfully recorded for 20 years they have not become widely used in a standard manner intraoperatively. Variability under anesthesia, questions of safety, and even questions as whether they are purely motor responses have hampered their acceptance. They would appear most indicated in surgeries involving Harrington rod placement where false negative SSEPs would seem a particular problem. We do not perform motor evoked potentials recording (MEPs) and refer the reader to the following source (19,20).

Conclusions

Electrophysiological monitoring is a safe and at least qualitatively effective method of reducing inadvertent damage to the spinal cord or nerve roots during spinal surgery. Keeping paradigms simple and maintaining clear communication among the monitoring team, surgeon, and anesthesia staff are important elements in making monitoring successful.

References

1. Epstein NE, Danto J, Nardi D. Evaluation of intraoperative somatosensory-evoked potential monitoring during 100 cervical operations. *Spine* 1993;18:737–747.
2. Lesser RP, Raudzens P, Luders H, et al. Postoperative neurological deficits may occur despite unchanged intraoperative somatosensory evoked potentials. *Ann Neurol* 1986;19:22–25.
3. Worth RM, Markand ON, DeRosa GP, et al. Intraoperative somatosensory evoked response monitoring during spinal cord surgery. In: Mauguiere CF, Revol M, eds. *Clinical applications of evoked potentials in neurology.* New York: Raven Press, 1982.
4. Moller AR. *Intraoperative neurophysiologic monitoring.* Harwood Academic Publishers, 1995.
5. Swets JA, Pickett RM. *Evaluation of diagnostic systems, methods from signal detection theory.* New York: Academic Press, 1986.
6. Spehlmann R. *Evoked potential primer. Visual, auditory and somatosensory evoked potentials in clinical diagnosis.* Boston: Butterworth, 1985.
7. Stegeman DF, Dimitru D, King JC, et al. Near- and far-fields: source characteristics and the conducting medium in neurophysiology. *J Clin Neurophysiol* 1997;14:429–442.
8. Jasper HH. The ten-twenty system of the International Federation of EEG. *Clin Neurophysiol* 1958;10:371–375.
9. Guideline nine: guidelines on Evoked Potentials. American Electroencephalographic Society. *J Clin Neurophysiol* 1994;11:40–73.
10. Tyner FS, Knott JR, Mayer WB. *Fundamentals of EEG technology.* New York: Raven Press, 1983.
11. Nuwer MR. *Evoked potential monitoring in the operating room.* New York: Raven Press, 1986.
12. Sloan TB. Anesthetic effects on electrophysiologic recordings. *J Clin Neurophysiol* 1998;15:217–226.
13. Nuwer MR. Spinal cord monitoring with somatosensory techniques. *J Clin Neurophysiol* 1998;15:183–193.
14. Toleikis JR, Sloan TB. Comparison of major nerve and dermatomal somatosensory evoked potentials in the evaluation of patients with spinal cord injury. In: Barber C, Blum T, eds. *Evoked potentials III.* Boston: Butterworth, 1987:309–316.
15. Calancie B, Madsen P, Lebwohl N. Stimulus-evoked monitoring during transpedicular lumbosacral spine instrumentation. *Spine* 1994; 19:2780–2786.
16. Owen JH, Bridwell KH, Lenke LG. Innervation pattern of dorsal roots and their effects on the specificity of dermatomal somatosensory evoked potentials. *Spine* 1993;18:748–754.
17. Isley MR, Pearlman RC, Wadsworth JS. Recent advances in intraoperative neuromonitoring of spinal cord function: pedicle screw stimulation techniques. *Am J END Technol* 1997;37:93–126.
18. Maguire J, Wallace S, Madiga R, et al. Evaluation of intrapedicular screw position using intraoperative evoked electromyography. *Spine* 1995;20:1068–1074.
19. Burke D, Hicks RG. Surgical monitoring of motor pathways. *J Clin Neurophysiol* 1998;15:194–205.
20. Russell GB. Motor evoked potentials. In: Russell GB, Rodichok LD. *Primer of intraoperative neurophysiologic monitoring.* Boston: Butterworth-Heinemann, 1995:159–169.

139. Image-Guided Spinal Surgery

Dean G. Karahalios and Sean A. Salehi

Frameless stereotactic image-guided techniques in neurosurgery initially were pioneered for use in cranial procedures. They were based on fundamental stereotactic principles used in neurosurgery for many years. With the advent of high-speed computer processing capabilities, the ability to rapidly compare stereotactic data with preoperative imaging data led to the evolution of a practical instrument that provided the surgeon with simultaneous multiplanar images depicting the precise location of a target intraoperatively. This instrument has become an indispensable component within our surgical armamentarium; its utility in cranial procedures has been well established for some time (1,2). However, its efficacy in spinal procedures has been realized only recently (3–34). As in cranial procedures, frameless stereotactic guidance can be used in spinal surgery for the precise localization of anatomical structures and pathological lesions. In addition, instrumentation can be implanted with greater precision and safety than without the assistance of image guidance.

Spinal image guidance differs from its use in cranial surgery in several important ways. First, the spine is not fixed during surgery. It is somewhat mobile within the body and must be tracked by attaching a reference frame directly onto it. Second, instead of registering fiducial markers on the body surface, the spine is registered by an anatomical point-to-point comparison and/or surface fit algorithm. Third, each level in the spine represents a separate and distinct anatomical structure that ideally should be individually registered and tracked during surgery. These differences make image guidance in the spine a bit more challenging than in cranial surgery. With experience, however, the process can be performed with reasonable efficiency. Certainly, the increased precision, safety, and confidence afforded by the technique far outweigh the additional time and inconvenience.

Conventional intraoperative localization in spinal surgery is accomplished by marking structures with radiopaque instruments and then using plain radiography or fluoroscopy. There are advantages to this type of localization. Chiefly, the information is gathered in real time, which means that the image displayed represents the concurrent status of the patient's anatomy. Real-time feedback is especially important if the relevant information relates to a change that one expects to occur intraoperatively. Examples of this include gauging the extent of decompression, the advancement of an implant, or the reduction of a fracture or subluxation. Although some of this information can be inferred with image guidance, the true status of the patient's anatomy intraoperatively can only represented by real-time imaging. This is limited to plain radiography or fluoroscopy in most centers. The paramount disadvantage of these modalities is that the information conveyed to the surgeon is limited to sagittal, coronal, or oblique planes.

Image guidance adds axial, three-dimensional (3D), and trajectory views, which markedly enhance the surgeon's ability to conceptually appreciate and navigate through the anatomy. The information conveyed, however, is not in real time. The images are based on preoperative radiographic studies and therefore do not necessarily reflect the concurrent state of the patient's anatomy. In most cases, the lack of real-time feedback is of little consequence. The degree of decompression or position of instrumentation, can be inferred safely if the patient's anatomy is accurately registered to the preoperative imaging data set. Another major advantage image guidance technology offers is the ability to significantly reduce or eliminate radiation exposure to the patient and operating room staff. This is especially important to the spine surgeon, who is otherwise exposed to much higher levels of radiation than other specialists using conventional intraoperative imaging (35).

A new hybrid technology has been developed recently that incorporates the advantages of both real-time modalities and frameless stereotactic guidance. Fluoroscopic navigation allows the surgeon to use guidance data (position of instruments or implants) superimposed simultaneously onto multiplanar fluoroscopic images obtained intraoperatively (25,33,34,36,37). This allows for real-time updating during a procedure. It also eliminates the need for a preoperative scan. The amount of radiation used is markedly reduced because "snapshots" are used for guidance, obviating the need for continuous fluoroscopy. Finally, there is no need to register the patient's anatomy to a preoperative imaging data set because you are navigating from an image obtained with the patient fixed in the operating position. This is a major advantage in cases where the patient's anatomy may be distorted (secondary to pathology or previous surgery), or where access to the patient's anatomy for registration purposes is limited (as in ventral approaches where the anatomy is nondescript and coplanar, or in minimally invasive percutaneous/endoscopic approaches). As with conventional fluoroscopy, a relative disadvantage is the inability to obtain an axial or trajectory view of the anatomy.

Intraoperative computed tomography (CT) and/or magnetic resonance imaging (MRI) offers an alternative to frameless stereotactic image guidance. Advantages include the ability to obtain real-time images with enhanced bone and soft-tissue detail in any plane of view required. However, the additional time required to obtain and subsequently update the images makes this technology impractical for most spinal applications. Furthermore, the high cost and marginal usefulness of these systems limits their implementation outside academic and research institutions.

The most common use for frameless stereotactic guidance in the spine is to place pedicle screws (5–9,12–15,17,20,23,24, 28,29,31,32,38). Another procedure for which it is particularly useful is the placement of posterior transarticular screws to fixate the atlas and axis (3,9,13,15,31). The technique also facilitates the resection of spinal neoplasms in cases where the bone–tumor interfaces are indistinct (4,13,31). In short, almost any spinal procedure performed from a dorsal approach can be performed with the advantage of image guidance.

Ventral approaches to the spine do not yet lend themselves well to conventional image guidance technology because of the difficulties in registration. The anterior spine lacks clear landmarks, precluding an accurate anatomical point-to-point registration. It is also relatively flat or coplanar as compared to the posterior elements. The anterior spine cannot be adequately registered using the surface fit algorithm without a 3D structure. Nonetheless, the successful use of this technology for ventral approaches to the spine has been described (13,15,16,18,19). A noteworthy exception to this is the transoral odontoidectomy, because a cranial algorithm may be used for registration purposes (30,31,39). Fluoroscopic navigation is also a useful solution for anterior/ventral approaches, because a registration process is not required (25,33,34,36,37).

Equipment and Methods

HARDWARE AND SOFTWARE. A number of image-guided and frameless stereotactic systems are available commercially. The most commonly used systems all share certain basic elements (Fig. 1). The first element is a method for transferring data from the CT or MR scanner to the computer workstation. These data can be transferred via a digital storage medium (e.g., tape, disk) or directly through a local area network (LAN) or ethernet. The transfer requires appropriate interfaces between the radiographic equipment and transferring modality.

Once downloaded into the workstation's computer (Fig. 1A), the data sets are manipulated using the system's software. The software program displays the imaging data sets both in a conventional manner (axial views, sagittal, and coronal reconstructions), and also provides a 3D model and trajectory views, which are particularly useful for preoperative planning and intraoperative navigation. The ability to identify a single anatomical point simultaneously displayed in any combination of views defines the powerful utility of this technology.

Currently, most of the systems used in spinal surgery are based on infrared tracking technology, which has three important elements. First, the infrared camera serves as the computer's eye, localizing the position of instruments, which are fitted with light emitting diodes (LEDs) (Fig. 1B). Second, a reference frame is attached to the spine so that the computer knows where the spine is in 3D space at any given time (Fig. 1C). Finally, a number of tools (e.g., pointers, awls, drill guides) are also fitted with infrared LEDs, which are tracked by the computer, comparing their position to that of the reference frame (Fig. 1D–F).

Virtually any instrument commonly used in spinal surgery

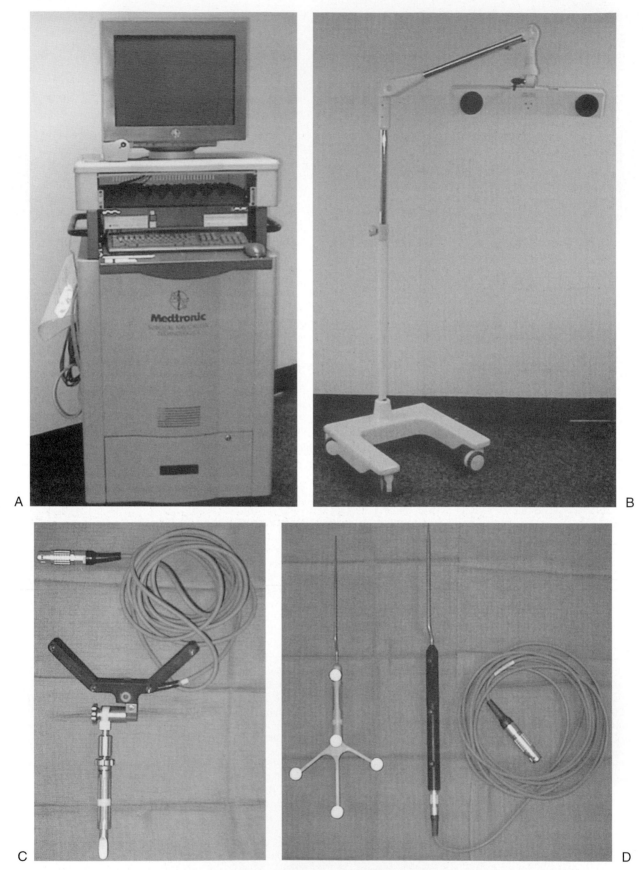

Fig. 1. Medtronic Sofamor Danek Stealth System (Minneapolis, MN) for frameless stereotactic image-guided surgery. **A:** Workstation with CPU, monitor, drives, and instrument interfaces. **B:** Infrared camera. **C:** Dynamic reference arc attaches to the spine. **D:** Passive *(left)* and active *(right)* pointing tools.

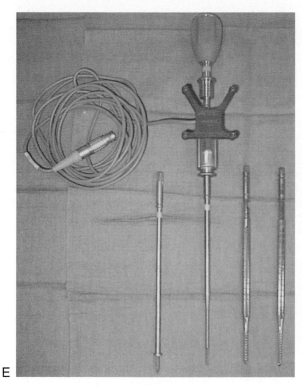

E

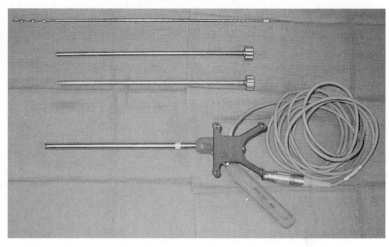

F

Fig. 1. (continued). **E:** Interchangeable image-guided tools (e.g., awls, taps). **F:** Image-guided universal drill-guide.

can be tracked, and its precise location on the patient's anatomy can be correlated with the multiplanar and 3D reconstructed views displayed on the workstation. Some systems incorporate the microscope as a pointing tool. The microscope fitted with advanced optical equipment is used to sight the target. The distance from the microscope to the target is precisely measured either based on the focal distance or by a convergent laser targeting system. The microscope itself is fitted with infrared LEDs that are tracked by the camera. In some microscope-integrated systems, a "heads-up" feature displays the image guidance information into one of the oculars that eliminates the need to look away from the microscope to view the workstation monitor. Image-injection technology, which is available with some systems, superimposes an outline of the target contours onto the surgical filed as viewed though the microscope (Medtronics, Memphis, TN; Carl Zeiss, Germany). The utility of this technology in spine surgery has not been clearly established because the microscope is not used in many spinal procedures.

The LED/infrared-based systems as described above are considered *active*. The instruments used are attached to wires connected to the workstation. They actively emit infrared signals from LED arrays, which are detected by the camera, which is also connected to the workstation. A second *passive* infrared-based system also is available. This system uses wireless instruments with reflective spheres on their distal ends (Fig. 1D). The camera emits an infrared signal that reflects off the spheres on the instruments. The camera then detects the reflected light.

IMAGING. Imaging for frameless stereotaxis begins by acquiring a digital radiographic study, usually either a CT scan or MRI. Typically, CT is best for spinal surgery because the detail of the bony elements is best defined with this modality. MR imaging is especially useful for neoplasms. Systems that permit the simultaneous superimposed display or fusion of CT and MR imaging studies provide the highest level of detail of both soft tissue and bone (40).

Thin cuts through the appropriate levels are obtained. No contrast media are needed unless an enhancing mass lesion must be localized. Unlike cranial stereotactic guidance, where fiducial markers are placed on the head before scanning, no external markers are typically placed on the spine. There are exceptions to the rule, however. In staged spinal procedures, radiopaque markers can be implanted during the first procedure, facilitating rapid and very precise registration during the second surgery (22). For transoral odontoidectomy, a cranial protocol is performed for registration. Thus, cranial fiducial markers are placed, and the entire head is scanned along with the atlas and axis (30,31).

PREOPERATIVE PLANNING. A patient may be scanned several days before an operative procedure because surface fiducials are not typically used in image-guided spinal surgery. This provides ample time for a surgeon to carefully review the imaging data and create a preoperative plan.

Once the patient has been scanned, the data are transferred to the workstation, and the software is used to reconstruct the images. As discussed, the images can be displayed in two-dimensional (2D) multiplanar and/or 3D views. The 3D view can be rotated. The planes of the simultaneous 2D views can be selected, and areas of interest can be highlighted to improve understanding of a particular anatomical structure or pathological lesion. The sizes of the images also can be manipulated. Other functions provided by some systems include drop-down menus with tools that enable precise measurements of structures.

Lending even more power and functionality to these systems is the capability to superimpose precisely scaled cursors with the same relative dimensions as instruments that will be used in surgery, or instrumentation that will be implanted. For example, if planning to place a pedicle screw, the surgeon can choose a virtual screw cursor and attempt to place it within the pedicle on the reconstructed image. The entry point, trajectory, or the dimensions of the screw can be manipulated to obtain an appropriate fit. This preoperative plan can be stored and used intraoperatively. The surgeon has the option of following the plan as established before surgery, or may revise it to accommodate a different appreciation of the anatomy or change in the anatomy intraoperatively. Some systems integrate all of the imaging data into a targeting view, or target and cross hairs, so that the surgeon need not cognitively process or integrate all of the critical views during the actual placement of the instrumentation.

OPERATING ROOM SET-UP AND PATIENT POSITIONING. The patient is positioned on the operating room table as for a conventional spinal procedure. The workstation monitor is placed in a location that will enable the surgeon to view it without having to turn his head away from the operative field. This positioning is less critical if a microscope with a heads-up image guided display is used. Some systems also have a lightweight flat color liquid crystal display (LCD) that can be mounted on a boom over the operative field. These displays also have touch-sensitive screens that the surgeon can activate during the procedure if they are covered by a clear sterile drape.

The positioning of the infrared camera is critical. It must be placed in the line of sight of the instruments to be tracked so that straight path of light traveling between the two is not blocked. The best location usually is near the foot or head of the table. The camera can be moved if the line of sight is obstructed during the procedure. During the positioning and preparation of the patient, obscuring the line of sight between the camera the operative field should be avoided.

REGISTRATION. Registration involves matching the patient's anatomy to the imaging data set stored in the computer. The first step is to place a reference frame onto the spine. If the spine moves during the procedure, then the computer knows and adjusts for the movement accordingly, keeping the patient's anatomy aligned or correlated with the imaging data set. Be-

cause the spine is comprised of multiple mobile segments, the reference frame optimally should be placed at the same level that is to be registered and operated on. If multiple levels are to be operated on, then the reference frame should be moved to each of the levels. This process is very time consuming and cumbersome. It is also impractical, because the reference frame is often placed on the spinous process, which is removed during most spinal operations. This may require a change in the way a particular procedure is performed. Typically, the decompression portion of a procedure is performed prior to the implantation of instrumentation. For image-guided spinal procedures, the portion of the procedure requiring stereotaxis, usually the implantation of hardware, can be performed first. In this way, the anatomical structures required for registration and anchoring the reference frame are still present. The problem also can be circumvented by placing the reference frame at a level above or below the level to be registered and operated on.

By definition, there is motion between adjacent spinal segments. Thus, movement of the registered segment may not be reflected accurately at the adjacent level where the reference frame is located. Theoretically, this error could be exacerbated by pathological instability between segments and by working several segments away from the reference frame. For example, this error could affect cases where a reference frame is placed at L1 and pedicle screws are placed at L2-4. The error should increase progressively, reaching its maximum at L4.

Practically, however, we have noted no significant loss of accuracy using this paradigm. A certain elastic memory exists, even though the spine is mobile. Consequently, if the spine is temporarily deflected or deformed, it will return to its previous position once the applied force is removed. We tested this theory by registering segments distal to the reference frame, performing a decompression, and then re-registering, and have found no significant differences in position (Karahalios and co-workers, unpublished data, 1996). Nonetheless, excessive force on the spine should be avoided while using image guidance for localization to avoid deflecting the spine beyond its elastic tolerance. Image guidance should be performed with the spine in its relaxed or nondeformed state.

The next step in the registration process is to register the individual spinal segments. First, a point-to-point registration is performed (Fig. 2A). This process involves finding a point

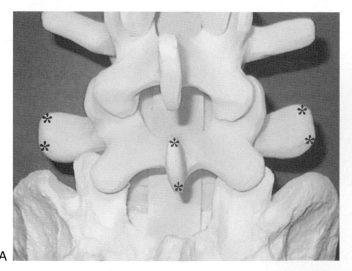

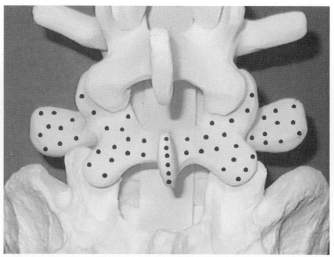

A   B

Fig. 2. Registration. **A:** Anatomic point-to-point. A number of well-defined points can be identified and registered for lumbar procedures, including the superior and inferior aspects of the transverse and spinous processes *(asterisk).* **B:** Surface fit algorithm. A number of points are chosen randomly along the surface of the segment to be registered to create a three-dimensional contour map *(black dots).*

on the patient's anatomy and matching it to the same point on the workstation's display. The target may be viewed in multiple planes and 3D to insure that the proper point is chosen. Registration points chosen preoperatively can be moved on the display to better reflect the anatomy seen intraoperatively. If a particularly prominent anatomical point is discovered intraoperatively, then one may search for this point on the display. In general, the more points that are chosen, the better is the accuracy. For a typical pedicle screw case, six points are chosen: the superior and inferior aspects of the distal transverse process bilaterally, and the superior and inferior aspects of the spinous process. Additional points (e.g., facet, pars interarticularis) can be added to increase accuracy or if an anatomical landmark is absent or distorted by disease or previous surgery. However, these points are less distinct and seldom chosen as the primary localizing points.

Next, a surface fit algorithm may be performed (Fig. 2B). This process involves touching multiple points over the surface of the dorsal spinal elements to create a 3D contour of the structure. Usually 40 points are chosen. Then, through a mathematical transformation, the computer matches the contour to its own imaging data set for that level.

Both registration techniques may be used together to decrease the error (8). Points that the computer determines are beyond their expected positions and that have high error values can be removed individually to increase the overall accuracy of the registration.

Holes can be placed in the bone that will remain after decompression. These holes can be included in the registration process so that once the midline bony elements are removed, the segment can be reregistered quickly if there is concern about accuracy or shift. These holes are small divots placed into the transverse process, pars interarticularis, or facets. Also, as mentioned, small metallic markers can be implanted for staged procedures. The patient is scanned again between the two procedures. Once reopened, the patient can be quickly and accurately reregistered using the implanted fiducials (22).

It is important to register each level independently before any bone is removed. Great care should be taken so that the same level for the patient and the IGS display are registered, because they can be confused easily. Labeling the levels during the reconstruction process can alleviate any potential confusion.

As mentioned, the registration process can be difficult or impossible if the patient's anatomy is distorted (by pathology or prior surgery), if one is operating anteriorly/ventrally were the anatomy is relatively coplanar and nondescript, or if one is attempting to operate in a minimally invasive fashion (percutaneously or endoscopically).

TRACKING. The operative procedure can proceed as usual once the appropriate levels have been registered. The camera tracks the movement of the reference frame and instruments. An unobscured line of sight should be established and maintained between the camera and operative field. Instruments fitted with LED emitters or reflective spheres such as pointing probes or the microscope then can be used to localize lesions and their margins.

For the placement of instrumentation, tools similar to their conventional counterparts have been similarly modified for tracking. For pedicle screw placement, either a spatula-tipped or pointed awl can be used for sounding the pedicle (Fig. 1E). Guides are available for drilling through the pedicle (Fig. 1F). The drill guides are also useful in other areas such as for placement of transarticular screws at C1-2, or lateral mass screws at other cervical levels. These guided tools not only serve as pointers to find the correct entry point, but also demonstrate the best angle or trajectory through the bony structure.

LED emitters also can be mounted on the drill, tap, and screwdriver (with screw) so that the tip of the instrument can be tracked as it passes through the bone. Alternatively, the depth of the target can be determined based on measurements made from the workstation images once the entry point and trajectory are chosen. The depth of the instrument to be advanced can be determined visually (manually) based on graduated marks or physical measurements made on the instruments.

FLUOROSCOPIC NAVIGATION. The equipment needed for fluoroscopic navigation varies slightly from that used in conventional image-guided spinal surgery (Fig. 3). The principal difference is the addition of an image acquisition device, in this case a fluoroscope, which obviates the need for preoperative imaging. It is mounted with a detector, which captures and digitizes

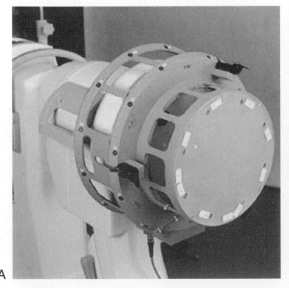

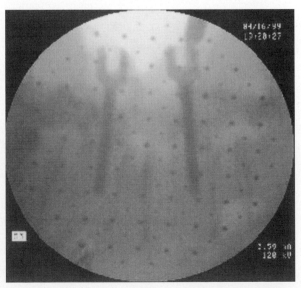

A   B

Fig. 3. Medtronic Sofamor Danek Fluoronav system for fluoroscopic image-guided navigation. **A:** Fluoroscope mounted with detector. **B:** Digitized lateral fluoroscopic image. (Courtesy of Medtronic Sofamor Danek, Minneapolis, MN.)

the images. The images are transferred to the workstation where they can be stored and manipulated. Several images in multiple planes can be stored and viewed simultaneously, simulating biplanar or multiplanar fluoroscopy (25,33,34,36,37).

A reference frame is fixed to the patient's anatomy. An infrared camera then tracks the movement of the patient's anatomy, and the position of instruments in relation to the anatomy as in conventional frameless stereotaxis. The position of a particular instrument is displayed on the selected stored images. Planning tools also are available to measure structures and plan trajectories. There is no need for a registration process because the images are obtained during surgery or in real time. Registration is automatic or instantaneous in a sense; hence, this technology is particularly well suited for anterolateral or ventral procedures where the coplanar and nondescript anatomy of the spine make conventional registration more difficult and less accurate (13,16,19,25,33,34,36,37). Because exposure of the spine is not necessary for registration, this technology is particularly useful for facilitating transcutaneous or minimally invasive procedures (25).

The fluoroscope can be moved out of the field once the images have been captured. If no further images are to be obtained, the surgeon and operating room staff have the advantage of removing their protective lead garments because there will be no further radiation exposure. Alternatively, additional images can be obtained to intermittently update the status or progress of a surgical procedure. This ability to obtain real-time information distinguishes this technology from conventional frameless stereotaxis. In select centers, intraoperative CT and/or MRI provide similar advantages, although the image acquisition process is much more laborious and time consuming, which limits its efficacy for most spinal procedures.

Clinical Applications

PEDICLE SCREWS. The placement of pedicle screws in the lumbar region is a relatively straightforward process. Most spine surgeons are comfortable with placing screws in the lumbar region with relatively few radiographic cues. Nonetheless, it has been demonstrated that the breakout rate can be surprisingly high (41–43), and image guidance can significantly decrease this rate (32). Using conventional frameless stereotaxis, one has the benefit of axial and trajectory views, which may be advantageous in situations where the anatomy may be distorted (6–9,12,13,17,23,28,31,32,38). Alternatively, fluoroscopic navigation can be used, which limits radiation exposure. Sagittal and coronal views are provided, which in most cases provide enough information to safely place pedicle screws (25,33,34, 36,37).

The use of conventional CT-based frameless stereotaxis becomes more important in the thoracic and cervical regions, where pedicles are smaller and vary significantly in shape, orientation, and angle (14,15,20). These are areas where the information gleaned from axial and trajectory views is critical for the safe placement of screws. These are also areas that are difficult to image well with the fluoroscope.

For example, a patient with a fracture-dislocation underwent thoracic pedicle screw fixation using conventional image guidance (Fig. 4). As discussed, the appropriate points were used for registration. Two 2D views were used during the sounding of the pedicle with an awl. The most informative views for this procedure were the axial view, which aligns the trajectory mediolaterally, and the sagittal view, which aligns the trajectory

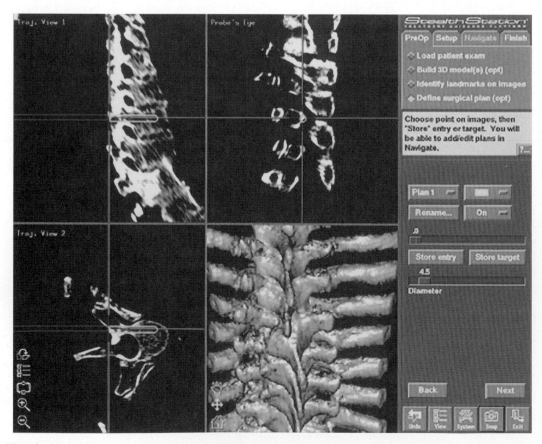

Fig. 4. Thoracic pedicle screw fixation. The axial and sagittal views on the Stealth display were instrumental in safely navigating through the narrow T2 pedicle.

cephalocaudally. The depth of the instrument tip was tracked as it was driven into the pedicle.

POSTERIOR TRANSARTICULAR ATLANTOAXIAL SCREW FIXATION. Posterior transarticular screw fixation for atlantoaxial fusion places a number of anatomical structures at risk (i.e., vertebral artery, spinal cord, and C2 nerve root). The procedure requires the placement of the screw through the pars interarticularis, which is quite narrow in many cases. The structure at highest risk for injury is the vertebral artery, which can take an extremely variable path through the axis. In some cases, the vertebral artery runs too high and medial, precluding the safe passage of transarticular screws. Algorithms based on preoperative CT analysis of C2 can be used to identify patients with anatomy that is not conducive for the placement of screws

(i.e., narrow pars, aberrant course of vertebral artery) (44). Using these algorithms, up to 18% of pars may be unsuitable for screw placement. The yield can be increased by 75% with the use of conventional image-guidance techniques (Karahalios and co-workers, unpublished data, 1998).

Conventional image-guided techniques using preoperative CT scanning are particularly well suited for this procedure (3, 9,13,15,31). Preoperative planning is essential to determine if the pars interarticularis is of a large enough diameter to accommodate a transarticular screw safely. In addition, one can determine if a safe trajectory can be established through the axis. This plan can be stored and then used in surgery.

The posterior elements are exposed once in surgery. The reference frame is attached to the spinous process of C2. The posterior elements are registered using a point-to-point (Fig. 5A) and surface fit algorithm. An important concept to understand is that the error is lowest within the volume that is regis-

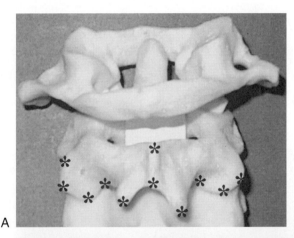

A

Fig. 5. Atlantoaxial transarticular screw fixation. **A:** Points chosen for anatomical point-to-point registration *(asterisks)*. **B:** Trajectory and "probe's eye" views are used to safely navigate through the pars interarticularis.

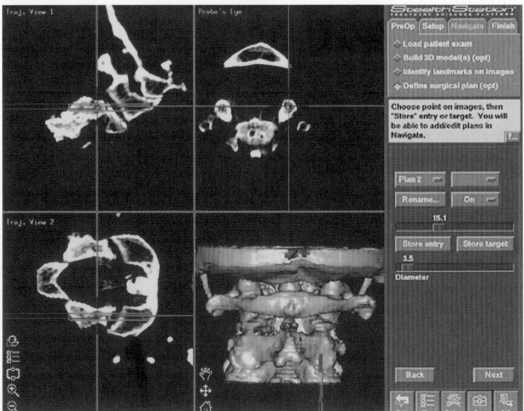

B

tered. Error increases as you advance an instrument deeper into the patient's anatomy and outside the radius that is registered. A maximum error of 1 to 2 mm should be attained prior to proceeding.

The planned entry point is localized based on the preoperative plan. An image-guided drill guide is then positioned over the entry point. The hole may then be drilled, or a K-wire may be advanced if using a cannulated screw system. The trajectory views are particularly useful for navigating the pars. These consist of modified sagittal and axial views, as well as a "probe's eye view" down the axis of the planned trajectory (Fig. 5B). Some surgeons prefer a targeting view, or target and cross hairs, which integrates all of the views into one dynamic schematic representation.

It is important to note that one is not tracking C1 during this process. The position of C1 on C2 should be confirmed intraoperatively using fluoroscopy or plain radiography to ensure that they are in proper alignment or reduced. All navigation that takes place is through C2 only. The path through C1 can be inferred if the atlas and axis are appropriately aligned. It is not typically important to track through C1 as well, because the critical portion of the procedure, or that associated with the highest risk, occurs when passing through C2. Technology is being developed that will allow simultaneous tracking of multiple independently mobile segments; however, this is not in wide clinical use at this time.

As an example of this technique, a patient is presented with a failed odontoid screw fixation for a type II fracture. A nonunion resulted in persistent atlantoaxial instability. The patient then underwent posterior transarticular screw fixation using image-guided techniques (Fig. 5B). The anatomical points used for the point-to-point registration were identified. A surface fit registration also was performed. Preoperative planning confirmed that a 4.0-mm screw could be placed safely, avoiding the vertebral artery and spinal canal. The drill guide was tracked, and multiplanar trajectory views were used for drilling along the planned screw trajectory. An excellent result was achieved.

SPINAL DECOMPRESSION. Image-guided techniques can be used to facilitate spinal decompression for degenerative and neoplastic processes (3,4,10,13,15,16,18,19,30,31). Posteriorly, one can use either conventional image-guided techniques or fluoroscopic navigation to gauge the extent of decompression. Using CT guidance, one can precisely outline the margins of a tumor to be resected preoperatively, then follow these highlighted margins intraoperatively to confidently achieve a gross total resection. For anterolateral or ventral approaches, one can also use conventional image-guided techniques, but again, registration can be difficult given the relatively coplanar and nondescript anatomy. Nonetheless, the successful use of these techniques anteriorly has been described (13,15,16,18,19). Fluoroscopic navigation is particularly well-suited for anterior techniques because registration is not required (25,33,34,36,37). One is limited by the absence of axial or trajectory views; however, typically these views are not needed for decompression. Image guidance for decompression anteriorly not only provides critical feedback when approaching the spinal canal, but also helps to gauge the mediolateral extent of decompression. This is especially important in the cervical region where an eccentric decompression may jeopardize the vertebral arteries.

TRANSORAL ODONTOIDECTOMY. Transoral decompressions typically are performed under lateral fluoroscopic guidance. This provides information regarding the cephalocaudal extent of the exposure and the depth of the decompression. Biplanar fluoroscopy adds an AP view, which allows one to gauge the mediolateral orientation, but is excessively obtrusive to the surgeon. One could use fluoroscopic navigation, which is less obtrusive, circumvents the problem with ventral registration, and limits radiation exposure. Alternatively, one could immobilize the patient in an external orthosis or halo (as would be needed in most cases in which an odontoidectomy is to be performed), which effectively eliminates significant motion between the cranium and C2, then scan the patient's head and upper cervical spine using a cranial protocol (3,30,31,39). In preparing for surgery, the halo is secured to the operating table using the Mayfield adapter. The reference frame is attached to the halo or adapter. The patient's head then is registered using surface landmarks and fiducials, which effectively registers the atlas and axis. Navigation then proceeds as in the other applications, using probes to gauge cephalocaudal and mediolateral orientation as well as depth. Because CT or MR are used, one is able to identify the location of the spinal cord/brainstem, which becomes especially important when these structures are displaced by pannus or tumor, which are also readily discernible.

As an example, a case is presented of an elderly woman with a chronic odontoid fracture and associated pannus deforming the cervicomedullary junction. She was placed in a halo brace and subsequently underwent an image-guided transoral odontoidectomy followed by posterior occipitocervical fixation (Fig. 6). Preoperatively, fiducial markers were placed on the scalp and the patient was scanned using a cranial protocol. The patient was positioned supine with the head fixated in a Mayfield head holder. The head was then registered using the fiducial markers and anatomical structures for a point-to-point registration. A surface fit registration was performed. Intraoperatively, multiplanar views provided more localizing information than would be available using a conventional single lateral fluoroscopic view.

Future Trends

Frameless stereotactic image-guidance technology is rapidly evolving. It will likely continue to change in a number of areas. Improvements in workstation hardware and software will increase the speed and functionality of these systems. Preoperative planning will become more sophisticated, allowing one to perform "virtual" surgery prior to the actual procedure. This ability to rehearse will allow both residents in training and attending surgeons to learn new techniques faster, and will make the actual procedures safer.

The ability to coregister fluoroscopic images obtained intraoperatively with 3D imaging data sets (CT or MRI) obtained preoperatively promises to provide a rapid and noninvasive means of registering multiple spinal levels without exposing the spine (25,36,37). This will allow us to use CT and/or MRI data more precisely and effectively for anterior approaches. Because the spine can be registered without exposure, it will also facilitate minimally invasive percutaneous techniques and make them safer (25,27).

Infrared-based tracking systems are now the industry standard. However, line of sight interference remains a significant source of frustration during image-guided procedures. Other tracking technologies, including magnetic field-based systems, are being developed to eliminate these problems.

Magnetic field-based systems work by creating a magnetic field around the spine. Instruments with small receiving antennae at their tips are tracked by sensing their relative positions in the field. Because this modality does not require line of sight, tracking and localization can occur transcutaneously. The sen-

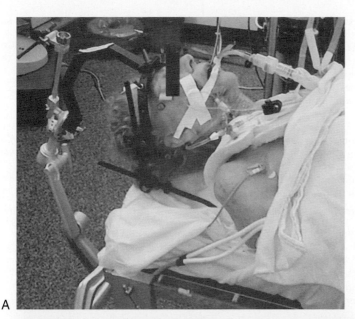

Fig. 6. Transoral odontoidectomy. **A:** The patient is positioned supine on the operating room table. An adaptor is used to secure the halo ring to the table. The anterior posts of the halo are removed to facilitate access for surgery. The reference frame for image guidance is connected to the Mayfield apparatus. **B:** Multiplanar views are used for localization, and to gauge the extent of decompression.

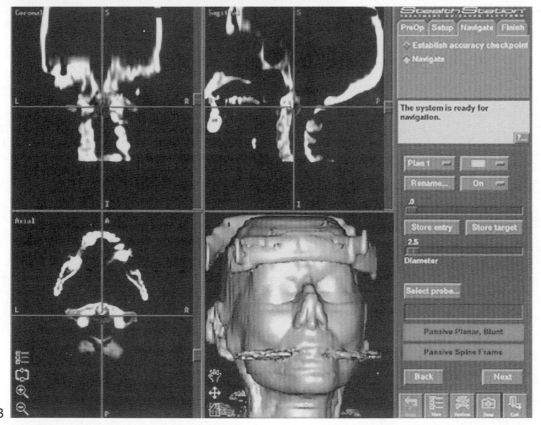

sors are quite small and unobtrusive (about the size of a pencil tip) compared to the LED arrays currently used in the infrared-based systems. They can be implanted percutaneously easily and used to track multiple vertebral motion segments simultaneously. Furthermore, because tracking occurs at the tip of the instrument rather than at the distal end, as in the infrared/LED-based systems, one can use flexible instruments such as endoscopes for guidance and localization. Presently there are some disadvantages to these systems, such as interference with adjacent metal instruments or implants. Once these current limi-

tations are resolved, this technology may become the new tracking standard.

Viewing the monitor is still a major source of frustration during surgery because the eyes must deviate from the surgical field to view the image guidance data. The use of the microscope has alleviated this problem by projecting the images through the oculars. Some systems go one step further and provide "image injection" or the superimposition of images over the exposed anatomy. This technique is optimal for avoiding eye deviation. Similar technology can be applied without microscopy. Images could be projected directly onto the patient's anatomy (45), or onto a live video image of the anatomy (46). Alternatively, using technology similar to that used by fighter pilots for weapons targeting applications, semitransparent images could be projected onto a visor worn by the surgeon. The visor and the surgeon's head would be tracked like any other image-guided tool. Two-dimensional and/or 3D images highlighting important anatomical structures or entry or target points for instrumentation would be superimposed onto the patient's anatomy as viewed through the visor. This would eliminate any need to deviate the head or eyes from the surgical field.

Finally, surgical robotic devices are being developed to allow a surgeon to perform intricate procedures more quickly and precisely (11,25). These devices, operated remotely from a workstation, dampen normal excessive physiological movements or tremor. The integration and application of noninvasive transcutaneous registration and tracking technologies, in conjunction with minimally invasive surgical techniques and automated robotic instrument carrier technology, will likely lead to faster operating times, enhanced precision, and decreased morbidity. In the future, surgeons may practice a virtual procedure on a computer workstation. Once the planning has been perfected, they can then perform the actual procedure on the patient remotely, without ever leaving the workstation.

Conclusion

Image-guided frameless stereotactic techniques have been successfully applied to spinal surgery. Advantages of this technology include enhanced localizing capability with respect to anatomical structures and pathology, added precision and safety for the implantation of instrumentation, and less radiation exposure for the patient and operating room staff. Future advances will likely further expand the utility of image guidance, allowing many or all spinal procedures to be performed in a minimally invasive fashion.

References

1. Golfinos JG, Fitzpatrick BC, Smith LR, et al. Clinical use of a frameless stereotactic arm: results of 325 cases. *J Neurosurg* 1995; 83:197–205.
2. Lawton MT, Golfinos JG, Geldmacher T, et al. A comparative clinical evaluation of current frameless stereotactic systems: accuracy, performance, and surgeon preference. *Perspect Neurosurg* 1998;9: 47–62.
3. Welch WC, Subach BR, Pollack IF, et al. Frameless stereotactic guidance for surgery of the upper cervical spine. *Neurosurgery* 1997;40: 958–964.
4. Patel N, Sandeman DR, Cobby M, et al. Interactive image-guided surgery of the spine—use of the ISG/Elekta viewing wand to aid intraoperative localization of a sacral osteoblastoma. *Br J Neurosurg* 1997;11:60–64.
5. Nolte LP, Zamorano LJ, Jiang Z, et al. Image-guided insertion of transpedicular screws. A laboratory set-up. *Spine* 1995;20:497–500.
6. Nolte L, Zamorano L, Arm E, et al. Image-guided computer-assisted spine surgery: a pilot study on pedicle screw fixation. *Stereotact Funct Neurosurg* 1996;66:108–117.
7. Kalfas IH, Kormos DW, Murphy MA, et al. Application of frameless stereotaxy to pedicle screw fixation of the spine. *J Neurosurg* 1995; 83:641–647.
8. Glossop ND, Hu RW, Randle JA. Computer-aided pedicle screw placement using frameless stereotaxis. *Spine* 1996;21:2026–2034.
9. Foley KT, Smith MM. Image-guided spine surgery. *Neurosurg Clin North Am* 1996;7:171–186.
10. Brodwater BK, Roberts DW, Nakajima T, et al. Extracranial application of the frameless stereotactic operating microscope: experience with lumbar spine. *Neurosurgery* 1993;32:209–213.
11. Abdel-Malek K, McGowan DP, Goel VK, et al. Bone registration method for robot assisted surgery: pedicle screw insertion. *Proc Inst Mech Eng (H)* 1997;211:221–233.
12. Lavallee S, Sautot P, Troccaz J, et al. Computer-assisted spine surgery: a technique for accurate transpedicular screw fixation using CT data and a 3D optical localizer. *J Image Guide Surg* 1995;1:65–73.
13. Kalfas IH. Image-guided spinal navigation. *Clin Neurosurg* 2000;46: 70–88.
14. Kamimura M, Ebara S, Itoh H, et al. Cervical pedicle screw insertion: assessment of safety and accuracy with computer-assisted image guidance. *J Spinal Disord* 2000;13:218–224.
15. Bolger C, Wigfield C. Image-guided surgery: applications to the cervical and thoracic spine and a review of the first 120 procedures. *J Neurosurg* 2000;92(suppl 2):175–180.
16. Bolger C, Wigfield C, Melkent T, et al. Frameless stereotaxy and anterior cervical surgery. *Comput Aided Surg* 1999;4:322–327.
17. Girardi FP, Cammisa FP Jr, Sandhu HS, et al. The placement of lumbar pedicle screws using computerised stereotactic guidance. *J Bone Joint Surg Br* 1999;81:825–829.
18. Klein GR, Ludwig SC, Vaccaro AR, et al. The efficacy of using an image-guided Kerrison punch in performing an anterior cervical foraminotomy. An anatomic analysis. *Spine* 1999;24:1358–1362.
19. Albert TJ, Klein GR, Vaccaro AR. Image-guided anterior cervical corpectomy. A feasibility study. *Spine* 1999;24:826–830.
20. Ludwig SC, Kramer DL, Vaccaro AR, et al. Transpedicle screw fixation of the cervical spine. *Clin Orthop* 1999;(359):77–88.
21. Kim KD, Johnson JP, Masciopinto JE, et al. Universal calibration of surgical instruments for spinal stereotaxy. *Neurosurgery* 1999;44: 173–177.
22. Salehi SA, Ondra SL. Use of internal fiducial markers in frameless stereotactic navigational systems during spinal surgery: technical note. *Neurosurgery* 2000;47:1460–1462.
23. Carl AL, Khanuja HS, Gatto CA, et al. In vivo pedicle screw placement: image-guided virtual vision. *J Spinal Disord* 2000;13:225–229.
24. Cammisa FP Jr, Parvataneni HK, Girardi FP, et al. Computerized frameless stereotactic image-guided spinal surgery. *Bull Hosp Joint Dis* 2000;59:17–26.
25. Cleary K, Anderson J, Brazaitis M, et al. Final report of the Technical Requirements for Image-Guided Spine Procedures Workshop, April 17–20, 1999, Ellicott City, MD. *Comput Aided Surg* 2000;5:180–215.
26. Barrick EF, O'Mara JW, Lane HE III. Iliosacral screw insertion using computer-assisted CT image guidance: a laboratory study. *Comput Aided Surg* 1998;3:289–296.
27. Tonetti J, Carrat L, Lavallee S, et al. Percutaneous iliosacral screw placement using image guided techniques. *Clin Orthop* 1998;Sep: 103–110.
28. Merloz P, Tonetti J, Pittet L, et al. Pedicle screw placement using image guided techniques. *Clin Orthop* 1998;Sep:39–48.
29. Carl AL, Khanuja HS, Sachs BL, et al. In vitro simulation. Early results of stereotaxy for pedicle screw placement. *Spine* 1997;22: 1160–1164.
30. Pollack IF, Welch W, Jacobs GB, et al. Frameless stereotactic guidance. An intraoperative adjunct in the transoral approach for ventral cervicomedullary junction decompression. *Spine* 1995;20:216–220.
31. Karahalios DG, Apostolides PJ, Geldmacher TR, et al. Image-guided spinal surgery. In: Sonntag VK, Spetzler RF, eds. *Operative techniques in neurosurgery*. Philadelphia: WB Saunders, 1998:104–112.
32. Steinmann JC, Herkowitz HN, el Kommos H, et al. Spinal pedicle fixation. Confirmation of an image-based technique for screw placement. *Spine* 1993;18:1856–1861.
33. Nolte LP, Slomczykowski MA, Berlemann U, et al. A new approach to computer-aided spine surgery: fluoroscopy-based surgical navigation. *Eur Spine J* 2000;9(suppl 1):S78–S88.
34. Hofstetter R, Slomczykowski M, Sati M, et al. Fluoroscopy as an imaging means for computer-assisted surgical navigation. *Comput Aided Surg* 1999;4:65–76.
35. Rampersaud YR, Foley KT, Shen AC, et al. Radiation exposure to the spine surgeon during fluoroscopically assisted pedicle screw insertion. *Spine* 2000;25:2637–2645.
36. Hamadeh A, Lavallee S, Cinquin P. Automated 3 dimensional com-

puted tomographic and fluoroscopic image registration. *Comput Aided Surg* 1998;3:11–19.

37. Weese J, Penney GP, Desmedt P, et al. Voxel-based 2D/3D registration of fluoroscopy images and CT scans for image-guided surgery. *IEEE Trans Inf Technol Biomed* 1997;1:284–293.

38. Schulze CJ, Munzinger E, Weber U. Clinical relevance of accuracy of pedicle screw placement. A computed tomographic-supported analysis. *Spine* 1998;23:2215–2220.

39. Welch WC, Subach BR, Pollack IF, et al. Frameless stereotactic guidance for surgery of the upper cervical spine (comments). *Neurosurgery* 1997;40:958–963.

40. Hemler PF, Sumanaweera TS, van den Elsen PA, et al. A versatile system for multimodality image fusion. *J Image Guide Surg* 1995; 1:35–45.

41. George DC, Krag MH, Johnson CC, et al. Hole preparation tech-

niques for transpedicle screws. Effect on pull-out strength from human cadaveric vertebrae. *Spine* 1991;16:181–184.

42. Gertzbein SD, Robbins SE. Accuracy of pedicular screw placement in vivo. *Spine* 1990;15:11–14.

43. Weinstein JN, Spratt KF, Spengler D, et al. Spinal pedicle fixation: reliability and validity of roentgenogram-based assessment and surgical factors on successful screw placement. *Spine* 1988;13: 1012–1018.

44. Paramore CG, Dickman CA, Sonntag VK. The anatomical suitability of the C1-2 complex for transarticular screw fixation. *J Neurosurg* 1996;85:221–224.

45. Gleason PL, Kikinis R, Altobelli D, et al. Video registration virtual reality for nonlinkage stereotactic surgery. *Stereotact Funct Neurosurg* 1994;63:139–143.

46. Gildenberg PL, Labuz J. Stereotactic craniotomy with the exoscope. *Stereotact Funct Neurosurg* 1997;68:64–71.

140. General Principles of Anesthesia in Spine Patients

**Patrick T. Healey and
William T. Monacci**

Preoperative Evaluation

HISTORY AND PHYSICAL EXAMINATION

Overall Medical Condition of the Patient. The preoperative evaluation of the patient begins with a history and physical examination. Age, gender, height and weight, drug allergies, medications, and previous surgical, anesthetic, and medical histories are documented (1). The patient is assessed for any chronic (2) or acute (3) conditions associated with spinal injury. A review of organ systems is performed to identify any significant organ disease that will impact on the anesthetic management (4). A physical examination complements this history. Particular emphasis is placed on assessing for signs of cardiopulmonary dysfunction, ease of vascular access, and evaluation of the patient's airway.

Directed History and Physical of the Cervical Spine. Although a standard component of the anesthesiologist's history and physical examination is in preparation to safely assume control of the patient's airway, patients for spine surgery as a group have three characteristics that warrant additional consideration of the airway realm.

First, some spine patient's have an airway that because of poor range of motion or some other anatomical abnormality, is predictably difficult or impossible to intubate by direct laryngoscopy (5). These patients' airways should be managed as recommended in the American Society of Anesthesiologists' (ASA) difficult airway algorithm (Fig. 1) (6).

Second, some spine patients by their primary disease process have a likelihood of having an asymptomatic unstable cervical spine. The cervical spine extension inherent in attempting intubation of these patients by direct laryngoscopy can cause neurological injury or death (7,8). These diseases include congenital disease such as Klippel-Feil syndrome (9), acquired disease such as rheumatoid arthritis (10), and traumatic injury (11–13).

Third, some spine patient's manifest signs and symptoms of compression of neural structures with motion of the cervical spine. This dynamic component to the patient's disease implies that care must be taken to preclude damage or compression to the neural structures during intubation, or more likely, positioning.

Dynamic cervical myelopathy, that is, signs and symptoms produced by spinal cord compression that worsen with cervical spine motion, must be distinguished from dynamic cervical radiculopathy. Cervical radiculopathy comprises the signs and symptoms of cervical nerve root compression. Even when this cervical radiculopathy is dynamic, the patient generally can be safely positioned after induction of anesthesia. However, the patient's cervical spine should be placed in a position that was without dynamic symptoms while awake.

In contrast, positioning the patient with dynamic cervical myelopathy should be done awake. A neurological examination performed several minutes after positioning the patient should demonstrate no change in baseline prior to general anesthesia being induced (14). As a practical matter, this implies that the patient is intubated awake as well, after appropriate topicalization (15) and/or airway blocks with local anesthetics (16). However, it is likely that the far greater risk to the myelopathic patient lies not with the brief position change necessary for direct laryngoscopy, but being placed for hours of surgery in a position that, because of the patient's unique pathology, precludes adequate perfusion to the spinal cord.

ANCILLARY STUDIES. For the purposes of the anesthetic evaluation of a patient for spine surgery, an appropriate starting point is that a history and physical examination (H&P) suffices for the young male patient without pertinent positive findings. Women of child-bearing age should have a urine or blood test to rule out pregnancy.

From this starting point, ancillary studies are based on posi-

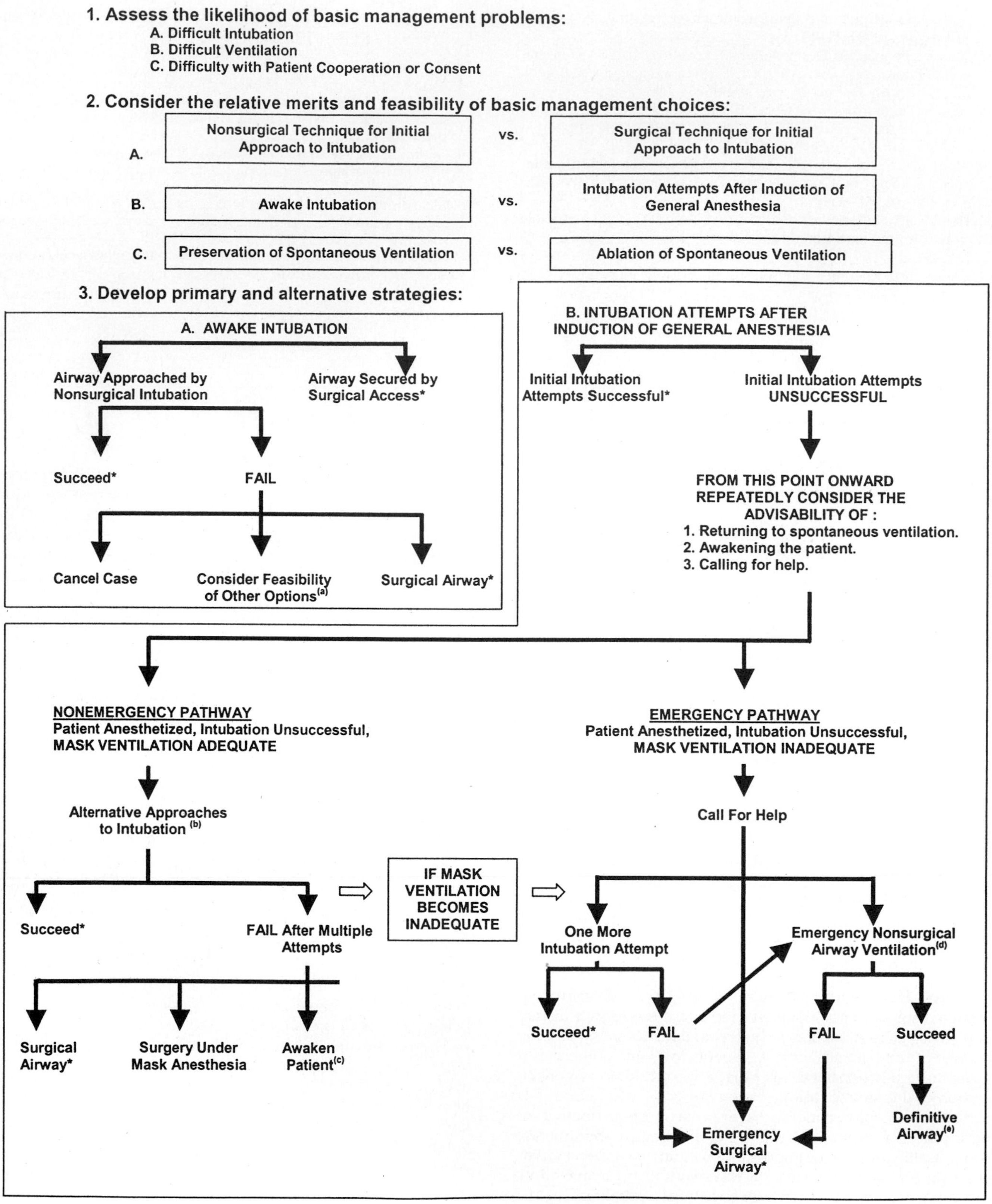

1. **Assess the likelihood of basic management problems:**
   A. Difficult Intubation
   B. Difficult Ventilation
   C. Difficulty with Patient Cooperation or Consent

2. **Consider the relative merits and feasibility of basic management choices:**

   A. | Nonsurgical Technique for Initial Approach to Intubation | **vs.** | Surgical Technique for Initial Approach to Intubation |

   B. | Awake Intubation | **vs.** | Intubation Attempts After Induction of General Anesthesia |

   C. | Preservation of Spontaneous Ventilation | **vs.** | Ablation of Spontaneous Ventilation |

3. **Develop primary and alternative strategies:**

A. AWAKE INTUBATION

- Airway Approached by Nonsurgical Intubation
- Airway Secured by Surgical Access*

- Succeed*
- FAIL
  - Cancel Case
  - Consider Feasibility of Other Options[a]
  - Surgical Airway*

B. INTUBATION ATTEMPTS AFTER INDUCTION OF GENERAL ANESTHESIA

- Initial Intubation Attempts Successful*
- Initial Intubation Attempts UNSUCCESSFUL

FROM THIS POINT ONWARD REPEATEDLY CONSIDER THE ADVISABILITY OF :
1. Returning to spontaneous ventilation.
2. Awakening the patient.
3. Calling for help.

NONEMERGENCY PATHWAY
Patient Anesthetized, Intubation Unsuccessful, **MASK VENTILATION ADEQUATE**

- Alternative Approaches to Intubation [b]
  - Succeed*
  - FAIL After Multiple Attempts
    - Surgical Airway*
    - Surgery Under Mask Anesthesia
    - Awaken Patient[c]

IF MASK VENTILATION BECOMES INADEQUATE

EMERGENCY PATHWAY
Patient Anesthetized, Intubation Unsuccessful, **MASK VENTILATION INADEQUATE**

- Call For Help
  - One More Intubation Attempt
    - Succeed*
    - FAIL
  - Emergency Nonsurgical Airway Ventilation[d]
    - FAIL
    - Succeed
      - Definitive Airway[e]
  - Emergency Surgical Airway*

Fig. 1. American Society of Anesthesiologists' difficult airway algorithm. *a:* Other options include (but are not limited to): surgery under mask anesthesia, surgery under local anesthesia infiltration or regional nerve blockade, or intubation attempts after induction of general anesthesia. *b:* Alternative approaches to difficult intubation include (but are not limited to): use of different laryngoscope blades, awake intubation, blind oral or nasal intubation, fiberoptic intubation, intubating stylet or tube changer, light wand, retrograde intubation, and surgical airway access. *c:* See awake intubation. *d:* Options for emergency nonsurgical airway ventilation include (but are not limited to): transtracheal jet ventilation, laryngeal mask ventilation, or esophageal–tracheal Combitube ventilation. *e:* Options for establishing a definitive airway include (but are not limited to): returning to awake state with spontaneous ventilation, tracheotomy, or endotracheal intubation.

tive findings on H&P. Furthermore, ancillary studies are appropriate in this case only if there is a potential to alter the patient's management based on the results.

Inasmuch as age is a risk factor for coronary artery disease, a screening electrocardiogram (EKG) is appropriate for patients over 50 years of age. Findings on H&P and EKG suspicious for cardiac disease should be pursued in accordance with the American College of Cardiology/American Heart Association Guidelines for Perioperative Cardiovascular Evaluation for Noncardiac Surgery (Fig. 2) (17).

In addition, scoliosis patients commonly present for spine surgery and are at risk for cardiac disease. These patients are at increasing risk for pulmonary hypertension, cor pulmonale, and right heart failure as their Cobb angle increases beyond 60 degrees. Furthermore, subgroups of these patients have congenital diseases with the additional risks of cardiac disease, including cardiomyopathy, valvular disease, and rhythm abnormalities (18–21). A cardiac workup beginning with a preoperative electrocardiogram is warranted.

Spine patients commonly present with baseline pulmonary disease. Scoliosis patients are at risk for restrictive pulmonary disease. Spinal surgery patients also include a proportionate representation of the relatively common obstructive pulmonary diseases of reactive airway disease (RAD) and chronic obstructive pulmonary disease (COPD).

Identification of Anesthetic Considerations

Surgery on the spine spans a wide spectrum of interventions. These range from, for example, the single level laminectomy, on the one extreme, to multiple-level anterior and posterior fusions with hardware placement on the other.

The former operation is generally completed within an hour or two through a small, midline incision with the patient positioned prone. Blood loss is usually minimal. For the average laminectomy patient, the anesthetic considerations revolve around issues inherent to prone positioning (22).

PRONE PROCEDURES. First, there is the obvious lack of ready access to the patient's airway. In the event of airway compromise, a gurney on which to turn the patient supine must be available.

Second, pronating the patient on a convex frame causes cephalad displacement of abdominal contents and increased intrathoracic pressure. As a consequence, there is increased ventilatory pressures and decreased cardiac stroke volume and cardiac index (23). The morbidly obese patient, for these reasons, may not tolerate prone positioning on the Wilson frame.

Third, there are numerous potential positioning injuries, including, but not limited to, the eyes, nose, cervical spine, brachial plexus, nipples, genitalia, and peripheral nerves (24). Patients with coronary artery bypass grafts may suffer cardiac ischemia owing to compression of the grafts (25). Visceral hypoperfusion and rhabdomyolysis also are reported complications of the prone position (26). Safeguarding the patient from positioning injuries requires not only meticulous positioning at the start of the case, but also vigilance during the case.

Local and Regional Anesthesia. Local and regional anesthesia in selected patients for selected prone procedures may an option.

Local anesthesia for posterior cervical surgery may offer the

advantage of an awake patient who can provide timely feedback to the surgeon during periods of spinal manipulation (27, 28). Permanent neurological injury might thus be averted. Local anesthesia has been used to avoid airway intervention yet accomplish release of cervical ligaments in a patient with rigid spine syndrome (29).

Spinal or epidural anesthesia for lumbar surgery can offer excellent surgical conditions, while decreasing the incidence of nausea and vomiting compared to general anesthesia (30). This may be particularly valuable in the same-day surgery population.

At the opposite end of the patient spectrum, regional anesthesia has been successfully employed for patients who it was felt would face excessive perioperative risks undergoing a general anesthetic. These have included ex-premature infants at risk for postoperative apnea (31) and patients with severe scoliosis (32).

General Anesthesia. In general, however, as the complexity, and typically the duration, of the prone operative procedure increases, selection of general anesthesia becomes likewise increasingly indicated. Additional anesthetic considerations come with more surgical complexity.

Inherent to inducing general endotracheal anesthesia comes the task of safely intubating the trachea of the patient who may have a difficult airway, as alluded to in the preceding. This intubation may need to be accomplished awake with airway topicalization and/or nerve blocks. Likewise, awake pronation may be indicated in the cervical myelopathy patient.

As the length of the operation and the amount of bone that is dissected increases, the greater is the potential for loss of blood. Similarly, the more venous sinuses opened in the dissected bone, the greater the risk that the operative area can be a source of venous air embolism. An additional consideration as the length of the operation increases is the increasing risk of hypothermia. Finally, hypothermia can exacerbate the problem of coagulopathy that can attend significant blood loss.

SITTING POSITION. An alternate position for approach to the posterior cervical spine or high thoracic spine is the sitting position (33). It offers better surgical exposure with less venous bleeding, but comes at the cost of increased risk of venous air embolism. Intraoperative monitoring for venous air embolism becomes more compelling, and placement of a multi-orifice right atrial catheter should be considered. Other considerations in the sitting patient is greater hemodynamic lability and the risk that excessive flexion of the head can cause spinal cord ischemia and macroglossia.

SUPINE POSITIONING. Supine positioning allows surgical exposure of the anterior as well as lateral aspects of the cervical spine. Although unlike the posterior position where the patient must be turned supine for access to the airway, nonetheless, access to the airway during supine cervical surgery can be problematic. The proximity of the surgical field and the encroachment of the surgical drapes can impede intraoperative airway interventions, which is an anesthetic consideration. Likewise, the proximity of surgery to the trachea and great vessels and the fact that the arms are tucked and unavailable, are anesthetic considerations.

Transoral. The transoral surgical approach provides access to the anterior craniocervical region (34). In this approach the surgeon and anesthesiologist share the airway. These patients frequently have unstable cervical spines and difficult airways. Intubation of the trachea may be achieved by the oral, nasal,

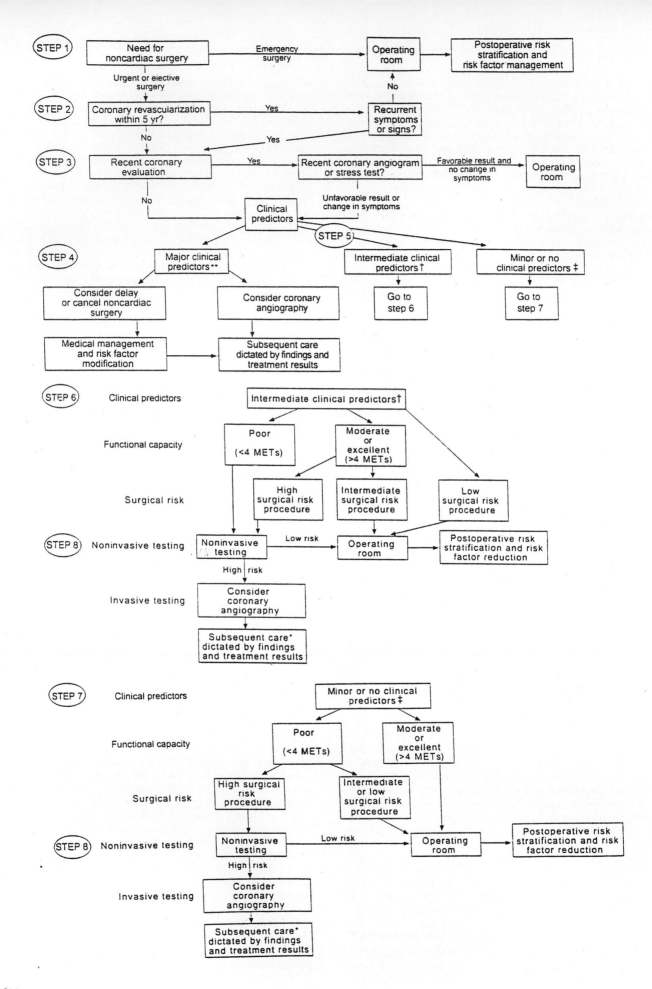

or tracheostomy route. Unrecognized blood loss into the esophagus, and pharyngeal swelling that requires continued intubation into the postoperative period, are anesthetic considerations.

Transabdominal. The supine position is also employed for access to the anterior aspects of the lower thoracic, lumbar, and sacral spine via a transabdominal approach. Inherent in this approach are the anesthetic considerations of the increased fluid requirements that accompany intraabdominal surgery and the surgeon's proximity to great vessels and retraction of visceral organs.

LATERAL POSITIONING. The lateral position is used when access to both the anterior and posterior aspects of the spine are desired, or when the spine is approached via a thoracotomy. Once the hemithorax is opened, the nondependent lung may be packed out of the way or selectively nonventilated. This invokes a host of anesthetic considerations for thoracic surgery, including placement and maintenance of a means of one lung ventilation, such as a double lumen endotracheal tube (35).

Physiology of an awake, spontaneously ventilating patient in the lateral position is such that the dependent lung is the better perfused and better ventilated lung. Unfortunately, when a patient is anesthetized, while the dependent lung is still the better perfused lung, it is no longer the better ventilated lung. This alteration is owing to a decrease in functional residual capacity. The net effect of muscle relaxation and the surgical opening of the nondependent hemithorax further diminishes the dependent lung volume. The mediastinum sags downward and abdominal contents press cephalad against the now-flaccid diaphragm (Fig. 3). Hence, intraoperative hypoxemia must be anticipated and preempted. Interventions such as continuous positive airway pressure (CPAP) to the nonventilated lung and positive end expiratory pressure (PEEP) to the dependent lung require prior preparation. Preoperative placement of an intraarterial cannula allows serial blood gas analysis. Likewise, in light of the pain associated with a thoracotomy, preoperative placement of a lumbar or thoracic epidural catheter or intrathecal narcotic injection should be considered.

Formulation of the Anesthetic Plan

Having conducted the preoperative evaluation, and having identified the anesthetic considerations inherent in the surgeon's intended procedure, the anesthesiologist formulates an anesthetic plan. This plan spans preoperative preparation, intraoperative management, and transition to postoperative care.

PREMEDICATION. Sedation may be appropriate in the anxious patient when its benefits outweigh its risks. Aspiration prophylaxis may be appropriate for the patient at risk. Beta blockade may be indicated in the patient with ischemic heart disease (36). An antisialagogue allows more effective topicalization of the airway when an awake intubation is intended (37).

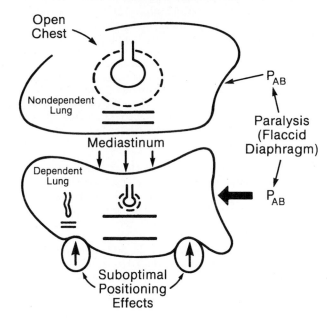

Lateral Decubitus Position Anesthetized

Fig. 3. Lateral decubitus position—anesthetized. Schematic summary of ventilation–perfusion relationships in the anesthetized patient in the lateral decubitus position who has an open chest and is paralyzed and suboptimally positioned. The nondependent lung is well ventilated *(large dashed lines)* but poorly perfused *(small perfusion vessel)*, and the dependent lung is poorly ventilated *(small dashed lines)* but well perfused *(large perfusion vessel)*. In addition, the dependent lung may also develop an atelectic shunt compartment *(left side of lower lung)* because of circumferential compression of this lung. P_{AB}, pressure of the abdominal contents. (Modified from Benumof JL. Physiology of the open chest and one-lung ventilation. In: Kaplan JA, ed. *Thoracic anesthesia.* New York: Churchill Livingstone, 1983, with permission.)

AIRWAY MANAGEMENT. Even when a natural airway is the plan, such as during lumbar procedures under spinal anesthesia, a backup plan must exist to expeditiously assume control of the patient's airway. A transition to controlled ventilation must be possible should some unforeseen intraoperative event render the patient unable to ventilate or protect his own airway.

On those occasions when on preoperative evaluation an elective awake intubation is indicated, the patient must be counseled and prepared for the procedure. It is not safe to attempt intubating an awake patient who is not cooperative, or on the other hand, is oversedated. Although a preferred intubation technique, for example, fiberoptic nasopharyngeal, may be initially selected, other modalities, such as intubating through a mask laryngeal airway (38) or over a retrograde wire (39), also should be immediately available. Prior to initiating the intubation, an abort threshold should be determined, such as five or six attempts. There are those patients that by virtue of trauma, tumor, congenital abnormalities, or degenerative changes are not possible to intubate by nonsurgical means. It is important to insure that trauma from repeated intubation attempts does not foreclose the patient's ability to ventilate.

Fig. 2. Stepwise approach to preoperative cardiac assessment. Steps are discussed in text. Subsequent care may include cancellation or delay of surgery, coronary revascularization followed by noncardiac surgery, or intensified care.

SELECTION OF MONITORING MODALITIES. Noninvasive monitors of oxygenation, ventilation, circulation, and temperature required for all anesthetics are specified in the ASA's Standards for Basic Anesthetic Monitoring (40). Invasive monitoring including intra-arterial, central venous, and pulmonary artery pressures, transesophageal echocardiography, and a Foley catheter are based on the patient's medical condition and the nature of the surgical procedure. Inasmuch as each invasive monitor is associated with some finite complication rate, the benefits accrued from placing the monitor must outweigh the risks. Neurological monitoring is selected based on the neural tissue at risk, and likewise is implemented when its potential benefits justify its risks and costs (Chapter 59).

PLACEMENT OF INTRAVASCULAR ACCESS AND INVASIVE MONITORS. After placement of an initial intravenous catheter, invasive devices can most commonly be inserted after anesthesia is induced. An exception is when the hemodynamic data an invasive monitor provides are required to safely induce anesthesia. Another exception is when a patient with cervical myelopathy must be intubated awake and pronate himself or herself. In this case arterial and central venous access and urinary catheters must be placed prior to pronation.

INDUCTION AND MAINTENANCE. The intravenous anesthetic agents for induction of general anesthesia are all rapid in onset but have differing side-effect profiles (41). An induction agent is selected for a given patient based on the patient's underlying medical conditions.

Agents commonly selected for maintenance of a general anesthesia serve the goals of providing the surgeon a patient who is free from sensation of pain, amnestic, motionless, and in good hemodynamic control. This often is achieved with some combination of volatile anesthetic, nitrous oxide, narcotic, and muscle relaxant. Additional considerations that may attend a spine procedure can require further refinements in this technique.

Neurological monitoring is one such consideration. Somatosensory evoked potentials (SSEPs) are progressively altered by increasing concentrations of inhalational anesthetics (42). It is imperative to avoid mistaking SSEP changes resulting from increasing anesthetic depth, from SSEP changes resulting from surgical intervention. This requires close coordination among anesthesiologist, surgeon, and neuromonitoring technician and, as much as possible, modest, steady-state levels of inhalational anesthetic. Monitoring electromyography (EMG) requires less than total blockade of the neuromuscular junction with muscle relaxants. Conducting an intraoperative wake-up test requires an anesthetic that allows rapid emergence and compliance with command (43).

TEMPERATURE MANAGEMENT. Unless deliberate hypothermia is part of the plan of spinal cord protection, normothermia should be maintained. It is easier to maintain a patient's temperature than to rewarm him once he is significantly hypothermic. Normothermia is most readily maintained by using a combined approach of active measures (e.g., forced air and water blankets), and passive measures (e.g., low fresh gas flows and increasing the room temperature). Hyperthermia should be avoided.

FLUID AND COAGULATION MANAGEMENT. A principal focus of the anesthesiologist's efforts during major spine surgery normally is the maintenance of an appropriate intravascular milieu. Although rapid blood loss is unusual, extensive bony dissection and lengthy procedures can result in a continuous ooze that adds up to multiple liters. The patient must be kept normovolemic in order to avoid inadequate perfusion. However, the fluid the anesthesiologist selects to maintain this intravascular volume is a balance between the patient's risks from transfusion with the patient's need for adequate oxygen-carrying capacity and coagulative function. There are no absolute triggers for transfusing blood products. Each patient's presenting condition and intraoperative course must be considered. Specific recommendations are found in the ASA's Practice Guidelines for Blood Component Therapy (44).

A number of strategies have been employed, individually and in combination, to help diminish the need for homologous transfusion. Among these are preoperative autologous donation (45), intraoperative scavenging, hemodilution (46), controlled hypotension (47), normotensive epidural blockade (48), and pharmacological adjuncts such as erythropoietin (49), and Premarin (50). None is without risks (51).

It is important that a transfusion management plan acceptable to the patient, surgeon, and anesthesiologist be agreed on prior to embarking on elective surgery likely to require transfusion.

Other issues include the need to maintain a normal electrolyte status and avoid hyperglycemia that could worsen ischemic damage to neural tissue (52).

TRANSITION TO POSTOPERATIVE MANAGEMENT. Part of the focus of preoperative preparation and intraoperative management is to be able to deliver to the postoperative care team a patient who is in the best condition he or she can be in considering the surgical procedure just undergone. Facilitating a smooth transition from operating room to recovery room or intensive care unit is inherent in the ASA Standards for Postanesthesia Care (53).

A major contribution the anesthesiologist can make to the patient's postoperative comfort is to provide for a means of postoperative analgesia appropriate to the magnitude of the surgery, as described in the ASA's Practice Guidelines for Acute Pain Management in the Perioperative Setting (54). Numerous options are possible, including wound infiltration by the surgeon with local anesthetic (55,56), placement of epidural morphine (57,58), or local anesthetic via a catheter.

Orderly transport from the operating room should be followed by a complete yet concise report to the accepting team that clearly identifies active issues requiring continued attention.

References

1. Roizen MF. Preoperative evaluation. In: Miller RD, ed. *Anesthesia,* 4th ed. New York: Churchill Livingstone, 1994:827–882.
2. Hambly PR, Martin B. Anaesthesia for chronic spinal cord lesions. *Anaesthesia* 1998;53:273–289.
3. Lam AM. Acute spinal cord injury: monitoring and anaesthetic implications. *Can J Anaesthesiol* 1991;38:pR60–R67.
4. Roizen MF. Anesthetic implications of concurrent diseases. In: Miller RD, ed. *Anesthesia,* 4th ed. New York: Churchill Livingstone, 1994:903–1014.
5. Popitz MD. Anaesthetic implications of chronic disease of the cervical spine. *Anesthesiol Analg* 1997;84:672–683.
6. Practice Guidelines for Management of the Difficult Airway. A report by the American Society of Anesthesiologists Task Force on management of the difficult airway. *Anesthesiology* 1993;78:597–602.
7. Sawin PD, Todd MM, Traynelis VC, et al. Cervical spine motion

with direct laryngoscopy and orotracheal intubation. *Anesthesiology* 1996;85:26–36.

8. Yaszemski MJ, Shepler TR. Sudden death from cord compression associated with atlanto-axial instability in rheumatoid arthritis. *Spine* 1990;15:338–341.

9. Black S. Surgical procedures of the cervical and thoracic spine: an overview. In: Porter SS, ed. *Anesthesia for surgery of the spine.* New York: McGraw-Hill, 1995:79–100.

10. Macarthur A, Kleiman S. Rheumatoid cervical joint disease: a challenge to the anaesthetist. *Can J Anaesth* 1993;40:154–159.

11. Hastings RH, Marks JD. Airway management for trauma patients with potential cervical spine injuries. *Anesthesiol Analg* 1991;73:471–482.

12. Suderman VS, Crosby ET, Lui A. Elective oral tracheal intubation in cervical spine-injured adults. *Can J Anaesthesiol* 1991;38:785–789.

13. Criswell JC, Nolan JP. Emergency airway management in patients with cervical spine injuries. *Anaesthesia* 1994;49:900–903.

14. Mahla ME. Cervical spine in anesthesia: evaluation and approach. In: Cucchiara RF, Black S, Michenfelder JD, eds. *Clinical neuroanesthesia,* 2nd ed. New York: Churchill Livingstone, 1998:389–402.

15. Sidhu VS, Whitehead EM, Ainsworth QP, et al. A technique of awake fiberoptic intubation. *Anaesthesia* 1993;48:910–913.

16. Reasoner DK, Warner DS, Todd MM. A comparison of anesthetic techniques for awake intubation in neurosurgical patients. *J Neurosurg Anesthesiol* 1995;7:94–99.

17. American Heart Association and American College of Cardiology. Guidelines for perioperative cardiovascular evaluation for noncardiac surgery. *Circulation* 1996;93:1278–1317.

18. Smith CL, Bush GH. Anaesthesia and progressive muscular dystrophy. *Br J Anaesthesiol* 1985;57:1113–1118.

19. Jensen V. The anaesthetic management of a patient with Emery-Dreifuss muscular dystrophy. *Can J Anaesthesiol* 1996;43:968–971.

20. Campbell AM, Bousfield JD. Anaesthesia in a patient with Noonan's syndrome and cardiomyopathy. *Anaesthesia* 1992;47:131–133.

21. Lee JJ, Imrie M, Taylor V. Anesthesia and tuberous sclerosis. *Br J Anaesthesiol* 1994;73:421–425.

22. Anderton JM. The prone position for the surgical patient: a historical review of the principles and hazards. *Br J Anaesthesiol* 1991;67:452–463.

23. Yokoyama M, Ueda M, Hirakawa M, et al. Hemodynamic effect of the prone position during anesthesia. *Acta Anaesthesiol Scand* 1991;35:741–744.

24. Hoski JJ, Eismont FJ, Green BA. Blindness as a complication of intraoperative positioning. *J Bone Joint Surg Am* 1993;75:1231–1232.

25. Weinlander CM, Coombs DW, Plume SK. Myocardial ischemia due to obstruction of an aortocoronary bypass graft by intraoperative positioning. *Anesthesiol Anal* 1985;64:933–936.

26. Ziser A, Friedhoff RJ, Rose SH. Prone position: visceral hypoperfusion and rhabdomyolysis. *Anesthesiol Analg* 1996;82:412–415.

27. Rao S, Yadav A, Galvan R. Posterior spinal stabilization under local anesthesia. *J Spinal Disord* 1990;3:250–254.

28. Nygaard OP, Romner B, Thoner J, et al. Local anesthesia in posterior cervical surgery. *Anesthesiology* 1997;86:242–243.

29. Kitayama M, Ohtomo N, Tetsuhiro S, et al. Airway management and rigid spine syndrome. *Anesthesiol Analg* 1997;84:690–691.

30. Pai-Yu T, His-Cheng T, Chih-Cheng C, et al. Epidural anesthesia for spine surgery. *Ma Tsui Hsueh Tsa Chi Anaesthesiol Sinica* 1990;28:203–207.

31. Aronsson DD, Gemery JM, Abajian JC. Spinal anesthesia for spine and lower extremity surgery in infants. *J Pediatr Orthop* 1996;16:259–263.

32. Dalens BJ, Khandwala RS, Tanguy A. Staged segmental scoliosis surgery during regional anesthesia in high risk patients: a report of six cases. *Anesthesiol Analg* 1993;76:434–439.

33. Matjasko J, Petrozza P, Cohen M. Anesthesia and surgery in the seated position: analysis of 554 cases. *Neurosurgery* 1985;17:695–702.

34. Marks RJ, Forrester PC, Calder I, et al. Anaesthesia for transoral craniocervical surgery. *Anaesthesia* 1986;41:1049–1052.

35. Benumof JL. *Anesthesia for thoracic surgery,* 2nd ed. Philadelphia: W.B. Saunders, 1995:123–151.

36. Wallace A, Layug B, Tateo I, et al. Prophylactic atenolol reduces postoperative myocardial ischemia. *Anesthesiology* 1998;88:7–17.

37. Watanabe L, Lindgren P, Rosenberg P, et al. Glycopyrronium prolongs topical anaesthesia of oral mucosa and enhances absorption of lignocaine. *Br J Anaesthesiol* 1993;70:94–95.

38. Benumof JL. Laryngeal mask airway and the ASA difficult airway algorithm. *Anesthesiology* 1996;84:686–699.

39. Barriot P, Riou B. Retrograde technique for tracheal intubation in trauma patients. *Crit Care Med* 1988;16:712–713.

40. American Society of Anesthesiologists. Standards for Basic Intraoperative Monitoring.

41. Van Hemelrijck J, Gonzales JM, White PF. Pharmacology of intravenous anesthetic agents. In: Rogers MC, Tinker JH, Covino BG, et al, eds. *Principles and practice of anesthesiology.* St. Louis: Mosby-Year Book, 1993:1131–1154.

42. Mahla ME, Horhocker TT. Vertebral column and spinal cord surgery. In: Cucchiara RF, Black S, Michenfelder JD, eds. *Clinical neuroanesthesia,* 2nd ed. New York: Churchill Livingstone, 1998:403–448.

43. Marshall WK, Mostrom JL. Neurosurgical diseases of the spine and spinal cord: anesthetic considerations. In: Cottrell JE, Smith DS, eds. *Anesthesia and neurosurgery,* 3rd ed. Mosby-Year Book, 1994:569–603.

44. American Society of Anesthesiologists Task Force on Blood Component Therapy. Practice guidelines for blood component therapy. *Anesthesiology* 1996;84:732–747.

45. Toy PT, Strauss RG, Stehling LC, et al. Predeposited autologous blood for elective surgery. *N Engl J Med* 1987;316:517–520.

46. Hur S, Huizenga BA, Major M. Acute normovolemic hemodilution combined with hypotensive anesthesia and other techniques to avoid homologous transfusion in spinal fusion surgery. *Spine* 1992;17:867–873.

47. Fox HJ, Thomas CH, Thompson AG. Spinal instrumentation for Duchenne's muscular dystrophy: experience of hypotensive anaesthesia to minimize blood loss. *J Pediatr Orthop* 1997;17:750–753.

48. Kakiuchi M. Reduction of blood loss during spinal surgery by epidural blockade under normotensive general anesthesia. *Spine* 1997;22:889–894.

49. Goodnough LT, Rudnick S, Price TH, et al. Increased preoperative collection of autologous blood with recombinant human erythropoietin therapy. *N Engl J Med* 1989;321:1163–1168.

50. McCall RE, Bilderback KK. Use of intravenous Premarin to decrease postoperative blood loss after pediatric scoliosis surgery. *Spine* 1997;22:1394–1397.

51. Katz DM, Trobe JD, Cornblath WT, et al. Ischemic optic neuropathy after lumbar spine surgery. *Arch Ophthalmol* 1994;112:925–931.

52. Drummond JC, Moore SS. The influence of dextrose administration on neurological outcome after temporary spinal cord ischemia in the rabbit. *Anesthesiology* 1989;70:64–70.

53. American Society of Anesthesiologists. Standards for postanesthesia care. In: Stoelting RK, Miller RD. *Basics of anesthesia.* New York: Churchill Livingstone, 1994:501–502.

54. American Society of Anesthesiologists Task Force on Pain Management. Practice guidelines for acute pain management in the perioperative setting. *Anesthesiology* 1995;82:1071–1081.

55. Milligan KR, Macafee AL, Fogarty DJ, et al. Intraoperative bupivacaine diminishes pain after lumbar laminectomy. *J Bone Joint Surg* 1993;75-B:769–771.

56. Cherian MN, Mathews MP, Chandy MJ. Local wound infiltration with bupivacaine in lumbar laminectomy. *Surg Neurol* 1997;47:120–123.

57. Joshi GP, McCarroll SM, O'Rourke K. Postoperative analgesia after lumbar laminectomy: epidural fentanyl infusion versus patient-controlled intravenous morphine. *Anesthesiol Analg* 1995;80:511–514.

58. Rainov NG, Gutjahr T, Burkert W. Intraoperative epidural morphine, fentanyl, and droperidol for control of pain after spinal surgery. A prospective, randomized, placebo-controlled, and double-blind trial. *Acta Neurochir (Wien)* 1996;138:33–39.

141. Pathophysiology of Degenerative Disc and Joint Disease

Sun H. Lee and
Frederick A. Simeone

Pathophysiology of Degenerative Disc and Joint Disease

The underlying pathophysiological mechanisms of disc herniation and degenerative joint disease of the spine are still not completely understood. However, there seems to be a consistent anatomical pattern of disc degeneration in the spine, with most changes occurring in the regions where mechanical stresses caused by spine movement take place. Midcervical, thoracolumbar, and lower lumbar regions show degenerative changes frequently with the aging process. A number of research studies on this subject over the past several years have contributed to an understanding of the pathophysiology of degenerative changes of disc and spinal stenosis, and the mechanism of pain secondary to this change.

The spinal motion segment can be visualized as a tripod joint complex, composed of the intervertebral disc and two facet joints. The three-joint intervertebral motion segment concept underscores the fact that disease in each component affects the others. Any alteration in one of these joints, which usually develops primarily at the disc, can lead to abnormal biomechanical stresses and may lead to progressive changes in the other segmental units (1). This results in degenerative changes in the facets and further deterioration of the disc itself. These changes are associated with the degeneration of discs, facets, and spurs or osteophyte formation at the end plates, ligament buckling, or hypertrophy and/or spondylolisthesis. This causes nerve root compression and/or spinal cord compression, and ensuing pain and neurological deficits, depending on the pathological level of the spine.

PATHOPHYSIOLOGY OF DISC DEGENERATION. The intervertebral disc consists of three components: the nucleus pulposus, annulus fibrosus, and cartilaginous end plates. The ventral annulus is usually wider and more organized than the dorsal annulus, which may even have discontinuous lamellae. The nucleus pulposus, derived from the notochord, has a higher proteoglycan and water content than the annulus fibrosus. The hyaline cartilage end plates contain collagen similar to the inner annulus fibrosus and nucleus pulposus.

The degenerative process in the intervertebral disc usually begins by the third decade of life and is characterized by a gradual decrease in the water content. In a collected autopsy series, disc degeneration first appeared in the second decade in males and in the third decade in females, with 97% of discs demonstrating degeneration by age 50. Annulus and nucleus pulposus borders become indistinct after the second decade. The first stage in the degenerative process of the spine in most patients is disc degeneration. However, facet arthritis precedes evidence of disc degeneration in 20% of degenerative spines (2).

STRUCTURAL COMPONENTS OF INTERVERTEBRAL DISCS. Water, collagen, and proteoglycans are the major structural components of intervertebral discs, together making up 90% to 95% of the volume of normal discs. The normal intervertebral disc is highly hydrated. The nucleus pulposus is composed of 85% water, and the annulus fibrosus 78% water. Water content decreases with degeneration, especially in the nucleus pulposus (3,4).

The collagen network provides the intervertebral connection, whereas its lamellar structure permits motion. The collagen content is higher in the outer portions of the annulus than in the inner annulus and nucleus pulposus. The intervertebral disc contains type I and II collagen. The collagen content of the annulus is composed of about 60% type II and 40% type I collagen. The nucleus pulposus contains only type II collagen. The type II fibrils from the nucleus pulposus have more intermolecular spacing than type I. Highly hydrated type II fibrils deform easily and absorb compressive forces. The collagen content increases as well as a change in the proportion of type I to type II, with type I increasing in content with age (5,6).

Proteoglycans of intervertebral discs are homologous to those from articular cartilage. They contain a core protein as well as glycosaminoglycans of chondroitin sulfate (CS) and keratin sulfate (KS). Glycosaminoglycans are attached to the core and are able to aggregate with hyaluronic acid. Link proteins stabilize the structure. The nucleus pulposus is richer in proteoglycan than the annulus. Proteoglycans imbibe water and maintain hydration of the disc tissues and provide tissue turgor with their hydrodynamic and electrostatic properties. With age and degeneration, total proteoglycan content as well as aggregation with hyaluronic acid decreases. The ratio of KS to CS and extractability increases with age (7).

Link proteins are the glycoproteins that stabilize the noncovalent bonding of aggregating proteoglycan to hyaluronate. There is an increase in smaller and fragmented link proteins with age and degeneration. The smallest link proteins accumulate along with fragmentation products. Activation of proteolytic activity in the disc may play a role in degenerative changes (8,9).

DEGENERATIVE PROCESS AND HERNIATION OF DISCS. In the intact disc, the nucleus of the disc is gelatinous and the annular material is distinct and lamellated. The annular contour is smooth and separate from the nucleus pulposus. Prior to actual displacement of disc material, the nucleus and annulus undergo certain well-defined structural changes. The disc receives its nutrients through small vessels in the cartilage end plates from the periphery of the annulus. The end plates calcify and vessel loss occurs with aging until nearly the entire disc is avascular. This causes increased lactic acid production and cellular necrosis. Loss of water and proteoglycan in the region of the inner annulus and nucleus pulposus is discussed in the preceding.

As the patient ages, there is a less well defined border between the nucleus pulposus and annulus, with fibrocartilage replacing the nuclear area. Nests of chondrocytes can be observed. The lamellae of the annulus become coarser and hyalinized with age. Radiating cracks in the annulus fibrosus develop in the most centrally situated lamellae and extend outward toward the periphery. These radiating clefts in the annulus weaken its resistance to nuclear herniation (10). With progression, there are also biomechanical and biochemical alterations in the annulus fibrosus and nucleus pulposus that cause narrowing of the intervertebral disc space. There is more bulging and herniation of nucleus pulposus as collapse and fissuring occur. These changes usually occur in more mobile disc segments such as L5-S1 and L4-5. The large disc herniations causing acute disc syndromes are more common in individuals between the ages of 30 and 50 because they have good turgor in the nucleus compared to the elderly whose nucleus is desiccated and fibrotic.

PATHOPHYSIOLOGY OF PAIN IN DISC HERNIATION.

Neurological dysfunction such as motor, sensory, reflex changes, and pain develop with the disc protrusion and spinal stenosis. Recent research has been done for defining pathophysiological events of pain at the cellular or subcellular levels. Two specific mechanisms of pain at the tissue level can be defined; mechanical deformation of the nerve roots and biochemical effects of the disc tissue on the roots (Fig. 1).

The spinal nerve roots are more susceptible to mechanical deformation than peripheral nerves because the nerve roots do not possess the same amounts and organization of protective connective tissue sheaths as do the peripheral nerves.

There have been several experimental nerve root compression studies. The results have shown that mechanical compression of the nerve root induces the changes in the microcirculation of the nerve tissue by venular and capillary stasis. A pressure of 5 to 10 mm Hg was found to cause acute changes in venular blood flow (11). Vascular impairment also induces an increase in the vascular permeability, leading to intraneural edema formation, which subsequently increases the endoneural fluid pressure, and compromises the nutrition of the nerve roots. Edema may negatively affect the nerve root for a longer period than the compression itself and also it may cause subsequent formation of intraneural fibrosis. The sensory fibers are slightly more susceptible to compression than the motor fibers.

According to animal experiments, a rapid compression of the nerve root induces more pronounced effects on edema formation. This may be related clinically to spinal trauma or acute disc herniation. Multiple level compression (e.g., multiple-level spinal stenosis) produces more pronounced symptoms than a single-level compression. There are no regional nutritive arteries from surrounding structures to the intraneural vascular system in the spinal nerve roots. There is experimental evidence that suggests that the nutrition to the nerve segment located between two compression sites in nerve roots is severely impaired, although this nerve segment itself is uncompressed. The nutrition to the uncompressed nerve segment located between two compression sites is affected almost to the same extent as at the compression sites, regardless of the distance between the compression sites (12,13).

There is an increase in substance P in the nerve root and dorsal root ganglion following nerve root compression that may provide evidence of pain (14). Mechanical deformation per se may induce impulses that could be interpreted by the central nervous system as pain.

Experimental studies demonstrated that the nucleus pulposus has significant properties to injure the nerve roots after local application, even though the mechanisms for the nucleus pulposus-induced nerve root injury are not yet fully understood. Several studies also demonstrated that autologous nucleus pulposus may elicit inflammatory reactions when it is applied outside the intervertebral disc space. McCarron and collaborators (15) applied autologous nucleus pulposus from dog's tail discs in the epidural space of the animal to elucidate biological effect of nucleus pulposus. They observed that there was an epidural inflammatory reaction that did not occur when saline was injected as a control. Olmarker and co-workers (16,17) presented a study that demonstrated that autologous nucleus pulposus may induce a reduction in nerve conduction velocity and light microscopic structural changes in a pig cauda equina model. There were significant injuries of the Schwann cells with vacuolization and disintegration of the Schmidt-Lanterman incisures, which are essential for the normal exchange of ions between

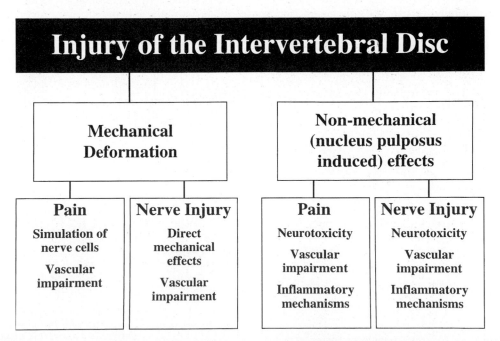

Fig. 1. The pathophysiological events in disc herniation. The two mechanisms at the tissue level—mechanical deformation and non-mechanical nucleus pulposus-induced effects—may both induce pain and nerve injury. (From Olmarker K. Experimental basis of sciatica. *J Orthop Sci* 1996;1:230–242, with permission.)

the axon and surrounding tissues (18). Minimal leakage of nucleus pulposus was enough to induce significant changes in structure and function of the adjacent nerve root (19). Epidural application of autologous nucleus pulposus induces an intraneural edema within 2 hours and it leads to a reduction of the intraneural blood flow within 3 hours. Histological changes of the nerve roots are present after three hours, and subsequent reduction of the nerve conduction velocity begins between 3 and 24 hours after application (16).

A potent antiinflammatory agent, methylprednisolone (MP), was administered intravenously at various times after the application of nucleus pulposus. The results showed clearly that the nucleus pulposus-induced reduction in nerve conduction velocity was eliminated if methylprednisolone was administered within 24 hours of application. This may result from the antiinflammatory properties of the MP or some other property (20). This may be an indication that inflammatory reactions were present.

The proteoglycans have been suggested to have a direct irritating effect on nerve tissues. Also, the cells of the nucleus pulposus have shown that these cells are capable of producing metalloproteases (e.g., collagenase or gelatinase) as well as interleukin-6 and prostaglandin-E2. The associated substances are probably membrane-bound. Substances such as immunoglobulin G, hydrogen ions, and phospholipase A2 also have been suggested to be responsible for the pathophysiological reactions. Furthermore, tumor necrosis factor (TNF) may induce both thrombus formation and increased vascular permeability (21), and seems to be closely related to neuropathic pain (22). It produces histological changes similar to those seen in nerve roots exposed to nucleus pulposus when injected into nerve fascicles. TNF also initiates local inflammatory reactions by stimulation and recruitment of inflammatory cells of the host. Cyclosporin is an immunosuppressant that acts by interfering with TNFα; it has been reported to block the reduction of nerve conduction velocity induced by incising lumbar discs in dogs.

DEGENERATIVE CHANGES OF FACET JOINTS. The degenerative process of facet joints and intervertebral discs was described well based on the three-joint intervertebral motion segment concept by Kirkaldy-Willis and co-workers to explain the development of multilevel spinal stenosis (Fig. 2).

The neuroforamen is bounded by the facet joints posteriorly, pedicles superiorly and inferiorly, and vertebral body and disc anteriorly. Any change in these structures with degenerative processes can lead to a compromise of the space available for the spinal nerve root. Degenerative changes in the facet joints, degenerative spondylolisthesis, and osteophyte formation contribute to the stenotic pattern both dynamically and statically.

The cartilage has a well-contoured, gliding surface in well-preserved facet joints, and the joints are covered with synovium and a capsule. When the disc space narrows as a result of loss of hydration of the nucleus pulposus, there is increased stress on the facet joints with concomitant erosion of the facet joints. The porosity of the bone in the facet increases with loss of joint space and decrease in subchondral sclerosis, suggesting an alteration in the stress distributions across the facet joints. The subsequent hypermobility of the intervertebral joint leads to marginal osteophyte formations and the cartilage surface begins to erode further. As the cartilage fails, the bone loses its mass and normal function. The joint surfaces become markedly irregular and override each other. The consequence of the narrowing of the disc is subluxation of the facet joints. With subluxation of the facet joint both in an axial and sagittal plane, joint erosion, recurrent joint effusion, degenerative changes, and osteophyte formation take place. The ligamentum flavum shortens with narrowing of the disc and subluxation of the facet joint. The thickened ligamentum is passively pushed into the neural space by the subluxed hypertrophied facet joints. Also, narrowing of the disc with displacement of the pedicle in an axial direction kinks the nerve root. It is also noted that lamina may overlap one another and that the major weight-bearing characteristics of the spine may shift posteriorly onto the subluxed hypertrophied facets and shingled lamina in central stenosis syndromes. Rotational subluxation may occur and affect the inferior facet on one side and the superior facet on the contralateral side, causing them to protrude into the spinal canal.

If the disc collapse exceeds the facet arthritis changes, then there may be some retrolisthesis of the superior vertebral body on the subjacent one, with posterior overriding of the facet joints. In the early stages of degeneration, there frequently is a subtle retrolisthesis of the superior vertebral body on the subjacent one, coupled with overriding facet and bulging disc spaces. If anterior and posterior column degeneration occurs relatively

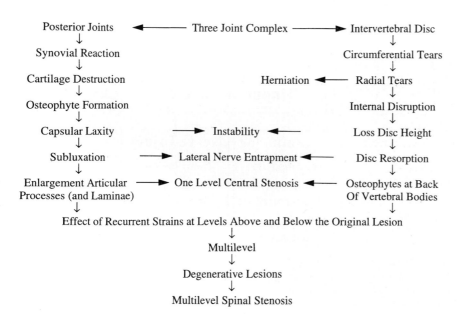

Fig. 2. Recurrent rotational strains (compression injury). Degenerative process of facet joints and intervertebral discs in the lumbar spine. (From Kirkaldy-Willis WH, Wedge JH, Yong-Hing K, et al. Pathology and pathogenesis of lumbar spondylosis and stenosis. *Spine* 1978;3:320, with permission.)

concurrently, then the facet joint begins to erode, hypertrophic changes develop, and a gradual realignment and redistribution of forces across the facet joint can occur. This may allow anterior subluxation of the vertebra (10,23–28).

At the cervical region, disc and facet joint degeneration as well as apophyseal joint degeneration can cause radiculopathy and/or myelopathy. Typical cervical lordosis is caused by increased thickness of the intervertebral disc anteriorly compared with posteriorly. The upper surface of each cervical vertebral body is concave; this is accentuated by a bony shelf that projects upward from the posterolateral aspect of each side of the body. This is called the uncinate process. The boundaries of the neural foramen are formed by the inferior and superior surfaces of the adjacent pedicles: posterolaterally, by the medial aspect of the facet joint and adjacent part of the articular column; and anterolaterally, by the posterolateral aspect of the uncinate process, intervertebral disc, and inferior part of the superior adjacent vertebrae. Osteophytes originate from the uncovertebral joints and/or the facet joints (29).

PATHOPHYSIOLOGY OF PAIN IN SPINAL STENOSIS. The pathophysiology of the symptoms and signs of spinal stenosis have not been fully elucidated. The degenerative processes can be related to chemical and mechanical changes that can affect and inflame the neural elements in the lumbar spine. Static and dynamic compression, vascular occlusion, ischemia, and metabolic–nutritional effect may lead to pain and neurological dysfunction.

It is unlikely that pure mechanical instability or isolated nerve root compression can explain the pain by themselves in spinal stenosis. Mechanical compression of the nerve roots in the lumbar spine can create a number of intraneural tissue reactions that may lead to pain or neurological alterations. Even low pressure (5 to 10 mm Hg) on the nerve root may lead to venous congestion of the intraneural microcirculation. Solute transport decreases and intraneural edema develops. Chronic inflammatory changes in and around the nerve tissue enhance and prolong mechanical compression. It may lead to demyelination combined with metabolic alterations. However, experimental studies also showed that constriction of the cauda equina in the midlumbar spine requires narrowing to approximately 50% of normal before it is significant (30).

This pain can be relieved when the patient flexes the spine by sitting or leaning forward. The symptomatic improvement results from increased spinal canal size, because flexion results in stretching of the protruding ligamentum flavum and posterior longitudinal ligament, as well as the reduction of overriding facets. During ambulation, some patients experience the onset of symptoms owing to increased metabolic demand in nerve roots that have become ischemic because of stenotic compression. With ambulation, edema and ischemia develop on the nerve roots owing to mechanical irritation and entrapment.

Venous hypertension and venous stasis, the disturbed vascular supply and nutritional support systems of the cauda equina, can cause pain in spinal stenosis (31). Notably, this vascular supply, coupled with the permeability of the microvessels in the dorsal root ganglion, suggests an increased metabolic demand. Several essential substances are synthesized at the dorsal root ganglion; therefore, any compromise in the blood supply and flow may lead to alterations in solute transport or manufacture and be a focus for pain. Chronic compression, inflammation, fibrosis, ischemia, and diminution in protein synthesis and metabolism may slow the diffusion process of cerebrospinal fluid that is also one of the nutritional transport systems. This can further contribute to the symptoms and signs of spinal stenosis. Sensory symptoms occur more frequently than motor symptoms and can be paresthesias, hypesthesia, or hyperalgesia.

Cell bodies of the primary afferent neurons contained in the dorsal root ganglion produce various neuropeptides that are transported to central and peripheral terminals. Substance P causes vasodilatation and release of histamine, leading to the inflammatory cascade and pain. Calcitonin gene-related peptide is found in primary sensory neurons and has been implicated in mediating sensory modalities such as nociception and mechanoreception. Other pain producing chemicals (non-neurogenic) released during tissue damage that sensitize pain fibers include bradykinin, serotonin, histamine, potassium ions, and prostaglandins (32–34).

Summary

Disc herniation and degenerative joint disease of the spine occur in the regions where mechanical stresses caused by spine movement take place. The spinal motion segment can be visualized as a tripod joint complex, composed of the intervertebral disc and two facet joints. The three-joint intervertebral motion segment concept underscores the fact that disease in each component affects the others. Any alteration in one of these joints, which usually develops primarily at the disc, can lead to abnormal biomechanical stresses and progressive changes in the other segmental units. The first stage in the degenerative process of the spine in most patients is disc degeneration. However, facet arthritis precedes evidence of disc degeneration in 20% of degenerative spines.

There is a less well-defined border between the nucleus pulposus and annulus, with fibrocartilage replacing the nuclear area as the patient ages. The annulus weakens its resistance to nuclear herniation, which causes narrowing of the intervertebral disc space as well as nerve root compression.

There is increased stress on the facet joints with concomitant erosion of the facet joints as degeneration of the disc takes places. Degenerative changes in the facet joints, degenerative spondylolisthesis, and osteophyte formation contribute to the stenotic pattern, both dynamically and statically. The consequence of the narrowing of the disc is subluxation of the facet joints. The ligamentum flavum shortens with narrowing of the disc and subluxation of the facet joint. The thickened ligamentum is passively pushed into the neural space by the subluxed hypertrophied facet joints. Also, narrowing of the disc with displacement of the pedicle in an axial direction kinks the nerve root.

The underlying pathophysiological mechanisms of disc herniation and degenerative joint disease of the spine are still not completely understood. However, there seems to be a consistent anatomical pattern of disc degeneration in the spine, with most changes occurring in the regions where mechanical stresses caused by spine movement take place.

References

1. Kirkaldy-Willis WH, Farfan HF. Instability of the lumbar spine. *Clin Orthop* 1982;165:110–123.
2. Videman T, Malmivaara A, Mooney V. The value of axial view in assessing diskograms. An experimental study with cadavers. *Spine* 1987;12:299–304.
3. Adams P, Eyre DR, Muir H. Biochemical aspects of development and aging of human lumbar intervertebral discs. *Rheumatol Rehab* 1977;16:22–29.
4. Lyons G, Eisenstein SM, Sweet MBE. Biochemical changes in in-

tervertebral disc degeneration. *Biochem Biophys Acta* 1981;673: 443–453.

5. Grynpas MD, Eyre DR, Kirschner DA. Collagen type II differs from type I in native molecular packing. *Biochem Biophys Acta* 1980;626: 346–355.

6. Brickley-Parsons D, Glimcher MJ. Is the chemistry of collagen in intervertebral discs an expression of Wolff's law? A study of the human lumbar spine. *Spine* 1984;9:148–163.

7. Garfin SR, Rydevik BL, Lipson SJ, et al. Spinal stenosis: pathophysiology. In: Herkowitz HN, Gartfin SR, Balderston RA, et al, eds. *Rothman-Simeone: The Spine*. Philadelphia: WB Saunders, 1999: 779–796.

8. Adams P, Muir H. Quantitative changes with age of proteoglycans of human lumbar disc. *Ann Rheum Dis* 1976;35:513–519.

9. Donohue PJ, Jahnke MR, Blaha JD, et al. Characterization of link proteins(s. from human intervertebral-disc tissues. *Biochem J* 1988; 251:739–747.

10. Kirkaldy-Willis WH, Wedge JH, Young-Hing K, et al. Pathology and pathogenesis of lumbar spondylosis and stenosis. *Spine* 1978;3: 319–328.

11. Rydevik B, Lundborg G, Bagge U. Effects of graded compression on intraneural blood flow. An in vivo study on rabbit tibial nerve. *J Hand Surg* 1981;6:3–12.

12. Rydevik B, Brown M, Lundborg G. Pathoanatomy and pathophysiology of nerve root compression. *Spine* 1984;9:7–15.

13. Rydevik B, Holm S, Brown MD, et al. Diffusion from the cerebrospinal fluid as a nutritional pathway for spinal nerve roots. *Acta Physiol Scand* 1990;138:247–248.

14. Cornefjord M, Olmarker K, Farley D, et al. Neuropeptide changes in compressed spinal nerve roots. *Spine* 1995;20:670–673.

15. McCarron RF, Wimpee MW, Hudkins P, et al. The inflammatory effect of nucleus pulposus; A possible element in the pathogenesis of low-back pain. *Spine* 1987;12:760–764.

16. Olmarker K, Rydevik B, Nordborg C. Autologous nucleus pulposus induces neurophysiologic and histological changes in porcine cauda equina nerve roots. *Spine* 1993;18:1425–1432.

17. Olmarker K. Experimental basis of sciatica. *J Orthop Sci* 1996;1: 230–242.

18. Olmarker K, Rydevik B, Nordborg C. Untrastructural changes in spinal nerve roots induced by autologous nucleus pulposus. *Spine* 1996;21:411–414.

19. Kayama S, Konno S, Olmarker K, et al. Incision of the annulus fibrosus induces nerve root morphologic, vascular and functional changes. *Spine* 1996;21:2539–2543.

20. Olmarker K, Byrod G, Cornefjord M, et al. Effects of methyl-prednisolone on nucleus pulposus-induced nerve root injury. *Spine* 1994; 19:1803–1808.

21. Rowlinson-Busza G, Maraveyas A, Epenetos AA. Effects of tumor necrosis factor on the uptake of specific and control monoclonal antibodies in a human tumor xenograft model. *Cr J Cancer* 1995; 71:660–665.

22. Myers RR. The pathogenesis of neuropathic pain. *Reg Anesthesia* 1995;20:173–184.

23. Posner I, White AA, Edwards WT, et al. A biomechanical analysis of the clinical stability of the lumbar and lumbosacral spine. *Spine* 1982;7:374–389.

24. Spengler D. Degenerative stenosis of the lumbar spine. Current concepts review. *J Bone Joint Surg Am* 1987;69:305–308.

25. Engel R, Bogduk N. The menisci of the lumbar zygapophyseal joints. *J Anat* 1982;135:795–809.

26. Taylor JR, Twomey LT. Age changes in lumbar zygapophyseal joints: observations on structure and function. *Spine* 1986;11:739–745.

27. Watanabe R, Parke WW. Vascular and neural pathology of lumbosacral spinal stenosis. *J Neurosurg* 1986;64:64–70.

28. Pennal GF, Schatzker J. Stenosis of the lumbar spinal canal. *Clin Neurosurg* 1971;18:86–105.

29. Lestini WF, Wiesel SW. The pathogenesis of cervical spondylosis. *Clin Orthop* 1989;239:69–93.

30. Schonstrom NS, Bolender NF, Spengler DM. The pathomorphology of spinal stenosis as seen on CT scans of the lumbar spine. *Spine* 1985;10:806–811.

31. Parke WW, Watanabe R. The intrinsic vasculature of the lumbosacral spinal nerve roots. *Spine* 1985;10:508–515.

32. Ahmed M, Bjurholm A, Kreicbergs A, et al. SP and CGRR-immunoreactive nerve fibers in the rat lumbar spine. *Neuro-Orthopedics* 1991; 12:19–28.

33. Cavanaugh J. Neural mechanisms of lumbar pain. *Spine* 1995;20: 1804–1809.

34. Chatani K, Kawakami M, Weinstein JN, et al. Characterization of thermal hyperalgesia, C-fos expression, and alterations in neuropeptides after mechanical irritation of the dorsal root ganglion. *Spine* 1995;20:277–290.

142. Acute Cervical Disc Herniation

Seth M. Zeidman

Acute disc herniation can occur with a tear in the annulus fibrosus. Deterioration of the nucleus leads to alterations in load distribution. This, in turn, alters the mechanics of the annulus, which may weaken, tear, and allow the nucleus to herniate or protrude. The degree of herniation ranges from slight bulging through a torn annulus to overt herniation through the posterior longitudinal ligament (PLL) with sequestration of nuclear material in the spinal canal or neural foramen. Herniation is most commonly posterolateral, causing nerve root compression, but may occur directly posteriorly, producing myelopathy.

Degenerative changes at a cervical disc level usually impinge on the nerve root exiting at the foramen bounded anteriorly by the disc (e.g., a C6-7 disc abnormality affects the C7 root). Compression occurs most commonly at the entrance or just medial to the foramen where the nerve roots pass immediately ventral to the superomedial edge of the superior articular process. Occasionally a herniated disc migrates laterally into the intervertebral foramen. The C5-6 and C6-7 disc levels are the most commonly involved sites causing radiculopathy; C4-5 and C7-T1 lesions are seen less frequently; and C3-4 lesions are distinctly uncommon.

The symptoms and signs produced are the result of nerve root compression, spinal cord compression, or both. Patients with cervical disc herniation typically present with one or more of the following symptoms: (a) neck pain, (b) brachialgia (i.e., root pain), (c) symptoms of upper-extremity nerve root neurological dysfunction, and (d) symptoms of spinal cord compression and dysfunction. Annual incidence of cervical radiculopathy is 83.2 per 100,000 population (1).

The natural history of radiculopathy and discogenic neck pain is less well defined. It has been suggested that many patients with radiculopathy improve with time and that devastating neurological consequences are distinctly uncommon. Most patients with neck pain (as many as 80%) improve with time; however, a subset of patients fail to improve. Acute radiculopathy from soft disc herniation are less likely to show spontaneous improvement, with as many as two-thirds of such patients having persistent symptoms.

Etiology

Cervical problems, particularly disc herniation, are not usually associated with a particular injury. Although acute trauma may play a role in the development of symptoms owing to an acutely herniated cervical disc and patients often attribute the onset of their symptoms to some particular event, many patients with neck or radicular pain but without recognized trauma develop unremitting symptoms, seemingly awakening one morning with pain. Most commonly, patients report awakening from sleep with noticeable neck and or arm pain, without identifiable trauma or other precipitating event.

Chronic injury caused by heavy labor also can result in cervical spine problems, although more often this is degenerative and less frequently acute disc herniation. In such a case, either the patient's history or imaging appearance of an older lesion leads the physician to postulate that the patient had an asymptomatic disc or osteophyte that became symptomatic because of some awkward posture during sleep or because of some minor, unnoticed event such as carrying a heavy load that transmitted traction to a nerve root.

Clinical Presentation

Root compression secondary to extruded disc material has the potential to result in neck and arm pain, motor weakness, sensory loss, and paresthesias. The most common symptom of a cervical disc herniation is neck pain that limits motion and is aggravated by extension. Looking up is avoided and bending the head down usually gives some relief. Pain also may radiate into one arm, in a pattern characteristic of the particular root involved. Patients often hold the arm elevated and behind the head, presumably because this maneuver reduces the tension on the nerve root and lessens the pain. Patients find relief with rotation of the head away from the symptomatic side.

Pain is commonly distributed proximally within the affected dermatome, and paresthesias more distally. Associated neck pain and decreased neck mobility generally are present. Diminished sensation in the appropriate dermatome and weakness and hyporeflexia in the appropriate myotome may be detected.

Sensory and motor deficits usually but not always are of equivalent severity.

Symptoms of myelopathy again may result from acute disc herniation. Uncommonly, severe spinal cord compression results in a complete lesion below the level of the herniation. Incomplete lesions are more frequent and include spastic paraparesis, central cord syndrome (painless weakness in the upper limbs with intact lower limbs), Brown-Séquard syndrome, and anterior cord syndrome (loss of motor and sensory function below the lesion, with preservation of dorsal column function) (2).

Other clinical manifestations of cervical disc disease may occur in addition to compression of neural structures. A syndrome of chronic neck pain, which also may include occipital, shoulder, and scapular region pain, has been described. Anteriorly projecting disc herniations can impinge on the esophagus and cause dysphagia.

Most of the symptoms of a disc herniation are related to pressure on a particular nerve roots (Table 1).

Diagnosis

As always, a careful history and physical examination are the first steps in diagnosis. The symptoms of a cervical disc herniation are always on the same side as the disc herniation. Some signs may help in aiding the physical diagnosis. These are very suggestive of cervical disc herniation when present, but frequently are absent in the presence of the disease. Spurling's sign refers to the reproduction or exacerbation of pain when downward pressure is applied to the head with the neck tilted toward the painful side and extended. This test is deemed positive if this reproduces the pain. With acute disc herniation, the test usually is positive, but it may be negative in more chronic cases. The reduction of pain when axial traction is applied to the head is also suggestive of a disc. Finally, in the shoulder abduction test raising the affected arm above the head reduces the pain.

Neck pain preceding the other symptoms helps distinguish this from shoulder pathology, thoracic outlet syndrome, cubital tunnel syndrome, tennis elbow, and de Quervain disease.

Myelopathy may result if the disc herniation compresses the spinal cord. Weakness in the hands and arms may be more generalized or bilateral, rather than confined to a root distribution. In addition, there may be leg weakness, usually manifested initially by a feeling of heaviness in the legs and noticeable difficulty in walking usual distances or up stairs. Examination

Table 1. Clinical Manifestations of Cervical Disc Herniation

Manifestation	Level of disc herniation			
	C4–5	C5–6	C6–7	C7-T1
Root	C5	C6	C7	C8
Motor Weakness	Deltoid (Biceps)	Biceps (Deltoid)	Triceps, wrist Extension	Hand intrinsics, wrist flexion ring, and little fingers
Sensory loss	Lateral shoulder	Lateral arm and forearm, thumb, and lateral aspect of index finger	Middle finger	
Diminished Reflex	Deltoid, Pectoralis	Biceps	Triceps	Finger flexion
Neck pain	Suprascapular	Suprascapular	Scapular/interscapular	Scapular/interscapular
Arm pain	None/Lateral upper arm	Lateral arm	Posterior arm	Medial arm

may show hyperactive reflexes, pathological reflexes, and a spastic gait. Finally, sphincter and sexual function may be compromised, usually later in the progression of myelopathy.

Lhermitte's sign refers to a sudden electrical sensation down the neck and back triggered by neck flexion. This was originally described in a patient with multiple sclerosis and dorsal column dysfunction. The conditions that can produce a Lhermitte's sign include: multiple sclerosis, cervical spondylotic disease, cervical disc herniation, spinal cord tumor, Chiari malformation, radiation myelopathy, and subacute combined degeneration (caused by vitamin B12 deficiency).

Electrodiagnostic studies are not essential for patients with a classic radicular syndrome, (e.g., pain in a roughly dermatomal distribution) and, when present, motor as well as sensory deficits in the same nerve root distribution. However, many patients do not present with a classic clinical syndrome, or the imaging studies do not match the clinical picture completely. Electrodiagnostic studies may be particularly helpful for diagnosing patients presenting in an atypical fashion. These patients include those presenting with weakness and atrophy in the absence of pain and patients who have spondylosis in addition to evidence of thoracic outlet compression or peripheral nerve entrapment (i.e., overlapping syndromes of the upper extremities). Evidence of denervation in a root distribution, with corresponding findings in the paravertebral axial musculature, is extremely helpful in confirming the diagnosis of radiculopathy. Appropriate studies also may help in the evaluation of peripheral nerve entrapment or thoracic outlet involvement.

Electromyography and nerve conduction studies are useful adjuncts in defining the extent and distribution of abnormalities and differentiating radiculopathy from other peripheral nerve lesions. Root lesions often cause limited clinical deficits, and electromyography can better define the extent and distribution of the abnormality. Noncompressive radiculopathies cannot be identified with radiological procedures. Similarly, the degree of physiological disturbance created by an apparent radiological deficit can be determined only with electromyography, because such defects may be relatively asymptomatic. Finally, certain peripheral nerve lesions clinically mimic radiculopathies, and this procedure is useful in differentiating these two entities.

Pathophysiologically, discogenic radiculopathies are compressive lesions that produce focal demyelination as well as wallerian degeneration in a portion of the fibers. Classic features of demyelination such as focal slowing and conduction block cannot be demonstrated because the roots are not amenable to stimulation above and just below the compressed segment.

Rather, the diagnosis of a radiculopathy depends primarily on needle examination findings related to wallerian degeneration (i.e., the occurrence of fibrillations and later motor unit potential changes suggestive of denervation occurring in a myotomal distribution). A reduction in the recruitment of motor unit potentials in the same distribution is caused by such axonal interruption and also by demyelination that results in conduction block.

Nerve conduction studies help exclude more peripheral lesions. Nerve conduction velocities rarely are abnormal in isolated radiculopathy. The demonstration of normal sensory responses is useful in localizing the lesion to the root level. In this regard, the useful sensory responses are the median with C6 and C7 symptoms; the ulnar with C8 symptoms; and the lateral antebrachial cutaneous with C6 symptoms. An appropriate response is not available for C5 fibers, and it may be difficult to distinguish a C5 root lesion from a lesion of the upper trunk of the brachial plexus. With severe C8 root lesions, conventional compound motor action potentials recorded from hand muscles may be of low amplitude (because of wallerian degeneration) and the motor nerve conduction velocities of these nerves be-

tween elbow and wrist may be mildly slowed. Root lesions at other levels cause no abnormalities of standard motor nerve conduction studies.

Similarly, measures of proximal conduction, such as F-wave analysis, also are of limited use. In a standard study, F waves are elicited only from the hand muscles and allow evaluation of the C8 root. Additionally, the abnormality in a short segment of nerve (i.e., the root) is diluted by the long stretch of nerves through which the F waves are conducted. Finally, although isolated abnormalities of F waves can occur with mild radiculopathies, they cannot be construed as definite evidence of a radiculopathy.

The earliest abnormality on needle examination is a reduction in recruitment in a myotomal distribution that occurs from the day of onset of symptoms. Fibrillations and positive waves develop after an appropriate interval (2 to 6 weeks), earlier in proximal than distal muscles of the myotome.

The occurrence of fibrillations in paraspinal muscles is evidence of a proximal location of the lesion, at the level of the roots or anterior horn cells. However, such activity tends to disappear over a short period of time (weeks or months). Thus, absence of fibrillations in paraspinal muscles does not preclude radiculopathy. Later in the course of a radiculopathy, the motor unit potentials show the characteristic denervation.

Radiographic Studies

If symptoms do not improve with nonoperative treatment or are very severe, an imaging study should be ordered. For the

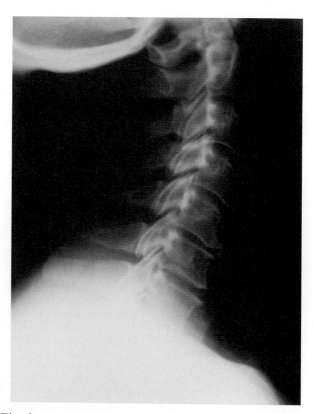

Fig. 1. Plain radiographs are the initial screening tools for evaluating a cervical disc herniation.

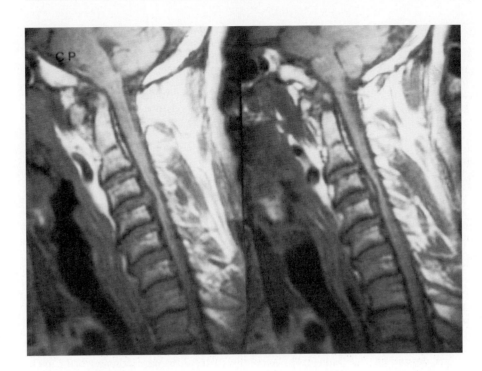

Fig. 2. MRI is the standard screening tool today for evaluating a cervical disc herniation.

evaluation of a patient with cervical radiculopathy or myelopathy, it is best to obtain plain x-rays of the cervical spine first, followed by magnetic resonance imaging (MRI) or myelography with a computed tomography (CT) scan.

The radiographic evaluation of a suspected spine disorder begins with plain radiographs. A herniated disc cannot be directly imaged radiographically; however, other associated changes may be seen, such as the bony ridges of cervical spondylosis. Plain cervical radiographs screen for pathology other than degenerative changes and reliably reveal abnormalities in sagittal alignment, canal narrowing, and congenital abnormalities, including cervical ribs and any other deformity. Lateral spinal x-rays can be obtained in a "dynamic mode," and the physician should request x-rays with flexion and extension views, as well as neutral position views. Oblique views should be included in every cervical spine x-ray study. The degree of facet arthropathy and uncovertebral joint abnormalities, size of the canal and neuroforamina, and extent of osteoporosis all can be assessed with plain radiographs (Fig. 1); however, if surgery is contemplated, then a more definitive study is required.

MRI is a very sensitive test for cervical disc herniation and has become the study of choice in most cases (3). Its superior resolution of soft tissues gives good definition of disc material, cord compression, and root compression. MRI provides physicians with a clearer understanding of the neural pathological processes associated with cervical disc herniation; however, physicians also have come to understand that abnormal MRI studies are not always associated with clinical abnormality. Although valuable in showing evidence of spinal cord and nerve root compression, MRI is less satisfactory for demonstrating abnormalities of bone, except for neoplasms or inflammatory processes (Fig. 2).

When bony detail is required, a CT myelogram should be obtained. This is more invasive than MRI and may produce effects such as headache, but in some cases may be essential in defining the anatomy. The CT myelogram allows more accurate delineation of the relationship between the neural elements and bony anatomy (4). It provides complementary data and is often essential in surgical planning. CT scanning should follow myelography. It provides the most accurate view of the spine in axial section; thin-section bone windows show the extent of neuroforaminal narrowing, facet joint disease, and osteophytic formation, whereas soft-tissue windows delineate disc and neural structures (Fig. 3). CT is most useful for detecting bony spondylitic spurs. The slice just cranial to the disc space generally is the most informative. Myelography should be considered in all instances in which the clinical picture and noninvasive diagnostic studies do not correlate anatomically. However, myelography is an invasive procedure involving the instillation of a foreign substance; therefore, it should be used only when the physician clearly determines its necessity.

It always should be remembered that disc protrusions are seen in 20% of asymptomatic patients 45 to 54 years old and in 57% in those over 64.

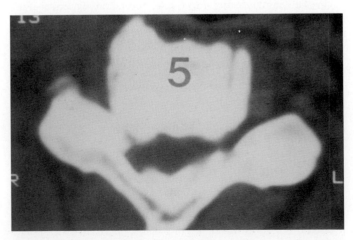

Fig. 3. CT myelography allows more accurate delineation of the relationship between the neural elements and the bony anatomy.

Treatment

The treatment of cervical disc herniation can be divided into two categories, nonoperative (conservative) and operative. In some rare cases of very large disc herniation causing significant pressure on the spinal cord, surgery may be considered the more conservative option.

NONOPERATIVE TREATMENTS. Nonoperative treatment modalities should be tried for every patient, unless the patient meets any of the absolute criteria for urgent surgery. In general, nonoperative management consists of maneuvers to reduce pressure on the nerve root. Immobilization with the neck in a flexed forward position may be helpful. Tethering of a nerve root over a protruded disc or osteophyte results in continued nerve root irritation and presumably increases the degree of root inflammation and edema, which can result in prolongation of pain and symptomatology. Root irritation will be minimized to the extent that a cervical collar restricts neck motion. Some collars or braces are more effective than others; soft collars provide little support or restriction of movement.

Physical therapy can include traction, stretching, strengthening maneuvers, exercise, heat, ice, gentle massage, and ultrasound. These can be using in various combinations, depending on the patient and all help to relieve neck and shoulder pain secondary to nerve root irritation. Physical therapy facilitates restoration of motor function following root compression treated with or without surgery. Straining and forceful neck manipulation should be avoided.

A course of home cervical traction often is beneficial. Daily home traction is more effective than traction administered only in conjunction with physical therapy, which most patients attend no more than three times per week. Cervical traction immobilizes the neck and decompresses the nerve roots by increasing the volume of the neural foramina. Traction can be very effective in relieving both axial and radicular pain, especially when the symptoms are acute. Improper use of the traction apparatus can result in failure or even exacerbation of pain. Traction should place the head and neck in a neutral or slightly flexed position; neck extension narrows the foramina and can aggravate symptoms. Twelve pounds of traction applied for 20 minutes three times a day are generally necessary to provide a fair test of the benefits of traction.

With rest and nonsteroidal antiinflammatory drugs (NSAIDs), the overwhelming majority of patients (up to 95%) with acute cervical radiculopathy from disc herniation experience improvement or resolution of pain without the need for surgical intervention.

Epidural steroid injections can be performed in the cervical region using a posterior approach through the ligamentum flavum. However, this procedure is not widely used because the spinal cord occupies the cervical vertebral canal, and most practitioners are unwilling to risk cord injury. Nevertheless, the procedure can be undertaken safely in well-trained hands, more so if done with radiographic guidance.

The literature on cervical epidural steroids is limited, however. The procedure was first mentioned anecdotally in 1972 (5), but no literature appears to follow until the 1980s. One brief report claims excellent to complete pain relief for over 4 months in 14 out of 95 patients (6). Subsequent reports have all been uncontrolled, retrospective reviews of experience. In patients with cervical pain, greater than 75% relief of pain has been reported in "most" of 45 patients (7), 16 of 25 cases (8), 18% of 96 patients reviewed out of an original sample of 155 (9), 38% of 40 patients (10), and 42% of 33 patients (11).

No controlled studies have been conducted on cervical epidural steroids; and in the absence of any greater documented clinical experience, the value of this procedure remains unproved. The striking aspect of these figures is the low percentage of patients obtaining substantial relief in the majority of studies; sometimes less than would be expected as a placebo response.

Repeated use of corticosteroids is not recommended; most practitioners who inject corticosteroids epidurally limit these injections to at most three over a given period, as dictated by the recurrence of pain. Finally, although a relatively safe procedure in experienced hands, serious complications have been reported, including epidural hematoma, root injury, and spinal cord injury (7,9,11).

MEDICATIONS. Four major categories of medications are useful in the treatment of patients with neck and radicular pain: analgesics, NSAIDs, muscle relaxants, and corticosteroids. These medications may be used together; the specific type of medication and frequency of use are determined by the severity of the patient's pain.

In the acute situation, analgesics are best used on a continuous rather than an "as-needed" basis. The amount of medication used should be sufficient to produce pain relief; incomplete relief may result in muscle splinting, which can then produce further pain. According to the physician's judgment of the intensity of pain, acetaminophen without or with codeine, hydrocodone, or oxycodone with acetaminophen may be used at recommended doses. Rarely, the physician needs to prescribe oral hydromorphone or meperidine either because of a patient's sensitivity to medication or the severity of pain. It is preferable to substitute non-narcotic medications for narcotics as soon as feasible.

NSAIDs often are an important adjunct in the management of pain associated with cervical radiculopathy. The patient's previous experience with these medications sometimes is a helpful guide to a specific drug. Many of these drugs produce gastric irritation, and an H2-receptor antagonist (e.g., ranitidine) should be prescribed for the sensitive patient along with NSAIDs.

Muscle relaxants are particularly useful for the relief of neck muscle spasm. Methocarbamol, cyclobenzaprine, and low doses of diazepam are useful alternatives; diazepam is reserved for more severe or protracted muscle spasm. These medications tend to have some central depressant effects; therefore, appropriate precautions regarding activity should be instituted.

A trial of oral corticosteroid therapy may be helpful for patients with very severe radicular pain. Either dexamethasone or methylprednisolone can be given in rapidly decreasing daily oral dose levels; methylprednisolone is available in a diminishing daily dosage formulation (Medrol Dose Pak). Use of an H2-receptor antagonist generally is recommended to prevent gastric ulcer formation.

TRANSCUTANEOUS ELECTRICAL NERVE STIMULATION. Patients with chronic neck and cervical nerve root pain may be helped by a transcutaneous electrical nerve stimulation (TENS) unit. The exact mechanism of action of the TENS unit is unknown. One theory is that it activates analgesia-producing areas in the brainstem; another proposes that the spinal gating mechanism is activated. A TENS unit also may inhibit peripheral small myelinated nerve fibers that are believed to be important in pain conduction. The unit generally may be rented for a trial period and initially should be applied by someone experienced with the device. Optimum placement of the electrodes by trial and error is very important. A trial of 2 weeks is recommended to determine whether a patient responds. No adverse side effects from this form of pain therapy are recognized, except for local irritation of skin from the conducting jelly or the adhesive tape holding the contact pads.

SURGICAL THERAPY

Indications. In general terms, surgical treatment for cervical radiculopathy is indicated if symptoms and signs correspond to a radiographically demonstrable site of nerve root compression in a patient whose symptoms have been refractory to a reasonable period of conservative therapy (e.g., 3 months). Because nonoperative therapy is applicable only in the elective situation, it is desirable to define the criteria for surgical intervention more precisely. In most patients, cervical disc disease is not life threatening, and surgery for the neurological conditions related to this spinal disorder is considered elective. Situations in which little, if any, disagreement exists regarding the necessity for surgery, provided that there is no major medical contraindication include the following.

It is impossible to state categorically when conservative treatment should be abandoned and surgery undertaken, and each patient should be assessed individually. When the physician recommends traction, physical therapy, and medical therapy, a time frame should be agreed on with the patient. In general, if a trend to improvement is not evident within 4 to 6 weeks of intensive therapy, a patient probably will not improve with further nonsurgical treatment, and surgery should be considered. However, if an acute disc herniation has occurred, causing unbearable pain, significant motor weakness, or progressive sensory deficit, earlier surgery may be warranted.

Surgery is reserved for patients who exhibit the signs and symptoms that require urgent decompression, patients who cannot or do not wish to spend the time to allow nonoperative approaches to work, and patients who have failed nonoperative management after a reasonable amount of time (6 to 8 weeks). Certainly, surgery is unwarranted if improvement is occurring. The presence, severity, and rate of progression of any neurological deficit, along with the duration of symptoms, are considerations when surgery is contemplated. Surgery is only indicated when symptoms worsen or fail to improve, but it also should be considered when there is significant compression of the spinal cord with signs of cord dysfunction. The best surgical results for myelopathy and radiculopathy have been reported to occur when symptoms have been of relatively short duration.

Operative intervention for radiculopathy has a low risk of serious sequelae (1%), but still must be balanced against the natural history. When nerve root compression has been demonstrated radiologically, a favorable surgical outcome can be expected in more than 90% of patients. Favorable surgical results also are reported for myelopathy. A favorable result from an isolated central disc herniation is obtained in 80% of patients.

If pain, weakness, or the sensory deficit is not severe, the indications for surgical intervention may be less obvious. Indications include: (a) chronic or frequently recurrent episodes of pain, motor, or sensory symptoms; (b) unacceptable lifestyle owing to activity restrictions necessary to minimize symptoms; (c) unacceptable lifestyle because of the need for medication, which may have undesirable side effects; and (d) failure of nonoperative therapy.

Pain that is disabling, requiring levels of medication that interfere with a person's work and personal life, or pain that does not respond to physical measures such as bed rest and traction usually leads a patient to seek relief as soon as possible. The response of such patients to appropriate surgical intervention often is immediate and dramatic.

Recovery of lost motor function owing to nerve root compression often is slow and may be incomplete. The prognosis for recovery of motor function is worse the longer the weakness has been allowed to persist, the more severe the weakness (particularly when associated with muscle atrophy), and in older patients. Because recovery may be incomplete and leave a patient with severe physical disability (e.g., hand weakness or inability to abduct the shoulder), evidence of progressive or significant weakness that shows no trend toward improvement indicates surgical decompression of the involved nerve root or roots.

Severe sensory impairment, particularly if it involves the hands, similarly can be very disabling, with respect to both a person's work and his or her activities of daily living. The same considerations regarding duration and severity of deficit that were just noted apply to sensory impairment. Persistent and significant deficits of pain sensation, light touch, and joint sensation should not be left untreated for too long, lest they become permanent.

The refractory nature of impaired sphincter control function and other manifestations of spinal cord compression, such as spasticity, is well known. In spondylotic cervical myelopathy, disabling spasticity may involve not only the lower limbs, but also the hands. Fortunately, prompt and effective decompression of the spinal cord often is followed by some improvement, although complete reversal of symptoms frequently does not occur depending on the severity of symptoms.

VERY ACUTE ONSET OF SEVERE DEFICIT. The recovery potential of neural tissue subjected to acute compression is significantly worse than the potential for recovery with equally severe but very gradual compression. Thus, severe motor and sensory deficits of acute onset may reflect an acute compressive mechanism, such as an acute disc herniation. Decompressive surgery is indicated unless prompt evidence of improvement appears following institution of generally effective treatment measures. This is especially true with myelopathic rather than radiculopathic deficits.

Surgical Approaches. A range of surgical options is available to treat cervical disc disease. Carefully delineating the patient's clinical problem and its causes, carefully selecting criteria for surgery, and matching the procedure to the disease for each patient obtain optimum results.

The surgeon must decide between an anterior and posterior approach and among several options with either approach. A number of factors must be considered in selecting the appropriate operative procedure, including the site of maximal neural compression, presence of deformity or instability, potential morbidity, and experience of the surgeon. Surgery for cervical disc herniation generally is divided into two approaches, anterior and posterior.

ANTERIOR VERSUS POSTERIOR APPROACHES. Whether to selection an anterior or a posterior approach is one of the most vigorously debated topics in neurosurgery. The results of surgical treatment of radiculopathy caused by a soft lateral disc herniation appear equally favorable for both anterior discectomy and posterior foraminotomy, with success rates of more than 90% for each (12).

However, in most patients with cervical disc disease, the compressive lesion lies anterior to the nerve root or spinal cord. because the disc is located in front of the spinal cord, the anterior approach often is more direct. Selection of the optimal technique to surgically treat a herniated cervical disc should be based on the location and type of the lesion. In general, soft lateral discs easily can be removed by a posterior approach; more paramedian discs should be removed via an anterior approach.

For anterior procedures, the patient is supine, with the neck neutral slightly extended. Posterior procedures may be performed with the patient either prone or sitting. The sitting position has fallen out of favor, principally because of concerns regarding air embolism and cardiovascular instability; however, this position offers significant advantages, including diminished venous engorgement and drainage of blood from the operative field (13). The neck is held in a neutral or slightly flexed position with the head held firmly with cranial pin fixation.

ANTERIOR APPROACHES. The most common anterior procedure is the anterior cervical discectomy and fusion (ACDF) (14). A transverse incision is made in the neck, usually just to the left of the midline. For a one- or two-level procedure, a transverse incision usually suffices, in a skin crease at the appropriate level extending from the midline to the body of the sternocleidomastoid muscle. For more extensive procedures, a vertical or "carotid" incision along the medial border of the sternocleidomastoid muscle may facilitate exposure.

The location of the incision can be determined by palpating the cricoid cartilage, which lies at the level of the C6 vertebral body, and Chassaignac's tubercle on the transverse process of C6; alternatively, use of intraoperative fluoroscopy allows precise location of the incision.

The approach may be from either the right or left side. The right side usually is more comfortable for right-handed surgeons, although the recurrent laryngeal nerve is at greater risk than when the approach is from the left side, particularly at lower levels (C6-7, C7-T1). The skin incision should be continued through the platysma, which is elevated and divided sharply. The anterior border of the sternocleidomastoid muscle must be identified and the fascia investing this muscle incised. A combination of blunt and sharp dissection allows formation of an atraumatic plane to be developed between the strap muscles and sternocleidomastoid, with entrance into the middle cervical fascia. This should be carried down to the prevertebral fascia. Identification of the paired longus colli muscles allows identification of the anterior surface of the cervical spine. However, intraoperative identification with an x-ray or fluoroscope to localize a beaded or bent spinal needle in a disc space is mandatory. Once the proper level is identified, the longus colli is mobilized laterally with subperiosteal dissection to allow placement of self-retaining retractors and facilitate complete discectomy. The disc is removed in its entirety with complete resection of the cartilaginous end plates but preservation of the bony end plates. Magnification should be used for decompression; the microscope is recommended, but a headlight and loupes are acceptable. The posterior longitudinal ligament should be opened and resected from one uncovertebral joint to the other to allow identification of disc fragments that have penetrated the PLL. Opening of the PLL is the only way to visualize the dura and ensure complete decompression with removal of all sequestered disc fragments. Any bleeding should be controlled with bipolar coagulation of the PLL edges or tiny pieces of hemostatic agents. The end plates should be either burred enough to allow slight bleeding or punctured with a curette to allow blood vessels to grow into the graft. Placement of pin distractors allows gentle disc space distraction that facilitates discectomy and allows placement of a precisely sized graft that is under compression. A precisely sized graft of either iliac crest autograft or allograft should be placed and countersunk 2 or 3 mm. It is essential not to place the graft too far posterior so that it does not impinge on the thecal sac or spinal cord. Generally cervical plate fixation is used to facilitate fusion (Fig. 4). After graft and/or plate placement, the wound should be irrigated and the platysma and skin closed. Immediately postoperatively, the patient should be checked for any new neurological deficits, and an x-ray should be taken to confirm graft and plate placement. Usually, the patient can return to work 3 to 4 weeks postoperatively. Follow-up x-rays should be performed at 1, 3, and 6 months postoperatively to confirm incorporation of the bone graft. Patients may be placed in a fitted cervical collar for up to 4 weeks.

Postoperatively, patients are ambulatory on the evening of surgery. Discomfort in swallowing, from esophageal retraction, occurs commonly and is mild and transient. Patients are usually discharged home that evening or the next day.

Some surgeons perform anterior cervical discectomy without fusion. Nonfusion prevents complications such as graft extrusion, absorption, nonunion, and donor site problems. However, these patients are prone to angulation deformity, disc space collapse with nerve root compression, and increased postoperative and interscapular pain.

Although the probability of serious complications after anterior procedures is low (less than 2%), a number can occur (15). Structures at risk include the recurrent laryngeal nerve, particularly with right-sided approaches, although this is nearly always transient. The esophagus, trachea and larynx, carotid artery, jugular vein, and cervical sympathetic chain are at risk for retraction injury. A dural tear and CSF leak may occur. This can usually be treated with a small piece of thrombin soaked Gelfoam. If this does not work, patching the defect with fat or fascia, and fibrin glue, and a period of lumbar drainage are recommended. Wound infection may occur, but this is uncommon with the use of perioperative antibiotics.

The vertebral artery may be injured if disc or osteophyte removal, particularly with the high-speed burr, is carried too far laterally. Spinal cord or nerve root injury is the most serious complication. Fortunately, this type of injury is rare, and the occurrence of permanent neurological damage is less than .2%. Improvement in symptoms of neck and arm pain is seen in about 90%.

POSTERIOR APPROACH. A small amount of bone is removed from the back of the spine over the affected nerve root in this operation. The patient is positioned prone with face in a headrest, and the neck flexed. The shoulders are retracted inferiorly with tape. Gentle retraction of the involved root often may allow removal of a soft disc (16).

LAMINOFORAMINOTOMY. Nerve root decompression may be accomplished by laminoforaminotomy at the appropriate level. Initially beginning with removal of one or more hemilaminae, Scoville developed the keyhole approach, which is generally in use today. This is performed in the sitting position for the reasons outlined in the preceding.

We use a posterior paramedian approach to perform a laminoforaminotomy. This approach uses a muscle-splitting incision, with dissection of the muscles from the region of the laminae and facet. The incision for a single-level laminoforaminotomy is only a few centimeters long, and is essential a localizing radiograph (Fig. 5). The laminae and facet joints are exposed at the appropriate level on the side being decompressed, and a self-retaining retractor is placed. A high-speed drill is used to burr away one third to one half of the superior and inferior laminae adjacent to the facet joint. Fine curettes and 1- and 2-mm Kerrison punches remove the thin shelf of bone. The medial one third to one half of the facet joint is then drilled away, followed by fine curettes and punches. Preserving half of the facet joint prevents instability. The ligamentum flavum is opened with a fine sharp blade and excised, exposing the lateral edge of the dural sac and nerve root. An overlying layer of epidural "pseudodura," which may contain a network of veins, often must be coagulated and swept away. The axilla of the nerve root is identified and gently retracted in a cephalad direction. A blunt nerve hook is used to explore beneath the nerve root. Any free disc fragments can be mobilized and extracted. Toothed forceps usually are adequate to remove the disc fragments. If the problem is a disc protrusion without herniation through the PLL, we incise the PLL with a sharp, pointed blade while the nerve root is retracted superiorly, always cutting away

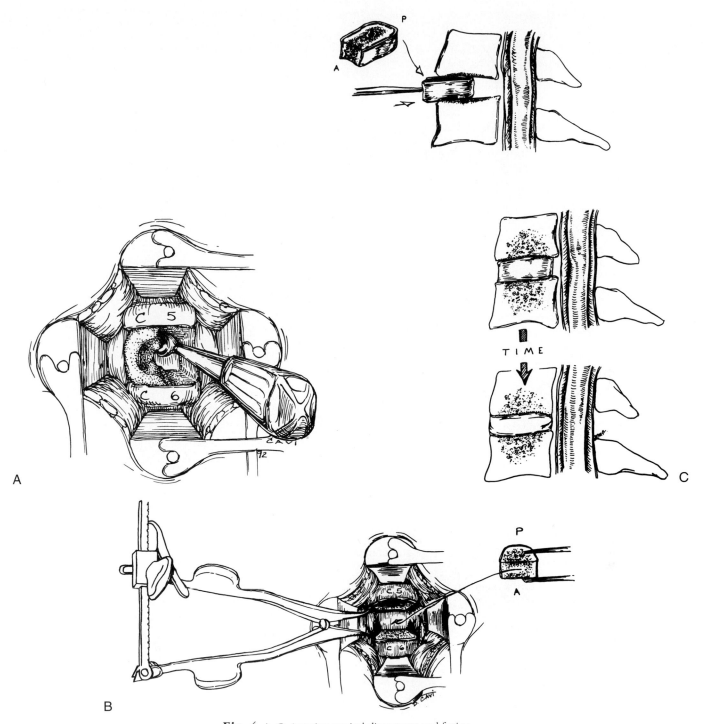

Fig. 4. A–C: Anterior cervical discectomy and fusion.

from the nerve root and dura. Disc fragments can be swept out with a blunt nerve hook. It is unnecessary to remove large amounts of disc material or to curette the disc space, as would be done with a lumbar discectomy, although the surgeon must be satisfied that no compressive fragments are left behind. Following the decompression, the wound is closed in multiple layers.

The patient is ambulatory the night of surgery. Narcotic analgesia and muscle relaxers may be required for the first 24 to 48 hours after surgery. After laminoforaminotomy, most patients can be discharged the next day and can return to work

in 2 to 3 weeks. Heavy manual work and sports can be resumed after 6 to 8 weeks.

Results of Treatment of Cervical Disc Disease and Spondylosis

No systematic review comparing the effects of conservative treatment and surgery has been performed for patients with

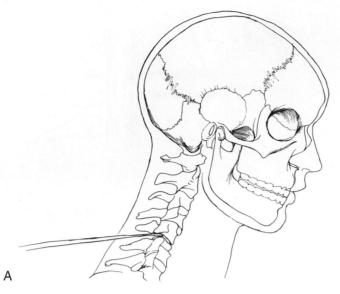

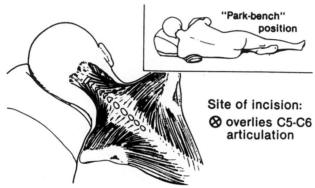

Fig. 5. **A–C:** Laminoforaminotomy.

"Park-bench" position

Site of incision:
⊗ **overlies C5-C6 articulation**

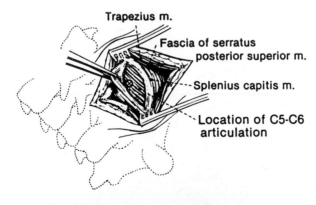

Trapezius m.

Fascia of serratus posterior superior m.

Splenius capitis m.

Location of C5-C6 articulation

Laminotomy site

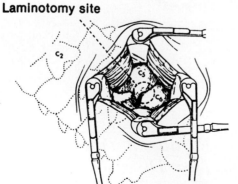

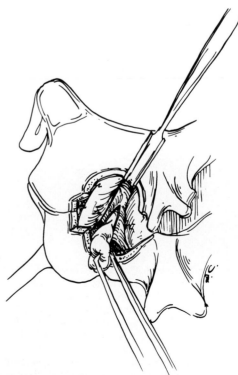

A

B

C

neck pain and radiculopathy. One nonblinded randomized clinical trial compared surgery with physical therapy or cervical immobilization with a collar. Participants were reassessed at 12 months. Although the surgery group had more rapid pain reduction, there was no difference between the groups at 1-year follow-up (17).

Patients with radiculopathy caused by nerve root compression demonstrable by imaging techniques respond well to surgical treatment, regardless of whether the approach is anterior or posterior. Numerous other series report the same outcome in more than 90% of their patients, both with anterior and posterior approaches (12,14).

Matsumoto and co-workers evaluated the outcome of conservative treatment for patients with mild myelopathy caused by cervical soft disc herniation. Twenty-seven patients with mild cervical myelopathy secondary to cervical soft disc herniation were treated nonoperatively with cervical bracing and restriction of daily activities. Of the 27 patients, 17 underwent nonoperative treatment only, which improved their neurological deficits, whereas the other 10 ultimately underwent decompression surgery because of neurological deterioration. Conservative treatment proved to be an effective treatment for mild cervical myelopathy caused by cervical soft disc herniation (18).

References

1. Radhakrishnan K, Litchy WJ, O'Fallon WM, et al. Epidemiology of cervical radiculopathy. A population-based study from Rochester, Minnesota, 1976 through 1990. *Brain* 1994;117:325–335.
2. Rumana CS, Baskin DS. Brown-Sequard syndrome produced by cervical disc herniation: case report and literature review. *Surg Neurol* 1996;45:359–361.
3. Van de Kelft E, van Vyve M. Diagnostic imaging algorithm for cervical soft disc herniation. *J Neurol Neurosurg Psychiatry* 1994;57:724–728.
4. Sprung C, Fabian A. Pitfalls in computed tomography of the cervical and lumbar spine. *Neurosurg Rev* 1994;17:19–28.
5. Winnie A, Hartman J, Meyers H, et al. Pain clinic 11: intradural and extradural corticosteroids for sciatica. 1972. *Anesthesiol Analg* 1972;51:990–1003.
6. Shulman M, Nimmagadda U, Valenta A. Cervical epidural steroid injection for pain of cervical spine origin. *Anesthesiology* 1984;61:A223.
7. Catchlove R, Braha R. The use of cervical epidural nerve blocks in the management of chronic head and neck pain. *Can Anaesth Soc J* 1984;31:188–191.
8. Rowlingson J, Kirschenbaum L. Epidural analgesic techniques in the management of cervical pain. *Anesthesiol Analg* 1986;65:938–942.
9. Shulman M. Treatment of neck pain with cervical epidural steroid injection. *Regional Anesthesiol* 1986;11:92–94.
10. Mangar D, Thomas P. Epidural steroid injections in the treatment of cervical and lumbar pain syndromes. *Regional Anesthesiol* 1991;16:246.
11. Purkis I. Cervical epidural steroids. *Pain Clin* 1986;1:3–7.
12. Rushton SA, Albert TJ. Cervical degenerative disease: rationale for selecting the appropriate fusion technique (anterior, posterior, and 360 degree). *Orthop Clin North Am* 1998;29:755–777.
13. Zeidman SM, Ducker TB. Posterior cervical laminoforaminotomy for radiculopathy: review of 172 cases. *Neurosurgery* 1993;33:356–362.
14. Whitecloud TS. Modern alternatives and techniques for one-level discectomy and fusion. *Clin Orthop* 1999;359:67–76.
15. Zeidman SM, Ducker TB, Raycroft J. Trends and complications in cervical spine surgery: 1989–1993. *J Spinal Disord* 1997;10:523–526.
16. Ducker TB, Zeidman SM. The posterior operative approach for cervical radiculopathy. *Neurosurg Clin North Am* 1993;4:61–74.
17. Persson LC, Moritz U, Brandt L, et al. Cervical radiculopathy: pain, muscle weakness and sensory loss in patients with cervical radiculopathy treated with surgery, physiotherapy or cervical collar. A prospective, controlled study. *Eur Spine J* 1997;6:256–266.
18. Matsumoto M, Chiba K, Ishikawa M, et al. Relationships between outcomes of conservative treatment and magnetic resonance imaging findings in patients with mild cervical myelopathy caused by soft disc herniations. *Spine* 2001;26:1592–1598.

143. Cervical Spondylosis with Radiculopathy and Myelopathy

Donald A. Smith, Evan M. Packer, and David W. Cahill

Cervical radiculopathy and myelopathy is a common clinical problem usually defined by stereotypic patterns of pain referral and neurological deficit conforming to the distribution of an affected nerve root or spinal cord level. The pathophysiology is unclear but mechanical deformation, inflammation, and vascular insufficiency are factors that have been implicated in its pathogenesis (1,2). Neuroimaging studies frequently reveal a putative cause: nerve root or cord impingement by a cervical disc herniation or osteophytic "spur." Osteophytic spurs are typical of the degenerative changes in the spine encountered in cervical spondylosis. Spondylosis is characterized by disc space narrowing and the formation of bony overgrowth at the vertebral endplates and facet joints, which may compress the exiting nerve root either within the lateral spinal canal or neural foramen (2–6). When accompanied by appropriate signs and symptoms this condition is termed cervical spondylotic radiculopathy (CSR). CSR exists on a continuum of degenerative disc pathology. At one end of this continuum is the so-called acute "soft" disc herniation. At the other end of this continuum CSR merges with the condition of cervical spondylotic myelopathy (CSM). CSM exists when spinal cord compression results in long track signs of disinhibition and spinal cord dysfunction. In this chapter we review the pertinent pathological anatomy, clinical presentation, and diagnosis of CSR and CSM.

History

The pathoanatomical description of cervical spondylosis and delineation of stenosis-associated clinical syndromes of radiculopathy and myelopathy were thoroughly detailed in the reports of Brain and Frykholm in the 1940s and 1950s (3,5). Pioneering neurosurgeons of that era proposed laminoforaminotomy as the primary surgical treatment of cervical disc disease with radiculopathy and myelopathy (7). By the late 1950s a significant clinical experience with these procedures had been amassed (8–10). At this same time surgical techniques were rapidly evolving, and anterior approaches to the cervical spine emphasizing restitution of intervertebral height and interbody fusion were advocated (11,12). Revolutionary advances in microprocessor technology in the 1970s and 1980s fostered development of computed tomography (CT) and magnetic resonance imaging (MRI). CT and MRI have significantly advanced our knowledge of the pathological anatomy of spondylosis in both symptomatic and asymptomatic populations and have enhanced the accuracy of clinical diagnosis (13). Whether by an anterior or posterior approach, the surgical treatment of CSR and CSM is among the most commonly performed spinal procedures.

Pathological Anatomy

Paired neural foramina are at each intervertebral level. In the cervical spine these transmit the nerve roots that correspond numerically with the inferior adjacent vertebra; therefore, the C4-5 foramen transmits the C5 nerve root. The neural foramen is bounded superiorly and inferiorly by the pedicles of the adjacent vertebrae. Anteriorly it is bordered by the cervical disc, uncovertebral joints (joints of Luschka), and portions of the vertebral bodies. Posteriorly it is framed by the facet (zygapophyseal) joint and adjacent lateral masses. Lying just medial to the neural foramen within the spinal canal proper is the thecal sac. Cervical nerve roots take a nearly horizontal course from the thecal sac to transit the neural foramen. Approximately one-third of the cross-sectional area of the foramen is occupied by the nerve root and radicular vessels that course with it; the remainder is filled with epidural fat.

Cervical spondylosis is a degenerative process thought to originate from degradation of the hydrophilic proteoglycan matrix of the nucleus pulposus of the intervertebral disc (2). The pathophysiology of spondylosis is reviewed elsewhere in this volume. It appears to be a nearly universal age-related phenomenon in Western populations (3,13–15). Desiccation of the nucleus leads to disc space narrowing and annular bulging. Over time marginal osteophyte formation develops at the point of Sharpey's fiber insertion into the vertebral endplates. Exuberant osteophytic "spurs" may also arise in relation to the uncovertebral joints. With loss of intervertebral height, the neural foramen becomes narrowed in a rostral-caudal dimension, and a larger burden of axial load-bearing may simultaneously shift posteriorly onto the facet joint complexes. In time this may lead to facet degeneration, spur formation, ligamentous thickening, and instability. The nerve root or spinal cord may be compressed within the neural foramen or canal by bulging disc material, marginal osteophytes, uncovertebral spurs, facet arthropathy, hypertrophic ligamentum flavum, or as the result of degenerative instability (3,4). The likelihood of symptomatic compression on the basis of these acquired factors is increased in the presence of an underlying congenital spinal stenosis (16).

Clinical Presentation and Diagnosis

Cervical spondylosis is nearly universal in the aging population. Analysis of neuroimaging studies in asymptomatic individuals

suggests a prevalence of disc degeneration of almost 60% after the age of 40 (13). "Major findings" of discal or foraminal stenosis were detected in 28% of asymptomatic individuals above the age of 40 in that study. A retrospective population-based study from Rochester, Minnesota with high levels of case ascertainment defined an overall annualized age-adjusted incidence of cervical radiculopathy of .83% (17). Peak incidence occurred at 50 to 55 years with an annual incidence more than twice that defined for the general population. Acute disc herniations and spondylosis are by far the leading causes of cervical radiculopathy and myelopathy, although the relative contribution of each is less clear. In the Rochester study 22% of cases were attributed to "disc protrusions," and nearly 70% resulted from "cervical spondylosis, disc, or both." Males accounted for about 60% of cases.

Cervical radiculopathy is characterized clinically by familiar patterns of cervical-brachial pain and neurological deficit. Multiple reports indicate that the C7 root is most commonly affected (40% to 70%); C6 is implicated in about 20% to 40% of cases; C5 and C8 individually and combinations of C5-6 or C6-7 are involved in 5% to 10% of cases each (8,17–20). These studies do not systematically distinguish cervical radiculopathy caused by acute disc herniations from that caused by spondylosis. Apart from the acuity of onset, little information exists to distinguish the pain caused by "soft disc" herniations from that associated with spondylosis. Because spondylosis is often bilateral and affects multiple levels of the spine (2,18), pain in CSR may be more diffuse than in symptomatic acute disc herniations, which are overwhelmingly confined to one level. The onset of pain may be either acute or insidious, and may or may not be triggered by an obvious trauma (2–4).

Nonspecific pains are commonly referred to the neck, shoulder, scapula, interscapular region, anterior chest wall, or breast, and may be aggravated by the assumption of particular neck postures. Although the source of these pains is indefinite, provocation studies reveal that stimulation of nociceptors within the disc annulus, vertebral periosteum, joint capsules, and ligaments as well as pressure on the cervical nerve roots themselves can reproduce or intensify pre-existing pains of like quality in similar distributions. However, annoying such complaints may be, they are not specific for cervical radiculopathy and lack dependable localizing value. The musculoskeletal examination often reveals nonspecific reduced range of motion in the cervical spine and tenderness or spasm of the paraspinal muscles

The clinical suspicion of cervical radiculopathy is strengthened by symptoms suggesting a "radiating" quality to the pain, projecting proximally from the neck or shoulder into the humerus or forearm in a stereotypic fashion. Radiating pains of this sort frequently signify nerve root irritation and have localizing value. The pain itself lacks a specific character apart from its distribution, and descriptors such as "sharp," "shooting," "aching," "electric," "knifelike," and even "burning" are reported commonly. The pain accompanying a C5 radiculopathy is frequently referred to the lateral humerus. C6 pain often is reported in the radial forearm; C7 pain is experienced in the posterior humerus and forearm; C8 pain is referred to the medial humerus and forearm. Rarely does the pain extend to the hand. Paresthesiae also may have localizing significance and overlap the brachial pain distributions, respecting well-characterized dermatomal patterns. Paresthesiae in the lateral humerus speak for C5 root irritation. Paresthesiae in the radial forearm and hand usually are associated with a C6 lesion, whereas paresthesiae of the central fingers refer to C7, and ulnar hand paresthesiae indicate a C8 radiculopathy. A positive neck compression test ("Spurling maneuver") is said to have high specificity, although relatively low sensitivity in the diagnosis of cervical radiculopathy. This test is performed by extending the neck and rotating the head toward the side of the symptomatic limb. A positive

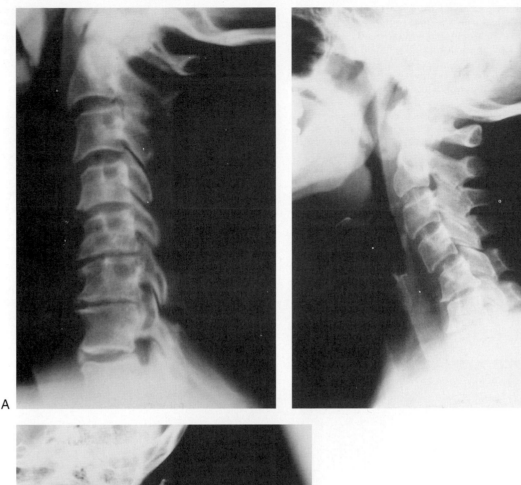

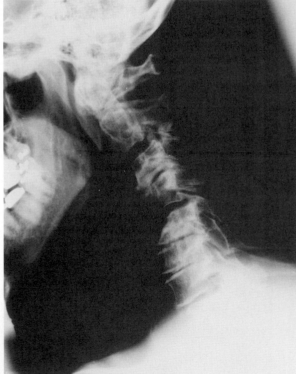

Fig. 1. Although plain radiographs sometimes do not correlate with clinical suspicion, they are very useful for surgical planning. The patient with a loss of lordosis secondary to collapse of the C5-6 and C6-7 disc spaces **(A)**, the patient with frank kyphosis and multisegmental disease **(B)**, and the patient with the swan neck deformity **(C)** all presented with C6 radiculopathy. Plain film information, often with dynamic films, is complementary to MRI and CT data.

result consists of intensification of radiating pain or paresthesiae in a dermatomal distribution on manual application of light axial compression to the head. Spontaneously occurring pain sometimes is alleviated by abduction of an affected limb over the head.

Motor involvement is stated to be the strongest localizing sign. Weakness concentrated in the deltoid, supraspinatus and infraspinatus, and to a lesser degree in the biceps and brachioradialis implies a C5 radiculopathy. The sixth cervical myotome dominates biceps and brachioradialis function, and also contributes strongly to functional wrist extension. C6 radiculopathy usually is associated with reduced biceps and brachioradialis reflexes. C7 radiculopathy causes weakness of triceps muscle, reduced wrist and finger extensors, and a diminished triceps reflex. Both C6 and C7 radiculopathy may present with scapular "winging." C8 and T1 roots are implicated by involvement of the intrinsic hand musculature. In advanced cases atrophy and fasciculations of involved muscles may become evident. Deviations from these "classic" patterns of radiculopathy are not infrequent and have been ascribed to anomalous innervation, overlapping cervical dermatomal and myotomal anatomy, and a pre- or post-fixed brachial plexus (2,19,20). Clinically recognizable radiculopathy of the C3 and C4 nerve roots rarely is encountered.

Cervical spondylotic myelopathy is characterized by a clinical syndrome that includes gait instability, hand clumsiness, numbness, or bowel/bladder disturbances. This is often insidious in its progression. Gait disturbance and instability also can accompany the syndrome of CSM. The level of cord compression determines the level of motor dysfunction.

The clinical diagnosis of cervical radiculopathy and myelopathy is founded on careful history and physical examination and is corroborated by radiographic evaluation. The value of plain films of the cervical spine in CSR and CSM as a definitive examination is somewhat limited given the high rate of false-positive and -negative results (3,15,21). Nonetheless plain x-rays continue to enjoy wide usage as a readily available and relatively low-cost screening measure and as a method of evaluating spinal alignment, instability, and congenital anomaly in symptomatic individuals (Fig. 1). The assessment of osteophytic compression as judged by plain film analysis correlates poorly with clinical localization because plain x-rays are unable to directly visualize neural tissue, intervertebral discs, or ligamentous structures.

The degree of overlap between CSR and CSM is controversial. Some maintain that CSR and CSM are largely distinct clinical entities, whereas others report that myeloradiculopathy is the most common neurological presentation of cervical spon-

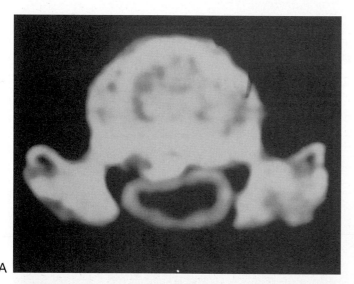

A

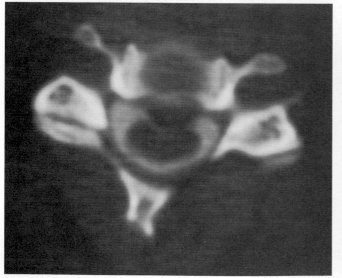

B

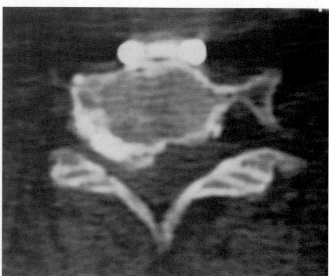

C

Fig. 2. **A:** Intrathecally enhanced CT scans after laminectomy done for spondylotic myeloradiculopathy failed to relieve radicular symptoms. Persistent ventral deformation is evident. CT scans offer better definitions of bony structures than do MRI scans. **B:** Persistent soft disc rupture after laminotomy for radiculopathy is evident on this CT scan. **C:** Plain CT scan reveals persistent foraminal osteophyte after cervical discectomy and fusion failed to relieve radicular symptoms.

dylosis (14). Cases that are atypical, associated with myelopathy or a major motor deficit, or that are refractory to a course of "conservative management" should have a more definitive neuroimaging study. Myelography, CT-myelography, and MR scanning address some of the limitations of plain film examination by direct or indirect visualization of the neural elements subject to compression. Cervical spondylosis causes extradural deformation of the subarachnoid space and neural elements at characteristic loci adjacent to disc spaces and facet joints. During myelography the subarachnoid space is opacified with contrast media, thereby outlining the spinal cord and exiting nerve roots and revealing any incongruities in the subarachnoid space. Water-soluble myelography has significantly enhanced sensitivity and specificity as compared with plain film examinations

(22). CT scans obtained after intrathecal contrast administration add further diagnostic specificity through more detailed imaging of the osteophytic and discal anatomy, especially in the lateral neural foramen where even the normal root sleeve may fill only sparsely with dye (Fig. 2). Disadvantages of myelography and post-myelographic CT include the necessity of subarachnoid puncture, possibility of neurological deterioration related to neck hyperextension during myelography, and occasional adverse reactions to the contrast media.

MRI scanning is currently accepted as the mainstay of imaging diagnosis in CSR and CSM (Fig. 3) (23). It provides direct visualization of the spinal cord and nerve roots and the supporting soft-tissue structure of the spine in multiplanar views. Brown and co-workers report an 88% concordance of MRI and surgical

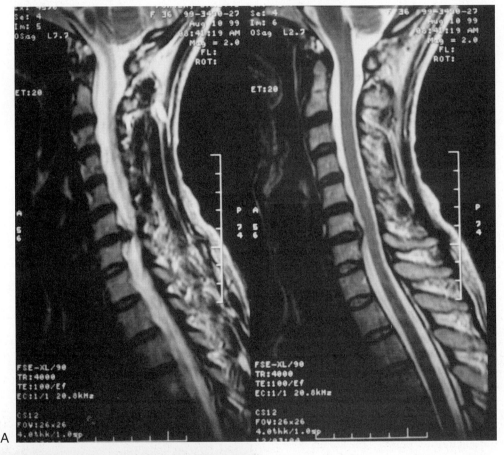

A

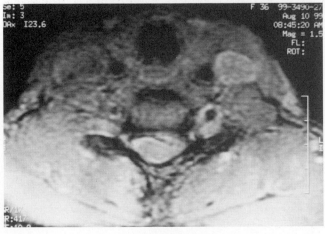

B

Fig. 3. A: Sagittal MRI of the cervical spine in a 36-year-old actress with acute C6 radiculopathy. Midline *(right)* and paramedian *(left)* images large posterolateral disc rupture. **B:** Axial MRI documents both cord and foraminal compromise.

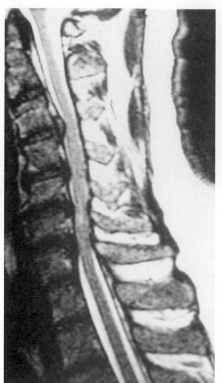
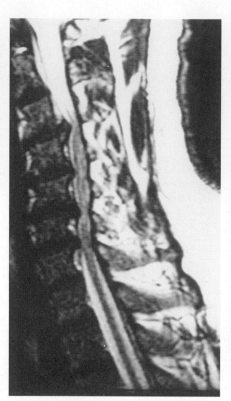
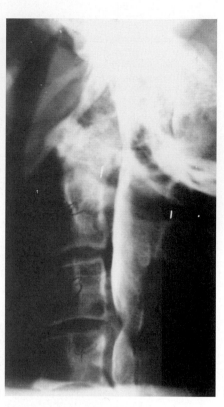

A,B

C

Fig. 4. MRI scans, myelogram, and intrathecally enhanced CT scans in a 46-year-old man with cervical myeloradiculopathy. Midline **(A)** and paramedian **(B)** sagittal MRI images reveal multisegmental stenosis, kyphosis, and multiple ventral bulges at the levels of the C3-4, C4-5, C5-6, and C6-7 disc spaces. **C:** Lateral radiograph after myelography reveals ventral defect in the dye column at C3-4. Shoulders precluded visualization below C5 because the intrathecally enhanced CT provides more information with a much smaller dye load. We no longer obtain plain radiographs after cervical myelography.

findings, exceeding the diagnostic accuracy of myelography, plain CT, and CT-myelography (24). Because MR does not define bony anatomy with the same clarity as CT, many practitioners use MRI and plain CT together as complimentary examinations (Fig. 4).

The differential diagnosis of CSR and CSM is potentially extensive and may include spinal tumors, trauma, infection, sarcoidosis, and arteritis. When there is accompanying myelopathy, processes such as syringomyelia, multiple sclerosis, basilar invagination, and motor neuron disease (ALS) must be ruled out (25). In routine cases of CSR alone, the principal alternative diagnostic considerations include peripheral entrapment neuropathy, thoracic outlet syndrome (TOS), and intrinsic shoulder pathology. Entrapment neuropathies are usually distinguished by characteristic sensory and motor involvements conforming to the distribution of a peripheral nerve (median, ulnar, or radial). This contrasts with the dermatomal and myotomal patterns of involvement encountered in radiculopathy which typically overlap the domain of two or more peripheral nerves. In unclear cases, electromyography and nerve conduction studies can be helpful in differentiating these entities. Radiculopathy and peripheral nerve entrapment can coexist as the syndrome of the "double crush," although the frequency of such occurrences is a matter of dispute (26). Intrinsic shoulder pathology such as rotator cuff tear usually is manifested through the local pain and tenderness to direct palpation and by limited passive range of motion. Neurological deficit is also unanticipated in conditions limited to the shoulder joint.

Treatment

The treatment of degenerative spinal conditions including CSR and CSM has never been subjected to a scientifically valid clinical trial. Conservative modalities may include various forms of physiotherapy, chiropractic manipulation, immobilization, traction, electrical stimulation, activity modification, local injections, acupuncture, exercise, biofeedback, hypnosis, and local heating or cooling, among others. Commonly prescribed medications include analgesics, muscle relaxants, antidepressants, and both steroidal and nonsteroidal antiinflammatory drugs (NSAIDs). The efficacy of such conservative interventions ideally would be measured against the natural history of the untreated condition. Published information concerning untreated CSR and CSM is limited. Studies purporting to address the natural history of CSR in fact describe outcomes of various forms of nonoperative therapy (27).

Multiple uncontrolled, nonrandomized, retrospective reports have described the results of nonoperative therapy (17,19, 27–31). These are flawed methodologically, employing inconsistent methods of case ascertainment, variable case management, and record very limited or incomplete follow-up. Issues of referral bias and selection factors are largely unaddressed. Diagnostic criteria generally lack rigor and radiculopathy or myelopathy caused by acute disc herniation is inconsistently distinguished from that caused by spondylosis. Outcome measures are poorly characterized and lack independent assess-

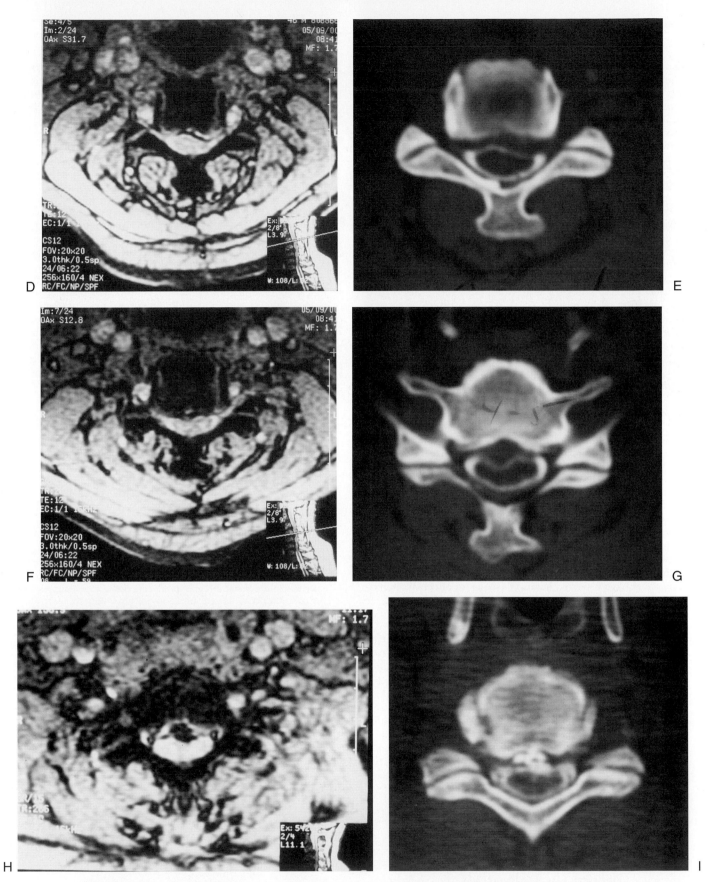

Fig. 4. (continued). **D–I:** MR images may fail to differentiate soft disc material from calcified ligaments, "hard disks," or osteophytes. In this case, the ventral mass noted at C3-4 proved to be a paramedian soft disc rupture **(D,E)**. At C4-5, a mass which appeared to be calcified on MRI proved to be another soft disc **(F,G)**. Conversely, at C6-7, a mass which appeared similar on sagittal MRI proved to be a heavily ossified posterior longitudinal ligament as demonstrated on CT scans **(H,I)**.

ment. Success is often vaguely defined by "excellent" or "good" relief of symptoms, with or without continuing need for medication or ongoing therapy. Employment and functional status are poorly delineated, and issues of patient satisfaction and sense of well-being are rarely addressed. Successful resolution of acute episodes is often given in the 70% to 95% range (17,19,28). Clinical relapse of CSR and CSM mandating renewed treatment seems to occur in about 10% to 20% of patients within 1 year and up to 20% cross over to surgery (28). Not surprisingly, surgically based series are much more pessimistic in appraising the results of nonoperative therapy (31,32).

An exception to these reports includes an early effort at a prospective multicenter trial comparing several nonoperative modalities organized and reported by the British Association of Physical Medicine in 1966 (28).

Operation often is advised for those individuals who present with a major motor weakness or who continue to suffer from "intractable pain" after some arbitrary period of conservative management in the case of CSR. In CSM, surgery is recommended for patients who show progression of myelopathy either during a period of observation or historically. The patient history, physical examination, and definitive neuroimaging study should be concordant, depicting a coherent picture of root or cord dysfunction. Neurological symptomatology should predominate over axial pain. A variety of anteriorly and posteriorly directed procedures with or without fusion or instrumentation have been employed in the treatment of CSR and CSM. The literature is replete with retrospective case series describing surgical "success rates" of 70% to 95% in patient populations who have already failed at some form of conservative management. Laminoforaminotomy and laminectomy enjoyed wide popularity in the surgical management of CSR and CSM into the 1970s (8–10,18,33–36). Following the early reports of Cloward and Smith a variety of anterior discectomy and corpectomy procedures, with and without osteophytectomy, interbody fusion, vertebral replacement, and instrumentation evolved. Anterior approaches also appear to be very effective in the surgical treatment of CSR and CSM. They currently enjoy a large measure of popularity (20,37–41). Recently Herkowitz and others have reported laminoplasty as an effective alternative in cases of multilevel CSR (42).

None of these operations has been compared to an alternative procedure or to nonoperative therapy in a scientifically valid clinical trial. Operator-evaluated case series reports with limited follow-up are apt to overestimate the benefits of surgery. In a recent prospective survey two thirds of surgically treated patients regarded themselves as being disabled in their everyday activities 5 years postoperatively (30). Although individual surgeons may express dogmatic beliefs about the optimal surgical management of CSR and CSM, the available literature suggests relatively equivalent rates of pain relief and sensorimotor restoration for both anterior and posterior procedures. Retrospective reviews do not indicate a clear outcome advantage for one particular operation over another (4,43).

Conclusion

We have amassed a huge body of individual and collective experience in the treatment of CSR and CSM. There is a general consensus that the majority of CSR patients respond well to "conservative" measures such as activity modification, NSAIDs, physiotherapy, and the passage of time. Operation is reserved for those individuals with genuinely severe or intractable symptoms and in whom the history, physical examination, and a definitive neuroimaging study are concordant. Anterior cervical

discectomy or corpectomy and posterior laminoforaminotomy or laminectomy appear to be highly effective procedures in appropriately selected individuals. However, it is often a temptation to mistake familiarity with a common condition such as CSR/CSM for knowledge of that condition, and our management decisions in CSR and CSM are not currently informed by scientifically valid clinical trials. The overwhelming preponderance of the literature published on both the conservative and surgical treatment of CSR and CSM is categorized as class 3 evidence; that is, uncontrolled, retrospectively organized case series and "expert opinion."

It is ironic that common conditions such as CSR and CSM often have been so poorly studied from a scientific perspective. The beliefs and biases of treating physicians, patient expectations, medicolegal considerations, and the difficulty in objectifying the pain experience all pose significant obstacles to the organization of a definitive study of this and other common surgical conditions. At present both anterior and posterior procedures appear to be valid and relatively equivalent treatment options. Perhaps the greatest challenge is to properly select patients for operation. Once this commitment has been made, the contemporary spinal surgeon should be facile with a variety of techniques so that the technical procedure can be tailored to individual clinical and anatomical circumstances as they arise.

References

1. Braakman R. Management of cervical spondylotic myelopathy and radiculopathy (editorial). *J Neurol Neruosurg Psychiatry* 1994;57: 256–263.
2. Lesini WF, Wiesel SW. The pathogenesis of cervical spondylosis. *Clin Orthop Rel Res* 1989;239:69–93.
3. Brain WR, Northfield D, Wilkinson M. The neurological manifestations of cervical spondylosis. *Brain* 1995;75:187–225.
4. Dillin W, Booth R, Cuckler J, et al. Cervical radiculopathy, a review. *Spine* 1986;11:988–991.
5. Frykholm R. Deformities of dural pouches and strictures of dural sheaths in the cervical region producing nerve root compression. A contribution to the etiology and operative therapy of brachial neuralgia. *J Neurosurg* 1947;4:403–413.
6. Parke WW. Correlative anatomy of cervical spondylotic myelopathy. *Spine* 1988;13:831–837.
7. Semmes RE, Murphey MF. The syndrome of unilateral rupture of the sixth cervical intervertebral disc with compression of the seventh cervical nerve root. A report of four cases with symptoms simulating coronary disease. *JAMA* 1943;121:1209–1214.
8. Odom GL, Finney W, Woohall B. Cervical disc lesions. *JAMA* 1958; 166:23–38.
9. Murphey F, Simmons J. Ruptured cervical disc: experience with 250 cases. *Am Surg* 1966;32:83–88.
10. Scoville WB. Types of cervical disc lesions and their surgical approaches. *JAMA* 1966;196:479–481.
11. Cloward R. The anterior approach for removal of ruptured cervical discs. *J Neurosurg* 1958;15:602–617.
12. Smith GW, Robinson RA. The treatment of certain cervical spine disorders by anterior removal of intervertebral disc and interbody fusion. *J Bone Joint Surg Am* 1958;40:607–624.
13. Boden SD, McCowin PR, Davis DO, et al. Abnormal magnetic resonance scans of the cervical spine in asymptomatic subjects: a prospective investigation. *J Bone Joint Surg (Am)* 1990;72:1178–1184.
14. Clark E, Robinson PK. Cervical myelopathy: complication of cervical spondylosis. *Brain* 1956;79:483–510.
15. Friedenberg ZB, Miller WT. Degenerative disease of the cervical spine; a comparative study of asymptomatic and symptomatic patients. *J Bone Joint Surg (Am)* 1963;45:1171–1178.
16. Debois V, Herz R, Berghmans D, et al. Soft cervical disc herniation: influence of cervical spinal canal measurements on development of neurological symptoms. *Spine* 1999;24:1996–2002.17 Radhakrishnan K, Litchy WJ, O'Fallon M, et al. Epidemiology of cervical radicu-

lopathy: a population-based study form Rochester, Minnesota, 1976 through 1990. *Brain* 1994;117:325–335.

18. Henderson CM, Hennessy RG, Shuey HM, et al. Posterior-lateral foraminotomy as an exclusive operative technique for cervical radiculopathy: a review of 846 consecutively operated cases. *Neurosurgery* 1983;13:504–512.
19. Honet JC, Puri K. Cervical radiculitis: treatment and results in 82 patients. *Arch Phys Med Rehabil* 1976;57:12–16.
20. Lunsford LD, Bissonette DJ, Jannetta PT, et al. Anterior surgery for cervical disc disease. Part 1: Treatment of lateral cervical disc herniation in 253 cases. *J Neurosurg* 1980;53:1–11.
21. Gore DC, Sepic SB, Gardner GM. Roentgenographic findings of the cervical spine in asymptomatic people. *Spine* 1986;11:521–524.
22. Nakagawa H, Okumura T, Sugiyama T, et al. Discrepancy between metrizamide CT and myelography in the diagnosis of cervical disc protrusions. *Am J Neuroradiol* 1983;4:604–606.
23. Wibar DW, Pezzuti RT, Place JN. Magnetic resonance imaging in the preoperative evaluation of cervical radiculopathy. *Neurosurgery* 1991;28:175–179.
24. Brown BM, Schwartz RH, Frank E, et al. Prospective evaluation of cervical radiculopathy and myelopathy by surface coil MR imaging. *AJNR* 1988;151:1205–1212.
25. Dvorak J, Janssen B, Brob D. The neurological workup in patients with cervical spine disorders. *Spine* 1990;15:1017–1022.
26. Wilbourn AJ, Gilliat RW. Double-crush syndrome: a critical analysis. *Neurology* 1997;49:22–29.
27. Lees F, Turner JW. Natural history and prognosis of cervical spondylosis. *Br Med J* 1963;2:1607–1610.
28. British Association of Physical Medicine. Pain in the neck and arm: a multicentre trial of the effects of physiotherapy. *Br Med J* 1966;1:253–258.
29. Martin GM, Corbin KB. An evaluation of conservative treatment for patients with cervical disc syndrome. *Arch Phys Med Rehabil* 54;35:87–92.
30. Heckmann JG, Lang CJ, Zobelein I, et al. Herniated cervical interver-
tebral discs with radiculopathy: an outcome study of conservatively or surgically treated patients. *J Spinal Disord* 1999;12:396–401.
31. Rothman R, Simeone S. *The spine.* Philadelphia: WB Saunders, 1982.
32. Arnasson O, Carlsson CA, Pellettieri L. Surgical and conservative treatment of cervical spondylotic radiculopathy and myelopathy. *Acta Neurochir (Wien)* 1987;84:48–53.
33. Davis RA. A long-term outcome study of 170 surgically treated patients with compressive cervical radiculopathy. *Surg Neurol* 1996;46:523–530.
34. Gregorius FK, Estrin T, Crandall PH. Cervical spondylotic radiculopathy and myelopathy: a long term study. *Arch Neurol* 1976;33:618–625.35 Williams RW. Microcervical foraminotomy: a surgical alternative for intractable radicular pain. *Spine* 1983;8:708–716.
36. Zeidman SM, Ducker TB. Posterior cervical laminoforaminotomy: review of 172 cases. *Neurosurgery* 1993;33:356–362.
37. Maurice-Williams RS, Dorward NL. Extended anterior cervical discectomy without fusion: a simple and sufficient operation for most cases of cervical disc disease. *Br J Neurosurg* 1996;10:261–266.
38. Bohlman HH, Emery SE, Goodfellow DB, et al. Robinson anterior cervical discectomy and arthrodesis for cervical radiculopathy: a long term follow up of 122 patients. *J Bone Joint Surg Am* 1993;75:1298–1307.
39. George B, Gauthier N, Lot G. Multisegmental cervical spondylotic myelopathy and radiculopathy treated by multilevel oblique carpectomies without fusion. *Neurosurgery* 1999;44:81–90.
40. Hadley MN, Sonntag VK. Cervical disc herniations: the anterior approach to symptomatic interspace pathology. *Neurosurg Clin N Am* 1993;4:45–52.
41. Robertson JT. Anterior removal of cervical discs without fusion. *Clin Neurosurg* 1973;20:259–261.
42. Herkowitz HN. Cervical laminoplasty: its role in the treatment of cervical radiculopathy. *J Spinal Disord* 1988;1:179–188.
43. Herkowitz HN. A comparison of anterior cervical fusion, cervical laminectomy, and cervical laminoplasty for the surgical management of multiple level spondylotic radiculopathy. *Spine* 1988;13:774–780.

144. Ossification of the Posterior Longitudinal Ligament

Nancy E. Epstein

Ossification of the posterior longitudinal ligament (OPLL) is seen in up to 27% of Japanese and 25% of North American patients exhibiting cervical myelopathy on examinations based on magnetic resonance imaging (MRI) or computed tomography (CT) (1–6). Anterior surgical options include the anterior discectomy/fusion (ADF) or anterior corpectomy/fusion (ACF), while posterior options are comprised of the laminectomy with/without fusion or laminoplasty (1–8). In this chapter we explore the etiology, clinical and radiographic presentation, and surgical management and outcomes of patients with OPLL.

cation of the anterior longitudinal ligament (OALL), and 0.5% have ossification of the yellow ligament (OYL). Genetic links to human leukocyte antigen haplotypes (HLAH), elevated levels of circulating growth and other hormones, as well as an autosomal-dominant mode of inheritance have emerged from studies of patients with OPLL and their probands.

Pathology

OPLL begins as a microscopic mineralization and proliferation of cartilaginous cells that infiltrate into periosteal tissues surrounding the posterior longitudinal ligament. This results in increased fibrosis of a hypervascular posterior longitudinal ligament, the coalescence of calcific foci into bone islands, the production of lamellar bone, and mature haversian canals actively engaged in bone marrow production. Cephalad/caudad

Epidemiology

Ossification of the cervical and thoracic spinal ligaments is observed in 34.4% of symptomatic Japanese patients over the age of 50 (7). Of these, 3.2% have cervical OPLL, 30.7% have ossifi-

extension of OPLL reportedly occurs at the rate of several milli-meters per year, the anteroposterior diameter expanding by slightly more than one-half millimeter per year. When OPLL occupying more than 30% of the spinal canal correlates with the onset of myelopathy, severe myelopathic syndromes will occur once 50% or more of the canal becomes compromised (1). Inherent cord changes differentially affect the gray matter more than the white matter. Those exhibiting reversible stage 0 to 1 cord changes defined by Mizuno and colleagues (i.e., edema, neurons intact) stand to benefit from surgical interven-tion, while those with irreversible stage 2 to 3 disease (i.e., myelomalacia, neuronal necrosis) do not (8).

Classification of Ossification of the Posterior Longitudinal Ligament

Hirabayashi was the first to define four *classic types* of OPLL (1–6,9,10). In descending order of frequency these are:

1. The *continuous type*, which crosses multiple vertebral bodies and their intervening interspaces.
2. The *segmental type*, located behind the vertebral bodies themselves.
3. The *mixed type*, consisting of both *continuous* and *segmental* elements with intervening skip areas.
4. The *other type*, confined to the disc spaces.

A fifth *early variant of OPLL* consists of hypertrophied posterior longitudinal ligament with punctate calcification/ossification (2–6,10).

Neurodiagnostic Studies

MAGNETIC RESONANCE IMAGING. On MRI, classic OPLL appears as a hypointense mass, while early OPLL projects a more inhomogeneous isointense signal (1–6,9–11). (Fig 1). Both separate the ventral vertebral marrow from the more dor-sal thecal sac and nerve roots (11). Whereas simple disc hernia-tions are confined to an interspace, the pathognomonic finding of OPLL is its retrovertebral extension that parallels the normal contour of the ligament: wider at the disc spaces, and narrower behind the vertebrae. On enhanced T1-weighted MRI studies, classic OPLL remains hypointense, while the hypertrophied posterior longitudinal ligament of early OPLL becomes hyperin-tense. However, even though MRI evaluations offer an excellent transaxial, coronal, and sagittal overview of the cervical spine, especially of the cervicothoracic junction, CT-based studies (CT, two-dimensional and three-dimensional CT, myelogram/CT) more directly demonstrate the full extent of OPLL (1–6, 10) (Figs. 2 and 3).

Clinical Data

AGE/SEX. Patients with early OPLL are typically in their mid-40s, while those with classic OPLL are typically over a decade

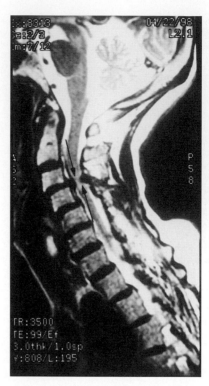

Fig. 1. Preoperative T2-weighted MRI of ossification of the posterior longitudinal ligament (OPLL), ossification of the yellow ligament (OYL), and stenosis. This MRI shows a normal-sized cord, maximally com-pressed at the C3-4 level *(arrows)* where a high intrinsic signal is seen due to OPLL, OYL, and stenosis.

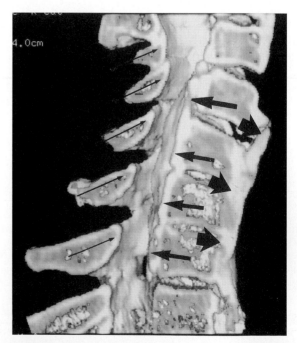

Fig. 2. Three-dimensional midline sagittal CT scan of ossification of the posterior longitudinal ligament (OPLL) and ossification of the ante-rior longitudinal ligament (OALL). Cord compromise on this CT scan was due to OPLL *(four smaller arrows)*, OALL *(three larger arrows)*, congenital stenosis, and laminar shingling *(thin arrows)*.

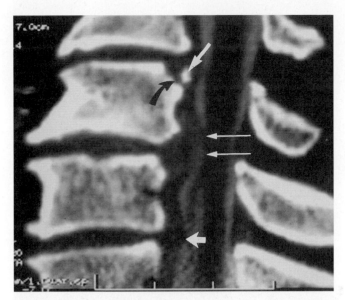

Fig. 3. Midline sagittal myelogram/CT reconstruction of early ossification of the posterior longitudinal ligament (OPLL). Early OPLL, consisting of hypertrophied posterior longitudinal ligament with pearls of ossification *(angled white arrow)* extends behind the C3-7 vertebrae *(all other arrows)*.

older, in their mid-to-late 50s (1–6,9,10). Gender is split equally between men and women.

NURICK AND JAPANESE ORTHOPEDIC ASSOCIATION

SCALES. Neurological function is graded using the Nurick scale (2–6). On this scale, Nurick grade 0 indicates radiculopathy without myelopathy; grade 1, mild myelopathy; grade 2, mild-to-moderate myelopathy; grade 3, moderate myelopathy; grade 4, moderate-to-severe myelopathy; and grade 5, severe myelopathy (5,6,10). The Japanese Orthopedic Association (JOA) grading system is assigned using a 17-point scale (1,9).

PATIENT SELECTION. Younger patients (under 65 years of age) with short-term and less severe preoperative deficits and without cord atrophy or myelomalacia exhibit better outcomes following surgery for OPLL (1–6,10). Older patients (over 65 years of age) with long-term and more severe preoperative deficits, cord atrophy, and myelomalacia demonstrate poorer postsurgical results. Other poor prognostic factors negatively impacting surgical outcomes include absent preoperative somatosensory evoked potentials (SSEPs), and the presence of significant medical comorbidities (i.e., diabetes, alcoholism, cardiac disease).

Surgery

SOMATOSENSORY EVOKED POTENTIAL MONITORING. Continuous intraoperative SSEP monitoring may eliminate the 2% or greater frequency of cervical spinal cord injuries, and limit the 1 to 3% to 17% incidence of root injuries reported in patients with unmonitored OPLL (12–14).

Significant medical/anesthetic or surgery-induced SSEP changes mandate immediate resuscitative maneuvers. On the medical/anesthetic front, the most commonly encountered hypotension (i.e., either supine or sitting) may be addressed by inducing hypertension, other efforts concentrating on the reduction of Forane or N_2O level, warming irrigating solutions, or increasing oxygen concentration (2–6,10,12,13). When the surgeon is at fault, as with inadvertent manipulation, retraction, distraction, or application of an oversized graft promoting cord ischemia, he or she may stop the dissection and retraction, release the distraction, or remove the oversized graft, allowing SSEP changes to normalize.

ANTERIOR DISCECTOMY/FUSION OR ANTERIOR CORPECTOMY/FUSION

Exposure. For any of the anterior surgical approaches (ADF, ACF), the patient's head is first immobilized on a padded head rest (2–6,10,14,15). An awake, nasotracheal fiberoptic intubation in a hard collar, with awake positioning under SSEP monitoring follows.

It should be remembered that in patients with OPLL with marked cord/nerve root compression, distraction is avoided until the decompression is complete. The use of distraction prior to the resection of pathology risks immediate SSEP deterioration and potentially permanent neurological sequelae.

Trough Width. Although 12- to 16-mm troughs suffice for medial/lateral dissection of OPLL in the Japanese population, North American patients are generally larger, and often require 16- to 20-mm troughs based on the interpedicular distance measured on preoperative CT studies. Trough dissection is best carried out in a methodical cephalad/caudad fashion. Careful attention is paid throughout to maintaining parallel planes of exposure: medial/lateral, cephalad/caudad, and inferior.

For patients with one- or two-level OPLL extending beyond the interspace, partial cephalad/caudad resection of cortical end plates or corpectomy may be performed under magnified vision using variously sized high- or low-speed burrs, without the use of distraction.

A clean dural plane is often present below the involved posterior longitudinal ligament, but must be carefully defined using a micronerve hook to avoid inadvertent entry into the thecal sac. This maneuver is most critical to operative success, as leaving the ligament behind fails to adequately decompress the neural elements. If left behind, distraction associated with graft placement will tether the cord/nerve roots over this residual pathology and likely contribute to neural injury. The operating microscope is essential to avoid a cerebrospinal fluid (CSF) fistula, although in our experience only one anticipated CSF leak occurred out of more than 200 patients undergoing OPLL surgery.

On occasion, profuse bleeding arises from the residual posterior vertebral cortex/OPLL mass, and may be controlled with bone wax, a diamond drill, or homeostatic agent. Bleeding from hypertrophied posterior longitudinal ligament may require bipolar cautery on a very low setting.

Graft Placement. The Caspar normal length or specially-machined, elongated, 1.5× distractors (designed especially for multilevel corpectomies) are only applied after OPLL dissection has been completed. As autogenous Smith-Robinson or iliac crest (rarely fibula) strut grafts are impacted in place, SSEP changes are closely monitored. Where oversized grafts, just like distraction, promote SSEP dropout due to ischemia, they must be removed, downsized, and reapplied.

Plate Instrumentation. As the application of anterior cervical plates carries a 5% morbidity (screw malplacement) and 1%

reoperation rate (back-out of plates/screws, dysphagia), they should only be selectively applied (16). They do not appear to be necessary for ADF or single level ACF (2–6,10). However, their routine addition to multilevel circumferential cervical surgery (anterior corpectomy with fusion/posterior wiring/fusion) has, thus far, eliminated vertebral fracture/graft extrusion (15).

CIRCUMFERENTIAL CERVICAL SURGERY WITH AND WITHOUT ANTERIOR PLATES. From 1989 to 1997, 22 patients with moderate-to-severe myelopathy (average Nurick grade 3.5) had circumferential cervical procedures for multilevel OPLL/stenosis (15). The patients included 13 men and 9 women, with an average age of 57 years (range 30 to 70 years). They were followed an average of 36 postoperative months. Anterior corpectomy with fusion (average 2.5 levels) was performed without plate instrumentation, but was supplemented with posterior wiring and fusion (average 5 levels, 5 also with laminectomies) and halo devices. The average operative time was 10 hours, requiring an average of 3.5 units of blood (range 1 to 8 units). Postoperatively, all patients improved neurologically (+3.0 Nurick grades) from moderate-to-severe preoperative myelopathic baselines to postoperative mild-to-moderate myelopathy. However, three (14%) patients developed vertebral fractures/graft extrusions less than 24 hours postoperatively, requiring anterior graft revision, with the application of salvage plates in two of the three patients. Nevertheless, 100% of the patients fused within an average of 4 postoperative months.

To avoid vertebral fractures/graft extrusions in the future, anterior cervical plates were routinely added to otherwise comparable circumferential cervical procedures performed in the most recently treated 17 patients (September 1997 through July 1998) (16). These 12 men and 5 women with an average age of 55 years (range 42 to 70 years), exhibited moderate-to-severe preoperative myelopathy (average Nurick grade 3.3). Similarly, extensive ACF (average of 2.8 levels), posterior wiring/fusions (5.4 levels), and halo bracing were supplemented with anterior plates. Plated circumferential procedures were completed over an average of 8 hours, using 3 (range 0 to 6) units of blood. In short, plating neither increased or decreased the duration blood loss associated with circumferential surgery. The average neurological improvement observed with plates (+2.8 Nurick grades) was equivalent to that seen without plates; all patients improved to show mild-to-moderate residual myelopathy. Thus far, and most important, anterior cervical plates have eliminated vertebral fractures/graft extrusions while maintaining a 100% fusion rate over a shorter average 3-month period (16) (Fig. 4).

POSTERIOR SURGERY

Laminectomy. Laminectomy effectively decompresses cervical OPLL/stenosis in older individuals (over 65 years of age) with cervical hyperlordosis without instability (2–6,10,17). Following awake nasotracheal or endotracheal fiberoptic intubation, patients may be positioned awake (sitting or prone). The head is immobilized in a three-pin Mayfield head holder, using 5 cc of local anesthetic (lidocaine hydrochloride) at each pin site. Once SSEP baselines have been reestablished, anesthesia may be induced (2–6,12,13).

Using a high-speed diamond air drill (Midas Rex diamond No. 8) bit laminae are removed just medial to the facet joint, and down to the yellow ligament (2–4). Next, laminae are sequentially elevated; a small Kerrison rongeur is used to remove ligament adherent to the overlying bone. At no time is the rongeur introduced beneath intact laminae, thus avoiding inadvertent spinal cord/nerve root compression. A small Kerrison rongeur is then employed to complete multilevel medial

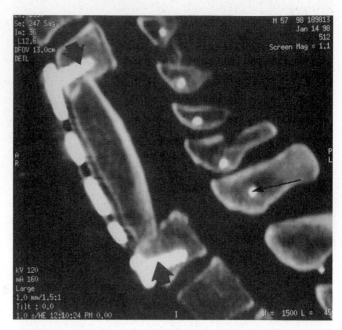

Fig. 4. Three-month postoperative midline sagittal CT following C3-7 anterior corpectomy/fusion, Orion plating, and C3-T1 posterior wiring/fusion. Fusion of the iliac strut graft, an intact Orion plate *(large arrows)* and braided cables *(long arrow)*, and solid fusion were seen.

facetectomies with foraminotomies. No attempts are made to excise OPLL through this dorsal exposure, as this is extremely dangerous and will likely damage the neural elements. Rather, if significant ventral disease is present, the patient should undergo a combined circumferential procedure (anterior discectomy/corpectomy with fusion, laminectomy, and facet/wiring/fusion). Success rates for laminectomy in carefully selected patients approach and occasionally exceed 80% (1–6,9,17). Nevertheless, major complications of laminectomy do include the risk of delayed neurological deterioration with progressive instability/kyphosis requiring multilevel anterior, posterior, or combined reconstructions (10,18).

Laminectomy with Posterior Wiring and Fusion. Cervical laminectomy combined with a posterior wiring and fusion may be an appropriate surgical alternative for the management of OPLL/stenosis/instability in older patients (over 65 years of age) with severe preoperative myelopathy (Nurick grades 4 through 5). In this instance, fusion should halt the more rapid progression of OPLL while avoiding the evolution of postlaminectomy kyphosis and attendant neurological dysfunction (9,17). To be successful, a hyperlordotic cervical curvature is essential as is MRI evidence of a normal-sized, not atrophic, cervical spinal cord. Here, an increased signal on T2-weighted images at the site of maximal cord compression should indicate the presence of edema rather than myelomalacia (8,11) (Fig. 5).

Once the laminectomy is completed in the routine fashion, a posterior wiring and fusion are performed. The braided titanium cable is passed between the spinous processes (above/below) and/or facet joints. The cable is then test-tightened under SSEP monitoring, and crimped after SSEPs have stabilized. Lateral decortication of the facets is completed with a cutting burr, the fusion being now supplemented with autologous laminectomy bone, and iliac crest autograft or cancellous autograft, plus 10 cc of demineralized bone matrix (Fig. 6). The average total operative time is 2.5 hours, requiring an average of 2 units of transfused blood. Patients immobilized in cervico-

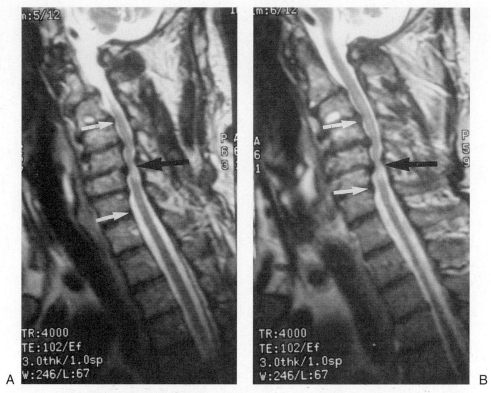

Fig. 5. Midline and paramedian sagittal T2 weighted MRI study of C3-7 cord compression due to ossification of the posterior longitudinal ligament (OPLL)/kyphosis. **A:** Midline C3-7 cord compression *(white arrows)* from C3-7, maximal at C5-6 where a high signal was seen in the cord *(black arrow)*, was due to both OPLL and kyphosis. **B:** This paramedian study showed the same findings *(white arrows, black arrow).*

thoracic orthoses fuse an average of 3 to 4 months later, and improve to show mild-to-moderate myelopathy (average improvement of +3 Nurick grades).

Laminoplasty. Patients with OPLL/stenosis treated with laminoplasty have demonstrated similar frequencies (63% to 80%) of good-to-excellent outcomes (9,17,19,20). Arguable advantages of the laminoplasty technique include reduced operating time, greater safety, enhanced stability with preserved flexibility, and the absence of a postlaminectomy membrane with delayed deterioration. Expansive open-door laminoplasty yielded a 63% incidence of good outcomes, the frequency significantly declining in patients over 65 years of age with more severe myelopathy (9,20). Indications favoring laminoplasty include OPLL over three or more levels; some authors maintain that better results are achieved following laminoplasty (good-to-excellent outcomes greater than 80%) as compared with laminectomy (greater than 70%) or anterior surgery (greater than 60%).

Complications

ANTERIOR SURGERY. Complications of anterior surgery include neural trauma, vascular compromise, Horner syndrome, hoarseness/dysphagia, esophageal fistulae, and graft complications (fractures/extrusions, pseudarthrosis, donor site complications) (1–6,9,10,14,15,17,18,21–24). CSF fistulae, reported in up to one-fourth of some OPLL series, should be avoided with the routine use of the operating microscope (25). When fistulae occur, direct dural repair is difficult. However, fascial grafts and

cryo-glue should be applied and supplemented with lumbar drains, or preferably, lumboperitoneal shunts. Vertebral fracture/graft extrusions, particularly following multilevel corpectomies, should be avoided with the addition of anterior plates and simultaneous performance of a posterior wiring and fusion (15,16,23,24). Plates may also limit the pseudarthrosis rate, but this is more likely dependent on the technique of fusion (i.e., better perforation of end plates, improved fashioning of the graft itself) (16,21,22).

The frequency of cord injuries in unmonitored series varies from 2% to 10%, while root injuries, particularly involving the C-5 root, are seen in up to 17% of patients (14,26). While cord damage is more likely caused by direct surgical trauma or overdistraction, lateral nerve root damage probably reflects traumatic lateral dissection expanded over 15 mm resulting in rapid untethering of the nerve root (14). Yet, if lateral decompression is restricted to 15 mm, inadequate root decompression or rapid OPLL regrowth/recurrence can both be responsible for short- and long-term nerve root compromise.

POSTERIOR SURGERY. Both unique and overlapping complications are observed in patents with OPLL/stenosis treated with laminectomy with/without fusion, or laminoplasty. Laminectomy alone may result in progressive kyphosis/swan neck deformity, and increased neurological deterioration with progressive draping of the cord over the more rapidly growing OPLL mass. Laminectomy with fusion risks are the same if pseudarthrosis occurs, or with a substantially reduced frequency should adequate fusion take place. Finally laminoplasty, like the laminectomy with fusion, has minimal risks of kyphosis and delayed deterioration but "closing of the door"

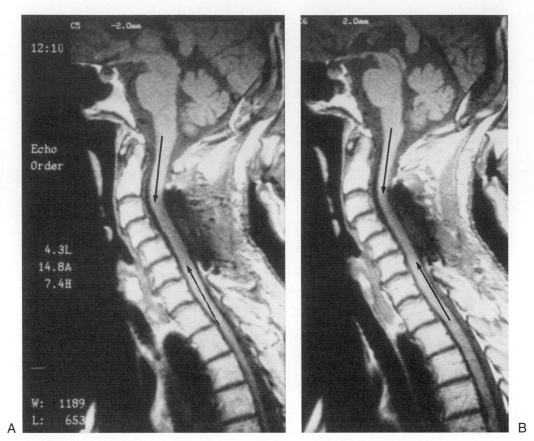

Fig. 6. Three-month postoperative sagittal T1-enhanced MRI study of C3-6 laminectomy/C3-7 posterior wiring/fusion. **A:** This study demonstrates a normal-sized cord that had been adequately decompressed *(long arrows)* following a C3-6 laminectomy with C3-7 posterior wiring and fusion. **B:** The paramedian view confirmed the same as the sagittal view *(arrows).*

may heighten the latter risk. Both cord and root injuries may occur due to rapid untethering of both structures following any of these three procedures, the C-5 nerve root being most often affected (1–6,9).

Bracing

ANTERIOR SURGERY. Patients undergoing one-to-four level ADF or one level corpectomy with fusion are immobilized for 3 months or until fusion has occurred in hard collars with extension braces. Halos are reserved for those undergoing two or more level circumferential procedures.

POSTERIOR SURGERY. Hard collars are employed 1 week following cervical laminectomy or laminoplasty. Patients are quickly weaned to soft collars and no collars within the first postoperative month. Those undergoing posterior wiring and fusion are kept in cervicothoracic orthoses with extension braces until fusion has been documented (typically 3 months) on flexion and extension radiographs, and confirmed with three-dimensional CT studies.

Outcomes of Anterior or Posterior Surgery

Success rates of 70% to 90% have been observed for patients with OPLL/stenosis managed with either anterior or posterior surgical procedures. However, younger patients (those in their mid-to-late 50s) with shorter symptom intervals and less severe preoperative deficits exhibit better outcomes with direct anterior excision of OPLL masses (1–6,10,15). In a study by Goto and associates of OPLL patients followed for over 10 years, better outcomes were observed after anterior surgery, although one-third demonstrated delayed deterioration due to residual/recurrent OPLL or kyphosis (27). Others including this author have observed an approximate 12% reoperation rate for OPLL patients managed anteriorly (10,28). On the other hand, laminectomy with/without fusion or laminoplasty is effective for older patients with hyperlordotic cervical curvatures.

References

1. Abe H, Tsuro M, Ito T et. al. Anterior decompression for ossification of the posterior longitudinal ligament of the cervical spine. *J Neurosurg* 1989;55:108–116.
2. Epstein NE. Diagnosis and surgical management of ossification of

the posterior longitudinal ligament. *Contemp Neurosurg* 1992;22: 1–6.

3. Epstein NE. Ossification of the posterior longitudinal ligament: diagnosis and surgical management. *Neurosurg Q* 1992;2:223–241.

4. Epstein NE. The surgical management of ossification of the posterior longitudinal ligament in 51 patients. *J Spinal Disord* 1993;6:432–454.

5. Epstein NE. The surgical management of ossification of the posterior longitudinal ligament in 43 North Americans. *Spine* 1994;19: 664–672.

6. Epstein NE. Ossification of the posterior longitudinal ligament tin evolution in 12 patients. *Spine* 1994;19:673–681.

7. Sakou T, Taketomi E, Matsunga S. Genetic study of ossification of the posterior longitudinal ligament in the cervical sine with human leukocyte antigen haplotype. *Spine* 1991;16:1249–1252.

8. Mizuno J, Nakagawa H, Iwata K, et al. Pathology of spinal cord lesions caused by ossification of the posterior longitudinal ligament, with special reference to reversibility of the spinal cord lesion. *Neurol Res* (England) 1992;14:312–314.

9. Hirabayashi K, Bohlman H. Multilevel cervical spondylosis. Laminoplasty versus anterior decompression. *Spine* 1995;10:1732–1734.

10. Epstein NE. Advanced cervical spondylosis with ossification into the posterior longitudinal ligament and resultant neurological sequelae. *J Spinal Disord* 1996;9:477–484.

11. Yamashita Y, Takashi M, Matsuno Y. Spinal cord compression due to ossification of ligaments: MR imaging. *Radiology* 1990;175:843–848.

12. Epstein NE, Danto J, Nardi D. Evaluation of intraoperative somatosensory evoked potential monitoring in 100 cervical operations. *Spine* 1993;18:737–747.

13. Epstein NE. Somatosensory evoked potential monitoring (SSEPs) in 173 cervical operations. *Neuro-Orthopedics* 1996;20:3–21.

14. Saunders RL. On the pathogenesis of the radiculopathy complicating multilevel corpectomy. *Neurosurgery* 1995;37:408–413.

15. Epstein NE. Circumferential surgery for the management of ossification of the posterior longitudinal ligament. *J Spinal Disord* 1998;11: 200–207.

16. Kostuik JP, Connolly J, Esses A. Anterior cervical plate fixation with the titanium hollow screw plate system. *Spine* 1993;18:1273–1278.

17. Herkowitz H. A comparison of anterior cervical fusion, cervical laminectomy, and cervical laminoplasty for the surgical management of multiple level spondylotic radiculopathy. *Spine* 1988;13:774–780.

18. Sonntag VK, Herman JM. Reoperation of the cervical spine for degenerative disease and tumor. *Clin Neuorsurg* 1992;39:244–269.

19. Morimoto T, Matsuyama T, Hirabayashi H, et al. Expansive laminoplasty for multilevel cervical OPLL. *J Spinal Disord* 1997;10: 296–298.

20. Satomi K, Nishu Y, Kohna T, et al. Long-term follow-up studies for cervical stenotic myelopathy. *Spine* 1994;19:507–510.

21. Epstein NE. Vertebral body fractures following extensive anterior cervical surgical procedures for ossification of the posterior longitudinal ligament. *Neuro-Orthopedics* 1997;21:1–11.

22. Epstein NE. Evaluation and treatment of clinical instability associated with pseudarthrosis following anterior cervical surgery for ossification of the posterior longitudinal ligament. *Surgical Neurology* 1998;49:246–252.

23. McAfee P, Regan JJ, Bohlman HH. Cervical cord compression from ossification of the posterior longitudinal ligament in non-Orientals. *J Bone Joint Surg Br* 1987;69:569–575.

24. McAfee PC, Bohlman HH, Ducker TB, et al. One-stage anterior cervical decompression and posterior stabilization. A study of one hundred patients with a minimum of two years of follow-up. *J Bone Joint Surg Am* 1995;77:1791–1800.

25. Smith MD, Bolesta MJ, Leventhal M, et al. Postoperative cerebrospinal-fluid fistula associated with erosion of the dura. Findings after anterior resection of ossification of the posterior longitudinal ligament in the cervical spine. *J Bone Joint Surg Am* 1992;74:270–277.

26. Harsh GR 4th, Sypert GW, Weinstein PR, et al. Cervical spine stenosis secondary to ossification of the posterior longitudinal ligament. *J Neurosurg* 1987;67:349–357.

27. Goto S, Mochizuki M, Watanabe T, et al. Long-term follow-up study of anterior surgery for cervical spondylotic myelopathy with special reference to the magnetic resonance imaging findings in 52 cases. *Clin Orthop* 1993;291:142–153.

28. Shinomiya K, Okamoto A, Kamikozuru M, et al. An analysis of failures in primary cervical anterior spinal cord decompression and fusion. *J Spinal Disord* 1993;6:277–288.

145. *Thoracic Disc Degeneration with Pain*

Richard A Gullick, Jr. and Kaveh Khajavi

Pain is real when you get other people to believe in it. If no one believes in it but you, your pain is madness or hysteria.
                              Naomi Wolf, *The Beauty Myth,* 1990.

The purpose of this chapter is to discuss the process of disc degeneration and lay out a rational approach to the assessment and treatment of patients with painful degenerative thoracic disc disease. In recent years, enormous strides have been made in the management of disorders of the spinal column. These advances have come in every aspect of diagnosis, evaluation, and treatment. New tools and concepts have given the spine surgeon an unprecedented ability to intercede in the disease processes affecting his or her patient. Despite the impact of modern technological advances there are still disorders that greatly affect the lives of our patients on whom we, as specialists, have only meager impact. One such area is the neurologi-

cally intact patient with degenerative disc disease and intractable pain. The mere existence of "discogenic" pain is a matter of some controversy in the spine community. The debate surrounding the evaluation and treatment of "discogenic" pain is heated to say the least (1).

The incidence of symptomatic and asymptotic thoracic disc degeneration and herniation has been better defined with the advent of magnetic resonance imaging (2,3). The incidence of degenerative changes in asymptotic individuals may be as high as 73% (4,5). The overall incidence of thoracic disc herniations is small, 0.25% to 0.75% of all disc herniations (6) and many are asymptotic (7). The vast majority of thoracic disc disease occurs below the level of the mid thoracic spine (6). Most patients are middle aged with no strong sex predilection (2). Pain and weakness are the most common presenting complaints (2, 6,8).

Pathophysiology

The mechanisms by which the human intervertebral disc ages and degenerates are incompletely understood. The means by which the degenerated disc may generate pain is even less well characterized. The pathophysiology of this degenerative process has been best studied in the lumbar and cervical spine. Although little has been published on the degeneration processes unique to the thoracic disc, useful analogies may be garnered from the data available from studies of the lumbar and cervical spine. Biologically all human intervertebral discs reasonably may be regarded as similar even if they are exposed to different stresses. A brief description of the normal development and anatomy of the human intervertebral disc lays the foundation for further discussion of the pathophysiology.

The human intervertebral disc arises from the embryological notochord and perichordal disc. The disc has three major anatomical divisions—the nucleus pulposus, annulus fibrosus, and cartilaginous end plate. The nucleus pulposus is thought to arise from the remnants of the notochord. The perichordal disc is believed to give rise to the remainder of the intervertebral disc. The nucleus pulposus is a complex gelatinous matrix of proteoglycans, collagen, and cells (notochordal cells, chondrocytes, and fibroblasts). The extensive negative charge on the proteoglycan molecules confers the ability to adsorb and hold water in the matrix. This hydrated matrix acts to transmit the stress of axial loads laterally to the annulus. The annulus is constructed of concentric lamellae of dense collagenous tissue anchored at the margins of the vertebral body. The fibers of the lamellae are oriented at approximately 60 degrees to the spinal axis and alternating lamellae are oriented in opposite directions. This confers great strength to resist the lateral forces transmitted by the nucleus pulposus during axial loading. The cartilaginous end plates are made up of hyaline cartilage. Nutrient vessels are found in the end plates and outer annulus but are absent from the nucleus pulposus (9).

The vascular supply to the thoracic intervertebral disc derives from the adjacent segmental radicular arteries. The arterial supply enters the disc proper from the adjacent vertebral bodies through the cartilaginous end plates and periosteum. Small feeders enter the annulus fibrosus but none enter the nucleus pulposus. The nucleus pulposus is dependent on diffusion of nutrients from the end plates and annulus. The human intervertebral disc is most richly supplied with arteries at birth and thereafter shows a steady decline in the number of feeding blood vessels. In adulthood, arterial input only can be found at the very margins of the disc (9).

The innervation of the intervertebral disc is derived from the sinuvertebral nerve, ventral ramus, and gray rami communicantes of the adjacent segmental spinal nerve. These neural inputs give off nociceptive fibers to the annulus fibrosus and the cartilaginous end plate, as well as associated structures such as the longitudinal ligaments, ligamentum flavum, and facet joints. Nerve endings normally can only be found in the outer third of the annulus. The inner two thirds and nucleus pulposus are devoid of neural tissue. Histological morphology of the nerve endings supports nociceptive function. This is corroborated by immunohistochemical studies that demonstrate neuropeptides associated with nociception in the nerve endings (10,11).

At birth, the intervertebral disc is characterized by luscious hydration of the proteoglycan matrix and a well-developed vascular network in the end plates and annulus. The nucleus pulposus comprises approximately half the disc volume and is nearly 90% water at birth. The matrix is rich in hydrated proteoglycan aggregates and aggrecan clusters with small amounts of collagen and elastin. The cellular content is that of residual notochordal cell (12).

Through childhood into adulthood, there is a steady increase in the overall size of the disc accompanied by a decline in the number and size of nutrient vessels in the end plates and annulus. The overall effect is to greatly lengthen the distance that nutrients must diffuse across to supply the central disc. During this time, the components of the matrix are undergoing change. The number of notochordal cells steadily decreases, whereas chondrocyte-like cells begin to appear. The proteoglycan components begin to form fewer and smaller aggregates and aggrecan clusters. This appears to mirror a decline in the concentration of the functional link protein responsible for aggregate formation (12) as well as an overall decline in biosynthesis (13). With the decline in proteoglycans, there is a concomitant decline in the hydration of the matrix of the nucleus pulposus. Similar declines in biosynthesis and matrix degeneration have been demonstrated to occur in the end plate (14). The composition of collagen in the annulus, matrices of the nucleus pulposus and end plates likewise show age-related changes. There is an overall shift in the relative proportions of the collagen subtypes as well as early oxidative posttranslational modifications and cross-linking alterations (15–17). These changes act to lessen the compliance and structural integrity of the disc.

The process of aging and degeneration progresses from the period of skeletal maturity onward. The decline in nutrient vessels continues and the surviving cellular components of the nucleus pulposus decline with them. The notochordal cells all but disappear and the remaining chondrocyte-like cells are left in an environment of falling oxygen tension, falling pH, and rising lactate levels (12). The matrix of the nucleus pulposus continues to lose proteoglycan aggregates, aggrecan clusters, and with them water of hydration. Noncollagenous protein concentrations increase in the nucleus pulposus. The matrix becomes firmer and less fluid and the disc loses height. This loss of fluid character alters the ability of the disc to effectively absorb and dissipate axial load. This leads to a shift of stress load from the nucleus to the annulus (18). The altered geometry and stress loading of the affected segment leads to increased stress on the facets, ligaments, and paraspinal muscles. Meanwhile, the annulus is undergoing changes in collagen composition and integrity. The inner lamella effectively increase in volume as the nucleus decreases. Fine cracks and fissures begin to appear and expand under the increased stress (19). Fissuring and buckling of the annulus may play a role in pain generation by stimulation of the nociceptive fibers in the outer third of the annulus. Examination of degenerated lumbar discs in patients with chronic low back pain has shown evidence of nerve ingrowth into the inner annulus and degenerated nucleus pulposus. These nerves showed immunohistochemical evidence of substance P expression, suggesting nociceptive function. Normal control discs showed no such ingrowth of nerves (20). These data, although limited, suggest plausible mechanisms by which degenerated discs may produce pain.

Principles of Treatment

The goals of treatment in painful thoracic disc degeneration are straightforward and central to spine surgery in general. The goals are alleviation of pain, correction of deformity, if present, stabilization if instability is present, and preservation or improvement of function. Failure to keep these goals foremost in mind when approaching the problem dooms the surgeon's efforts to failure. Removal of a pain-generating disc without addressing concomitant issues of deformity and/or instability leaves open the avenue for persistent or recurrent pain. Instability begets deformity begets pain. Likewise, a solid well-aligned fusion is no guarantee of pain relief if the pain generator is left untouched. Micromotion, even in a seemingly solid fusion, may stimulate pain (21). To achieve the goal of pain relief the pain generator or generators must be clearly identified and eliminated.

Assessment

Patients with symptomatic degenerative thoracic discs often suffer with the undiagnosed disease for prolonged periods. This is not infrequently the result of the often vague, ill-defined pain patterns that fail to conclusively point to an anatomical source and an absence of objective physical findings. In addition, to delay in diagnosis, the unclear nature of the patients' complaints too often earn them the label of hysteria, neurosis, or drug-seeking behavior. The history typically given by patients with thoracic degenerative disc disease follows three general patterns: axial pain, radiculopathy, and myelopathy. Of course, patients commonly present with a mixture of these complaints. Additionally, patients not uncommonly have atypical pain patterns involving the ribs, chest, sternum, abdomen, and viscera (22–24). Extraspinal causes for such complaints must be sought and eliminated. A history of antecedent trauma frequently is lacking.

Axial back and paraspinal pain is common and may point to the problem, but often the pain is not seen as clearly emanating from the disc. The pain may be described as dull, aching, burning, stabbing, or cramping. Pain often is localized to the region of the involved disc but may be difficult for the patient to discretely localize. Activity, load bearing, and cough or sneezing often exacerbates such pain. Recumbent posture often offers some relief. Atypical pain patterns may demonstrate similar patterns of exacerbation and relief. Objective physical findings may be totally lacking. Often there will be local pain on palpation and/or focal muscle spasm, but the physical examination typically is unhelpful in localizing the symptomatic level. Differentiation of lower thoracic disc pain from upper lumbar pain is difficult because there are often no reliable physical findings.

Thoracic radicular pain typically follows a bandlike pattern in the appropriate dermatome. Often it is unilateral, but may be bilateral. Descriptions of the pain vary; stabbing, electric shocks, burning, tearing, and so on. Radicular pain components often share exacerbating and alleviating factors with the axial pain patterns. A dermatomal band of hypesthesia may be present, but is often quite subtle and not infrequently absent. No motor deficit is evident in the absence of cord compression. Local palpation may reveal focal tenderness and/or spasm. Cough or a Valsalva maneuver may reproduce the pain. In the upper thoracic spine a Horner's syndrome rarely may result from disc herniation.

Myelopathy from degenerative thoracic disc disease presents in a myriad of ways. Infrequently the presentation is one of rapidly evolving paraparesis with or without pain. More commonly there is a history of vague complaints of lower extremity numbness, paresthesias, weakness, heaviness, stiffness, or easy fatigability. Motor and sensory symptoms may be unilateral or bilateral. Often such symptoms are dismissed by unwary clinicians because they fail to follow clear nerve root or peripheral nerve patterns. Bowel and bladder complaints are not infrequent. Physical examination reveals long tract signs: increased motor tone, hyperreflexia, clonus, and/or Babinski's sign. Variable degrees of motor weakness and sensory disturbances are present. The patients gait may be normal to profoundly spastic. Rectal tone may be decreased.

RADIOGRAPHIC EVALUATION. Plain film radiographs of the thoracic spine are of use in the evaluation of patients with painful degenerative disc disease. The radiographs may appear normal, but more commonly demonstrate nonspecific degenerative changes. Marginal osteophytes, facet arthropathy, ligamentous calcification, calcification of the disc space, and end plate sclerosis are not infrequently seen. Loss of disc height may give a clue to the symptomatic level, but is far from definitive. Vacuum disc phenomenon is indicative of disc degeneration but not specific to pain generating discs. Kyphosis, scoliosis, osteoporosis, and/or compression fractures may indicate possible sources for pain beyond the disc. Obviously lytic lesions, pedicle erosion, neuroforaminal expansion, and other potential indications of neoplasm or infection must be thoroughly examined.

Contrast myelography is quite sensitive in identifying disc herniations in the thoracic spine. Until recently it was the best imaging modality for evaluation of thoracic disc disease, particularly when coupled with computed tomography (CT). Impingement of the thecal sac is readily identified. It does, however, fail to demonstrate degenerated discs that have not herniated. In patients with myelopathic or radicular symptoms myelography is likely to demonstrate the source. The myelogram is likely to be uninformative in patients with predominantly axial pain from degenerative discs.

CT is quite good at imaging the osseous structures of the spine. Disc herniations may be identified, particularly when calcified. Degenerative changes of the facet joints and rib head articulations are readily apparent. Primary degenerative changes of the disc are often beyond the sensitivity of CT. Secondary changes such as osteophytes, annular bulge and calcification, vacuum phenomenon, and end plate sclerosis are imaged quite nicely. Unfortunately, nothing demonstrable on CT is specific to pain generating discs.

Nuclear medicine offers a range of radionucleotide imaging modalities for application in the spine. These modalities are exquisitely sensitive to even mild metabolic alterations in bone but suffer from lack of specificity and limited resolution. Their use in identifying symptomatic degenerative disc disease currently is limited by these factors.

Magnetic resonance imaging (MRI) has revolutionized imaging of the spine. Technological innovations that go beyond the scope of this chapter are improving the ability of MRI to offer anatomical and pathological/biochemical information. Detailed discussion of MRI may be found in Chapter 11. MRI offers exquisite soft-tissue detail, multiplanar imaging, and the ability to differentiate subtle alterations in tissue fluid content and consistency. It demonstrates in great detail the hydration state of the discs and the fine detail of the neural structures within the thecal sac. It does, however, poorly image osseous structures including osteophytes. Degenerative changes in the disc are easily seen on MRI. Most notably the loss of hydration leads to decrease signal intensity on both T1- and, more obviously, T2-weighted images. Loss of disc height is readily apparent as is bulging of the annulus, end plate irregularities, Schmorl's nodes, and frank herniations. Characteristic signal changes in the vertebral body marrow adjacent to the end plates have been correlated with pathological changes in degenerated discs (25, 26). The addition of gadolinium diethylenetriamine pentaacetic acid (DTPA) enhancement has been reported to reveal enhancement of granulation tissue adjacent to tears of the annulus fibrosus (27) and can help differentiate scar tissue from disc material in the previously operated patient (28).

Thoracic discography has been described and used to identify pain generating thoracic discs (23,29). The use of discography to identify the symptomatic level of disease is based on the observation that discography generally elicits pain in radiographically degenerated discs and is usually painless in radiographically normal discs (29–31). The utility of discography in the assessment of spinal disc pathology is controversial and is not without potential complications (23,32,33). Although there is no definitive study to prove or refute its utility, there is support for the use of discography in selected patients to guide therapy (34). Only a brief discussion of discography is given here because it is amply covered in a separate chapter.

MRI generally is used to identify morphologically abnormal discs to be studied by discography. Discography is performed by injecting contrast material into the nucleus pulposus of the disc to be studied. The morphology of the disc is assessed via fluoroscopy as the injection is performed. Resistance to injection also is noted. Additionally, evidence of annular tears, herniations, disc height, and end plate appearances are noted. Post-discography CT can give additional anatomical detail. As the injection is performed, the patient is asked to characterize the pain produced, if any. A variety of descriptors can be used, but in general they should discretely describe the degree of concordance. For example, exactly concordant, strongly concordant, nonconcordant, and no pain can be used. The patient also is asked to describe the intensity of the pain produced, typically via a 0 to 5- or 0 to 10-point scale. Each suspicious level is investigated as well as at least one morphologically normal disc as a control. The reliability of pain provocation during discography in predicting response to surgical intervention is unproved. The magnitude and concordance of the elicited pain with the patients presenting pain pattern is of great importance. Minimal pain that is strongly concordant is not reassuring and any pain, however severe, that is clearly nonconcordant argues against surgical intervention. The injection of local anesthetics into the disc space has been suggested to improve the specificity of cervical discography if the patients typical pain pattern is relieved (35) and may similarly apply to thoracic discography.

Preoperative Management

The preoperative management of patients with thoracic disc disease depends on the presenting history, physical examination, and supporting imaging studies. The rare patient who presents with acute paraparesis and/or sphincter dysfunction from an acute disc herniation presents no great management dilemma. Urgent surgical decompression is required. The patient with clear thoracic radicular pain, appropriate radiographic confirmation, and failure to improve with conservative measures is straightforward. Unfortunately, few patients with purely degenerative disc disease present with such clear indications for intervention. These remaining patients may be divided into two groups for consideration: the patient with a neurological deficit and the neurologically intact patient with pain.

Patients who present with a stable or slowly progressive myelopathy from thoracic disc disease warrant timely imaging of the thoracic spine with MRI. Identification of spinal cord compression in this setting is a clear indication for nonurgent surgical intervention. Multilevel disease without clear identification of a discrete level of compression on MRI suggests myelography for clarification of the symptomatic level(s). Conservative therapies have little role in the management of these patients other than the possible benefits of general strengthening and increased stamina afforded by a physical therapy program.

The patient presenting neurologically intact with pain man-

dates a more detailed evaluation and judicious management. In general, conservative measures may be undertaken even before going to diagnostic imaging. Obviously any "red flags" for potential serious underlying etiologies (i.e., history of cancer, advanced age, symptoms or history of infectious disease, acute onset or rapidly worsening pain, and so on) mandate timely imaging. However, the typical patient with a long history of stable or slowly worsening pain and no deficit may be given an initial trial of conservative therapy prior to or while awaiting imaging. Conservative measures may include any of the following; nonsteroidal antiinflammatory drugs (NSAIDs), physical therapy for trunk and back strengthening and stamina, epidural steroids, facet or nerve blocks, general exercise and weight loss (in the obese patient), smoking cessation, and even chiropractic manipulation. Although a minority of patients have complete relief with conservative therapies, a number derive sufficient relief to forestall surgical intervention (36). Incapacitating pain that fails to respond to prolonged (6 to 12 months) of conservative therapy or progresses despite therapy may be an indication for surgical intervention. During the period of conservative therapy every effort should be made by the surgeon to build a strong therapeutic relationship with the patient. The decision to proceed with surgery is often based as much on the "feel" for the patient built during this period as on the more objective data.

Prior to surgical intervention, the exact source or sources of the patient's pain must be clearly identified. Careful evaluation of all imaging (plain films, CT, MRI, myelography, discography) usually identifies focal degenerative levels as the likely source of pain. Patients with radicular pain often have obvious focal herniation on MRI. Patients with only axial pain or atypical pain syndromes require more detailed evaluation. Discography may be a useful tool in sorting out the symptomatic level in patients with multilevel degenerative disease and in confirming the pain source in patients with only one apparent level of involvement (29). To be of value a discogram must reproduce significant strongly or exactly concordant pain at one or two levels and clearly negative at normal control levels. Patients with pain at multiple levels, even if strongly concordant should be treated with great circumspection.

General preoperative medical evaluation is straightforward. The patient is evaluated for general medical condition and suitability to undergo a major surgical procedure. Special consideration is given to cardiopulmonary function, particularly when a transthoracic approach is planned. Preoperative pulmonary function tests may be helpful in determining a patient's likelihood of tolerating one lung ventilation should it be necessary. In cases where blood loss is expected to be significant preoperative autologous donation may be considered.

Preoperative Planning

Adequate preoperative planning is paramount to surgical safety and success. Preoperative planning begins with the careful patient assessment as described in the preceding. Selection of appropriate patients obviously is critical. Selection of the surgical approach is no less critical. In addressing "discogenic" pain, aggressive discectomy is mandatory and the surgical approach must facilitate that end. Patients with simple radicular pain may not require the extensive exposure required for total discectomy. The anatomical level of disease, patient body habitus, and considerations for fusion and instrumentation critically affect the selection of a specific approach. Likewise comorbid medical conditions may limit the available approaches (i.e., significant pulmonary disease negates transthoracic approaches).

Planning for intraoperative patient care includes consultation with the anesthetic team to ensure the complete operative plan is understood by all involved. Such consultation should include expected blood loss and plan for replacement (i.e., cell-saver, autologous donation, and so on), special anesthetic considerations (one lung ventilation, agent impact on monitoring, and so on) and neurophysiological monitoring.

Intraoperative monitoring is discussed in detail in the appropriate chapter and is dealt with only superficially here. Neurophysiological monitoring during thoracic spine surgery is strongly recommended. The method of monitoring is largely based on surgeon preference and available resources. Generally somatosensory evoked potentials (SSEP), motor evoked potentials (MEP), or dermatomal evoked potentials (DEP) are used. SSEPs commonly are used and are familiar to most surgeons. The function of the dorsal columns is monitored and can give early warning to any insult to the cord. MEPs monitor the ventral motor pathways and are less commonly used but often of more interest to the surgeon. DEPs are useful in monitoring the function of individual segmental nerves and are rarely used in spine surgery. One circumstance in which DEPs may be of particular use is in the parascapular extrapleural approach where the critical C8 and T1 nerve roots are at increased risk of injury.

Surgical Technique

The detailed description of surgical approaches is beyond the scope of this chapter and is amply dealt with in other chapters of this textbook. Here we confine ourselves to a brief description of various approaches and the general advantages and disadvantages of each.

The dorsal midline approach, although familiar and technically easy, is unacceptable for addressing discogenic disease of the thoracic spine because of its poor exposure of the disc and well-described risk of neurological injury (37). A variety of surgical exposures have been developed for various uses because of these limitations. The transpedicular approach (38) is technically easy and can be used to gain exposure to any thoracic disc level. Very limited exposure of the disc space for complete disc excision and fusion limits its use in treating painful disc disease in the thoracic spine. The transfacet approach (2,39) is quite similar to the transpedicular approach and suffers from the same limitations but requires less bone resection. Dorsolateral approaches, costotransversectomy (40,41), and lateral extracavitary (42,43) can be used to great advantage for exposure of the entire thoracic spine. They offer the distinct advantage over more dorsal approaches of giving lateral access to the disc space and vertebrae for discectomy and fusion. Dorsolateral approaches provide the opportunity for dorsal instrumentation and possible ventral instrumentation. Purely ventral approaches offer the most direct access to the pathology for total extirpation of the disc, provide excellent exposure for ventral instrumentation, and possibly better outcomes (44). In general, such approaches can be used to reach all but the most superior thoracic levels. The transthoracic approach gives excellent multilevel exposure from T2 to T10 where the diaphragm intervenes. This approach is quite amenable to complete disc excision and ventral instrumentation (45). Dorsal instrumentation is precluded without a second approach and often requires the placement of a thoracostomy tube. Thoracic retropleural approaches offer the advantage of avoiding the thoracostomy tube. The need for exposure of the lower thoracic levels and thoracolumbar junction can be accomplished via various thoracoabdominal approaches (41,43).

Exposure of the cervicothoracic junction and upper thoracic spine offers special challenges because of the tight packing of vital anatomical structures in the region. Fortunately, disc disease at these levels is uncommon. A trans-sternal approach to the upper thoracic spine has been described (46,47). This approach offers exposure from the lower cervical vertebrae to the level of T2. The great vessels hamper lower exposure. This approach suffers from the risks of injury to the mediastinal vessels, carotid sheath, thoracic duct, and the morbidity of detaching the sternoclavicular joint and manubrium. Additionally the removal of the discs suffers from late visualization of the thecal sac. The transaxillary approach (41) offers exposure from T1 to T4 from a lateral view. This facilitates direct visualization of the thecal sac during removal of the discs. The approach, however, involves violation of the pleura and requires a thoracostomy tube postoperatively. The lateral parascapular extrapleural approach (48) spares the patient a thoracostomy tube and offers a more lateral exposure of C7 to T2 than does the transsternal approach. The risk of injury to the C8 and T1 nerve roots is a disadvantage.

Perhaps the most exciting recent area of development in the treatment of thoracic disc disease is that of minimally invasive thoracoscopic surgery (49–54). These approaches require special equipment, are unfamiliar to most spine surgeons, and have a steep learning curve. Advantages include direct exposure of the pathology, minimal invasiveness, and subsequent rapid recovery.

General Rehabilitation and Postoperative Principles

The goal of postoperative care and rehabilitation is to maximize the patients' functional recovery, return him or her to normal function as quickly as possible, and circumvent potential postoperative complications. The approach to each patient's rehabilitation must be individualized. The patient's preoperative functional status and the surgical approach used greatly determine the path of rehabilitation. Only general principles are given here.

Early postoperative care centers on complication avoidance. Prevention of deep venous thrombosis begins in the OR with sequential compression devices (SCD). SCDs are continued in the early postoperative period and supplemented with subcutaneous heparin or similar anticoagulant on postoperative day two. Pulmonary care is begun immediately after surgery and is of particular importance in patients undergoing a transthoracic approach. Incentive spirometry complements deep breathing exercises, coughing, and chest physiotherapy. Early mobilization is emphasized where practical. Mobilization facilitates pulmonary toilet, increases stamina, decreases the risk of deep venous thrombosis and, importantly, increases confidence and a sense of progress. Adequate analgesia greatly facilitates pulmonary effort and mobilization. A bowel protocol is instituted immediately following surgery to avoid undue constipation. Bracing generally is not necessary in most cases. Appropriate orthoses may be used in patients undergoing procedures at the cervicothoracic or thoracolumbar junctions where bracing is needed.

Pitfalls and Complications

The complications commonly associated with thoracic spine surgery are well described (37) and beyond the scope of this chapter. General complications include vascular injury, infection, neural injury (spinal cord, roots and sympathetic trunk), intercostal neuralgia, pneumothorax, atelectasis, pneumonia, pulmonary embolism, and so on. Obviously each surgical approach is associated with its own array of unique potential complications. More detailed discussions of the potential complications may be found in the chapters dealing with individual approaches.

Author's Perspective

Patients with painful degenerative thoracic disc disease represent major diagnostic and therapeutic challenges. The often vague symptoms and paucity of hard physical findings too often lead to their being dismissed without serious evaluation. Thankfully the majority of patients with painful degenerative thoracic disc disease respond well to conservative therapy alone. Surgery may benefit those few patients whose suffering is inadequately alleviated by conservative measures. Such patients in whom the clinical history, physical examination, and radiographic and provocative studies are in agreement may be legitimately considered for surgical intervention with a real hope of symptomatic improvement. The establishment of a strong therapeutic relationship with the patient prior to any consideration for surgical intervention cannot be overemphasized.

References

1. Nachemson A, Zdeblick TA, O'Brien JP. Lumbar disc disease with discogenic pain. What surgical treatment is most effective? *Spine* 1996;21:1835–1838.
2. Stillerman CB, et al. Experience in the surgical management of 82 symptomatic herniated thoracic discs and review of the literature. *J Neurosurg* 1998;88:623–633.
3. Sward L, et al. Disc degeneration and associated abnormalities of the spine in elite gymnasts. A magnetic resonance imaging study. *Spine* 1991;16:437–443.
4. Wood KB, et al. Magnetic resonance imaging of the thoracic spine. Evaluation of asymptomatic individuals. *J Bone Joint Surg Am* 1995; 77:1631–1680.
5. Williams MP, Cherryman GR, Husband JE. Significance of thoracic disc herniation demonstrated by MR imaging. *J Comput Assist Tomogr* 1989;13:211–214.
6. Arce CA, Dohrmann GJ. Herniated thoracic disks. *Neurol Clin* 1985; 3:383–392.
7. Wood KB, et al. The natural history of asymptomatic thoracic disc herniations. *Spine* 1997;22:525–529; discussion 529–530.
8. Simpson JM, et al. Thoracic disc herniation. Re-evaluation of the posterior approach using a modified costotransversectomy. *Spine* 1993;18:1872–1877.
9. Rogers MA, Larson SJ. The normal and aging intervertebral disk. In: *Neurosurgery: the scientific basis of clinical practice.* Boston: Blackwell, 1992:705–716.
10. Bogduk N, Windsor M, Inglis A. The innervation of the cervical intervertebral discs. *Spine* 1988;13:2–8.
11. Bogduk N. The lumbar disc and low back pain. *Neurosurg Clin North Am* 1991;2:791–806.
12. Buckwalter JA. Aging and degeneration of the human intervertebral disc. *Spine* 1995;20:1307–1314.
13. Antoniou J, et al. The human lumbar intervertebral disc: evidence for changes in the biosynthesis and denaturation of the extracellular matrix with growth, maturation, ageing, and degeneration. *J Clin Invest* 1996;98:996–1003.
14. Antoniou J, et al. The human lumbar end plate. Evidence of changes in biosynthesis and denaturation of the extracellular matrix with

15. growth, maturation, aging, and degeneration. *Spine* 1996;21: 1153–1161.
15. Nerlich AG, Schleicher ED, Boos N. 1997 Volvo Award winner in basic science studies. Immunohistologic markers for age-related changes of human lumbar intervertebral discs. *Spine* 1997;22: 2781–2795.
16. Pokharna HK, Phillips FM. Collagen crosslinks in human lumbar intervertebral disc aging. *Spine* 1998;23:1645–1648.
17. Olczyk K. Age-related changes in collagen of human intervertebral disks. *Gerontology* 1992;38:196–204.
18. Adams MA, McNally DS, Dolan P. 'Stress' distributions inside intervertebral discs. The effects of age and degeneration. *J Bone Joint Surg Br* 1996;78:965–972.
19. Osti OL, et al. Annular tears and disc degeneration in the lumbar spine. A post-mortem study of 135 discs. *J Bone Joint Surg Br* 1992; 74:678–682.
20. Freemont AJ, et al. Nerve ingrowth into diseased intervertebral disc in chronic back pain. *Lancet* 1997;350:178–181.
21. Weatherley CR, Prickett CF, O'Brien JP. Discogenic pain persisting despite solid posterior fusion. *J Bone Joint Surg Br* 1986;68:142–143.
22. Whitcomb DC, et al. Chronic abdominal pain caused by thoracic disc herniation. *Am J Gastroenterol* 1995;90:835–837.
23. Skubick JK. Thoracic pain syndromes and thoracic disc herniation. In: Freymoyer J, ed. *The adult spine: principles and practice.* New York: Raven, 1991:1443–1461.
24. Eleraky MA, et al. Herniated thoracic discs mimic cardiac disease: three case reports. *Acta Neurochir* 1998;140:643–646.
25. Modic MT, et al. Degenerative disk disease: assessment of changes in vertebral body marrow with MR imaging. *Radiology* 1988;166: 193–199.
26. Lenz GP, et al. New aspects of lumbar disc disease. MR imaging and histological findings. *Arch Orthop Trauma Surg* 1990;109:75–82.
27. Ross JS, Modic MT, Masaryk TJ. Tears of the anulus fibrosus: assessment with Gd-DTPA-enhanced MR imaging. *AJNR Am J Neuroradiol* 1989;10:1251–1254.
28. Ross JS, et al. MR imaging of the postoperative lumbar spine: assessment with gadopentetate dimeglumine. *AJR Am J Roentgenol* 1990; 155:867–872.
29. Schellhas KP, Pollei SR, Dorwart RH. Thoracic discography. A safe and reliable technique (see comments). *Spine* 1994;19:2103–2109.
30. Vanharanta H, et al. Pain provocation and disc deterioration by age. A CT/discography study in a low-back pain population. *Spine* 1989; 14:420–423.
31. Walsh TR, et al. Lumbar discography in normal subjects. A controlled, prospective study. *J Bone Joint Surg Am* 1990;72:1081–1088.
32. Zeidman SM, Thompson K, Ducker TB. Complications of cervical discography: analysis of 4400 diagnostic disc injections. *Neurosurgery* 1995;37:414–417.
33. Guyer RD, et al. Complications of cervical discography: findings in a large series. *J Spinal Disord* 1997;10:95–101.
34. Guyer RD, Ohnmeiss DD. Lumbar discography. Position statement from the North American Spine Society Diagnostic and Therapeutic Committee (see comments). *Spine* 1995;20:2048–2059.
35. Osler GE. Cervical analgesic discography. A test for diagnosis of the painful disc syndrome. *South Afr Med J* 1987;71:363.
36. Brown CW, et al. The natural history of thoracic disc herniation. *Spine* 1992;17:S97–102.
37. Fessler RG, Sturgill M. Review: complications of surgery for thoracic disc disease. *Surg Neurol* 1998;49:609–618.
38. Patterson RH Jr, Arbit E. A surgical approach through the pedicle to protruded thoracic discs. *J Neurosurg* 1978;48:768–772.
39. Stillerman CB, et al. The transfacet pedicle-sparing approach for thoracic disc removal: cadaveric morphometric analysis and preliminary clinical experience (see comments). *J Neurosurg* 1995;83: 971–976.
40. Garrido E. Modified costotransversectomy: a surgical approach to ventrally placed lesions in the thoracic spinal canal. *Surg Neurol* 1980;13:109–113.
41. Watkins R. *Surgical approaches to the spine.* New York: Springer-Verlag, 1983.
42. Larson SJ, et al. Lateral extracavitary approach to traumatic lesions of the thoracic and lumbar spine. *J Neurosurg* 1976;45:628–637.
43. Graham AW 3rd, Mac Millan M, Fessler RG. Lateral extracavitary approach to the thoracic and thoracolumbar spine. *Orthopedics* 1997;20:605–610.

44. Mulier S, Debois V. Thoracic disc herniations: transthoracic, lateral, or posterolateral approach? A review. *Surg Neurol* 1998;49:599–606; discussion 606–608.
45. Currier BL, Eismont FJ, Green BA. Transthoracic disc excision and fusion for herniated thoracic discs. *Spine* 1994;19:323–328.
46. Sundaresan N, et al. An anterior surgical approach to the upper thoracic vertebrae. *J Neurosurg* 1984;61:686–690.
47. Sundaresan N, Shah J, Feghali JG. A transsternal approach to the upper thoracic vertebrae. *Am J Surg* 1984;148:473–477.
48. Fessler RG, et al. Lateral parascapular extrapleural approach to the upper thoracic spine. *J Neurosurg* 1991;75(3):349–355.
49. Dickman CA, et al. Thoracic vertebrectomy and reconstruction using a microsurgical thoracoscopic approach. *Neurosurgery* 1996;38:279–293.
50. Dickman CA, Karahalios DG. Thoracoscopic spinal surgery. *Clin Neurosurg* 1996;43:392–422.
51. Dickman CA, Mican CA. Multilevel anterior thoracic discectomies and anterior interbody fusion using a microsurgical thoracoscopic approach. Case report. *J Neurosurg* 1996;84:104–109.
52. Karahalios DG, et al. Thoracoscopic spinal surgery. Treatment of thoracic instability. *Neurosurg Clin North Am* 1997;8:555–573.
53. Rosenthal D, Dickman CA. Thoracoscopic microsurgical excision of herniated thoracic discs. *J Neurosurg* 1998;89:224–235.
54. Visocchi M, et al. Thoracoscopic approaches to the thoracic spine. *Acta Neurochir* 1998;140:737–743.

146. Herniated Lumbar Disc

Allan Jorge and Gregory J. Przybylski

The original description of sciatica is attributed to Hippocrates in 400 BC. Although this referred pain along the course of the sciatic nerve (L4-S3) is often related to a displaced lumbar disc, it was more than two thousand years later before Mixter and Barr reported in 1934 the surgical treatment of a herniated disc (1). Subsequently, the surgical treatment of the herniated lumbar disc has become one of the most common procedures performed by neurosurgeons. Consequently, familiarity with the diagnosis and treatment of symptomatic lumbar intervertebral disc displacement is critical to the practice of neurosurgery. This chapter summarizes the anatomy, epidemiology, and diagnosis of a displaced lumbar disc as well as comparing the natural history of displaced discs with various treatment options used to manage this common problem.

Anatomy

The primary curvatures of the spine can be identified during early fetal life as concave thoracic and sacrococcygeal curves, providing rigidity and limited mobility (2). During development, the secondary convex curves of the cervical and lumbar regions can be identified, coinciding with the ability to maintain the head erect and ambulate, respectively. The transitional zones between the mobile cervical and lumbar spinal regions and the more rigid thoracic and sacral regions sustain greater degrees of stress, which may be related to the greater frequency of disc displacements seen at the lower cervical and lumbar levels.

The intervertebral disc separates the vertebrae and is composed of outer ligamentous layers termed the annulus fibrosis, a viscoelastic inner core termed the nucleus pulposus, and the end plate cartilage. The annulus is comprised of concentric layers of diagonally oriented collagen fibers bridging adjacent vertebrae and arranged in opposite directions within alternating layers. Although the annular fibers attach to the cartilaginous end plates centrally, direct attachments via Sharpey's fibers to the vertebral bone are observed peripherally. Repetitive mechanical forces of the outer annular fibers are thought to cause osteophytes, termed traction spurs of MacNab. The centrally located nucleus pulposus is a remnant of the notochord and is comprised of a collagen mesh filled with proteoglycan molecular aggregates. A central core of hyaluronic acid serves as the backbone to which proteoglycan monomers attach via link proteins. Although the nucleus is predominantly comprised of water in childhood, progressive desiccation is observed with aging. The nucleus helps to distribute axial loads peripherally by stretching the annular fibers. Finally, the cartilaginous end plates are deformable as well, further helping to dissipate axial loads.

Disc displacements typically are observed earlier in the aging process before significant disc degeneration has occurred. The reduction in water content of the gelatinous nucleus pulposus reduces the ability of the intervertebral disc to dissipate axial loads. This leads to progressive fibrosis and alteration in the collagen components of both the annulus and nucleus. As a result, there is a gradual disappearance of the previously defined border between these two structures. Subsequently, radial fissures between annular fibers develop through which nuclear material can migrate. Autopsy examinations have demonstrated the onset of disc degeneration in the second decade of life in men and the third decade in women, whereas nearly all humans have degenerated lumbar discs in their sixth decade, typically at L3-4 and L4-5 (3).

The outermost dorsal annular fibers additionally are supported centrally by the posterior longitudinal ligament. This elastic ligament is approximately 10 mm wide at the intervertebral disc and may contribute to the posterolateral rather than central displacement of many disc herniations. Asymmetric bulging of the annulus beyond the borders of the end plates has been termed a protruded or contained disc displacement (Fig. 1). Disc extrusion is observed if further annular fissuring allows nuclear displacement beyond the outer annular fibers. Delimitation by the posterior longitudinal ligament is termed a sequestered or subligamentous disc displacement (Fig. 2), whereas complete separation of the displaced fragment from the intervertebral space is called a "free fragment."

The anatomy of the nervous system protected within the spinal canal also must be appreciated to understand the clinical syndromes associated with displaced lumbar intervertebral

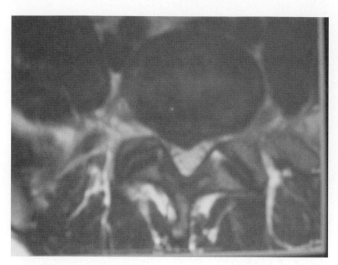

Fig. 1. Axial T2-weighted MRI of a protruded right L5-S1 intervertebral disc displacement causing an S1 radiculopathy in this 30-year-old man.

discs. The caudal extent of the spinal cord, termed the conus medullaris, typically extends to the L1 level and should not be found beyond the inferior L2 vertebral body. The nerve roots emanating from the lower spinal cord form the cauda equina. These paired sensory and motor rootlets combine and exit at each vertebral level in close proximity to its respective pedicle. Because the intervertebral disc is located caudal to the pedicle, a posterolateral L5-S1 disc displacement typically spares the exiting L5 nerve root rostrally but deforms the S1 nerve root as it passes the disc space. In contrast, the less common far lateral (foraminal) disc displacement may effect the exiting L5 nerve root (Fig. 3). Central disc displacements may cause a wide range of symptoms including bilateral radiculopathy and urinary symptoms.

Although the cause of radicular pain is unknown, mechanical compression of the dorsal root ganglion may in part be responsible for the development of radiculopathy. Increased endoneurial fluid pressure has been associated with edema and hemorrhage in the nerve root ganglion (4). Moreover, afferent sensory nerve conduction may be more severely impaired with mechanical compression in comparison to efferent motor conduction,

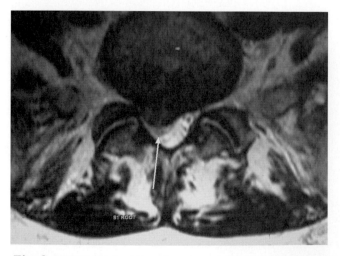

Fig. 2. Axial T2-weighted MRI of a sequestered right L5-S1 intervertebral disc displacement causing an S1 radiculopathy in this 34-year-old woman.

supporting the clinical observation of motor recovery before sensory recovery. Alternatively, certain biochemical substances such as neural proteinases, cytokines, nitric oxide, and prostaglandins may be released by the intervertebral disc and may contribute to radiculopathy as well (5).

Epidemiology

The risk factors associated with the occurrence of disc displacement are similar to those associated with low back pain. For example, low back pain is the second most common reason for medical evaluation. Moreover, lumbago accounts for 15% of all sick-leave time and is the leading cause of disability in patients younger than 45 years of age (6). The annual incidence of low back pain is estimated to be 5%, with a lifetime prevalence ranging from 60% to 90% (7). Despite its frequency, an etiological diagnosis is made in only 15% of patients. Fortunately, symptomatic improvement without treatment is common, because spontaneous recovery is observed in 90% of patients within 1 month of symptom onset (8).

Yet, only 1% of patients with lumbago develop radiculopathy. The lifetime prevalence of disc displacement is approximately 2%, representing a significant minority of patients with low back pain (9). However, spontaneous recovery from radiculopathy also is quite common, with improvement with or without surgical intervention in 80% of patients (8). In fact, fewer than 2% of symptomatic patients may undergo operative treatment (10).

The most commonly identified risk factors associated with lumbar intervertebral disc displacement include young age, male gender, familial association, environmental factors, trauma, and cigarette smoking. In contrast to the increasing prevalence of low back pain with aging, the highest occurrence of lumbar disc displacement occurs in patients between 30 and 50 years of age, with initial symptoms occurring in patients during their third decade of life (11). The progressive desiccation and fibrosis of the annulus may be responsible for the reduced frequency of disc displacement seen beyond the sixth decade. Although a large European study found a 1.6-fold greater incidence of lumbar disc displacement in men, others have found equal distribution among men and women (12). Twin studies have revealed similarities in juvenile disc displacements (13,14). In addition, environmental factors including exposure to excessive mechanical forces, a predominantly sedentary lifestyle, and repetitive vibrational exposure are associated risk factors for disc displacement (15). However, a single traumatic event is an infrequent cause of disc herniation. Finally, the incidence of intervertebral disc degeneration, low back pain, and intervertebral disc displacement is greater among cigarette smokers when compared with nonsmokers (13).

Clinical History and Neurological Examination

The symptoms and signs of lumbar disc displacement are quite variable. The typical patient describes intermittent low back pain of varying severity. However, low back pain usually is a minor component of pain when compared with radiating leg pain. Most patients predominantly complain of pain in a radicular distribution that follows the sensory distribution of the compressed nerve root. Movement or Valsalva often aggravate the pain, whereas bed rest may improve the pain. The pattern of

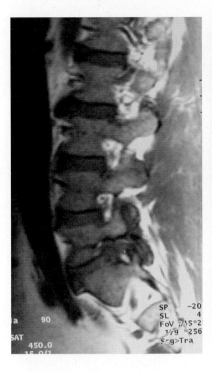
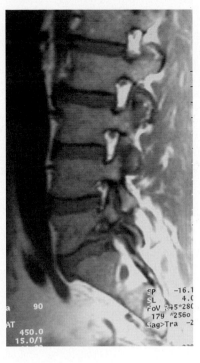

Fig. 3. Parasagittal T1-weighted MRI of a far lateral right L5-S1 intervertebral disc displacement causing an L5 radiculopathy in this 37-year-old man.

pain distribution usually prompts identification of the symptomatic disc level (Table 1). However, a complete history should be obtained to identify symptoms that may require urgent surgical treatment and to identify risk factors of neoplastic or infectious diseases that might also cause radicular symptoms.

The neurological examination should confirm the neurological level suspected from the clinical history. The pattern of motor, sensory, and reflex change in a particular nerve root distribution allows identification of the symptomatic level (Table 1). Moreover, 95% of lumbar disc displacements are observed at L5-S1 and L4-5. In contrast, only 4% occur at L3-4 and rarely at more rostral intervertebral levels (9).

Nonspecific maneuvers such as nerve root tension signs may support the diagnosis of disc displacement. For example, Lasegue described the development of radicular leg pain with less than 60 degrees of leg extension at the hip ipsilateral to the disc displacement. This physical sign is 80% sensitive but only 40% specific for a disc displacement (8). A more specific sign may be the crossed straight leg raise described by Fajerszdahn. Ipsilateral radicular pain with extension of the contralateral leg may be associated with a disc displacement at the axilla. Although less sensitive than the Lasegue maneuver at 25%, the crossed straight leg raise is 90% specific. A bowstring test results in symptom alleviation with knee flexion, potentially differentiating radicular pain from hip pain.

Among patients with sciatica, the predictive value of the straight leg raise and crossed straight leg raise are .67 and .79, respectively (16). Although both are better than the .65 predictive value of an absent ankle jerk, none of these signs is particularly helpful in predicting disc displacement among patients with low back pain alone. Moreover, patients with mid- or high lumbar or far lateral disc displacements do not typically have these nerve root tension signs. A reverse straight leg raise performed either in the prone position or in lateral bending ipsilateral to the disc displacement potentiates the radicular pain in most patients (17).

Certain clinical syndromes should be differentiated from lumbar radiculopathy. Although a foot drop may result from lumbar root compression, a peroneal nerve palsy may cause similar weakness. The common peroneal nerve lies superficially along the fibular head where it is vulnerable to compressive injuries. In addition to the dorsiflexion and external hallices longus weakness seen with L5 radiculopathy, impairment of foot eversion is seen with peroneal nerve palsy. Sensory impairment may be minimal or affect the lateral calf and dorsum of the foot. Although an acute foot drop from L5 nerve root compression may warrant rapid surgical decompression, acute surgery for weakness of longer duration may not provide additional benefit (11,18,19). Large central intervertebral disc displacement, typically at the L4-5 level, may result in cauda equina syndrome

Table 1. Lumbar Nerve Root Compression Patterns

Disc	Nerve Root	Pain	Sensory	Motor	Reflex
L3-4	L4	Anterior thigh	Anterior thigh to medial ankle	Knee extension	Patellar
L4-5	L5	Posterolateral leg	First web space and dorsum of foot	Extensor hallicus longus and dorsiflexion	Medial hamstring
L5-S1	S1	Posterior calf and plantar foot	Lateral and plantar foot	Plantar flexion	Achilles

EHL, extensor hallicus longus.

(20). Rapid symptom onset is associated with poorer recovery patterns when compared with a slowly progressive presentation. Neurological signs include sensory loss in a saddle distribution, unilateral or bilateral leg weakness, and urinary sphincter dysfunction. Although urinary retention is common, overflow incontinence also may be observed. Fewer than half of the patients with bladder dysfunction regain control after treatment of the displaced intervertebral disc (21). Additionally, reduction in rectal tone with stool incontinence also may be observed. Although urgent decompressive surgery usually is recommended, delaying treatment to within 48 hours may not result in a worse neurological outcome (22).

The history and physical examination should also focus on signs of trauma, neoplastic disease, or infection. Even minor trauma may result in vertebral fractures among older patients with steroid use and osteoporosis. Back pain in patients older than 50 years of age with a personal history of cancer is associated with metastatic spinal disease. Several neoplasms including prostate, breast, kidney, thyroid, and lung cancer are associated with bony metastases. The pain may occur at night and is often persistent with recumbency. In contrast, a history of fever, prior cutaneous infection, diabetes, and intravenous drug abuse may suggest the presence of pyogenic discitis, prompting blood tests such as an erythrocyte sedimentation rate and C-reactive protein and contrast imaging studies.

Diagnostic Imaging Studies

The diagnosis of a displaced intervertebral disc with current imaging modalities is reasonably straightforward. However, correlating the imaging findings with a patient's symptomatic complaints often proves much more difficult. For example, symptoms may not correlate with imaging abnormalities in 85% of patients (23). Moreover, the wide interobserver variability further limits the reliability of imaging reports (24). In fact, interobserver agreement among three neuroradiologists in one study of normal volunteers was only 25% (25). In addition, another study of 52 asymptomatic patients revealed imaging abnormalities in 20% of participants younger than 40 years of age and in half over 40 years old (23). Because spontaneous improvement in low back pain and sciatica occurs in the majority of patients within 1 month, imaging studies are not recommended during the first month of symptoms unless significant risk factors for other diseases are present.

Plain radiographs are inadequate for the diagnosis of intervertebral disc displacement, although these can be helpful in the setting of trauma, neoplastic disease or infection. In contrast, lumbar computed tomography (CT) has a sensitivity of 80% to 95% and a specificity of 68% to 88% (26,27). The natural history of lumbar disc displacements has been examined with serial CT imaging, demonstrating reduction or disappearance of displaced and sequestered discs over time (28). The specificity of CT can be improved with myelography performed before the CT study. Extradural filling defects and with impaired filling of the clinically suspected nerve root strongly support the presence of a disc displacement. Magnetic resonance imaging (MRI) has become the gold standard test for the diagnosis of intervertebral disc displacement (Fig. 1); however, many asymptomatic disc displacements are identified with MRI (25).

Treatment

The natural history of sciatica has shown that the majority of patients improve, typically with a few months of symptom onset. Consequently, initial nonoperative management is recommended for patients with new onset of radiculopathy but without significant neurological impairment or risk factors. This conservative approach may extend for at least 6 weeks but not more than 6 months (8). During this conservative management treatment, activity recommendations may include brief bed rest, modification of types of movement, and gradual introduction of an exercise program. Prolonged immobilization may cause deconditioning and prolong the recovery phase, whereas early activity is associated with more rapid pain resolution and functional recovery (29). Avoidance of heavy lifting, with particular attention to bending and twisting restriction may be recommended. Instead, a program of low impact aerobic exercise consisting of walking, bicycling, or swimming may limit deconditioning and allow sufficient symptom reduction before introducing back strengthening exercises focusing on low back and abdominal muscles.

In addition, a variety of medications have been utilized to reduce symptom intensity with some success. Nonsteroidal anti-inflammatory agents are the mainstay of treatment and have demonstrated successful reduction in back pain (30). Other medications have included oral and epidural steroids. However, no differences in outcome at 1 week and 1 year were observed in a randomized study of patients receiving placebo or oral dexamethasone (31). Similarly, epidural steroids have not shown persistent improvement in symptoms at 3 months (32).

Similarly, several surgical treatments have been explored in the management of persistent radicular symptoms related to a lumbar intervertebral disc displacement. Percutaneous procedures have been used with mixed results. Chemonucleolysis using intradiscal injection of chymopapain results in improvement of only 63% of patients at 1 year (33). The risks of anaphylaxis, neurological injury, and iatrogenic discitis have limited broader use of this technique. Percutaneous laser disc decompression, automated percutaneous discectomy with a nucleotome, and intradiscal electrothermal therapy are other minimally invasive techniques that have been explored.

The microdiscectomy remains the gold standard treatment for patients with persistent symptoms caused by lumbar intervertebral disc displacement. In fact, nearly 80% of patients achieve complete relief of sciatic pain at 1 year after surgery (34). Although one randomized study comparing discectomy with nonoperative treatment showed no differences in back pain or sciatica at 4- and 10-year follow-up, 25% of patients failing to improve with nonoperative treatment subsequently underwent discectomy (19). The surgical group had better reported symptom relief at 1 year, suggesting that surgical treatment may facilitate recovery faster than nonoperative management. Percutaneous endoscopic techniques have also been developed to reduce postoperative incisional discomfort. However, fewer than half of the patients treated in this manner among 326 patients treated for lumbar disc displacements reported a good result after endoscopic discectomy (35).

In conclusion, low back pain is a common malady affecting most people as they age. Lumbar intervertebral disc displacement occurs less commonly. However, both low back pain and lumbar radiculopathy have a relatively benign natural history, with most patients improving in a short duration without surgical intervention. Knowledge of intervertebral disc and nerve root anatomy can facilitate diagnosis and localization of intervertebral disc disorders. Various surgical techniques are available for patients who have persistent symptoms despite nonoperative management.

References

1. Mixter W, Barr JS. Rupture of the intervertebral disc with involvement of the spinal canal. *N Engl J Med* 1934;211:210–215.

2. Kieth L Moore. *Clinically oriented anatomy,* 3rd ed. Baltimore: Williams & Wilkins, 1992.
3. Miller JA, Schmartz C, Schultz AB. Lumbar disc degeneration: correlation with age, sex, and spine level in 600 autopsy specimens. *Spine* 1988;13:173–178.
4. White A, Panjabi M. *Clinical biomechanics of the spine,* 2nd ed. Philadelphia: JB Lippincott, 1990.
5. Kang JD, Stefanovic-Racic M, McIntyre LA, et al. Toward a biochemical understanding of human intervertebral disc degeneration and herniation. Contributions of nitric oxide, interleukins, prostaglandin E2, and matrix metalloproteinases. *Spine* 1997;22:1065–1073.
6. Cunningham LS, Kelsey JL. Epidemiology of musculoskeletal impairments and associated disability. *Am J Public Health* 1984;74: 574–579.
7. Frymoyer JW. Back pain and sciatica. *N Engl J Med* 1988;318: 291–300.
8. Bigos S, Bowyer O, Braen G, et al. Acute low back pain problems in adults. Clinical Practice Guideline No. 14, AHCPR Publication No. 95-0642. Agency for Health Care Policy and Research, Public Health Care Service, U.S. Department of Health and Human Services, Rockville, MD, 1944.
9. Hanley E. Surgical indications and techniques. The International Society for the Study of the Lumbar Spine. *The lumbar spine,* 2nd ed. Philadelphia: WB Saunders, 1996:492–524.
10. Deyo RA, Tsui-Wu YJ. Descriptive epidemiology of low-back pain and its related medical care in the United States. *Spine* 1987;12: 264–268.
11. Weber H. Lumbar disc herniation. A prospective study of factors including a controlled trial. *J Oslo City Hosp* 1978;28:33–64, 89–120.
12. Heliovaara M, Knekt P, Aromaa A. Incidence and risk factors of herniated lumbar intervertebral disc or sciatica leading to hospitalization. *Chronic Dis* 1987;40:251–258.
13. Battie MC, Videman T, Gill K, et al. Smoking and lumbar intervertebral disc degeneration: an MRI study of identical twins. *Spine* 1991; 16:1015–1021.
14. Videman T. Epidemiology of disc disease. The International Society for the Study of the Lumbar Spine. *The lumbar spine,* 2nd ed. Philadelphia: WB Saunders, 1996:16–25.
15. Ljunggren A. Epidemiology of disc disease. The International Society for the Study of the Lumbar Spine. *The lumbar spine,* 2nd ed. Philadelphia: WB Saunders, 1996:475.
16. Deyo RA, Rainville J, Kent DL. What can the history and exam tell us about low back pain? *J Am Med Assoc* 1992;268:760–765.
17. Abdullah AF, Wolber PGH, Warfield JR. Surgical management of extreme lateral lumbar disc herniations: review of 138 cases. *Neurosurgery* 1988;22:648–653.
18. Saal JA, Saal JS. Nonoperative treatment of herniated lumbar intervertebral disc with radiculopathy: an outcome study. *Spine* 1989; 14:431–437.
19. Weber H. Lumbar disc herniation. A controlled prospective study with ten years of observation. *Spine* 1983;8:131–140.
20. Shapiro S. Cauda equina syndrome secondary to lumbar disc herniation. *Neurosurgery* 1993;32:743–747.
21. Kostuik JP, Harrington I, Alexander D. Cauda equina syndrome and lumbar disc herniation. *J Bone Joint Surg Am* 1986;68:386–391.
22. Shapiro S. Medical realities of cauda equina syndrome from lumbar disc herniation. *Spine* 2000;25:348–351.
23. White AA, Gordon SL. Synopsis: workshop on idiopathic low-back pain. *Spine* 1982;7:141–149.
24. Deyo RA, Diehl AK, Rosenthal M. How many days of bed rest for acute low back pain? A randomized clinical trial. *N Engl J Med* 1986; 315:1064–1070.
25. Boden SD, Davis DO, Dina TS. Abnormal magnetic-resonance scans of the lumbar spine in asymptomatic subjects. *J Bone Joint Surg Am* 1990;72:403–408.
26. Bosacco SJ, Berman AT, Garbarino JL. A comparison of CT scanning and myelography in the diagnosis of lumbar disc herniation. *Clin Orthop* 1984;190:124–128.
27. Moufarriji NA, Hardy RW, Weinstein MA. Computed tomography, myelographic, and operative findings in patients with suspected herniated lumbar discs. *Neurosurgery* 1983;12:184–188.
28. Cowan NC, Bush K, Katz DE, et al. The natural history of sciatica: a prospective radiological study. *Clin Radiol* 1992;46:7–12.
29. Gilbert JR, Taylor DW, Hildebrand A, et al. Clinical trial of common treatments for low back pain in family practice. *Br Med J Clin Res* 1985;291:791–794.
30. Amlie E, Weber H, Holme I. Treatment of acute low-back pain with piroxicam: results of a double-blind placebo-controlled study. *Spine* 1987;12:473–476.
31. Haimovic IC, Beresford HR. Dexamethasone is not superior to placebo for treating lumbosacral radicular pain. *Neurology* 1986;36: 1593–1594.
32. Carette S, Leclaire R, Marcoux S. Epidural corticosteroid injection for sciatica due to herniated nucleus pulposus. *N Engl J Med* 1997; 336:1634–1640.
33. Van Alphen HA, Braakman R, Bexemer PD. Chemonucleolysis versus discectomy: a randomized multicenter trial. *J Neurosurg* 1989; 70:869–875.
34. Tulberg T, Isacson J, Weidenhielm L. Does microscopic removal of lumbar disc herniation lead to better results than the standard procedure? Results of a one-year randomized study. *J Neurosurg* 1993;70:869–875.
35. Klienpeter G, Markowitsch MM, Bock F. Percutaneous endoscopic lumbar discectomy: minimally invasive, but perhaps minimally useful? *Surg Neurol* 1995;43:534–541.

147. Far Lateral and Foraminal Lumbar Disc Herniations

Nancy E. Epstein

Four different degrees of facet resection are required for the removal of far lateral disc herniations. These include the medial facetectomy, intertransverse approach, full facetectomy, and extreme lateral approach. Each procedure must be accompanied by bony dissection varying from a laminotomy to multilevel laminectomy with or without fusion depending on the underlying pathology; that is, stenosis, spondyloarthrosis, degenerative spondylolisthesis, degenerative scoliosis, and limbus vertebral fractures. However, there are pros and cons for each technique, and the operative approach chosen must be tailored to the individual's needs (1).

Definition of Far Lateral Discs

The far lateral compartment is located lateral to the pedicle beyond the neural foramen. Borders include the pedicle superiorly, disc anteriorly, vertebral body and leading edge of the superior articular facet medially, and fat laterally (2). Far lateral discs, comprising between 7% and 12% of all lumbar disc herniations, are typically sequestrated fragments that have migrated both superiorly and laterally into the foramen or far lateral compartment, where they compress the superiorly exiting nerve root and ganglion (3–6). However, far lateral herniations frequently are accompanied by foraminal lesions located in the subarticular region bordered by the medial and lateral pedicles. Siebner and Faulhauer found that 3% of 694 herniated lumbar discs were both foraminal and far lateral in their location, whereas 4% were isolated extraforaminal herniations (2).

Even in the absence of spinal stenosis, little room is available for a compressed, swollen ganglion in this far lateral compartment because spontaneous decompression may only occur laterally into the fat. When short pedicle stenosis is present, the degree of narrowing is further heightened by spondyloarthrosis, degenerative scoliosis, limbus fractures, degenerative spondylolisthesis, and spondylolytic spondylolysis. Far lateral disc herniations extending medial to the pedicle and beneath the superior articular facet, may simultaneously compromise both the superiorly and inferiorly exiting nerve roots or cauda equina.

LEVELS. The L4-5 (59%), L3-L4 (31%), and L5-S1 (7%) levels were the most commonly involved sites of far lateral disc herniations in Donaldson's series; Maroon's patients showed similar distributions (7,8). More cephalad involvement at the L1-2 or L2-3 levels was rare, except in An's series (3).

Neurological Presentation

Patients presenting with far lateral pathology average 55 years of age (range, 50 to 78 years old) (1–9). Half are men and half women. They usually complain of exquisite radicular pain, a finding attributed to compromise of the dorsal nerve root ganglion in the far lateral compartment. Leg pain is intense, although there may be minor back pain (4).

Because far lateral disc herniations compress the superior nerve root they exhibit cephalad root syndromes (6,7). Proximal far lateral discs (L1-2 through L4-5) produce hip, groin, and proximal thigh and knee pain. These symptoms may be confused with those observed for hip disease. Neurological findings include a positive reversed Laségue maneuver (femoral stretch test), iliopsoas and/or quadriceps weakness, diminished patellar responses, and appropriate sensory changes to pin appreciation in the L1-4 dermatomes. Alternatively, those with L5-S1 far lateral disc herniations affecting the L5 root exhibit sciatica radiating to the calf and ankle, associated with positive Laségue maneuvers, extensor hallicus longus/dorsiflexors weakness, decreased or absent Achilles responses, and decreased pin appreciation in the L5 distribution.

Pathology Accompanying Far Lateral Disc Herniations

LIMBUS VERTEBRAL FRACTURES. Limbus fractures, defined as disc herniations combined with cartilage, and cortical/cancellous bone, may occur in conjunction with far lateral disc herniations. Although more common in younger individuals (twenties to forties), they are also observed in older individuals (fifties to sixties) (10).

There are four types of vertebral fractures. Type I fractures, consisting of a central shelf of cortical bone crossing the base of the spinal canal, may contribute to thecal sac compression and cauda equina syndromes. Type II square-chip fractures also

may produce cauda equina compression because they occur centrally beneath the thecal sac. Type III limbus lateral chip fractures are more likely to impinge on nerve roots laterally, foraminally, or far laterally, whereas Type IV limbus fractures, involving the entire posterior vertebral cortex, extending from interspace to interspace, most frequently result in cauda equina dysfunction.

If a foraminal or far lateral limbus fracture accompanies a far lateral disc herniation, a full facetectomy often will be required to afford adequate exposure and decompression of the involved nerve root (10). Resection techniques typically include the initial creation of an underlying trough in the disc space itself, followed by gentle piecemeal resection of the limbus fracture using a downbiting curette, tamp, and mallet technique. Once the bony fragments are delivered into the underlying interspace, they may then be removed with pituitary forceps.

STENOSIS AND SPONDYLOSIS. Lumbar stenosis, congenital or acquired, further limits the available space in the far lateral compartment, and more frequently requires the completion of a full facetectomy to safely remove a far lateral disc. Short pedicles and vertically oriented thickened lamina make the technical removal of a far lateral disc more difficult, as hypertrophied or massively arthrotic facet joints overlay not only the foramen but a significant part of the lateral recess and portions of the far lateral compartment as well. The need for a full facetectomy and obscuration of anatomy resulting from stenosis requires clear identification of the appropriate disc space on a cross table lateral x-ray. Out of 857 patients treated for lumbar stenosis, 40 had far lateral disc herniations, the remaining had five combinations of far lateral spondylostenosis, degenerative spondylolisthesis, scoliosis, and limbus fractures (7–9). Here, multilevel laminectomies with single-level facetectomies adequately addressed the pathology. In our own and An's experience, patients with far lateral disc herniations and stenosis required more extended decompressions (3,9). Myelo-CT examinations often demonstrating the full expanse of disease to be addressed (9).

DEGENERATIVE SPONDYLOLISTHESIS. Grade I degenerative spondylolisthesis is most often encountered at the L4-5 level, followed in descending frequency by the L3-4, L2-3, and L5-S1 interspaces (11–13). Grade I olisthy is limited to one quarter of the vertebral body width as the more sagittally oriented hugely arthrotic facet joints lock at this point. Although routine disc herniations may accompany the slip 4.3% to 20% of the time, those located far laterally at the level of the slip often should be addressed with decompressive laminectomy, full unilateral facetectomy, and instrumented fusion to avoid future instability (1,14). Good to excellent outcomes are observed over 80% of the time.

SPONDYLOLISTHESIS WITH LYSIS. In spondylolisthesis with lysis, the superiorly exiting nerve root is compressed as it slips below the pedicle making its way through the neural foramen toward the far lateral compartment. Here the free-floating lamina and fibrotic lytic area must be excised to decompress this nerve root and should be followed by an instrumented fusion if instability has been demonstrated. Outcomes are good to excellent from 76% to more than 80% of the time (14–16).

DEGENERATIVE SCOLIOSIS. Older patients with degenerative scoliosis may exhibit far lateral pathology often reflecting rotational and conformational facet and foraminal productive changes rather than far lateral herniated discs. Most changes occur on the concave side where the pedicles converge, further constricting the foramen.

Neurodiagnostic Evaluation

MAGNETIC RESONANCE SCANS. Magnetic resonance axial and parasagittal foraminal images show isointense to hypointense densities obliterating the normal fat, lying lateral to the pedicle in the far lateral compartment (5,6). When supplemented with gadolinium diethylenetriamine-pentaacetic acid, MRs help differentiate between tumor, scar (enhancing), and recurrent disc (nonenhancing).

COMPUTED TOMOGRAPHY. These studies should be supplemented with computed tomography (CT) based examinations that better define both the far lateral disc itself, appearing as an isolated focus of isointense tissue, and accompanying far lateral bony pathology; that is, scoliosis, spondyloarthrosis, degenerative or lytic olisthy, or limbus fractures (4,17).

MYELO-COMPUTED TOMOGRAPHY. Although Myelo-CT scans do not show abnormalities with isolated far lateral discs herniations (18) because the subarachnoid space tapers off in the neural foramen, they do modify the operations performed in these patients by defining significant attendant pathology (8,9).

Conservative Management

The management of far lateral disc herniations should include initial conservative treatment (bed rest, antiinflammatory medication, etc.), except in the presence of significant neurological deficits, because approximately 10% of patients improve without surgical intervention. In the presence of an extruded disc, epidural steroid injections are minimally effective and can result in significant cerebrospinal fluid fistulas, which make surgical intervention more difficult.

Surgical Techniques

MEDIAL FACETECTOMY. The medial facetectomy with the laminotomy, hemilaminectomy, or complete laminectomy provides access to proximal foraminal and far lateral disc herniations particularly at the least stenotic L5-S1 level (Figs. 1 and 2). Multiple sequestrated disc fragments and far lateral stenosis owing to spondyloarthrosis, degenerative spondylolisthesis, scoliosis, and limbus fractures warrant the more extended intertransverse or full facetectomy procedures. One risks retained disc fragments, incomplete decompression, and inadvertent nerve root injury with medial facetectomy (1,8,9).

INTERTRANSVERSE TECHNIQUE. The intertransverse technique (ITT), requiring both medial (laminotomy/laminectomy) and far lateral extraforaminal exposure, offers removal of a far lateral disc while preserving the pars interarticularis and facet joint (11,19) (Fig. 3). At any level, the cephalad nerve root may

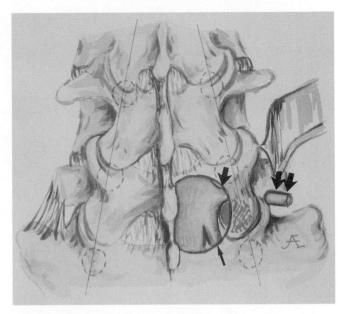

Fig. 1. Extended right L5 laminotomy with medical facetectomy and foraminotomy for excision of foraminal L5-S1 disc. This exposure provides access both to the proximal L5 *(single large arrow)* and S1 nerve roots *(small single arrow)*, but not to the lateral foraminal or far lateral L5 root sleeve *(double arrows)*. (From the American Association of Neurological Surgeons Publications Committee, with permission.)

be followed into the proximal neural foramen, and again exposed far laterally by removing the superolateral most aspect of the facet joint and intertransverse ligament/fascia (6,19). An advantage of the ITT approach is the ability to simultaneously resect the far lateral sequestrated fragment while emptying the medial portion of the disc to avoid disc recurrence (1,4). Five out of Deckler's 15 patients treated with the ITT technique showed no recurrent disc herniations, whereas three of 10 managed with the isolated extraforaminal (EF) exposure developed recurrent herniations (4). However, the residual intraforaminal portion of the nerve root may be injured during disc resection, although the ITT technique does preserve stability.

FULL FACETECTOMY. When spondylosis, arthrosis, degenerative spondylolisthesis, scoliosis, far lateral stenosis, or limbus fractures accompany far lateral disc herniations, the complete facetectomy allows for full visualization of the nerve root throughout its intracanalicular, foraminal, and extracanalicular course (Fig. 4). Blind manipulation, retained disc fragments, and residual stenosis are avoided at the potential expense of stability. However, in Garrido and Connaughton's experience, most enjoyed good to excellent outcomes in 38 of 41 cases, with only one in 41 patients requiring secondary fusion (17). Fusion requirements following full facetectomy in the author's experience varied from one in 60 (9) to four in 170 (1). At the other extreme, some uniformly fuse these patients (20).

EXTRAFORAMINAL (EXTREME LATERAL) APPROACH. The extreme lateral (EF) extraforaminal approach may be used alone or as part of the trans pars and intertransverse techniques (2,5,8,17) (Fig. 5). The far lateral compartment may be exposed using either a midline or paramedian muscle splitting approach. Dissection, carried out lateral to the facet joint, requires resection of the intertransversarius ligament and fascia and removal

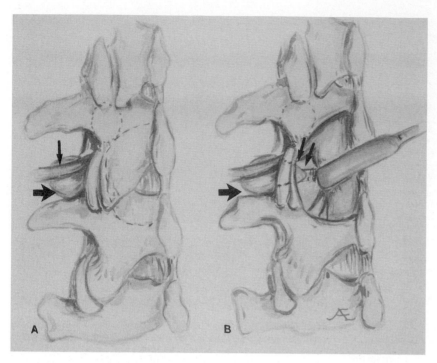

Fig. 2. Left L4-5 medial facetectomy and foraminotomy for excision of foraminal and far lateral disc herniation. **A:** Far lateral disc L4-5 *(left)*. The planned extended L4-5 laminotomy *(dotted line)* with medial facetectomy and foraminotomy should provide access to the proximal foraminal "tail" of this sequestrated fragment *(large arrow)* located far laterally where it impinges on the L4 root *(small arrow)*. **B:** Foraminal "tail" of L4-5 sequestrated far lateral disc following the decompression, the medial "tail" of the far lateral disc *(double arrows)* may be seen in the proximal neural foramen, but the far lateral portion of the disc *(large single arrow)* and L4 nerve root are not visualized. (From the American Association of Neurological Surgeons Publications Committee, with permission.)

of only the superolateral most aspect of the facet joint. Outcomes have been reported as good to excellent in up to 85% of patients using this technique (2,5,8). The minimal bony decompression and facet excision markedly limited postoperative instability, whereas the lack of medial exposure eliminates medial scarring but increases chances of disc recurrence (4).

TRANS PARS TECHNIQUE. Performance of the trans pars approach first requires at minimum a laminotomy one level above the far lateral disc herniation (Fig. 6). The cephalad nerve root is then followed caudally as it crosses the cephalad disc space, and dips beneath the pars interarticularis and inferior pedicle, extending to and through the neural foramen into the far lateral compartment (1,7,9). Advantages include visualization of the nerve root along its entire course, and arguable preservation of the facet joint that remains supported by the residual lamina, but without access to the medial portion of the disc, thereby increasing the chances of a disc recurrence.

PERCUTANEOUS TECHNIQUES. Few patients are appropriate candidates for the varied percutaneous techniques (success

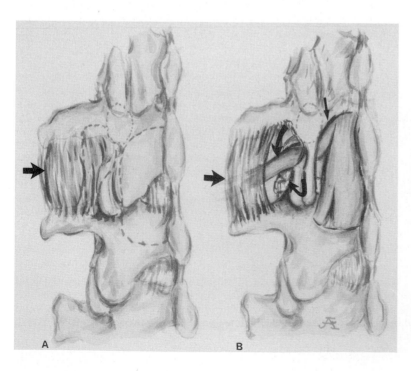

Fig. 3. **A,B:** Intertransverse approach to left L4-5 far lateral disc. **A:** Preoperative view. The medial and extreme lateral exposures facilitate resection of this L4-5 far lateral disc herniation. The medial dotted line outlines the laminotomy, the lateral red dotted line outlines the resection of the superolateral most aspect of the L4-5 facet joint made possible following removal of the intertransversarius ligament and fascia *(large arrow)*. **B:** Postoperative view. Intertransverse approach to left L4-5 far lateral disc where the L4-5 laminotomy with medial facetectomy and foraminotomy exposed the L4 nerve root in the canal and proximal neural foramen *(small single arrow)*. The extreme lateral approach, requiring removal of the intertransversarius ligament and fascia *(large straight arrow)* and superior-lateral-most portion of the L5 superior articular facet provided visualization of the far lateral nerve root *(mildly curved arrow)* and disc *(very curved arrow)*. (From the American Association of Neurological Surgeons Publications Committee, with permission.)

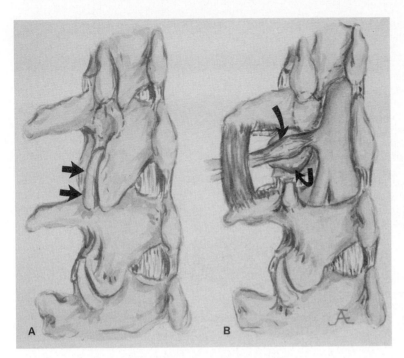

Fig. 4. Full facetectomy for excision of lateral, foraminal, and far lateral left L4-5 disc. **A:** Preoperative view. The full L4-5 facetectomy *(double arrows)* addresses the foraminal and far lateral spondylostenosis and far lateral disc herniation. **B:** Postoperative view: left L4 hemilaminectomy with L4-5 full facetectomy for resection of far lateral disc following the discussed exposure, supplemented with the removal of the intertransversarius ligament and fascia, the full course of the L4 nerve root *(mildly curved arrow)* and sequestrated lateral, foraminal, and far lateral disc *(very curved arrow)* is visualized. (From the American Association of Neurological Surgeons Publications Committee, with permission.)

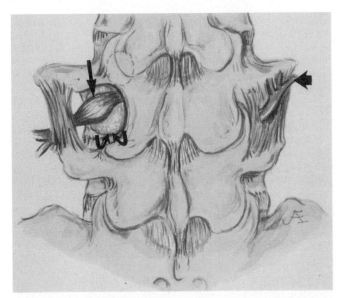

Fig. 5. Extreme lateral approach to a left L4-5 far lateral disc. This approach may be initiated through a midline or paramedian multifidus longissimus muscle splitting approach. Note how resection of the superior/lateral aspect of the facet joint allows for adequate visualization of the far lateral disc fragment *(double very curved arrows)* and L4 nerve root/ganglion *(long single arrow)* as long as the patient is not stenotic. The ramus dorsalis of the lumbar artery *(short single arrow)* seen on the right far laterally can bleed vigorously. (From the American Association of Neurological Surgeons Publications Committee, with permission.)

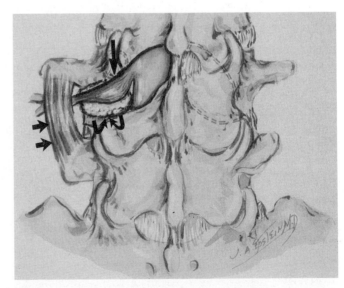

Fig. 6. Trans pars resection of left L4-5 lateral, foraminal, and far lateral disc. This exposure requires an L3-4 laminotomy *(dotted lines)*, resection of the L4 pars interarticularis *(long single arrow)* with sparing of the L4-5 facet joint, and removal of the lateral ligaments/fascia *(double arrows)*. (From the American Association of Neurological Surgeons Publications Committee, with permission.)

rates of less than 70%), especially in the presence of spondylostenosis, leaving direct microsurgery the procedure of choice.

FUSION REQUIREMENTS. Each of the techniques of facet resection offered for far lateral disc resection may be associated with some degree of postoperative spinal instability. The most destabilizing procedure is the full facetectomy, followed in descending order by the trans pars, intertransverse, and isolated extraforaminal exposures. Clinical data show that instability is uncommon (1.6% to 2.4%) irrespective of the technique of facet resection employed (1,9,17). However, when instability is present, particularly in patients with degenerative spondylolisthesis requiring a unilateral full facetectomy for far lateral disc/stenosis excision, pedicle screw or rod fixation techniques best provide for immediate stabilization while reducing the risk of postoperative pseudarthrosis (21).

OUTCOMES. Success rates for the different approaches to far lateral discs varied from 70% to 100% (2–4,7). Our results were similar, demonstrating comparable good to excellent outcome using three different facet resection techniques (1,9,22).

PITFALLS OF FAR LATERAL DISC SURGERY. Pitfalls common to far lateral disc surgery include operating at the wrong level or wrong side, and making the wrong diagnosis. In extremely difficult cases, placing a Penfield elevator in the interspace to reconfirm the correct level and converting to a full facetectomy is the best salvage maneuver.

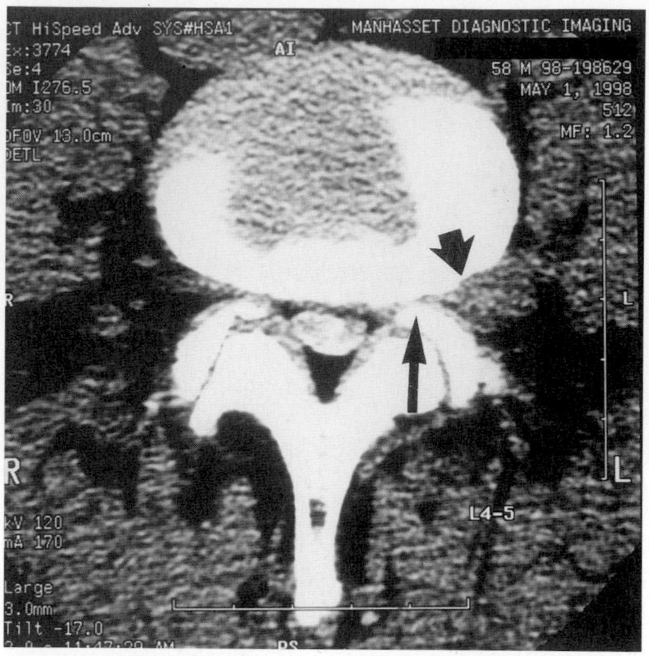

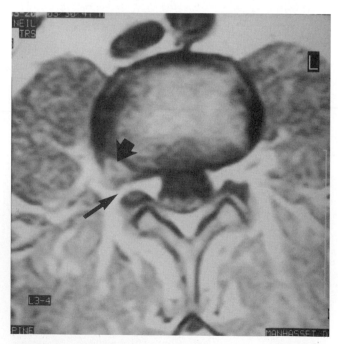

Fig. 7. Full left L4-5 facetectomy for removal of myelo-CT documented lateral recess/foraminal stenosis and a far lateral disc. Here, an L4 hemilaminectomy with L4-5 full left facetectomy must decompress the marked lateral recess and foraminal stenosis *(long arrow)* identified along with the foraminal and far lateral disc *(short arrow)*.

Personal Series

Between 1984 and 1994, 170 patients had far lateral disc surgery (1). Patients averaged 55 years of age, included 112 males and 58 females, and were followed an average of 5 years. Neurological findings included positive mechanical signs (84%), motor dysfunction (74%), reflex abnormalities (98%), prominent sensory deficits (79%), and rare sphincter dysfunction (2.4%).

Preoperative MR, CT, or myelo-CT studies demonstrated far lateral disc herniations at L4-5 (68), L3-4 (63), L5-S1 (33), L2-3 (4), and L1-2 (2). Far lateral spondylostenosis and scoliosis accompanied far lateral disc herniations in 30 patients, whereas degenerative spondylolisthesis was noted in another 23 individuals. Three months postoperatively, routine flexion and extension x-rays were performed, instability being documented where there was greater than 4 mm of motion.

SURGERY. The 36 patients requiring laminectomy for decompression of significant stenosis with their far lateral disc herniations, required the more extensive full facetectomies, whereas those undergoing laminotomies or hemilaminectomies (134) were managed more readily with the ITT or medial facetectomy approaches (Figs. 7–10).

FUSION REQUIREMENTS. Four of the 170 patients with L4-5 degenerative spondylolisthesis and an L4-5 far lateral disc requiring full facetectomy developed instability and required pedicle screw/rod instrumented fusions. Four months postoperatively all showed good outcomes and had successfully fused.

Fig. 8. Transaxial T1-weighted MRI of right L3-4 far lateral sequestrated disc treated with intertransverse technique. The right L3-4 far lateral disc herniation *(short arrow)* shown on this MR study, with minimal stenosis, confirmed by the presence of fat within the foramen *(long arrow)* was removed using an intertransverse exposure.

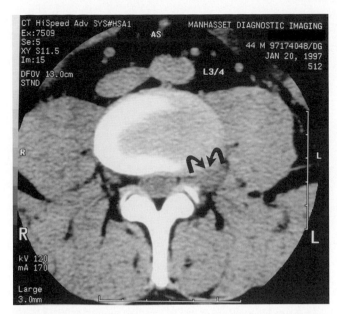

Fig. 9. Transaxial CT of left-sided L3-4 foraminal and far lateral disc requiring intertransverse approach. Adequate exposure of this far lateral disc required an L3 hemilaminectomy with L4 laminotomy, medial facetectomy, and foraminotomy plus extreme lateral exposure for far foraminal and lateral disc excision *(arrows)*.

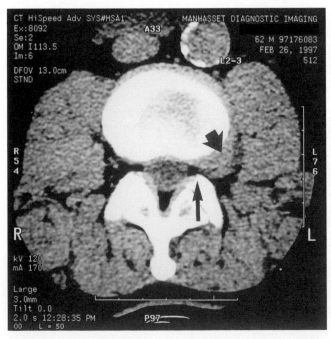

Fig. 10. Noncontrast transaxial CT study showing left L2-3 stenosis and far lateral disc herniation managed with full facetectomy. The foraminal and far lateral disc fragment *(short arrow)*, lodged beneath the large, medially impinging arthrotic facet joint *(long arrow)* consistent with stenosis, had to be resected using a full L2-3 facetectomy and L2 hemilaminectomy/L3 laminotomy.

OUTCOMES. Postoperatively, outcomes were ranked as excellent (no deficit), good (mild residual radiculopathy requiring minimal analgesia), fair (moderate residual radiculopathy or unchanged requiring moderate analgesia), and poor (increased radiculopathy requiring increased analgesia) using Odom's criteria (18,23,24). Excellent outcomes were achieved in 73, good outcomes in 51, fair in 26, and poor results in 20 patients. Of interest, good to excellent outcomes using any of the three facet resection techniques did not significantly differ: 79% for the intertransverse approach, 70% for those undergoing full facetectomy, and 68% having medial facetectomy.

Surgeon- Versus Patient-Based Outcome Analysis (SF-36) of Far Lateral Disc Surgery

Patient-based outcome studies are becoming more prominent in clinical research and are increasingly influencing surgical policy or surgeon-based outcome measures (25). The Medical Outcomes Trust Short Form (SF-36), which measures physical function, role physical, bodily pain, general health, vitality, social function, role–emotional, and mental health using 36 generic questions, has been used successfully over the last two decades in over 260 medical and surgical outcome studies (26). The SF-36 was retrospectively administered to 76 (45%) of patients having far lateral disc surgery, and the results were then compared with the surgeon's (Odom's criteria) assessment of outcome (1,26). Overall, correlations between the surgeon's assessment and SF-36 responses were modest. For patients seen within the last 4.5 years, the surgeon's assessment was a relatively good predictor of mean SF-36 outcome scores, varying from .187 to .378 , all but General Health and Social Function Scales passing statistical significance. Physical Function, Role Physical, and Bodily Pain best correlated on a descending scale with the surgeon's assessment of physical function. In Kantz, Harris, and Levitsky and associates' study, the surgeon's assessment also was best correlated with Physical Function and Role Physical Scales (27). The SF-36, used in a cardiac surgery series, demonstrated that a minimum of six postoperative months was required before patients demonstrate adequate postoperative improvement (28). In the future, SF-36 outcome studies applied to far lateral disc surgery should serve as an inexpensive way of assessing short- and long-term outcome, allowing us to better compare the relative efficacy of different surgical techniques.

References

1. Epstein NE. Evaluation of varied surgical approaches used in the management of 170 far-lateral lumbar disc herniations: indications and results. *J Neurosurg* 1995;83:648–656.
2. Siebner HR, Faulhauer K. Frequency and specific surgical management of far lateral lumbar disc herniations. *Acta Neurochir (Wien)* 1990;105:124–131.
3. An HS, Vaccaro A, Simeone FA, et al. Herniated lumbar disc in patients over the age of fifty. *J Spinal Disord* 1990;3:143–146.
4. Deckler R, Hamburger C, Schmiedek P, et al. Surgical observations in extremely lateral lumbar disc herniation. *Neurosurg Rev* 1992;15:255–258.
5. Faust SE, Ducker TB, Van Hassent JA. Lateral lumbar disc herniations. *J Spinal Disord* 1992;5:97–103.
6. Hood RS. Far Lateral lumbar disc herniations. *Neurosurg Clin North Am* 1993;4:117–124.

7. Donaldson WF, Star MJ, Thorne RP. Surgical treatment of far lateral herniated lumbar disc. *Spine* 1993;18:1263–1267.

8. Maroon JC, Kopitnik TA, Schulhof LA, et al. Diagnosis and microsurgical approach to far-lateral disc herniation in the lumbar spine. *J Neurosurg* 1990;73:642–643.

9. Epstein NE, Epstein JA, Carras R, et al. Far lateral lumbar disc herniations and associated structural abnormalities. An evaluation in 60 patients of the comparative value of CT, MRI, and myelo-CT in diagnosis and management. *Spine* 1990;15:534–539.

10. Epstein NE. Lumbar surgery for 56 limbus fractures, emphasizing non calcified type II lesions. *Spine* 1992;17:1489–1496.

11. Wiltse LL, Spencer CW. New uses and refinements of the paraspinal approach to the lumbar spine. *Spine* 1988;13:696–706.

12. Epstein NE. Decompression in the surgical management of degenerative spondylolisthesis: advantages of a conservative approach in 290 patients. *J Spinal Disord* 1998;11:116–122.

13. Tsou PM, Hopp E. Postsurgical instability in spinal stenosis. In: Hopp E, ed. *Spine: state of the art reviews.* Philadelphia: Hanley and Belfus, 1987:533–550.

14. Epstein NE. Primary fusion for the management of "unstable" degenerative spondylolisthesis. *Neuro-Orthop* 1998;23:45–52.

15. Markwalder TM, Saager C, Reulen HJ. Isthmic spondylolisthesis: an analysis of the clinical and radiological presentation in relation to intraoperative findings and surgical results in 72 consecutive cases. *Acta Neurochir* 1991;110:154–159.

16. Boos N, Marchesi D, Aebi M. Treatment of spondylolysis and spondylolisthesis with Cotrel-Dubousset instrumentation: a preliminary report. *J Spinal Disord* 1991;4:472–479.

17. Garrido E, Connaughton PN. Unilateral facetectomy approach for lateral lumbar disc herniation. *J Neurosurg* 1992;76:342–343.

18. Epstein NE, Epstein JA. Lumbar decompression for spinal stenosis: surgical indications and techniques with and without fusion. In: Frymoyer JW, Ducker TB, Kostuik JP, et al, eds. *The adult spine,* 2nd ed. Philadelphia: Lippincott–Raven Publishers, 1997: 2055–2088.

19. Jane JA, Haworth CS, Broaddus WC. A neurosurgical approach to far-lateral disc herniation. technical note. *J Neurosurg* 1990;72: 143–144.

20. Kunogi J, Hasue M. Diagnosis and operative treatment of intraforaminal and extraforaminal nerve root compression. *Spine* 1991;16: 1312–1320.

21. Matsuzaki H, Tokuhashi Y, Matsumoto F, et al. Problems and solutions of pedicle screw plate fixation of the lumbar spine. *Spine* 1990; 15:1159–1165.

22. Epstein NE. Review article: different surgical approaches to far lateral lumbar disc herniations. *J Spinal Disord* 1995;8:383–394.

23. Epstein NE, Epstein JA. Surgery for spinal stenosis. In: Wiesel SW, Weinstein JN, Herkowitz H, et al, eds. *The lumbar spine,* 2nd ed. Philadelphia: WB Saunders, 1996:737–757.

24. Epstein JA, Epstein NE. Lumbar spondylosis and spinal stenosis. In: Wilkins RH, Rengachary SS, eds. *Neurosurgery,* 2nd ed. New York: McGraw-Hill, 1996:3831–3840.

25. Epstein NE, Hood DC. A comparison of surgeon's assessment to patient's self analysis (short form 36) after far lateral lumbar disc surgery: an outcome study. *Spine* 1997;22:2422–2428.

26. Ware JE Jr, Snow KK, Kosinski M, et al. *SF-36 health survey: manual and interpretation guide.* Boston: Nimrod Press, 1993:1–12.

27. Kantz ME, Harris WJ, Levitsky K, et al. Methods for assessing condition-specific and generic functional status outcomes after total knee replacement. *Med Care* 1992;30:MS240–M252.

28. Phillips RC, Lansky DJ. Outcomes management in heart valve replacement surgery: early experience. *J Heart Valve Dis* 1992;1: 42–50.

148. Failed Back Surgery Syndrome

Seth M. Zeidman

Failed back surgery syndrome (FBSS), or the "failed back syndrome," is a clinical condition in which patients who undergo one or more surgical procedures for lumbosacral disease obtain unsatisfactory long-term relief of symptoms, with persistent or recurrent low back pain (1–3).

Failed back syndrome is characterized by a constellation of pain, psychological disturbances, and incapacitation from low back and/or leg pain secondary to lumbar spinal disease. The major etiologies of FBSS include inappropriate patient selection, diagnosis, poor operative technique, iatrogenic instability, and surgical complications. Failed back syndrome most often occurs in those patients inappropriately selected for surgery who are then left with residual pain and neurological deficits. Most FBSS patients have undergone multiple surgical procedures in attempts to relieve intractable and incapacitating sciatica and/or low back pain. Appropriate therapeutic decision making in FBSS patients depends on two factors: (a) establishment of an accurate diagnosis that considers underlying medical problems and related comorbidities; and (b) a rational, individualized therapeutic regimen that addresses the diagnosed abnormalities.

Prevention of FBSS is more important and helpful than any available treatment. It requires an understanding of the natural history of spinal traumatic and degenerative disease as well as the complications from psychological, social, and economic factors. In this chapter, we define FBSS, detail the causes of failure in patients who have had lumbosacral spine surgery, and outline the clinical presentations of FBSS patients. We also delineate the therapeutic regimens available when specific failures have occurred, and provide an algorithm for the evaluation and treatment of this complex clinical entity (Table 1).

History and Epidemiology

Mixter and Barr first recognized lumbar disc herniation as a distinct surgical entity in 1934. Operations to correct disc herniation rapidly gained acceptance, and by the early 1950s reports of the first series of reoperations on the lumbar spine were published (4). Each year more than 250,000 patients undergo lumbosacral operative procedures (5,6). The response of 207 patients to a questionnaire indicate that success rates from lumbosacral surgery depend on the design of the questionnaire, with satisfactory results ranging from 97% to 60% (7). Burton and co-workers (8) report that conservative treatment including complete bed rest with analgesics or gravity traction is frequently inadequate in patients with low back pain. Failure to identify and treat patients with lateral spinal stenosis could increase the high incidence of FBSS (8).

Table 1. Algorithm for the Treatment
of Failed Back Surgery Syndrome

Diagnosis: history and physical examination
    History
        Number of previous back operations
        Length of pain-free interval(s)
        Distribution of pain
        Exacerbating/relieving factors
    Physical examination
        Neurological examination
        Tension signs
        Functional signs
        Thorough general medical examination and review of systems
    Determine if pain has nonspinal cause: diabetes, abdominal aortic
    aneurysm, pancreatitis
        Psychiatric evaluation (if any hint of psychosocial abnormality)
        Radiographic evaluation
    Plain radiographs
    Flexion-extension films
    CT myelogram
    MRI with gadolinium
Therapeutic intervention
    Nonsurgical
        Rehabilitation
        Detoxification as needed
        Multidisciplinary pain treatment center
    Surgery
        Reoperation (minority)
        Ablative procedures other than facet denervations are not helpful
        Spinal cord stimulation (particularly for radicular pain)

Etiology and Pathogenesis

Multiple factors that contribute to the failure of lumbar surgery to relieve symptoms and effect a favorable outcome from surgery include: (a) incorrect preoperative diagnosis, (b) improper patient selection, (c) inadequate surgical decompression, (d) complications from the procedure, and (e) psychosocial factors. Biological and iatrogenic factors also contribute to FBSS. Spinal stenosis, recurrent disc herniation, fusion overgrowth, development of mechanical pain, pseudarthrosis, and neuropathic pain all may follow lumbar spine surgery. Neuropathic pain may result from nerve root injury, pseudomeningocele formation, adhesive arachnoiditis, epidural fibrosis, and reaction to a retained foreign body. Patient populations and author biases often are poorly defined, which increases the problem of identifying FBSS.

Complaints of pain are subjective phenomena, and clinicians can only observe pain-related behavior. Pain does not necessarily denote active tissue damage or injury, and chronic pain behaviors rarely correlate with active tissue irritation or damage. In general, FBSS patients are not malingerers. Many of the factors that contribute to the chronicity and incapacity are on a subconscious level, and failure is likely when inadequate preoperative assessment is combined with incomplete comprehension of the impact of psychosocial problems on outcome.

Most clinicians gain insight into a patient's psychological status during the history and physical examination. Personality dysfunction is the most common psychological problem complicating FBSS. Over 50% of patients referred to the Johns Hopkins chronic paint treatment center suffer from substantial personality dysfunction (9). Questions relating to interactions with family and friends, marital history, military and vocational history, problems with the law, and substance abuse (including misuse of narcotics and psychotropics) often provide relevant information.

The role of psychological factors in FBSS is difficult to assess, but these factors, which include unresolved compensation issues, should be considered in patient selection. Many patients who present with intractable back pain are incapacitated by personality and psychosocial factors. The degree of incapacitation should reflect demonstrated pathology and the degree of physical impairment. Patients should be observed carefully for signs of exaggerated pain and disability during the history and physical examination. Skilled clinicians learn to recognize these behaviors that other patients do not display and that are always related to psychosocial dysfunction. Several studies indicated that patients diagnosed with psychological problems have poor outcomes for reoperation (1,10). Psychological testing may be affected by organic disease, reflecting the underlying diagnosis. Standardized psychological testing explains only a portion of the variance in treatment outcome and should be used as one of several patient-selection criteria.

Before selection for any procedure, FBSS patients with drug habituation problems should undergo a behavioral program with an emphasis on detoxification. Patients with substance "addiction" should not be denied necessary therapy because of psychosocial symptomatology; however, they should be encouraged to seek assistance with their substance abuse before direct intervention is initiated (9).

Clinical Findings

CRITERIA. The American Association of Neurological Surgeons, and the American Academy of Orthopedic Surgeons developed criteria for the selection of patients for lumbosacral spine surgery that include: (a) failure of extended conservative therapy; (b) an abnormal myelogram, computed tomography (CT) scan, and/or magnetic resonance imaging (MRI) study that demonstrates nerve root compression and/or segmental instability consistent with the patient's symptoms and signs; (c) conformity of radicular pain complaints to physiological, dermatomal, or sclerotomal patterns; and (d) one or more of the following: sensory loss, motor loss, and deep tendon reflex abnormalities in corresponding segment(s). These criteria apply to both reoperation and primary procedures. Analyses of the initial preoperative imaging studies of patients with FBSS commonly fail to meet standard criteria for surgical intervention (6, 8). The probability of a successful outcome is small in these circumstances even if criteria for reoperation are met.

PATIENT HISTORY AND PHYSICAL EXAMINATION. Clinical evaluation of FBSS patients does not differ substantially from that of other patients who suffer from intractable and incapacitating low back pain. It is important to obtain the complete details of the patient's original presentation, previous examinations, prior neurodiagnostic imaging studies, and reports of interventional therapy. These data should be reviewed before the patient's initial visit, because these provide technical details of which the patient may be unaware as well as an overview of prior interactions with the health care system. They also make the initial appointment more directed and revealing. Pain behavior, postural abnormalities, impairment of range of motion, and elements of neurological deficit often are evident even before formal examination begins.

A general medical history and physical examination can rule out extraspinal causes of pain that include abdominal aortic aneurysm, gynecological disease, prostate tumor, renal disease, or rectosigmoid disease. Entities such as meralgia paresthetica, acetabular pain, and sacroiliac joint pain should form part of a working differential diagnosis. Patients should be examined for evidence for local myositis, fasciitis, or bursitis, and also indications of arthritic or autoimmune disease. The possibility of undiagnosed disease, including Paget disease, metastatic neoplasia, and rheumatoid/acromegalic spondylitis, also should be considered.

The combination of history and physical examination often provides a reasonable idea of both instability and nerve root compression. Straight leg raising can be useful to identify root compression. The interpretation of neurological findings may be difficult because of residual deficits from prior surgery. Long-term follow-up studies have shown that 40% to 50% of patients with prior successful disc excision have residual alterations in deep tendon reflexes and sensation corresponding to the original level of root involvement (11,12). Fixed neurological deficits suggest root injury but may result from ongoing compression, although nerve root tension signs rarely persist after surgery and are very useful when positive (13). It is unlikely that surgical intervention will be useful in the absence of symptoms suggesting nerve root compression or instability.

One goal of examination is to determine physical impairment as well as exaggeration of impairment. Waddell and associates (14) proposed the use of clinical tests that provide a simple means of identifying patients who have inappropriate pain responses.

Diagnosis

The physician must distinguish between the patient with a mechanical lesion such as recurrent disc herniation, spinal instability, or spinal stenosis, and one with nonmechanical conditions, including intradural scar tissue and systemic medical disease. Surgery benefits patients with mechanical lesions, but surgical intervention rarely helps patients with nonmechanical lesions.

The probability of a favorable outcome diminishes with each procedure, regardless of diagnosis. Finnegan and co-workers (15) emphasized the importance of the postoperative pain-free interval and identified three typical syndromes: (a) no initial relief or symptoms immediately worse, (b) initial relief followed by increased numbness or weakness, and (b) patient receives complete relief but develops recurrent radiculopathy months or years later. Persistent radicular pain in the immediate postoperative period suggests inadequate nerve root decompression, irreversible nerve root injury, or improper patient selection. If the pain-free interval is between 1 and 6 months and the recurrent symptoms occur gradually, scar tissue may be responsible. Recurrent pain 6 months postoperatively may result from disc herniation at the same or different level. Frymoyer and colleagues (13) stressed the importance of long-term failures, which are usually the manifestation of an ongoing degenerative process. Predominant leg pain suggests disc herniation or spinal stenosis, although scar tissue also can produce this. Instability, infection, and scar tissue are all possible causes if back pain is the major component.

Imaging and Diagnostic Studies

Precise correlation of clinical findings with diagnostic imaging studies is necessary because of the high incidence of clinically false-positive myelograms, discograms, CT scans, and MRI scans in asymptomatic individuals or at asymptomatic levels (9–21). Imaging studies of asymptomatic postoperative patients often reveal significant abnormalities. Frymoyer reported that 40% of CT scans, myelograms, and discograms show abnormalities in asymptomatic individuals (13). The combination of clinical history, physical examination, and radiologic imaging studies should provide an excellent correlation between anatomical abnormalities and the patient's complaints. Nonspecific spondylotic changes do not necessarily correlate with pain, and these changes do not always indicate the need for surgery.

Modern diagnostic imaging techniques have improved the definition of both primary and postsurgical lumbosacral spine disease. Radiologic evaluation is particularly important in excluding surgically correctable lesions.

PLAIN RADIOGRAPHS. Radiographic evaluation should begin with plain radiographs to determine the extent and level of previous surgery. Lateral flexion-extension radiographs may demonstrate abnormal motion and instability and detect the presence of primary bone tumors. The degree of disc degeneration, facet joint arthritis, spinal misalignment, and spondylolisthesis with or without motion all can be identified from plain radiographs. MRI and/or CT are usually satisfactory and plain myelography generally is unnecessary for those patients who have had a single surgical procedure.

MYELOGRAPHICALLY ENHANCED CT. CT myelography is perhaps the most important diagnostic technique in evaluating the patient with FBSS. Patients who have undergone previous operations often are difficult to evaluate without intrathecal contrast. However, CT myelography permits determination of canal size, bony defects, and hypertrophic bony changes as well as bony encroachment on the neural elements and evaluation of the lateral recesses and neural foramina. Contrast allows evaluation of the cauda equina by demonstrating the presence or absence of nerve root compression and the relationship of the nerve roots to the lateral recesses, foramina, and discs. Lesions such as far lateral disc herniations still can be missed (22–24).

Myelography with enhanced multiplanar CT provides the most powerful modality to assess the possibility of lateral or central stenosis as a cause of continued nerve root symptomatology after lumbar decompression. CT with three-dimensional reconstruction is a significant advancement that benefits examinations of the neural foramina and remainder of the bony anatomy.

MRI. The enhanced MRI scan is very sensitive to inflammatory and neoplastic conditions and is the most sensitive technique for differentiating scar tissue from recurrent pathology. In the immediate postoperative period, the area of bone and ligament resection shows edematous soft tissues isointense to muscle on T1-weighted images that increase on T2-weighted images and replace normal tissue signal. In the absence of postoperative hematoma, significant mass effect on the thecal sac is unusual. Gradual replacement of the immediate postoperative changes from scar tissue occur 6 months postsurgery (8,25). The signal intensity of posterior scar tissue is variable on T2-weighted images.

Changes from discectomy are visible immediately after surgery. T1-weighted images show increased signal anterior to the thecal sac, with an indistinct posterior annular margin. This soft-tissue signal may blend smoothly into the disc space and increase on T2-weighted images. Anterior epidural edema combined with posterior annular disruption caused by disc incision and curettage, can mimic preoperative disc herniation and produce mass effect. These changes within the anterior epidural space involute in the months after surgery, with a corresponding normalization of the thecal margin.

The interpretation of MRI within the first 6 weeks postoperatively requires caution because of the tremendous changes in the epidural soft tissues and intervertebral disc after surgery. Tissue disruption and edema can impinge on the thecal sac. MRI in the immediate postoperative period provides a gross overview of the thecal sac and epidural space and can often exclude significant hemorrhage, pseudomeningocele, or disc space infection. Small posterior fluid collections are common after laminectomy.

ELECTROPHYSIOLOGY. Electromyography (EMG), thermography (TMG), and spinal evoked potentials are of limited use in the evaluation of the patient with FBSS. The major benefit of these diagnostic tools is in differentiating cauda equina compression from peripheral nerve entrapment syndromes. Electromyography can corroborate root injury but cannot differentiate injury from compression. Thermography may help diagnose a secondary sympathetic dystrophy syndrome and can be useful in differentiating root from peripheral nerve injury. Both electrophysiological studies and TMG have a role in certain clinical settings, although their sensitivity is limited. Equivocal neurological deficits may be objectively demonstrated and quantitated clinically. Paraspinous EMG typically demonstrates nonspecific postsurgical changes in the patient with FBSS.

LUMBAR DISCOGRAPHY. Lumbar discography has undergone a resurgence as a physiological rather than an anatomical study. Injection of fluid into the disc is postulated to reproduce pain originating in the same disc (9). Subsequent injection of local anesthetic provides relief. Pain provocation by injection and relief with local anesthetic constitutes a positive study. However, no controlled study has verified the hypothesis underlying this procedure.

FACET AND NERVE BLOCKS. Facet blockade has been unsatisfactory for defining the role of anatomical structures that cause pain, although in one series it did prove useful (26). Selective nerve root injections under radiographic control are helpful in more difficult cases in which radiculopathy predominates (27). No definitive scientific evidence exists that peripheral blockade that produces pain relief predicts a successful outcome from surgery. The role of blockade of the lumbar zygapophyseal joints remains unproved.

Patients selected for facet blockade should have back pain exacerbated by rotation and lateral bending, and improved with bracing. The block technique described by Bogduk and Long includes blocking the medial branch of the posterior primary ramus on the transverse process or the sacrum with a small amount of local anesthetic. A positive block provides total pain relief for the duration expected from the procedure. Patients with radicular pain and those with partial pain relief from blockade rarely respond satisfactorily to permanent neurotomy (28).

Incorrect Diagnosis/Inappropriate Surgery

As many as 50% of patients with FBSS are found on review of their original history, physical examination, and diagnostic studies not to have met generally accepted criteria for the primary surgical procedure.

Inappropriate stabilization procedures in patients with mechanical etiology for their pain are another source of FBSS. Although inadequate surgery often is cited, inappropriate surgery is the major factor. Operations at the wrong level, wrong side, and for the wrong pathology are rare but often quite dramatic and memorable.

Psychosocial Causes

Psychogenic factors are the single most common cause of failure to relieve pain by discectomy. Long states that "patients suffering from failed back syndrome are incapacitated by psychiatric, psychologic and social/vocational factors which relate to the back complaint only indirectly" (3). In a study of 266 patients with FBSS, 15% of these patients were diagnosed with psychiatric disorders before the onset of low back pain (3).

Data from Brown indicate that poor or fair results were twice as common in workers' compensation cases, whereas good to excellent results were one third more common in the non-workers' compensation group (28). Sorenson and co-workers attempted to predict the outcome of disc surgery by preoperative testing with a modification of the Minnesota Multiphasic Personality Inventory (MMPI) (29). Some patients can be expected to do poorly for reasons unrelated to the surgery. The important factors in predicting failure are workers' compensation, job dissatisfaction, low education and income, heavy job requirements, cigarette smoking, psychological disturbances, and litigation (2,30,31).

Discogenic Pain and Internal Disc Disruption

Internal disc disruption (IDD) is a condition marked by alterations in the internal structure and metabolic functions of one or more discs, usually after significant trauma. The clinical syndrome includes axial and extremity pain exacerbated by any physical activity that compresses affected discs. The pain typically is deep, does not rapidly abate with rest, and worsens over time. Profound energy loss occurs, sometimes in conjunction with significant weight loss and psychological disturbances. It is not associated with herniation of the disc fragment. Disc degeneration with loss of disc height and osteophyte formation is rare.

Discography, which was the principal diagnostic tool for IDD, has been supplanted by MRI. Patients with IDD show changes in the signal generated from the affected intervertebral disc and often from adjacent vertebral levels. Once the diagnosis of disc disruption is made and surgical intervention is considered appropriate, disc excision with anterior interbody fusion is the most effective operation for persistent disabling symptoms. Disc excision also is indicated for patients who do not respond to nonoperative therapies, including analgesics, nonsteroidal antiinflammatory drugs, and psychotropic agents.

Inadequate Surgery

Inadequate surgery (i.e., inadequate decompression) has been suggested as a frequent cause of FBSS. Lateral recess stenosis and persistent disc herniation usually are cited as the responsible pathologies for inadequate decompression. One of the most common pitfalls is failure to recognize the contribution of lateral foraminal or extraforaminal compression to the patient's radiculopathy, with initial disc removal without adequate decompression of the bony component. Burton analyzed the data of 800 FBSS patients and reported that concomitant lateral recess and/or central stenosis account for 71% of failures. MacNab concluded that lateral recess stenosis was the most common source of failure after lumbar disc surgery (32). Spengler and colleagues reported a 30% incidence of lateral recess stenosis that required medial foraminotomy at surgery in his series of discectomy patients (30). Nerve root decompression should provide an excursion of at least 5 mm, so that a blunt probe can be passed into the foramen easily. Further bony decompression to uncover a laterally herniated disc or hypertrophic superior facet in the foramen should be necessary if nerve root decompression is not accomplished. In some cases, the entire joint or even the pedicle must be sacrificed. Fusion is indicated in these patients with a destabilized spine.

Temporary Relief (Days to Weeks) with Early Failure of Relief or Infection

In 1936 Milward described the clinical and radiographic characteristics of interspace infection after the inadvertent introduction of microorganisms into a disc space during lumbar puncture (33). Ramirez and Thisted reported infection rate of .3% in an analysis of 28,395 patients who underwent lumbar laminectomy for radiculopathy in the United States in 1980 (34). Patients with aseptic necrosis of interspace infection typically are asymptomatic immediately after surgery but within 2 weeks begin to experience excruciating spasms in the lower back with or without radiation into the legs. The white blood cell count and temperature of these patients often are normal but the sedimentation rate is elevated, often higher than 100 mm per hour. Lumbosacral radiographs may reveal erosion of the cartilaginous plates as the disease progresses. Needle aspirations of the interspace may reveal the offending organisms, although such aspirations often are negative (33). Patients with a clear-cut infectious syndrome should be placed on intravenous antibiotics. The persistence of an elevated temperature for several days postoperatively may indicate an infection. The wound should be examined for erythema, selling, tenderness, and drainage. Management of the infection should include Gram stain and culture with antibiotics if the clinical indication is strong. The patient should be returned to the operating room, the wound reopened, thoroughly débrided, and irrigated if the infection continues despite antibiotic treatment. The wound can be managed open with frequent dressing changes.

Postoperative intervertebral disc space infection (discitis) has rates ranging from .1% to 3.8% (34–38). Postoperative discitis typically produces persistent intense back pain with unremarkable associated physical findings 2 weeks to 3 months after discectomy. Patients with discitis often have elevated erythrocyte sedimentation rates. Bone scan, CT, and MRI are sensitive for detecting discitis and can identify changes associated with discitis earlier than plain radiographs.

Early diagnosis and prompt treatment are important to prevent chronic infection. Immobilization often is effective for pain relief, and 4 to 6 weeks of intravenous antibiotic therapy is recommended. Uncomplicated discitis should not require surgery, and most patients undergo spontaneous interbody fusion. Paresis may develop from lumbar epidural abscesses that then require immediate decompressive laminectomy.

Infection may be introduced directly into the intervertebral disc space during surgery and spread to the adjacent vertebral bodies, producing osteomyelitis. Any patient with increasing back pain more than 2 weeks postoperatively and an erythrocyte sedimentation rate greater than 50 mm per hour should be considered to have discitis until proven otherwise. Percutaneous disc biopsy can be helpful in the diagnosis of postoperative discitis but often is falsely negative.

Epidural abscess after decompression is rare but should be considered in a patient with increasing neurological symptoms and signs in the early postoperative period. It may be difficult to differentiate from an expanding hematoma in the absence of systemic evidence of infection.

MRI can localize the site of infection and provide more information than CT regarding the extent of abscess involvement and degree of cord compromise.

Decompression and aggressive antibiotic management are the cornerstones of therapy. Epidural abscess often arises in association with vertebral osteomyelitis and is an indication for early decompression.

MENINGEAL CYST OR PSEUDOMENINGOCELE. Meningeal cysts rarely cause early recurrent radiculopathy after disc excision and are reported in less than 1% of patients. Incidental durotomy during disc excision does not compromise the later results if the dural leak is recognized and closed; durotomy that is unrecognized or incompletely repaired can produce a slowly expanding mass. Nerve roots can become trapped in the meningeal cyst and cause pain. Physical examination occasionally reveals soft-tissue bulging that may or may not be recognized as fluctuant, but often increases when the patient stands. Myelography or MRI are important diagnostic studies to identify meningeal cysts. Removal of the meningeal cyst requires careful dissection around the cyst and identification of the dural opening. The cyst should be opened to avoid injury to involved nerve roots prior to excision. Closure can be accomplished by closing the dura with or without duraplasty.

Midterm Failures (Weeks to Months)

HERNIATED INTERVERTEBRAL DISC. There are many explanations for persistent pain caused by disc herniation. An inadequate discectomy produces pain because of continued nerve root irritation. Patients do not report any pain-free interval and sometimes awaken from surgery complaining of their preoperative pain. Recurrent intervertebral disc herniation at the previously decompressed level also may occur. Patients with this problem often have a pain-free interval of more than 6 months. Those patients with a herniated disc that ruptures at a different level usually benefit from a repeat operation. Patients may describe persistent severe pain and paresthesias in a radicular distribution after unsuccessful lumbar disc surgery. The pain is superimposed on an area of residual numbness that is constant and described as either burning or ice cold. Often it is more distressing than the original disc herniation pain. These patients with pain of nerve injury or deafferentation sometimes respond to spinal cord stimulation (SCS) (6,9).

RECURRENT DISC FRAGMENT. The incidence of recurrent rupture after laminectomy has been reported to range from a low rate of .26% for ruptures that occur within the first 6 weeks after surgery (on the same side and level), to a rate of 18% for recurrences that take place at any time or any level after the initial operation. Recurrent disc herniation may occur on the same side and at the same level as the prior operation, on the opposite side at the same level, or at an entirely new level. Vigorous disc space evacuation does not prevent recurrent disc herniation. In some cases, the patient is pain free for years after surgery, and then back and sciatic pain suddenly return. MRI with gadolinium-DTPA (Gd-DTPA) and CT myelography can confirm a diagnosis of disc herniation but may be difficult to interpret because of postoperative changes. Physical examination reveals signs of disc herniation with positive tension signs. Surgery is indicated for intractable pain once the diagnosis is established and nonsurgical treatment fails. Previous back surgery does not preclude an excellent result: Some patients feel better after the second operation than the first. Frymoyer and co-workers have shown that the outcome from surgery after recurrent disc herniation and primary disc excision is identical (11).

BATTERED ROOT SYNDROME AND PERINEURAL SCARRING. Perineural scarring is a common occurrence after spinal decompression, although clinical failure from perineural scarring occurs in only 1% to 2% of patients who undergo disc excision (11). Nerve root scarring may be caused by excessive bleeding, conjoined nerve roots, ad the use of cottonoid patties. The immediate postoperative course generally is benign but may be associated with incomplete resolution of sciatica, sometimes accompanied by an increased sensory or even motor deficit. Sciatica and back pain gradually increase over 3 to 6 months. A variety of surgical therapies have been advocated, including scar removal with membrane interposition, radical decompression, longitudinal sectioning of scar over nerve root, spinal fusion, and electrical stimulator implantation (39).

EPIDURAL SCARRING. Scar tissue around the dura and nerve roots can cause recurrent sciatica. Prevention is essential owing to the lack of effective surgical therapy for epidural fibrosis. In this difficult patient population, the differentiation of recurrent disc herniation from scar is critical, because reoperation on scar often produces a poor surgical result and additional scarring. CT with intravenous contrast, which has an accuracy of 67% to 100% in distinguishing scar tissue from disc, is technically demanding, involves a large contrast load, and includes only single-plane imaging. Intravenous contrast increases the diagnostic accuracy of CT from 43% to 74%, which makes differentiating between recurrent herniated disc fragments and postsurgical scar tissue more likely (8,40). Recurrent disc fragments are avascular and enhance only at the periphery, whereas postsurgical scar tissue demonstrates uniform enhancement after infusion of intravenous contrast material. The peripheral enhancement observed in recurrent disc herniation is thought to result from a thin layer of surgical scar tissue or vascularity in the annulus fibrosus or epidural venous plexus.

MRI allows differentiation of recurrent disc herniation from epidural scar. MRI has 100% sensitivity, 71% specificity, and 89% accuracy in distinguishing recurrent disc herniation from epidural scar. Bundschuh evaluated 20 patients with MRI, 14 of whom underwent exploration. MRI diagnosis was confirmed in 12 patients at surgery. Eight of nine of these patients also had CT findings confirmed at surgery.

Epidural fibrosis can be differentiated from disc by signal intensity and the configuration and margination of the extradural mass on unenhanced MRI scans. Recurrent disc hernia-

tions are seen at or near the disc space, exhibit mass effect, and on T1-weighted image are slightly hyperintense compared to fibrosis. Free fragments are hyperintense on T2-weighted images. Unenhanced epidural scar, which lacks mass effect, is not contiguous with the disc space and is hypointense or isointense on T1-weighted images. Fibrotic scar has higher signal intensity than disc material or annulus on T2-weighted images. Sotiropolous compared the diagnostic accuracy of contrast CT to unenhanced MRI in 25 patients and found that unenhanced MRI is equivalent to contrast-enhanced CT for identifying scar from disc (40).

MRI with intravenous Gd-DTPA administration is the most accurate technique to distinguish scar from disc. Hueftle and associates analyzed the role of Gd-enhanced MRI in the differentiation of scar tissue versus disc. Enhanced MRI was able to predict operative findings with 100% accuracy in 30 patients evaluated with MRI before and after administration of .1 mmol/kg Gd. Hueftle and associates reported uniform scar enhancement on early postcontrast T-weighted images, whereas recurrent discs exhibited peripheral enhancement on delayed postcontrast images.

Although limited data are available on the use of contrast in the immediate postoperative period, enhancement is visible in the epidural space within the first 4 days of surgery. Pathological changes are difficult to differentiate from the tremendous changes that normally occur after any surgical procedure, which creates a problem in identifying enhancement.

ARACHNOIDITIS. Although arachnoiditis originally was described as a complication of infection, we prefer the term *chronic adhesive arachnoiditis.*

Clinical Syndrome. Most patients diagnosed with arachnoiditis have low back and lower extremity symptoms; recurrent symptoms often are similar to those that occurred originally. A neurogenic claudication syndrome has been diagnosed in some patients who complain of leg weakness and burning pain that is affected by sitting or standing. Bowel or bladder dysfunction is common in these patients. The burning character of the pain, associated with hyperpathia and claudication, suggests arachnoiditis but cannot be differentiated from other forms of spinal stenosis.

Etiology. Any agent injected into the lumbar subarachnoid space has the potential to cause arachnoiditis. All of the contrast agents cause a severe inflammatory reaction in the subarachnoid space. Oil-based agents were used for years with minimal problems. Although early water-soluble contrast agents were extremely noxious, improvements to these agents have reduced the potential for inflammation. Little evidence is available that use of the common clinical contrast materials causes a significant incidence of arachnoiditis. Traumatic or repeated myelography, particularly with multiple surgeries, may affect the incidence of arachnoiditis.

All authors stress the fact that the new syndrome of chronic adhesive arachnoiditis is quite different from the rapidly progressive arachnoiditis that complicates infection. The patients are stable, neurological deterioration occurs but is rare, and pain is the predominant issue.

Diagnosis and Treatment. The diagnosis of arachnoiditis usually occurs in the course of repeat myelography. In our experience, clear-cut abnormalities that would otherwise be candidates for reparative surgery should be treated even if arachnoiditis is diagnosed. Arachnoiditis does not detract from the potential success of reparative surgery. Direct surgery on the arachnoiditis should not be considered unless the patient has a progressive neuralgic deficit. Surgery to correct arachnoiditis is a delicate and dangerous operation, and the surgeon must be very familiar with this highly technical procedure. Pain relief occurs in less than half of the patients and the risk of a substantial new neurological deficit is high.

Alternatives to Direct Therapy. SCS is the most effective therapy to relieve the pain in those patients with arachnoiditis and FBSS who are not candidates for any other procedure. Brain stimulation and intrathecal narcotic pumps have both successfully reduced pain in severely disabled patients. The use of chronic oral narcotic administration is undergoing investigation in a select group of patients. Improved myelographic techniques, the newest water-soluble agents, and improved surgical techniques may all contribute to reduce the incidence of this difficult complication.

Long-Term Failures (Months to Years)

Instability is defined as abnormal or excessive movement of one vertebra on another, which may cause pain. The patient's intrinsic back disease or excessively wide bilateral laminectomies may be responsible for the instability. Patients complain predominantly of back pain, and physical examination often is unremarkable. Relative flexion-sagittal plane translation of more than 8% of the AP diameter of the vertebral body or a relative flexion-sagittal plan rotation of more than 9% or degrees between adjacent segments are the most commonly cited radiographic guidelines for instability of the lumbar spine.

Spinal fusion should be considered for symptomatic patients with evidence of instability. The incidence of post-decompression spondylolisthesis ranges from 2% to 10%, whereas the incidence of progressive slippage after decompressive laminectomy in patients with preoperative degenerative spondylolisthesis is even higher. The factors that contribute to post-decompression slippage include patients less than 40 years of age with normal disc heights, and those who have undergone extensive surgery. The extent of surgery is an important contributor in the development of postoperative instability. Discectomy at the time of laminectomy may cause additional instability. Complete laminectomy and bilateral facetectomies also create spinal instability.

Symptoms sufficient to require later stabilization occur in only 3% of patients following simple discectomy. It is possible to excise 50% of both facets or 100% of one facet without significantly altering the stiffness of human intervertebral segments. After extensive spinal decompression, accentuation of preexistent deformity occasionally occurs but often is asymptomatic. Radical facetectomy for degenerative spondylolisthesis always produces increased deformity but frequently is asymptomatic. Greater disc space height at the time of decompression, the absence of osteophytes, discectomy at the time of decompression, and a younger age may predispose the patient to later deformity. Presence of any or all of these factors can indicate the need for fusion at the time of decompression. Younger patients who undergo multilevel decompressive laminectomies for congenital or mixed spinal stenosis commonly develop a new deformity after the laminectomy.

PSEUDOARTHRITIS OF PRIOR FUSION. Pseudarthrosis is a complication that may stem from technical faults by the surgeon or from biological deficiency of the patient. The incidence of pseudarthrosis depends on the number of levels fused, the techniques involved, and whether the patient smokes. The overall rate of pseudarthrosis is higher in two-level compared to one-level fusion, with the lumbosacral junction presenting a special challenge. The variety of therapeutic options for FBSS emphasizes the lack of a uniform method of treatment.

Nonsurgical Treatment Options

Certain general principles should be followed in treating FBSS, irrespective of the pathological process. Rehabilitation is an important component in the management of FBSS patients, and programs specializing in this are proliferating. The ultimate goal of rehabilitation is restoration of the patient to a functional status. Psychiatric and psychosocial comorbidities must be identified and treated. The effect of economic issues must be addressed. Psychological dysfunction affects the patient's ability to cope as well as the rehabilitation process. Detrimental pain behaviors can be modified by appropriate therapies, and it is important to use these psychotherapeutic techniques within the context of an overall program.

The psychological needs of each patient must be identified and treated specifically because stereotyped programs are generally of little value. Professional assessment of patients' physical therapy needs and an individualized regimen of graduated exercise are essential. Formal evaluation and treatment sessions allow the patient to understand the techniques and rationale for physical therapy. Patients with FBSS must be urged to translate the short-term pain relief resulting from effective application of therapies into increased productive activity.

In some cases, hospitalization in a multidisciplinary pain treatment program may be necessary. Abuse of medications, including narcotics and benzodiazepines, must be curtailed. Pain-management centers focus on increasing the quality of life and physical function in spite of residual pain that maximal therapy cannot relieve. The pain treatment center also educates the patient about physical and nonphysical factors in chronic pain and realistic expectations from therapy.

Patients initially require therapy to stretch muscles back to a functional length; they also need coordinated muscle activity with intensive physical reconditioning to improve strength and endurance. Some patients require specific therapy to address myofascial pain and careful instruction in body biomechanics to prevent further insults.

The concept of productive rehabilitation or work hardening with work site-style conditioning has been both practical and popular. Work-hardening programs specify when patients are fit to return to work and what practical work restrictions are necessary. Patients should gain the physical capacity and confidence to do their jobs, and lead a more normal life once they have completed the program.

Surgical Treatment and Reoperation

The physician is obliged to rule out a persistent surgical problem as part of the surgical history. Surgery should be viewed as part of a continuum of care rather than as the sole event leading to functional restoration of the patient.

Surgery should only be considered if the patient suffers from either compression and/or instability, particularly if the disease is progressive or associated with major neurological deficits. Stereotyped procedures applied without considering the physical and psychological components of each patient are virtually guaranteed to fail. Patients with spondylotic disease characterized by disc herniation, canal and foraminal stenosis, and instability benefit the most from surgery. Radicular pain, back pain related to activity and relieved by rest, improvement with stabilization, and neurogenic claudication will improve with surgical intervention.

The initial decision to operate is most important; once recurrent pain occurs after surgery, the potential for relief is limited at best. It is no longer acceptable to consider exploratory surgery of the lower back when objective criteria are not met. The residual effects of abnormalities already treated definitively (e.g., disc herniation causing root injury before its removal) may be difficult to differentiate from untreated and iatrogenic abnormalities, in patients considered for reoperation.

Prior to reoperation, the surgeon should review the contrast studies to be certain of the location of the original disc injury. Fragments that are lateral or in the axilla of the nerve root often are overlooked. Repeat surgery is relatively easy within days of the first operation, but is more difficult several weeks later, when adhesions are present. We prefer to extend the bone removal above and below the original laminotomy, which increases the exposure and allows identification of normal structures prior to removing epidural scar at the original operative site.

Interventional or surgical therapy can only achieve two objectives: neural decompression and spinal stabilization. Interventional therapy is ineffective and may lead to FBSS if the patient's underlying problem is not a neural compressive lesion or incapacitating mechanical instability. Of the degenerative processes where reparative surgery is the only reasonable alternative to leaving the patient untreated, neurogenic claudication cannot be treated by any other technique.

Decompressive surgery is indicated when the patient's complaints of pain are compatible with demonstrated compression. The other problem for which surgery generally is indicated is overt, serious instability. Although the patient may be temporarily relieved by bracing, nothing will correct the problem except stabilization. Spinal fusion is used to stabilize segments that have been damaged to such a degree that normal physiological forces will cause damage to neural structures or progressive loss of biomechanical integrity.

Loss of stability may occur following operative decompression and destabilization of a spinal motion segment. *Stability* is a mechanical term that is often used without a clear or precise definition. Clinical instability does not necessarily indicate mechanical instability. Patients with clinical instability have abnormal symptomatic motion, whereas patients with mechanical instability do not necessarily of these symptoms. Patients with symptomatic instability are able to function, although minor changes in motion may precipitate severe symptomatic back and/or leg pain. Symptoms and signs that may be indicative of clinical instability include low back pain exacerbated with standing and lifting and relieved by lying down. A sudden catch when extending from the flexed to the straight posture as well as a feeling of disconnection in the lumbar spine accentuated by motion are helpful in identifying instability. Lumbar bracing may provide some relief in these patients. Clinical instability is frequently present in patients who have had previous surgery for back disorders.

Ablative Procedures

Ablation of the involved primary afferent neurons is expected to provide pain relief whether pain originates in a joint, disc, or ligament as a nociceptive mechanism or as abnormal activity in an injured peripheral nerve, root, or dorsal root ganglion. After nerve injury, activity signaling pain may originate in neuromas or dorsal root ganglia. Large myelinated afferents, which do not normally conduct pain sensation, may transmit postinjury hyperalgesia. Primary afferent ablation should address any of these mechanisms.

Dorsal rhizotomy may reduce persistent radicular pain after lumbosacral surgery. More proximal radiofrequency thermocoagulation of the primary spinal nerve trunk and ganglion has been described. Uematsu and coworkers described percutaneous spinal rhizotomy to relieve nociceptive pain in the affected limbs. This procedure can result in a motor and sensory deficit if performed at a functioning root level. Dorsal rhizotomy does not interrupt all afferent input, because numerous ventral root afferents with cell bodies in the dorsal root ganglia exist, and these convey pain from peripheral receptors even after dorsal rhizotomy. Dorsal root ganglionectomy has also not been effective for FBSS.

Incomplete primary afferent ablation after dorsal root ganglionectomy could be the cause of disappointing results of dorsal rhizotomy. Authors for a century have described cell bodies in the ventral root and peripheral nervous system that escape ganglionectomy. The central pathophysiology of pain after nerve injury and deafferentation may be another reason for the failure of primary afferent ablation to relieve pain.

Percutaneous radiofrequency lumbar facet denervation (medical branch posterior primary ramus neurotomy) is a simple peripheral ablative procedure for patients with mechanical low back syndrome. North and coworkers report that facet denervations are successful on a long-term basis in just under one half of the patients interviewed. This result compares favorably with that of reoperation, with the advantage that the morbidity of facet denervation is negligible. Failure of prior disc surgery suggests that significant symptomatic disc disease is absent at the initial procedure. Failure can also result from poor clinical selection of patients who may be nonspecifically refractory to any treatment.

Rehabilitation

Because rehabilitation is an important part of the management of FBSS, rehabilitation programs specializing in this area are proliferating. Patients who completed such programs have a high rate of reported functional improvement and return to work, although pain ratings are not reduced. These programs complement surgical management for selected patients, but the roles of these different therapies awaits prospective study.

Conclusion

Because FBSS comprises a wide range of primary pathologies, the determination of precise treatments and outcomes is difficult. It is difficult to assess treatment options or outcomes accurately until clarifications with subsets of diagnoses is achieved.

The FBSS diagnosis is too broad to be meaningful and should be eliminated.

The overall goal in the management of the patient with FBSS is to maximize quality of life, using a treatment program that is highly effective yet poses the smallest amount of risk. The diagnosis and management of FBSS often requires sophisticated diagnostic imaging and multidisciplinary input. Many patients are best served by a comprehensive pain treatment program. The cornerstone of any successful program for patients with FBSS is accurate diagnosis, allowing precisely targeted therapy. The inherent complexity of these cases necessitates a diagnostic and therapeutic protocol that is precise and cost efficient.

References

1. Burton CV. Causes of failure of surgery on the lumbar spine: ten-year follow-up. *Mt Sinai J Med* 1991;58:183.
2. Fager CA, Freidberg SR. Analysis of failures and poor results of lumbar spine surgery. *Spine* 1980;5:87.
3. Long DM. Failed back surgery syndrome. *Neurosurg Clin North Am* 1991;2:899.
4. Greenwood J, McGuire T, Kimball F. A study of causes of failure in the herniated disc operation: an analysis of 67 repeated cases. *J Neurosurg* 1952;9:15.
5. Frymoyer JW, Cats-Barfl BW. An overview of the incidences and costs of low back pain. *Orthop Clin North Am* 1991;22:263.
6. North R, Zeidman S. Failed back surgery syndrome. *Contemp Neurosurg* 1993;16:1.
7. Howe J, Frymoyer JW. The effects of questionnaire design on the determination of end results in lumbar spinal surgery. *Spine* 1985;10:804.
8. Burton CV, Kirkaidy WW, Yong HK, et al. Causes of failure of surgery on the lumbar spine. *Clin Orthop* 1981;157:191.
9. Long DM. Decision making in lumbar disc disease. *Clin Neurosurg* 1992;39:36.
10. Frymoyer JW, Rosen JC, Clements J, et al. Psychologic factors in low-back-pain disability. *Clin Orthop* 1985;195:178.
11. Frymoyer JW, Matteri RE, Hanley EN, et al. Failed lumbar disc surgery requiring second operation: A longterm follow-up study. *Spine* 1978;3:7.
12. Nashold BJ, Hrubec A. *Lumbar disc disease: a twenty-year clinical follow-up study.* St. Louis: Mosby, 1971.
13. Frymoyer JW, Nelson RM, Spangfort E, et al. Clinical tests applicable to the study of chronic low-back disability. *Spine* 1991;16:681.
14. Waddell G, Somerville D, Henderson L, et al. Objective clinical evaluation of physical impairment in chronic low back pain. *Spine* 1992;17:617.
15. Finnegan W, Fentin J, Marvel J, et al. Results of surgical intervention in the symptomatic multioperated back patient. *J Bone Joint Surg Am* 1979;61:1077.
16. Waddell G, Kummel EG, Lotto WN, et al. Failed lumbar disc surgery and repeat surgery following industrial injuries. *J Bone Joint Surg Am* 1979;61:201.
17. North RB, Campbell JN, James CS, et al. Failed back surgery syndrome: 5-year follow-up in 102 patients undergoing repeated operation. *Neurosurgery* 1991;28:685.
18. Barrios C, Ahmed M, Arrotegui JI, et al. Clinical factors predicting outcome after surgery for herniated lumbar disc: an epidemiological multivariate analysis. *J Spinal Disord* 1990;3:205.
19. Bems DH, Blaser SI, Modic MT. Magnetic resonance imaging of the spine. *Clin Orthop* 1989;244:78.
20. Bobman SA, Atlas SW, Listerud J, et al. Postoperative lumbar spine: contrast-enhanced chemical shift MR imaging. *Radiology* 1991;179:557.
21. Brodsky AE, Kovalsky ES, Khalil MA. Correlation of radiologic assessment of lumbar spine fusions with surgical exploration. *Spine* 1991;16:5261.
22. Bundschuh CV, Stein L, Slusser JH, et al. Distinguishing between scar and recurrent herniated disc in postoperative patients: value of contrast-enhanced CT and MR imaging. *AJNR* 1990;11:949.
23. Neill S. Computed tomography in failed back syndrome. *Radiography Today* 1991;57:9.
24. Patrick BS. Extreme lateral ruptures of lumbar intervertebral discs. *Surg Neurol* 1975;3:301.
25. Crock HV. Anterior lumbar interbody fusion: indications for its use and notes on surgical technique. *Clin Orthop* 1982;165:157.
26. Fairbank J, Park W, McCall L. Apophyseal injection of local anesthetic as a diagnostic aid in primary low-back pain syndromes. *Spine* 1981;6:598.
27. Krempen J, Smith B. Nerve root injection: a method for evaluating the etiology of sciatica. *J Bone Joint Surg Am* 1974;56:1435.
28. Bogduk N, Long DM. Percutaneous lumbar medial branch neurotomy: a modification of facet denervation. *Spine* 1980;5:193.
29. Walsh T, Weinstein JN, Spratt KF, et al. Lumbar discography in normal subjects: a controlled, prospective study. *J Bone Joint Surg Am* 1990;72:1081.
30. Spengler DM, Freeman C, Westbrook R, et al. Low-back pain following multiple lumbar spine procedures: failure of initial selection? *Spine* 1980;5:356.
31. Long DM, Filtzer DL, BenDebba M, et al. Clinical features of the feedback syndrome. *J Neurosurg* 1988;69:61.
32. MacNab L. Negative disc exploration: an analysis of the causes of nerve root involvement in 68 patients. *J Bone Joint Surg Am* 1971;53:891.
33. Gieseking H: Lokalisierte Spondylitis nach operiertern Bandscheibenvorfall. *Zenti-albi Chii* 1951;76:1470.
34. Ramirez L, Thisted R. Complication and demographic characteristics of patients undergoing lumbar discectomy in community hospitals. *Neurosurgery* 1989;25:226.
35. Roberts M. Complications of lumbar disc surgery. *Spinal Surg* 1988;2:13.
36. Hudgins W. The role of microdiscectomy. *Orthop Clin North Am* 1983;14:589.
37. Bircher M, Tasker T, Crawshaw C, et al. Discitis following lumbar surgery. *Spine* 1988;13:98.
38. Ford L, Key L. Postoperative infection of the intervertebral disc space. *Sotith Med J* 1955;48:1295.
39. Braun L, Hoffman J, David P. Contrast enhancement in CT differentiation between recurrent disc herniation and postoperative scar: prospective study. *AJR* 1985;145:785.
40. Sotiropoulos S, Chaftez N, Lang P, et al. Differentiation between postoperative scar and recurrent disc herniation: prospective comparison of MR, CT, and contrast enhanced CT. *AJNR* 1989;10:639.

149. Lumbar Spinal Stenosis and Laminectomy

Ivan Ciric, Sean A. Salehi, and
Lance E. Gravely

Anatomical Structure of the Spinal Canal

The spinal canal is bordered ventrally by the vertebral bodies and intervertebral discs, laterally by the pedicles, dorsolaterally by the facet joints, and dorsally by the ligamentum flava and laminae. The position of the laminae usually resembles a pitched roof with the two laminae approaching each other at a 45- to 65-degree angle. Lateral recesses are lateral compartments of the spinal canal bordered laterally by the pedicle, ventrally by the lateral portion of the posterior surface of the vertebral body, and dorsally by the superior facet of the same vertebra (Fig. 1). The interrupted nature of the ligamentum flava and their attachments to the mid-undersurface of the laminae positioned rostrally and the upper border of the laminae positioned caudally, respectively, is well known. Laterally, the ligamentum flava attach to the medial border as well as to the undersurface of the superior facet, reaching as far lateral as the pedicle and the intervertebral foramen where they merge imperceptibly with the facet joint capsule (Fig. 2). This particular anatomical detail plays a role in the development of spinal and lateral recess stenosis. In patients with a congenital narrowing of the anteroposterior (AP) diameter of the spinal canal, usually due to short pedicles, the position of the laminae usually resemble a domed roof with the laminae approaching each other at a greater than 90-degree angle.

Pathology

The term stenosis derives from the Greek word *stenos*, or narrow. Spinal and lateral recess stenosis refer to an AP narrowing of the spinal canal either in a median or paramedian location dorsally to the neural elements. Narrowing of the AP diameter of the spinal canal due to a central disc herniation or a ventral osteoarthritic ridge formation is usually not considered as spinal stenosis.

The narrowing of the AP diameter of the spinal canal can occur as a consequence of changes in the facet joint, ligamentum flava, intervertebral foramina, and alignment of the spinal canal (scoliosis, spondylolisthesis). These changes include hypertrophy of the ligamentum flava (Fig. 3), degenerative osteoproliferative processes involving the facet (Fig. 4), and spinal stenosis due to spondylolisthesis. In this chapter we will not consider common causes for spinal stenosis. A host of pathological processes (dorsally situated osseous tumors, both primary and metastatic, extradural infectious processes, etc.) and a variety of iatrogenic causes (bony overgrowth due to spinal fusion, malpositioned instrumentation, etc.) should also be considered when a patient presents with symptoms of stenosis.

Pathophysiology

The pathological process responsible for a symptomatic spinal stenosis, such as joint or ligament hypertrophy and spondyloli-

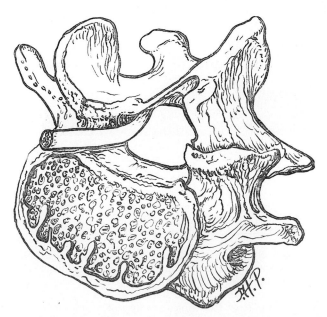

Fig. 1. Lateral recess anatomy. The height of the lateral increases in a rostrocaudal direction. Distal lateral recess merges with the intervertebral foramen. (From Ciric I, Mikhael MA, Tarkington JA, et al: The lateral recess syndrome: a variant of spinal stenosis. *J Neurosurg* 53:433–443, 1980, with permission.)

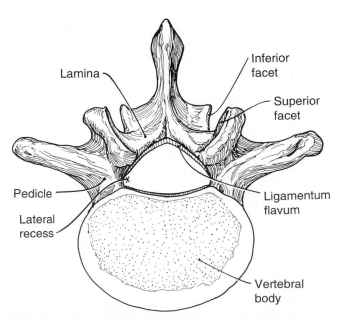

Fig. 2. Anatomy of the ligamentum flava. (©2002, Thomas H. Weinzerl.)

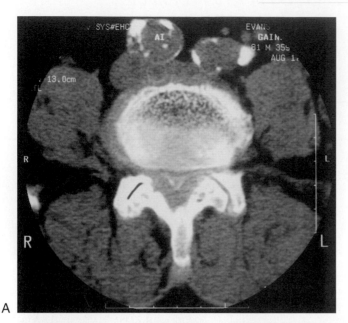

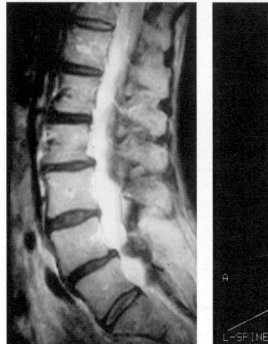

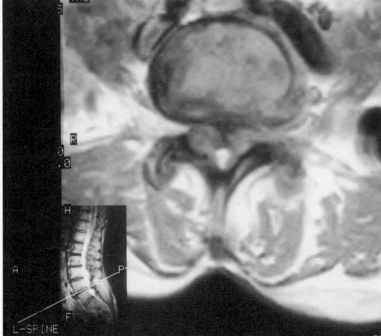

Fig. 3. CT scan **(A)** and MRI **(B)** in a patient with spinal stenosis due to ligament hypertrophy.

sthesis with or without joint or ligament hypertrophy, is always situated dorsally to the thecal sac and lumbar nerve roots (1). This explains why spinal stenosis is more symptomatic when the patient is erect, either standing or walking. With an individual upright, the lumbar lordosis becomes more prominent and the pathological process responsible for spinal stenosis moves forward, compressing the neural elements in the spinal canal and increasing radicular symptoms. In contrast, sitting down, leaning forward, or even squatting will result in a spinal kyphosis causing the pathological process to move away from the neural elements and bring about symptomatic relief. This is also true in patients with foraminal disc herniations.

Clinical Presentation

Patients with lumbar spinal stenosis are typically older adults. Patients with spondylolisthesis and some individuals with a congenitally narrow, gracile spinal canal who may go on to develop symptoms of spinal stenosis earlier in life are exceptions to this rule. The clinical picture of symptomatic spinal stenosis is characterized by claudication-like symptoms in the buttocks and lower extremities that are usually provoked and aggravated by standing and walking. Back pain alone, while often associated with the imaging appearance of a lumbar spinal stenosis, should not be considered as an expression of a symp-

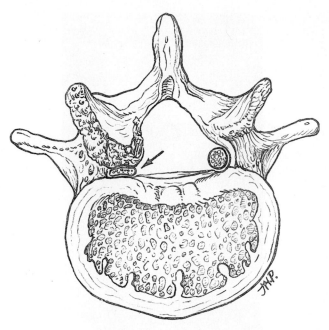

Fig. 4. Artist's drawing of lateral recess stenosis secondary to hypertrophy of superior articular facet. (From Ciric I, Mikhael MA, Tarkington JA, et al: The lateral recess syndrome: a variant of spinal stenosis. *J Neurosurg* 53:433–443, 1980, with permission.)

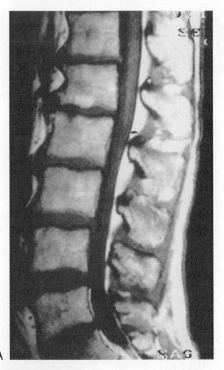

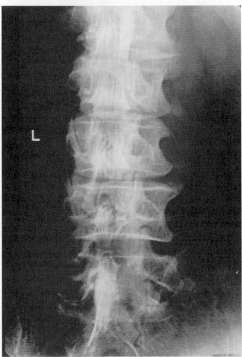

Fig. 5. MRI **(A)** and myelogram **(B)** of a patient with bilateral neurogenic claudications. Note the relatively mild stenosis demonstrated on the MRI. In contrast, the myelogram shows a high-grade obstruction at multiple levels in conjunction with edematous and tortuous nerve rootlets.

tomatic spinal stenosis. Instead, the etiology of a low back pain is invariably related to a structural abnormality of the lumbar spine and is, therefore, not the consequence of a neural compression. Symptoms of lumbar spinal stenosis associated with the buttocks and lower extremities can vary from true radicular pain to feelings of achiness in the buttocks, tightness in the hamstrings or calves, and heaviness, fatigue or even weakness in the legs to a point where the individual has to sit down so as not to fall. A feeling of numbness and tingling in the lower extremities can be experienced. Patients also describe paresthesias associated with a cold sensation in their legs. A true imbalance and unsteadiness is rare as are the symptoms of a neurogenic bladder. A typical flat-footed gait is seen with the weight redistributed primarily toward the heels.

The neurological examination is oftentimes negative for any significant abnormality. The most common finding can be bilaterally absent ankle jerk reflex. This can be a normal finding in older adults even under physiological circumstances. If present, the neurological deficit is usually mild with a plantar or dorsiflexion weakness being one of the earliest neurological deficits. Patients are often unaware of their deficits.

A number of pathological entities should be considered in the differential diagnosis of neurogenic claudications (Fig. 5). These include vascular claudications, a herniated lumbar disc, spinal neoplasms, peripheral neuropathies, hip-related pathologies, and cervical myelopathy.

The main differential diagnostic feature between neurogenic and vascular claudications is that while the former are caused by both standing and walking, the latter are usually precipitated only by exertion, that is to say by walking and not by standing. The presence of examination findings such as poor peripheral pulses and abnormal vascular studies assists in making the correct diagnosis.

Radicular symptoms in patients with a herniated disc are usually precipitated by sitting and leaning forward, rather than by standing and walking, thus quite the opposite from the pain pattern in patients with spinal stenosis. When asked what they would rather do, sit, stand, or walk to alleviate their pain, patients with spinal stenosis will invariably state that they prefer to either sit down or lean against objects such as a shopping cart, kitchen sink, and so forth. Patients with a herniated lumbar disc will state that they prefer to stand.

Patients with intradural lumbar spinal neoplasms, who are often younger, usually complain of a radicular pain that is worse when they are recumbent, especially at night. Patients with a peripheral neuropathy may complain of painful dysesthesias in their lower extremities, usually distally, as well as of a numbness in a stocking-like distribution unrelated to standing and walking. They may also complain of unsteadiness, especially without a visual cue. A constellation of these symptoms should raise a suspicion for a peripheral neuropathy leading to an electromyogram/nerve conduction velocity study and a correct diagnosis. Of course, there are individuals who may have both, a spinal stenosis and peripheral neuropathy. These patients pose a challenging diagnostic and indications problem.

Hip-related pathology is probably the most common differential diagnostic stumbling block in the daily practice of clinicians other than neurosurgeons who have a peripheral knowledge of spinal stenosis. Patients with hip-related pathology, especially when the pathology is incipient, often complain of a pain in and around the hip joint, in the buttocks, and especially in the groin, although the pain may radiate to some degree along either the lateral or inner aspect of the thigh. This is often made worse with weight bearing. There is a relatively fine difference in the presentation of pain between a patient with spinal stenosis and a hip-related pathology. Pain related to hip pathology is oftentimes at its peak when the patient first gets up from a recumbent or sitting position and initiates ambulation with the pain actually improving as the patient continues to ambulate, especially in the early stages of the abnormality. A very careful history with emphasis on all the patterns surrounding the pain syndrome will help in distinguishing neurogenic claudications of spinal stenosis from a hip-related pathology, weight-bearing–induced pain. One of the features in the history that can identify the hip as the primary pathological site is a history of bursitis. This is worse when the patient retires to bed at night and especially if the patient lies on the involved side. On examination, patients suffering from pain related to a hip pathology will often have a characteristic antalgic gait, limping, waddling, and a general favoring of the involved side. In addition, maneuvers such as external or internal rotation of the thigh in conjunction with abduction or adduction, respectively, will often cause pain usually experienced in the groin region. The neurological examination is otherwise typically negative for any abnormality. Hip radiographs are often negative in such patients; a bone scan or a magnetic resonance image (MRI) of the hip should be obtained as indicated.

Patients with a cervical myelopathy may have lower extremity symptoms. A careful history and neurological examination should easily be able to determine the source of these symptoms.

Imaging Diagnosis of Spinal Stenosis

While an MRI is the mainstay of the imaging diagnosis of lumbar spinal stenosis, plain radiographs of the lumbar spine and a myelogram/computed tomography (CT) scan continue to have an important role in imaging patients with spinal stenosis. For example, an MRI may be less than revealing, indeed, at times deceiving, in patients with a grade I spondylolisthesis. A mild

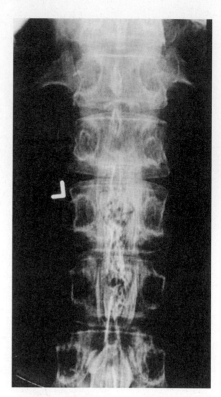

Fig. 6. Myelographic demonstration of engorged and tortuous nerve rootlets at multiple levels in a patient whose MRI shows severe stenosis at L4-5 and apparently mild stenosis at L2-3 and L3-4 levels.

spondylolisthesis or segmental instability may be missed on the MRI in such patients or a misdiagnosis of a central disc herniation may be made, when, in fact, the patient has spondylolisthesis and a pseudodisc phenomenon. Thus, lumbar spine radiographs with flexion and extension views should be part of the imaging diagnosis in these patients. At times, the MRI may also not correlate well with the symptoms. A myelogram/CT scan may be more revealing in such cases. An example of an MRI showing relatively moderate stenosis while the myelogram/CT scan disclosed a high-grade blockage to contrast flow is seen in Fig. 6. A demonstration of engorged, tortuous intradural rootlets is usually an indication that a stenosis is symptomatic at that level (Fig. 7). Thus, while the MRI may suggest a one- or two-level stenosis, the myelogram/CT scan can show that the stenosis is more extensive than anticipated.

Nonoperative Treatment

Some controversy still remains in the literature as to the use of conservative treatment of lumbar spinal stenosis, with some considering it superior to surgical therapy (2,3), some advocating the reverse (4–6) and then again, claiming no lasting difference between the two. The differences of opinions stem largely from poorly defined outcome measures (7,8).

Nonoperative treatment for spinal stenosis, however, has only limited options. These include avoidance of activities that cause pain. Exercises done sitting (bicycle, rowing, etc.), done upright with the individual leaning against handlebars (treadmill), and aquatic exercises may prove useful and comfortable to these patients. Structured physical therapy is usually of lim-

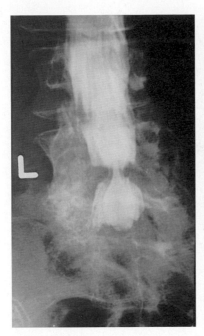 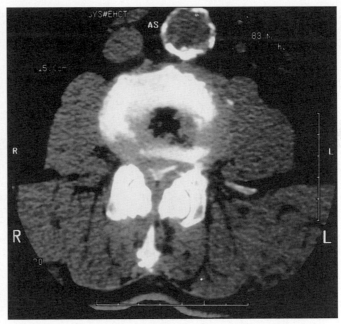

Fig. 7. Single-level stenosis due to facet arthropathy and ligament hypertrophy, without spondylolisthesis, is usually associated with excellent surgical outcomes following a decompression of the central canal and lateral recesses.

ited benefit. A lumbosacral back support corset-brace may help diminish the symptoms in a patient with a spondylolisthetic spinal stenosis. Nonsteroidal antiinflammatory medication is often helpful on a chronic basis. The mainstay of conservative treatment of these patients consists of epidural steroid injections. The predictability of the response to these injections, however, is rather low.

Surgical Indications

Surgical indications are usually based on quality of life issues. The surgical indications, therefore, are rarely placed because of a potentially threatening loss of neurological functions due to the spinal stenosis. Even in patients in whom a myelogram/CT scan shows evidence of a high-grade blockage in the lumbar spinal canal, the possibility of a devastating neurological sequela is quite low. The surgeon should explain to the patient the nature and implications of spinal stenosis, available treatment options, including a thorough discussion of the surgical option and its expectations, limitations, and possible, although fortunately uncommon, risk (9–11).

A review of the literature on the surgical treatment of spinal stenosis reveals a significant difference of opinions as to the use and benefits derived from surgery as well as the appropriate surgical technique. On balance though, certain trends and consensus do emerge from such a review. It is generally thought that surgical treatment is superior to nonsurgical therapy with immediate to intermediate follow-up results showing good to excellent patient-based satisfaction outcomes ranging from 50% to 98% in various reports (4–7,12–17). The incidence of good outcomes tends to decrease with long-term follow-ups (7,13, 16,18). Predictors of good outcomes usually relate to patient selection (13,19,20) (neurogenic claudications, absence of back pain, severe constriction on imaging studies) and appropriate patient expectations and motivation (9,21) and less so to any

evidence of sagittal instability (12,17). Axial instability usually portends a poorer prognosis (22) as does an operation for a recurrent lumbar spinal stenosis (23) due to bony overgrowth (24). Other favorable surgical prognostic factors are good health of the patient and absence of any concurrent causes for pain, such as hip arthropathy (11,25). Ample evidence for excellent outcomes following decompressive surgery in older adults is also found in the literature (16,26,27).

The prevailing thinking on treatment is supported by what appears to be a valid statistical analysis. A simple decompression is probably superior to a fusion in the majority of patients (10,14,28), although this opinion is not unanimous (29). This appears to be true not only for short- and long-term outcomes but also in terms of complication rate, downtime, and cost-effectiveness of these two fundamentally different operative approaches (30). As far as the type of decompression is concerned, all procedures, from the minimally invasive to the tailored decompression to the standard laminectomy, are represented in the literature, with the authors claiming superiority of their respective techniques over others (17,28,31–33). A trend toward less invasiveness, however, is evidenced in more current literature.

Clearly, patients with neurogenic claudications require a decompressive procedure designed to decompress the spinal canal, especially the lateral recesses and, if necessary, the foramina. Lumbar fusion is not indicated in the majority of patients. In fact, in our experience with close to 1,500 patients with symptomatic spinal stenosis, a spinal fusion is indicated in approximately 5% to 8% of patients. Younger patients with a significant or predominant low back pain, in whom one also anticipates removal of a degenerated disc and, on the imaging studies, has vertically oriented facet joints with a rudimentary developed horizontal portion of the superior facets, may be considered as candidates for spinal fusion. As suggested, by the literature, we also believe that the presence of a grade I spondylolisthesis is not necessarily an indication for fusion unless the above described criteria are fulfilled. As an example, a patient with neurogenic claudications secondary to a spondylolisthetic spinal stenosis who has no back pain and whose imaging studies show evidence of well-developed horizontal segments of the superior facets, in all likelihood does not require a fusion. We also agree with the reports in the literature that prior conservative treatment (4) does not mitigate against a good outcome, although patients with shorter history tend to fare better.

Surgical Treatment: Laminectomy

The hallmark of the surgical treatment continues to be a decompressive laminectomy in conjunction with a release of the lateral recesses at the involved sites. Intraoperative electrophysiological monitoring is still controversial as to its value during operations for lumbar spinal stenosis. We typically perform our operations without such monitoring.

Under general anesthesia, the patient is positioned prone on the operating table with the chest and abdomen supported by a well-padded laminectomy frame or special operating table that allows for an easy respiratory exchange and avoids abdominal compression. During the positioning of the patient, greatest care should be exercised to avoid neck extension and pressure against the dependent eye and the exposed peripheral nerves. Quadriparesis due to neck extension in older patients who often suffer from cervical spondylosis with stenosis, possibly even a concurrent myelopathy, is one of the most devastating complications associated with the surgical treatment of lumbar spinal stenosis. Positioning should be the responsibility of the operating surgeon.

With the patient prepared and draped sterilely and after a localizing radiograph is obtained, the desired posterior elements are exposed through a midline incision and subperiosteal dissection of the paraspinal muscles. A second, positive radiographic localization of the desired levels should be obtained with the posterior elements exposed and before the self-retaining retractors are inserted. With the self-retaining retractors in place, the exposed dorsal elements should be inspected for any pathology. More often than not, the inspection will reveal evidence of joint hypertrophy of the facet joint synovia that has extended in a redundant fashion outside the joint and between the spinous processes. The laminectomy is performed by removing the spinous processes and lamina that were first thinned out with a microsurgical drill, preferably a cone-shaped one that is less injurious to the dura, and burr under continuous irrigation-suction technique so that only the ventral cortices of the exposed lamina are still intact. The drilling is usually carried out into the medial, overhanging segments of the inferior facets without entering into the facet joints. The thinned out lamina and the thinned out medial segments of the hypertrophied inferior facets are then removed with a fine, thin-lipped punch rongeur.

It is our technique to leave the ligamenta flava in place until the laminectomy is completed. Hypertrophied ligamenta flava are often significant contributors to a dorsolateral compression of the thecal sac and of the nerve roots in their corresponding lateral recesses. Thus, removal of these ligaments as far lateral as their insertion along the medial margin of the corresponding superior facets and the facet joint interface is necessary. A liberal rotation of the operating table in either direction will allow the surgeon to tangentially view the ligaments and remove them in their entirety. It has been our experience that in the majority of patients with neurogenic claudications secondary to spinal stenosis, the lumbar nerve roots are significantly compressed in their corresponding lateral recesses by an enlarged and redundant superior facet. Such an enlarged superior facet can be

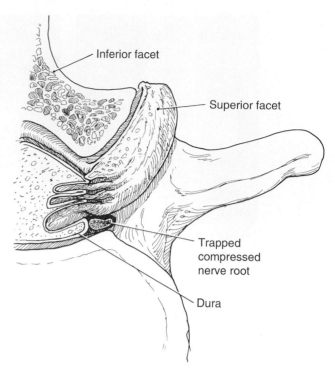

Fig. 8. The medial aspect of the superior facet can hypertrophy in such a way as to not only cause a lateral recess stenosis, but also to interdigitate with and trap the dura along the equatorial plane of the thecal sac. (©2002, Thomas H. Weinzerl.)

deeply imbedded in the lateral aspect of the thecal sac to a point where the dura of the thecal sac can be intimately inherent to various indentations and overgrowths of the medial margin of the superior facets (Fig. 8). An attempt to free and separate this superior facet–dura interface may result in dural tears of some significance. Consequently, our technique is to undercut the protruding, enlarged horizontal segment of the superior facets laterally as it reaches the pedicle and thin it out from lateral to medial in order to gain additional exposure and maneuvering room before the medial extension of the superior facet can be separated from the dural sac.

A nerve root is decompressed when it can be visualized in its entirety from the point of its emergence from the thecal sac to the point where it exits the spinal canal just inferior to the pedicle (Fig. 9). The lateral recess is unroofed as far lateral as the corresponding pedicle. The number of lateral recesses decompressed will depend on the preoperative imaging studies. At the completion of the procedure, the thecal sac should be decompressed dorsally and laterally, the lateral recesses should be opened, and the corresponding nerve roots visualized in their entirety at the levels predetermined by the preoperative imaging studies.

During the laminectomy and removal of the medial, overhanging segments of the facet joints that narrow the lateral recesses, great care should be exercised to leave enough of a bony bridge along the isthmus of the inferior facet where it approximates the pars. This can be accomplished by undercutting the inferior facet obliquely from mediodorsal to ventrolateral. The previously described removal of the medially enlarged horizontal segments of the superior facets does not lead to an instability in close to 85% to 95% of patients. There is sufficient ventral support by the residual superior facet and the inferior facet if the pars remains intact.

After irrigating the operative site thoroughly with an antibiotic

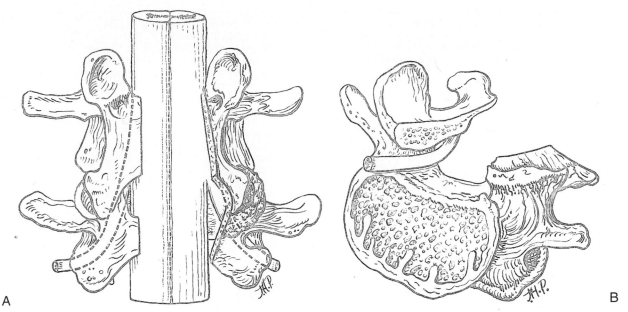

Fig. 9. A,B: Artist's representation of an accomplished decompression of the central canal and of the lateral recess. Note that the lateral recess should be decompressed as far lateral as the pedicle. (From Ciric I, Mikhael MA, Tarkington JA, et al: The lateral recess syndrome: a variant of spinal stenosis. *J Neurosurg* 53:433–443, 1980, with permission.)

solution, the incision is closed in anatomical layers using resorbable suture material for the subcutaneous layers and surgical staples for skin. The patient is usually ambulated on the first postoperative day and discharged home on the second or third postoperative day.

Results

A good surgical outcome depends on the correct diagnosis, appropriate indications, adequacy of the decompression, and avoidance of complications. Excellent results with resolution of preoperative neurogenic claudications and return to premorbid activities can be achieved in close to 90% of properly selected patients if the previously described surgical criteria are observed closely. Postoperative instability occurs in approximately 5% to 15% of patients. Therefore, few patients subsequently require a fusion. Postoperative complications such as a neurological deficit, cerebrospinal fluid leak, neuropathic pain, and so forth, are rare in conjunction with a properly executed surgery that should include microsurgical techniques, especially during the release of the lateral recesses. Approximately 5% to 8% of patients may develop a recurrence of symptoms due to a subsequently acquired stenosis at a level above the previous decompression. Indeed, the surgical outcomes in patients treated for central or lateral recess stenosis in a select group of patients that have been deemed suitable for such a procedure, are among the most favorable in our surgical practice.

References

1. Ciric I, Mikhael MA, Tarkington JA, et al: The lateral recess syndrome. A variant of spinal stenosis. *J Neurosurg* 53:433–443, 1980.
2. Gibson JN, Grant IC, Waddell G: The Cochrane review of surgery for lumbar disc prolapse and degenerative lumbar spondylosis. *Spine* 24:1820–1832, 1999.
3. Radu AS, Menkes CJ: Update on lumbar spinal stenosis. Retrospective study of 62 patients and review of the literature. *Revue Du Rhumatisme* (English ed) 65:337–345, 1998.
4. Amundsen T, Weber H, Nordal HJ, et al: Lumbar spinal stenosis: conservative or surgical management? A prospective 10-year-study. *Spine* 25:1424–1435, 2000.
5. Atlas SJ, Deyo RA, Keller RB, et al: The Maine Lumbar Spine Study, Part III. 1-year outcomes of surgical and nonsurgical management of lumbar spinal stenosis. *Spine* 21:1787–1794, 1996.
6. Atlas SJ, Keller RB, Robson D, et al: Surgical and nonsurgical management of lumbar spinal stenosis: four year outcomes from the Maine Lumbar Spine Study. *Spine* 25:556–562, 2000.
7. Fox MW, Onofrio BM, Hanssen AD: Clinical outcomes and radiological instability following decompressive lumbar laminectomy for degenerative spinal stenosis: a comparison of patients undergoing concomitant arthrodesis versus decompression alone. *J Neurosurg* 85:793–802, 1996.
8. Fritz JM, Delitto A, Welch WC, et al: Lumbar spinal stenosis: a review of current concepts in evaluation, management, and outcome measurements. *Arch Phys Med Rehabil* 79:700–708, 1998.
9. Iversen MD, Daltroy LH, Fossel AH, et al: The prognostic importance of patient pre-operative expectations of surgery for lumbar spinal stenosis. *Patient Educ Couns* 34:169–178, 1998.
10. Katz JN, Lipson SJ, Lew RA, et al: Lumbar laminectomy alone or with instrumented or noninstrumented arthrodesis in degenerative lumbar spinal stenosis. Patient selection, costs, and surgical outcomes. *Spine* 22:1123–1131, 1997.
11. Katz JN, Stucki G, Lipson SJ, et al: Predictors of surgical outcome in degenerative lumbar spinal stenosis. *Spine* 24:2229–2233, 1999.
12. Iguchi T, Kurihara A, Nakayama J, et al: Minimum 10-year outcome of decompressive laminectomy for degenerative lumbar spinal stenosis. *Spine* 25:1754–1759, 2000.
13. Jonsson B, Annertz M, Sjoberg C, et al: A prospective and consecutive study of surgically treated lumbar spinal stenosis. Part II: five-year follow-up by an independent observer. *Spine* 22:2938–2944, 1997.
14. Kalbarczyk A, Lukes A, Seiler RW: Surgical treatment of lumbar spinal stenosis in the elderly. *Acta Neurochir* 140:637–641, 1998.
15. Postacchini F: Surgical management of lumbar spinal stenosis. *Spine* 24:1043–1047, 1999.

16. Scholz M, Firsching R, Lanksch WR: Long-term follow up in lumbar spinal stenosis. *Spinal Cord* 36:200–204, 1998.
17. Tsai RY, Yang RS, Bray RS Jr: Microscopic laminotomies for degenerative lumbar spinal stenosis. *J Spinal Disord* 11:389–394, 1998.
18. Rompe JD, Eysel P, Zollner J, et al: Degenerative lumbar spinal stenosis. Long-term results after undercutting decompression compared with decompressive laminectomy alone or with instrumental fusion. *Neurosurg Rev* 22:102–106, 1999.
19. Deen HG Jr, Zimmerman RS, Lyons MK, et al: Analysis of early failures after lumbar decompressive laminectomy for spinal stenosis. *Mayo Clinic Proc* 70:33–36, 1995.
20. Katz JN, Lipson SJ, Brick GW, et al: Clinical correlates of patient satisfaction after laminectomy for degenerative lumbar spinal stenosis. *Spine* 20:1155–1160, 1995.
21. Herno A, Saari T, Suomalainen O, et al: The degree of decompressive relief and its relation to clinical outcome in patients undergoing surgery for lumbar spinal stenosis. *Spine* 24:1010–1014, 1999.
22. Frazier DD, Lipson SJ, Fossel AH, et al: Associations between spinal deformity and outcomes after decompression for spinal stenosis. *Spine* 22:2025–2029, 1997.
23. Herno A, Airaksinen O, Saari T, et al: Surgical results of lumbar spinal stenosis. A comparison of patients with or without previous back surgery. *Spine* 20:964–969, 1995.
24. Guigui P, Barre E, Benoist M, et al: Radiologic and computed tomography image evaluation of bone regrowth after wide surgical decompression for lumbar stenosis. *Spine* 24:281–288, 1999.
25. Airaksinen O, Herno A, Turunen V, et al: Surgical outcome of 438 patients treated surgically for lumbar spinal stenosis. *Spine* 22:2278–2282, 1997.
26. Clinchot DM, Kaplan PE, Lamb JF: Lumbar spinal stenosis in an elderly patient. *J Gerontol* 53:M72–75, 1998.
27. Vitaz TW, Raque GH, Shields CB, et al: Surgical treatment of lumbar spinal stenosis in patients older than 75 years of age. *J Neurosurg* 91(2 suppl):181–185, 1999.
28. Kleeman TJ, Hiscoe AC, Berg EE: Patient outcomes after minimally destabilizing lumbar stenosis decompression: the "port-hole" technique. *Spine* 25:865–870, 2000.
29. Yone K, Sakou T, Kawauchi Y, et al: Indication of fusion for lumbar spinal stenosis in elderly patients and its significance. *Spine* 21:242–248, 1996.
30. Niggemeyer O, Strauss JM, Schulitz KP: Comparison of surgical procedures for degenerative lumbar spinal stenosis: a meta-analysis of the literature from 1975–1995. *Eur Spine J* 6:423–429, 1997.
31. DiPierro CG, Helm GA, Shaffrey CI, et al: Treatment of lumbar spinal stenosis by extensive unilateral decompression and contralateral autologous bone fusion: operative techniques and results. *J Neurosurg* 84:166–173, 1996.
32. Eule JM, Breeze R, Kindt GW: Bilateral partial laminectomy: a treatment for lumbar spinal stenosis and midline disc herniation. *Surg Neurol* 52:329–337, 1999.
33. Mackay DC, Wheelwright EF: Unilateral fenestration in the treatment of lumbar spinal stenosis. *Br J Neurosurg* 12:556–558, 1998.

150. Surgical Management of Spondylolisthesis and Spondylolysis

J. Keith Preston and Gregory R. Trost

Classification of Spondylolisthesis

Spondylolisthesis is the lumbosacral spine disorder in which failure of the pars interarticularis or other vertebral elements allows abnormal motion, usually in the anterior-posterior direction, between two adjacent vertebral levels. The lumbosacral spine is the most common spinal level affected by spondylolisthesis, and patients often present with symptoms of back pain owing to the abnormal mechanical forces present within the spinal column. A defect in the pars interarticularis may be present at the same level as the slip, which is referred to as spondylolysis. Compression of neural elements owing to lateral recess stenosis, or central spinal stenosis in more severe cases, may lead to radiculopathy and associated leg pain. Occasionally, bowel and bladder dysfunction may be noted along with the presence of pain, but rarely is observed alone.

A plethora of underlying etiologies for spondylolisthesis have been discovered and analyzed with respect to their causative nature, effect on disease progression, and the likelihood of eventual surgical intervention. Classification schemes have been proposed by different authors based on the broad variety of causative entities of spondylolisthesis. These methods of classification have value in clinical decision making regarding patients with this disorder by predicting the natural history of patients with different types of spondylolisthesis. The most common method of classifying spondylolisthesis recognizes five or six types of causative etiologies of the disorder, and was first proposed by Newman in 1963 (1) then further revised by Wilse and co-workers in 1976 (2). Iatrogenic postoperative spondylolisthesis is now considered a separate entity by many authorities, resulting in the extra classification category. Brief descriptions of the categories of spondylolisthesis are presented in the following.

DYSPLASTIC. Dysplastic spondylolisthesis, also known as congenital spondylolisthesis, results from abnormalities of vertebral facets and neural arches, usually at L5 and S1, allowing anterior slip of the L5 vertebral body in relation to the sacrum. A female predominance over males of about two to one has been noted, and 15% to 20% of spondylolisthesis cases are attributed to congenital factors. Hypoplastic facets are usually present along with rounded superior end plates, and spina bifida occulta may be present. Type a is a subtype in which the dysplastic articular facets are axially oriented and type b is represented by sagittally oriented facets (Fig. 1). Progressive listhesis may result in pars elongation or a pars defect, though the neural arch usually remains intact and therefore results in a higher incidence of neurological compression symptoms as compared to isthmic spondylolisthesis (3). Patients with dysplastic spondylolisthesis may present with the "tight hamstring

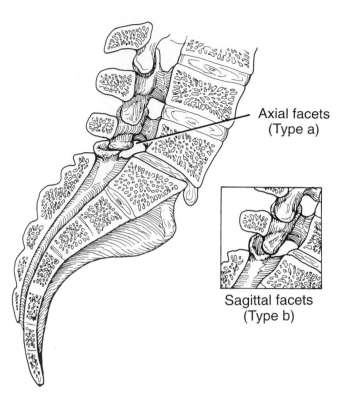

Fig. 1. Axially oriented dysplastic facets (type a) and sagittally oriented facets (type b). (©2002, Thomas H. Weinzerl.)

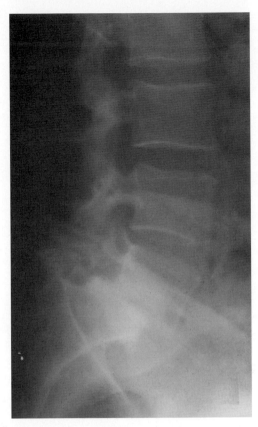

Fig. 2. Grade II (type a) L5-S1 spondylolisthesis and spondylolysis.

syndrome," characterized by a posture of slight hip and knee flexion and variable pain (4). Generally, a subluxation of 35% or greater is present before neurological symptoms occur.

ISTHMIC. Incompetence of the pars interarticularis, such as might result from a stress fracture, allows anterior translational movement of the superior vertebral body in relation to the inferior element. Facet orientation in this subtype remains normal. This is the most commonly observed type of spondylolisthesis in the young (5), and usually occurs at the L5-S1 level, resulting in neural compression owing to fibrocartilage proliferation at the fracture site (Fig. 2). Further classification has been proposed, with type a representing a distinct pars fracture that has filled with fibroelastic tissue; type b being an elongated pars owing to repeated micro fractures and healing; and type c occurring when an acute pars fracture is present, usually associated with fracture of another part of the vertebral body (Fig. 3). The abnormal forces on the annulus result in its eventual failure, and a localized kyphosis thus may be seen, sometimes accompanied by hyperlordosis or retrolisthesis at adjoining superior level. Bulging of the disc may compress the nerve root against the more cephalad pedicle, contributing to or causing radicular symptoms that may be present because of lateral recess or central spinal stenosis. Evidence of chronicity of the malalignment often is seen, such as sclerotic margins around the site of pars fracture. Some authors suggest cumulative trauma is the most common cause of healed pars interarticularis fractures seen on imaging studies rather than an acute traumatic event. The majority of patients with isthmic spondylolisthesis progress to only a low-grade slip, and remain asymptomatic from a neurological standpoint (6).

DEGENERATIVE. In the early 1900s, a form of spondylolisthesis resulting from zygapophyseal joint dysfunction allowing

anterior movement of L5 in relation to the sacrum was noted and termed pseudospondylolisthesis (7). No evidence of neural arch incompetence and absence of pars defect was exhibited by patients with this disorder. More recently this form of spondylolisthesis has been termed degenerative type, because it results from osteoarthritic changes of the spinal column. It is seen almost exclusively in individuals more than 40 years of age, with a female to male predominance of about four or five to one (8). Degenerative spondylolisthesis occurs most often at the L4-5 level but may be seen at L3-4 and L5-S1 as well. The posterior elements remain intact with this type of slip and spinal stenosis with neurogenic claudication is a frequent result, along with varying degrees of lower back pain. The neurological examination often is normal in these patients.

TRAUMATIC. This type of spondylolisthesis occurs with traumatic fractures of vertebral posterior elements, is seen with relatively low frequency, and may be accompanied by fracture of the pars interarticularis at the affected level. It is similar to subtype c of isthmic spondylolisthesis. Hyperextension of the lumbar spine in the setting of major traumatic injury is thought to be the most usual mode of injury in this setting, and severe disruption of the bony and ligamentous elements including facets, disc, and body are usually present in the patient with acute traumatic spondylolisthesis (9,10).

PATHOLOGICAL. This is a form of spondylolisthesis that may occur in patients owing to invasion and subsequent destruction of vertebral bony elements by neoplastic or infectious processes. Involvement of the pars interarticularis or the pedicle

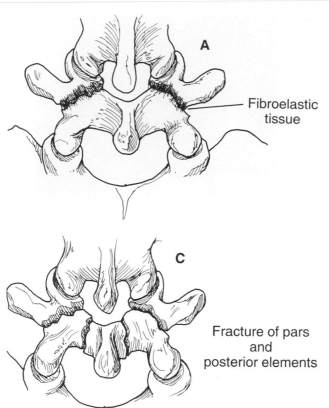

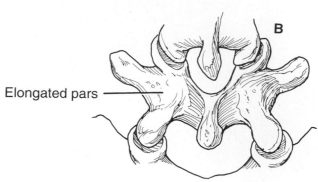

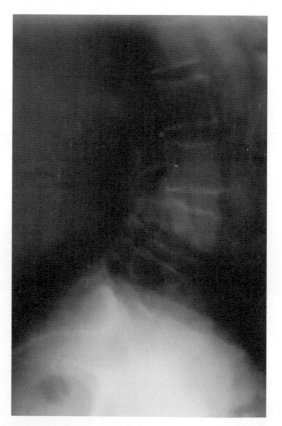

Fig. 3. **A–C:** Three types of isthmic spondylolisthesis: Chronic pars interarticularis fracture associated with fibroelastic tissue (type a), elongated pars interarticularis *(type b),* and acute pars fracture associated with posterior elemental fractures (type c). (©2002, Thomas H. Weinzerl.)

may sufficiently destabilize the spine and allow translational movement between two levels; osteoporosis and other rare bone diseases have been reported to result in this type of spondylolisthesis as well (11).

POSTSURGICAL. Now considered a separate entity by most authorities, iatrogenic spondylolisthesis is seen following extensive removal of stabilizing posterior elements, usually in a decompressive procedure for spinal degenerative disease (Fig. 4). A low-grade slip most often is seen, but associated symptoms can be quite prominent, consisting of back or leg pain that develops months after surgery. Extensive removal of the facet complex bilaterally may predispose a patient to development of postoperative spondylolisthesis, most commonly following a decompression procedure for central spinal stenosis. Reports of postsurgical spondylolisthesis following simple laminectomy and discectomy are present in the literature, as well as a condition referred to as acquired spondylolisthesis, which represents development of a slip at a level adjacent to a surgically fused level (2,12). Preoperative risk for the development of a postsurgical spondylolisthesis may be quantified by evaluating the amount of vertebral body slippage on flexion-extension radiographs (13). Increasing levels of decompression also have been associated with increased risk of postsurgical spondylolisthesis development (14).

Nonoperative Management of Spondylolisthesis

A majority of patients with spondylolisthesis and spondylolysis should be managed conservatively on initial presentation (15,

Fig. 4. Postsurgical spondylolisthesis in a 53-year-old woman who had undergone decompressive laminectomies at L4 and L5 three months earlier.

16). Patients with a low-grade slip who are asymptomatic should always be managed nonoperatively and followed serially with radiographs, the time course of follow-up dependent on the patient's risk of progression to a more severe slip. Children and adolescents with spondylolisthesis and/or spondylolysis rarely develop severe symptoms and often can be adequately managed with activity modification, brace immobilization, physiotherapy, or a combination of these interventions (17,18). The prognosis for patients with degenerative spondylolisthesis treated conservatively is good as well, with most studies reporting eventual spontaneous fusion rates of 10% to 20% in this subgroup of patients. The presence of significant or debilitating neurological deficit, such as urinary or fecal incontinence, warrants consideration of early operative intervention in any patient with spondylolisthesis.

Pain is an important issue for patients with spondylolisthesis and spondylolysis and, as such, it merits attention from a psychosocial standpoint with regard to narcotic addiction, unemployment and disability status, and potential secondary gains through pain behavior. Most authors believe nonsteroidal antiinflammatory drugs and muscle relaxants are adequate for oral pain control in patients with spondylolisthesis, and that narcotics are rarely indicated and usually best avoided. Strengthening exercises and physiotherapy often are helpful and should be a part of the initial management plan for spondylolisthesis. Several studies indicate flexion exercises to be more effective than extension exercises, with a higher number of patients using flexion exercises returning to work sooner and experiencing less pain than patients using extension exercises. Training in posture control, lifting techniques, and use of heat are also important factors to be included in the physical therapy regimen of this disorder.

Surgical Management of Spondylolisthesis and Spondylolysis

PATIENT SELECTION. As alluded to in prior sections, most patients with spondylolisthesis can be managed adequately without operative intervention (15,16,19). Because most patients present with back or leg pain, or a combination of the two, conservative therapy is frequently appropriate in order to attempt pain relief. Those patients with significant neurological deficits on initial presentation and patients with persistent back or leg pain following a trial of conservative management should be offered spinal fusion, accompanied by a decompressive procedure if the degree of symptomatology from spinal stenosis is significant. In the absence of radiculopathy and neurogenic claudication, spinal fusion may be performed successfully without decompression in an attempt to relieve mechanical back pain (15,20,21).

Spinal fusion procedures involve potential for significant blood loss and a careful preoperative evaluation should be conducted with regard to the overall medical condition and ability of the patient to withstand the proposed surgery. Although some patients may be treated with an anterior approach for fusion, most undergo posterior spinal surgery and may require prone positioning for several hours during the procedure. Consideration should be given to preoperative blood donation for autotransfusion along with screening for coagulation and bleeding abnormalities. Preoperative evaluation of the spine should include plain flexion and extension films in order to assess the degree of movement between the affected levels.

SURGICAL TECHNIQUES WITHOUT FUSION OF MOTION SEGMENTS

The Gill Procedure. The Gill procedure is mainly of historical interest. When performed alone, it is a laminectomy and the removal of loose posterior elements in order to decompress affected nerve roots in patients with lytic spondylolisthesis (22). Several long-term follow-up reports suggest satisfactory outcome with this type of surgical treatment in patients over 40 years of age (23,24). Most authorities recommend avoiding the Gill procedure in patients less than 30 years of age because of the high incidence of slip worsening over time in younger patients (23).

Direct Repair of Pars Defect in Spondylolysis. If the pars interarticularis is the source of pain, its repair theoretically could alleviate mechanical pain symptoms without the lost motion segments and increased operative morbidity associated with spinal fusion (25). Repair of the pars defect may be accomplished by screw fixation of the lamina to the pedicle, or by wiring of the transverse processes and lamina. Operative time and blood loss are reduced with pars repair alone and satisfactory outcomes have been published, although only a small amount of outcome data are available (26,27).

NONREDUCTIVE FUSION. *In situ* fusion without reduction results in excellent outcome in many patients with spondylolisthesis (28,29). Consideration of the patient's symptom complex with regard to the etiology of pain is important in determining if reduction of the spondylolisthesis is necessary when performing spinal fusion. Because a majority of patients with spondylolisthesis experience mechanical pain in their back or buttocks, eliminating motion in the segment with the abnormal slip often improves or eliminates the discomfort in the lumbar area. Pain referable to compression of nerve roots and presenting as radiculopathy often is adequately treated with solid fusion of the offending segment, but major symptoms of neural compression usually should be treated with decompression before fusion is performed (29).

REDUCTIVE FUSION. Operative reduction of spondylolisthesis followed by spinal fusion is attractive from an aesthetic standpoint, but each procedure must be carefully evaluated and compared to the usual excellent results obtained with nonreductive fusion. Improvement of radiographic appearance and technical satisfaction do not always correlate with improved patient outcome (30). Increased complexity and length of the operative procedure may warrant a reductive procedure impractical, despite its technical possibility, and neural elements may not well tolerate prolonged elongation after reduction.

Some authors have proposed criteria for the indication of operative reduction, including a slip greater than 75% with angle greater than 45°, relative skeletal maturity, and rigid deformity (31). Other proposed criteria include cauda equina syndrome, progressive slip of greater than 40% to 50%, presence of major deformity, and major pain or deficit with two or more risk factors (32).

References

1. Newman PH. The etiology of spondylolisthesis. *J Bone Joint Surg Br* 1963;45:39–59.

2. Wiltse LL, Newman PH, MacNab I. Classification of spondylolysis and spondylolisthesis. *Clin Orthop* 1976;117:23–29.
3. Wenger DR, Lee CS. Spondylolisthesis in children and adolescents. *Semin Spine Surg* 1993;5:308–319.
4. Baldwin NG. Lumbar spondylolysis and spondylolisthesis. In: Menezes AH, Sonntag VKH, eds. *Principles of spinal surgery.* New York: McGraw-Hill, 1996:681–703.
5. Newman PH. Stenosis of the lumbar spine in spondylolisthesis. *Clin Orthop* 1976;115:116–121.
6. Fredrickson BE, Baker D, McHolick WJ, et al. The natural history of spondylolysis and spondylolisthesis. *J Bone Joint Surg Am* 1984; 66:699–707.
7. Junghanns H. Spondylolisthesis ohne spalt im zwischengelenkstuck. *Arch Orthop Unfallchir (Munchen)* 1930;29:118.
8. Rosenberg NJ. Degenerative spondylolisthesis: predisposing factors. *J Bone Joint Surg Am* 1975;57:467–474.
9. Bennett GJ. Spondylolysis and spondylolisthesis. In: Youmans JR, ed. *Neurological surgery,* 4th ed. Philadelphia: WB Saunders, 1995: 2416–2431.
10. Levine AM, Bosse M, Edwards CC. Bilateral facet dislocations in the thoracolumbar spine. *Spine* 1988;13:630.
11. Elghazawi AK. Clinical syndromes and differential diagnosis of spinal disorders. *Radiol Clin North Am* 1991;117:121–128.
12. Lee CK. Accelerated degeneration of the segment adjacent to a lumbar fusion. *Spine* 1988;13:375.
13. Johnsson KE, Redlund-Johnell I, Uden A, et al. Preoperative and postoperative instability in lumbar spine stenosis. *Spine* 1989;13: 591.
14. Shenkin HA, Hash CJ. Spondylolisthesis after multiple bilateral laminectomies and facetectomies for lumbar spondylosis. *J Neurosurg* 1979;50:45.
15. Wiltse LL, Jackson DW. Treatment of spondylolisthesis and spondylolysis in children. *Clin Orthop* 1976;117:92.
16. Nachemson AL. Newest knowledge of low back pain: a critical look. *Clin Orthop* 1992;279:8–20.
17. Gupta M, Boachie-Adjei O. Conservative treatment of spondylolysis and spondylolisthesis. *Semin Spine Surg* 1994;6:1–11.
18. Micheli LJ, Hall JE, Miller ME. Use of modified Boston brace for back injuries in athletes. *Am J Sports Med* 1980;8:351–356.
19. Rombold C. Treatment of spondylolisthesis by posterolateral fusion, resection of the pars interarticularis, and prompt mobilization of the patient. An end-result study of seventy-three patients. *J Bone Joint Surg Am* 1966;48:1282–1300.
20. Laurent LE, Osterman K. Operative treatment of spondylolisthesis in young patients. *Clin Orthop* 1976;117:85.
21. Johnson JR, Kirwan EO. The long-term results of fusion in situ for severe spondylolisthesis. *J Bone Joint Surg Br* 1983;65:43.
22. Gill GG, Manning JG, White HL. Surgical treatment of spondylolisthesis without spine fusion. *J Bone Joint Surg Am* 1955;37:493–520.
23. Osterman K, Lindholm TS, Laurent LE. Late results of removal of the loose posterior element (Gill's operation) in the treatment of lytic lumbar spondylolisthesis. *Clin Orthop* 1976;117:121–128.
24. Cedell CA, Wiberg G. Long-term results of laminectomy in spondylolisthesis. *Acta Orthop Scand* 1969;40:773–776.
25. Suh PB, Esses SI, Kostuik JP. Repair of pars interarticularis defect: the prognostic value of pars infiltration. *Spine* 1991;16:S445–S448.
26. Pedersen AK, Hagen R. Spondylolysis and spondylolisthesis: treatment by internal fixation and bone-grafting of the defect. *J Bone Joint Surg Am* 1988;70:15–24.
27. Nicol RO, Scott JH. Lytic spondylolisthesis: repair by wiring. *Spine* 1986;11:1027–1030.
28. Hanley EN, Levy JA. Surgical treatment of isthmic lumbosacral spondylolisthesis: analysis of variables influencing results. *Spine* 1989; 14:48–50.
29. Zindrick MR, Lorenz MA, Hodges SD. The nonreductive treatment of spondylolisthesis. *Semin Spine Surg* 1994;6:12–21.
30. Heller JG, Schimandle JH, Garfin SR. The operative reduction of spondylolisthesis: indications, results, complications. *Semin Spine Surg* 1994;6:22–23.
31. Bradford DS. Management of spondylolysis and spondylolisthesis. Instructional Course Lectures XXXII. American Academy of Orthopaedic Surgeons. St. Louis, Mosby 1983, 151–162.
32. Amundson G, Edwards CC, Garfin SR. Spondylolisthesis. In: Rothman RH, Simeone FA, eds. *The spine,* 13th ed. Philadelphia: WB Saunders, 1992:913–969.

151. Osteoporosis and Percutaneous Vertebroplasty

Dino Samartzis and John C. Liu

Osteoporosis

Bone is a connective tissue responsible for hematopoiesis, mechanical and structural support, and mineral storage of inorganic salts and organic material. Bone is constantly broken down and architecturally rebuilds to provide optimal mechanical support for its various functions. If bone turnover (the breakdown and formation of new bone) is unbalanced, then progression of bone loss develops. However, peak bone mass is achieved at 35 years of age and is in decline thereafter; thus, bone loss is expected in adulthood and consequently in old age. Although various other factors also contribute to progressed bone loss, an increase in bone resorption and decrease in new bone formation are the hallmarks of osteoporosis.

Osteoporosis, the most common debilitating metabolic bone disease, is marked by a reduction in bone mass per unit volume with normal bone chemical composition, decreased skeletal function, progressive spinal deformity, and vulnerability to fractures. Also dubbed porous bone disease or brittle bone disease, osteoporosis is a universal disease with a common language of improper bone remodeling posing an array of complications.

Spine surgery concerns in osteoporotic patients are abundant. Decreased bone mass density (BMD) provides the foundation for numerous intraoperative and postoperative complications. Proper surgical approach and instrumentation constructs and application must be selected to cater to the spine's altered persona.

Osteoporosis increases the risk for fracture, leading to discomfort and pain that often are difficult to manage. Vertebral fractures often provide excruciating pain and ensuing deformity. Thorough knowledge of diagnosis and therapeutic treatment is imperative to manage an osteoporotic patient. Although avenues exist that aid in the prevention and conservative treatment of the disease, percutaneous vertebroplasty is a technique that offers immediate vertebral pain relief to combat the effects of vertebral compression fractures.

PREVALENCE. Metabolic diseases of the skeletal system are either congenital or secondary in nature. The primary affect on bone in lieu of osteoporosis is a decrease in bone mass owing to improper bone remodeling. As is often the case, the disease has a penchant to affect more women than men because women possess 10% to 25% less total bone mass at maturity. Moreover, osteoporosis has a high predilection to occur in white and Asian women than any other race, with a high risk of developing an osteoporotic fracture owing to low bone mineral density (1). In the United States, 35% of women over the age of 65 and 15% of white postmenopausal women are osteoporotic (2). In the United States, this debilitating disease amasses 1 million individuals with fractures per year, and 14 billion dollars are spent for treatment (3). Hip and vertebral fractures occur in women at rates of 250,000 and 500,000, respectively; an additional 250,000 fractures are experienced by men yearly (4,5). Vertebral fractures in women increase in menopause and old age, with a female to male ratio of 2 to 1.

BONE BIOLOGY. Bone is the grand architect of the human body, providing structure, stability, protection, and movement via muscular assistance. The primary structure of bone is distinguished by cortical bone (compact bone) and trabecular bone (cancellous or spongy bone). Trabecular bone has many interconnecting cavities, consisting of red bone marrow forming red blood cells and yellow bone marrow composed of fat cells. Conversely, cortical bone is generally on the surface and is characterized by its dense composition without cavities. The extent of trabecular and cortical bone varies depending on the location of bone. Bone is composed of osteoprogenitor cells, osteoblasts, osteocytes, osteoclasts, neurovascular cells of external origin, bone surface-lining cells, and an array of inorganic and organic constituents. Furthermore, two types of bone are evident: primary and secondary. Primary or woven bone first appears in early embryonic development characterized by its low mineral content, higher abundance of osteocytes, and increased presence of collagen fibers. Although primary bone still remains in adulthood (as is evident at cranial bone sutures, tooth sockets, and tendon insertions), secondary bone is primarily present. Secondary or lamellar bone consists of parallel collagenous fibrils know as lamellae.

The bone matrix is the extracellular mineralized component of bone that contains 10% to 20% water (6) and inorganic and organic constituents that account for 65% to 70% and 30% to 35% of its dry weight, respectively (6,7). Proportions of hydrated and dry weight of bone varies with age, location, sex, and metabolic prowess. Furthermore, an immature or demineralized bone matrix in the process of bone formation is referred to as an osteoid.

The inorganic constituents or bone crystals are electrodense and become more abundant with age, whereas water content decreases. Bone crystals are small with large surfaces and are interconnected with narrow gaps containing water and organic macromolecules. The majority of bone ions are calcium, phosphate, hydroxy, and carbonate. However, citrate, copper, boron, aluminum, sodium, magnesium, potassium, chloride, iron, zinc, lead, strontium, silicon, and fluoride also exist in smaller amounts. The main mineral formed by bone crystals is hydroxyapatite ($Ca_{10}(PO_4)_6(OH)_2$). Ninety-nine percent of the body's calcium deposit is harvested by bone, which is found in hydroxyapatite and provides a constant interchange between calcium reserve in the bone and that in the periphery. Calcified bone matrix prohibits diffusion of metabolites into peripheral tissue. However, canaculi are used for transporting material between blood vessels and osteocytes. Various Group II ions, such as lead, radium, and strontium, are bone-seeking cations

and could replace calcium, posing hazardous toxic effects to bone marrow's hematopoietic tissue.

The bone matrix also is composed of organic constituents. Type I collagen is the most abundant material in the organic bone matrix that provides strength and mineral deposition, primarily of hydroxyapatite. Collagen present in bone is synthesized from osteoblasts and forms strong covalent cross-links with enlarged fibrillar transverse spacing that inorganic minerals inhabit. The collagen is located within the inner and outer bone and forms parallel fibers in secondary lamellar bone.

Less abundant organic constituents also are present. Growth factors, such as proteases and protease inhibitors produced by osteoblasts, also make up the organic matrix. Sialoproteins, osteoporotin, and thrombospondin are responsible for bone–cell adhesion and are found in the organic matrix in addition. Glycoproteins, such as Sparc/osteonectin and osteocalcin, are also present in the organic matrix with biglycan and decorin proteoglycans.

Osteoblasts and osteoclasts are the main bone cells integral in bone remodeling. According to Frost in 1964, osteoclasts are multinucleated cells responsible for bone resorption and osteoblasts are bone-forming cells (8). Bone cells possess a plasticity that provide remodeling capabilities in response to bone cell-derived growth factors, local factors, and varying degrees of stress that induce osteogenesis (7,9). Parathyroid hormone (PTH), 1-25-dihydroxyvitamin, prostaglandins E2, and interleukin (IL-1) are some of the hormones and local factors that influence bone turnover. Therefore, these factors stimulate the activation of osteoclasts, which further require osteoblast and osteoclast precursors for a fully operable osteoclast. Osteoprotegerin ligand (OPGL), osteoclast differentiating factor (ODF), and RANK or TRACE ligands alter the molecular surface of osteoblast precursors allowing interaction with osteoclast precursors. As a result, osteoprogenitor cells, derived from pluripotential stem cells, are thoroughly involved in intramembranous and endochondral bone formation by proliferating and differentiating into osteoblasts. Osteoblasts further proliferate and develop into osteocytes that remain in primary or secondary bone. Osteocytes and osteoblasts can therefore "revert to osteoprogenitor" cells to adapt to changing conditions.

Bone resorption begins once complete osteoclast differentiation is accomplished. Osteoclasts then form erosive cavities at the bone surface, priming migration of mononuclear cells to occupy that area. Of these cells, osteoblasts arise and fill the cavities made by the osteoclasts over a process of 3 to 4 weeks. Bone resorption equals bone formation in the young adult. With age, osteoblasts activity decreases priming an increased bone resorption. The resorptive activity seems to increase with age because of prevention of cell apoptosis by interleukins and tumor necrosis factor, as is noted in postmenopausal women who are estrogen deficient. Trabecular or cancellous bone weakens if cavities still remain. Trabecular bone becomes more perforated, allowing limited surface for new bone to build on if widespread bone resorption is present and progresses. Trabecular bone is largely targeted because bone turnover is dependent on surface area. Therefore, vertebrae in postmenopausal women are more susceptible to decreased bone mass and ensuing fracture because of their abundant cancellous bone.

GENETIC FACTORS. Various factors influence osteoporotic low BMD. Age-related effects are a major public health problem and the catalyst to suspect the involvement of genetic factors. Although various genes, such as interleukin-6, interleukin-1, estrogen receptors, and receptor 2, have been suggested to be involved in osteoporosis, the vitamin D receptor (VDR) and the collagen I alpha I (COLIAI) genes have received the most attention. However, gene–environment interactions, improper sampling, linkage disequilibrium, and population selection could affect the basis of genetic influence.

In 1994, Morrison and co-workers discovered a single gene that plays a role in determining an individual's risk for developing osteoporosis—coined the VDR gene (10). Two versions of the VDR gene have been unearthed and are believed to allow cells to absorb calcium. Stronger skeletons are linked with the first gene "b," whereas weaker ones are linked with the "B" gene. Researchers believe that risk for osteoporosis is based on which version of the VDR gene an individual inherits. Although the VDR gene could be responsible for creating a cell's vitamin D receptor sites, whether it plays a role in BMD and predicts the risk for osteoporosis is controversial.

The COLIAI gene is another candidate for genetic influence for osteoporotic low BMD. COLIAI and COLIA2 genes are responsible for translating type I collagen. Polymorphism of the COLIAI gene has been researched concerning the "S" and "s" alleles. Various studies have been conducted and indicate that both alleles have shown a risk for fracture and osteoporosis (11).

BONE MARKERS. The assessment of bone turnover has been greatly facilitated with the advent of biochemical tests that measure serum or urinary enzyme bone markers of spillover osteoblast synthesized matrix proteins and osteoclast degradation products. Although bone densitometry catalogs BMD, bone markers furnish a biochemical index of the rate of bone remodeling. As a primary advantage of monitoring the short-term effectiveness of antiresorptive therapy, bone markers coupled with BMD measurements complement the evaluation of a patient's risk of osteoporosis and fracture, and aid in monitoring therapeutic response. In addition, alkaline phosphatase and osteocalcin serum levels are considered more reliable forms of bone formation. Alternatively, collagen degradation products measured in urine are regarded as representative bone resorption markers. Whichever biochemical bone marker is preferred to assess bone remodeling, limitations of their efficacy exist, demanding further evaluation and study of their precise role.

BONE FORMING MARKERS

Alkaline Phosphatase. Alkaline phosphatase is an enzyme found in the kidneys, placenta, intestines, and abundantly in bone and liver. Alkaline phosphatase is a cell membrane enzyme, a product of osteoblasts. Although various isoenzymes are present, one predominant isoform exists for each of the tissue sources mentioned as a result of post-translation. An increase in serum alkaline phosphatase is largely accredited to isoforms of the liver or bone, with an elevation also seen in germ and placental cells in cancer patients. It often is difficult to obtain specificity and sensitivity to born turnover because various isoenzymes of alkaline phosphatase are present throughout the body. However, it is possible to measure the expressed alkaline phosphatase enzyme and its correlation to increased rates of bone mineralization because of various techniques available to distinguish among the array of isoforms, such as lectin neuraminidase or immunoassay (12,13). Parathyroid hormone, calcitriol, growth hormones, glucocorticoids, and various steroid hormones influence the expression of alkaline phosphatase (13,14).

Osteocalcin. Osteocalcin, a noncollagenous protein also called bone Gla-protein (BGP), forms 1% of the organic matrix in bone and is expressed by osteoblasts. Osteocalcin is synthesized by osteoblasts integrated within the extracellular matrix and is inherently bound to hydroxyapatite (13,15,16). Osteocal-

cin acquired the name BGP because of the presence of 3-gamma-carboxy glutamic amino acid residues that are negatively charged and bind to a calcium cation within hydroxyapatite, which in turn binds to bone. The precise function of osteocalcin is yet to be determined, but is believed to act as an inhibitor for growth factor activity and leucocyte elastase and as a second messenger in bone resorption for calcitriol (15). Nevertheless, serum osteocalcin reflects osteoblast synthetic activity spillover and is degraded into fragments on resorption (17,18). Thyroid hormone, glucocorticoids, insulin, estrogen, vitamin D, and growth factors have been found to aid in the production of osteocalcin; whereas Calcitrol and vitamin K assist in expressing the protein.

Although osteocalcin is predominantly found in bone, a small proportion is released into the circulation. As a result, fragments of the molecule are found in the serum and measured by immunoassays via monoclonal antibodies or polyclonal antisera. However, impaired renal function (which could increase osteocalcin concentration) or the natural circulatory concentration of osteocalcin could misconstrue the rate of bone formation. Also, serum osteocalcin concentration increases in various bone mineralization conditions. In addition, osteocalcin serum concentration does not parallel the level of alkaline phosphatase in bone (19,20), which also could be attributed to its late expression.

Procollagen I Extension Peptides. Type I collagen is the major component of the bone matrix and is considered a marker for bone formation (21–25). Assuming a triple helical shape, type I collagen is formed from a procollagen I precursor molecule possessing propeptide amino and carboxy-terminals and are evident in serum as collagen synthesis byproducts. Before collagen fibrils become incorporated into the extracellular matrix, the terminals are removed by hydrolysis. Thereby, bone formation can be assessed by evaluating the rate of formation of type I procollagen by measuring serum concentrations of procollagen I carboxypeptide (PICP). PICP has a large molecular weight that is not affected by the glomerular filtration rate. Increases in serum PICP represent cancellous bone formation during high activity, but not in faint remodeling conditions.

BONE RESORPTION MARKERS

Hydroxyproline. Bone tissue contains 50% of the total body collagen mainly possessing a rich supply of Type I collagen. Hydroxyproline represents 13% of the amino acid content in collagen, and its urinary excretion could be used as an indicator for bone resorption (22,26). The hydroxyproline molecule is formed on the peptide chain by post-translational hydroxylation and cannot be reused in collagen synthesis. Hydroxyproline excreted in the urine represents 10% from collagen breakdown, of which the rest is excreted by the kidney as a free amino acid and reabsorbed by the liver and further oxidized. However, alterations in renal and hepatic functioning as well as diet could influence the amount of urinary hydroxyproline excretion and improper technique specificity could prove inaccurate representation of bone resorption (22,27).

Hydroxylysine Glycosides. Hydroxylysine glycosides residues are present on collagenous proteins and excreted in urine as a result of collagen catabolism (28). Hydroxylysine glycosides are amino acids with two residues: galactosyl- and glucosyl-galactosyl-hydroxylysine, of which the former is more present in urine. Overall, hydroxylysine glycosides are present in lesser amounts in urine than hydroxyproline, but could offer insight in the bone resorption rate.

Collagen Cross-links. The physical and chemical characteristics of collagen are determined by the collagen cross-links. These cross-links provide tensile strength and support indicative of collagen primarily in bone. Pyridinoline, a major collagen cross-link, is largely present in cartilage, with a lesser amount in bone. Alternatively, deoxypyridinoline comprises 21% of total cross-links in bone. Nevertheless, further free collagen cross-links and peptide fragments are found in urinary excretion, but all are derived from mature collagen. With age, collagen cross-links urinary excretion increases twofold or threefold in post-menopausal women and is unaffected by diet, exercise, or renal function (29). However, increase in urinary collagen cross-links as a measure of bone resorption also is indicative of osteoarthritis, rheumatoid arthritis, Paget disease, hyperthyroidism, and primary hyperparathyroidism.

Acid Phosphatase. Tartrate-resistant acid phosphatase (TRAP) is an osteoclastic product also involved in other cell types that marks bone resorption when tested for osteoclastic-specific enzyme molecule by immunoassays (30). Six structural forms of acid phosphatase are present in the body and can be distinguished by electrophoresis. Of the more prominent types of inhibition sensitive isoenzymes, TRAP is present on the osteoclast's border and released into lacunae for resorption. Presence of TRAP indicates bone resorption activity. Parathyroid hormone increases the presence of TRAP in osteoclasts and calcitonin inhibits it (31).

Osteoporotic Fractures. Also dubbed "porous bone disease" or "brittle bone disease," osteoporosis is associated with an increased risk of fractures. Fractures are more prone to occur at the hip, ribs, wrists, and vertebrae. In 1990, it was estimated that 1.66 million osteoporotic individuals worldwide suffered hip fractures. An increased risk of mortality exists among osteoporotic patients who experience a hip fracture, with 25% of patients dying in the first year (32–36). Of those who survive, 50% are unable to resume their previous independent lifestyle (37). Such complications as pneumonia, blood clots in the lungs, and heart failure contribute to the complications of an osteoporotic hip fracture. Vertebral compression fractures (VCFs) can decrease height up to 15 cm and result in a kyphotic deformity called "dowager's hump." VCFs in women result in 15% higher mortality compared to women with no disruption (38). Furthermore, VCFs increase with age, affecting 40% of women in their eighties.

VCFs occur because of the inability for the osteoporotic vertebra to sustain internal stresses applied from vertebral load from daily life or minor or major traumatic events. Trabecular bone is largely responsible for the majority of the axial forces and inherited extraaxial stress and strains. The architecture of trabecular bone becomes altered with the cascade of osteoporotic effects and aging. This is characterized by increased spaces, thinness, disorientation, and weakened connectivity. Although trabecular bone network maintains both horizontal and vertical framework, a decrease in density and loss of structural strength compromise the vertebra's mechanical prowess, integrity, and spinal column stability, predisposing it to trabecular buckling. Therefore, alteration of trabecular bone as seen in osteoporotic individuals and with age is accompanied by a decrease in bone density (39–41) and a propensity for fracture (42).

Diagnosis of vertebral fracture is difficult to assess compared to peripheral fractures. Decrease in height and vertebral deformities are indications of vertebral fractures. According to Cooper and associates, 16% of vertebral fractures are diagnosed radiographically when the initial investigation is for another problem (43). VCFs maintain an axis of rotation at the middle column. As a result, anterior column disruption is seen with intact middle and posterior columns. Neurological deficits are not as common because the neural arch remains intact. Bioconcave VCFs manifest as a central vertebral deformity because a crush fracture involves anterior, posterior, and central aspects. Wedge fractures are the most common VCFs, affecting anterior elements more often than posterior. Whatever morphology VCFs adopt, fractures occur more often at the thoracolumbar and mid-thoracic region (43–45). The penchant of VCFs to occur at these regions could be attributed to alterations of stiffness from thoracic spine to the more mobile lumbar region and transitory curvature from kyphosis to lordosis.

Multiple VCFs develop a hyperkyphotic or dowager's hump at the thoracic level with a stooped posture decreasing abdominal and thoracic cavities. Multiple lumbar VCFs further increase lordosis, creating a protruding abdomen. Decrease in axial height is a result of reduction of intervertebral and vertebral loss of height. Also, stooped posture progresses to the point where ribs rest on the iliac crest with circumferential pachydermal skin folds developing at the pelvis and ribs. As this posture becomes more severe, eating becomes difficult and the patient eats less, feeling full and bloated. The cauda equina or spinal cord-related symptoms are uncommon and are secondary to other conditions, such as Paget disease, lymphoma, primary or metastatic bone tumors, myeloma, and infection (46). The abdomen appears normal on awakening, only to distend throughout the day. Nonrestorative sleep or trouble getting to sleep often is the case with patients. Lifestyle changes occur, such as difficulty driving a car, getting dressed, and fear of large crowds; then depression develops. Self-esteem also is compromised as a result of a socially unacceptable body image. After a second vertebral fracture, women report high levels of anxiety because of fear of future recurrences (47) and accompanying stress (48). Time progression and continued osteoporotic problems (signs of depression) develop in women. Social support and roles are affected by decreased function and progressed disease-related problems of osteoporotic VCFs and deformity.

Most VCFs are asymptomatic with unknown origin of injury. Nonetheless, pain could occur abruptly. Initially, pain is acute, lasting 2 to 3 months and comprising deep back pain, with or without unilateral or bilateral radiculopathy and/or segmental costal nerve symptoms and paravertebral muscle spasms. Spinal movement is restricted with flexion primarily decreased. Pain is experienced when standing from a seated position, bending, lifting, and after prolonged seating and standing. Walking is sluggish, but gait is normal. Coughing, sneezing, and bowel exertion exacerbate pain. A succession of VCFs could follow the first initial fracture with discontinued pain between each period of disruption or present continually. However, cluster VCFs have a string of fractures with severe and persistent pain. Pain is relieved by recumbent positioning and bed rest.

DIAGNOSIS. Osteoporosis, as noted by Riggs and Melton, is categorized into two types (37). Type I osteoporosis (also known as postmenopausal osteoporosis) occurs six times more frequently in women than men 51 to 65 years old. Primarily it involves trabecular bone and presents no calcium deficiency. Estrogen deficiency is present and associated vertebral and Colles fractures are prevalent. Whereas Type II osteoporosis (senile osteoporosis) occurs in twice as many women as men 75 years or older, involves cortical bone, is related to calcium intake, and is void of estrogen deficiency. Moreover, fractures of Type II osteoporosis entail the pelvis, hip, proximal tibia, and proximal humerus. Also, decrease in vitamin D and increased PTH activity and impaired bone formation are indicated in Type II osteoporosis. Type I osteoporosis risk factors are low calcium intake, low-weight–bearing regime, cigarette smoking, and excessive alcohol consumption.

Iatrogenic osteoporosis greatly affects trabecular bone and

BMD, depending on the dose and duration of therapy. Corticosteroid-induced osteoporotic affects bone loss within the first 6 to 12 months of use. Corticosteroids increase urinary excretion of calcium and interfere with its gastrointestinal absorption. These events reduce serum calcium levels and influence the parathyroid hormone to compensate for the loss by stimulating osteoclasts to increase bone resorption in an effort to increase serum calcium levels. On the other hand, BMD is reduced, progressing to osteoporosis and fractures. Furthermore, corticosteroids inhibit osteoblasts, which in turn decrease bone formation and reduce the release of gonadal hormones. Furosemide, a loop diuretic, increases renal calcium excretion and decreases serum calcium levels. Thyroid supplements suppress the production of TSH and decrease BMD. Also, anticonvulsants enhance the hepatic degradation of calcium, vitamin D, and vitamin D receptors. Heparin inhibits osteoblast formation and stimulates osteoclasts. Antacids containing aluminum interact with gastrointestinal calcium and decrease calcium absorption. Hyperparathyroidism can be increased with an increase of PTH as a result of Lithium use. In addition, cytotoxic agents also could inhibit bone remodeling.

The best indication of osteoporosis is low bone mass. However, numerous secondary causes that effect bone mass must be excluded before rendering a diagnosis of primary, idiopathic, or iatrogenic osteoporosis. Such secondary causes include Paget disease, osteomalacia hypogonadism, malabsorption syndrome, primary hyperparathyroidism, multiple myeloma, and hyperthyroidism. Prolonged drug therapy also could affect bone mass. Medication has been shown to affect bone mass as well as age, gender, early menopause, genetics, and race. Moreover, inadequate nutrition, smoking, excessive alcohol consumption, and sedentary lifestyle lower BMD and increase fracture risk (5).

Medical evaluation requires thorough investigation of family and medical history as well as physical and gynecological assessment. As is often the case, secondary causes or coexisting diseases may be the catalyst or exacerbate bone loss. Various measures are required in order to eliminate extraneous factors and properly develop a therapeutic regime. A complete blood cell count, serum chemistry group, and urinalysis (including a pH count) should followed. Further tests should be undertaken if the physician has reason to suspect other underlying causes. These tests include thyrotropin, a 24-hour urinary calcium excretion, erythrocyte sedimentation rate, parathyroid hormone, and 25-hydroxyvitamin D concentrations, dexamethasone suppression, acid-base studies, serum or urine protein electrophoresis, bone biopsy and/or bone marrow examination, and an undecalcified iliac bone biopsy.

Radiographic assessment in diagnosing osteoporosis is difficult to confirm because a minimum of 30% bone mass loss is necessary for the condition to surface (2–4). Osteopenia is a term used to denote visible radiographic changes of decreased bone mass. Osteoporosis is more commonly diagnosed when a fracture occurs and when CT or bone densitometry measures bone mass and indicates low BMD. Because osteoporosis is a disease characterized by low bone mineral density, dual-energy x-ray absorptiometry (DXA) measures bone density of the axial skeleton, hip, trochanter, wrist, and heel. In 1994, the World Health Organization (WHO) established diagnostic criteria to designate the presence of osteoporosis based on DXA measurements (49). Normal individuals possess a bone mineral density of 1 SD of the mean of young adults. Osteopenia is indicated if the SD of bone mineral density is between 1.0 and 2.5 below the mean of a young adult population. If bone mineral density is measured 2.5 or more SD below the mean of a young adult population, then osteoporosis is present. Furthermore, severe osteoporosis is denoted when one or more accompanying fragility fractures is present. Low BMD has been associated with an increased likelihood of developing a fracture (1). Based on this criteria, it is estimated that 38% of white females in their mid-seventies have osteoporosis and 94% of that population have low bone mass (50). However, these criteria set forth by the WHO are a measure of the prevalence of osteoporosis and are not intended as a guideline for therapeutic course. An individual assessment of the patient is required that not only measures bone mass, but also accounts for risk factors that guide diagnosis and proper treatment modalities.

Radiographic Techniques. Certain calibration methods can be employed on plain radiographs to measure the cortical thickness of bone at various sites, such as the metacarpal shafts and phalanges of the hand. Although plain radiographic assessment and monitoring of osteoporosis is difficult (because 30% of bone mass must be lost for radiographic changes to become evident), the use of bone densitometry allows assessment of cortical and trabecular bone with greater ease, accuracy, precision, low radiation exposure, and reasonable cost.

One of the first techniques used to assess peripheral bone mass was radiographic absorptiometry (RA). This technique used an aluminum film wedge incorporated on hand x-rays and an optical densitometer to assess the presence of bone loss. In the 1960s, single photon absorptiometry (SPA) was introduced and widely used to measure wrist and heel BMD until the advent of single x-ray absorptiometry (SXA). Although these methods provided some insight into BMD, the presence of composition and variable thickness in soft tissue in such areas as the hip, spine, and the whole body in general ushered in dual photon absorptiometry (DPA) in the 1980s. However, in 1987 dual x-ray absorptiometry (DXA) was established, affording improved spatial resolution, more precision, and decreased examination time. Equipped with a C-arm, DXA assessment allows for AP and lateral evaluation of the spine's trabecular and cortical bone with the patient in a supine position. Peripheral dual x-ray absorptiometry (pDXA) also is available for assessing BMD at the heel and proximal and distal forearm. Recently, an innovative method called instant vertebral assessment (IVD) revealed existing vertebral deformities that could contribute to the risk of fracture and affect the treatment modality.

A CT scanner implementing low doses could perform quantitative computed tomography (QCT) images primarily to determine vertebral trabecular bone density. Three-dimensional images of the volumetric density of trabecular bone and metabolic activity can be ascertained through QCT that provide discriminatory criteria among osteoporosis disease progression, aging, therapy, and fracture. Moreover, peripheral quantitative computed tomography (pQCT) scanners have been developed that also operate with reasonable precision and accuracy as QCT. However, a portable and low-cost method of monitoring BMD and the risk of fracture called quantitative ultrasound (QUS) has been designed. Ultrasound transmission velocity or broadband ultrasound attenuation is measured by QUS at the toes, heel, knee, tibia, and fingers.

PREVENTION AND CONSERVATIVE TREATMENT. Antiresorptive therapy and preventative measures are essential considerations in managing and preventing osteoporotic manifestations. Slowing bone loss is of utmost concern. Bone mass is ever-changing, with peak levels obtained in the mid-thirties. Because more women than men are osteoporotic and are at greater risk for developing osteoporosis, various factors are at play accounting for the variable rates in bone loss. Women lose 3% to 7% of BMD around the onset of menopause, followed by a 1% to 2% decline yearly in the postmenopausal period. Men also lose bone with age, but at similar levels as postmenopausal women. Yet, men seem to continue to increase cortical surface by gaining cortical bone through periosteal deposition until the age of 75 (40). Nevertheless, numerous factors must be considered before administering an appropriate regime of preventative and therapeutic measures to combat osteoporosis.

Calcium and Vitamin D. The use of calcium in preventing and reestablishing bone mass for osteoporotic conditions has been questioned. However, proper calcium intake in childhood could establish optimal peak bone mass in adulthood and decrease the risk of fracture. Obviously, age dictates appropriate calcium intake. Children younger than 10 years of age require 700 mg of calcium intake daily, whereas youth 10 to 25 need 1,300 mg of calcium daily to provide the foundation for peak bone mass. Particular attention must be directed toward teenage girls, who have a propensity for improper calcium intake. Afterward, adults sustain adequate calcium concentrations with 800 mg daily. Furthermore, daily calcium intake must be increased to 1,500 mg for pregnant women and 2,000 mg for lactating women. Also, caffeine, alcohol, heparin, tetracycline, furosemide, isoniazid, corticosteroids, drugs detoxified by the P-450 hydrolase system, and high-fiber foods containing oxalic acid have a tendency to interfere with the body's calcium retention and absorption.

Premenopausal women lose approximately 0.3% of bone mass yearly; and menopausal women lose 2% yearly. This rapid succession of bone loss is addressed with an increase of calcium intake to 1,200 mg and 1,500 mg daily for premenopausal and menopausal women, respectively. An increase in calcium slows down or prevents bone loss in premenopausal and postmenopausal women and has shown an increase in femoral bone mass by 3% to 5% after the first year of use.

Although appropriate calcium can be obtained from a daily calcium-rich diet, supplement intervention offers sufficient substitution and possibly a more reliable route to increase and maintain an appropriate calcium intake. The two most common forms of calcium supplementation are calcium citrate and calcium carbonate. Calcium carbonate increases the risk of kidney stones, is not preferred for patients with constipation, requires gastric acidity, and H blockers may interfere with its absorption. However, calcium citrate is preferred over calcium carbonate because absorption is easier (especially for individuals with increased gastric pH) and the risk for kidney stones is decreased. In addition, calcium supplements could cause constipation, and hypercalciuric patients should not receive calcium supplementation.

The recommended daily allowance of vitamin D is 400 to 800 IU daily. Its role in bone deposition and calcium absorption is essential. The most common compound belonging to the vitamin D family is D3 (cholecalciferol). Vitamin D3 is obtained from the skin as a result of irradiation of 7-dehydrocholesterol by ultraviolet rays from the sun or from food. However, vitamin D3 is not the active substance actively employed in osteoporotic prevention. Vitamin D3 must be converted to 1,25-dihydroxycholecalciferol (1,25-dihydroxyvitamin), which is accomplished with the aid of the liver and kidney. In the kidney, cholecalciferol first is converted to 25-hydroxycholecalciferol and later to 1,25-dihydroxycholecalciferol by parathyroid hormone in the proximal tubules in the kidney. In the intestinal epithelium over 2 days, 1,25-dihydroxycholecalciferol increases calcium-binding proteins located on brush borders that transport calcium ions by facilitated diffusion through the cell membrane and is absorbed and deposited in bone and various other tissue. Calcium-binding proteins remain in the intestine for several weeks after removal of 1,25-dihydroxycholecalciferol. Although individuals usually obtain vitamin D through food and sun exposure, supplemented daily allowances is recommended for those with a vitamin D-deficient diet and who remain in-

doors. Serum and urine calcium levels should be monitored if more than 800 IU are administered daily.

Sources of calcium and vitamin D are present in various food sources, but supplementation is available. Usually, suitable doses of vitamin D are accompanied with calcium supplements or are present in multivitamins. The combination of calcium and vitamin D always should be used when calcitonin or bisphosphonates are implemented. The combination of calcium and vitamin D has been shown to lower the fracture rate, primarily hip fractures (51,52).

Bisphosphonates. Presently, bisphosphonates are the most influential class of antiresorptive agents implemented for the treatment of metabolic bone diseases encompassing osteoporosis, Paget disease, hypercalcemia, and tumor-associated osteolysis. These compounds, which possess a low bioavailability with less than 1% absorption when taken orally, target bone mineral owing to their high affinity for calcium and inhibit osteoclast function by binding to osteoclast-resorbing cells. The molecular mechanism of action of bisphosphonates involves a nitrogen-containing class that inhibits a rate-limiting step in the cell's mevalonic acid pathway preventing prenylation of GTPase signaling proteins that are crucial for osteoblast function (53). In addition, bisphosphonates have been shown to promote osteoclast apoptosis (54,55).

Alendronate is the first bisphosphonate approved by the Food and Drug Administration (FDA) for the treatment of osteoporosis. Although other bisphosphonates, such as clinodrate, pamidronate, risedronate, and tiludronate are being investigated for osteoporosis treatment (56), since the early 1990s alendronate has been heralded as improving bone mass quality by increasing forearm, hip (1% to 2% per year), and spine (2% to 3% per year) BMD; and reducing the risk of fractures by 50% after the first year (57,58). In men, Orwoll and co-workers conducted a double blind study of 244 osteoporotic men over a 2-year period and found that alendronate has been shown to reduce the risk of vertebral fractures; increase hip, spine, and total body BMD; and reduce the loss of vertebral height (59). A DXA value of 0 to 2 SD below peak recommends a dosage of 5 mg a day of alendronate for preventative measures; whereas, 10 mg a day is preferred as treatment for a SD greater than 2. However, alendronate may not be ideal for newly developed fractures, but is recommended for the typical postmenopausal nonfractured patient with accompanied estrogen replacement therapy. Also, a patient with a family history of breast cancer, a normal cardiolipid profile, manageable postmenopausal symptoms, and a history of thrombophlebitis would benefit from alendronate therapy (60). With prolonged use or improper use the patient may experience esophagitis from oral alendronate. Dosage may be reduced or the patient must take the drug in an upright position and remain so for at least a half hour before laying down to eliminate the problem.

Of the longest used bisphosphonates, etidronate enjoyed success in treating Paget disease and has been used to treat osteoporosis patients in Canada. Although not approved by the FDA for treatment of osteoporosis in the United States, cyclic etidronate with a dosage of 400 mg daily for 14 days for 2 months has been reported to decrease vertebral fractures and increase BMD (61,62). Also, etidronate is effective in patients with long-term glucocorticoid use (63). The long-term effects of etidronate for treatment of osteoporosis are still debatable and require extensive testing and observation.

Calcitonin. Calcitonin is a large polypeptide secreted by the parafollicular or C cells of the thyroid gland. The C cells comprise .1% of the thyroid gland. Besides reducing plasma concentration of calcium ions, calcitonin redirects calcium deposition and decreases osteoclasts' formation and absorptive properties, thereby preventing osteolytic effects. Originally approved to treat Paget disease, synthetic calcitonin has been marketed and widely used to decrease osteoclast activity, thereby increasing spine bone density and vertebral fracture reduction (64,65). A subcutaneous injection of calcitonin (approved in 1984) and a nasal spray (approved in 1995) are available; the latter has greater acceptance and fewer side effects. Also, calcitonin provides an analgesic effect by increasing the brain's B-endorphins, decreasing prostaglandin E2, calcium flux interference, neuromodulator effect, involvement of cholinergic or serotoninergic systems, or direct central nervous system receptor effects (65, 66). The nasal spray helps increase the body's calcitonin level through a daily dosage of one spray of 200 IU.

Hormone Replacement Therapy. The role of hormones in the development of osteoporosis has been studied extensively. Estrogens has been widely used since the conception of laboratory isolation in 1929. In 1941 Fuller Albright reported the presence of postmenopausal osteoporosis and its clinical manifestations. Oral estrogens became available between 1942 and 1943 and have remained so over the years. Estrogen replacement therapy (ERT) has been indicated for the treatment and prevention for atrophic vaginitis and vasomotor symptoms. Further preventative uses of estrogen include delay of Alzheimer disease and macular degeneration, coronary heart disease, and tooth decay. Although many uses were indicated for ERT, eventually it was used for the treatment and prevention of osteoporosis in postmenopausal women by increasing BMD and decreasing the risk of fracture (67–70). Currently, ERT is present with dosage as conjugated equine estrogen, 17B-estradiol, and transdermal estrogen. ERT decreases bone loss of the hip and spine (67) and increases BMD in patients 60 years and older if initiated within 10 years of menopause (71). Moreover, the efficacy of ERT in increasing BMD is enhanced when calcium and vitamin D accommodate low-dose estrogen (72–75).

The precise mechanism of how estrogen functions is not yet well understood; however, it is believed that the presence of estrogen inhibits the levels of cytokine activity associated with osteoclast stimulation, thus reducing bone resorption (76). Possibly, estrogen decreases the formation of osteoclasts by lowering the production of osteoclast precursors, interleukin-1, interleukin-6, tumor necrosis factor, monocytes, and granulocytes. Moreover, estrogen is involved in calcium absorption. However, ERT benefits cease when therapy is terminated (67, 77), use has been shown to increase the risk of breast and uterine cancer (78), and it increases the incidence of venous thromboembolism (79). Low compliance has been observed because of the effects of estrogen use, and as many as 70% of women refuse ERT (80). As a result, selective estrogen receptor modulators (SERMs) have been developed as an alternative therapeutic method to provide the benefit of estrogen without its many complications for postmenopausal women. SERMs bind to estrogen receptors and produce an agonist or antagonistic effect depending on the tissue and type of SERM.

Various SERMs exist, including benzothiophenes, benzopyrans, tetrahydronaphthylenes, and triphenylethylenes, which vary in safety and clinical prowess. Tamoxifen, a triphenylethylene, is the first SERM and has been widely employed in the treatment and reduction of risk for breast cancer (81). Tamoxifen, which has antiestrogen effects on the breast, has estrogen-like effects in the prevention of bone loss and build-up of BMD in postmenopausal women (82). However, tamoxifen users are at risk of developing endometrial cancer and thromboembolism. Alternatively, raloxifene hydrochloride, a benzothiophene-derived SERM, has prominent skeletal antiresorptive prowess and estrogen antagonistic effects on breast and uterine tissue for postmenopausal women (83). According to Cummings and associates, raloxifene decreases the risk of breast cancer by 76% in postmenopausal osteoporotic women. Furthermore, after a period of 12 to 24 months of raloxifene use by postmenopausal women, BMD increased at various sites by 2.5% (84) and the risk of vertebral fractures decreased (85).

Postmenopausal women enjoy the availability of ERT or selected SERMs to reduce bone turnover, increase BMD, and decrease the risk of fracture. Osteoporotic men with hypogonadism or low levels of testosterone owing to age are unable to achieve peak bone mass but have the luxury of testosterone replacement therapy (TRT). TRT in men is indicated if testosterone deficiency (86), vertebral fracture without established testosterone deficiency (87), or corticosteroid therapy is present (88). Studies have shown that 59% to 70% of men with hip fractures had low levels of testosterone (89). Furthermore, an increase of 5% spine BMD in 6 months is noted when testosterone is administered to osteoporotic agonadal men (87).

Parathyroid Hormone. The use of parathyroid hormone (PTH) and its various peptides and analogues in the treatment and prevention of osteoporosis has been an issue of heated debate and vigorous study. PTH has been employed since the 1920s for its role in bone mass. Four parathyroid glands are present in the human body. Chief and oxyphil are the main cells of the parathyroid gland; chief cells predominantly secrete PTH. Naturally, PTH—a hormone produced by the body's parathyroid glands—is instrumental in calcium and phosphate absorption in bone, excretion by the kidneys, intestinal absorption, and interplay with vitamin D.

Synthetic PTH is not FDA approved, but is believed to play a therapeutic role in the treatment and prevention of osteoporosis (90–93). Rat studies have indicated that continuous administration of PTH increases bone turnover in favor of bone formation. Over a 2-week period, PTH-related protein (PTHrP) has shown to increase bone mass in rats *in vivo* (94). PTH treatment has been shown to increase cancellous vertebral bone volume at the first lumbar vertebra and fifth caudal vertebra by 67% and 37%, respectively, in ovariectomized rats with an equally impressive increased bone formation of 635% and 359% at the same locale (95). Lindsay and associates reported that postmenopausal women on HRT receiving 25 μg subcutaneous injections daily of PTH for 3 years increased lumbar bone mineral content by 18.9%, as opposed to a 3% increase in HRT alone, of which 50% was noted in the first year (96). Furthermore, PTH and HRT therapy increased vertebral area 5.5% as compared to a 2% increase with HRT solely. Of further interest, an anabolic synergistic or additive strength increasing effect of PTH and growth hormone also has shown promise in ovariectomized osteopenic rats (97). Moreover, PTHrP (1–36) administered to humans for 2 weeks has been associated with suppression of bone resorption and stimulation of bone formation in postmenopausal women (98). Other studies indicate that hPTH (1–34) treatment for 1 to 3 months has a potent effect on increasing lumbar BMD in osteoporotic postmenopausal women (91) and in corticosteroid-induced osteoporosis (99).

Sodium Fluoride. Initial insight in the role of fluoride on the musculoskeletal system was reported in 1937 by Roholm. His observations of industrial workers exposed to fluoride resulted in tendon and ligament calcification and periosteal new bone formation contingent on the duration and amount of fluoride exposure. Almost a quarter of a century later, Rich and Ensinck conducted the first clinical experiments with sodium fluoride in an attempt to substantiate Roholm's claims. They concluded that a positive calcium balance was achieved in patients with postmenopausal or steroid-induced osteoporosis, including patients with Paget disease at a dosage of 60 mg daily for 14 weeks or more. In the ensuing years, radiographic changes were noted from sodium fluoride use.

Sodium fluoride alters bone remodeling by stimulating osteoblast proliferation (100). Fluoride ions have an affinity for apatite ions and form fluorapatite by replacing the hydroxyl group. Fluorapatite crystals become more stable by being deposited along collagen fibrils, thus establishing more resistance to osteoclastic resorptive activity. A dose of 80 mg daily or more of sodium fluoride could induce osteomalacia by altering bone matrix and transferring it from lamellar to woven and irregularly fibrosed poorly mineralizing the osteoid (101). Fluoride-induced osteomalacia is not dependent on vitamin D; vitamin D therapy does not resolve the developed disease; and calcium supplementation may not be sufficient to prevent formation of the disease. Bone formation rates and osteoblast aptitude are impaired after 3 years of continuous sodium fluoride therapy; however, this alteration is rectified after continued therapy for more than 3 years.

Fluoride commonly is found in water, food processed with fluoridated water, toothpaste, and mouthwash. Oral fluoride is absorbed 75% to 90% in the stomach as hydrofluoride; however, absorption decreases with age. Various factors, such as aluminum, calcium, and magnesium, reduce fluoride absorption to 20% to 35% (102,103). Because calcium is used in the treatment and prevention of osteoporosis and can interfere with fluoride absorption, it is recommended that these two substances be administered 1 hour apart. Also, fluoride consumption should be limited in individuals who have renal impairment to avoid toxicity.

The effects of sodium fluoride on increasing BMD and decreasing fracture risk remain controversial, and demand further controlled studies. However, sodium fluoride at 30 mg daily has been found to increase spinal bone mass with a linear relationship between duration of therapy and bone mass (104). Therapy response is established 12 to 24 months after initial treatment. However, not all patients benefit from sodium fluoride therapy; 70% of treated patients increase in bone mass and volume (105).

Various side effects accompany sodium fluoride use. Painful lower extremity syndrome, gastrointestinal discomfort, frank hematemesis, and melena are known complications of sodium fluoride. Symptoms subside after 12 to 48 hours of therapy interruption. Therapy can be restarted 6 to 8 weeks after interruption, and side effects are minimized further by taking sodium fluoride with food or calcium.

Exercise. Fracture rate is related to falls, which increase with age. Over 90% of falls result in hip or wrist fracture (106). Thirty percent of patients over 65 years suffer at least one fall per year. Muscle strength, postural stability, and adequate BMD are factors that prevent falls and subsequent fracture.

Bone remodeling relies a great deal on bone mechanical loading through exercise or daily activity. Bone cellular activity changes in response to loads that fall below or above the threshold by adjusting bone mass and strength to accommodate strain (107). Once loads stop falling outside the threshold, bone remodeling is not required. Yet, changes in BMD are highly correlated with changes in calcium balance. Healthy subjects placed in bed rest loss approximately .5% of total body calcium per month and subsequently develop a negative calcium balance.

Muscle mass and strength decrease with age (108). A decline of muscle fibers, motor units, and metabolic capacity are characteristic of aged muscle. Although decrease in muscle performance is expected with aging, physical activity limits the degree of age-related muscle decline. Strength training increases muscle size, improves aerobic activity, and enhances metabolic rate.

Inactivity and aging results in parallel decline of BMD and muscle mass and strength (109). For example, weight bearing in paralyzed patients with the absence of muscle activity is an ineffective measure for prevention of osteoporosis. The micro-

gravity of space flight is known to reduce BMD and produce a negative calcium balance in astronauts (110). In immobilized conditions, bone loss is localized at the site of immobilization; therefore, bone strengthening is contingent on normal muscular forces. However, recovery from bone loss transpires at a rate less than initial bone loss itself (111–113).

Participation in an exercise program improves mobility and balance in an attempt to reduce the likelihood of a fall. A proper weight-bearing and strength-training program should be tailored to prevent bone loss. Sports, dancing, and various other exercise routines have advantages for balance training. For example, 15 weeks of participation in Tai Chi Chuan classes result in a decreased risk of falling (114); however, frail, disabled, and chronically diseased individuals may not have the capacity to tolerate certain strenuous exercise programs.

Various factors related to exercise influence BMD. Maximum oxygen uptake from cardiorespiratory fitness is a predictor for BMD. Although maximum oxygen uptake is found to relate to femoral and vertebral BMD, the latter is significantly correlated in elderly men and premenopausal women (115). Also, perimenopausal and postmenopausal women who were active in sports during their adolescence display a greater amount of vertebral BMD than women whose youth was sedentary (116). However, amenorrheic female athletes have lower vertebral BMD than menstruating athletes (117,118). Furthermore, reduced progestogen levels in female athletes may contribute to reduced BMD.

Modifiable Risk Factors. Various risk factors contributing to osteoporosis are unavoidable. For example, history of fracture, family history, poor health, gender, early menopause, genetics, and race and ethnic background could account for a reduction of BMD and an increased risk of fracture. However, certain risk factors could be modified to reduce the rate of bone loss, increase BMD, and prevent fractures. Elimination of excess alcohol intake; use of cigarettes, anticonvulsants, and long-acting benzodiazepines; excess thyroid; and prolonged use of glucocorticoids could drastically affect the rate of bone loss. Nonetheless, the minimal effective dosage should be administered if medication is required with intermittent use and increased nutritional intake (e.g., calcium and vitamin D); also, appropriate exercises to prevent bone demineralization and subsequent fractures should be instituted. Furthermore, monitoring BMD with bone densitometry measurements every 6 months could prove invaluable to prevent the dire effects of the aforementioned risk factors.

OPERATIVE MANAGEMENT. Spine surgery coupled with severe osteoporotic manifestations is a recipe for intraoperative and postoperative complications. The vertebral body is rich in trabecular bone and more susceptible to osteoporotic invasion. Tackling an osteoporotic spine during surgery requires consideration of the biomechanical alterations inherited by the disease and alternative modalities to reduce surgical complications and ascertain beneficial results.

Various factors contribute to poor surgical outcome. For example, pseudoarthrosis, subluxation, fracture risk, and hardware pullout are some of the complications associated with an osteoporotic spine. A simple laminectomy often results in vertebral collapse. Fusion failure is high as a result of poor bone stock to accommodate instrumentation and should be avoided, especially threaded cage constructs. Intraoperatively, spinal osteoporosis creates difficulty obtaining proper screw placement and achieving adequate bone purchase. Often, an alternative site or alteration in instrumentation is pursued, as well as accepting less deformity correction and opting for circumferential fixation. If the anterior approach is selected, then bicortical bone purchase must be obtained and posterior stabilization performed. Moreover, supplementation of screws with cement, bone stimulator, and bone matrix also provides advantages. Postoperatively, hardware prominence may be observed; and radiographic hardware pullout or loosening, pain, and neurological deficits may arise. Radiographically, screws develop a halo effect, indicating poor bone–screw incorporation. Revision surgery with additional release is required in such a case in order to decrease excessive forces and provide greater flexibility.

Autogenous bone grafting, which offers optimal fusion rates, is used commonly in spine surgery. However, osteoporotic bones possess poor bone stock for autogenous grafting because of decreased trabeculae and increased fatty marrow content, which offers fewer osteoconductive and osteoinductive factors for proper bone fusion. Alternatively, allograft substrates are used to compensate for poor quality autograft. Fusion rates are not as successful as autograft, although allograft is an appropriate supplement.

Pedicle screw implementation has been used for many years for spinal stabilization. Pedicle screw pullout strength is correlated with BMD (119–122). The efficacy of pedicle screws are threatened with the presence of osteoporosis. Screw augmentation doubles pullout strength. Proper screw hole preparation and implementing larger and longer screws provides a quick fix without the addition of more hardware (123). However, larger screws could increase the risk of pedicle fracture. In lieu of osteoporosis, trabecular bone stock and cortical thickness further contribute to fracture risk in addition to malposition or inappropriate screw size. According to Misenheimer and co-workers, a screw diameter exceeding 80% of the pedicle's outer diameter developed plastic pedicle deformation followed by fracture (124). Sjostrom and co-workers also reported that 85% of pedicles expanded with a pedicle size 60% of the outer pedicle diameter (125). Furthermore, Hirano and colleagues concluded that a vertebral BMD less than .7 g/cm^2 dictates a screw diameter not to exceed 70% of the outer pedicle diameter to prevent fracture (126). Possible bicortical purchase, polymethylmethacrylate (PMMA), or other bioactive cement (127), transverse connections, and laminar hooks (120,128) accompanying pedicle screws could enhance fixation and decrease osteoporotic-associated complications.

Laminae are considered to possess more cortical than trabecular bone compared to other spinous structures (119); thus, osteoporotic effects are less common or slow to manifest than in other vertebral regions. As a result, laminae are more capable to accommodate greater posterior resistance forces. Likewise, laminae could increase screw stiffness by 50% and could accommodate screw augmentation. Use of laminar hooks allows multiple purchase points and rigid fixation.

Sublaminar wires also have been employed for segmental fixation. This type of fixation commonly is used for neuromuscular deformities. Nevertheless, sublaminar wiring in an osteoporotic spine is advantages at thoracic segments because of the unpopular use of laminectomy and pedicle screw fixation at this region, multiple segment fixation dexterity, and tightening capabilities to achieve desired fixation. However, passage of sublaminar wires often is associated with neurological injury mainly occurring at extreme kyphotic or lordotic segments (129). Axial control is limited in the absence of rod fixation. In addition, junctional kyphosis (130) is a concern when a construct ends proximally with sublaminar wires at a kyphotic segment. Use of proximal hooks and increasing instrumentation past the site of fusion can diminish the probability of such an occurrence.

VCFs have the potential to dramatically affect vertebral integrity by decreasing axial height throughout the spine resulting in possible gross deformity. A thoracic hyperkyphosis or dowa-

ger's hump is a physical manifestation that commonly manifests as a result of VCFs. This spinal deformity could be asymptomatic or present with pain, neurological deficit, pulmonary dysfunction, and physical abnormality. Usually, VCFs are treated nonsurgically with bracing, bed rest, analgesics, and often calcitonin. However, immobilization could contribute further to bone demineralization, chronic back pain may exist, neurological deficit continues to persist because of spinal or foraminal canal compromise, and gross spinal instability could offset the prowess of nonsurgical management. In such an osteoporotic kyphotic spine, certain stresses are present at various sites dictating various vertebral segment correction. Multiple segmental fixation is dictated to correct for an osteoporotic kyphotic spine. Sublaminar wiring, hooks, and transpedicular screw fixation are various internal instrumentation used to correct for spinal deformity and pain relief secondary to osteoporosis. However, such instrumentation is also accompanied with numerous pitfalls, most importantly poor hardware–bone incorporation and resulting pullout. Recently, percutaneous vertebroplasty has become an alternative method avoiding internal spinal instrumentation and providing immediate pain relief.

Percutaneous Vertebroplasty

Percutaneous vertebroplasty (PV) is a radiographic guided procedure for injection of PMMA bone cement into the vertebral body to relieve pain owing to fractured or neoplastic manifestation at the vertebral body. Furthermore, PV provides bone strengthening, offers decompression, increases mobility, decreases analgesic dependency, and ultimately improves the quality of life. Since its inception in 1984 in France by Galibert and colleagues (131), PMMA has been used for treatment of giant cell tumors of long bones, vertebral hemangiomas (131–133), osteolytic metastasis, multiple myelomas, and vertebral collapse caused by osteoporotic compression fractures. Although PMMA injection via PV gathered a following, international fame escaped it until it was introduced in the United States in 1988 at the annual meeting of the Radiological Society of North America (134). Nevertheless, it is a fairly new procedure that has managed to ascertain a following for its invasive nature. However, PMMA bone cements are not presently approved by the FDA, most health insurance companies in the United States are skeptical of its efficacy, and attract eager physicians searching to expand their repertoire who lack the clinical expertise to rule out alternative appropriate measures to treat the patient. At any rate, understanding the procedure is essential to obtain beneficial outcome and avoid further injury.

INDICATIONS FOR PROCEDURE

Vertebral Neoplasms. Osteolytic metastases or myeloma are the main indicators for PV. Multiple myelomas are the most common primary malignant tumors of the bony spine that rarely affect the posterior elements. These tumors are rare radiosensitive lesions occurring in two to three cases per 100,000. Diffuse multiple myeloma presents reoccurring lesions at previously radiated levels and offers poor prognosis. Initially, patients report severe pain and disability and are unresponsive to drug treatment. The disease is usually multifocal in nature and surgical consolidation is not advantageous. In spite of this, single-level lesions are treated with vertebrectomy and strut grafting with some success. Nonetheless, radiation therapy alone or as an adjunct to surgery to address the painful manifestation of malignant lesion offers partial or complete pain relief in 90% of patients. Then again, this pain relief is delayed 10 to 14 days after initial radiotherapy. Also, initiation of spine strengthening begins 2 to 4 months after initial radiotherapy. Thus, delayed reconstruction predisposes the spine to vertebral collapse and ensuing neural compromise. PV offers an alternative route for immediate pain relief, bone strengthening, and mobility. Although PV semi-restores the mechanical integrity of the vertebral body and provides a degree of pain relief, tumor growth is not prevented. Therefore, radiotherapy accompanying PV is appropriate because it does not affect the properties of the bone cement, affects tumor growth, compliments pain relief and spine strengthening.

Hemangiomas are benign bony spine lesions whose detection is dubious because of its asymptomatic disposition. Often, hemangiomas are detected during evaluation of back pain and subsequent routine plain radiographs. Soft-tissue extension of the lesion may compress the spinal cord and nerve roots and produce neurological symptoms and even epidural hemorrhage (135). If extensive growth of the hemangioma transpires, vertebral integrity may be compensated resulting in fracture with pain associated at the level of the lesion (136). Hemangioma aggressiveness is indicative on clinical symptoms and radiological evaluation. Vertebral collapse, neural arch invasion, and soft-tissue mass extensions are signs of the aggressive nature of hemangiomas and their candidacy for PV. Furthermore, lymphomas and eosinophilic granulomas also are candidates for PV treatment.

Osteoporotic Vertebral Body Collapse. Osteoporotic individuals are susceptible to VCFs because of the low bone mass that could adequately sustain mechanical forces. Sixteen percent of postmenopausal osteoporotic women experience VCFs (137). However, 65% of individuals presenting with compression fractures are asymptomatic (46,138). These fractures lead to decreased height, back pain, neurological compromise, and disability. Analgesics, bed rest, and external bracing could offer some relief, but conservative therapy may fail and demand alternative intervention. PV is preferred for immediate pain relief and decompression of the neural elements.

CONTRAINDICATIONS. Severe cardiopulmonary disease and uncorrectable coagulopathy are contradictory and could pose complications intraoperatively. Also, preexisting neurological symptoms could be exacerbated by cement leakage. Severe vertebral collapse less than one third remaining height may not adequately relieve symptoms if cement injected. Moreover, PV should be avoided if the patient is not able to lie prone for several hours and if emergency decompressive surgery cannot be performed.

PREOPERATIVE ASSESSMENT. Physical examination is conducted to correlate pain to the level of involvement. The patient usually presents poor mobility and deep focal pain with or without radicular and myelopathic symptoms unresponsive to oral analgesics or bracing. Presence of malnutrition should be evaluated and compensated.

Following a thorough physical assessment of the patient, preoperative radiographic evaluation is necessary to establish the patient's present condition and plan a course of action. However, osteoporotic invasion of the spine handicaps accurate assessment of the integrity of the vertebrae and location of the lesion. Even so, certain radiographic aspects must be considered to obtain optimal surgical outcome. Evaluation of the lesion accounting for vertebral collapse and effected structures is crucial. Magnetic resonance imaging and computed tomogra-

phy scans are performed to rule out further causes of pain resulting in canal and foraminal compromise. Plain radiographs are conducted to assess presence of scoliosis and evaluate sagittal balance. Also, a bone scan is performed to further localize and validate the "active" level(s). Generally, if one third of the vertebral height remains and posterior vertebral elements are affected, then PV is avoided and open surgical decompression and stabilization are performed. Furthermore, stenotic effects, pedicle integrity to accommodate needle diameter, and visibility of concerned structures on radiograph also are accounted.

MATERIALS USED. Location of the lesion dictates appropriate surgical instrumentation used to acquire appropriate depth and vertebral insertion. A 14- to 15-gauge needle 7 cm in length is used for the cervical spine. For the thoracic and lumbar spine a 10- to 11-gauge needle 10- to 15-cm long is implemented. The bone cement is loaded in a 1- to 3-mL Luer-Lok syringe.

Bone liquid cement containing methyl methacrylate (MMA) is contained in a sterile ampule. Bone cement powder containing PMMA and barium sulfate as the radiopaque agent are enclosed in a sterile polyethylene bag. Tantalum or tungsten powder is added to PMMA to improve visualization under intraoperative imaging.

TECHNIQUE

Imaging. Proper intraoperative imaging is essential to properly assess paravertebral vascularity, needle guidance to avoid neurovascular damage, and appropriate bone cement placement. Moreover, radiographic assessment is imperative to detect bone leakage and hematoma development because of inability to assess the patient's neurological level when under general anesthesia. As a response to these concerns, a biplane C-arm fluoroscopy commonly is used.

Although fluoroscopy alone is adequate, scapular obstruction could prevent sufficient view of the upper thoracic vertebrae. Nevertheless, a combined CT and fluoroscopy is preferred (139). CT guidance is advantageous for transpedicular needle placement, especially for the thoracic spine. Pedicle dimensions are more elaborated with CT and avoid pedicle fracture, dictating appropriate needle size. Epidural leakage is identified on CT, which decreases injury to the spinal cord, ganglion, and nerve root. Also, CT monitoring is employed postinjection to detect bone cement excavation and development of a hematoma. Then again, fluoroscopy could detect bone cement leakage, but a hematoma on fluoroscopy is radiolucent.

Polymethylmethacrylate Preparation. Methyl methacrylate is mixed with bone cement powder to achieve a paste or liquid consistency. However, a liquid may leak into the paravertebral tissue and venous leakage could occur in highly vascular regions. The temperature and quantity of the solvent determine the viscosity of the mixture into a liquid or paste consistency. Proceed to mix 20 cm^3 PMMA powder with 1 g tantalum powder in a sterile, clean, and dry mixing bowel (140). The contents are then mixed with .5 mL MMA liquid for less then 1 minute to obtain a homogenous mixture. The mixture is then allowed to polymerize to obtain a paste-like consistency. The paste is inserted into 2- to 3-mL syringes and is prepared for implementation.

Vertebral Puncture Approach. Surgical approach is based on location and characteristics of the lesion and extent of vertebral destruction. Moreover, needle size is established by the location of the lesion on the spine, as was previously noted. The patient is placed in a prone position under general or local anesthesia.

However, treating the patient with PV in hyperextension for kyphotic reduction and height restoration is an alternative route (132). At the cervical spine, an anterolateral approach is preferred with lateral vessel finger manipulation directing the needle between the vessels and the pharyngolarynx. A posterolateral approach is used at the thoracic and lumbar levels with preference at the lumbar vertebrae. Although risk of pneumothorax is present at the thoracic level, in general this approach could injure segmental nerves and predispose paravertebral tissue to PMMA leakage, whereas a transpedicular approach reduces paravertebral tissue leakage and decreases risk of segmental nerve injury. Half the vertebral body can be reached via a transpedicular approach without anatomical compromise of the pedicle. However, the transpedicular approach is detrimental if osteolytic invasion affects the pedicles and poor imaging visualization is present.

The patient is placed prone on a CT scanner table, which facilitates segmental needle guidance by providing segmental images. If desired, a C-arm fluoroscopy could provide a lateral view to assist in pedicle needle insertion. Then again, a biplane fluoroscopy is preferred to allow imaging of two planes of the stylet tip positioning. The needle is inserted at the level of the lesion whatever the choice of image guidance.

Venography should be performed before injection of PMMA in order to highlight direct anastomosis of the epidural, central veins, and inferior vena cava. This provides an outline of the venous drainage, delineates vertebral cortex fractures, and confirms needle placement within the bony trabeculae (141). Furthermore, shunting is avoided from bone to venous structures and epidural space. If needle injection risks compromise as indicated on the venogram, repositioning is immediately performed with gradual injection. However, in the presence of metastatic tumors, injection of contrast media diffuses into the tumoral tissue and stains it causing interference of proper fluoroscopic guidance of needle insertion and PMMA injection. Also, spinal biopsy could be obtained by inserting a biopsy needle into the vertebroplasty needle. Spinal biopsy is recommended for spinal metastases and osteoporotic vertebral body collapse because of metastatic lesion, but is not recommended for angiomas.

Once proper needle placement is obtained crossing the midline one or multiple injections are performed under pressure to obtain desired stability. Depending on the extent of the lesion, 2 to 10 mL of bone cement can be used per level avoiding the posterior cortex. However, injection is terminated if leakage occurs at the foraminal, epidural, or vascular structures to prevent pulmonary embolism and further neural compression. The procedure also is terminated if leakage migrates to the intervertebral disc or the anterior internal venous plexus that could compress the spinal cord. Furthermore, proper needle placement and removal is essential to avoid proximal needle breakage. Therefore, minimal force must be applied to the needle when inserted and on removal the needle must be rotated on its axis to avoid adhering to the intravertebral cement.

POSTOPERATIVE. Immediately following PV procedure a CT scan is administered to determine leakage of the bone cement and hematoma development. Avoid axial loading for 3 hours to allow settling of the PMMA, observe the patient overnight, and administer analgesics and NSAIDs for 1 to 2 days depending on the clinical status of the patient. Prophylactics are continued if the patient is immunosuppressive or immunodeficient.

COMPLICATIONS. The complication rate for PV is 0% to 10% (131,139,141,142) varying depending on the initial indication for the procedure. Vertebral malignant tumors pose the greatest complication of PV (10%) as compared to vertebral angiomas (2% to 5%) and osteoporotic lesions (1% to 3%). Of primary concern in the cervical spine is to avoid injury to the carotid and jugular vein. Pleural injury and rib fracture with ensuing radicular symptoms in the thoracic region is an ever-present concern. Pedicle disruption by the transpedicular approach could occur in the thoracic and lumbar spine with inner cortex disruption and following PMMA leakage into the foramina and spinal canal. Also, proper needle placement is essential to avoid epidural and nerve root injury. Furthermore, accidental bone cement injection into venous structures could result in pulmonary embolism. Nevertheless, needle track leakage and leakage from primary cortical hole as a result from secondary injection are complications that could arise regardless the approach. Antibiotic powder mixed within the PMMA bone cement could reduce such a risk, although infection could occur regardless of procedure.

In 1997, Jensen and associates were the first in the United States to report their experience with PV by treating 29 patients (141). In their 3 years of performing PV, two patients who had thoracic vertebral puncture experienced a nondisplaced rib fracture producing limited chest pain. Two patients had cement leakage to the inferior vena cava with pulmonary embolism and leakage into the lumbar internal venous plexus compressing the thecal sac was noted in one patient. Furthermore, nine patients experienced adjacent disc leakage with no clinical symptoms.

Similar findings have been reported regarding PV since 1997. Cortet and co-workers reported that 13 of 20 (65%) vertebrae treated with PV experienced cement leakage (143). Leakage was noted in six cases in the paravertebral soft tissue, three cases in the peridural space seen only in tumoral lesions (not osteoporotic vertebral collapse), three cases involved adjacent disc infiltration, and one venous plexus. Barr and co-workers noted that 6.4% of patients treated by PV who also had osteoporotic fractures had complications, such as dermatome radicular neuritis, nonbacterial urethritis owing to catheter placement, and ulnar fracture possibly not related to the procedure (132). According to Barr and associates, osteoporotic patients with one level treated by PV are predisposed to secondary vertebral fractures because of added mechanical forces posed by the strengthened vertebra. Therefore, Barr and associates advocate prophylaxis to avoid adjacent vertebral fractures following PV.

The chemical affects of PMMA also have been an issue. Thermal reaction caused by polymerization generates a certain amount of heat that could harm adjacent neural structures and be responsible for postoperative transitory radicular pains. However, Wang and colleagues postulate that ligamentous structures and dural rich vascularity are insulators and impede heat dissipation (144).

OUTCOME. Results of PV are welcoming, although leakage of bone cement is of utmost concern. Debussche-Depriester and colleagues reported 90% pain relief in myeloma (145). Jensen and co-workers noted 90% pain relief within 24 hours in 29 osteoporotic patients with 47 vertebral fractures treated by PV and two patients experiencing immediate pain relief (141). Furthermore, Barr and associates reported that 95% of 38 patients treated by PV reported initial pain relief and maintained relief at 18 months follow-up (132).

FUTURE VERTEBRAL COMPRESSION FRACTURE MANAGEMENT. The past decade has posed an array of alternative methods in treating and managing osteoporosis and its ill effects. Of the most debilitating aspects of osteoporosis, VCF is a worldwide concern that has led to innovative internal fixation and minimally invasive techniques. The future promises a continuation of such thought with newly developed bioactive substances, bone growth hormones, and other natural bone materials that may very well be the new wave of VCF management. Of further interest, direct endoscopic visualization or sterotactic guidance one day may be routine for PV.

Recently, kyphoplasty has been introduced that attempts to eliminate pain and spinal deformity caused by VCFs (146–148). Although a fairly new procedure, kyphoplasty promises dramatic vertebral height correction with height correction reported at 39% to 71%. The procedure operates along the same principle as PV, but introduces an inflatable bone temp transpedicularly into the fractured vertebra that expands the body with a balloon; bone cement is inserted as an internal cast. However, such procedures as kyphoplasty, new bone cement, hormones, or newly developed bioactive substances demand further testing and established clinical results in order to deem their use fit.

Conclusion

Osteoporosis is a worldwide disease affecting millions. The advent and evolution of preventative and therapeutic modalities provide new routes of management of the disease. The effects of VCFs usually are asymptomatic, but threaten the integrity of the vertebral body, resulting in decreased height and possible neurological deficit. PV is a minimally invasive option for painful fractures providing an overall safe, effective, and immediate therapeutic outcome as opposed to the alternative of long-term bracing, bed rest, and chemotherapeutic treatment. However, the risk of complications requires accurate localization of the pain segment, proper screw placement, and intraoperative and postoperative radiographic monitoring to avoid cement excavation. PV is not intended to substitute for spinal canal and foraminal compromise, nor for correction of deformity; it is implemented to reduce pain. In addition, managing an osteoporotic spine in spine surgery requires an alternative approach from traditional modalities to avoid complications and obtain a beneficial outcome.

References

1. Mosekilde L, Bentzen SM, Ortoft G, et al: The predictive value of quantitative computed tomography for vertebral body compressive strength and ash density. *Bone* 10:465–470, 1989.
2. World Health Organization: Assessment of fracture risk and its application to screening for postmenopausal osteoporosis: report of a World Health Organization Study Group. *World Health Organ Tech Rep Ser* 843:1–129, 1994.
3. Riggs BL, Khosla S, Melton LJ: A unitary model for involutional osteoporosis: Estrogen deficiency causes both Type I and Type II osteoporosis in postmenopausal women and contributes to bone loss in aging men. *J Bone Miner Res* 13:763–773, 1998.
4. Burger H, de Laet CE, van Daele PL, et al: Risk factors for increased bone loss in an elderly population: the Rotterdam Study. *Am J Epidemiol* 147:871–879, 1998.
5. Kenny AM, Prestwood KM: Osteoporosis: pathogenesis, diagnosis, and treatment in older adults. *Rheum Dis Clin North Am* 26:569–591, 2000.
6. Recker RR: Embryology, anatomy, and microstructure of bone. In: Coe FL, Favus MJ, eds. *Disorders of Bone and Mineral Metabolism*. New York: Raven Press, 1992:219–240.
7. Prolo DJ.: Biology of bone fusion. *Clin Neurosurg* 36:135–146, 1988.
8. Frost HM: Dynamics of bone remodeling. In: Frost HM, ed. *Bone Biodynamics*. Boston: Little, Brown, 1964:315–333.
9. Burchardt H: Biology of bone transplantation. *Orthop Clin North Am* 18:187–196, 1987.
10. Morrison NA, Qi JC, Tokita A, et al: Prediction of bone density from vitamin D receptor alleles. *Nature* 367:284–287, 1994.
11. Grant SFA, Reid DM, Blake G, et al: Reduced bone density and osteoporosis associated with a polymorphic Sp1 binding site in the collagen type I (alpha) 1 gene. *Nat Genet* 14:203–205, 1996.
12. Behr W, Barnert J: Quantification of bone alkaline phosphatase in serum by precipitation with wheat-germ lectin: a simplified method and its clinical plausibility. *Clin Chem* 32:1960–1966, 1986.
13. Price CP: Multiple forms of human serum alkaline phosphatase: detection and quantitation. *Ann Clin Biochem* 30:355–372, 1993.
14. Weiss MJ, Henthorn PS, Lafferty MA, et al: Isolation and characterization of a cDNA encoding a human liver/bone/kidney-type alkaline phosphatase. *Proc Natl Acad Sci USA* 83:7182–7186, 1986.
15. Power MJ, Fottrell PF: Osteocalcin: diagnostic methods and clinical applications. *Crit Rev Clin Lab Sci* 28:287–335, 1991.
16. Price PA: Vitamin K-dependent bone proteins. In: Cohn DV, Martin TJ, Meunier PJ, eds. *Calcium Regulation and Bone Metabolism: Basic and Clinical Aspects*. Amsterdam: Elsevier, 1987:419–426.
17. Gundberg CM, Lian JB, et al: Urinary g-carboxy glutamic acid and serum osteocalcin as bone markers: studies in osteoporosis and Paget disease. *J Clin Endocrinol Metab* 57:1221–1225, 1983.
18. Price PA, Nishimoto SK: Radioimmunoassay for the vitamin K-dependent protein of bone and its discovery in plasma. *Proc Natl Acad Sci USA* 77:2234–2238, 1980.
19. Deftos LJ: Bone protein and peptide assays in the diagnosis and management of skeletal disease. *Clin Chem* 37:1143–1148, 1991.
20. Diaz-Diego EM, Diaz-Martin MA, de la Piedra C, et al: Lack of correlation between levels of osteocalcin and bone alkaline phosphatase in healthy control and postmenopausal osteoporotic women. *Horm Metab Res* 27:151–154, 1995.
21. Calvo MS, Eyre DR, Gundberg CM: Molecular basis and clinical application of biological markers of bone turnover. *Endocr Rev* 17:333–338, 1996.
22. Delmas PD: Clinical use of biochemical markers of bone remodeling in osteoporosis. *Bone* 13:S17–S21, 1992.
23. Ebeling PR, Petersen JM, Riggs BL: Utility of type I procollagen propeptide assays for assessing abnormalities in metabolic bone disease. *J Bone Miner Res* 7:1243–1250, 1992.
24. Eriksen EF, Brixen K, Charles P: New markers of bone metabolism: clinical use in metabolic bone disease. *Eur J Endocrinol* 132:251–263, 1995.
25. Parfit AM, Simon LS, Villanueva AR, et al: Procollagen type I carboxyy-terminal extension peptide in serum as a marker of collagen biosynthesis in bone: correlation with iliac bone formation rates and comparison with total alkaline phosphatase. *J Bone Miner Res* 2:427–436, 1987.
26. Kivirikko KI: Urinary excretion of hydroxyproline in health and disease. *Int Rev Connect Tissue Res* 5:93–163, 1970.
27. Teerlink T, Tavernier P, Netelenbos JC: Selective determination of hydroxyproline in urine by high performance liquid chromatography using precolumn derivatisation. *Clin Chim Acta* 183:309–316, 1989.
28. Segrest JP, Cunningham LW: Variation in human urinary O-hydroxylysyl glycoside levels and their relationship to collagen metabolism. *J Clin Invest* 49:1497–1509, 1970.
29. Seibel MJ, Robins SP, Bilezikian JP: Urinary pyridinium crosslinks of collagen: specific markers of bone resorption in metabolic bone disease. *Endocrin Metab* 3:263–270, 1992.
30. Minikin C: Bone acid phosphatase: tartrate resistant acid phosphatase as a marker of osteoclast function. *Calcif Tissue Int* 34:285–290, 1982.
31. Miller SC: The rapid appearance of acid phosphatase at the developing ruffled border of parathyroid hormone activated medullary bone osteoclasts. *Calcif Tissue Int* 37:526–529, 1985
32. Browner WS, Pressman AR, Nevitt MC, et al: Mortality following fractures in older women: the study of osteoporotic fractures. *Arch Intern Med* 156:1521–1525, 1996.
33. Conference CD: Diagnosis, prophylaxis and treatment of osteoporosis. *Am J Med* 94: 646–650, 1993.
34. Cummings SR, Kelsey JL, Nevitt MC, et al: Epidemiology of osteoporosis and osteoporotic fractures. *Epidemiol Rev* 7:178–208, 1985.

35. Jacobsen SJ, Goldberg J, Miles TP, et al: Race and sex differences in mortality following fracture of the hip. *Am J Public Health* 82: 1147–1150, 1992.

36. Lu-Yao GL, Baron JA, Fisher ES: Treatment and survival among elderly Americans with hip fractures: a population-based study. *Am J Public Health* 84:1287–1291, 1994.

37. Riggs BL, Melton LJ: Involutional osteoporosis. *N Engl J Med* 9: 1005–1010, 1986.

38. Cooper C, Atkinson EJ, Jacobsen SJ, et al: Population-based study of survival after osteoporotic fractures. *Am J Epidemiol* 137: 1001–1005, 1993.

39. Mosekilde L: Age-related changes in vertebral trabecular bone architecture. *Bone* 9:247–250, 1988.

40. Mosekilde L, Mosekilde L: Sex differences in age-related changes in vertebral body size, density and biomechanical competence in normal individuals. *Bone* 11:67–73, 1990.

41. Snyder BD, Piazza S, Edwards WT, et al: Role of trabecular morphology in the etiology of age-related vertebral fractures. *Calcif Tissue Int* 53:S14–S22, 1993.

42. Ross PD, Wasnich RD, Heilbrun LK, et al: Definition of a spine fracture threshold based on prospective fracture risk. *Bone* 8: 271–278, 1987.

43. Cooper C, Atkinson EJ, O'Fallon WM, et al: Incidence of clinically diagnosed vertebral fractures: a population based study in Rochester, Minnesota, 1985–1989. *J Bone Miner Res* 7:221–277, 1992.

44. Hedlund LR, Gallagher JC, Meeger C, et al: Change in vertebral shape in spinal osteoporosis. *Calcif Tissue Int* 44:168–172, 1989.

45. Krolner B, Pors-Nielsen S: Bone mineral content of the lumbar spine in normal and osteoporotic women: cross-sectional and longitudinal studies. *Clin Sci* 62:329–336, 1982.

46. Glaser DL, Kaplan FS: Osteoporosis: definition and clinical presentation. *Spine* 22 (Suppl 24):12S–16S, 1997.

47. Gold DT, Bales CW, Lyles KW, et al: Treatment of osteoporosis: the psychological impact of a medical education program on older patients. *J Am Geriatr Soc* 37:417–422, 1989.

48. Roberto KA: Stress and adaptation patterns of older osteoporotic women. *Women Health* 14:105–119, 1988.

49. Assessment of fracture risk and its application to screening for postmenopausal osteoporosis. Report of a World Health Organization Study Group. *World Health Organ Tech Rep Ser* 843:1–129, 1994.

50. Riggs BL, Wahner HW, Dunn WL, et al: Differential changes in bone mineral density of the appendicular and axial skeleton with aging: relationship to spinal osteoporosis. *J Clin Invest* 67:328–335, 1981.

51. Chapuy MC, Arlot ME, Duboeuf F, et al.: Vitamin D3 and calcium to prevent hip fractures in the elderly woman. *N Engl J Med* 327: 1637–1642, 1992.

52. Dawson-Hughes S, Harris SS, Krall EA, et al: Effect of calcium and vitamin D supplementation on bone density in men and women 65 years of age and older. *N Engl J Med* 337:670–676, 1997.

53. Rogers MJ, Gordon S, Benford HL, et al: Cellular and molecular mechanisms of action of bisphosphonates. *Cancer* 88(12 Suppl): 2961–2978, 2000.

54. Coxon FP, Benford HL, Russel RGG, et al: Protein synthesis is required for caspase activation and induction of apoptosis by bisphosphonate drugs. *Mol Pharmacol* 54:631–638, 1998.

55. Luckman SP, Coxon FP, Ebetino FH, et al: Heterocycle-containing bisphosphonates cause apoptosis and inhibit bone resorption by preventing protein prenylation: evidence from structure-activity relationships in J774 macrophages. *J Bone Miner Res* 13:1668–1678, 1998.

56. Ott SM: Clinical effects of bisphosphonates in involutional osteoporosis. *J Bone Miner Res* 8 (Suppl 2):S597–S606, 1993.

57. Cummings SR, Black DM, Thompson DE, et al: Effect of alendronate on risk of fracture in women with low bone density but without vertebral fractures. *JAMA* 280:2077–2082, 1998.

58. Lieberman UA, Weiss SR, Broll J, et al: Effect of oral alendronate on bone mineral density and the incidence of fracture in postmenopausal osteoporotic women. *N Engl J Med* 333:1437–1443, 1995.

59. Orwoll E, et al.: Alendronate for the treatment of osteoporosis in men. *N Engl J Med* 343:604–610, 2000.

60. Lane JM, Bernstein J: Metabolic bone disease of the spine. In: Herkowitz HN, Garfin SR, Balderston RA, eds. *The Spine*. Philadelphia: W.B. Saunders, 1999:1259–1280.

61. Storm T, Thamsborg G, Steinich T, et al: Effect of intermittent cyclical etidronate therapy on bone mass and fracture rate in women with postmenopausal osteoporosis. *N Engl J Med* 32:1265–1271, 1990.

62. Watts NB, Harris ST, Genant HK, et al: Intermittent cyclical etidronate treatment of postmenopausal osteoporosis. *N Engl J Med* 323: 73–79, 1990.

63. Adachi JD, Bensen WG, Brown J, et al: Intermittent etidronate therapy to prevent corticosteroid induced osteoporosis. *N Engl J Med* 337:382–387, 1997.

64. Overgaard K, Hansen MA, Nielsen VAH, et al: Discontinuous calcitonin treatment of established osteoporosis-effects of withdrawal of treatment. *Am J Med* 89:1–6, 1990.

65. Silverman SL: Calcitonin. *Am J Med Sci* 313:13–16, 1997.

66. Lyritis GP, Tsakalakos N, Karachalios T, et al: Analgesic effect of salmon calcitonin in osteoporotic vertebral fractures: a double-blind placebo-controlled clinical study. *Calcif Tissue Int* 49: 369–372, 1991.

67. Cauley JA, Seeley DG, Ensrud K, et al: Estrogen replacement therapy and fractures in older women. Study of Osteoporotic Fractures Research Group. *Ann Intern Med* 122:9–16, 1995.

68. Kiel DP, Felson DT, Anderson JJ, et al: Hip fracture and the use of estrogens in postmenopausal women. The Framingham Study. *N Engl J Med* 317:1169–1174, 1987.

69. Lindsay R, Tohme JF: Estrogen treatment of patients with established postmenopausal osteoporosis. *Obstet Gynecol* 76:290–295, 1990.

70. Weiss NS, Ure CL, Ballard JH, et al: Decreased risk of fractures of the hip and lower forearm with postmenopausal use of estrogen. *N Engl J Med* 303:1195–1198, 1980.

71. Schneider DL, Barrett-Connor EL, Morton DJ: Timing of postmenopausal estrogen for optimal bone mineral density: the Rancho Bernardo Study. *JAMA* 277:543–547, 1997.

72. Naessen T, Berglund L, Ulmsten U: Bone loss in elderly women by ultralow doses of parenteral 17B estradiol. *Am J Obstet Gynecol* 177:115–119, 1997.

73. Prestwood KM, Fall PM, Pilbeam CC, et al: Estrogen and calcium have an additive effect on bone turnover in older women. *J Bone Miner Res* 11(Suppl 1):450, 1996.

74. Prestwood KM, Pilbeam CC, Fall PM, et al: Low dose conjugated estrogen reduces biomechanical markers of bone turnover in older women (abstract). *J Bone Min Res* 10 (Suppl 1):256, 1995.

75. Reckers RR, Davies KM, Dowd RM, et al: The effect of low-dose continuous estrogen and progesterone therapy with calcium and vitamin D on bone in elderly women: a randomized, controlled trial. *Annal Int Med* 130:897–904, 1999.

76. Jilka RL: Cytokines, bone remodeling, and estrogen deficiency. *Bone* 23:75–81, 1998.

77. Felson DT, Zhang Y, Hannan MT, et al: The effect of postmenopausal estrogen therapy on bone mineral density in elderly women. *N Engl J Med* 329:1141–1146, 1993.

78. Beresford SA, Weiss NS, Voigt LF, et al: Risk of endometrial cancer in relation to use of estrogen combined with cyclic progestagen therapy in postmenopausal women. *Lancet* 349:458–461, 1997.

79. Jick H, Derbey LE, Myers MW, et al: Risk of hospital admission for idiopathic venous thromboembolism among users of postmenopausal estrogens. *Lancet* 348:981–983, 1996.

80. Ravnikar VA: Compliance with hormone replacement therapy preventative health benefits? *Women's Health Issues* 2:75–82, 1992.

81. Osborne CK: Tamoxifen in the treatment of breast cancer. *N Engl J Med* 339:1609–1618, 1998.

82. Love RR, Mazess RB, Barden HS, et al: Effects of tamoxifen on bone mineral density in postmenopausal women with breast cancer. *N Engl J Med* 326:852–856, 1992.

83. Khovidhunkit W, Shoback DM: Clinical effects of raloxifene hydrochloride in women. *Ann Intern Med* 130:431–439, 1999.

84. Lufkin EG, Whitaker MD, Nickelsen T, et al: Treatment of established postmenopausal osteoporosis with raloxifene: a randomized trial. *J Bone Miner Res* 13:1747–1754, 1998.

85. Ensrud K, Black DM, Recker R, et al: For the MORE study group: the effect f2 and 3 years of raloxifene on vertebral and non-vertebral fractures in postmenopausal women with osteoporosis. *Bone* 23: S174(abstract 1105), 1998.

86. Katznelson L, Finkelstein JS, Schoenfeld DA, et al: Increase in bone density and lean body mass during testosterone administration in

men with acquired hypogonadism. *J Clin Endocrin Metab* 81: 4358–4365, 1996.

87. Anderson FH, Francis RM, Peaston RT, et al: Androgen supplementation in eugonadal men with osteoporosis: effects of six months treatment on markers of bone formation and resorption. *J Bone Miner Res* 12:472–478, 1997.
88. Reid IA, Wattie D, Evans MC, et al: Testosterone therapy in glucocorticoid -treated men. *Arch Intern Med* 156:1173–1177, 1996.
89. Stanley HL, Schmitt BP, Poses RM, et al: Does hypogonadism contribute to the occurrence of a minimal trauma hip fracture in elderly men? *J Am Geriatr Soc* 39:766–771, 1991.
90. Finkelstein JS, Klibanski A, Schaefer EH, et al: Parathyroid hormone for the prevention of bone loss induced by estrogen deficiency. *N Engl J Med* 331:1618–1623, 1994.
91. Hodsman AB, Fraher LJ, Watson PH, et al: A randomized controlled clinical trial to compare the efficacy of cyclical parathyroid hormone versus cyclical parathyroid hormone and sequential calcitonin to improve bone mass in postmenopausal women with osteoporosis. *J Clin Endocrinol Metab* 82:620–628, 1997.
92. Lindsay R, Hodsman A, Genant HK, et al: A randomised clinical trial of the 1-84 hPTH for treatment of postmenopausal osteoporosis. *Bone* 23(Suppl):1109, 1998.
93. Lindsay R, Nieves J, Formica C, et al: Randomised clinical trial of the effect of parathyroid hormone on vertebral bone mass and fracture incidence among postmenopausal women with osteoporosis. *Lancet* 350:550–555, 1997.
94. Hock JM, Fonseca J, Gunness-Hey M, et al: Comparison of the anabolic effects of synthetic parathyroid hormone-related protein (PTHrP) 1-34 and PTH 1-34 on bone in rats. *Endocrinology* 125: 2022–2027, 1989.
95. Li M, Liang H, Shen Y, et al: Parathyroid hormone stimulates cancellous bone formation at skeletal sites regardless of marrow composition in ovariectomized rats. *Bone* 24:95–100, 1999.
96. Lindsay R, Cosman F, Nieves J, et al: Does treatment with parathyroid hormone increase vertebral size? (Abstract). *Osteoporosis Int* Suppl 2: S206, June 2000.
97. Mosekilde L, Tornvig L, Thomsen JS, et al: Parathyroid hormone and growth hormone have additive or synergetic effect when used as intervention treatment in ovariectomized rats with established osteopenia. *Bone* 26:643–651, 2000.
98. Plotkin H, Gundberg CM, Mitnick M, et al: Dissociation of bone formation from resorption during two-week treatment with hPTHrP(1-36) in humans: potential as an anabolic therapy for osteoporosis. *J Clin Endocrinol Metab* 83:2786–2791, 1998.
99. Lane NE, Sanchez S, Modin GW, et al: Parathyroid hormone treatment can reverse corticosteroid-induced osteoporosis. *J Clin Invest* 102:1627–1633, 1998.
100. Farley JR, Wergedal JE, Baylink DJ: Fluoride directly stimulates proliferation and alkaline phosphatase activity of bone forming cells. *Science* 222:330–332, 1983.
101. Parfit AM: Osteomalacia and related disorders. In: Avioli LV, Krane SM, eds. *Metabolic Bone Disease and Clinically Related Disorders*. Philadelphia: W.B. Saunders, 1990:329–396.
102. Jowsey J, Riggs BL: Effect of concurrent calcium ingestion on intestinal absorption of fluoride. *Metabolism* 27: 971–974, 1978.
103. Shulman ER, Vallejo M: Effect of gastric contents on the bioavailability of fluoride in humans. *Pediatr Dent* 12:237–240, 1990.
104. Riggs BL, Hodgson SF, O'Fallon WM, et al: Effect of fluoride treatment on the fracture rate in postmenopausal women with osteoporosis. *N Engl J Med* 322:802–809, 1990.
105. Briancon D, Meunier PJ: Treatment of osteoporosis with fluoride, calcium and vitamin D. *Orthop Clin North Am* 12:629–648, 1981.
106. Grisso JA, Kelsey JL, Strom BL, et al.: Risk factors for falls as a cause of hip fracture in women. *N Engl J Med* 324:1326–1331, 1991.
107. Lanyon L: Control of bone architecture by functional load bearing. *J Bone Miner Res* 7(suppl):369–375, 1992.
108. Rogers MA, Evans WJ: Changes in skeletal muscle with aging: effects of exercise training. *Exerc Sport Sci Rev* 21:65–102, 1993.
109. Cohn SH, Vartsky D, Yasumura S, et al: Compartmental body composition based on total-body nitrogen, potassium, and calcium. *Am J Physiol* 239:524–530, 1980.
110. Rambaut PC, Goode AW: Skeletal changes during space flight. *Lancet* 2:1050–1052, 1985.
111. Kannus P, Leppala J, Lehto M, et al: A rotator cuff rupture produces permanent osteoporosis in the affected extremity, but not in those

with whom shoulder function has returned to normal. *J Bone Miner Res* 10:1263–1271, 1995.

112. Lane NE, Kaneos AJ, Stover SM, et al: Bone mineral density and turnover following forelimb immobilization and recovery in young adult dogs. *Calcif Tissue Int* 59:401–406, 1996.
113. Uhthoff H, Jaworski Z: Bone loss in response to long-term immobilisation. *J Bone Joint Surg Br* 60:420–429, 1978.
114. Wolf SL, Barnhart HX, Kutner NG, et al: Reducung frailty and falls in older persons: an investigation of tai chi and computerized training. *J Am Geriatr Soc* 44:489–497, 1996.
115. Kirk S, Sharp CF, Elbaum N, et al: effect of long-distance running on bone mass in women. *J Bone Miner res* 4:515–522, 1989.
116. Puntilla E, Kroger H, Lakka T, et al: Physical activity in adolescence and bone density in peri- and postmenopausal women: a population-based study. *Bone* 21:363–367, 1997.
117. Drinkwater B, Nilson K, Chestnut C, et al: Bone mineral content of amenorrheic and eumenorrheic athletes. *N Engl J Med* 311: 277–281, 1984.
118. Marcus R, Cann C, Madvig P, et al: Menstrual function and bone mass in elite women distance runners. *Ann Intern Med* 102: 158–163, 1985.
119. Coe JD, Warden KE, Herzig MA, et al: Influence of bone mineral density on the fixation of the fixation of thoracolumbar implants: a comparative study of transpedicular screws, laminar hooks, and spinous process wires. *Spine* 15:902–907, 1990.
120. Halvorson TL, Kelley LA, Thomas KA, et al: Effects of bone mineral density on pedicle screw fixation. *Spine* 19:2415–2420, 1994.
121. Okuyama K, Sato K, Abe E, et al: Stability of transpedicle screwing for the osteoporotic spine: An in vitro study of the mechanical stability. *Spine* 19:2240–2245, 1993.
122. Soshi S, Shiba R, Kondo H, et al: An experimental study on transpedicular screw fixation in relation to osteoporosis in the lumbar spine. *Spine* 16:1335–1341, 1991.
123. Zdeblick TA, Kunz DN, Cooke ME, et al: Pedicle screw pullout strength. *Spine* 18:1673–1676, 1993.
124. Misenheimer GR, Peek RD, Wiltse LL, et al: Anatomic analysis of pedicle cortical and cancellous diameter as related to screw size. *Spine* 14:367–372, 1988.
125. Sjostrom L, Jacobsson O, Karlstrom G, et al: CT analysis of pedicles and screw tracts after implant removal in thoracolumbar fractures. *J Spinal Disord* 6:225–231, 1993.
126. Hirano T, Hasegawa K, Washio T, et al: Fracture risk during pedicle screw insertion in osteoporotic spine. *J Spinal Disord* 11:493–497, 1998.
127. Moore DC, Maitra RS, Farjo LA, et al: Restoration of pedicle screw fixation with an in situ setting calcium phosphate cement. *Spine* 22:1696–1705, 1997.
128. Hasegawa K, Hirano T, Hara T, et al: An experimental study of a combination method using pedicle screw and laminar hook for osteoporotic spine. *Spine* 22:958–962, 1997.
129. Wilber RG, Thompson SH, Shaffer JW, et al: Postoperative neurological deficits in segmental instrumentation. A study using spinal cord monitoring. *J Bone Joint Surg Am* 66:1178–1187, 1984.
130. Reinhardt P, Bassett GS: Short segmental kyphosis following fusion for Scheuermann's disease. *J Spinal Disord* 3:162–168, 1990.
131. Galibert P, Deramond H, Rosat P, et al: Preliminary note on the treatment of vertebral angioma by percutaneous acrylic vertebroplasty. *Neurochirurgie* 33:166–168, 1987.
132. Barr JD, Barr MS, Lemley TJ, et al: Percutaneous vertebroplasty for pain relief and spinal stabilization. *Spine* 25:923–928, 2000.
133. Cotten A, Deramond H, Cortet B, et al.: Preoperative percutaneous injection of methyl methacrylate and N-butyl cyanoacrylate in vertebral hemangiomas. *AJNR* 17:137–142, 1996.
134. Bascoulergue Y, Duquesne JR, et al.: Percutaneous injection of methyl methacrylate in the vertebral body for treatment of various diseases: percutaneous vertebroplasty (abstr). *Radiology* 169:372, 1988.
135. Fox M, Onofrio B: The natural history and management of symptomatic and asymptomatic vertebral hemangiomas. *J Neurosurg* 78: 36–45, 1993.
136. Foley K: The treatment of cancer pain. *N Engl J Med* 313:84–95, 1985.
137. Melton LJ: Epidemiology of spinal osteoporosis. *Spine* 22:2S–11S, 1997.

138. Lane JM, Riley EH, Wirganowicz PZ: Osteoporosis: diagnosis and treatment. *J Bone Joint Surg Am* 78:618–632, 1996.

139. Gangi A, Kastler BA, Dietemann JL: Percutaneous vertebroplasty guided by a combination of CT and fluoroscopy. *AJNR* 15:83–86, 1994.

140. Deramond H, Depriester C, Galibert P, et al: Percutaneous vertebroplasty with polymethylmethacrylate. *Radiol Clin North Am* 36:533–546, 1998.

141. Jensen ME, Evans AJ, Mathis JM, et al: Percutaneous polymethylmethacrylate vertebroplasty in the treatment of osteoporotic vertebral body compression fractures: technical aspects. *Am J Neuroradiol* 18:1897–1904, 1997.

142. Weill A, Chiras J, Simon J, et al.: Spinal metastases: indications for and results of percutaneous injection of acrylic surgical cement. *Radiology* 199:241–247, 1996.

143. Cortet B, Cotten A, Boutry N, et al: Percutaneous vertebroplasty in the treatment of osteoporotic vertebral compression fractures: an open prospective study. *J Rheumatol* 26:2222–2228, 1999.

144. Wang GW, Wilson CS, Hubbard SL, et al.: Safety of anterior cement fixation in the cervical spine: in vivo study of dog spine. *South Med J* 77:178–179, 1984.

145. Debussche-Depriester C, Deramond H, Fardellone P, et al.: Percutaneous vertebroplasty with acrylic cement in the treatment of osteoporotic vertebral crush fracture syndrome. *Neuroradiology* 33:149–152, 1991.

146. Dudeney S, Lieberman IH, Phillips F: Kyphoplasty for vertebral compression fractures. *Osteoporosis Int* Suppl 2:S178, June 2000.

147. Lane JM, Girardi F, Parvataneni H, et al: Preliminary outcomes of the first 226 consecutive kyphoplasties for the fixation of painful osteoporotic vertebral compression fractures. *Osteoporosis Int* Suppl 2: S206, June 2000.

148. Yuan HA, Garfin SR, Lieberman IH, et al: Early clinical outcomes with kyphoplasty, the minimally-invasive reduction and fixation of painful osteoporotic vertebral body compression fracture (VCF) (Abstract). *Presented at the 2000 AANS/CNS Section of Disorders of the Spine & Peripheral Nerves Annual Meeting*, February, 2000.

152. Abnormalities of the Craniovertebral Junction

Geoffrey P. Zubay and Stephen L. Ondra

The atlas, axis, and occipital bones surrounding the foramen magnum represent the craniovertebral junction (CVJ). The unique osseous architecture of the CVJ is the product of its complex embryological development and affords this region its unique biomechanical properties. Abnormalities may arise from congenital, developmental, and acquired conditions.

Developmental and acquired conditions typically present with an insidious onset of disease related symptoms, although most congenital CVJ abnormalities remain clinically silent for extended periods of time before becoming symptomatic. Symptoms usually are the consequence of acquired biomechanical derangements that arise secondary to the underlying structural abnormalities; such biomechanical derangements include basilar invagination and impression, atlantoaxial instability, or a combination of these processes. These conditions frequently require surgical correction and stabilization. Understanding the biomechanical and structural properties of the abnormality is the first step in: (a) understanding the possible complications and consequences that may arise, and (b) being able to identify the proper indications for surgical management.

The Craniovertebral Junction

The craniovertebral junction (CVJ) harbors two motion segments: the occipital-atlantal segment and the atlanto-axial segment. These two motion segments are responsible for a large part of the range of motion of the head and neck. The large displacements that are able to occur at these joints place considerable stress on the supporting ligaments. Structural and mechanical instability can result from either an acute or chronic process.

Acute compromise of the CVJ motion segments typically is the result of trauma. Trauma can compromise the osseous and ligamentous structures of these motion segments, resulting in instability. Many of the ligaments that bolster the CVJ are very strong; subsequently, the large forces needed to impair these ligaments and joints frequently result in neurological injury and mortality. One retrospective review of 1,915 cervical spine injuries showed that occipital-atlantal dislocation was associated with a 100% incidence of neurological injury and 82% incidence of mortality on presentation (1,2).

Chronic compromise of the CVJ motion segments can occur from either developmental anomalies or chronic disease processes. The abnormal architecture of the occipital-atlantal and atlantoaxial joints associated with developmental dysplasias and segmentation anomalies can place excessive stress and strain on these motion segments, resulting in malalignment and instability (3). In contrast, chronic disease processes typically occur in the setting of normal architecture with failure of the CVJ motion segments occurring as the result of disease-related compromise of the supporting ligamentous structures or compromise of the normal load-bearing features of the bone. Failure of the occipital-atlantal and atlantoaxial joints results from a gradual process in either case.

Development dysplasias, segmentation abnormalities, and chronic disease processes frequently result in gradual vertical translocation of the cervical spine into the foramen magnum, whereas trauma typically results in glacial instability of the occipital-atlantal joint. Vertical translocation causes crowding of the foramen magnum with prolapse of the odontoid process. The condition is called basilar invagination when prolapse occurs from architectural alterations of the CVJ; this occurs in congenital dysplasias and segmentation anomalies typically. The condition is called basilar impression when prolapse occurs from a settling phenomenon related to altered load-bearing features of the skull base or compromised ligamentous structures (4,5).

Chronic compromise of the atlanto-axial joints can result in instability. Because of the unique osseous architecture at this motion segment, the integrity of the numerous supporting ligaments has a significant role in maintaining normal anatomical alignment. Glacial instability results when the supporting ligaments are absent or fail, causing abnormal horizontal displacements that may compromise of the spinal cord.

Understanding the embryological development, biomechanics, and different disease processes that can affect the CVJ is instrumental in understanding why different conditions lead to vertical translocation and atlanto-axial instability.

Embryology

Forty-two somites are formed during the forty-second week of gestation. Each somite differentiates into an outer dermatome, inner myotome, and medial sclerotome (6). The medial sclerotome is responsible for the development of the vertebral body. The superior half of one sclerotome unites with the inferior half of another sclerotome in the spine to form the vertebral body. The first four sclerotomes do not follow this pattern of development. Instead, they unite to form the base of the occiput and foramen magnum. From a rostral caudal orientation, the first four sclerotomes are designated the O1-3 and proatlas, respectively (7,8).

The first and second occipital sclerotomes are responsible for the development of the basiocciput. The third occipital sclerotome forms the jugular tubercles. The development of the proatlas is more complicated because it acts as the interface between the cranial spinal axis. The proatlas has three embryological centers of development: the hypocentrum, centrum, and neural arch. The hypocentrum forms the anterior tubercle of the clivus. The centrum forms the apical ligament and apex of the dens. The neural arch forms the occipital condyles, foramen magnum, alar and cruciate ligaments, superior portions of the posterior arch of C1, and lateral atlantal masses.

The first spinal sclerotome contributes to the formation of the transitional vertebrae, the atlas. The first spinal sclerotome's development is divided into three embryological centers like the proatlas. The hypocentrum forms the anterior arch of the atlas; the centrum forms the dens; and the neural arch forms the posterior inferior portions of the atlas arch.

The proper development of the craniovertebral junction depends not only on the presence of the individual sclerotomes, but also on the subsequent development of the proper and appropriate union of individual ossification centers. Most of these processes are completed near the advent of skeletal maturity, with the ossification and union of the ossiculum terminale occurring last at the age of 12. Ligamentous anatomy helps to maintain the appropriate alignment of the individual components during development. With age the relationships among the occiput, atlas, and axis become more rigid, with reduced laxity of the ligaments. Understanding the biomechanics of the normal CVJ is essential in the understanding of the importance of the individual components.

Biomechanics of the Craniovertebral Junction

The complex ligamentous and bone anatomy at the craniovertebral junction makes analysis in this region difficult (9). Neither the C0-1 nor the C1-2 joint has an intervertebral disc. The C0-1 is a ball and socket joint, and the C1-2 is made of two biconvex articular surfaces. The unique anatomy of these joints allows complex movements to occur. The ball socket joint of C0-1 affords a wide range of flexion and extension, and the biconvex articular joint of C1-2 affords a wide range of axial rotation. Motion typically is described in an x-, y-, and z-axis. Frequently, motion in one axis results in a concomitant but lesser degree of motion in another axis. When this occurs, the secondary motions are said to be coupled. The lateral bending at the C0-1 joints and axial rotation at the C1-2 joints are strongly coupled to one another (9).

The allowed range of motion that may occur at these joints has been quantified using *in vitro* cadaveric spine models. Range of motion is a measure of the normal physiological motion able to be tolerated by a joint. It is the sum of motion that may occur through the neutral and elastic zones before failure of the joint occurs. The neutral zone is the range of motion where small loads produce large displacements with minimal stress to the surrounding supporting ligaments (10). The elastic zone is the range of motion where larger displacements are required to produce small deformations before resulting in failure of supporting ligaments. Supporting ligaments are placed under maximal tension when reaching the limits of the elastic range of motion.

Based on contemporary experimentation, there are estimates of the allowed range of motion at these joints when flexion, extension, axial rotation, and lateral bending occur. At C0-1, the range of motion during flexion, extension, axial rotation, and lateral bending is 21, 3.5, 7.2, and 5.5 degrees, respectively. At C1-2, the range of motion during flexion, extension, axial rotation, and lateral bending is 12.5, 9.9, 38.8, and 6.7 degrees, respectively (9,11). Normal load distribution during range of motion at these motion segments depends on normal osseous and ligamentous anatomy; however, normal range of motion primarily is limited by the complex ligamentous anatomy.

Numerous ligamentous structures join the axis, atlas, and occipital bone. The atlas and axis are bonded by four synovial joints: two that surround the odontoid's articulation with the atlas, and two that enclose the biconvex articular joints of the lateral masses. In front, the anterior longitudinal ligament exists as a wide ligamentous band connecting the atlas and axis. In the spinal canal, the posterior longitudinal ligament continues to the clivus as the tectorial membrane. are Numerous supporting ligaments that secure the relationship of the dens to the atlas and skull base between the anterior and posterior longitudinal ligaments. Anteriorly, the apical ligament extends from the tip of the dens to the anterior margin of the foramen magnum. The alar ligaments extend from either side of the dens to the medial surface of the occipital condyles. The cruciate ligament interconnects the three segments of the CVJ. The rostral aspect of the cruciate ligament extends to the tip of the clivus. The caudal aspect inserts on the body of the axis. The transverse part, also known as the transverse ligament, interconnects the medial tubercles of the lateral masses of the atlas posterior to the dens.

The importance of individual ligamentous structures is underscored by biomechanical studies that have elucidated their role in normal joint motion. The capsular ligaments supporting the synovial joints of the lateral masses limit range of motion during axial rotation. Failure of these ligaments can lead to an increase in axial rotation leading to rotatory subluxation. The alar ligaments stabilize the CVJ during coupled flexion-extension motion, and help limit range of motion during axial rotation and lateral bending. Unilateral compromise of the alar ligament leads to a small increase in C1-2 axial rotation, whereas bilateral compromise of the alar ligament leads to more significant changes in stability during coupled movements in all vectors at the CVJ (12). The transverse ligament secures the dens' relationship to the atlas by preventing posterior displacement of the odontoid into the spinal canal (13). Compromise of the transverse ligament leads to instability at the atlantoaxial motion segment, allowing posterior translation of the dens into the spinal cord.

Normal biomechanics at the occipital cervical junction depends on normal osseous architecture and ligamentous anatomy. Minor derangements are able to be tolerated by the motion segments; however, more significant derangements can compromise the biomechanical stability of the motion segment. A developmental dysplasia or segmentation abnormality may be intrinsically unstable because of altered anatomy. More commonly, a developmental dyplasia or segmentation abnormality acquires instability over time. The altered osseous architecture and malformed ligamentous structures cause unfavorable redistribution of loads during cyclic loading, which can accelerate failure of the segment. Understanding the biomechanics of congenital anomalies requires an understanding of normal mechanics and the associated complex aberrant architecture.

Congenital Anomalies of the Craniovertebral Junction

There are numerous anomalies of the CVJ that can form as a result of abnormal embryological development. Errors in development either can be the result of formation or segmentation abnormalities (4,5,14,15). Some are biomechanically stable, some are frankly unstable, and others accelerate the acquisition of instability. Instability frequently is demonstrated either by basilar invagination or atlantoaxial instability.

Congenital anomalies that affect the more rostral sclerotomes result in abnormal development of the skull base and are more likely to be associated with basilar invagination. There are four occipital sclerotomes. The first two occipital sclerotomes are responsible for the development of the normal basiocciput. Dysplasia of any of the occipital sclerotomes can lead to basilar invagination. Basilar invagination may occur as a result of anterior or paramedian prolapse of the cervical spine into the foramen magnum. The type of prolapse that occurs is a function of the underlying architectural abnormality (4,5). Hypoplasia of the basiocciput leads to shortening of the clivus, platybasia, and development of a small posterior fossa, which can lead to anterior invagination. In contrast, hypoplasia of the exoccipital bones and occipital condyles can lead to paramedian invagination.

Congenital anomalies that affect the normal embryological development of the first and second cervical vertebrae are not associated with basilar invagination but are more likely to be associated with atlantoaxial instability. Dysplastic abnormalities are more frequently associated with instability from intrinsic ligamentous abnormalities. Segmentation abnormalities are more frequently associated with acquired instability as a result of increased joint stress from altered load distributions (16). The following is a description of some of the more commonly cited abnormalities affecting the occiput, atlas, and odontoid.

ANOMALIES OF THE OCCIPUT. Vertebralization of the occiput may result from vertebralization of the third occipital somite and proatlas. This abnormality is distinguished from atlas assimilation by the absence of the normal foramen through which the vertebral artery and suboccipital nerve pass. Incomplete vertebralization of the third occipital somite and proatlas may manifest by the genesis of transverse clefts or fissures in the clivus. An ossified remnant is present at the distal end of the clivus called the condylus tertius when the proatlas completely fails to integrate with the clivus (3). When present there may be numerous ossicles that may form a joint or pseudojoint with the odontoid process or anterior arch of the atlas limiting normal range of motion at the craniovertebral junction. Hypermobility at this segment may lead to pathological accumulation of reactive granulation tissue that may act as a mass compressing the cervicomedullary region of the spinal cord.

Frequently associated with vertebralization of occiput are a wide range of atlanto-occipital ossifications. Some of these are thought to represent a vestigial transverse process from the proatlas (17). They may be identified as a paracondylar mass that forms an osseous bridge connecting the paracondylar region with the transverse process of C1. These paracondylar lesions typically are asymptomatic and incidental in nature.

The association of a persistent ossiculum terminale and os odontoideum is unclear. The osseous abnormalities identified in patients with vertebralization of the occiput may be classified as such; however, the preceding terms usually are reserved for isolated abnormalities of the odontoid.

Occipital condylar hypoplasia can result from incomplete development of the proatlas. The relative flattening of the occipital condyles results in relative elevation of the atlas with respect to the skull base. This may present unilaterally or bilaterally and result in paramedian basilar invagination. Although dysgenesis of the occipital condyles may occur sporadically, it has been associated with Morquio disease, Conradi syndrome, and spondyloepiphyseal dysplasia (3,4,15).

ANOMALIES OF THE ATLAS. Aplasia or hypoplasia of the atlas also may result. Aplasia of the atlas is rare and is probably the result of incomplete sclerotome development. Hemiaplasia of the atlas also may occur. Hypoplasia of the atlas is identified more commonly. Hypoplasia of the atlas typically is manifested as a cleft in the ring of the atlas. Because the atlas forms from both the proatlas and first vertebral sclerotomes, clefts in the atlas are more likely the result of incomplete ossification occurring later in development. Primary ossification centers first develop in the lateral masses during the seventh week of gestation. Incomplete development of these ossification centers can lead to aplasia or hemiaplasia of the atlas. Ossification proceeds with these lateral ossification centers during normal ossification of the atlas. Frequently, secondary ossification centers form in the anterior and posterior arches. Closure of the anterior and posterior arches occurs later, with fusion completing by 6 to 10 and 3 to 5 years of age, respectively. Posterior arch defects are more common, being identified in .5% to 5% of anatomical specimens (17). Midline defects are much more common than lateral defects (18). These anomalies usually are sporadic but also may be associated with spina bifida and Klippel-Feil syndrome. Rarely, they are symptomatic and result in instability (19,20).

Atlantooccipital assimilation occurs when there is normal development of the individual sclerotomes but a failure of segmentation between the occiput and first cervical vertebrae. This a commonly identified radiographic abnormality, reportedly affecting .14% to 2.76% of individuals (4,5). The abnormality is manifested by assimilation of the anterior arch of C1 with the base of the clivus. The lateral masses of the atlas may be fused directly to the overlying hypoplastic condyles. Less frequently, portions of the posterior arch are involved; usually, a remnant of the posterior arch is identified along the posterior rim of the foramen magnum. This abnormality also frequently is associated with congenital fusion of the second and third cervical vertebrae. These segmentation anomalies may place increased load on the remaining motion segments. Although not intrinsically unstable, this abnormality may lead to gradual loosening of the atlantodental joint over time, with atlantoaxial subluxation occurring in approximately 50% of cases (3). Hypermobility at the affected segments also may lead to the accumulation of space-occupying granulation tissue.

ANOMALIES OF THE ODONTOID. Congenital abnormalities of the odontoid also may occur. The odontoid is formed by three ossification centers (4). The tip of the odontoid develops from an ossification center from the proatlas called the ossiculum terminale (17). The base of the odontoid develops from two paramedian ossification centers from the C1 sclerotome that extend below the superior slopes of the C2 facets and interface with the C2 body through the neural central synchondrosis.

The spectrum of abnormalities that can affect the dens arise either from malunion of the ossification centers or incomplete formation of the ossification centers responsible for the normal development of the odontoid (21–29). Incomplete fusion of the two main ossification centers can produce a bicornuate dens (23). Incomplete fusion of the third ossification center can lead to the development of an ossiculum terminale persistens also called the Bergman ossicle (3). Incomplete development of the ossification centers can lead to dens hypoplasia or aplasia.

The os odontoideum is less well understood. The os odontoideum originally was described as a congenital anomaly arising from incomplete fusion of the centrum component of C1 with C2 resulting from persistence of the neural central synchondrosis (30). However, because the neural central synchondrosis lies in a plane below the superior plane of the C2 facet and the abnormality that is frequently described as an os odontoideum is frequently a hyperplastic nodule of bone above this plane, it is believed that this abnormality probably is not the result of an incomplete fusion process but rather is the result of occult trauma occurring during childhood that results in separation of the tip of the dens (29,31–33). Trauma probably results in separation of the tip of the dens, which retracts away from the remaining portions of the dens because of its attachments to the apical and alar ligaments. The fragment persists and hypertrophies with age because the tip of the dens receives its blood supply separately from a branch of the occipital artery (34). Associated abnormalities of surrounding ligamentous structures may produce instability at this segment, endangering the spinal cord.

SYNDROMES ASSOCIATED WITH CONGENITAL ANOMALIES OF THE CRANIOVERTEBRAL JUNCTION. Numerous syndromes and genetic disorders can present with derangements in the normal architecture of the CVJ secondary to compromised ligamentous structures. Connective tissue disorders and syndromes that result in the production of lax ligaments can result in instability of the CVJ. Down syndrome, mucopolysaccharidoses (Morquio), and Marfan are all examples of disorders that result in the development of ligaments with impaired tensile properties that predispose patients to atlantoaxial instability or incidental rotatory subluxation of the atlantoaxial joint. In contrast, fewer conditions result in the actual dysgenesis of the osseous components of the craniovertebral junction.

Klippel-Feil syndrome is a disorder defined by the presence of congenitally fused vertebrae (35). Patients with Klippel-Feil syndrome typically present with a triad of clinical findings including a short neck, low posterior hair line, and restricted range of motion in the neck. Klippel-Feil patients also may have a myriad of abnormalities affecting other organ systems, but this is beyond the focus of this chapter. Common vertebral column abnormalities are congenital fusions of the spine, hemiverte-

brae, atlas assimilation, basilar invagination, and scoliosis. Less common spine-associated abnormalities are iniencephaly, spina bifida, and Chiari malformations.

Down syndrome is a common chromosomal abnormality that has a frequent association with spinal column abnormalities. Atlantoaxial instability secondary to ligamentous laxity is the most common abnormality, occurring in as many as 31% of patients with Down syndrome (36,37). Spitzer and colleagues were the first to describe occipitoatlantal dislocation and atlantal hypoplasia in Down syndrome in 1961 (38). Patients infrequently are symptomatic, although atlantoaxial instability frequently is present on radiographic studies. Aside from instability arising from pure ligamentous laxity, numerous dysplastic abnormalities of the craniovertebral junction are associated with Down syndrome. Frequently cited abnormalities are os odontoideum, odontoid hypoplasia, and bifid or hypoplastic atlantal arches. Other malformations identified are brachycephaly, basilar invagination, and occipital vertebrae (7,36). Many of these dysplastic abnormalities in combination with the intrinsic ligamentous laxity associated with Down syndrome may produce highly unstable conditions predisposing the patient to neurological injury (36,38).

Chiari I malformations also are associated with frequent abnormalities of the CVJ. Basilar invagination is identified in as many as 5% to 31% of patients with Chiari I malformations (4, 5,39–41). Menezes proposes that atlas assimilation and segmentation failures of the upper cervical spine may contribute to ligamentous laxity and proliferation of granulation tissue, leading to irreducible basilar invagination (5). Enlargement of the foramen magnum, scoliosis, shallow posterior fossa, widening of the cervical canal, pedicle atrophy, scalloping of vertebral bodies, atlas assimilation, and Klippel-Feil syndrome and associated anomalies are all described (40,41).

Acquired Anomalies of the Craniovertebral Junction

After normal osseous development has occurred, numerous processes can occur to a patient that may result in derangements of the normal CVJ architecture. The condition is described as basilar invagination when congenitally inherited anomalies result in prolapse of the odontoid process into the skull base. To distinguish this process from acquired conditions, basilar impression is a term used to describe states in which acquired changes to the load-bearing features of the craniovertebral junction lead to prolapse of the spinal column into the skull base. Numerous systemic conditions compromise the integrity of the normal load-bearing features of bone that can lead to basilar impression. These include Paget disease, osteomalacia, Hurler syndrome, rickets, hyperparathyroidism, skull base infections, and osteogenesis imperfecta (4,5,7). Trauma is a rare cause of basilar impression. Malunion and long-term changes associated with an occult Jefferson fracture has been associated with basilar impression (42). Last, although the changes that occur in rheumatoid arthritis are pathogenetically similar, the term "cranial settling" typically is used to describe the changes associated with this condition.

Clinical Presentation

Many of the complex CVJ abnormalities previously described are associated with either instability or lead to complications from basilar impression, basilar invagination, and atlantoaxial instability. Because these abnormalities frequently present in the setting of a complex syndrome or congenital dysplastic condition, patients present with symptoms that are typically predicated by their underlying condition.

Patients who have instability at the craniovertebral junction may have neck pain on initial presentation. Instability may lead to chronic compression of the cervicomedullary junction leading to clinical symptoms of chronic myelopathy. Persistent compression of the cervicomedullary junction may also lead to the pathogenesis of syringomyelia. Dynamic instability may elicit a Lhermitte sign of examination. Clinical signs of myelopathy on examination are pathological reflexes, generalized weakness, bowel and bladder incontinence, and gait instability. When injury occurs acutely to the cervicomedullary junction, Bell cruciate palsy may result (43–45). Bell cruciate palsy is manifested by proximal weakness in the arms with relative preservation of strength in the legs.

Basilar invagination and impression may cause a unique constellation of symptoms in addition to those related to chronic cervicomedullary compression. These symptoms are not only the consequence of vertical translocation of the odontoid peg but also the result of cranial–caudal migration of the brainstem accompanying this process (39,41,46). On postmortem examination of patients with basilar invagination, the relationship of cranial and spinal nerves to the clivus and nerve root foramen may be deranged with nerves traveling upward to reach their respective foramen. Stretch on these nerves may result in palsies or dysfunction. Chronic compression of the vertebrobasilar system from the translocated odontoid peg may cause intermittent or chronic vertebrobasilar ischemia and even neurogenic hypertension (47). Direct compression of the medulla may lead to derangements in respiratory drive and place tension on exiting cranial nerves (48). Vertigo, dysphagia, facial paralysis, decreased hearing, and tongue atrophy are common phenomena probably related to direct medullary compression.

Radiographic Evaluation

The use of plain radiographs in the evaluation of the craniovertebral junction requires the visualization of several anatomical landmarks that are not typically provided for on plain radiographs of the cervical spine. Frequently, radiographs of the skull that include the craniovertebral junction need to be acquired. Furthermore, the appropriate visualization of these structures frequently is obscured if any there is an obliquity when the film is obtained. Typical landmarks required on a plain lateral radiograph of the skull are nasion, tuberculum sella, basion, opisthion, the posterior pole of the hard palate, anterior arch of the atlas, posterior arch of the atlas, and odontoid. Typical landmarks required on an anteroposterior view of the craniovertebral junction are the occipital condyles, lateral masses of the atlas, odontoid process, axis body, and tips of the mastoid processes.

Chamberlain's line extends from the posterior pole of the hard palate to the posterior margin of the foramen magnum (opisthion). The tip of the odontoid should not extend more than 2.5 mm above the line in the absence of vertical translocation. Because opisthion frequently is difficult to visualize, the McGregor line was developed (49). This line is drawn from the posterior pole of the hard palate and extends tangentially to the base of the occiput. Because this line as drawn is lower than Chamberlain's line, the tip of the odontoid should not extend more than 4.5 mm above it (50). Wackenheim's line may be used if the hard palate is unable to the easily visualized (51). This is a line constructed by drawing a line along the angle

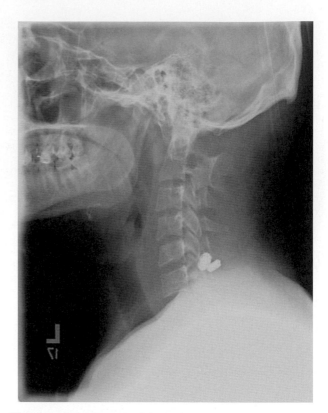

Fig. 1. Lateral radiograph of the cervical spine in a patient with Klippel-Feil syndrome with congenital fusion of C2 and C3 and basilar invagination. The radiograph demonstrates how the odontoid extends above the line of the clivus (Wackenheim's line), indicating basilar invagination.

of the clivus and extending it inferiorly into the upper cervical spine region. The tip of the odontoid normally intersects with this line tangentially. Vertical translocation is presumed whenever the tip of the odontoid extends above this line (Fig 1).

The craniovertebral junction can be visualized from an anteroposterior view by using an open mouth odontoid view. A line connecting the tip of both mastoid processes is known as Fishgold's digastric line (Fig 2) (3). Extension of any portion of the odontoid is considered abnormal. The sensitivity and specificity of such measurements often is poor because the consistent identification of different anatomical landmarks often is difficult when using plain radiographs. Using multiple methods to confirm the presence of basilar invagination increases the sensitivity and specificity of such methods.

Assessment of atlantoaxial instability is a feat more easily achieved with plain radiographs. A plain lateral radiograph affords the ability to measure the atlantodental interval (ADI) in most patients. The ADI should not exceed 3 mm in normal adults and 5 mm in normal children (9). The ADI can be misleading when used as a criterion for identifying instability in cases that are also complicated by basilar impression or invagination. An abnormal ADI may be reduced with vertical translocation, a phenomenon known as pseudostabilization.

Today computed tomography (CT) and magnetic resonance imaging (MRI) provide superior imaging of the craniovertebral junction. Detailed anatomy of the osseous components is provided for with CT and three-dimensionally reconstructed images. MRI techniques provide high-resolution images in the sagittal and axial planes that may demonstrate compromised neural structures and detect compromise of individual ligamentous structures (Fig. 3). When MRI techniques are unable to be per-

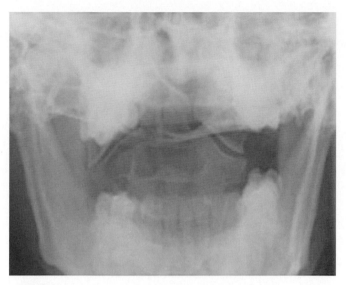

Fig. 2. Anteroposterior radiograph of the cervical spine in a patient with Klippel-Feil syndrome with basilar invagination. The radiograph illustrates how the tip of the odontoid extends superior to the line connecting the tips of the mastoid processes bilaterally (Fishgold's digastric line).

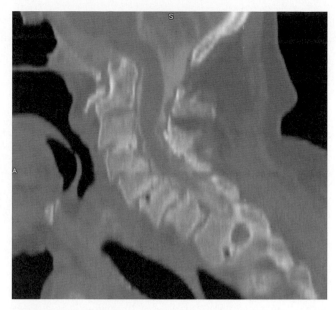

Fig. 4. CT myelogram of a patient with rheumatoid arthritis. The sagittally reconstructed CT myelographic image demonstrates the pathological compression of the adjacent neural structures.

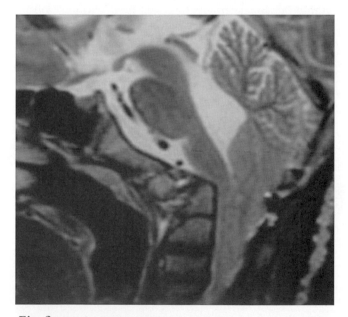

Fig. 3. MRI of a patient with rheumatoid arthritis and cranial settling. The upward migration of the odontoid has resulted in compression of the brainstem and cervical medullary junction. The MRI demonstrates the pathological compression of the neural structures, effacement of the cerebrospinal fluid space anterior to the brainstem, and pathological erosion of the related joints.

formed, CT myelographic techniques can be used to detect the extent of neural compression resulting from abnormalities at the CVJ (Fig. 4).

Treatment

Surgical treatment is necessitated when any of the aforementioned conditions leads to instability and compression of the underlying neural structures. Symptomatic unstable anomalies deserve surgical stabilization to protect the patient from further neurological deterioration. Prophylactic surgical stabilization is controversial. Routine screening should be performed in patients with congenital disorders to monitor deformity progression in the absence of any symptomatic progression. The Committee on Sports Medicine of the American Academy of Pediatrics recommends screening all patients with Down syndrome prior to participation in sports activities (52). Routine screening and aggressive early surgical stabilization sometimes is recommended in patients with chronic conditions. Some argue that asymptomatic patients with rheumatoid arthritis who have significant radiographic evidence of CVJ disease should be considered for early surgery because of: (a) the poor functional recovery that occurs in patients who have surgery after clinical deterioration, and (b) the possible prevention of disease progression with early surgery (53).

Occipital cervical fusion is required to restore stability when instability bridges the occipito-atlantal joint. Numerous techniques are used to perform this operation. Most differ based on how the instrumentation and hardware are affixed to the base of the skull and the posterior aspect of the cervical spine. The distance the fusion needs to be extended along the posterior aspect of the cervical spine depends on the strength of the used fixation points and presence or absence of any adjacent pathology.

A C1-2 fusion is required when instability spares the occipital-atlantal joint but affects the atlantoaxial joint. A C1-2 fusion is best achieved with transarticular screws, which provide rigid immobilization and adequate resistance to rotational stresses; however, many individuals with congenital and developmental dysplasias may not have a C2 pars large enough to allow safe passage of transarticular screws. Interspinous wiring with an interlaminar bone strut is a good alternative. These patients may need to be maintained in a halo for immobilization to optimize the likelihood of a stable fusion.

The cause of the compression needs to be appreciated before treatment when neural structures are compromised as a result of the pathology. Compression of neural structures may be the result of a growing or migrating abnormal osseous structure, a growing soft-tissue pannus, or misalignment of structures.

Manual reduction prior to surgical fusion often achieves the needed results when the cause of neural compression is misalignment. Stenosis from glacial instability at the atlantal axial joint and the occipital-atlantal joint frequently are reducible abnormalities. Fusion at the C1-2 motion segment and occipital cervical junction can be achieved easily. Intraoperative reduction typically restores the needed alignment when preoperative manual reduction may not be performed.

In contrast, compression from basilar invagination and impression is inconsistently able to be manually reduced. A surgical decompression often is necessitated when the cause of neural compression is a nonreducible misalignment. This surgical decompression may require a posterior laminectomy or transoral odontectomy. Frequently, such surgical procedures in the setting of surrounding abnormal osseous and ligamentous development necessitate a fusion to prevent any complications from iatrogenic induced instability.

Surgical resection of the structure frequently is required when the cause of neural compression is a growing abnormal osseous structure or slowly migrating osseous structure (Fig. 5). Sometimes resection of the osseous mass can be achieved without compromising the underlying stability of the motion segment. For example, some investigators report that patients with congenital bone malformations have only a 50% chance of acquired instability after a transoral odontoid resection. Presumably this

is because surrounding ligamentous and bone structures are not intrinsically compromised. In contrast, degenerative and inflammatory arthropathies such as rheumatoid arthritis can change the normal kinematics of the spine by global compromise of the normal ligamentous anatomy; subsequently, patients with rheumatoid arthritis have a greater likelihood (90%) of acquired instability after a transoral odontectomy and uniformly should have a posterior occipital cervical fusion performed at the time (9,54). Understanding the global disease process is important when considering the repercussions of performing a local decompression.

Resection of the pannus is the most common treatment when the cause of neural compression is a growing soft-tissue pannus. A soft-tissue pannus can form anywhere, but in the occipitocervical junction it most frequently forms in the periodontoid region. The pannus is typically a combination of fibrous and inflammatory tissue. It can result from a chronic malunion of an odontoid fracture or chronic inflammatory process. Basilar impression frequently is a concomitant problem when associated with an inflammatory arthropathy. A transoral resection of the pannus frequently is required when the patient is actively deteriorating from direct compression of neural structures by the pannus. Prior to transoral resection of the pannus, reduction with manual traction can be attempted to facilitate exposure of the pannus from the transoral route and minimize the need for resection of the soft palate and clivus. The transoral resection of the pannus allows immediate decompression of the underlying neural structures.

One can consider fusing the involved motion segments alone when the patient is not actively deteriorating. Fusion and stabilization should theoretically result in elimination of the inciting process because the pannus forms as a result of chronic inflammation and instability. The pannus should resolve over time after surgical fusion. Fusion without transoral resection of a large pannus with long-term follow-up demonstrating resolution of the pannus has been demonstrated only in patients with rheumatoid arthritis (55). Whether the same phenomenon will

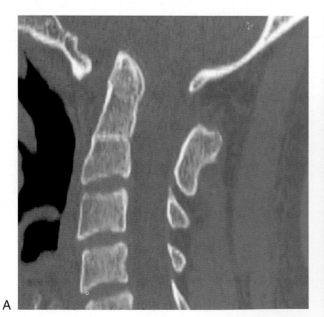
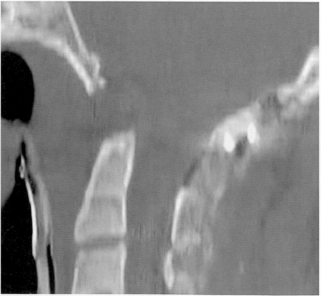

A   B

Fig. 5. **A:** A CT sagittal reconstructed image of the craniovertebral junction in a patient with Klippel-Feil syndrome with a congenital fusion of C2 and C3 and basilar invagination. The image illustrates how the tip of the odontoid extends above Wackenheim's line. **B:** An image of the same patient after a transoral odontectomy illustrating how the pathological portion of the odontoid has been surgically resected.

occur in patients with a pannus from a chronic odontoid fracture malunion is unknown.

Appropriate surgical treatment begins and ends with understanding the underlying pathological process. This ensures that the surgeon is able to most aptly address the biomechanical and neurological needs of the patient.

Conclusion

Numerous congenital and acquired conditions can result in derangement of the CVJ. Congenital dysplasias and segmentation anomalies may be intrinsically unstable or acquire instability from abnormal load distributions. Chronic disease processes may alter the normal load-bearing features of the bone and ligaments leading to instability. When instability occurs in these processes the integrity of the occipito-atlantal joint and the atlanto-axial joint frequently are compromised. Basilar invagination, basilar impression, and atlanto-axial instability may result. Many of these abnormalities are associated with congenital syndromes and particular diseases; therefore, patients identified with underlying anomalies of the CVJ should be scrutinized for underlying congenital syndromes or disease states. Neurological impairment may be avoided by early identification of instability and its early surgical stabilization. The biomechanical requirements for adequate surgical stabilization often are predicated by the underlying disease process; therefore, understanding the conditions that lead to these abnormalities is important.

References

1. Dickman CA, Papadopoulos SM, Sonntag VKH. Traumatic occipitoatlantal dislocations. *J Spinal Disord* 1993;6(4):300–313.
2. Dickman CA, Green KA, Sonntag VKH. Traumatic injuries of the craniovertebral junction. In: Dickman CA, et al, ed. *Surgery of the craniovertebral junction.* Stuttgart: Thieme, 1998:175–196.
3. Smoker WRK. Craniovertebral junction: normal anatomy, craniometry, and congenital anomalies. *Radiographics* 1994;14.255–277.
4. Menezes AH. Normal and abnormal development of the craniovertebral junction. In: Crockard A, Hayward R, Hoff JT, eds. *Neurosurgery: the scientific basis of clinical practice.* Boston: Blackwell, 1992:63–83.
5. Menezes AH, Ryken TC. Abnormalities of the craniovertebral junction. In: Cheek WR, ed. *Pediatric neurosurgery,* 3rd ed. Philadelphia: WB Saunders, 1994:139–158.
6. Arey LB. *Developmental anatomy: a textbook and laboratory manual of embryology,* 7th ed. Philadelphia: WB Saunders, 1965: 404–407.
7. Piper JG, Traynelis VC. Congenital malformations of craniovertebral junction. In: Dickman CA, et al, ed.*Surgery of the craniovertebral junction.* Stuttgart: Thieme, 1998:123–150.
8. Menezes AH. Embryology, development, and classification of disorders of the craniovertebral junction. In: Dickman CA, et al, ed. *Surgery of the craniovertebral junction.* Stuttgart: Thieme, 1998:3–12.
9. Dickman CA, Crawford NR. Biomechanics of the craniovertebral junction. In: Dickman CA, et al, ed. *Surgery of the craniovertebral junction.* Stuttgart: Thieme, 1998:59–80.
10. Panjabi MM. The stabilizing system of the spine. Part II. Neutral zone and instability hypothesis. *J Spinal Disord* 1992;5(4):390–396.
11. White AA, Panjabi MM. *Clinical biomechanics of the spine,* 2nd ed. Philadelphia: JB Lippincott, 1990.
12. Panjabi MM, Dvorak J, Crisco JJ III, et al. Effects of alar ligament transection on upper cervical spine rotation. *J Orthop Res* 1991;9(4): 584–593.
13. Fielding JW, Cochran GVB, Lawsing JF III, et al. Tears of the trans-verse ligament of the atlas. A clinical and biomechanical study. *J Bone Joint Surg Am* 1974;56:1683–1691.
14. Garber JN. Abnormalities of the atlas and axis vertebrae: congenital and traumatic. *J Bone Joint Surg Am* 1964;47:1782–1790.
15. Gray SW, Romaine CB, Skandalakis JE. Congenital fusion of the cervical vertebrae. *Surg Gynecol Obstet* 1964;118:373–380.
16. Crockard HA, Stevens JM. Craniovertebral junction anomalies in inherited disorders: part of the syndrome or caused by the disorder? *Eur J Pediatr* 1995;154:504–512.
17. Naidich TP, McClone DG, Harwood-Nash DC. Malformations of the craniocervical junction. In: Newton TH, Potts DG, eds. *Computed tomography of the spine and the spinal cord.* San Anselmo, CA: Clavadel Press, 1983:355–366.
18. Dorne HL, Just N, Lander PH. CT recognition of anomalies of the posterior arch of atlas vertebrae: differentiation from fracture. *AJNR* 1986;7:176–177.
19. Logan WW, Stuard ID. Absent posterior arch of the atlas. *Am J Roentgenol* 1973;118:431–434.
20. Schulze PJ, Buurman R. Absence of the posterior arch of the atlas. *Am J Roentgenol* 1980;134:178–180.
21. Davis D, Guttierrez FA. Congenital anomaly of the odontoid in children. A report of four cases. *Childs Brain* 1977;3:219–229.
22. Gillman EL. Congenital absence of the odontoid process of the a six. Report of a case. *J Bone Joint Surg Am* 1959;41:345–348.
23. Hensinger RN, MacEwen GD. Congenital anomalies of the spine. In: Rothman RH, Simeone FA, eds. *The spine,* 2nd ed. Philadelphia: WB Saunders, 1982:205–215.
24. Shiraski N, Okada K, Oka S, et al. Os odontoideum with posterior atlantoaxial instability. *Spine* 1991;16:706–715.
25. Nagashima C. Atlantoaxial dislocation due to agenesis of the os odontoideum or odontoid. *J Neurosurg* 1970;33:270–280.
26. Dyck P. Os odontoideum in children: neurological manifestations and surgical management. *Neurosurgery* 1978;2:93–99.
27. Fielding JW, Hensinger RN, Hawkins RJ. Os odontoideum. *J Bone Joint Surg Am* 1980;62:376–383.
28. Spierings ELH, Braakman R. The management of os odontoideum. Analysis of 37 cases. *J Bone Joint Surg Br* 1982;64:422–428.
29. Freiberger RH, Wilson PD Jr, Nicholas JA. Acquired absence of the odontoid process. A case report. *J Bone Joint Surg Am* 1965;47: 1231–1236.
30. Wollin DG. The os odontoideum: separate odontoid process. *J Bone Joint Surg* 1963;45:1459–1471.
31. Hawkins RJ, Fielding JW, Thompson WJ. Os odontoideum: congenital or acquired. A case report. *J Bone Joint Surg Am* 1976;58:413–414.
32. Riccardi JE, Kaufer H, Louis DS. Acquired os odontoideum following acute ligament injury. *J Bone Joint Surg Am* 1976;58:410–412.
33. Menezes AH. Os odontoideum-pathogenesis, dynamics and management. In: Marlin AE, ed. *Concepts in pediatric neurosurgery.* Basel: Karger, 1988:133–145.
34. Schiff DCM, Parke WW. The arterial supply of the odontoid process (dens). *Anat Rec* 1972;172:399–410.
35. Klippel M, Feil A. Un cas d'absence des vertebras cervicales. Avec cage thoracique remontant jusqu'a la base du crane (cage thoracique cervicale). *Nouv Icon Salpetriere* 1912;25:223–250.
36. Taggard DA, Menezes AH, Ryken TC. Treatment of Down syndrome-associated craniovertebral abnormalities. *J Neurosurg Spine* 2000;93;(2):205–213.
37. Tishler J, Martel W. Dislocation of the atlas in mongolism: preliminary report. *Radiology* 1965;84:904–906.
38. Spitzer R, Rabinowitch JY, Wybar KC. A study of the abnormalities of the skull, teeth, and lenses in mongolism. *Can MA J* 1961;84: 567–672.
39. Milhorat TH, Chou MW, Trinidad EM, et al. Chiari I malformation redefined: clinical and radiographic findings for 364 symptomatic patients. *Neurosurgery* 1999;44(5):1005–1017.
40. Dyste GN, Menezes AH. Presentation and management of pediatric Chiari malformations without myelodysplasia. *Neurosurgery* 1988; 23:589–597.
41. Grabb PA, Mapstone TB, Oakes WJ. Ventral brain stem compression in pediatric and young adult patients with Chiari I malformations. *Neurosurgery* 1999;44:520–528.
42. Day GL, Jacoby CG, Dolan KD. Basilar invagination resulting from untreated Jefferson's fracture. *AJR* 1979;133:529–531.
43. Bell HS. Paralysis of both arms from injury of the upper portion of

the pyramidal decussation: "cruciate paralysis." *J Neurosurg* 1970; 33(4):376–380.

44. Coxe WS, Landau WM. Patterns of Marchi degeneration in the monkey pyramidal tract following small discrete cortical lesions. *Neurology* 1970;20(1):89–100.
45. Lassek AM, Rasmussen GL. Comparative fiber and numerical analysis of the pyramidal tract. *J Comp Neurol* 1940;72:417–428.
46. Menezes AH, Vangilder JC, Clark CR, et al. Odontoid upward migration in rheumatoid arthritis. *J Neurosurg* 1985;63:500–509.
47. Dickinson LD, Papadopoulos SM, Hoff JT. Neurogenic hypertension related to basilar impression. *J Neurosurg* 1993;79:924–928.
48. Hirose Y, Sagoh M, Mayanagi K, et al. Abducens nerve palsy caused by basilar impression associated with atlanto-occipital assimilation. *Neurol Med Chir (Tokyo)* 1998;38:363–366.
49. McGregor M. The significance of certain measurements of the skull in the diagnosis of basilar impression. *Br J Radiol* 1948;21:171.
50. Chamberlain WE. Basilar impression (platybasia): bizarre developmental anomaly of the occipital bone and upper cervical spine with striking and misleading neurological manifestations. *Yale J Biol Med* 1939;11:487–496.
51. Wackenheim A. *Roentgen diagnosis of the craniovertebral region.* New York: Springer-Verlag, 1974:660.
52. Shaffer TE, Dyment PG, Luckstead EF, et al. Atlantoaxial instability in Down syndrome. *Pediatrics* 1984;74:152–154.
53. Agarwal AK, Peppelman WC, Kraus DR, et al. Recurrence of cervical spine instability in rheumatoid arthritis following previous fusion: can disease progression be prevented by early surgery. *J Rheumatol* 1992;19(9):1364–1370.
54. Dickman CA, Crawford NR, Brantley AGU, et al. Biomechanical effects of transoral odontoidectomy. *Neurosurgery* 1995;36(6): 1146–1153.
55. Zygmunt S, Saveland H, Brattstrom H, et al. Reduction of rheumatoid periodontoid pannus following posterior occipito-cervical fusion visualized by magnetic resonance imaging. *Br J Neurosurg* 1988;2: 315–320.

153. Paget Disease

Ross R. Moquin

Paget disease is a disorder of skeletal remodeling first described as "osteitis deformans" by Sir James Paget in 1877. He described patients with the mid to late stages of the chronic debilitating polyostotic forms of the disease. He believed the condition to be a chronic inflammation of unknown etiology because of its asymmetrical skeletal distribution, chronicity, and gross appearance of the bones. Fractures were common, and poor healing resulted in deformities of the limbs and spine (1).

Pathophysiology

Paget disease is a focal disorder of the metabolic process of bone remodeling or turnover. Bone is a metabolically active tissue. Bone renews or remodels itself in response to routine physiological stresses. Osteoclasts break down older or unneeded bone and the osteoblast forms new bone. Under normal conditions there is a balance between the actions of the osteoclasts and osteoblasts, resulting in no net increase or decrease in the size or the shape of the bone. This balance is altered in Paget disease, usually resulting in larger deformed bones. Paget disease does not affect all of the bones simultaneously. Discrete lesions are present on one bone (monostotic) or multiple bones (polyostotic) throughout the body.

Pathogenesis

No clear consensus exists for the etiology of Paget disease. In 1974, Rebel and co-workers were the first to find abnormalities in the ultrastructure of the osteoclasts (2). In 1976, Mills and Singer found nuclear inclusion bodies within the osteoclasts (3). These findings were thought to be consistent with a viral cause of the disease. More recently, genetic etiologies also are being invoked (chromosome 18) (4). Furthermore, a frequent association with the HLA-B27 antigen has been found.

Most authors agree that the causative agent is a slow virus, possibly a paramyxovirus such as measles or respiratory syncytial virus. Features of Paget disease that are suggestive of a slow virus include a long clinical latency period, involvement of a single organ, and lack of an inflammatory response.

The presumed pathogenesis of the disease begins with the infection of the bone by the slow virus. A prolonged latency period ensues leading to a mutation that incites increased cytokine production that stimulates osteoclast enlargement, proliferation, and increased activity. This causes an increased osteoclastic resorption of bone (lytic phase) followed by a compensatory increase in the osteoblastic formation of bone (sclerotic phase). The net result of this aggressive disorganized turnover is a highly vascular abnormal bone that then enters the final phase where there is little further abnormal cellular activity (5). The architecture of the final abnormal bone is an enlarged disorganized mosaic pattern of irregular lamellar and cement lines having normal mineralization.

Pagetic bone has poor mechanical strength and is prone to fractures. The disorganized architecture and callous formation from the resulting pathological fractures lead to discrete areas of bone enlargement. Long bones of the leg, pelvis, spine, and skull are the most frequent sites for Pagetic lesions.

Paget disease can lead to other pathological conditions. Juxta-articular deformity and enlargement of the bone alters joint mechanics leading to osteoarthritis. Hypervascularity of the abnormal bone results in increased surface skin temperature over the affected area and high output cardiac failure in extreme cases (5). Accelerated nucleic acid turnover from the rapid bone remodeling cause increased uric acid levels, which increases the likelihood for gout.

Malignant degeneration also can occur. Osteosarcoma, chondrosarcoma, fibrosarcoma, giant cell tumors (6), and secondary metastasis have been found at the sites of Pagetic lesions. Paget sarcoma occurs in less than 1% of cases, usually in patients over the age of 70, and is associated with an extremely poor prognosis (7).

One-third of patients with Paget disease have lesions that affect the spine. Radiographic evidence of spinal involvement is frequently seen in more than one vertebral segment. The most frequent site for spinal involvement is the lumbar spine (60%), followed by the thoracic spine (45%). The cervical spine is the least likely site for involvement (15%) (8).

Structural enlargement of the vertebral segment encroaches on the spinal canal, resulting in spinal stenosis. Direct involvement of the facet or mechanical alteration of the joint lead to facet arthropathy. One-third of patients with spinal involvement are symptomatic with neurogenic claudication from nerve root or spinal cord compression and one-half have back pain from facet arthropathy (9). Neurological symptoms also can be present without compressive lesions. Douglas and colleagues postulated that the hypervascular Pagetic lesions create a steal phenomenon, thus compromising the nearby spinal cord or nerve roots (10).

Tissue other than bone can be invaded by Pagetic tissue as well. Disc space involvement is found in 10% of patients with spinal involvement and usually is not symptomatic (11). Paget disease can affect the spine in other less common ways, such as epidural hematoma, extramedullary hematopoiesis, and ossification of the epidural fat (12).

Epidemiology

Paget disease is the second most common metabolic bone disease in most developed countries. It is second only to osteoporosis in the United States, Australasia, and most areas of western Europe (13). The disease is rarely found in Asia, Africa, or Scandinavia. In areas where it is common, the disease is found in 3% to 4% of those over 50 years of age and in 10% to 15% of those over 90 years. It is almost never found before the age of 30. Most series report a slightly higher incidence of occurrence in men (8).

Clinical Presentation

Many patients with Paget disease are asymptomatic. When symptoms are present, the hallmark of Paget disease is bone pain and deformity. The pain usually is slow and progressive in onset and not relieved by rest. Likewise, the deformities are gradual in onset except when a pathological fracture occurs. The most common deformities are found in the long bones of the lower leg, especially bowing of the tibia. Patients report warmth over the site of involved bone; joints near the lesions can be painful.

Patients with skull involvement report increase in hat size, tinnitus, vertigo, or headaches. Back pain is the most common complaint with spinal involvement. One-third of patients with spinal involvement complain of neurogenic claudication or some neurological deficit. In one series, 10% had neurological deficits without back pain (14). Pathological fractures can lead to acute neurological deterioration.

Radiographic Findings

The radiologic findings in Paget disease follow the different phases of the disease process. Radiolucent areas appear in the long bones or skull during the initial phase of increased osteoclast activity (lytic phase). In the long bones, a characteristic V-shaped line clearly demarcates involved bone from the normal bone. Skull involvement demonstrated a radiographically characteristic appearance termed *osteoporosis circumscripta*. Like the long bones, there are radiolucent areas, with clear delineation between the normal and Pagetic bone. The frontal and occipital bones are the most frequently involved and some larger lesions may have islands of normal-appearing bone within them. Spinal involvement usually is not specifically evident on radiographic evaluation during the initial phase.

Hyperdense or osteoblastic lesions are found in all involved bones during the phase of increased osteoblastic activity (sclerotic phase). At this point, long bone deformity occurs and becomes clearly evident radiographically. The skull also begins to show evidence of deformity with expansion of the normal cranial outline (Fig. 1). The borders between the inner and outer table are lost in an irregular pattern, leading to the descriptive term *cotton wool* appearance (15). The vertebral bodies are enlarged in the spine, especially in the anterior posterior dimension, and assume a square shape. The cortex becomes thickened, whereas the central portions remain relatively radiolucent. This gives what has been described as a *picture frame* appearance (Fig. 2). Vertebral bodies also can become homogeneously hyperdense leading to an *ivory* vertebra. The absence of syndesmophyte formations differentiates Paget from ankylosing spondylitis and the overall enlargement of the vertebral body differentiates Paget from blastic neoplastic lesions (16).

During the final phase, the Pagetic bone can go through degenerative changes similar to those found in other states of weakened bone physiology. The long bones are prone to pathological fractures and further deformities. Osteoarthritic changes occur at joint spaces. The long-term effects on the skull from Paget disease include cranial nerve compression from hyperostosis. In long-standing cases, a gradual infolding of the basi-occiput leads to basilar impression in one-third of patients (17). MRI is the study of choice to evaluate the degree of

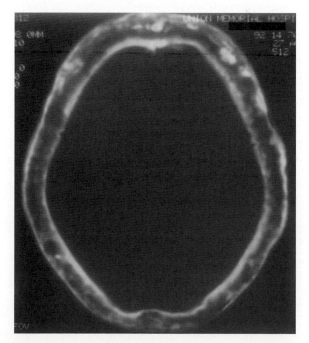

Fig. 1. CT scan of the skull of an elderly woman with Paget disease. Notice the marked thickening of the diffuse thickening of the cranial bone.

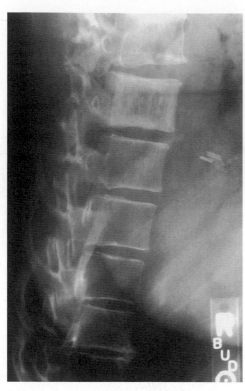

Fig. 2. Elderly man with "picture frame" appearance of the body of L3.

compression on the brainstem. Collapse of the vertebral bodies, either partially or completely, indicate weakened structural integrity of the spine. Secondary degeneration such as osteophyte formation and disc space narrowing are accelerated at and near the areas involved. Multiple contiguous levels of degeneration and collapse can lead to kyphotic deformity.

Quantitative bone scans using Tc 99m-EHDP have been found to be more sensitive in finding pagetic sites than plain roentgenograms (8).

Laboratory Findings

Elevated alkaline phosphatase and urine hydroxyproline are the most characteristic laboratory markers for the disease. The more active the osteoclasts, the higher the level of alkaline phosphatase and urine hydroxyproline. These biochemical markers can be used to track the progression of the disease and its response to medical management. Normally serum and urine calcium levels are normal in Paget disease patients. If there are other factors, such as hyperparathyroidism or immobilization, then the calcium levels are elevated.

Treatment

MEDICAL MANAGEMENT. Most patients with Paget disease are asymptomatic. Paget lesions often are found incidentally in the course of evaluation for other conditions. Indications for treatment include pain, neural compression, progressive defor-

mity, fractures or impending fracture, and high output cardiac failure (17).

Medical management is the first line when it is determined that the patient is a candidate for treatment. The rationale of therapy is to inhibit the abnormal osteoclastic activity. Until recently medical treatment consisted of calcitonin, which inhibits the activity of the normal and hyperactive osteoclast of Paget disease and mithramycin, which is an antibiotic toxic to osteoblasts. Recent pharmacological advances have substantially improved the treatment of Paget disease (18). Bisphosphonates have superseded calcitonin as the first-line treatment agent. Bisphosphonates are potent inhibitors of osteoclastic activity. They are synthetic analogues of pyrophosphate that bind to the hydroxyapatite at the site of bone reabsorption, directly inhibiting the action of the mature osteoclasts. Bisphosphonates then are incorporated into the newly formed bone and are made unavailable; thus, continual dosing is required to maintain the balance of bone formation. The bisphosphonates maintain a longer remission period than calcitonin. Currently etidronate, pamidronate, and alendronate are the most used of these agents.

Medical treatment does not reduce the size of the expanded bone but arrests further deformity and guard against fractures. Development of abnormal hypervascular bone halts and may decrease vascular steal from neural tissue. Long-term treatment is required because the imbalanced bone metabolism can return with drug cessation.

SURGICAL TREATMENT. Surgical treatment is rarely indicated but quite effective when medical management has failed. The most common surgical misadventures in Paget disease surgery are excessive bleeding and inadequate bone healing. Any surgical intervention is made safer and more effective by medical suppression therapy before and after the surgery. Preoperative treatment with bisphosphonates or calcitonin should decrease the vascularity and improve the healing of the pagetic bone. The most common indication for surgery in Paget disease is painful gait caused by hip or joint deformities. Osteotomies and joint replacements are effective in increasing pain-free ambulation.

Surgical indication for basilar impression include cranial neuropathies and upper cervical myelopathy. Anterior decompression of the brainstem and upper cervical spinal cord has become much more popular with improvement in technique and instrumentation (19). Very few patients with spinal involvement require surgical decompression; thus, there is a paucity of reported experience in the literature. Indications for spinal surgery include severe neurological deficit from stenosis or acute fracture, instability, or intractable pain. In performing decompressive spinal surgery, the surgeon should proceed deliberately and with great attention to hemostasis of the cut bone edges. Bone wax should be used liberally. The use of cell salvage techniques and preoperative autologous blood donation should be strongly considered. Careful selection and preparation of implant and bone graft sites is extremely important if deformity correction or spinal fusion is indicated. Iatrogenic instability owing to poor bone quality must be kept in mind when planning for the need and extent of fusion after decompressive surgery. Suppression therapy should continue for the entire period of the fusion healing and consolidation.

References

1. Mirra JM. Pathogenesis of Paget disease based on viral etiology. *Clin Orthop* 1987;217:162–170.

2. Rebel A, Malkani K, Basle M, et al. Particularities ultrastructure des osteoclasts de la maladie de Paget. *Rev Rheum Mal Ostoeartic* 1974; 41:767–771.
3. Mills BG, Singer FR. Nuclear inclusions in Paget disease of bone. *Science* 1976;194:201–202.
4. Haslam S, Van Hul W, Morales-Piga A, et al. Paget disease of the bone: evidence for a susceptibility locus on chromosome 18q and for genetic heterogeneity. *J Bone Min Res* 1998;13:911–917.
5. Kaplan FS, Singer FR. Paget disease of bone, pathophysiology, diagnosis and treatment. *J Amer Acad Orthop Surg* 1995;3:336–344.
6. Gebhart M, Vandeweyer E, Nemec E. Paget disease of bone complicated by giant cell tumor. *Clin Orthop Rel Res* 1998;352:187–193.
7. Price CHG, Goldie W. Paget sarcoma of bone. *J Bone Joint Surg Br* 1969;51:205–224.
8. Meunier P, Salson C, Mathiev L, et al. Skeletal distribution and biomechanical parameters of Paget disease. *Clin Orthop* 1987;217: 37–44.
9. Altman RD, Brown M, Gargano F. Low back pain in Paget disease of bone. *Clin Orthop Rel Res* 1987;217:152–161.
10. Douglas DL, Duckworth T, Kanis JA. Spinal cord dysfunction in Paget disease of the bone. *J Bone Joint Surg Br* 1981;63:495–503.
11. Hadjipavlou A, Lander P, Srolovitz H. Pagetic arthritis: pathophysiology and management *Clin Orthop* 1986;208:15–19.
12. Ryan MD, Taylor TK. Spinal manifestations of Paget disease. *Aust NZ J Surg* 1992;62:33–38.
13. Kanis JA. *Pathophysiology and treatment of Paget disease of bone.* London: Martin Dunitz, 1992.
14. Hadjipavlou A, Lander P. Paget and osteoporosis clinic, McGill University. *J Bone Joint Surg Am* 1991;73:1376–1381.
15. Harkey HL. Osteoporosis, osteomalacia and Paget disease. In: Menezes A, Sonntag V, eds. *Principles of spinal surgery.* New York: McGraw-Hill, 1996:500–502.
16. Booth RE, Simpson JM, Herkowitz HN. Arthritis of the spine. In: Herkowitz H, Garfin S, Balderston R, et al, eds. *Rothman-Simeone, the spine,* 4th ed. Philadelphia: WB Saunders, 1999:427–453.
17. White B, Wilson J. Metabolic diseases. In: Benzel E, Stillerman C, eds. *The thoracic spine.* St Louis: Quality Medical Publishing, 1999: 549–574.
18. Hosking D, Meunier PJ, Ringe JD, et al. Advances in the management of Paget disease of bone: diagnosis and management. *Br Med J* 1996; 312:491–494.
19. Crockard HA, Johnston F. Development of transoral approaches to the skull base and craniocervical junction. *Neurosurg Q* 1993;3:61.

154. *Ankylosing Spondylitis*

Dino Samartzis and John C. Liu

Historical Perspective

Ankylosing spondylitis (AS), a chronic progressive form of arthritis, is a systemic inflammatory disease with a possible genetic disposition. AS affects primarily the spine and sacroiliac joints, but can manifest in peripheral joints. The origin of AS has been found in the skeletal remnants of an Egyptian mummy dated 2,900 BC (1–3). In 1559, Realdo Columbo mentioned the first historical description of abnormalities typical of AS in two skeletons in his book, *De Re Anatomica.*

Although Bechterew and Strumpell contributed greatly toward describing AS, Marie gave a complete description of the disease (4).

AS is the third most common form of chronic arthritis in the United States (5). Since 1973, the major histocompatibility antigen HLA-B27 has been associated with AS; therefore providing a genetic component and additional insight in the pathogenesis of the disease.

Overview

AS belongs to a group of rheumatoid factor-negative disorders known as seronegative spondyloarthropathies (SNSA). This group is composed of Behçet disease, Crohn disease, juvenile chronic arthropathy, Reiter syndrome, ulcerative colitis, uveitis, Whipple disease, and *Salmonella*- and *Yersinia*-reactive arthropathies (6). SNSAs present peripheral inflammatory arthritis, sacroiliac joint inflammation, primary spinal involvement, and extraskeletal manifestations. It is estimated that 1.4% of the general population suffers from AS (7). However, incidence of the disease varies based on gender, race, and severity of symptoms or progressive disease characteristics that serve as catalysts to seek medical attention (8–10).

Population

The etiology of the AS is still unknown. Stages of the disease vary between individuals as well as remission and exacerbation periods. It is believed that AS occurs much later in life with slower progression for women compared to men. Recent reports state the male to female ratio to be more realistic, around 5:1 (11).

CHARACTERISTICS. Characteristics of AS are spinal rigidity and back pain as a result of calcification or ossification of joints and entheses. Enthesopathy or inflammation of bone attachment of tendon, joint capsule, and ligament mainly occurs at the axial skeleton. Vertebral body end plates and the annulus fibrosis are primarily involved. Inflammatory response and subsequent bone turnover produce ossification of paravertebral ligaments and intervertebral disc, and syndesmophyte formation. AS also produces fusion, erosion, and narrowing of the apophyseal joints and destruction of the anterior vertebral body concavity. Fusion of the spine occurs mainly at the thoracolumbar region with possible cervical progression producing a fixed-flexion deformity or a "bamboo spine" appearance on radiographic imaging. The spine mimics a long bone and becomes susceptible to fracture. Progressed condition results in fusion of the costovertebral joints, limiting chest wall expansion and reducing vital pulmonary capacity.

Destruction of the vertebral body's subchondral bone and

resultant sclerotic effects contribute to the kyphotic deformity of the spine. Furthermore, in order to minimize back and chest pain, individuals with AS seek a more pronounced spinal flexion. As a result, long-term sufferers develop loss of cervical and lumbar lordosis and an increase in thoracic kyphosis. Such a posture contributes to pain in the lower extremities when standing or sitting (12). Decreased activity and lack of exercise also contribute to the spine becoming more flexed. The abnormal posture increases the risk of a fall or injury leading to a fracture. Furthermore, progressive kyphosis or inflammation at the spinal canal could result in the development of radiculopathic, myelopathic, or myeloradiculopathic manifestations. Prolonged sufferers could also develop anorexia, fatigue, spinal stenosis, and cauda equina syndrome. In addition, psychological implications also exist because of the individual's dissatisfaction with external appearance and feelings of inadequacy (13). Functional embarrassment and pain in sufferers of AS also seems to lead to alcohol abuse, which may contribute to a greater risk of death as a result of accidents or violence (14).

Osteoporosis is also a manifestation with undetermined onset, although believed to exist at the early stages, and severity affecting many AS patients. In 1877, Fagge was the first to report osteoporotic manifestations from cadaveric examination of an AS patient (15). Since then, the presence of osteoporosis in an AS patient has been confirmed by various studies (16–18). Osteoporosis is a complicating feature of AS (19) increasing the risk of vertebral fractures (16–18,20,21) and contributing to impending surgical instrumentation complications. It is estimated that 4% to 18% of AS osteoporosis patients have vertebral fractures (16,22) and are more prevalent in AS patients (22,23).

Diagnostic Criteria

Timely and accurate diagnosis of AS is a task left to the experienced clinician because of its insidious nature. Herniated disc, back strain, degenerative spinal changes, and metabolic effects could disguise the correct diagnosis of AS. As a result, several criteria have been established to measure and evaluate the prevalence of the disease. Further diagnostic measures need to be accompanied, although much discussion has arisen regarding the accuracy of these criteria.

AS mainly occurs in individuals between the age of 20 to 40 who present with progressive limited range of motion, chronic back pain lasting more than 3 months, early morning stiffness, pain decreasing throughout the day, and improvement of condition with exercise. Sacroiliitis is predominantly the fist sign of AS. The disease initially manifests as pain in the low back region and buttocks area, with or without radiating lower extremity pain. In 1977 Calin and associates developed a screening method for AS composed of five items that have proven useful (24). An individual is considered positive for the disease if four of the five criteria are met (Table 1).

Table 1. Calin's Screening Test

Back pain:
1. Commences <40 years
2. Insidious onset
3. Persists >3 months
4. Associated morning stiffness
5. Improves with exercise

Inflammatory ankylosing spondylitis if 4/5 criteria met.

Table 2. Rome Criteria for the Diagnosis of Ankylosing Spondylitis

Clinical criteria	Radiological criteria

Low back pain and stiffnesss
  Greater than 3 months
  Does not subside with rest
	Bilateral sacroiliac changes
	(excluding bilateral
	osteoarthritic changes)

Pain and stiffness in thoracic region	
Limited lumbar motion	
Limited chest expansion	

Ankylosing spondylitis if 4/5 clinical criteria met without sacroiliitis or sacroiliitis with any clinical criteria.

Other diagnostic criteria have been established also that consider physical and radiographic findings in diagnosing AS. The first, is a set of measures called the Rome criteria established in Rome in 1961 (Table 2) (25). This framework requires one of five clinical criteria with the presence of bilateral radiographic sacroiliitis or four criteria met without sacroiliitis. The New York criteria were first reported in 1966 and offered similar standards as the Rome criteria, but more elaborate requiring the presence of radiological sacroiliitis as a major component in the diagnosis of AS (Table 3) (26). Later in 1982, van der Linden presented in his doctoral thesis a more modified version of the New York criteria that became known as the Modified New York criteria (Table 3) (27).

Recently, new criteria for scoring radiologic change in the spine have been developed. The Bath Ankylosing Spondylitis Radiology Index (BASRI) scores changes in the SI joints, and lumbar and cervical spine (Table 4) (28). The BASRI has been reported as a "reliable and rapid method" to grade radiographic changes in AS. Other systems gaining recent popularity in evaluating physical function in AS is the Bath Ankylosing Spondylitis Functional Index (BASFI) (29) and the Dougados Functional Index (DFI) (30).

Physical assessment includes evaluation of back pain and tenderness in the sacroiliac joints. Palpation of the iliac crest, spinous processes, costotransverse joints, and peripheral joints is essential to determine the degree of involvement of the disease. Further tests include Schober's test, which accounts for limitation for lumbar motion through flexion, Mennell's sign, occiput to the wall test to determine loss of cervical flexion, Patrick's test (which accounts for positive sacroiliac stress), and chest expansion measurements to determine progression of the disease in the costovertebral joints. Chest expansion less than 5 cm is uncommon for young adults and may raise suspicion of AS involvement. Gaenslen's test also is performed to investigate sacroiliac enthesopathy. Radiographic evaluation and measurement of spinal kyphosis by using the Cobb method also is followed. Furthermore, onset of pain during the day and duration is accounted for as well as finger–floor distance.

In assessing a patient, the physician should be aware of certain disorders that could mimic the symptoms of AS. For example, diffuse idiopathic skeletal hyperostosis (DISH) often is confused with AS. However, individuals with DISH who pose normal ESR usually do not present the HLA-B27 antigen, and their radiographic impressions exhibit no activity in the sacroiliac, apophyseal, and intervertebral joints, as do sufferers of AS. Another disease that could mimic the effects of sacroiliitis is fibromyalgia. Fibromyalgia, which can present with tender points throughout the body, could easily mislead the clinician. In addition, neoplasms, infection, acro-osteolysis, Paget disease, fluorosis, and ochronosis should be considered and dismissed.

Individuals with AS could develop extraspinal abnormalities.

Table 3. Comparison between New York and Modified New York Criteria

	New York	Modified New York

Clinical criteria	Dorso lumbar junction or lumbar pain	Low back pain
		  Greater than 3 months
		  Improved with exercise

	Limited lumbar motion
	  Sagittal
	  Frontal
		Limited lumbar motion
		  Sagittal
		  Frontal

	Limited chest expansion	Limited chest expansion below 2.5 cm
Radiological criteria	*Definite* Grade 3–4 bilateral with one clinical criterion Grade 3–4 unilateral or Grade 2 bilateral with either limited back motion and pain plus limited chest expansion *Probable* Grade 3–4 bilateral sacroiliitis with no clinical criteria	Grade 2 bilateral or Grade 3 unilateral

Uveitis is an ocular inflammatory condition that has been observed in 10% to 30% of individuals with AS (31,32). Other manifestations, including iridocyclitis, pulmonary fibrosis, myocardial fibrosis, aortitis, cardiac conduction abnormalities, cauda equina syndrome, and renal failure could develop, increasing the risk of death. Ankylosing spondylitis also is associated with multiple sclerosis, psoriasis, ulcerative colitis, enteritis, and other diseases belonging to the SNSA group mentioned in the preceding. Prolonged sufferers also develop anorexia, fatigue, and spinal stenosis. Inflammation at the level of the spinal canal could result in radiculopathy and myelopathy.

LABORATORY TESTS. Various laboratory tests are useful in monitoring and contributing to the diagnosis of AS. Among their many uses, C-reactive protein (CRP) and erythrocyte sedimentation rate (ESR) (33,34) are considered in the differential diagnosis of AS. Although clinical trials examining the reliability of these two disease markers are limiting, some type of association with AS exists (35–37).

Erythrocyte sedimentation rate increases 24 to 48 hours after exposure to inflammation and the level may take weeks to return to normal (33). C-reactive protein responds to inflammatory stimulus within hours and returns to normal shortly after the stimulus has been removed (33). Elevated levels of ESR have been reported in 75% of AS patients (35,37). Alternatively, CRP is considered to be a direct measure of inflammation and implemented in monitoring chronic disease anemia that affects the hematopoietic system., but is not considered superior in assessing AS activity (38). Moreover, ESR is sensitive to immunoglobulins and rheumatoid factor (RF), but is doubtful in its reliability in assessing disease activity of AS (33,35,37). Sheehan

Table 4. BASRI Spine Criteria for Scoring Radiological Change

Score	Grade	Application to lumbar and cervical spine
0	Normal	No change
1	Suspicious	No definite change
2	Mild	Any number of erosions, squaring, sclerosis with or without syndesmophytes on <2 vertebrae
3	Moderate	Syndesmophytes on >3 vertebrae with or without fusion involving 2 vertebrae
4	Severe	Fusion involving >3 vertebrae

BASRI, Bath Ankylosing Spondylitis Radiology Index.

and associates (39) and Laurent and Panayi (40) indicate that elevated ESR and CRP levels are more prevalent in the peripheral involvement of AS patients and are not a direct measure of axial activity.

Researchers have indicated that various biochemical markers of bone metabolism provide insight of AS activity, although the efficacy of AS disease activity and the correlation between ESR and CPR is continuously debated. Toussirot and colleagues reported that levels of pyridinium cross-links, independent from sex, disease duration, and not related to the peripheral skeleton are elevated in AS patients with raised ESR levels, but not CRP. These findings suggest that AS patients are at a higher risk for bone loss or that urinary excretion of pyridinium cross-links maybe because of cartilage collagen breakdown. Macdonald and colleagues (41) and Marhoffer and associates (42) reported similar findings, except that Marhoffer and associates also noted a correlation with CRP. Furthermore, serum amyloid A (SAA) also is considered indicative in monitoring disease activity of AS. SAA circulation is also increased with elevated ESR, CRP, and BASDAI, and usually appears in rheumatoid arthritis (43).

GENETIC MARKERS. Calin and Fries first reported that 90% of U.S. whites with AS tested positive for the HLA-B27 antigen (28). However, recent studies have showed that the presence of the HLA-B27 antigen is a weaker indicator of AS than first thought. Jajic found 128 of 276 individuals with chronic back pain of more than 3 months who were positive for the HLA-B27 antigen to have AS (44). The and co-workers found in 1985 that 51% of 43 patients who were negative for HLA-B27, but presented with back pain, had AS (26). Furthermore, it has been reported that the risk of HLA-B27-positive individuals with HLA-B27-positive relatives are 16 times more likely to develop AS than HLA-B27-positive individuals in the general population (45).

Although the role of HLA-B27 as a marker for developing AS still is under debate, the recent emergence of various Class II encoded factors of HLA could be responsible for the phenotype of the disease. In 1995, Maksymowych and co-workers reported that a gene called LMP2 linked to HLA may be responsible for developing extraspinal manifestations in individuals with AS (46). Maksymowych and his group believed that the polymorphism of LMP2 at the site of the HLA affects certain peptides at the extraspinal regions that induce autoreactivity. Nevertheless, Maksymowych and co-workers further investigated the effects or disease expression that LMP2 has in individuals with AS. Therefore, in 2000 they determined that the LMP2 gene is associated with disease phenotype in HLA-B27-negative and -positive individuals with AS (47).

RADIOGRAPHIC FINDINGS

Plain Radiographs. Sacroiliitis is the predominant feature at the beginning stages of AS. Eventually, bilateral osteoporosis develops, followed by widening of the joint space accompanied with poorly defined joint margins. Subsequently, subchondral sclerosis occurs and spinal changes take effect.

Destruction of the corners of the vertebral body occurs, developing a "square" vertebral body and loss of anterior vertebral concavity as a result of the inflammatory response on the insertion of ligament or tendon to the site. As the disease progresses, a bony bridge or a syndesmophyte develops across the intervertebral space, connecting the superior to the inferior vertebra. The syndesmophyte formation produces ossification of the outer border of the annulus fibrosis, resulting in the appearance of a "bamboo spine." Osteophytes also develop in proximity to the discovertebral margins as a result of disc degeneration as well as bone and fibrous command of the intervertebral disc. Osteophyte formations initially develop projection in a horizontal direction perpendicular to the axial skeleton, but later are positioned vertically

The apophyseal joints are affected as the disease progresses. On the anteroposterior radiograph view, "train track" lines are evident because of the calcification of the capsular ligaments. Further erosion, narrowing, and fusion of the apophyseal joints originates in the lumbar region and progresses cephalically, eventually incorporating the costovertebral joints. Fusion of the interfacet joints is noticeable on lateral projection. In addition, osteoporotic conditions develop in the vertebral bodies and further contribute to the instability and vulnerability of the spine. Lateral imaging also is essential to determine sagittal balance, especially in kyphotic individuals.

MRI and CT. Other methods have been sought to provide more lucent and early diagnosis of the disease because of the potential misinterpretation that plain radiographs pose in establishing early stages of AS. Use of magnetic resonance imaging (MRI) and computed tomography (CT) to facilitate differential diagnosis of AS is beneficial, and possibly more advantages in identifying early signs of sacroiliitis. Recent studies suggest that MRI (48,49) and CT (48) can detect early cartilaginous changes of sacroiliitis than plain radiography; however, many practitioners prefer to rely on plain radiographs because of the economic pitfalls of MRI and CT.

Management

MEDICATION. Nonsteroidal antiinflammatory drugs (NSAIDs) are an integral component of nonsurgical treatment to help decrease the pain, stiffness, and discomfort associated with the inflammatory response of AS. A wide variety of NSAIDs are available, but efficacy varies between individuals. Indomethacin (50), naproxen (51), and phenylbutazone (50) are widely used among AS sufferers. Sulfasalazine, (52,53), diclofenac, fenoprofen calcium, and salicylates also have been effective in relieving symptoms of AS. Although salicylates and aspirin initially are sought to relieve symptoms of AS, sufferers tend to depart from this therapy and seek other, more potent regiments, as mentioned in the preceding (50,54). Gastrointestinal bleeding, development of ulcers, and other adverse reactions

are associated with the majority of NSAIDs, but are not commonplace with selective Cox2 inhibitors.

Although the goal of drug therapy is to reduce or manage pain and stiffness in AS patients, optimal outcome is ascertained with proper exercise and physical therapy. Medication coupled with exercise are beneficial because inflammation is reduced and progressive or fixed fusion associated with AS leading to maladaptive curvature is hindered because of avoidance of long periods of rest. Prevention of poor posture is further avoided by increasing the body's range of motion.

Fracture Management

ATLANTOAXIAL SPINE. Ankylosing spondylitis initiates an abnormal fusion cascade that often affects the subaxial spine, but rarely the atlantoaxial region. Tremendous stress is applied on the atlantoaxial junction as a consequence of rigid kyphotic cervical deformity, subjecting the region to a risk of subluxation. Sharp and Pursar highlighted the severity of atlantoaxial subluxation (AAS) in AS patients, noting the occurrence of ASS in 17 out of 1,000 consecutive AS cases (55). Ramos-Remus and associates evaluated 81 cases of AAS and reported 74% anterior AAS, 13% vertical AAS, 11% rotatory instability, and 2% presented with mixed forms (56). Of these patients, 60% underwent surgery and 38% were handled with traction.

Atlantoaxial AS involvement could affect the odontoid by initiating erosive changes, allowing it to sink and move beneath an intact transverse ligament (57). Synovitis could cause laxity and rupture of the transverse ligament (55,57,58).

AS patients with atlantoaxial instability usually develop occiput pain that could follow with myelopathic and myopathic symptoms. Surgery is required if pain persists, and the prognosis is optimistic (56). At any rate, lateral neutral, flexion, and extension plain radiographs as well as axial and sagittal CT or MRI views must be examined to accurately account for canal and neurovascular compromise.

Transarticular screw fixation, initially reported by Magerl and Seeman, is an effective technique for posterior fixation in treating atlantoaxial instability (59). This technique has shown immediate obliteration of rotational motion, and with the adjunct of posterior graft-cable constructs has eliminated the need for discomforting and prolonged external postoperative immobilization by halo.

Atlantoaxial posterior fusion and wiring via the Gallie method has proven beneficial in AS patients (60). The Gallie method prevents atlantoaxial internal fixation, preserves occipitocervical motion, avoids neurovascular injury, and sufficiently relieves symptoms.

Odontoid involvement could further complicate the atlantoaxial region of an AS cervical spine. Superior migration of the odontoid could compress the spinal cord and brainstem. Surgical intervention then is sought to stabilize the odontoid process and the atlantoaxial vertebrae by occipitocervical fusion. Management of severe spinal cord, brainstem compression, or a fracture of the odontoid process usually justifies an anterior transoral approach to decompress the elements and remove fractured odontoid fragments (61).

SUBAXIAL CERVICAL SPINE

Preassessment. Cervical spine fracture is a serious condition and detrimental to the AS patient, demanding immediate attention. Cervical fractures in AS patients has been reported to result from minor trauma (62–64) or no apparent trauma (20,65). Multiple one segment fractures are not common in AS patients; however, simultaneous disruptions of cervical and thoracic regions have been reported (66–68). In AS patients, 75% of spinal fractures occur in the cervical spine (20). Cervical fracture increases distraction and angulation of the brittle AS spine, which contributes to an increased risk of morbidity and mortality (63, 69–71). It is estimated that 35% of cervical fractures in patients with AS lead to death as compared to 20% in spines without the disease (72). In fact, threat of neurological complications after injury occurs in 57% of patients with AS (72). The physician should be highly speculative of a cervical fracture when an individual with AS has suffered a minor trauma and immediately pursue necessary diagnostic and therapeutic intervention.

Ankylosing spondylitic patients who develop a progressed cervical kyphotic deformity present a deterioration of their visual field and are more prone to fall and fracture as a result. The AS spine adopts a long-bone characteristic, assuming the characteristics of a long lever arm, which attracts forces at the weakest point. The cervical AS spine is susceptible to stress fractures largely because of its osteoporotic persona and grossly adopted rigid kyphotic deformity. Although various traumatic episodes could attribute to a cervical fracture, hyperextension usually is at fault (20,62–64,66,69,71–73,75–77). Usually, fractures occur at the level of the intervertebral disc (62). The intervertebral disc is more vulnerable because of its tardy ossification of the nucleus pulposus. Furthermore, fractures at the cervical spine usually are complete and unstable because of the inability of the fused immobile facet joints and ligamentous structures to adequately inherit stress, pressure, and maintain segmental motion as does a normal spine.

Usually, plain radiographs are insufficient and other avenues of detection should be sought. For example, tomography, CT scan, and/or myelogram could prove useful in identifying and interpreting a fracture. Delicate attention needs to be administered when positioning an AS patient for such diagnostic imaging. Moreover, fractures are usually present in the lower cervical spine (72,78,79), which also could pose problematic radiographic detection because of scapular hindrance and porous manifestations.

Nonoperative Management. Often, individuals who suffer a cervical fracture are found in a paralytic condition in which urgent attention is sought. A common flaw when first addressing immobilization of the cervical spine is placing a collar or a type of external orthosis that usually benefit an individual without AS. An AS spine in a neutral position is kyphotic; therefore, placing a collar to immobilize the fracture would only complicate the condition. Application of a halo vest is appropriate to reduce the fracture and place the cervical spine in its "normal" alignment to obtain its preexisting kyphotic curvature.

One school of thought in treating an AS patient with a cervical fracture is the application of a halo brace or collar to avoid open reduction of the fracture, hoping that the closed reduction and fixation will allow the fracture to rapidly fuse, given the nature of the disease. However, it may be more beneficial to avoid conservative treatment and opt for open fracture reduction by using internal instrumentation. In this fashion, the internal fixation may avoid pseudoarthrosis; discomfort and hospital time by eliminating the vest, brace, or collar; and any motion with the external fixation, which could result in an improper fracture reduction and prolonged neurological complications. Plating the spine is quick, efficient, and benefits the patient in many aspects; however, plating may not be optimal in AS patients with osteoporosis because of poor screw acceptance by the bone construct. Also, AS patients who have multiple cervical fractures may not benefit from plating.

Surgical Management. A halo vest apparatus provides external immobilization and attempts to avoid surgical intervention, subluxation recurrences, failure of ligamentous healing, neurological deficits, prolonged bed rest, and external wear discomfort contribute to the appeal of surgery.

Some report high mortality rates from open reduction. Various factors are at play that could contribute to such a complication. For example, positioning the patient for radiographs could increase neural compromise. Also, transporting the patient or operating room table positioning could enflame the situation and promote displacement and neurological deficit. Therefore, rigid external immobilization must be applied immediately. Immobilization with a halo vest to prevent further compression must be performed before an AS patient with cervical pain is moved.

Surgery could decompress and stabilize the fractured cervical spine, but certain factors need to be considered. The halo vest should be used for immobilization and positioning with univariate traction along the axis of the neck. Some contend that a simultaneous bivariate intraoperative traction directed by ventral and cranial vectors provides greater stability. However, such an apparatus imparts limited positioning by the surgeon and increases patient discomfort.

Anesthetic choice and operative positioning are variables that could contribute detrimental effects if not addressed. General anesthesia with intubation is hazardous in a fractured AS cervical spine. Moreover, the nature of the deformity and risk of displacement limits positioning preference.

Although variations in open reduction exist, we advocate a combined anterior and posterior approach. In a fractured, long lever arm, and stiff AS cervical spine, movement is contained only at the fracture site. Therefore, two-sided fixation is preferred to avoid the strong stress forces applied on sole internal fixation devices and remove possible formation of granulation tissue. As a response, an anterior plate is applied at the level of fracture with possible interbody or strut grafting dependent on fracture recurrence and neurological compromise followed by lateral mass plating.

THORACOLUMBAR SPINE. The effects of AS are numerous, as noted. The propensity for fracture occurrence in the spine is greater than with than without AS—even with minor trauma, because of altered biomechanics and mass ossification of the AS spine coupled with possible osteopenic or osteoporotic manifestations. The thoracic and lumbar regions, as in the cervical spine, are susceptible to stress or compression fractures. Although cervical spine fractures appear more common in AS patients, a fracture in the thoracic and lumbar regions may occur, with the majority located at the thoracolumbar junction. Three types of fractures are observed in thoracic and lumbar regions: shearing or slice fracture (80), wedge compression injury (74,81), and fractures associated with pseudoarthrosis (82, 83).

The thoracolumbar junction in an AS patient inherits a great amount of stress. Because of the progressive loss of lumbar lordosis, the apex of a normal kyphosis is relocated distally and assumes the role of a fulcrum between two long lever arms—the thoracic region with its rib attachments and the lower lumbar and pelvic elements. The increased stress assumed by the biomechanically altered spine coupled with metabolic alterations increase the risk of fracture dramatically.

A common clinical characteristic is localized back pain, aggravated by movement, and pain not relieved by rest (84). Owing to the nature of AS, any patient with acute onset of back pain must be treated with the suspicion of fracture until proven otherwise. The fracture may occur through the intervertebral disc, near the end plate, or through the vertebral body. Spine fractures in the AS spine usually entail three-column involvement, rendering the spine susceptible to displacement. Kyphotic or lordotic angulation may ensue if the fracture is left untreated, causing displacement and possible spinal cord injury. Thus, cord compression is caused by the altered alignment of the spinal canal and fracture reduction must be performed.

Initial radiographic evaluation is crucial, but often difficult to access and misleading because of osteoporotic invasion and mass inflammatory manifestations associated with AS. CT imaging and bone scans may prove useful if plain radiographs fail to elucidate. Timely radiographic fracture diagnosis is imperative to avoid dreadful neurological compromise (84). Neurological injury was noted in 75% of presenting fractures in AS patients, according to Hunter and Dubo (20). A study based on the experience of treating thoracolumbar spine fractures in AS patients by Trent and colleagues illustrated that 20 of 25 fractures occurred between T9 and L2, with 25% involving neurological deficit on initial presentation (84).

Some physicians may attempt nonoperative management of fractures in this region by plaster casting or brace; however, external immobilization may be counterintuitive and predispose the spine to neural injury, instability, and progressed spinal deformity because the involvement of fracture typically involves three columns and is unstable. In the past, Harrington distraction rods have been implemented as well as a countered Luque rods with segmental wiring to reduce the fracture and obtain stability (84). Nonetheless, to obtain adequate fracture reduction and reestablish spinal curvature, posterior Cotrel-Dubousset instrumentation is applied with fusion. Use of instrumentation should not end at the apex of kyphosis or an open disc space because of the risk of stress fractures above and below the fusion (85). The fusion should consist of one or two segments above and below to cover these areas (84). An anterior and posterior fusion and instrumentation is performed if the fracture displacement is radical and the amount of kyphotic deformity is greatly pronounced. In any case, proper intraoperative positioning and movement are essential to avoid further exacerbation of the spinal condition.

Deformity Correction

CERVICAL OSTEOTOMY. Severe flexion deformity of the cervical spine is a disabling manifestation with often grotesque and embarrassing morphology. Individuals with such a condition often have difficulty chewing, swallowing, and breathing. They undergo excessive weight loss, skin care maintenance is handicapped, field of vision is decreased compensating horizontal gaze, and are at greater risk for trauma. Avenues for correction exist, although severe cervical deformity arrests a milieu of normal daily functioning activities. However, correction of cervical kyphotic deformity of AS via surgical intervention is generally a tactic not widely sought in lieu of various complications associated with spinal operative correction.

Several criteria should be considered before pursuit of surgical correction of cervical kyphotic deformity in AS. Extent of cervical deformity is measured by the chin-brow technique and Cobb angle. Modification of horizontal gaze, sagittal balance, and symptomatic relief is primarily accomplished through thoracolumbar osteotomy. However, if thoracolumbar fixed-flexion deformity is not pronounced initially, then lumbar osteotomy correction achieves inadequate results. In turn, severity of deformity is greater in the cervical spine and cervical osteotomy is warranted.

Technique Considerations. Surgical prowess of cervical osteotomy is largely credited to Simmons' 1977 report of his experi-

ence of 42 AS patients who underwent surgical correction (86). Of 42 patients, Simmons noted one postoperative death owing to myocardial infarction and one incident of pulmonary embolism. Simmons cervical osteotomy approach mimicked Urist's (87) method. Preoperatively, the patients were fitted with a plaster jacket for 2 to 3 days in which a halo apparatus was applied the day before surgery. Patients were operated under local anesthesia in a sitting position with C7-T1 levels as the site of correction. Intraoperatively, the halo was used to apply traction and control head positioning. After the osteotomy was closed by halo extension, the patient continued to don the apparatus. Sensation and movement of extremities was examined and the patient was able to walk from the operating room to the circoelectric bed. The patient then was instructed to wear the halo cast unit for 4 months and was later placed in a cervical brace for 2 months. However, Simmons did experience two cases of postoperative nonunion. To correct this condition, Simmons conducted a second operation of anterior cervical fusion at C7-T1 with a Keystone technique resulting in solid union.

In 1999, Mehdian and co-workers proposed a method of cervical osteotomy with internal rigid screw-rod fixation (88). General anesthesia with fiberoptic endotracheal intubation was administered followed by application of a halo ring and positioning of the patient in a prone position with a horseshoe head rest to accommodate the deformity. A midline incision was made and anatomical landmarks were identified. Lateral mass hole drilling commenced at C3-6 with additional holes at T2-5 pedicles. The osteotomy was performed as described by Simmons with addition of screw insertion at the lateral masses and pedicles. A temporary malleable rod was inserted on the left as a hinge of sagittal motion during extension. When a desired position was achieved, the rod was replaced with a titanium-contoured rod on both sides and autologous iliac crest bone was positioned posteriorly. Postoperatively, the halo was removed and the patient was placed in an occipito-cervical thoracic orthosis for three months. The patient was followed up for 18 months and exhibited no signs of neurological complication, presented good correction and fusion, and horizontal gaze had improved.

Complications. Compression of the nerve roots at the osteotomy site is always a risk. Neural structures could be stretched if the osteotomy is miscut. In order to minimize nerve root compression, it is recommended that adequate pedicle removal be performed above and below the nerve root to prevent deficit when the spine adopts a newly angulated form owing to extension osteotomy. Additional indication of neural structure compression is evident during closing extension osteotomy when the dura is observed not wrinkled, but stretched. Also, placement of bone graft material in the midline of the osteotomy subjects the cord to compression. In addition, improper positioning of internal instrumentation, such as screws or sublaminar wires could compress neural structures or tear the underlying dura. Furthermore, somatosensory evoked potential monitoring and periodic extremity functioning should be assessed intraoperatively to reduce the risk of neurological compromise (89,90).

Although in many instances a halo jacket or cervical brace is used postoperatively to maintain the cervical alignment of the newly osteotomized extended spine, risk of loss of correction does exist. Internal instrumentation greatly reduces the occurrence of loss of correction and further stabilizes the spine.

THORACOLUMBAR SPINE

Indications for Surgery. Surgical intervention is sought when intractable axial pain develops or excruciating pain is overwhelming, neurological deterioration manifests, nonresponsive conservative therapy, reduction in horizontal gaze contributing to the risk of trauma, and when spinal deformity inhibits daily activity. Although many operative risks are associated with surgical intervention to correct for the delicate state of fixed-flexion deformity, operative treatment can prove beneficial by reducing or eliminating pain, improving function and mobility, and softening aesthetic embarrassment. A timeline for surgical management is dependent on the severity of the deformity and effects on daily functioning because expressivity of AS varies among individuals.

Various factors must be assessed to determine the viability of operative treatment and include the following: age, sex, occupation, deterioration of quality of life, location of pronounced deformity, feasibility of the surgical procedure, and postoperative rehabilitation measures. Spinal deformity is assessed by radiographic measurements, such as the Cobb angle and the visual brow-chin method. In this technique, the vertical axis is intersected by a line drawn from the brow to the chin and the resultant angle is measured. Periodic assessment of the brow–chin measurement is essential to monitor the patient's progressive spinal changes and establish a baseline. As the angle increases, spinal deformity is more pronounced warranting operative intervention. Optimal sagittal balance should attempt to recreate the plumb line's intersection of the C7 vertebra and body of the sacrum.

Surgical correction for spinal kyphotic deformity of AS has been investigated as well as scrutinized since the 1940s. No universal consensus has been established as to the appropriate technique for spinal deformity correction largely owing to the precarious nature of the disease and surgical technical prowess of the surgeon. Selection of the vertebral level for correction is imperative. Pronounced thoracolumbar deformity warrants surgical correction at the lumbar level; whereas, marked thoracic deformity with an intact lumbar lordosis demands thoracic correction.

In 1945, Smith-Petersen and associates introduced vertebral osteotomy to correct for spinal deformity in AS (12). Since then, numerous accounts highlighting operative technique to correct kyphotic deformity, the role if internal instrumentation, appropriate depth of osteotomy, approach selection, and use of bone graft have been explored. Nevertheless, the majority of deformity correction is accomplished through lumbar relordosation.

In the technique illustrated by Smith-Petersen and associates, monosegmental or multisegmental posterior V-shaped wedge osteotomy provides the foundation for correction of pronounced kyphotic deformity associated with AS. Their initial experience with five patients illustrated the importance of selecting the appropriate operative vertebral level because the less ossified segment(s) based on radiographic evaluation present the greatest ease for manipulation. This approach entails positioning the patient prone intraoperatively under general anesthesia. A midline incision is performed extending one level above and below the main vertebral osteotomy site in the lumbar region. Retraction of muscle attachment from the spinous processes and lamina is performed and the spinous processes are excised. The ligamentum flavum is removed and an osteotome is employed to create a V-shaped wedged osteotomy with a 45-degree angle from the frontal plane through the superior articular processes of the inferior vertebra and inferior articular processes of the superior vertebra (12). Bone graft from the excised spinous processes is inserted between the lamina for support and as an anchor to achieve desired lordosis. The osteotomy then is closed by manual means or raising the head or lower extremities by manipulating the operating table to obtain the desired spinal curvature.

In efforts to prevent elongation of the anterior column and reduce the risk of injury to proximal vascular and neural struc-

tures, Thomasen in 1885 advocated a posterior monosegmental wedge osteotomy with partial dorsal vertebral corpectomy (91). In his initial experience, Thomasen's method, similar to a previous technique performed by Scudese and Calabro in 1963, (92) achieved 12- to 50-degree kyphotic correction in 11 patients. Thomasen's osteotomy site was L2. After a midline incision was performed at T11 to L4 and proper muscle retraction accomplished at L1-4, a posterior wedge osteotomy was performed that removed the tips of the spinous processes of L2 and L3, and proceeded to remove L2's pedicles, laminae, transverse processes, superior articular processes, and the upper portion of the L3 lamina. The dural sac was retracted accordingly to facilitate resection of the posterior vertebral wall by an osteotome. Rongeur then was implemented to remove cancellous vertebral bone to create the partial corpectomy. Closing osteotomy was achieved by manual and operative table manipulation. Postoperatively, a plaster jacket was worn for 3 months to aid bone fusion, and positive outcome was reported by patients. Thomasen also implemented plates and metallic wires posteriorly in some patients. The nature of Thomasen's osteotomy technique heightens visibility of neural structures to avoid peripheral compression, and decreases stretching of the cauda equina, aorta, and intraabdominal muscles. Solid bone fusion is facilitated by an intact anterior longitudinal ligament and anterior cortex of the vertebra acting as hinges as well as the richly vascularized cancellous vertebral body site.

Although many have contributed possible avenues for correction of thoracic or lumbar fixed-flexion deformity in AS, no one method is superior to the others. The patient's overall condition must be evaluated, accounting for the apex of the deformity and desired sagittal correction. It is common to combine a Thomasen vertebral monosegmental osteotomy at L2-3 or L3-4 with transpedicular screw fixation (93,94). However, a two-staged anterior-posterior approach under general anesthesia is feasible to rupture the ossified anterior longitudinal ligament, create posterior wedge-shaped osteotomies, and perform an anterior osteotomy and fusion. For that matter, multilevel thoracic posterior osteotomies could be performed to obtain the desired curvature if progressed thoracic kyphosis is present.

The osteotomy should be performed at the apex of the curve with the amount of osteotomies performed in accordance with degree of pronounced kyphotic deformity and desired spinal curvature. Employ segmental instrumentation with posterior transpedicular screw fixation. Afterward, multiple posterior osteotomies are recommended to aid in shortening the posterior column; anterior strut grafts are implemented for additional support if needed.

Our main objective is to help the spinal surgeon to grasp the concept of thoracolumbar osteotomy and understand the various benefits and complications that pertain to the preceding approaches. The goal of deformity correction is to obtain a more erect posture, increase horizontal gaze, increase pulmonary capabilities, reduce or eliminate pain, and obtain a more physically aesthetic appearance.

Complications. Although surgical innovations and technique enhancement have decreased the risk of neurological, vascular, and pulmonary complications associated with operative treatment of spinal fixed-flexion deformity (93–96), mortality rates as high as 10% are reminders of the high-risk stigma associated with surgical correction of AS (13,97–100). Avenues to decrease operative complications are essential. Aortic rupture in AS operative correction was first reported in 1956 by Lichtblau and Wilson, when rupture of the anterior longitudinal ligament ruptured an aorta that failed to give, leading to death (101). Further cases were also noted by Klems and Friedebold (102) and Weatherley and associates (103). The latter study highlighted two cases of aortic rupture leading to death where cardiovascular collapse was preceded by retroperitoneal hematoma development owing to lumbar extension osteotomy. Fibrosis of cardiac vessels and the aorta are potential disease-related inflammatory manifestations that increase the risk of intraoperative complications by weakening, and dispose to rupture by aneurysms. Fibrosis also may affect the myocardium, causing arrhythmia or other altered cardiac conduction, cardiomegaly, and angina (31). Furthermore, pulmonary fibrosis may invade the upper lobe, causing edema.

Intraoperative complications also may stem from anesthetization methods. Respiratory complications may arise from inappropriate intubation positioning owing to the abnormal cervical curvature found in progressed stages of AS (86,104,105). Accumulation of mucus in the respiratory tract as a result of improper intubation may prevent proper postoperative coughing. Pulmonary restriction also has been noted to occur in patients with progressed kyphotic cervical spine. Therefore, proper patient intraoperative positioning is essential to reduce possible complications (86,93,94,104–107).

Further complications also are present. Elongation of the anterior spinal column may contribute to complications associated with operative spinal correction of AS. Gastric dilation may develop from elongation of the anterior column by stretching the superior mesenteric artery over the duodenum (86). As a result, patients may vomit with further complications of obstruction from intubation. Moreover, thrombosis (100) and possible aortic rupture may develop from vascular vessel elasticity (13, 101–103). Furthermore, insufficient bone removal (94), subluxation, and impingement may cause cord compression and ensuing neuropraxia or paraplegia (96,106). In addition, retrograde ejaculation also is a potential risk (108,109). Instrumentation failure could ensue because of inappropriate application or improper screw tightening to establish proper compressive forces (94–96,109,110). Furthermore, shock (97), amyloidosis (97), pneumonia (97), pulmonary embolism (110), deep wound infection (96,110), dural leak (95,110,111), deep venous thrombosis (106), nonunion (109), and overcorrection could surface as well.

Spondylodiscitis

Spondylodiscitis is an uncommon inflammatory or mechanical manifestation in AS patients affecting the vertebral end plates and intervertebral disc space. Andersson, in 1937, first reported spondylodiscitis and its radiographic manifestations characterized by sclerotic and erosive changes in vertebral end plates adjacent to the disc (112). In 1940, Endstrom further described the clinical manifestations of spondylodiscitis (113). However, Cawley and co-workers in 1972 established the classical description of clinical manifestations of spondylodiscitis by noting the following: localized central discovertebral lesions, localized peripheral discovertebral lesions, or a combination of both (114). Moreover, intervertebral disc space narrowing or widening was noted, producing a "vacuum phenomenon" or "blown-up" affect of the disc space.

Radiographic evaluation of spondylodiscitis may be obtained through plain radiographs. However, confirmation is skeptical and requires execution of MRI and skeletal scintigraphy to substantiate spondylodiscitis detection. Diagnosis varies between individuals, but usually presents in longer duration AS patients (114–119). Rasker and associates reported only six patients (1.5%) with spondylodiscitis from a pool of 400 AS patients (120). Kabasakal and colleagues reported a slightly higher amount—8% of 147 consecutive AS patients with spondylodiscitis (115). Five to eight percent (115,121,122) of AS patients

with symptoms for 10 years or more are prone to develop spondylodiscitis. Multilevel lesions also are common in spondylodiscitis, mainly occurring in the lower thoracic and lumbar region (115,116,123,124). Lesions, either single or multilevel, are accompanied with fused apophyseal joints and syndesmophytes (115).

Patients usually are asymptomatic, although spondylodiscitis alters an already deformed spine (116). However, Rivelis and Freiberger noted that all five AS patients with spondylodiscitis were symptomatic with pain at the level of the lesion (117). Alternatively, Kabasakal and co-workers only noted two from six AS patients with spondylodiscitis who presented back pain at the lesion site. Nevertheless, spinal cord damage could develop because of granulation tissue proliferation within the epidural space at the lesion (21,119,125). Symptomatic relief is obtained through conservative treatment by NSAIDs, therapy, rest, and corset application. Surgical intervention is pursued if instability and neurological complications are persistent and not relieved with conservative treatment. If approached anteriorly, the disc is excised, and strut grafts replace the void accompanied with posterior Harrington compression system or by extension osteotomy at the lesion site simultaneously, correcting the deformity followed by external thoracolumbar support until fusion is obtained.

Conclusion

Ankylosing spondylitis is a chronic inflammatory condition that arrests a multitude of normal bodily functions and affects the patient's quality of life. Sadly, there is no known cure; however, an understanding of the disease, precautionary measures, and conservative medicinal therapy can offer tremendous relief and improve daily functioning.

Spinal involvement is largely prevalent, although peripheral joints are involved. Severe spinal deformity owing to AS could radically affect the body. Fracture disruptions could render the patient a quadriplegic or lead to death if not properly managed. Immobilization in the preinjured cervical curvature is key; however, proper progression of the disease must be assessed in order to properly execute correct fixation. Correction of fixed-flexion spinal deformity is a difficult and strenuous task that demands the capabilities of a highly trained and knowledgeable spine surgeon. Reduction of the kyphotic deformity is an aesthetically pleasing outcome. However, risk of complications and the threat of death are aspects of surgical intervention that require awareness by both physician and patient.

References

1. Calin A. Ankylosing spondilitis. Clin Rheum Dis 11:41–60, 1985.
2. Calin A. Ankylosing spondylitis. In: Kelly WN, Harris EDJ, Rudy S, et al, eds. Textbook of rheumatology. Philadelphia: WB Saunders, 1985:993–1006.
3. Rogers J, Watt I, Dieppe P. Paleopathology of spinal osteophytosis, vertebral ankylosis, ankylosing spondylitis, and vertebral hyperostosis. Ann Rheum Dis 44:113–120, 1985.
4. Benoist M. Historical perspective Pierre Marie. Spine 20:849–852, 1995.
5. Shah BC, Khan MA. Review of ankylosing spondylitis. Comp Ther 13:152–159, 1987.
6. Fox MV, Onofrio BM. Ankylosing spondylitis. In: Menezes AH, Sonntag VH, eds. Principles of spinal surgery. New York: McGraw-Hill, 1996:735.

7. Cruickshank B. Histopathology of diarthrodial joints in ankylosing spondylitis. *Ann Rheum Dis* 10:393–404, 1951.
8. Carbone LD, Cooper C, Michet CJ. Ankylosing spondylitis in Rochester, Minnesota, 1935–1989: is the epidemiology changing? *Arthritis Rheum* 35:1476–1482, 1992.
9. Gran JT, Husby G. The epidemiology of ankylosing spondylitis. *Semin Arthritis Rheum* 22:319–334, 1993.
10. Kahn MA. An overview of clinical spectrum and heterogeneity of spondyloarthropathies. *Rheum Dis Clin North Am* 18:1, 1992.
11. Apple DF, Anson C. Spinal cord injury occurring in patients with ankylosing spondylitis: a multicenter study. *Spinal Cord Injury* 18:1005–1011, 1995.
12. Smith-Petersen MN, Larson CB, Aufranc OE. Osteotomy of the spine for correction of flexion deformity in rheumatoid arthritis. *J Bone Joint Surg Am* 27:1–11, 1945.
13. Camargo FP, Cordeiro EN, Napoli MM. Corrective osteotomy of the spine in ankylosing spondylitis. Experience with 66 cases. *Clin Orthop* 208:157–167, 1986.
14. Myllykangas-Luosujarvi R, Aho K, Lehtinen K, et al. Increased incidence of alcohol-related deaths from accidents and violence in subjects with ankylosing spondylitis. *Br J Rheumatol* 37:688–690, 1988.
15. Fagge CH. Diseases of the osseous system. Case No. 1. *Trans Path Soc Lond* 28:201–206, 1877.
16. Hanson CA, Shagrin JW, Duncan H. Vertebral osteoporosis in ankylosing spondylitis. *Clin Orthop Rel Res* 74:59–64, 1971.
17. Mullaji AB, Upadhyay SS, Ho EKW. Bone mineral density in ankylosing spondylitis. *J Bone Joint Surg Br* 76:660–665, 1994.
18. Will R, Palmer R, Bhalla AK, et al. Osteoporosis in early ankylosing spondylitis: a primary pathologic event? *Lancet* 2:1483–1485, 1989.
19. Toussirot E, Wendling D. L'osteoporose de la spondylarthrite ankylosante. *Presse Med* 25:720–724, 1996.
20. Hunter T, Dubo H. Spinal fractures complicating ankylosing spondylitis. *Ann Intern Med* 88:546–549, 1978.
21. Hunter T, Dubo H. Spinal fractures complicating ankylosing spondylitis: a long-term study. *Arthritis Rheum* 26:751–759, 1983.
22. Cooper C, Carbone L, Michet CJ, et al. Fracture risk in patients with ankylosing spondylitis: a population based study. *J Rheumatol* 21:1877–1882, 1994.
23. Ralston SH, Urquhart GDK, Brzeski M, et al. Prevalence of vertebral compression fractures due to osteoporosis in ankylosing spondylitis. *Br Med J* 300:563–565, 1990.
24. Calin A, Porta J, Fries JF, et al. Clinical history as a screening test for ankylosing spondylitis. *JAMA* 237:2613–2614, 1977.
25. Kellgren JH, Jeffrey MR, Ball J. *The epidemiology of chronic rheumatism*. Oxford, UK: Blackwell Scientific, 1963.
26. The HSG, Steven MM, Van der Linden SM, et al. Evaluation of diagnostic criteria for ankylosing spondylitis: a comparison of the Rome, New York, and Modified New York criteria in patients with a positive clinical history screening test for ankylosing spondylitis. *Br J Rheumatol* 24:242–249, 1985.
27. van der Linden S. *Spondylitis ankylopoetica. Een famile en bevolkingsonderzoet en toetsing van diagnostische criteria*. Leiden: University of Leiden, 1982.
28. Calin A, Fries JF. The striking prevalence of ankylosing spondylitis in healthy W27 positive males and females: a controlled study. *N Engl J Med* 293:835, 1975.
29. Calin A, Garrett S, Whitelock H, et al. A new approach to defining functional ability in ankylosing spondylitis: the development of the Bath Ankylosing Spondylitis Functional Index. *J Rheumatol* 21:2281–2285, 1994.
30. Dougados M, Gueguen A, Nakache JP, et al. Evaluation of a functional index and an articular index in ankylosing spondylitis. *J Rheumatol* 15:302–307, 1988.
31. Calabro JJ. Clinical aspects of juvenile and adult ankylosing spondylitis. *Br J Rheumatol* 22(suppl 2):104–109, 1983.
32. Correia J, et al. Uveitis. *Acta Med Port* 11:877–881, 1998.
33. Wolfe F. Comparative usefulness of C-reactive protein and erythrocyte sedimentation rate in patients with rheumatoid arthritis. *J Rheumatol* 24:1477–1485, 1997.
34. Wolfe F, Michaud K. The clinical and research significance of the erythrocyte sedimentation rate. *J Rheumatol* 21:1227–1237, 1994.
35. Bessette L, Katz N, Liang MH. Differential diagnosis and conservative treatment of rheumatic disorders. In: Frymoyer JW, ed. *The adult spine*. Philadelphia: Lippincott-Raven, 1997:804–809.
36. Ruof J, Stucki G. Validity aspects of erythrocyte sedimentation rate and c-reactive protein in ankylosing spondylitis: a literature review. *J Rheumatol* 26:966–970, 1999.
37. van der Linden S. Ankylosing spondylitis. In: Kelley WN, Ruddy S, Harris ED, et al, eds. *Textbook of rheumatology*. Philadelphia: WB Saunders, 1997:969–982.
38. Spoorenberg A, van der Heijde D, de Klerk E, et al. Relative value of erythrocyte sedimentation rate and C-reactive protein in assessment of disease activity in ankylosing spondylitis. *J Rheumatol* 26:980–984, 1999.
39. Sheehan NJ, Slavin BM, Donovan MP, et al. Lack of correlation between clinical disease activity and erythrocyte sedimentation rate, acute phase proteins or protease inhibitors in ankylosing spondylitis. *Br J Rheumatol* 25:171–174, 1986.
40. Laurent MR, Panayi GS. Acute-phase proteins and serum immunoglobulins in ankylosing spondylitis. *Ann Rheum Dis* 42:524–528, 1983.
41. Macdonald AG, Birkinshaw G, Durham B, et al. Biomechanical markers of bone turnover in seronegative spondyloarthropathy: relationship to disease activity. *Br J Rheumatol* 35:50–53, 1997.
42. Marhoffer W, Stracke H, Masoud I, et al. Evidence of impaired cartilage/bone turnover in patients with active ankylosing spondylitis. *Ann Rheum Dis* 54:556–559, 1995.
43. Lang U, Boss B, Teichmann J, et al. Serum amyloid A—an indicator of inflammation in ankylosing spondylitis. *Rheumatol Int* 19:119–122, 2000.
44. Jajic I. The role of HLA—B27 in the diagnosis of low back pain. *Acta Orthop Scand* 50:411–413, 1979.
45. van der Linden SM, Valkenburg HA, De Jongh BM, et al. The risk of developing ankylosing spondylitis in HLA-B27–positive individuals. *Arthritis Rheum* 27:241–249, 1984.
46. Maksymowych WP, Suarez–Almazor M, Chou C, et al. Polymorphism in the LMP2 gene influences susceptibility to extraspinal disease in HLA-B27 positive individuals with ankylosing spondylitis. *Ann Rheum Dis* 54:321–324, 1995.
47. Maksymowych WP, Tao S, Vaile J, et al. LMP2 polymorphism is associated with extraspinal disease in HLA—B27 negative Caucasian and Mexican Mestizo patients with ankylosing spondylitis. *J Rheumatol* 27:183–189, 2000.
48. Oostvee J, Prevo R, den Boer J, et al. Early detection of sacroiliitis on magnetic resonance imaging and subsequent development of sacroiliitis on plain radiography. A prospective, longitudinal study. *J Rheumatol* 26:1953–1958, 1999.
49. Yu W, Feng F, Dion E, et al. Comparison of radiography, computed tomography and magnetic resonance imaging in the detection of sacroiliitis accompanying ankylosing spondylitis. *Skel Radiol* 27:311–320, 1998
50. Calabro JJ. Sustained—released Indomethacin in the management of ankylosing spondylitis. *Am J Med* 79(suppl 4C):39–51, 1985.
51. Wasner C, Britton MC, Kraines G, et al. Nonsteroidal anti-inflammatory agents in rheumatoid arthritis and ankylosing spondylitis. *JAMA* 246:2168–2172, 1981.
52. Clegg DO, et al. Comparison of sulfasalazine and placebo in the treatment of ankylosing spondylitis. A Department of Veterans Affairs Cooperative Study. *Arthritis Rheum* 39:2004–2012, 1996.
53. Ferraz MB, Tugwell P, Goldsmith CH, et al. Meta-analysis of sulfasalazine in ankylosing spondylitis. *J Rheumatol* 17:1482–1486, 1990.
54. Godfrey RG, Calabro JJ, Mills D, et al. A double-blind crossover trial aspirin, indomethacin and phenylbutazone in ankylosing spondylitis. *Arthritis Rheum* 15:110, 1972.
55. Sharp J, Purser DW. Spontaneous atlanto-axial dislocation ankylosing spondylitis and rheumatoid arthritis. *Ann Rheum Dis* 20:47–77, 1961.
56. Ramos-Remus C, Gomez-Vargus A, Hernandez-Chavez A, et al. Two year follow-up of anterior and vertical atlantoaxial subluxation in ankylosing spondylitis. *J Rheumatol* 24:507–510, 1997.
57. Martel W. The occipito-atlanto-axial joints in rheumatoid arthritis and ankylosing spondylitis. *AJR* 86:223–240, 1961.
58. Weinstein PR, Karpman RR, Gall EP, et al. Spinal cord injury, spinal fractures, and spinal stenosis in ankylosing spondylitis. *J Neurosurg* 57:609–616, 1982.
59. Magerl F, Seeman P. Stable posterior fusion of the atlas and axis by transarticular screw fixation. In: Kehr P, Weidner A, eds. *Cervical spine I. Strasbourg*. New York: Springer-Verlag, 1987:322–327.

60. Coyne TJ, Fehlings MG, Wallace MC, et al. C1-C2 posterior cervical fusion: long-term evaluation of results and efficacy. *Neurosurgery* 37:688–692; discussion 692–693, 1995.
61. Fang HSY, Ong GB. Direct anterior approach to the upper cervical spine. *J Bone Joint Surg* 44:1588–1604, 1962.
62. Graham B, Van Peteghem PK. Fractures of the spine in ankylosing spondylitis: diagnosis, treatment, and complications. *Spine* 14:803–807, 1987.
63. Lemmen LJ, Laing PG. Fracture of the cervical spine in patients with rheumatoid arthritis. *J Neurosurg* 16:542–550, 1959.
64. Woodruff FP, Dewing SB. Fracture of the cervical spine in patients with ankylosing spondylitis. *Radiology* 80:17–23, 1963.
65. Kanefield D, Mullins BP, Freehafer A, et al. Destructive lesions of the spine in rheumatoid ankylosing spondylitis. *J Bone Joint Surg* 51:1369–1375, 1969.
66. Kewalramani LS, Taylor RG, Albrand OW. Cervical spine injury in patients with ankylosing spondylitis. *J Trauma* 15:931–934, 1975.
67. Lieberg OU, Spengler DM, Bailey RW. Two-level disruption of the ankylosed spine: a case report. *J Trauma* 15:1064–1066, 1975.
68. Osgood C, Abbasy M, Matthews T. Multiple spine fractures in ankylosing spondylitis. *J Trauma* 15:163–166, 1975.
69. Bohlman H. Acute fractures and dislocations of the cervical spine. *J Bone Joint Surg* 61:1119–1142, 1979.
70. Olerud C, Frost A, Bring J. Spinal fractures in patients with ankylosing spondylitis. *Eur Spine J* 5:51–55, 1996.
71. Osgood C, Martin LG, Ackerman E. Fracture-dislocation of the cervical spine with ankylosing spondylitis. *J Neurosurg* 39:764–769, 1973.
72. Murray GC, Persellin RH. Cervical fracture complicating ankylosing spondylitis. *Am J Med* 70:1033–1041, 1981.
73. Bergman EW. Fractures of the ankylosed spine. *J Bone Joint Surg Am* 31:669–671, 1949.
74. Grisolia A, Bell RL, Peltier LF. Fractures and dislocations of the spine complicating ankylosing spondylitis. *J Bone Joint Surg Am* 49:339–344, 1967.
75. Janda WE, Kelly PJ, Rhoton AL, et al. Fracture dislocation of the cervical part of the spinal column in patients with ankylosing spondylitis. *Mayo Clin Proc* 43:714–721, 1968.
76. Surin VV. Fractures of the cervical spine in patients with ankylosing spondylitis. *Acta Orthop Scand* 51:79–84, 1980.
77. Young JS, Cheshire DJE, Pierce JA, et al. Cervical ankylosis acute spinal cord injury. *Paraplegia* 15:133–146, 1977.
78. Harding JR, McCall IW, Park WM, et al. Fracture of the cervical spine in ankylosing spondylitis. *Br J Radiol* 58:3–7, 1985.
79. Kiwerski J, Wieclarvek H, Garwacka I. Fractures of the cervical spine in ankylosing spondylitis. *Int Orthop* 8:243–246, 1985.
80. Gelman MI, Unber JS. Fractures of the thoracolumbar spine in ankylosing spondylitis. *AJR* 130:485, 1978.
81. Hanson CA, Shagrin JW, Duncan H. Vertebral osteoporosis in ankylosing spondylitis. *Clin Orthop* 74:59, 1971.
82. Heywood AWB, Smith P, Majoos F. Spinal pseudoarthrosis in ankylosing spondylitis. *J Bone Joint Surg Br* 64:146, 1982.
83. Lorber A, Pearson CM, Rene RM. Osteolytic vertebral lesions as a manifestation of rheumatoid arthritis and related disorders. *Arthritis Rheum* 4:514, 1961.
84. Trent G, Armstrong GWD, O'Neil J. Thoracolumbar fractures in ankylosing spondylitis. *Clin Orthop* 227:61–66, 1988.
85. Hansen ST, Taylor TKF, Honet JC, et al. Fracture dislocations of the ankylosed thoracic spine in rheumatoid spondylitis. *J Trauma* 7:827, 1967.
86. Simmons EH. Kyphotic deformity of the spine in ankylosing spondylitis. *Clin Orthop* 128:65–77, 1977.
87. Urist MR. Osteotomy of the cervical spine. *J Bone Joint Surg Am* 40:833–843, 1958.
88. Mehdian SMH, Freeman BJC, Licina P. Cervical osteotomy for ankylosing spondylitis: an innovative variation on an existing technique. *Eur Spine J* 8:505–509, 1999.
89. May DM, Jones SJ, Crockard HA. Somatosensory evoked potential monitoring in cervical surgery: identification of pre and intraoperative risk factors associated with neurological deterioration. *J Neurosurg* 85:566–573, 1996.
90. Shimizu K, Matsushita M, Fujibayashi S, et al. Correction of kyphotic deformity of the cervical spine in ankylosing spondylitis using general anesthesia and internal fixation. *J Spinal Disord* 9:540–543, 1996.
91. Thomasen E. Vertebral osteotomy for correction of kyphosis in ankylosing spondylitis. *Clin Orthop* 194:142–146, 1985.
92. Scudese V, Calabro JJ. Vertebral wedge osteotomy. *JAMA* 186:627, 1963.
93. Jaffray D, Becker V, Eisenstein S. Closing wedge osteotomy with transpedicular fixation in ankylosing spondylitis. *Clin Orthop* 279:122–126, 1992.
94. van Royen B, Slot GH. Closing-wedge posterior osteotomy for ankylosing spondylitis. *J Bone Joint Surg Br* 77:117–121, 1995.
95. Danisa OA, Turner D, Richardson WJ. Surgical correction of lumbar kyphotic deformity:posterior reduction "eggshell" osteotomy. *J Neurosurg* 92:50–56, 2000.
96. Hehne HJ, Zielke K, Bohm H. Polysegmental lumbar osteotomies and transpedicled fixation for correction of long-curved kyphotic deformities in ankylosing spondylitis. *Clin Orthop* 258:49–55, 1990.
97. Law WA. Lumbar spinal osteotomy. *J Bone Joint Surg Br* 41:270–278, 1959.
98. Law WA. Osteotomy of the spine. *J Bone Joint Surg Am* 44:1199–1206, 1962.
99. Law WA. Osteotomy of the spine. *Clin Orthop* 66:70–76, 1969.
100. Law WA. Surgical treatment of the rheumatic diseases. *J Bone Joint Surg Br* 34:215–225, 1952.
101. Lichtblau PO, Wilson PD. Possible mechanism of aortic rupture in orthopaedic correction of rheumatoid spondylitis. *J Bone Joint Surg* 38:123–127, 1956.
102. Klems H, Friedebold G. Ruptur der Aorta abdominalis nach Aufrichtungsoperation bei Spondylitis ankylopoetica. *Z Orthop* 108:554–563, 1971.
103. Weatherley C, Jaffray D, Terry A. Vascular complications associated with osteotomy in ankylosing spondylitis: a report of two cases. *Spine* 13:43–46, 1988.
104. Adams JC. Technique, dangers and safeguards in osteotomy. *J Bone Joint Surg Br* 34:226, 1952.
105. La Chapelle EH. Osteotomy of the lumbar spine for correction of kyphosis in a case of ankylosing spondyloarthritis. *J Bone Joint Surg* 28:851–858, 1946.
106. Bohm H, Harms J, Donk R, et al. Correction and stabilization of angular kyphosis. *Clin Orthop* 258:56–61, 1990.
107. Halm H, Metz-Stavenhagen P, Zielke K. Results of surgical correction of kyphotic deformities of the spine in ankylosing spondylitis on the basis of the modified arthritis impact measurement scales. *Spine* 20:1612–1619, 1995.
108. Stybo K, Bossers GT, Slot GH. Osteotomy for kyphosis in ankylosing spondylitis. *Acta Orthop Scand* 56:294–297, 1985.
109. Weal AE, Marsh CH, Yeoman PM. Secure fixation of lumbar osteotomy. *Clin Orthop* 321:216–222, 1995.
110. Ohlin A, Karlsson M, Duppe H, et al. Complications after transpedicular stabilization of the spine. *Spine* 19:2774–2779, 1994.
111. Thiranont N, Netrawichien P. Transpedicular decancellation closed wedge vertebral osteotomy for treatment of fixed flexion deformity of spine in ankylosing spondylitis. *Spine* 18:2517–2522, 1993.
112. Andersson O. Rontgenbilden vid spondylarthritis ankylopoetica. *Nordisk Medicinsk Tidskr* 14:2000–2002, 1937.
113. Endstrom G. Is spondylarthritis ankylopoetica an independent disease or a rheumatic syndrome? *Acta Med Scand* 104:396, 1940.
114. Cawley MID, Chalmers TM, Kellgran JH, et al. Destructive lesions of vertebral bodies in ankylosing spondylitis. *Ann Rheum Dis* 31:345–358, 1972.
115. Kabasakal Y, Garrett SL, Calin A. The epidemiology of spondylodiscitis in ankylosing spondylitis—a controlled study. *Br J Rheumatol* 35:660–663, 1996.
116. Little H, Urowitz MB, Smythe HA, et al. Asymptomatic spondylodiscitis. An unusual feature of ankylosing spondylitis. *Arthritis Rheum* 17:487–493, 1974.
117. Rivelis M, Freiberger RH. Vertebral destruction at unfused segments in late ankylosing spondylitis. *Radiology* 93:251–256, 1969.
118. Sutherland IL, Matheson D. Inflammatory involvement of vertebrae in ankylosing spondylitis. *Rheumatology* 2:296–302, 1975.
119. Wise CM, Irby WR. Spondylodiscitis in ankylosing spondylitis: variable presentations. *J Rheumatol* 10:1004–1006, 1983.
120. Rasker JJ, Prevo RL, Lanting PJH. Spondylodiscitis in ankylosing spondylitis, inflammation or trauma? *Scand J Rheumatol* 25:52–57, 1996.

121. Rosen PS, Graham DC. Ankylosing (Strümpell-Marie) spondylitis. (A clinical review of 128 cases). *Arch Int Rheumatol* 5:158–233, 1962.
122. Schulitz KP. Destruktive Veranderungen an Wirbelkorpern bei der Spondylarthritis Ankylopoetica. *Arch Orthop Unfall Chir* 64: 116–134, 1968.

123. Loyout P, Gaucher A, Mathieu J, et al. La spondylodiscite de la spondylarthrite ankylosante. *Rev Rhum* 30:263, 1963.
124. Streda A. Inflammatory destructive changes in the spinal column in ankylosing spondylitis. *Radiol Diagn* 5:43, 1964.
125. Hunter T. The spinal complications of ankylosing spondylitis. *Semin Arthritis Rheum* 19:172–182, 1989.

155. Initial Evaluation and Treatment of Patients with Spinal Trauma

Michael P.B. Kilburn,
Donald P. Smith III, and
Mark N. Hadley

An alarming number of individuals sustain trauma each year in the United States, the majority related to motor vehicle accidents, falls, and violent assault. Approximately 200,000 of these traumatic incidents result in human vertebral column injury, and roughly 10% to 15% of these result in injury to the spinal cord with neurological deficit (1–6). Most investigators will argue that the majority of spinal injuries are preventable, and virtually all will agree that once a spinal column injury does occur, the initial management of that injury has a major impact on neurological outcome and long-term survival (1,2,7–12). Despite this consensus, there is a remarkable variability in the timing, intensity, and completeness of the initial management of patients who have sustained spinal trauma from clinician to clinician and from institution to institution across North America. This chapter attempts to bring together the best elements from a variety of management schemes and provide the most up-to-date, contemporary management paradigm for patients with spinal column and spinal cord injury available today (10, 12–14).

A variety of pioneers have contributed to the medical foundations of the management of patients who have sustained acute spinal column and spinal cord injuries. As we learn from the lessons of the past and continue clinical and basic science investigation into the dilemmas of the present, treatment for future spinal column/spinal cord injury will be optimized.

in a given year. It is predicted that by the year 2025, 24% of patients who sustain spinal column trauma will be over 60 years of age (5).

The incidence of spinal column injury has been on the rise in recent years. Motor vehicle accidents (MVAs) continue to be the most common cause. Despite mandatory seat belt and occupant restraint legislation in nearly all 50 states, the majority of MVA-related spinal injuries occur among passengers who are unrestrained at the time of their accident. A review by Huelke and colleagues (4) finds that if an accident is severe enough to disable one or more vehicles, restrained passengers have a 1 in 300 likelihood of severe cervical spinal injury. His group notes, however, that if passengers are unrestrained and ejected from the vehicle, the likelihood of severe spinal injury soars to 1 in 14 individuals.

Following MVAs, falls, violence, and sports- or leisure-related trauma (diving) account for the next most common causes of vertebral column injury (15–21). Athletic-related spinal column and spinal cord injuries have been on the wane over the last decade, mainly due to equipment modifications and rules changes, except in the sport of hockey, in which the incidence of injury has increased despite equipment and rules changes (22). Diving accidents as a cause of spinal column and spinal cord injuries remain an important cause of quadriplegia among individuals 12 to 25 years old. The incidence of these injuries in North America has diminished somewhat over the last 10 years, in part due to public education and injury awareness programs like "Think First", offered in schools to adolescents.

Epidemiology

Approximately 200,000 traumatic vertebral column injuries occur each year in the United States. Roughly 10% to 15% of these injuries result in spinal cord injury with neurological deficit (1,2,3,5). There are probably an additional 10,000 victims of acute spinal column trauma who do not survive their initial injuries, individuals believed to have succumbed at the scene of their accident due to high spinal cord transection, paralysis, and respiratory failure (6).

Males between the ages of 15 and 25 years are most likely to sustain traumatic spine and spinal cord injury. Older adults, an ever-increasing portion of the U.S. population, currently account for 11% of patients who sustain traumatic spinal injuries

Field Management

The diagnosis of a traumatic vertebral column or spinal cord injury is made by history, physical examination, and radiological investigation. This process must begin at the scene of the trauma and must be initiated by the rescue personnel who first attend to the victim. The importance of recognizing the potential for a vertebral column injury, particularly of the cervical spine, cannot be overstated. Emergency medical personnel must maintain a high index of suspicion for a potential spinal injury among any victim of trauma they respond to. Immobilization of the spinal column as outlined by the Advanced Trauma Life Support (ATLS) protocol of the American College of Surgeons must accompany ongoing extrication and resuscitative efforts (23).

Removal of the victim from risk of further injury is the first priority at any accident scene, followed by the ABC's of resuscitation in order to restore or maintain the injured individual's vital functions. Immediate immobilization of the patient "as they lie" followed by protection and maintenance of the airway are primary concerns. Victims encountered by trained emergency medical personnel should be log rolled into the supine position on a long rigid backboard. The victim's head and neck must be held immobile with respect to their torso (Fig. 1). One care provider can accomplish this by two distinct means. The solo care provider can kneel to the victim's right side, hold the victim's head with their left hand, using the right hand to grasp the victim's mandible near the genu on either side (one can provide upward lift of the jaw to improve the victim's airway with this maneuver as well). The muscular side of the forearm can be pressed against the victim's chest to immobilize the head and neck with respect to the torso. If the victim attempts to sit up or roll, the rescuer is mechanically well positioned to resist these maneuvers while maintaining relative immobility of the victim's head and both the cervical and thoracic spinal segments. If the rescuer is one of several, they can be positioned at the head of the victim, immobilizing the head and neck of the victim in the neutral position between the forearms. The rescuer's hands should be firmly attached to the victim's shoulder girdle musculature at the base of the neck on either side. This maneuver not only serves to immobilize the victim's head and cervical spinal segment but allows other rescuers access to the airway, access for intravenous (i.v.) line placement, assessment of other injuries, and so forth.

Supplemental oxygen should be provided to the injury victim early in the resuscitation. Assistance with ventilation may be required. Orotracheal intubation using the chin-lift method with in-line axial traction and immobilization of the head and neck may be required. Nasotracheal intubation is the preferred method of securing the victim's airway but the patient must be breathing spontaneously and the rescuer needs some degree of experience in performing the maneuver (24). It is far better to intubate a severely injured patient with possible spinal injury prior to transport than for the patient to experience ventilatory/respiratory failure in transit. The insertion of two large-bore i.v. lines running 0.9% saline or Ringer's lactate solution must occur early in the resuscitation process. A mean arterial blood pressure (MAP) of 85 mm Hg via bolus infusion should be the target of hemodynamic resuscitation, especially if a spinal cord injury is suspected (10). Hypotension, even neurogenic shock, are not uncommon sequelae to multisystem trauma, particularly if the patient has sustained a severe spinal cord injury, and must be dealt with aggressively with the use of crystalloid, colloid, and when necessary, vagolytics such as atropine and glycopyrrolate (25,26). The use of sympathomimetics, such as dopamine and norepinephrine, can help maintain MAP early in the resuscitation and transport process in patients who are hypotensive but not volume deficient. This, however, requires direct physician assessment, administration, and monitoring.

Clues to the pattern of potential spinal injury may often be discerned from the victim or from the scene of the trauma. Every effort should be made to question anyone who may have been witness to the accident to assist in determining the likely mechanisms of injury. Survivors of motor vehicle trauma often have coexistent moderate to severe traumatic brain injury (TBI), which can further complicate their clinical assessment and management (1,26). Indeed TBI, or even less severe external injuries to the scalp or skull, can suggest to an experienced clinician the potential of an occult neck injury and the means by which it may have occurred. This can be especially helpful in the circumstance of serious TBI and in situations where intoxication is present, when no direct patient history can be provided. It must be remembered that the incidence of spinal column/spinal cord injury in the presence of TBI may approach 60% (1,27). In unconscious patients other clinical examination clues may suggest co-existent spinal injury. The presence of a mandibular fracture may suggest an upper cervical spine injury. Clavicle or high rib fractures may coexist with lower cervical spine or upper thoracic spine injury. Ecchymosis, abrasions, and supra-prominent spinous processes identified on the initial clinical survey may overlie thoracic, thoracolumbar, or lumbar fractures.

At any scene of accident or trauma, time is of the essence. Emergency medical personnel must assess, extricate, immobilize, provide essential resuscitation, tamponade hemorrhage, place i.v. lines, ensure or provide an airway, and prepare the patient for timely transport to a definitive care facility. The victim should be strapped to a long, rigid spine board, with the

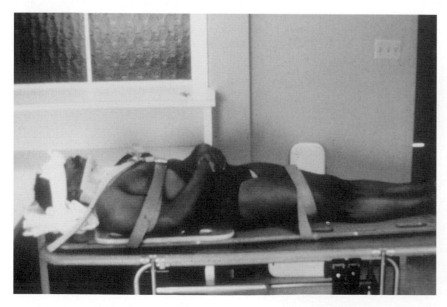

Fig. 1. Trauma victim immobilized on long spine board for transport purposes. Collar and short board were used by emergency medical technicians initially during extrication. Note immobilization of entire patient head, neck, thorax, and lower extremities until injury can be excluded.

extremities immobilized in addition to the entire spinal column. A collar is not a definitive immobilization device for cervical spine fracture injuries (1,28). Too often, once a collar is placed, the cervical spine is considered "immobilized." While collars provide some external support, they must be used in conjunction with active immobilization and observation from care providers. They can obscure important clinical findings such as tracheal deviation and untoward jugular venous distention. If used, collars must be reassessed often. The head and torso must be immobilized with tape, straps, or caregiver restraint (1,29, 30). Sandbag immobilization of the head and cervical spine has been advocated as a transport immobilization adjunct. Its use requires strict attention from care providers. Sandbags are heavy and if the long extrication board is tipped side to side during evacuation and transport, they can slide, resulting in lateral displacement of the victim's head and neck with respect to their torso. Sandbags can be taped in proper position to a long board, but because they are small compared to the patient, this can be difficult and/or ineffective. Finally, sandbags must be removed prior to initial lateral cervical spine x-ray assessment because they can obscure the radiographic bony anatomy of the cervical spine.

We prefer use of lightweight, compressible, rolled fire blankets as immobilization adjuncts for the transport of patients with potential cervical spinal injuries, rather than sandbags. Fire blankets can be rolled tight, placed next to the victim's head and neck, from the top of the shoulder upward. They can be built up higher than the ventral surfaces of the victim's head and neck and can be strapped to the long board and secured to the victim with tape, aiding true immobilization (1,31). Fire blankets are lightweight, will not create lateral neck displacement if the long board is tipped from one side to another, and they can be used in the emergency department and imaged through during the initial x-ray assessment of the cervical spine, if necessary.

Emergency Department Care and Triage

Once the injury victim arrives in the emergency department (ED), the medical priorities change from removing the victim from further harm, resuscitation, evacuation, and transport, to saving the victim's life, more thorough, complete resuscitation, and determination of the nature and extent of injury. Both the intensity and sophistication of this process magnifies. In most medical facilities, a "trauma team" comprised of a general surgeon, neurosurgeon, orthopedic surgeon (if long bone fractures are present), and an experienced staff of nurses and assistants will simultaneously assess the victim. The adequacy of the initial resuscitation efforts, i.v. lines, and airway adjuncts are reassessed and refortified as indicated. Unintubated patients with respiratory distress or severe injuries for which airway control and assisted ventilation will be an advantage should be intubated. Large bore central venous catheters and bladder catheters should be inserted. Volume resuscitation will be guided by blood pressure, central venous pressure, and other perfusion parameters. Before the patient is removed from restraints, three rapid initial portable radiographs should be obtained; an anterior-posterior (AP) view of the chest, an AP view of the abdomen, and a lateral view of the cervical spine.

During the initial ED assessment, the patient should be examined in detail. The presence or absence of bilateral breath sounds should be ascertained. Open wounds should be briefly examined, tamponaded as needed, and covered with saline-soaked sterile gauze. Jugular venous distention, tracheal deviation, and tympany over the chest wall or abdomen should be looked for and acted upon if noted. The patient's functional status and neurological examination must be assessed and recorded. If the patient's level of consciousness permits, a complete, reproducible neurological assessment, including level of consciousness and mentation assessment, motor, sensory, and reflex examination testing abdominal and cremasteric reflexes, and a rectal examination, must be performed and documented during this initial phase. We prefer the American Spinal Injury Association (ASIA) impairment scale for this purpose. It allows definitive assessment of neurological abilities with respect to spinal cord function, both motor and sensory, and provides a benchmark assessment against which all further examinations can be compared (10,32).

Patients who have sustained TBI or who are intoxicated cannot cooperate with this complete assessment, but reflex examination, sphincter tone assessment, and provocation testing (withdrawal to painful stimuli) can assist in determining segmental spinal function and integrity. Patients who have sustained significant spinal cord injury may not be able to provide characteristic clinical clues to serious chest and abdominal injuries due to muscular paralysis or sensory loss below the level of cord compromise. Chest and abdominal computed tomography (CT) assessment and/or peritoneal lavage should be readily considered in these patients. In addition to potential chest or abdominal traumatic injury, long-bone fractures are often missed in the presence of spinal column injury. It is estimated that 10% to 15% of fractures not involving the spine are missed under these circumstances (27,33).

Once the initial ED assessment by the trauma team and/or neurosurgeon is complete, a complete spinal x-ray assessment is mandatory. This should include AP and lateral views of the cervical spine through the T1 level (a swimmer's view may be required), an open mouth view of C1-2 articulations and the odontoid process (an oblique "pillar view" of the dens is an alternative), and AP and lateral views of the thoracic and lumbar spine and of the pelvis. Radiographic assessment for noncontiguous spinal fracture injuries must be undertaken as their incidence approaches 15% in this multiple injury population (33–35). Any radiographic evidence of fracture or dislocation injury on these radiographs should prompt thin-section CT assessment of the region in question (1,3,36,37).

If the cervicothoracic junction cannot be visualized well with standard radiographic techniques, CT assessment with sagittal reconstruction can be of great help in assessment of this important potential site of spinal injury. Patients with neurological deficits from potential spinal cord injury must also be assessed with thin-section CT, the specific spinal examination to be directed by the level of potential cord dysfunction, irrespective of the plain x-ray appearance of that spinal segment (1,2,3,37).

Multiple injury patients may require CT assessment of TBI, chest and abdominal injury, as well as vertebral column injury. The priority of these examinations will be dictated by the coordinated efforts of the neurosurgeon and trauma surgeon and the patient's condition. As a general rule, head and abdominal CT studies are obtained first depending on the neurological status and hemodynamic stability of the victim. Spinal and chest CT studies are obtained next. Any and all of these studies can be obtained while the patient remains restrained and immobilized on a long spine board. Emergent brain operations and/or laparotomies as necessary to save the patient's life can effectively be accomplished with close neurosurgical and anesthetic attention to the immobilization of the spinal column and adequate perfusion of the spinal cord, even if a cervical or thoracic spinal fracture-dislocation injury is present.

Definitive Early Care

If the resuscitated patient has a spinal fracture without spinal cord or nerve root injury, the radiographic features of the fracture and the mechanism of injury dictate its initial care. A lumbar transverse process fracture, a nondisplaced lamina fracture, a slight vertebral body compression fracture, or a small anterior-inferior chip fracture of a cervical vertebra may require little or no care other than symptomatic musculoskeletal therapy, analgesics, and clinical follow-up (3,38,39). Most other fractures of the vertebral column are more serious and have the potential of being associated with acute spinal instability, delayed spinal instability with deformity, and/or neural compression without overt initial neurological injury. Patients with traumatic spinal fractures should be kept immobilized until definitive radiographic and CT assessment can be accomplished. Flexion-extension radiographs can provide early clues about spinal stability if a gross fracture injury or malalignment is not present on initial films. CT studies can identify multiple contiguous fractures (combination C1 and C2 fractures, for example), multiple fractures through the same vertebral segment (body fracture with a lateral mass, pars, lamina, or facet fracture), and can document the presence or absence of spinal canal compromise due to retropulsed bony fragments (compression fracture), or imploded laminar fractures. Ultimately, magnetic resonance imaging (MRI) should be considered to assess cord or root compression, disc herniation, and/or ligamentous injury (interspinous ligament disruption or transverse atlanto-ligament injury, are but two examples) in selected patients with spinal fractures (1,2,40–47). Definitive care for patients with spinal fracture injuries must be individualized based on the presence or absence of neural compression, and the anatomy, biomechanics, and natural history of the specific bony-ligamentous injury the patient has sustained.

At our institution, a patient with a cervical fracture dislocation injury is rapidly transferred from the ED or radiology suite to the neurosurgical intensive care unit (NICU) for MRI-compatible halo ring placement and invasive hemodynamic monitoring (e.g., central venous line, arterial line, Foley catheter) (Fig. 2). We proceed rapidly through attempted closed reduction with halo-ring traction using real-time fluoroscopy, beginning at 5 lbs per superior level and ceasing at realignment, a change in neurological status, overdistraction at a noninjured level, or the limit of 15 lbs per superior level. Whether we accomplish reduction or not, the patient is then secured in a halo-ring vest orthosis. We then proceed with MRI assessment. Patients with reduced, realigned injuries without cord compression are treated in the halo device or are offered nonurgent stabilization and fusion, as appropriate for their injury. Patients with irreducible injuries or with cord compression or distortion from disc blood or bone are treated with early surgical decompression, realignment, stabilization, and fusion (1,2,11,13,48–54). The principles that guide this treatment philosophy are:

1. Thoroughly assess and identify the spinal fracture injury.
2. Immobilize the patient until the severity of injury can be determined based on fracture and ligamentous injury characteristics.
3. Realign the malaligned spinal column to restore anatomical position and/or curvature.
4. *Most important*, protect, reduce, and decompress underlying neural structures.
5. Provide definitive care to allow protection and healing in as ideal an anatomical and biomechanical means as possible, using bracing, bony fusion, and internal fixation devices as necessary.

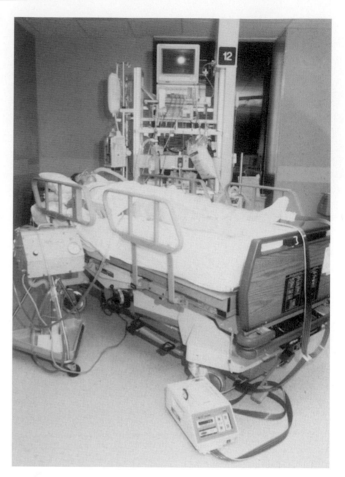

Fig. 2. The neurological intensive care unit setting allows for aggressive, acute management of the multiple-injury trauma patient. This patient has multiple rib fractures, hemothorax, and a 40% T12 compression fracture without neurological injury.

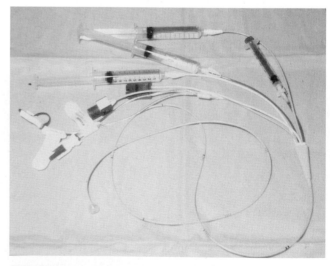

Fig. 3. The Swan-Ganz catheter is an important adjunct in the assessment and management of the patient with multiple-injury trauma, those with acute spinal cord injuries, and/or patients with cardiac dysfunction in whom aggressive resuscitation is needed.

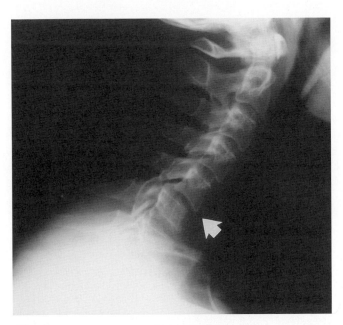

Fig. 4. Patient with acute C5-6 fracture-dislocation injury with incomplete spinal cord injury. Note facet dislocation injury and subluxation (*arrow*).

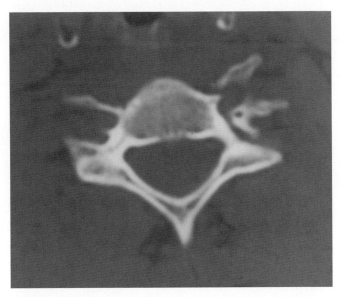

Fig. 6. CT of C6 vertebra after closed reduction of facet dislocation at C5-6. Note fracture through transverse foramen on left.

If a traumatic spinal cord injury is present, we recommend early, aggressive medical intervention to maintain spinal cord perfusion. The use of steroids within 8 hours of acute spinal cord injury is controversial (1,2,12,55–57). We attempt to maintain the patient's MAP at 85 mm Hg or better from the time of arrival. If the clinician elects to treat with steroids, a bolus infusion of methylprednisolone of 30 mg per kg over 45 minutes is administered to selected patients. A 23-hour infusion of 5.4 mg per kg is administered 15 minutes after the bolus infusion to patients who sustained spinal cord injury within 3 hours. A 47-hour infusion is recommended to those patients who sus-

tained injury between 3 and 8 hours prior to arrival. No methylprednisolone, neither bolus nor infusion, should be offered to victims who sustained spinal cord injury 8 hours or more prior to arrival. These therapeutic maneuvers are initiated in the ED as the patient is prepared for radiographic and CT examination, or as soon as possible thereafter. The implementation of these procedures may include the placement of a central venous line, an arterial line, a Foley catheter, and the administration of crystalloid, colloid, and pressors, if necessary (depending on the patient's volume status), in addition to the steroid bolus, to maintain a MAP of 85 mm Hg to bolster spinal cord perfusion (1,10). Swan-Ganz catheters are used when comprehensive hemodynamic assessment and treatment are required (Fig. 3).

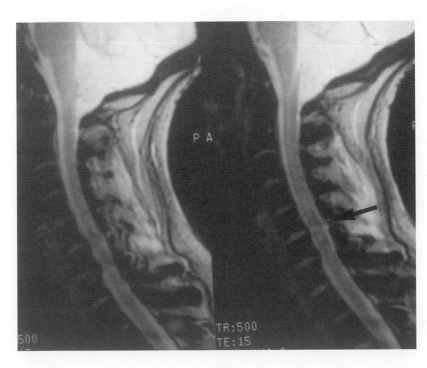

Fig. 5. MRI of the same patient as in Fig. 4, following successful closed reduction with halo-ring traction. Note signal change in cord behind C5-6 level (*arrow*).

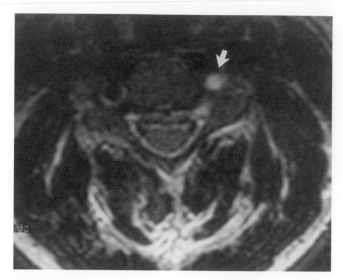

Fig. 7. Axial MRI reveals acute left vertebral artery occlusion (*arrow*).

We then follow the same treatment paradigm as described previously for the spinal fracture injury patient, but with even greater minute-to-minute attention to ventilation, oxygenation, blood pressure management, and spinal cord perfusion. Our view is that patients with spinal cord injury deserve the same early aggressive resuscitation, medical and pharmacological therapy, and surgical treatment (if indicated) as patients with acute brain injury (1,2,10,58–67) (Figs. 4–8). Not all acute spinal cord injuries, even complete injuries, are fixed and unrecoverable. We have had considerable success with this early, aggres-

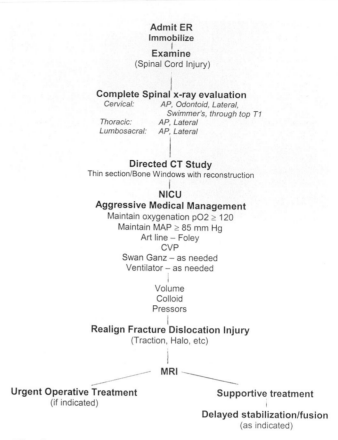

Admit ER
Immobilize
|
Examine
(Spinal Cord Injury)
|
Complete Spinal x-ray evaluation
Cervical: AP, Odontoid, Lateral,
                 Swimmer's, through top T1
Thoracic: AP, Lateral
Lumbosacral: AP, Lateral
|
Directed CT Study
Thin section/Bone Windows with reconstruction
|
NICU
Aggressive Medical Management
Maintain oxygenation pO2 ≥ 120
Maintain MAP ≥ 85 mm Hg
Art line – Foley
CVP
Swan Ganz – as needed
Ventilator – as needed
|
Volume
Colloid
Pressors
|
Realign Fracture Dislocation Injury
(Traction, Halo, etc)
|
—— **MRI** ——
Urgent Operative Treatment   **Supportive treatment**
(if indicated) |
                             Delayed stabilization/fusion
                                       (as indicated)

Fig. 9. Contemporary acute spinal column/spinal cord injury algorithm used at the University of Alabama Medical Center.

sive, combined medical-surgical treatment paradigm (Fig. 9) at our institution, and believe this approach offers the best potential for neurological recovery of any spinal cord injury treatment scheme currently available (1,2,10).

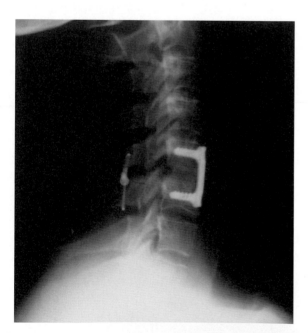

Fig. 8. Postoperative cervical spine radiograph reveals dorsal/ventral reduction, internal fixation, and fusion. Patient required dorsal approach as primary procedure due to failure to achieve anatomical reduction at facet fracture site. Marked instability required ventral approach as well. Following early surgery the patient was treated with anticoagulants for 6 months for vertebral artery injury. The patient's neurological recovery has been complete. Follow-up angiography at 6 months revealed reconstitution of injured vertebral artery.

References

1. Hadley MN, Argires PJ. The acute/emergent management of vertebral column fracture/dislocation injuries. In: *Neurological emergencies.* Vol II. The American Association of Neurological Surgeons, 249–262, 1994.
2. Hadley MN, Bishop RC. Management of craniocervical junction and upper cervical spine injuries. In: *The practice of neurosurgery.* Vol II. Baltimore: Williams & Wilkins, 1687–1701, 1996.
3. Sonntag VKH, Hadley MN. Management of upper cervical spinal instability. In: Wilkins RH, Rengadnay SS, eds. *Neurosurgery update II.* New York: McGraw-Hill, 222–233, 1991.
4. Huelke DF, et al. Cervical injuries suffered in automobile crashes. *J Neurosurg* 54:316–322, 1981.
5. Lasfargues JE, et al. A model for estimating spinal cord injury prevalence in the United States. *Paraplegia* 33:62–68, 1995.
6. Hadley MN, Sonntag VKH, Grahm TW, et al. Axis fractures resulting from motor vehicle accidents: the need for occupant restraints. *Spine* 11:861–864, 1986.
7. Ducker TB, Lucas JT, Wallace CA. Recovery from spinal cord surgery. *Clin Neurosurg* 30:495–513, 1983.
8. Frankel HL, Hancock DU, Hyslop G, et al. The value of postural reduction in the initial management of closed injuries of the spine with paraplegia and tetraplegia. *Paraplegia* 7:179–192, 1969.

9. Gillingham J. Early management of spinal cord trauma [Letter]. *J Neurosurg* 44:766–767, 1976.

10. Vale FL, Burns J, Jackson AB, et al. Combined medical and surgical treatment after acute spinal cord injury: results of a prospective pilot study to assess the merits of aggressive medical resuscitation and blood pressure management. *J Neurosurg* 87:239–246, 1997.

11. Duh M-S, Shepard MJ, Wilberger JE, et al. The effectiveness of surgery on the treatment of acute spinal cord injury and its relation to pharmacological treatment. *Neurosurgery* 35:240–249, 1994.

12. Bracken MB, Shepard MJ, Holford, TR, et al. Administration of methylprednisolone for 24 or 48 hours or tirilazad mesylate for 48 hours in the treatment of acute spinal cord injury. Results of the Third National Acute Spinal Cord Injury Randomized Controlled Trial (NASCIS III). *JAMA* 277:1597–1604, 1997.

13. Schlegel J, Bayley J, Yuan H, et al. Timing of surgical decompression and fixation of acute spinal fractures. *J Orthopaed Trauma* 10:323–330, 1996.

14. Dolan EJ, Tator CH. The effect of blood transfusion, dopamine and gamma-hydroxybutyrate on post traumatic ischemia of the spinal cord. *J Neurosurg* 56:350–358, 1982.

15. Taylor M, Thomas A, Jackowski A. Missed cervical spine injury following barflying. *J Accident Emerg Med* 13:222–223, 1996.

16. Ladd AL, Scranton PE. Congenital cervical stenosis presenting as transient quadriplegia in athletes. *J Bone Joint Surg Am* 68:1371–1374, 1986.

17. Mueller FO. Fatalities from head and cervical spine injuries occurring in tackle football: 50 years' experience. *Clin Sports Med* 17:169–182, 1998.

18. Torg JS. Epidemiology, pathomechanics, and prevention of athletic injuries to the cervical spine. *Med Sci Sports Exercise* 17:295–303, 1985.

19. Prall JA, Winston KR, Brennan R. Spine and spinal cord injuries in downhill skiers. *J Trauma: Injury Infect Crit Care* 39:1115–1118, 1995.

20. Torg JS, Das M. Trampoline-related quadriplegia: review of the literature and reflections on the American Academy of Pediatrics' Position Statement. *Pediatrics* 74:804–812, 1984.

21. Kip P, Hunter RE. Cervical spinal fractures in alpine skiers. *Orthopedics* 18:737–741, 1995.

22. Tator CH, Carson JD, Edmonds VE. Spinal injuries in ice hockey. *Clin Sports Med* 17:183–194, 1998,

23. American College of Surgeons. Spine and spinal cord trauma. In: *Advanced trauma life support instructor manual.* Chicago: American College of Surgeons, 263–300, 1997.

24. Sellick BA. Cricoid pressure to control regurgitation of stomach contents during induction of anesthesia. *Lancet* 2:404–406, 1961.

25. Troll, GF, Dohrmann GJ. Anesthesia of the spinal cord injured patient: cardiovascular problems and their management. *Paraplegia* 13:162–171, 1975.

26. Meyer, GA, Berman, IR, Poty, DB, et al. Hemodynamic responses to acute quadriplegia with or without chest trauma. *J Neurosurg* 34:168–177, 1971.

27. Galard, DE, Rhoades, ME. Orthopedic management of brain injured adults, part II. *Clin Orthoped* 131:111–122, 1978.

28. White AA, Punjabi MM. *Clinical biomechanics of the spine.* Philadelphia: JB Lippincott Co, 345–359, 1978.

29. Bodolsky S, Baraff LJ, Simon RR, et al. Efficacy of cervical spine immobilization methods. *J Trauma* 23:461–465, 1983.

30. Johnson RM, Owen BA, Hart DL, et al. Cervical orthoses: a guide to their selection and use. *Clin Orthopaed Rel Res* 154:34–45, 1981.

31. Walton R, DeSalvo JF, Ernst AA. Padded vs unpadded spine board for cervical spine immobilization. *Acad Emerg Med* 2:725–728, 1995.

32. Tator CH, Raved, DW, Schwartz ML. Sunnybrook cord injury scales for assessing neurological injury and neurological recovery. In Tator CH, ed. *Early management of acute spinal cord injury.* New York: Raven Press, 7–24, 1982.

33. Bentley G, McSweeney T. Multiple spinal injuries. *Br J Surg* 55:565–570, 1968.

34. Kewalramani L, Taylor RG. Multiple non-contiguous injuries to the spine. *Acta Orthoped Scand* 47:52–58, 1976.

35. Calenoff L, et al. Multiple level spine injuries: importance of early recognition. *AJR* 130:665–669, 1978.

36. Brant-Zawaclzki M, et al. CT in the evaluation of spinal trauma. *AJR* 136:369–375,1981.

37. Sonntag VKH, Hadley MN. Non-operative management of cervical spine injuries. *Clin Neurosurg* 34:630–649, 1986.

38. Sypert GW. Management of lower cervical spinal instability. In: Wilkins RH, Rengadnay SS, eds. *Neurosurgery update II.* New York: McGraw-Hill, 234–243, 1991.

39. Ray-Camille R, et al. Traumatismes recente descing dernieres vertebres cervicales chez l'adulte. *Hup Sem Paris* 59:1479–1488, 1983.

40. Betz RR, Gelman AJ, DeFilipp GJ, et al. Magnetic resonance imaging in the evaluation of spinal cord injured children and adolescents. *Paraplegia* 25:92–99, 1987.

41. Chakeres DW, Flickinger F, Bresnahan J, et al. MR imaging of acute spinal cord trauma. *AJNR* 8:5–10, 1987.

42. Goldberg AL, Rothfus WE, Deeb ZL. The impact of magnetic resonance on the diagnostic evaluation of acute cervicothoracic spinal trauma. *Skeletal Radiol* 17:89–95,1988.

43. Hackney DB, Asato R, Joseph PM. Hemorrhage and edema in acute spinal cord compression: demonstration by MR imaging. *Radiology* 161:387–390, 1987.

44. Kadoya S, Nakamura T, Kobayashi S, et al. Magnetic resonance imaging of acute spinal cord injury. *Neuroradiology* 29:252–255, 1987.

45. Kalfas I, Wilberger J, Goldberg A, et al. Magnetic resonance imaging in acute spinal cord trauma. *Neurosurgery* 23:295–299, 1988.

46. Pan G, Kulkarni M, MacDougall DJ, et al. Traumatic epidural hematoma of the cervical spine: diagnosis with magnetic resonance imaging. *J Neurosurg* 68:798–801, 1988.

47. Schaefer DM, Flanders A, Northrup BE, et al. Magnetic resonance imaging of acute cervical spine trauma. *Spine* 14:1090–1095, 1989.

48. Heiden JS, Weiss MH, Rosenberg AW, et al. Management of cervical spinal cord trauma in Southern California. *J Neurosurg* 43:732–736, 1975.

49. Tator CH, Duncan EG, Edmonds VE, et al. Comparison of surgical and conservative management in 208 patients with acute spinal cord injury. *Can J Neurol Sci* 14:60–69, 1987.

50. Benzel EC, Larson SJ. Functional recovery after decompressive spine operation for cervical spine fractures. *Neurosurgery* 20:742–746, 1987.

51. Wagner FC, Chehrazi B. Early decompression and neurological outcome in acute cervical spinal cord injuries. *J Neurosurg* 56:699–705, 1982.

52. Dolan EJ, Tator CH, Endrenyi L. The value of decompression for acute experimental spinal cord compression injury. *J Neurosurg* 53:749–755, 1980.

53. Guha A, Tator CH, Endrenyi L, et al. Decompression of the spinal cord improves recovery after acute experimental spinal cord compression injury. *Paraplegia* 25:324–339, 1987.

54. Ducker TB, Bellegarrigue R, Salcman M, et al. Timing of operative care in cervical spinal cord injury. *Spine* 9:525–531, 1984.

55. Bracken MB, Shepard MJ, Collins WF, et al. A randomized, controlled trial of methylprednisolone or naloxone in the treatment of acute spinal cord injury. Results of the Second National Acute Spinal Cord Injury Study (NASCIS II). *N Engl J Med* 322:1405–1411, 1990.

56. Bracken MB, Shepard MJ, Collins WF, et al. Methylprednisolone or naloxone treatment after acute spinal cord injury: 1-year follow-up data. Results of the Second National Acute Spinal Cord Injury Study (NASCIS II). *J Neurosurg* 76:23–31, 1992.

57. Bracken MB, Shepard MJ, Holford TR, et al. Methylprednisolone or tirilazad mesylate administration after acute spinal cord injury: 1 year follow up. Results of the Third National Acute Spinal Cord Injury Study (NASCIS III). *J Neurosurg* 89:699–706, 1998.

58. Levy ML, Day JD, Zelman V, et al. Cardiac performance enhancement and hypervolemic therapy. *Neurosurg Clin North Am* 5:725–739, 1994.

59. Anthes DL, Theriault E, Tator CH. Ultrastructural evidence for arteriolar vasospasm after spinal cord trauma. *Neurosurgery* 39:804–814, 1996.

60. Tator CH, Koyanagi I. Vascular mechanisms in the pathophysiology of human spinal cord injury. *J Neurosurg* 86:483–492, 1997.

61. Wallace MC, Tator CH, Frazee P. Relationship between posttraumatic ischemia and hemorrhage in the injured rat spinal cord as shown by colloidal carbon angiography. *Neurosurgery* 18:433–439, 1986.

62. Koyanagi I, Tator CH, Lea PJ. Three-dimensional analysis of the vascular system in the rat spinal cord with scanning electron microscopy of vascular corrosion casts. Part 1: Normal spinal cord. *Neurosurgery* 33:277–284, 1993.

63. Koyanagi I, Tator CH, Lea PJ. Three-dimensional analysis of the vascular system in the rat spinal cord with scanning electron microscopy of vascular corrosion casts. Part 2: acute spinal cord injury. *Neurosurgery* 33:285–292, 1993.
64. Kobrine AI, Doyle TF, Rizzoli HV. Spinal cord blood flow as affected by changes in systemic arterial blood pressure. *J Neurosurg* 44: 12–15, 1976.
65. Fried LC, Goodkin R. Microangiographic observations of the ex-perimentally traumatized spinal cord. *J Neurosurg* 35:709–714, 1971.
66. Wolf LL, Belzberg H. Hemodynamic parameters in patients with acute cervical cord trauma: description, intervention and prediction of outcome. *Neurosurgery* 33:1007–1016, 1993.
67. Fehlings MG, Tator CH, Linden RD. The effect of nimodipine and dextran on axonal function and blood flow following experimental spinal cord injury. *J Neurosurg* 71:403–416, 1989.

156. Radiological Considerations in Spine Trauma

Lisa P. Mulligan, James M. Ecklund, and John B. Stockel

Although the need to evaluate spine trauma is a daily requirement at many hospitals, the choice of imaging modality used to evaluate a patient with potential acute spinal column injury remains controversial. There are a host of imaging modalities available including plain film radiography, computed tomography (CT), and magnetic resonance imaging (MRI). Each modality has strengths and weaknesses that must be considered in a particular clinical circumstance. Specifically, one must consider the mechanism of injury, the patient's level of alertness, the neurological status, and the other associated injuries. The radiological evaluation may also be limited by the immediate availability of services at the individual medical treatment facility. In this chapter, we will discuss many of the considerations in the radiographic examination, with a particular emphasis on the evidence justifying the use of various studies. It is important to note that radiographic clearance of the cervical spine in the acute, posttraumatic setting does not exclude the possibility of a significant spinal cord injury.

Plain Film Radiography

Plain film radiography is an excellent screening tool in the evaluation of acute cervical spine trauma. Disagreement exists even with plain film radiography, however, as to what constitutes an adequate trauma series. Most authors agree that a cross-table lateral (CTL) alone is not sufficient. False-negative rates ranging from 15% to 32% have been reported (1–3). A study by Woodring and Lee looked at the accuracy of a one-view versus a three-view series [CTL, anteroposterior (AP), and open-mouth view] (3). This case series retrospectively evaluated the records of 216 consecutive patients with traumatic cervical subluxations, fractures, or dislocations at a single institution. The authors reported the initial readings by the trauma team as a prospective arm. Two radiologists later reviewed all the films establishing a retrospective arm. The retrospective arm of their study showed that the CTL radiograph alone had a 15% false-negative rate, but when viewed prospectively, the false-negative rate was actually 32%. The addition of the anterior-posterior and open mouth view increased accuracy to 94% retrospectively and 77% prospectively.

Some physicians believe that the addition of supine oblique views improve the sensitivity of the trauma series. Turetsky and colleagues (4) conducted a retrospective review of 83 trauma patients with confirmed cervical spine injuries. Each patient underwent a five-view series and a CT scan. The standard three-view was initially reviewed by three neuroradiologists followed by the obliques and CT scans. Of the 83 patients, five were found to have fractures or ligamentous injuries on the five-view series that were missed on the three-view series. Two others were found to have fractures better defined on the oblique projections. The obliques provided better visualization of the pedicles, laminae, articular pillars, and the neural foramina. Obliques may also be valuable in cases where the cervicothoracic junction is poorly visualized on standard projections especially if CT augmentation is not available.

An alternative opinion is offered by Freemyer and associates (5). These authors prospectively studied 58 high-risk patients of whom 33 had a fracture, subluxation, or dislocation. The evaluation first included only a three-view series reviewed by two radiologists and a senior emergency department physician. Next, the same reviewers were given two obliques. In that study no fractures were found on the obliques that were not already identified from the three-view series. They did acknowledge, however, that those reading the films for the study were very experienced, suggesting that in less experienced hands the five-view series may prove to be more helpful. The final recommendation, based on this small series, was for a standard three-view series to be used for the initial screening study.

The value of the plain film anterior-posterior (AP) view has also been disputed. Over a 3-year period, at a level I trauma center, Holliman and co-workers retrospectively reviewed 60 cases of spine fracture or dislocation (6). They found that no cases of cervical spine injury were detected on the AP view that were not also revealed on the lateral or odontoid view.

Plain film radiography has limitations. The injuries that are most commonly missed on plain film are at the craniocervical and cervicothoracic junctions (1-4,7–10). Several factors come into play when accounting for these false-negative readings. Image quality is often an issue in the trauma setting. Factors that can compromise success in obtaining good quality films include lack of patient cooperation, decreased mental status, intubation, and unfavorable body habitus. A good quality image however does not guarantee accurate findings. In a prospective study of 253 patients with 274 spine injuries, Reid and colleagues (11) report that 20 patients had a misinterpretation of the initial films. Only 20% of these misinterpretations were due to poor quality images. A number of the missed injuries in that study resulted from inadequately visualizing the cervicothoracic junction.

Particular attention must be paid to obtaining views that clearly demonstrate the C7-T1 junction (Fig. 1). If that is not possible with an assistant pulling down on the arms, then a swimmer's view should be obtained. If that is inadequate, then CT should be performed through the area. Even when abnormalities are identified, plain film radiography may underestimate the extent of the injuries. In the study by Woodring and Lee (3), the radiographs often misdiagnosed the extent of injury. In several patients, multiple fractures were found despite the suggestion of a single injury on initial radiographs. Therefore, a physician treating trauma patients must have a high index of suspicion for spine trauma and must be prepared to pursue other imaging modalities as appropriate to make the correct diagnosis.

The role of flexion and extension views has also been reviewed. Lewis and associates (12) retrospectively reviewed 141 patients who underwent flexion and extension views in the course of their trauma evaluation. They discovered eleven patients with spinal instability. Four of eleven had a three-view series interpreted as normal. Ten of eleven had persistent neck pain with the eleventh being intoxicated. In alert, sober patients who complain of neck pain but have normal initial plain films, flexion/extension radiographs may identify those with instability resulting from ligamentous injuries. In these situations, the patients perform flexion/extension actively so that pain can limit excessive motion. However, muscle spasm can inhibit the patient's range of motion and possibly mask a subluxation. It is therefore recommended that patients complaining of posttraumatic neck pain who are neurologically intact and have had normal radiographs but poor flexion-extension efforts, should remain in a hard collar. The films can be repeated in 1 to 2 weeks when the spasm has resolved, at which point the need for the collar can be readdressed.

Dynamic studies under fluoroscopy are sometimes used to evaluate the stability of an obtunded patient. Davis and coworkers (13) evaluated 116 patients with normal three-view cervical spine series and a Glasgow Coma Scale score less than 13 with dynamic flexion-extension views. One demonstrated a subluxation and none had neurological deterioration as a result of the examination. The chief benefit of early clearance is the prevention of decubiti from the collar. This technique, however, has an inherent risk, and must be performed by experienced

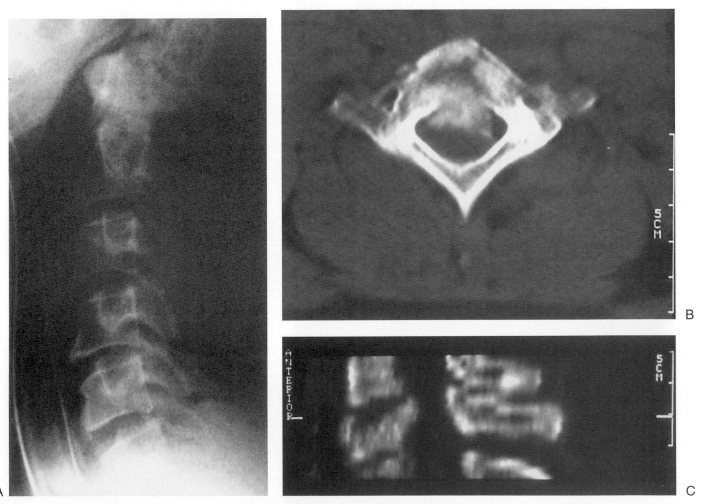

Fig. 1. A: Plain c-spine radiograph of a 43-year-old man who presented with neck pain and C8 dermatomal paresthesias after diving into shallow water. This patient's body habitus made visualization below C6 inadequate despite shoulder distraction. **B,C:** CT with reconstructed views through C7 demonstrate a C7 compression fracture with significant retropulsion into the canal.

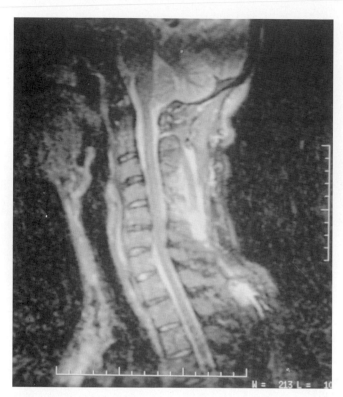

Fig. 2. T2-weighted sagittal MRI of a patient with a hyperflexion injury. Plain films were unremarkable except for the loss of normal cervical lordosis. Note the increased signal in the interspinous space at C3-4 and C4-5, suggesting disruption of the interspinous ligament.

personnel. The need for flexion-extension studies in the comatose patient may be reduced by MRI, which can also diagnose acute ligamentous injury in the absence of fracture (Fig. 2).

With regard to thoracic and lumbar injuries, a screening AP and lateral is usually sufficient (14). This study may be reserved for patients with specific complaints referable to those areas, and in patients in whom the clinical examination is compromised. In their review of 99 patients who had thoracolumbar films during their workup for blunt trauma, Samuels and Kerstein (15) report that all 58 patients who were asymptomatic had negative films. Meek (16) published the results of a retrospective study that involved 594 patients less than 40 years of age who had sustained significant blunt trauma. A 10% frequency of thoracolumbar fractures was found in that group. Meek also reports on the circumstances of six patients who had missed thoracolumbar fractures. None of those six complained of back pain or tenderness to palpation. Each, however, had either a slightly decreased mental status or another severe "distracting" injury. Likewise, patients with cervical injuries can have thoracic or lumbar injuries that can easily be missed because of their inability to perceive symptoms referable to those areas. In one study 4% of patients with cervical spine injuries had an associated thoracic spine injury, 4% had a lumbar spine injury, and 1% had both (17).

CT

CT is useful both in the diagnosis of unrecognized fractures and in the further evaluation of fractures diagnosed on plain radiographs. It provides detailed bony information of higher resolution than plain films and is especially helpful in evaluating the central bony canal and the neural foramina. Additionally, it proves useful in better visualizing fixed subluxations.

Most controversy surrounding CT revolves around its scope of use in the trauma setting. Some authors advocate limited CT evaluation (i.e., the craniocervical junction or the cervicothoracic junction), while others recommend full cervical spine CT. Several studies have been done to address the efficacy of CT in certain circumstances. Link and others (18) performed craniocervical junction CT on 202 patients with head injury. Eight occipital condyle fractures and eleven C1-C2 fractures were identified that were not discovered on the plain films. Likewise, Blacksin and Lee (19) performed craniocervical junction CT on 100 patients with head injury and found 8% to have a fracture of the occipital condyles, C1, or C2.

Similarly, CT has been studied for its usefulness in evaluating the cervicothoracic junction. Tehranzadeh and associates (20) retrospectively reviewed the records of 100 trauma patients who underwent cervicothoracic junction CT due to inadequate visualization on plain films. Of those 100, three demonstrated fractures.

Scheelhauf and co-workers (21) performed a prospective study on 104 trauma patients who underwent CT. Four groups of patients were included in the study: those with inadequate plain films, those with films suspicious for an unstable injury, those with plain films positive for an unstable injury, and those with persistent pain. Patients were also examined with conventional tomography, video cineradiography, bone scan, and flexion-extension views as dictated by their clinical scenario. Of the 56 patients in the first group, four had a scan positive for injury, one of which was found to be falsely positive by other confirmatory examinations. If we assume their final clinical diagnosis to be correct, CT has a sensitivity of 1.0 and a specificity of 0.98. These data suggest CT is a valuable tool when plain films are suboptimal. Of interest, however, when data from the other three groups were added, the sensitivity of CT dropped to 78%. This provides an argument against its use as a screening study, but the numbers in each subgroup were small. The false-negative studies all involved ligamentous injuries at the occipitocervical and atlantoaxial junctions.

Borock and colleagues (22) performed a similar prospective study in 179 traumatized patients. They used the same categories of patients as the Scheelhauf group. They report that of the 123 patients with inadequate plain films, one had a fracture. They then combined the positive and suspicious plain film categories, which totaled 54 patients. Of those, 39 were confirmed to have pathology on CT. Based on these data, the authors assigned a 28% false-positive rate to plain film examination. Two patients in this study had negative plain films with a neurological deficit. Both of these patients had abnormal findings on CT. CT was also falsely negative in one patient with a transversely oriented fracture visualized well on plain film. Based on their data, CT alone demonstrated 98% of the fractures, and in combination with a standard three-view plain film series, 100% of the injuries were demonstrated. However, no mention of follow-up was made so it is unclear if any injuries were discovered in a delayed fashion. Additionally, other tests to evaluate ligamentous stability were not reported.

Quencer and co-workers (2) propose a wide application of CT. Based on their experiences in a major trauma center, they found combining a standard plain film series and limited CT often required multiple attempts at x-rays and often more than one trip to the CT scanner. They advocate C1-7 helical CT in all high-risk patients following the CTL radiograph. These authors define patients as high risk when sustaining a mechanism of injury associated with spine trauma (i.e., high-speed motor vehicle accident), having other severe associated injuries, or having a diminished mental status. They argue that this significantly reduces the time necessary to evaluate the cervical spine radiographically. To evaluate ligamentous stability, they recommend flexion-extension films if CTL and CT are normal.

At our institution, we have found optimum cervical spine CTs are obtained by the following protocol. Axial CTs are obtained using 3-mm collimation progressing by 2-mm increments. If an abnormality is identified, the area is reimaged using 1 mm × 1 mm. If helical scanning is performed, 3-mm helical slices are used with 1:1 pitch. Images should be acquired using a detail or bone algorithm. The data can then be reprocessed to a soft tissue or standard algorithm allowing better evaluation of the paravertebral soft tissues and contents of the spinal canal. In all cases sagittal and coronal images are reconstructed from the axial data. Images reconstructed in the coronal plane are particularly useful in the evaluation of the craniocervical junction and the atlantoaxial relationship. Images reconstructed in the sagittal plane are particularly useful evaluating the relationship between the odontoid and the anterior arch of C1. Evaluating these relationships on a workstation also allows for accurate documentation of important traditional plain film measurements such as the atlantodental interval (ADI), the basion-axial interval (BAI), and the occipitoatlantal relationship using the Powers ratio or X-line method.

CT is also very useful for the further evaluation of thoracolumbar fractures (23). It is particularly helpful for determining the degree of canal compromise from retropulsed fragments from a burst fracture (Fig. 3). When imaging the T-spine on axial acquisition, 5-mm slices with 4-mm progression are used. For helical acquisition, 5-mm increments are used. If three-dimensional reconstruction is required most software packages require a zero gantry angle during image acquisition. The level above and below the fracture should be included at a minimum.

Obtaining a CT is now relatively affordable and straightforward. The scans have become very fast over the last decade. A helical cervical CT from skull base to T1 takes one minute. Axial scans require two minutes. Most seriously injured patients will require other CT studies (i.e., head, chest, abdomen, and pelvis). It is therefore relatively easy to obtain the cervical studies without requiring an additional trip out of the trauma bay. No special nonferrous, patient-stabilizing or life-support equipment is needed as is the case with MRI.

CT does have limitations, however. Noncontrasted CT provides no information about the cord, disc herniations, or ligamentous injuries. Certain types of fractures are also often missed on CT. Pech and colleagues (24) performed a cadaveric study in which six cadavers were dropped 1 to 2 M head first to simulate a diving accident. The cadavers were then scanned and subsequently sectioned on a cryotome. Two neuroradiologists reviewed the CT scans and their results were compared to the anatomical sections. CT was very accurate for body fractures, Jefferson and hangman fractures, and bilateral locked facets. However, the CTs did not reveal a transverse fracture through C2, nondisplaced spinous process fractures and certain posterior element fractures. Additionally, isolated superior articular process fractures were not visualized, but a widening in the facet secondary to hemarthrosis was consistently demonstrated.

CT and plain film myelography using intrathecal, nonionic-iodinated contrast continues to play a role in the evaluation of the acutely injured patient. It is extremely sensitive in detecting nerve root avulsions, pseudomeningoceles, and dural lacerations (9,25–27) (Fig. 4). Walker and associates (27) prospectively studied the efficacy of CT myelography in eight patients, seven of whom were trauma victims (the eighth was a birth injury). They evaluated CT myelography against surgical findings and found it 95% sensitive and 98% specific for complete avulsions. All three partial avulsions were not detected. Kline and Hudson (26), however, caution that CT myelography can miss 2- to 3-mm gaps and that plain film myelography with AP and oblique views remains essential for nerve root evaluation.

CT myelography also accurately depicts extrinsic spinal cord compression and spinal cord edema, although MRI currently tends to be the first-line study of choice. Generally the adult dose of intrathecal contrast should not exceed 300 mg (iodine)

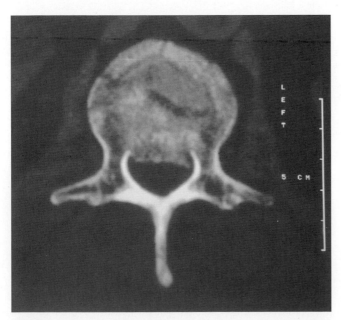

Fig. 3. Axial CT scan of a patient who sustained an L2 burst fracture in a motor vehicle accident. This imaging technique provides excellent visualization of fragment apposition and extent of bony canal compromise.

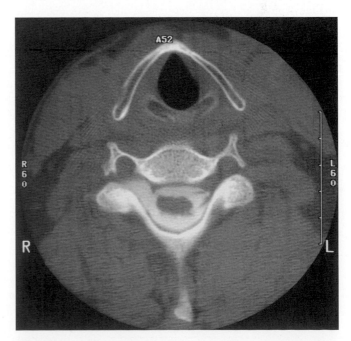

Fig. 4. CT myelogram of a soldier who sustained a brachial plexus avulsion injury when his tracked vehicle was run over by tank. Note the pseudomeningocele and absence of nerve rootlets on the right.

of a nonionic contrast approved for intrathecal administration. Certain factors that may limit the use of this technique in certain patients are the presence of increased intracranial pressure, a known hypersensitivity to iodinated contrast, and a history of a convulsive disorder.

MRI

MRI is the newest addition to the diagnostic armamentarium for imaging the traumatized spine. It surpasses CT and plain films in its ability to comprehensively image acute intrinsic spinal cord pathology such as edema, contusion, or hematoma. Surrounding soft-tissue structures such as the paravertebral soft tissues, the discs, and the structural ligaments are well visualized by MRI (1,2,9,28–33). Additionally, it is helpful in evaluating the sequelae of traumatic cord injury (myelomalacia and syrinx) for prognostic purposes (34,35).

Much effort has been directed at developing the best combinations of imaging sequences. One set of recommendations comes from Flanders and colleagues (34). They recommend that two orthogonal views, in the sagittal and axial plane, be obtained using spin-echo T1-weighted and T2-weighted sequences. The axial images may be targeted to the levels of pathology discovered on the sagittal images. These authors note that T1-weighted sagittal images provide the most accurate evaluation of the spinal cord dimensions. T1-weighted axial images provide the best visualization of nerve roots. T2-weighted images are useful for delineating hemorrhage and edema within the cord. Deoxyhemoglobin, an acute phase blood product, produces an isointense to hypointense signal on T1-weighted images and a markedly hyperintense signal on T2-weighted images. Disc herniations are best evaluated on that sequence due to the "myelographic effect" provided by the hyperintense CSF. Ligamentous injuries are also evaluated well on T2 images, manifesting as an increased signal at the site of disruption (Fig. 2).

In addition to T1- and T2-weighting, the Flanders group also recommends a gradient-echo sequence. This type of sequence allows for acquisition of a T2-weighted image in a shorter period of time without the need for cardiac gating. The gradient echo images are most useful in the thoracic and cervical spines and are particularly good for evaluating thecal sac compression. They also provide a sharp contrast at the interface between cortical bone and the adjacent soft tissues. Gradient-echo images are also sensitive for detecting hemosiderin. However, when compared with spin-echo T2-weighted images, gradient-echo images are less sensitive in detecting abnormal signal from edema within the substance of the spinal cord. A three-dimensional multiplanar gradient recall sequence allows for multiplanar reformatting of the data.

The fast spin-echo (FSE) technique used for MRI acquisition has many properties similar to a true T2-weighted sequence but takes far less time to acquire. It is an excellent sequence for identifying edema and is valuable for imaging those patients who already have instrumentation in place as it is subject to less metallic artifact. While FSE T2 images have many advantages over traditional T2-weighted images, they are not as sensitive in detecting acute hemorrhage.

At our institution, we use a conventional T1-weighted sequence and a FSE T2-weighted sequence. The three-dimensional FSE T2-weighted sequence is particularly sensitive for

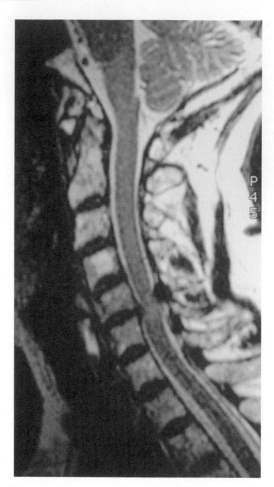

Fig. 5. A 66-year-old woman developed paresthesias in both upper and lower extremities following a forced extension injury. A three-dimensional, fast spin-echo T2-weighted (TR/TE/NEX:2000/139Ef/2NEX) volume acquisition partitioned into thin-section images revealed a soft disc herniation at a level of focal stenosis with malacic changes in the spinal cord.

the detection of soft disc herniations (Fig. 5). It also allows for multiplanar reformatting of the data into very thin sections.

MRI has been slow to gain acceptance in the evaluation of the trauma patient. There are many practical reasons for this resistance. The study is far slower than CT and even with newer, faster sequences, still isolates the critically ill patient for an extended period of time. While an open MRI may make this less of a concern, many trauma centers do not have ready access to this equipment. MRI is also more sensitive than CT to image degradation consequent to patient motion. Standard precautions regarding the use of items susceptible to high field strength magnets must be abided (36). All monitors, ventilators, and devices used to immobilize the patient must be MRI-compatible. In patients who have undergone closed reduction, MRI-compatible Gardner-Wells tongs or halo rings must be used and water bags must replace standard weights. There are also several implantable medical devices that, if present, would preclude MRI. MRI is contraindicated in patients with pacemakers, implanted medicine pumps, nerve stimulators, older aneurysm clips, and ferrous bullet fragments. Since a medical history is often difficult to attain in the trauma setting, attention must be paid to identifying these devices either by physical or radiographic examination. The routine trauma films of the chest, abdomen, and skull (as part of the lateral c-spine film) can be reviewed for the presence of metallic implants if an MRI is to be obtained. If unfamiliar devices are identified, it would be prudent to bypass MRI in favor of a safer imaging modality.

Despite the difficulties, the information MRI provides can alter surgical management and often provides better prognostic information than other modalities. Several studies have been performed to evaluate the frequency of disc herniations in patients with spine injury. Pratt and co-workers (32) retrospectively reviewed 48 patients with unstable spine injuries who underwent an MRI scan in the course of their evaluation. This included 19 cervical injuries, 6 thoracic injuries, and 23 thoracolumbar injuries. Disc herniations were identified by MRI in 47% of the patients with cervical injuries, 50% of those with thoracic injuries, and 13% with thoracolumbar injuries. All of these were later confirmed at surgery.

Rizzolo and associates (33) reviewed the MRI results of 55 patients with spine injuries. Of note, all patients requiring closed reduction were reduced prior to MRI. Twenty-three (42%) had an acute disc disruption. Of the patients requiring closed reduction, it is uncertain whether the retropulsed disc material was present prior to the reduction, but there were no cases of neurological deterioration following closed reduction. The patients with the highest rates of disc herniation were those with bilateral facet dislocations (80%) and anterior cord syndrome (100%). Hypertension injuries (60%), unilateral facet dislocation (40%), and central cord syndrome (47%) were other factors associated with high rates of disc herniation in this small series.

Hall and colleagues (28) described their experiences with MRI and surgical planning in a series of six patients with facet injuries. Of those six, three had surgery-proven disc herniations, one had a probable herniation, and two did not have disc herniations. In the four patients where MRI suggested a herniated disc, the surgeon selected an anterior surgical approach.

MRI can also augment the determination of spinal stability (28,29,37). Halliday and others (29) report the results of a retrospective study of 24 patients with unilateral facet fractures aimed at determining which patients would need surgery. Although their numbers were small, their data suggest that injuries involving three or four of the major ligaments (anterior longitudinal ligament, posterior longitudinal ligament, facet capsule, or interspinous ligaments) require surgical intervention.

Benzel and associates (37) studied a group of 174 patients with a clinical history of potential spinal instability and equivocal plain films. Criteria for obtaining an MRI and inclusion in the study were neck pain, loss of lordosis, subtle abnormalities of alignment, or an inability to communicate. Any patients with obvious neurological or plain film radiographic abnormalities were excluded. Soft-tissue injuries visualized on MRI were divided into ventral ligamentous, dorsal ligamentous, or disc injuries. Sixty-two of 174 patients had abnormalities in one or more of the soft-tissue areas. All patients with abnormalities were placed in either a semi-rigid cervical collar or a Minerva jacket. One patient with injuries in all three regions underwent surgical fusion. All but one patient was seen in follow-up 1 to 3 months later and none had evidence of excess instability on flexion-extension plain films. Although no control arm was present, Benzel's management strategy with these patients led to good results. As further studies are done to correlate MRI results with clinical course, MRI may become very helpful in determining the stability of patients.

Patients with neurological deficits but no abnormalities on plain films or CT are also excellent candidates for an MRI. MRI can evaluate the status of the spinal cord and distinguish between operable lesions causing spinal cord compromise such as an epidural hematoma, retropulsed bone fracture fragments, or an acutely herniated disc versus inoperable lesions, such as spinal cord contusion. ·

Several authors have also sought to establish the value of MRI in determining prognosis for patients with spinal cord injury (34,35). Schaefer and co-workers (35) evaluated MRI examinations of 57 patients with closed cervical injuries. Twenty-one patients had intramedullary hematomas, 17 had intramedullary edema extending greater than one spinal segment and 19 had edema extending less than one spinal segment. The American Spinal Injury Association total motor scores were averaged for each group on admission and at follow-up examination (ranging from 2 to 18 months). Statistical analysis showed that the first group had the least improvement while the third group showed the greatest improvement.

MRI is also sensitive in the detection of a posttraumatic syrinx. Patients with spinal cord injury, particularly with thoracolumbar trauma, are at risk to undergo a decline several months after their injury as a consequence of a posttraumatic syrinx (34). Because MRI is very sensitive in identifying those lesions, early imaging and interval screening can reveal development of a posttraumatic syrinx. This information can assist the surgeon in determining both the need and the optimum timing of any surgical intervention.

Some authors recommend that every cervical MRI be accompanied by a magnetic resonance angiogram (MRA) with particular attention paid to the vertebral arteries (9). The vertebral arteries travel in the foramina transversarium from C6 to C1. Vertebral artery dissections or transections are well-documented complications of cervical spine trauma. Carotid artery dissections can also occur with forceful rotation of the neck. MRA is a noninvasive imaging evaluation of intravascular blood flow. MRA and MRI can reveal a tapered narrowing of a vessel caused by dissection. Axial spin-echo images may also demonstrate the abnormal signal of degrading blood products contained within a false lumen adjacent to a vascular flow void. Since there is normal anatomical variability in the caliber of the vertebral arteries, the presence of a uniformly narrow vertebral artery in the absence of other MRI findings or neurological deficits does not suggest a dissection. There are two basic types of MRA, both of which can be acquired using two-dimensional and three-dimensional techniques. For imaging the carotid and vertebral arteries, two-dimensional MRA is favored over three-dimensional MRA because of a greater sensitivity for detecting flow perpendicular to the imaging plane. Three-dimensional techniques are favored when there is complex or turbulent flow parallel to the acquisition plane. The technique of phase-contrast (PC) MRA is based on the dynamics of intravascular flow. The signal produced is proportional to intravascular flow contrasted to the static background soft tissue contained in the interrogated volume. This technique allows for determination of flow velocity and direction and is highly sensitive to slow flow states. Time-of-flight (TOF) MRA is a gradient-echo sequence based on the principle that unsaturated protons enter into a volume of tissue, the signal of which has been suppressed by a series of radio frequency pulses. Since TOF MRA is sensitive to the T1 properties of all tissues contained in the imaged volume, any tissue (including extravascular blood products) exhibiting increased signal on T1-weighted images may be visualized and mistaken for intravascular blood flow. This difficulty is not encountered with PC MRA.

Although there are studies assessing standard arteriography and MRA independently (38–42), little data exist directly comparing results of both techniques. Consequently, it is difficult to establish the false-negative rate of MRA versus the gold standard. At our institution, we recommend MRA with the spinal MRI for all patients with significant spine trauma, especially when there are fractures through the foramen transversarium. We proceed to conventional arteriography in cases were an abnormality is identified on the MRA or if the patient has a clinical examination highly suggestive of a vertebral or carotid artery injury. Although little data exist on the role of CT angiography in the trauma setting, it may emerge as an excellent alternative to conventional arteriography. It is, however, very time- and labor-intensive, and as a result will not likely have a role as a screening study.

Despite the many imaging modalities available and the marked improvements in cross-sectional imaging that have occurred over the last 10 to 15 years, there is no substitute for sound clinical judgment. For patients who have significantly diminished level of consciousness or who are comatose, there is no definitive radiographic study done in the acute setting that can definitively clear the spine. Those patients should be maintained in a cervical collar until the patient becomes alert enough to render a reliable neurological examination or more definitive examinations can be performed. Nearly every patient who comes to a trauma center will arrive in a collar and on a backboard, but not all of those patients may need to be extensively imaged. Several studies have evaluated the need for imaging in trauma (17,43–45). In 1987, Bachulis and co-workers (43) published their experience with 1,823 trauma patients who had radiographs taken of their c-spines. Of that number, 94 were found to have spinal injury (5%); 65 of those patients were alert. Each of the 65 either complained of neck pain or had tenderness to palpation on examination. Similarly, Ringenberg and associates (17) published their data in 1988 of 312 patients with traumatic c-spine injuries, 257 of whom were alert in the emergency department; 215 (84%) had neck pain and tenderness; 34 had motor and/or sensory abnormalities, and the remaining 8 patients had other severely painful injuries that may have masked pain elsewhere. Kreipke and others (44) also examined this issue and found that of 324 asymptomatic patients, none had positive cervical spine radiographs. They also noted that patients with abnormal respiratory patterns (arrest or agonal breathing), motor changes, or an altered sensorium had a statistically significant likelihood of having a cervical spine abnormality. Certainly any patient with diminished mental status needs a full radiographic evaluation. Likewise, any patient with a complaint of neck pain, tenderness on examination, abnormal neurological examination, or a mechanism of injury with a high risk for cervical injury merits a full evaluation as do patients with other severe injuries that may mask cervical pain.

References

1. El-Khoury GY, Kathol MH, Daniel WW. Imaging of acute injuries of the cervical spine: value of plain radiography, CT, and MRI. Am J Radiol 1995;164:43–50.
2. Quencer RM, Nunez D, Green BA. Controversies in imaging acute cervical spine trauma. Am J Neuroradiol 1997;18:1866–1868.
3. Woodring JH, Lee C. Limitations of cervical radiography in the evaluation of acute cervical trauma. J Trauma 1993;34:32–39.
4. Turetsky DB, Vines FS, Clayman DA, et al. Technique and use of supine oblique views in acute cervical spine trauma. Ann Emerg Med 1993;22:685–689.
5. Freemyer B, Knopp R, Piche J, et al. Comparison of five-view and three-view cervical spine series in the evaluation of patients with cervical trauma. Ann Emerg Med 1989;18:818–821.
6. Holliman CJ, Mayer JS, Cook RT, et al. Is the anterior cervical spine radiograph necessary in initial trauma screening? Am J Emerg Med 1991;9:421–425.
7. Clark CR, Igram CM, El-Khoury GY, et al. Radiographic evaluation of cervical spine injuries. Spine 1988;13:742–747.
8. Harris, JH. Radiographic evaluation of spinal trauma. Orthoped Clin North Am 1986;17:75–86.
9. Harris JH, Mirvis SE. The radiology of acute cervical spine trauma, 3rd ed. Baltimore: Williams & Wilkins, 1996.
10. Harris MB, Waguespack AM, Kronlage S. 'Clearing' cervical spine injuries in polytrauma patients: is it really safe to remove the collar? Orthopedics 1997;20:903–907.
11. Reid C, Henderson R, Soboe L, et al. Etiology and clinical course of missed spine fractures. J Trauma 1987;27:980–986.
12. Lewis LM, Docherty M, Ruoff BE, et al. Flexion-extension views in the evaluation of cervical-spine injuries. Ann Emerg Med 1991;20:117–121.
13. Davis JW, Parks SN, Detlefs CL, et al. Clearing the cervical spine in obtunded patients: the use of dynamic fluoroscopy. J Trauma: Injury Infect Crit Care 1995;39:435–438.
14. Brandser EA, El-Khoury GY. Thoracic and lumbar spine trauma. Radiol Clin North Am 1997;35:533–556.
15. Samuels LE, Kerstein MD. 'Routine' radiologic evaluation of the thoracolumbar spine in blunt trauma patients: a reappraisal. J Trauma 1993;34:85–89.
16. Meek S. Fractures of the thoracolumbar spine in major trauma patients. BMJ 1998;317:1442–1443.
17. Ringenberg BJ, Fisher AK, Urdaneta LF, et al. Rational ordering of cervical spine radiographs following trauma. Ann Emerg Medicine. 1988;17:792–796.
18. Link TM, Schuierer G, Hufendiek A, et al. Substantial head trauma: value of routine CT examination of the cervicocranium. Radiology 1995;196:741–745.
19. Blacksin MF, Lee HJ. Frequency and significance of fractures of the upper cervical spine detected by CT in patients with severe neck trauma. AJR 1995;165:1201–1204.
20. Tehranzedeh J, Bonk T, Ansari A, et al. Efficacy of limited CT for non-visualized lower cervical spine in patients with blunt trauma. Skeletal Radiol 1994;23:349–352.
21. Schleenhauf K, Ross S, Civil ID, et al. Computed tomography in the initial evaluation of the cervical spine. Ann Emerg Med 1989;18:815–817.
22. Borock EC, Gabram SGA, Jacobs LM, et al. A prospective analysis of a two-year experience using computed tomography as an adjunct for cervical spine clearance. J Trauma 1991;31:1001–1006.
23. Saifuddin A, Noordeen H, Taylor BA, et al. The role of imaging in the diagnosis and management of thoracolumbar burst fractures: current concepts and review of the literature. Skeletal Radiol 1996;25:603–613.
24. Pech P, Kilgore DP, Pojunas KW, et al. Cervical spinal fractures: CT detection. Radiology 1985;157:117–120.
25. Carvalho GA, Nikkhah G, Matthies C, et al. Diagnosis of root avulsions in traumatic brachial plexus injuries: value of computerized tomography myelography and magnetic resonance imaging. J Neurosurg 1997;86:69–76.
26. Kline DG, Hudson AR. Diagnosis of root avulsions [Letter]. J Neurosurg 1997;87:483–484
27. Walker AT, Chaloupka JC, deLotbiniere AC, et al. Detection of nerve rootlet avulsion on CT myelography in patients with birth palsy and brachial plexus injury after trauma. AJR 1996;167:1283–1287.
28. Hall AJ, Wagle VG, Raycroft J, et al. Magnetic resonance imaging in cervical spine trauma. J Trauma. 1993;34:21–26.
29. Halliday AL, Henderson BR, Hart BL, et al. The management of unilateral lateral mass/facet fractures of the subaxial cervical spine. Spine 1997;22:2614–2621.
30. Kathol MH. Cervical spine trauma. Radiol Clin North Am 1997;35:507–532. 30.
31. Mirivs SE, Geisler FH, Jelinek JJ, et al. Acute cervical spine trauma: evaluation with 1.5-T MR imaging. Radiology 1988;166:807–816.
32. Pratt ES, Green DA, Spengler DM. Herniated intervertebral discs associated with unstable spinal injuries. Spine 1990;15:662–666.
33. Rizzolo SJ, Piazza MR, Cotler JM, et al. Intervertebral disc injury complicating cervical spine trauma. Spine 1991;16:187–189.
34. Flanders AE, Tartaglino LM, Friedman DP, et al. Magnetic resonance imaging in acute spinal injury. Semin Roentgen 1992;27:271–298.
35. Schaefer DM, Flanders AE, Osterholm JL, et al. Prognostic significance of magnetic resonance imaging in the acute phase of cervical spine injury. J Neurosurgery 1992;76:218–223.
36. Shellock FG. Pocket guide to MR procedures and metallic objects: update 1997. New York: Lippincott–Raven Publishers, 1997.
37. Benzel EC, Hart BL, Ball PA, et al. Magnetic resonance imaging for the evaluation of patients with occult cervical spine injury. J Neurosurg 1996;85:824–829.
38. Bok AP, Peter JC. Carotid and vertebral artery occlusion after blunt

cervical injury: the role of MR angiography in early diagnosis. *J Trauma: Injury Infect Crit Care* 1996;40:968–972.

39. Deen HG, McGirr SJ. Vertebral artery injury associated with cervical spine fracture. *Spine* 1992;17:230–234.
40. Friedman D, Flanders A, Thomas C, et al. Vertebral artery injury after acute cervical spine trauma: rate of occurrence as detected by MR angiography and assessment of clinical consequences. *AJR* 1995; 164:443–447.
41. Louw JA, Mafoyane NA, Small B, et al. Occlusion of the vertebral artery in cervical spine dislocations. *J Bone Joint Surg Br* 1990;15: 662–666.

42. Willis BK, Greiner F, Orrison WW, et al. The incidence of vertebral artery injury after midcervical spine fracture or subluxation. *Neurosurgery* 1994;34: 435–441.
43. Bachulis BL, Long WB, Hynes GD, et al. Clinical indications for cervical spine radiographs in the traumatized patient. *Am J Surg* 1987;153:473–477.
44. Kreipke DL, Gillespie KR, McCarthy MC, et al. Reliability of indications for cervical spine films in trauma patients. *J Trauma* 1989;29: 1438–1439.
45. Saddison D, Vanek VW, Racanelli JL. Clinical indications for cervical spine radiographs in alert trauma patients. *Am Surg* 1991;57:366–9.

157. Occipital Cervical Junction Injury and Dislocation

**Derek A. Taggard and
Vincent C. Traynelis**

The clinical relevance of injury to the atlanto-occipital segment has increased remarkably over the last few decades. This is in part due to enhanced emergency medical response services and resuscitation. Additionally, advances in imaging modalities have made the diagnosis of craniovertebral junction (CVJ) injury easier, and perhaps more common.

The CVJ is often injured in patients who die following trauma to the head and/or neck (1,2). Atlanto-occipital dislocation (AOD) is associated with 6% to 8% of all traumatic fatalities (1, 2). It is the most common cervical spine injury found at autopsy of vehicular fatality victims (2). However, reports of successful management of AOD with good neurological recovery emphasize the importance of prompt diagnosis and management. One can expect AOD to account for about 1% of presenting traumatic cervical spine injuries (3,4).

Historically, diagnosis of an occipital condyle fracture (OCF) has been uncommon, and even more rarely suspected as they are rarely visible on plain radiographic studies. OCFs are now becoming an increasingly common diagnosis with the common use of computed tomography (CT) as a diagnostic tool in the patient with significant craniocervical trauma (5,6). Understanding the potential instability associated with some of these injuries can enable the clinician to appropriately address these "incidentally" found fractures.

Anatomy and Biomechanics

The ligaments that maintain the craniocervical articulation can be divided into two groups (Fig. 1). The first set attaches the skull to the atlas and includes the articular capsule ligaments, the anterior and posterior atlanto-occipital ligaments, and two lateral atlanto-occipital ligaments. The anterior atlanto-occipital ligament is a continuation of the anterior longitudinal ligament, and the posterior atlanto-occipital ligament spans between the posterior border of the foramen magnum and the atlanto-posterior arch. The cruciate ligament (a longitudinally oriented structure associated with the transverse ligament of the atlas) also contributes to the stability of this articulation.

A second set of ligaments secures the cranium to the axis, and is the primary source of stability across the CVJ. These ligaments include the apical dental ligament, the alar ligaments, the tectorial membrane, and the ligamentum nuchae (7,8). The alar ligaments are paired structures with two components each: the atlantal alar and the occipital alar. These ligaments connect the tip of the odontoid to the occipital condyles and the lateral masses of the atlas, respectively (9). The alar ligaments are the main restraints for axial rotation, which occurs mostly across the C1-2 articulation. To a lesser degree, the alar ligaments also limit lateral flexion (7).

The tectorial membrane is a continuation of the posterior longitudinal ligament. It reaches from the dorsal surface of the odontoid to insert on the ventral surface of the foramen magnum (10,11). The tectorial membrane resists hyperextension (7). If the tectorial membrane is incompetent, contact between the posterior arch of the atlas and the occiput will limit hyperextension (12). Flexion is restricted by contact of the odontoid process with the anterior foramen magnum (7). The apical dental ligament and the ligamentum nuchae contribute only slightly to the stability of the CVJ.

Atlanto-Occipital Dislocation

INJURY MECHANISMS. AOD occurs following complete or near complete disruption of the ligamentous structures between the occiput and the upper cervical spine. Extreme forces in hyperextension, hyperflexion, and lateral flexion or in combination can result in this injury (13–15). Most likely, the prominent force responsible for producing AOD is hyperextension that results in rupture of the tectorial membrane (16,17). Incompetence of the alar ligaments and tectorial membrane allows for anterior dislocation of the cranium with respect to the upper cervical spine (7). Other authors have suggested that hyperflexion forces may also be involved in some cases of AOD (14) based on the observation that the posterior elements of C1 and C2 are commonly separated in the setting of AOD. Another

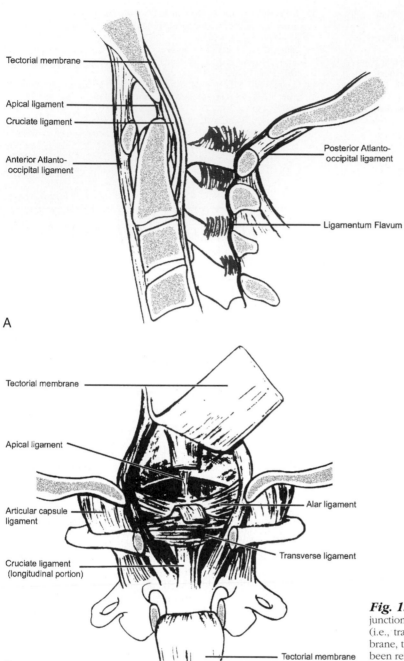

A

B

Fig. 1. Lateral (**A**) and posterior (**B**) views of the craniovertebral junction. Note the cruciate ligament is composed of horizontal fibers (i.e., transverse ligament) and vertical fibers. The tectorial membrane, the rostral extent of the posterior longitudinal ligament, has been reflected in **B** to allow for visualization of more ventral structures.

theory focuses on damage to the alar ligaments through extreme lateral flexion (18–20).

An increased incidence of AOD in children (3,14,16) may be related to the relatively high incidence of automobile-pedestrian accidents, immaturity of the CVJ, or both (7,14). Anatomically, children have shallow, horizontally oriented surfaces at O-C1 that are less biomechanically stable than the deep-seated, vertically oriented articulation of the adult. Also, children's ligaments are not as stiff as their adult counterparts and are required to support a proportionately larger head than the adult for a given body size.

CLINICAL PRESENTATION. The most common causes of AOD are high-speed motor vehicle accidents or pedestrians

struck by motor vehicles (3,14). Devastating brainstem injury at the time of dislocation probably accounts for the high mortality rate seen with AOD (19). Patients who survive may be neurologically intact or show dysfunction of the brainstem, cranial nerves, spinal cord, or cervical nerve roots (20–22). Coexistent head injury is common and can confound the clinical examination.

A survivor's motor examination may be normal or may display deficits including vegetative posturing responses, cruciate paralysis, or quadriparesis. Additionally, patients commonly present with hemiparesis that may result from unilateral pyramidal injury, though more rostral structures in the brainstem may also be involved. Cranial nerves commonly injured include VI followed by the lower group of IX through XII. Vascular struc-

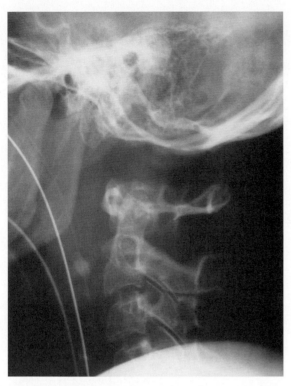

Fig. 2. Lateral radiograph of a man with type II atlanto-occipital dislocation. Note the gross separation of the occiput from C1 as well as widening of the posterior elements of C1 and C2.

tures at risk for compression, dissection, or stretch injury include the anterior spinal, vertebral, and carotid arteries.

RADIOLOGY. Radiographic findings of AOD may be quite dramatic (Fig. 2), but are commonly subtle or even absent on initial films (18–21). When alignment of bony structures appears preserved, one must appreciate suggestive indicators that dislocation has occurred. An increase in the prevertebral soft tissue should raise suspicion of serious spinal injury. In the case of AOD, a retropharyngeal hematoma is invariably present. Other signs include retropharyngeal emphysema (16,23) or increase in the interval between the posterior elements of C1 and C2 (14).

Several criteria that can be applied to plain lateral cervical radiographs to secure the diagnosis of AOD have been developed. The basilar line of Wackenheim is drawn as a caudal extension of the posterior surface of the clivus in the midsagittal plane (Fig. 3A) (24). In a normal individual, the line of Wackenheim lies tangential to the posterior tip of the odontoid process and is not altered by flexion or extension. The line will intersect the dens if the occiput is displaced anterior to the atlantoaxial segment. If the skull is displaced posteriorly then the line will not intersect any portion of the odontoid process.

In the neutral position, the interval between the odontoid tip and the basion remains constant (Fig. 3B) (25). Measurements of greater than 5 mm in adults and 10 mm in infants have been suggested as abnormal (24,25). However, the applicability of the dens-basion interval was challenged when 100 adult and 50 pediatric cervical spine radiographs were reviewed and 85% of individuals exceeded the proposed limits. With a reported average distance of 9 mm, as many as 50% of patients with

known AOD might fall within the range spanned by the normal population (4).

Subsequently, Powers and colleagues suggest the ratio of two measurements could be used to define normal craniovertebral relationships (Fig. 3C) (4). The first distance is measured between the basion (B) and the inner aspect of the atlanto-posterior arch (C) and the other represents the distance between the opisthion (O) and the inner aspect of the atlanto-anterior arch (A). The mean BC/OA ratio in normal subjects is 0.77 and a value greater than 1.0 may indicate AOD. Unreliable results may be obtained if the landmarks are difficult to identify, congenital anomalies are present, or if the atlas is fractured. Additionally, if the occiput is dislocated posteriorly or purely longitudinally then a value less than one may be obtained (26–28).

Lee and colleagues suggest the use of the x-line method to detect AOD (Fig. 3D) (26). The first line is the distance between the basion to the midpoint of the C2 spinolaminar line (BC2Sl) and the second denotes the distance from the opisthion to the posteroinferior edge of the axis body (C2O). The BC2Sl line should tangentially intersect the posterosuperior aspect of the dens in normal individuals over the age of 5 years. The C2O line should tangentially cross the most rostral edge of the C1 spinolaminar line. While one of the relationships defined by these lines may not be properly aligned in normal subjects, alteration of both of these relationships should lead one to be highly suspicious of AOD. Appropriate use of this method requires a normal atlantoaxial relationship—a segment that can be abnormal in over half of cases of AOD (14).

While each of the methods described here was developed to improve the accuracy of diagnosis, none are sufficiently sensitive to warrant independent usage. Suspicion of AOD should prompt further imaging techniques. High-resolution CT is an accurate means of diagnosing AOD (14,26,29,30) and should include sagittal and coronal reconstructed images. The best means of assessing ligamentous and other soft-tissue injury is with magnetic resonance imaging (MRI), though CT may allow one to infer the degree of ligamentous injury when avulsion induces bony damage. In a limited number of cases, AOD has been diagnosed by MRI findings alone (3). Additionally, spinal cord signal abnormalities can be correlated with the clinical examination and vertebral artery injury and/or thrombosis may be discovered.

Three specific types of AOD have been suggested that can easily be classified according to plain radiographic appearance (Fig. 4) (14). A type I dislocation consists of anterior displacement of the occiput with respect to the atlas. Type II is primarily a longitudinal distraction with separation of the occiput from the atlas. Type III AOD exists when the occiput is dislocated in a posterior direction relative to C1. Additionally, rotatory atlanto-occipital dislocation has also been described (3).

TREATMENT CONSIDERATIONS. Maintaining awareness of the possibility of AOD is critical to making the diagnosis. In addition to appropriate cardiopulmonary support and spinal immobilization, medical therapy of patients who may have a spinal cord injury includes intravenous methylprednisolone (31). Surgical hematomas at the CVJ in the setting of AOD are rare but may require emergent decompressive procedures if associated with neurological deficit.

The use of traction is controversial when treating patients with AOD. Some authors have concluded that traction should not be employed because the injury is highly unstable (3,19, 22,28). Others have documented its benefits toward achieving a successful outcome (4,18,20,21,32,33). The goal of traction, if used, is to decompress the neural elements by realigning the bony structures.

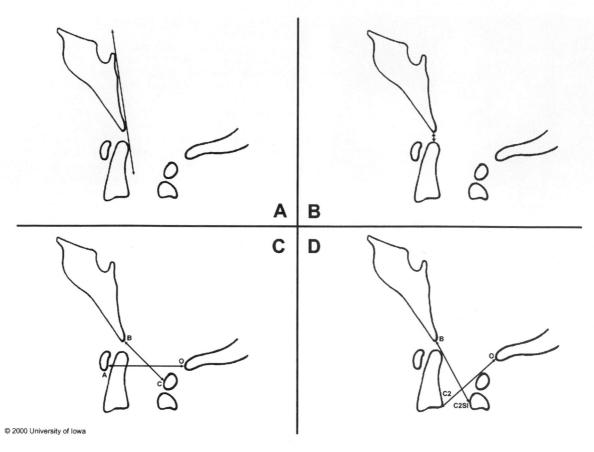

© 2000 University of Iowa

Fig. 3. Schematic diagrams depicting various criteria developed to assess the craniovertebral junction (CVJ). Wackenheim's line **(A)** is drawn as a caudal extension of the clivus and should tangentially intersect the tip of the dens in a normal individual. A normal dens-basion interval **(B)** should not exceed 5 mm in an adult and 10 mm in an infant. The distance between the basion *(B)* and inner surface of the posterior arch of C1 *(C)* divided by the distance from the opisthion *(O)* to the inner surface of the anterior arch of C1 *(A)* defines the Powers ratio **(C)**. The mean value in normal subjects is 0.77. **D:** The x-line method for evaluating the CVJ. The line between the basion *(B)* and midpoint of the C2 spinolaminar line *(C2Sl)* should tangentially intersect the dens. The line defined by the opisthion *(O)* and the posteroinferior edge of the axis body *(C2)* should cross the rostral limit of the C1 spinolaminar line.

Recognition of the dislocation type (I, III, or III), as described earlier, has been suggested as a means of guiding this decision (14). Consideration of traction is best reserved for instances of type I (anterior), type III (posterior), and lateral AOD that is associated with neurological deficit (14,34). Traction in the setting of a type II dislocation is contraindicated as the pathology is primarily a result of longitudinal distraction, which would only be worsened by traction. Even in rotatory subluxations, small amounts of traction have resulted in a dangerous amount of distraction (3).

A reasonable approach to patients with only minor malalignment or slight neurological deficits is to attempt manual realignment with fluoroscopic guidance. Thus, the use of traction is reserved for instances of grossly abnormal alignment accompanied by significant neurological deficit. The use of fluoroscopy during initial application of traction is strongly recommended. The amount of weight required should not exceed 5 lbs. Frequent clinical and radiographic monitoring is essential. Neurological worsening or an increase in distraction or subluxation should prompt a reduction or discontinuation of the traction. Once the end point of improving neurological status or radiographic realignment has been achieved, then traction may be reduced to 1 to 2 lbs or discontinued and the patient immobilized in a halo vest.

AOD often heals poorly with strictly conservative measures because it is primarily a ligamentous injury with severe instability. Though external immobilization in a halo vest has may allow the injury to heal, maintaining reduction may prove difficult (3, 17,18,35). A more definitive approach is to proceed with posterior fusion once the patient is medically stable (3,14,22,36). In fact, Dickman and colleagues recommend bypassing traction and performing acute internal reduction and fixation (3). A dorsal fusion with rigid internal fixation incorporating at least the occiput to C2 is required for an adequate construct.

Whether due to immediate neurological devastation or other organ system trauma, AOD remains a highly lethal injury. However, patients surviving 48 hours from the traumatic event may have a good outcome. Up to one-fourth of surviving patients are ultimately intact neurologically, and in another one-fourth only minor neurological deficits remain (14).

Occipital Condyle Fractures

CLINICAL PRESENTATION. The clinical presentation of patients with OCFs is variable. Concomitant head injury is common in the patient with an OCF (6,37,38). Subjects whose sensorium is preserved may complain of pain and tenderness in the

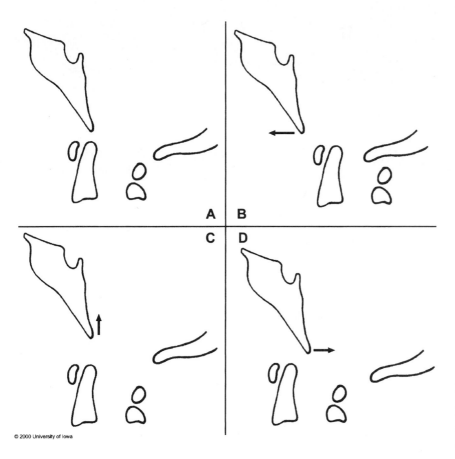

Fig. 4. Classification of atlanto-occipital dislocation as proposed by Traynelis and colleagues (14). **A:** The normal craniovertebral junction. Dislocations may occur through anterior displacement (**B**), longitudinal distraction (**C**), or posterior displacement (**D**) of the occiput relative to the atlas.

© 2000 University of Iowa

posterior occipitocervical region (39). From a neurological standpoint, patients may be intact or have profound deficits including lower cranial nerve palsies and varying degrees of hemiparesis or quadriparesis.

The proximity of numerous neurovascular structures to the occipital condyles explains many of the symptoms encountered with this injury. Structures at risk include the brainstem, lower cranial nerves, and venous and arterial vessels. The jugular foramen is just lateral to the condyle and contains cranial nerves IX, X, and XI as well as the jugular vein. On the anteromedial aspect of the base of the occipital condyle is the hypoglossal canal. More medially, within the foramen magnum, are the cervicomedullary junction and the vertebral arteries.

Lower cranial nerve palsies occur in nearly a third of patients with an OCF (40). Dysfunction will develop in a delayed manner in approximately one-third of these patients with the others suffering acute palsies (40). Delayed palsies may occur secondary to bone fragment migration or fibrous tissue proliferation producing an insidious, progressive compression of the lower cranial nerves (41,42). Alternatively, progressive edema within the cranial nerve(s) may account for a delayed presentation (43).

RADIOLOGY. Most OCFs occur as isolated injuries of the CVJ (24,37,38,39). Plain radiographs are inadequate to diagnose an OCF. As with AOD, the presence of a retropharyngeal hematoma may be the only clue on a plain film that serious craniovertebral insult has occurred. Tomography, or more commonly CT, provides the definitive diagnostic images (6,37,38,44). At one institution, 14 of 15 cases of OCF were diagnosed using bone windows of the trauma head CT and none were found on plain radiographs (44).

A classification scheme of OCFs was proposed by Anderson and Montesano in 1988 based on CT morphology, probable mechanisms of injury, and potential for instability (Fig. 5) (38). A type I fracture is produced by axial loading and results in comminution of the occipital condyle with little or no displacement of fragments into foramen magnum. If the ipsilateral alar ligament is incompetent then instability may result (22). However, stability is usually preserved by an intact tectorial membrane and contralateral alar ligament. Type II fractures occur as an extension of a linear basilar skull fracture through the occipital condyle. No ligamentous injury occurs so stability is maintained. Excessive loading in rotation and/or lateral bending can result in condylar avulsion, or a type III OCF, as seen in the CT in Fig. 6. Similar to type I fractures, potential for instability exists, particularly as these injuries may be associated with increased load on the tectorial membrane.

TREATMENT CONSIDERATIONS. A clinically useful alternative to the radiographic groupings of Anderson and Montesano is a management-based classification proposed by Tuli and co-workers (40). If the fractured condyle is nondisplaced, it is a type I fracture and no immobilization is required. Type II fractures exhibit displacement of the condyle. Further subdivision of type II fractures is based on O-C1-C2 instability demonstrated by conventional radiography, CT criteria, or evidence of ligamentous disruption on MRI. Suggested treatment for stable fractures with intact ligaments (type IIA) is immobilization in a hard collar. If instability and/or ligamentous disruption is detected, the fracture is then classified as type IIB and treated either with a halo vest or internal fixation. Surgical intervention is rare and conservative management of all isolated OCFs is

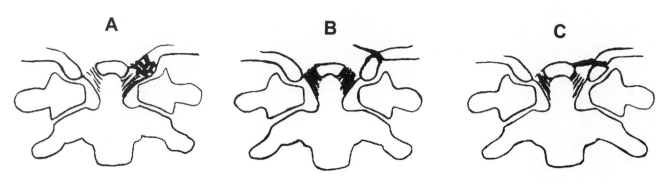

© 2000 University of Iowa

Fig. 5. Occipital condyle fracture classification as proposed by Anderson and Montesano. **A:** Comminuted fractures of a condyle with minimal or no displacement of bone fragments defines a type I fracture. **B:** Type II fractures result from extension of a linear basilar skull fracture into an occipital condyle. **C:** A condylar avulsion is defined as a type III fracture.

generally supported, even in cases of brainstem compression with neurological injury (40,45).

The limited number of cases discussed in the literature, lack of clinical follow-up in some series, and variability of fracture descriptions and treatment approaches combine to make outcome assessments difficult. Consistent with other bony injuries, the fractures usually heal well with a conservative approach. In general, patients make reasonable neurological recoveries, though not necessarily complete (43,45). The prognosis of cranial nerve paralysis of a delayed presentation is more favorable than those of an acute nature (16).

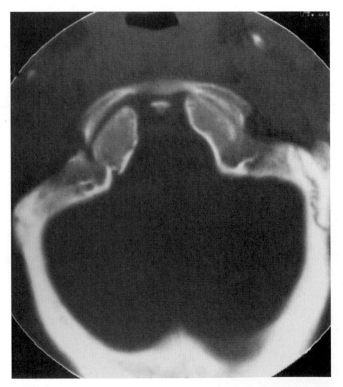

Fig. 6. Axial CT scan of a type III occipital condyle fracture with minimal displacement of the condyle into foramen magnum. The outline of the anterior arch of C1 can be seen anterior to the occipital condyles.

References

1. Bucholz RW, Burkhead WZ, Graham W, et al. Occult cervical spine injuries in fatal traffic accidents. *J Trauma: Injury Infect Crit Care* 1979;19:768–771.
2. Alker GJ Jr, Oh YS, Leslie EV. High cervical spine and craniocervical junction injuries in fatal traffic accidents: a radiological study. *Orthop Clin North Am* 1978;9:1003–1010.
3. Dickman CA, Papadopoulos SM, Sonntag VK, et al. Traumatic occipitoatlantal dislocations [Review; 51 refs]. *J Spinal Disord* 1993;6: 300–313.
4. Powers B, Miller MD, Kramer RS, et al. Traumatic anterior atlantooccipital dislocation. *Neurosurgery* 1979;4:12–17.
5. Blacksin MF, Lee HJ. Frequency and significance of fractures of the upper cervical spine detected by CT in patients with severe neck trauma. *Am J Roentgenol* 1995;165:1201–1204.
6. Link TM, Schuierer G, Hufendiek A, et al. Substantial head trauma: value of routine CT examination of the cervicocranium. *Radiology* 1995;196:741–745.
7. Werne S. Studies in spontaneous atlas dislocation. *Acta Orthop Scand Suppl* 1957;23:1–150.
8. White AA III, Panjabi MM. The clinical biomechanics of the occipitoatlantoaxial complex. *Orthop Clin North Am* 1978;9:867–878.
9. Dvorak J, Schneider E, Saldinger P, et al. Biomechanics of the craniocervical region: the alar and transverse ligaments. *J Orthop Res* 1988;6:452–461.
10. Wiesel S, Kraus D, Rothman RH. Atlanto-occipital hypermobility. *Orthop Clin North Am* 1978;9:969–972.
11. Wiesel SW, Rothman RH. Occipitoatlantal hypermobility. *Spine* 1979;4:187–191.
12. Harris MB, Duval MJ, Davis JA Jr, et al. Anatomical and roentgenographic features of atlantooccipital instability. *J Spinal Disord* 1993; 6:5–10.
13. Davis D, Bohlman H, Walker AE, et al. The pathological findings in fatal craniospinal injuries. *J Neurosurg* 1971;34:603–613.
14. Traynelis VC, Marano GD, Dunker RO, et al. Traumatic atlantooccipital dislocation. Case report [Published erratum appears in *J Neurosurg* 1987;66(5):789]. *J Neurosurg* 1986;65:863–870.
15. Bohlman HH, Ducker TB, Lucas JT. *Spine and spinal cord injuries*, 2nd ed. Vol 2. Philadelphia: WB Saunders, 1982, 661–756.
16. Bucholz RW, Burkhead WZ. The pathological anatomy of fatal atlanto-occipital dislocations. *J Bone Joint Surg Am* 1979;61:248–250.
17. Page CP, Story JL, Wissinger JP, et al. Traumatic atlantooccipital dislocation. Case report. *J Neurosurg* 1973;39:394–397.
18. Gabrielsen TO, Maxwell JA. Traumatic atlanto-occipital dislocation; with case report of a patient who survived. *Am J Roentgenol Radium Ther Nucl Med* 1966;97:624–629.
19. Pang D, Wilberger JE Jr. Traumatic atlanto-occipital dislocation with survival: case report and review. *Neurosurgery* 1980;7:503–508.

20. Woodring JH, Selke AC Jr, Duff DE. Traumatic atlantooccipital dislocation with survival. *Am J Roentgenol* 1981;137:21–24.
21. Eismont FJ, Bohlman HH. Posterior atlanto-occipital dislocation with fractures of the atlas and odontoid process. *J Bone Joint Surg Am* 1978;60:397–399.
22. Levine AM, Edwards CC. Traumatic lesions of the occipitoatlantoaxial complex. *Clin Orthop* 1989;53–68.
23. Alker GJ, Oh YS, Leslie EV, et al. Postmortem radiology of head neck injuries in fatal traffic accidents. *Radiology* 1975;114:611–617.
24. Wackenheim A. *Roentgen diagnosis of the craniovertebral region.* Berlin: Springer-Verlag, 1974.
25. Wholey JH, Bruwer AJ, Baker HLJ. The lateral roentgenogram of the neck (with comments on the atlanto-odontoid-basion relationship). *Radiology* 1958;71:350–356.
26. Lee C, Woodring JH, Goldstein SJ, et al. Evaluation of traumatic atlantooccipital dislocations [See comments]. *AJNR* 1987;8:19–26.
27. Kaufman RA, Carroll CD, Buncher CR. Atlantooccipital junction: standards for measurement in normal children. *AJNR* 1987;8:995–999.
28. Kaufman RA, Dunbar JS, Botsford JA, et al. Traumatic longitudinal atlanto-occipital distraction injuries in children. *AJNR* 1982;3:415–419.
29. DiBenedetto T, Lee CK. Traumatic atlanto-occipital instability. A case report with follow-up and a new diagnostic technique. *Spine* 1990;15:595–597.
30. Gerlock AJ Jr, Mirfakhraee M, Benzel EC. Computed tomography of traumatic atlantooccipital dislocation. *Neurosurgery* 1983;13:316–319.
31. Bracken MB, Shepard MJ, Collins WF, et al. A randomized, controlled trial of methylprednisolone or naloxone in the treatment of acute spinal-cord injury. Results of the Second National Acute Spinal Cord Injury Study [See comments]. *New Engl J Med* 1990;322:1405–1411.
32. Watridge CB, Orrison WW, Arnold H, et al. Lateral atlantooccipital dislocation: case report. *Neurosurgery* 1985;17:345–347.
33. Evarts CM. Traumatic occipito-atlantal dislocation. *J Bone Joint Surg Am* 1970;52:1653–1660.
34. Jevtich V. Traumatic lateral atlanto-occipital dislocation with spontaneous bony fusion. A case report. *Spine* 1989;14:123–124.
35. Ramsay AH, Waxman BP, O'Brien JF. A case of traumatic atlanto-occipital dislocation with survival. *Injury* 1986;17:412–413.
36. Collalto PM, DeMuth WW, Schwentker EP, et al. Traumatic atlanto-occipital dislocation. Case report. *J Bone Joint Surg Am* 1986;68:1106–1109.
37. Spencer JA, Yeakley JW, Kaufman HH. Fracture of the occipital condyle. *Neurosurgery* 1984;15:101–103.
38. Anderson PA, Montesano PX. Morphology and treatment of occipital condyle fractures. *Spine* 1988;13:731–736.
39. Desai SS, Coumas JM, Danylevich A, et al. Fracture of the occipital condyle: case report and review of the literature. *J Trauma: Injury Infect Crit Care* 1990;30:240–241.
40. Tuli S, Tator CH, Fehlings MG, et al. Occipital condyle fractures. *Neurosurgery* 1997;41:368–376.
41. Orbay T, Aykol S, Seckin Z, et al. Late hypoglossal nerve palsy following fracture of the occipital condyle. *Surg Neurol* 1989;31:402–404.
42. Deeb ZL, Rothfus WE, Goldberg AL, et al. Occult occipital condyle fractures presenting as tumors. *J Comput Tomogr* 1988;12:261–263.
43. Urculo E, Arrazola M, Arrazola M Jr, et al. Delayed glossopharyngeal and vagus nerve paralysis following occipital condyle fracture. Case report. *J Neurosurg* 1996;84:522–525.
44. Noble ER, Smoker WR. The forgotten condyle: the appearance, morphology, and classification of occipital condyle fractures. *AJNR* 1996;17:507–513.
45. Young WF, Rosenwasser RH, Getch C, et al, Diagnosis and management of occipital condyle fractures. *Neurosurgery* 1994;34:257–260.

158. Diagnosis and Treatment of Atlas Fractures

Geoffrey P. Zubay and Curtis A. Dickman

History

Despite the lack of radiographic imaging, several fractures of the atlas were described in the 19th century. In 1817, Bell (1) described a C1-C2 combination fracture in a man who fell 50 feet onto his shoulders and died instantly. In 1822, Cooper (2) described an anterior and posterior arch fracture in a 3-year-old boy who fell and died 1 year later. In 1922, Sir Geoffrey Jefferson (3) gave the first systematic description of atlas fractures. He described a variety of fracture patterns based on his review of two patients with C1 fractures whom he had treated, two museum specimens that he examined, and 42 previously reported cases of C1 fractures. Because of his contributions, the four-part burst fracture of C1 was given the eponym Jefferson fracture. In his original monograph, Jefferson proposed axial loading as the mechanism of injury. He was essentially correct, but the biomechanics of C1 fractures have been elaborated on further over the years by numerous investigators using both *in vitro* and *in vivo* models.

Increased awareness of the importance of the transverse ligament has been paramount in the understanding of C1 fractures. In 1970, Spence and colleagues (4) alluded to this issue in their experiment with cadaveric specimens. They concluded that more than 6.9 mm of total bilateral displacement of the C1 lateral masses indicated disruption of the transverse ligament and instability requiring surgical fusion. Because of magnetic resonance imaging (MRI), numerous biomechanical and anatomical studies, and many retrospective clinical series, our understanding of the importance of the transverse ligament and when surgical fusion is needed has become more sophisticated.

Anatomy

The craniovertebral junction (CVJ) is comprised of the base of the skull, the atlas, and the axis. The biomechanical stability of the CVJ depends on the ligamentous anatomy and bony architecture. The interface of the CVJ is the atlas, which is a unique vertebral segment. It has no vertebral body and no adjacent discs. These features are critical to how the atlas affords the CVJ its unique range of motion.

Beginning around the seventh week of gestation, the atlas develops from three primary ossification centers. During intra-uterine life, the lateral masses form first. At birth, neither the anterior or posterior arches have formed. Typically, the anterior arch forms from either a single center representing the anterior tubercle or from multiple centers on each side of the tubercle, or it is a direct extension of the lateral masses. The anterior arch tends to be completely developed by 7 to 10 years of age. At birth the posterior halves of the posterior arch are separated by several millimeters of cartilage. The posterior arch usually fuses by the fourth year of life. In approximately 2% of the population, a fourth ossification center develops during the second year of life and forms the posterior tubercle between the two posterior arches (5,6).

Developmental abnormalities of the atlas tend to manifest as failure of the ossification centers to fuse (Fig. 1). Defects of the anterior arch are extremely rare. In his review of 2,749 specimens, Geipel (7) reports that the postmortem incidence of anterior arch clefts was 0.1%. Although posterior arch defects are also rare, they occur at least four times as often as anterior arch defects. Defects in the posterior arch range from a midline cleft to partial or complete absence of the posterior arch (8). Median clefts are the most common and have been estimated to occur in approximately 4% of the population and to represent 97% of posterior arch defects (9).

Other types of defects are less common (0.67% of the population) and consist of unilateral cleft defects, bilateral cleft defects, absence of the posterior arch with a persistent posterior tubercle, and total agenesis of the posterior arch. In the presence of these abnormalities, malrotation or instability at C1 or C2 is uncommon (10). They are usually detected by routine radiographic evaluation of the spine after minor trauma. Other congenital abnormalities tend to involve abnormal fusion centers, resulting in congenital fusion of C1, C2, and the occiput or occipitalization of the atlas. The most common findings are fusion between the anterior aspect of the atlas and the rim of the foramen magnum, posterior displacement of the odontoid process, and an abnormal size of the odontoid (10). Many of the abnormalities may be associated with systemic disorders such as Klippel-Feil syndrome, basilar impression, condylar hypoplasia, and occipital vertebrae.

Another abnormality, which is extrinsic to the atlas, involves the maldevelopment of an occipital vertebra. The occipital vertebra is similar to the proatlas, which is found in reptiles. It lies between the atlas and the occiput. When the odontoid is abnormally short, it is often referred to as an os odontoideum. In the absence of any disproportional abnormalities of the atlas and odontoid, the occipital vertebra is clearly a separate entity (11). Manifestations include a third condyle, a paracondylar process, a basilar process, accessory bone elements separate or fused to the foramen magnum, and a transverse fissure of the basioccipital bone. This abnormality is a manifestation of trisomy.

The normally developed atlas consists of a competent ante-

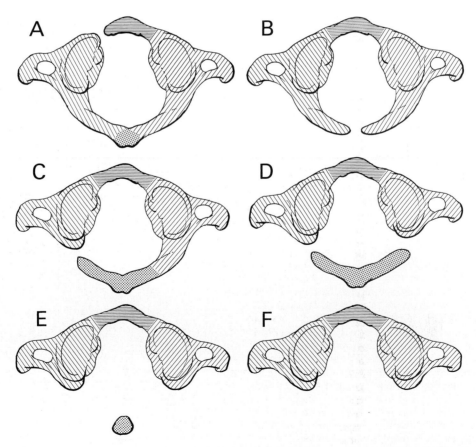

Fig. 1. Developmental abnormalities of the atlas. **A:** Unilateral anterior arch cleft. **B:** Median posterior arch cleft. **C:** Unilateral posterior arch cleft. **D:** Bilateral posterior arch cleft. **E:** Absence of posterior arch with persistent posterior tubercle. **F:** Total agenesis of the posterior arch. (From Barrow Neurological Institute, Phoenix, AZ, with permission.)

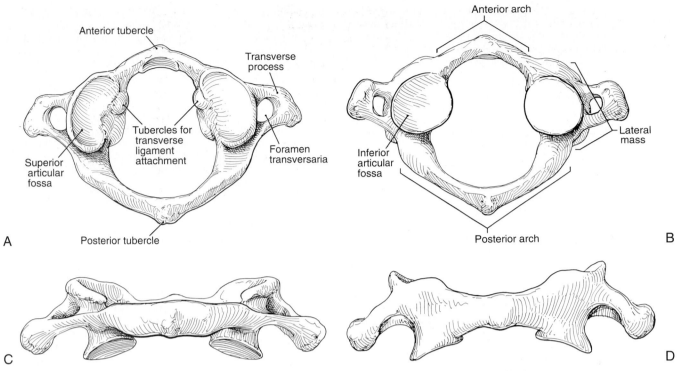

Fig. 2. Normal bony anatomy of the atlas: superior view **(A)**, inferior view **(B)**, posterior view **(C)**, and anterior view **(D)**. (From Barrow Neurological Institute, Phoenix, AZ, with permission.)

rior and posterior arch, lateral masses, and transverse processes with transverse foramina for passage of the vertebral arteries (Fig. 2). The anterior and posterior arches are narrow, curved cylinders. The cylinders are mostly made of thin cortical bone. With respect to their thinnest plane, the anterior arch is oriented horizontally and the posterior arch is oriented vertically. This configuration predicts the propensity for fractures and the orientation of fractures in the anterior and posterior arch.

The lateral masses are oval, and the transverse processes project laterally from the lateral surfaces. The medial surfaces of the lateral masses have a bony tubercle where the transverse ligament inserts. The superior and inferior articular surfaces of the lateral masses are concave and slightly convex, respectively. They articulate with the occipital condyles and the superior facets of C2, respectively. The occipital-C1 joint is a "ball-and-socket" joint that permits a small degree of flexion, extension, and lateral bending but no axial extension. The atlantoaxial joint consists of a bi-convex surface and permits a wide range of axial rotation as well as moderate flexion, extension, and lateral bending. The atlanto-occipital joint is more intimately fixed; therefore, the atlas follows the occiput more than C2.

Doherty and Heggeness (12) reviewed the anatomical proportions of 88 dried human cadaveric C1 vertebrae. The thickest bone was in the anterior arch (mean 1.8 mm), and the posterior arch was significantly thinner (mean 1.0 mm) than the anterior arch of C1. There was a constant relationship between the antero-posterior (AP) and lateral dimensions of the spinal canal but no particular alignment of the trabeculae in the lateral masses. Finally, the size and shape of the vertebral foramina were uniform. Their findings allowed some interpretation of the biomechanical function of the atlas. The thickness of the anterior arch is consistent with its load-bearing function. The absence of trabecular organization suggests that the load paths borne by the atlas are highly variable. However, uniformity of the vertebral canals was thought to be the result of selection error.

Other work by Panjabi and colleagues on the biomechanics of the atlas and an analysis of the bone architecture of the atlas implicates the propensity of fractures to occur where the cortical bone is the thinnest in the anterior and posterior arches (Fig. 3) (13,14). These conclusions correlate with clinical findings of atlas fractures. Furthermore, Panjabi alludes that the orientation of the thinnest portions of the cortex of the anterior and posterior arches plays a role in how they fracture. Specifically, the anterior arch can fracture as a result of an axial-loading mechanism that causes outward displacement of the lateral masses.

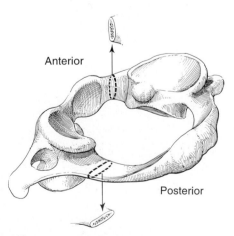

Fig. 3. Three-dimensional anatomy of the atlas depicting the vertical orientation of the anterior arch and the horizontal orientation of the posterior arch. This view demonstrates the orientation of the thinnest portion of the cortical bone in the anterior and posterior arches. (From Barrow Neurological Institute, Phoenix, AZ, with permission.)

Conversely, because of the orientation of the thinnest portion of the cortex, a fracture of the posterior arch usually requires hyperextension of the skull and load placed on the posterior arch by the occiput and posterior elements of C2.

Biomechanics of the Craniovertebral Junction

The normal atlas serves as a transition zone between the occiput and the cervical spine. It functions like a washer. The biomechanics of the normal atlas are limited by the complex ligamentous anatomy. Likewise traumatic instability at this joint is the result of disruption of the normal ligamentous anatomy or mechanical dissociation of the bony architecture with the surrounding ligamentous anatomy.

The normal ligamentous anatomy includes the apical ligament, anterior and posterior atlanto-occipital membranes, tectorial membrane, ligamentum flavum, anterior and posterior longitudinal ligaments, and capsular ligaments (Fig. 4). The principal ligaments of the atlas are the transverse ligament and the alar ligament. The transverse ligament is the principal stabilizing ligament of the atlas. Its primary function is to stabilize the orientation of the dens and to permit stable rotation. The synovium surrounding the dens facilitates this motion. The alar ligament indirectly stabilizes the atlas by fixing the dens to the skull base and thereby limits excessive rotation and lateral

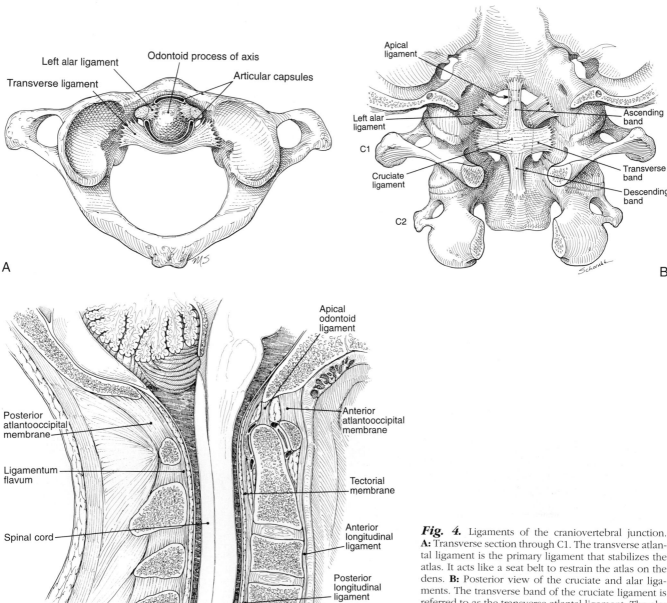

Fig. 4. Ligaments of the craniovertebral junction. **A:** Transverse section through C1. The transverse atlantal ligament is the primary ligament that stabilizes the atlas. It acts like a seat belt to restrain the atlas on the dens. **B:** Posterior view of the cruciate and alar ligaments. The transverse band of the cruciate ligament is referred to as the transverse atlantal ligament. The alar ligaments prevent excessive lateral bending and axial rotation of C1. **C:** Midline sagittal section demonstrating the ligaments of the upper cervical spine. (From Barrow Neurological Institute, Phoenix, AZ, with permission.)

bending. The remainder of the ligaments of the atlas are thought to provide additional support and to stretch with no significant limitation.

Normal range of motion has been studied in detail in both cadaveric models and normal subjects. Range of motion at the CVJ is complex and cannot be described in terms of one component. At the atlanto-occipital joint, there is no axial rotation, 10 degrees of flexion and extension, and 10 degrees of lateral bending. At the atlantoaxial joint, there are 40 degrees of unilateral axial rotation, 10 degrees of flexion and extension, and 10 degrees of lateral bending (13,14).

Biomechanics of Atlas Fractures

Most of what is understood about the biomechanical stability of the atlas fracture is the result of multiple cadaveric biomechanical studies. Because atlas fractures have not been reliably reproduced in whole cadavers, most studies have relied on the use of cadaveric specimens of the cervical spine stripped of their intrinsic musculature. The two most frequently cited studies are those led by Spence (4) and Panjabi (13). The extensive work of Panjabi and co-workers attempts to understand the biomechanics of the atlas fracture both qualitatively and quantitatively by reproducing the loading mechanism and assessing the biomechanical stability of the fracture after injury (13). In contrast, Spence and colleagues attempted to correlate the extent of lateral mass displacement with the incidence of ligament disruption as a model for predicting the probability of instability after injury (4). A review of their experimental models and findings is worthwhile.

The Panjabi group (13) did extensive *in vitro* work on atlas fractures. In their experimental model, cadaveric specimens of the cervical spine (C0-C3) were subjected to variable traumatic axial loads while the spine was in either a neutral or extended posture. They measured the posttraumatic instability of the specimen as a function of flexibility, range of motion, and the neutral zone. Flexibility was defined as the amount of deformation in response to a unit load. The neutral zone was defined as the range of motion that can occur when minimal force is applied and minimal stress is conferred to the restricting ligaments. The elastic zone, defined as the portion of the load-deformation curve during which ligaments become stretched and stiff, ultimately defines the limits of the range of motion. Instability was defined as the ratio of the posttraumatic range of motion to the intact specimen's range of motion (i.e., a statistically significant ratio greater than 1). The greatest instability resulted from flexion-extension. Compressive fractures caused a 90% increase in the neutral zone and a 40% increase in the range of motion. Lateral bending was also altered with a 20% increase in both the neutral zone and range of motion. The change in axial rotation, however, was not statistically significant—the increase in the neutral zone and range of motion was only 10% (13).

The experiment of Panjabi and colleagues (13) also elaborates on the mechanism of injury. Posterior arch fractures were more common in an extended resting state at the time of load application. This finding was hypothesized to be the result of the anatomical orientation of the architecture of the anterior and posterior arch. The anterior arch is most often fractured, probably because of the orientation of the thinnest portion or the arch's cortical bone (Fig. 3). The posterior arch was fractured less often when the spine was in the neutral orientation because the thinnest portion of the cortex has a perpendicular orientation. The posterior arch probably is fractured as a secondary event that involves translation of energy during outward displacement of the lateral masses or as a result of a secondary hyperextension injury (Fig. 5). Extension may allow the base of the skull or the posterior arch of C2 to strike the posterior arch with a bending moment strong enough to cause a fracture. Because energy often dissipates or no extension occurs during the injury, the posterior arch is often spared while the anterior arch is fractured. The extended posture of the spine also needed less load to fracture. Force and impulse were decreased by 31% and 50%, respectively, when the spine was moved from the neutral position to the extended position before load application.

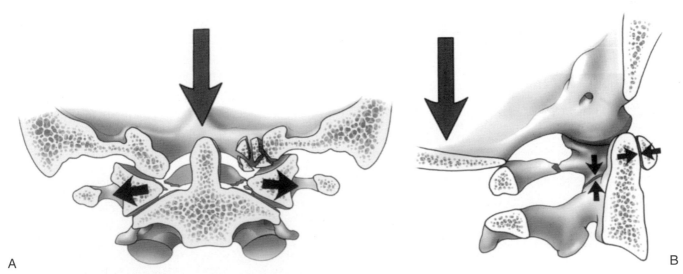

A   B

Fig. 5. Primary injury vectors involved in atlas fractures. **A:** A neutrally aligned axial compressive force causing outward displacement of the lateral masses leads to a four-part Jefferson fracture, which can occur with axial-loading injuries to the cervical spine. **B:** A posteriorly positioned compressive force can lead to fracture of the posterior ring. This fracture can occur with hyperextension injuries. (Adapted from White JJ, Panjabi MM. *Clinical biomechanics of the spine*, 2nd ed. Philadelphia: JB Lippincott Co, 1990, with permission.)

This work provides the best experimental evidence for the mechanism and load requirements underlying atlas fractures. However, the number of specimens was limited. Hence, conclusions about the frequency and extent of instability associated with different types of atlas fractures could not be drawn. It is interesting to note that Jefferson's early observations that no pain accompanied axial rotation after injury ("flexion of the head was possible through a few degrees only, and rotation was quite painless") are supported by Panjabi and co-workers' determination that atlas fractures are accompanied by no instability with axial rotation.

In the study by Spence and associates (4) 10 cadaveric cervical spines were stripped of their intrinsic musculature. The anterior and posterior arches were cut bilaterally to simulate a burst fracture. Rods were then drilled through both lateral masses, and a laterally distracting force was applied to the lateral masses until the transverse ligament ruptured. The transverse ligament ruptured when the lateral masses were distracted 4.8 mm to 7.6 mm (mean 6.3 mm). They concluded that disruption of the transverse ligament was unlikely when radiographic displacement of the lateral mass was less than 5.7 mm and likely when it was greater than 6.9 mm. The experiment was flawed because the mechanism used to disrupt the transverse ligament was not representative of the axial-loading mechanism that causes atlas fractures. Rather, they used a purely tension-based model. Nevertheless, their experimental findings, remembered as the Rule of Spence, are still often used as a crude predictor of instability during radiographic assessment of atlas fractures.

Epidemiology of Atlas Fractures

Atlas fractures are often the result of motor vehicle accidents, motorcycle accidents, and traumatic falls. They occur in men almost twice as often as in women and are most common during the second decade of life (15–18). Atlas fractures account for 4% to 15% of cervical spine fractures and 1% to 3% of all spinal column injuries. Because of the load requirements and the mechanism of injury, about half the cases of atlas fractures are accompanied by axis fractures. Atlas fractures only occur as an isolated injury to the spinal column in 39% to 56% of cases. From 1976 to 1993 at the Barrow Neurological Institute in Phoenix, 120 atlas fractures were identified, 50 (41%) of which were associated with axis fractures (Table 1) (19).

Atlas fractures are seldom associated with neurological deficits. The incidence of neurological deficits ranges between 4% to 17% of cases (15–17). When neurological deficits are present, they are usually the result of injury at other spinal levels. This observation is partly artifactual because patients with atlas fractures and severe neurological impairment rarely survive to reach a hospital for assessment. Autopsy studies demonstrate that upper cervical spine injuries account for 20% of fatal spine injuries (20,21). Steele's Rule of Thirds, however, predicts that

the likelihood of neurological injury at the level of the atlas is reduced because the mechanism of injury is axial loading, which causes centripetal spread of the fracture fragments, and because the volumetric space occupied at C1 is divided equally by the odontoid, cerebrospinal fluid, and the spinal cord (Fig. 4A).

Patients with atlas fractures usually report pain and dysphagia. The pain occurs in the distribution of the greater occipital nerve, which is prone to injury as it exits through the atlantoaxial membrane posteriorly. Dysphagia tends to be the consequence of a retropharyngeal hematoma. Vertebral artery symptoms are reported less often and may be the result of transient arterial compression from lateral mass displacement. The incidence of vertebral arterial dissection is unknown, but the diagnosis should be considered when C1 is fractured.

Diagnosis of Atlas Fractures

In Jefferson's original monograph, patients with atlas fractures were described as having a limited capacity to flex because of pain, but they were able to rotate their head effortlessly. In awake and alert patients who have been placed in cervical spine precautions, these characteristics may be useful clinical markers for raising suspicion of an atlas fracture. However, because most atlas fractures are incurred traumatically, most patients present in cervical spine precautions as a level 1 or 2 trauma. The new Advanced Trauma Life Support protocol allows surgeons to clear the cervical spine in patients who are awake, not intoxicated, and neurologically intact, and who have a Glasgow Coma Scale score of 15 and no cervical spine discomfort in the absence of any distracting injuries. In our experience, such patients are few. Consequently, the error rate associated with attempts to clear the cervical spine in the absence of any radiographic studies would likely be higher. We therefore recommend radiographic studies for all trauma patients. Certainly, radiographic studies should be obtained from all neurologically intact patients who are awake and cooperative and who complain of a stiff neck, neck discomfort, occipital anesthesia, or suboccipital tenderness. Furthermore, an injury of the occipitocervical junction should be suspected and ruled out with plain AP and lateral radiographs. However, plain radiographs can fail to visualize the atlas and occipitocervical junction adequately, and computed tomography (CT) is often needed.

A subset of patients will present with dysarthria and dysphagia from a retropharyngeal injury. These symptoms should also raise suspicion of a vertebral artery injury from a posterior circulation stroke. Cerebrovascular studies should include magnetic resonance angiography (MRA) or conventional angiography. The timing of such studies relative to stabilization of the patient depends on the severity of the symptoms and the radiographic evidence for a compromised vertebral foramen.

For unconscious patients, a cervical spine injury should be

Table 1. Demographics of Upper Cervical Spine Fractures in 414 Patients (1976–1993)

Fracture type	Total no. of injuries	No. of neurological injuries (%)	No. of deaths (%)	Patients requiring surgical stabilization (%)
Isolated C1 fracture	70	3 (4)	1 (1)	3 (4)
Isolated C2 fracture	294	24 (8)	20 (7)	51 (17)
Combination C1-C2 fractures	50	10 (20)	3 (6)	13 (26)

From Dickman CA, Greene KA. Treatment of atlas fractures. In: Sonntag VKH, Menezes AH, eds. *Principles of spinal surgery.* New York: McGraw-Hill, with permission.

suspected until proven otherwise. Because these patients are often intubated, adequate open-mouth odontoid views can seldom be obtained. In such cases, a CT scan of the occipitocervical junction should be obtained.

When a fracture is identified by conventional radiography, CT is needed to delineate the three-dimensional anatomy of the fracture. For reasons discussed later in this chapter, MRI should also be performed to assess the integrity of the ligaments and the spinal cord.

PLAIN RADIOGRAPHY. Both lateral and AP open-mouth radiographs should be obtained (Fig. 6). Multiple studies have indicated that about 25% of plain radiographs fail to identify atlas fractures. Consequently, patients with relevant clinical symptoms or an enlarged shadow associated with the retropharyngeal soft tissue should undergo CT (15,22,23). The retropharyngeal shadow at C1-2 should be less than 5 mm in adults (24, 25). No reliable measurement is available to screen pediatric patients.

On AP views, the symmetry of the lateral masses should be assessed with respect to their orientation to the odontoid. An asymmetrical or offset lateral mass can indicate an atlas fracture, although unilateral offset of the lateral mass over C2 can be an artifact of rotation. Pseudospread (defined as greater than 2-mm total overlap of the two C1 lateral masses on an AP open-mouth view) is present in most children between 3 months and 4 years of age. During the second year of life, its prevalence is evident in 91% to 100% of children (26). Pseudospread is probably the result of disproportionate growth of C1 on C2 and is usually the cause of radiographic C1 abnormalities in children. Atlas fractures are rare in preteens, who are protected by their flexible necks, body weight, skull plasticity, and shock-absorbing synchondroses of C1.

Lateral radiographs can help identify posterior ring fractures

and compromise of the transverse ligament from an anterior ring fracture. The atlantodental interval (ADI) is a useful radiographic landmark for detecting compromise of the anterior arch and transverse ligament in the absence of any visible fracture lines (27,28). The ADI is measured from the middle of the posterior cortex of the anterior arch of C1 to the adjacent anterior cortex of the dens. The normal ADI is not mobile and does not exceed 3 mm in adults or 5 mm in children. When the ADI is widened, compromise of the anterior arch and transverse ligament should be suspected.

CT. CT with three-dimensional reconstructions allows a more precise assessment of the two- and three-dimensional anatomy of C1 (Fig. 7). Axial slices 1.5 mm-thick are usually needed to assess the anatomy adequately. As mentioned earlier, CT often reveals fractures that plain radiographs are unable to demonstrate. Furthermore, CT permits precise assessment of the occiput and C2, which may be important for the assessment of associated injuries such as C1-C2 combination fractures, atlantooccipital dislocations, and occipital condyle fractures.

The exceptional detail of the bone anatomy as visualized with CT can provide additional useful clinical information. Disruption of the bony tubercle on which the transverse ligaments insert can identify disruption of the transverse ligament in the absence of an MRI study and can indicate instability. The precise orientation of the fractured atlas fragments can also help determine the stability of the fracture. Compromise of the vertebral foramen from fracture lines or fragments warrants further radiographic investigation to rule out dissection or compromise of the vertebral artery.

MRI. The usefulness of MRI lies in its ability to assess the condition of the surrounding soft tissue, the associated ligamentous anatomy, and the spinal cord (Fig. 8). Furthermore, MRA can

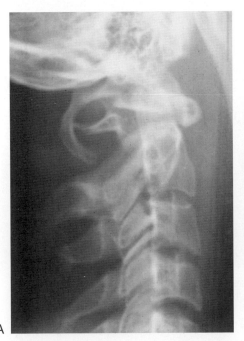
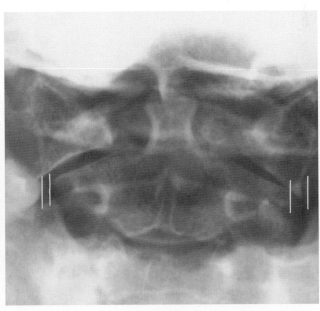

Fig. 6. **A:** Lateral cervical radiograph of a posterior arch fracture of C1 in a 42-year-old man. **B:** An open-mouth radiographic view of a 23-year-old man with a comminuted fracture of the left lateral mass of C1. Bilaterally, the margins of the C1 lateral masses are offset from the lateral margins of C2 *(white lines)*. (From Dickman CA, Greene KA. Treatment of atlas fractures. In: Sonntag VKH, Menezes AH, eds. *Principles of spinal surgery*. New York: McGraw-Hill, 1996, with permission.)

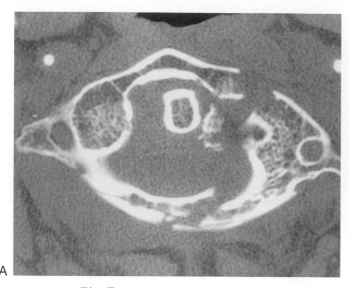
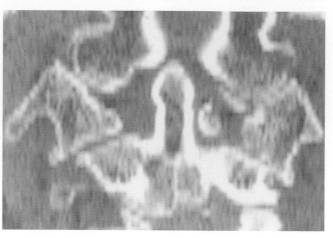

Fig. 7. A: CT scan of the patient whose plain radiographs were shown in Fig. 6B. The left lateral mass is disconnected from C1. The bone is fractured where the anterior arch joins the lateral mass and through the posterior C1 ring. The tubercle for transverse ligament insertion is sheared off the C1 lateral mass. This comminuted fracture represents an "unstable" injury. It can heal only if the bone fragments unite. **B:** The reconstructed coronal view of the CT shows the bony detail better than the plain radiographs in Fig. 6B. (From Dickman CA, Greene KA. Treatment of atlas fractures. In: Sonntag VKH, Menezes AH, eds. *Principles of spinal surgery.* New York: McGraw-Hill, 1996, with permission.)

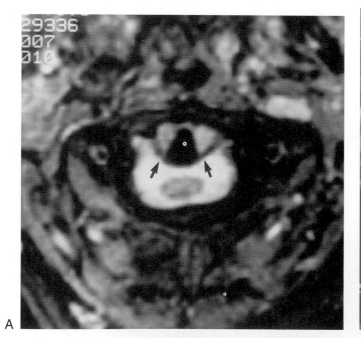
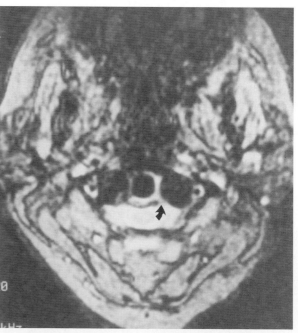

Fig. 8. Gradient-echo MRI of the transverse atlantal ligament obtained in a high-resolution MRI unit. (Signa, GE, 1.5 T unit with a surface coil; imaging parameters: TE, 18 milliseconds; flip angle, 20 degrees; and 3-mm slices). Images were obtained parallel to the C1 ring. **A:** The normal transverse atlantal ligament has a homogeneous low-intensity signal *(arrows)* that extends between the tubercles of the lateral masses of C1. The ligament is contrasted by a high-intensity signal anteriorly by the synovial space that surrounds the dens and posteriorly by the high-intensity signal from the cerebrospinal fluid. **B:** Disrupted transverse atlantal ligament shows the loss of anatomical continuity. Blood *(arrow)* separates the ligament from the tubercle of C1. (From Dickman CA, Greene KA. Treatment of atlas fractures. In: Sonntag VKH, Menezes AH, eds. *Principles of spinal surgery.* New York: McGraw-Hill, 1996, with permission.)

be used in place of conventional angiography to assess the integrity of the vertebral arteries.

The condition of the transverse ligament is critical to determining the stability of an atlas fracture. Disruption of the transverse ligament precludes atlanto-axial stability with healing of the fracture fragments and may indicate the need for surgical stabilization.

In 1991, the MRI technique used at the Barrow Neurological Institute to assess the integrity of the transverse ligament was described (27). Sagittal and axial images of the upper cervical spine and transverse ligament were acquired using a multiplanar gradient-echo technique (TR 733 milliseconds, TE 18 milliseconds, flip angle 20 degrees, with 3-mm slices). An additional three-dimensional volume-acquisition technique with axial reconstructions is used (TR 35 milliseconds, TE 15 milliseconds, flip angle 5 degrees, with 2-mm slices). The ligament's high degree of contrast with the surrounding structures permits it to be visualized. The low-intensity signal evident on gradient-echo images with small flip angles reflects the dense structure of the ligaments. The circular zone of high-intensity signal surrounding the dens is a result of the long relaxation time on T2-weighted images of the synovium and the synovial fluid. Tears of the ligament appear as the loss of anatomical continuity. A high-intensity signal is usually visible within the ligament at the site of injury.

Classification of Atlas Fractures

Atlas fractures are often mislabeled as Jefferson fractures. The term Jefferson fracture is reserved for four-part fractures involving the anterior and posterior rings in an almost symmetrical fashion. Few atlas fractures fall into this category.

A review of the literature combined with the collective experience with C1 fractures at the Barrow Neurological Institute revealed six basic fracture patterns (Fig. 9). Atlas fractures can be classified as anterior arch fractures, posterior arch fractures, simple lateral mass fractures, comminuted lateral mass fractures, multiple ring burst fractures (Jefferson fractures), and anteroposterior ring fractures. This classification has an important bearing on the stability of the fracture and the need for immobilization and stabilization.

At our institution, injuries to the transverse ligament have also been classified based on anatomical variations of injury and their impact on long-term stability. Four basic injuries can occur (Fig. 10) (29). Type I injuries involve disruption of the ligament in its midportion (IA) or its periosteal insertion (IB). Type I injuries are incapable of healing, are unstable, and require surgical fixation of C1 and C2. Type II injuries disconnect the tubercle from its insertion on the adjacent lateral mass as a result of an avulsion injury (IIB) or involvement of a comminuted lateral mass fracture (IIA). Type II injuries usually heal with a rigid orthosis (halo brace).

Management of Acute Atlas Fractures

Initial management should always consist of reduction and immobilization (Fig. 11). If axial traction is to be used, 2 to 10 lbs of weight should be used, and neurological monitoring should be meticulous. Distraction can be harmful if done carelessly in the presence of atlanto-occipital instability. More often realignment and reduction can be achieved with gentle distraction and subsequent halo immobilization with either plain radiographic or fluoroscopic-assisted visualization of the bone anatomy.

Most atlas fractures are stable and heal properly with external orthotic immobilization alone. Isolated anterior or posterior ring fractures, minimally displaced burst fractures, and linear lateral mass fractures can all be treated with a Philadelphia collar or a sternal-occipital-mandibular immobilization (SOMI) brace. Soft collars are not recommended because they do not restrict movement sufficiently. Although the halo vest is the most effective device for immobilizing the upper cervical spine, it is not an absolute necessity in these cases (30–35). Lee and co-workers report successful treatment of 12 patients with a Miami J collar alone for 10 to 12 weeks (36). However, most prefer the use of the halo vest because there are fewer complications related to patient compliance. Widely displaced or comminuted fractures require a stable orthosis such as a halo brace because the displaced fracture fragments or comminuted lateral masses are usually accompanied by compromise of the transverse ligament.

In our experience, atlas fractures should be screened with MRI of the transverse ligament. Other authors choose to assess the ligament by features on plain radiography, flexion and extension radiographs, and CT, and they rely on Spence's criterion of 7 mm of lateral distraction of the lateral masses as an indication of ligamentous disruption. However, the Rule of Spence does not accurately reflect whether the transverse ligament has been injured. Even in single-ring fractures, the ligament could have been disrupted by the initial axial loading and distracting forces of the injury even though the fracture fragments returned to their resting positions.

Review of the literature definitively identifies type IA and IB transverse ligamentous injuries as unstable and requiring operative reduction and fixation. In contrast, type IIA and IIB transverse ligament injuries have the ability to heal with external orthosis alone. In a review of 39 patients with traumatic disruption of the transverse atlantal ligament (29), 16 of 20 patients with type IIA fractures healed with halo fixation alone. Only four patients had type IIB fractures, two of which had malunion of the ligament as evidenced by instability. The failure rate of type IIA fractures to heal with halo fixation alone was 30%. No generalizations could be made about type IIB fractures because there were too few patients. These fractures, however, may have a tendency for malunion.

Because type I ligament injuries will not heal, all patients with these injuries should be reduced and fixated surgically, regardless of the anatomy of the fracture. Patients with type II ligament injuries should be considered for a trial of halo fixation. Because judicious follow-up and care are needed, patients with type II ligament injuries at risk of poor compliance with the treatment should probably be surgically stabilized first.

C1-C2 combination fractures deserve further consideration and involve a more complicated management scheme. They are discussed separately in the following section.

C1-C2 COMBINATION FRACTURES. Because of the intimate relationship between C1 and C2, concomitant fractures of C2 are common (Table 1). Depending on the morphology of the C2 fracture and the displacement of fractured fragments, a C1-C2 combination fracture may be intrinsically unstable and require open reduction internal fixation or may be amenable to closed external reduction and orthotic immobilization. Most are of the latter type and as many as 95% of C1-C2 fractures are successfully managed in this fashion.

If the transverse ligament is disrupted, regardless of the type of ligamentous injury, surgery for internal fixation should be the primary treatment. The combined intrinsic instability of the

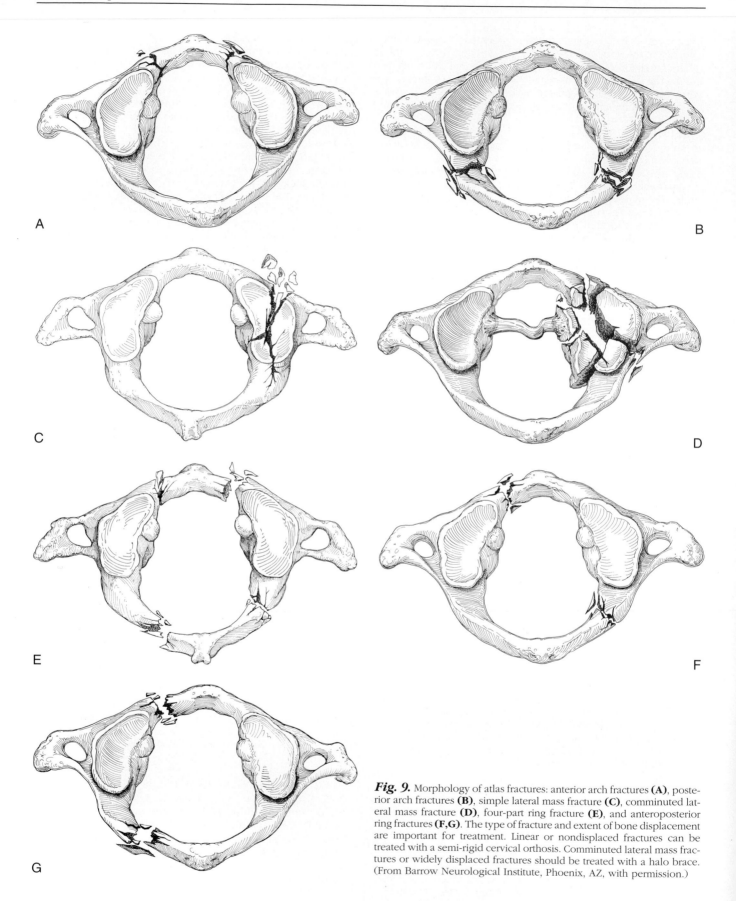

Fig. 9. Morphology of atlas fractures: anterior arch fractures **(A)**, posterior arch fractures **(B)**, simple lateral mass fracture **(C)**, comminuted lateral mass fracture **(D)**, four-part ring fracture **(E)**, and anteroposterior ring fractures **(F,G)**. The type of fracture and extent of bone displacement are important for treatment. Linear or nondisplaced fractures can be treated with a semi-rigid cervical orthosis. Comminuted lateral mass fractures or widely displaced fractures should be treated with a halo brace. (From Barrow Neurological Institute, Phoenix, AZ, with permission.)

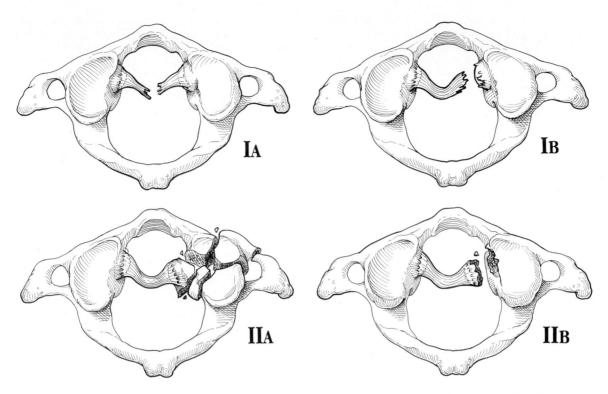

Fig. 10. Classification of injuries of the transverse atlantal ligament. Type I injuries disrupt the substance of the ligament in its midportion *(IA)* or at its periosteal insertion *(IB)*. Type II injuries disconnect the tubercle, where the transverse ligament inserts, from the C1 lateral mass and involve a comminuted C1 lateral mass *(IIA)* or the tubercle avulsed from an intact lateral mass *(IIB)*. (From Barrow Neurological Institute, Phoenix, AZ, with permission.)

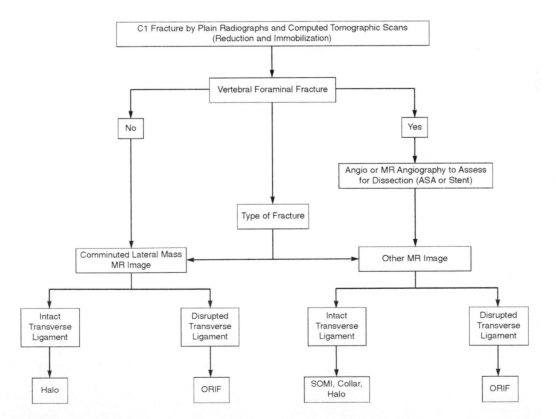

Fig. 11. Treatment algorithm for C1 fractures. *ORIF*, open reduction with internal fixation; *ASA*, aspirin; *SOMI*, sterno-occipital mandibular immobilizer.

disrupted C1 transverse ligament and the C2 fracture leads to higher malunion rates with external orthosis alone.

Type I odontoid fractures are extremely rare and are thought to be related to either avulsion of the alar ligament or atlanto-occipital dislocation. They are intrinsically stable fractures and heal well with external orthosis alone. In combination with a stable C1 fracture, external orthotic immobilization should be the first line of treatment.

Type II odontoid fractures are typically treated based on the extent of the displacement of the dens. More than 6 mm of displacement, regardless of direction, may indicate transverse ligament instability and subsequent need for surgical repair. In their review of 107 cases of axis fracture, Hadley and associates found that patients with more than 6 mm of displacement experienced a 67% nonunion rate compared to 26% for those with less than 6 mm of displacement (37). Likewise, in a C1-C2 combination fracture with more than 6 mm of displacement of the dens, the rules that apply to C1 fractures associated with disruption of the transverse ligament may also apply. In the absence of any clinical or radiographic signs of transverse ligament disruption, a halo brace may suffice.

Type III odontoid fractures, hangman's fractures, and C2 miscellaneous fractures in combination with C1 fractures may be treated with external orthosis alone (38). The management of these fractures is based on the intrinsic stability of the C2 fracture in the presence of a C1 fracture with an intact transverse ligament.

Subsequently, surgery for C1-C2 combination fractures should be reserved for patients who have a disrupted transverse ligament. For patients with an intact transverse ligament but who have high-risk factors for malunion or who fail external orthotic immobilization, surgery may also be appropriate. The type of surgery depends on the morphology of the fractures, which often dictates which instrumentation can be applied.

The goal of surgery is to restore C1-C2 stability. Odontoid screw fixation can be used if the transverse ligament is intact (39). If the pedicles are intact and the lateral masses of C2 are not comminuted, transarticular screws from a posterior approach or facet screws from an anterior approach can be used. If the posterior arch and posterior spinous process of C2 are intact, posterior cervical wiring or a Halifax clamp (Codman, Raynham, MA) can be used. However, when C1 cannot be directly fixated to C2, fusion may have to extend to the occiput or lower cervical levels.

Conclusions

Extensive experience with atlas fractures has indicated that treatment should be based upon the ligamentous stability associated with the fracture. Atlas fractures are seldom isolated injuries; therefore, concomitant injuries need to be considered. C1-C2 combination fractures are often unstable and require open reduction and fixation. Typically, occipital fractures (condylar fractures) are stable and require only moderate immobilization with a cervical orthosis such as a Miami J collar. Occipital condylar fractures in combination with C1 fractures have not been reviewed as a separate clinical entity. Given the stability of condylar fractures, however, it would be reasonable to assume that stable C1 fractures associated with condylar fractures could be treated much like C1-C2 fractures.

At our institution, isolated but stable C1 atlas fractures, as determined by the integrity of the transverse ligament, are typically treated with halo immobilization or a cervical collar. Halo immobilization affords patients with displaced fractures the best opportunity for nonoperative closed reduction and osseous union. We also prefer halo immobilization in patients who may fail to comply with treatment, although the Miami J collar or SOMI also provides adequate immobilization. Typically, we treat patients with 8 to 12 weeks of immobilization in the brace with periodic radiographic assessments (every 4 weeks) to confirm alignment before challenging them with flexion-extension studies when the halo brace is removed.

For patients with a compromised transverse ligament, open reduction and fixation are usually achieved with occipitocervical fusion, C1-C2 fusion with transarticular screws, or C1-C2 wiring, depending on the anatomy of the fracture.

References

1. Bell C. *Surgical observations: a quarterly report of cases in surgery treated in Middlesex Hospital* London: 1817.
2. Cooper A. *A treatise on dislocations and on fractures of the joints,* London: 1822.
3. Jefferson G. Fracture of the atlas vertebra: report of four cases, and a review of those previously recorded. *Br J Surg* 1920;7:407–422.
4. Spence KF Jr, Decker S, Sell KW. Bursting atlantal fracture associated with rupture of the transverse ligament. *J Bone Joint Surg Am* 1970; 52:543–549.
5. Truex RC Jr, Johnson CH. Congenital anomalies of the upper cervical spine. *Orthop Clin North Am* 1978;9:891–900.
6. Gehweiler JA Jr, Daffner RH, Roberts L Jr. Malformations of the atlas vertebra simulating the Jefferson fracture. *AJR* 1983;140:1083–1086.
7. Geipel P. Zur Kenntnis der spaltbidungen das atlas und epistopheus. Teil IV. *Zantralbl Allg Pathol* 1955;94:19–84.
8. Wadia NH. Myelopathy complicating congenital atlanto-axial dislocation. (A study of 28 cases.) *Brain* 1967;90:449–472.
9. Phan N, Marras C, Midha R, et al. Cervical myelopathy caused by hypoplasia of the atlas: two case reports and review of the literature. *Neurosurgery* 1998;43:629–633.
10. Brinker MR, Weeden SH, Whitecloud TS III. Congenital anomalies of the cervical spine. In: Frymoyer JW, Ducker TB, Hadler NM, et al, eds. *The adult spine. Principles and practice.* Philadelphia: Lippincott-Raven, 1997;1205–1221.
11. Martel W, Uyham R, Stimson CW. Subluxation of the atlas causing spinal cord compression in a case of Down's syndrome with a "manifestation of an occipital vertebra." *Radiology* 1969;93:839–840.
12. Doherty BJ, Heggeness MH. The quantitative anatomy of the atlas. *Spine* 1994;19:2497–2500.
13. Panjabi MM, Oda T, Crisco JJ III, et al. Experimental study of atlas injuries. I. Biomechanical analysis of their mechanisms and fracture patterns. *Spine* 1991;16:460–465.
14. Oda T, Panjabi MM, Crisco JJ III, et al. Experimental study of atlas injuries. II. Relevance to clinical diagnosis and treatment. *Spine* 1991;16:466–473.
15. Dickman CA, Hadley MN, Browner C, et al. Neurosurgical management of acute atlas-axis combination fractures. A review of 25 cases. *J Neurosurg* 1989;70:45–49.
16. Lee C, Woodring JH. Unstable Jefferson variant atlas fractures: an unrecognized cervical injury. *AJNR* 1991;12:1105–1110.
17. Landells CD, Van Peteghem PK. Fractures of the atlas: classification, treatment and morbidity. *Spine* 1988;13:450–452.
18. Fowler JL, Sandhu A, Fraser RD. A review of fractures of the atlas vertebra. *J Spinal Disord* 1990;3:19–24.
19. Dickman CA, Greene KA. Treatment of atlas fractures. In: Menezes AH, Sonntag VKH, eds. *Principles of spinal surgery.* New York: McGraw-Hill, 1996;855–869.
20. Bucholz RW, Burkhead WZ, Graham W, et al. Occult cervical spine injuries in fatal traffic accidents. *J Trauma* 1979;19:768–771.
21. Alker GJ Jr, Oh YS, Leslie EV. High cervical spine and craniocervical junction injuries in fatal traffic accidents: a radiological study. *Orthop Clin North Am* 1978;9:1003–1010.
22. Gehweiler JA, Osborne RL, Becker RF. *The radiology of vertebral trauma.* Philadelphia: WB Saunders, 1980.
23. Hadley MN, Dickman CA, Browner CM, et al. Acute traumatic atlas fractures: management and long term outcome. *Neurosurgery* 1988; 23:31–35.

24. Templeton PA, Young JW, Mirvis SE, et al. The value of retropharyngeal soft tissue measurements in trauma of the adult cervical spine. Cervical spine soft tissue measurements. *Skeletal Radiol* 1987;16:98–104.
25. Penning L. Prevertebral hematoma in cervical spine injury: incidence and etiologic significance. *AJR* 1981;136:553–561.
26. Suss RA, Zimmerman RD, Leeds NE. Pseudospread of the atlas: false sign of Jefferson fracture in young children. *AJR* 1983;140:1079–1082.
27. Dickman CA, Mamourian A, Sonntag VKH, et al. Magnetic resonance imaging of the transverse atlantal ligament for the evaluation of atlantoaxial instability. *J Neurosurg* 1991;75:221–227.
28. Fielding JW, Cochran GVB, Lawsing JF III, et al. Tears of the transverse ligament of the atlas. A clinical biomechanical study. *J Bone Joint Surg Am* 1974;56:1683–1691.
29. Dickman CA, Greene KA, Sonntag VKH. Injuries involving the transverse atlantal ligament: classification and treatment guidelines based upon experience with 39 injuries. *Neurosurgery* 1996;38:44–50.
30. Koch RA, Nickel VL. The halo vest: An evaluation of motion and forces across the neck. *Spine* 1978;3:103–107.
31. Johnson RM, Hart DL, Simmons EF, et al. Cervical orthoses. A study comparing their effectiveness in restricting cervical motion in normal subjects. *J Bone Joint Surg Am* 1977;59:332–339.
32. Nickel VL, Perry J, Garrett A, et al. The halo. A spinal skeletal traction fixation device. *J Bone Joint Surg Am* 1968;50:1400–1409.
33. Prolo DJ, Runnels JB, Jameson RM. The injured cervical spine. Immediate and long-term immobilization with the halo. *JAMA* 1973;224:591–594.
34. Thompson H. The "halo" traction apparatus. A method of external splinting of the cervical spine after injury. *J Bone Joint Surg Br* 1962;44:655–661.
35. Zwerling MT, Riggins RS. Use of the halo apparatus in acute injuries of the cervical spine. *Surg Gynecol Obstet* 1974;138:189–193.
36. Lee TT, Greene BA, Petrin DR. Treatment of stable burst fracture of the atlas (Jefferson fracture) with rigid cervical collar. *Spine* 1998;23:1963–1967.
37. Hadley MN, Browner C, Sonntag VKH. Axis fractures: a comprehensive review of management and treatment in 107 cases. *Neurosurgery* 1985;17:281–290.
38. Clark CT, Apuzzo MLJ. The evaluation and management of trauma to the odontoid process. In: Cooper PR, ed. *Management of post-traumatic spinal instability.* Park Ridge, IL: American Association of Neurological Surgeons, 1990;77–97.
39. Dickman CA, Sonntag VKH, Marcotte P. Techniques of screw fixation for the cervical spine. *BNI Quarterly* 1992;8:9–26.

159. Fractures of the Second Cervical Vertebra

Mark Gerber, A. Giancarlo Vishteh, Jonathan J. Baskin, Curtis A. Dickman, and Volker K.H. Sonntag

Fractures of the second cervical vertebra have an interesting history. As a result of the unique anatomy of and biomechanical forces on this joint, several distinct fracture patterns are common. Over the years, investigators have classified fractures of the second cervical vertebra into three distinct groups. The grouping of these fractures has improved communication about the type of fracture incurred as well as treatment for these injuries.

The recognition and treatment of cervical spine injuries are exceedingly important. Since the advent of motorized transportation, injuries to the cervical spine have undoubtedly become more prevalent. In a 1997 study, 340 of 1,820 cervical spine fractures treated at a single institution involved C2 (1). Additionally, high cervical spinal cord injuries associated with these fractures necessitate rapid intervention in an effort to optimize neurological outcomes and to minimize potentially disastrous complications.

Embryology

It is difficult to discuss the anatomy of the axis without reviewing the embryology of the craniovertebral junction. During the fourth week of gestation, cells of mesenchymal origin align themselves in the midline to form 42 somites (2). The four occipital somites and the first two cervical spinal somites ultimately differentiate to form the craniovertebral junction including the clivus, basiocciput, C1, and C2 (3).

The proatlas is the fourth occipital sclerotome (Fig. 1) (4–6). This somite is unique because it contributes to the formation of the anterior tubercle of the clivus, apical ligament, apex of the dens, occipital condyles, foramen magnum, alar and cruciate ligaments, posterior arch of C1, and the lateral masses of C2 (2, 7). Additional contributions to the formation of C2 include the first spinal sclerotome, which forms the dens, and the second spinal sclerotome, which forms the body and posterior arch of C2.

The developmental complexity of the axis subjects it to congenital aberrations. True os odontoideum is a rare condition defined as hypoplasia of the odontoid process. The odontoid process appears as an unfused oval ossicle and lies above the superior facets of the axis. This condition is thought to develop as a result of failure of the dens (C1 sclerotome) to fuse with the body of C2 (C2 sclerotome) (6). More recent explanations include traumatic distraction/separation of these two sclerotomes before the age of 4 years (8–10). Radiographic imaging can help distinguish congenital os odontoideum from a traumatic etiology.

Ossiculum terminale is another congenital abnormality in which the apex of the dens (proatlas) does not fuse with the dens (C1 sclerotome). Os odontoideum is at risk for being unstable and may require fixation whereas ossiculum terminale is considered stable. Congenital anomalies of the odontoid process are associated with Down syndrome, skeletal dysplasias, and mucopolysaccharidoses such as Morquio disease.

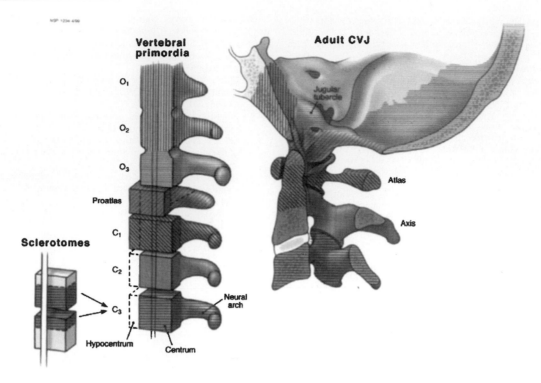

Fig. 1. In mammals, the neural arch of the proatlas splits into a rostral and caudal segment; the former is fused into the occipital bone to form the paired occipital condyles. The caudal portion of the proatlas neural arch is incorporated into the atlas and is represented by the paired rostral articulation facets of the atlas and a small portion of the lateral mass. The hypocentrum of the proatlas is reduced into the vestigial condylus tertius or the thin ridge-like anterior prominence of the basicranium. The core of the proatlas centrum transforms into the apical ligament of the dens. The apical ligament may contain notochordal tissue and can be regarded as a rudimentary intervertebral disc. The paired alar or check ligaments and the transverse ligament of the atlas are derived from the proatlas as unossified tissue. *CVJ,* craniovertebral junction. (From Barrow Neurological Institute, Phoenix, AZ, with permission.)

Anatomy and Biomechanics

The craniocervical junction is perhaps the most unique region of the axial spine. The forces of evolution have led to its unusual architecture, which provides humans with a stable platform on which to support the heavy cranium and its contents while simultaneously allowing a great degree of mobility. Multiple biomechanical studies of the atlantoaxial junction have demonstrated on average 40 degrees of axial rotation (unilateral), 20 degrees combined flexion/extension, and 5 degrees of lateral bending (unilateral) (11).

Ligamentous attachments to the odontoid process provide most of the stability of the atlantoaxial joint (Fig. 2). In particular, the transverse ligament and anterior arch of the atlas create a ring structure around the dens, providing rotational mobility yet significant stability to this articulation. As proof of this stability, studies have demonstrated that the failure strength of the transverse ligament exceeds 350 N (12,13). Other ligamentous structures, including the alar ligaments, superior and inferior longitudinal fibers of the cruciform ligament, and the tectorial membrane, provide secondary stability.

The bony anatomy of the atlantoaxial junction bears discussion as well. The atlas, with its rostral extension, the odontoid process, is like no other element of the axial spine. The lateral masses are attached to the short stout pedicles and the superior articular facets are on their rostral surfaces. The superior articular facets of the axis are actually convex as are the inferior facets of the lateral masses of the atlas. This arrangement permits a sliding motion along this surface. Projecting caudally and posteriorly from either lateral mass is the pars interarticularis, which ultimately joins the lamina to complete the ring.

C2 Fractures and Their Management

Axis fractures can be divided into odontoid fractures, bilateral spondylolisthesis of the pars interarticularis ("hangman's fracture"), and miscellaneous fractures. Depending on the pattern, angulation, and displacement of the fracture, investigators have developed widely accepted algorithms for treatment (Fig. 3). The primary goals of managing fractures of the axis are to maximize the chance of bony fusion, to restore stability to allow early ambulation, and to prevent further neurological deterioration.

ODONTOID FRACTURES. Of traumatic axis injuries, fractures of the dens are the most common, representing approximately 55% of all C2 fractures (14).

Type I Fractures. Anderson and D'Alonzo (15) initially divided odontoid fractures into three types. The least common of these fractures, type I, is a fracture through the tip of the odontoid (1,16). The fracture line is usually oblique. Type I fractures are

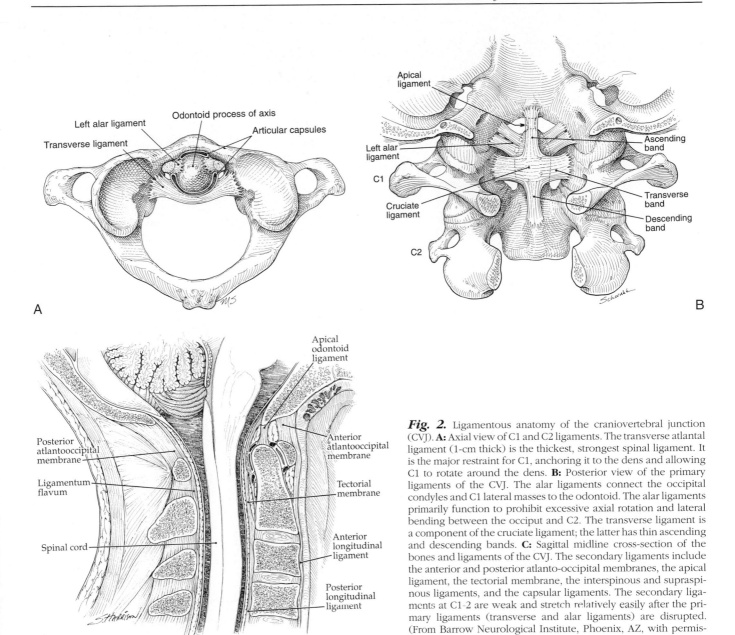

Fig. 2. Ligamentous anatomy of the craniovertebral junction (CVJ). **A:** Axial view of C1 and C2 ligaments. The transverse atlantal ligament (1-cm thick) is the thickest, strongest spinal ligament. It is the major restraint for C1, anchoring it to the dens and allowing C1 to rotate around the dens. **B:** Posterior view of the primary ligaments of the CVJ. The alar ligaments connect the occipital condyles and C1 lateral masses to the odontoid. The alar ligaments primarily function to prohibit excessive axial rotation and lateral bending between the occiput and C2. The transverse ligament is a component of the cruciate ligament; the latter has thin ascending and descending bands. **C:** Sagittal midline cross-section of the bones and ligaments of the CVJ. The secondary ligaments include the anterior and posterior atlanto-occipital membranes, the apical ligament, the tectorial membrane, the interspinous and supraspinous ligaments, and the capsular ligaments. The secondary ligaments at C1-2 are weak and stretch relatively easily after the primary ligaments (transverse and alar ligaments) are disrupted. (From Barrow Neurological Institute, Phoenix, AZ, with permission.)

thought to be secondary to avulsion of the alar ligament from the tip of the dens. Despite their rarity, type I odontoid fractures are thought to be stable fractures and are treated with a hard collar.

Type II Fractures. Type II odontoid fractures, the most common of this group, involve a horizontal break through the base of the dens where it joins the body of C2. Type II odontoid fractures are typically managed based on the magnitude of the displacement of the dens. Hadley and colleagues (17) found that type II fractures with more than 6 mm of displacement had a 78% chance of nonunion when managed with halo-vest immobilization. Patients older than 60 years with type II fractures had three times (39%) the nonunion rate of those younger than 60, although the finding was not statistically significant. Consequently, early surgical intervention is advocated for all patients with more than 6 mm dislocation on their initial imaging studies. Methods of surgical fixation include posterior atlan-

toaxial fusion with wiring or Halifax clamps, atlantoaxial facet screw fixation and fusion, or anterior odontoid screw fixation. Otherwise, type II fractures with less than 6 mm can be treated nonsurgically with halo vest immobilization or semi-rigid orthosis. Union rates range between 87% and 93%.

Hadley and colleagues (17) also describe type IIA odontoid fractures, which have either anterior or posterior chip-fracture fragments at the base of the dens. This subclassification has clinical significance because these fractures are unstable and require surgical intervention to insure bony fusion (Fig. 4). They are often widely displaced and have a nonunion rate of 75% to 85% when treated conservatively with rigid external orthosis. Early surgical intervention is therefore recommended for this fracture type.

Type II odontoid fractures may also involve ligamentous and soft tissues. Magnetic resonance imaging is often necessary to assess the competence of the transverse ligament adequately, although the ligament can sometimes be visualized on fine-cut

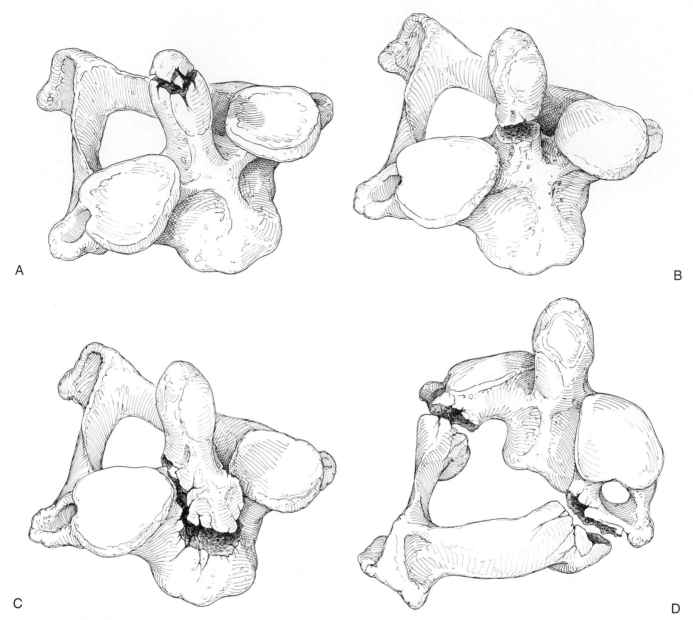

A

B

C

D

Fig. 3. Classification of fractures of the second cervical vertebra. Types I **(A)**, II **(B)**, and III **(C)** odontoid fractures are, respectively, through the apex of the dens, across the base of the dens, and into the body of C2. **D:** Hangman's fractures involve spondylitic fractures bilaterally across the pars interarticularis. Miscellaneous C2 fractures include the laminae, facets, spinous process, or body of C2 (i.e., nonodontoid, non-hangman's fractures). (From Barrow Neurological Institute, Phoenix, AZ, with permission.)

computed tomography, especially if it is calcified. When the transverse ligament is disrupted, odontoid screw fixation is contraindicated and C1-C2 fixation must be performed.

Type III Fractures. Type III odontoid fractures are similar to type II fractures except that the fracture line continues down into the cancellous bone of the C2 body. Most type III odontoid fractures fuse satisfactorily with external immobilization. Despite involving a greater bony surface area, including the body of C2, several reviews corroborate that surgical intervention is unnecessary to treat these fractures. Surgery, however, may be necessary if nonunion persists after 12 weeks of halo immobilization.

HANGMAN'S FRACTURES. Traumatic spondylolisthesis of the axis, popularly referred to as the "hangman's fracture", occupies a unique position in the history of vertebral column injuries.

Historical Perspective. Preliminary investigations into the nature and pathomechanics of this fracture during the late 19th and early 20th centuries were the result of the judicial initiative to achieve reproducibly "humane" executions by hanging. To this end, Marshall (18) first observed the effectiveness of a submental knot for inducing death rapidly through a high cervical spinal cord injury. In contrast, the historically favored subaural (mandibular angle) knot most often produced death by strangulation or decapitation. Through postmortem examinations,

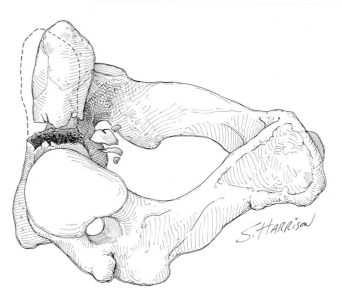

Fig. 4. Artist's representation of an odontoid type IIA fracture. Fracture fragments at the base of the dens may be anterior or posterior. (From Hadley MN, Browner CM, Liu SS, et al. New subtype of acute odontoid fractures (type IIA). *Neurosurgery* 22:67–71, 1988, with permission.)

Paterson (19) detailed the bony and ligamentous injuries associated with hangings performed with the submental knot. These injuries included bilateral fractures of the C2 pars interarticularis, rupture of the anterior and posterior longitudinal ligaments, and disruption of the C2-3 disc space. In the first study of the clinical biomechanics involving the cervical spine, Wood-Jones (20,21) identified hyperextension and distraction as the vectors responsible for this type of injury (22).

In 1965, Schneider and associates (23) reported eight patients who sustained bilateral avulsion fractures of the axial neural arch in motor vehicle accidents. Given the comparable appearance of these lesions to the axial fracture incurred by judicial hanging, they coined the term "hangman's fracture" to describe them. Despite their radiographic similarities, however, the judicial and "civilian" derived hangman's fracture have different biomechanical etiologies and, consequently, different associated neurological morbidities.

Cervical hyperextension is fundamental to both the civilian and judicial mechanisms of traumatic C2 spondylolisthesis, but contemporary injuries responsible for hangman's fractures (i.e., vehicular, fall, diving) typically involve a component of axial loading rather than pure axial distraction inherent to hanging. Whereas the latter vector results in a uniformly fatal disruption of the cervical spinal cord, axial loading is thought to produce a fracture configuration that functionally "decompresses" the vertebral canal and thereby averts permanent neurological injury in most cases.

Before hangman's fractures can be considered a neurologically benign entity, however, it is important to recognize that as many as 40% of patients who die at the scene of their trauma harbor acute fractures involving either the axial vertebra or the craniovertebral junction (20,21,24,25). Some of the fatalities may be the result of high cervical myelopathy. Thus, although several clinical series have corroborated a low incidence of neurological injury associated with hangman's fractures produced by axial loading, the studies share an inherent selection bias due to inclusion of only those patients who survive their accident.

Classification of Hangman's Fractures. The works of groups led by Effendi (26) and Francis (27) were simultaneously intro-

duced as a framework upon which hangman's fractures could be classified and compared in terms of pathoanatomical appearance, potential instability, and risk for osseous nonunion. The Effendi classification subdivided these fractures into three groups based upon qualitative radiographic criteria that included the presence of fracture displacement, the integrity of the C2-3 disc space, and the integrity of the C2-3 facet complex. The Francis classification system stratified fracture type based on quantitative measurements of the displacement and angulation of the C2 fragment relative to the C3 body and was based on biomechanical criteria of White and co-workers (28).

A modified system, described by Levine and Edwards (29) and incorporating aspects of the qualitative system of Effendi and colleagues (26) and the quantitative system of Francis and associates (27), has emerged as a popular grading scheme for hangman's fractures (Table 1). The four-fracture classification corresponds to different mechanisms of injury (23). Type I hangman's fractures are thought to occur secondary to axial loading and hyperextension. These are associated with less than 3 mm of subluxation of C2 on C3 and no angulation. Type II fractures are caused by axial loading and extension with rebound flexion. They disrupt the C2-3 disc and posterior longitudinal ligament, leading to more than 4 mm of subluxation and more than 11 degrees of angulation. Type IIA fractures are associated with more severe angulation than type II fractures. Type III fractures result from primary flexion and are associated with C2-3 facet fractures with significant subluxation and angulation.

Management of Hangman's Fractures. Several retrospective series have demonstrated that permanent neurological injury (myeloradiculopathy) associated with this lesion is rare. The outcome data from several sources, including a recent retrospective review of 74 hangman's fractures from this institution (1), demonstrate that most hangman's fractures are amenable to nonoperative management. Moreover, the ability to achieve osseous union with the hangman's fracture, despite incomplete or nonanatomical closed fracture reduction, is well recognized (9,18,19,23,26,30–33) and has been documented even with extreme fracture displacements (34).

Although the halo brace has been the orthosis of choice for producing and maintaining closed reduction and for stabilizing hangman's fracture, these injuries have also been treated successfully with nonrigid immobilization. Most recently, the clinical experience with nonrigid immobilization of hangman's fractures has been expanded by a series of 39 patients with noncontiguous, "stable" hangman's fractures in whom bony fusion was attained after immobilization in a Philadelphia collar (32). In that study, fractures were defined as "stable" if the radiographic fragment displacement measured on initial presentation and after flexion-extension maneuvers was less than 6 mm.

Attention has since been directed toward a subset of "atypical" hangman's fractures in which the fracture line involves the posterior cortex of C2. This morphology causes a potentially "canal-compromising" fracture that is associated with a greater risk of myelopathy than that anticipated with the classic hangman's fracture (9,28,35). Consequently, some authors believe that these variants of hangman's fracture primarily require surgical fixation rather than risking neurological injury from inadequate stabilization with external bracing.

MISCELLANEOUS FRACTURES OF THE AXIS. In 1994, Benzel and co-workers (12) classified miscellaneous C2 body fractures into three types. Fifteen patients were included in their analysis, which included clinical and radiographic correlations. The first fracture described, type I, demonstrated a coronally oriented vertical fracture. Sagittally oriented vertical fractures

Table 1. Comparison of Francis, Effendi, and Levine Grading Systems for Hangman's Fractures

Type of grade	I	II	IIa	III	IV	V[a]
Francis						
Displacement	<3.5 mm	<3.5 mm	NA	>3.5 mm but <50% C3 body length	>3.5 mm but <50% C3 body length	>50% C3 body length
Angulation	< 11°	> 11°	NA	< 11°	> 11°	Disc space widening > central height of the next normal disc
Effendi	Isolated hairline fracture of axis ring with "minimal" displacement of the body of C2 and normal C2-C3 disc space	Displaced anterior fracture fragment with abnormal C2-C3 disc space	NA	Anteriorly displaced fragment in flexion with bilaterally locked C2-C3 facets	NA	NA
Levine	≤3 mm displacement of fracture fragment and no angulation	"Significant" angulation and displacement of fragment	Minimal fragment displacement but "severe" angulation	"Severe" angulation and displacement of fragment and concomitant facet disruption (unilateral or bilateral)	NA	NA
Mechanism of injury	Hyperextension-axial loading	Hyperextension-axial loading followed by flexion-compression	Flexion-distraction	Flexion-compression	NA	NA

NA, not applicable
[a] Disc disruption per Francis.
From Baskin JJ, Greene KA, Vishteh AG, et al. Operative management of unstable hangman's fractures. In: Zdeblick T, Benzel E, Stillerman C, et al., eds, *Controversies in spine surgery.* St. Louis: Quality Medical, 1999, with permission.

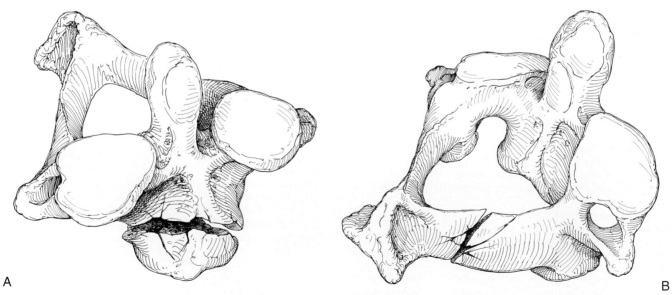

A   B

Fig. 5. Illustrations of the six types of miscellaneous axis fractures. **A:** Anterior inferior C2 body fracture. **B:** Laminar fracture.

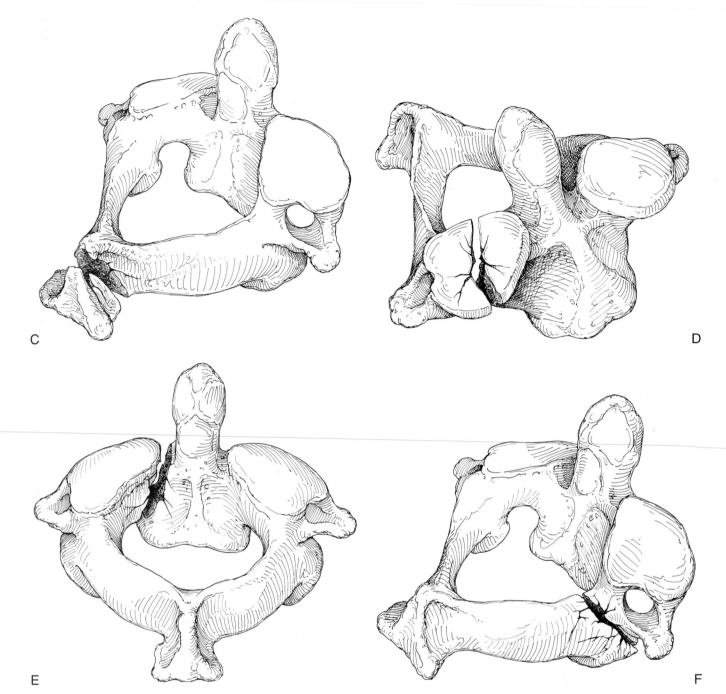

Fig. 5. (continued). **C:** Spinous process fracture. **D:** Lateral mass fracture. **E:** Pedicle fracture. **F:** Unilateral pars interarticularis fracture. (From Barrow Neurological Institute, Phoenix, AZ, with permission.)

were also identified and categorized as type II fractures. The last variant of C2 body fractures was the horizontal rostral fracture, which the Benzel group (12) classified as a type III fracture. In fact, this fracture is the previously described type III odontoid fracture of Anderson and D'Alonzo (15).

Although Benzel and colleagues (12) made no treatment recommendations in their paper, they reviewed the mechanism of injury and associated fracture pattern comprehensively. A full appreciation for the complex anatomy and biomechanical forces of the atlantoaxial joint greatly enhances understanding of the mechanisms leading to these fractures.

Hadley and associates (14) describe six other miscellaneous

fractures of the axis. In their review of 107 acute C2 fractures, 23 (22%) fell into this category. They included (in order of frequency) fractures of the anterior inferior vertebral body, lateral mass, lamina, pedicle, spinous process, and unilateral pars interarticularis (Fig. 5). Initial treatment of these fractures included 3 to 5 lbs of traction with Gardner-Wells tongs and, in most cases, subsequent halo placement. Others were managed with either hard collars or a sternal-occipital-mandibular immobilization brace. One patient developed a nonunion and was ultimately fixated surgically.

Evaluation of traumatic injuries of the atlantoaxial junction should also heighten surgeons' awareness of the potential for vertebral artery injuries. At our institution, patients sustaining fractures that include the foramen transversarium or significant subluxation undergo vascular study either by magnetic resonance angiography or digital subtraction angiography. This generalization holds true even in patients without localizing vascular findings. Traumatic vertebral artery dissection and occlusions have been identified in multiple cases.

In general, treatment of miscellaneous fractures must be individualized. Patients with more significant injuries, including major vertebral body, pedicle, or lateral mass fractures, subluxation, or other cervical spine fractures, should be treated with halo immobilization.

Barrow Neurological Institute Series

In a review that spanned 17 years (1975–1993) (1), 340 consecutive acute axis fractures were catalogued retrospectively and their management and outcome were described. The incidence of neurological injury attributable to C2 fractures of all types was 8.5%, and 20.3% sustained concomitant moderate to severe head injuries (Table 2) (1). Also of note, 34% of the patients had concomitant fractures elsewhere in their axial spine.

ODONTOID FRACTURES. There were 199 odontoid fractures, overwhelmingly the most common fracture in this cohort. Type II odontoid fractures were the most common subtype of odontoid fractures, representing 60% (120 of 199) of all odontoid fractures. Five patients died from severe head injuries or pulmonary complications within the first week of admission. Twenty patients underwent early surgery. Eight of these patients had type II odontoid fractures with dislocations in excess of 6 mm and halo immobilization failed to maintain alignment. Four patients in the surgical group had type IIA fractures. These patients were also unstable with halo immobilization although a fifth patient with a type IIA fracture developed a solid fusion after wearing a halo brace for 13 weeks. The remaining seven patients, each with less than 6-mm dislocation, chose elective surgical fixation instead of halo vest immobilization. Surgical fusion techniques used to treat type II and IIA fractures included posterior atlantoaxial fusion with wiring or Halifax clamps, atlantoaxial facet screw fixation and fusion, or anterior odontoid screw fixation.

The remaining 95 patients with type II odontoid fractures were initially managed with external fixation for 10 to 28 weeks.

A solid fusion failed to develop in 26 (28.4%) of the 88 patients available for follow-up. Prolonged external fixation was successful in seven of these patients. The remaining 18 patients required surgical intervention and demonstrated no further instability after posterior atlantoaxial autologous iliac crest bone graft fusion. Patients with a dens displacement in excess of 6 mm had a statistically significant nonunion rate of 86% compared to an 18% nonunion rate in patients with less than 6 mm displacement.

Seventy-seven patients presented with type III odontoid fractures, two of whom died early from severe head injuries. Six patients underwent early surgical fusion. Halo immobilization failed to maintain alignment in five; the sixth patient had a significant C2-3 subluxation that warranted surgical intervention. Posterior fusion techniques were used in four patients while the other two were treated with odontoid screw fixation. All six patients developed satisfactory fusions. External immobilization was used to treat the remaining 69 patients with type III odontoid fractures, and only one patient demonstrated instability after 13 weeks in a halo. He subsequently underwent a posterior fusion with excellent results.

HANGMAN'S FRACTURES. Overall, hangman's fractures accounted for about 4% of cervical spinal fractures and 22% (74 of 340) of axial fractures. Traumatic spondylolisthesis of the axis was identified in patients as young as 2 months old and as old as 92 years. The distribution of hangman's fractures according to the Effendi and Francis classifications is depicted in Table 3.

Of the 74 patients who presented with hangman's fractures, two patients died from severe concomitant traumatic brain injuries. Of the remaining 72 patients, seven demonstrated instability on upright and supine plain lateral radiographs despite preliminary management with closed reduction using gentle traction and rigid external immobilization with a halo brace. Of these seven fractures, six were Effendi type II. The only Effendi type III fracture within the series was the seventh unstable fracture in the operative cohort. Alternatively, one of these fracture types corresponded to Francis grade I, one to Francis grade II, two to Francis grade III, and three to Francis grade IV (Table 4).

Of the seven patients with unstable fractures, five had concomitant disruption of the posterior elements (C1, C3, or both) and underwent an anterior approach for stabilization. Surgery entailed an anterior cervical discectomy at the level of C2-3,

Table 2. Neurological Injuries Concomitant with 340 Axis Fractures

Neurological injury type	n (%)[a]
Associated head injuries	89 (26)
Mild	20 (6)
Moderate to severe	69 (20)
Spinal cord injuries	67 (20)
Quadriplegia	64 (19)
Paraplegia	3 (1)
Spinal root	9 (3)

[a] Percentage of 340 patients.
From Greene KA, Dickman CA, Marciano FF, et al. Acute axis fractures. Analysis of management and outcome in 340 consecutive cases. *Spine* 1997;22(16):1843–1852, with permission.

Table 3. Distribution of 74 Hangman Fractures by Effendi Type and Francis Grade

Classification	n_{Total} (%)[a]	$n_{Unstable}$ (%)
Effendi type		
I	53 (72)	0 (0)[b]
II	20 (27)	6 (30)[b]
III	1 (1)	1 (100)[b]
Francis grade		
I	48 (65)	1 (2)[c]
II	12 (16)	1 (8)[c]
III	11 (15)	2 (18)[c]
IV	3 (4)	3 (100)[c]
V	0 (0)	0 (0)[c]

[a] Percentage of 74 hangman fractures.
[b] Percentage of Effendi type (26).
[c] Percentage of Francis grade (27).
From Greene KA, Dickman CA, Marciano FF, et al. Acute axis fractures. Analysis of management and outcome in 340 consecutive cases. *Spine* 1997;22(16):1843–1852, with permission.

Table 4. Fracture Classification and Clinical Data for Seven Patients Undergoing Early Surgery for Hangman Fracture

Age (y)	Sex	Effendi type[a]	Francis grade[b]	Surgery on postinjury day
35	F	II	I	8
54	F	II	II	8
26	M	II	III	6
36	F	II	III	10
35	M	II	IV	8
64	F	II	IV	5
35	M	III	IV	4

[a] Criteria established by Effendi, et al. (26).
[b] Criteria established by Francis, et al. (27).
From Greene KA, Dickman CA, Marciano FF, et al. Acute axis fractures. Analysis of management and outcome in 340 consecutive cases. *Spine* 1997;22(16): 1843–1852, with permission.

placement of an autologous iliac crest bone graft, and internal fixation with a screw-plate across the C2-3 interspace. The two patients with intact posterior elements underwent posterior fixation with a C1-3 wire/autologous graft construct. Currently, however, our preference is to manage these patients by an anterior surgical approach to spare the atlantoaxial motion segment. All patients within the operative group demonstrated stable bony fusions throughout a follow-up period longer than 3 years.

MISCELLANEOUS FRACTURES. Miscellaneous C2 fractures occurred in 20% of the 340 patients. Most of these fractures involved the vertebral body or lateral mass of C2. Sixty-one patients were managed with external immobilization. One patient with a lateral mass fracture and 5-mm subluxation (C2 to C3) underwent early surgery. The overall nonunion rate for miscellaneous odontoid fractures managed nonoperatively was 1.6%, as one patient demonstrated instability 15 weeks after halo vest placement.

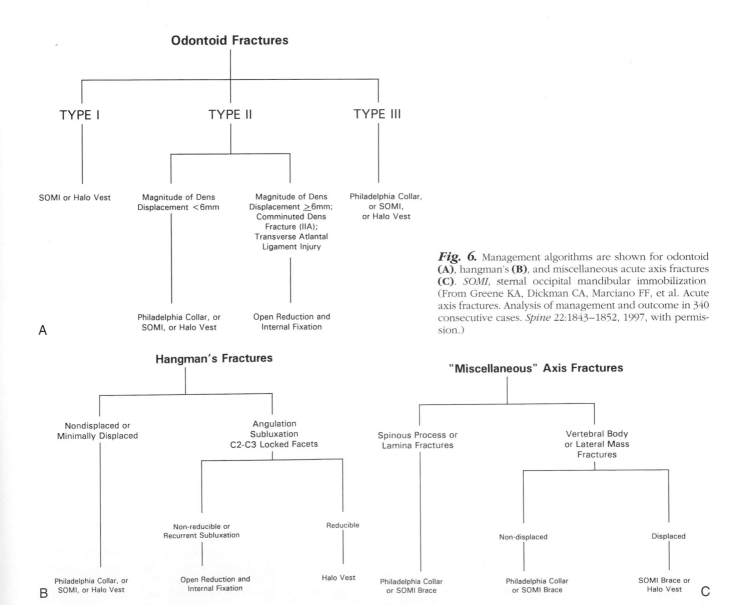

Fig. 6. Management algorithms are shown for odontoid **(A)**, hangman's **(B)**, and miscellaneous acute axis fractures **(C)**. *SOMI*, sternal occipital mandibular immobilization. (From Greene KA, Dickman CA, Marciano FF, et al. Acute axis fractures. Analysis of management and outcome in 340 consecutive cases. *Spine* 22:1843–1852, 1997, with permission.)

Conclusion

As dependence on motorized transportation and time for recreational activities increase, fractures of the axis will continue to occur. Advances in radiographic imaging have made diagnosis of C2 fractures easier and have allowed surgeons to classify fractures with greater accuracy. These classification systems have enabled the generation of treatment protocols and algorithms that can be used safely and effectively (Fig. 6). It must be emphasized, however, that a fundamental knowledge of the complex anatomy and biomechanics of the atlantoaxial junction is required to treat these injuries appropriately, especially when surgical intervention is indicated.

References

1. Greene KA, Dickman CA, Marciano FF, et al. Acute axis fractures. Analysis of management and outcome in 340 consecutive cases. *Spine* 1997;22:1843–1852.
2. Ganguly DN, Roy KK. A study on the cranio-vertebral joint in the man. *Anat Anz* 1964;114:433–452.
3. Dickman CA, Spetzler RF, Sonntag VKH. *Surgery of the craniovertebral junction*. New York: Thieme Medical Publishers, 1998.
4. Garber JN. Abnormalities of the atlas and axis vertebrae—congenital and traumatic. *J Bone Joint Surg Am* 1964;46–A:1782–1791.
5. Gray SW, Romaine CB, Skandalakis JE. Congenital fusion of the cervical vertebrae. *Surg Gynecol Obstet* 1964;118:373–385.
6. Wolin DG. The os odontoideum. Separate odontoid process. *J Bone Joint Surg Am* 1963;45:1459–1471.
7. Gladstone RJ, Wakeley CP. Variation of the occipitoatlantal joint in relation to the metameric structure of the craniovertebral junction. *J Anat (London)* 1924;59:195–216.
8. Fielding JW, Cochran GVB, Lawsing JFI, et al. Tears of the transverse ligament of the atlas. A clinical and biomechanical study. *J Bone Joint Surg Am* 1974;56:1683–1691.
9. Fielding JW, Francis WR Jr, Hawkins RJ, et al. Traumatic spondylolisthesis of the axis. *Clin Orthop* 1989;239:47–52.
10. Fielding JW, Hensinger RN, Hawkins RJ. Os odontoideum. *J Bone Joint Surg Am* 1980;62:376–383.
11. Panjabi MM, White AA III. *Clinical biomechanics of the spine*. Philadelphia: JB Lippincott Co, 1978.
12. Benzel EC, Hart BL, Ball PA, et al. Fractures of the C-2 vertebral body. *J Neurosurg* 1994;81:206–212.
13. Benzel EC. *Biomechanics of spine stabilization, principles and clinical practice*. New York: McGraw-Hill, 1995.
14. Hadley MN, Browner C, Sonntag VKH. Miscellaneous fractures of the second cervical vertebra. *BNI Quarterly* 1985;1:34–39.
15. Anderson LD, D'Alonzo RT. Fractures of the odontoid process of the axis. *J Bone Joint Surg Am* 1974;56:1663–1674.
16. Greene KA, Dickman CA, Marciano FF, et al. Transverse atlantal ligament disruption associated with odontoid fractures. *Spine* 1994; 19:2307–2314.
17. Hadley MN, Browner CM, Liu SS, et al. New subtype of acute odontoid fractures (type IIA). *Neurosurgery* 1988;22:67–71.
18. Marshall JJ. Judicial hanging. *Br Med J* 1888;2:779–782.
19. Paterson AM. Fracture of cervical vertebrae. *J Anat (London)* 1890; 24:9.
20. Wood-Jones F. The ideal lesion produced by judicial hanging. *Lancet* 1913;1:53.
21. Wood-Jones F. The examination of the bodies of 100 men executed in Nubia in Roman times. *Br Med J* 1908;1:736–737.
22. Mollan RA, Watt PC. Hangman's fracture. *Injury* 1982;14:265–267.
23. Schneider RC, Livingston KE, Cave AJE, et al. "Hangman's fracture" of the cervical spine. *J Neurosurg* 1965;22:141–154.
24. Francis WR, Fielding JW. Traumatic spondylolisthesis of the axis. *Orthop Clin North Am* 1978;9:1011–1027.
25. Coric D, Wilson JA, Kelley DL Jr. Treatment of traumatic spondylolisthesis of the axis with nonrigid immobilization: a review of 64 cases. *J Neurosurg* 1996;85:550–554.
26. Effendi B, Roy D, Cornish B, et al. Fractures of the ring of the axis. A classification based on the analysis of 131 cases. *J Bone Joint Surg Br* 1981;63:319–327.
27. Francis WR, Fielding JW, Hawkins RJ, et al. Traumatic spondylolisthesis of the axis. *J Bone Joint Surg Br* 1981;63:313–318.
28. White AA III, Johnson RM, Panjabi MM, et al. Biomechanical analysis of clinical stability in the cervical spine. *Clin Orthop* 1975;109:85–96.
29. Levine AM, Edwards CC. The management of traumatic spondylolisthesis of the axis. *J Bone Joint Surg Am* 1985;67:217–226.
30. Alker GJ Jr, Oh YS, Leslie EV. High cervical spine and craniocervical junction injuries in fatal traffic accidents: a radiological study. *Orthop Clin North Am* 1978;9:1003–1010.
31. Huelke DF, O'Day J, Mendelsohn RA. Cervical injuries suffered in automobile crashes. *J Neurosurg* 1981;54:316–322.
32. Govender S, Charles RW. Traumatic spondylolisthesis of the axis. *Injury* 1987;18:333–335.
33. Marar BC. Fracture of the axis arch. "Hangman's fracture" of the cervical spine. *Clin Orthop* 1975;106:155–165.
34. Borne GM, Bedou GL, Pinaudeau M. Treatment of pedicular fractures of the axis. A clinical study and screw fixation technique. *J Neurosurg* 1984;60:88–93.
35. Bucholz RW, Burkhead WZ, Graham W, et al. Occult cervical spine injuries in fatal traffic accidents. *J Trauma* 1979;19:768–771.

160. *Subaxial Cervical Fractures*

Gregory J. Przybylski

The management of subaxial cervical spinal injuries remains controversial. A recent survey of spinal surgeons demonstrated the variability of treatment recommendations for several common cervical spine injuries (1). For example, appropriate management of a reduced unilateral facet dislocation included maintenance of halo vest immobilization, less rigid external immobilization, and posterior instrumentation with or without decompression. The study highlighted both the importance of reviewing the available literature examining management strategies for various cervical injuries as well as directing future

clinical research at identifying ideal treatment protocols. This chapter will review the practical application of mechanistic classification schemes to evaluating subaxial cervical fractures. In addition, the results of several biomechanical studies supporting the conclusions of the classification methods will be examined. Moreover, the radiographic evaluation of the injuries will also be considered. Finally, treatment algorithms for common types of subaxial cervical fractures will be suggested.

In order to compare treatment options for subaxial fractures, the mechanisms of injury have been studied through biomechanical testing as well as radiographic imaging. These efforts have led to a variety of classification systems to guide therapeutic interventions. In 1960, biomechanical testing of fresh postmortem spinal segments was reported by Roaf (2). He observed that vertical compression distorted the vertebral end plates rather than causing intervertebral disc injury. As a result, he suggested that the disc resists compression better than the vertebral body and that expression of blood from within the cancellous bone is an important mechanism of force dissipation. However, older specimens with impaired nucleus pulposus function behaved differently. In contrast, annular tearing and buckling of the vertebral body side walls was seen. In fact, this was reproduced in younger specimens in which the nucleus was removed. Typically, vertebral compression preceded posterior ligamentous disruption. Similarly, neural arch fracture preceded anterior ligamentous disruption. However, the intervertebral discs were more vulnerable to rotational and shear injuries, often without concurrent vertebral fracture. These observations provided a foundation for the development of a mechanistic classification of spinal injuries.

In 1968, Kelly and Whitesides proposed evaluation of thoracolumbar spinal injuries in terms of anterior and posterior columns (3). The anterior column was comprised of the vertebral body, intervertebral disc, and longitudinal ligaments, whereas the posterior column consisted of the remaining structures. Instability was likely if the components of one column and an additional structure of the other column were injured. Holdsworth applied these concepts to the cervical spine as well and suggested several mechanisms of spinal injury (4,5). He grouped together three relatively stable injuries, including wedge fractures, burst fractures, and extension injuries. Traction, bed rest, and various durations of external immobilization were recommended. In contrast, dislocations, rotational-fracture dislocations, and shear fractures were considered unstable injuries. Treatment included traction, immobilization, and arthrodesis.

Subsequently, Denis proposed a three-column injury model for thoracolumbar fractures based on imaging and treatment results in a series of more than 400 spinal injuries (6). He suggested dividing the anterior column of Kelly and Whitesides (3) in half, creating a middle column comprised of the posterior half of the vertebra, the posterior annulus, and the posterior longitudinal ligament. Instability was likely if the components of two columns were injured. He drew particular attention to the middle column as having a strong influence upon spinal stability.

Around the same time, Allen and colleagues proposed a mechanistic classification of subaxial cervical fractures and dislocations (7). Based upon a study of 165 spinal injuries, the authors suggested six patterns of injury. Compressive flexion injuries, such as the "tear drop" fracture described by Schneider and Kahn (8), were subdivided into five stages of progressive injury. The first stage consists of blunting of the anterior-superior aspect of the vertebral body, whereas the second stage additionally consists of anterior vertebral height loss and anterior-inferior beaking. In the third stage, a "tear drop" fracture of the beak is observed. Finally, the fourth stage involves posterior displacement of the posterior-inferior vertebral body, while the fifth stage includes separation of the facet joints and spinous processes.

In contrast, distractive flexion injuries, such as bilateral facet dislocation described by Beatson (9), were observed most often and were subdivided into four stages of progressive injury. The first stage consists of posterior ligamentous "strain," with facet subluxation and interspinous widening as well as rounding of the anterior-superior aspect of the caudal vertebral body. The second stage consists of unilateral facet dislocation, with varying degrees of posterior ligamentous injury. Bilateral facet dislo-

cations were included in the third stage in which 50% anterior displacement of the rostral vertebral body was seen. Finally, complete anterior subluxation of the rostral vertebral body was seen in the fourth stage.

Similarly, extension injuries were observed in either compression or extension. Compressive extension injuries consisted of posterior element fracture. Five stages of injury were proposed, including unilateral laminar fractures (stage 1), bilateral laminar fractures (stage 2), additional facet or pedicular fractures without body displacement (stage 3) or with partial displacement (stage 4), and with complete body displacement (stage 5). In contrast, distractive extension injuries, previously described by Taylor and Blackwood (10), were subdivided into two stages. The first stage consists of anterior ligamentous injury without posterior displacement, whereas the second stage consists of additional posterior ligamentous injury with some posterior vertebral body displacement of the rostral vertebra.

Two other forms of vertebral injuries were also described. Vertical compression fractures, often termed "burst" fractures, were subdivided into three stages of progressive vertebral body injury. The first two stages involve single or paired end-plate fractures with a "cupped" appearance on lateral radiographs. Fragmentation of the vertebral body centrum is seen in the third stage, with centripetal dispersion of fragments. Finally, lateral flexion injuries were observed the least. Two stages of injury included asymmetrical compression of the body with accompanying laminar or other posterior bony fracture and the addition of distractive injury on the contralateral side.

Application of engineering principles to evaluation of spinal mechanics has provided additional insight into the effects of load upon the cervical spine. For example, Maiman and associates demonstrated the resistance of the cervical column to axial loads. In fact, axial compression failure required twice the load necessary to cause flexion or extension injuries (11). This may be related to the load-sharing capacity of the facet joints (12). Perhaps this explains the infrequency of vertical compression injuries reported by Allen and colleagues (7) in comparison to compressive flexion or extension injuries. However, this study also demonstrates that the direction of force application only partially correlated with the resulting injury observed. Another study by Yoganandan and co-workers demonstrates the ability of the cervical spine to dissipate applied loads (13). For example, forces measured distally were substantially less than the applied force to the head-neck complex. During progressive force application, the cervical spinal components will change position to best accommodate the load until failure occurs (14).

Other dynamic biomechanical studies have highlighted the limitations of inferring the degree of canal compromise during the injury in comparison to postinjury examination. Based upon the absence of significant correlation between canal diameter and degree of neurological deficit, Carter and colleagues compared the degree of canal occlusion during injury with that measured after injury (15). In a study of 12 cervical cadaveric spines, fast axial loading produced burst fractures, whereas slow loading produced wedge compression fractures. The amount of canal occlusion was significantly smaller after a burst fracture occurred in comparison to the canal diameter during the injury process.

The radiographic assessment of cervical spine injury has been subjected to substantial study over the past few decades. Although most physicians agree that three-view cervical radiographs can be helpful in identifying fractures, the conditions that should prompt initial imaging as well as supplementary imaging are less understood. Several studies have examined the use of clinical history and examination in identifying patients with possible cervical injuries. For example, a prospective study of more than 2,000 consecutive blunt trauma patients without altered consciousness (Glasgow Coma Scale scores of

14 or 15) evaluated the presence of neck pain and physical examination of the neck as predictors of cervical injury (16). Of the 33 patients (1.6%) with cervical injuries, three had a negative clinical examination. Two of these patients had fractures on cervical radiographs, including a spinous process fracture and a vertebral body fracture. No injuries were missed in patients with elevated blood alcohol levels. The authors concluded the plain radiographs did not increase the sensitivity of the clinical examination in identifying awake blunt trauma victims with cervical spine injuries.

A multicenter prospective study of more than 34,000 blunt trauma patients identified 818 patients with cervical spine injuries (17). Using the criteria of normal alertness, no intoxication, no cervical pain, absence of distracting injury, and no cervical tenderness, only eight patients were not diagnosed. Only two of these patients had a significant injury, one of which was treated surgically. The authors recommend application of the criteria to blunt trauma patients for evaluation of possible cervical injuries.

The risk of cervical spinal cord injury has been related to sagittal diameter of the spinal canal observed on radiographic imaging. In a series of nearly 300 patients, Kang and associates examined the sagittal canal diameters in patients with subaxial cervical fractures and dislocations (18). Although the severity of neurological injury was not significantly related to canal narrowing, smaller diameters were identified in patients with spinal cord injuries compared with those without cord injury.

Although plain radiographs are imperative in patients with risk factors of neck pain, neck tenderness, or neurological deficits referable to the cervical spine, this type of imaging may fail to identify some injuries. Woodring and Lee demonstrated the limitations of plain radiographs and computed tomography (CT) in identifying cervical fractures (19). For example, plain radiographs identified 93% of subluxations and dislocations, but only 58% of fractures. In contrast, CT identified 90% of fractures, but only 54% of subluxations and dislocations. Overall, both studies alone missed 6% to 8% of cervical injuries. However, the combination of studies identified all cervical injuries in this series of more than 200 patients. In a smaller series of obtunded patients, plain radiographs missed eight injuries, three of which were unstable, whereas helical CT missed only two injuries, both of which were stable (20). Finally, a cost-effectiveness analysis of CT imaging of the nonvisualized cervicothoracic junction (21) or in trauma patients with moderate to high risk of cervical injury (22) supported use of CT evaluation. Factors predicting higher risk included severe head injury, higher energy trauma, and focal neurological deficits (23).

More frequent application of magnetic resonance imaging (MRI) to trauma patients has led to additional evaluation of this technique for identifying other injuries missed on static plain radiographs and CT. Although MRI was less sensitive to acute fractures than conventional imaging, soft-tissue hemorrhage, longitudinal ligament injuries, disc displacement, and cord contusion or hemorrhage were identified with MRI (24). Similarly, a retrospective study of MRI showed failure to reliably identify cervical spine fractures in comparison to CT, but was superior in showing evidence of spinal cord injury, disc disruption, and soft-tissue injury (25). Application of implied ligamentous injury seen on MRI to treatment of cervical injuries has been suggested (26). For example, the presence of at least three injured ligaments among the facet capsule, interspinous ligament, and either longitudinal ligament may be related to instability in unilateral facet fractures (27).

Finally, magnetic resonance angiography has been used to evaluate concurrent vertebral artery injuries associated with subaxial cervical fractures and dislocations (28). Although the frequency of vertebral injury may range from 20% to 50% with certain cervical injuries (29), most patients are asymptomatic.

In fact, the majority of vertebral artery occlusions do not reconstitute during the subsequent 2 years (30). Although treatment with anticoagulation is recommended only for symptomatic vertebral injuries, identification of these injuries may alter surgical treatment of cervical injuries in which screw insertion places the remaining vertebral artery at risk of iatrogenic injury.

In order to apply the mechanistic classification and radiographic assessment to the treatment of subaxial cervical spine fractures, the various types of common injuries will be examined individually. First, compressive injuries will be discussed, including flexion-induced wedge fractures, axial-induced burst fractures, and extension-induced posterior arch fractures. Next, distractive injuries will be evaluated, including flexion-induced unilateral and bilateral facet dislocations and extension-induced intervertebral disc injuries. It is important to be familiar with normal measurements of the cervical spine on lateral radiographs as well as the normal range of motion observed at a segmental level. More than 11 degrees of additional angulation observed when comparing the injured segment with adjacent segments has been associated with flexion instability related to posterior ligamentous injury (31). Likewise, subluxation beyond 3.5 mm also suggests instability (32). Normal segmental ranges of motion are 8 to 15 degrees in flexion-extension, 6 to 10 degrees in lateral bending, and 5 to 10 degrees in axial rotation (33,34). These characteristics were combined into a rating scale for predicting instability (31). Points were attributed to various abnormalities including two points for anterior injury, posterior injury, excess translation, excess angulation, a positive stretch test, and spinal cord injury. In contrast, one point was given for root injury, abnormal intervertebral disc space narrowing, congenital spinal stenosis, or anticipation of dangerous loads. The accumulation of more than five points was associated with instability.

Compressive injuries in flexion are managed based upon the degree of deformity and the association of posterior ligamentous injury from tension. Many of these fractures are not associated with neurological injury. Mild wedge fractures with little loss of vertebral height (Fig. 1) may be managed with rigid collar immobilization, whereas those with greater vertebral height loss may be managed in a halo orthosis (35).

In contrast, vertical compression injuries causing burst fractures may be more often associated with neurological injury. Since the ligamentous structures are typically undamaged, these injuries can often be reduced with traction and treated with external immobilization alone in the neurologically intact patient (35). However, patients with incomplete neurological injury related to the level of burst fracture may benefit from surgical decompression. Typically, an anterior cervical corpectomy with interbody reconstruction and anterior plate fixation can restore canal diameter, spinal alignment, and provide sufficient stability, even in the setting of concurrent posterior arch fracture.

Compressive injuries in extension were the second most common injury observed by Allen and colleagues (7). Patients often have a normal neurological examination or systems or radiculopathy. However, central cord injuries and complete spinal cord injuries are occasionally seen. Unless significant vertebral displacement is observed, most of these injuries may be treated with external immobilization alone in patients without neurological dysfunction.

Flexion-distraction injuries such as unilateral or bilateral facet dislocations are also often associated with neurological injury (Fig. 2). Reduction in axial skeletal traction is typically recommended first. Significant controversy remains regarding the type of imaging required prior to reduction with traction. In 1990, Eismont and associates reported six patients with displaced intervertebral discs among 68 patients with facet subluxations or dislocations (36). The first patient had a radicular deficit refer-

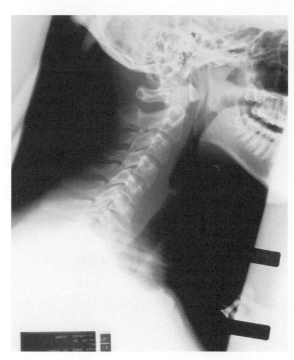

Fig. 1. A 25-year-old man sustained a C6 flexion-compression fracture without neurological injury after a fall while skiing. Plain lateral cervical radiograph reveals reduction in height of the vertebral centrum, blunting of the anterior-superior vertebral body angle, as well as cupping of the inferior end plate.

able to bilateral facet dislocation at C6-7. After unsuccessful attempts at closed reduction, she underwent a posterior open reduction and internal fixation with wiring. The patient awoke with quadriplegia; an emergent myelogram demonstrated a displaced cervical disc with complete block associated with slight penetration of the spinous process wire through the lamina posteriorly. Although she underwent emergent anterior cervical decompression and fusion, she did not recover neurological function. Subsequent patients were evaluated preoperatively with myelography or MRI, or intraoperatively with ultrasonography if successful closed reduction could not be achieved. Imaging of patients with increasing symptoms or new deficits after injury was recommended, particularly if neurological changes developed during attempted reduction. Preoperative imaging was recommended if closed reduction could not be achieved prior to surgical treatment.

Similarly, Hadley and co-workers report a series of 68 patients with either unilateral or bilateral facet dislocations (37). Although only 58% were successfully reduced with closed traction, seven patients deteriorated during unsuccessful attempts at closed reduction. Six of these patients eventually recovered. Yet, successful closed reduction resulted in improved neurological function in most patients, including one with complete quadriplegia.

More frequent disc displacements were reported by Harrington and colleagues in a series of 37 patients with fracture subluxations (38). Although nearly all patients were successfully reduced in traction and none sustained neurological deterioration, nine patients were subsequently diagnosed with displaced cervical discs at the level of injury. A higher frequency of disc displacement was reported by Rizzolo and colleagues, particularly in patients with bilateral facet dislocations or anterior cord syndromes (39). Although closed reduction, when necessary, was performed before MRI, none of their patients deteriorated

during closed reduction. A larger retrospective series of 82 patients undergoing MRI after closed reduction revealed disc displacement or disruption in nearly 25% (40). No patient sustained neurological deterioration during closed reduction.

These studies suggest that neurological deterioration with closed reduction is infrequent. Consequently, closed reduction of facet dislocations in nonobtunded patients in whom a neurological examination can be performed can be followed safely without MRI before reduction. High weight reduction to 140 lbs has been used successfully to realign the cervical spine after facet dislocation (41). Failure to achieve reduction with traction should prompt additional imaging to determine the condition of the disc and its relationship to the spinal cord before proceeding to open reduction and internal fixation.

The recommended management of unilateral facet dislocations is likewise controversial. Hadley and co-workers report treatment with halo immobilization in 16 patients with successful closed reduction (37). Three patients who failed closed reduction were also treated with halo immobilization because severe concurrent injuries precluded open reduction. Similarly, halo immobilization was used in 15 patients with bilateral facet dislocations successfully reduced with traction. Of the combined 31 patients, bony union was achieved in 24. Seven had recurrent subluxation in the halo and underwent surgical stabilization. Five of these patients did not have concurrent facet fractures. In contrast, Shapiro and associates report a series of 51 patients with unilateral facet dislocations, half of whom had concurrent facet fractures (42). Two patients placed in halo immobilization after closed reduction had recurrent subluxation. All patients underwent surgical fixation, most with neurological improvement at follow-up. Persistent pain in patients with unreduced unilateral dislocations treated with immobilization has prompted recommendation of open reduction in patients failing closed treatment (43).

Most spinal surgeons recommend surgical stabilization after closed reduction for bilateral facet dislocations. Typically, a posterior approach is chosen with either wiring techniques or lateral mass plate fixation for internal stabilization. Occasionally, unilateral plating with interspinous wiring may be used in the setting of a unilateral facet fracture to obviate extension to an adjacent level. Two series encompassing 80 patients demonstrated successful treatment with surgical stabilization of these injuries (44,45). Although most patients were treated posteriorly, 10 patients underwent either an anterior approach alone or with additional posterior fusion. Since the mechanism of injury involves distractive flexion with predominant posterior ligamentous injury, a posterior tension band would seem to be the most prudent method of internal fixation. However, patients with disc displacement who fail closed reduction may require anterior decompression before reduction. An anterior decompression, open reduction, and internal plate fixation may be sufficient to treat these injuries, despite the posterior ligamentous failure. Vital and associates describe a treatment protocol for unilateral and bilateral facet dislocations in a series of 168 patients (46). The regimen failed in only five patients, each of whom had a chronic unilateral dislocation. Among patients with bilateral dislocations, three-fourths were reduced with either closed traction or closed manipulation with general anesthesia. In contrast, surgical reduction was required in more than one-third of patients with unilateral dislocations. Anterior treatment was successful for reduction and stabilization. The absence of facet fracture and the type of postoperative immobilization may be factors to consider if anterior arthrodesis and fixation alone are performed.

Distractive extension injuries are less common, and often difficult to diagnose. Many patients have no neurological deficits and have only subtle signs of abnormality on plain cervical

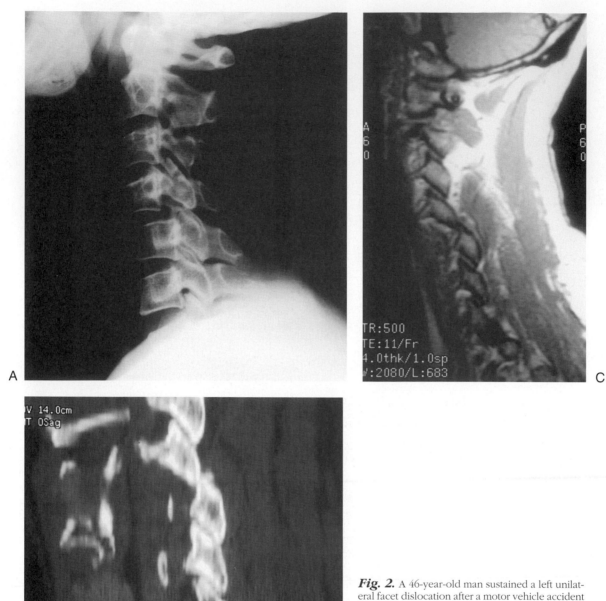

Fig. 2. A 46-year-old man sustained a left unilateral facet dislocation after a motor vehicle accident with radiculopathy. **A:** Lateral radiograph reveals less than 50% anterior subluxation. Sagittal CT reconstruction **(B)** and sagittal T1-weighted MRI **(C)** reveal the jumped facet.

radiography (Fig. 3). This injury may be more commonly seen in older adult patients who have arthrosis of one or more cervical interspaces from spondylosis, ankylosing spondylitis, diffuse idiopathic skeletal hyperostosis, or Klippel-Feil syndrome (47–50). Since the predominant mechanism of injury results in primarily discoligamentous disruption with preservation of posterior ligamentous support, anterior cervical fusion with plate fixation may be preferred. However, easy distractibility of the interspace during interbody arthrodesis may suggest occult posterior ligamentous laxity that may require additional posterior fixation as well.

Despite the success of cervical arthrodesis in achieving stability after subaxial cervical spine injuries, the long-term consequences of arthrodesis in young patients typically sustaining these injuries is unknown. For example, there is growing evidence that cervical arthrodesis increases the frequency of osteoarthrosis at adjacent unfused spinal segments. McGrory and

Klassen report successful management of cervical fractures and dislocations in a pediatric population with arthrodesis (51). Yet, more than one-third of patients developed extension of the fusion mass across uninjured segments. Moreover, radiographs after prolonged follow-up showed a significantly increased frequency of osteoarthrosis of the adjacent interspaces.

In conclusion, subaxial cervical fractures comprise a variety of injuries that require identification of the mechanism of failure to facilitate the most appropriate treatment. Instability develops along a continuum, with greater degrees of displacement or angulation suggesting progressive failure of supporting ligamentous structures. External immobilization with rigid collars or halo vest is often successful in treating predominantly osseous injuries not associated with significant ligamentous injuries. However, it is important to identify evidence of concurrent injury in the opposite spinal column, which may suggest the potential for progressive instability despite external immobiliza-

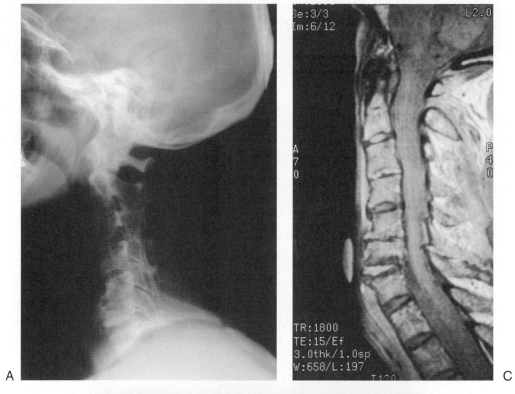

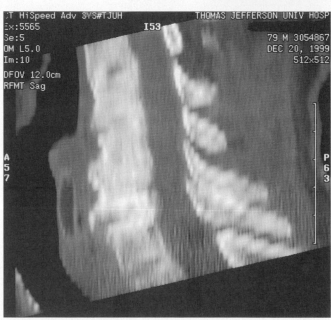

Fig. 3. A 79-year-old man sustained a C6-7 distractive extension injury without neurological injury after a motor vehicle accident. **A:** Lateral radiograph reveals severe spondylosis of C5-6 as well as widening and irregularity of the end plates at C6-7. **B:** Sagittal CT reconstruction reveals spontaneous arthrosis of C5-6 and widening of the C6-7 interspace. **C:** Sagittal MRI demonstrates increased signal intensity in the C6-7 intervertebral disc with a "fish-mouth" appearance confirming the distractive extension injury.

tion. Future investigations should focus on developing treatment protocols that allow safe and effective treatment for the more common injuries.

References

1. Glaser JA, Jaworski BA, Cuddy BG, et al. Variation in surgical opinion regarding management of selected cervical spine injuries. A preliminary study. *Spine* 23:975–983, 1998.
2. Roaf R. A study of mechanics of spinal injuries. *J Bone Joint Surg Br* 42:810–823, 1960.
3. Kelly RP, Whitesides TE. Treatment of lumbodorsal fracture-dislocations. *Ann Surg* 167:705–717, 1968.
4. Holdsworth FW. Fractures, dislocations, and fracture-dislocations of the spine. *J Bone Joint Surg Br* 45:6–20, 1963.
5. Holdsworth F. Fractures, dislocations, and fracture-dislocations of the spine. *J Bone Joint Surg Am* 52:1534–1551, 1970.
6. Denis F. The three column spine and its significance in the classification of acute thoracolumbar spinal injuries. *Spine* 8:817–831, 1983.
7. Allen BL, Ferguson RL, Lehmann TR, et al. A mechanistic classification of closed, indirect fractures and dislocations of the lower cervical spine. *Spine* 7:1–21, 1982.
8. Schneider RC, Kahn EA. Chronic neurological sequelae of acute trauma to the spine and spinal cord. Part 1. The significance of the acute-flexion or "tear-drop" fracture-dislocation of the cervical spine. *J Bone Joint Surg Am* 38:985–997, 1956.
9. Beatson TR. Fractures and dislocations of the cervical spine. *J Bone Joint Surg Br* 45:21–35, 1963.
10. Taylor AR, Blackwood W. Paraplegia in hyperextension cervical injuries with normal radiographic appearances. *J Bone Joint Surg Br* 30:245–248, 1948.
11. Maiman DJ, Sances A, Myklebust JB, et al. Compression injuries of the cervical spine: a biomechanical analysis. *Neurosurgery* 13:254–260, 1983.
12. Yoganandan N, Sances A, Maiman DJ, et al. Experimental spinal injuries with vertical impact. *Spine* 11:855–860, 1986.
13. Yoganandan N, Sances A, Pintar F, et al. Injury biomechanics of the human cervical column. *Spine* 15:1031–1039, 1990.
14. Yoganandan N, Pintar F, Sances A, et al. Strength and motion analysis of the human head-neck complex. *J Spinal Disord* 4:73–85, 1991.
15. Carter JW, Mirza SK, Tencer AF, et al. Canal geometry changes associated with axial compressive cervical spine fracture. *Spine* 25:46–54, 2000.
16. Gonzalez RP, Fried PO, Bukhalo M, et al. Role of clinical examination in screening for blunt cervical spine injury. *J Am Coll Surg* 189:152–157, 1999.
17. Hoffman JR, Mower WR, Wolfson AB, et al. Validity of a set of clinical criteria to rule out injury to the cervical spine in patients with blunt trauma. National Emergency X-Radiography Utilization Study Group. *New Engl J Med* 343:94–99, 2000.
18. Kang JD, Figgie MP, Bohlman HH. Sagittal measurements of the cervical spine in subaxial fractures and dislocations. An analysis of two hundred and eighty-eight patients with and without neurological deficits. *J Bone Joint Surg Am* 76:1617–1628, 1994.
19. Woodring JH, Lee C. The role and limitations of computed tomographic scanning in evaluation of cervical trauma. *J Trauma* 33:698–708, 1992.
20. Berne JD, Velmahos GC, El-Tawil Q, et al. Value of complete cervical helical computed tomographic scanning in identifying cervical spine injury in the unevaluable blunt trauma patient with multiple injuries: a prospective study. *J Trauma-Injury Infect Crit Care* 47:896–902, 1999.
21. Tan E, Schweitzer ME, Vaccaro A, et al. Is computed tomography of nonvisualized C7-T1 cost-effective? *J Spinal Disord* 12:472–476, 1999.
22. Blackmore CC, Ramsey SD, Mann FA, et al. Cervical spine screening with CT in trauma patients: a cost-effectiveness analysis. *Radiology* 212:117–125, 1999.
23. Blackmore CC, Emerson SS, Mann FA, et al. Cervical spine imaging in patients with trauma: determination of fracture risk to optimize use. *Radiology* 211:759–765, 1999.
24. Katzberg RW, Benedetti PF, Drake CM, et al. Acute cervical spine injuries: prospective MR imaging assessment at a level 1 trauma center. *Radiology* 213:203–212, 1999.
25. Klein GR, Vaccaro AR, Albert TJ, et al. Efficacy of magnetic resonance imaging in the evaluation of posterior cervical spine fractures. *Spine* 24:771–774, 1999.
26. Benzel EC, Hart BL, Ball PA, et al. Magnetic resonance imaging for the evaluation of patients with occult spine injury. *J Neurosurg* 85:824–829, 1996.
27. Halliday AL, Henderson BR, Hart BL, et al. The management of unilateral mass/facet fractures of the subaxial cervical spine. The use of magnetic resonance imaging to predict instability. *Spine* 22:2614–2621, 1997.
28. Friedman D, Flanders A, Thomas C, et al. Vertebral artery injury after acute cervical spine trauma: rate of occurrence as detected by MR angiography and assessment of clinical consequences. *Am J Radiol* 164:443–447, 1995.
29. Willis BK, Greiner F, Orrison WW, et al. The incidence of vertebral artery injury after midcervical spine fracture or subluxation. *Neurosurgery* 34:435–442, 1994.
30. Vaccaro AR, Klein GR, Flanders AE, et al. Long-term evaluation of vertebral artery injuries following cervical spine trauma using magnetic resonance angiography. *Spine* 23:789–795, 1998.
31. White AA, Panjabi MM. *Clinical biomechanics of the spine*, 2nd ed. Philadelphia: JB Lippincott Co, 1990.
32. White AA, Johnson RM, Panjabi MM. Biomechanical analysis of clinical stability in the cervical spine. *Clin Orthop Rel Res* 109:85–96, 1975.
33. Holmes A, Wang C, Han ZH, et al. The range and nature of flexion-extension motion in the cervical spine. *Spine* 19:2505–2510, 1994.
34. Lysell E. Motion in the cervical spine. *Acta Orthop Scand* (Suppl) 123:1–61, 1969.
35. An HS. Cervical spine trauma. *Spine* 23:2713–2729, 1998.
36. Eismont FJ, Arena MJ, Green BA. Extrusion of an intervertebral disc associated with traumatic subluxation or dislocation of cervical facets. *J Bone Joint Surg Am* 73:1555–1560, 1991.
37. Hadley MN, Fitzpatrick BC, Sonntag VKH, et al. Facet fracture-dislocation injuries of the cervical spine. *Neurosurgery* 31:661–666, 1992.
38. Harrington JF, Likavec MJ, Smith AS. Disc herniation in cervical fracture subluxation. *Neurosurgery* 29:374–379, 1991.
39. Rizzolo SJ, Piazza MR, Cotler JM, et al. Intervertebral disc injury complicating cervical spine trauma. *Spine* 16:S187–189, 1991.
40. Grant GA, Mirza SK, Chapman JR, et al. Risk of early closed reduction in cervical spine subluxation injuries. *J Neurosurg* 90:13–18, 1999.
41. Cotler JM, Herbison GJ, Nasuti JF, et al. Closed reduction of traumatic cervical spine dislocations using traction weights up to 140 pounds. *Spine* 18:386–390, 1993.
42. Shapiro S, Snyder W, Kaufman K, et al. Outcome of 51 cases of unilateral locked cervical facets: interspinous braided cable or lateral mass plate fusion compared with interspinous wire and facet wiring with iliac crest. *J Neurosurg* 91:19–24, 1999.
43. Rorabeck CH, Rock MG, Hawkins RJ, et al. Unilateral facet dislocation of the cervical spine. *Spine* 12:23–27, 1987.
44. Maiman DJ, Barolat G, Larson SJ. Management of bilateral locked facets of the cervical spine. *Neurosurgery* 18:542–547, 1986.
45. Wolf A, Levi L, Mirvis S, et al. Operative management of bilateral facet dislocation. *J Neurosurg* 75:883–890, 1991.
46. Vital JM, Gille O, Senegas J, et al. Reduction technique for uni- and biarticular dislocations of the lower cervical spine. *Spine* 23:949–954, 1998.
47. Karasick D, Schweitzer ME, Vaccaro AR. The traumatized cervical spine in Klippel-Feil syndrome: imaging features. *Am J Roentgenol* 170:85–88, 1998.
48. Le Hir PX, Sautet A, Le Gars L, et al. Hyperextension vertebral body fractures in diffuse idiopathic skeletal hyperostosis: a cause of intravertebral fluidlike collections on MR imaging. *Am J Roentgenol* 173:1679–1683, 1999.
49. Meyer PR. Diffuse idiopathic skeletal hyperostosis in the cervical spine. *Clin Orthop Rel Res* 359:49–57, 1999.
50. Taggard DA, Traynelis VC. Management of cervical spinal fractures in ankylosing spondylitis with posterior fixation. *Spine* 25:2035–2039, 2000.
51. McGrory BJ, Klassen RA. Arthrodesis of the cervical spine for fractures and dislocations in children and adolescents. A long-term follow-up study. *J Bone Joint Surg Am* 76:1606–1616, 1994.

161. Thoracolumbar Fracture Classification and Grading

Gregory J. Przybylski

A dramatic evolution in the management of thoracolumbar spine fractures has taken place over the past 30 years. Previously, these injuries were predominantly treated with posterior rod systems in distraction or compression, and gradually evolved to segmental fixation systems (1–3). Subsequently, technical advances in spinal instrumentation, improved familiarity with anterior thoracolumbar approaches, and enhanced cardiopulmonary anesthetic and critical care management further facilitated interest in the operative treatment of the injured patient (4,5). However, surgeons have also reported successful management of some of these fractures with external immobilization alone (6–8). The variable degree of instability that may be present supports establishment of a method to identify the mechanism of injury and estimate the likelihood of successful healing using a particular treatment scheme. In order to distinguish among a variety of techniques available for treating these injuries, several different classification systems have been proposed to guide the surgeon in treatment planning. This chapter will examine the historical evolution of classification schemes for thoracolumbar fractures in order to provide a foundation for evaluating images of thoracolumbar injuries and planning a treatment regimen.

The earliest classification of thoracolumbar fractures was proposed by Boehler in 1929 (9). He suggested the possibility of five primary spinal injuries, including (a) compression injury with vertebral body fracture, (b) anterior flexion injury with anterior compressive and posterior distractive injuries, (c) extension injury with discoligamentous disruption and posterior arch fracture, (d) shear injury with large displacements, and (e) torsional injuries with asymmetrical patterns of fracture. Although subsequent classifications have examined these categories in greater detail, most can be distilled into this rather succinct framework. In 1931, the concept of ligamentous injury was suggested by Watson-Jones (10) and further refined by Nicoll in 1949 (11). During management of these injuries, unexpected displacement while reducing a malaligned segment led to consideration of longitudinal ligament injury, annular tearing, and comminution of the vertebra as contributors to instability.

After inferring the mechanisms of force transmission suggested by such a classification, Roaf applied forces to fresh postmortem spine segments, predominantly from child or young adult decedents, in order to elucidate the magnitude and direction of forces required to reproduce clinically observed spinal injuries (12). With vertical compressive forces, he observed predominant distortion in the vertebral end plate rather than the annulus. As a result, blood is gradually expressed from the cancellous bone of the vertebral body. Roaf proposed that movement of blood out of the vertebra is an important mechanism of force dissipation. With increasing pressure, the end plate fractures, allowing displacement of disc material. He concluded that the disc resists compression better than the vertebral body. However, older specimens with impaired nucleus pulposus structure failed with annular tearing and buckling of the side walls of the vertebral body. Similar findings were reproduced in younger specimens in which the nucleus was experimentally removed. Roaf was unable to cause posterior ligament disruption after spinal flexion without initial compression of the vertebral body. He suggested that the pressure developed in the nucleus exceeded the tolerance of the vertebral end plate. Similarly, he was unable to tear the anterior longitudinal ligament

without initially fracturing the neural arch. In contrast, the intervertebral discs and supporting ligaments were vulnerable in rotation and shear. With loss of nuclear turgor, rotational ligamentous injuries occurred more easily, sometimes without an accompanying fracture. Roaf concluded that fractures result from compressive forces, whereas dislocations result from rotational forces.

Based on observations accumulated over two decades in 1,000 patients, Holdsworth proposed a six-tiered classification system to help predict the results of treatment (13,14). He described simple wedge fractures with intact end plates but without interspinous widening that could be treated with several weeks of bed rest initially, followed by external immobilization for 8 to 12 weeks. Burst injuries were characterized by end-plate and vertebral body fracture with outward displacement but without interspinous widening. Holdsworth likewise believed that these fractures were essentially stable, given that spontaneous fusion would be expected secondary to comminution of the body and the end-plate fracture. Treatment with immobilization on a plaster bed and subsequent external immobilization in a jacket for 12 weeks was recommended. The last "stable" injury was described with extension, and rarely occurred in the thoracolumbar spine. For this, he recommended 12 weeks of immobilization. This author also identified three groups of unstable injuries. Dislocations were accompanied by posterior ligamentous failure in which healing did not reliably occur. Operative reduction with posterior fusion followed by plaster bed immobilization for 12 to 14 weeks was suggested. Fracture-dislocations were estimated to be the most unstable injuries. Either prolonged bed rest or internal fixation was used to treat these injuries. Finally, shear injuries with large displacements and fractures typically occurred in the thoracic spine and were treated with open reduction only if the displacement was substantial.

The concept of "columns" of injury was initially suggested by Kelly and Whitesides in 1968 (15). They divided the spinal axis into an anterior column composed of the vertebral bodies and intervening annular and longitudinal ligaments that resisted compression, and a posterior column of ligaments that resisted tension. The authors identified retropulsion of bone into the spinal canal with comminuted burst fractures that might warrant surgical removal through an anterior approach.

In 1970, Roy-Camille and Lelievre (16) suggested the presence of an intermediate spinal segment composed of the posterior annulus, posterior longitudinal ligament, pedicles, and facet complexes. Subsequently, Louis and Goutallier described a three-column system that divided the posterior column proposed by Kelly and Whitesides into paired lateral columns composed of the facet complexes, linked to the anterior column by pedicles and to each other posteriorly by the neural arch (17). The three columns were valued with one point, whereas each pedicle and each lamina were valued with half a point. Louis defined instability based on an injury score of two or more.

A different three-column structure was proposed by Denis one decade later (18). Based on a retrospective examination of more than 400 thoracolumbar injuries, some with computed tomography (CT) imaging, the anterior column of Kelly and Whitesides was bisected into an anterior and middle column respectively composed of the anterior and posterior halves of the annular and longitudinal ligaments. He described four pri-

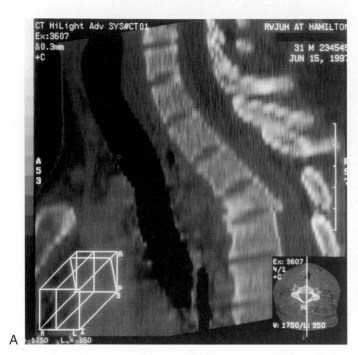
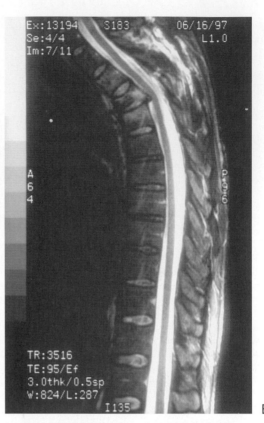

Fig. 1. A 31-year-old man sustained a T3 fracture without neurological injury after improperly landing while mountain biking. **A:** Sagittal CT reconstruction reveals a flexion-compression fracture with kyphosis. **B:** Sagittal MRI shows the anterior proximity of the spinal cord to the area of kyphosis.

mary injury types, including compression, burst, seat belt, and fracture-dislocation. Compression injuries were sustained from anterior or lateral flexion forces (Fig. 1). Fractures were divided into four subcategories, including superior end-plate, coronal plane, anterior buckling, and inferior end-plate fractures in decreasing order of frequency. Preservation of the posterior vertebral body cortex was observed and mild interspinous widening commensurate with the degree of angulation was seen.

Burst fractures caused by axial forces (Fig. 2) were subdivided into five different mechanisms, based on accompanying secondary forces of anterior or lateral flexion or rotation. These included fractures of the superior end plate, both end plates, fracture of the inferior end plate, fracture of both end plates accompanied by rotational displacement, and coronal plane asymmetry from lateral flexion in decreasing order of frequency. Seat-belt injuries resulted from failure of the middle and posterior columns in tension, but near preservation of the anterior column. Both osseous Chance fractures (19) and discoligamentous injuries (Fig. 3) through one or two vertebral segments were described. Finally, fracture-dislocations (Fig. 4) were subdivided into flexion-distraction, flexion-rotation, and shear forces. The former injury was least common, representing tension failure of the middle and posterior columns seen in seat-belt injuries with additional anterior column failure in tension with annular ligament disruption. In contrast, flexion-rotation injuries were most often seen in this subgroup, representing similar tension injury of the middle and posterior columns but additionally failure of the anterior column in compression and rotation beyond that observed in the seat-belt injury. Finally, shear injuries represented complete failure of all three columns.

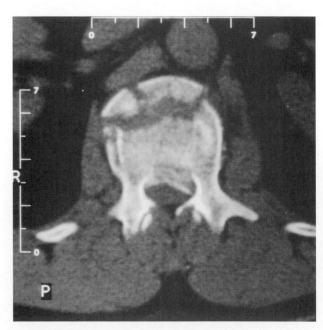

Fig. 2. A 35-year-old firefighter sustained a fall without neurological injury. Axial CT reveals an L1 burst fracture.

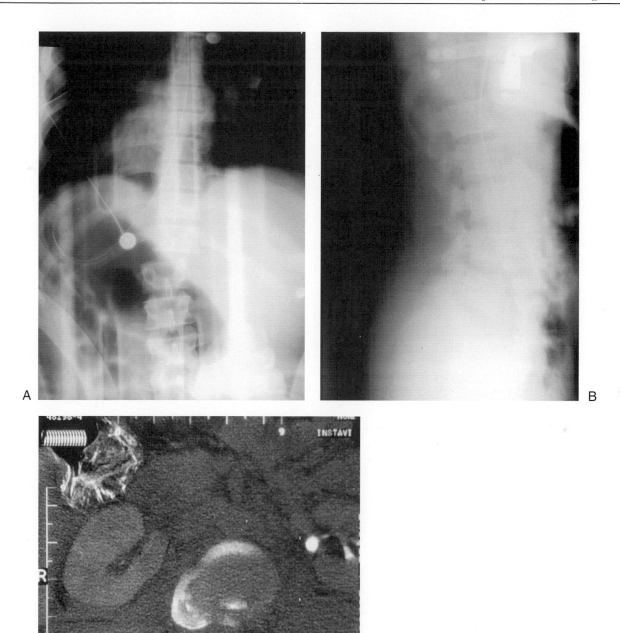

Fig. 3. A 17-year-old boy sustained paraplegia after a motor vehicle accident. Anteroposterior **(A)** and lateral **(B)** thoracolumbar radiographs reveal a T12-L1 discoligamentous Chance injury. **C:** Axial CT shows the lateral displacement without accompanying fracture.

Denis summarized a treatment algorithm based on degrees of instability (18). Compression fractures contained an intact posterior column and were treated with or without external immobilization. The first degree of instability (mechanical) was observed in severe compression fractures and seat-belt injuries. Failure in flexion was seen around the hinge of the middle or anterior columns, respectively. Either external immobilization in extension or internal fixation was recommended. Second-degree instability (neurological) was observed in burst fractures. Although many patients were neurologically normal initially, neurological worsening in some nonoperatively treated patients suggested the risk of progressive displacement of fragments with axial loading. Finally, third-degree instability

(mechanical and neurological) characterized the fracture dislocation injuries; surgical decompression and stabilization were recommended.

Alternative classification schemes have been suggested which use variations of the compression, flexion, seat belt, and fracture-dislocation categories. Argenson and Boileau describe a modification that defines unstable injuries in all four categories (20). For example, compressive injuries with intact middle column function but posterior ligamentous disruption were associated with late kyphosis, suggesting potential instability. Similarly, progressively increasing posterior displacement was associated with late neurological impairment and pseudoarthrosis. In addition, only the osseous subtype ("Chance" frac-

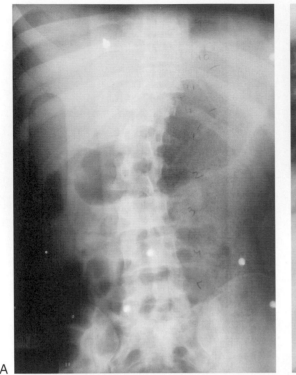
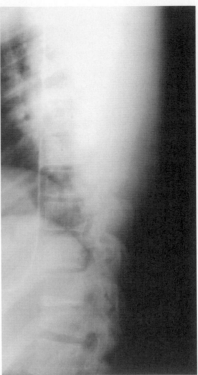

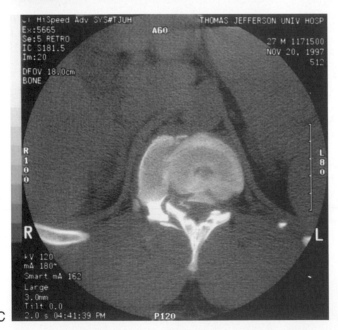

Fig. 4. A 27-year-old man fell off of scaffolding, sustaining paraplegia. Anteroposterior (**A**) and lateral (**B**) thoracolumbar radiographs reveal a T11-12 fracture dislocation. **C:** Axial CT shows the lateral dislocation and accompanying fracture.

ture) of seat-belt injuries could be treated with immobilization alone without risk of late pseudoarthrosis.

In contrast, a 3 × 3 matrix was suggested based upon 1,445 patients organized under the AO Fracture Classification System (21). Primarily three injury types were noted, including vertebral body compression (type A), anterior and posterior element distraction (type B), and anterior and posterior element injury with rotation (type C). Three levels of severity were described in each of the three types of injury. Vertebral injuries alone or accompanied by posterior column injury without disc disruption constituted type A injuries. The presence of disc disruption identified type B injuries, whereas additional rotational injuries defined type C.

After Denis proposed the importance of middle column injury in assessing thoracolumbar fracture stability, several investigators have used radiological or biomechanical examinations of fractures to test this hypothesis. McAfee and colleagues examined CT imaging in 100 consecutive patients, offering a classification scheme with treatment based on an assessment of middle column injury (22). They implicitly suggest three primary mechanisms of injury, which include axial compression, axial distraction, and translation in the transverse plane. Although they considered six different classes of thoracolumbar fractures, it was believed that combinations of these three mechanisms sufficiently described the range of these injuries. In fact, the presence of a translational injury alone or in combination with axial compression or distraction often defined instability. Wedge compression fractures developed from anterior column injury in flexion, whereas stable burst fractures resulted from anterior and middle column failure in compression. Both injuries were treated with external immobilization, except when a significant deformity associated with mild neurological deficit was present secondary to multiple contiguous level injuries.

In contrast, unstable burst fractures included compressive failure of the anterior and middle columns along with posterior column failure in distraction, compression, lateral flexion, or rotation. Chance fractures involved flexion distraction forces around an axis anterior to the anterior longitudinal ligament, whereas forces posterior to the anterior longitudinal ligament led to flexion distraction injuries. Three of four Chance injuries were treated with immobilization, whereas most flexion distraction injuries underwent stabilization with a compression rod system. The authors concluded that the mode of failure of the middle column was associated with the degree of neurological deficit, degree of instability, and the type of instrumentation required. Finally, translational injuries with malalignment of the spinal canal result from shear forces. These injuries were typically treated with segmental stabilization.

Alternatively, a biomechanical examination of thoracolumbar junction fractures in six cadaveric spine segments by James and associates (23) implies that the disruption of the posterior ligamentous complex plays a larger role in predicting failure of nonoperative treatment than injury of the middle column as suggested by Denis (18). Failure in flexion from posterior ligamentous injury was observed. A sequential column disruption technique was used. Added injury to the middle column resulted in much less incremental angulation, whereas additional posterior ligamentous disruption significantly increased angulation in flexion. In fact, the posterior column contributed twice as much as the middle column in flexion stability. Given that middle column failure was observed in both stable and unstable injuries treated by McAfee and colleagues (22), perhaps the critical injury identifying potential instability involves concurrent tension failure of the posterior column.

In order to identify patients who may develop progressive deformity, Farcy and co-workers (24) measured the degree of sagittal plane kyphosis relative to the normal segmental angulation. The sagittal index measures the difference between the angle of segmental kyphosis and the normal kyphotic or lordotic segmental angle. A sagittal index of less than 15 degrees was not associated with progressive deformity. The authors surgically treated patients with a sagittal index of greater than 15 degrees, but recommended consideration of conservative treatment for a sagittal index between 20 and 25 degrees.

Concerns about the order of severity in this classification system however led to a modification by a committee formed from members of several national spine societies (25). Injuries were grouped in order of increasing severity based on the primary mechanism of injury including compression, distraction, or multidirectional with translation. Each category was subdivided into three additional classes. Compression injuries included wedge fracture, coronal or sagittal split fractures, and burst fractures. Distraction injuries were divided among posterior ligamentous injury, additional neural arch injury, and anterior disc injury (in order of progressive distraction from posterior to anterior). Finally, translational injuries were grouped into anteroposterior, lateral, or rotational directions. Using this classification, a treatment algorithm was recommended based upon the failure mechanism similar to McAfee's scheme (22). Unstable compressive injuries were treated with distraction, distraction injuries with compression, and translational injuries with multisegmental fixation. Torsional injuries in particular were associated with delayed neurological deterioration (26).

A more complex classification system was suggested by Fer-

guson and Allen (27). Seven injury types were described including compressive flexion, distractive flexion, lateral flexion, translational, torsional flexion, vertical compression, and distractive extension. The "three-column" concept was modified, such that the middle column comprised the posterior third of the intervertebral disc, thereby locating the transition between anterior and middle columns closer to the instantaneous axis of rotation. Compressive flexion was subdivided into the stable anterior wedge compression fracture with isolated anterior column failure, the more unstable anterior column injury accompanied by posterior column injury in tension, and finally additional middle column failure. In contrast, distractive flexion occurs after tension failure of all three columns. Lateral flexion injuries may involve isolated, unilateral anterior and middle column compression fracture or additional failure of the contralateral posterior column in tension. Translational injuries were often associated with other injury mechanisms. Torsional flexion injuries add rotation to anterior column compression failure and posterior column distraction. Vertical compression injuries occur after all three columns fail in compression. Finally, distractive extension injuries are anterior column injuries in extension with posterior column failure in compression.

A somewhat different concept of classification was proposed by McCormack and co-workers to define the ability of short-segment posterior fixation to allow successful treatment of three-column thoracolumbar injuries (28). Three characteristics were identified including the degree of vertebral body comminution seen on sagittal CT reconstruction, the dispersion of fragments on axial CT, and the degree of correction of kyphosis when comparing preoperative and postoperative plain radiographs. One to three points were given for comminution (less than 30%, 30% to 60%, greater than 60%), dispersion (minimal, greater than 2 mm of less than half of the cross-sectional area, greater than 2 mm displacement of more than half of the cross-sectional area), and kyphotic correction (less than 3 degrees, 4 to 9 degrees, and greater than 10 degrees). A score of seven to nine points was associated with screw fracture.

In conclusion, an understanding of the evolution of classification systems for describing thoracolumbar fractures can assist the surgeon in assessing the degree of instability as well as to guide treatment of these often complex injuries. Although the methods used for classifying these injuries have varied, the fractures can be summarized into the three basic categories of compression, distraction, and rotational injuries. Further subclassification, often considering accompanying middle and posterior column injuries, facilitates differentiation among those injuries that may be successfully treated with external immobilization and those that may require internal fixation.

References

1. Daniaux H, Seykora P, Genelin A, et al. Application of posterior plating and modifications I thoracolumbar spine injuries. Indication, techniques, and results. *Spine* 16:S125–133, 1991.
2. Tasdemiroglu E, Tibbs PA. Long-term follow-up results of thoracolumbar fractures after posterior instrumentation. *Spine* 20:1704–1708, 1995.
3. Vornanen MJ, Bostman OM, Myllynen PJ. Reduction of bone retropulsed into the spinal canal in thoracolumbar vertebral body compression burst fractures. A prospective randomized comparative study between Harrington rods and two transpedicular devices. *Spine* 20:1699–1703, 1995.
4. Haas N, Blauth M, Tscherne H. Anterior plating in thoracolumbar spine injuries. Indication, technique and results. *Spine* 16:S100–111, 1991.
5. Kaneda K, Abumi K, Fujiya M. Burst fractures with neurologic defi-

cits of the thoracolumbar-lumbar spine. Results of anterior decompression and stabilization with anterior instrumentation. *Spine* 9:788–795, 1984.

6. Cantor JB, Lebwohl NH, Garvey T, et al. Nonoperative management of stable thoracolumbar fractures with early ambulation and bracing. *Spine* 18:971–976, 1993.

7. Mumford J, Weinstein JN, Spratt KF, et al. thoracolumbar burst fractures: the clinical efficacy and outcome of nonoperative management. *Spine* 18:955–970, 1993.

8. Weinstein JN, Collalto P, Lehmann TR. Thoracolumbar "burst" fractures treated conservatively: a long-term follow-up. *Spine* 13:33–38, 1988.

9. Boehler L. *Technique de traitment des fractures de la colonne dorsale et lombaire.* Paris: Masson, 1944; 149.

10. Watson-Jones R. *Fractures and other bone and joint injuries.* Edinburgh: E & S Livingstone Ltd, 1940.

11. Nicoll EA. Fractures of the dorsolumbar spine. *J Bone Joint Surg Br* 31:376–394, 1949.

12. Roaf R. A study of mechanics of spinal injuries. *J Bone Joint Surg Br* 42:810–823, 1960.

13. Holdsworth FW. Fractures, dislocations, and fracture-dislocations of the spine. *J Bone Joint Surg Br* 45:6–20, 1963.

14. Holdsworth F. Fractures, dislocations, and fracture-dislocations of the spine. *J Bone Joint Surg Am* 52:1534–1551, 1970.

15. Kelly RP, Whitesides TE. Treatment of lumbodorsal fracture-dislocations. *Ann Surg* 167:705–717, 1968.

16. Roy-Camille R, Lelievre JF. [Pseudarthrosis of the dorso-lumbar vertebrae.] *Rev Chir Orthop Reparatrice Appar Mot* 61:249–257, 1975.

17. Louis R, Goutallier D. Fractures instables du rachis. *Symp Rev Chir Orthop* 63:415–481, 1977.

18. Denis F. The three column spine and its significance in the classification of acute thoracolumbar spinal injuries. *Spine* 8:817–831, 1983.

19. Chance GO. Note on a type of flexion fracture of the spine. *Br J Radiol* 21:452–453,1948.

20. Argenson C, Boileau P. Classification of thoracolumbar spine fractures. In: Floman Y, Farcy JPC, Argenson C, eds. *Thoracolumbar spine fractures.* New York: Raven Press, 1993; 131–156.

21. Magerl F, Aebi M, Gertzbein SD, et al. A comprehensive classification of thoracic and lumbar injuries. *Eur Spine J* 3:1–18, 1994.

22. McAfee PC, Yuan HA, Fredrickson BE, et al. The value of computed tomography in thoracolumbar fractures. An analysis of one hundred consecutive cases and a new classification. *J Bone Joint Surg Am* 65:461–473, 1983.

23. James KS, Wenger KH, Schlegel JD, et al. Biomechanical evaluation of the stability of thoracolumbar burst fractures. *Spine* 19:1731–1740, 1994.

24. Farcy JPC, Weidenbaum M, Glassman SD. Sagittal index in management of thoracolumbar burst fractures. *Spine* 15:958–965, 1990.

25. Gertzbein SD. Spine update. Classification of thoracolumbar fractures. *Spine* 19:626–628, 1994.

26. Gertzbein SD. Neurologic deterioration in patients with thoracic and lumbar fractures after admission to the hospital. *Spine* 19:1723–1725, 1994.

27. Ferguson RL, Allen BL. A mechanistic classification of thoracolumbar spine fractures. *Clin Orthop* 189;77–88, 1984.

28. McCormack T, Karaikovic E, Gaines RW. The load sharing classification of spine fractures. *Spine* 19:1741–1744, 1994.

162. Lumbar Fractures

Naresh P. Patel, Michael S. Hahn, and J. Patrick Johnson

Some 60,000 spinal column injuries are sustained in the United States annually. Fractures to the lower lumbar spine comprise only 4% of these, while the majority of injuries occur in the midcervical region and thoracolumbar (TL) junction (1–3). TL junction (i.e., T10-L1) fractures are distinctly different from fractures occurring in the L2-5 region with regard to anatomical, biomechanical, and neurological considerations. Consequently, the surgical techniques for stabilization and fixation of lumbar fractures differ from those for more rostral injuries. Additionally, spinal injuries may occur at two or more at levels in the same patient, as 20% of spinal fracture patients have multiple sites of injury. This chapter focuses on the management of patients with lower lumbar fractures (L2-5).

Anatomy and Biomechanics

The vertebral column consists of multiple bony components coupled by strong ligamentous attachments providing both strength and flexibility while protecting the contents of the spinal canal (Fig. 1). The vertebral bodies and intervertebral discs support approximately 80% of spinal loading. Vertebral body height is maximal at L2, and the width of the lumbar vertebral bodies increases caudally. Vertebral body size increases with caudal progression and corresponds with a decreasing incidence of fractures in the lumbar spine secondary to greater load resistance (4,5) (Fig. 2).

The facet joints provide minimal axial loading support but play a significant role in the complex mobility of the lumbar spine. The facets are apophyseal joints with a loose capsule and synovial lining that bear more axial load in extension and less in flexion. The superior articular facet surface faces medially in the upper lumbar spine and articulates with the inferior articular facet surface. Progressing caudally, the facets are located farther apart and face more anteriorly (6,7). The lumbar spine facet joint angle increases in cephalocaudal progression (Fig. 3). It is the sagittal facet orientation that limits rotation, but allows significant flexion and extension in the upper lumbar segments. The converse occurs in the lower lumbar levels, where the L5-S1 facets have the most coronal orientation, allowing more translational movement. Lumbar fractures are uncommon with flexion-extension injuries but are much more common with rotatory injuries (8). Lumbar facet dislocations from disruption of capsular ligaments are rare compared to those in the cervical and upper thoracic regions due to the very strong ligamentous attachments. Complex spinal motion can occur in two directions and three different planes that are important in understanding the force vectors, classification of injury mechanisms, and relative instability.

The anterior longitudinal ligament (ALL), posterior longitudinal ligament (PLL), interspinous ligaments (IL), ligamentum flavum (LF), and capsular ligaments (CL) provide intersegmental stability throughout the lumbar spine. The ALL is the strongest ligament. It resists extension and progressively increases in strength caudally. The PLL primarily resists flexion and is comparatively weaker than the ALL. The interspinous ligaments resist flexion but are often very thin from L4 to S1. The ligamentum flavum is discontinuous, extending between each lamina, and is usually taut except in extreme extension (9) (Fig. 4).

The lumbar region normally has a lordotic curve. The transition occurs at the TL junction with the T12-L1 disc space oriented at −3 degrees lordosis and the L1 vertebral body at +3 degrees kyphosis. Injuries at the TL junction are uniquely different from those in the caudal lumbar spine and are described in another chapter. The L3-4 interspace is the lumbar lordotic apex. Normal lordosis is −20 degrees at L4-5 and −28 degrees at L5-S1 (10–13). The lumbar spine is markedly mobile between the relatively immobile thoracic spine and the sacrum. There

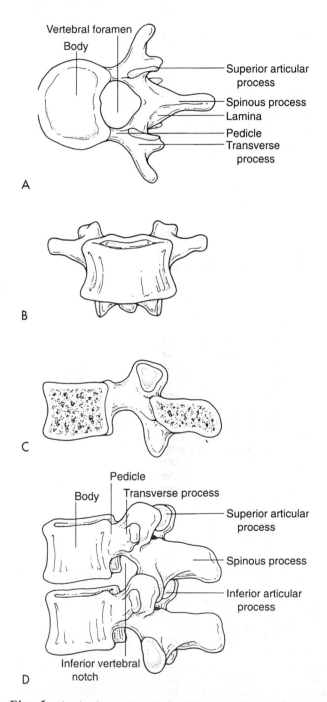

Fig. 1. The lumbar spine. **A:** Superior view. **B:** Anterior view. **C:** Cross-sectional midline lateral view. **D:** Lateral view.

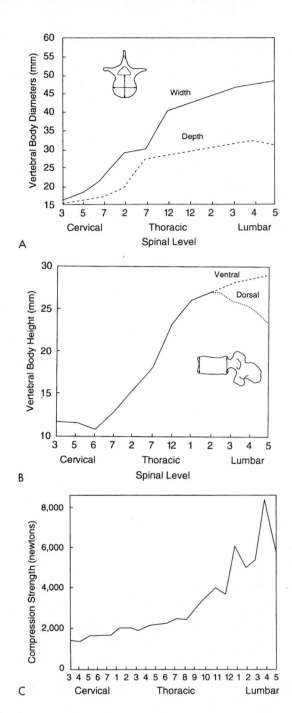

Fig. 2. Vertebral body size and strength. **A:** Vertebral body diameter. **B:** Vertebral body height. **C:** Compression strength.

are 20 degrees of flexion and extension at the L5-S1 level and this progressively decreases in more rostral segments. The greater lordosis and larger vertebral bodies in the lower lumbar region result in more axial loading forces that can cause burst fractures. Additionally, vertebral body strength decreases from a loss in trabecular bone associated with age and osteoporosis starting after 40 years of age (14,15).

Because the conus medullaris most commonly ends at the L1 level in adults, adjacent fractures may result in injuries to the conus. Fractures below this level often involve the cauda equina. The lumbar spinal canal is usually capacious with the

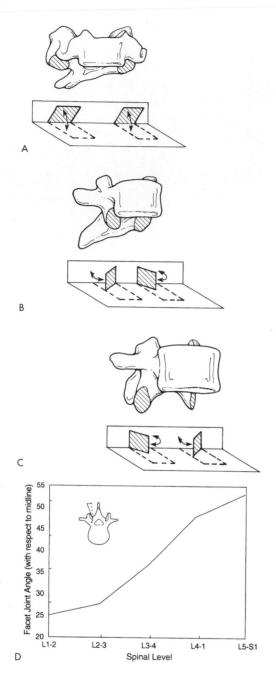

Fig. 3. Facet joint orientation. **A:** Coronal plane orientation of the cervical spine. **B:** Intermediate orientation of the thoracic spine. **C:** Sagittal orientation of the lumbar spine. **D:** Lumbar facet joint angle increases in caudal progression.

sagittal diameter remaining relatively constant and the transverse diameter increasing from 20 mm at T12 to 26 mm at L5 resulting in a 25% increase in cross-sectional area (3,10,11). This intraspinal large volume coupled with the resilience of the cauda equina reduces the incidence of neurological injury resulting from lumbar spine fractures. Since approximately 30% of the spinal canal in the lower lumbar spine is occupied by the cauda equina, burst fractures with 60% canal compromise are less likely to cause significant neurological injury when compared to similar fractures at the TL junction (10–12,16,17).

Emergency Diagnosis and Management

Lumbar spine fractures often occur in multiple trauma patients and should be managed with appropriate Advanced Trauma Life Support (ATLS) protocol. Patients with a lumbar spine injury often have associated cranial, thoracic, and/or abdominal injuries requiring emergency management that may necessarily delay definitive treatment of the lumbar fracture. A detailed neurological examination should occur concurrently with a major injury assessment and should include testing of the mental status, motor, reflex, and sensory examinations. Motor strength is assessed and graded based on a 0 to 5 scale using the American Spinal Injury Association (ASIA) scoring system. Similarly, reflexes are scored on a scale from 0 to 4. Detailed sensory examination should include light touch, pinprick, and proprioception that includes the sacral dermatomes. Rectal tone and bulbocavernosus reflexes, when applicable, should be assessed and the spine should be visually inspected and palpated. Spinal precautions should be employed until fractures have been excluded. The mechanism of injury can often be determined from the history of the injury, as the treatment of lumbar fractures requires knowledge of anatomy and biomechanics. Although most lumbar fractures can be categorized, the management of each case requires individualization based on the patient's overall condition. The goals of treatment are to: (a) preserve, maintain, or restore neurological function; (b) restore spinal stability; and (c) prevent late deformity and chronic pain.

Plain lumbar spine radiographs can demonstrate obvious alterations of spinal alignment with subluxation or rotatory displacement, or vertebral disruption causing loss of body height or widening of the interpedicular distance. Any suspected fractures should be evaluated by computed tomography (CT) scan with two-dimensional sagittal reconstructions to provide detailed anatomy of fractures and alignment. CT scans can identify the severity of comminution, spinal canal compromise, and posterior element fractures to assess overall stability. Three-dimensional CT reconstruction in multiple views may aid in further understanding the bony anatomy for surgical planning. The presence of soft-tissue injury, herniated disc, or hematoma associated with fractures is poorly visualized on CT and is better evaluated with magnetic resonance imaging (MRI). Myelography with axial CT scanning can be used to enhance visualization of subtle alterations of spinal canal anatomy but is not routinely used in trauma patients due to the need for lumbar puncture and the availability of MRI.

Spinal Stability

The definition of spinal stability, as described by White and Panjabi using a point scale, is "the ability of the spine under physiological loads to limit patterns of displacement so as not to damage or irritate the spinal cord or nerve roots, and in addition, to prevent incapacitating deformity or pain due to structural changes" (9). Spinal stability has also been described with two-column and three-column models by Houldsworth and Denis, respectively (9,18,19). The Three-column model forms our current basis of understanding spinal fractures (Fig. 5). Disruption of two or more columns, with emphasis on the middle column, is generally considered unstable. Ligamentous disruption of the ALL which allows hyperextension, or the PLL

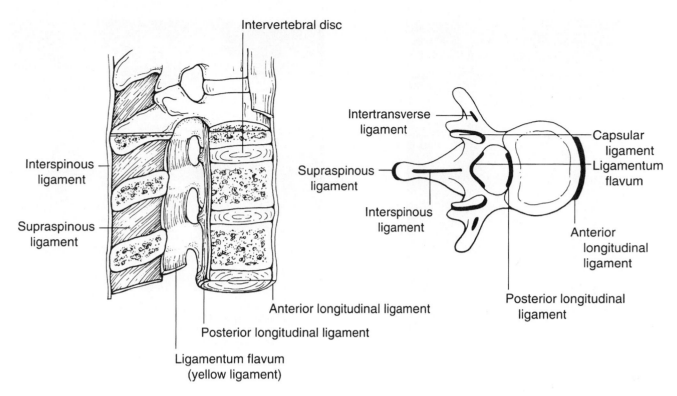

Fig. 4. Lumbar sagittal and axial sections demonstrating the associated ligaments.

which allows hyperflexion is also important in the assessment of overall stability.

Types of Fractures

COMPRESSION FRACTURES. Axial loading is a common mechanism in many lumbar spine injuries, including compression fractures. Fractures with less than 50% loss of height of the vertebral body are usually not considered clinically significant (Fig. 6). The middle column and pedicles are not involved by definition, but posterior ligamentous disruption may be evidenced with MRI. These fractures are most frequent in the lower lumbar spine and result from heavy axial loading. They are usually considered stable and are treated with bracing, analgesics, and medical management of osteoporosis if present (20). For compression fractures that demonstrate progressive loss in vertebral body height over time, vertebroplasty may be considered.

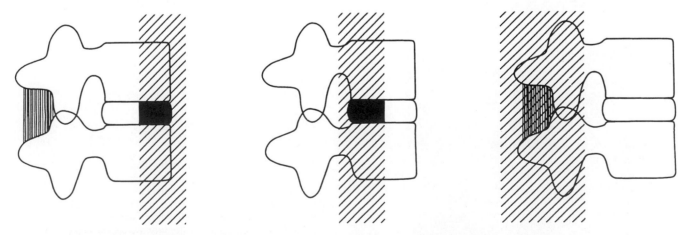

Fig. 5. Schematic representation of the three-column model. **Anterior column:** Anterior disc, ligaments, and vertebrae. **Middle column:** Posterior longitudinal ligament, posterior vertebra, and pedicle. **Posterior column:** Lamina, pars, facets, spinous processes, and posterior ligamentous complex.

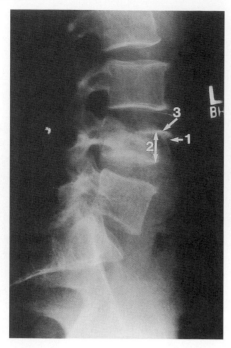

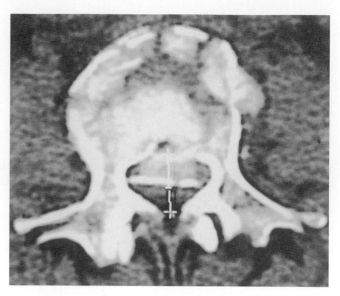

Fig. 8. Axial CT scan of a lumbar burst fracture. The retropulsed bone fragment causes significant canal compromise.

Fig. 6. Lateral radiograph of an L4 compression fracture: *1,* anterior cortex buckling; *2,* wedge deformity; *3,* an increase in bone density beneath the affected end plate with an associated end-plate fracture.

BURST FRACTURES. Burst fractures result from severe axial loading injuries that involve the anterior and middle columns in varying severity. These fractures typically widen the interpedicular distance due to a vertical fracture in the sagittal plane of the vertebral body. A fracture in the upper and posterior aspect of the vertebral body is also present, which is variably retropulsed into the spinal canal (Figs. 7 and 8). Burst fractures show variable loss of vertebral body height and varying degrees

of comminution. Excluding the TL junction, burst fractures are more frequent in the lumbar spine due to increased vertebral body axial loading. Denis divides these injuries into five subtypes: (a) involvement of the superior end plate alone, (b) involvement of both the superior and inferior end plates, (c) involvement of the inferior end plate alone, (d) a burst fracture with a rotatory component, and (e) a lateral burst fracture (21). Posterior element involvement is also variable involving laminar, facet, and spinous process fractures that may result in nerve root injuries and dural tears. Less severe burst fractures are stable, not requiring operative intervention, and can be managed with bracing and analgesics with good outcomes (22,23). These patients must be selected carefully for surgical treatment based upon the degree of vertebral comminution, angulation, spinal canal compromise, and posterior element involvement.

CHANCE FRACTURES. Chance fractures are also known as translational-shear or "seat-belt" injuries that commonly occur in the lower lumbar spine and are now less frequent due to the use of vehicle shoulder belts that prevent upper torso flexion during deceleration (19,24). These fractures are often associated with intraabdominal injuries. Flexion and distraction are the mechanism of injury, which results in a horizontal fracture extending from the vertebral body through the posterior bony elements involving all three columns, often resulting in neurological injury (Fig. 9). These fractures are highly unstable, necessitate surgical stabilization, and may require decompression and correction of spinal alignment.

FRACTURE DISLOCATIONS. Fracture dislocations, also known as fracture subluxations, are unstable and require surgical stabilization. These are relatively uncommon three-column injuries that result primarily from disruptions of the ligamentous structures and the disc space. They can, however, also involve bony element disruption, with a rotatory component associated with facet and transverse process fractures. The neural arch is often fractured and disconnected from the vertebral body with significant displacement. Dural lacerations and neurological injury are not uncommon with these fractures.

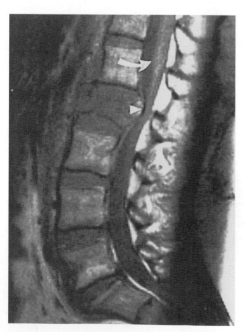

Fig. 7. Sagittal T1-weighted MRI of an L2 burst fracture. The level of the conus medullaris is rostral to the injury site *(arrow).* The retropulsed fragment is known to cause canal compromise *(arrowhead).*

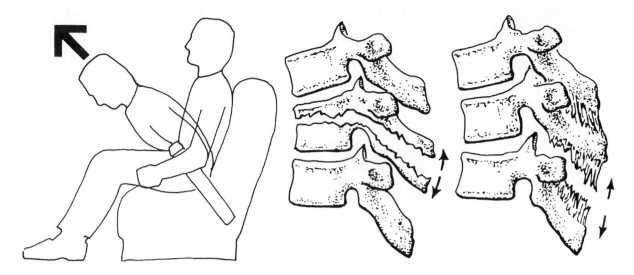

Fig. 9. The Chance fracture. **Left:** Mechanism of injury: use of a lap belt without a shoulder harness. **Center:** Diastasis (fracture cleavage) through the pedicles. **Right:** Fracture cleavage through the vertebral end plate and intervertebral disc.

UNCOMMON FRACTURES. Other fractures include isolated posterior column injuries that are uncommon because of the size and strength of the posterior lumbar elements (25). Hyperextension injuries are the most common cause of laminar and pars interarticularis fractures. Isolated facet dislocations, unilateral facet fractures, and dislocations are rare in the lumbar spine (26,27).

Surgical Management

COMPRESSION FRACTURES. The most common compression fractures have less than 50% loss in height and less than 30 degrees angulation and are successfully managed nonoperatively with adequate analgesics, bracing, and immobilization. Follow-up radiographs are necessary to evaluate for progression of loss of vertebral body height as well as angulation. Most patients have satisfactory outcomes with minimal progression of sagittal plane angulation.

If operative intervention is necessary, an anterolateral extraperitoneal approach provides access to the fractured vertebral body for reconstruction. The adjacent disc spaces are removed with careful preservation of the adjoining end plates and the vertebra is removed with a drill or sharp curettage. Reconstruction is achieved with a femoral shaft allograft, iliac crest autograft, or titanium mesh cage filled with autologous bone. Careful carpentry is necessary in order to place the graft in compression with matching of end-plate surfaces for equal load distribution. Instrumentation with either a plate or rod-screw construct spanning the graft on the lateral aspect of the vertebral column provides stability while bone fusion occurs. Postoperative management includes bracing, analgesics, and mobilization. Some patients with severe persistent back pain from osteoporotic compression fractures have been treated with percutaneous vertebroplasty using methylmethacrylate injected through the pedicle into the fractured vertebral body under fluoroscopic guidance. This potentially provides immediate stabilization of the vertebral segment, reduces pain, and allows for early mobilization.

BURST FRACTURES. Treatment of burst fractures remains somewhat controversial, however the decision-making process depends upon a combination of factors that include the number of columns injured, amount of vertebral body comminution, and degree of kyphotic angulation. Additional factors include the presence or absence of neurological injury, the patient's body habitus, and the surgeon's experience. This spectrum of factors and severity makes a simple treatment algorithm difficult to apply (28). Therefore, the surgeon must be well versed in both anterior and posterior reconstructive procedures. Neurological injuries resulting from burst fractures range from spinal cord damage to cauda equina injury to isolated nerve root deficit. Early surgical intervention attempting to improve neurological outcome is preferable, but the efficacy remains unclear and requires further studies. Patients with progression or worsening of incomplete deficits, however, should undergo urgent surgery to prevent further neurological deficit. The classic indications for surgical treatment of burst fractures are: (a) loss of more than 50% of vertebral body height, (b) retropulsed bony fragments narrowing the canal by more than 50%, and (c) kyphotic angulation of 25 degrees or more. In patients without neurological deficits and less severe burst fractures, successful outcomes can often result from bracing with an external orthosis. Fracture healing with satisfactory alignment, as well as remodeling and resorption of the bony fragments in the spinal canal, occur without significant differences in outcomes on operated and nonoperated patients regarding back pain and degree of kyphosis (22,29). However, some authors have demonstrated significant increases in kyphosis during nonoperative burst fracture healing (23). In another study, Denis and colleagues reported on 104 patients with 52 treated nonoperatively and found only 25% were able to return to work and 17% had delayed neurological deficits (30). These studies represent significant diversity in fracture severity, which makes it difficult to stratify and predict which fractures will progress. The Gaines classification of defining burst fractures in terms of severity of comminution, angulation, and posterior element disruption was used to define the success of short segmental posterior pedicle fixation (28). This type of scheme may be useful in determining treatment for individual fractures, but it does not constitute a complete algorithm. Currently, the management trend is toward early surgical intervention, and most authors agree on decompression and stabilization for patients with partial or progressive deficits. Timing of surgery for patients with neurological deficits remains unclear.

The decision making for anterior versus posterior reconstruction is also controversial but should take into the account the severity of comminution, degree of kyphosis, and posterior element disruption as well as the presence of neurological injury and spinal canal compromise. The surgeon's experience can be a factor but optimal management will require skills necessary to perform either (or both) procedures as deemed necessary. A simplified approach for treatment of burst fractures is to reconstruct severe anterior defects with anterior procedures and severe posterior fractures with posterior stabilization. Fractures with both extensive anterior and posterior involvement may require combined anterior-posterior procedures. The Gaines classification scheme employs a three-point grading system for the percentage of vertebral body comminution, the spreading of vertebral fragments, and the severity of kyphotic deformity to determine which patients can be treated with posterior instrumentation alone or whether they would require anterior and posterior fusion. One to three points are designated in each of the three categories resulting in a score between 3 and 9. Patients with scores of 7 or more should be treated with both anterior and posterior procedures while those with a score of 6 or less could be treated with posterior instrumentation alone (28). Other factors that need consideration with this scheme include body habitus, age, smoking history, osteoporosis, and presence of neurological injury.

CHANCE FRACTURES AND FRACTURE DISLOCATIONS. Posterior stabilization procedures are usually adequate for Chance fractures and fracture-dislocations. Neurological injury is common due to extensive vertebral body injury resulting in severe instability with malalignment of the spinal column. However, these fractures do not result in retropulsion of bony fragments into the spinal canal. A bilateral posterior long rod construct alone for this type of fracture is biomechanically sufficient to provide an adequate lever arm to maintain reduction of the fracture while bony fusion occurs. Long segmental posterior fixation is preferable to short segmental fixation, which is inadequate for these extremely unstable fractures. However, posterior short segment fixation combined with an anterior fixation would provide adequate reconstruction for severe instability, but requires a lengthy and possibly two-staged procedure.

Posterior Approaches

Posterior stabilization procedures involve decompression and fusion with either long- or short-segment instrumentation using titanium pedicle screws, hooks and rods, or a combination of screws and hooks to achieve successful fixation. Somatosensory evoked potentials (SEPs) are useful for posterior spinal procedures as positioning, decompression, and reconstruction can all result in potential neurological injury. A laminectomy over the fracture can be performed to decompress the spinal canal and repair dural tears. Decompression of ventral fragments in burst fractures from a posterior approach can be facilitated with a wide laminectomy that allows fragments to be impacted anteriorly from the spinal canal with a reverse-angle curette or similar instrument. The fracture line may need to be drilled adjacent to the pedicle to allow the fragments to be pushed anteriorly from the spinal canal. Intraoperative ultrasound may be benefi-

cial in visualizing the spinal canal in some of these cases. Various types of instrumentation strategies can be used to reduce and maintain a fracture deformity. These include hook-rod constructs, pedicle screw and hook-rod combination, or short-segment pedicle screw constructs. The current trend is toward shorter segmental fixation using pedicle screws. However, this may be inadequate in severe anterior column fractures (i.e., burst fractures) as the instrumentation often cannot sufficiently maintain reduction of severe anterior and middle column fractures. The instrumentation provides only temporary immobilization of spinal fractures while bony fusion is proceeding. Therefore, careful and extensive decortication of the fractured segments with bone grafting is important in order to achieve a successful fusion. Cortical-cancellous autologous bone graft is packed into the decorticated facet joints and along the transverse processes.

Anterior Approaches

Anterior reconstruction alone can be performed when there are relatively intact posterior elements. Ventral lumbar reconstruction is performed through a left anterior or lateral retroperitoneal approach. Exposure from L1 to L5 can be achieved depending on the level of the incision, which should provide a perpendicular view of the vertebra(e) of interest. The patient is placed in a semi-lateral position for a standard retroperitoneal approach by mobilizing the abdominal contents anteriorly and the great vessels to the contralateral side. This is performed through the left side with a general or vascular surgeon mobilizing the aorta and iliac vessels, rather than through the right side which would require retracting the vena cava and the liver. Once the appropriate levels are localized, resection of the vertebra is accomplished with the use of the high-speed drill, rongeurs, and curettes. The pedicle and foramen are the anatomical landmarks that are used to identify the spinal canal for decompression. Bone screws can be placed transversely in the adjacent vertebrae of the midlumbar region down to L4 for distraction that improves visualization of the spinal canal during decompression and are used later for instrumentation. The ALL can be left intact to provide graft compression, but the PLL is typically removed to ensure complete spinal canal decompression. The vertebral end plates are carefully decorticated with a high-speed drill, ensuring preservation of their integrity, which provides structural support for load-bearing grafts and prevents graft settling into adjacent vertebral bodies. Vertebral body reconstruction is usually performed with either a femoral allograft filled with iliac autograft or a titanium cage similarly filled with autologous bone. This vertebral strut is then inserted into the defect while distraction is applied to the adjacent vertebrae to restore sagittal alignment. If adequate distraction is achieved, the tensile retraction of the soft tissues around the adjacent vertebra will naturally place the graft in compression. Spinal instrumentation with a lateral fixation plate or screw-rod construct is placed in the vertebral body above and below and secured (with additional compression if needed) to assure that the graft is loaded in compression. The major advantage of this approach is that it allows direct treatment of vertebral fractures through reconstruction of the anterior and middle columns. Ventral bone fragments can be removed safely and completely ensuring an adequate decompression. Disadvantages include a relatively unfamiliar exposure and mobilization of major abdominal and vascular structures.

Another anterior approach is the lateral extracavitary technique described by Capener and popularized by Larson and colleagues. This technique allows a minimal approach to the vertebral spine, but includes exposure and access to the posterior elements laterally. Advantages include the ease of dissection at L1 and L2, preservation of the psoas muscle, and the ability to perform posterior instrumentation simultaneously. Disadvantages include the need for careful nerve root dissection from the iliopsoas muscle, as well as the possibility of lumbar plexus injury (31,32).

Postoperative Care

Postoperative care requires adequate analgesia and early mobilization. A closed suction wound drain is usually placed to keep the dressing dry and reduce the chance of a wound infection or hematoma. In the case of a dural rent that cannot be repaired in its entirety a lumbar drain may be considered. In these cases, a self-suction wound drain should be avoided. External bracing with a lumbar corset or thoracolumbar spinal orthosis (TLSO) should be used for 2 to 4 months when the patient is sitting or ambulating. Many patients with lumbar fractures will need rehabilitation, particularly those with neurological injuries. Plain radiographs are obtained at 1- to 2-month intervals postoperatively to evaluate fusion progression and maintenance of spinal alignment.

Complications

The anatomical location of these injuries and surgical reconstruction carry the attendant risks to the spine, spinal cord, and adjacent soft tissues. Spinal complications include worsening of neurological deficits and cerebrospinal fluid leaks. Dural tears can be repaired primarily with suture repair and fibrin glue, with possible lumbar subarachnoid drain placement, if necessary. Vascular complications with injuries to the great vessels require immediate repair. Thrombotic events, particularly in the lower extremities of patients with neurological injuries, are common and may require vascular surgical assistance and postoperative anticoagulation or both. Retroperitoneal chylous leakage is a rare complication but can occur after inadvertent division of lymphatic channels located on the anterior aspect of the vertebral column. Primary ligature intraoperatively and/or total parenteral nutrition postoperatively if discovered postoperatively provides effective treatment.

Failed fusion, pseudarthrosis, or hardware failure can result in progressive spinal deformity, pain, or neurological deficit. These are treated by revision of the failed construct or supplemental fixation, or both.

Conclusion

Lumbar fractures below the TL junction have several unique aspects that distinguish them from their more rostral counterparts. The mechanisms of injury are often the key to diagnosis and management of neural compression, restoration, and maintenance of spinal alignment. Each case requires an individual approach with attention paid to neurological status and biomechanics; stabilization and reconstruction may be required from anteriorly, posteriorly, or both.

References

1. Riggins RS, Kraus JF: The risk of neurologic damage with fractures of the vertebrae. *J Trauma* 1977;17:126–133.
2. An HS, Simpson JM, Ebraheim NA, et al: Low lumbar burst fractures: comparison between conservative and surgical treatments. *Orthopedics* 1992;15:367–373.
3. Levine AM: The surgical treatment of low lumbar fractures. *Semin Spine Surg* 1990;2:41–53.
4. White AA, Panjabi MM: *Clinical biomechanics of the spine*, 2nd ed. Philadelphia: Lippincott-Raven Publishers, 1990:1–125.
5. Perry O: Resistance and compression of the lumbar vertebrae. In: *Encyclopedia of medical radiology.* New York: Springer-Verlag, 1974:215–221.
6. Van Schaik JPT, Verbeist H, Van Schaik FDJ: The orientation of the laminae and facet joints in the lower lumbar spine. *Spine* 1985;10:59–63.
7. Ahmed AM, Duncan NA, Burke DL: The effect of facet geometry on the axial torque-rotation response of lumbar motion segments. *Trans Orthop Res Soc* (Atlanta) 1988:1–10.
8. Benzel EC: *Biomechanics of spine stabilization: principles and clinical practice.* New York: McGraw-Hill, 1995:55–71.
9. Benzel EC: *Biomechanics of spine stabilization: principles and clinical practice.* New York: McGraw-Hill, 1995:1–16.
10. Bernhardt M, Bridwell KH: Segmental analysis of the sagittal plane alignment of the normal thoracic and lumbar spines and thoracolumbar junction. *Spine* 1989;14:717–721.
11. Scoles PV, Linton AE, Latimer B, et al: Vertebral body and posterior element morphology: the normal spine in middle life. *Spine* 1988;13:1802–1806.
12. White AA III, Panjabi MM: The basic kinematics of the human spine: a review of past and current knowledge. *Spine* 1978;3:12–20.
13. Wamboldt A, Spencer DL: A segmental analysis of the distribution of lumbar lordosis in the normal spine. *Orthop Trans* 1987;11:92–93.
14. Gertzbein SD: *Fractures of the thoracic and lumbar spine.* Baltimore: Williams & Wilkins, 1992.
15. Dickman CA, Fessler RG, MacMillan M, et al: Transpedicular screw-rod fixation of the lumbar spine: operative technique and outcome in 104 cases. *J Neurosurg* 1992;77:860–870.
16. McAfee PC, Yuan HA, Frederickson BE, et al: The value of computed tomography in thoracolumbar fractures: an analysis of one hundred consecutive cases and a new classification. *J Bone Joint Surg Am* 1983;65:461–473.
17. Atlas SW, Regenbogen V, Rogers LF, Kim KS: The radiographic characterization of burst fractures of the spine. *AJR* 1986;147:575–582.
18. Denis F: Spinal instability as defined by the three-column concept in acute spinal trauma. *Clin Orthop* 1984;189:65–76.
19. Denis F: The three column model and its significance in the classification of acute thoracolumbar spinal injuries. *Spine* 1983;8:817–831.
20. White AA, Panjabi MM: *Clinical biomechanics of the spine*, 2nd ed. Philadelphia: Lippincott-Raven Publishers, 1990:30–342.
21. Court-Brown CM, Gertzbein SD: The management of burst fractures of the fifth lumbar vertebrae. *Spine* 1987;12:308–312.
22. Chan DPK, Seng NK, Kaan KT: Non-operative treatment in burst fractures of the lumbar spine (L2-L5) without neurologic deficit. *Spine* 1983;18:320–325.
23. Krompinger WJ, Frederickson BE, Mino DE, et al: Conservative treatment of fractures of the thoracic and lumbar spine. *Orthop Clin North Am* 1986;17:161–170.
24. Smith WS, Kaufer H: Patterns and mechanisms of lumbar injuries associated with lap seat belts. *J Bone Joint Surg Am* 1969;51:239–254.
25. Bucholz RW, Gill K: Classification of injuries to the thoracolumbar spine. *Orthop Clin North Am* 1986;17:67–83.
26. Kramer VM, Levine AM: Unilateral facet dislocation of the lumbosacral junction: a case report and review of the literature. *J Bone Joint Surg Am* 1989;71:1258–1261.
27. Levine AM, Bosse MJ, Edwards CC: Bilateral facet dislocations in the thoracolumbar spine. *Spine* 1988;13:630–640.
28. McCormack T, Karaikovic E, Gaines RW: The load sharing classification of spine fractures. *Spine* 1994;19:1741–1744.
29. Weinstein JN, Collato P, Lehmann TR: Long-term follow-up on non-operatively treated thoracolumbar spine fractures. *J Spinal Disord* 1987;1:152–159.

30. Denis F, Armstrong GWD, Searls K, et al: Acute thoracolumbar burst fractures in the absence of neurologic deficit: a comparison between operative and non-operative treatment. *Clin Orthop Rel Res* 1984; 189:149.
31. Larson SJ, Holst RA, Hemmy DC, et al: Lateral extracavitary approach

to traumatic lesions of the thoracic and lumbar spine. *J Neurosurg* 1976;45:628.
32. Maiman DJ, Larson SJ: Lateral extracavitary approach to the thoracic and lumbar spine. In: Rengachary SS, Wilkins RM, eds. *Neurosurgical operative atlas*. Baltimore: Williams & Wilkins, 1992.

163. Sacral Fractures

Jongsoo Park and J. Patrick Johnson

"Os sacrum" originated from ancient Roman belief of the sacred protection of genitals and was used in sacrificial rituals for its resilience (1). The sacrum is intrinsically rigid with multiple fused vertebrae, and fractures only occur from high-energy impact. Subsequently, the incidence and survival of patients with sacral fractures was low and they received little attention in the early literature (2,3). In modern times sacral fractures usually resulting from high-velocity automobile accidents or falls from significant height have become relatively common (4). Sacral fractures still occur in less than 1% of reported injuries, however, the incidence of patients with sacral fractures requiring treatment appears to be increasing (5,6).

Since sacral fractures may injure sacral nerves and cause longterm neurological deficits (7), the relationship between the sacral nerves and the osseous sacrum is important in the diagnosis, clinical decision making, and operative treatment. Sacral fractures are associated with pelvic fractures in nearly half of the cases and should be suspected in all patients with pelvic fractures (8). This chapter will review the anatomy of the sacrum as it pertains to clinical assessment, diagnosis, and treatment of patients with pelvic trauma. The classifications of sacral fractures are reviewed in comparison with types of neurological injuries observed in various subgroups.

Anatomy of the Sacrum

The sacrum is a triangular, wedge-shaped bone consisting of five fused vertebrae. It forms the posterior wall of the pelvic ring and articulates between the ilia forming two synchondrosed sacroiliac (SI) joints. The SI ligamentous attachments are the sacrospinous, sacrotuberous, and iliolumbar ligaments (Fig. 1). The SI joints extend from S1 to S2 in females and S1 to S3 in males (9). Superiorly, the sacrum articulates with lumbar vertebrae via the lumbosacral intervertebral disc and inferiorly with the coccyx via the sacrococcygeal joint. Posteriorly, the spinous processes are fused to form the prominent median sacral crest (Fig. 2). There are four paired anterior and posterior sacral foramina which communicate with the sacral spinal canal where the sacrum is weakest and most fractures occur (9,10). The horizontal prominence between the foramina is called transverse ridge and is the remnant of intervertebral disc space. Lateral to the foramina lie the lateral sacral crest which consists of a series of tubercles. The ventral aspect of the body of S1 is the sacral promontory and lateral to the sacral promontory are the wing-shaped alae (Fig. 3).

Variations in sacral anatomy include the number of sacral vertebrae, development of the dorsal sacrum, and male–female variations that can be important in the understanding the management of relevant injury patterns as they apply to surgical treatment of sacral fractures.

NEURAL ANATOMY. The sacral canal contains the caudal extent of the dural sac which includes the sacral and coccygeal nerves and ends at S2. The filum terminale extends distally through the dural sac and continues into the coccyx (Fig. 4). The cauda equina arises from the spinal cord in the upper lumbar region traveling a significant distance to the sacrum and forms loose bundles that accommodate the excursion created by normal range of motion. Dorsal and ventral roots of S1-4, each contained within arachnoid and dural coverings, exit the dural sac separately while the S5 root emerges below the sacrum and superior-lateral to the coccyx. Unlike any other spinal levels, the dorsal root ganglia of the sacrum are found within the sacral canal.

The lumbosacral plexus (L4-S1) innervates the distal lower extremities, and the lower sacral roots (S2-4) control sphincter and sexual function (Fig. 5). The sciatic nerve exits the pelvis through the sciatic notch, and the first two lateral branches from the lumbosacral plexus are the superior and inferior gluteal nerves which exit through greater sciatic foramen along with smaller nerves to the quadratus femoris, gemelli, and obturator internus muscles that all originate from sacral plexus. Rootlets from the S2 to S4 levels join to form the pudendal nerve.

Extensive autonomic innervation occurs throughout the sacrum and pelvis. The sympathetic chain continues from its thoracolumbar origins on the ventral surface of the sacrum forming the superior hypogastric trunk. Parasympathetic innervation arises from the S2 to S4 nerve roots which form the pelvic splanchnic nerves. These autonomic fibers are distributed distally via the pelvic plexus to the various pelvic organs.

VASCULAR ANATOMY. Numerous anatomical variations of vascular supply to the sacrum exist; this chapter however will focus only on the most common variations. The middle sacral artery originates from the aortic bifurcation at the L4-5 level and descends on the ventral surface of the sacrum to the coccyx. It gives rise to several anastomotic branching arteries on both sides of the sacrum. The lateral sacral artery arises from the internal iliac artery and forms anastomotic arteries that penetrate through the sacral foramina (Fig. 6). The iliolumbar artery usually arises from the common iliac artery which branches

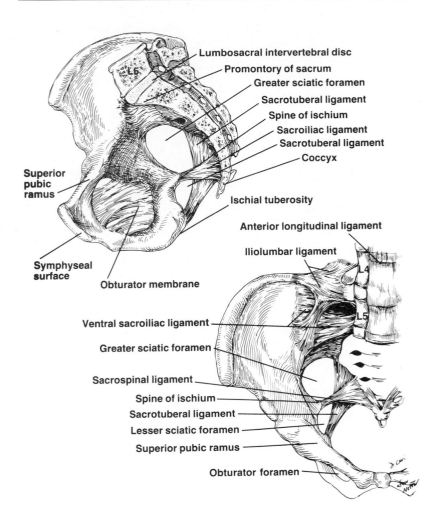

Lumbosacral intervertebral disc
Promontory of sacrum
Greater sciatic foramen
Sacrotuberal ligament
Spine of ischium
Sacroiliac ligament
Sacrotuberal ligament
Coccyx

Superior pubic ramus

Ischial tuberosity

Anterior longitudinal ligament

Iliolumbar ligament

Symphyseal surface

Obturator membrane

Ventral sacroiliac ligament

Greater sciatic foramen

Sacrospinal ligament

Spine of ischium

Sacrotuberal ligament

Lesser sciatic foramen

Superior pubic ramus

Obturator foramen

Fig. 1. Anatomy of the sacrum and pelvis: bone and ligaments. (Courtesy of F.H. Netter, with permission.)

Dorsal surface

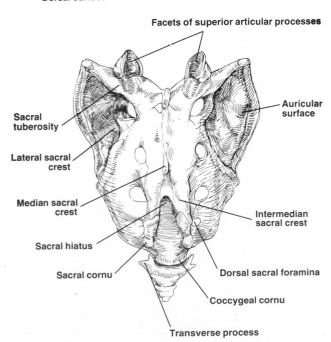

Facets of superior articular processes

Sacral tuberosity

Lateral sacral crest

Median sacral crest

Sacral hiatus

Sacral cornu

Auricular surface

Intermedian sacral crest

Dorsal sacral foramina

Coccygeal cornu

Transverse process

Fig. 2. Posterior sacrum and coccyx. (Courtesy of F.H. Netter, with permission.)

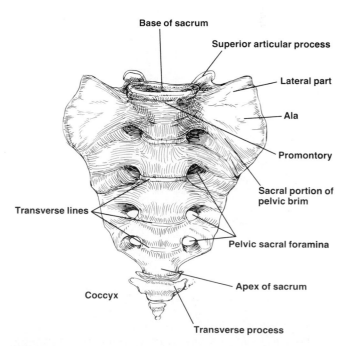

Base of sacrum

Superior articular process

Lateral part

Ala

Promontory

Sacral portion of pelvic brim

Transverse lines

Pelvic sacral foramina

Coccyx

Apex of sacrum

Transverse process

Fig. 3. Anterior sacrum and coccyx. (Courtesy of F.H. Netter, with permission.)

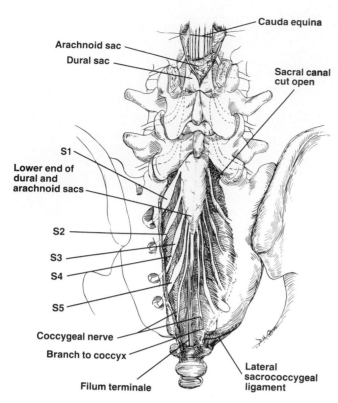

Fig. 4. Lumbosacral neural elements. (From Frymoyer JW, ed. *The adult spine.* New York: Lippincott–Raven Publishers, 1997, with permission.)

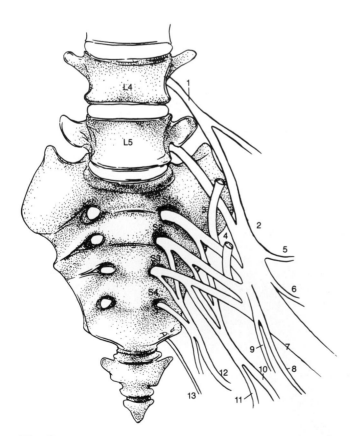

Fig. 5. Lumbosacral plexus. (From Frymoyer JW, ed. *The adult spine.* New York: Lippincott–Raven Publishers, 1997, with permission.)

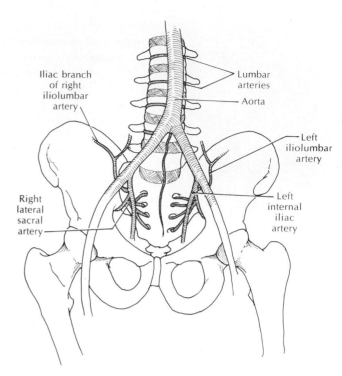

Fig. 6. Arterial anatomy of the lumbosacrum. (From Frymoyer JW, ed. *The adult spine.* New York: Lippincott–Raven Publishers, 1997, with permission.)

superiorly and laterally. Other major arteries include the superior and inferior gluteal arteries that arise from the internal iliac arteries. The venous anatomy is also extensive and parallels arterial anatomy. Due to the extensive blood supply to the sacrum, fractures or dislocation may cause major arterial and venous injury with massive retroperitoneal bleeding resulting in hypovolemia, shock, and death (11).

Classifications

Several different classifications of sacral fractures have been suggested based on the location, extent of the fracture, and the mechanisms of injury. These systematic approaches for clinical situations provide a framework for assessment and appropriate treatment. The first classification was described by Bonnin in 1945 (4), but more recent classifications have been proposed based upon the type and degree of bony disruption of sacral elements. Most of these classification systems describe fractures that occur along the stress flow lines and sacral foramina (3,4, 9,10).

The most common classification in current use is the Denis classification based upon the analysis of 236 sacral fractures (10). This classification categorizes sacral fractures into three zones. Zone I is defined by a vertical fracture through the ala that does not involve the foramina or the central sacral canal (Fig. 7). These fractures are not usually associated with neurological deficits and are considered stable unless there is a component of vertical displacement causing compression of the L5 nerve root between the ala and the transverse process. Pelvic traction can reduce the L5 entrapment, but a persistent neurological deficit may warrant surgical intervention.

Denis zone II fractures occur through one or more sacral

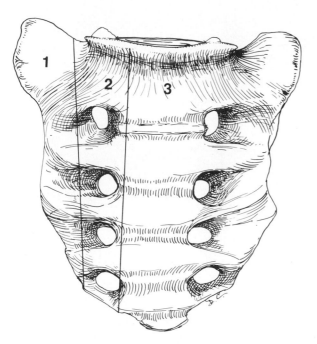

Fig. 7. Denis sacral fracture classification. *1,* Zone I; *2,* Zone II; *3,* Zone III. (From Denis F, Steven D, Comfort T: Sacral fracture: an important problem: retrospective analysis of 236 cases. *Clinic Orthop* 27:67–81, 1988, with permission.)

foramina (Fig. 7). These fractures are usually vertical, however, the fracture line may diverge and exit laterally at any level. Neurological injury is more frequent in this group due to fractures through the foramen (12). Denis and colleagues report that 57% of these fractures resulted in a neurological deficit, and 28% occurred in the distribution of L5, S1, and S2 nerve roots (10). Bowel and bladder dysfunction are not unusual but usually are recovered in patients with unilateral zone II fractures (12).

Denis zone III fractures have multiple areas of fracture involvement that include any type of fracture through the central canal (Fig. 7). Both low and high transverse fractures and penetrating injuries are also included. Neurological injury is very common and occurs in more than 80% of zone III fracture cases (13). High transverse zone III sacral fractures have the highest frequency of neurological involvement with a highly variable combination of nerve root injuries, cauda equina injuries, and bowel and bladder dysfunction. Although, the Denis classification is simple and useful in predicting neurological outcomes corresponding to the different zones of fractures it has limitations, as it does not consider the mechanisms of injury or degree of bony disruption.

The other widely used classification has been described by Schmidek and associates (9) (Table 1). This system classifies sacral fractures into two main categories: direct and indirect trauma. Penetrating and low transverse fractures are included in the direct trauma group, and the most common penetrating sacral fractures are gunshot wounds (14). Although gunshot wounds cause extensive tissue damage, they are usually considered stable because the majority of the bony injury is confined to the posterior pelvic ring. Direct blunt trauma to the sacrum, usually resulting from falls onto the buttocks, typically causes low transverse fractures near the kyphus of sacrum below the S3 (14). Variable anterior displacement of the distal segment occurs, but these fractures are often structurally stable and neurological deficits are uncommon (7).

Schmidek's classification of the indirect trauma includes verti-

Table 1. Classification of Sacral Fractures

1. Direct trauma
Penetrating
Low-transverse fracture (S-3 and below)
2. Indirect trauma
High-transverse fracture (S-1 and S-2)
Lumbosacral fracture dislocation
Lateral mass fracture
Juxtaarticular fracture   ⎫
Cleaving fracture   ⎬ Associated with pelvic
Avulsion fracture   ⎭   ring disruption
Combination fracture

From Schmidek HH, Smith DA, Kristiansen TK. Sacral fractures. *Neurosurgery* 1984;15:735–746, with permission.

cal and high transverse fractures (9). These injuries are caused by indirect forces acting on the sacrum transmitted through the pelvis or lumbar spine as occurs with lateral impact in motor vehicle accidents (4). Vertical sacral fractures are commonly associated with pelvic fractures in up to 90% of cases (15), where transverse sacral fractures are often isolated injuries. There are four different types of vertical fractures described in the literature: lateral mass fracture, juxtaarticular fracture, cleaving fracture, and avulsion fracture (6,16) (Fig. 8).

The lateral mass fracture is defined by extension of a fracture along the side of the ventral foramen (i.e., zone II of Denis classification) that exits laterally into the ipsilateral SI joint at any level. The juxtaarticular fractures involve a single-level sacral foramen and its lateral sacral mass adjacent to the SI joint where the fragmented bone is dissociated from the body of the sacrum. Cleaving fractures extend from the proximal sacral foramen down to the coccyx and may or may not involve multiple foramina. Avulsion fractures are located at the margins of the insertion of the sacrotuberous and sacrospinous ligaments (3,9).

High transverse sacral fractures are the other type of indirect injuries that occur in flexion injuries (6). They are infrequent and occur as isolated injuries but have a high frequency of neurological injuries. Roy-Camille and colleagues divided these fractures into three types (16). The type I fracture has anterior displacement of the upper segment resulting from flexion forces. The type II fracture occurs from posterior displacement of the upper segment from flexion forces. The type III fracture results from anterior displacement of the upper segment due to extension forces resulting in lumbar hyperlordosis. In younger patients traumatic spondylolisthesis may occur from incomplete intersegmental ossification of the sacrum. The most significant neurological deficits are associated with high transverse fractures (6,9,16).

Diagnostic Assessment

Sacral fractures are often overlooked due to the presence of multiple other injuries in polytraumatized patients (17). After Advanced Trauma Life Support (ATLS) protocol of the American College of Surgeons has secured the immediately life-threatening issues, a careful secondary survey and neurological assessment must follow. When sacral and pelvic fractures are present, clinical examination of neurological function related to sacral fractures from L4 to S5 is required and includes dorsiflexion, plantar flexion, anal sphincter tone, anal wink, and bulbocavernosus reflexes. Cystometrogram assessment of sacral root injury and neurogenic bladder was previously emphasized in the literature (10,18), however, it has limited practical use in the emer-

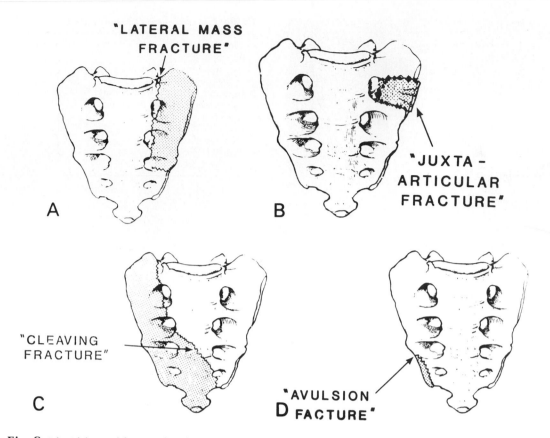

Fig. 8. Schmidek sacral fracture classification. **A:** Lateral mass fracture. **B:** Juxtaarticular fracture. **C:** Cleaving fracture. **D:** Avulsion fracture. (From Schmidek HH, Smith DA, Kristiansen TK: Sacral fractures. *Neurosurgery* 15:735–746, 1984, with permission.)

gency setting and acute injury. Similarly, electromyography is not helpful in acute injuries since the abnormalities are not detectable for several weeks.

Sacral fractures are associated with pelvic fractures in nearly half of the cases and should be suspected in all patients with pelvic fractures. Anteroposterior (AP) pelvic radiographs are mandatory in the assessment of all multiple trauma patients and all others with a high index of suspicion for sacral and pelvic fractures (17). Conventional radiographs are not optimal for the diagnosis of subtle fractures of the sacrum because of the curvature and lordosis of the sacral surface and overlying intestinal gas often interfere with interpretation of radiological details (9). Thin-cut computed tomography (CT) scans with sagittal reconstructions of the sacrum are most useful for confirming these subtle fractures. In the presence of neurological injury, it is recommended to obtain both tomography and CT scan (19). Magnetic resonance imaging has become valuable in the evaluation of soft tissues associated with sacral fractures.

Management and Treatment

Treatment of sacral fractures is similar to the management of other spine fractures and includes: (a) overall general medical status of the patient, (b) the stability and degree of displacement of the fracture, (c) type and extent of neurological deficit, (d) stabilization of fractures (open versus closed), and (e) rehabilitation potential (9).

The majority of sacral fractures are Denis zone I fractures which result from axial loading injuries. In the absence of pelvic ring injuries, these fractures are considered structurally stable and are treated symptomatically with analgesics, a pelvic sling, and bed rest. These patients can be mobilized early with partial weight bearing on the uninjured side. However, in zone I fractures associated with multiple fractures and disruption of the pelvic ring, the hemipelvis may migrate and result in a vertical shear pattern displacement (15). This type of injury is considered to be highly unstable and requires definitive treatment with internal or external fixation (10,14,20). Initially, external reduction can be attempted with a pelvic sling. Anterior stabilization of the pelvic ring can be achieved by using external fixation to stabilize the pelvis and control acute hemorrhage in an emergency situation (14,20). Similarly, open reduction and internal fixation of anterior pelvic fractures have the same result (21). If posterior fracture displacement persists after anterior fixation and external pelvic traction, then open posterior reduction and internal fixation is necessary (14).

Zone II fractures involve sacral foramina, and neurological deficits occur in more than 50% of cases (9,22). If the CT scan shows narrowing of the sacral foraminal size by 50% or more, then early surgical decompression is indicated (7). Comminuted zone II fractures associated with pelvic ring disruption are considered unstable and open reduction posteriorly in conjunction with anterior pelvic stabilization may be required (23,24).

Zone III fractures involve the central sacral canal and cause neurological injuries in highly variable patterns (13,21–23). Denis and colleagues recommend early decompressive laminectomy and foraminotomy in these patients in the absence of

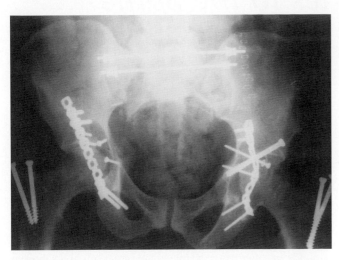

Fig. 9. Open reduction internal fixation of sacrum and pelvis with iliac tension band and pelvic reconstruction plates (From Frymoyer JW, ed. *The adult spine.* New York: Lippincott–Raven Publishers, 1997, with permission.)

structural instability (10). The treatment of zone III fractures without neurological deficit is aimed at structural stabilization (8,23).

The primary strategy of sacral stabilization is to indirectly stabilize posterior pelvic ring fixation of the sacrum using the posterior iliac crests (25). Iliosacral screw fixation is used in SI joint dislocations, unstable vertical sacral fractures (types I and II), and juxtaarticular fractures of ilium (15,19). However, the sacral body must be intact for good iliosacral screw-plate fixation (26). The posterior tension banding technique connects the bilateral posterior iliac crests with a threaded metal rod posterior to the sacrum to sandwich the sacrum in between. Anterior-posterior bar and pelvic reconstruction plates are useful in stabilization of both focal and extensive fractures of sacrum (21,27) (Fig. 9).

Conclusion

Most sacral fractures are not associated with neurological injury and can be treated conservatively; however, sacral fractures associated with neurological deficits or pelvic ring disruption require reduction and stabilization (28). Emergency nerve root decompression in sacral fractures is rarely needed (12), since closed reduction can achieve satisfactory decompression in many cases. However, if the nerve root compression persists, then early decompression may result in the best clinical outcome (22).

References

1. Sugar O: How the sacrum got its name. *JAMA* 257:2061–2063, 1987.
2. Kristiansen, TK: Fracture of the sacrum and coccygodynia. In: Frymoyer JW, ed. *The adult spine.* New York: Lippincott–Raven Publishers, 1997.
3. Sabiston CP, Wing PC. Sacral fractures: classifications and neurologic implications. *J Trauma* 26:1113–1115, 1986.
4. Bonnin JG. Sacral fractures and injuries to the cauda equina. *J Bone Joint Surg* 27:113–127, 1945.
5. LaFollette BF, Levine MI, McNiesh LM: Bilateral fracture-dislocation of the sacrum. A case report. *J Bone Joint Surg Am* 68:1099–1101, 1896.
6. Phalen ST, Jones DA, Bishay M: Conservative management of transverse fractures of the sacrum with neurological features. A report of four cases. *J Bone Joint Surg Br* 73:969–971, 1991.
7. Fisher RG: Sacral fracture with compression of cauda equina: surgical treatment. *J Trauma* 28:1678–1680, 1988.
8. Isler B: Lumbosacral nerve injury associated with pelvic ring injuries. *J Orthop Trauma* 4:1–6, 1990.
9. Schmidek HH, Smith DA, Kristiansen TK: Sacral fractures. *Neurosurgery* 15:735–746, 1984.
10. Denis F, Steven D, Comfort T: Sacral fracture: an important problem: retrospective analysis of 236 cases. *Clin Orthop* 27:67–81, 1988.
11. McMurtry R, Walton D, Dickinson D, et al: Pelvic disruption of the polytraumatized patient: a management protocol. *Clin Orthop* 151: 22–30, 1980.
12. Epstein NE, Epstein JA, Carras R: Unilateral S1 root compression syndrome caused by fracture of the sacrum. *Neurosurgery* 19: 1025–1027, 1986.
13. Bucknill TM, Blackburne JS: Fracture-dislocation of the sacrum: report of three cases. *J Bone Joint Surg Br* 58:467–470, 1978.
14. Froman C, Stein S: Complicated crushing injuries of the pelvis. *J Bone Joint Surg Br* 49:24–32, 1967.
15. Northrop CH, Eto RT, Loop JW: Vertical fractures of the sacral ala: significance of non-continuity of the anterior superior sacral foraminal line. *AJR* 124:102–106, 1975.
16. Roy-Camille R, Saillant G, Gagna G, et al: Transverse fracture of the upper sacrum. Suicidal jumper's fracture. *Spine* 10:838–845, 1985.
17. Resnik CS, Stackhouse DJ, Shanmuganahan K, et al: Diagnosis of pelvic fracture in patients with acute pelvic trauma: efficacy of plain radiographs. *AJR* 158:109–112, 1992.
18. Fountain SS, Hamilton RD, Jameson RM: Transverse fractures of the sacrum: a report of six cases. *J Bone Joint Surg Am* 59:486–489, 1977.
19. Nelson DW, Duwelius PJ: CT-guided fixation of sacral fractures and sacroiliac joint disruption. *Radiology* 180:527–532, 1991.
20. Mears DC, Fu FH: Modern concepts of external skeletal fixation of the pelvis. *AJR* 42:65–72, 1980.
21. Ferris B, Hutton P: Anteriorly displaced transverse fracture of the sacrum at the level of the sacroiliac joint: a report of two cases. *J Bone Joint Surg Am* 65:407–409, 1983.
22. Goodell CL: Neurological deficits associated with pelvic fractures. *J Neurosurg* 24:837–842, 1966.
23. Fardon DF: Displaced transverse fracture of the sacrum with nerve root injury: report of a case with successful operative management. *J Trauma* 19:119–122, 1979.
24. Raf L: Double vertical fractures of the pelvis. *Acta Chir Scand* 131: 298–305, 1966.
25. Meyer TL, Wiltberger B: Displaced sacral fracture. *Am J Orthop* 4: 187, 1962.
26. Kellam JF, Mc Murtry RY, Paley D, et al: The unstable pelvic fracture. Operative treatment. *Orthop Clin North Am* 18:25–41, 1987.
27. Mears DC, Capito CP, Deleeuw H: Posterior pelvic disruptions managed by the use of the Double Cobra Plate. *Instr Course Lect* 37: 143–150, 1988.
28. Gibbons KJ, Soloniuk DS, Razack N: Neurological injury and patterns of sacral fractures. *J Neurosurg* 72:889–893, 1990.

164. Penetrating Injuries to the Spine

Eric P. Sipos, Leon E. Moores, and James M. Ecklund

Penetrating trauma is the third most common cause of spinal cord injury in North America after motor vehicle accidents and falls (1–3). Together, gunshot wounds and stab wounds accounted for 14.6% of all spinal cord injuries reported in two large multicenter epidemiological studies in North America and constitute a major source of morbidity and mortality, primarily among young males (1,2). The mean age reported in these studies was 33.5 and 29.7 years. Eighty percent of the victims were male. Although the preponderance of penetrating spinal cord trauma in the United States is due to gunshot wounds, stab injuries to the spinal cord occur with greater frequency outside of the United States. One South African study, for example, reported over 25% of more than 1,600 spinal cord injuries were due to stab wounds (4).

Mortality rates following both penetrating and blunt spinal cord injuries have been reported to be 3 to 21 times higher than matched patient groups without spinal injury (5). Additionally, the economic costs of caring for patients with spinal cord injuries are tremendous. In one study of 22 patients with neurological deficits from spinal cord injuries, the average intensive care unit (ICU) stay was 13.5 days, the average hospital stay was 45 days, and the average hospital charges exceeded fifty thousand dollars (6).

Although penetrating spinal injuries are a major source of mortality and neurological morbidity and pose a significant economic burden to our society, there is a paucity of compelling experimental evidence upon which to base therapeutic recommendations. Therefore, the clinical evaluation and management of patients with penetrating spinal injuries remains controversial. Standards or guidelines regarding the role of antibiotic therapy or steroids in the treatment of these patients, for example, have not been established. Furthermore, indications and techniques for surgical intervention have yet to be resolved conclusively. In this chapter, we will review the evidentiary basis in the modern literature for clinical decision making in the management of penetrating spine injuries.

Pathophysiology

The pathophysiology of penetrating wounds of the spine is dependent upon the mechanism of injury and the velocity of the penetrating foreign object. The lowest velocity mechanism of injury occurs with stab wounds and impalements. These are typically associated with tissue disruption only along the direct path of the instrument involved, and associated vascular and visceral injuries are limited to this region.

The wounding and ballistic characteristics of firearms are related to the mass (m) of the bullet, the velocity (v) of the bullet at the time of impact, the shape and metallic composition of the bullet, and the energy absorption characteristics of the tissue encountered. The kinetic energy (Ek) transmitted by a projectile is defined by the equation $Ek = \frac{1}{2}mv^2$. A penetrating projectile may create tissue injury through direct transmission of kinetic energy to tissues in the path of the bullet and, in the case of high-velocity missiles, through explosive temporary cavitation forces with stretching of body tissues (7). Thus, intermediate levels of regional tissue damage are created with low-velocity gunshot wounds typical of civilian trauma and neurological def-

icits are usually the result of direct injury to the neural elements and adjacent vertebral structures. Military weapons, however, may create extensive regional tissue damage due to extraordinary energy transmission by high-velocity projectiles, and temporary cavitation forces may cause neurological deficits even when the spinal column is not directly violated. Shrapnel injuries from fragments of explosive devices produce unpredictable injury patterns due to the variable size, shape, velocity, and aerodynamic instability of the fragments.

Information regarding the identity, metallic composition, and ballistic characteristics of projectiles used to inflict penetrating wounds are often not available to the physicians and surgeons treating trauma victims. Therefore, treatment must proceed from an assessment of the end result rather than the inciting cause.

Initial Clinical Evaluation and Management

Initial evaluation and management of victims of penetrating spinal injury should follow the guidelines for Advanced Trauma Life Support (ATLS) of the American College of Surgeons (8). The first priorities for emergent intervention are the establishment of a secure airway, adequate ventilation, and hemodynamic support while providing for immobilization and stabilization of the spinal column to prevent secondary neurological injury.

Maintenance of adequate perfusion of the spinal cord and other tissues is achieved through aggressive efforts to maintain systemic oxygenation and hemodynamic stability. The incidence of associated injuries to surrounding vessels and viscera is between 21% and 64% (9–11). Often, management of these wounds will take priority over treatment of the spinal injury.

Hypotension in the setting of penetrating injury is usually due to acute blood loss and requires intravascular volume replacement; however, in the presence of cervical or upper thoracic spinal cord injuries, autonomic instability (i.e., neurogenic shock) may compound the problem. In these patients, hypotension may be exacerbated by loss of vasomotor tone and sympathetic innervation to the heart. In this situation, hemodynamic resuscitation may require judicious use of vasopressors and vagolytics such as atropine (8).

Spinal instability as a direct consequence of penetrating trauma is unusual (9,12,13), but does occur when the penetrating object causes adequate bony or ligamentous disruption. Also, gunshot and stab wounds do not always occur in isolation. A patient may have been subjected to another mechanism of injury such as blunt trauma or a fall from a height at the time of the penetrating injury. Standard emergency medical service (EMS) spinal immobilization protocols are appropriate until additional trauma has been ruled out and the degree of vertebral disruption and spinal instability has been defined radiographically.

Neurological examination to establish a clinical baseline should be completed early. Progressive neurological deficit can only be diagnosed with serial examinations. Complete motor assessment with strength grading of all major muscle groups bilaterally, sensory examination including light touch, pinprick, and proprioception, and examination for evidence of autonomic instability should be completed within moments of the patient's arrival. A well-defined and reproducible clinical grading scale such as that of the American Spinal Injury Association (ASIA) should be used in this assessment (14). The neurological level of the spinal cord injury should be defined and characterized as complete (i.e., no preservation of sensory or motor function below the level of neurological injury) or incomplete. In busy trauma settings it is important to document this information quickly, as multiple patients with similar examinations may present in rapid succession.

Diagnostic Imaging

Radiographic evaluation beyond the initial trauma screen should diagnose associated systemic or vascular injuries, locate retained fragments, ascertain the presence of neural element compression, and demonstrate spinal instability.

Plain radiographic examination and computed tomography (CT) are helpful for the localization of fragments, the study of bony anatomy, and assessment of the path of a penetrating missile (Fig. 1). Often, the presence of a large bone or foreign body fragment within the neural canal will be enough to diagnose persistent compression of the neural elements.

The high incidence of associated injuries to major blood vessels or other structures within the neck, thorax, or abdominal cavity (9–11,15) should guide the initial diagnostic evaluation of patients with penetrating spinal trauma since management of these injuries will usually take precedence over treatment of the spinal injury. Angiography should be performed if external bleeding or the presence of a hematoma suggesting vascular injury is encountered. Similarly, if the path of a bullet as defined by plain radiographs or CT is such that important vascular structures may have been disrupted, angiography is required (Fig. 2).

Occasionally, magnetic resonance imaging (MRI) or myelography with CT may be desirable to further define the anatomy of a penetrating spinal injury. Case reports (class III data) have demonstrated the use of MRI for evaluation of gunshot wounds (16,17); however, laboratory studies characterizing the ferromagnetic properties of typical ballistic materials (18–21) support a more cautious and limited role for MRI in the presence of retained metallic fragments. In a study of the most commonly used air gun pellets, 2 of 6 pellets tested were strongly ferromagnetic and were deflected within the magnetic field of an MRI system (18). Another study demonstrated 5 of 22 commonly used bullets and shotgun pellets were markedly ferromagnetic, rotating within ballistic gelatin and deflecting when exposed to a magnetic field (20,21). Similarly, in a study of the 28 most common types of ballistic materials encountered in the urban setting by the Cleveland Police Department, all steel-containing bullets and one copper-jacketed, nonsteel bullet were deflected within the magnetic field of an MRI system (19).

Although lead shotgun pellets are usually nonferromagnetic and pose no significant risk within the magnetic field of an MRI scanner, recent federal legislation mandates the use of steel rather than lead shotgun pellets because of environmental concerns. Clinicians must be aware of this new policy when imaging victims of shotgun wounds (21,22).

The use of MRI in penetrating spinal trauma should therefore be restricted unless retained metallic fragments are known to be nonferromagnetic and MRI-compatible, particularly if these foreign bodies are located near vital and vulnerable anatomical structures. Contrast myelography with CT may be used as an alternative to MRI when the specific composition of a retained foreign body is unknown, the presence of neural element compression is not clear from other studies, and the data obtained from the imaging study could affect patient management.

Medical Management

ANTIBIOTIC THERAPY. The use of antibiotics in penetrating spinal injury remains controversial.

All of the available published data regarding the role of antibiotic therapy in the management of penetrating spinal injury is class III. The best published reports available are uncontrolled case series. Since these data support conflicting conclusions, it is not possible to make scientifically well-substantiated therapeutic recommendations regarding antibiotic choice, duration of therapy, or even whether antibiotic therapy is warranted at all (23–27). The clinical practice reported by Heary and associates (23) seems most reasonable, however, since excellent results were achieved in a large number of patients using uniform, rational, and reproducible methods.

Heary and associates report 239 patients with gunshot wounds to the spine who were treated with broad-spectrum antibiotics for 48 hours, but whose antibiotic coverage was extended to 7 days if the alimentary canal was perforated. Surgery was performed for any abdominal injury, progressive neurological deficit, or persistent cerebrospinal fluid leak. Only five patients developed spinal or paraspinal infections, including three cases of meningitis (23).

STEROID THERAPY. The use of high-dose methylprednisolone therapy in patients with nonpenetrating spinal cord injuries has become standard since publication of the second National Acute Spinal Cord Injury Study (NASCIS II) (28). Although this study did not address the potential benefit of glucocorticoid therapy for penetrating spinal cord injuries, some institutions have extrapolated the findings of NASCIS II to justify use of high-dose methylprednisolone for these patients as well. In response to this trend, two retrospective nonrandomized clinical studies were reported comparing clinical outcomes for penetrating spinal cord injury patients with and without steroid therapy (29,30).

In 1996, Levy and colleagues (29) reported a series of 55 patients with penetrating missile injuries to the spinal cord treated with the NASCIS II protocol (28) compared to 181 historical controls treated without steroid therapy. Frankel scores (31) were used at admission and discharge to determine improvement in functional outcome. In this series, there was no significant outcome benefit or increase in complication rate in the steroid treatment group (29).

In 1997, Heary and associates reported the results of 254 patients followed for a mean duration of 56 months (30). Sixty-one patients received steroids, all at outside institutions prior to transfer to the study institution. Thirty-one patients received steroids according to the NASCIS II protocol (28) and 30 received Decadron with variable initial doses ranging from 10 to 100 mg. ASIA scores were compared and no statistically significant improvement was noted in the steroid groups. The complication rate, however, was increased in patients treated with steroids. There was an increase in infections in these patients, although this difference was not statistically significant. Additionally, there was a statistically significant increase in gastrointestinal complications such as bleeding in the Decadron group and a statistically significant increased incidence of acute pan-

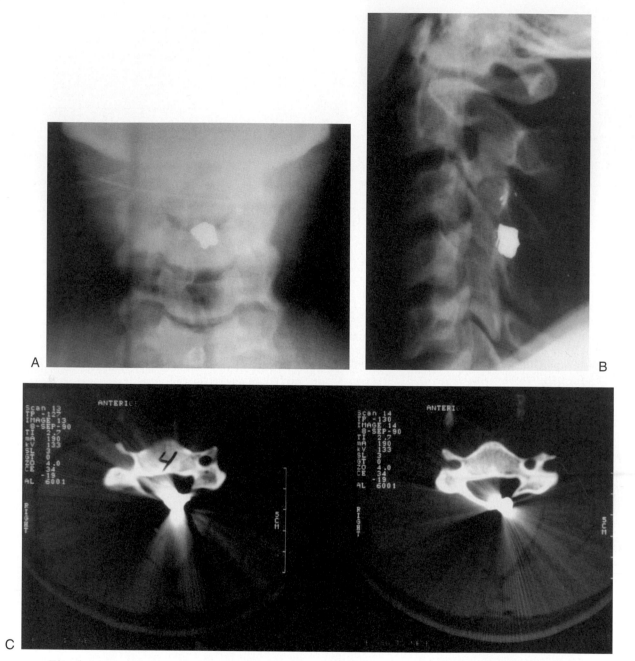

Fig. 1. A,B: Anteroposterior and lateral plain radiographs of a patient who sustained a gunshot wound to the neck. The position of the bullet at C3-4 is well demonstrated. This information, along with the location of the entrance wound in the left posterior neck, permit one to deduce the approximate path of the projectile. **C:** More precise anatomical assessment of the location and trajectory of the bullet may be possible using information from CT scans.

creatitis in the Solumedrol group (30). Since all patients who received steroids were transferred to this level one trauma center after initial resuscitation at another institution, a selection bias resulted from the potential for increased complications from transfer or from varying levels of trauma management expertise.

Although the data reported in these two studies are class III, the conclusions are in agreement: no therapeutic benefit of high-dose corticosteroids was identified. A practice option to avoid the use of steroids in penetrating spinal trauma therefore is reasonable.

Surgical Management

The role of surgery in the management of penetrating spinal injuries remains controversial. Many potential indications for surgical intervention have been proposed, including neurological considerations (i.e., incomplete spinal cord injury with canal compromise, nerve root compression, cauda equina injuries, and progressive neurological deficits), retained foreign body fragments, spinal instability, prevention of infectious complications, and cerebrospinal fluid fistulae. The following sections

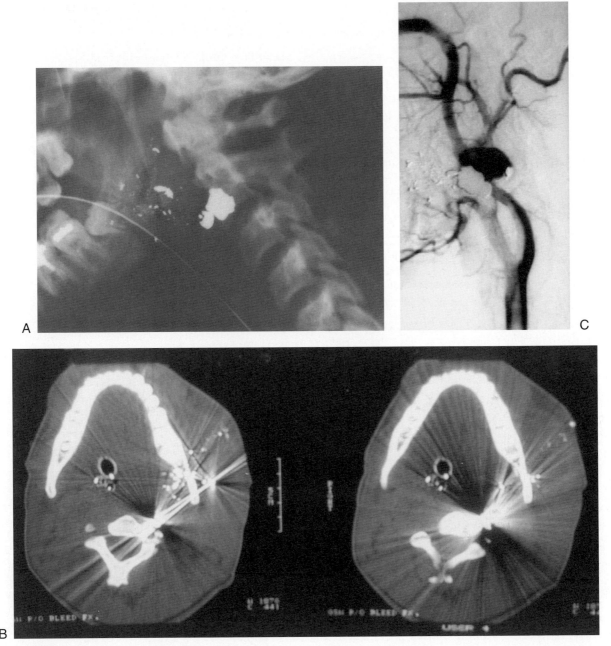

Fig. 2. **A:** Lateral radiograph of a patient who sustained a gunshot wound to the neck. The entrance wound was near the angle of the jaw. **B:** A CT scan confirmed the path of tissue destruction from the bullet and its proximity to the carotid and vertebral arteries. **C:** An angiogram was therefore performed and revealed a pseudoaneurysm of the left internal carotid artery.

will review the significance of each of these potential indications in surgical decision making.

NEUROLOGICAL CONSIDERATIONS. The principal objective in treatment of any neurologically injured patient is reversal or improvement of neurological deficits and prevention of secondary neurological injury. In order to make well-reasoned decisions regarding the need for surgical intervention in any given patient, it is imperative that surgeons have meaningful data comparing neurological outcomes with surgical and nonsurgical management. Although a number of studies have addressed

this topic, a review of the literature yields only class III data. The more frequently cited studies on this topic reveal that these data are inconclusive and often contradictory (10,11,32–34).

In the largest modern series of military penetrating spinal injuries, Aarabi and colleagues report a retrospective review of 205 casualties from the Iran-Iraq conflict in 1996 (35). Of these patients, 138 suffered shrapnel injuries and 60 sustained high-velocity injuries from assault rifles. The type of projectile was not defined in 7 victims. In this series, 145 of the original 205 patients were available for outcome assessment. Eighty-seven of these patients had been treated surgically and 58 received nonoperative management; however, it is clear from the description of surgical indications and myelographic findings that important differences existed between these two groups. Although the neurological and functional outcomes for patients in the two groups were the same, the incidence of complications (including cerebrospinal fistulae, meningitis, and local infections) was highest in the surgical treatment group (35). Unfortunately, because of the retrospective, uncontrolled design of this study, the two treatment groups are not equivalent. Additional selection bias resulted from the prolonged time period between injury and initial assessment.

Regardless of the level of injury (spinal cord or cauda equina), degree of neurological deficit (complete or incomplete), or the presence or absence of spinal canal compromise from retained ballistic fragments or bony elements, the available clinical data do not clearly resolve the question of whether surgical intervention improves neurological outcome. The central issue to be considered in each individual case relates to the extent of irreversible neurological damage imparted by the penetrating foreign body. If secondary injury can potentially be averted with intervention, then that intervention is indicated. In the case of a patient with a deteriorating neurological condition and radiographic evidence of persistent mass effect upon the spinal cord or cauda equina, surgical decompression seems most appropriate. Surgical intervention may however be of less benefit in patients with fixed neurological deficits. Further clinical investigation (ideally in the form of a prospective, randomized clinical trial) will be required to establish meaningful therapeutic recommendations to assist clinicians in selecting patients who may benefit neurologically from surgical intervention.

RETAINED FOREIGN BODY FRAGMENTS. In addition to the neurological considerations discussed above, a variety of other potential complications from retained foreign body fragments have been cited as justification for surgical intervention, including migration of bullet fragments within the central nervous system, radicular pain, and lead toxicity.

Bullet Migration. Several authors have reported spontaneous migration of ballistic fragments within the central nervous system (36–38). Migrating bullets have been reported most commonly between midthoracic and sacral levels where the spinal canal is widest; however, isolated case reports of more distant migrations also exist. This may result in transient radicular symptoms that require no further treatment (38); however, persistent neurological symptoms referable to the location of a migrating foreign body might be effectively treated with removal of the bullet.

Radicular Pain. In the prospective series reported by Waters and Adkins in 1991, 22 of 66 patients with penetrating spinal injuries had gunshot wound-related pain at their initial evaluation. Of those patients, 14 had persistent pain one year later. Eight patients subsequently had the retained bullet fragments removed with resolution of the pain in only three. Six patients did not have the bullet removed, and the pain subsequently resolved in three (10). Although it would appear from this report that bullet removal did not effect resolution of pain, the character and location of the pain and the location of the retained fragments was not reported. Thus, no evidence-based conclusions can be drawn from these data.

The potential benefit of bullet removal for treatment of radicular pain is illustrated in the series of patients with penetrating cauda equina injuries reported by Robertson and Simpson: all patients with radicular pain at the time of admission had relief after decompressive laminectomy and fragment removal (11). In this series, however, there were no nonsurgically treated controls. These and similar class III data support the treatment

option of considering surgical removal of retained bullets when their anatomical location correlates with the distribution of persistent radicular symptoms.

Lead Poisoning. Although rare, lead poisoning has been reported (39,40) and is a potentially fatal delayed complication of retained bullet fragments (40). Bullets lodged within a disc space, a synovial cavity, or a pseudocyst where they are continually bathed by body fluids are more likely to cause lead intoxication (39,40). One might therefore conjecture that a patient with a bullet in the subarachnoid space could also potentially develop lead poisoning. Radiographic studies and elevated serum and urine lead levels may help establish this diagnosis. When lead toxicity from retained bullet fragments is recognized, treatment with a chelating agent should precede removal of the lead source (40). These treatment options are supported by class III data.

SPINAL INSTABILITY. Although it is a widely held belief that most penetrating spinal injuries are biomechanically stable, some clinical series have included reports of patients with acute or delayed spinal instability resulting from gunshot wounds to the spine (9,15,41,42). This may be of special concern in the presence of extensive vertebral body disruption, or when the bullet passes transversely, destroying both facets or both pedicles (42). Although it may be intuitively reasonable to surmise that localized trauma produced by penetrating spinal injury should not create as much ligamentous disruption as is commonly seen with nonpenetrating spine trauma, careful consideration must be given to the anatomical structures disrupted by the path of the missile and the impact this disruption will have on spinal stability (Fig. 3). Additionally, one should not assume

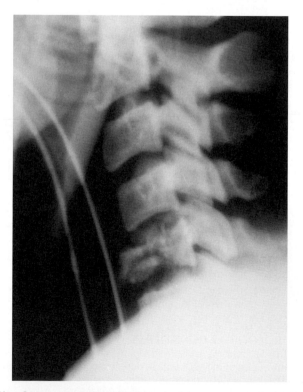

Fig. 3. The destabilizing destruction of the C5 vertebral body seen in this lateral radiograph resulted from a through-and-through gunshot wound of the neck. This injury was treated with anterior cervical corpectomy and fusion with iliac crest bone graft and anterior cervical plating, facilitating early mobilization of the patient.

that a penetrating injury occurred in isolation: the possibility of associated injuries from blunt trauma or falls should be considered as well.

The criteria of White and colleagues for cervical spine instability (43) and the Denis three-column lumbar spine model (44) commonly used in the assessment of nonpenetrating spinal injuries also provide useful conceptual frameworks for assessing spinal stability from plain radiographs, flexion-extension studies, and CT scans in the setting of penetrating injuries. Using these criteria, Isiklar and co-workers discovered four cases of instability (three cervical and one lumbar) in their series of 37 civilian gunshot wounds to the spine (9). These criteria may also be useful in predicting which patients are at risk for postsurgical instability following decompressive laminectomies, a commonly reported complication of spinal surgery for gunshot wounds (13,32,33). Once spinal instability has been recognized, standard techniques for stabilization, including external orthoses and/or surgical fusion may be considered (Fig. 3).

PREVENTION OF INFECTIOUS COMPLICATIONS. The importance of surgery for removal of retained bullet fragments that have passed through pelvic, abdominal, thoracic, or cervical viscera prior to striking the spine has long been the subject of debate. Some have postulated that surgical debridement of the spinal injury should be performed in addition to exploration and repair of the visceral injury by a general surgeon (45). Considerable data from retrospective case series have been collected by a number of authors suggesting that routine spinal surgery for debridement and removal of bullet fragments in patients with gunshot wounds to the spine associated with injury to hollow viscera is unnecessary (15,23–26,46,47). These patients were effectively managed with broad-spectrum antibiotics and general surgical exploration and repair of visceral injuries. Data from retrospective case series have documented an increased incidence of complications, including meningitis and wound infections, among patients treated with surgical debridement of spinal penetrating wounds (11,15,33,35,41).

In a retrospective case series of 160 civilian patients with penetrating spinal injuries and neurological deficits reported in 1989, Venger and associates found associated injuries to the esophagus, trachea, bronchi, or bowel in 107 cases (67%). Surgical exploration and repair of visceral injuries were performed in all patients, but surgical decompression of neural elements and debridement of the spinal injury were performed in only 19. The indications for selecting these 19 patients who underwent spinal surgery are not specified. In the group of 117 patients with associated injuries, infectious complications occurred in 2 of 19 patients (11%) who underwent spinal surgery and 4 of 88 patients (5%) treated without spinal surgery (15).

In a South African series of 153 patients with gunshot wounds to the spine, the overall incidence of septic complications was 9.8%. Local wound infections were seen in 7.4% of 81 patients with retained bullet fragments. In 72 patients, the bullet exited the body or was removed surgically. The local wound infection rate in this group was 12.5%. Among patients with associated colonic injuries, the overall incidence of infectious complications was 8.4% (47).

On the basis of these class III data, one may conclude that retained bullet fragments do not pose an increased risk for infectious complications. A treatment option is suggested that, even in the presence of visceral injury, routine spinal debridement for the purpose of preventing infectious complications is not necessary.

CEREBROSPINAL FLUID LEAK. Fundamental principles of wound closure and management of cerebrospinal fluid leaks

apply. There are no data in the literature that specifically examine the efficacy of closure of cerebrospinal fluid leaks, the timing of closure of cerebrospinal fluid leaks, or the role of conservative management of cerebrospinal fluid leaks in the setting of penetrating spinal trauma. Nevertheless, there is widespread agreement that persistent cerebrospinal fluid leaks are an indication for surgical intervention. A treatment option in favor of surgical repair of persistent cerebrospinal fluid fistulae is therefore suggested.

Summary of Recommendations

The first priorities for emergency management of patients with penetrating injuries to the spine are the establishment of a secure airway, adequate ventilation, and hemodynamic support in accordance with ATLS protocols while providing for immobilization and stabilization of the spinal column to prevent secondary neurological injury.

Plain films are used to demonstrate bony anatomy and the presence and location of retained fragments. CT scan is used for detailed anatomy of localized pathology based upon neurological examination and plain film findings. If clinically indicated, angiographic evaluation of adjacent vascular structures should be performed. In the presence of an incomplete or progressive deficit, and when previous imaging studies do not conclusively demonstrate compression of neural elements, myelography with CT may be helpful. MRI may be used if the absence of retained ferromagnetic fragments near vital and vulnerable structures is assured.

The use of high-dose corticosteroids in penetrating spinal injury does not appear to be of benefit. The complication rate is higher in patients treated with steroids and there is no demonstrated improvement in neurological outcome.

The best published data regarding the role of antibiotic therapy in the management of penetrating spinal injury are from uncontrolled retrospective case series that support conflicting conclusions. It is therefore not possible to make scientifically, well-substantiated therapeutic recommendations regarding antibiotic choice, duration of therapy, or treatment indications. One reasonable and appropriate clinical practice is to administer a 48-hour course of broad-spectrum antibiotics to all patients with penetrating spinal injuries and extend this coverage to 7 days if the alimentary canal is perforated. Routine surgical debridement of the spinal injury and removal of bullet fragments are not necessary for the prevention of infectious complications.

The surgical management of penetrating spinal trauma may be fashioned to meet the needs of each individual patient according to the following principles. Associated injuries are treated according to standard general surgery protocols. Wounds that are grossly clean in appearance and have cerebrospinal fluid leakage are locally debrided and closed. Grossly contaminated wounds leaking cerebrospinal fluid are debrided until clean, healthy tissue is reached. During this procedure, the source of cerebrospinal fluid leakage may be identified, debrided, and closed with autologous tissue patch graft and fibrin glue if necessary. Patients with progressive neurological deficits and persistent mass effect are surgically decompressed; however, the benefits of surgery for patients with stable incomplete neurological injuries and persistent mass effect are not as well established. Laminectomy, removal of bone and projectile fragments, and dural closure using autologous patch graft and fibrin glue are performed. When spinal instability is demonstrated radiographically, spinal stabilization using external orthoses and/or surgical fusion is performed. Symptomatic bullet migration or radicular pain attributable to the presence of retained foreign bodies may be effectively treated by removal of these foreign bodies. No attempt is made to remove retained fragments for the purpose of preventing long-term complications. Lead intoxication from retained bullet fragments rarely occurs. If this is diagnosed, treatment with chelating agents should be initiated prior to surgical removal of the bullet fragments.

These evidence-based clinical practice recommendations for management of penetrating spine trauma are derived from class III data. These data are often contradictory; therefore, most of the clinical issues reviewed in this chapter warrant further, more definitive clinical investigation.

References

1. Burney RE, Maio RF, Maynard F, et al. Incidence, characteristics, and outcome of spinal cord injury at trauma centers in North America. *Arch Surg* 1993;128:596–599.
2. Stover SL, Fine PR. The epidemiology and economics of spinal cord injury. *Paraplegia* 1987;25:225–228.
3. Young JS, Burns PE, Bowen AM, McCutchen R. *Spinal cord injury statistics: experience of the regional spinal cord injury systems.* Phoenix: Good Samaritan Medical Center, 1982.
4. Peacock WJ, Shrosbree RD, Key AG. A review of 450 stabwounds of the spinal cord. *S Afr Med J* 1977;51:961–964.
5. DeVivo MJ, Kartus PL, Stover SL, et al. Seven-year survival following spinal cord injury. *Arch Neurol* 1987;44:872–875.
6. Roye WPJ, Dunn EL, Moody JA. Cervical spinal cord injury—a public catastrophe. *J Trauma* 1988;28:1260–1264.
7. Fackler ML. Ballistic injury. *Ann Emerg Med* 1986;15:1451–1455.
8. Committee on Trauma of the American College of Surgeons. *Advanced Trauma Life Support student manual.* Chicago: The American College of Surgeons, 1993.
9. Isiklar ZU, Lindsey RW. Low-velocity civilian gunshot wounds of the spine. *Orthopedics* 1997;20:967–972.
10. Waters RL, Adkins RH. The effects of removal of bullet fragments retained in the spinal canal. A collaborative study by the National Spinal Cord Injury Model Systems. *Spine* 1991;16:934–939.
11. Robertson DP, Simpson RK. Penetrating injuries restricted to the cauda equina: a retrospective review. *Neurosurgery* 1992;31:265–269.
12. Arishita GI, Vayer JS, Bellamy RF. Cervical spine immobilization of penetrating neck wounds in a hostile environment. *J Trauma* 1989;29:332–337.
13. Kupcha PC, An HS, Cotler JM. Gunshot wounds to the cervical spine. *Spine* 1990;15:1058–1063.
14. American Spinal Injury Association. *Standards for neurological classification of spinal cord injury patients.* Chicago: American Spinal Injury Association, 1992.
15. Venger BH, Simpson RK, Narayan RK. Neurosurgical intervention in penetrating spinal trauma with associated visceral injury. *J Neurosurg* 1989;70:514–518.
16. Ebraheim NA, Savolaine ER, Jackson WT, et al. Magnetic resonance imaging in the evaluation of a gunshot wound to the cervical spine. *J Orthop Trauma* 1989;33:19–22.
17. Bashir EF, Cybulski GR, Chaudhri K, et al. Magnetic resonance imaging and computed tomography in the evaluation of penetrating gunshot injury of the spine. *Spine* 1993;18:772–795.
18. Oliver C, Kabala J. Air gun pellet injuries: the safety of MR imaging. *Clin Radiol* 1997;52:299–300.
19. Smith AS, Hurst GC, Duerk JL, et al. MR of ballistic materials: imaging artifacts and potential hazards. *AJNR* 1991;12:567–572.
20. Teitelbaum GP, Yee CA, VanHorn AS, et al. Metallic ballistic fragments: MR imaging safety and artifacts. *Radiology* 1990;175:855–859.
21. Teitelbaum GP. Metallic ballistic fragments: MR imaging safety and artifacts [Letter]. *Radiology* 1990;177:883.
22. Lufkin RB. MR imaging of firearm projectiles [Letter]. *Radiology* 1991;179:285.
23. Heary RF, Vaccaro AR, Mesa JJ, et al. Thoracolumbar infections in penetrating injuries to the spine. *Orthop Clin North Am* 1996;27:69–81.
24. Lin SS, Vaccaro AR, Reich SM, et al. Low-velocity gunshot wounds to the spine with an associated transperitoneal injury. *J Spinal Disord* 1995;8:136–144.
25. Roffi RP, Waters RL, Adkins RH. Gunshot wounds to the spine associated with a perforated viscus. *Spine* 1989;14:808–811.
26. Kihtir T, Ivatury RR, Simon R, et al. Management of transperitoneal gunshot wounds of the spine. *J Trauma* 1991;31:1579–1583.
27. Romanick PC, Smith TK, Kopaniky DR, et al. Infection about the spine associated with low-velocity-missile injury to the abdomen. *J Bone Joint Surg* 1985;67-A:1195–1201.
28. Bracken MB, Shepard MJ, Collins WF, et al. A randomized controlled trial of methylprednisolone or naloxone in the treatment of acute spinal cord injury. *N Engl J Med* 1990;322:1405–1411.
29. Levy ML, Gans W, Wijesinghe HS, et al. Use of methylprednisolone as an adjunct in the management of patients with penetrating spinal cord injury: outcome analysis. *Neurosurgery* 1996;39:1141–1148.
30. Heary RF, Vaccaro AR, Mesa JJ, et al. Steroids and gunshot wounds to the spine. *Neurosurgery* 1997;41:576–584.
31. Frankel HL, Hancock DO, Hyslop G, et al. The value of postural reduction in the initial management of closed injuries of the spine with paraplegia and tetraplegia. *Paraplegia* 1969;7:179–192.
32. Heiden JS, Weiss MH, Rosenberg AW, et al. Penetrating gunshot wounds of the cervical spine in civilians. *J Neurosurg* 1975;42:575–579.
33. Stauffer ES, Wood RW, Kelly EG. Gunshot wounds of the spine: the effects of laminectomy. *J Bone Joint Surg* 1979;61:389–392.
34. Benzel EC, Hadden TA, Coleman JE. Civilian gunshot wounds to the spinal cord and cauda equina. *Neurosurgery* 1987;20:281–285.
35. Aarabi B, Alibaii E, Taghipur M, et al. Comparative study of functional recovery for surgically explored and conservatively managed spinal cord missile injuries. *Neurosurgery* 1996;39:1133–1140.
36. Karim NO, Nabors MW, Golocovsky M, et al. Spontaneous migration of a bullet in the spinal subarachnoid space causing delayed radicular symptoms. *Neurosurgery* 1986;18:97–100.
37. Young WFJ, Katz MR, Rosenwasser RH. Spontaneous migration of an intracranial bullet into the cervical canal. *South Med J* 1993;86:557–559.
38. Rajan DK, Alcantara AL, Michael DB. Where's the bullet? A migration in two acts. *J Trauma* 1997;43:716–718.
39. Grogan DP, Bucholz RW. Acute lead intoxication from a bullet in an intervertebral disc space: a case report. *J Bone Joint Surg* 1981;63:1180–1182.
40. Linden MA, Manton WI, Stewart RM, et al. Lead poisoning from retained bullets: pathogenesis, diagnosis, and management. *Ann Surg* 1982;195:305–313.
41. Simpson RKJ, Venger BH, Narayan RK. Treatment of acute penetrating injuries of the spine: a retrospective analysis. *J Trauma* 1989;29:42–46.
42. Yoshida GM, Garland D, Waters RL. Gunshot wounds to the spine. *Orthop Clin North Am* 1995;26:109–116.
43. White AAr, Johnson RM, Panjabi MM, et al. Biomechanical analysis of clinical stability in the cervical spine. *Clin Orthop* 1975;109:85–96.
44. Denis F. The three column spine and its significance in the classification of acute thoracolumbar spinal injuries. *Spine* 1983;8:817–831.
45. Flint LMJ, Voyles CR, Richardson JD, Fry DE. Missile tract infections after transcolonic gunshot wounds. *Arch Surg* 1978;113:727–728.
46. Maier RV, Carrico CJ, Heimbach DM. Pyogenic osteomyelitis of axial bones following civilian gunshot wounds. *Am J Surg* 1979;137:378–380.
47. Velmahos G, Demetriades D. Gunshot wounds of the spine: should retained bullets be removed to prevent infection? *Ann R Coll Surg Engl* 1994;76:85–87.

165. Spine Injuries in Athletes

Julian E. Bailes and Vincent J. Miele

Spinal cord injury is perhaps the most feared complication of athletic activities. Minor spinal column injury or damage to the musculotendinous supporting structures is common in sports. Each participant in nearly every sporting or recreational activity is at potential risk for sustaining an injury to the spine. The vertebral column may be solely involved, either with or without the spinal cord itself suffering neurological damage. An entire spectrum, therefore, of soft tissue, bony structural elements, or spinal cord injury can be seen. There is no other sports-related injury that is potentially more catastrophic than a cervical spinal cord lesion. In contrast to other injuries encountered in sports medicine, spinal injuries at the least usually result in significant disability or time lost from competition, and can become the source of chronic pain with functional limitation. There are many facets of an optimal response to the athlete with suspect or proven neck injuries that are unique and important, which will be detailed in this chapter.

Incidence and Classification

The categorization of spinal injuries in athletes is facilitated by analysis of two different types of activities. Injuries commonly occur during participation in recreational, nonsupervised sports such as diving, surfing, skiing, and other activities. In these sports there are limited degrees of training, rules, participation, and supervision, which makes it difficult to achieve improvement in injury patterns. There is also a limited ability to enforce safety guidelines and manufacturing standards in nonsupervised recreational activities. The second category of injuries includes those occurring in supervised, organized sports with a higher level of bodily contact, velocity or torque forces, competition, and team participation. These injuries happen primarily in athletes participating in football, wrestling, ice hockey, gymnastics, rugby, and others.

Each year, there are approximately 10,000 cases of spinal cord injury in the United States, approximately 10% of which occur during athletic events. The majority of spinal trauma, which constitutes 2% to 3% of all sports-related injuries, occurs during activities such as diving, surfing, skiing, and "sandlot" games (1). Much more visible, however, are those injuries that occur during football, wrestling, soccer, rugby, ice hockey, and gymnastics (1–3). Spinal injuries among professional football players are the most highly profiled. For the thousands of physicians and athletic trainers who are responsible for the medical care of these athletes, no situation is fraught with more danger or elicits more anxiety than that of the injured player who manifests symptoms of a cervical fracture and/or spinal cord dysfunction.

The ongoing risk is emphasized, however, by the four high school football players in Louisiana who sustained cervical spinal cord injuries during the 1989 football season alone (4). These accidents occurred in a state where, based on the national average, only one such injury would be expected during a 14.5-year period.

At the high school, college, and professional levels over the last 20 years, there has been a decrease in the incidence of permanent catastrophic injuries to the cervical spine in terms of fracture, dislocations, and irreversible spinal cord injuries. Over this same time period, however, there has been an increased awareness of sports-related injuries with newly recognized syndromes associated with quadriplegia, quadriparesis, and central cord abnormalities that involve two or more extremities (5).

Water Sports

Diving injuries tend to occur in teenage males who are involved in recreational, unsupervised activities in the summer months (6). Diving accidents have been reported to comprise between 2% and 22% of all spinal injuries, with the incidence increasing when the reporting center lies in close proximity to an area of high water-sport activity frequented by younger age groups or in times of seasonal droughts (7). Up to 75% of recreation-related spinal cord injuries are due to diving mishaps (8,9). Although diving injuries usually contribute to the majority of all sports-related spinal injuries, the true incidence is thought to be even higher, because many are likely to have occurred in drowning victims. In addition, many of the diving injury patients have alcohol consumption as a contributing factor in their injury and presentation.

In reviewing the medical literature, it is seen that flexion, often with axial compression, is the usual mechanism of diving injuries; others include lateral flexion or hyperextension. Divers may occasionally enter the water in an unconventional manner, producing a mechanism that is essentially that of a fall (10). The most common method of injury in diving is when the diver strikes his head on the bottom of a pool, lake, or ocean after having miscalculated the depth of the water. Diving injuries have also been reported after one swimmer strikes another swimmer or a submerged object. For example, several patients sustained broken necks when they dove into murky water, striking their heads on a submerged object such as a nonvisible picnic table or boulder that had been thrown in during the winter months. Surfing-related cervical injuries usually entail a variety of impact positions, as surfers are propelled by falls or tidal action, striking their heads and necks. This initiates different mechanisms of injury to the vertebral column (11).

Diving injuries occur almost exclusively in the cervical spine and usually cause quadriplegic injury. The C5 level has the highest frequency of injury, 70% in our series; this is attributed to the range of motion that occurs in association with the relatively smaller size of the vertebral canal at the midcervical level. Most multilevel injuries also have involvement at the C5 level. In addition, in four patients, the C1 vertebra was also fractured due to an axial load, resulting in a Jefferson fracture in each case. In only two patients were odontoid fractures identified, emphasizing the relative rarity of diving injuries of the upper cervical spine (3).

Diving injuries constitute a unique entity for several reasons. First, they are essentially completely isolated cervical spine injuries. They are ideal for preventive programs, and in fact were the impetus for the "Think First" injury prevention program sponsored by organized neurosurgery. Prevention can occur along several lines, including warnings about diving in shallow water and above-ground pools or in places where there may be submerged objects, use of improper technique, diving while under the influence of alcohol, and so on. It is calculated that when a person is diving from deck level or higher, it takes almost double the diver's height in water depth to cause complete deceleration (12). It is believed that just as the public is cautioned against the dangers of drinking and driving, it should be warned against drinking and diving (3).

Football

Football players are the most likely athletes to sustain cervical trauma and are the group for whom the most reliable records of the frequency and incidence of injury are available, although reporting in the past has varied. There are approximately 1.4 million athletes participating in junior and senior high school football, 75,000 in college football, and 1,000 in professional play. This contrasts to roughly 60,000 rugby players in the United States. With the innumerable high-velocity collisions that occur every year during practice and games, football is the most dangerous sport for spinal cord injury in terms of exposure. Although more than 1 million preadolescents and early adolescents participate in organized football programs such as Pop Warner leagues, disabling spinal injuries are almost nonexistent among them. This is due to their small size and the relative lack of high-velocity collisions.

The vast majority (83%) of cervical spinal cord injuries are sustained by high school players. This may be largely explained by discrepancies in player size, age, maturity, and speed among those on the high school field of competition. Most football players are injured during the course of tackling, and thus defensive players are usually involved (Fig. 1). Defensive backs,

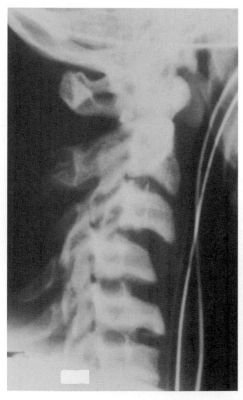

Fig. 1. Lateral cervical radiograph demonstrating C3-4 fracture dislocation resulting in quadriplegia in a college football player. This injury was sustained during the course of making a tackle.

members of the kickoff and receiving teams, and linebackers constitute the majority of those injured. The annual incidence since 1977 of fewer than 10 cases reported by Cantu and Mueller (13) represents a 50% reduction from the rate reported by Torg and co-workers (14) in the 1970s.

Apart from position, players with long, slender necks in high school appear to be the most vulnerable. Almost all cervical spine injuries occur with high-velocity impact, usually with the player striking the opponent by using the vertex of the helmet or with the head down (2,15). This results in an axial loading mechanism, often with a minor or major component of flexion. In football, impacts with the head may involve hyperflexion, hyperextension, lateral flexion, rotation, axial compression, or a combination of these. The cervical musculature that is responsible for maintaining such extension is much stronger than that used in maintaining flexion. A player who lowers his head in blocking or tackling places his cervical spine in a position that is less able to absorb the opponent's energy, and he therefore is vulnerable to cervical injury. Recent laboratory and clinical evidence has shown that in almost every sport where collisions occur, axial loading is the primary method of sustaining cervical fracture or fracture dislocation.

Baseball/Softball

In the sports of baseball and softball, minor injuries are fairly common and catastrophic injuries do occur. According to the National Spinal Cord Injury Data Research Center (NSCIDRC), baseball accounted for 1% of all sports-related spinal cord injuries between 1973 and 1981 (16). The head-first slide into a base seems to cause the most risk for a baseball player of catastrophic spinal cord injury. If the hands of the runner separate, the top of his head can collide with the leg of the defensive player, creating a great deal of axial load transmission to the vertebral column. While the use of breakaway bases substantially decreases the risk for occurrence of sliding-related injuries, serious injuries can still occur. The use of low-profile bases and the outlawing of sliding have also been suggested (17).

Basketball

The most common neurological risk in basketball is to the player's spine. According to the NSCIDRC, basketball accounted for 1% of all sports-related spinal cord injuries between 1973 and 1981 (16).

Acute back injuries associated with basketball include lumbosacral sprains, contusions, facet joint and pars interarticularis injuries, spinal stenosis, and lumbar disc injuries or fractures (18–22). Herniated discs are usually posterior or posterolateral. While in the nonactive young population discogenic disease is rare, its incidence increases with involvement in sporting activity. Clark (23) reported a case of a 12-year-old athlete incurring a lumbar disc herniation with apophyseal fracture during athletic activity. Disc herniation in athletes is a consequence of numerous microtraumas of the intervertebral disc, which are further compounded by the syndrome of chronic overstraining. Basketball is a leading cause of sports-related disc disease and was the second most common cause of disc herniation among a series of 55 athletes reported by Kovac et al. (24). Other injuries can resemble disc disease. Garth and Van Patten (25) reported

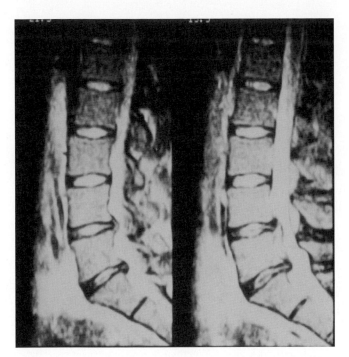

Fig. 2. Lumbar disc herniation at L4-5 and L5-S1 in a high school basketball player resulting in active lumbar radiculopathy. This was managed successfully with rest, antiinflammatory medication, and physiotherapy allowing the athlete to return to full activity within 6 weeks.

a fracture of the lumbar lamina with epidural hematoma simulating herniation of a disc. Facet syndrome can cause lower back pain in the basketball player. It is often associated with disc disease or injury, and recurrent pain while playing the game (18,26,27). Pain from this source is greatest with hyperextension or twisting of the spine and may be unilateral (Fig. 2).

Because the sport involves rapid changes in direction and explosive movements, repeated stress on the vertebrae of the spine can result in spondylolysis. Pars interarticularis defects can cause areas of spinal instability and low back pain in the player (18–20,26,28). Secondary to the athletes' rapid growth, adolescent players with these defects are at a higher risk of vertebral slippage and spondylolisthesis (29). Early detection in the adolescent is critical to reverse this degenerative process. Patients with spondylolysis or spondylolisthesis with less than 50% slippage can be treated with rest. More severe injuries require bracing of the lumbosacral spine or surgical fusion (18, 20,30). If the injury is not corrected early, spinal stenosis and narrowing of the foramen can result in chronic lower back pain and radiculopathy.

Fractures of the lumbar spine are rare occurrences in basketball (18,28). If a fracture does occur, timely diagnosis and treatment is essential (28). Fractures of the spinous or transverse processes can occur secondary to trauma or from strong muscular contraction (18,28). These more commonly affect the lumbosacral area rather than the cervical spine.

Cervical cord neurapraxia has been reported in basketball players. It is a transient neurological phenomenon usually not associated with any permanent neurological injury. No permanent morbidity has occurred in patients who returned to contact activities. Once a player experiences it, however, they have over a 50% chance of recurrence. This risk of recurrence is strongly and inversely correlated with sagittal canal diameter (31).

Cycling

Cycling-related injuries to the spine can be secondary to acute trauma or overuse. According to the NSCIDRC, the mean age of cycling-related spinal cord injury between 1980 and 1981 was found to be 24, with a range of 14 to 57; 100% of the injuries occurred in men and 43% occurred in individuals considered adept at the sport. Forty-three percent resulted in quadriplegia. Eighty-six percent of the injuries occurred to an individual not participating in an organized class or team (16). Over half of the total cycle injuries result from contacts with motor vehicles. A study by Rivara et al. (32), found that the risk of neck injury was increased in cyclists struck by motor vehicles or hospitalized for any injury.

Pain in the neck and back is extremely common in cyclists, occurring in up to 60% of participants (33). Its etiology is the combination of increased load on the arms and shoulders required to support the cyclist and hyperextension of the neck in the horizontal, bent forward position of riding. If the bicycle is not properly fitted to the cyclist and he or she must reach forward to the handlebars, these stresses are aggravated by the resultant hyperextension of the neck and extreme flexion of the back. Wilber et al. (34) analyzed overuse injuries among cyclists. The most common anatomical site for overuse injuries was the neck (48.8%), and the back accounted for 30.3% of complaints. The odds of female cyclists developing neck and shoulder overuse problems have been reported to be 1.5 and 2.0 times more, respectively, than their male counterparts (34). Lower back pain in these athletes is partially the result of hyperextension of the pelvic/spine angle, which results in an increase in stress at the promontorium (35).

Equestrian Sports

Between 1997 and 1998, 465 spinal cord injuries related to equestrian sports were reported (36). Approximately 20% of the injuries sustained in the young rider occur to the central nervous system (37,38). According to the NSCIDRC, equestrian sports accounted for 2% of all sports-related spinal cord injuries between 1973 and 1981. This represented less than 0.5% of all spinal cord injuries at the time (16).

A case series by Hamilton and Tranmer (39) reviewed horseback-riding accidents occurring over a 6-year period. It demonstrated that 13% ($n = 19$) of the patients had injury to the spinal cord. When this occurred, it was associated with a head injury in nearly half the cases. The cervical region was affected in six of the spinal cord injury patients. These included fractures and dislocations. Two of the spinal injury patients required surgery to stabilize these fractures and dislocations of the cervical spine. Eleven injuries to the thoracic and lumbar spine occurred. Of the injuries to the spinal cord, there were three incomplete cervical cord injuries, two spinal cord concussions, one case of cervical radiculopathy, and two cases of cauda equina syndrome. Outcome from the spinal cord injuries was also assessed using the Glasgow Outcome Scale (GOS). Good outcome was determined in 16 of the cases and moderate disability was found in three patients. In the Hamilton and Tranmer study (39), the average age of the patient was 25, with a range of 1 to 72 years. Grossman et al. (40) prospectively studied 110 injured equestrians. They found no correlation between injury and age, sex, or experience. Equipment failure was shown to be a cause of several injuries.

There is no question that rodeo rough-stock riding, which consists of bull riding, bareback bronco riding, and saddle bronco riding, is high on the list of dangerous sports. According to the NSCIDRC, rodeo sports accounted for 1% of all sports-related spinal cord injuries between 1973 and 1981 (16). Nebergall et al. (41) evaluated 6 years of injuries sustained at the elite professional level; 11.7% of the 738 participants sustained significant injuries. Spinal injuries included cervical and lumbar sprain, acute torticollis secondary to being thrown, and cervicothoracic strain secondary to missing the animal in the steer wrestling competition.

Gymnastics

The back is an area of the body that is very often injured by gymnasts. Alexander (42) reported that gymnastics (along with weight lifting and football) is a sport with the greatest risk of back injury (42). A National Registry of Gymnastic Catastrophic Injury was established in 1978 (43). Twenty gymnastic injuries of the cervical spine occurred in the first 4 years. Of these, 17 remained quadriplegic and three died secondary to the injury. Notably, most of the injuries occurred in experienced gymnasts during practice. Between 1997 and 1998, 325 spinal cord injuries related to gymnastics sports were reported (36). According to the NSCIDRC, gymnastics accounted for 6% of all sports related spinal cord injuries between 1973 and 1981. This represented 1% of all spinal cord injuries at the time (16). Kolt and Kirkby (44) reported a back injury rate of 14.9% in an 18-month study of elite and subelite female gymnasts. Silver et al. (45) reported 31 gymnastics-related spinal injuries between 1954 and 1984. Of these, 28 were in the cervical region and three in the thoracolumbar region. Clarke (46), in a study of quadriplegic injuries in high school and college athletes between 1973 and 1975, found gymnastics the only sport with female representatives.

The most common etiologies of back injury in this sport are the repeated hyperextensions of the back that are performed, which are compounded by impact loading from tumbling and landing from height (47). Spondylolysis is a relatively common injury in the gymnast. If the condition is not recognized early, it can evolve into spondylolisthesis. Letts et al. (48) reported that gymnastics and hockey are the sports most commonly associated with stress fractures of the pars interarticularis.

Rugby

Spinal injuries are common in the traditional tackle games that include rugby union, rugby league, and Australian-rules football. These activities commonly result in injuries to the neck. Kew et al. (49) performed a retrospective study of spinal cord injuries in rugby from 1960 thru 1989 and identified 117 catastrophic neck injuries. The authors also reported that for every serious rugby-associated spinal cord injury, 10 severe neck injuries occur that do not involve the cord (49). The NSCIDRC reported the mean age of rugby-related spinal cord injury to be 21 with a range of 20 to 22 (16). While rugby-associated spinal cord injuries have declined over the last decade in England, Australia, and New Zealand, their incidence has remained constant in South Africa (50–52). An average of 5.4 players/year were admitted to the Spinal Cord Injury Center in Cape Town between 1981 and 1987. This figure rose to 8.7 players/year (53) between 1987 and 1996.

Three specific activities during the game of rugby—the tackle, tight scrum, and loose play (ruck and maul)—result in the majority of injuries to the cervical spine (54). Kew et al. (49) found that 21% of spinal cord injuries occurred while tackling and 30% occurred while being tackled. The greatest cause of injury in the tackler is poor technique. Scher (55,56) analyzed tackling injuries and discovered three common mechanisms of injury. These are injury of the tackler secondary to head impact, injury to the recipient from a high tackle, and injury from a double tackle. Injury from impact to the tackler's head occurs when his head suddenly stops forward progress from contact with the ground or the body of the opponent (usually the thigh). This can result in compression fractures of the vertebral bodies from axial forces transmitted down the spine. These forces are increased significantly if the player's neck is flexed, as if diving, which eliminates the normal lordosis of the cervical spine. As in American football, if a tackler's first point of contact with an opponent is the vertex of his head, there is a substantial risk of injury (15). Injuries secondary to high tackles can be from behind or to the side of the recipient. If the tackle is from behind, hyperextension injuries are likely secondary to the head being pulled back and down. If the tackle is from the side, hyperflexion injury often results. Rotational forces are also a factor in these injuries, especially if the tackle is performed with only one arm. Double tackles, often referred to as sandwich or high-low tackles, occur both intentionally and by chance. They are more common near the goal with a concentration of defenders merging on the ball carrier. This tackle can cause injury to both the offensive and defensive player. If the defensive players miss their target, they can collide into each other with considerable force at unexpected angles. If the tackle is successful, the offensive player's body is forced in two directions. This inhibits the player from moving with either force completely, increasing rotational and shearing stresses to the spine.

Wrestling

The sport of wrestling has been associated with severe trauma to the cervical spine and spinal cord. According to the NSCIDRC, wrestling accounted for 3% of all sports-related spinal cord injuries between 1973 and 1981 (16). Jarret et al. (57) evaluated National Collegiate Athletic Association (NCAA) Injury Surveillance System data on collegiate wrestling during an 11-year period. The authors found that most injuries occurred during takedowns and sparring. The most common cause of these injuries in wrestling today is landing with the body twisted on the head and neck, because, although the intervertebral discs, joints, and ligaments are resistant to compression stresses, they are very susceptible to injury by rotational and shearing forces (58). Bailes et al. (2) analyzed 63 patients who sustained cervical spine injuries while participating in organized sporting events. Forty-five patients suffered permanent injury to the vertebral column and/or spinal cord, while 18 suffered only transient spinal cord symptoms. Wrestling accounted for the second highest number of injuries, preceded only by football. Leidholt (59) studied sports injuries, excluding football, over a 1-year period at the Air Force Academy. He reported a total of 31 spinal cord injuries, of which 11 were related to wrestling. Wu and Lewis (60) presented cases of three young athletes suffering quadriparesis and quadriplegia. Two of the victims suffered fracture-dislocations of the cervical spine resulting in quadriplegia. The third athlete suffered quadriparesis without any damage or disruption to the vertebrae. The first athlete's injury was a fracture-dislocation of the C5-6 vertebrae secondary to a full nelson applied during high school wrestling practice. The second patient was injured during a regulation high school wrestling match when he was thrown and landed on the right side of his neck in a twisted position. He became immediately quadriplegic with a sensory level of C4. Radiography revealed a fracture-dislocation of C3 anteriorly onto C4. The final athlete in the series was also injured by being thrown during a regulation match. As in the previously cited injury, he landed in a twisted configuration on his head, neck, and shoulders. Although radiography revealed no bony deformities, myelography revealed a block at C7-T1. An emergent laminectomy was performed revealing petechial hemorrhage and edema of the epidural fat. Various combinations of radiologic abnormalities of the thoracolumbar spine have been found to be more prevalent in wrestlers than in other athletes and the general population (61). Spondylolysis is a common occurrence in the competitive wrestler. Rossi and Dragoni (62) reported 390 cases found in 3,132 randomly selected competitive athletes. This prevalence is much higher than found in the general public. Slightly over 29% of wrestlers have been shown to suffer this condition, making the sport one of the highest risk athletic activities for this injury.

Injury Patterns

The musculotendinous structures of the cervical and lumbar spine are commonly injured in athletic activities. A strain is the result of mechanical overloading with forces that exceed the extensor musculature capacity. There is a characteristic response of the muscle to injury. Initially, there is localized pain, tenderness, and diminution or inhibition of voluntary muscle contraction. Weakness may be the only initial sign. Within several hours there is usually swelling of musculature and limitation of motion. Stretching of the musculature by flexing the neck to the opposite side may cause pain.

Injury to the ligaments or capsular structures of the spine is termed a *sprain* and may occur without muscular strain. The pain is located in the neck, interscapular area, and occasionally the upper arm in cervical injuries. Lumbar ligamentous sprain is usually located in the lumbar paraspinal and midline positions. In all true sprain syndromes, the pain is nonradicular and there is no sensory disturbance.

The ligamentous supporting structures of the spine may be damaged by repeated insult, leading to chronic tears, calcification, and the development of fibrous tissue. A cumulative effect of ligamentous hemorrhage causes fibrous tissue reaction that may lead to restricted motion and chronic pain. In both strain and sprain syndromes, vertebral column and neurological injury must be excluded. With sprain injuries, one must be certain to exclude ligamentous damage resulting in spinal instability.

The mechanism of spinal injuries in football was initially felt to be primarily hyperflexion. Research has shown that axial loading is a leading factor in placing the cervical spine at risk. Often an athlete will improperly flex his neck, eliminating the cervical lordosis and making the spine a straight segmented column. If he strikes an opponent or some other rigid surface, energy is transmitted directly to the osseous spine. With improper neck positioning, this energy transfer cannot be absorbed by the cervical musculature and supporting structures, which are the ordinary buffers for such energy. Forces of sufficient magnitude may cause failure of the intervertebral discs, ligaments, and vertebrae, resulting in neurological injury in the majority (58% in our series) of athletes. The C5 level is the most common region involved in athletic spinal injury, both vertebral and neurological. Fracture dislocation injury is seen in 33% and anterior compression fracture in 22%. As observed not only for football, but also wrestling, ice hockey, and diving, the C5 level is the most commonly involved because of the greater degree of motion here.

Syndromes of Spinal Cord Injury

Trauma to the spinal column may cause a variety of clinical syndromes depending on the type and severity of the impact and bony displacement as well as secondary insults such as hemorrhage, ischemia, and edema. Complete spinal cord injury results in a transverse myelopathy with total loss of spinal function below the level of the lesion. This insult is caused by either anatomic disruption of the spinal cord or hemorrhagic or ischemic injury at the site of injury. Complete injury patterns are rarely reversible, although, with long-term follow-up, improvement of one spinal level may be seen as a result of resolution of initial segmental traumatic spinal cord swelling. There are several patterns of incomplete spinal cord injury, usually produced on a vascular basis.

In addition to the classic syndromes of spinal cord injury, there are many patients who have an incomplete injury not classifiable into any certain pattern. These injuries usually consist of loss of all or nearly all useful motor function below the level of injury, with a sensory loss that does not fit any specific pattern. This sensory preservation, however, does portend a better recovery than does complete functional loss. The burning hands syndrome is characterized by burning dysesthesias and paresthesias in both hands, commonly seen in athletes who participate in contact sports, especially football and wrestling, with repeated cervical trauma. It was proposed that the burning hands syndrome was a variant of central cord syndrome in which there was selective injury to the central fibers of the spinothalamic tract that subserve pain and temperature sensation to the upper limbs (63).

In addition to persons with syndromes caused by blunt trauma directed to the spinal column and underlying neural structures, there is a small group of patients at risk for neurological injury on the basis of vascular involvement. The carotid and vertebral arteries are at risk from direct compression or as a result of traumatic fracture-subluxation. However, a patient with a vascular injury may radiographically show only chronic degenerative changes or have a normal spine (64). The carotid arteries are rarely injured in athletic competition, but it must be kept in mind whenever signs or symptoms suggest cerebral hemispheric dysfunction (hemiparesis, hemiplegia, hemianesthesia, dysphasia, homonymous visual fields defects). A delay in the appearance of the neurological defect, even up to several days, is most characteristic. Transient ischemic attacks (TIAs) in the territories of the anterior or middle cerebral arteries may occur secondary to distal embolization of the thrombotic material forming at a site of intimal tear in the vessel (65).

Types of Injuries

The senior author has designed and prospectively applied a classification system for the management of athletic spinal injuries (2). This classification consists of three types of athletic cervical spine injuries. Each type is observed often by physicians and may cause difficulty in diagnosis and management.

TYPE I. Type I injuries cause permanent spinal cord damage, which may vary from immediate and complete paralysis below

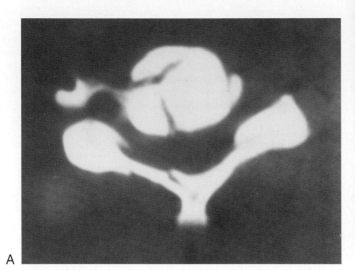

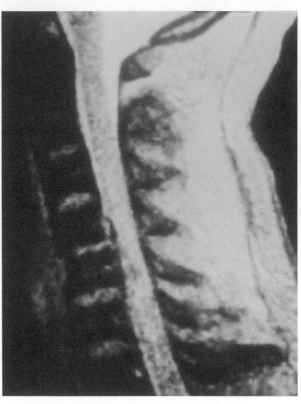

Fig. 3. A: Computed tomography (CT) scan demonstrating a C5 fracture, which occurred while this high school football player was making a tackle, resulting in complete quadriplegia. **B**: Sagittal magnetic resonance imaging (MRI) scan demonstrating the appearance of the spinal cord several days after this athlete was injured. No recovery was subsequently attained.

the level of injury to various patterns of incomplete spinal cord injury syndromes (Fig. 3). As discussed above, with patients who have anterior spinal cord syndrome there is preservation of only posterior column function. Patients with central cord injury syndrome experience selective weakness of the upper extremities with relative preservation of lower extremity function. Often seen is an overlap of spinal cord injury syndromes, however, rather than the classic anatomical presentation. A central cord/Brown-Séquard combination, which consists of motor/sensory deficit on different sides of the body with a relatively greater weakness in the upper extremities, often is diagnosed on neurological examination.

At times the athlete may have symptoms that are minor but are associated with radiological evidence of spinal cord injury. Typically the latter is documented by a magnetic resonance imaging (MRI) scan or myelogram suggestive of intrinsic spinal cord contusion, which is seen most clearly on intermediate MRI images as a high-intensity lesion within the spinal cord. Usually documentation of spinal cord injury, either clinically or radiologically, contraindicates the athlete's return to contact sports (1,2) (Fig. 4).

TYPE II. Type II injuries exist transiently after athletic trauma and are related to the spinal cord, but occur in individuals whose neurological examinations and radiological surveys, including MRI, yield normal results. Transient spinal cord injuries tend to happen in the cervical spine (90%), may have a pure motor, sensory, or combined sensorimotor deficit, and resolve within minutes to hours (2,66). Because there is no evidence of vertebral fracture, spinal column instability, or intrinsic cord

injury or contusion, the physician may have serious difficulty judging whether or not to recommend return to sports activities.

Symptoms of spinal cord involvement in a patient must be actively sought by the physician (51,67). A diagnostic problem often involves a distinction between the "burner" or "stinger" injury and spinal cord injury. The former is a common injury that, in some studies, is seen in as many as 50% of collegiate football players during the course of a season (68). A burning, dysesthetic pain is usually present and begins in the region of the shoulder and radiates unilaterally into the arm and hand; at times it is associated with numbness and/or weakness, usually in the C5 and C6 distribution. Several mechanisms for the burner or stinger injury have been proposed; the most common etiology is believed to be traction on the upper trunk of the brachial plexus occurring when a force is applied that depresses the ipsilateral shoulder when the neck is laterally flexed to the contralateral side (68,69). These injuries usually resolve within several minutes, but may persist for days or weeks. Burners usually leave no residual neurological damage unless they become a chronic injury. All radiological studies yield normal results, and there are no findings suggestive of spinal cord involvement such as bilaterality, lower extremity symptoms, long tract findings, sphincter disturbance, or sexual dysfunction. Electromyography may be useful several weeks after the injury in confirming brachial plexus involvement by showing denervation potential (68). It is also believed that some players with repetitive trauma to the nerve root within the neural foramen may develop a chronic burner syndrome (70).

The burner or stinger injury is different from the "burning hands" syndrome that is thought to be a mild variant of the central cord syndrome. The burning hands syndrome causes a

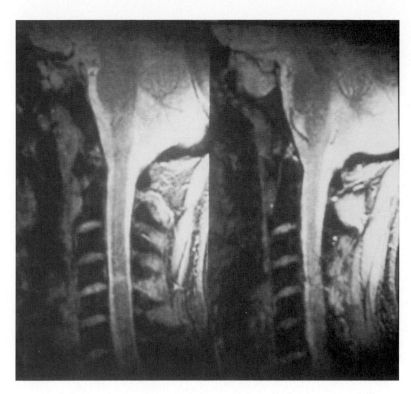

Fig. 4. Sagittal intermediate weighted MRI scan demonstrating a high signal intensity indicative of spinal cord contusion at the C4-5 level.

burning dysesthesia and associated weakness in arms and hands. It is believed that the anteroposterior compressive forces result in injury to the corticospinal and spinothalamic tracts, both of which are somatotopically arranged; the latter accounts for the dysesthetic pain. Reversible abnormalities documented by MRI and electrophysiology have been described in conjunction with the burning hands syndrome (71). In the authors' experience, most of these patients have a normal radiographic workup and complete resolution of symptoms within 24 hours. Athletes who experience burning hands syndrome are allowed to return to competition once they are asymptomatic (63,71).

Temporary spinal cord dysfunction, including transient quadriplegia, is not completely understood on a pathophysiological basis (31). It has been referred to as "neurapraxia," a term that ordinarily implies peripheral nerve dysfunction secondary to a physiological block in conduction, with no anatomical axonal interruption. Peripheral nerve neurapraxia is usually caused by mild degrees of compression or contusion. Gross inspection reveals a healthy peripheral nerve, whereas microscopically the nerve may have segmental demyelination and preservation of continuity of the axis cylinder (72). The term *spinal cord concussion* was first used by Obersteiner in 1879 to describe spinal cord injuries that resulted in complete neurological recovery within 24 to 48 hours. Since then, few experimental models of reversible spinal cord injury have been developed. It has been postulated that spinal cord concussion could be secondary to a prolongation of the absolute refractory period of long tract axons, which exaggerates the normal time during which axonal segments are unresponsive to any subsequent impulse (66).

Available data indicate that athletes who experience spinal cord concussion usually have no significant spinal abnormalities that predispose the spinal cord to a direct compressive effect, nor does this transient dysfunction secondary to athletic injury necessarily predispose them to subsequent permanent spinal cord injury. The combined results of studies by Zwimpfer and Bernstein (66) and Torg et al. (51) showed that 49 patients with transient spinal cord dysfunction experienced recurrent

symptoms but did not have permanent neurological sequelae. Conversely, in interviews with 117 athletes who sustained permanent spinal cord injuries from football, none recalled a prodromal experience of transient motor paresis (51). Transiently injured athletes, therefore, have a good prognosis, but must be highly scrutinized before being allowed to resume competition. They often may be allowed to return to full participation in contact sports if there is no neurological deficit or radiologically demonstrable injury or congenital cervical spine anomaly. If the athlete becomes a "repeat offender," however, with multiple episodes of spinal cord dysfunction, he or she is considered to be at high risk for catastrophic injury, and thought should be given to curtailing future participation in contact sports.

TYPE III. Solely radiographic abnormalities are termed type III injuries. In athletes with an unstable fracture or fracture/dislocation, surgical stabilization or external orthosis is required. Further participation in contact sports by these patients ordinarily should not be allowed. A skeletal injury that appears to be stable on dynamic radiographs and during normal physiological ranges of motion may not be stable under stress. A more difficult management issue is posed by bony injuries involving other portions of the vertebrae that have healed and appear stable during physiological range of motion testing (flexion-extension radiographs), but exist in an area of the spine that normally contributes significantly to spinal column stability (73).

The ability of the vertebral column and associated musculature to withstand and absorb the large amount of linear and angular forces involved in contact sports is not well quantitated. In addition, there are few experimental or clinical data that can be used to assess the degree of stability of a healed fracture or ligament injury of the cervical spine when it is placed under extreme degrees of stress. It is known that the cervical posterior ligamentous structures contribute more to stability in flexion, whereas the anterior ligaments are most important in extension

(74). It has been generally accepted that cervical instability exists when there is a more than 3.5-mm horizontal or 11-degree angular displacement between adjacent vertebrae (74,75). There are no definitive data concerning the contribution of individual vertebral components to the stability of the cervical spine, especially when one includes variables such as the possibility of either partial or complete ligament injuries, the healing process, the insertion of a bone graft, and the exceptional stress forces to which the athlete may be subjected (74).

Other spinal fractures, however, are considered inherently stable. Fractures that occur with no neurological injury need not necessarily prevent the athlete from further participation in contact sports. These fractures include isolated lamina or spinous process fractures. Depending on the given situation, a healed minor vertebral body fracture that is stable according to flexion-extension films also may be considered stable, and further participation by the patient in contact sports may be allowed.

Injuries showing radiological evidence of abnormality other than fracture are included among the type III injuries. An example of a type III injury is one that results in evidence of spinal motion on dynamic radiographs, which suggests a ligamentous injury requiring an orthosis or surgical stabilization. In such a case the authors usually would not recommend further participation in contact sports because the likelihood of injury would be significantly higher than in a healthy patient (75). Other type III injuries include radiological abnormalities that ordinarily would not be considered unstable, but which assume a greater importance in individuals who participate in contact sports. Compromise by the posterior ligaments, most commonly diagnosed with myelography or MRI, is considered to functionally narrow the size of the cervical canal, especially under high degrees of motion or stress forces. Combined with a congenitally narrow or relatively narrow cervical canal, this finding would place the athlete at a higher risk for further injury.

Historically, a diagnosis of congenital stenosis of the cervical spine has been made when the anteroposterior (AP) diameter of the spinal canal is less than 14 mm, a finding believed by some to predispose athletes to injury (51,76). Torg (77), however, related the ratio of the AP diameter of the spinal canal to the AP size of the vertebral body and concluded that a canal-to-body ratio of 0.80 or less, which indicates congenital cervical spine stenosis, is not a contraindication to participation in contact activities by otherwise asymptomatic athletes (Fig. 5). Torg further concluded that football players with narrowed cervical canals are not predisposed necessarily to subsequent injury if they return to contact sports after an episode of transient sensory symptoms of cord origin.

Torg et al.'s (31) report of 110 cases of athletic transient cervical cord injury associated with canal stenosis cites the latter as a causative factor. Permanent spinal cord injury was not seen with return to contact sports, although 56% of these had recurrent episodes that were best predicted by sagittal canal diameter. However, there was no correlation with subsequent spinal cord injury, and Torg et al. recommended that an athlete with an uncomplicated transient cord injury and canal stenosis ordinarily be allowed to return to contact sports (31). The canal/body ratio sometimes is still used as a sensitive screening device for stenosis; however, there are two major pitfalls in relying on such a ratio. Athletes have been shown to have significantly larger vertebral bodies than those of control individuals, which gives an abnormal ratio in at least one cervical level (78). Also, a bone measurement does not elucidate the relative size and accommodation of the cervical spinal cord. A "functional" MRI is relied on to clarify the spinal canal–to-cord relationship. In summary, the available medical literature indicates that cervical spinal canal stenosis per se does not indicate a high probability that catastrophic spinal cord injury will occur. On the contrary,

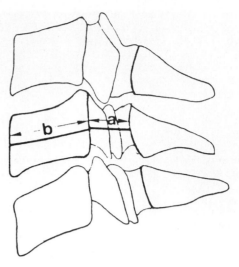

Fig. 5. Diagram demonstrating the calculation of vertebral canal to body forming the ratio. Although not as accurate as MRI scanning, this does give some indication of the magnification of the relative size of the canal during screening with cervical radiographs.

it appears that there is not an increased risk that the spinal cord is unusually susceptible, just as most athletes who have had a cord injury have not had prior warning episodes (31). In the absence of complicating factors, instability, existing neurological deficit, and repetitive episodes, most athletes with canal stenosis who have had transient or "neurapraxic" spinal cord symptomatology may be individually considered for return to contact participation.

Also common among type III injuries are herniated intervertebral cervical discs, which are frequently difficult to manage. The symptoms of a herniated intervertebral cervical disc are usually radiculopathy, cervical pain, and occasional myelopathic signs, regardless of whether the injury occurs spontaneously or traumatically. There is little controversy about treatment because most symptomatic herniated cervical discs are surgically removed, either by an anterior approach if they are central or a posterior or anterior approach if they are lateral. There are no absolute guidelines that indicate whether a bony fusion should be performed. It has been suggested, however, that healed anterior interbody fusion results in a preservation of strength in the cervical spine when tested in flexion and extension (79). A posterior surgical approach maintains the integrity of the anterior and posterior longitudinal ligaments. In such a case, it may be possible for the patient to return to contact sports after 6 to 12 months of recuperation and demonstration of stability on flexion-extension radiographs. If the patient has congenital spinal fusion, some increase in movement at the motion segments above and below the fused level would be expected. Unless congenital spinal fusion is associated with more widespread abnormalities consistent with Klippel-Feil syndrome, a narrowed spinal canal, multilevel fusion, motion on flexion-extension radiographs, or recurrent neurological symptoms, this entity alone should not preclude engagement by the patient in contact sports.

Spear Tackler's Spine

Torg et al. (67) described a group of athletes who are at high risk for cervical quadriplegic injury with the clinical term *spear tackler's spine.* Spear tackler's spine is thought to be a contraindication for participation in contact sports activities. Torg et al. found that football players with (a) developmental cervical canal stenosis; (b) persistent straightening or reversal of the normal cervical spine lordotic curve; (c) evidence of preexisting, posttraumatic radiographic abnormalities of the cervical spine; and (d) documentation of having previously used spear tackling techniques are predisposed to injury from cervical spine axial energy forces. When a spine with a congenitally narrowed canal is straightened, impact at the top or crown of the helmet causes buckling of the neck because the movement of the head is momentarily stopped while the trunk continues to accelerate forward. Radiographic documentation of prior traumatic cervical spine injuries, such as healed cervical compression fractures, ligamentous instability, and intervertebral cervical disc bulge or herniation, indicates that athletes with these injuries are habitual users of spear tackling techniques. In their study, Torg et al. (67) reported a series of 15 athletes whose playing techniques were examined because the athletes had cervical spine or brachial plexus symptoms; four of these athletes sustained permanent neurological injuries. It was concluded that axial loading impact to the persistently straightened cervical spine, which occurs when athletes deliberately engage in frequent head impact, resulted in permanent spinal cord injury in these athletes. Occasionally, if no significant bone or ligamentous instability is present, the cervical lordosis is restored through physiotherapy. If the player can be coached against using head vertex impact, a return to competition may be allowed. Otherwise, the authors of this study concur with the recommendation that individuals with symptoms of tackler's spine be withheld from participation in contact sports.

On-Field Evaluation and Management

Perhaps the most important fact in dealing with potentially injured athletes is that an unstable spine injury can be easily converted into an injury with permanent neurological deficit if the athlete is mishandled. Since severe athletic-related injuries are relatively rare, the experience of the on-site medical staff is usually limited. Thus, everyone who shares responsibility for managing spine-injured athletes should be adequately trained and frequently refreshed in the care of any situation that may arise. Prior preparation should ensure that all of the proper equipment, such as a spine board, cervical collars or immobilization devices, and stretcher, is available. There should be a clear hierarchy among the medical staff, indicating one member as the "captain" who directs the efforts of the team. In addition, arrangements should be made in advance to have ambulance services on site or close at hand. Preparation allays discomfort among providers and fosters efficiency and good decision making on behalf of the injured participant (72). It should also be mentioned that those who would manage injured athletes place themselves into legal responsibility for their actions, and precedent exists for legal action against team physicians and trainers who fail to properly handle those players (80).

The prevailing goal among the medical team members should be the prevention of secondary neurological injury as a result of improper handling of the fallen athlete. Cervical spine injury should be suspected, and the athlete managed as if the injury were present whenever the mechanism of injury involves forced movement of the head and neck, even in the absence of neurological deficit. The head and neck of the player should be immediately immobilized in a neutral position. As in any

resuscitation, assessment of airway, breathing, and circulation should proceed, as well as evaluation of the athlete's level of consciousness. Unless players are unconscious or airway or breathing considerations exist, they should be left in the position in which they lie, until they can be safely transferred onto a spine board. If the player is wearing a helmet, it should be left in place until adequate immobilization of the head and neck can be instituted. Then the helmet can be gently removed in line with the neck without flexion or extension, but only in conjunction with simultaneous shoulder pad removal. The occiput should be firmly supported during and after helmet removal (66). It is ordinarily not necessary to remove the helmet for airway access.

Treatment and Return to Competition

The treatment of the various forms of cervical spine injury has been previously summarized by Bailes et al. (81) and others, and follows established guidelines (2,77). As mentioned, the emphasis must be on preventing secondary or further neurological injury through suboptimal management. Proper management begins with immobilization of the spine and withdrawal of the player from competition until the exact nature of the injury is delineated. When a vertebral column or a neurological injury is identified, the athlete must be transferred promptly to a facility for definitive management (75).

The initial caregivers of the spine and spinal cord–injured athlete must be aware of the potential for respiratory failure and hemodynamic instability, as well as associated lesions, such as head injuries, which may affect the timing and order of needed treatments. Because of these concerns, patients with acute neurological deficit from spinal cord injuries usually are initially managed in an intensive care environment. The neurological deficits from spinal cord injury may be improved by methylprednisolone administration that has been felt to be beneficial if given in the first 8 hours from the time of injury (78).

After initial resuscitation and radiographic evaluation of the player has been accomplished, informed decisions concerning management of the specific injuries can be made. Some bony injuries, such as spinous process fractures or unilateral laminar fractures, may require no treatment or only immobilization in a cervical collar. Others, such as the bilateral pars interarticularis fracture of C2 ("hangman's fracture") often may be treated with a cervical collar, or in some cases halo vest immobilization. Unstable injuries should initially be reduced and temporarily stabilized with cervical traction using Gardner-Wells tongs or a halo ring device. Contrast-enhanced computed tomography (CT) scan or MRI of the cervical spine often should be obtained before fracture reduction to rule out the presence of retropulsed intervertebral disc material. Unrecognized retropulsed disc material has been implicated in the sudden neurological deterioration of patients undergoing reduction of their cervical fractures. Surgical treatment may subsequently be required for severe comminuted vertebral body fractures, unstable posterior element fractures, type 2 odontoid fractures, incomplete spinal cord injuries with canal or cord compromise, and in those patients with progression of their neurological deficit to higher levels of spinal cord function (Fig. 6).

Any athlete with a permanent neurological injury should be prohibited from further competition. However, those without cord injury who have stable fractures as evidenced by flexion-extension radiographs should be allowed to return to their normal daily activities. Athletes with burning hands syndrome or

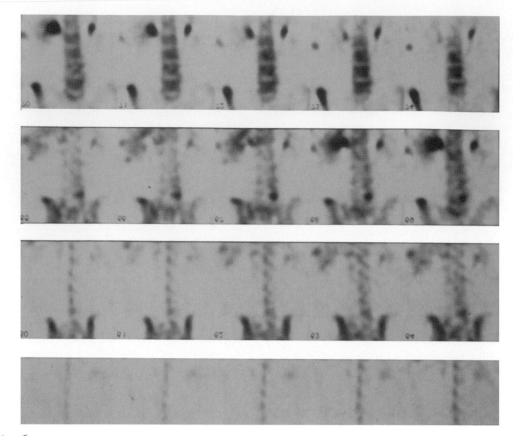

Fig. 6. Radionuclide scan demonstrating increased activity at the L5 pars region explaining this professional football player's continued low back pain. This was successfully managed conservatively.

brachial plexus injuries may be considered healed and safe for return to play when their neurological examination returns to normal and they are symptom free (69). Those whose fractures require halo vest or surgical stabilization are usually considered to have insufficient spinal strength to safely return to contact sports, although there may be exceptions. Even after the fracture has healed, the altered biomechanics in surrounding spinal segments and loss of normal motion produce high risk of future sports-related injury.

Managing athletes with traumatic spine or spinal cord injury presents unique challenges for the spinal surgeon. The classification scheme previously described is useful in decision making regarding optimal treatment and ultimate playing status of these athletes. Type I athletic injuries are those with permanent neurologic injury and preclude the player from further participation in contact sports. Type II injuries consist of transient neurologic disturbances with normal radiographic studies. If the complete workup reveals no injury, these players may return to competition once they are symptom free. Type III injuries are heterogeneous, including all players with radiographic abnormalities. Those athletes with bony or ligamentous spinal instability, or spinal cord contusion, are advised not to return to contact sports. Other radiographic abnormalities, such as spear-tackler's spine, posterior ligamentous injury, congenital fusion or stenosis, herniated discs, or degenerative spondylitic disease require consideration on an individual basis.

References

1. Bailes JE, Maroon JC. Management of cervical spine injuries in athletes. *Sports Med Clin North Am* 1989;8:43–58.
2. Bailes JE, Hadley MN, Quigley MR, et al. Management of athletic injuries of the cervical spine and spinal cord. *Neurosurgery* 1991; 29:491–497.
3. Bailes JE, Herman JM, Quigley MR, et al. Diving injuries of the cervical spine. *Surg Neurol* 1990;4:155–158.
4. CDC Communication. Football-related spinal cord injuries among high school players—Louisiana, 1989. *MMWR* 1990;39:586–587.
5. Clarke KS. Epidemiology of athletic neck injury. *Clin Sports Med* 1998;17:83–97.
6. Scher AT. Diving injuries to the cervical spinal cord. *S Afr Med J* 1981;59:603–605.
7. Raymond CA. Summer's drought reinforces diving's dangers. *JAMA* 1988;260:1199–1200.
8. Frankel HL, Montero FA, Penny PT. Spinal cord injuries due to diving. *Paraplegia* 1980;18:118–122.
9. Good RP, Nickel VL. Cervical spine injuries resulting from water sports. *Spine* 1980;5:502–506.
10. Kewalramini LS, Kraus JF. Acute spinal cord lesions from diving—epidemiological and clinical features. *West J Med* 1977;126: 353–361.
11. Steinbruck K, Paeslack V. Analysis of 139 spinal cord injuries due to accidents in water sports. *Paraplegia* 1980;18:86–93.
12. Albrand OW, Watter J. Underwater deceleration curves in relation to injuries from diving. *Surg Neurol* 1975;4:461–464.
13. Cantu RC, Mueller FO. Catastrophic spine injuries in football. *J Spinal Disord* 1990;3:227–231.
14. Torg JS, Truex R Jr, Quedenfeld TC, et al. The national football head and neck injury registry. *JAMA* 1979;241:1477–1479.
15. Torg JS, Truex RC Jr, Marshall J, et al. Spinal injury at the level of the third and fourth cervical vertebrae from football. *J Bone Joint Surg* 1977;59A:1015–1019.
16. Clarke K. National Spinal Cord Injury Data Research Center, Phoenix, 1983.
17. Nadeau MT, Brown T, Boatman J, et al. The prevention of softball injuries: the experience at Yokota. *Mil Med* 1990;155:3–5.

18. Jackson D, Mannarino F. Lumbar spine in athletes. In: Scott W, ed. *Principles of sports medicine*. Baltimore: Williams & Wilkins, 1984: 212–215.

19. Jackson D, Wiltse L. Low back pain in athletes. *Phys Sports Med* 1983;2:53.

20. Micheli L, Hall J, Miller E. Use of modified Boston brace for back injuries in athletes. *Am J Sports Med* 1980;8:351.

21. Smith C. Physical management of muscular low back pain in the athlete. *Can Med Assoc J* 1977;177:632.

22. Sward L, Hellstrom M, Jacobsson B, et al. Back pain and radiologic changes in the thoraco-lumbar spine of athletes. *Spine* 1990;15: 124–129.

23. Clark JE. Apophyseal fracture of the lumbar spine in adolescence. *Orthop Rev* 1991;20:512–516.

24. Kovac D, Negovetic L, Vukic M, et al. [Surgical treatment of lumbar disc hernias in athletes]. *Reumatizam* 1998;46:35–41.

25. Garth WP Jr, Van Patten PK. Fractures of the lumbar lamina with epidural hematoma simulating herniation of a disc. A case report. *J Bone Joint Surg* 1989;71A:771–772.

26. Hirish D, Inglemark B, Miller M. The anatomical basis of low back pain. *Acta Orthop Scand* 1963;33:1.

27. Mooney V, Robertson J. The facet syndrome. *Clin Orthop* 1976;115: 149.

28. Ellison A. *Training and sports medicine*. Chicago: American Academy of Orthopedic Surgeons, 1984.

29. Wiltse L, Widell E, Jackson D. Fatigue fracture: the basic lesion in isthmic spondylolisthesis. *J Bone Joint Surg* 1975;57:27.

30. Micheli L. Back injuries in dancers. *Clin Sports Med* 1983;2:473.

31. Torg JS, Corcoran TA, Thibault LE, et al. Cervical cord neurapraxia: classification, pathomechanics, morbidity, and management guidelines. *J Neurosurg* 1997;87:843–50.

32. Rivara FP, Thompson DC, Thompson RS. Epidemiology of bicycle injuries and risk factors for serious injury. *Inj Prev* 1997;3:110–114.

33. Weiss BD. Nontraumatic injuries in amateur long distance bicyclists. *Am J Sports Med* 1985;13:187–192.

34. Wilber CA, Holland GJ, Madison RE, et al. An epidemiological analysis of overuse injuries among recreational cyclists. *Int J Sports Med* 1995;16:201–206.

35. Salai M, Brosh T, Blankstein A, et al. Effect of changing the saddle angle on the incidence of low back pain in recreational bicyclists. *Br J Sports Med* 1999;33:398–400.

36. Wilberger JE Jr. Athletic spinal cord and spine injuries. *Clin Sports Med* 1998;17:113.

37. Bernhang A, Winslet G. Equestrian injuries. *Phys Sports Med* 1983; 11:90.

38. Brooks W, Bixby-Hammett D. Prevention of neurologic injuries in equestrian sports. *Phys Sports Med* 1988;16:84–95.

39. Hamilton M, Tranmer B. Nervous injuries in horseback-riding accidents. *J Trauma* 1993;34:227–231.

40. Grossman JA, Kulund DN, Miller CW, et al. Equestrian injuries. Results of a prospective study. *JAMA* 1978;240:1881–1882.

41. Nebergall R, Bauer J, Eimen R. Rough rides: how much risk in rodeo. *Phys Sports Med* 1992;20:85–92.

42. Alexander MJ. Biomechanical aspects of lumbar spine injuries in athletes: a review. *Can J Appl Sport Sci* 1985;10:1–20.

43. Clarke K. An epidemiological view. In: Torg J, ed. *Athletic injuries to the head, neck and face*. St. Louis: Mosby-Yearbook, 1991:19–21.

44. Kolt GS, Kirkby RJ. Epidemiology of injury in elite and subelite female gymnasts: a comparison of retrospective and prospective findings. *Br J Sports Med* 1999;33:312–318.

45. Silver JR, Silver DD, Godfrey JJ. Injuries of the spine sustained during gymnastic activities. *Br Med J (Clin Res Ed)* 1986;293:861–863.

46. Clarke K. Spinal cord injuries in organized sports. *SCI Digest* 1980; 16.

47. Wadley GH, Albright JP. Women's intercollegiate gymnastics. Injury patterns and "permanent" medical disability. *Am J Sports Med* 1993; 21:314–320.

48. Letts M, Smallman T, Afanasiev R, et al. Fracture of the pars interarticularis in adolescent athletes: a clinical-biomechanical analysis. *J Pediatr Orthop* 1986;6:40–46.

49. Kew T, Noakes T, Scher A. A retrospective study of spinal cord injuries in Cape Province rugby players. *S Afr Med J* 1991;80: 127–133.

50. Silver JR, Gill S. Injuries of the spine sustained during rugby. *Sports Med* 1988;5:328–334.

51. Torg JS, Pavlov H, Genuario SE, et al. Neurapraxia of the cervical spinal cord with transient quadriplegia. *J Bone Joint Surg* 1986;68: 1354–1370.

52. Burry H, Calcinai C. The need to make rugby safer. *BMJ* 1988;296: 149–150.

53. Scher A. Rugby injuries to the cervical spine and spinal cord: a ten year review. *Clin Sports Med* 1998;17:197.

54. Scher A. Rugby injuries of the spine and spinal cord. *Clin Sports Med* 1987;6:87–99.

55. Scher A. The high rugby tackle—an avoidable cause of cervical spinal cord injury. *S Afr Med J* 1978;53:1015–1018.

56. Scher A. The "double" tackle—another cause of serious cervical spinal injury in rugby players. *S Afr Med J* 1983;64:595–596.

57. Jarret GJ, Orwin JF, Dick RW. Injuries in collegiate wrestling. *Am J Sports Med* 1998;26:674–680.

58. Roaf R. A study of the mechanics of spinal injuries. *J Bone Joint Surg* 1960;42B:810–823.

59. Leidholt J. Spine injuries to athletes: be prepared. *Orthop Clin North Am* 1973;4:691–707.

60. Wu WQ, Lewis RC. Injuries of the cervical spine in high school wrestling. *Surg Neurol* 1985;23:143–147.

61. Hellstrom M, Jacobsson B, Sward L, et al. Radiologic abnormalities of the thoraco-lumbar spine in athletes. *Acta Radiol* 1990;31:127–132.

62. Rossi F, Dragoni S. Lumbar spondylolysis: occurrence in competitive athletes. Updated achievements in a series of 390 cases. *J Sports Med Phys Fitness* 1990;30:450–452.

63. Maroon JC. "Burning hands" in football spinal cord injuries. *JAMA* 1977;238:2049–2051.

64. Lyness SS, Simcone FA. Vascular complications of upper cervical spine injuries. *Orthop Clin North Am* 1978;9:1029.

65. Hart GR, Easton JD. Dissection of cervical and cerebral arteries. *Neurol Clin North Am* 1983;1:155.

66. Zwimpfer TJ, Bernstein M. Spinal cord concussion. *J Neurosurg* 1990;72:894–900.

67. Torg JS, Sennett B, Pavlov H, et al. Spear tackler's spine. *Am J Sports Med* 1993;21:640–649.

68. Clancy WG, Brand RL, Bergfield JA. Upper trunk brachial plexus injuries in contact sports. *Am J Sports Med* 1977;5:209–216.

69. Poindexter DP, Johnson EW. Football shoulder and neck injury: a study of the "stinger." *Arch Phys Med Rehabil* 1984;65:601–602.

70. Levitz CL, Reilly PJ, Torg JS. The pathomechanics of chronic, recurrent cervical nerve root neurapraxia. The chronic burner syndrome. *Am J Sports Med* 1997;25:73–76.

71. Wilberger JE, Abla A, Maroon JC. Burning hands syndrome revisited. *Neurosurgery* 1986;19:1038–1040.

72. Kline DG, Hudson AR. Acute injuries of peripheral nerves. In: Youmans JR, ed. *Neurological surgery*. Philadelphia: WB Saunders, 1990;2423–2510.

73. Torg JS, Ramsey-Emrhein JA. Suggested management guidelines for participation in collision activities with congenital, developmental, or postinjury lesions involving the cervical spine. *Med Sci Sports Exerc* 1997;29:S256–S272.

74. White AA 3rd, Johnson RM, Panjabi MM, et al. Biomechanical analysis of chemical stability in the cervical spine. *Clin Orthop Relat Res* 1975;109:85–96.

75. Meyer PR Jr, Heim S. Surgical stabilization of the cervical spine. In: Meyer PR Jr, ed. *Surgery of spine trauma*. New York: Churchill Livingstone, 1989:397–523.

76. Torg JS, Narayan RJ Jr, Pavlov H, et al. The relationship of developmental narrowing of the cervical spinal canal to reversible and irreversible injury of the cervical spinal cord in football players: an epidemiological study. *J Bone Joint Surg* 1996;78A:1308–1314.

77. Torg JS. *Athletic injuries to head, neck and face*. St. Louis: Mosby-Yearbook, 1991.

78. Herzog RJ, Wiens JJ, Dillingham MF, et al. Normal cervical spine morphometry and cervical spinal stenosis in asymptomatic professional football players. *Spine* 1991;16:S178–S186.

79. Johnson RM, Wolf JW Jr. Stability. In: Bailey RW, ed. *The cervical spine*. Philadelphia: Lippincott, 1983:35–53.

80. Schneider RC, Gosch HH, Norrell H, et al. Vascular insufficiency and differential distortion of brain and cord caused by cervicomedullary football injuries. *J Neurosurg* 1970;33:363–375.

81. Bailes JE, Cerullo LJ, Engelhard HH. Injuries. In: Meyer PR Jr, ed. *Surgery of spine trauma*. New York: Churchill Livingstone, 1989: 137–156.

166. Metastatic Disease of the Cranial Cervical Junction

John Martin and William T. Monacci

Metastatic cancer to the cranial-cervical junction remains a formidable challenge for those caring for patients with malignant disease. For the purposes of this chapter the cranial-cervical junction is defined as the most cephalad two cervical vertebrae, the atlas and axis, the foramen magnum, and the caudal clivus. Involvement at this level is usually osseous in nature, although extension from metastatic sarcoma to the local soft tissues is possible. Histological types of metastatic disease that most commonly affect this area are those that have a predilection for osseous spread: breast, prostate, lung, and hemopoietic neoplasms. Other rarer tumors include renal and metastatic bony neoplasms such as osteosarcoma.

Spread of malignant cells to the spine is thought to occur through one of several possible routes. The most common is through the valveless basivertebral or Batson's plexus that leads to involvement primarily of the anterior and middle columns. Direct extension to this region from solid tumors such as lymphoma through the intervertebral foramen cancers can also occur. Seventy-three percent of patients with breast cancer are found to have spinal metastases at autopsy. One-third of patients with common solid tumors such as soft tissue sarcomas and lung carcinomas have spinal metastases. Approximately 5% to 10% of patients with advanced cancer present with epidural spinal cord compression as an initial manifestation. This comprises approximately 18,000 cases. The ratio of involvement of the different segments of the spine is roughly equivalent to their sagittal length, with the cervical spine involved in approximately 10% of cases and the cranial-cervical junction in 3% of patients (1). The median survival in these patients is generally poor, although longevity is improving owing to advances in cancer therapy.

Age of onset is typically in the sixth and seventh decade of life, with incidence evenly divided between the sexes, thus reflecting the site of origin. In one large study of metastatic spinal disease, 47% of patients presenting with symptoms and signs of epidural compression had no previous diagnosis of malignancy. The site of origin was subsequently identified in 70% of cases, of which 50% was pulmonary in origin. In large tertiary medical centers the number of patients presenting with manifestations of spinal cord compression as the initial sign was significantly lower (2).

Early recognition in the management of cancer involving the spinal column is important in maintaining the ability to reconstruct and stabilize effectively. The hallmark of clinical presentation is intractable pain occurring day and night that is unrelieved with conventional pain management techniques. Studies have concluded this symptom is frequently present many months prior to changes on plain radiographs (3). Patients with a known history of malignancy and new or progressive neck and/or back pain warrant aggressive imaging by their health care providers. Patients with thoracic pain, pain worsened by recumbency, and pain refractory to conservative measures should receive a radiographic evaluation. Symptoms of spinal cord compression including myelopathy and/or radiculopathy occur in most cases long after the onset of pain. Pain has been found to be a good localizer for site of involvement (3).

Progressive growth of metastases can lead to focal neurological deficits from either spinal instability with osseous collapse/ listhesis or epidural disease with direct compression of neural structures. At the cranial-cervical junction this can lead to one of several presentations. Atlantoaxial subluxation may produce spastic quadriparesis or cruciate paralysis due to compression of the descending medullary pyramids (4). Basilar impression may lead to various signs of brainstem dysfunction (5). Compression of the exiting C2 root leads to cephalgia in the distribution of the greater occipital nerve. Patients exhibiting these signs warrant immobilization and prompt imaging.

Principles of Treatment

Management of metastatic spinal disease should be directed toward achieving the following goals: (a) alleviation of pain, (b) preservation/restoration of neurological function, (c) restoration of biomechanical stability, and (d) local cure when possible (6). Clinical decision making in these patients is complex. The unique anatomy of the cranial-cervical junction obviates comparison to the remainder of the axial skeleton for the incidence of instability or neurological compromise from epidural compression. Due to the infrequent involvement of this region with metastatic disease, clinical data from the literature is limited. While case reports and small case series exist, the natural history of cervical metastasis has been poorly delineated to date (7). Management decisions should be predicated on the patient's present neurological status, level of pain, degree of structural instability, medical and nutritional status, prior therapy, and life expectancy.

Nonoperative treatment of metastatic disease is indicated in those patients whose life expectancy is short, less than 3 to 6 months, as well as those whose cardiovascular and/or pulmonary status prohibit general anesthesia. Complete loss of neurological function for longer than 24 hours is also a relative contraindication. In the absence of significant neurological deficit, bracing using a hard cervical collar is justified with the patients followed closely for either increasing neurological deficit or deteriorating structural support. Surgical intervention can be offered if these signs of progression occur. A series of odontoid fractures in patients with breast cancer were treated in this manner at Sloan-Kettering, with six of 18 patients necessitating fusion at some point during their treatment (8). A hard collar with or without a thoracic extension is preferred over the use of a halo fixation device because of the additional morbidity introduced with pin fixation and the vest, which can restrict chest movement particularly in the elderly and pulmonary compromised.

Preoperative Evaluation and Management

Management of the patient with cranial cervical junction metastatic disease is dependent on several key factors including the specific tumor biology and stage of disease, the stability of the spine, location of the tumor, overall health of the patient, as well as the current neurological status. The major factor in determining a course of treatment is the nature of the patient's primary malignancy and what the patient's life expectancy is. Oncological colleagues who are familiar with the course of the disease and the patient's comorbidities may approximate life expectancy with some accuracy. Some patients harboring less aggressive breast or prostate malignancies can live an extended period of time and may warrant aggressive treatment. If the patient has a poor nutritional status or a history of tobacco use, wound healing and bone formation may be impaired. The degree of instability plays a role in whether bracing and observation versus surgical intervention should be utilized.

Radiation therapy plays a major role in the management of cranial-cervical junction metastatic disease, just as it does in other areas of the spine. For radiosensitive tumors from the prostate and breast in patients who do not have a rapid loss of function, gross instability, or bony compression, radiation therapy is usually the preferred means of initial treatment. Bracing, usually a hard cervical collar, is used until after the completion of radiation, to be followed by dynamic imaging of the cranial-cervical junction to assess any resulting loss of stability. Even tumors such as colon, kidney, and adenocarcinoma of lung origin, which are relatively radioresistant tumors, can be palliated effectively with radiotherapy alone in the patient with a short life expectancy (9). Depending on the method of fractionation, cord tolerance is thought to be between 45 and 50 Gy. Radiotherapy varies depending on the institution; however, a typical regimen is 30 Gy over 10 fractions (9). If latent instability develops, surgical stabilization may be required depending on the patient factors previously discussed.

Preoperative Planning and Preparation

Cranial-cervical arthrodesis restricts motion significantly and may significantly impair a patient's activities. Occipitoatlantoaxial fixation results in a loss of approximately 25 degrees of flexion/extension and 40 degrees of lateral rotation. This can have a significant impact on ambulation, particularly in patients with impaired proprioception or balance function.

Contrast triplaner magnetic resonance imaging (MRI) remains the standard for evaluating the osseoligamentous integrity of the cranial-cervical junction, and is a noninvasive means of identifying neural compression by epidural metastases (Fig. 1). For patients who are unable to have an MRI, contrast myelography and follow-up computed tomography (CT) scanning is helpful. The patient should be assessed for stability at the cranial-cervical junction with dynamic plain film imaging supplemented with thin-section helical CT scanning with reconstructions in the sagittal and coronal planes. This modality exquisitely demonstrates the bony anatomy of the region, and allows for the assessment of the integrity of elements that could be used for fixation (Fig. 2). It has largely replaced the use of thin-section tomography in most centers; however, the latter remains quite useful.

Plain film imaging continues to play a role in both diagnosis and treatment of metastatic disease. Vertebral collapse, focal osteopenia, and pedicle dropout are classic findings in metastatic spinal disease. Though plain film lacks the sensitivity of other modalities, its relative ease and low expense allow for several applications. Serial imaging allows for detection of progressive deformity. Dynamic films can provide information on the relative stability and plastic deformity of the spinal column. Flexion-extension films reveal instability not assessed by static images. Traction films provide information on the relative re-

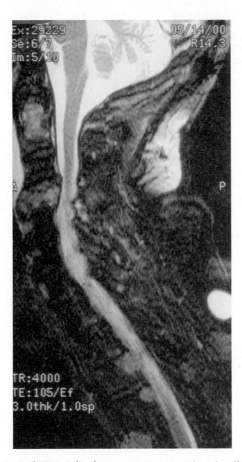

Fig. 1. Sagittal T2-weighted magnetic resonance imaging (MRI) demonstrating metastatic disease of the prostate to C1-2 as well as osseous destruction from involvement of the subaxial cervical spine.

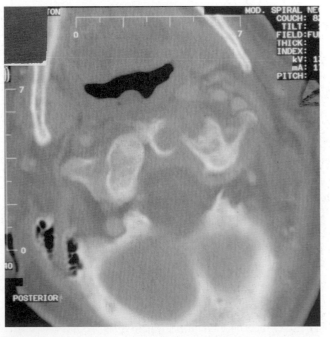

Fig. 2. Axial computed tomography (CT) scan demonstrating osseous involvement of C2 by metastatic prostate cancer.

ducibility of pathology. Angiography is indicated in vascular tumors or those with suspected involvement of the vertebral artery and/or foramen transversarium. Assessment of tumor vascular supply and the relative contributions of an involved vertebral artery to the cerebral circulation can be directly assessed (10). When indicated, endovascular techniques can be utilized to embolize blood supply to the tumor (11). Balloon test occlusion should be considered if vertebral sacrifice is likely.

Bone scanning plays a limited role in the evaluation of symptomatic metastatic disease. Though capable of detecting subclinical metastatic disease, it lacks specificity and provides nonanatomical information on localized disease. Its utility lies in its ability to localize additional foci of metastatic disease to assist in the clinical decision-making process. Up to 50% of patients presenting with a diagnosis of spinal metastasis are not known to have a primary malignancy at the time of presentation. In the absence of a known diagnosis, biopsy of an accessible spinal lesion can provide diagnostic information that can be utilized to guide further therapy. CT-guided biopsy of cervical spine pathology has been demonstrated in small series to have a diagnostic accuracy of greater than 85% (11).

Cervical traction with either Gardner-Wells tongs or a halo ring may be necessary to reduce deformities resulting from osseous collapse or ligamentous laxity. In cases where C1-2 transarticular screws are going to be used, frameless stereotaxis may be helpful in both preoperative planning as well as operative placement of the screws.

The patient's medical and nutritional status should be optimized prior to surgical therapy if possible to maximize wound healing and bone formation. The use of corticosteroids to improve neurologic status perioperatively is well documented (12).

Operative Stategies

The goals of surgical intervention are to provide stabilization, relieve compression of the neuroaxis, and alleviate pain. Surgical treatment also promotes early mobilization and relief from pain in approximately 80% of patients (13). The method of decompression and fixation depends on the location and extent of involvement of the cranial-cervical articulation. Spinal cord compression from tumor bulk is rare in comparison to the rest of the spinal axis at this level given the relatively large diameter of the spinal canal. The majority of patients' disease is found secondary to pain prior to the onset of significant neurological deficit. Most patients who are found to have spinal metastases are in an advanced stage of the disease, and thus the majority of procedures will be directed toward providing stabilization. In those cases where decompression is required, the approaches used are the same as those for benign pathology or primary neoplasms such as osteoma or chordoma.

If anterior decompression is warranted in the C1-2 region, a choice of transcervical/parapharyngeal approaches or a transoral route may be used. The advantages and disadvantages of each method warrant discussion. The high cervical parapharyngeal approach yields a primarily unilateral exposure to the C1-2 region without violating the gastrointestinal (GI) tract (14). The transoral route allows for good exposure of the midline but is limited laterally and opens the wound to GI flora. Fixation methods through this exposure are difficult and prone to infection. When postoperative radiotherapy is employed, not opening the GI tract is a definite advantage, as wound breakdown after a transoral procedure is a very difficult situation to manage.

Determining whether to incorporate the occiput in the patient with malignant involvement of C1-2 is usually straightforward. The amount of osseous destruction necessary to cause bony collapse and ligamentous laxity requires the incorporation of the occiput the majority of the time, particularly when the base of skull is involved. Rigid fixation with a contoured titanium ring/loop can be secured in a number of ways depending on the availability of involved bone. If the posterior elements are intact, sublaminar wires at C1-2 with occipital wires can be used. Screw fixation both at the occiput and the C1-2 articulation can also provide immediate short-term stability. The routine use of autograft over methylmethacrylate in all but the shortest life expectancy patients is the method of choice. Methylmethacrylate can be used to augment a bone graft arthrodesis for more immediate stability (15).

Postoperative Principles

Postoperative efforts should be aimed at mobilizing the patient as soon as feasible in an appropriate orthosis, which in most cases is a hard collar or extended hard collar depending on the rigidity of the construct. Bracing is difficult because of the high degree of multiplanar movement allowed by the cranial-cervical junction complex. Of the options available only the cranial-thoracic fixation orthoses offer significant stability at the cranial-cervical junction (16). Most orthoses allow significant translational and capital flexion-extension. Use of a halo vest device in these frequently disabled patients can lead to poor mobilization and further complications such as infection, pin dislodgment, and calvarial penetration. Four to 6 months in an orthosis followed by dynamic imaging once a fusion mass is recognized is important to verify fusion and resulting stability. Postoperative radiotherapy can proceed once the wound is healed. Postoperative nutritional status should continue to be optimized.

References

1. Byrne TN. Spinal cord compression from epidural metastases. *N Engl J Med* 1992;327:614–619.
2. Grant R, Papadopoulus SM, Greenberg H. Metastatic epidural spinal cord compression. *Neurol Clin* 1991;9:825–839.
3. Black P. Spinal metastasis: current status and recommended guidelines for management. *Neurosurgery* 1979;5:726–734.
4. Zeidman SM, Ducker TB. Rheumatoid arthritis: neuroanatomy, compression, and grading of deficits. *Spine* 1994;19:2259–2266.
5. Rosenberg WS, Salame KS, Shumrick KV, et al. Compression of the upper cervical spinal cord causing symptoms of brainstem compromise: a case report. *Spine* 1998;23:1497–1500.
6. Sundaresan N, Scher H, Yagoda A. Surgical treatment of spinal metastases in kidney cancer. *J Clin Oncol* 1986;4:1851–1856.
7. Rao S, Badani K, Schildhauer T, et al. Metastatic malignancy of the cervical spine: a nonoperative history. *Spine* 1992;17:407–412.
8. Sundaresan N, Galicich JH, Lane JM, et al. Treatment of odontoid fractures in cancer patients. *J Neurosurg* 1981;54(2):187–192.
9. Seydel HH, ed. *Tumors of the nervous system.* New York: Raven Press, 1975.
10. Sen C, Eisenberg M, Casden AM, et al. Management of the vertebral artery in excision of extradural tumors of the cervical spine. *Neurosurgery* 1995;36:106–116.
11. Hess T, Kramann B, Schmidt E, et al. Use of preoperative vascular embolization in spinal metastasis resection. *Arch Orthop Trauma Surg* 1997;116:279–282.
12. Hillner BE, Ingle JN, Berenson JR, et al. American Society of Clinical Oncology guideline on the role of bisphosphonates in breast cancer. *J Clin Oncol* 2000;18:1378–1391.

13. Siegal T, Siegal T. Surgical decompression of anterior or posterior malignant epidural tumors compressing the spinal cord: a prospective study. *Neurosurgery* 1985;17:424–432.
14. McDonnell DE, Harrison SJ. Lateral approach to the craniocervical complex. *Tech Neurosurg* 1998;4:306–318.
15. Ransford AO, Crockard HA, Pozo JL. Craniocervical instability treated with contoured loop fixation. *J Bone Joint Surg* 1986;68B: 173–177.
16. Benzel EC. *Biomechanics of spine stabilization: principles and clinical practice.* New York: McGraw Hill, 1994:13.

167. Metastatic Disease of the Subaxial Cervical Spine

Anthony K. Frempong-Boadu and Paul R. Cooper

Cancer is the second leading cause of death in the United States (1). Two thirds of all cancer patients ultimately develop metastases (2,3). The most frequently encountered skeletal metastases are those that involve the spine (4,5). Evidence of vertebral body metastases is found in over one third of cancer patients in autopsy series (6). Although any systemic tumor can metastasize to the spine, the vast majority arise from breast, lung, prostate, kidney, thyroid, and the hematopoietic system (4, 7–9).

In most cases the spread of cancer to the spinal column is hematogenous. Although tumor may metastasize to any of the vertebral elements, the vertebral body is more commonly involved than the posterior elements, presumably because the highly vascular red marrow of the vertebral body promotes metastatic growth and because the mass of the body is large in comparison to the posterior elements. As the tumor grows, bone resorption occurs due to the influence of osteoclast activating factors and prostaglandins (10).

The distribution of metastatic disease in the spine is directly proportional to the volume of the vertebrae (11). Because the cervical spine contains a small volume of bone compared to the lumbar and thoracic spine, metastatic disease of the cervical spine is distinctly less common than to the thoracic and lumbar regions (5).

Because of differences in regional anatomy, the potential for instability and neurological dysfunction depends on the level of the affected vertebra (12). In the upper cervical spine, the involvement of the atlas and axis by osseous metastases poses a risk of rotatory instability or craniocervical dislocation. Similarly neoplastic destruction of the dens can lead to atlantoaxial instability (13).

The subaxial cervical spine (C3-7) undergoes a wide range of motion under physiological conditions; in this location destruction of a vertebral body with concomitant involvement of the posterior elements will lead to instability and loss of the structural integrity of the cervical spine. The kyphotic deformity that results from destruction of both anterior and posterior elements produces pain and direct impingement of the thecal sac and spinal cord by bone or tumor.

Clinical Presentation

Metastasis to the spine frequently represents a manifestation of advanced systemic disease. However, the wide spectrum of clinical presentations underscores the need to individualize treatment plans in these patients. The therapeutic goals are to obtain an accurate diagnosis, control pain, preserve or restore neurological function, and maintain alignment and stability of the bony spine.

Neck pain in a cancer patient should be considered to be the result of metastatic disease until proven otherwise. The most common sites of pain in a patient with osseous metastases to the subaxial cervical spine are the neck and interscapular region. Most often the pain begins slowly and at a low level of intensity but is usually progressive and may be exacerbated by movement or changes in position. When neck pain begins acutely it is often the result of pathologic compression fractures associated with vertebral body destruction and development of instability.

Pain and paresthesias in a radicular distribution are present in 20% of patients with cervical metastases (14). Weakness, sensory loss, and sphincter dysfunction secondary to spinal cord compression may follow within weeks to months depending on the growth rate of the tumor and the extent of bony involvement. Acute symptoms of spinal cord compression are usually associated with pathological cervical fracture/dislocation.

A careful history and physical examination will provide a baseline for assessing progression of disease and the effect of therapy. The neck should be examined for tenderness to palpation, paraspinous muscle spasm, and localized kyphotic deformity. Motor function is graded using a standard five-point scale. Sensory examination is directed toward eliciting the presence of a sensory level or radicular sensory changes. Deep tendon reflexes, pathological reflexes, and rectal tone are recorded. A postvoid residual is obtained in patients with suspected sphincter dysfunction (15).

Diagnostic Imaging

The goal of imaging evaluation is to define the presence of neural compression, assess the extent of bony destruction, and provide information about stability. In patients with primary tumors of unknown origin it may provide information about etiology. Complete evaluation will usually include plain films, computed tomography (CT) scan, and magnetic resonance imaging (MRI).

PLAIN FILMS. Plain films are a useful screening examination and should be obtained on any patient with a history of systemic malignancy who complains of neck pain. Evaluation of plain radiographs should include an assessment of the following: qualitative bony alterations (i.e., lytic, blastic, or sclerotic abnormalities); the site of involvement (vertebral body, pedicles, or posterior elements); and assessment of the structural integrity of the spinal column (i.e., level of involvement, vertebral body height, presence of pathological fractures/dislocations or malalignment).

The earliest and most common radiological abnormality seen on plain radiographs in the thoracic and lumbar spine is pedicle erosion. In the cervical spine vertebral body collapse and destruction by tumor is easier to see and is more common. In the thoracic and lumbar spine neoplastic vertebral body destruction may sometimes be difficult to distinguish from spontaneous compression fractures due to osteoporosis. However, the cervical spine supports little weight, and compression fractures are uncommon in the absence of a history of trauma. Neoplastic vertebral body destruction may be differentiated from pyogenic osteomyelitis by preservation of the disc spaces. The intervertebral disc is highly resistant to tumor invasion and will maintain its height despite significant vertebral body involvement. On the other hand in patients with pyogenic processes involving the vertebral bodies, the intervening discs are collapsed and destroyed early in the course of the disease (16,17).

The sensitivity of plain radiographs in detecting early metastases is low; 30% to 50% of trabecular bone must be destroyed before changes are evident on plain radiographs (18). Although plain radiographs are frequently employed as an initial screening tool, normal plain films do not necessarily indicate the absence of metastatic disease.

BONE SCAN. Technetium (Tc) 99 bone scintigraphy is an effective screening tool for detecting lesions in patients with suspected bony metastases because it shows evidence of metastatic bone disease at an earlier stage than plain radiographs (19,20). Limitations of bone scanning include false-positive results in patients with nonmalignant disease (degenerative processes, trauma, metabolic bone disease) and false-negative results in patients with plasmacytoma. Although bone scans lack specificity, their sensitivity makes them a valuable tool in assessing symptomatic patients with negative or equivocal radiographs, in determining the extent of systemic dissemination (21), and in directing subsequent imaging studies.

COMPUTED TOMOGRAPHY. Computed tomography (CT) is highly sensitive to alterations in bone density and will identify the extent of bony destruction and the distribution of a lesion (vertebral body, pedicles, or posterior elements) in the axial plane. It is the preferred modality for demonstrating the extent of bony involvement of metastatic lesions in the cervical spine. Soft tissue compression of neural elements may sometimes be inferred from a good CT, but compression by retropulsed bone or kyphotic deformity is usually obvious when appropriate bone windows are obtained.

CT/MYELOGRAPHY. Myelography with and without CT was formerly the preferred imaging modality for patients with neurological deficits secondary to compressive lesions of the spinal cord prior to the advent of MRI.

Patients with an unstable spine may experience neurological deterioration when tilted on a myelography table or their neck is manipulated to prevent the intracranial passage of contrast (22,23). Lumbar puncture in the presence of a high-grade extra-dural block may result in neurological deterioration. If the level of a block identified on lumbar myelography is inconsistent with a patient's neurological examination, a second cervical puncture is necessary to determine the extent of a single lesion or to identify multiple lesions (24–26).

CT myelography is now used only when MRI is unavailable or cannot be used because of patient size or the presence of certain implanted metallic objects such as pacemakers or aneurysm clips.

MAGNETIC RESONANCE IMAGING. Magnetic resonance imaging (MRI) is the imaging modality of choice for the evaluation of neural compression by bone or tumor in patients with suspected metastatic neoplasms of the cervical spine (27–29). It provides excellent delineation of tumor extent and involvement of paravertebral structures. Furthermore the entire spinal column can be visualized in the sagittal plain to identify noncontiguous areas of spinal involvement, an important consideration as multiple sites of spinal cord compression are present in as many as 19% of patients with metastatic bone disease (30).

The vast majority of metastatic lesions appear hypointense relative to marrow on T1-weighted images and hyperintense on T2-weighted images (31). Gadolinium enhancement is unnecessary for the evaluation of spine metastases and should not be used because it may obscure metastatic bone lesions. This occurs when the involved vertebrae enhances and becomes isointense with the marrow in the normal vertebrae.

FINE-NEEDLE ASPIRATION/BIOPSY. Fine-needle aspiration/biopsy performed using CT guidance can provide a histological diagnosis without the need for operation. This technique is particularly useful in patients who present without a known primary lesion or have other nonosseous metastatic lesions that are not readily accessible for biopsy. While the exact tissue diagnosis is generally not essential in patients who will need operative decompression or stabilization, knowledge of the presence of a hypervascular tumor (hypernephroma, thyroid, melanoma) requiring embolization is important in patients who will likely need operative resection. Needle biopsy is also useful in establishing the diagnosis of lymphoreticular tumors, which may be treated with chemotherapy and radiation without the need for surgery.

However, because only a small amount of tissue is obtained for evaluation, fine-needle aspiration/biopsy is subject to sampling errors. Although the diagnostic accuracy of fine-needle aspiration/biopsy has been quoted to be as high as 80% (32–34), in our experience aspiration/biopsy has been nondiagnostic in at least half of all patients.

ANGIOGRAPHY AND EMBOLIZATION. In hypervascular tumors such as melanoma, hypernephroma, and thyroid carcinomas, preoperative angiography and embolization is advisable to minimize intraoperative blood loss (35–37). We prefer to perform embolization within 48 hours of the definitive surgical procedure to preclude the possibility of revascularization of the lesion through recruitment of adjacent nonembolized feeding vessels (38). Most metastatic cervical spine tumors receive their blood supply from branches of the vertebral artery, making embolization more difficult to perform than with is the case tumors that metastasize to the thoracic and lumbar spine (Fig. 1).

Even when complete occlusion of tumor vessels is not possible, reduction of the blood supply by embolization makes operation easier for the surgeon. When a nondominant vertebral artery is surrounded by tumor that has destroyed the vertebral body and obscured anatomical landmarks, endovascular occlu-

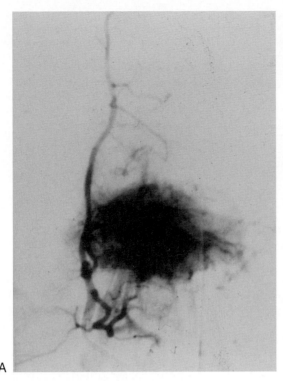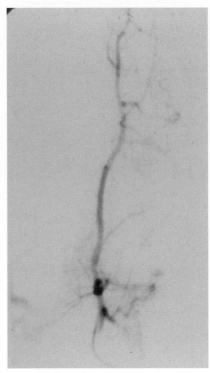

A   B

Fig. 1. **A**: Preoperative arteriogram of a patient with a highly vascular metastatic hemangiopericytoma of C7 supplied by the deep cervical branches of the vertebral artery. **B**: Postembolization angiogram shows obliteration of the blood supply to the tumor.

sion of the vertebral artery will prevent massive hemorrhage from inadvertent operative transection of the vessel during tumor resection.

Management Decision Making

In all but a few lucky patients, complete removal or eradication of tumor metastasizing to the cervical spine is not possible. In the few cases where complete removal is possible, it is likely that other systemic metastases will eventually result in the patient's demise. Therefore, the goal of treatment is improvement in the quality of the patient's remaining life. Operative decompression and stabilization or treatment with chemotherapy and radiation may achieve this by preserving or restoring neurological function, relieving pain, and allowing ambulation.

Before deciding on treatment, the clinician should ask the following questions:

1. What is the patient's current neurological status and how long has the patient been symptomatic? (If the patient has complete neurological deficit, how long has this been present?)
2. Is the neurological examination stable?
3. Is the diagnosis known?
4. Is the tumor radiosensitive (breast, lung, prostate) or radioresistant (melanoma, renal cell)?
5. Has the patient undergone previous radiation therapy (i.e., is the patient a radiation failure)?
6. Is there evidence of cervical spine instability?
7. If spinal cord compression is present, is it caused by tumor or bone?

8. Is the primary lesion controlled and what is the patient's life expectancy?
9. What is the overall health and nutritional status of the patient?

Pretreatment neurological status has been shown to correlate with postoperative outcome (4,39–42). Patients with severe motor dysfunction greater than 24 hours' duration generally will not have any functional recovery with therapy (43). In one study, 79% of patients who were ambulatory at the time of diagnosis remained ambulatory, whereas only 18% of nonambulatory patients regained ambulation (4).

Radiation Therapy

Radiation therapy is the initial treatment in the majority of patients with cervical metastases (44–47). It is recommended for patients with widespread metastases with poor systemic control whose survival is measured in weeks. It is also an appropriate initial treatment for patients with minimal or no neurological findings with soft tissue compression and no evidence of instability.

HISTOLOGICAL DIAGNOSIS. The nature of the tumor is important in predicting the likely response to radiation therapy. Breast, prostate, and hematopoietic tumors are typically radiation sensitive. Metastases from lung and thyroid tumors are intermediate in their radiation responsiveness. Melanoma, hypernephroma, and gastrointestinal tumors are often radioresistant, and unless the tumor is quite small and without significant neural compression, radiation therapy without surgical decompression is likely to fail (46,47).

NEUROLOGICAL STATUS. The patient's pretreatment neurological status is an important predictor of response to radiation therapy. If a patient has severe neurological compromise, it is unlikely that radiation therapy alone will restore neurological function (44–47). The nature of spinal cord compression is also an important predictor of the success of radiation therapy. Patients with neurological deficit from bony compression or instability require operation and will not be helped by radiation therapy.

TREATMENT IN SELECTED PATIENTS. In appropriately selected patients, over half of those treated with radiation therapy will show an improvement in neurological examination and pain control (44–47). The usual dose of radiation depends on the nature of the tumor and length of time over which treatment is given but 3,000 cGy delivered in 300-cGy fractions over 10 days is typical. To avoid radiation injury to the spinal cord, the total dose should be limited to a maximum of 4,500 cGy. The field of treatment should extend at least one vertebral body above and below the lesion. If serial neurological examinations show that the patient is deteriorating, the patient should be considered a radiation failure and treated with surgery.

Operative Management

INDICATIONS. Indications for surgery include patients with (a) an unknown primary who cannot undergo needle biopsy; (b) progressive neurological dysfunction despite treatment with radiation, corticosteroids, and chemotherapy; (c) radioresistant tumors or tumors that have recurred following radiation therapy; (d) instability and dislocations due to bony destruction by tumor; and (e) spinal cord compression by destroyed bone (17, 48,49).

The numbers of patients undergoing operative treatment for metastatic disease of the spine has increased considerably in the past decade for two main reasons. Conceptual advances in the understanding of the biomechanics of the spine and the availability of sophisticated instrumentation for stabilization have greatly improved the neurological outcome from what had been reported in the 1960s and 1970s (8,50–53). In addition, improved survival of patients with a variety of neoplasms has resulted in increased number of patients who present with spinal metastases.

CONTRAINDICATIONS. We do not believe that operation is appropriate in patients with an expected survival of <12 weeks or in those who are so debilitated that operation is likely to result in their demise. Patients who are severely immunocompromised from their disease or recent chemotherapy and those with abnormal clotting studies that cannot be corrected with appropriate replacement therapy are not candidates for operation. Surgical contraindications also include a very radiosensitive tumor (lymphoma, myeloma) in a patient with minimal symptoms, who has not been previously irradiated. Patients with absence of motor or sensory function of greater than 12 hours are unlikely to have neurological improvement with operation and are not candidates for operative decompression unless cervical instability or deformity results in intractable pain.

PREOPERATIVE MANAGEMENT. Preoperatively patients with spinal instability should be placed in cervical traction. Patients who are experiencing severe pain or who have severe bony destruction without instability are treated with a cervical collar. All patients should be placed on high-dose steroids (125 to 250 mg of methylprednisolone or its equivalent q.i.d.). Patients with vascular lesions (renal cell, thyroid, hepatoma, and melanoma) should undergo preoperative angiography and embolization as discussed in a preceding section.

All patients are evaluated with Doppler studies of the lower extremity venous system preoperatively and have placement of intermittent compressive boots preoperatively. If venous thrombosis is detected in the perioperative period, a vena caval filter is placed.

Anesthetic Considerations and Preoperative Preparation. A major concern in patients with osseous metastases to the cervical spine is the pre- and postoperative stability of the spine. In patients with instability who arrive at the operating room in external fixation devices or traction, flexion and extension movements must be minimized during intubation. An awake fiberoptic intubation is preferable because it limits neck manipulation (54,55) and minimizes the risk of iatrogenic spinal cord injury while securing the airway. Prior to induction, the patient should be examined to document movement of the extremities. If the patient is in cervical traction, it is critical to reduce the traction weight to 5 lbs prior to induction of anesthesia, to avoid distraction injury to the spinal cord. In patients who are undergoing anterior operation, traction with the reduced weight is left in place and the head is placed on a doughnut or horseshoe head holder. An x-ray is taken to confirm alignment.

Posterior approaches require a postintubation turn to the prone position. The surgeon should supervise all aspects of the turn and is directly responsible for maintaining a neutral position throughout the entire positioning process using a cervical collar or by maintaining traction on the halo ring or tongs. After the patient is turned to the prone position the cervical tongs or halo ring is removed and the head is secured in a three-pin head holder fixed to the operating table. An x-ray is taken to confirm satisfactory alignment and plan the location of the skin incision.

Although we use neurophysiological monitoring in patients with preservation of neurological function, there is no convincing data in the literature that the use of either somatosensory evoked potentials (SSEPs) or motor evoked potentials (MEPs) beneficially affects outcome. While they may *predict* an adverse neurological outcome, it is not clear that they can prevent neurological disaster (56,57).

SURGICAL MANAGEMENT

Anterior Approach. The primary site of tumor involvement dictates the surgical approach. The majority of osseous metastases to the cervical spine involve the vertebral body and compression by retropulsed bone or tumor is from an anterior location. Therefore, an anterior approach with vertebral body resection and stabilization is appropriate for most patients with metastatic cervical spine disease.

We routinely use the operating microscope; intraoperative fluoroscopy is also used if anterior plates are to be placed. We utilize a standard anterior approach to the spine with a transverse skin incision. A right- or left-sided approach can be used. The choice of side depends on the site of major paraspinal component, the side of previous surgery, or evidence of preoperative unilateral vocal cord paresis. If the patient has had prior anterior cervical surgery, we make an incision on the contralateral side because scarring can make surgery more difficult.

Tumor involvement usually results in a vertebral body that is soft and may be removed with curettes or pituitary rongeurs. After the vertebral body has been removed, we resect the posterior longitudinal ligament for a more complete tumor removal and easier mobilization of retropulsed bone fragments. Because bone may be destroyed in the region of the foramen transversarium, care should be taken not to extend the tumor resection too far laterally lest the vertebral artery be injured. It must be emphasized that operative treatment is palliative and the goal is not cure but decompression and prevention of recurrence within the patient's expected lifetime.

Vertebrectomy should be followed by reconstruction of the anterior load-bearing support structures with either bone graft or methylmethacrylate. If the patient's expected survival is less than 2 years, if postoperative radiation is anticipated, or if multilevel decompression is required, reconstruction with methylmethacrylate is recommended (58–60).

The discs adjacent to the area of resection are removed and a 2- to 3-mm right-angle drill is used to make a hole in the cortical bone of the end plates of the superior and inferior vertebral bodies. Two Steinmann pins are cut to an appropriate length; one is inserted into the upper vertebral body and the other into the lower one through the holes previously drilled into the end plates. The pins should extend 1 to 2 cm into each vertebral body and protrude by the same amount into the area of vertebral body resection so that they overlap each other. Semisolid methylmethacrylate is then poured into the bony defect and is secured in place by the pins (Fig. 2). Care must be taken to avoid contact between the cement and the dura. The use of a Gelfoam sheet can help prevent contact. Because polymerization of the methylmethacrylate occurs through an exo-

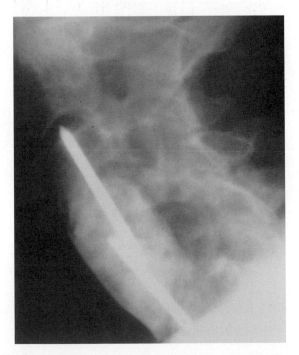

Fig. 2. Postoperative lateral roentgenogram in a patient with metastatic carcinoma destroying the C4 and C5 vertebral bodies. After resection of the involved vertebral bodies, Steinmann pins were advanced into the vertebral bodies of C3 and C6. Methylmethacrylate impregnated with barium was allowed to harden slightly and was then poured into the area of the vertebrectomy around the pins. The methylmethacrylate reconstructs the anterior column, precluding the development of kyphotic deformity, and the pins prevent movement of the methylmethacrylate after it hardens.

thermic reaction, the methylmethacrylate should be irrigated continuously with cool saline as it hardens.

Alternatively, methylmethacrylate may be poured into the defect and stability maintained by anterior cervical plates fixed by screws to the vertebral bodies above and below the resected destroyed vertebral body (Fig. 3). Because methylmethacrylate does not fuse to adjacent bone, we have had concerns about screw and plate loosening in patients with unexpectedly long survival and have preferred to use the technique using Steinmann pins as described above. Backout of the pins through the methylmethacrylate is not possible, and extrusion of the pins through the anterior aspect of the vertebral bodies has not been seen.

If long-term survival is anticipated, anterior column reconstruction with bone graft can be performed. If bone is used, anterior cervical plating should also be performed because it provides immediate stability and helps maintain postreconstruction alignment (61,62).

Posterior Approach. Isolated posterior compression by tumor is less common than anterior compression. When present, laminectomy is appropriate for resecting tumor and decompressing the spinal cord and nerve roots. Care must be taken when dissecting the muscle off the posterior elements to avoid entering the spinal canal inadvertently if the laminae are destroyed by tumor. If the facet joints are intact, laminectomy alone is sufficient and will not result in instability. If there is destruction of the facet joints, instability is likely and posterior instrumentation and fusion should be utilized.

There are a variety of posterior fixation methods and techniques available for subaxial cervical spinal fusion. The authors prefer the use of lateral mass fixation because it can be used for single or multilevel fixation, and does not require intact posterior elements for application as does spinous process or sublaminar wiring. Furthermore, lateral mass plates provide superior rotational stability as they fix the spine close to the facet joint, the site of the instability.

The technique has been well described for patients with trauma (62–66), and there are only minor variations for patients with instability due to neoplastic disease. As a general principle, the plates should be placed bilaterally and symmetrically and include the lateral masses of the unstable vertebrae. If the lateral masses are involved by tumor, the plates should be extended to the next uninvolved level above or below. We prefer to place the screw holes in the lateral masses prior to the laminectomy so that the laminae will protect the spinal cord in case the awl or drill slips while making the holes. Similarly the facets are curetted and packed with bone from uninvolved spinous processes prior to the laminectomy. Patients are placed in a soft cervical collar postoperatively for 8 weeks.

Combined Anterior and Posterior Approach. A combined anterior and posterior approach is used when there is circumferential spinal cord compression by tumor or when kyphotic deformity is present as a result of extensive vertebral body destruction by tumor (Fig. 4). In patients with kyphotic deformities, we prefer to perform the anterior decompression and reconstruction first to allow for correction of the kyphotic deformity. Patients are positioned on the operating table and the traction is adjusted to maximize extension and reduce the deformity. If methylmethacrylate is used for vertebral body replacement, distraction must be maintained until the methylmethacrylate has completely hardened.

After completion of the anterior operation, the patient is placed in the three-pin head holder and turned to the prone position with the head holder fixed to the table. In patients with kyphotic deformity without posterior compression by tumor, lateral mass plates are placed to include the vertebral levels

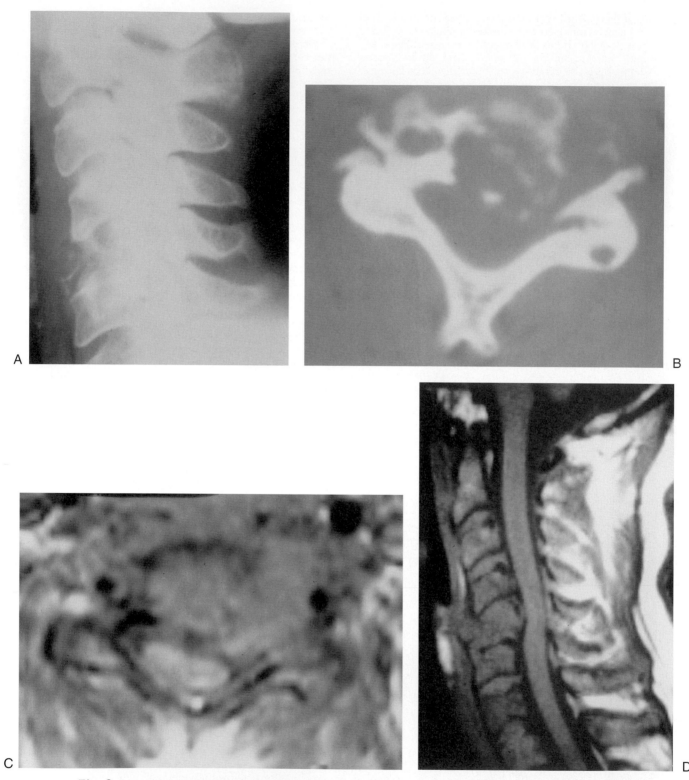

Fig. 3. **A**: Lateral cervical roentgenogram shows vertebral body destruction from metastatic carcinoma of the breast to C5 without significant kyphotic deformity. **B**: Axial computed tomography (CT) shows almost complete destruction of the C5 vertebral body with destruction of bone forming the left foramen transversarium. **C,D**: Axial and sagittal magnetic resonance imaging (MRI) shows the extent of spinal cord compression.

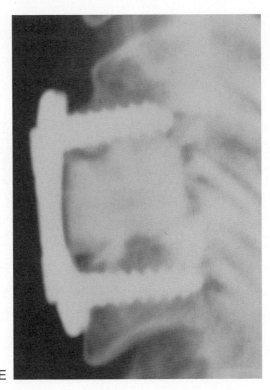

Fig. 3. (continued). **E**: Postoperative lateral roentgenogram shows the bone defect filled by methylmethacrylate with an anterior cervical plate from C4 to C6.

above and below the vertebral body resection. If there is posterior compression by tumor, holes are first drilled in the lateral masses after which laminectomy and tumor resection is carried out. The lateral mass plates are then placed. If a bone graft has been placed anteriorly, we do not pack the facet joints with bone, as anterior fusion will provide sufficient stability. If methylmethacrylate has been placed anteriorly, we place bone in the facet joints, as this will be the only site of bony fusion.

POSTOPERATIVE MANAGEMENT

Wound Management. Long-term corticosteroid use, poor nutritional status, prior surgery, and prior chemotherapy and radiation therapy have been reported to result in wound infection and dehiscence in upward of 30% of patients with spinal metastases (49,60,67). Pressure should be kept off wounds and wound care should be meticulous. Superficial sutures should be kept in place for an extended period of time, and, if possible, radiation therapy should be delayed for at least 2 weeks to allow for wound healing (67).

Prevention of Thromboembolic Disease. Rapid mobilization and early postoperative involvement of physiatrists and physical therapists is desirable in these patients to diminish the risks of postoperative thromboembolic complications. Cancer patients are often hypercoagulable, and decreased postoperative mobility further adds to the risk of postoperative deep venous thrombosis (DVT) or pulmonary embolization (68,69). Early mobilization, physical therapy, and sequential compression stockings aid in reducing the incidence of postoperative lower extremity venous thrombosis and pulmonary embolus. We routinely use Lovinox in low dose in the postoperative period beginning ≥4 hours after surgery.

Corticosteroids. Corticosteroids are administered preoperatively to all patients with spinal metastases because they protect the spinal cord, improve neurological function, and reduce lesional edema (70,71). They also have a direct cytotoxic effect on lymphoreticular tumors (70). We utilize methylprednisolone in a dose of 125 to 250 mg q6h or an equivalent dosage of other corticosteroids and rapidly taper the dose postoperatively.

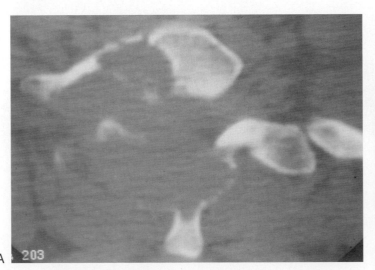
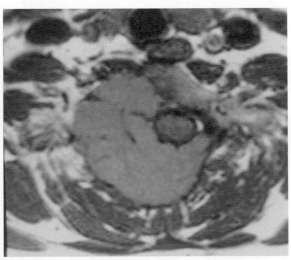

Fig. 4. A: Axial CT of a patient with extensive destruction of C7 by metastatic tumor. **B**: Axial MRI at the same level shows nearly circumferential involvement of the C7 vertebral body. (*Figure continues.*)

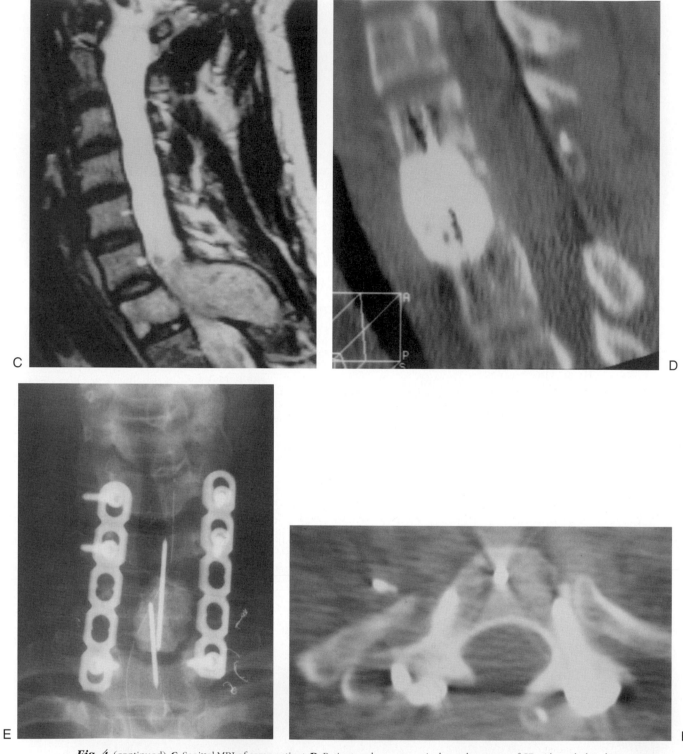

Fig. 4. (continued). **C**: Sagittal MRI of same patient. **D**: Patient underwent cervical vertebrectomy of C7 with methylmethacrylate and Steinmann pin reconstruction. **E**: After laminectomy, lateral mass plates were placed from C5 to T1. **F**: Pedicle screws were placed at T1.

Gastrointestinal Prophylaxis. Prolonged use of corticosteroids is associated with an increased incidence of gastrointestinal bleeding and perforation (70,71). All patients on corticosteroids should be placed on H_2-receptor antagonists.

Postoperative Imaging Surveillance. Lateral plain films are useful to show the cervical alignment, position, and integrity of the anterior and posterior reconstruction and instrumentation. If the lower cervical spine is obscured by the shoulders on plain films, CT scans done with 1-mm axial cuts with sagittal reformatting will provided excellent assessment of bony anatomy and alignment. The use of titanium alloys has done much to improve the quality of postoperative imaging. Postoperative artifact on MRI is a function of both the size of the metallic implants and its ferromagnetic content. In general, excellent assessment of soft tissue compression can be obtained using MRI in patients who have had cervical instrumentation with titanium implants. This is frequently not true in patients who have thoracic or lumbar instrumentation. If necessary, myelography may always be used to assess the presence of spinal cord compression (24–26).

We follow patients with spinal reconstruction for neoplastic disease closer than patients who have had reconstruction for nonneoplastic conditions. Tumor recurrence with loss of stability, destruction of adjacent previously unaffected bony levels, and local regrowth of tumor is a more frequent and distressing problem, as the life span of these patients has been prolonged by newer chemotherapy regimens. Tumor recurrence is especially common in patients with hypernephroma and melanoma and other tumors that are poorly responsive to radiation and chemotherapy.

We therefore study these patients with plain films on a routine basis every 3 to 6 months and with plain films and MRI if they should have an otherwise unexplained increase in pain, or recurrence of neurological deficit.

RESULTS AND COMPLICATIONS. The prognosis for patients with symptomatic spinal metastases is variable, given the heterogeneity of this patient population. But appropriate surgical treatment can have a dramatic impact on function and outcome. Functional recovery and pain relief can be expected in 80% of properly selected patients (8,50–53,60). However, overall patient survival is determined by the patient's systemic disease and tumor biology.

Several factors give rise to increased operative morbidity in patients with metastatic spine disease: advanced age, chronic corticosteroid use, immobility, poor medical condition, poor nutritional status, coagulation abnormalities, prior surgery, and prior chemotherapy or radiation therapy.

Conclusions

The management of metastatic tumors to the subaxial cervical spine requires a multidisciplinary approach involving the surgeon, medical and radiation oncologists, and physiatrists. In appropriately selected patients, the goals of preserving/improving neurological function, restoring spinal alignment and stability, and relieving pain can usually be achieved with an improvement in the quality of life.

References

1. Silverberg E. Cancer statistics, 1984. *J Clin Cancer* 1984;34:7–23.
2. Jaffe W. *Tumors and tumorous conditions of the bones and joints.* Philadelphia: Lea and Febiger, 1958.
3. Willis RA. *The spread of tumours in the human body,* 3rd. London: Butterworths, 1973.
4. Harrington K. Current concepts review: metastatic disease of the spine. *J Bone Joint Surg* 1986;68A:1110–1115.
5. Tubiana-hulin M. Incidence, prevalence and distribution of bone metastases. *Bone* 1991;12:S9–S10.
6. Fornasier VL, Horne JG. Metastases to vertebral column. *Cancer* 1975;36:590–594.
7. Constans JP, deDevitiis E, Donzelli R, et al. Spinal metastases with neurologic manifestations: review of 600 cases. *J Neurosurg* 1983;59:111–118.
8. Dunn RC, Kelly WA, Whons RNW, et al. Spinal epidural neoplasia. A 15 year review of the results of surgical therapy. *J Neurosurg* 1980;52:47–51.
9. Fontana M, Pompili A, Cattani F, et al. Metastatic spinal cord compression. Follow-up study. *J Neurosurg* 1980;24:141–146.
10. Berrettoni BA, Carter JR. Mechanisms of cancer metastasis to bone. *J Bone Joint Surg* 1986;68A:308–312.
11. Perrin RG, McBroom RJ. Metastatic tumors of the cervical spine. In: Block P, ed. *Clinical neurosurgery.* Baltimore: Williams & Wilkins 1991:740–755.
12. Atanasiu JP, Badatcheff F, Pidhorz L. Metastatic lesions of the cervical spine. *Spine* 1993;18(10):1279–1284.
13. Phillips E, Levine AM. Metastatic disease of the upper cervical spine. *Spine* 1989;14(10):1071–1077.
14. Weinstein JN, McLain RF. Primary tumors of the spine. *Spine* 1987;12:843–851.
15. Welch WC, Jacobs GB. Surgery for metastatic spinal disease. *J Neurooncol* 1995;23:163–170.
16. An HS, Vaccaro AR, Dolinskas CA, et al. Differentiation between spinal tumors and infections with magnetic resonance imaging. *Spine* 1991;16:S334–338.
17. Black P. Spinal metastasis: current status and recommended guidelines for management. *Neurosurgery* 1979;5:726–746.
18. Edelstyn GA, Gillespie PJ, Grebbell ES. The radiologic demonstration of osseous metastases: experimental observations. *Clin Radiol* 1967;18:158–162.
19. Belliveau RE, Spencer RP. Incidence and sites of bone lesions detected by 99m Tc-polyphosphate scans in patients with tumors. *Cancer* 1975;36:359–363.
20. McNeil B. Rationale for the use of bone scans in selected metastatic primary bone tumors. *Semin Nucl Med* 1978;8:336–345.
21. Citrin DL, Bessent RG, Greig WR. A comparison of sensitivity and accuracy of the 99m Tc phosphate bone scan and skeletal radiographs in the diagnosis of bone metastases. *Clin Radiol* 1977;28:107–111.
22. Corcoran RJ, Thrall JH, Kyle RW. Solitary abnormalities in bone scans of patients with extraosseous malignancies. *Radiology* 1976;121:663–667.
23. Bruckman JE, Bloomer WD. Management of spinal cord compression. *Semin Oncol* 1978;5:135–140.
24. Fink IJ, Garra BS, Zabell A, et al. Computed tomography with metrizamide myelography to define the extent of spinal canal block due to tumor. *J Comput Assist Tomogr* 1984;86:1072–1075.
25. Hagenau C, Graosh W, Currie M, et al. Comparison of spinal magnetic resonance imaging and myelography in cancer patients. *J Clin Oncol* 1987;5:1663–1669.
26. Overby MC, Rothman AS. Anterolateral decompression for metastatic epidural spinal cord tumors. Results of a modified costotransversectomy approach. *J Neurosurg* 1985;62:344–338.
27. Aichner F, Poewe W, Rogalsky W, et al. Magnetic resonance imaging in the diagnosis of spinal cord diseases. *J Neurol Neurosurg Psychiatry* 1985;48:1220–1229.
28. Harnsberger HR, Dillon WP. The radiologic role in diagnosis, staging, and follow-up of neoplasia of the brain, spine, and head and neck. *Semin Ultrasound CT MR* 1989;10:431–452.
29. Jones JM, Schwartz RB, Mantello MT, et al. Fast spin-echo MR in the detection of vertebral metastases: comparison of three sequences. *AJNR* 1994;15:401–407.
30. Lien HH, Blomlie V, Heimdal K. Magnetic resonance imaging of malignant extradural tumors with acute spinal cord compression. *Acta Radiol* 1990;31:187–190.
31. Hackney DB. Neoplasms and related disorders. *Top Magn Reson Imaging* 1992;4:37–61.

32. Fyfe IS, Henry APJ, Mulholland RC. Closed vertebral biopsy. *J Bone Joint Surg* 1983;65:140–143.

33. Ghelman B, Lospinuso MF, Levine DB, et al. Percutaneous computed-tomography-guided biopsy of the thoracic and lumbar spine. *Spine* 1991;16:736–739.

34. Sundaresan N, Schmidek HH, Schiller AL, et al. *Tumors of the spine: diagnosis and clinical management.* Philadelphia: WB Saunders, 1990.

35. Fidler M. Anterior and posterior stabilization of the spine following vertebral body resection. A postmortem investigation. *Spine* 1986;11:362–366.

36. Olerud C, Jonsson H, Lofberg AM, et al. Embolization of spinal metastases reduces preoperative blood loss. 21 patients operated on for renal cell carcinoma. *Acta Orthop Scand* 1993;64:9–12.

37. Sundaresan N, Scher H, Digiacinto GV, et al. Surgical treatment of spinal cord compression in kidney cancer. *J Clin Oncol* 1986;4:1851–1856.

38. Broddus WC, Grady MS, Delashaw JB Jr, et al. Preoperative superselective arteriolar embolization: a new approach to enhance resectability of spinal tumors. *Neurosurgery* 1990;176:755–759.

39. Byrne TN, Desorges JF. Spinal cord compression from epidural metastases. *N Engl J Med* 1992;327:614–619.

40. Harper GR, Rodichuk LD, Prevosti L. Early diagnosis of spinal metastases leads to improved treatment outcome. *Proc Am Soc Clin Oncol* 1982;11:6(abst).

41. Harrington K. Anterior decompression and stabilization of the spine as a treatment for vertebral body collapse and spinal cord compression from metastatic malignancy. *Clin Orthop* 1988;233:177–197.

42. Manabe S, Tateishi A, Abe M, et al. Surgical treatment of metastatic tumors of the spine. *Spine* 1989;14:41–47.

43. Sorensen PS, Borgesen SE, Rohde K, et al. Metastatic epidural spinal cord compression. Results of treatment and survival. *Cancer* 1990;65:1502–1508.

44. Calkins AR, Olson MA, Ellis JH. Impact of myelography on the radiotherapeutic management of malignant spinal cord compression. *Neurosurgery* 1986;19:614–616.

45. Gilbert RW, Kim JH, Posner JB. Epidural spinal cord compression from metastatic tumor: diagnosis and treatment. *Ann Neurol* 1978;3:40–51.

46. Sundaresan N, DiGiacinto GV, Hughes JEO. Surgical treatment of spinal metastases. *Clin Neurosurg* 1986;33:503–522.

47. Tomita T, Galicich JH, Sundaresan N. Radiation therapy for spinal epidural metastases with complete block. *Acta Radiol Oncol* 1983;22:135–143.

48. Ratanatharathorn V, Powers RE. Epidural spinal cord compression from metastatic tumor: diagnosis and guidelines for management. *Cancer Treat Rev* 1991;18:55–71.

49. Seigal T, Seigal T. Current considerations in the management of neoplastic spinal cord compression. *Spine* 1988;14:223–228.

50. Hellar M, McBroom RJ, MacNab T, et al. Treatment of metastatic disease of the spine with postero-lateral decompression and Luque instrumentation. *Neuroorthopedics* 1986;2:70–74.

51. Seigal T, Seigal T. Surgical decompression of anterior and posterior malignant epidural tumors compressing the spinal cord: a prospective study. *Neurosurgery* 1985;17:424–432.

52. McClain RF, Weinstein JN. Tumors of the spine. *Semin Spine Surg* 1990;2:157–180.

53. Martenson JA, Evans RG, Lie MR, et al. Treatment outcome in patients treated for malignant epidural spinal cord compression (SCC). *J Neurooncol* 1985;3:77–84.

54. Meschino A, Devitt JH, Koch JP, et al. The safety of awake tracheal intubation in cervical spine injury. *Can J Anesth* 1992;39:114–117.

55. Lee C, Barnes A, Nagel EL. Neuroleptanalgesia for awake pronation of surgical patients. *Anesth Analg* 1977;56:276–278.

56. Russel GB, Rodichok LD. *Primer of intraoperative neurophysiologic monitoring.* Boston: Butterworth-Heinemann, 1995.

57. Ginsburg HH, Shetter AG, Raudzens PA. Postoperative paraplegia with preserved intraoperative somatosensory potentials. *J Neurosurg* 1985;63:296–300.

58. Kostuik JP, Errico TJ, Gleason TF, et al. Spinal stabilization of vertebral column tumors. *Spine* 1988;13:250–256.

59. Rao S, Davis R. Cervical spine metastases. In: Clark C, ed. *The cervical spine*, 3rd ed. Philadelphia: Raven Press, 1998:603–609.

60. Sundaresan N, Krol G, Hughes J, et al. Tumors of the spine: diagnosis and management. In: Tindal GT, Cooper PR, Barrow DL, eds. *The practice of neurosurgery.* Baltimore: Williams & Wilkins, 1996:1303–1322.

61. Caspar W, Barbier DD, Klara PM. Anterior cervical fusion and Caspar plate stabilization for cervical trauma. *Neurosurgery* 1989;25:491–502.

62. Cooper PR, Cohen A, Rosiello A, et al. Posterior stabilization of cervical spine fractures and subluxations using plates and screws. *Neurosurgery* 1988;23:300–306.

63. Cooper P. Stabilization of fractures and subluxations of the lower cervical spine. In: Cooper P, ed. Management of posttraumatic spinal instability. Park Ridge, IL: AANS, 1990:111–134.

64. Fehlings MG, Cooper PR, Errico TJ. Posterior plates in the management of cervical instability: long-term results in 44 patients. *J Neurosurg* 1994;81:341–349.

65. Grob D, Magerl F. Dorsale Spondylodese der Halswirbelsaule mit der Hakenplatte. *Orthopade* 1987;16:55–61.

66. Roy-Camille R, Saillant G, Mazel C. Internal fixation for the unstable cervical spine by posterior osteosynthesis with plates and screws. In: Committee CSRSE, ed. *The cervical spine*, 2nd ed. Philadelphia: Lippincott, 1989:390–403.

67. Lawrence W. Wound healing in the cancer patient: effect of the disease and its treatment. In: Moosa AR, Schimpff SC, Robson MC, eds. *Comprehensive textbook of oncology*, vol 2. Baltimore: Williams & Wilkins, 1991:1697–1707.

68. Schafer A. The hypercoagulable states. *Ann Intern Med* 1985;102:814–828.

69. Kaelin WG, Mayer RJ. Hematologic complications of cancer and cancer therapy. In: Moosa AR, Schimpff SC, Robson MC, eds. *Comprehensive textbook of oncology*, vol 2. Baltimore: Williams & Wilkins, 1991:1754–1769.

70. Coleman R. Glucocorticoids in cancer therapy. *Biotherapy* 1992;4:37–44.

71. Ikeda H, Ushio Y, Hayakawa T, et al. Edema and circulatory disturbance in the spinal cord by epidural neoplasms in rabbits. *J Neurosurg* 1980;52:203–209.

168. Metastatic Disease of the Thoracolumbar Spine

David W. Cahill and Bret B. Abshire

With rare exception, secondary malignant neoplasms that involve the thoracolumbar spine arrive via hematogenous dissemination from a noncontiguous source (1–4). Occasionally the thoracolumbar vertebrae may become directly invaded by an expanding lung carcinoma with pleural extension, a renal cell carcinoma with retroperitoneal spread, or an expanding retroperitoneal sarcoma (3) (see below). In childhood, the thoracolumbar spine is commonly involved by neuroblastomas (5), Wilms' tumors, lymphoreticular tumors, and leukemia, but these lesions are generally treated with radiation and chemotherapy and rarely come to the attention of surgeons. Similarly, in adults, lymphomas/leukemias rarely require surgery. Myeloma in the spine needs surgery only for posttreatment lytic collapse and not for the tumor per se.

In children, the majority of metastatic thoracolumbar tumors that come to surgery are sarcomas. Ewing's sarcomas, osteosarcomas, rhabdomyosarcomas, and chondrosarcomas are the usual culprits (5,6). In children with neurofibromatosis type I, neurofibrosarcomas and various other malignant spindle cell neoplasms occasionally arise (7) (Fig. 1). In adults, the secondary tumors that affect the thoracolumbar spine are the same as for the spine as a whole. Lung, breast, and prostate tumors account for half. If renal, gastrointestinal, and thyroid carcinomas are added, fully 70% are included. The remaining third include many other carcinomas, sarcomas, and lymphoreticular neoplasms (6,8–12).

In most of the cases that come to surgeons, the primary tumor is known. On our services today, only about 10% of metastatic spinal tumors present de novo. Fewer still have an undiagnosed primary at the time of spinal surgery. Modern magnetic resonance imaging (MRI) and computed tomography (CT) scanning techniques make "unknown primary" a progressively less common diagnosis. This chapter discusses those aspects of metastatic disease to the spine that are specific to the thoracolumbar region and the tumors that are most commonly found there.

Diagnosis

In the 21st century, MRI is rapidly becoming the sine qua non for all aspects of spinal tumor diagnosis (13,14). Screening MRI is displacing isotope scanning for this purpose. MRI scans are now replacing CT scans in the guidance of percutaneous needle biopsies. However, we still prefer CT scanning with "bone windows" for surgical planning (Fig. 2), but this too may soon be replaced by newer MRI sequences that improve bone visualization (15). Multisequence MRI with and without enhancing agents and sometimes coupled with MR angiography are often the only preoperative studies needed. In many institutions, however, the MR hardware and software necessary to accom-

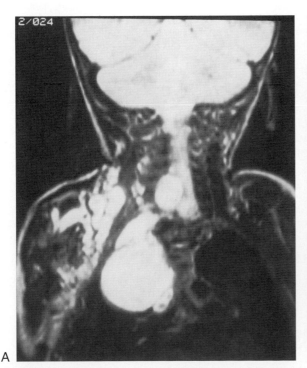
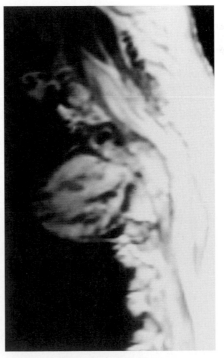

A   B

Fig. 1. **A**: A 4-year-old girl with neurofibromatosis type I. Coronal magnetic resonance imaging (MRI) reveals extensive neurofibrosarcoma extending from a dumbbell tumor in the right lower subaxial cervical spine into the right brachial plexus and chest. **B**: Paraspinal cut from sagittal MRI of a 13-year-old with metastatic rhabdomyosarcoma involving the thoracic spine T5-9.

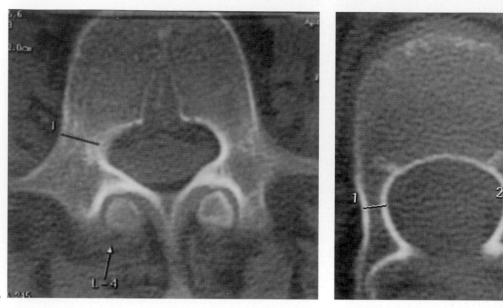

Fig. 2. **A**: Axial computed tomography (CT) scan of L3 vertebra in a child with metastatic osteosarcoma in L2 and L3. Pedicle width is suitable for screw placement. **B**: Axial CT scan of T12 vertebra in the same child. Pedicle width at this level is too narrow to allow even 5-mm screws. Bone-window CT scans are very useful for preoperative planning. See also Fig. 3.

plish multiplanar visualization of bony and soft-tissue structures, cerebrospinal fluid (CSF) flow, and surrounding vasculature are not yet available. One can never have too much information preoperatively; therefore, we strongly encourage the use of multiple imaging modalities to visualize a given tumor in multiple planes, both bony and soft tissue components, within the spinal canal, within the bony spine, and paraspinally (16).

Currently, we use biplanar plain radiographs and MRI before every case. CT and isotope screening studies are used selectively. The frequency of CT scan usage is inversely proportional to the quality of the MR images with particular reference to bony dimensions. For surgical planning, it is mandatory to know the degree of spinal canal and foraminal compromise, the alignment of the spine in three planes, and the extent of paraspinal tumor encroachment. The relative vascularity of the tumor is a useful but not mandatory bit of accessory information sometimes available noninvasively. If the tissue type of the tumor is known, relative vascularity can be predicted with acceptable accuracy in most cases.

Tumor Biology for Common Metastatic Lesions

Thankfully, metastatic spinal tumors requiring surgery are quite rare in childhood. Most are sarcomas and behave like highly malignant spindle cell tumors. Spinal metastases from Ewing's sarcomas are usually seen in conjunction with widespread visceral and bony metastatic disease. Surgery in such patients usually offers very temporary palliation. Children with isolated single metastases from primary osteosarcomas or rhabdomyosarcomas in the extremities may survive for many months to years with modern chemotherapy regimens. In the absence of visceral (lung, liver, adrenal, brain) metastatic deposits, a vigorous surgical approach to isolated spinal disease is warranted

as such tumors are often radioresistant and may produce rapid paraplegia if left untreated (17–19) (Fig. 3).

Metastatic childhood sarcomas have usually been irradiated before the surgeon is consulted. Not uncommonly, they involve both anterior and posterior spinal elements and usually require circumferential resection and reconstruction. In such cases, small, thin anatomy and previous radiation make the use of very low profile hardware desirable. If possible, incisions should overlap irradiated skin minimally, anterior hardware should be as rigid as possible, and posterior hardware should be no higher than the spinous processes of instrumented segments. This is discussed further below.

Of the six common adult cancers mentioned above, some are more likely than others to affect the thoracolumbar junction and come to the attention of surgeons. Compared to lung, breast, prostate, and colon carcinomas, thyroid tumors are relatively rare. They surely do metastasize to the thoracolumbar junction, but many respond nicely to radioiodine and do not come to surgery (20). Of those that do, most are hypovascular and lytic in nature, and present with kyphotic collapse after iodine (I) 125 or external radiation therapy.

Colon carcinomas occasionally metastasize to the thoracolumbar junction, but in most cases have diffuse peritoneal metastatic disease and widespread liver metastases by the time the spinal disease is diagnosed. In our experience, it is rare for a spine surgeon to be consulted in such cases.

Renal cell carcinomas are unique in several respects. First, they arise in the retroperitoneum just anterolateral to the thoracolumbar spine. They may spread to the spine from direct invasion or by true vascular metastasis (21) (Fig. 4). Second, almost without exception, they are extremely vascular tumors. In most cases, the surgery benefits significantly from preoperative embolization of such lesions (22–24). Third, not uncommonly, the primary tumor and the subjacent spinal metastasis are diagnosed at the same time (25,26). The pain from the thoracolumbar metastasis is the presenting symptom. The primary renal mass is often visualizable on MR or CT scans obtained to evaluate the thoracolumbar spine (Fig. 4). Fourth, renal cell carcino-

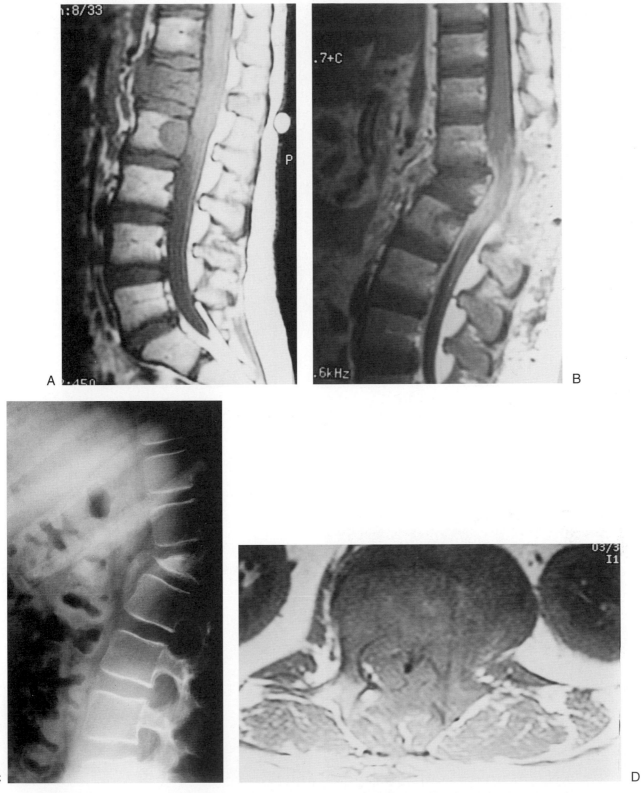

Fig. 3. **A**: A 12-year-old girl with isolated metastatic osteosarcoma to L1 and L2 visualized on preoperative sagittal T1-weighted MRI. **B**: Patient underwent laminectomy at referring institution with secondary kyphotic collapse and conus medullaris compression as visualized on this MRI 3 months after surgery. **C**: Plain radiograph just prior to second surgery reveals vertebral body collapse with 40-degree relative kyphosis status post–posterior element resection. **D**: Axial MRI reveals tumor in all three columns of the L1 vertebra with left paraspinal extension as well.

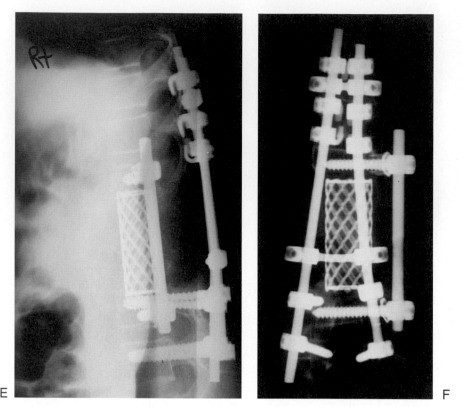

Fig. 3. (continued). **E,F**: Anteroposterior (AP) and lateral radiographs after total spondylectomies at L1 and L2 reconstructed with interbody cage packed with cancellous allograft. Circumferential stabilization is provided after the correction of deformity by anterolateral staple fixated rod and posterior double rod construct fixated with screws caudally and hooks rostrally (see also Fig. 2).

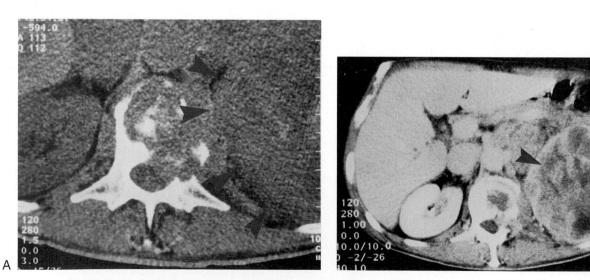

Fig. 4. A 58-year-old man with renal cell carcinoma. **A**: Axial CT scan of lumbar spine through the L2 vertebra. The patient had no known tumor. CT was obtained to evaluate back pain. The tumor in the lumbar vertebra is extending directly from the large left renal mass noted first on this study (*arrowheads*). **B**: Subsequently, this CT scan of the abdomen visualized a large renal carcinoma with direct invasion into the spine.

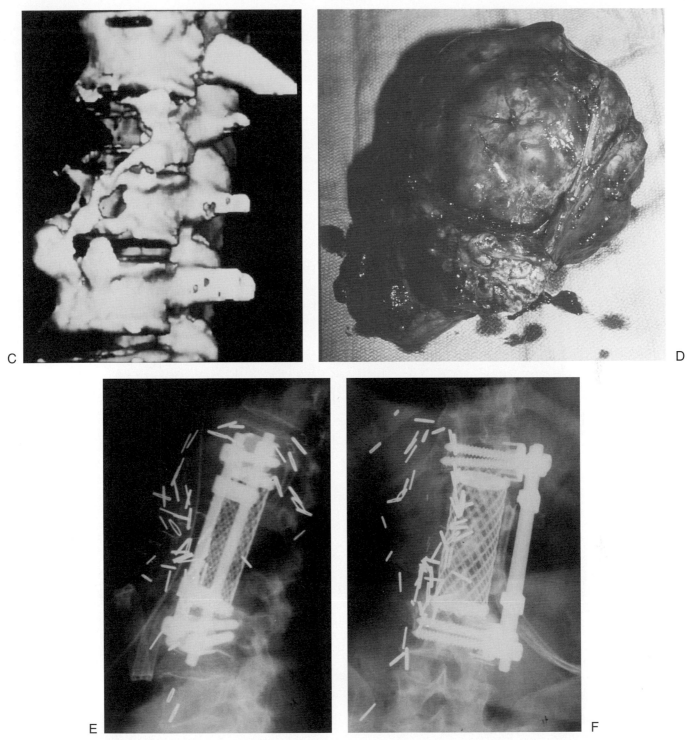

Fig. 4. (continued). **C:** Three-dimensional (3D) CT reconstruction of the upper lumbar spine reveals the extent of bony involvement in L1, L2, and L3. **D:** Intraoperative specimen after resection of large (16 cm) renal tumor and adjacent anterior lumbar vertebrae. **E,F:** AP and lateral radiographs after reconstruction with interbody cage, allograft, and rigid anterolateral device. Uninvolved posterior elements (**A**) were left intact. Therefore no posterior hardware was necessary.

mas are the most likely tumors to have the primary and metastatic lesions resected simultaneously, often through the same flank incision. The percentage of metastatic renal cell carcinomas that comes to surgery in the thoracolumbar spine exceeds the relative percentage of metastatic tumors as a whole.

Virtually all types of lung carcinomas metastasize to the thoracolumbar spine, but some are more likely to come to surgery than others. Small cell carcinomas (oat cell tumors) are virtually always widely metastatic at the time of diagnosis of thoracolumbar disease. The metastatic deposits usually respond initially to external radiotherapy, and the patients usually succumb to the disease before spine surgery could be done (6,26). Like small

cell tumors, squamous cell carcinomas of the lung are usually widely disseminated when the thoracolumbar disease is diagnosed (6). Visceral metastases often precede symptomatic spinal disease. Unlike small cell tumors, however, squamous cell metastases are often radioresistant. Such cases usually come to surgery as a last-ditch effort to prevent paraplegia rather than for pain control or in an effort to control grossly visualizable disease (27). Widespread noncontiguous metastatic deposits in the spine may make reconstruction especially difficult.

Adenocarcinomas of the lung are the pulmonary primaries most likely to present with isolated spinal metastases in the absence of known visceral or noncontiguous spinal disease.

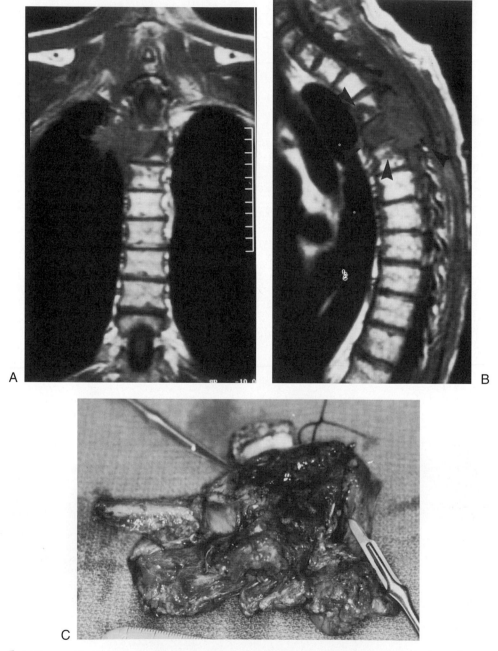

Fig. 5. A 39-year-old woman with adenocarcinoma of the lung after biopsy and irradiation. **A**: Coronal MRI reveals primary pleural-based lung tumor directly invading the upper thoracic spine on the right. **B**: Sagittal MRI reveals circumferential involvement of T3 as well as portions of T2 and T4. **C**: Operative specimen after resection of primary tumor and involved portions of ribs and vertebrae.

Though the patient's life expectancy with these tumors is much worse than with adenocarcinomas of the breast or prostate, they are more likely to present with the type of spinal disease for which surgery is most beneficial. After renal cell carcinomas, they are the next most common tumor in which the presenting symptoms may arise from the spinal metastatic lesion. Also like renal cell tumors, adenocarcinomas of the lung may involve the thoracolumbar spine by direct transpleural extension (28). On rare occasion the primary and secondary lesions may be resected simultaneously (Fig. 5).

Metastatic carcinomas of the breast and prostate make up a disproportionately high percentage of the spine oncologist's practice (10). In many cases, these tumors are less virulent than lung, colon, renal, or thyroid lesions. Hence, the victim's life expectancy is much longer. The majority of metastatic breast and prostate carcinomas involve the spine before death. Both tumors are often hormone sensitive, and sometimes enjoy long-term survival without cytotoxic chemotherapy. All of these factors make the spine surgeon's involvement with these tumors more likely.

Presumably on the basis of contiguity or, perhaps, venous spread, breast carcinomas commonly involve the thoracic spine and, not uncommonly, the thoracolumbar junction. Previous chest wall and axillary surgery as well as previous primary irradiation fields may complicate the spine surgeon's job. Spine metastases from breast carcinomas are often multiple and may be noncontiguous. We have patients who have come to surgery for three separate spinal metastases over 5 to 7 years. Most breast metastases respond to radiotherapy initially, but subsequently recur if the patient enjoys long-term survival. Antiestrogenic hormone therapy often used in breast cancer patients may lead to severe osteoporosis, greatly increasing the risk of spinal hardware pullout or fracture. All of these factors must be considered as surgical procedures are planned (29).

As breast cancers drift down from the thoracic spine to the thoracolumbar junction, prostate cancers usually present first in the lumbosacral spine but may later involve the thoracolumbar junction. Also like breast lesions, prostate metastases usually respond initially to radiotherapy, only to recur later if the patient survives. Primary surgical incisions and radiation portals for prostate carcinomas are usually not an issue at the thoracolumbar junction. Multiplicity and caudal segment disease often are. Prostate carcinomas are usually seen in men over 70 years of age (10). Age-related osteoporosis and cardiopulmonary disease further complicate the surgeon's task.

Therefore, not all thoracolumbar metastases are alike. Each tumor type brings unique features to challenge or benefit the spine surgeon. Each case is unique and many factors must be considered. The 10 most important factors are summarized in ref. 6 (also see ref. 30).

Biomechanical Considerations at the Thoracolumbar Junction

As with other junctional regions in the spine, the thoracolumbar junction joins a relatively mobile (lumbar) segment to a relatively immobile (thoracic) segment. Fusion constructs crossing the junction must resist motion across a pathologic axis of rotation with a long moment arm consisting of the rib-fixated thoracic vertebrae on the cephalad side of the axis. Normal postoperative mobilization produces significant pullout strain on fixation devices on the caudal side of any construct. This is the first consideration in choice of construct (6,31).

In the sagittal plane, the thoracolumbar junction is normally

sigmoid. It is where the lumbar lordosis reverses to the thoracic kyphosis. In general, metastatic tumors produce an exaggerated thoracic kyphosis and loss of lumbar lordosis. Successful reconstruction demands restoration of anterior height in most cases and reconstruction of a posterior tension band in those cases in which tumor or surgery have resulted in posterior element disruption (32) (Fig. 3). Undercorrection leaves persistent kyphosis with bow-stringing of the underlying cord. Overcorrection produces a flat back and chronic pain (6).

The great majority of metastatic thoracolumbar junction tumors destroy the anterior and middle columns of the spine; 20% to 30% may also involve the posterior column. In tumors with only anterior and middle column involvement, resection is usually accomplished via an anterior approach (33–35). Reconstruction must restore alignment and anterior weight-bearing capacity. In many cases this may be accomplished with an anterior weight-bearing strut or cage stabilized with a rigid lateral device (Fig. 6).

In cases with circumferential involvement and in those in whom a posterolateral approach to resection of anterior elements was chosen, a posterior tension band construct (compression rods) must be added to the anterior weight-bearing construct (32,36) (Fig. 3). The same reconstructive principles that we use as guides in the repair of thoracolumbar trauma may be applied to thoracolumbar tumors. The additional complications of osteoporosis, noncontiguous disease in segments to be instrumented, previous local irradiation, and paraspinal extension of tumor make the choices of reconstructive technique more critical in tumor patients than is usually the case in the young, healthy trauma victim.

Reconstructive Techniques in Thoracolumbar Tumors

The overlying aorta, vena cava, and esophagus above the diaphragm and the intraperitoneal and retroperitoneal viscera below it make a direct anterior approach to the thoracolumbar junction undesirable. Therefore, the junction may be approached laterally or posteriorly. Posterior approaches to the laminae and underlying spinal canal are straightforward and familiar to all spine surgeons. Such approaches may be extended posterolaterally to resect anterior spinal elements (see below). Anterolateral approaches must protect the lung and the great vessels on the cephalad side of the diaphragm, and the psoas muscle with its contained lumbar plexus, the retroperitoneum (particularly the ureter), and great vessels on the caudal side. Salvage of the ipsilateral sympathetic chain is often impossible.

In most cases, tumors that involve only the anterior and middle columns of the junctional vertebrae are best approached anterolaterally. This allows preservation of the intact posterior elements and allows single-stage resection and reconstruction with a short segment construct (Fig. 6). Exceptions to this approach may include patients with previous thoracoabdominal surgery or those considered too frail to withstand a thoracoabdominal procedure (6,37).

In approaching the thoracolumbar junction anterolaterally, either the left or right side is feasible. The left side is usually preferable, as the aorta is easier to see and easier to repair than the vena cava and because the liver is on the right. The right side is usually chosen if there is a large right-sided tumor extension paraspinally or the primary tumor is to be resected and is on the right side. If there was previous right-sided surgery (Fig. 7), the right side is chosen so as to preserve contralateral segmental

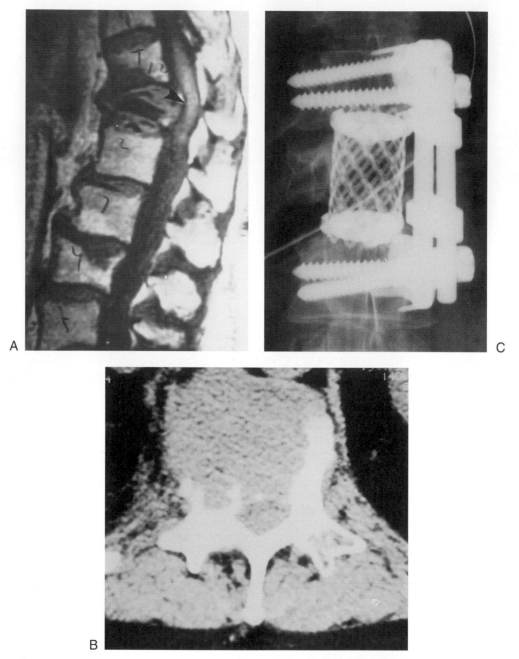

Fig. 6. A 77-year-old man with metastatic prostate carcinoma to L1 vertebra. **A:** Sagittal MRI reveals obvious kyphosis and conus medullaris compression. **B:** Axial CT scan through L1 reveals tumor involves entire body and right pedicle but spares the posterior column. **C:** After resection via corpectomy and pediculectomy, reconstruction used an interbody cage stabilized with a rigid anterolateral device.

vessels. [The only cases of paraplegia attributable to segmental vessel sacrifice are in cases in which the contralateral segmentals had been previously taken (6,37).]

The skin incision should follow the course of a rib two segments above the vertebra to be resected. Below T10, an extrapleural dissection is usually feasible, and it is rarely necessary to collapse the ipsilateral lung with a double-lumen tube. Only the most medial attachments of the diaphragm need to be taken down. Below the diaphragm, the psoas attachments are dissected off the lateral margins of the vertebrae to expose the ipsilateral pedicles of all levels to be resected or instrumented. Segmental vessels are isolated, coagulated, and clipped or tied

at each level to be resected or instrumented. The ipsilateral sympathetic chain is usually lost to the tumor. No effort is made to save it, as dissection has the same effect as resection and is in both cases transient.

Resection of the involved vertebra or vertebrae is preceded by placement of transverse bicortical screws in the vertebrae to be instrumented above and below. This allows use of temporary distractors to prevent malalignment during tumor resection. In these usually osteoporotic individuals, we prefer bicortical screws anchored through multipoint staples in an effort to minimize the risk of screw cut out or extrusion (Figs. 4 and 6). Unicortical devices and plate devices dependent on single stress

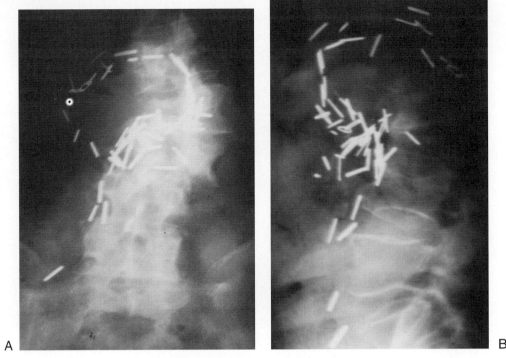

Fig. 7. A 68-year-old man status–right nephrectomy for renal cell carcinoma 5 years previously. AP (**A**) and lateral (**B**) radiographs reveal right concave kyphoscoliotic deformity secondary to direct invasion from the old resection margin. A right-sided approach is preferable under these circumstances (see text).

bearing bolts are more likely to fail in osteoporotic patients, particularly if significant force is to be applied for correction.

Resection begins with discectomies above and below the vertebrae to be resected. This allows careful visualization and preservation of the vertebral end plate that will subsequently hold the anterior weight-bearing graft (38). End-plate preservation is important in tumor-ridden osteoporotic spines in which anterior graft compression and telescoping with recurrent kyphosis is always a risk. Resection proceeds through the entire vertebral body or bodies to be taken including the proximal pedicles, the disc annulus on both sides, and both anterior and posterior longitudinal ligaments (ALL and PLL). The PLL is taken to guarantee dural decompression. The ALL is taken to ensure tumor resection and allow unimpeded distraction anteriorly to correct kyphotic deformity.

After complete corpectomy and resection of any paraspinal tumor, slight overdistraction is applied between the transverse screws. A longitudinal titanium cage is cut to the desired length and packed with cancellous allograft bone. End rings are applied to the cage to further decrease the risk of telescoping. The cage is then fit into position and checked fluoroscopically in two planes. Double rods are applied between the previously placed screws, mild compression is applied across the cage, and then the construct is torqued and cross-links applied between the rods.

We prefer to avoid autograft bone in patients with metastatic lesions both to avoid graft site morbidity and to avoid potential surgical metastasis. Weight-bearing allograft struts at the thoracolumbar junction should usually be at least the diameter of a human humerus. We find longitudinal cages easier to use and less likely to telescope or extrude (38) (Fig. 8). It must be remembered that fusion is usually not the goal in most palliative operations for metastatic disease.

In patients in whom there is posterior element involvement or in whom the posterior elements of involved vertebrae have

been previously resected, a posterior approach to reconstruction is mandated. Resection of tumor bearing posterior elements after previous anterior resection and reconstruction is straightforward. The laminae, spinous process, facets, pars, pedicles, and transverse processes of involved vertebrae should be resected completely. Note that to resect the superior facets and pedicles of an involved thoracolumbar vertebrae requires resection of the caudal laminae of the cephalad vertebra. All involved portions of the ribs should also be taken.

Posterior reconstruction should include placement of bilateral compression rods a minimum of two levels above and two levels below the resected vertebrae. In large individuals, pedicle screws may be used at both cephalad and caudal ends of the rods (up to about T8). In smaller individuals hooks should be used to fixate the rods at least at the cephalad end (Fig. 3). Down-going sublaminar and up-going pedicle hooks are stronger than screws in pullout resistance. Hooks require no fluoroscopy or image guidance for placement and are therefore less time-consuming. In the face of a rigid anterior construct, stability in extension is not required of the posterior construct. For all of these reasons, we generally employ compression hooks only for the fixation of posterior rods for tension banding. In the absence of a double rod anterior construct, screw fixation of the posterior construct becomes more desirable (6,31).

In patients with three-column tumor involvement in whom an anterior transcavitary operation is undesirable due to frailty or previous surgery, it is quite possible to resect the entire vertebra or vertebrae from a purely posterior approach (39–41). The technique is an expansion of a bilateral costotransversectomy and involves anterior reconstruction by posterolateral insertion of anterior intervertebral cages or struts. This technique is greatly facilitated by sacrifice of the exiting nerve roots on one side, and therefore is most applicable to the thoracic spine (Fig. 9). At the thoracolumbar junction, it is usually desirable to preserve all nerve roots below T11. It is quite possible to resect

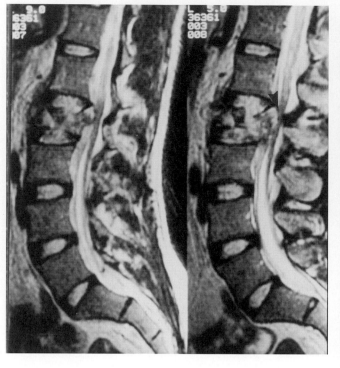

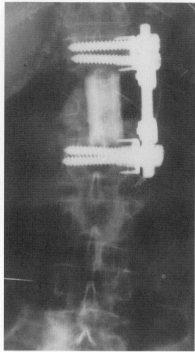

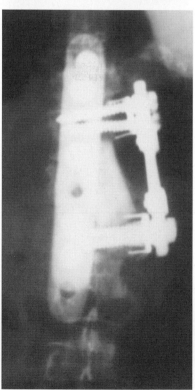

Fig. 8. An osteoporotic 46-year-old woman with metastatic breast carcinoma to L2 vertebra after 5 years of antiestrogenic therapy. **A**: Sagittal T2-weighted MRI demonstrates obvious cauda equina compression. **B**: Initial postoperative radiograph after L2 corpectomy and reconstruction using an allograft humeral strut fixated with a rigid anterolateral device. **C**: Two weeks later, the strut has telescoped and the lower end screws have partially extruded despite rigid internal fixation and external orthosis. We currently perform intraoperative vertebroplasties of the vertebrae to be instrumented in an effort to decrease the risk of this complication in osteoprotic patients.

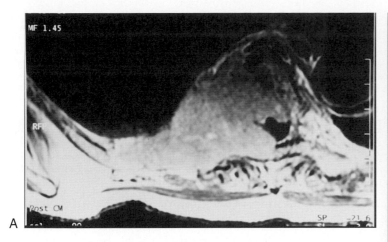

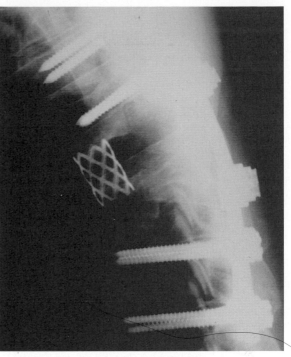

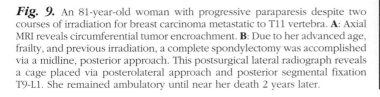

Fig. 9. An 81-year-old woman with progressive paraparesis despite two courses of irradiation for breast carcinoma metastatic to T11 vertebra. **A**: Axial MRI reveals circumferential tumor encroachment. **B**: Due to her advanced age, frailty, and previous irradiation, a complete spondylectomy was accomplished via a midline, posterior approach. This postsurgical lateral radiograph reveals a cage placed via posterolateral approach and posterior segmental fixation T9-L1. She remained ambulatory until near her death 2 years later.

any thoracolumbar vertebra from a solely posterior approach, but the restoration of anterior height and placement of weight-bearing struts is problematic if the nerve roots are to be saved. In very frail individuals in whom realignment is less important and decompression is the primary goal of surgery, posterior spondylectomy and anterior reconstruction with methylmethacrylate may be adequate. If a posterior spondylectomy is performed, it is very important to place a temporary unilateral posterior rod after dorsal arch resection and before vertebral body resection to prevent sagittal and rotational translation prior to anterior reconstruction (6,31) (Fig. 10).

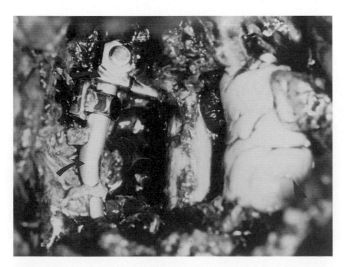

Fig. 10. Interoperative photograph demonstrating short, temporary posterior rod (*curved arrows*) placed after dorsal arch resection and before anterior element resection to prevent kyphotic or rotational dislocation prior to anterior element reconstruction. After interbody strut (*arrowhead*) is placed (in this case a methylmethacrylate block), the temporary rod is removed and large, permanent posterior rods applied.

Conclusions

Current reconstructive techniques have dramatically improved the surgeon's ability to restore structural and neurological function after the radical resection of metastatic tumors of the thoracolumbar spine. Though surgery for metastatic disease remains palliative, the duration and functional success of the palliation are far beyond the state of affairs 20 years ago when Posner and colleagues found radiation alone more effective than surgery in the management of metastatic spinal disease. Significant problems remain with osteoporosis-induced hardware failure, radiation-induced wound failure, and with the cost of surgery with short-term goals. Nonetheless, there can be little question that biomechanically informed surgical procedures are finally improving the lives of the unfortunate victims of secondary malignancy in the spine.

References

1. Onuigbo WI. Batson's theory of vertebral venous metastasis: a review. *Oncology* 1975;32(3–4):145–150.
2. Vider M, Maruyama Y, Narvaez R. Significance of the vertebral venous (Batson's) plexus in metastatic spread in colorectal carcinoma. *Cancer* 1977;40(1):67–71.
3. Yuh WT, Quets JP, Lee HJ, et al. Anatomic distribution of metastases in the vertebral body and modes of hematogenous spread. *Spine* 1996;21(19):2243–2250.
4. Geldof AA. Models for cancer skeletal metastasis: a reappraisal of Batson's plexus. *Anticancer Res* 1997;17(3A):1535–1539.
5. Bouffet E, Marec-Berard P, Thiesse P, et al. Spinal cord compression by secondary epi- and intradural metastasis in childhood. *Childs Nerv Syst* 1997;13(7):383–387.
6. Cahill DW. Malignant Tumors of the Bony Spine. In: Menezes A, Sonntag J, Benzel E, et al., eds. *Principles of spinal surgery.* New York: McGraw-Hill, 1996:1401–1421.

7. Kett-White R, Martin JL, Jones EW, et al. Malignant spinal neurofibro-sarcoma. *Spine* 2000;25(6):752–755.

8. Onimus M, Papin P, Gangloff S. Results of surgical treatment of spinal thoracic and lumbar metastases. *Eur Spine J* 1996;5(6):407–411.

9. Rao S, Badani K, Schildhauer T, et al. Metastatic malignancy of the cervical spine. A nonoperative history. *Spine* 1992;17(10 suppl):S407–412.

10. Sioutos PJ, Arbit E, Meshulam CF, et al. Spinal metastases from solid tumors. Analysis of factors affecting survival. *Cancer* 1995;76(8):1453–1459.

11. Schaberg J, Gainor BJ. A profile of metastatic carcinoma of the spine. *Spine* 1985;10(1):19–20.

12. Nottebaert M, von Hochstetter AR, Exner GU, et al. Metastatic carcinoma of the spine. A study of 92 cases. *Int Orthop* 1987;11(4):345–348.

13. Schiff D, O'Neill BP, Wang CH, et al. Neuroimaging and treatment implications of patients with multiple epidural spinal metastases. *Cancer* 1998;83(8):1593–1601.

14. Layer G, Steudel A, Schuller H, et al. Magnetic resonance imaging to detect bone marrow metastases in the initial staging of small cell lung carcinoma and breast carcinoma. *Cancer* 1999;85(4):1004–1009.

15. Uchida N, Sugimura K, Kajitani A, et al. MR imaging of vertebral metastases: evaluation of fat saturation imaging. *Eur J Radiol* 1993;17(2):91–94.

16. Algra PR, Bloem JL, Tissing H, et al. Detection of vertebral metastases: comparison between MR imaging and bone scintigraphy. *Radiographics* 1991;11(2):219–232.

17. Yang RS, Eckardt JJ, Eilber FR, et al. Surgical indications for Ewing's sarcoma of the pelvis. *Cancer* 1995;76(8):1388–1397.

18. Vlasak R, Sim FH. Ewing's sarcoma. *Orthop Clin North Am* 1996;27(3):591–603.

19. Bauernhofer T, Stoger H, Kasparek AK, et al. Combined treatment of metastatic osteosarcoma of the spine. *Oncology* 1999;57(4):265–268.

20. Scarrow AM, Colina JL, Levy EI, et al. Thyroid carcinoma with isolated spinal metastasis: case history and review of the literature. *Clin Neurol Neurosurg* 1999;101(4):245–248.

21. King GJ, Kostuik JP, McBroom RJ, et al. Surgical management of metastatic renal carcinoma of the spine. *Spine* 1991;16(3):265–271.

22. Olerud C, Jonsson H Jr, Lofberg AM, et al. Embolization of spinal metastases reduces preoperative blood loss: 21 patients operated on for renal cell carcinoma. *Acta Orthop Scand* 1993;64(1):9–12

23. Roscoe MW, McBroom RJ, St Louis E, et al. Preoperative embolization in the treatment of osseous metastases from renal cell carcinoma. *Clin Orthop* 1989;238:302–307.

24. Broaddus WC, Grady MS, Delashaw JB Jr, et al. Preoperative super-selective arteriolar embolization: a new approach to enhance resectability of spinal tumors. *Neurosurgery* 1990;27(5):755–759.

25. Durr HR, Maier M, Pfahler M, et al. Surgical treatment of osseous metastases in patients with renal cell carcinoma. *Clin Orthop* 1999;367:283–290.

26. Giehl JP, Kluba T. Metastatic spine disease in renal cell carcinoma—indication and results of surgery. *Anticancer Res* 1999;19(2C):1619–1623.

27. Weigel B, Maghsudi M, Neumann C, et al. Surgical management of symptomatic spinal metastases. Postoperative outcome and quality of life. *Spine* 1999;24(21):2240–2246.

28. Grunenwald D, Mazel C, Girard P, et al. Total vertebrectomy for en bloc resection of lung cancer invading the spine. *Ann Thorac Surg* 1996;61(2):723–725; discussion 725–726.

29. Okuyama T, Korenaga D, Tamura S, et al. Quality of life following surgery for vertebral metastases from breast cancer. *J Surg Oncol* 1999;70(1):60–63.

30. Tokuhashi Y, Matsuzaki H, Toriyama S, et al. Scoring system for the preoperative evaluation of metastatic spine tumor prognosis. *Spine* 1990;15(11):1110–1113.

31. Benzel EC. *Biomechanics of spine stabilization principles and clinical practice*. New York: McGraw-Hill, 1994.

32. Kanayama M, Ng JT, Cunningham BW, et al. Biomechanical analysis of anterior versus circumferential spinal reconstruction for various anatomic stages of tumor lesions. *Spine* 1999;24(5):445–450.

33. McLain RF, Bell GR. Newer management options in patients with spinal metastasis. *Cleve Clin J Med* 1998;65(7):359–366.

34. Bell GR. Surgical treatment of spinal tumors. *Clin Orthop* 1997;335:54–63.

35. Hopf C, Heine J. Operative therapy in metastases and primary tumors of the spine. *Neurosurg Rev* 1990;13(3):205–210.

36. Oda I, Cunningham BW, Abumi K, et al. The stability of reconstruction methods after thoracolumbar total spondylectomy. An in vitro investigation. *Spine* 1999;24(16):1634–1638.

37. Kostuik JP. Differential diagnosis and surgical treatment of metastatic spine tumors. In: Frymoyer JW, ed. *The adult spine: principles and practice*, 2nd ed. New York: Lippincott-Raven, 1997:989–1014.

38. Hollowell JP, Vollmer DG, Wilson CR, et al. Biomechanical analysis of thoracolumbar interbody constructs. How important is the endplate? *Spine* 1996;21(9):1032–1036.

39. Abe E, Sato K, Tazawa H, et al. Total spondylectomy for primary tumor of the thoracolumbar spine. *Spinal Cord* 2000;38(3):146–152.

40. Tomita K, Kawahara N, Baba H, et al. Total en bloc spondylectomy for solitary spinal metastases. *Int Orthop* 1994;18(5):291–298.

41. Cahill DW, Kumar R. Palliative subtotal vertebroplasty with anterior and posterior reconstruction using a single posterior approach. *J Neurosurg Spine* 1999;90(1):42–47.

169. Primary and Metastatic Disease of the Sacrum and Lumbar–Sacral Junction

Stephen L. Ondra, Sean A. Salehi, and Aruna Ganju

Diseases of the sacrum and lumbar–sacral junction can be divided into two broad pathological categories The tumors that most commonly involve the sacrum are metastatic lesions. The tumors of the second group, seen far less frequently, are the primary bone tumors, such as chordoma, sarcoma, myeloid, and giant cell tumors. The treatment and prognosis for these two categories of disease are fundamentally different. Therefore, the proper treatment of patients with bony disease of the sacrum depends on an accurate diagnosis, treatment based specifically on that diagnosis, and a consideration of the biomechanical consequences of the disease and its treatment.

Primary Tumors of the Sacrum

Primary bone tumors of the sacrum can be divided into two general groups. In the first group are the primary malignant tumors, such as chordoma, sarcoma, and giant cell tumor. In the second are the so-called round cell tumors. This group of lesions includes myeloma, plasmacytoma, lymphoma, and, in children, Ewing sarcoma.

Primary malignant tumors of the sacrum respond best to multimodal treatment. The cornerstone of treatment remains en bloc resection when possible (1–3). This is typically combined with radiation and chemotherapy for the best clinical result. The exact combination and timing of the different treatment modalities vary according to the type of lesion.

Chordoma is a rare tumor that arises from notochord remnant cells. The male-to-female ratio is 2:1. Peak occurrence is in the fifth to seventh decades, with a smaller peak seen in children and adolescents. Half of these lesions develop in the sacrum. They are typically lytic on roentgenograms and have a locally aggressive soft-tissue component (4). Despite their locally aggressive behavior, the rate of metastasis for these tumors is low. Rates as low as 5% and as high as 40% have been quoted. In patients whose lesions are successfully resected en bloc with negative margins, the recurrence rate is about 25%. If an en bloc resection cannot be achieved, radiation and chemotherapy can still be administered, but the benefit is limited. Recurrence and eventual death are the rule. As a group, patients with chordoma have a 10-year survival rate of 50% to 75% (4–7).

Giant cell tumor is the most common benign tumor of the sacrum (3). A female-to-male predominance of 2:1 is noted. This lesion is typically an expansile lytic mass that involves the vertebral body. Cortical breakthrough is commonly seen, but the soft-tissue component is typically less aggressive than that of chordoma (Fig. 1). Giant cell tumors most often occur proximally in the sacrum, whereas chordomas generally arise more distally. A 10% incidence of sarcomatous degeneration has been

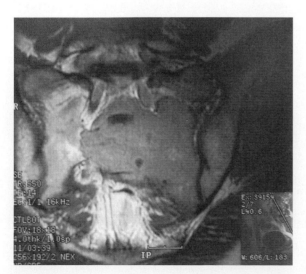

Fig. 1. Giant cell tumor of the sacrum. This lesion is characteristically located more cephalad and eccentrically in the sacrum.

reported. En bloc resection is the primary treatment. Radiation and chemotherapy are typically reserved for patients in whom an en bloc resection is not possible or who have recurrence. The recurrence rate varies from 10% to 50%, depending on the success of resection.

Osteosarcoma is a malignant bone-forming tumor that occurs throughout the appendicular skeleton; 3% of all osteosarcomas arise in the sacrum. These blastic lesions have a bubble-like appearance on both plane roentgenography and computed tomography (CT). Their metastatic rate is high, and they also exhibit locally aggressive behavior. Treatment typically consists of preoperative chemotherapy to induce tumor involution (1, 8). En bloc resection is followed by radiation therapy. Despite this aggressive multimodal approach, the prognosis remains dismal, with patients typically surviving for 6 to 12 months.

Chondrosarcomas are cartilage-forming tumors that occur more commonly in the appendicular skeleton and rarely affect the spine (3,9). When the sacrum is involved, the only effective therapy is surgical excision. Chemotherapy has little effect. Radiation seems primarily palliative. These lesions are rare enough that true survival rates are difficult to determine. With en bloc resection, it appears that 5-year survival rates of 60% to 80% are possible. Survival depends somewhat on tumor grade.

Myeloid Tumors of the Sacrum

Unlike primary and malignant solid tumors of the sacrum, myeloid tumors typically respond well to primary treatment with radiation and chemotherapy. Surgery is generally combined with the primary medical treatments or reserved as a salvage or stabilization technique. Again, the prognosis depends on pathology.

The myeloid tumors most commonly involving the spine include plasmacytoma, myeloma, and lymphoma. Plasmacytoma is a tumor composed of malignant marrow plasma cells. It is an exquisitely radiosensitive lesion (9). The 5-year survival rate is approximately 70%. Multiple myeloma is a diffuse disease of the bone that is seen most often in patients more than 50 years old (10). The spine is diffusely involved in virtually all cases. Lymphoma is a malignant lesion of white blood cells that affects the spine in 10% to 20% of cases and can result in spinal cord compression. Patients with this systemic disease have a 10-year survival rate of 30% when bony involvement occurs.

Each of the myeloid lesions discussed above is radiosensitive. Because most are systemic, radiation is typically combined with chemotherapy for primary treatment. Surgery is generally used for structural stabilization or for neurological salvage and decompression when necessary. It is not utilized as a primary treatment for this group of diseases.

Ewing Sarcoma

Ewing sarcoma is a rare, highly malignant neoplasm of adolescents and children. The mean age of patients presenting with this round cell lesion is 16 to 17 years; it can be seen rarely later in life. Ewing sarcoma is an aggressive lytic lesion that can metastasize, and bone scan and chest CT are part of the initial evaluation. On roentgenography, some peripheral areas of sclerosis and soft-tissue extension may be seen. Aggressive surgical debulking is combined with postoperative radiation and

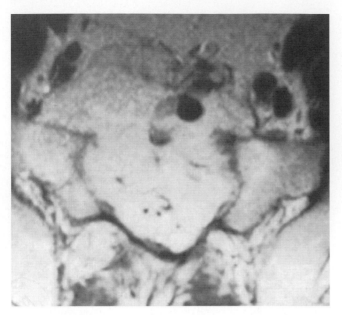

Fig. 2. Metastatic lesion (paraganglioma) with extensive destruction of the sacrum and lumbar sacral junction resulting in gross instability.

chemotherapy. Some have recommended preoperative radiation or chemotherapy to induce tumor involution before surgery. Regardless, the prognosis is poor. The overall 5-year survival remains at 20% (2,11).

Metastatic Disease of the Sacrum

Metastatic disease is rare in the sacrum in comparison with other sites, but metastatic disease in this region is still 40 times more frequent than primary bone tumors (Fig. 2). The survival rate of such patients despite gross total resection remains dismal (12). Radiation and chemotherapy are the treatments of choice when structural stability is not an issue. If the structural integrity of the lumbosacral junction is compromised, surgical stabilization and tumor debulking should be performed before adjuvant therapy is administered. This arrangement results in better wound healing and reconstruction. The medical treatment is of course based on the primary disease.

Presentation of Sacral Tumors

The most common presenting symptom of all sacral tumors is pain, which is typically lumbar or pelvic. It generally increases with weight bearing but can occur at rest. Pain at night is not uncommon. Neurological symptoms are related to compression of the sacral roots, which causes pain in the posterior leg, groin, or gluteal region. Bowel and bladder disturbances are common. L5 root dysfunction is also frequently seen with lesions of the proximal sacrum and lumbar–sacral junction. More extensive pelvic disease may lead to diffuse involvement of the lum-

bar–sacral plexus and additional symptoms of the lower extremities.

Treatment

For patients with metastatic or primary tumors of the sacrum and lumbar–sacral junction, three separate issues must be addressed. The first is tumor treatment. As we have seen, this depends greatly on tumor pathology. The second is neural decompression. This can be accomplished medically with chemosensitive or radiosensitive lesions and surgically when the lesion is not responsive. The third is the potential instability that results from bony destruction, which can lead to mechanical instability and pain. This structural issue is a surgical problem if the patient has an expected survival of 6 months or more.

A discussion of the nonsurgical treatments of sacral tumors is beyond the scope of this chapter. The two primary goals of surgery in patients with sacral lesions are treatment of the primary disease and spinal stabilization.

Surgical lesions of the sacrum can be divided into two groups, based on the anatomical location of the lesion. Lesions below S1 are considered caudal sacral lesions. Those within S1 are considered proximal sacral lesions. These two locations are fundamentally different biomechanically.

CAUDAL SACRAL LESIONS. In general, caudal lesions are structurally stable and require no reconstruction. Surgery is performed for primary treatment of the tumor when medical therapy is ineffective or not indicated as a primary treatment. It can also be undertaken for salvage and pain control. With primary bony tumors for which en bloc resection is required, we prefer to perform a single-stage posterior resection.

Gluteal flaps are turned and the spine is exposed. A margin of muscle is left over the lesion (Fig. 3). The rectum is mobilized from the sacrum and bluntly dissected anteriorly. An osteotomy

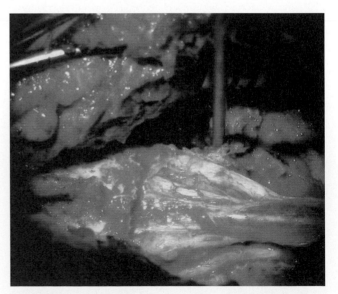

Fig. 3. The resection of caudal sacral chordoma begins with elevation of gluteal flaps to expose the sacrum. The rectum is then mobilized anteriorly to allow the insertion of lap pads between the sacrum and pelvic structures to the level of S1-2 and occasionally the sacral promontory.

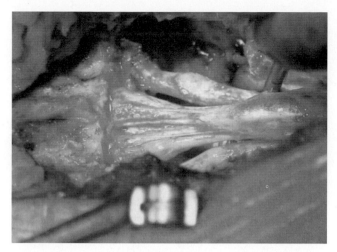

Fig. 4. En bloc resection and removal of the sacrum. Note the osteotomy at the level of the S2 body.

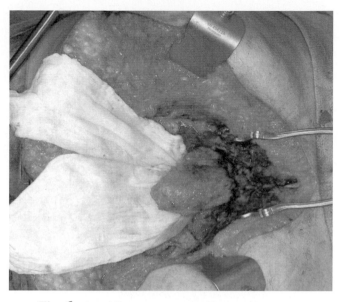

Fig. 6. Gluteal flap reconstruction after sacral resection.

is performed with a drill proximal to the lesion, and the sacral roots involved in the lesion are doubly ligated with 2-0 silk ties. The sacral roots are then cut. With a lap pad inserted anterior to the sacrum to protect the rectum and soft tissues, an osteotome is used to separate the sacrum proximal to the lesion, then at the sacroiliac joint bilaterally. The sacrum and roots are then lifted out as an en bloc specimen (Figs. 4 and 5). The gluteal flaps are reconstructed and the rectum reincorporated (Fig. 6). If the lesion invades the rectum or the rectum must be resected, a colostomy is performed. If the rectum is not affected, colostomy is not always necessary.

In caudal metastatic disease, en bloc resection is not necessary. When radiation and chemotherapy are ineffective in relieving neurological symptoms or pain, surgery can be utilized to debulk the tumor and relieve symptomatic neural compression. A simple midline incision is performed. The sacrum is unroofed, and the Cavitron ultrasonic aspirator can be used to debulk the lesion with sparing of the neural elements. Resection

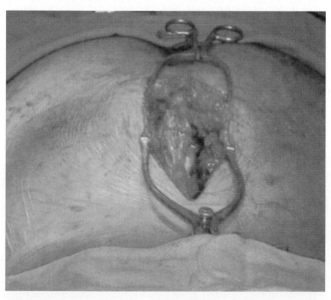

Fig. 5. Resection bed after removal of the sacrum. Shown are the pelvic fascia, residual sacrum above mid-S2, and resected cauda equina. The preserved nerves of the cauda equina are also visualized.

can be carried out to the pelvic fascia. Reconstruction is not necessary.

PROXIMAL SACRAL TUMORS. The treatment of primary tumors of the proximal sacrum requires en bloc resection through an anterior–posterior technique. Therefore, the neural structures below the level of the lesion, typically L4 or L5, are sacrificed (5,13–18), with the inevitable result of lower-extremity weakness and loss of bowel and bladder control.

The initial approach is anterior. A midline incision is utilized, and the rectum, iliac vessels, and soft-tissue structures are mobilized. An osteotome is utilized to begin separation of the sacrum lateral to the lesion or at the sacroiliac joints. Another cut is made caudal to the lesion. The L5-S1 disc is removed. After anterior closure, the posterior portion of the procedure is begun.

A midline posterior incision is performed from L3 to the caudal sacrum. An L5 laminectomy (occasionally L4-5) is performed in addition to a sacral undoming if the lamina is not involved with tumor. The cauda equina nerves that transit the portion of the sacrum involved with tumor are doubly ligated with 2-0 silk ties and transected. Posterior osteotomies are then performed laterally and caudally to match the anterior cuts created during the anterior stage of the procedure. The posterior annulus of the L5-S1 disc is removed, and the sacrum is lifted out posteriorly en bloc. We have not found it practical to reverse this procedure because it is very difficult to lift out the sacrum anteriorly with all the soft-tissue structures in the way.

After neural sacrifice and en bloc tumor resection with a negative margin have been accomplished, reconstruction is carried out. The strategies for treating metastatic disease of the proximal sacrum have traditionally been similar to those for treating primary tumors. Such an approach is not reasonable for metastatic disease.

Because of the limited life expectancy of patients with metastatic cancer, an approach that preserves and maintains quality of life is required. The preservation of neurological function, control of pain, and early mobilization are all necessary. Additionally, patients with metastatic disease typically are offered a variety of chemotherapy/radiation therapy options for disease control. By definition, such patients are not surgically curable regardless of the results of local resection. Therefore, the goals

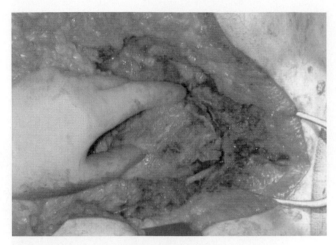

Fig. 7. Metastatic lesion resection begins with undoming of the sacrum. This fully exposes the cauda equina.

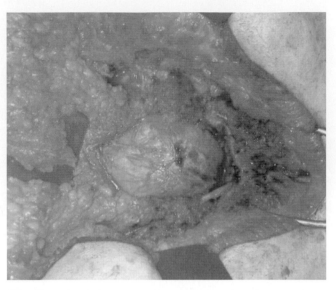

Fig. 8. Gross total resection of metastatic tumor to the pelvic fascia with preservation of all neural structures. This resection includes all of S1, so that reconstruction is required.

of surgery and the management plans are radically changed. Patients are typically first treated with chemotherapy or radiation. If this fails, decompression and any necessary stabilization are carried out.

The goal of surgical decompression is to control pain and preserve neurological function. Surgical decompression can be carried out from either an anterior or a posterior approach. The choice depends on the pathology. We prefer an anterior approach when disease is penetrating the pelvic fascia and a significant intrapelvic mass is present. Another circumstance in which an anterior approach is preferred would be a highly vascular tumor that has recruited pelvic vessels. In this situation, the better vascular control, visualization, and pelvic access make the anterior approach preferable. It can be combined with a second-stage posterior decompression and reconstruction.

In all other circumstances, we prefer a one-stage posterior approach, which allows a single-stage decompression and reconstruction. Additionally, the thecal sac and lumbar–sacral nerves can be followed from normal to abnormal anatomy, so that the risk for neurological injury is minimized. This is accomplished by a laminectomy of L5. If disease extends widely in the sacrum (in particular near the end plate), a facetectomy is performed. An L4 laminectomy is required only if significant associated L5 disease is present. An undoming of the entire sacral canal to the pedicles is then performed (Fig. 7). The thecal sac is identified, and the sacral roots are followed into the tumor or the anterior sacrum. The tumor is removed by means of loop or microscopic dissection. Standard microtechniques are employed. We typically use an ultrasonic aspirator. Access is gained by working between and retracting the nerve roots and thecal sac. Complete resection of tumor and, if desired, bone infiltrated with disease can be carried out to the pelvic fascia anterior to the sacrum (Fig. 8). Care must be taken not to violate this region to avoid injury to the pelvic contents. The rectum, ureters, and iliac vessels are of particular concern. Resection may extend out to but not through the sacroiliac joint if reconstruction that allows mobilization is to be considered.

Stability and Reconstruction of the Lumbar–Sacral Junction

STABILITY OF THE LUMBAR–SACRAL JUNCTION. Instability should be assessed in terms of the anterior column, axial

load transfer to the pelvis from the anterior column, and posterior tension band competence. The anterior column is rendered unstable when resection of the sacrum or erosion resulting from the primary disease process extends to 1 cm below the sacral promontory in more than two thirds of the sacral end-plate surface (19). When such a resection is necessitated by tumor growth, a 50% reduction in pelvic strength and incompetence of the anterior spinal column result. In this situation, it is necessary to restore anterior column stability and load transfer to the pelvis to allow mobilization, prevent deformity, and decrease pain. Pelvic ring competence must also be restored to avoid structural pelvic failure, which can result in such problems as fracture of the pubic symphysis.

If the sacrum is structurally competent, with more than 1 cm of bone preserved below the promontory over at least one third to one half the S1 end plate, no anterior column reconstruction is required after tumor resection.

The posterior tension band is always affected by the large laminectomy required for resection. It may also be rendered functionally weak by tumor extension into the posterior elements. In cases in which the facet joints and pars interarticularis are preserved, it is reasonable to defer reconstruction. If the facets or pars is violated, a tension band reconstruction is required. Additionally, we recommend tension band restoration with segmental instrumentation in cases in which the patient has significant preoperative back pain or a significant anterior column defect. Such an anterior column structural defect places additional stress on the posterior construct regardless of whether it meets the criteria for an independent anterior column reconstruction. Removal of the sacrum results in a loss of anterior column support for the spine and an unstable axial load transfer from the spinal column to the pelvis. Additionally, removal of the sacrum renders the pelvic ring incompetent. To correct these two structural problems, reconstruction has typically been performed with two distinct goals: restoration of the pelvic ring and load transfer of the spine to the pelvis.

Pelvic ring stability is typically restored by placement of a transiliac bar. The spinal load is transferred to the pelvis by pedicle screws and rods connecting the lumbar spine to the residual ilium. This reconstruction does not allow anterior column axial support or load.

RECONSTRUCTION OF THE ANTERIOR COLUMN AND PELVIS. Reconstruction can be carried out by means of the more traditional methods described previously. Unfortunately, they do not result in immediate axial stability of the spine and do not allow early ambulation. Posterior column reconstruction alone does not allow transfer of the anterior column axial load to the pelvis. Because this is where 80% of the axial load is carried, posterior column load transfer alone is insufficient for weight bearing, and prolonged periods of bed rest ranging from 3 to 6 months have been described (16,20). For these reasons, we prefer a reconstruction method for the anterior column that allows both axial support of the spine and load transfer to the pelvis. It also restores the pelvic ring, so that early mobilization is possible.

This is accomplished by fitting a titanium mesh cage against the fused end plate of L5. The cage, packed with bone graft and having a hole that allows passage of a 0.25-in titanium rod, is introduced between the retracted nerve roots. A Kirschner wire is then passed through a stab incision in the skin on the lateral aspect of the hip. The Kirschner wire is passed under fluoroscopic guidance through the cage and contralateral ilium and out through the contralateral hip. A 0.25-in cannulated reamer is passed over the Kirschner wire, and the ilium is perforated bilaterally. A 0.25-in titanium rod is passed through the ilium bilaterally and the cage (Fig. 9). Connectors are affixed to the rod to prevent movement.

The cage does not rock because of its broad surface contact with L5. Additional bone and graft material can be packed around the cage and rod to allow fusion or dense scar to give added support to the construct. In this way, the anterior column is given axial support and load transfer to the pelvis. The pelvic ring is also reconstituted.

POSTERIOR TENSION BAND RECONSTRUCTION AND SPINAL PELVIC LOAD SHARING. The posterior tension band can be established when mechanically necessary with or without an anterior column reconstruction. Pedicle screws are placed at L4 and L5. Attachment to the ilium can then be accomplished by means of a Galveston rod technique, in which a rod is placed into the ilium and connected to the pedicle screws.

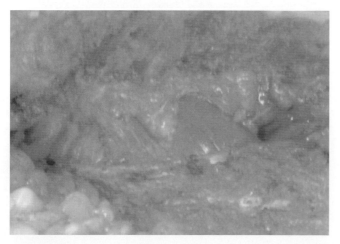

Fig. 9. Initial reconstruction begins with the insertion of a rod through each ilium and a titanium cage filled with bone graft. This establishes axial support of the spine with load transfer to the pelvis. The rods are cut off at the ilium after connectors have been placed at the ends. These connectors prevent rod migration. In addition to axial support, this part of the reconstruction allows reconstitution of the pelvic ring.

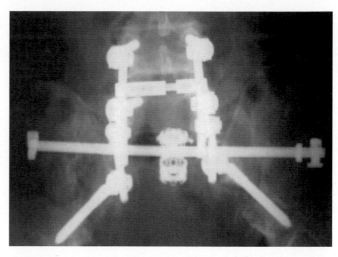

Fig. 10. Final reconstruction after sacral resection. The cage is seated against L5, providing axial support. Load transfer and pelvic ring reconstruction are provided by the transiliac bar. A posterior tension band and additional axial load transfer are provided by the posterior rod system, which reconnects the spine and ilium through a combination of pedicle screws and iliac bolts in a modified Galveston technique.

An alternative is to place an iliac bolt and affix the rod to this and the pedicle screws to restore the posterior tension band between the spine and ilium. It also allows some posterior column axial load transfer to the pelvis (Fig. 10).

Arthrodesis and grafting can be carried out along the posterior elements and ilium. An iliac crest graft is not possible because of the need for iliac fixation. If the patient is likely to be a long-term survivor, alternative graft sources, such as rib, can be considered. In other patients, allograft or no graft are reasonable options. Cross-linking is performed to provide added stability, especially for torsion. Additional pelvic ring stability may also be provided by the cross-linked rods.

Surgical Results in Patients with Proximal Sacral Metastatic Disease

This combined anterior–posterior reconstruction has been performed successfully in four patients. All patients had metastatic disease that resulted in pain and instability when evaluated by the previously discussed criteria (Table 1).

Resection achieved an 80% to 90% removal of tumor. This was accomplished with excellent preservation of neurological function (Table 2). The patients were mobilized within 1 to 2 weeks of surgery (mean, 10 days), whereas in other reported experiences, surgery resulted in significant neurological impairment, prolonged bed rest, or both (5,12,14,16,20–22). The reconstruction can be accomplished with acceptable morbidity given the magnitude of the problem (Table 3).

Conclusions

Tumors of the sacrum remain among the most challenging and controversial management problems in spinal disease. Treatment can be categorized according to tumor location and type.

Table 1. Preoperative Symptoms of Patients with Proximal Sacral Metastatic Disease

Case no.	Age	Diagnosis	Preoperative symptoms	Pertinent examination findings
1	52	Fibrosarcoma (metastatic)	Low-back pain, left S1 radiculopathy, urinary incontinence	5/5 Motor all groups
2	52	Adenocarcinoma	Low-back pain, right-foot weakness	Right 3/5 plantar flexor
3	35	Paraganglioma	Low-back pain, left S1 radiculopathy, urinary incontinence	Bilateral 4/5 dorsiflexor
4	46	Adenocarcinoma	Low-back pain, left S1 and S2 radiculopathy, urinary retention	

Table 2. Postoperative Symptoms of Patients with Proximal Sacral Metastatic Disease

Case no.	Postoperative symptoms	Pertinent examination findings
1	Resolved radiculopathy, normal bladder function	5/5 Motor all groups
2	Normal bladder function	Right 4/5 plantar flexor
3	Normal bladder function	Bilateral 3/5 dorsiflexor
4	Normal bladder function	Transient radiculopathy left L5

Table 3. Postoperative Non-neurologic Complications

Case no.	Postoperative non-neurologic complications
1	Internal iliac vein thrombosis, return to operating room for instrumentation failure
2	None
3	Disseminated intravascular coagulation
4	None

Proximal lesions that result in instability are surgical problems first, with adjuvant therapy administered after healing; the sole exception is osteosarcoma, for which involutional chemotherapy is given first. Proximal lesions that do not cause instability are typically treated medically; surgery is performed as a salvage procedure because it is understood that resection of proximal primary bone tumors results in instability.

Lesions of the caudal sacrum do not require reconstruction, and initial treatment is based on pathology. Primary tumors are surgically resected as initial treatment. Myeloid and metastatic lesions are treated medically first, with surgical salvage.

Despite the progress that has been made, the treatment of sacral tumors is still debilitating to the patient, and the prognosis remains poor.

References

1. Barwick KW, Huvos AG, Smith J. Primary osteosarcoma of the vertebral column: a clinical pathologic correlation of 10 patients. *Cancer* 1989;46:595.
2. Rosen G, Caparros B, Nirenberg A, et al. Ewing's sarcoma: ten-year experience with adjuvant chemotherapy. *Cancer* 1981;47:2204.
3. Weinstein JN, McLain RF: Primary tumors of the spine. *Spine* 1987;12:843.
4. Rosenthal DI, Scott JA, Mankin HJ, et al. Sacrococcygeal chordomas: magnetic resonance imaging and computed tomography. *Am J Radiol* 1985;145:143.
5. Samson I, Springfield D, Suit H, et al. Operative treatment of sacrococcygeal chordoma. *J Bone Joint Surg Am* 1993;75:1476–1484.
6. Kaiser TE, Pritchard DJ, Unni KK. Clinical pathologic studies of sacrococcygeal chordoma. *Cancer* 1984;54:2574.
7. Sundaresan N, Huvos AG, Krol G, et al. Spinal chordoma: results of surgical treatment. *Arch Surg* 1987;122:1478.
8. Sundaresan N, Rosen G, Huvos AG, et al. Combined modality treatment of osteosarcoma of the spine. *Neurosurgery* 1988;23:714.
9. Merryweather R, Middlemiss JH, Sanerkin NG. Malignant transformation of osteoblastoma. *J Bone Joint Surg Am* 1981;63:381.
10. Bataille R, Sany J. Solitary myeloma: clinical and prognostic features of a review of 114 cases. *Cancer* 1981;48:845.
11. Wilkens RM, Pritchard DJ, Burgert EO, et al. Ewing's sarcoma of bone: experience with 140 patients. *Cancer* 1986;58:2551.
12. Huth J, Dawson E, Eliber F. Abdominosacral resection for malignant tumors of the sacrum. *Am J Surg* 1984;148:157–161.
13. Gokaslan ZL, Romsdahl MM, Kroll SS, et al. Total sacrectomy and Galveston L-rod reconstruction for malignant neoplasms. Technical note. *J Neurosurg* 1997;87:781–787.
14. Localio SA, Eng K, Ranson J. Abdominosacral approach for retrorectal tumors. *Ann Surg* 1980;191:555–560.
15. Ozdemir MH, Gurkan I, Yildia Y, et al. Surgical treatment of the malignant tumors of the sacrum. *Eur J Surg Oncol* 1999;25:44–49.
16. Sung HW, Shu WP, Wang HM, et al. Surgical treatment of primary tumors of the sacrum. *Clin Orthop* 1987;215:91–98.
17. Tomita K, Tsuchiya H. Total sacrectomy and reconstruction for huge sacral tumors. *Spine* 1990;15:1223–1227.
18. Wuisman P, Harle A, Matthiab HH, et al. Two-stage therapy in the treatment of sacral tumors. *Arch Orthop Trauma Surg* 1989;108:255–260.
19. Gunterberg B, Romanus B, Stener B. Pelvic strength after major amputation of the sacrum. *Acta Orthop* 1976;47:635–642.
20. Stener B, Gunterberg B. High amputation of the sacrum for extirpation of tumors. *Spine* 1977;3:351–366.
21. Jackson RJ, Gokaslan ZL. Spinal–pelvic fixation in patients with lumbosacral neoplasms. *J Neurosurg* 2000;1(suppl):61–70.
22. Shikata J, Yamamuro T, Kptoura Y, et al. Total sacrectomy and reconstruction for primary tumors. *J Bone Joint Surg Am* 1988;70:122–125.

170. Primary Bone Tumors of the Spine and Nonosseous Primary Tumors of the Spine and Facets

**W. Bradley Jacobs and
Michael G. Fehlings**

Primary osseous and nonosseous tumors of the spinal column are uncommon. Neoplastic invasion of the vertebral axis most often represents metastasis of systemic tumors, such as those of the lung, breast, and prostate, or of hematopoietic neoplasms, such as multiple myeloma and lymphoma. Such metastasis reflects not only the prevalence of these systemic neoplasms, but also their predilection for the spinal column. In contrast, primary osseous and nonosseous tumors of the spine account for only 0.4% of all tumors (1), and only 11% of tumors involving bone (2). They are approximately 40 times less common than spinal column metastases (3). Because they are uncommon, individual neurosurgeons are not likely to encounter many primary spinal column tumors in the course of their practice. However, to ensure that patients harboring a primary neoplasm of the vertebral axis receive a correct treatment plan that utilizes modern spinal surgical techniques in an appropriate manner, neurosurgeons must have a thorough understanding of the clinical presentation and natural history of the different tumors within this broad category, and be familiar with the viable treatment options.

Clinical Evaluation

SIGNS AND SYMPTOMS. Pain is the most common presenting symptom, but primary neoplasms of the spinal column may also present as a deformity, a painless mass, neurological deficit, or an incidental finding on a neuroimaging study. The pain associated with neoplasms of the vertebral axis is classically unremitting, worse in the supine position, and often more noticeable when the patient is at rest or in bed during the night (3,4). The pain can be radicular, secondary to compression or invasion of nerve structures, or it can be local, secondary to neoplastic erosion and infiltration of bony structures. Although the pain of a bone tumor can be similar to that of a herniated disc, in comparison with muscular, fascial, discogenic, or spondylitic pain, the pain of a bone tumor is more persistent and less likely to be relieved by positional changes. Pain may also develop in conjunction with the new onset of a deformity, such as torticollis or scoliosis. Thus, painful scoliosis in a young patient should not be considered idiopathic before a detailed etiological search is undertaken. Bone tumors may also result in painful instability of the spine secondary to pathological fractures or facet instability.

Primary spine tumors may also present with neurological deficit. Neurological deficit occurs more commonly in conjunction with malignant neoplasms (~50%), the specific deficit depending on the level of involvement (4) and the structure compressed. Compression of a nerve root, the spinal cord, or the cauda equina produces the corresponding neurological findings of radiculopathy, myelopathy, or cauda equina syndrome. Physical examination of the patient with a primary spine tumor often reveals local pain, paraspinal spasm, and rarely a localized mass extending into the posterior soft tissues, in addition to potential neurological deficits, signs of instability, and deformity.

The age of the patient is very important when a vertebral axis tumor is being considered because different lesions with different clinical implications are characteristic of each age group (5). In general, children harbor benign spine tumors, adults have malignant primary spine tumors, and elderly patients have metastatic spine lesions (5,6).

CLINICAL INVESTIGATIONS. Besides a thorough history and physical examination, the clinical investigation of any patient with back pain should consist of routine laboratory investigations, including a complete blood cell count and determination of the erythrocyte sedimentation rate. These tests help to suggest or rule out infectious etiologies. In appropriate patients, serum and protein electrophoresis and levels of prostate-specific antigen can help in the diagnosis of multiple myeloma and metastatic prostate carcinoma, respectively (7). The diagnosis of a primary neoplasm of the vertebral axis requires detailed imaging of the region of the spine in question. Although modern neuroimaging methods have greatly facilitated the diagnosis of these lesions, the plain radiograph remains a useful first test. It can provide an abundance of information regarding lytic destruction of bone, vertebral collapse, kyphosis, and subluxation. Further imaging with computed tomography (CT), CT–myelography, and magnetic resonance imaging (MRI) adds greatly to the clinical evaluation. CT provides important information about the status of the cortical bone, whereas MRI is superior in delineating epidural and bone marrow tumor infiltration and separates the extraosseous soft-tissue component of a neoplasm from the normal paraspinal soft tissues and neural structures (8). When MRI is contraindicated, CT–myelography provides excellent visualization of the thecal sac and demonstrates spinal canal compromise by invading neoplasm. Patients suspected of having either multifocal primary or metastatic disease should also undergo a technetium bone scan. This test is invaluable in quantifying the extent of bone involvement over the entire skeletal structure and provides information about bone-forming and bone-destroying neoplastic entities. In those patients whose bone tumor is likely a metastasis, chest radiography and abdominal ultrasonography are useful first tests to aid in identifying of a primary lesion.

Classification of Primary Spinal Tumors

The most intuitive way to develop a classification system for primary spine tumors is according to embryological tissue of origin. In this manner, it is possible to distinguish between true osseous neoplasms and those tumors derived from tissues intimately associated with the vertebrae, but not from bone per se

Table 1. Primary Tumors of the Spine

Cell of origin	Benign	Malignant
Osseous	Osteoid osteoma[a] Osteoblastoma[a]	Osteosarcoma[a]
Cartilaginous	Osteochondroma[a] Enchondroma	Chondrosarcoma[a]
Marrow		Solitary plasmacytoma[a] Ewing sarcoma[a] Lymphoma Multiple myeloma
Fibrous	Fibroma	Fibrosarcoma Malignant fibrous histiocytoma
Vascular	Hemangioma[a] Aneurysmal bone cyst[a]	
Notochordal		Chordoma[a]
Other	Giant cell tumor[a] Eosinophilic granuloma[a]	

[a]Discussed in the text.

(Table 1). The axial skeleton is composed of osseous, fibrous, and cartilaginous elements, and both benign and malignant neoplasms may evolve from these structures. Primary neoplasms of the spinal column may also arise from the abundant vascular structures, bone marrow, and notochordal remnants that are present in the vertebral axis. The vertebral bodies are rich in red marrow, reflecting the predilection of systemic metastases and hematopoietic neoplasms for these structures.

BENIGN TUMORS

Osteoid Osteoma. Osteoid osteomas are benign bone tumors found predominantly in adolescents and young adults (Fig. 1). Almost all patients present with pain that is worse at night and that is dramatically relieved with salicylates or nonsteroidal antiinflammatory medications (9). Other common presenting symptoms include a limited range of motion of the spine and painful torticollis or scoliosis (9). Osteoid osteoma is the most frequent cause of painful scoliosis in adolescents. Osteoid osteomas tend to affect the posterior elements of the spine, with 75% located posteriorly, and are slightly more common in the lumbar spine (10).

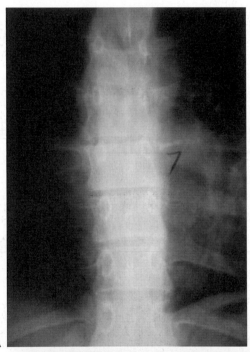

A

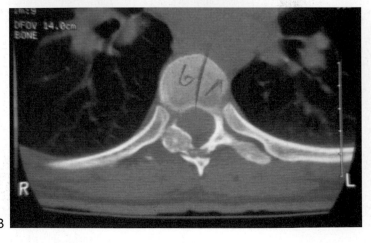

B

Fig. 1. Osteoid osteoma. This 22-year-old woman presented with a several-year history of unremitting back pain that was initially responsive to nonsteroidal inflammatory medications. Plain films (**A**) and computed tomography (CT) (**B**) show a well-circumscribed ovoid lesion with peripheral sclerosis and a radiolucent center involving the lamina/pedicle at T7. The lesion was treated by complete excision with an excellent outcome. Histologically (**C**), the lesion is characterized by osteoblasts and osteoid in a highly vascularized stroma.

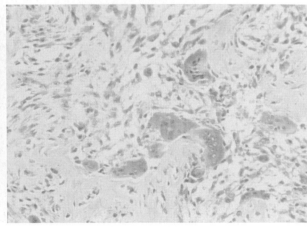

C

Radiologically, this lesion consists of a discrete radiolucent nidus surrounded by a variable degree of sclerosis. An arbitrary maximal diameter of 1.5 cm is used to differentiate osteoid osteoma from the larger but pathologically identical osteoblastoma. Bone scans demonstrate increased uptake of radionuclide in the area surrounding the lesion, with a "cold" nidus. On CT, the imaging modality of choice for these lesions, the nidus is a well-defined lesion with low attenuation and with or without central calcification (10). Pathologically, osteoid osteomas are composed of well-organized, interconnected trabecular bone with a background of vascularized fibrous connective tissue (10). Reactive bone invariably forms a pseudocapsule around the lesion. Surgery is the treatment of choice for these tumors and usually relieves pain and corrects spontaneous deformity, especially if the deformity has been present for less than 15 months (9). Grossly, osteoid osteoma is very similar to normal cortical bone, so that it is difficult to determine when total surgical extirpation has been achieved. Numerous strategies, including preoperative radionuclide labeling of the nidus and CT-guided needle placement, have been used to avoid this problem. Recurrence is unlikely if the lesion has been totally removed. Radiation therapy is not indicated in the treatment of osteoid osteoma.

Osteoblastoma. Osteoblastoma and osteoid osteoma are similar but distinct lesions. The two are histologically identical, with lesions larger than 1.5 cm in diameter arbitrarily defined as osteoblastomas. Like osteoid osteomas, osteoblastomas tend to involve the posterior elements, occur frequently in young patients, and most commonly present with pain. Forty-five percent of osteoblastomas are located in the spine (11), but a predilection for a specific region of the spine is not noted. Unlike the pain of osteoid osteoma, the pain associated with osteoblastoma is relieved with salicylates in only a minority of cases (12). Neurological deficit is also more commonly associated with osteoblastomas, occurring in 25% of cases (11,12), a finding that is likely attributable to the larger size and somewhat more invasive nature of these tumors. Except for their larger size, osteoblastomas are very similar to osteoid osteomas in radiological appearance. An aggressive appearance has been noted in some osteoblastomas, consisting of osseous expansion, bone destruction, and infiltration of surrounding soft tissues (10). The histology of osteoblastoma is usually similar to that of osteoid osteoma. However, an aggressive subgroup of osteoblastomas have been described that appear similar to osteosarcoma and consist of prominent epithelioid osteoblasts (13).

Surgical resection remains the mainstay of treatment. Because of the larger size of osteoblastomas, it is occasionally necessary to destabilize the spine to achieve complete excision. In such cases, spinal instrumentation and fusion are required. Despite surgical resection, recurrence rates are somewhat higher than for osteoid osteomas, approaching 10% (14). Invasion of the epidural space is not an uncommon finding at surgery (9) and necessitates careful dissection of tumor away from the dura mater.

Osteochondroma. Although osteochondromas are common bone tumors, only 4% occur in the vertebral axis (15). These are benign cartilaginous tumors that arise during development when physeal cartilage is trapped outside the physeal plate. In very rare instances, an osteochondroma can undergo malignant transformation to a chondrosarcoma. Osteochondromas have a predilection for the cervical spine and are more commonly found in the posterior elements of the vertebrae. Reflecting their developmental origin, osteochondromas are usually discovered in patients less than 30 years of age. The male-to-female sex ratio is greater than 2:1.

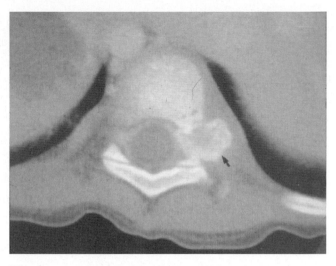

Fig. 2. Osteochondroma. Axial CT through T9 shows an exophytic lesion in a 4-year-old child with back pain. This was successfully treated by resection through a posterolateral approach.

The radiographic appearance is nonspecific, although occasionally plain radiographs or CT reveal the exostosis and its cartilaginous cap (Fig. 2). Histologically, osteochondromas are composed of normal bone with a cartilaginous cap, from which the growth occurs. The pathological hallmark is continuity of the lesion with the marrow and cortex of the underlying bone.

Asymptomatic lesions can be followed conservatively, but surgery should be considered whenever the diagnosis is in question, if the patient is in pain, or in the rare case of progressive neurological deficit (16). Symptoms are relieved after surgical extirpation. The recurrence rate is extremely low, but rare documentation of regrowth after subtotal excision has been reported (3).

Hemangioma. The hemangioma, a benign vascular tumor, is the most common neoplasm affecting the spinal column; it is found in 11% of spines at autopsy, with the vast majority of cases having been asymptomatic (Fig. 3, Color Plate 33). Hemangiomas are found more often in the thoracolumbar and lumbar spine and usually involve the vertebral body. Hemangiomas usually become symptomatic only after vertebral collapse, pathological fracture, or rarely compression of neural structures has occurred. Clinical presentation peaks in the fifth decade. Rare cases of exacerbation of hemangioma symptomatology during pregnancy, secondary to either hormonal or hemodynamic influences, have been documented (17).

Hemangiomas have a characteristic appearance on plain radiography, demonstrating a hypertrophic vertical trabeculation that develops in response to the neoplastic destruction of horizontal trabeculae. Because of their high content of adipose and vascular tissue, hemangiomas are bright on both T1-weighted and T2-weighted MRI sequences. Histologically, hemangiomas are composed of endothelium-lined capillary and cavernous sinuses. The former consist of thin-walled vessels separated by normal bone, whereas the latter consist of dilated blood vessels without intervening bone stroma.

Given the real risk for exsanguinating hemorrhage at surgery, the vast majority of symptomatic hemangiomas can be treated conservatively with external bracing. Radiation therapy and endovascular embolization are also therapeutic options, although the efficacy of these as stand-alone therapies is debatable. Surgery should be reserved for those cases of neurological deficit that are secondary to significant kyphosis and vertebral canal

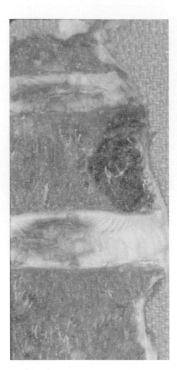

Fig. 3. Postmortem specimen of hemangioma.

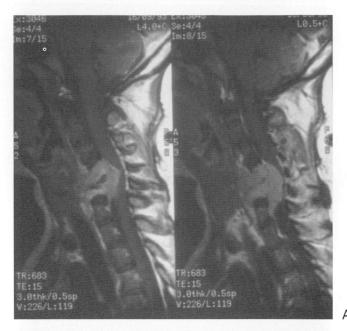

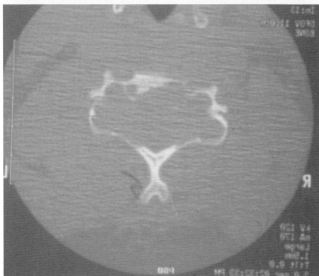

Fig. 4. Giant cell tumor. This 25-year-old woman presented with neck pain and progressive tetraparesis. Magnetic resonance imaging (MRI) (**A**) and CT (**B**) show an expansile lesion arising from the vertebral bodies of C5 and C6 with involvement of the transverse foramina and posterior elements. The lesion was successfully treated with a combined anterior/posterior resection and reconstruction.

compromise. In these situations, therapy must be directed at restoration of the correct anatomical relationships and spinal alignment. Preoperative embolization is imperative to avoid massive blood loss during tumor resection.

Aneurysmal Bone Cyst. The aneurysmal bone cyst (ABC) is another benign vascular lesion that commonly presents in the first three decades of life. The spine is involved in approximately 20% of cases (18). Like most other benign primary lesions of the spinal column, ABCs tend to involve the posterior elements. Patients most commonly present with pain; however, neurological deficit is a relatively frequently presenting feature, occurring in up to 50% of cases (19), and is likely related to the marked expansile nature of ABCs, with resultant epidural compression.

Although neuroimaging studies often are not definitive in the diagnosis of ABCs, marked expansile remodeling centered on the posterior elements is a typical feature. CT and MRI frequently show the cystic nature of the lesion, and multiple fluid levels, indicative of old hemorrhage and sedimentation, can be appreciated on MRI (10). Grossly, ABCs are often described as a "blood-filled sponge," consisting of multiloculated, blood-filled spaces that are not lined by endothelium. Although the vast majority of ABCs are primary lesions, up to 30% occur in association with other neoplasms, such as giant cell tumor (GCT), osteoblastoma, and osteosarcoma (8).

Surgical resection is the treatment of choice for ABCs. Complete resection is often not possible without excessive morbidity because the lesions are often quite large at the time of presentation (20). Preoperative embolization can be used to minimize operative blood loss. Recurrence rates are low, ranging from 10% to 25% at 10 years (19,20). Radiation therapy, although carrying inherent risks, is a viable adjuvant treatment option for refractory ABCs that cannot be excised completely.

Giant Cell Tumor. GCTs are histologically benign but aggressive lesions of unknown cell origin (Fig. 4, Color Plate 34). They

occur throughout the skeleton, with tumors of the vertebral column accounting for 5% of these lesions. Although most commonly located in the sacrum, GCTs of the mobile spine are equally divided among the cervical, thoracic, and lumbar segments. GCTs tend to involve the vertebral body. A definite female preponderance is noted, with most lesions presenting between the third and fifth decades of life (21).

Characteristically, imaging studies demonstrate an expansile destructive lesion within the vertebral body. Unlike other spinal neoplasms, GCTs may involve and extend across the intervertebral disc space, simulating infectious entities on neuroimaging studies (10). On CT and MRI, heterogeneous signal characteristics are common because of the hemorrhage and necrosis that are often present in GCTs (8). Histologically, GCTs consist of numerous osteoclastic giant cells admixed in a vascular and fibrous stroma. Regions of necrosis and hemorrhage are frequent. Although cytologically benign, GCTs are locally invasive and can even metastasize.

Surgical resection is the treatment of choice for GCTs of the axial skeleton; these tumors are relatively resistant to radiation therapy and chemotherapy. En bloc resection is always desirable but rarely possible in the vertebral axis. Because of the locally invasive nature of GCTs, recurrence rates as high as 50% have been reported in instances of subtotal resection, such as after intralesional curettage (22). Given this high recurrence rate, local radiation therapy has been advocated as a useful adjuvant to facilitate local control (23). However, sarcomatous degeneration of radiated GCT is well documented, and these patients require close follow-up.

Eosinophilic Granuloma.
Eosinophilic granuloma (EG) is the most common and benign form of Langerhans cell histiocytosis. EG is a tumorlike collection of eosinophils and histiocytes. The proliferation of hematopoietic cells arises from the marrow elements of the vertebral body in the vertebral column. EG is largely a pediatric ailment, with more than 75% of cases presenting in the first two decades of life. Approximately 15% of cases of EG involve the spine, with the calvarium, mandible, and long bones accounting for the remaining cases (8). Spinal EG occurs mainly in the thoracic and lumbar segments.

An acute onset of back pain is the typical presentation; neurological deficit is extremely rare. The classical radiographic finding is that of a symmetrically flattened vertebral body, in conjunction with preservation of the disc space, sparing of the posterior elements, and an absence of kyphosis, known as *vertebra plana*. Vertebra plana can be associated with other spinal tumors and should not be considered pathognomonic for EG. The natural history of EG is one of a self-limiting disease. Partial restitution of vertebral height generally occurs. Treatment should consist of pain control and external orthosis to maintain spinal alignment during the acute episode. Surgery is rarely indicated and should be reserved for rare cases with progressive neurological deficit or structural deformity.

MALIGNANT TUMORS.
Systemic lymphoproliferative neoplasms such as multiple myeloma and lymphoma commonly affect the vertebral axis of middle aged and elderly persons and are the most common malignant neoplasms of the spinal column. Clinically, radiologically, and pathologically, these spinal column neoplasms are identical to their systemic counterparts. In general, both are amenable to radiotherapy and chemotherapy, with surgery reserved for cases of acute neurological deterioration. Given their systemic nature, these entities are not discussed further here.

Solitary Plasmacytoma.
Solitary plasmacytoma, which is histologically indistinguishable from multiple myeloma, consists of a collection of B-cell–derived neoplastic plasma cells. However, unlike multiple myelomas, which are systemic neoplasms frequently associated with widespread bone marrow involvement and a resultant normocytic, normochromic anemia, an elevated erythrocyte sedimentation rate, and a monoclonal proteinemia, plasmacytomas are isolated neoplasms without systemic manifestations. Although multiple myeloma of the vertebral axis is quite common, solitary plasmacytoma remains relatively rare. As with all other bone neoplasms, the presentation is quite nonspecific and often consists of local pain or neurological compromise secondary to root or cord compression. Radiographically, plasmacytomas are lytic lesions with occasional sclerosis. The posterior elements of the vertebrae are typically spared (8). The results of radionuclide bone scans are generally negative. All patients suspected of having a plasmacytoma should undergo a skeletal survey to rule out multiple myeloma.

Radiotherapy is the treatment of choice for histologically proven solitary plasmacytoma. A recent case series demonstrated excellent local control (96%) and a median survival of 11 years after radiotherapy (24). Surgical therapy is reserved for cases of neural compression or instability. Patients with solitary plasmacytoma require close follow-up because multiple myeloma eventually develops in more than 50% of cases (24).

Osteosarcoma.
Primary osteosarcomas of the vertebral column are extremely rare, accounting for fewer than 3% of osteosarcomas and only 5% of primary malignant tumors of the spine (25). Spinal column osteosarcoma more commonly occurs as a result of secondary spread from another skeletal osteosarcoma, against the backdrop of a preexisting bony lesion (e.g., Paget disease), or in previously irradiated bone. The patients presenting with spinal osteosarcoma are slightly older than those with appendicular lesions; the mean presentation is in the fifth decade. Although pain is often the initial symptom, most patients (~80%) have neurological deficit at presentation (25).

Osteosarcoma of the spine tends to involve the vertebral bodies, and, like most spinal neoplasms, spares the adjacent intervertebral discs. Radiographs often demonstrate a combination of osteoblastic and osteolytic bone destruction, whereas CT and MRI are very useful in evaluating the extent of the lesion and involvement of the adjacent paraspinal soft tissues (10). Pulmonary metastases commonly occur with osteosarcoma; thus, chest radiography should also be performed to stage the lesion. Histologically, osteosarcomas are characterized by highly anaplastic osteoblasts admixed in a vascular stroma (26).

Unfortunately, the prognosis for patients with osteosarcoma of the spine is poor. Because of the inability to achieve radical surgical resection in the vertebral axis, in combination with the highly radiation-resistant nature of these lesions, treatment is often less than satisfactory. Partial surgical resection is warranted for cases of neural element compression and structural instability. Although efficacy is poor, adjuvant chemotherapy and local irradiation should be administered. Few patients survive longer than 1 year (25).

Chordoma.
After the lymphoproliferative neoplasms, chordoma is the second most common primary malignant neoplasm of the adult vertebral axis. Chordomas arise from embryological remnants of the primitive notochord. Developmentally, the notochord extends from the Rathke pouch to the coccyx. Chordomas arise in a parallel distribution where notochordal rests are thought to exist. (A notochordal rest is known as *ecchordosis physaliphora*.) Fifty percent are located in the sacro-coccygeal region, 35% in the region of the clivus, and the remaining 15% in the mobile spine. Most chordomas of the mobile spine occur in the cervical segment, especially the axis, and chordomas are exceedingly uncommon in the thoracic spine (27). Although the nucleus pulposus is the sole persisting anatomical derivative of the notochord, chordomas do not appear to originate from this structure but instead arise from the vertebral body. The presence of notochordal remnants in the vertebral body has not been confirmed. The incidence of chordoma peaks in middle age, with men affected twice as frequently as women (27). The typical clinical presentation of pain and progressive myeloradiculopathy is nonspecific. Cervical chordomas may also present with airway obstruction and dysphagia or as an oropharyngeal mass because of the extensive soft-tissue component that is often present.

Chordomas are slow-growing but locally aggressive invasive lesions. Typically, radiographs reveal a destructive lesion centered about a vertebral body in association with a large soft-tissue mass. Bony expansion and associated calcification are also seen in the majority of lesions (10). Like GCTs, and unlike most other tumors of the spinal column, chordomas often involve the intervertebral disc space as they spread to adjacent bodies. MRI provides excellent delineation of the anterior soft-tissue extension and the extent of vertebral canal compromise. Chordoma is isointense on T1-weighted images and hyperintense on T2-weighted images, enhances with gadolinium, and often has foci of low signal attenuation secondary to calcification (8). Histological analysis reveals a microstructure composed of vacuolated clear cells, known as *physaliphorous cells,* and abundant intracellular and extracellular mucin.

Because of the locally invasive nature of chordoma and the late occurrence of metastases, the natural history is one of local relapse. Given this pattern, it is generally agreed that aggressive en bloc surgical resection is the treatment of choice. Although this is often possible in cases of sacrococcygeal chordoma, when the mobile spine is involved this goal is rarely achieved because of the inherent anatomical constraints (28). Conventional radiotherapy is not effective in eradicating residual tumor, although it can promote local control in a subgroup of patients. For this reason, various new strategies, including radiosurgery, are being explored. Because of the difficulties encountered in treating chordoma, only a small portion of patients are rendered disease-free. Recent series suggest that overall survival rates following relapse at 2 and 5 years are 63% and 6%, respectively (29).

Chondrosarcoma. After chordoma, chondrosarcoma is the most common nonlymphoproliferative tumor of the spinal column (Fig. 5, Color Plate 35). Chondrosarcomas account for 10% to 20% of primary bone tumors, with approximately 10% of them occurring in the mobile spine (30). Seventy-five percent arise as a primary lesion, but secondary lesions also develop as a consequence of malignant degeneration of a preexisting enchondroma or osteochondroma. The peak incidence of chondrosarcoma is in the fifth to sixth decade, with men more commonly affected. Radiographically, few features distinguish chondrosarcoma from other bony tumors. Bone destruction is evident, with involvement of the anterior and posterior elements occurring equally often. Chondrosarcomas display a wide range of malignant potential, varying from low-grade lesions with slow growth to highly aggressive lesions with a tendency to metastasize. Because a significant number of chondro-

sarcomas of the spine are low-grade lesions, survival is protracted; the median survival approaches 6 years.

Chondrosarcomas should be treated by en bloc excision with wide or marginal histological margins (30). These lesions are largely resistant to radiotherapy and chemotherapy, and adjuvant radiotherapy does not appear to alter the disease-free interval (31).

Ewing Sarcoma. Ewing sarcoma (ES) is the most common primary malignant tumor of the spinal column in children. Primary ES of the spinal column accounts for approximately 10% of cases (Fig. 6); secondary foci involving the spine are much more common. ES of the vertebral axis rarely presents after the age of 30. Pain and progressive neurological deficit herald the onset of disease. Most commonly, ES is centered in the vertebral body but often extends to involve the posterior elements. Sacrococcygeal disease is most frequent, followed by disease in thoracic and lumbar locations. The cervical spine is rarely involved. Sclerosis and osseous expansion are frequent findings on radiographs, whereas CT and MRI demonstrate the soft-tissue component, which is often prominent (10). Microscopically, ES is composed of sheets of small blue cells and abundant glycogen. Cytogenetic studies facilitate the diagnosis; ES contains a characteristic translocation of chromosomes 11 and 22.

ES is sensitive to both radiotherapy and chemotherapy, so that surgical excision of primary ES of the spinal column should be reserved for cases of progressive neurological compromise or structural deformity (32). Despite sensitivity to both radiation and chemotherapy, ES remains an aggressive tumor. In the Mayo Clinic series, with multimodal therapy the median survival was 2.9 years and 5-year survival was 33% (33).

Management of Primary Spine Tumors

The management of a primary tumor of the spinal column requires a thorough preoperative workup. A detailed clinical history and physical examination in addition to laboratory investigations and imaging studies are essential to this process. After an evaluation of the local and systemic extent of the lesion,

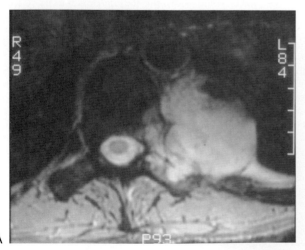 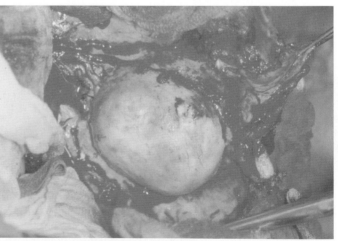

A   B

Fig. 5. Chondrosarcoma. This 38-year-old man presented with severe back and left thoracic radicular pain. MRI (**A**) shows the lesion at T9, with invasion of the vertebral body and chest wall. Radical resection of the lesion via a transthoracic approach (**B**) was followed by radiotherapy.

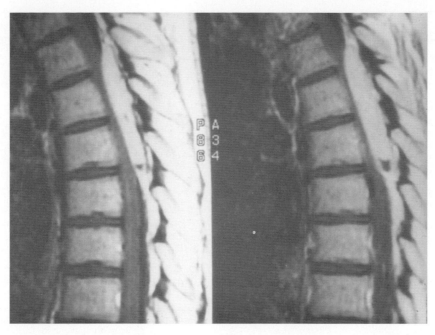

Fig. 6. Ewing sarcoma. This 26-year-old woman had progressive paraparesis and an extradural lesion extending from T5 to T7. The lesion was managed with posterior resection followed by chemotherapy and radiation.

appropriate oncological and surgical staging can be performed. This in turn allows a surgical procedure to be planned, when indicated, that is adequate for the specific tumor (34).

Biopsy of the tumor is the final stage in the planning process. Three options are available when neoplastic lesions are suspected: percutaneous needle biopsy, open incisional biopsy, and excisional biopsy. To avoid seeding healthy tissue with neoplastic cells, it is imperative that the biopsy route be placed such that the tumor can be excised with adequate margins at the time of definitive resection. If this tenet is to be followed, vertebral body lesions, whether the biopsy is performed in an open procedure or percutaneously, must be approached anteriorly or via a transpedicular route to avoid contamination of the epidural space, as would occur in a laminectomy.

ONCOLOGICAL AND SURGICAL STAGING. Appropriate therapy for patients with primary tumors of the vertebral axis

can be achieved only through correct oncological staging. Enneking (2) developed an oncological staging system for primary bone tumors that defines their biological behavior. It has been effective in guiding surgical therapy for limb lesions and has also been successfully applied in the treatment of primary tumors of the spinal column (35). The Enneking system is very useful in developing the most effective treatment plan for individual primary spinal tumors (Table 2).

Surgical staging is appropriate after the diagnosis has been established and the oncological staging is complete. The unique anatomy of the spinal column and the restrictions that the contents of the thecal sac place on surgical resection in the vertebral axis have mandated the formulation of a surgical staging system specific to the spine. The Weinstein-Boriani-Biagini (WBB) system divides the vertebrae into 12 radiating zones and five layers (35). It allows for a rational and logical approach to surgical planning and takes into account the limitations to marginal en bloc excision in the spinal column.

Table 2. Enneking System of Oncologic Staging

	Stage	Description	Ideal management
Benign	S1 (latent/inactive): tumor not growing	Well-defined capsule; few symptoms	Conservative (unless decompression or stabilization required)
	S2 (active): slow growth	Confined to bone; thin capsule with reactive pseudocapsule	Intralesional curettage
	S3 (aggressive): rapid growth	Capsule thin, incomplete, or absent; wide reactive pseudocapsule	Marginal *en bloc* excision
Malignant	Low-grade (I): IA (confined to vertebra) IB (paravertebral extension)	No capsule; wide pseudocapsule containing islands of tumor	Wide *en bloc* excision
	High-grade (II): IIA (confined to vertebra) IIB (paravertebral extension)	Pseudocapsule infiltrated by tumor; island of tumor found in vertebra remote from tumor mass	Wide *en bloc* excision and adjuvant therapy
	High-grade with metastases (III)	Distant metastases	Palliative surgery and adjuvant therapy

References

1. Weinstein JN. Surgical approaches to spine tumors. *Orthopedics* 1989;12:897–905.
2. Enneking WF. *Musculoskeletal tumor surgery.* New York: Churchill Livingstone, 1983.
3. Camins MB, Oppenheim JS, Perrin RG. Tumors of the vertebral axis: benign, primary malignant, and metastatic tumors. In: Youmans JR, ed. *Neurological surgery,* 4th ed. Philadelphia: WB Saunders, 1996: 3134–3167.
4. Fehlings MG, Rao SC. Spinal cord and spinal column tumors. In: Bernstein M, Berger MS, eds. *Neuro-oncology: the essentials.* New York: Thieme Medical Publishers, 2000:445–464.
5. Friedlaender GE, Southwick WO. Tumors of the spine. In: Rothman RH, Simeone FA, eds. *The spine.* Philadelphia: WB Saunders, 1982: 1022–1040.
6. Weinstein JN, McLain RF. Primary tumors of the spine. *Spine* 1987; 12:843–851.
7. Mallon WJ, Harrelson JM. Primary neoplasms of the spine. In: Wilkins RH, Rengachary SS, eds. *Neurosurgery,* 2nd ed. New York: McGraw-Hill, 1996:1805–1814.
8. Keogh C, Bergin D, Brennan D, et al. MR imaging of bone tumors of the cervical spine. *Magn Reson Imaging Clin N Am* 2000;8:513–527.
9. Raskas DS, Graziano GP, Herzenberg JE, et al. Osteoid osteoma and osteoblastoma of the spine. *J Spinal Disord* 1992;5:204–211.
10. Murphey MD, Andrews CL, Flemming DJ, et al. Primary tumors of the spine: radiologic-pathologic correlation. *Radiographics* 1996;16: 1131–1158.
11. Boriani S, Capanna R, Donati D, et al. Osteoblastoma of the spine. *Clin Orthop* 1992;278:37–45.
12. Nemoto O, Moser RP Jr, Van Dam BE, et al. Osteoblastoma of the spine. A review of 75 cases. *Spine* 1990;15:1272–1280.
13. Mayer L. Malignant transformation of benign osteoblastoma. *Bull Hosp Jt Dis* 1967;28:4–13.
14. Lucas DR, Unni KK, McLeod RA, et al. Osteoblastoma: clinicopathologic study of 306 cases. *Hum Pathol* 1994;25:117–134.
15. Albrecht S, Crutchfield J, SeGall G. On spinal osteochondromas. *J Neurosurg* 1992;77:247–252.
16. Khosla A, Martin DS, Awwad EE. The solitary intraspinal vertebral osteochondroma. An unusual cause of compressive myelopathy: features and literature review. *Spine* 1999;24:77–81.
17. Schwartz TH, Hibshoosh H, Riedel CJ. Estrogen and progesterone receptor-negative T11 vertebral hemangioma presenting as a postpartum compression fracture: case report and management. *Neurosurgery* 2000;46:218–221.
18. DiCaprio MR, Murphy MJ, Camp RL. Aneurysmal bone cyst of the spine with familial incidence. *Spine* 2000;25:1589–1592.
19. Papagelopoulos PJ, Currier BL, Shaughnessy WJ, et al. Aneurysmal bone cyst of the spine. Management and outcome. *Spine* 1998;23: 621–628.
20. de Kleuver M, van der Heul RO, Veraart BE. Aneurysmal bone cyst of the spine: 31 cases and the importance of the surgical approach. *J Pediatr Orthop B* 1998;7:286–292.
21. Sanjay BK, Sim FH, Unni KK, et al. Giant-cell tumours of the spine. *J Bone Joint Surg Br* 1993;75:148–154.
22. Campanacci M, Boriani S, Giunti A. Giant cell tumors of the spine. In: Sundaresan N, Schmidek H, Schiller A, eds. *Tumors of the spine: diagnosis and clinical management.* Philadelphia: WB Saunders, 1990:163–180.
23. Khan DC, Malhotra S, Stevens RE, et al. Radiotherapy for the treatment of giant cell tumor of the spine: a report of six cases and review of the literature. *Cancer Invest* 1999;17:110–113.
24. Liebross RH, Ha CS, Cox JD, et al. Solitary bone plasmacytoma: outcome and prognostic factors following radiotherapy. *Int J Radiat Oncol Biol Phys* 1998;15:1063–1067.
25. Barwick KW, Huvos AG, Smith J. Primary osteogenic sarcoma of the vertebral column: a clinicopathologic correlation of ten patients. *Cancer* 1980;46:595–604.
26. Kebudi R, Ayan I, Daredelier E, et al. Primary osteosarcoma of the cervical spine: a pediatric case report and review of the literature. *Med Pediatr Oncol* 1994;23:162–165.
27. Bjornsson J, Wold LE, Ebersold MJ, et al. Chordoma of the mobile spine: a clinicopathologic analysis of 40 patients. *Cancer* 1993;71: 735–740.
28. Boriani S, Chevalley F, Weinstein JN, et al. Chordoma of the spine above the sacrum. Treatment and outcome in 21 cases. *Spine* 1996; 21:1569–1577.
29. Fagundes MA, Hug EB, Liebsch NJ, et al. Radiation therapy for chordomas of the base of skull and cervical spine: patterns of failure and outcome after relapse. *Int J Radiat Oncol Biol Phys* 1995;33: 579–584.
30. Boriani S, De Iure F, Bandiera S, et al. Chondrosarcoma of the mobile spine: report on 22 cases. *Spine* 2000;25:804–812.
31. York, JE, Berk RH, Fuller GN, et al. Chondrosarcoma of the spine: 1954 to 1997. *J Neurosurg* 1999;90(1 suppl):73–78.
32. Sharafuddin MJ, Haddad FS, Hitchon PW, et al. Treatment options in primary Ewing's sarcoma of the spine: report of seven cases and review of the literature. *Neurosurgery* 1992;30:610–618.
33. Grubb MR, Currier BL, Pritchard DJ, et al. Primary Ewing's sarcoma of the spine. *Spine* 1994;19:309–313.
34. Abdu WA, Provencher M. Primary bone and metastatic tumors of the cervical spine. *Spine* 1998;23:2767–2777.
35. Boriani S, Weinstein JN, Biagini R. Primary bone tumors of the spine: terminology and surgical staging. *Spine* 1997;22:1036–1044.

171. *Vascular Lesions of the Spine*

Howard Morgan and Kevin Morrill

This chapter deals with vascular disorders of the bony spine and excludes entities usually classified as spinal cord arteriovenous malformations (AVMs) and fistulae (i.e., types I through IV spinal AVMs and cavernous malformations of the spinal cord), which are discussed elsewhere. Included in this chapter is a discussion of the vertebral vascular lesions that primarily involve bone—hemangiomas, aneurysmal bone cysts, and AVMs of the bone and epidural space. Tumors of the vertebrae may be highly vascular but are not discussed herein.

Vascular lesions of the bony spine usually become clinically apparent when they cause pain in the area of the spine involved; the discomfort may be of a mechanical nature. Radiculopathic and myelopathic signs and symptoms occur as the nerve roots, cauda equina, and spinal cord become affected, usually by compression. Plain roentgenography of the spine is often the first study undertaken and may suggest the diagnosis. The judicious use of additional imaging studies, especially computed tomography (CT) and magnetic resonance imaging (MRI), is invaluable in helping to establish the likely diagnosis and extent of involvement. Radioactive bone scanning may be useful, especially to exclude multiple lesions. Vertebral angiography is necessary to identify the blood supply of those lesions that appear highly vascular and also to determine whether or not preoperative neurointerventional devascularization (hereafter termed simply *embolization*) may be of assistance. CT-guided needle biopsy may establish the tissue diagnosis for those lesions in which the diagnosis is questionable but should not be used as a "routine" measure.

Some bony vascular lesions of the spine, especially vertebral hemangiomas, are discovered incidentally and require no treatment or follow-up. Those causing pain and especially those producing neurological signs and symptoms usually require treatment, which may be nonsurgical or surgical. When surgical treatment is undertaken and cure is the goal, an extensive procedure with reconstruction and stabilization, perhaps both anteriorly and posteriorly, may be indicated (e.g., see the cases discussed in Figs. 7 and 8). A simple decompressive laminectomy alone will not be sufficient to treat many of these lesions adequately.

Vertebral Hemangiomas

Vertebral hemangiomas are common, benign vascular lesions of bone that usually are of no clinical significance. Based on large autopsy and radiographic series, a 10% to 12% incidence is estimated in the population at large, with a higher rate noted in middle-aged persons and the elderly. The majority of vertebral hemangiomas are clinically silent (Fig. 1A,B); perhaps 1% become symptomatic. Of the symptomatic lesions, half are characterized by pain only, and half are associated with variable neurological manifestations (1,2). Three histological types have been described: cavernous, capillary, and mixed. The cavernous type consists of large dilated blood vessels clustered closely together with little intervening stroma. In the capillary type, thin-walled vessels of varying degrees of maturity and size are separated by normal bone tissue. Capillary loops tend to spread outward in a "sunburst" fashion. The mixed type exhibits characteristics of both the cavernous and the capillary types. In most reported series, pathological typing is not mentioned as clinically significant, but in one series from the Ukraine, the pathological type was clinically relevant (2). Vertebral hemangiomas occur most frequently in the lower thoracic and lumbar areas, are somewhat more common in women, and seldom appear before the middle decades; however, those lesions that produce myelopathy tend to occur in younger patients (3). When seen in the early stages, the process may involve only a quadrant of the vertebral body or pedicle (4). Although an individual patient may have multiple lesions, hemangiomas in adjacent vertebral bodies are unusual. When two or more contiguous vertebral bodies are involved in a benign-appearing osteolytic process, the diagnosis is far more likely to be aneurysmal bone cyst than hemangioma (5).

Today, most vertebral hemangiomas are diagnosed incidentally on spinal imaging studies. The plain roentgenographic appearance is characteristically a striated pattern in the vertebral body, representing alternating coarse trabeculae interspersed with areas of low density (Fig. 1D). The terms "corduroy cloth" and "honeycomb" are appropriately descriptive. One third of the vertebral body must be involved before this radiographic finding becomes apparent (6). Consequently, smaller lesions that are apparent on CT or MR scans are not seen on plain spinal roentgenograms. Axial CT typically shows a "polka-dot" or "honeycomb" appearance (Figs. 1C and 2A). Vertebral hemangiomas usually display an increased signal on T1-weighted and T2-weighted MRI when the process is not evolving. An isodense signal on the T1-weighted image and an increased signal on the T2-weighted image suggest that the hemangioma

is evolving and more likely to be or become symptomatic (1). The radiographic appearance of Paget disease and slowly growing neoplasms, such as chordoma and multiple myeloma, may be confused with that of hemangiomas (4).

Vertebral hemangiomas are thought to be congenital and derived from embryonic rests. The vertebral body is the most common site, although the pedicles or posterior elements may be involved. Occasionally, vertebral hemangiomas are circumferential, and these are the ones most likely to result in spinal cord compression. Female sex and location of the lesion in the thoracic area also are predisposing factors for spinal cord involvement (3). Although neurological signs and symptoms are usually caused by direct compression resulting from hemangiomatous or bony growth into the epidural space (Fig. 2), epidural hemorrhage, bony collapse, and a diversion of blood flow ("steal phenomenon") may produce neurological manifestations (6,7). Spinal hemangiomas occasionally are confined to the epidural space (Fig. 3).

The treatment of spinal hemangiomas varies widely according to the severity of symptoms, age and general health of the patient, whether or not spinal cord or nerve root compression has occurred, location of the lesion, extent of the destructive disease process, and whether or not the lesion is estimated to be progressive. Those incidental lesions that produce no symptoms need not be treated at all. An asymptomatic patient with an extensive lesion may warrant follow-up; however, a lesion that is discovered incidentally rarely becomes symptomatic (1). For patients who have only pain and no neurological signs or symptoms, nonsurgical treatment is indicated in most cases, especially as initial therapy. In addition to pain control measures, nonsurgical treatment options include radiation therapy and embolization. Radiation therapy and embolization also may be useful in the case of a postoperative surgical patient who has had an incomplete excision, and sometimes in preoperative situations in an effort to lessen the blood supply to a highly vascular lesion and so make surgical resection less hazardous. Surgery is indicated for the infrequent patient with neurological signs and symptoms resulting from compression secondary to epidural extension of the lesion, vertebral collapse, or epidural hematoma, and for the patient who has severe pain that is refractory to nonsurgical treatment. The successful treatment of spinal hemangiomas with embolization and no subsequent surgery has been reported (8,9). Sudden paraplegia occurs rarely in patients with spinal hemangiomas and is caused by spinal cord compression by either hemorrhage resulting in epidural hematoma or collapse of the weakened vertebral body, perhaps in association with trauma (Fig. 3). Pregnancy and the menstrual cycle have been reported to be contributing factors to the onset and exacerbation of symptoms (2,3) (Figs. 2 and 4).

Aneurysmal Bone Cysts of the Spine

Aneurysmal bone cysts (ABCs) are benign, expansile, lytic lesions of bone of unknown cause that occur in young patients, more commonly in the first two decades. Although no gender preference is noted in some series, an increased incidence in female patients is reported in others. ABCs are neither aneurysms nor cysts. Large, blood-filled channels under pressure without a normal endothelial lining are characteristic and may so affect the bone that it resembles a sponge (5). ABCs are composed of multiple cavities containing unclotted blood under pressure. Fibrous septa lined with fibrovascular

(text continues on p. 1851)

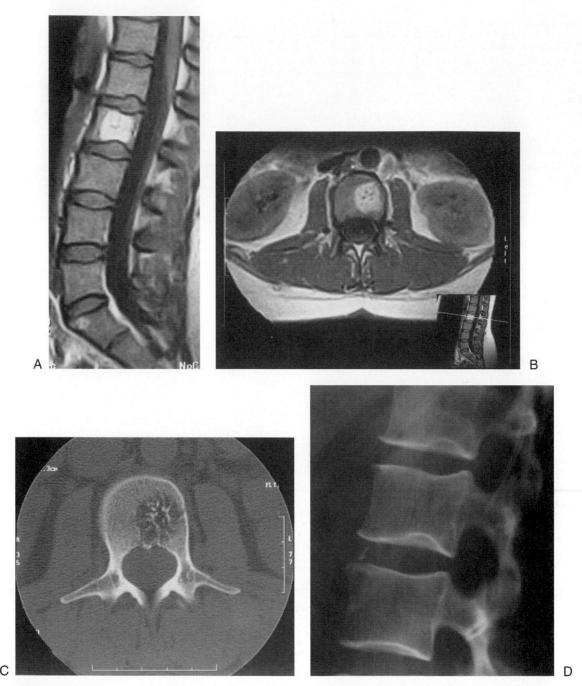

Fig. 1. Asymptomatic hemangioma of the L2 vertebral body in a middle-aged woman who underwent spinal magnetic resonance imaging (MRI) for evaluation of an unrelated condition. Hemangioma was discovered in the L2 vertebral body (**A,B**). Computed tomography (CT) (**C**) and lateral spine roentgenography (**D**) confirm the diagnosis. Note the faint vertical striations in the vertebral body in the center of **D**, and note that the involvement is much less marked on the roentgenogram than on CT and MRI.

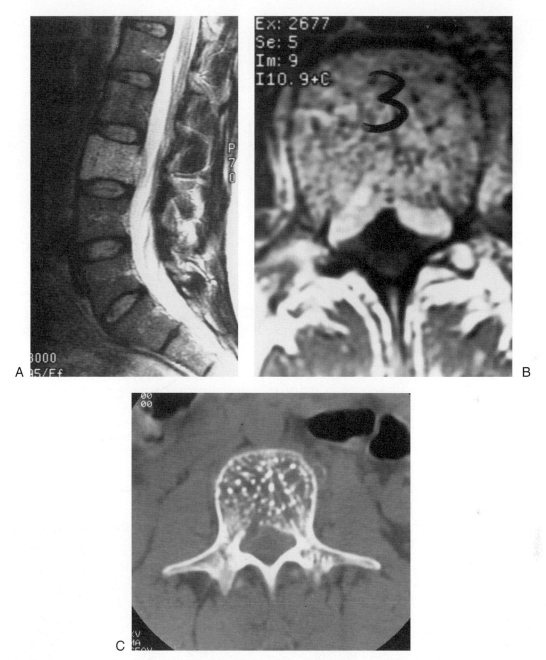

Fig. 2. L3 vertebral hemangioma with epidural extension in a 41-year-old woman with long-standing pain in the low back and left lower extremity. She began to experience worsening pain with bilateral lower-extremity numbness and weakness, especially when walking up stairs. Note the "polka-dot" CT appearance of the L3 vertebral body (**A**) and extension of the hemangioma on MRI into the epidural space (**B,C**). She required anterior and posterior decompression/ reconstruction from L2 to L4, and 5 years later she has no symptoms except occasional back stiffness and soreness.

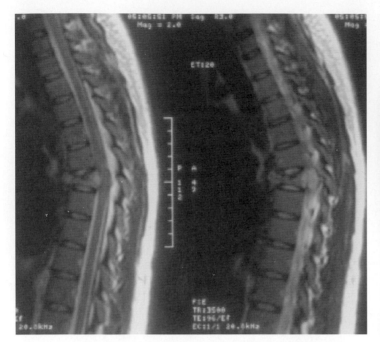

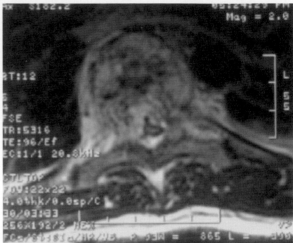

Fig. 3. MRI of a T6 hemangioma causing paraplegia in a 22-year-old woman. During late pregnancy, the patient experienced progressively severe back pain and paraparesis. After a fall, she rapidly became paraplegic with a complete midthoracic motor and sensory level. She was near term and delivered a healthy baby by emergency cesarean section. Treatment consisted of embolization followed by anterior decompression/reconstruction. At 18 months after surgery, the patient had regained continence and was able to ambulate with braces.

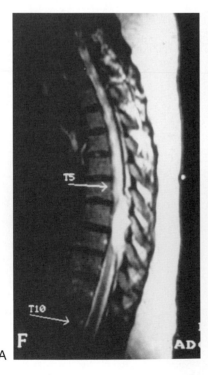

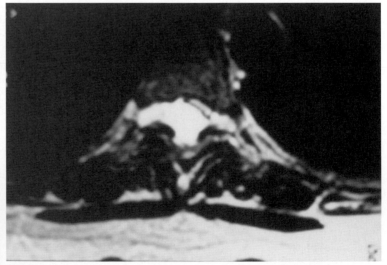

Fig. 4. A: MRI of a thoracic epidural hemangioma in a 36-year-old woman. This patient had a 3-month history of progressive thoracolumbar pain and lower-extremity numbness and mild spastic paraparesis. Fourteen months earlier, during the latter stages of pregnancy, she had noted the onset of lower-extremity numbness, which resolved after delivery. At surgery, a bloody, partially collapsible, fleshy mass in the epidural space was removed, and the patient made a complete recovery. Note the marked displacement of the ribbon-thin spinal cord in the axial scan (**B**).

endothelium compartmentalize the cavities. Bleeding during surgery usually "is brisk, but spurting is noticeably absent" (10). ABCs may occur in any part of the skeleton, but metaphyses of the long bones are the most common site. Of all ABCs, 10% to 20% occur in the spine; the lumbar region and the posterior elements are most frequently affected. A conspicuous and little understood feature of ABCs of the spine is their capacity to advance from one vertebra to another (5). They may appear pernicious in their capacity for osseous destruction and can be mistaken for primary or metastatic bony malignancy or a benign neoplastic process (e.g., giant cell tumor), and on occasion, malignant lesions of the vertebrae may appear similar to an ABC (Fig. 5). Other differential diagnostic possibilities include fibrous dysplasia, eosinophilic granuloma, and tuberculosis.

Mechanical back pain is the typical presenting symptom. The pain often becomes more intense at night and disturbs the patient's sleep. Swelling and tenderness may accompany the back pain. ABCs may advance rapidly and can cause local hemorrhage. As an ABC progresses, nerve root, cauda equina, and spinal cord compression can result in radiculopathic and myelopathic signs and symptoms. Roentgenography and CT of a spinal ABC typically show an expanded, osteolytic cavity with strands of bone forming a bubbly appearance. The cortical bone is often eggshell thin and "blown out." MRI typically shows a high-density signal on T2-weighted and T1-weighted images surrounded by a rim of low intensity. Within the areas of high-density signal are fluid-filled cavities containing septa that produce a mottled appearance. Mottling and fluid layering within the cavities are clues to the diagnosis of ABC but can also be associated with other pathological processes (Fig. 5).

Treatment should be designed to eliminate pain, decompress the neural structures if necessary, stabilize the spine if deformity or instability is present, and halt progression of the disease.

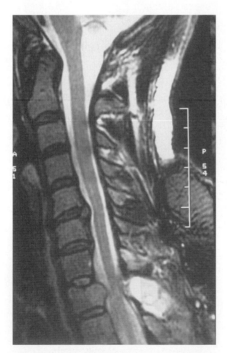

Fig. 5. A 37-year-old woman with a lytic process at T1 radiographically diagnosed as an aneurysmal bone cyst (ABC). The patient had excruciating pain in the upper back and left arm and myeloradiculopathy. Note the apparent fluid layering within the posterior elements of T1, which is highly suggestive of ABC. However, the lesion on angiography was not highly vascular, and the pathological diagnosis was metastatic carcinoma.

Complete resection is desirable but may be impossible without risking catastrophic hemorrhage or injury to important adjacent structures. When total resection is not possible, curettage and packing the cavity with bone graft is probably the best alternative. Incomplete excision has been reported to result in a high recurrence rate during the first year after surgery by some authors (11,12), but not by others (10,13). Depending on the degree of bony involvement and extent of surgical resection, internal or external stabilization with reconstruction and arthrodesis may be indicated (Fig. 6). Nonsurgical treatment has been advocated in some circumstances and seems best suited for those lesions causing pain but no neurological compression. ABCs are usually considered sensitive to radiation therapy, but when the spine is involved, the risk for radiation myelopathy, disturbance of growth, and recurrence as sarcoma should be considered in the evaluation of treatment options, especially as these patients are usually young (10,12). Fortunately, low doses of radiation (<30 Gy) have been reported to be successful in controlling the disease (14,15); however, in one series, treatment with radiation alone had a 50% failure rate (13). When surgery results in an incomplete resection, radiation therapy is often recommended as a means of controlling advancement of the disease, but Capanna et al. (13) found radiotherapy to be of no value in such circumstances. Although arterial embolization is usually considered an adjunct to surgical treatment to reduce hemorrhage at the time of surgery, embolization without surgery has been reported to be successful in treating ABCs (9,16).

Arteriovenous Malformations of the Spine Involving the Bone and Epidural Space

Outside the usual classification scheme of spinal AVMs (types I through IV and cavernous malformations) is a group of lesions that have been termed *spinal epidural* or *extradural AVMs* by some authors (17,18) and *metameric spinal AVMs* by others (19,20). Some of these lesions have extensive bony, paraspinous soft-tissue, and extraparaspinous soft-tissue components in addition to cutaneous manifestations. Thus, the embryological term *metameric* is used; however, because *metameric* connotes involvement of the entire somite, we suggest reserving that term for a small subgroup of extradural vertebral AVMs in which the malformation is present in all layers of tissue derived from the somite. Extradural vertebral AVMs typically are outside the spinal cord and dura, although dilated vessels in the epidural space may compress the neural elements. Features of most of these lesions include prominence in the epidural space and extension of the epidural AVM into or erosion of bone by large, dilated vessels; the epidural component may be so extensive as to act as an epidural mass and compress the spinal cord or nerve roots (Figs. 7 and 8). These lesions also may become symptomatic when they cause vascular "steal" or venous engorgement of the spinal cord. Isolated cases of epidural AMVs with little or no bony involvement have been reported (21–25). These epidural lesions are prone to spontaneous hemorrhage, sometimes during pregnancy (24), producing a compressive epidural hematoma. Additionally, epidural AVMs with bony involvement similar to our cases in Figs. 7 and 8 have been reported (26,27).

Our preoperative neurointerventional experience with patients having extradural vertebral AVMs has been similar to that mentioned by other authors (20,21); these lesions are ideally

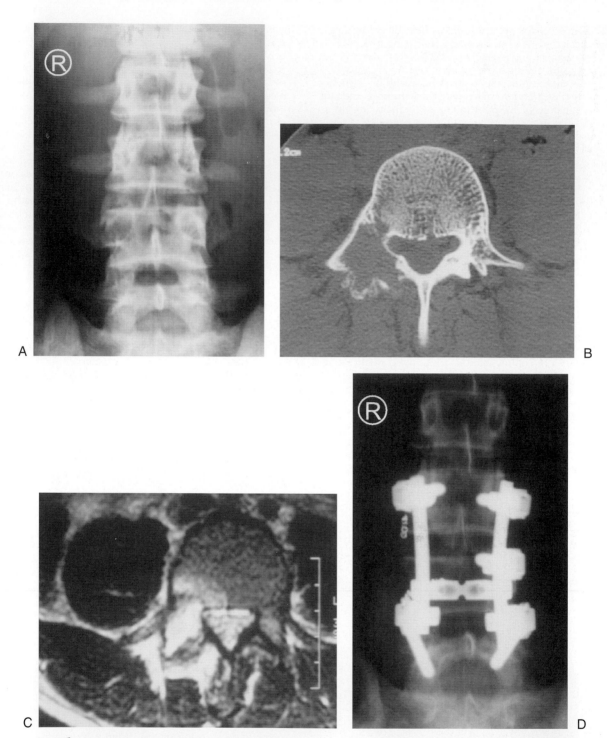

Fig. 6. ABC of the lumbar spine in a 14-year-old boy with severe, progressive pain of the low back. Note the expanded right L4 pedicle on the roentgenogram (**A**), corresponding to the appearance on CT (**B**) and MRI (**C**). The patient underwent excision of the lesion followed by posterior–lateral fusion and instrumentation (**D**). Preoperative embolization resulted in manageable blood loss (note the coil in D just superior and to the right of the L4-5 disc space). By 1 year after surgery, the patient had resumed playing golf and baseball. (Courtesy of Dr. Michael J. Bolesta, Department of Orthopedic Surgery, University of Texas Southwestern Medical Center at Dallas.)

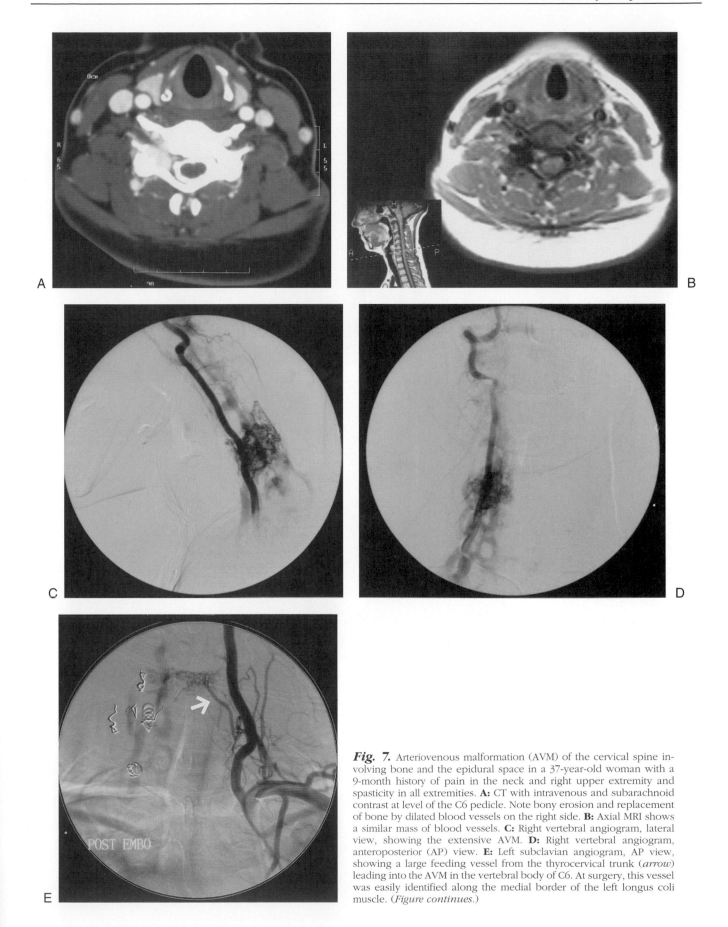

Fig. 7. Arteriovenous malformation (AVM) of the cervical spine involving bone and the epidural space in a 37-year-old woman with a 9-month history of pain in the neck and right upper extremity and spasticity in all extremities. **A:** CT with intravenous and subarachnoid contrast at level of the C6 pedicle. Note bony erosion and replacement of bone by dilated blood vessels on the right side. **B:** Axial MRI shows a similar mass of blood vessels. **C:** Right vertebral angiogram, lateral view, showing the extensive AVM. **D:** Right vertebral angiogram, anteroposterior (AP) view. **E:** Left subclavian angiogram, AP view, showing a large feeding vessel from the thyrocervical trunk (*arrow*) leading into the AVM in the vertebral body of C6. At surgery, this vessel was easily identified along the medial border of the left longus coli muscle. (*Figure continues.*)

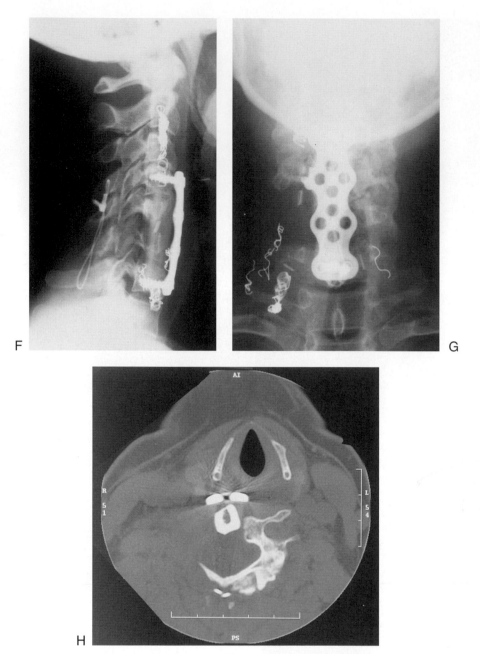

Fig. 7. (continued). **F,G:** Lateral and AP roentgenographic view of the reconstruction 3 months after surgery. Note the embolization coils. **H:** CT 3 months after surgery at level of the C6 pedicle. Note absence of bone on the right side because of the AVM and surgery. Also note the arthrodesis (iliac graft) on the left side.

suited for preoperative embolization because the vascular supply to the AVM is separate from the blood supply to the spinal cord (Figs. 7 and 8). We do not consider embolization alone sufficient to cure the majority of these lesions, but embolization should be considered as a part of the overall treatment plan. Surgical resection of these lesions may require extensive or even multiple exposures, followed by reconstruction and stabilization to prevent postoperative instability. Although vessels from the AVM may extend inside the dura, they are thought to be dilated draining veins that resolve after the AVM is resected, and consequently the dura need not be opened in the majority of cases (18,20).

We argue that vertebral AVMs involving the bone, epidural

space, and adjacent tissues are a distinct group and suggest the designation *spinal AVM type V* as an extension of the commonly accepted classification. That these AVMs are distinct from the usually recognized lesions—spinal AVMs types I through IV and cavernous malformations—is obvious. Within this fifth group are two subtypes, which we label *A* and *B*. Examples of subtype VA are those AVMs seen in Figs. 7 and 8. Type VA spinal AVMs vary along a continuum from small, isolated lesions in the epidural space to epidural AVMs with bony erosion to AVMs invading the bone and paraspinous tissues in addition to the epidural space. Type VB spinal AVMs are rare—true metameric lesions with epidural, bony, paraspinous, and extra-paraspinous involvement.

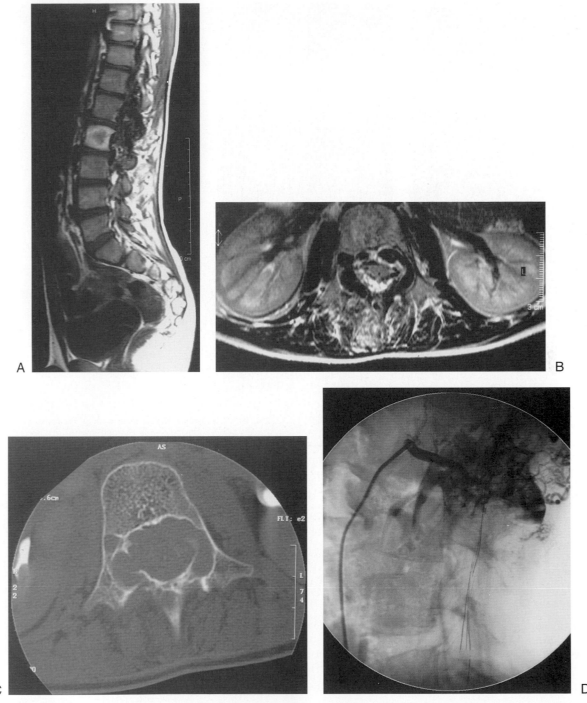

Fig. 8. A 9-year-old boy had a 2-year history of back pain and an unusual gait. He had an exaggerated lumbar lordosis, markedly limited range of motion in the low back, and lower-extremity spasticity. After multiple embolization procedures, the lesion was excised posteriorly. Because of the extensive destruction by disease and surgery of the posterior elements and pedicles, stabilization was performed from L3 to T12 with the use of a rod-hook-screw-cable construct and autologous rib bone graft. **A,B:** Lateral and axial MRI showing circumferential dilated blood vessels on the dorsal aspect of the spine and hyperemia in the L2 vertebral body. **C:** CT demonstrating bony erosion of L2. **D:** Angiogram of the left L2 segmental artery. Note that the AVM extends into the paraspinous tissues. (*Figure continues.*)

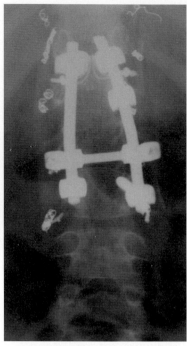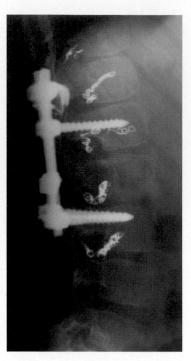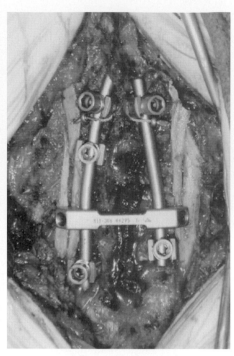

E,F   G

Fig. 8. (continued). **E,F,G:**. Postoperative AP and lateral roentgenograms and operative photograph showing the reconstruction, embolization coils, and rib bone grafts.

References

1. Fox MW, Onofrio BM. The natural history and management of symptomatic and asymptomatic vertebral hemangiomas. *J Neurosurg* 1993;78:36–45.
2. Pastushyn AI, Slin'ko EI, Mirzoyeva GM. Vertebral hemangiomas: diagnosis, management, natural history and clinicopathological correlates in 86 patients. *Surg Neurol* 1998;50:535–547.
3. Fox MW, Onofrio BM. Medical and surgical management of vertebral hemangiomas. *Contemp Neurosurg* 1993;15:1–6.
4. Traveras JM, Wood EH. *Diagnostic neuroradiology,* 2nd ed. Baltimore: Williams & Wilkins, 1976.
5. Luck JV, Monsen DCG. Bone tumors and tumor-like lesions of vertebrae. In: Ruge D, Wiltse LL, eds. *Spinal disorders. Diagnosis and treatment.* Philadelphia: Lea & Febiger, 1977:274–286.
6. Healy M, Herz DA, Pearl L. Spinal hemangiomas. *Neurosurgery* 1983;13:689–691.
7. Reizine D, Laredo JD, Riche MC, et al. Vertebral hemangiomas. In: Jeanmart, ed. *Radiology of the spine. Tumors.* Berlin: Springer-Verlag, 1986:73–80.
8. Gross CE, Hodge CJ Jr, Binet EF, et al. Relief of spinal block during embolization of a vertebral body hemangioma. *J Neurosurg* 1976;45:327–330.
9. DeCristofaro R, Biagini R, Boriani S, et al. Selective arterial embolization in the treatment of aneurysmal bone cyst and angioma of bone. *Skeletal Radiol* 1992;21:523–527.
10. MacCarty CS, Dahlin DC, Doyle JB Jr, et al. Aneurysmal bone cysts of the neural axis. *J Neurosurg* 1961;18:671–677.
11. Dietel KM, Fehlings MG. Primary bone tumors. In: Benzel EC, Stillerman CB, eds. *The thoracic spine.* St. Louis: Quality Medical Publishing, 1999:379–391.
12. Vandertop WP, Pruijs JEH, Snoeck IN, et al. Aneurysmal bone cyst of the thoracic spine: radical excision with use of the Cavitron. *J Bone Joint Surg Am* 1994;76:608–611.
13. Capanna R, Albisinni U, Picci P, et al. Aneurysmal bone cyst of the spine. *J Bone Joint Surg Am* 1985;67:527–531.
14. Birdwell KH, Ogilvie JW. Primary tumors of the spine (benign and malignant). In: Birdwell KH, DeWald RL, eds. *The textbook of spinal surgery.* Philadelphia: JB Lippincott Co, 1991:1143–1185.

15. Ohry A, Lipschitz M, Shemesh Y, et al. Disappearance of quadriparesis due to a huge cervicothoracic aneurysmal bone cyst. *Surg Neurol* 1988;29:307–311.
16. Berlin O, Vaughan LM. Spinal and axial tumors. *Curr Opin Orthop* 1991;2:801–810.
17. Barrow DL, Johnson WD. Historical perspective and classification of spinal vascular malformations. In: Barrow DL, Awad IA, eds. *Spinal vascular malformations.* Park Ridge, IL: American Association of Neurological Surgeons, 1999:1–7.
18. Malis LI. Arteriovenous malformations of the spinal cord. In: Youmans JR, ed. *Neurological surgery,* 2nd ed. Philadelphia: WB Saunders, 1982:1850–1874.
19. Hamilton MG, Anson JA, Spetzler RF. Arteriovenous and other vascular malformations of the spine. In: Menezes AH, Sonntag VKH, eds. *Principles of spinal surgery.* New York: McGraw-Hill, 1996:1423–1451
20. Merland JJ, Reizine D. Embolization techniques in the spinal cord. In: Dondelinger RF, Rossi P, Kurdziel JC, et al., eds. *Interventional radiology.* New York: Thieme Medical Publishers, 1990:433–442.
21. Sharma RR, Selmi F, Cast IP, et al. Spinal extradural arteriovenous malformation presenting with recurrent hemorrhage and intermittent paraplegia: case report and review of the literature. *Surg Neurol* 1994;41:26–31.
22. D'Angelo V, Bizzozero L, Talamonti G, et al. Value of magnetic resonance imaging in spontaneous extradural spinal hematoma due to vascular malformation: case report. *Surg Neurol* 1990;34:343–344.
23. Emery DJ, Cochrane DD. Spontaneous remission of paralysis due to spinal extradural hematoma: case report. *Neurosurgery* 1988;23:762–764.
24. Olivero WC, Hanigan WC, McCluney KW. Angiographic demonstration of a spinal epidural arteriovenous malformation. Case report. *J Neurosurg* 1993;79:119–120.
25. Foo D, Rossier AB. Preoperative neurological status in predicting surgical outcome of spinal epidural hematomas. *Surg Neurol* 1981;15:389–401.
26. Bradac GB, Simon RS, Schramm J. Cervical epidural AVM. Report of a case of uncommon location. *Neuroradiology* 1977;14:97–100.
27. Han SS, Love MB, Simeone FA. Diagnosis and treatment of a lumbar extradural arteriovenous malformation. *AJNR Am J Neuroradiol* 1987;8:1129–1130.

172. Spinal Meningiomas

Paul R. Cooper, Robert J. Wienecke, and Benjamin T. White

Intradural extramedullary tumors of the spinal cord comprise approximately 70% of all intradural tumors; they include meningiomas, schwannomas, and neurofibromas. In Nittner's review of 4,885 spinal cord tumors, the most common tumors in the intradural extramedullary compartment were noted to be meningiomas and schwannomas. Spinal meningiomas represent only 3% of all central nervous system meningiomas. Despite this, it is the most common benign tumor when located at or below the foramen magnum.

The first successful surgical removal of a spinal meningioma is credited to Sir Victor Horsely in 1887 (1). Advances in microsurgical techniques, spinal instrumentation, fusion, and radiographic imaging have allowed for early diagnosis and easier removal of such lesions in the present day. Today spinal meningiomas can be successfully resected with minimal risk of morbidity to the patient.

Epidemiology

INCIDENCE. Approximately 70% of spinal intradural tumors in adults are extramedullary. Of these extramedullary lesions, virtually all are nerve sheath tumors or meningiomas. The ratio of nerve sheath tumors to meningiomas in the spine is approximately 6:5 (2). Nevertheless, spinal meningiomas are distinctly less common than intracranial ones and represent approximately 3% of all central nervous system meningiomas.

AGE AND SEX. Spinal meningiomas are distinctly more common in women than men, as 70% to 80% of patients in most reports are females (3–11). The female preponderance may be due to the presence of progesterone receptors in a high proportion of tumors (3). In support of hormonal control of meningiomas is the fact that meningiomas frequently increase in size during pregnancy (12,13).

Spinal meningiomas are a lesion of the middle aged and elderly. Occurrence before the age of 40 is unusual (14). In one large retrospective review, two thirds of patients presented after the sixth decade (9). The mean age of patients in the series of Levy et al. (5) was 53 years. Meningiomas in childhood have been reported but are rare (7,15–17).

LOCATION. Of spinal meningiomas, 66% to 86% originate in the thoracic region and the remainder are in the cervical location (5–8). Lumbar lesions have been reported but are unusual (5,17,18). The presumed site of origin of spinal meningiomas from arachnoidal cap cells at the spinal nerve root exit zones accounts for their location lateral to the spinal cord; the absence of arachnoid cap cells in the lumbar spine may explain the infrequency of meningiomas in this location. In the cervical region, meningiomas are more likely to be anterolateral to the spinal cord, and in the thoracic region meningiomas are more likely to be in a posterolateral location. A direct dorsal location is unusual. Unlike their intracranial counterpart, spinal meningiomas typically do not disrupt the pia and are infrequently adherent to the spinal cord.

Extradural spinal meningiomas are unusual. Their incidence among all spinal meningiomas is reported to be 2.7% to 15% (4,5,10,16,17,19–25). They are more common in men, originate in the root exit zone, may grow both intradurally and extradurally, and may extend into the thoracic cavity (26). They are typically noted to be more aggressive, have a shorter time course, and frequently invade adjacent bone and soft tissues.

HISTOLOGY. There are numerous histological subtypes of meningiomas. They can be classified as meningothelial, fibroblastic, transitional, psammomatous, and angiomatous. Immunohistochemical staining is typically positive for vimentin and epithelial membrane antigen (27). Progesterone receptor activity is not infrequently found in meningiomas. The presence of progesterone receptors is thought to account for both the female preponderance of meningiomas and their association with breast cancer (28,29).

Lekanne Deprez et al. (14) describes a translocation involving chromosome 22 in a meningioma. This translocation involves the area of chromosome 22 also known to harbor the gene responsible for neurofibromatosis type 2 (NF2). The gene predisposing to NF2 and the meningioma tumor-suppressor gene located at t(4;22) may be the same according to some researchers (14).

Most spinal meningiomas are either of the psammomatous or meningothelial subtype. Malignancy is large and is noted when invasion of adjacent tissue, nuclear pleomorphism, and mitosis are identified on histological staining. In a large retrospective study of spinal meningiomas by Levy et al. (5), meningothelial and psammomatous meningiomas represented respectively 59% and 21% of the tumors. In another series, 57% of the tumors were noted to be psammomatous meningiomas.

Signs and Symptoms

The signs and symptoms of spinal meningiomas depend on the spinal level of origin and the tumor location with respect to the spinal cord. Because these tumors are slow growing, they can reach considerable size and cause severe compression of the spinal cord before the patient's symptoms cause him or her to seek medical attention. Even when symptoms are present, they are insidious in onset and development, and they are frequently present for 1 to 2 years at the time of presentation (5,9).

Midline thoracic pain and nocturnal exacerbation of back pain is a common presentation among patients with thoracic meningiomas. In the cervical region, neck pain and headache are common. Radicular symptoms in thoracic and cervical region occur in 20% of patients, but are less common than in the case of nerve sheath tumors, where radicular symptoms predominate (5).

On examination, a sensory level is found in almost one half of patients. Posterior column dysfunction is relatively uncommon because spinal meningiomas are infrequently dorsal to the spinal cord. At the time of presentation, 75% to 80% of patients have upper motor neuron type motor deficits with spasticity and pathological reflexes, although two thirds are ambulatory (5,10). Because most tumors are located laterally or anterolaterally, they may produce asymmetric signs and symptoms with greater motor deficits ipsilateral to the side of the lesion and a sensory deficit beginning one or two levels below the level of the lesion. Sphincter dysfunction is less common and is seen in only 15% of patients.

Differential Diagnosis

In theory, the variety of lesions that produce spinal cord dysfunction produce specific patterns of neurological dysfunction that should suggest a specific etiology; in practice, it is difficult to make a definitive diagnosis of a meningioma based on clinical presentation and neurological examination alone. In addition, while the clinical examination and history are important in defining the presence and level spinal cord dysfunction, they are less important in suggesting a specific diagnosis because of the exquisite ability of magnetic resonance imaging (MRI) to define the nature and location of the lesion. Nevertheless, knowledge of typical features of the more common lesions is useful in directing the most appropriate MRI sequences and the use of contrast enhancement.

Cervical Spondylotic Myelopathy

Cervical spondylotic myelopathy (CSM) is the most common cause of cervical spinal cord dysfunction in adults over the age of 50. The onset tends to be insidious, as is also the case for benign intradural tumors, but symptoms and signs are more likely to be symmetrical. In addition, the bilateral sensory and motor dysfunction of the hands, which starts about the same time as lower extremity corticospinal dysfunction, is typical of CSM but unusual with meningiomas.

Nerve Sheath Tumors

Nerve sheath tumors (neurofibromas and schwannomas) are the most common intradural extramedullary lesion. They are infrequently indistinguishable from meningiomas on clinical grounds alone. Because they almost always originate from the dorsal root, they are most likely to produce sensory disturbances than are meningiomas. Radicular sensory symptoms caused by nerve sheath tumors will almost always precede the development of myelopathy, unlike meningiomas where radicular symptoms occur later, if at all.

Intramedullary Spinal Cord Tumor and Syringomyelia

The most common intramedullary lesions are ependymomas and astrocytomas. Ependymomas are always centrally located within the spinal cord; astrocytomas are also usually central, although they may grow eccentrically. Both may present with suspended sensory loss as a result of stretching or invasion of crossing fibers of the lateral spinothalamic tract. Cervical intramedullary tumors and syrinxes produce wasting of upper extremity musculature, particularly the hand intrinsic muscles, as

a result of injury to the centrally located anterior horn cells. This type of sensory and motor finding is not seen with meningiomas.

Extradural Tumors

Metastatic disease is the most common cause of extradural compression by a neoplasm. It usually occurs in patients with a known primary tumor and frequently in a setting of other metastatic lesions. Neck or mid-back pain is common and frequently severe, and neurological deterioration is rapid.

Imaging Evaluation

MAGNETIC RESONANCE IMAGING. MRI with and without gadolinium diethylenetriamine pentaacetic acid (DTPA) enhancement is the imaging modality of choice for the evaluation of spinal meningiomas. T1- and T2-weighted images should be obtained in both the sagittal and axial planes. On the unenhanced T1-weighted images meningiomas will appear iso- or hypointense in relation to the spinal cord, and on T2-weighted images they will be slightly hyperintense (30–32). They homogeneously enhance after the intravenous administration of gadolinium DTPA, whereas the enhancement of nerve sheath tumors is more heterogeneous (Fig. 1). Meningiomas are located intradurally, usually in the lateral quadrants of the spinal canal, most frequently anterolaterally in the cervical region and posterolaterally in the thoracic region. Unlike nerve sheath tumors, they usually do not extend into the neural foramen, although a small percentage may be located extradurally.

Multiple meningiomas of the spine are rare but have been reported (33–35). They occur in 2% of patients with spinal meningiomas (5). Their presence typically suggests an underlying diagnosis of neurofibromatosis. Multiple meningiomas outside an underlying diagnosis of neurofibromatosis have been noted. Patronas et al. (36) reported a case of multiple meningiomas in a patient who had undergone prior irradiation for mediastinal and thyroid masses. Solero et al. (10) reported one incidental case of multiple meningiomas in his surgical series of 174 patients. Levy et al. (5) reported two patients with multiple meningiomas in their series of 97 spinal meningiomas. Whether the presence of multiple meningiomas portends a poorer long-term prognosis is unknown.

COMPUTED TOMOGRAPHY/MYELOGRAPHY. Computed tomography (CT)/myelography was formerly the preferred diagnostic modality for imaging spinal tumors. Presently it is utilized primarily only when MRI is contraindicated because of the presence of pacemakers, ferromagnetic aneurysm clips, or metallic foreign bodies. The spinal cord will be seen displaced and the subarachnoid space widened on the side of the tumor rostrally and caudally.

PLAIN FILMS. Plain films of the spine are usually not helpful in the diagnosis of meningiomas, although occasionally they may show subtle calcifications within the spinal canal. In the patient with paraparesis or quadriparesis of unknown cause they are most useful in excluding the diagnosis of meningioma by showing bony abnormalities consistent with metastatic dis-

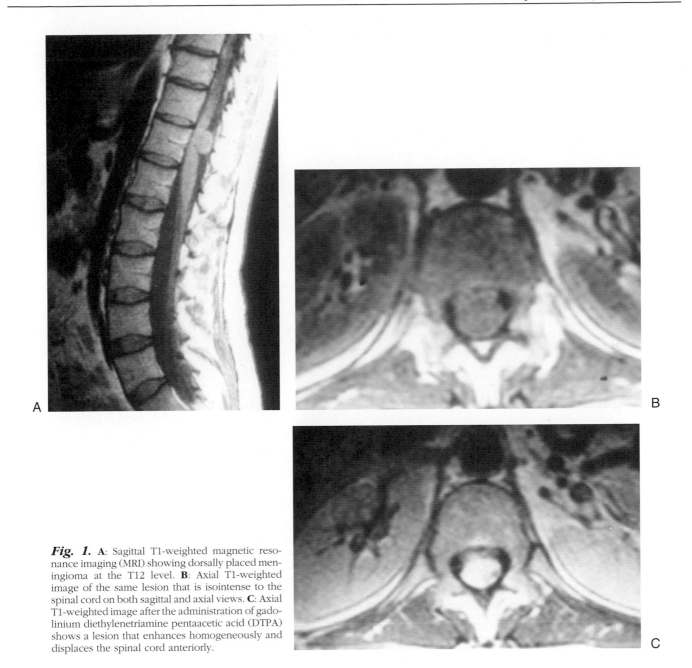

Fig. 1. **A**: Sagittal T1-weighted magnetic resonance imaging (MRI) showing dorsally placed meningioma at the T12 level. **B**: Axial T1-weighted image of the same lesion that is isointense to the spinal cord on both sagittal and axial views. **C**: Axial T1-weighted image after the administration of gadolinium diethylenetriamine pentaacetic acid (DTPA) shows a lesion that enhances homogeneously and displaces the spinal cord anteriorly.

ease. Neural foraminal enlargement strongly suggests the diagnosis of nerve sheath tumor.

Surgical Treatment

TIMING OF OPERATION. All patients with intradural tumors consistent with meningiomas and with signs or symptoms of spinal cord compression should undergo resection. The urgency of surgery depends on the severity and the rapidity of progression of the patient's neurological deficit. Occasionally, patients may deteriorate extremely rapidly and progress in spite of corticosteroid administration, and operative resection may have to be carried out on an emergency basis; however, more often, operation may be deferred for days to weeks.

The correct management of the asymptomatic patient with an incidentally discovered meningioma is not always clear. In the elderly patient it is appropriate to defer surgery and follow the patient's neurological examination. In younger patients, the growth of the tumor may be followed with serial MRI examinations on a yearly basis. Operation should be undertaken if there is clear evidence of tumor enlargement or the development of neurological signs and symptoms.

PERIOPERATIVE PREPARATION. The goal of treatment is complete removal of the tumor and restoration of normal neurological function. When initially evaluated, patients must be counseled that the extent of preoperative impairment is correlated with their ability to sustain neurological improvement after tumor removal. Patients with profound deficit (e.g., preservation of sensory function and absent or very slight motor function) are unlikely to walk postoperatively. They should also be advised that neurological deterioration, while unusual, is possible after surgery.

Patients are begun on high-dose corticosteroids (64 mg of methylprednisolone q.i.d. or its equivalent) 24 hours prior to surgery. They are advised to cease the use of aspirin and nonsteroidal antiinflammatory agents at least 1 week prior to the operation.

We use the prone position for all spinal meningiomas regardless of location. Patients are placed on chest rolls; for cervical and upper thoracic meningiomas, the head is fixed in a neutral position in a three-pin head holder; for thoracic tumors below T3, the head is turned to the side. Electrodes are placed for motor and somatosensory evoked potential monitoring for all spinal cord tumor surgeries.

OPERATIVE INCISION AND BONE EXPOSURE. In the thoracic region, the operative incision is localized using a preoperative thoracic spine x-ray correlated with radiopaque skin markers. Alternatively, an intraoperative localizing x-ray may be obtained. In the cervical spine, a localizing x-ray is taken when the spinous processes are exposed.

Laminectomy is performed over the site of the tumor and one level above and below. Because the spinal cord is already compressed by the bulk of a tumor mass, we avoid placing rongeurs within the spinal canal and favor performing the laminectomy using a high-speed drill with rough diamond bits. The wound is filled with saline and an ultrasound probe is used to image the tumor in the sagittal and axial planes. Additional bone is removed as necessary to gain exposure above and below the tumor.

Posterior or posterolaterally placed tumors offer little difficulty in exposure. For tumors anterior to the spinal cord or those in the anterolateral quadrant, ideal exposure is obtained by approaching the tumors through a trajectory that is as far lateral and anterior as possible. In the thoracic region this is accomplished by dissecting the muscle of the bone laterally to the head of the rib. The facet, pedicle, head of the rib, and the transverse process are all removed (Fig. 2). Because of the inherent stability of the thoracic spine, unilateral removal of bone as described is unlikely to cause instability. In the cervical spine the facet joint may be removed unilaterally to gain exposure to an anteriorly placed tumor. However, the entire contra-lateral facet must be preserved to increase the chance of stability and decrease the rate of postoperative kyphosis. If concern about instability exists, consideration should be given to instrumentation and fusion to restore the posterior tension band.

DURAL OPENING AND TUMOR REMOVAL. The dura mater should be incised in the midline above the tumor after which the arachnoid is opened and cerebrospinal fluid (CSF) is removed. If the dura mater is opened below the level of the tumor, the spinal cord may move against the tumor as CSF is removed, resulting in an increase in neurological deficit. The dural incision is continued above and below the tumor and the opening may be continued in a U-shaped fashion to retract the dura far laterally in order to visualize anteriorly placed lesions. The remainder of the intradural portion of the operation is performed using the operating microscope.

The dura mater is retracted to either side of the midline using 4-0 sutures and the arachnoid is opened over the tumor. For lateral and posterolaterally placed meningiomas, the lesion may be devascularized and then removed by progressively cauterizing and cutting its dural attachment. For ventral tumors, the dentate ligament is cut, improving visualization of the lesion. In the thoracic region below T1, a nerve root may be cut to gain additional exposure (Fig. 3).

The dural attachment of ventral tumors frequently cannot be visualized until the tumor bulk is reduced. The ultrasonic aspirator is extremely useful for resecting tumor and is used to debulk the center of the lesion, after which it may be rolled on itself and removed (Fig. 4). However, the use of the ultrasonic aspirator in vascular meningiomas may result in excessive bleeding. In this event, the bipolar forceps may be used to grasp the tumor and shrink and cauterize it. The tumor may then be retracted away from the spinal cord, after which the base of the tumor is cut and the tumor is removed. Although exposure can be improved by utilizing the edge of the cut dentate ligament to rotate the spinal cord, this maneuver is dangerous and may exacerbate spinal cord dysfunction.

Meningiomas en plaque (Fig. 5) are unusual, and total resection is not feasible because of the extensive dural attachment of these lesions (37). The bulk of the tumor is resected as described above, and the dura and residual tumor are extensively cauterized. Delayed neurological deficits may occur as a result of adhesive arachnoiditis.

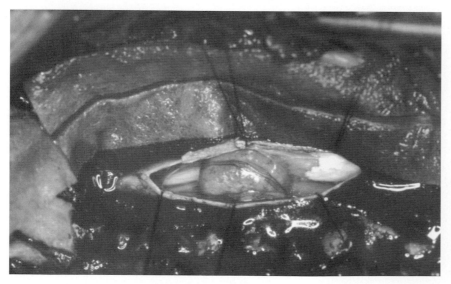

Fig. 2. Intraoperative photograph shows an anterolaterally placed thoracic meningioma displacing the spinal cord laterally and anteriorly. Removal of the pedicle and the head of the rib will allow excellent visualization of the tumor, its dural attachment, and the displaced spinal cord.

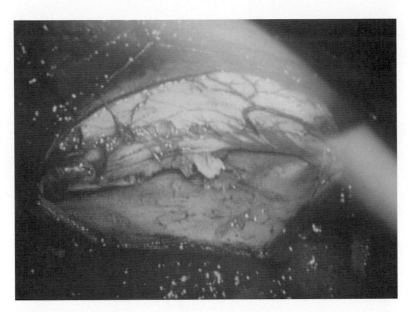

Fig. 3. Postoperative photograph taken after removal of a thoracic meningioma. Because the pedicle, head of rib, and facet have been resected, the area of the tumor could be approached quite laterally, allowing excellent visualization of the tumor and ventral dura well past the midline. A thoracic nerve root was cut, which provided additional exposure.

Calcified meningiomas present particular problems because they cannot be removed with either suction-aspiration or the ultrasonic aspirator. If they cannot be shrunk with the bipolar cautery, they may have to be removed without debulking by cutting them free from their dural attachment.

In patients younger than 60 with lateral or posterolateral tumors, the dural attachment of the tumor should be resected to minimize recurrence. Resection of the dural attachment may be difficult to achieve with tumors that originate from the ventral dura mater. Even if the dural attachment can be resected, watertight closure is not possible and blood may pass into the intradural space in the postoperative period from epidural bleeding. For this reason, we prefer to extensively cauterize the anterior dural attachment without resecting it.

CLOSURE. When possible, the dura mater should be closed primarily in a watertight fashion. If this cannot be achieved without putting pressure on the spinal cord, a patch graft of autogenous fascia is used. Alloderm (allogenic dermis) is easy to handle and is also useful for duroplasty. We no longer use duroplasties of Teflon (Preclude) as it is difficult to achieve a watertight closure with this material. The muscle and fascia are closed as separate layers with interrupted sutures spaced at intervals of 1 cm. Patients are kept flat in bed for 48 hours to minimize the chance of CSF fistula. Corticosteroids are tapered over 3 to 5 days.

Complications

NEUROLOGICAL DETERIORATION. Postoperative neurological deterioration is related to three factors: reoperation for recurrent tumor, calcified tumor precluding piecemeal removal, and lesions that are located directly anteriorly. Recurrent tumors tend to be adherent to the spinal cord because of prior surgical disruption of the arachnoid plane. While subtotal resection is less satisfying, leaving a small bit of tumor adherent to the cord may provide the patient with many years of palliation.

ASEPTIC MENINGITIS/ARACHNOIDITIS. Aseptic meningitis and arachnoiditis may occur as a result of blood left within the subarachnoid space. At the conclusion of tumor resection an attempt should be made to irrigate all blood from within the intradural space and to make certain that absolute hemostasis has been obtained. Although some authors do not close the dura, a watertight dural closure will prevent blood from entering the subarachnoid space (5). On two occasions we have observed shunt-dependent hydrocephalus from blood left in the cervical subarachnoid space after meningioma resection.

Aseptic meningitis is manifested by a stiff neck, fever, headache, and eosinophilia. It may occur as a result of placement of dural substitutes of animal origin such as bovine pericardium. CSF pleocytosis, negative bacterial cultures, and clinical improvement with steroids confirm the diagnosis. Symptoms also clear promptly with removal of the dural substitute.

PSEUDOMENINGOCELE/CEREBROSPINAL FLUID FISTULA. A watertight dural closure and meticulous muscle and fascial closure usually prevent a cutaneous fistula. A pseudomeningocele is usually prevented by a good dural closure. Small collections of CSF adjacent to the dura are frequently seen on postoperative MRI scans and are generally of no significance. On occasion, extradural collections of CSF may compress the spinal cord or be of such volume that secondary closure becomes necessary.

Tumor Recurrence

The recurrence rate of spinal meningiomas is lower than reported from intracranial meningiomas. Mirimanoff et al. (38) observed a recurrence rate of 3% after 5 years and 25% after 10 years for intracranial meningiomas. For spinal meningiomas there was no recurrence in 5 years and a 13% recurrence after 10 years. Levy et al. (5) reported a 4% recurrence rate with none occurring in the first 5 years after surgery. The reason for the discrepancy in recurrence rates between spinal and intracranial meningiomas is not clear but is probably due to a variety of factors. It is easier to achieve resection of the tumors dural origin in the spine than intracranially. Philippon and colleagues (39) postulate that spinal meningiomas are mostly slowly growing

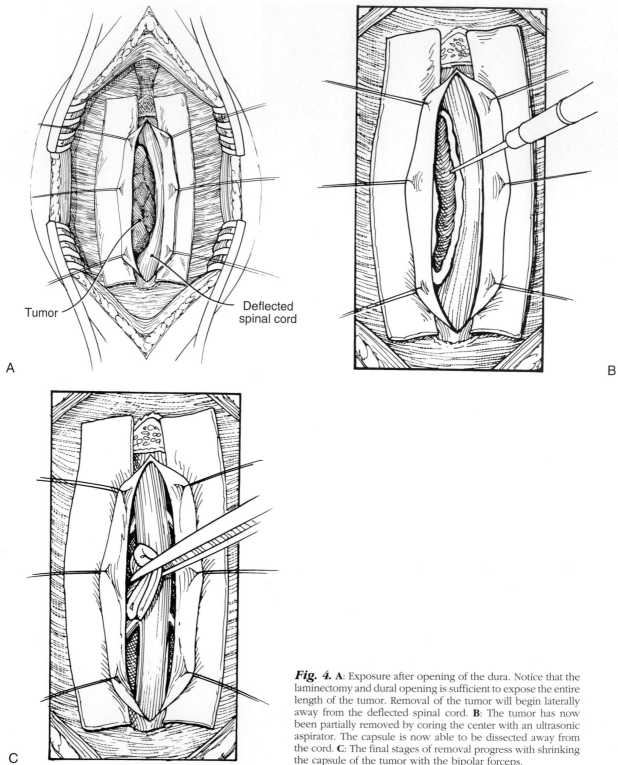

Tumor

Deflected
spinal cord

A

B

C

Fig. 4. **A**: Exposure after opening of the dura. Notice that the
laminectomy and dural opening is sufficient to expose the entire
length of the tumor. Removal of the tumor will begin laterally
away from the deflected spinal cord. **B**: The tumor has now
been partially removed by coring the center with an ultrasonic
aspirator. The capsule is now able to be dissected away from
the cord. **C**: The final stages of removal progress with shrinking
the capsule of the tumor with the bipolar forceps.

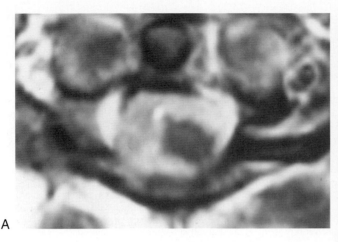

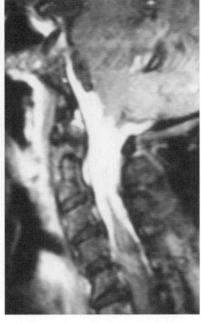

Fig. 5. **A**: An axial T1-weighted MRI at the C1 level after the administration of gadolinium DTPA shows a meningioma en plaque encircling the spinal cord. **B**: Sagittal T1-weighted MRI after the administration of gadolinium DTPA shows the tumor extending from the clivus down to the C3 level. This type of tumor cannot be completely resected.

psammomatous tumors occurring in an elderly population, many of whom will die before tumors recur.

The efficacy of dural resection at the point of tumor attachment in decreasing the incidence of recurrence is not clear. In one series, the authors reported no recurrence in any patient with an anteriorly placed tumor whose dura was coagulated but not resected (5). Solero and colleagues (10) concluded that there was no correlation between recurrence and the extent of dural resection.

When resection of the dural attachment of the tumor has not been accomplished, it is the authors' policy to perform a baseline MRI with and without gadolinium DTPA enhancement 6 months after operation and 3 to 5 years later (40). If recurrence of tumor is not visualized after 5 years, no further MRI examinations need be performed.

Histologically, malignant tumors are unusual and more likely to recur if residual tumor remains. Patients with such tumors should be studied with MRI earlier after surgery and at more frequent intervals. Patients with evidence of residual tumor or early recurrence on MRI should be considered candidates for radiotherapy. With the exception of patients with extensive en plaque meningiomas, we do not utilize radiotherapy for histologically benign spinal meningiomas.

Neurological Outcome

Neurological outcome is to a large extent related to the patient's preoperative neurological function. In most large series, over 90% of patients experience improvement or stabilization of neurological function (5,7,10). However, even patients with severe motor deficits will regain function. In one report, over one half of patients with severe preoperative deficits were able to ambulate after operation.

References

1. Gowers W, Horsely V: A case of tumor of the spinal cord. Removal. Recovery. *Med Chir Trans* 71:377–428, 1888.
2. Sloof JL, Kernohan JW, MacCarty C: *Primary intramedullary tumors of the spinal cord and filum terminale.* Philadelphia: WB Saunders, 1964.
3. Black PM: Hormones, radiosurgery and virtual reality: new aspects of meningioma management. *Can J Neurol Sci* 24:302–306, 1997.
4. Borghi G: Extradural spinal meningioma. *Acta Neurochir (Wien)* 29:195–202, 1973.
5. Levy WJ, Bay J, Dohn D: Spinal cord meningioma. *J Neurosurg* 57:804–812, 1982.
6. McCormick PC, Post KD, Stein BM: Intradural extramedullary tumors in adults. *Neurosurg Clin North Am* 1:591–598, 1990.
7. Namer IJ, Pamir MN, Benli K, et al.: Spinal meningiomas. *Neurochirurgia (Stuttg)* 30:11–15, 1987.
8. Ortaeskinazi H, Postalci L, Kepoglu U, et al.: Spinal meningiomas. *Chir Organi Mov* 83:191–195, 1998.
9. Rustichelli P, Scoditti U, Moretti G, et al.: Studio retrospettivo di 50 casi di meningioma spinale. *Acta Biomed Ateneo Parmense* 55:255–260, 1984.
10. Solero CL, Fornari M, Giombini S, et al.: Spinal meningiomas: review of 174 operated cases. *Neurosurgery* 25:153–160, 1989.
11. Torres LF, Madalozzo LE, Werner B, et al.: Meningiomas. Estudo epidemiologico e anatomo-patologico de 304 casos. *Arq Neuropsiquiatr* 54:549–556, 1996.
12. Bickerstaff ER, Small JM, Guest IA: The relapsing course of certain meningiomas in relation to pregnancy and menstruation. *J Neurol Neurosurg Psychiatry* 21:89–91, 1958.
13. Weyand RD, MacCarty CS, Wilson RB: The effect of pregnancy on intracranial meningiomas occurring about the optic chiasm. *Surg Clin North Am* 31:1225–1233, 1951.
14. Lekanne Deprez RH, Groen NA, van Biezen NA, et al.: A t(4;22) in a meningioma points to the localization of a putative tumor-suppressor gene. *Am J Genet* 48:783–790, 1991.
15. Chen HJ, Lui CC, Chen L: Spinal epidural meningioma in a child. *Childs Nerv Syst* 8:465–467, 1992.
16. Motomochi M, Makita Y, Nabeshima S, et al.: Spinal epidural meningioma in childhood. *Surg Neurol* 13:5–7, 1980.
17. Roux FX, Nataf F, Pinjaudeau M, et al.: Intraspinal meningiomas: review of 54 cases with discussion of poor prognosis factors and modern therapeutic management. *Surg Neurol* 46:458–463, 1996.
18. Tolias CM, Beale DJ, Sakas DE: Giant lumbar meningioma: common tumour in an unusual location. *Neuroradiology* 39:276–277, 1997.
19. Bull JWB: Spinal meningiomas and neurofibromas. *Acta Radiol* 40:283–300, 1953.
20. Cassinari V, Bernasconi V: Tumori e malformazione vasali spinali. *Acta Neurochir (Wien)* 9:612–658, 1961.

21. Early CB, Sayers MP: Spinal epidural meningioma. Case report. *J Neurosurg* 25:571–573, 1966.
22. Fortuna A, Gambacorta D, Occhipinti EMN: Spinal extradural meningiomas. *Neurochirurg (Stuttg)* 12:166–180, 1969.
23. Gambardella G, Toscano S, Staropoli C, et al.: Extradural spinal meningioma. Role of magnetic resonance in differential diagnosis. *Acta Neurochir (Wien)* 107:70–73, 1990.
24. Haft A, Shenkin HA: Spinal epidural meningioma. Case report. *J Neurosurg* 20:801–804, 1963.
25. Martinez R, Ramiro J, Montero C, et al.: Extradural spinal meningiomas with intrathoracic extension. Report of two cases. *J Neurosurg Sci* 32:179–181, 1988.
26. Calogero JA, Moossy J: Extradural spinal meningiomas. *J Neurosurg* 37:442–447, 1972.
27. Burger PC, Scheithauer BW, Vogel FS: *Surgical pathology of the nervous system and its coverings.* New York: Churchill Livingstone, 1991.
28. Blankenstein MA, Blaauw G, Lamberts SWJ: Presence of progesterone receptors and absence of oestrogen receptors in human intracranial meningioma cytosols. *Eur J Cancer Clin Oncol* 19:363–370, 1983.
29. Schoenberg BS, Christine BW, Whisnant JP: Nervous system neoplasms and primary malignancies of other sites. The unique association between meningiomas and breast cancer. *Neurology* 25:705–712, 1975.
30. Boisserie-Lacroix M, Kien P, Caille JM: L'imagerie des tumeurs intradurales et extra-medullaires: les neurinomes et les meningiomes. *J Neuroradiol* 14:66–81, 1987.
31. Parizel PM, Baleriaux D, Rodesch G, et al.: Gd-DTPA-enhanced MR imaging of spinal tumors. *AJR* 152:1087–1096, 1989.
32. Scotti G, Scialfa G, Colombo N, et al.: MR imaging of intradural extramedullary tumors of the cervical spine. *J Comput Assist Tomogr* 9:1037–1041, 1985.
33. Pagni CA, Canavero S, Cento A: Multiple spinal meningiomas: case report and review of the literature. *Zentralbl Neurochir* 51:225–228, 1990.
34. Rand RW: Multiple spinal cord meningiomas. *J Neurosurg* 9:310–314, 1952.
35. Rath S, Mathai KV, Chandy J: Multiple meningiomas of the spinal canal. Case report. *J Neurosurg* 26:639–640, 1967.
36. Patronas NJ, Brown F, Duda EE: Multiple meningiomas in the spinal canal. *Surg Neurol* 13{1}:78–80, 1980.
37. Stechison MT, Tasker RR, Wortzman G: Spinal meningioma en plaque: report of two cases. *J Neurosurg* 67:452–455, 1987.
38. Mirimanoff RO, Dosretz DE, Lingood RM, et al.: Meningiomas: analysis of recurrence and progression following neurosurgical resection. *J Neurosurg* 62:18–24, 1985.
39. Philippon J, Cornu PR, Grob R, et al.: Les méningiomes récidivantes. *Neurochirurgie* 32(suppl 1):54–62, 1986.
40. Weingarten K, Ernst RJ, Jahre C, et al.: Detection of residual or recurrent meningioma after surgery: value of enhanced vs unenhanced MR imaging. *AJR* 158:645–650, 1992.

173. Intramedullary Tumors of the Spinal Cord

Theodore H. Schwartz and Paul C. McCormick

The role of surgery in the management of intramedullary spinal cord tumors has evolved significantly in recent years. Once employed for diagnosis alone, surgery now represents the most effective treatment of benign well-circumscribed tumors (1–7). Since the majority of intramedullary spinal cord neoplasms are low-grade lesions, long-term tumor control or cure with preservation of neurological function can be achieved in most patients with microsurgical removal alone (1–7). Most surgical series indicate that the strongest predictor of postoperative functional outcome is preoperative functional ability (1–7). Significant improvement of a severe or long-standing preoperative neurological deficit rarely occurs following technically successful surgical excision. Surgical morbidity is also greater in patients with more significant preoperative deficits. As a result, early clinical diagnosis and definitive initial treatment are critical to successful clinical management of most intramedullary tumors.

Clinical Evaluation

The clinical features of intramedullary spinal cord tumors are variable. Early symptoms are usually nonspecific and may only subtly progress. Symptom duration prior to diagnosis is often in the range of 3 to 4 years (2,6). Malignant or metastatic neoplasms will present with a much shorter course, in the range of several weeks to a few months (2,6). Intratumoral hemorrhage may produce an abrupt deterioration that is more commonly associated with ependymomas.

Pain and weakness are the most frequent presenting symptom of intramedullary spinal cord tumors in adults (2,3,6–8). The pain typically localizes to the level of the tumor and is rarely radicular. The distribution and progression of the symptoms is related to tumor location. Upper extremity symptoms predominate with cervical neoplasms. Thoracic cord tumors produce spasticity and sensory disturbances. Numbness is a common complaint and typically begins distally in the legs with proximal progression. Tumors of the lumbar enlargement and conus medullaris often present with back and leg pain. The leg pain may be radicular in nature. Urogenital and anorectal dysfunction tend to occur early.

Differential Diagnosis

Although a wide variety of pathological processes may arise from or secondarily involve the spinal cord as a mass lesion, primary glial tumors account for at least 80% of intramedullary tumors in most published series (2–6). These include astrocytoma and ependymoma as well as the less common glial neoplasms such as ganglioglioma, oligodendroglioma, and sub-

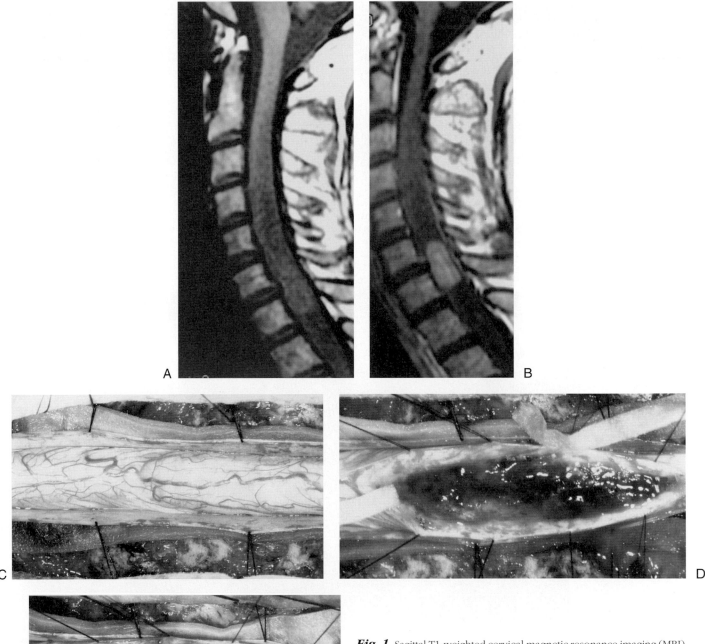

Fig. 1. Sagittal T1-weighted cervical magnetic resonance imaging (MRI) without (**A**) and with (**B**) gadolinium contrast demonstrates a homogeneously enhancing ependymoma with rostral and caudally extending syrinx. **C**: Intraoperative photograph demonstrates focal enlargement the spinal cord. Note the cottonoids, which maintain a dry surgical field. **D**: Following midline myelotomy, the entire rostrocaudal extent of the ependymoma is exposed. Note the pial traction sutures and the glistening appearance of the ependymoma. **E**: After removal of the ependymoma the tumor has been completely removed and hemostasis obtained.

ependymoma. Hemangioblastomas account for 3% to 8% of intramedullary neoplasms (9). Inclusion tumors and cysts, metastases, nerve sheath tumors, neurocytoma, and melanocytoma account for much of the remainder of intramedullary mass lesions. Metastatic lesions can also be found in an intramedullary location, with lung and breast being the most common sources.

EPENDYMOMA. Ependymomas are the most common intramedullary tumor in adults (10). They occur throughout life but more frequently in middle age. Men and women are equally affected. Approximately 65% will have associated syrinx, particularly when presenting in cervical locations (Fig. 1) (11). A variety of histological subtypes may be encountered. The cellular ependymoma is the most common but epithelial, tanacytic (fibrillar), subependymoma, myxopapillary, or mixed examples may occur. Nearly all are histologically benign (1,3,5,12,13). Although unencapsulated, these glial-derived tumors are usu-

ally well circumscribed and do not infiltrate adjacent spinal cord tissue.

ASTROCYTOMA. About 3% of central nervous system (CNS) astrocytomas arise within the spinal cord (14). These tumors occur at any age but seem most prevalent in the first three decades of life. Nearly 60% of these tumors occur in the cervical and cervicothoracic region (3) and 20% will have associated syrinx (Fig. 2) (11). Spinal cord astrocytomas represent a heterogeneous group with respect to histology, gross characteristics, biology, and natural history. These tumors include the low-grade fibrillary and pilocytic astrocytoma, malignant astrocytoma and glioblastoma, ganglioglioma, and the rare oligodendroglioma. Most of these are grade I or II fibrillary astrocytomas. Juvenile pilocytic astrocytomas and gangliogliomas are more common in the pediatric population. The designation of a pilocytic astrocytoma in the adult usually reflects an abundance of pilocytic features that occur as a secondary structure in an

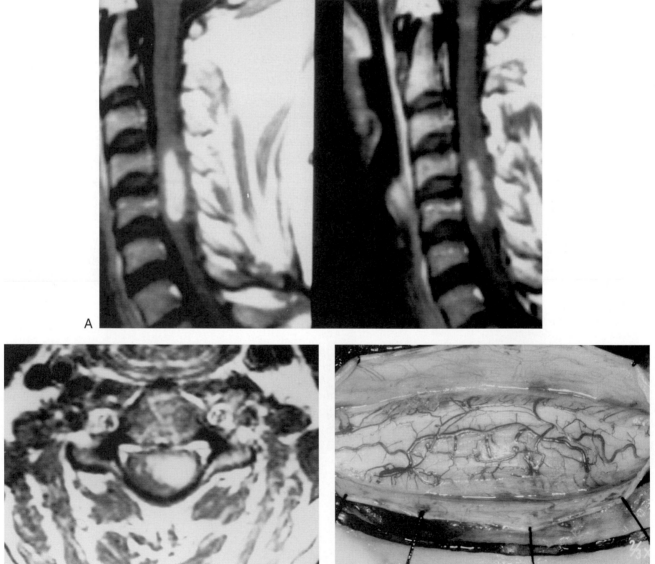

Fig. 2. Sagittal (**A**) and axial (**B**) T1-weighted cervical MRI with gadolinium contrast demonstrates a homogeneously enhancing astrocytoma. Note the irregular margin. **C:** Intraoperative photograph demonstrates focal enlargement of the spinal cord.

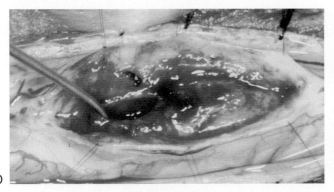

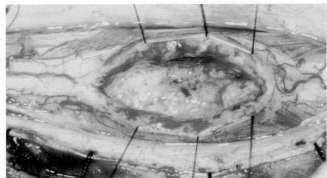

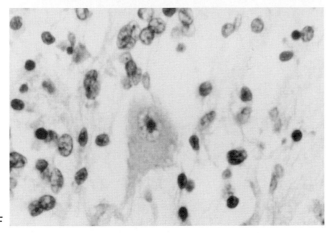

Fig. 2. (continued). **D**: Following midline myelotomy, the entire rostrocaudal extent of the astrocytoma is exposed. **E**: After removal, the tumor appears completely removed but residual cells certainly exist in the tumor bed. **F**: Histological specimen, 60×, H&E stain, reveals tumor around neuron, indicating neoplastic infiltration into parenchyma.

otherwise typical fibrillary astrocytoma (13). It is unclear whether these pilocytic features have prognostic significance. About 25% of adult astrocytomas are malignant (Fig. 3) (1,3).

HEMANGIOBLASTOMA. Hemangioblastomas account for 3% to 8% of intramedullary tumors (9); 15% to 25% occur in association with von Hippel–Lindau syndrome (VHL)—an autosomal-dominant trait with incomplete penetrance and incomplete expression (9). These tumors arise at any age but are rare in early childhood. Associated syringes are common (11). Hemangioblastomas are benign tumors of vascular origin that are sharply circumscribed but not encapsulated. Almost all have a pial attachment. Most are dorsal or dorsolaterally located (Fig. 4).

MISCELLANEOUS PATHOLOGY. Approximately 4% of apparent intramedullary spinal cord tumors will turn out to be nonneoplastic lesions (15). An acute or subacute clinical course is characteristic, and evidence of systemic involvement further suggests the diagnosis. The differential diagnosis of an intramedullary tumor also includes inflammatory or demyelinating conditions of the cord such as bacterial abscess, tuberculoma, inflammatory pseudotumor, sarcoidosis, multiple sclerosis, viral or parainfectious myelitis, paraneoplastic involvement, or an intermediate entity between multiple sclerosis and acute disseminated encephalomyelitis (15–17). Many of these conditions are grouped under the heading of transverse myelitis. These conditions generally present with an acute or subacute myelopathy that advances rapidly over several hours to a few days. An acute clinical course with significant neurological deficit in the absence of obvious spinal cord enlargement on magnetic reso-

nance imaging (MRI) generally distinguishes these medical myelopathies from surgical mass lesions (Fig. 5).

Inclusion tumors and cysts may rarely occur and have an intramedullary location. Lipomas are the most common dysembryogenic lesion and account for about 1% of intramedullary tumors. These lesions enlarge and produce symptoms in early adulthood and middle age through increased fat disposition in metabolically normal fat cells and are considered juxtamedullary because they occupy a subpial location. Metastases account for only about 2% of intramedullary tumors, which is probably due to the small size of the spinal cord and its remote vascular accessibility to hematogenous tumor emboli (18). Lung and breast are the most common primaries. Melanocytoma, melanoma, fibrosarcoma, and peripheral neuroectodermal tumor (PNET) can also arise in an intramedullary location (17,19). Cavernous malformations, amyloid angiopathy, and other isolated intramedullary vascular lesions may also present as an intramedullary mass (15,20).

Radiographic Evaluation

Gadolinium-enhanced MRI is the procedure of choice for imaging and preoperative evaluation of an intramedullary tumor (21). Spinal cord enlargement and tumor enhancement are the characteristic findings. Most intramedullary tumors are isointense or slightly hypointense for the surrounding spinal cord on T1-weighted images (21). Often there is only ill-defined spinal cord enlargement on T1-weighted images. T2-weighted images are more sensitive for tumor identification because most tumors are hyperintense to the spinal cord on T2-weighted im-

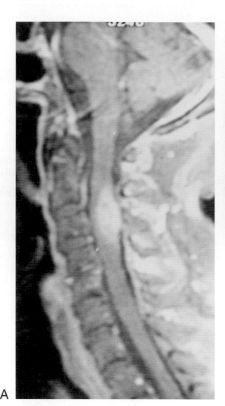

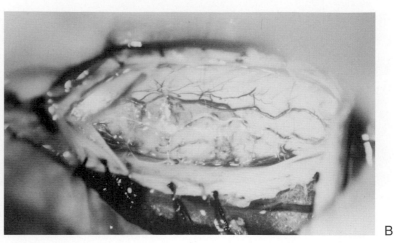

A

B

Fig. 3. **A**: Sagittal T1-weighted cervical MRI reveals a glioblastoma. **B**: Intraoperative photograph demonstrates tumor fungating through pia.

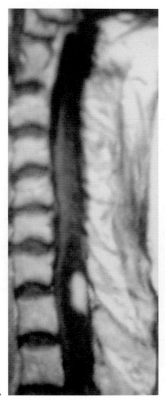

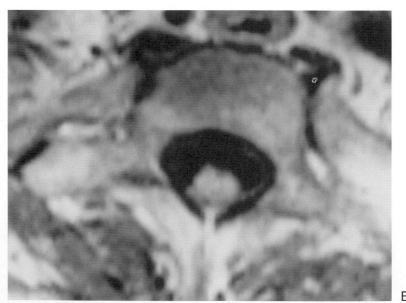

A

B

Fig. 4. T1-weighted gadolinium enhanced sagittal (**A**) and axial cervicothoracic (**B**) MRI demonstrates a dorsal homogeneously enhancing hemangioblastoma with associated syrinx.

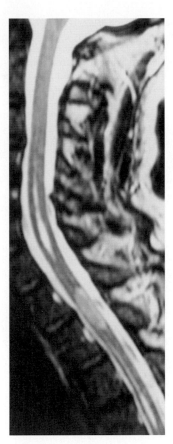

Fig. 5. T2-weighted sagittal cervicothoracic MRI demonstrates a multiple sclerosis plaque with associated rostral syrinx. Note that the spinal cord is not enlarged.

ages (21). Nearly all intramedullary neoplasms will demonstrate contrast uptake. Ependymomas usually demonstrate uniform contrast enhancement and are symmetrically located within the spinal cord (Fig. 1). Polar cysts are identified in the majority of cases, particularly in cervical and cervicothoracic locations (11). Heterogeneous enhancement from intratumoral cysts or necrosis can be seen with ependymomas.

The MRI appearance of astrocytomas is much more variable. These tumors tend to be less well defined than ependymomas on contrast-enhanced MRI because of their irregular tumor margins (Fig. 2). Contrast uptake may be minimal, uniform, or patchy (21). Heterogeneous uptake and patchy irregular margins is more commonly seen with astrocytomas because of intratumoral cysts or necrosis. Despite characteristic MRI patterns, however, there is enough variability and overlap MRI appearance of these tumors to preclude competent histological diagnosis of tumor type based on MRI characteristics alone.

The MRI appearance of inflammatory conditions is variable and probably related to the etiology (15). An acute multiple sclerosis plaque, for example, usually demonstrates focal homogeneous contrast enhancement, which may be confined to the white matter. There is minimal, if any, spinal cord enlargement (Fig. 5). Patchy contrast enhancement over several cord segments is more characteristic of viral or parainfectious myelitis. Leptomeningeal enhancement can be seen with lymphoma, metastases, and bacterial, fungal, or tuberculous myelitis (21).

Surgical Objective

The most important factor in determining the surgical objective is the plane between the tumor and the spinal cord. This interface can only be accurately assessed through an adequate myelotomy that extends over the entire rostral caudal extent of the tumor. Although the presence of a syrinx may improve the chances of a gross-total resection, it cannot be used as an independent predictor of outcome (11). Benign tumors such as ependymomas and hemangioblastomas, although unencapsulated, are noninfiltrative lesions that typically display a distinct plane. Gross-total removal is the treatment of choice in these cases. Astrocytomas are more variable. Although some benign astrocytomas are well circumscribed and allow gross total resection, most exhibit variable infiltration into the surrounding spinal cord. This is often reflected in a gradual transition zone between the tumor and spinal cord. More peripheral dissection beyond what is clearly tumor tissue risks neurological function from possible resection of infiltrative yet functionally viable spinal cord parenchyma. Thus, the surgical objective for spinal cord astrocytomas remains unclear. Specifically, a correlation between the extent of resection and tumor control has not been definitively established (3,8,11). Since preservation of neurological function, rather than complete tumor resection, is the more prudent treatment objective in these cases, tumor removal is limited to that which is clearly distinguishable from the surrounding spinal cord. The extent of tumor removal, therefore, will vary.

Management of less common intramedullary mass lesions is also dictated by the nature of the tumor/spinal cord interface. Metastatic spinal cord tumors, for example, usually present as a well-circumscribed focal mass amenable to gross total resection. Intramedullary lipomas are inclusion tumors that result from disordered embryogenesis, probably defective cleavage of germ cell layers. These are not true neoplasms but probably slowly enlarge through continued fat deposition of metabolically normal cells. Gross total resection is not possible because these lesions insinuate into functional spinal cord tissue at their margins. Conservative internal decompression results in long-term clinical stabilization in most cases.

Intraoperative biopsy can be useful in certain circumstances but should not be used as the sole criterion dictating the surgical objective. First, interpretation of tiny biopsy fragments often is inaccurate or nondiagnostic and may consist of only peritumoral gliosis, which may be erroneously interpreted as an infiltrating astrocytoma. Second, it is difficult, if not impossible, to accurately assess the nature of the tumor/spinal cord interface through a tiny myelotomy. Biopsy results, however, may be particularly helpful in some circumstances. Identification of a histologically malignant tumor, for example, independently signals an end to the procedure since surgery is of no benefit for malignant intramedullary neoplasms (3,22,23). In other cases in which the tumor/spinal cord interface may not be apparent, confident histological identification of an ependymoma reassures the surgeon that a plane must exist and that surgical removal should continue.

Surgical Technique

Following intubation and administration of perioperative steroids and antibiotics, the patient is placed in the prone position. A Mayfield skull clamp is utilized for cervical and upper thoracic lesions. Neck flexion and head elevation (i.e., military prone) reduces the spinal curvature at these levels. Sensory and motor evoked potentials (MEPs) are utilized throughout the procedure (24,25). Sensory potentials may be lost following midline myelotomy and are not predictive of postoperative motor function. Sub/epidural MEPs can be monitored in 60% of patients and provide real-time feedback. A 50% decline in amplitude may be an indication of a new, permanent postoperative weakness (25).

A midline incision and subperiosteal bony dissection is accomplished. A standard laminectomy is performed that should extend at least one segment above and below the solid tumor component. The facets are preserved. Delayed instability rarely occurs following laminectomy for intramedullary tumor removal in adults. While laminoplasty may be a reasonable option (6,7), it is not required in the adult population. Strict hemostasis must be secured prior to dural opening to prevent ongoing blood contamination into the dependent microsurgical field. Wide moist cottonoid wall-offs cover the exposed muscles. Surgicel is generously spread over the lateral gutters to prevent operative field blood contamination. The dura is opened in the midline and tented laterally to the muscles with sutures and the operating microscope is brought into the field (Figs. 1C and 2C). The arachnoid is opened separately. The spinal cord is inspected for any surface abnormality. Some authors have commented that even at first-time operations, encountering arachnoid scarring and pial tethering can complicate operative resection and predicts a poor functional outcome (7,11). We have not found this phenomenon to be a frequent occurrence. Most glial tumors present only localized spinal cord enlargement (Figs. 1C, 2C, and 3B). The spinal cord may be rotated. Occasionally the overlying spinal cord may be thinned or even transparent by a large or eccentrically located tumor or polar cyst. Ultrasound is useful for tumor localization and assurance of adequate bony exposure (26). Malignant neoplasms may replace surface spinal cord tissue and/or fungate through the pia into the subarachnoid space. Most hemangioblastomas arise from the dorsal half of the spinal cord with a visible pial attachment (Fig. 4).

A standard midline myelotomy is performed through the posterior median septum. The dorsal midline can be accurately estimated by noting the midpoint between the dorsal nerve root entry zones bilaterally. Small veins that exit from the septum may also assist in establishing the midline. Midline crossing vessels in the pia are cauterized and divided. The pia is a robust glistening white membrane with longitudinal striations. It requires sharp incision with a microknife or scissors. The myelotomy should extend over the entire rostrocaudal extent of the tumor. The myelotomy is deepened by gentle spreading of the posterior columns with microforceps or dissectors. The tumor is first encountered in the area of maximum cord enlargement. The dissection continues on the surface of the tumor until the entire rostrocaudal extent has been identified. Polar cysts are entered and drained when present. Once the entire dorsal extent of the tumor has been identified, 6-0 pial traction sutures are placed (Figs. 1D and 2D). Small mosquito clamps on the sutures provide constant superior and lateral spinal cord retraction. The technique of tumor removal is determined by the surgical objective, tumor size, and gross and histological characteristics of the tumor. If no plane is apparent between the tumor and the surrounding spinal cord, then it is likely that an infiltrative tumor is present. Biopsy is obtained to establish a histological diagnosis. If an infiltrating or malignant astrocytoma is identified and is consistent with the intraoperative findings, further tumor removal is not warranted. In most cases, however, a reasonably well-defined benign glial tumor will be identified. Ependymomas appear with a smooth reddish gray glistening tumor surface, which is sharply demarcated from the surrounding spinal cord (Fig. 1D). Variable blood vessels can be seen crossing the tumor surface that distinguish these tumors from astrocytomas, which rarely display these surface characteristics. Traction on the surface of the tumor is used against the countertraction provided by the pial sutures, which allows the development of the dissection plane. Small feeding blood vessels and fibrous adhesions between the spinal cord and tumor are cauterized and divided. Large tumors may require internal decompression with an ultrasonic aspirator or laser. Once significant tumor and debulking has been performed, dissection of the lateral and ventral margins may be accomplished. The ventral tumor margin is developed by applying traction to a tumor pole, perpendicular to the long axis of the spinal cord. Feeding arteries from the anterior spinal artery are easily identified, cauterized, and divided.

Most benign astrocytomas will present varying degrees of circumscription (Fig. 2D). About one third of adult patients have benign, infiltrative tumors without an identifiable tumor mass. Biopsy for diagnosis is all that can be established in these patients. Occasionally, an astrocytoma may be so well developed as to mimic an ependymoma. Nevertheless, there is rarely as defined a plane with astrocytomas as is typically seen with ependymomas. Dissection on the surface of an astrocytoma usually results in the development of laminated pseudo-planes (Fig. 2D). Decompression is achieved with an ultrasonic aspirator or laser, and proceeds systematically from the center of the tumor radially to the surface. Although a clean plane does not exist for the majority of astrocytomas, there is frequently a difference in the color of the tumor with respect to the spinal cord. The surgeon must rely on his own judgment and experience. Obviously, if gross tumor is easily identified, then continued removal is reasonable. Changes in motor sensory evoked potentials or uncertainty of spinal cord/tumor interface should signal an end to tumor resection. Removal of hemangioblastomas is facilitated by excision of the pial attachment as part of the tumor mass. Cauterization of the surface tumor vessels is followed by a circumscribing incision around the pial base. The buried portion of the tumor within the spinal cord is easily dissected and delivered with traction on the pial base. A small polar myelotomy may provide better visualization for larger tumors. Internal decompression cannot be performed with these neoplasms but cautery on the tumor surface will shrink the tumor into a more manageable size.

Following the removal of an intramedullary tumor, the resection bed is inspected and any bleeding points are controlled with warm saline or oxidized cotton (Figs. 1E and 2E). Pial traction sutures are removed, which allows the cord to assume its normal position. Closure of the myelotomy is not performed. The dura is usually closed primarily, although a dural patch graft may prevent dorsal tethering of the spinal cord at the operative site, which may be a potential cause of morbidity in the postoperative period. An autologous fascia lata or thoracodorsal fascia patch graft can be utilized. The remainder of the wound is closed in standard fashion. Meticulous closure techniques are especially important in reoperations and in previously radiated spines, which present a high risk of postoperative cerebrospinal fluid (CSF) fistula.

Postoperative Management

Early mobilization is encouraged to prevent complications of recumbency such as deep venous thrombosis and pneumonia. Paretic patients are particularly vulnerable to thromboembolic complications. Subcutaneous heparin 5,000 units b.i.d. is begun on the second postoperative day in these patients. Orthostatic hypotension may occasionally occur following removal of upper thoracic and cervical intramedullary neoplasms. This is usually a self-limiting problem that can be managed with liberalization of fluids and more gradual mobilization. A posterior fossa syndrome occasionally occurs following removal of a high cervical intramedullary neoplasm. This is effectively managed with steroids, although a spinal tap may be required to rule out meningitis. CSF fistulas are aggressively managed to prevent meningitis. An early return to the operating room for wound revision is recommended to prevent this complication.

Despite confident gross total resection, benign intramedullary tumors present a continued risk of recurrence. Long-term clinical and radiographic follow-up is warranted in these patients. An early postoperative MRI—6 to 8 weeks following surgery—establishes the completeness of resection and serves as a baseline against which further studies can be compared. Serial gadolinium-enhanced MRIs are obtained yearly because radiographic tumor recurrence usually precedes clinical symptoms.

Functional Outcome

The immediate results of surgery are related primarily to the patient's preoperative status and tumor location (1–3,6,7). In general, most patients note sensory loss in the early postoperative period, most likely as a result of the midline myelotomy, transient edema, or vascular compromise. These complaints are more subjective than objective in nature and can be significant even with little or no objective deficit. They usually resolve within 3 months (7). Additional surgical morbidity is directly related to the patient's preoperative status, the location of the tumor, and the presence of spinal cord atrophy and arachnoid scarring (2,3,6,7,11). Patients with significant or long-standing deficit rarely demonstrate any significant recovery and are more likely to worsen following surgery. A shorter duration of preoperative symptoms, however, may favor improvement even in patients with a significant preoperative deficit, particularly those with ependymomas (7). Thoracic location has also been correlated with a decline in postoperative function (4,6,7,27), perhaps due to a more tenuous blood supply in this region. Appreciation of spinal cord atrophy and arachnoid scarring may indicate chronic spinal cord compression and predict poor functional outcome (7,11). Preservation, rather than restoration, of neurological function is the reasonable expectation for intramedullary tumor surgery. The greatest benefit and least risk of surgery for intramedullary tumors, therefore, is derived in those patients who are only minimally symptomatic (2,3,7). This underscores the importance of early diagnosis and aggressive initial treatment prior to the onset of objective deficit. It is equally important in the follow-up period since periodic MRI evaluation will most likely demonstrate evidence of tumor recurrence prior to clinical recurrence.

Tumor Control

Long-term outcome and risk of recurrence are dependent primarily on tumor histology and, with the exception of malignant neoplasms and many low-grade astrocytomas, on the completeness of the original resection. It has become clear that gross total removal of benign intramedullary ependymomas more consistently provides long-term tumor control or cure than subtotal resection and radiation therapy (1,5–7,28). Nevertheless,

these tumors are friable and often are quite adherent to the spinal cord, particularly at their polar regions, which may not allow for a microscopic total resection. Long-term follow-up with periodic clinical evaluation and gadolinium-enhanced MRI is mandatory because of the continued risk of tumor recurrence. Depending on the patient's age and critical circumstances, reoperation may be undertaken if tumor recurrence is clearly established on MRI. The evidence to support postoperative radiation following subtotal resection is difficult to interpret because it is largely based on studies with small patient populations, limited follow-up, and inadequate numbers of or no matched controls treated without radiation therapy (reviewed in ref. 2). Despite these limitations, the accumulated data in these series suggest that radiation may be beneficial following subtotal resection. We recommend adjuvant radiation for malignant ependymomas and the rare benign lesion that cannot be totally resected.

The optimum treatment strategy for astrocytomas is less clear. With the exception of high-grade gliomas, which all authors agree do not benefit from surgery and progress rapidly, low-grade intramedullary spinal cord astrocytomas have been difficult to evaluate because of their rare occurrence and biological variability. Age appears to be the most significant prognostic factor. Pediatric astrocytomas are associated with a particularly indolent behavior that is partly explained by their predominantly benign histology (90%) and the high percentage of juvenile pilocytic astrocytomas and gangliogliomas (8,29,30). The influence of extent of resection on outcome remains controversial. While some authors have found that gross total resection may influence outcome (4,6), other authors find no such relationship (3,8).

Despite numerous interrelated factors that may correlate with clinical behavior such as age of presentation, histology, and extent of resection, it is usually not possible to predict outcome for a given astrocytoma, although in adults astrocytomas usually pursue a progressive course. Parameters that predict which patients will benefit from a more aggressive removal have not been identified. We strive for a gross total removal if it can be achieved safely because the possibility of surgical cure exists in a small subgroup of patients (4,8). Those lesions with favorable histology may lend themselves to a more complete resection. If only a subtotal resection is achieved, radiation therapy may be given, although the data on its efficacy for low-grade tumors is not conclusive. Recurrence within the irradiated volume following radiation therapy occurs in approximately 50% of patients and there is little agreement about the dose-response relationship (3,8,29,31,32). We do not routinely administer radiation therapy following subtotal resection since it complicates the prospects for future surgery, may require doses above the accepted tolerance of the spinal cord to be efficacious, and has been associated with an increased incidence of spinal deformity and secondary malignancy (27,31–33). The patient is followed clinically and with serial MRIs. Depending on the clinical circumstance, repeat surgery may be offered at the time of clinical recurrence, which is often several years after radiographic recurrence. Radiation therapy may then be considered, depending on the time of recurrence and the degree of resection accomplished. Surgery plays only a diagnostic role in patients who harbor malignant intramedullary astrocytic neoplasms. Radical resection does not prolong survival and is associated with greater surgical morbidity (2–4). Radiation therapy is recommended in these patients but survival is poor, with an average survival of 6 months to 1 year (3,4,6,23,32).

References

1. McCormick PC, Torres R, Post KD, et al. Intramedullary ependymoma of the spinal cord. *J Neurosurg* 1990;72:523–533.

2. McCormick PC, Stein BM. Intramedullary tumors in adults. *Neurosurg Clin North Am* 1990;1:609–630.
3. Cooper PR. Outcome after operative treatment of intramedullary spinal cord tumors in adults: intermediate and long-term results in 51 patients. *Neurosurgery* 1989;25:855–859.
4. Epstein FJ, Farmer J-P, Freed D. Adult intramedullary astrocytomas of the spinal cord. *J Neurosurg* 1992;77:355–359.
5. Epstein FJ, Farmer J-P, Freed D. Adult intramedullary spinal cord ependymomas: the result of surgery in 38 patients. *J Neurosurg* 1993; 79:204–209.
6. Cristante L, Herrmann H-D. Surgical management of intramedullary spinal cord tumors: functional outcome and sources of morbidity. *Neurosurgery* 1994;35:69–76.
7. Hoshimaru M, Koyama T, Hashimmoto N, et al. Results of microsurgical treatment for intramedullary spinal cord ependymomas: analysis of 36 cases. *Neurosurgery* 1999;44:264–269.
8. Sandler HM, Papadopoulos SM, Thuntan AF, et al. Spinal cord astrocytoma: results of therapy. *Neurosurgery* 1992;30:490–493.
9. Neumann HPH, Eggert HR, Weigel K. Hemangioblastomas of the central nervous system: a 10-year study with special reference to Von Hippel-Lindau syndrome. *J Neurosurg* 1989;70:24–30.
10. Helseth A, Mørk SJ. Primary intraspinal neoplasms in Norway, 1955–1986. A population-based survey of 467 patients. *J Neurosurg* 1989;71:842–845.
11. Samii M, Klekamp J. Surgical results of 100 intramedullary tumors in relation to accompanying syringomyelia. *Neurosurgery* 1994;35:865–873.
12. Mørk SJ, Løken AC. Ependymoma. A follow-up study of 101 cases. *Cancer* 1977;40:907–915.
13. Russell DS, Rubenstein LJ. *Pathology of tumors of the nervous system.* Baltimore: Williams & Wilkins, 1989.
14. Sloof JL, Kernohan JW, McCarthy CS. *Primarly intramedullary tumors of the spinal cord and filum terminale.* Philadelphia: WB Saunders, 1964.
15. Lee M, Epstein FJ, Rezzai AR, et al. Nonneoplastic intramedullary spinal cord lesions mimicking tumors. *Neurosurgery* 1998;43:788–795.
16. Kepes JJ. Large focal tumor-like demyelinating lesions of the brain: intermediate entity between multiple sclerosis and acute disseminated encephalomyelitis? a study of 31 patients. *Ann Neurol* 1993;3:18–27.
17. McCormick PC, Stein BM. Miscellaneous intradural pathology. *Neurosurg Clin North Am* 1990;1:687–700.
18. Costigan DA, Winkelman MD. Intramedullary spinal cord metastases. A clinicopathological study of 13 cases. *J Neurosurg* 1985;62:227–233.
19. Deme S, Ang L-C, Skaf G, et al. Primary intramedullary primitive neuroectodermal tumor of the spinal cord: case report and review of the literature. *Neurosurgery* 1997;41:1417–1420.
20. Schwartz TH, Chang Y, Stein BM. Unusual intramedullary vascular lesions: report of two cases. *Neurosurgery* 1997;40:1295–1301.
21. Bourgouin PM, Lesage J, Fontaine S, et al. A pattern approach to the differential diagnosis of intramedullary spinal cord lesions on MR imaging. *AJR* 1998;170:1645–1649.
22. Cohen AR, Wisoff JH, Allen JC, et al. Malignant astrocytomas of the spinal cord. *J Neurosurg* 1989;70:50–54.
23. Kopelson G, Linggood RM. Intramedullary spinal cord astrocytoma versus glioblastoma. The prognostic importance of histologic grade. *Cancer* 1982;50:732–735.
24. Adams DC, Emerson RG, Heyer EJ. Intraoperative evoked potential monitoring with controlled neuromuscular blockade. *Anesth Anal* 1993;77:913–918.
25. Morota N, Deletis V, Constantini S, et al. The role of motor evoked potentials during surgery for intramedullary spinal cord tumors. *Neurosurgery* 1997;41:1327–1336.
26. Epstein FJ, Farmer J-P, Schneider SJ. Intraoperative ultrasonography: an important surgical adjunct for intramedullary tumors. *J Neurosurg* 1991;74:729–733.
27. Brotchi J, Dewitte O, Leviver M, et al. A survey of 65 tumors within the spinal cord: surgical results and the importance of preoperative magnetic resonance imaging. *Neurosurgery* 1991;29:651–657.
28. Fisher G, Mansuy L. Total removal of intramedullary ependymomas: follow-up study of 16 cases. *Surg Neurol* 1980;14:243–249.
29. Rossitch E, Zeidman S, Burger PC, et al. Clinical and pathological analysis of spinal and astrocytomas in children. *Neurosurgery* 1990;27:193–196.
30. Epstein FJ, Farmer J-P. Pediatric spinal cord tumor surgery. *Neurosurg Clin North Am* 1990;1:569–590.
31. Garcia DM. Primary spinal cord tumors treated with surgery and postoperative irradiation. *In J Radiat Oncol Biol Phys* 1985;11:1933–1939.
32. Linstadt DE, Wara WM, Leibel SA, et al. Postoperative radiotherapy of primary spinal cord tumors. *Int J Radiat Oncol Biol Phys* 1989;16:1397–1403.
33. O'Sullivan C, Jenkin D, Doherty MA, et al. Spinal cord tumors in children: long-term results of combined surgical and radiation treatment. *J Neurosurg* 1994;81:507–512.

174. Spinal Deformity: Definitions and Indications for Correction

**Michael J. Rauzzino,
Christopher I. Shaffrey,
Aruna Ganju, and Russell P. Nockels**

The term *spinal deformity* implies some deviation from the normal, three-dimensional anatomy of the spinal column. Spinal deformities may be characterized according to location, plane, age at presentation, and etiology (Table 1).

The simple presence of a spinal deformity, either clinically or radiographically, is not necessarily a mandate for correction. When a patient with a spinal deformity is approached, two simple questions should be addressed: (a) What is the deformity to be treated? and (b) Why do we need to treat it (1)?

To answer these questions, one must understand the normal and pathological curvatures that define spinal deformities. In addition, the surgeon must have a knowledge of the natural

Table 1. Characterization of Deformity

DEFORMITY→LOCATION→PLANE →		AGE →	ETIOLOGY
Cervical	Sagittal	Infantile	Congenital
Thoracic	Coronal	Juvenile	Idiopathic
Lumbar	Axial	Adolescent	Traumatic
Sacral	Multiplanar	Adult	Degenerative
Junctional			Iatrogenic
			Neoplastic
			Infectious
			Metabolic

history of the untreated deformity in addition to realistic expectations of what goals may be achieved with either conservative or surgical measures.

Spinal Deformity: Definitions

NORMAL ANATOMY. The human axial skeleton is unique in that it allows for bipedal (upright) ambulation without an extravagant expenditure of energy. In utero, the spinal column comprises primarily two curves, a thoracic kyphosis and a lumbosacral kyphosis. As infants acquire the ability to support the head and ambulate, secondary curves develop: the cervical lordosis and lumbar lordosis.

In the sagittal plane, the adult spine comprises four curves: two primary (thoracic and sacral) and two secondary (cervical and lumbar). Whereas the thoracic curve is somewhat rigid, because of its articulation with the sternum and rib cage, the cervical and lumbar curves are flexible. These curves are dynamic and maintain balance in the upright position. This same flexibility, however, also makes these curves more vulnerable to the destabilizing effects of pathological processes.

In the coronal plane, the spine is essentially straight; a deviation in the coronal plane of 10 degrees or more is defined as scoliosis. Scoliosis can occur by itself or in combination with the previously mentioned deformities, lordosis and kyphosis. The resulting conditions, kyphoscoliosis and lordoscoliosis, imply a lateral curvature of the spine associated with a sagittal plane imbalance.

The spine should be aligned or balanced in both the sagittal and coronal planes. In the coronal plane, the spinous processes of all the vertebrae should line up with a point bisecting the sacrum (midsacral line). In the sagittal plane, a line can be drawn from the craniovertebral junction, through the bodies of T1 and T12, to the sacral promontory (Fig. 1). This line should be posterior to the cervical and lumbar lordoses and anterior to the thoracic kyphosis. The terms *positive balance* and *negative balance* imply angular deviations of the spine that affect this line (sagittal vertical axis). Specifically, in positive balance, the sagittal vertical axis lies anterior to the sacral promontory. An example of positive sagittal balance is a patient with the so-called flat-back syndrome, who has a forward posture secondary to hypolordosis of the lumbar curvature. In negative balance, the vertical axis lies posterior to the sacral promontory. An example of negative balance is hypokyphosis of the thoracic spine, which is often seen concurrently in patients with a severe thoracic scoliosis. Other factors to consider in the maintenance of sagittal balance are the status of the hips and the quality of the cervical curve. All these factors interact to maintain or hinder the balance needed for upright ambulation (2).

Normal quantitative values for each of the spinal curves have been determined. Curve angles are approximated via the Cobb method, which measures the angle formed by the intersection of two lines that are perpendicular to the end plates of the vertebrae at the upper and lower ends of a curve. The cervical curve is defined as extending from C1 to C6, with an apex at C4. The normal cervical lordosis ranges from 25 to 50 degrees. Extending from T2 to T11 is the thoracic curvature, with an apex at T7. The thoracic kyphosis ranges from 20 to 45 degrees. Finally, the lumbar lordosis extends from L1 to S1, with an apex at L3-4. The lumbar lordosis averages 40 to 70 degrees, with approximately two thirds of this total lordosis occurring between L4 and S1. In patients with pathological curves, such as kyphoscoliosis, these normal values may not apply. In the assessment of the overall sagittal balance of these patients, a good rule of thumb is that they should have at least 30 degrees more of lumbar lordosis than of thoracic kyphosis (3).

CURVE ANALYSIS. When more than one pathological curve is present, the surgeon must decide whether both curves need to be corrected. Typically, one of the curves is a structural curve, and the other is a compensatory curve that arises in response to the structural curve. A structural curve is a fixed, inflexible, lateral curvature that corrects minimally on supine side-bending radiographs. Nonstructural or functional curves, in contrast, are more flexible and may correct or overcorrect on supine side-bending radiographs. The terms *primary* and *major* have been used to describe the structural curve. The terms *secondary* and *minor* have been used to describe the compensatory curve. It is possible for a scoliotic deformity to comprise two structural curves; this is known as a *double major scoliosis* (4). In nonstructural scoliotic deformities, the curves are flexible and correctable. Examples of these are postural variations that develop when pain is generated by other conditions, such as a herniated lumbar disc or appendicitis. Supratentorial causes of nonstructural scoliosis can also be found; in hysterical scoliosis, the spinal deformity is a physical manifestation of a conversion reaction.

True pathological curves are defined by the radiographic location of their apical and end vertebrae. The apical vertebra is the one that is maximally rotated and farthest from the vertical axis (4). The end vertebrae are the most cephalic and caudal vertebrae of a curve; their superior and inferior end plates, respectively, tilt maximally into the concavity of the curve. Modifiers such as *dextro* (right), *levo* (left), *concave*, and *convex* should be used routinely to indicate the shape, direction, and affected segment of the spine.

Spinal deformities are most commonly classified according

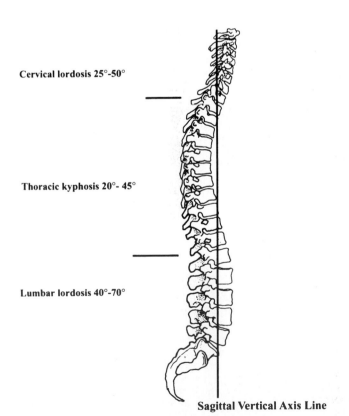

Cervical lordosis 25°-50°

Thoracic kyphosis 20°- 45°

Lumbar lordosis 40°-70°

Sagittal Vertical Axis Line

Fig. 1. Sagittal spinal profile.

Table 2. Classification of Structural Deformity

I. Scoliosis
  A. Congenital
    1. Failure of formation
    2. Failure of segmentation
    3. Mixed failure
  B. Idiopathic
  C. Neuromuscular
    1. Neuropathic
    2. Myopathic
  D. Iatrogenic
  E. Traumatic
  F. Malignancy
  G. Infectious
  H. Mesenchymal disorders
    1. Marfan syndrome
    2. Ehlers-Danlos syndrome
    3. Other
  I. Osteochondrodystrophies
    1. Mucopolysaccharidoses
    2. Epiphyseal dysplasia
    3. Other
  J. Metabolic disorders
    1. Rickets
    2. Osteogenesis imperfecta
    3. Other
  K. Nonstructural

II. Kyphosis
  A. Congenital
    1. Failure of formation
    2. Failure of segmentation
    3. Mixed failure
  B. Scheuermann disease
  C. Neuromuscular
  D. Iatrogenic
    1. Postsurgical
    2. Postirradiation
  E. Traumatic
  F. Malignancy
  G. Infectious/inflammatory
  H. Mesenchymal disorders
    1. Mucopolysaccharidoses
    2. Other
  I. Osteochondrodystrophies
  J. Metabolic disorders
    1. Osteoporosis
    2. Osteomalacia
    3. Osteogenesis imperfecta
  K. Nonstructural

III. Lordosis
  A. Congenital
  B. Neuromuscular
  C. Postsurgical
  D. Nonstructural

to their primary plane (scoliosis, kyphosis, and lordosis) and their cause. For example, a patient may have a scoliosis that is described as congenital, idiopathic, degenerative, neuromuscular (neuropathic and myopathic), traumatic, iatrogenic, and hysterical (Table 2).

Indications for Correction

Indications for correction of deformities include the following: (a) reduction of pain, (b) prevention/reduction of neurological deficits, (c) prevention of inexorable progression of deformity,

(d) correction of cardiac/pulmonary compromise, (e) cosmesis, and (f) correction of structural disabilities.

PAIN. The reduction of pain is a common indication for the correction of a deformity, particularly in adults with scoliosis (5–10). It is important to determine that the pain is actually being caused by the deformity in question, given that most people without any deformity experience low-back pain and radicular pain during their lifetime (11). The pain associated with deformity may arise from several sources. Radicular pain resulting from nerve root compression may be caused by foraminal collapse or nerve root traction secondary to vertebral rotation or displacement (12). Radicular pain may also develop in patients with spinal stenosis and a neurogenic claudication syndrome. Pain may be caused by abnormal motion and disc degeneration. Pseudoarthrosis from failed prior attempts at fusion may contribute to pain. Provocative discography may be helpful in identifying which discs are symptomatic and should be included in a potential fusion (9). Facet blocks and selective nerve root blocks are also useful in localizing generators of pain. Nonradicular, nonmechanical pain is often associated with deformity and presents the greatest challenge to the surgeon. Proposed mechanisms for generalized pain include muscular fatigue resulting from abnormal tension on muscles and joints (5).

Certain deformities produce characteristic patterns of pain, depending on their cause and location. Pain is typically absent as a presenting symptom in adolescent idiopathic scoliosis, whereas in adult scoliosis, pain is the most common presenting symptom (13). Pain is rare in thoracic curves and more common in lumbar or thoracolumbar curves. The pain is often located on the convexity of the curve and is an aching muscular pain that may be diffuse and worsen as the day goes on. Typically, the pain is relieved by lying flat. Later, as facet degeneration occurs, the pain may move to the concavity of the curve, and less upright activity is required to exacerbate the pain (14).

A specific example in which pain is frequently an indication for corrective surgery is the sagittal plane deformity known as *flat-back syndrome* (15–19). Flat-back deformities are caused by loss of the physiological lumbar lordosis and may be seen after posterior fusion for scoliosis, particularly with distraction Harrington instrumentation. Other causes include untreated scoliosis, ankylosing spondylitis, and kyphosis that develops following a thoracolumbar fracture. These patients present with back and leg pain. They typically adopt a forward posture and are unable to stand erect without hip and knee flexion. The loss of normal sagittal alignment results in a decreased lever arm for the paraspinal muscles, which leads to increased muscle work and fatigue. Additionally, the thighs and buttocks are under constant strain to maintain a corrective posture. These imbalances produce a dull aching pain that worsens during upright activity (15).

Surgical treatment for this condition includes osteotomies centered over the apex of the scoliosis and over the kyphotic segments to recreate lordosis (20). Typically, L3-4 is considered an ideal site for posterior osteotomy because it is at the usual physiological apex of the lordosis, below the rib cage, and well above the vascular bifurcations. Approximately 1 degree of sagittal correction is gained for each millimeter of bone resected. Typically, 10 to 15 mm of bone can be removed at each osteotomy level without the need for an anterior release if the disc height is at least 5 mm and no bridging osteophytes are present.

It cannot be overemphasized that before any surgical intervention is undertaken, the initial treatment of painful deformity should involve a series of conservative measures, including physical therapy and conditioning, weight loss, nonsteroidal analgesics, epidural steroids, facet or nerve root blocks, and occasionally bracing. It is always important in the surgical decision process to exclude other sources of pain that are unlikely to be relieved by surgery. Arachnoiditis, syrinx, and residual spinal cord injury are examples.

The results of surgery for pain in adults with scoliosis are variable. Kostuik et al. (18) reported that 70% of 350 patients with adult scoliosis experienced at least some relief from pain, but few prospective studies have been reported in which pain relief was objectively measured in surgical cases of adult scoliosis. Booth (15) reported relief from pain in an impressive 78% of 28 adult patients whose flat-back deformities were treated with osteotomies, but again, few large series have been reported in which relief from pain was quantifiably measured (21).

NEUROLOGICAL INJURY. Neurological dysfunction in cases of deformity is caused by compression of or traction on the spinal cord, nerve roots, or both. Progressive neurological dysfunction does not respond to conservative therapy and is an absolute indication for reduction of the deformity and decompression of the affected neural elements, followed by stabilization and fusion when indicated. The time course and severity of the neurological deficits dictate the urgency of the surgery.

The location and plane of the deformity partially determine the risk for neurological injury. Deformities in the coronal plane (i.e., adolescent idiopathic scoliosis) are less commonly associated with major neurological deficits than are deformities in the sagittal plane (i.e., congenital kyphosis or lordosis). The thoracic spinal cord is most susceptible to injury because of its vascular anatomy (22). A worst-case scenario is seen in patients with untreated type I congenital thoracic kyphosis (23). Such kyphosis is associated with an anterior failure of formation and produces a sharp, angulated deformity that if untreated is often associated with paraplegia. In North America, thoracic congenital kyphosis is the leading cause of paraplegia in patients with spinal deformity (24). Paralysis can develop in these patients after minor trauma, and neurological injury commonly occurs during the adolescent growth spurt. Neurological injury may also be iatrogenic or exacerbated by incorrect treatment, such as the use of traction to reduce the kyphotic deformity without a prior anterior release.

Nerve root injury can be seen in patients with high-grade lumbar spondylolisthesis, in which radicular symptoms and bowel and bladder dysfunction may be caused by traction on the lumbosacral nerves (25).

Lastly, if the deformity arises as the result of neural injury (i.e., neuromuscular scoliosis), neurological recovery is not associated with correction of the deformity (26).

PREVENTION OF PROGRESSION OF DEFORMITY. A severe deformity is easier to prevent than treat. Therefore, it is important to identify which deformities are likely to progress and manage them while they are smaller and easier to treat. In certain deformities, such as congenital and idiopathic scoliosis, the natural histories of both treated and untreated patients have been well established (27,28). The risk for progression of deformity depends on many factors, including the following: (a) cause of the deformity; (b) magnitude of the presenting deformity; (c) potential for further growth (skeletal maturity of the patient); (d) symmetry of growth potential; (e) location of the deformity (cervical, thoracic, lumbar, junctional); (f) number of vertebral segments involved; (g) plane of deformity; and (h) bone quality.

A brief discussion of congenital scoliosis will serve to illustrate some important points regarding the progression of deformity.

Congenital scoliosis is a lateral curvature of the spine produced by one or more congenital vertebral anomalies that result in an imbalance of longitudinal growth. Typically, the scoliosis is caused by defects in segmentation or formation, or a combination of the two (Fig. 2).

Defects of segmentation can be unilateral or bilateral. If the segmentation error is bilateral, a *block vertebra* is the result. This defect shortens the spine but is unlikely to cause deformity because the growth, although abnormal, is balanced. In contradistinction, a unilateral defect in segmentation causing a *unilateral unsegmented bar* is highly likely to progress to a significant deformity. No growth potential exists on the concave side of the curve, and with continued growth on the convex side of the curve, severe deformity invariably results. An unsegmented bar opposite a hemivertebra has the poorest prognosis in regard to rapid progression and should be surgically treated at an early stage to prevent severe deformity. In the series of McMaster and Ohtsuka (29), this specific deformity progressed at a rate of at least 6 degrees per year, and the deformities of all their patients exceeded 50 degrees by 4 years of age.

Defects in formation typically produce *hemivertebrae.* The patterns of hemivertebrae can range from mild wedging to complete absence of one side of the vertebra. Four types of hemivertebrae are known: *fully segmented,* with growth plates inferiorly and superiorly; *semisegmented,* with only one end plate open; *unsegmented,* with fusions or slit end plates; and *incarcerated,* in which a small, ovoid hemivertebra is tucked into the side of the spine. The prognosis varies according to the type, location, and number of hemivertebrae. Generally, 25% of hemivertebrae progress rapidly, 25% do not progress, and 50% progress slowly (30). The presence of open vertebral growth plates indicates a tendency to progress, so that a fully segmented hemivertebra, with a functional plate superiorly and inferiorly, is most likely to progress and is usually managed surgically. Unsegmented hemivertebrae, which do not have asymmetrical growth plates and therefore do not tend to progress, are typically managed nonsurgically. Thus, the potential for unbalanced growth can be used to guide surgical treatment (Table 3).

In cases of congenital scoliosis, the risk for the development of deformities of large magnitude is great. Not only is growth asymmetrical; potential growth is maximal. The growth of children with congenital kyphosis and congenital lordosis is similarly dramatically unbalanced, and they should be treated at presentation (23,31–33) (Fig. 3).

In patients with idiopathic scoliosis, the magnitude of the curve at presentation and the amount of remaining growth potential are the key determinants of curve progression. For example, among patients with moderate scoliosis (between 20 and 29 degrees), a 10-year-old child has a 60% chance of progression, whereas a 16-year-old with a curve of the same magnitude at presentation has only a 10% chance of progression. Similarly, if the Risser grade is used as a measure of skeletal maturity, a patient with a Risser grade of 0 to 1 (skeletally immature) has a 68% chance of progression, whereas a patient with a Risser grade of 2 to 4 (skeletally mature) has only a 23% chance of progression in (34,35).

Although skeletal growth is important in curve progression, it is not necessary. In patients with idiopathic scoliosis, a common misconception is that all curve progression stops with skeletal maturity and cessation of growth (27,36). In studies by Weinstein and colleagues (28,37), although most thoracic curves of less than 40 degrees were unlikely to progress during adulthood, larger curves (>50 degrees) could progress insidiously at a rate of 1 to 2 degrees a year. This means that in an adolescent with a curve of 55 degrees at cessation of skeletal growth who was not treated, a 100-degree curve could develop by age 50. Lumbar curves, which lack the additional stability of the rib cage, were even less stable, and similar progression could be

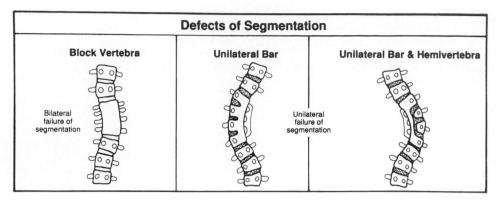

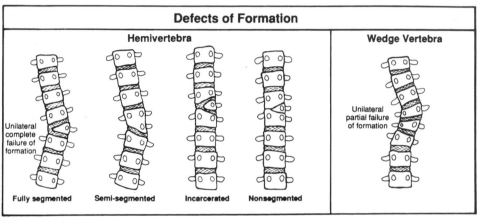

Fig. 2. Congenital vertebral anomalies. (Reprinted from Pehrsson K, Bake B, Larsson S, et al. Lung function in adult idiopathic scoliosis: a 20-year follow-up. *Thorax* 46:474–478, 1991, with permission.)

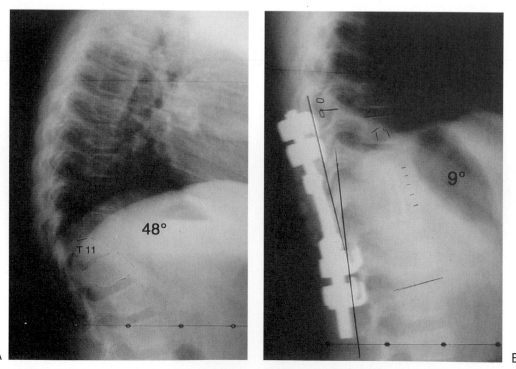

Fig. 3. Congenital kyphosis: **A:** Child with T11 hemivertebra causing 48-degree thoracic kyphosis. **B:** Postoperative radiograph of same patient following anterior resection of hemivertebra and stabilization.

Table 3. Management of Congenital Anomalies Producing Scoliosis

Location	Vertebra		Hemivertebrae		Unilateral unsegmented bar	Unilateral unsegmented bar and contralateral hemivertebrae
	Block	Wedge	Single	Double		
Upper thoracic	N	N	?	Y	Y	Y
Lower thoracic	N	?	?	Y	Y	Y
Thoracolumbar	N	N	?	Y	Y	Y
Lumbar	N	N	?	*	Y	*

N, No surgical treatment required; ?, may require spinal fusion; Y, spinal fusion indicated; *, too few patients studied.
Modified from Ascani E, Bartolozzi P, Logroscino CA, et al. Natural history of untreated idiopathic scoliosis after skeletal maturity. *Spine* 11:784–789, 1986.

documented for smaller curves (>30 degrees) that were beginning. In thoracic curves, apical vertebral rotation greater than 30% or a rib vertebral angle difference greater than 30 degrees was also associated with an increased risk for curve progression. In thoracolumbar or lumbar curves, apical vertebral rotation greater than 30% and the presence of translatory shifts were again associated with an increased risk for curve progression. Surgery is indicated for these curves to prevent further progression.

Predictable progression of deformity can be seen in patients with dysplastic spondylolisthesis with or without skeletal growth. Dysplastic spondylolisthesis and a slippage greater than 30% or a measured slip angle greater than 55 degrees have been associated with progression of deformity and neurological symptoms; surgical fusion is recommended in patients with these abnormalities (Fig. 4).

Spinal deformity with the possibility of progression may also occur after trauma. Patients sustaining thoracolumbar burst fractures often have some degree of resultant kyphotic deformity at the thoracolumbar junction. An early kyphosis of greater than 30 degrees is often associated with pain and progression and can be managed surgically (38–40).

CARDIOPULMONARY COMPROMISE. Patients with severe spinal deformities may present with pulmonary compromise, which in turn can lead to cardiac failure and death (41–46). Patients with untreated scoliosis and curves of large magnitude have been shown to have a higher mortality rate than controls, with death often related to pulmonary embarrassment. Surgery may be proposed to prevent or correct pulmonary dysfunction. Sagittal plane deformities, such as congenital lordosis, are typically associated with the greatest impairment of pulmonary function, and surgery is indicated for patients who present with these abnormalities (33,47). When patients with other deformities are being evaluated, it is crucial to recognize that the reduction in pulmonary vital capacity is directly related to the magnitude of the deformity. In adult patients with moderate curves of thoracic scoliosis (<35 degrees), the resting pulmonary function is normal, whereas studies have shown that larger curves (scoliosis >40 degrees, kyphosis >50 degrees) are associated with a reduction in vital capacity (48). Physiological changes include a high energy cost of breathing secondary to reduced pulmonary compliance, ventilation/perfusion mismatching, rapid shallow breathing with resultant hypoxia and respiratory acidosis secondary to hypercapnea, pulmonary arterial hypertension, and, in the final stages, right ventricular failure (cor pulmonale) and death.

Despite these changes, most patients are able to tolerate such dysfunction clinically until the curves have reached a large magnitude (>100 degrees). The pulmonary function and survival of patients with severe scoliosis from both idiopathic and neuro-

muscular causes are improved after surgery. It is important to manage these patients surgically while they are good operative candidates. In a series of 35 adult patients with deformity-related respiratory insufficiency (average scoliosis, 136 degrees; average kyphosis, 132 degrees; average lordosis, 15 degrees) treated at an experienced center, the mortality rate was 21% within the first postoperative year (49). Better outcomes after surgery are seen in younger patients, nonsmokers, patients who have a vital capacity of at least 30% before surgery, and patients with significant curve correction at surgery (≥30% correction of scoliosis, ≥40% correction of kyphosis).

Children with neuromuscular conditions resulting in deformity pose special problems in terms of cardiac and pulmonary function. They often present with larger, stiffer curves and are more likely to have significant pulmonary dysfunction than are patients with idiopathic scoliosis. Diseases such as Duchenne dystrophy and Friedreich ataxia are associated with myopathy (including cardiac myopathy) that is unrelated to the actual deformity. Because patients with spinal deformity often rely heavily on accessory muscles to assist ventilation, their pulmonary function is more severely impaired. Surgery may be considered for patients with smaller curves in this population (50).

COSMESIS. Cosmetic indications for the surgical management of deformity are the most difficult to clarify. Cosmetic issues affect the patient's self-image, self-confidence, and socialization skills (51). Although cosmesis is a subjective issue, a number of authors have proposed various scales for judging a patient's presurgical and postsurgical appearance (52,53). Still, objective data regarding cosmetic outcomes in the literature are scarce (54).

Clinical experience has demonstrated that scoliosis of up to 20 degrees is typically unnoticed by the patient, and obese patients may have even larger occult curves. Often, it is not the spinal deformity that causes the most distress to the patient but rather the compensatory changes of the body (e.g., rib hump and waist asymmetry). Curve magnitude does not necessarily correlate with poor cosmesis; for example, a double major scoliosis may comprise two large-magnitude but balanced curves that in combination cause only minor cosmetic distress for the patient.

Cosmetic issues are especially important in the management of adolescent idiopathic scoliosis. Patients present most commonly for cosmetic reasons; pain and neurologic compromise are rare in this population. The majority of these patients are adolescent girls, for whom issues of cosmesis are paramount. Whereas the treating surgeon may gauge success in terms of degrees of curve correction, the patients often are most pleased by the loss or reduction of the noticeable rib hump. Thoracoplasty has been shown to result in a greater degree of hump reduction than curve correction alone and should be consid-

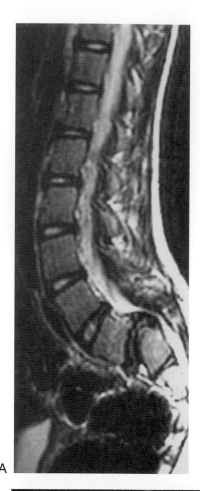

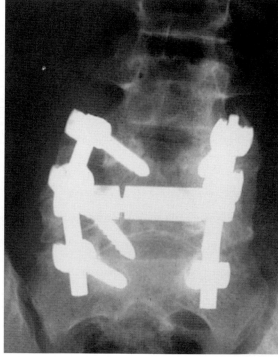

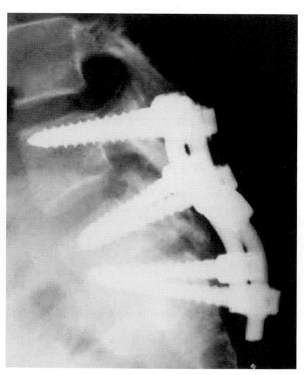

Fig. 4. L5-S1 dysplastic spondylolisthesis. **A:** Preoperative sagittal magnetic resonance image of an adolescent with L5-S1 dysplastic spondylolisthesis. **B:** Postoperative antero-posterior radiograph of same patient after L4-S1 fusion. **C:** Postoperative lateral radiograph.

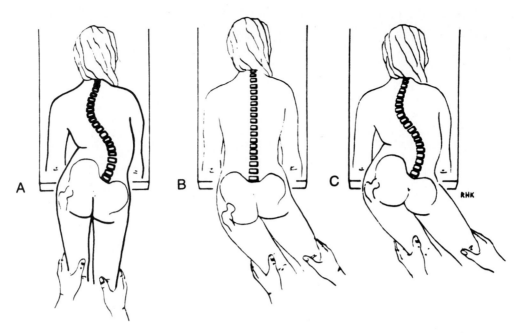

Fig. 5. Assessment of pelvic obliquity. **A:** Positioning of patient on examination table. **B:** Correction of obliquity with hip manipulation. **C:** Failure of hip manipulation to correct pelvic obliquity.

ered in the management of these patients (55,56). In adult patients with scoliosis, cosmetic issues are the second most common reason for presentation, after pain. Patients with Scheuermann kyphosis (round-back deformity) also typically seek surgery for correction of their deformity, and kyphosis of greater than 75 degrees is considered a surgical indication in these patients (57).

FUNCTIONAL DISABILITY. A functional disability is an alteration in daily activities necessitated by a deformity. Surgery may be considered in such cases to improve the functional quality of life (58). A good example is a wheelchair-bound patient with severe neuromuscular scoliosis. The spinal deformity may lead to pelvic obliquity, in which the pelvis fails to remain horizontal to the sitting surface and perpendicular to the spine in the frontal plane. With an unstable base for the trunk, patients may have to support themselves constantly with their arms to maintain an upright posture in the wheelchair, so that they are functionally reduced from a paraplegic level to a quadriplegic level. Additionally, the uneven sitting surface may lead to pain or to pressure sores in an area that is insensate. Pelvic obliquity may be caused by muscle contractures above (spinopelvic or spinofemoral) or below (pelvofemoral) the pelvis. In the case of a fixed spinopelvic obliquity, an anterior spinal fusion to shorten the spine and release the pelvis is indicated. In the case of a pelvofemoral obliquity, a smaller procedure to release the pelvofemoral muscles is indicated. To determine the cause of a pelvic obliquity, the patient is placed prone on the examining table with the hips flexed over the end of the table (Fig. 5A). If the pelvic obliquity is corrected with either abduction or adduction of the hips (Fig. 5B), then a simple release of the contracted pelvofemoral muscles may be all that is required. If the pelvic obliquity is not decreased with these maneuvers (Fig. 5C), then a true fixed spinopelvic obliquity is present, and an anterior spinal fusion to shorten the spine and release the pelvis is indicated (50).

Conclusions

The indications for the surgical management of spinal deformities continue to evolve. The most common indications for surgery are still to relieve pain and prevent the progression of deformity. Surgical procedures to relieve neurological deficit or cardiopulmonary compromise are less common because spinal deformities are being managed while they are still of relatively small magnitude. The issue of cosmesis as a sole indication for surgery to correct spinal deformity is still unresolved.

References

1. Dickson RA. Spinal deformity—adolescent idiopathic scoliosis. *Spine* 24:2601–2606, 1999.
2. Terminology Committee, Scoliosis Research Society. A glossary of scoliosis terms. *Spine* 1:57–58, 1976.
3. Bernhardt M, Bridwell K. Segmental analysis of the sagittal plane alignment of the normal thoracic and lumbar spines and the thoracolumbar junction. *Spine* 14:717–723, 1989.
4. Winter RB. Classification and terminology. In: Lonstein JE, Winter RB, Bradford DS, et al., eds. *Moe's textbook of scoliosis and other spinal deformities,* 3rd ed. Philadelphia: WB Saunders, 1995:39–43.
5. Bradford DS, Tay BK, Hu SS. Adult scoliosis: surgical indications, operative management, complications, and outcomes. *Spine* 24: 2617–2629, 1999.
6. Grubb SA, Lipscomb HJ. Diagnostic findings in painful adult scoliosis. *Spine* 17:518–527, 1992.
7. Grubb SA, Lipscomb HJ, Suh PB. Results of surgical treatment of painful adult scoliosis. *Spine* 19:1619–1627, 1994.
8. Kostuik JP, Bentivoglio J. The incidence of low back pain in adult scoliosis. *Spine* 6:268–273, 1981.
9. Kostuik JP. Decision making in adult scoliosis. *Spine* 4:521–525, 1979.

10. Pritchett JW, Bortel DT. Degenerative symptomatic lumbar scoliosis. *Spine* 18:700–703, 1993.
11. Jackson RP, Simmons EH, Stripinis D. Incidence and severity of back pain in adult idiopathic scoliosis. *Spine* 7:749–756, 1983.
12. Simmons EH, Jackson RP. The management of nerve root entrapment syndromes associated with the collapsing scoliosis of idiopathic lumbar and thoracolumbar curves. *Spine* 4:533–541, 1979.
13. Bridwell K. Surgical treatment of idiopathic adolescent scoliosis. *Spine* 24:2607–2616, 1999.
14. Lonstein JE. Adult scoliosis. In: Bradford DS, Lonstein JE, Moe JH, et al., eds. *Moe's textbook of scoliosis and other spinal deformities.* Philadelphia: WB Saunders, 1987:47–88.
15. Booth KC, Bridwell KH, Lenke LG, et al. Complications and predictive factors for the successful treatment of flat back deformity (fixed sagittal imbalance). *Spine* 24:1712–1720, 1999.
16. Cochran T, Irstam L, Nachemson A. Long-term anatomic and functional changes in patients with adolescent idiopathic scoliosis treated by Harrington rod fusion. *Spine* 8:576–584, 1983.
17. Farcy JP, Schwab FJ. Management of flat back and related kyphotic deformity syndromes. *Spine* 22:2452–2457, 1997.
18. Kostuik JP, Maurais GR, Richardson WJ, et al. Combined single stage anterior and posterior osteotomy for correction of iatrogenic lumbar kyphosis. *Spine* 13:257–266, 1988.
19. Lagrone MO, Bradford DS, Moe JH, et al. Treatment of symptomatic flat back after spinal fusion. *J Bone Joint Surg Am* 70:569–580, 1988.
20. Bridwell K. Osteotomies for fixed deformities in the thoracic and lumbar spine. In: Bridwell K, DeWald RL, eds. *The textbook of spinal surgery,* 2nd ed. Philadelphia: Lippincott–Raven Publishers, 1997: 821–835.
21. Simmons ED Jr, Kowalski JM, Simmons EH. The results of surgical treatment for adult scoliosis. *Spine* 18:718–724, 1993.
22. Lonstein JE, Winter RB, Moe JH, et al. Neurologic deficits secondary to spinal deformity: a review of the literature and report of 43 cases. *Spine* 5:331–355, 1980.
23. Winter RB, Moe JH, Wang JF. Congenital kyphosis: its natural history and treatment as observed in a population of 130 patients. *J Bone Joint Surg Am* 55:223–256, 1973.
24. Winter RB, Moe JH, Lonstein JE. The surgical treatment of congenital kyphosis. A review of 94 patients age 5 years or older with two years or more of follow-up in 77 patients. *Spine* 10:224–231, 1985.
25. Lonstein JE. Spondylolisthesis in children: cause, natural history and management. *Spine* 24:2640–2648, 1999.
26. McCarthy RE. Management of neuromuscular scoliosis. *Orthop Clin North Am* 30:435–449, 1999.
27. Collis DK, Ponseti IV. Long-term follow-up of patients with idiopathic scoliosis not treated surgically. *J Bone Joint Surg Am* 51: 425–445, 1969.
28. Weinstein SL, Ponseti IV. Curve progression in idiopathic scoliosis. Long-term follow-up. *J Bone Joint Surg Am* 65:447–456, 1983.
29. McMaster MJ, Ohtsuka K. The natural history of congenital scoliosis. A study of two hundred and fifty-one patients. *J Bone Joint Surg Am* 64:1128–1147, 1982.
30. McMaster MJ. Congenital scoliosis. In: Weinstein SL, ed. *The pediatric spine: principles and practice.* New York: Raven Press, 1994: 227–224.
31. Bradford DS, Blatt JM, Rasp FL. Surgical management of severe thoracic lordosis. A new technique to restore normal kyphosis. *Spine* 8:420–428, 1983.
32. Montgomery SP, Hall JE. Congenital kyphosis. *Spine* 7:360–364, 1982.
33. Winter RB, Moe JH, Bradford DS. Congenital chronic lordosis. *J Bone Joint Surg Am* 60:806–810, 1978.
34. Lonstein JE, Carlson JM. The prediction of curve progression in un-

treated idiopathic scoliosis during growth. *J Bone Joint Surg Am* 66: 1061–1071, 1984.
35. Weinstein S. Idiopathic scoliosis: natural history. *Spine* 11:780–786, 1986.
36. Ascani E, Bartolozzi P, Logroscino CA, et al. Natural history of untreated idiopathic scoliosis after skeletal maturity. *Spine* 11:784–789, 1986.
37. Weinstein SL, Zavala DC, Ponseti IV. Idiopathic scoliosis: long-term follow-up and prognosis in untreated patients. *J Bone Joint Surg Am* 63:702–712, 1981.
38. Lowe TG. Revision surgery for kyphotic deformity. In: Margulies JY, Aebi M, Farcy JPC, eds. *Revision spine surgery.* St. Louis: Mosby, 1999:480–507.
39. Malcolm BW, Bradford DS, Winter RB, et al. Post-traumatic kyphosis. A review of forty-eight surgically treated patients. *J Bone Joint Surg Am* 63:891–899, 1981.
40. Shaffrey CI, Shaffrey ME, Whitehill R, et al. Surgical treatment of thoracolumbar fractures. *Neurosurg Clin N Am* 8:519–540, 1997.
41. Aaro S, Ohlund C. Scoliosis and pulmonary function. *Spine* 9: 220–222, 1984.
42. Branthwaite MA. Cardiorespiratory consequences of unfused idiopathic scoliosis. *Br J Dis Chest* 80:360–369, 1996.
43. Kinnear WJ, Kinnear GC, Watson L, et al. Pulmonary function after spinal surgery for idiopathic scoliosis. *Spine* 17:708–713, 1992.
44. Lenke LG, Bridwell KH, Blanke K, et al. Analysis of pulmonary function and chest cage dimension changes after thoracoplasty in idiopathic scoliosis. *Spine* 20:1343–1350, 1995.
45. Nilsonne U, Lundgren KD. Long-term prognosis in idiopathic scoliosis. *Acta Orthop Scand* 39:456–465, 1968.
46. Pehrsson K, Larsson S, Oden A, et al. Long-term follow-up of patients with untreated scoliosis. A study of mortality, causes of death, and symptoms. *Spine* 17:1091–1096, 1992.
47. Ferris G, Servera-Pieras E, Vergara P, et al. Kyphoscoliosis ventilatory insufficiency: noninvasive management outcomes. *Am J Phys Med Rehabil* 79:24–29, 2000.
48. Pehrsson K, Bake B, Larsson S, et al. Lung function in adult idiopathic scoliosis: a 20-year follow-up. *Thorax* 46:474–478, 1991.
49. Rizzi PE, Winter RB, Lonstein JE, et al. Adult spinal deformity and respiratory failure. Surgical results in 35 patients. *Spine* 22: 2517–2530, 1997.
50. Shook J, Lubicky JP. Paralytic scoliosis. In: Bridwell K, DeWald RL, eds. *The textbook of spinal surgery,* 2nd ed. Philadelphia: Lippincott–Raven Publishers, 1997:839–880.
51. Nachemson AL. A long-term follow-up study of non-treated scoliosis. *Acta Orthop Scand* 39:466–476, 1968.
52. Iwahara T, Imai M, Atsuta Y. Quantification of cosmesis for patients affected by adolescent idiopathic scoliosis. *Eur Spine J* 17:12–25, 1998.
53. Theologis TN, Jefferson RJ, Simpson AH, et al. Quantifying the cosmetic defect of adolescent idiopathic scoliosis. *Spine* 18:909–912, 1993.
54. Edgar MA, Mehta MH. Long-term follow-up of fused and unfused idiopathic scoliosis. *J Bone Joint Surg Br* 70:712–716, 1988.
55. Geissele AE, Ogilvie JW, Cohen M, et al. Thoracoplasty for the treatment of rib prominence in thoracic scoliosis. *Spine* 19:1636–1642, 1994.
56. Harvey CJ Jr, Betz RR, Clements DH, et al. Are there indications for partial rib resection in patients with adolescent idiopathic scoliosis treated with Cotrel-Dubousset instrumentation? *Spine* 18: 1593–1598, 1993.
57. Wegner DR, Frick SL. Scheuermann kyphosis. *Spine* 24:2631–2639, 1999.
58. Lonstein JE, Akbarnia BA. Operative treatment of spinal deformities in patients with cerebral palsy or mental retardation: an analysis of one hundred and seven cases. *J Bone Joint Surg Am* 65:43–55, 1983.

175. Biomechanical Principles of Deformity Correction

Robert F. Heary and Christopher M. Bono

Spinal deformity can develop as a result of various etiologies, each with distinct natural histories. Curvatures can be described by their anatomical region and plane of imbalance. They are also distinguished by their propensity to progress as well as their intrinsic flexibility. Treatment must include consideration of these characteristics. Among other factors, the central component of corrective management must be a thoughtful strategy using sound biomechanical principles in regard to the overall benefit to the individual patient.

Curve correction can be operative or nonoperative. Nonoperative management includes bracing and casting. In appropriate cases, it can be planned to either correct or arrest curve progression. Operative approaches can be anterior, posterior, or combined anteroposterior (AP) and consists of soft tissue and/or bony procedures. Stabilization and fusion is paramount for effective surgical treatment of spinal deformity. Various fusion methods as well as instrumentation options are currently available, each with biomechanical advantages and limitations.

A functional understanding of vertebral biomechanics is a requisite for correction of spinal deformities. With knowledge of the forces contributing to an abnormal curvature, the practitioner can better determine the necessary mechanical elements of alleviating it. This chapter discusses general principles in reference to specific pathological conditions. In learning these principles, the spinal surgeon can more clearly formulate correction of any spinal deformity.

Etiology and Epidemiology

Spinal deformity occurs in varied age groups from numerous etiologies. Congenital deformity can be caused by a defect in vertebral formation, segmentation, or both. Partially formed or unfused segments of the vertebrae cause asymmetric spinal growth. Although present at birth, they may not become clinically evident until accelerated growth spurts exaggerate the deformity. Congenital scoliosis, though the most prevalent, carries the best prognosis. It is strongly progressive in only half of cases and has the least incidence of associated paralysis (1). Congenital kyphosis, the second most common, has a greater tendency to progress than congenital scoliosis. Interestingly, it is currently the most common cause of deformity-induced paraplegia in North America (1). Congenital lordosis is strongly progressive in nearly all cases and reliably creates life-threatening respiratory compromise if untreated.

Spinal deformity can be idiopathic, as in adolescent scoliosis or Scheuermann's disease. Despite a myriad of hypotheses, the etiologies of these conditions are still unclear and are most probably multifactorial. Despite the cause, resultant structural abnormalities of the vertebrae, discs and ligaments contribute to the abnormal curvature. Adolescent idiopathic scoliosis (AIS) occurs in approximately 0.5% of the population, with a 2 to 1 female preponderance (2). As a result of the initial treatment of scoliosis with purely distractive posterior constructs, surgeons have created spinal deformity. A loss of the normal thoracolumbar sagittal contour may occur with distractive constructs. This

may result in the "flat-back" syndrome, which is a frequent cause of low back pain (3). Scheuermann's disease is a primarily sagittal deformity with a male preponderance. The disease affects between 0.4% and 8.3% of the population and typically presents early in the second decade. Wedging of both the disc and vertebral body account for kyphosis, although kyphoscoliosis is present in some cases.

Paralysis, either from developmental or traumatic nerve dysfunction, can also lead to spinal deformity. Persistent gravitational forces on a muscularly unsupported vertebral column cause multiplanar curve progression. Neoplastic and infectious erosion can also imbalance the architecture of the vertebral column and lead to a variety of deformity types. Traumatic deformities are the result of high-energy forces displacing and damaging the vertebral elements. Acutely, traumatic deformities are readily correctable, whereas chronically they can develop following nonoperative or inadequate surgical stabilization (4).

Prevention

Deformity, dependent on etiology, is often not preventable. Congenital deformities are best treated by early diagnosis and intervention. The morbidity and mortality associated with pulmonary compromise is minimized by early correction. Early diagnosis of idiopathic curves is also efficacious. School screening with scoliometer parameter protocols can produce acceptable referral rates (5). This process may facilitate recognition of curves while still being amenable to bracing. Typically, bracing is utilized for scoliotic curves that measure greater than 25 degrees in adolescents. Fractures and medically managed bone infections must be monitored radiographically for curve progression. Employing sound biomechanical principles is the best way to prevent iatrogenic deformities after spinal surgery.

Structural Deforming Forces

The vertebral column consists of three components: bone, ligament, and intervertebral disc. Bone, a relatively inelastic component, comprises the vertebrae. Mechanically, ligaments are more elastic with relative tensioning depending on posture. The intervertebral discs are the most elastic component and are the site of movement between consecutive segments. Together, they form a flexible encasement of the spinal cord and roots that allows multiplanar segmental motion and supports the body.

ANATOMY. Vertebrae consist of a large cylinder-shaped body. At its posterolateral aspect, pedicles originate and span the spinal canal. At the pedicle's junction with the broader laminae, transverse processes reach laterally for paraspinal muscle attachment in addition to articulations with the ribs in the thoracic region. Laminae converge to form the posterior neural arch.

Extending dorsally from the union of bilateral laminae, a midline spinous process serves as a lever arm for paraspinal muscle insertion.

The anterior longitudinal ligament (ALL) spans the anterior surfaces of each vertebral body. It is intimately associated with the anterior aspect of the intervertebral disc at each level. The posterior longitudinal ligament (PLL) spans the posterior surface of the bodies. It is the anterior limit of the spinal canal and it may be a site of calcification in degenerative specimens. The ligamentum flavum connects adjacent laminae, completing the posterior limit of the canal. The interspinous ligaments tether consecutive spinous processes and are frequently referred to as the posterior ligamentous complex.

Each vertebra has six articulating joint surfaces. Adjacent inferior and superior end plates interact via the intervertebral disc. The annulus fibrosis is a thick circumferential fibrous band that serves to contain the viscous gel-like nucleus pulposus. Sharpey's fibers strongly bind the annulus to the vertebral bone, creating a volume-limited environment during compression of the nucleus. Bilateral superior and inferior articulating facets project from the pedicle–lamina junctions. The inferior facet of the superior vertebrae and the superior facet of the inferior vertebrae form a diarthrodial articulation stabilized by a strong fibrous joint capsule. Joint surfaces are oriented coronally in the cervical spine, sagittally in the lumbar spine, and obliquely in the thoracic spine. Additional articulations with the ribs are present in the thoracic spine. Notably, each costovertebral junction spans a motion segment.

MECHANICS. Functionally, the spine has been divided into three columns of stability: anterior, middle, and posterior (6). Though this delineation of columns was originally formulated in respect to spinal stability after fracture, it has been applied to numerous nontraumatic conditions of the spine. The anterior column is anatomically composed of the anterior two thirds of the vertebral body, the disc, and the ALL. The middle column is composed of the posterior vertebral body, the disc and the PLL. The posterior column encompasses the posterior arch (pedicles, laminae, spinous processes, transverse processes) and posterior ligamentous complex (interspinous ligaments, ligamentum flavum). In the thoracic spine, the ribs interact with both the middle and posterior columns. By definition, loss of at least two columns of support indicates spinal instability.

In spinal motion, columns move in relation to each other around instantaneous axes of rotation (IAR) (7–9). During flexion, the IAR is located at the anterior aspect of the disc (anterior column), with compressive forces being transmitted anteriorly and distractive energies posteriorly. In extension, the IAR is located at the posterior aspect of the disc (middle column), with compressive forces concentrated posteriorly and distractive energies anteriorly. In rotation, the IAR is located just posterior to the PLL at the junction of the posterior and middle column. Functionally, this minimizes the translational movement of the spinal canal and its contents. The intervertebral disc is the major stabilizer against rotational forces, although the facet joints also make a substantial contribution.

PATHOMECHANICS. Alterations of the vertebral column can change the location of the IAR. Simply, the IAR translates toward the stiffest aspect of the spine in any one plane of motion. For example, posterior instrumentation or anterior column destruction shifts the IAR posteriorly. Likewise, the IAR migrates anteriorly with either anterior instrumentation or posterior destruction.

Abnormal curvatures of the spine can arise from deformities of one or more its components. In Scheuermann's kyphosis, anterior vertebral or disc wedging represents anterior column deficiency and can shift the IAR forward, leading to continuously greater distractive forces on the posterior ligamentous complex (10). With progressive height loss, further shifts of the center of mass can sustain or even potentiate the deformity.

In congenital spine deformities, a failure of formation or segmentation can be manifested as a "hemivertebra" or a "bar," respectively, that may cause asymmetric growth. Depending on the location of the anomaly, deformity is created in the sagittal or coronal plane. For example, a left hemivertebra in the midthoracic spine may cause greater growth on that side forming a convexity or gibbus on the side of the anomaly (Fig. 1A). In contrast, a left unilateral bar will constrict longitudinal growth, producing a concavity on the side of the anomaly (Fig. 1B). A posterior hemivertebra may lead to a kyphotic gibbus deformity secondary to continued growth posteriorly and diminished de-

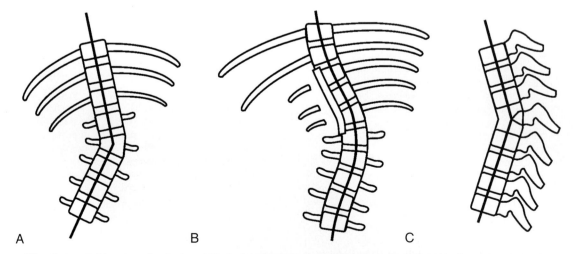

Fig. 1. **A**: A left hemivertebra in the midthoracic spine may cause greater growth on that side, forming a convexity or gibbus on the side of the anomaly. **B**: In contrast, a left unilateral bar will constrict longitudinal growth, producing a concavity on the side of the anomaly. **C**: A posterior hemivertebra may cause a kyphotic gibbus deformity secondary to continued growth posteriorly and diminished development anteriorly. (© 2002, Thomas H. Weinzerl.)

velopment anteriorly (Fig. 1C). Posterior column loss can result from trauma, neural arch defects, or a wide decompressive laminectomy. Theoretically, posterior destruction shifts the flexion IAR anteriorly, potentiating kyphotic deformities.

Rib deformities are commonly associated with AIS. Rib "humps" develop secondary to abnormal rotation of the vertebrae. Lateral rib offset (sagittal displacement) increases with greater sagittal spinal curvature. Likewise, rib cage rotation parallels apical vertebrae rotational deformity (11). Though not the primary cause, resection of the rib heads can facilitate correction during surgery (12).

With long-standing deformities, spinal ligaments act to maintain the deformity. Ligaments mechanically and histologically respond to their environment and stresses. With prolonged shortening and decreased stresses, they become more brittle and less fibrillar. In severe kyphotic deformities, the ALL becomes contracted and inelastic and can limit the amount of passive correction achievable with positioning. The PLL, the weakest of the spinal ligaments and closest to the IAR, contributes little to deformity maintenance (13).

Characterization of Deformity

Deformities are described by location, flexibility, and progressivity. Abnormalities can be located in the cervical, thoracic, or lumbar spines. Some diseases are more common in a particular region. Idiopathic scoliosis most commonly affects the thoracic spine, with secondary compensatory curves in the lumbar spine. In contrast, congenital lordosis most often occurs in the lumbar region.

Curves may be flexible or rigid. Flexible curves can be fully or partially passively correctable, whereas rigid curves are resistant to corrective maneuvers. Both can be present in the same spine simultaneously. In AIS, simultaneous rigid and flexible curves represent a primary structural curve and a compensatory nonstructural curve, respectively. In ankylosing spondylitis, rigid curves are maintained by bridging syndesmophytes that effectively arthrodese the involved segments. Forceful attempts at passive correction may lead to fracture and neurological injury. A flexible compensatory hyperlordotic posture of the lumbar spine can develop caudal to an ankylosed kyphotic thoracic deformity.

Progressivity must be noted in evaluating spinal deformities. In most cases, progression is documented on serial radiographic examinations. This is the case for adolescent scoliosis or Scheuermann's disease in which curves develop slowly. Most adult kyphotic or scoliotic deformities are slowly progressive, exhibiting 1 to 2 degrees of curve increase per year. In contrast, most congenital spinal deformities are aggressive and progressivity may be presumed from the type of defect. For example, congenital scoliosis from a unilateral unsegmented bar with a contralateral hemivertebra may progress 10 to 12 degrees per year, reaching up to 140 to 180 degrees of angulation by mid-adolescence (1).

Vertebral Balance

SAGITTAL BALANCE. The vertebral column is naturally contoured in the sagittal plane, while normally straight in the coronal plane. Sagittal contour is achieved by a combination of cervical and lumbar lordosis, with intervening thoracic kyphosis.

Although many authors document "normal" ranges for these curvatures, the actual ranges are quite variable. These curvatures are measured statically and represent the spine in a standing weight-bearing state. Average lumbar lordosis is approximately 50 degrees, with values ranging from 32 to 82 degrees. Thoracic kyphosis averages 37 degrees, ranging from 7 to 63 degrees (14).

Biomechanically, cervical, thoracic, and lumbar curvatures must be considered in concert. Together, they attempt to achieve vertebral balance. Sagittal balance can be assessed on a full-length lateral radiograph by dropping a vertical plumb line from the base of the occiput. Balance is realized if that line intersects the seventh cervical vertebral body cranially and lies within 1 cm of the sacral promontory of the first sacral segment caudally (Fig. 2). Mechanically, this ensures that the weight borne by the spine in the resting position is acting to maintain its position within space. Relatively hyperkyphotic segments can be balanced by compensatory hyperlordosis in other segments (Fig. 3). This carries the weight-bearing line more posterior to rest at its balanced position at the sacral promontory. The sacral promontory is centered over the hips.

Sagittal deformities sometimes progress to a point where the compensatory capability of the vertebral column is exceeded. The weight-bearing line can no longer return to its balanced position, resulting in self-propagating sagittal imbalance. To illustrate this, one can compare the hyperkyphotic spine to the Tower of Pisa. Balance is maintained if the center of mass lies within the boundaries of the base. Thus, the weight of the tower (or spine) functions to maintain its current position. However, if the tower leans over so much that the center of mass lies outside its base, the weight of the tower will cause it to fall (Fig. 4). Corrective measures in deformity treatment attempt to

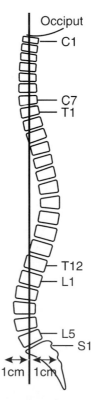

Fig. 2. Balance is realized if the line intersects the seventh cervical vertebral body cranially and lies within 1 cm of the sacral promontory of the first sacral segment caudally. (© 2002, Thomas H. Weinzerl.)

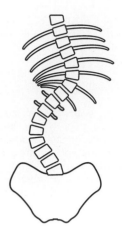

Fig. 3. Hyperkyphotic segments can be balanced by compensatory hyperlordosis in other segments. (© 2002, Thomas H. Weinzerl.)

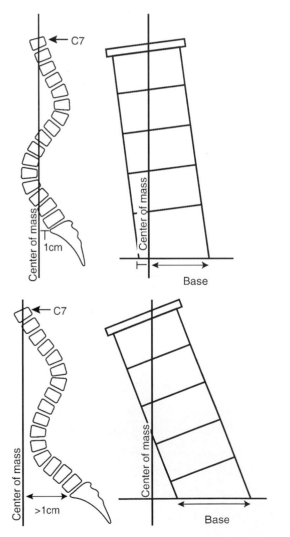

Fig. 4. To illustrate spinal balance, one can compare the hyperkyphotic spine to the Tower of Pisa. Balance is maintained if the center of mass lies within the boundaries of the base. Thus, the weight of the tower (or spine) functions to maintain its current position. If the tower leans over so much that the center of mass lies outside its base, the weight of the tower will cause it to fall. (© 2002, Thomas H. Weinzerl.)

restore the weight-bearing line or center of mass of the body to the anatomical base, which is the sacral promontory.

CORONAL BALANCE. In the coronal plane, the spine is normally straight. The weight-bearing line can be drawn to intersect the occiput, all spinous processes, and the midline sacrum. Any coronal curvature is abnormal, shifting the weight-bearing axis laterally. As in sagittal deformities, coronal deformities can be balanced by compensatory curves in other regions. For example, primary scoliotic thoracic curves can develop compensatory lumbar curves caudally. In addition, extravertebral compensation can also be present. Pelvic or shoulder obliquities may develop to balance coronal offset. In addition, scoliotic patients can exhibit unilateral toe walking to effectively compensate for pelvic obliquity.

ROTATIONAL BALANCE. Similar to coronal balance, the vertebral column is normally rotationally neutral. Spinous processes are midline to the vertebral bodies and pedicles in the axial plane. The vertebrae revolve around the rotational IAR located just posterior to the PLL. Functionally, this maintains a constant position for the spinal canal during rotatory motion.

COUPLED MOTION. Though sagittal motion is not normally associated with rotation, lateral flexion is coupled with vertebral rotation. In the cervical spine, the vertebrae rotate toward the contralateral side, while in the lumbar spine the vertebrae rotate toward the ipsilateral side. In the thoracic spine, abnormal coronal curvature is associated with rotational deformity. Postoperatively, iatrogenic rotational deformity, known as the crankshaft phenomenon, may develop after selective posterior fusion in a skeletally immature patient. Continued anterior growth along a posterior tether causes progressive rotation of the vertebrae.

Correction: Nonoperative

Correction of spinal deformities can be operative or nonoperative. Operative treatment involves direct bony manipulation, instrumentation, and fusion. Nonoperative measures rely on indirect manipulation of the curvature. Although numerous methods of nonsurgical treatment have been previously used, including traction, electrical stimulation, and stretching, only bracing and casting have had clinical efficacy.

Nonoperative deformity correction must achieve one of two goals. First, treatment must prevent or arrest progression of the curve. Second, it should restore and maintain physiologically compatible spinal balance and contour. Bracing and casting are the best nonoperative option. Bracing is indicated to treat AIS curves between 25 and 39 degrees in a skeletally immature patient. In this instance, cessation of curve progression is a positive result. In other conditions such as Scheuermann's kyphosis, bracing is effective in maintaining a corrected spine, especially with curves less than 60 degrees (15). External orthotic management has limited usefulness in congenital spinal deformities and is generally unsuccessful.

Spinal bracing attempts to position the vertebral column in a corrected or overcorrected position. Correction is obtained indirectly from externally applied forces. These forces must be applied to the skin and transmitted to subcutaneous skeletal structures that are confluent with the vertebrae. Posteriorly, the spinous processes are largely subcutaneous and accessible for brace contact. Anteriorly, thoracic and abdominal viscera cover the spine, creating a deficiency of direct contact points. Manipulation of pelvic structures, such as the iliac crest, and the rib cage influence spinal orientation through rigid articulations at the sacroiliac and costovertebral joints, respectively. Though not directly continuous, the mandible has also been a site of brace contact to enable better control of the upper thoracic column (Milwaukee-type brace). However, its use has been curtailed because of the development of dental deformities in young patients (16).

Conceptually, brace correction requires a three-point bending moment applied to a flexible deformity. An ipsilateral force is applied toward the apex of the convexity, while contralateral forces above and below are simultaneously applied in the same plane. Through contact areas, constant force vectors are applied to correct or overcorrect deformities in either the sagittal or coronal planes. Coronal vectors are produced at the lateral rib cage or iliac wing. Sagittal vectors are applied to the sternum, anterior iliac spines, and spinous processes. Rotational deformity is not directly controlled by bracing maneuvers. It is partially corrected by improving sagittal and coronal alignment and relies on reversal of coupled coronal-rotational motion.

Biomechanically, braces are limited by several factors. Force applied must be compatible with tissue survival. Skin breakdown and pressure necrosis can complicate brace treatment, especially in the insensate patient. This necessitates contact pads with large surface areas and frequent clinical monitoring of the integument. Large pads dissipate corrective forces over broader surfaces and relieve concentrated points of pressure. Braces are also limited in that forces are broadly applied and cannot be directed toward a specific vertebral level. Thus, correction is achieved by orienting the vertebral column as a whole to achieve functional balance. In addition, these vectors are applied at a significant lateral distance from the spinal column. Some of the corrective forces are dissipated into extravertebral structures.

Correction: Operative

The goals of surgical correction are similar to nonoperative methods. Restoration of balance and contour, in addition to prevention of progression of the deformity, are fundamental. Surgical treatment is achieved through a combination of techniques. Intraoperative positioning exploits the intrinsic flexibility of spinal curvatures, using similar biomechanical principles as bracing. In rigid curvatures, soft tissue releases or bony procedures are indicated if further correction is needed. Stabilization with structural graft and/or instrumentation facilitates solid osseous fusion of the involved levels.

RESTORATION OF SPINAL BALANCE. Functional balance, not necessarily anatomical curvature, is the fundamental goal. Imbalance can develop from abnormalities in the soft tissues, ligaments, or bone. Deforming forces must be countered to achieve proper correction. With adequate release and resection, the spinal elements are more freely manipulated. Spinal correction is directed toward biplanar restoration of the weight-bearing line to the sacral promontory.

Many curves exhibit intrinsic flexibility, while others are wholly rigid. Ankylosed spines are inherently inflexible, as scoliotic curves generally have components of varying flexibility. Preoperative bending films allude to the amount of passive intraoperative correction possible. Lateral flexion (on an AP radio-

graph) bending films are most useful for coronal plane deformities, while flexion-extension (on a lateral radiograph) bending films are helpful in preoperative evaluation of sagittal deformities. In scoliosis, structural curves must be distinguished from compensatory curves prior to surgery on both static and lateral bending radiographs. Bending films assess the relative flexibility of scoliotic curves. Structural curves have been defined as demonstrating a Cobb angle of 35 degrees or greater with no more than 20 degrees of correction on opposite side bending. On an AP roentgenogram, structural curves exhibit rotation of grade one or greater according to the Nash-Moe system (Fig. 5) (17). Compensatory curves can be presented cranial or caudal to structural curves. They are flexible and typically correct fully on bending films. Generally, they should be excluded from the fusion segment.

King et al. (18) popularized the concept of the stable vertebra in coronal spinal deformity. By definition, it is the first vertebra transected by a vertical line drawn from the center of the sacral body on an AP radiograph (Fig. 6). Biomechanically, it represents the caudal extent of fusion necessary for stable coronal correction. Fusion extending to levels above the stable vertebrae can lead to progressive recurrence of deformity.

In sagittal kyphosis, Lowe and Kasten (19) highlight the importance of spanning the apex of deformity. Specifically, fusion should include all wedged vertebrae, including the first adjacent lordotic vertebra distally. Proximal and distal junctional kypho-

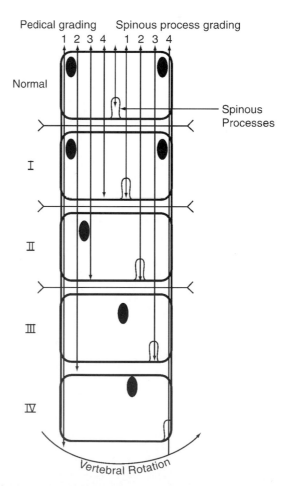

Fig. 5. On an anteroposterior roentgenogram, structural curves exhibit rotation of grade one or greater according to the Nash-Moe system. Rotation may be judged by the orientation of the spinous processes or the pedicles. (© 2002, Thomas H. Weinzerl.)

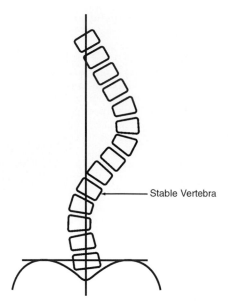

Stable Vertebra

Fig. 6. The stable vertebra is the first vertebra transected by a vertical line drawn from the center of the sacral body on an anteroposterior radiograph. The first vertebra in which the line intersects the pedicles is deemed the stable vertebra. In general, this should be the most caudal aspect of the fusion segment. (© 2002, Thomas H. Weinzerl.)

sis has been observed in rigidly kyphotic spines that were fused short of the first kyphotic segment or first lordotic segment, respectively.

Intraoperative positioning facilitates deformity correction but is influenced by the relative flexibilities of the curves (20). Prone positioning on a flat table utilizes body weight to reduce kyphosis, as some investigators believe it is responsible for the majority of intraoperative correction (20). Ninety-ninety degree positioning (hips and knees flexed to 90 degrees), though useful to distract the posterior ligamentous complex and widen the interlaminar spaces, can lead to loss of lumbar lordosis. Lateral decubitus positioning enables anterior surgery through a retroperitoneal or transthoracic approach. In this position, gravitational forces can help reduce coronal curvature. Four-poster operating tables can be utilized to reduce scoliotic curvatures in the prone position.

SOFT TISSUE RELEASES. Soft tissue constraints can be a significant limiting agent to effective correction. The ALL and the intervertebral disc can be contracted and deformed. Normally a restraint to distractive anterior forces, it limits sagittal plane extension. The ALL is the strongest of the spinal ligaments (13). With long-standing deformity, the ligament becomes shortened and contracted on the concave side. For example, kyphotic curves that do not passively correct to less than 50 to 60 degrees frequently require anterior release. Likewise, abnormally lordotic segments may be tethered by contracted posterior ligamentous structures.

The anterior annulus can also contribute to a shortened anterior column. In anterior approaches to scoliosis correction, discs are excised to allow full coronal and sagittal reduction. As the anterior two thirds are a major component of rotational resistance, disc excision also enables rotational correction.

BONY PROCEDURES. With severe and rigid curves, osseous procedures should be considered and these may be indicated

when soft tissue resection alone is not sufficient. Various bony maneuvers have been developed. Osteotomy or resection can increase or decrease the effective lengths of the anterior or posterior columns. Bony intervention for congenital deformity must be considered differently. Often the deformity arises from a single vertebral defect such as a unilateral bar or a hemivertebra. Excision of the defect should be the primary goal of surgery, as multiple soft tissue releases are not necessary (21).

Sagittal plane deformities can be addressed by posterior osteotomies. Multiple-level posterior osteotomies have been used to correct kyphotic deformities. Partial resection of adjacent laminae and posterior facet joints enables closing wedges to be formed (22). The effective length of the posterior column is decreased. Stabilization is then effected by standard methods of posterior instrumentation and fusion. The "eggshell" procedure, first described by Michele and Krudger (23), involves excavation of the cancellous bone from the vertebral body through a posterior portal in the pedicle. The decancellated body with the mechanical properties of an eggshell is then horizontally osteotomized via propagation of a small fracture line iatrogenically created at the lateral pedicle wall. After removal of the posterior elements, the posterior wall of the vertebral body is pushed forward into the decancellated cavity, which allows compression and shortening of the anterior and posterior columns through a single posterior approach.

The major component of rotational deformity is contained within the anterior intervertebral disc. In the thoracic spine, additional forces are contributed by the costal head articulation with the vertebrae. Resection of these heads has been found to increase rotational degree of freedom and enhance rotational deformity correction (12,24).

Spinal Reconstruction

ANTERIOR COLUMN RECONSTRUCTION. The anterior column of the spine can be reconstructed in several ways. Anterior structural bone grafting can be implanted for mechanical anterior support and as a conduit for bony arthrodesis. Large specimens of autogenous cortical strut graft can be harvested from the iliac crests, fibulae, or resected ribs. Allograft analogues are also available, although they carry the theoretical risk of disease transmission. There are no reported cases of human immunodeficiency virus (HIV) transmission following bony allograft transplant. Strut grafts are interposed between intervening vertebral bodies to maintain anterior column weight-bearing support. Maintenance of the end-plate integrity is recommended to minimize subsidence into the cancellous bone of the adjacent vertebral bodies.

Because purely bony grafts can be resorbed prior to solid fusion, some surgeons advocate the use of cylindrical metallic fusion cages to augment anterior column reconstruction. They are packed with autogenous cancellous graft and/or commercial osteoinductive substances and implanted between adjacent vertebral bodies in lieu of structural grafts. Fusion cages can be oriented vertically (Harms-type titanium mesh) or longitudinally. Longitudinal cages are designed to be oriented sagittally (Ray type) or laterally (BAK type). Using lateral cylindrical cages, some authors describe "dialing-in" correction by placing different-sized anterior and posterior cages implanted in the same intervertebral space. However, the efficacy of this practice remains to be proven.

ANTERIOR INSTRUMENTATION. Anterior instrumentation can be used to correct spinal deformities. Its primary utility is in the treatment of scoliotic deformity, although it may be useful in the treatment of other entities. Anterior instrumentation typically consists of vertebral screws placed lateral to medial into the vertebral body with a unilateral connecting rod. They are effective in providing compressive and rotational forces. In scoliotic curves, they are implanted on the convex side of the curve to correct coronal curvature. Anterior instrumentation can be effective in reducing rotational deformities through direct de-rotational maneuvers as well as coupled de-rotation (17).

Anterior stabilization is commonly used as an adjunct to posterior treatment of such disorders as Scheuermann's kyphosis. This practice may have some biomechanical advantages. Anterior load sharing decreases the demands placed on the posterior hardware and fusion mass and has been effective in decreasing the high rate of pseudarthrosis with posterior surgery alone (19). Long-term subsidence and loss of correction can be minimized with combined anterior and posterior fusion surgery.

POSTERIOR INSTRUMENTATION AND FUSION. Posterior instrumentation is the treatment of choice for many spinal deformities. Various implant options exist, including pedicle screws, plates, wires, hooks, and rods. Instrumentation can affect angulation, translation, and effective lengths of the three columns.

Hook designs are the most common type of instrumentation used in deformity correction. Spinal hooks may be inserted onto lamina, pedicles or transverse processes. Transverse process hooks shift the IAR posteriorly. Placed farther away from neurovascular structures, they are comparatively safer to implant than laminar or pedicle hooks. However, hooks in this position offer weaker support than other locations. Laminar hooks are inserted onto stronger bone and are relatively easy to implant. Mechanically, the IAR is moved more posteriorly than with transverse process hooks. Potential neural injury may arise from anterior migration of the hook into the spinal canal intra- or postoperatively. The hooks are readily placed in the lower thoracic and lumbar spine where interlaminar distances are greatest. Pedicle hooks are perhaps the most technically demanding, but they apply forces to the vertebrae closest to the natural IAR. The risk of neural damage is greatest due to the close proximity of the exiting nerve roots.

Hook constructs may act to distract or compress the posterior elements of the spine, increasing or decreasing the effective length of the posterior column. Distraction can be achieved by a simple rod construct of proximal up-going hooks and distal down-going hooks. This "claw" construct is the fundamental principle of scoliosis correction with Harrington instrumentation. Hook direction could be reversed to provide compression on the contralateral side. In this manner, the two proximal (or distal) hooks together form an interlocking claw.

Many advances in hook construct design have taken place since the development of Harrington rods. Presently, most hook systems rely on the stability of multiple proximal and distal claw configurations. A claw is composed of two oppositely oriented hooks compressing an individual vertebra (Fig. 7). Acting as a vise grip devise, it is a stable anchoring point of one end of a construct without relying on distraction or compression along the entire system to maintain position. Between claws the surgeon can provide compressive or distractive forces to influence alignment. Hook systems provide posterior column support only and rely on an intact or stable reconstructed anterior column.

Pedicle screw constructs are an alternative or adjunct to hook systems. Screws are placed from posterior to anterior through the posterior cortical surface at the junction of the transverse process and the midline of the pars interarticularis. They are generally safe in the lumbar and lower thoracic spinal vertebrae,

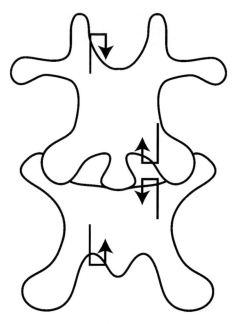

Fig. 7. A claw is composed of two oppositely oriented hooks compressing an individual vertebra. The claw may be formed by hooks on the same or contralateral sides of the vertebra. (© 2002, Thomas H. Weinzerl.)

although they may be cautiously implanted in the upper thoracic spine. Biomechanically, pedicle screws offer three-column support to the spine.

Multiple hooks or screws are statically linked by spanning rods. Through this rigid interaction, the rod exerts multiplanar forces on the deformed spinal column. Rods can be unilateral or bilateral. Bilateral rods are more stable and can be used to provide differential forces on either side of the spine. Larger diameter rods are stronger. Bilateral rods may be cross-linked to significantly increase torsional stability (25).

Longitudinal forces act to shorten, lengthen, translate, or rotate the segments. As in previous discussions, lengthening or shortening the posterior column has a kyphotic or lordotic effect, respectively. Posterior distraction increases the relative length of the posterior column over a fixed anterior column length. Conceptually, this maneuver influences sagittal balance while maintaining stable anterior length. This length differential has the overall effect of angulating the vertebral elements around a large anterior radius and effectively producing kyphosis. Posterior compression has the opposite effect, curving the vertebrae around a large posterior radius, producing relative lordosis. Biomechanically, forces are primarily in the vertical axis, transmitted via upward or downward pressures of the hooks or screws on the bony elements. Rotational deformity is not directly addressed by these forces but may be secondarily corrected by coupled motion.

Correction can be enhanced by rod contouring. Rods can be regionally bent to approximate zones of kyphosis and lordosis. Anterior or posterior forces are transmitted to the vertebrae via the rod–hook or rod–screw interaction. Anterior curvature (apex posterior) produces kyphosis, while posterior curvature (apex anterior) creates lordosis. With rod contouring, correction is achieved by changing the relative length of the anterior column. Posterior column length is maintained by static fixation to the posterior rod.

Rod contouring may be performed prior to implantation or *in situ*. *In situ* contouring, although advocated by some (26), requires slight "overbending" of the rod to achieve the desired correction. *In situ* contouring has been found to increase the cantilever stresses at pedicle screw–rod junctions, which may lead to early fatigue failure of the construct (27). Precontouring requires that an approximation of the desired correction be performed prior to rod implantation.

Precontouring can be combined with a technique of rod rotation for correction of sagittal and coronal deformities simultaneously. It has been most commonly used for cases of idiopathic scoliosis. The rod is precontoured to approximate the shape of the coronal spinal deformity. The rod is then securely fixed posteriorly via the hooks or screws. Ninety-degree *in situ* rod rotation in a sufficiently flexible deformity transforms the coronal deformity into sagittal contour. Additional correction can be effected by *in situ* bending.

Complications

Complications of spinal deformity correction may be divided into short-term and long-term. Short-term complications include intraoperative difficulties. Laminar, pedicle, and transverse process fractures can occur secondary to the large forces applied via the construct. Nerve or spinal cord compression from hooks or screws may be a result of improper hardware placement or translation of the hardware after rod manipulation. Spinal cord injury can also occur from excessive correction. Cerebrospinal fluid leaks from dural tears should be repaired intraoperatively. Immediate postoperative leaks may be managed by short-term subarachnoid drain placement and antibiotic administration. Failure to respond to such conservative measures necessitates operative repair. Hardware failure is a significant long-term complication. Implant breakage or dislodging can represent motion at the site of a pseudarthrosis.

References

1. Winter R, Lonstein J, Boachie-Adjei O. Congenital spinal deformity. In: Pritchard D, ed. *Instructional course lectures.* Rosemont, IL: American Academy of Orthopaedic Surgeons, 1996:117–127.
2. Chambers. 1985.
3. Willers U, Hedlund R, Aaro S, et al. Long-term results of Harrington instrumentation in idiopathic scoliosis. *Spine* 1993;18:713–717.
4. Sasso R, Cotler H. Posterior instrumentation and fusion for unstable fractures and fracture dislocations of the thoracic and lumbar spine. *Spine* 1993;18:450–460.
5. Soucacos P, Soucacos P, Zacharis K, et al. School-screening for scoliosis. A prospective epidemiological study in northwestern and central Greece. *J Bone Joint Surg* 1997;79A:1498–1503.
6. Denis F. The three columns of the spine and its significance in the classification of acute thoracolumbar spine injuries. *Spine* 1983;8: 817–831.
7. Haher T, O'Brien M, Felmly W, et al. Instantaneous axis of rotation as a function of the three columns of the spine. *Spine* 1992;17: S149–154.
8. Haher T, Tozzi J, Lospinuso M, et al. The contribution of the three columns of the spine to spinal stability: a biomechanical model. *Paraplegia* 1989;27:432–439.
9. Resnick D, Weller S, Benzel E. Biomechanics of the thoracolumbar spine. *Neurosurg Clin North Am* 1997;8:455–469.
10. Riina J, Merola A, Cerabona F, et al. The role of anterior column surgery in the treatment of kyphosis. In: Devlin V, ed. *Spine: state of the art reviews.* Philadelphia: Hanley and Belfus, 1998:639–645.
11. Closkey R. Rib cage deformities in scoliosis: spine morphology, rib cage stiffness, and tomography imaging. *J Orthop Res* 1993;11: 730–737.
12. Feiertag M, Horton W, Norman J, et al. The effect of different surgical release on thoracic spinal motion. A cadaveric study. *Spine* 1995; 15:1604–1611.
13. Pintar F, Yoganandan N, Myers T, et al. Biomechanical properties of human lumbar spine ligaments. *J Biomech* 1992;25:1351–1356.
14. Bernhardt M, Bridwell K. Segmental analysis of the sagittal plane alignment of the normal thoracic and lumbar spines and thoracolumbar junction. *Spine* 1989;14:717–721.
15. Sachs B, Bradford D, Winter R, et al. Scheuermann kyphosis. Follow-up of Milwaukee-brace treatment. *J Bone Joint Surg* 1987;69A: 50–57.
16. Logan W. The effect of Milwaukee brace on the developing dentition. In: *Transactions of the British Society of Orthod.* London: 1962: 1–8.
17. Lenke L, Bridwell K. Biomechanical consideration in the correction of adolescent idiopathic scoliosis. In: Haher T, Merola A, eds. *Spine: state of the art reviews.* Philadelphia: Hanley and Belfus, 1996: 409–432.
18. King H, Moe J, Bradford D, et al. The selection of fusion levels in thoracic idiopathic scoliosis. *J Bone Joint Surg* 1983;65A:1302–1313.
19. Lowe T, Kasten M. An analysis of sagittal curves and balance after Cotrel-Dubousset instrumentation for kyphosis secondary to Scheuermann's disease. A review of 32 patients. *Spine* 1994;19: 1680–1685.
20. Marsicano J, Lenke L, Bridwell K, et al. The lordotic effect of the OSI frame on operative adolescent idiopathic scoliosis patients. *Spine* 1998;23:1341–1348.
21. Bradford D, Hu S. Excision of hemivertebrae. In: Bradford D, ed. *Master techniques in orthopaedic surgery. The spine.* Philadelphia: Lippincott-Raven, 1997:185–197.
22. Ponte A. Scheuermann's kyphosis: Posterior shortening procedure by segmental closing wedge resection. *Orthop Trans* 1995;19: 603.
23. Michele A, Krudger F. A surgical approach to the vertebral body. *J Bone Joint Surg* 1949;31A:873–878.
24. Oda I, Abumi K, Lu D, et al. Biomechanical role of the posterior elements, costovertebral joints, and rib cage in the stability of the thoracic spine. *Spine* 1996;21:1423–1429.
25. Dick J, Jone M, Zdeblick T, et al. A biomechanical comparison evaluating the use of intermediate screws and cross-linkage in lumbar pedicle fixation. *J Spinal Disord* 1994;7:402–407.
26. Jackson R. Intrasacral fixation and in situ contoured spinal corrections: biomechanical considerations. In: Haher T, Merola A, eds. *Spine: state of the art reviews.* Philadelphia: Hanley and Belfus, 1996: 561–586.
27. Voor M, Roberts C, Rose S, et al. Biomechanics of in situ rod contouring of short-segment pedicle screw instrumentation in the thoracolumbar spine. *J Spinal Disord* 1997;10:106–116.

176. Special Anesthetic Considerations and Monitoring

Eugene S. Fu, Deborah A. Rusy, and David W. Cahill

In comparison with the anesthetic management of patients undergoing laminectomy and discectomy procedures, that of patients undergoing surgery to correct a spinal deformity is complicated and fraught with potential hazards to the spinal cord. The airway management of patients with kyphosis or severe flexion deformity of the cervical spine is challenging in that spinal cord damage associated with pathological motion of the unstable vertebrae must be prevented. Patients with scoliosis of the thoracic spine often present with cardiac and pulmonary compromise as a result of ventilation–perfusion abnormalities associated with mechanical and anatomic changes of the thoracic rib cage. Intraoperatively, the anesthesiologist is faced with the problem of administering anesthetic agents that are known to interfere with somatosensory and motor evoked potential monitoring of the spinal cord. This chapter focuses on special anesthetic considerations and the application of intraoperative neuromonitoring in patients undergoing surgery to correct spinal deformity.

Special Anesthetic Considerations

Spinal deformities may be classified as kyphotic, scoliotic, or rotational (1). Kyphosis is excessive flexion in the sagittal plane of the vertebral column. Scoliosis is excessive deviation in the coronal plane, with or without rotation. A noninclusive list of spinal deformities appears in Table 1. The anesthetic management of patients with kyphosis in the cervical spine or scoliosis in the thoracic spine who undergo surgery to correct their deformity presents unique challenges.

Table 1. Classification of Spinal Deformities

I. Cervical spine
  A. Kyphosis/flexion deformities
    1. Postlaminectomy
    2. Inflammatory (ankylosing spondylitis and rheumatoid arthritis)
    3. Infectious (tuberculous spondylitis)
II. Thoracic spine
  A. Kyphosis
    1. Postlaminectomy
    2. Inflammatory
    3. Infectious
    4. Traumatic
    5. Postirradiation
    6. Pathological fracture secondary to osteoporosis
  B. Scoliosis
    1. Idiopathic
    2. Myopathic (muscular dystrophy)
    3. Neuropathic (poliomyelitis, cerebral palsy, Friedreich ataxia)
    4. Congenital
    5. Inflammatory (rheumatoid arthritis)
    6. Infectious (vertebral osteomyelitis)
    7. Traumatic
    8. Postirradiation

CONSIDERATIONS FOR CERVICAL SPINAL PROCEDURES. Severe kyphotic or flexion deformities of the cervical spine are seen in patients with ankylosing spondylitis, rheumatoid arthritis, or posttraumatic deformity. The numerous problems of these patients include a restricted field of vision, difficulty in opening the mouth, an inability to care for the skin between the chin and the chest (2), and various degrees of myelopathy. Surgical procedures to correct flexion deformities in the cervical spine are associated with the potential hazard of spinal cord damage secondary to movement of the neck during endotracheal intubation and patient positioning. In the past, cervical osteotomy procedures were performed under local anesthesia with mild sedation to avoid manipulating the airway and to be able to monitor the neurological status with the patient awake (3). The development of the fiberoptic bronchoscope to perform endotracheal intubation and the monitoring of evoked potentials have made it feasible to perform cervical osteotomies under general anesthesia. It is often difficult to intubate patients with severe flexion deformities in the cervical spine by direct laryngoscopy because of the inability to align the oral, pharyngeal, and laryngeal axes properly for optimal exposure of the glottic opening. Moreover, the neck can move during direct laryngoscopy. Therefore, awake fiberoptic intubation is the technique of choice in securing the airway in these patients in that manipulation of the cervical spine is avoided and the patient can maintain an airway while the larynx is visualized with the fiberoptic bronchoscope. Topical anesthesia to the airway and the judicious use of sedation may be needed to facilitate awake fiberoptic bronchoscopy (3).

Patients with kyphotic deformities of the cervical spine may present with fractures requiring stabilization in the neutral position with in-line traction. Gardner-Wells tongs or a halo device is applied to reduce the dislocation. In-line traction immobilizes the neck in the event that direct laryngoscopy is used to secure the airway. If a patient is not cooperative for an awake fiberoptic intubation, the anesthesiologist may consider placing the endotracheal tube with direct laryngoscopy or other methods of intubation after inducing general anesthesia. For patients undergoing transoral surgical procedures involving odontoid resection, an oral endotracheal tube is placed, and a tonsillectomy retraction device is used to secure the tube out of the way. A nasal endotracheal tube is not acceptable because it obscures the surgical field. Because of concerns of swelling in the posterior pharynx during the postoperative period, these patients remain intubated for several days. If a posterior surgical procedure is planned in the next few days, the patient is not usually extubated until after the second procedure (4).

CONSIDERATIONS FOR THORACIC SPINAL PROCEDURES. Severe scoliosis in the thoracic spine is associated with restrictive rib cage deformities that result in decreased lung volumes and compliance. The vital capacity, total lung capacity, and functional residual capacity may be decreased 60% to 80% (5). The magnitude of the reduction in lung volumes and compliance appears to correlate with the angle of curvature (6). The severity of scoliosis is defined by the angle of curvature,

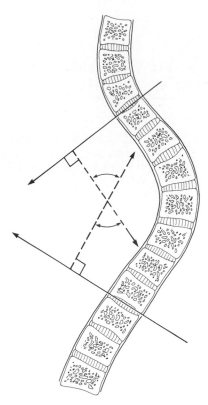

Fig. 1. The angle of curvature as measured by the Cobb method. *Solid lines* are drawn across the upper border of the highest vertebral body and the lower border of the lowest vertebral body of the curve. An angle of intersection is formed by *dotted lines* drawn perpendicular to the solid lines. (© 2002, Thomas H. Weinzerl.)

measured by the Cobb method. As shown in Fig. 1, one set of lines (*solid*) is drawn across the cephalic border of the highest vertebral body and the caudal border of the lowest vertebral body of the curve. Another set of lines (*dotted*) is drawn perpendicular to the solid lines to form a Cobb angle of intersection. A Cobb angle greater than 60 degrees increases the likelihood of cardiopulmonary complications, including respiratory failure, pulmonary hypertension, and failure of the right side of the heart (3). Therefore, some have advocated the surgical correction of deformities with a Cobb angle greater than 50 degrees (7).

The major abnormality of gas exchange in scoliosis is ventilation–perfusion mismatch, a consequence of abnormal chest wall anatomy and mechanics (4). Generalized alveolar hypoventilation and increased dead space ventilation are evidenced by increases in the ratio of dead space to tidal volume and in the alveolar oxygen difference. Initially, the arterial oxygen tension is decreased and the arterial carbon dioxide tension is normal. Further deterioration in the ventilation–perfusion relationship leads to an increase in ventilatory demand, manifested as hypercapnia (3,6). As a consequence of progressive hypoxia and hypercapnia, pulmonary hypertension and cor pulmonale may develop. Several mechanisms have been postulated to account for the increases in pulmonary arterial pressure and pulmonary vascular resistance (6). A decrease in the number of vascular units per lung volume is associated with abnormal development of the pulmonary vasculature secondary to rib cage deformity. Additionally, alveolar hypoxia causes vasoconstriction and hypertensive pulmonary vascular changes. Therefore, cardiorespiratory failure represents the culmination of the

effects of scoliotic rib cage deformity, which are impaired gas exchange and pulmonary vasculopathy (6).

The anesthetic management of patients undergoing transthoracic procedures may require placement of a double-lumen endotracheal tube to expose the anterolateral thoracic spine by isolating one lung for ventilation. In the double-lumen tube, a tracheal lumen is affixed to a bronchial lumen, each lumen having its own pilot balloon. The bronchial lumen is inserted a short distance into the right or left main bronchus until the tracheal lumen resides in the trachea. With right-sided double-lumen tubes, extreme caution is taken to prevent blockage of the right upper lobe, which is just past the carina. During two-lung ventilation, both lumina are ventilated, whereas during one-lung ventilation, one lumen is clamped. Fiberoptic examination after intubation with a double-lumen tube is essential to rule out herniation of the bronchial balloon cuff into the trachea and blockage of a lung bronchus as a result of tube malpositioning. If arterial desaturation during one-lung ventilation occurs, the anesthesiologist initially needs to rule out tube malposition before attributing the desaturation to increased shunting during one-lung ventilation. Moreover, the shunt effects of one-lung ventilation are compounded in patients with preexisting ventilation–perfusion mismatch resulting from rib cage deformities. The treatment of hypoxemia during one-lung ventilation involves the use of higher concentrations of inspired oxygen and the application of continuous positive airway pressure (CPAP) or positive end-expiratory pressure (PEEP).

Extensive fusion and instrumentation of the thoracic spine are also associated with significant blood loss, which often necessitates perioperative transfusion (8). Complications of homologous blood transfusions include transfusion reactions, hepatitis, and acquired immune deficiency syndrome (AIDS). Various forms of autologous blood transfusion are widely used to minimize the amount of homologous blood administered. Patients can donate several autologous units a few weeks before surgery. Iron supplements and recombinant erythropoietin may be administered preoperatively. Recently, intraoperative salvaging of autologous blood with a cell saver device has been increasingly used as an effective method to decrease the need for homologous transfusion (3,8). Scavenging lost blood entails the suctioning of heparinized blood from the surgical field to a reservoir in which cells are washed to create a red cell concentrate for reinfusion (8). Relative contraindications to administering cell saver blood include infection, malignancy, and the possibility of aspirating wound irritants, such as Betadine (povidone-iodine) and bacitracin, into the cell saver suction device.

Intraoperative Neuromonitoring

Neurological deficit is one of the most devastating complications that can occur following the surgical correction of spinal deformity. The mechanism of neurological injury may be spinal cord ischemia secondary to disruption of the arterial supply, direct compression of the spinal cord, or excessive stretching of the spinal cord during corrective distraction of the scoliotic spine (9). The goal of spinal cord monitoring is the rapid detection and treatment of any compromise in neurological function during the surgical procedure, before permanent damage occurs. Ideally, simultaneous recording of the ventral and dorsal spinal cord would indicate to the clinician that the integrity of the motor and sensory tracts has been preserved throughout the surgical procedure. The somatosensory pathway of the dorsal columns is depicted in Fig. 2. Afferent sensory information, including light touch, vibration, and proprioception, is transmitted via the ascending tracts to reach the somatosensory cortex. The motor pathway of the ventral spinal cord is depicted in Fig. 3. Efferent impulses from the motor cortex are transmitted to the anterior horn cells via the descending corticospinal tract. Current methods to monitor spinal cord functioning include the wake-up test, monitoring of the somatosensory evoked potential (SSEP), and monitoring of the motor evoked potential (MEP).

WAKE-UP TEST. A traditional method to assess intraoperative neurological function is the wake-up test, first described in 1973 by Vauzelle et al. (10). In this test, the patient is awakened to allow movement of the upper and lower extremities shortly after spinal instrumentation. If a deficit is observed, the instrumentation is removed immediately, with the hope that neurological functioning will be restored. An advance warning of 30 to 45 minutes should be sufficient to ensure that the anesthesiologist appropriately tapers the inhalational agent, muscle relaxant, and narcotics before the patient is to be awakened (4). The observation of limited movement with partial blockade is sufficient evidence for the clinician that the patient has not been paralyzed by the instrumentation. Therefore, some recommend the incomplete reversal of neuromuscular blockade to avoid the potential hazards of having the patient regain full muscular

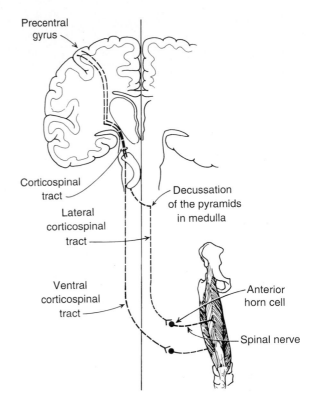

Fig. 3. Motor pathway (efferent or descending). (Redrawn from Ganong WF. *Review of medical physiology,* 18th ed. Norwalk, CT: Appleton & Lange, 1997. © 2002, Thomas H. Weinzerl.)

strength during the wake-up test (4). Awakening the patient entails certain risks, such as deep inspiration, which can lead to air embolism, and violent movements, which can dislodge the spinal instrumentation or endotracheal tube. Another limitation of the wake-up test is that it evaluates the integrity of the corticospinal tract (motor function) only, not that of the somatosensory tract (sensory function). Moreover, the wake-up test can detect neurological deficits only at the time it is applied. Ben-David et al. (11) described a patient who experienced postoperative neurological deficits despite normal findings during the wake-up test.

MONITORING OF THE SOMATOSENSORY EVOKED POTENTIAL. With electrophysiological monitoring of the spinal cord, the clinician can continuously assess the integrity of neural pathways at risk during spinal cord surgery. SSEPs are a measure of ascending neural activity following the stimulation of a peripheral sensory nerve (e.g., median, ulnar, posterior tibial, or peroneal nerve). As shown in Fig. 2, electrical stimulation of an upper extremity produces a propagated neural signal that enters the spinal cord via the dorsal root ganglion, ascends along the ipsilateral dorsal columns to synapse at the nucleus cuneatus, and crosses at the decussation to the contralateral thalamus and cortex. SSEP monitoring in an upper extremity assesses the integrity of the dorsal column pathways, which are primarily supplied by the posterior spinal arteries. Evoked stimulation of a lower extremity involves conduction not only along the dorsal column but also along the dorsal spinocerebellar tracts (12). Interestingly, the dorsal spinocerebellar tracts receive their blood supply from the anterior spinal artery, which also supplies the motor tracts. In fact, lower-extremity SSEPs correlate well with postoperative sensory and motor neurologi-

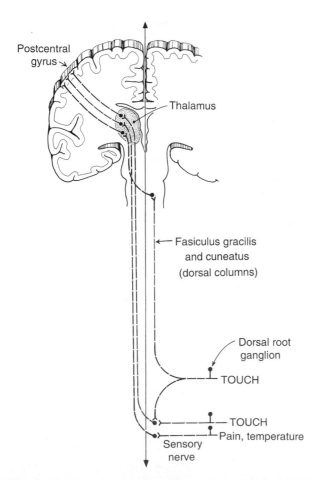

Fig. 2. Somatosensory pathway (afferent or ascending). (Redrawn from Ganong WF. *Review of medical physiology,* 18th ed. Norwalk, CT: Appleton & Lange, 1997. © 2002, Thomas H. Weinzerl.)

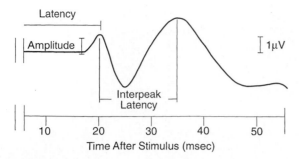

Fig. 4. Characterization of evoked potentials by latency and amplitude. (Redrawn from Cucchiara RF, Black S, Michenfelder JD, eds. *Clinical neuroanesthesia,* 2nd ed. New York: Churchill Livingstone, 1998. © 2002, Thomas H. Weinzerl.)

cal outcome; the false-negative rate is less than 1% (13). Nevertheless, SSEP monitoring to assess the integrity of the motor tract has limitations; the presence of postoperative motor deficits despite normal SSEP measurements in a lower extremity has been documented in several case reports (14,15). Ideally, SSEP monitoring should be used in conjunction with other modalities that assess motor function, such as the wake-up test or monitoring of the MEP.

Oscilloscopic SSEP waveforms are characterized by latency and amplitude. Latency is the time in milliseconds from the stimulus to the maximum amplitude of a positive or negative peak, and amplitude is the maximum height in microvolts of a positive or negative peak (Fig. 4). As shown in Fig. 5, evoked potential responses in SSEP monitoring are recorded in multiple sites, such as peripheral nerves, subcortical structures (e.g., cervical spinal cord/brainstem), and cortical structures in the brain.

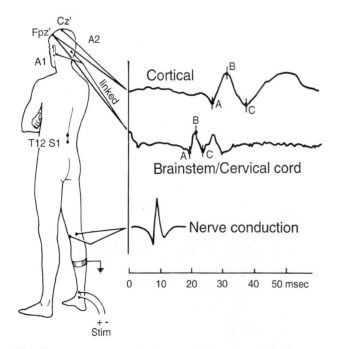

Fig. 5. Somatosensory evoked potentials (SSEPs) generated by stimulation of the posterior tibial nerve. Recording sites include the cerebral cortex, brainstem/cervical spinal cord, and peripheral nerve. (Modified from Misulis KE. *Spehlmann's evoked potential primer. Visual, auditory and somatosensory evoked potential in clinical diagnosis,* 2nd ed. Newton, MA: Butterworth-Heinemann, 1994. © 2002, Thomas H. Weinzerl.)

If changes in the SSEPs are noted, the clinician must determine whether they represent technical difficulties in recording waveforms or suppression by anesthetics, or whether they are truly related to surgical manipulation. For example, abnormal responses in the peripheral nerve site with normal subcortical and cortical recordings may indicate a technical problem, such as dislodged recording electrodes in the periphery. Normal peripheral nerve evoked responses indicate that the stimulus to the peripheral nerve is intact and may rule out technical failure when abnormal cortical evoked responses are detected. Normal recordings over the cervical spinal cord indicate that the stimulus is reaching the central nervous system (CNS). Spinal cord and subcortical responses are more resistant to the effects of anesthetics than are cortical responses. When it is possible to place surface electrodes near the spinal cord rostral to the site of surgery, the subcortical response may be more useful than the cortical site, allowing the anesthesiologist more flexibility in the choice of anesthetic (13).

Various electrical and nonelectrical factors other than surgical trauma and anesthesia may alter the SSEP response. Background electrical interference (60-Hz artifact) in the operating room can affect the ability to optimize recordings of SSEPs. Equipment with 60-cycle artifact that can interfere with SSEP measurements includes the electrocautery unit, Cavitron ultrasonic aspirator, fluid warmer, and cell saver centrifuge device. Evoked potential signals, which typically have amplitudes of less than 10 μV, are small in relation to background electrical noise. Signal averaging is a complex process involving the Fourier transformation of many evoked responses with a digital computer (16). The summation of the evoked responses to repetitive stimulation improves the signal-to-noise ratio by signal averaging and the effective subtraction of noise. SSEP averaging entails obtaining responses from several hundred to a thousand repetitive stimuli based on the principle that only the evoked responses are time-locked to the stimulus, whereas background noise occurs randomly. The standard use of high (2,000- to 3,000-Hz) and low (30- to 100-Hz) band pass filters to eliminate frequency components outside the range of the evoked potential frequencies being studied also minimizes noise to improve the signal-to-noise ratio.

Nonelectrical factors, such as changes in the patient's physiological status, may be confounding influences in the interpretation of the SSEP. Decreases in blood pressure, blood volume, and oxygen saturation can alter the SSEP (17,18). At temperatures below 34°C, moderate increases in latency and decreases in amplitude are seen, whereas more severe changes occur at temperatures below 31°C (19). Significant blood loss with rapid decreases in blood volume, hematocrit, and blood pressure can result in the attenuation or loss of SSEP recordings. Fig. 6A represents the baseline intraoperative SSEP tracings recorded in a patient during a circumferential spinal fusion with instru-

Table 2. Effects of Anesthetic Drugs on Somatosensory Evoked Potentials

Drug	Amplitude	Latency
Thiopental	Small/none	Increased
Etomidate	Increased	Increased
Fentanyl	Small/none	Modest or no increase
Diazepam	Decreased	Increased
Midazolam	Decreased	Increased
Ketamine	Increased	Increased
Propofol	None	Increased
Nitrous oxide	Decreased	No change
Volatile anesthetic	Decreased	Increased

mentation for correction of scoliosis. Fig. 6B represents the changes in SSEPs during rapid blood loss, with a decrease in the hematocrit from 28% to approximately 12%. These traces are shown against the baseline. Attenuation of the popliteal tracings (lines 3 and 7) was accompanied by the loss of cervical (lines 4 and 8) and brainstem (lines 2 and 6) tracings. After vigorous volume resuscitation, the SSEP tracings were restored (Fig. 6C), and no new neurological deficit was noted following surgery.

The effects of anesthetics on the latency and amplitude of cortical SSEPs are summarized in Table 2. Potent volatile inhalation agents (e.g, halothane, isoflurane, and desflurane) are known to cause dose-dependent suppression of the SSEP (17, 20,21). The practice of combining nitrous oxide with volatile agents is controversial. Pathak et al. (21) showed that a volatile agent at a minimum alveolar concentration (MAC) of less than 0.75 could be used with 60% nitrous oxide. However, in a recent study by Schwartz et al. (22), the administration of 60% to 65% nitrous oxide depressed SSEP responses by more than 50% without volatile inhalation agents. These authors concluded that the suppressive effects of nitrous oxide on SSEP values have been previously underestimated, and that the use of ni-

trous oxide should not be recommended for patients with compromised baseline amplitudes secondary to coexisting spinal cord or peripheral nerve disease. Fig. 7A shows the posterior tibial SSEP recordings obtained after completion of a scoliosis surgical procedure in which the patient received isoflurane anesthesia at a MAC of 0.5 to 0.8 without nitrous oxide. The patient had undergone successful instrumentation of the thoracolumbar spine without any changes in the evoked potential tracings throughout the procedure. After the surgical team decided that neuromonitoring was no longer indicated, 70% nitrous oxide was administered. Interestingly, a complete loss of amplitude in the cortical deflections occurred at P37 and N45 within 5 minutes after the addition of 70% nitrous oxide (Fig. 7B).

Generally, intravenous (IV) agents have a less suppressive effect than do inhalation agents. IV agents like sodium thiopental and propofol moderately depress the SSEP response when given as bolus injections during the induction of anesthesia (19). IV induction agents like ketamine and etomidate increase the SSEP amplitude. Opioids (e.g, fentanyl, sufentanil, alfentanil) are considered to be the maintenance agents of choice because narcotics have only modest effects on the early compo-

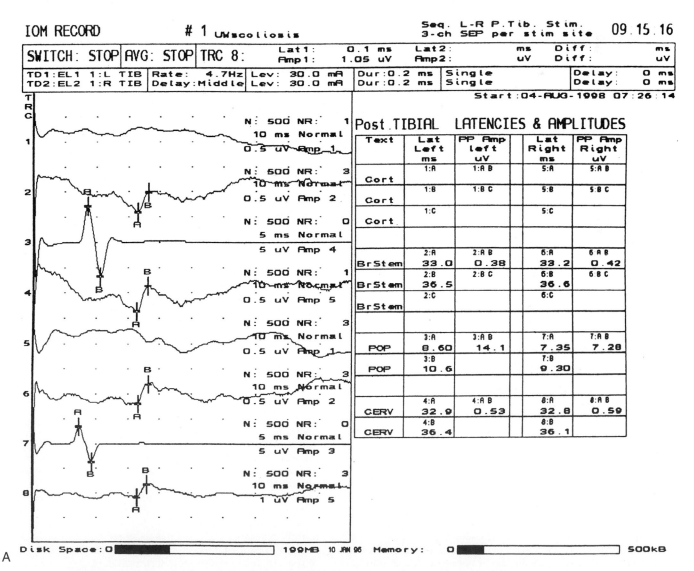

Fig. 6. Attenuation of the SSEPs following rapid blood loss. **A:** Baseline intraoperative tracings. (*Figure continues.*)

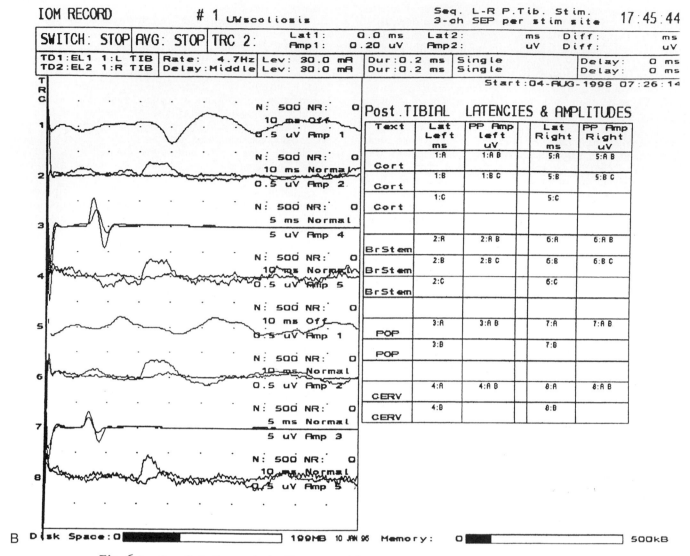

Fig. 6. (continued). **B:** Changes in the SSEP tracings following a drop in the hematocrit from 28% to 12%.

nent of the SSEP waveforms (19). Traditionally, a nitrous oxide–narcotic anesthetic technique has been used by many practitioners (4,23) during SSEP monitoring, but a total IV anesthesia (TIVA) technique may be more advantageous. In the study of Kalkman et al. (24), cortical and posterior tibial nerve SSEPs were preserved better during alfentanil–propofol anesthesia than during alfentanil–nitrous oxide anesthesia. Moreover, Schwartz et al. (22) showed that latency prolongation and amplitude reduction were two times greater with nitrous oxide–sufentanil anesthesia than with propofol–sufentanil anesthesia.

The patient's primary disease and physiological state may account for reductions in the amplitude and latency of baseline SSEP recordings. Patients with idiopathic or congenital scoliosis generally have intact CNS pathways in which spinal, brainstem, and cortical SSEPs are easily recorded. In patients with scoliosis secondary to neuromuscular disorders, hereditary degenerative neurological disorders, or preoperative paraplegia, it may be impossible to obtain any baseline evoked potential recordings. Patients with cerebral palsy or static encephalopathy may have normal spinal or brainstem evoked potentials, but cortical waveforms may not be obtainable. It is essential to determine before surgical incision that an easily interpreted, reproducible

SSEP waveform is present that will allow the accurate detection of intraoperative somatosensory changes (9).

Various studies (25–27) have shown that the results of SSEP monitoring may predict the neurological outcome in spinal surgery. However, none of these studies was prospectively randomized. The Scoliosis Research Society performed a multicenter survey in 1995 in which more than 51,000 surgical spinal cases were reviewed (25). They found 50% fewer postoperative neurological deficits in medical centers with experienced SSEP neuromonitoring teams than in medical centers with inexperienced teams. Meyer et al. (26) retrospectively reviewed 295 patients who underwent operative treatment for acute spinal injuries. Of the 295 patients, 150 had intraoperative SSEP monitoring, and one (0.7%) of these had a new postoperative neurological deficit. Of the remaining 145 patients, who did not have intraoperative SSEP monitoring, 10 (6.9%) had new postoperative neurological deficits. Epstein et al. (27) studied the incidence of quadriplegia following cervical spine surgery. They found no instances of quadriplegia in the 100 consecutive patients who had SSEP monitoring procedures, whereas 8 (3.7%) of the 218 patients who were historical controls and were not monitored had quadriplegia.

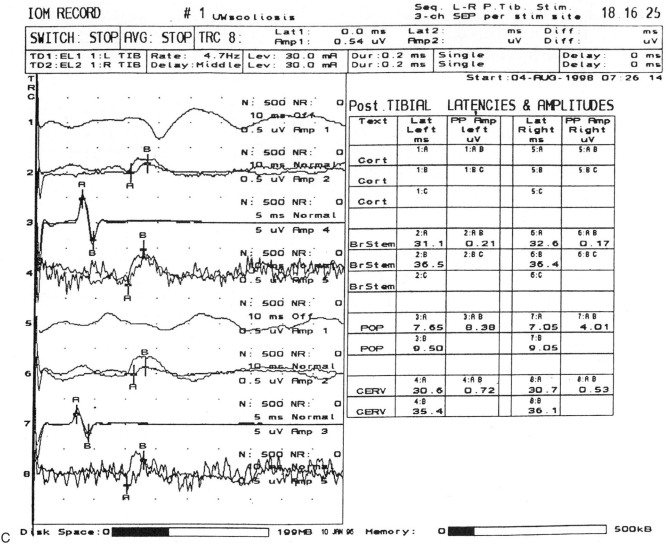

Fig. 6. (continued). **C:** Restoration of the SSEP tracings after vigorous volume resuscitation. (SSEP recordings from the University of Wisconsin Medical School.)

When SSEP changes are abrupt and irreversible, as in vascular injury, spinal cord contusion, or rarely epidural and subdural hematoma, it is highly likely that a new postoperative neurological deficit will develop. More often, alterations in SSEPs evolve gradually and usually occur during surgical manipulation or distraction of the spine, which may cause ischemia in the spinal cord. When the changes are gradual, the clinician can usually intervene in time and avert an adverse postoperative neurological outcome. In the study of York et al. (28), increases in latency up to 15% or decreases in amplitude of 50% or less were not associated with postoperative neurological deficits. Nuwer (9) found that if evoked potential amplitudes were attenuated by more than 50%, the patient was at high risk for postoperative neurological impairment. It is generally felt that when decreases in amplitude of more than 50% or increases in latency of more than 15% are seen, the surgeon should immediately be notified for possible reversal of recent manipulations (28). Should the surgeon decide before the procedure that the operative plan will not vary despite any changes seen in SSEP recordings, there is no clinical reason to perform intraoperative monitoring (9). The ultimate goal of SSEP monitoring during spinal surgery is

to decrease the risk for iatrogenic postoperative paralysis resulting from intraoperative procedures. With continuous SSEP monitoring, neurological compromise may be detected promptly, so that immediate intervention to alleviate the causes and attempts to reverse the neurological deficit can be undertaken. Nevertheless, false-negative outcomes in the detection of motor deficits will not be eliminated if SSEP monitoring is not supplemented with another technique to assess motor function. Moreover, SSEP monitoring may be further limited by the technical difficulties associated with preexisting spinal cord disease, interference from electrical noise in the operating room, and suppression associated with anesthesia.

MONITORING OF THE MOTOR EVOKED POTENTIAL.

Because SSEP monitoring does not directly assess the integrity of the anterior spinal cord, tests to assess the function of the motor tracts are needed. As mentioned previously, the wake-up test is associated with many potential hazards. Transcranial stimulation of the motor cortex can be performed electrically or magnetically to produce myogenic motor evoked potential

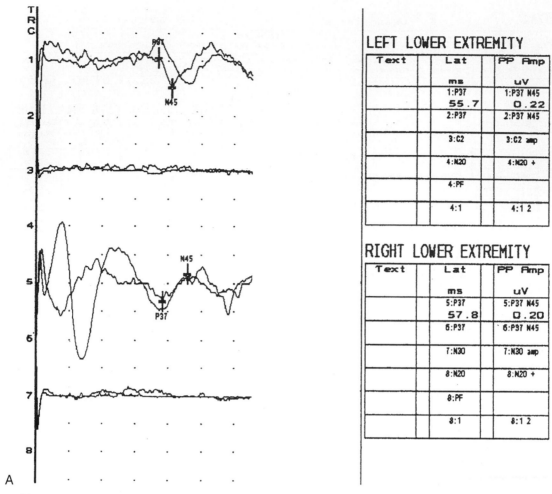

LEFT LOWER EXTREMITY

Text	Lat	PP Amp
	ms	uV
	1:P37	1:P37 N45
	55.7	0.22
	2:P37	2:P37 N45
	3:C2	3:C2 amp
	4:N20	4:N20 +
	4:PF	
	4:1	4:1 2

RIGHT LOWER EXTREMITY

Text	Lat	PP Amp
	ms	uV
	5:P37	5:P37 N45
	57.8	0.20
	6:P37	6:P37 N45
	7:N30	7:N30 amp
	8:N20	8:N20 +
	8:PF	
	8:1	8:1 2

Fig. 7. Posterior tibial nerve SSEP recordings during scoliosis surgery. **A:** Cortical SSEP tracings before the administration of nitrous oxide. Cortical deflections are present at P37 and N45.

(MEP) responses that are recorded over peripheral muscles in the upper or lower extremity. One problem with myogenic transcranial MEP monitoring is that electromyographic (EMG) recordings of the MEP are very sensitive to inhalation agents (19). Zentner et al. (29) demonstrated that MACs of volatile inhalation agents of more than 0.5 are capable of eliminating the EMG response during transcranial MEP recordings in rabbits. In a later study, Zentner et al. (30) showed that nitrous oxide concentrations above 50% without volatile agents significantly alter the EMG amplitude during myogenic transcranial MEP monitoring in rabbits. In a clinical study, Kalkman et al. (31) demonstrated that low concentrations of isoflurane abolish myogenic transcranial MEPs during opioid–nitrous oxide anesthesia. Another drawback to myogenic MEP monitoring is that muscle relaxants greatly reduce the MEP tracing from muscles. However, Lang et al. (32) suggested that the interpretation of myogenic MEP recordings is possible if only partial neuromuscular blockade is used.

Another method for monitoring the descending corticospinal tract is to record neurogenic activity instead of myogenic activity by placing the recording electrodes over the spinal cord and peripheral nerves. As previously mentioned, Zentner et al. (29) showed that a volatile inhalation agent (halothane, enflurane, or isoflurane) at a MAC of 0.5 abolishes the myogenic responses to transcranial electric motor cortex stimulation in animals. Sub-

sequently, these investigators found that descending MEP responses obtained from spinal cord electrode recordings following motor cortex stimulation were resistant to inhalational anesthetics. Peripheral nerve recordings following the electrical stimulation of cervical and lumbar nerve roots also were not affected by the administration of volatile anesthetic agents in MACs of up to 1.5. These authors concluded that monitoring of the descending motor pathway during inhalational anesthesia is feasible only when neurogenic activity is evaluated.

Neurogenic motor evoked potential (NMEP) monitoring via electrical stimulation of the spinal cord has been evaluated by various investigators (33–35). Spinal cord stimulation involves placing needle electrodes into the cancellous bone of the spinous processes of the vertebral bodies at levels just rostral to the site of surgery (Fig. 8) while recording electrodes are placed near peripheral nerves (e.g., sciatic nerve). Owen et al. (33) found that NMEP recordings were a more valid indicator of postoperative motor function than were SSEP recordings. Bernard et al. (34) showed that NMEP signals are well preserved in patients undergoing scoliosis surgery under general anesthesia with isoflurane or desflurane at MACs of up to 1. In a review of 116 cases involving concurrent NMEP and SSEP monitoring, Nagle et al. (35) concluded that for optimal monitoring during spinal surgery, both monitors must be used. These authors found that intraoperative spinal cord injury often involves con-

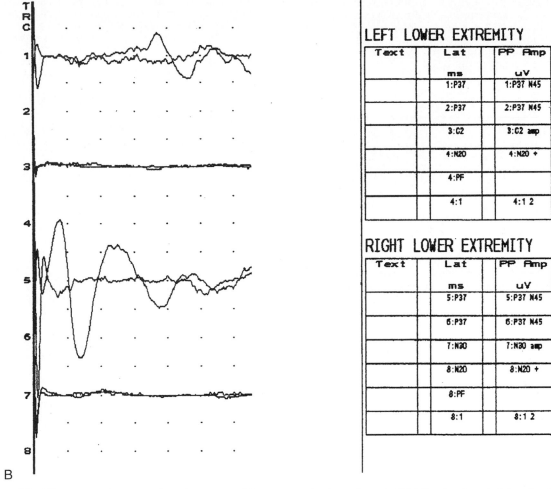

LEFT LOWER EXTREMITY		
Text	Lat	PP Amp
	ms	uV
	1:P37	1:P37 N45
	2:P37	2:P37 N45
	3:C2	3:C2 amp
	4:N20	4:N20 +
	4:PF	
	4:1	4:1 2

RIGHT LOWER EXTREMITY		
Text	Lat	PP Amp
	ms	uV
	5:P37	5:P37 N45
	6:P37	6:P37 N45
	7:N20	7:N20 amp
	8:N20	8:N20 +
	8:PF	
	8:1	8:1 2

B

Fig. 7. (continued). **B:** Complete elimination of the SSEP amplitude at P37 and N45 following the administration for several minutes of 70% nitrous oxide. (SSEP recordings from the University of South Florida College of Medicine.)

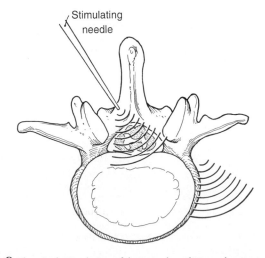

Fig. 8. Electrical stimulation of the spinal cord to produce neurogenic motor evoked potentials. Needle electrodes are embedded in the base of the spinous processes of vertebral bodies rostral to the site of surgery. (Redrawn from Cucchiara RF, Black S, Michenfelder JD, eds. *Clinical neuroanesthesia,* 2nd ed. New York: Churchill Livingstone, 1998. © 2002, Thomas H. Weinzerl.)

cordant deterioration in the NMEPs and SSEPs; however, occasional insults selectively involve one system.

Nevertheless, the application of NMEP monitoring with stimulation of the spinal cord is limited by the fact that these MEP recordings do not necessarily reflect selective activation of the motor tract. Descending evoked potentials generated by spinal cord stimulation appear to be mediated through multiple spinal pathways and probably represent mixed activation of motor and sensory tracts (36,37). In fact, Su et al. (36) demonstrated that following spinal cord stimulation, descending evoked potential signals recorded at the peripheral nerve can be generated through backfiring of the sensory pathways. This observation has been described as antidromic sensory conduction, in which neuronal impulses travel in a reverse direction along sensory fibers. Despite the controversy that NMEP signals may reflect antidromic sensory information rather than motor conduction, neurogenic MEP monitoring with spinal cord stimulation continues to be utilized by clinicians to predict motor neurological outcome when SSEP monitoring may be inadequate.

Only single-stimulus transcranial magnetic stimulation has been approved by the Food and Drug Administration as a low-risk procedure; transcranial electrical stimulation (singly or in trains) and multiple-stimulus transcranial magnetic stimulation have not been approved for use in humans (13). As previously mentioned, the EMG signal to single-twitch stimulation is very susceptible to the depressant effects of anesthetics, but multiple-twitch stimulation allows for temporal summation and augmentation of the EMG signal (19,38). However, repeated stimulation of the cerebral cortex may be undesirable because electrical stimulation may theoretically cause seizures, and magnetic stimulation may be problematic in patients with implanted metallic devices (e.g., aneurysm clips).

Conclusions

An understanding of the airway and respiratory conditions related to kyphosis of the cervical spine and scoliosis of the thoracic spine is of great importance in the preoperative preparation of patients undergoing corrective spinal surgery. Thus far, SSEP monitoring has been widely used intraoperatively to assess neurological function; the clinical application of MEP monitoring has had limited success. Future improvements in MEP monitoring technology may entail the use of signal averaging of multiple responses to multiple-twitch transcranial stimulation. The optimal management of patients undergoing surgery for spinal deformity involves combining SSEP monitoring with a more reliable modality to assess motor function.

References

1. Ogilvie JW. Scoliosis, kyphosis, and lordosis. In: Youmans JR, ed. *Neurological surgery,* 4th ed. Philadelphia: WB Saunders, 1996: 2475–2482.
2. Simmons EH. Ankylosing spondylitis: surgical considerations. In: Rothman RH, Simeone FA, eds. *The spine,* 3rd ed. Philadelphia: WB Saunders, 1992:1447–1511.
3. Concepcion M. Anesthesia for orthopedic surgery. In: Longnecker DE, Tinker JH, Morgan GE, eds. *Principles and practice of anesthesiology,* 2nd ed. St. Louis: Mosby, 1998:2113–2137.
4. Mahla ME, Horlocker TT. Vertebral column and spinal cord surgery. In: Cucchiara RF, Black S, Michenfelder JD, eds. *Clinical neuroanesthesia,* 2nd ed. New York: Churchill Livingstone, 1998:403–448.
5. Kafer ER. Idiopathic scoliosis: mechanical properties of the respiratory system and ventilatory response to carbon dioxide. *J Clin Invest* 1975;55:1153–1163.
6. Kafer ER. Respiratory and cardiovascular functions in scoliosis and the principles of anesthetic management. *Anesthesiology* 1980;52: 339–351.
7. Youngman PME, Edgar MA. Posterior spinal fusion and instrumentation in the treatment of adolescent idiopathic scoliosis. *Ann R Coll Surg Engl* 1985;67:313–317.
8. Murray DJ. Monitoring of hemostasis. In: Longnecker DE, Tinker JH, Morgan GE, eds. *Principles and practice of anesthesiology,* 2nd ed. St. Louis: Mosby, 1998:923–941.
9. Nuwer MR. *Evoked potential monitoring in the operating room.* New York: Raven Press, 1986.
10. Vauzelle C, Stagnara P, Jouvinroux P. Functional monitoring of spinal cord activity during spinal surgery. *Clin Orthop* 1973;93: 173–178.
11. Ben-David B, Taylor PD, Haller GS. Posterior spinal fusion complicated by posterior column injury: a case report of a false-negative wake-up test. *Spine* 1987;12:540–543.
12. Gaines R, York DH, Watts C. Identification of spinal cord pathways responsible for the peroneal evoked response in the dog. *Spine* 1984;9:810–814.
13. Mahla ME. Neurologic monitoring. In: Cucchiara RF, Black S, Michenfelder JD, eds. *Clinical neuroanesthesia,* 2nd ed. New York: Churchill Livingstone, 1998:125–176.
14. Ginsburg HH, Shetter AG, Raudzens PA. Postoperative paraplegia with preserved intraoperative somatosensory evoked potentials. *J Neurosurg* 1985;63:296–300.
15. Zornow MH, Grafe MR, Tybor C, et al. Preservation of evoked potentials in a case of anterior spinal artery syndrome. *Electroencephalogr Clin Neurophysiol* 1990;77:137–139.
16. Sloan TB. Evoked potential monitoring. *Int Anesthesiol Clin* 1996; 34:109–136.
17. Grundy BL. Monitoring of sensory evoked potentials during neurosurgical operations: methods and applications. *Neurosurgery* 1982; 11:556–575.
18. Nuwer MR, Daube J, Fischer C, et al. Neuromonitoring during surgery. Report to an IFCN committee. *Electroencephalogr Clin Neurophysiol* 1993;87:263–276.
19. McPherson RW. Intraoperative neurologic monitoring. In: Longnecker DE, Tinker JH, Morgan GE, eds. *Principles and practice of anesthesiology,* 2nd ed. St. Louis: Mosby, 1998:883–906.
20. McPherson RW, Mahla M, Johnson R, et al. Effects of enflurane, isoflurane, and nitrous oxide on somatosensory evoked potentials during fentanyl anesthesia. *Anesthesiology* 1985;62:626–633.
21. Pathak KS, Ammadio M, Kalamchi A, et al. Effects of halothane, enflurane, and isoflurane on somatosensory evoked potentials during nitrous oxide anesthesia. *Anesthesiology* 1987;66:753–757.
22. Schwartz DM, Schwartz JA, Pratt RE, et al. Influence of nitrous oxide on posterior tibial nerve cortical somatosensory evoked potentials. *J Spinal Disord* 1997;10:80–86.
23. Langeron O, Lille F, Zerhouni O, et al. Comparison of the effects of ketamine-midazolam with those of fentanyl-midazolam on cortical somatosensory evoked potentials during major spine surgery. *Br J Anaesth* 1997;78:701–706.
24. Kalkman CJ, Traast H, Zuurmond WWA, et al. Differential effects of propofol and nitrous oxide on posterior tibial nerve somatosensory cortical evoked potentials during alfentanil anaesthesia. *Br J Anaesth* 1991;66:483–489.
25. Nuwer MR, Dawson EG, Carlson LG, et al. Somatosensory evoked potential spinal cord monitoring reduces neurologic deficits after scoliosis surgery: results of a large multicenter survey. *Electroencephalogr Clin Neurophysiol* 1995;96:6–11.
26. Meyer PR, Cotler HB, Gireesan GT. Operative complications resulting from thoracic and lumbar spine fixation. *Clin Orthop* 1988;237: 125–131.
27. Epstein NE, Danto J, Nardi D. Evaluation of intraoperative somatosensory-evoked potential monitoring during 100 cervical operations. *Spine* 1993;18:737–747.
28. York DH, Chabot RJ, Gaines RW. Response variability of somatosensory evoked potentials during scoliosis surgery. *Spine* 1987;12: 864–876.
29. Zentner J, Albrecht T, Heuser D. Influence of halothane, enflurane, and isoflurane on motor evoked potentials. *Neurosurgery* 1992;31: 298–305.
30. Zentner J, Thees C, Pechstein U, et al. Influence of nitrous oxide on motor-evoked potentials. *Spine* 1997;22:1002–1006.
31. Kalkman CJ, Drummond JC, Ribberink AA. Low concentrations of isoflurane abolish motor evoked responses to transcranial electrical stimulation during nitrous oxide/opioid anesthesia in humans. *Anesth Analg* 1991;73:410–415.
32. Lang EW, Beutler AS, Chestnut RM, et al. Myogenic motor-evoked potential monitoring using partial neuromuscular blockade in surgery of the spine. *Spine* 1996;21:1676–1686.
33. Owen JH, Bridwell KH, Grubb R, et al. The clinical application of neurogenic motor evoked potential to monitor spinal cord function during surgery. *Spine* 1991;16:S385–S390.
34. Bernard J-M, Pereon Y, Fayet G, et al. Effects of isoflurane and desflurane on neurogenic motor- and somatosensory-evoked potential monitoring for scoliosis surgery. *Anesthesiology* 1996;85: 1013–1019.
35. Nagle KJ, Emerson RG, Adams DC, et al. Intraoperative monitoring of motor evoked potentials: a review of 116 cases. *Neurology* 1996; 47:999–1004.
36. Su CF, Haghighi SS, Oro JJ, et al. A backfiring in spinal cord monitoring. High thoracic spinal cord stimulation evokes sciatic response by antidromic sensory pathway, not motor tract conduction. *Spine* 1992;17:504–508.
37. Machida M, Weinstein SL, Yamada T, et al. Spinal cord monitoring: electrophysiological measures of sensory and motor function during spinal surgery. *Spine* 1985;10:407–413.
38. Taylor BA, Fennelly ME, Taylor A, et al. Temporal summation—the key to motor evoked potential spinal cord monitoring in humans. *J Neurol Neurosurg Psychiatry* 1993;56:104–106.

177. Sagittal Plane Deformity of the Cervical Spine

David W. Cahill, Mark Melton, and M. V. Hajjar

The cervical spine may be deformed in the axial, coronal, longitudinal, or sagittal axis. Axial deformity most commonly occurs with atlantoaxial or subaxial facet dislocation. Coronal plane deformity is most often seen as a secondary correction for thoracolumbar scoliosis or in the face of congenital occipitoatlantal dysplasia. Longitudinal deformity may rarely involve destructive trauma (i.e., atlanto-occipital dislocation) but is usually an incidental concomitant of degenerative disc collapse with foreshortening. Without question, however, the most common cervical deformity seen in the practice of spine surgery is in the sagittal plane and most often involves a loss of normal lordosis or true kyphosis secondary to degenerative disc collapse and spondylosis. Sadly, many such cases are created or exacerbated by ill-conceived surgical procedures that have disrupted anterior or posterior osteoligamentous structures without concomitant repair or reconstruction (1–5).

Epidemiologically, it is convenient to divide cervical sagittal deformity into adult and pediatric categories. Postlaminectomy kyphosis is very common among prepubertal children. Postlaminectomy hyperlordosis is largely limited to young children, often under the age of 5 years (6). Adult sagittal plane deformities may be iatrogenic, neoplastic, traumatic, or congenital, but the great majority of cases seen in clinical practice are degenerative in origin, frequently exacerbated by surgery (1,3,5).

Pediatric Deformity

Cervical sagittal plane deformity may accompany a variety of congenital dysplastic or dystrophic syndromes, including achondroplasia (Fig. 1A), spondyloepiphyseal dysplasia, mucopolysaccharidoses, and the more common Down syndrome (Fig. 1B) and von Recklinghausen disease (7–9). The chondrodysplasias often include anomalies of the craniocervical junction and are discussed elsewhere in this text. The mucopolysaccharidoses rarely come to surgical attention. Although kyphoscoliotic deformity may be seen in cases of neurofibromatosis type I in the absence of spinal tumors, cervical deformity most commonly occurs after neoplastic destruction of the vertebral elements or after surgical destruction at the time of tumor resection. The sagittal atlantoaxial instability seen in Down syndrome has certain unique characteristics and is discussed below.

Easily the most common cervical deformity seen in unoperated children is the atlantoaxial dislocation usually associated with os odontoideum (sometimes called *"type I" odontoid fracture*). Yet more common, unfortunately, is the kyphosis (or occasionally hyperlordosis in very young children) that follows laminectomy for Chiari malformation/syringomyelia or the resection of benign or malignant tumors (10,11).

ATLANTOAXIAL DEFORMITY IN CHILDREN. Down syndrome occurs in approximately 1 in 700 live births. Between 7% and 40% of patients with Down syndrome have radiographically demonstrable instability in the occipitoatlantoaxial com-

plex, apparently related in most cases to the generalized ligamentous laxity seen in this condition and, in relatively fewer cases, to dysplastic bony elements (12–15) (Fig. 1C). Luckily, only a small percentage of these patients ever become symptomatic and therefore warrant surgical consideration (16–19). Although sagittal atlantoaxial subluxation is most commonly noted, atlanto-occipital luxation and rotational deformity of the occiput-C1 and C1-2 articulations are not unusual (20–23).

Although earlier literature suggests that the surgical management of the deformities found in Down syndrome is associated with excessive morbidity and mortality, modern anesthetic and surgical techniques appear to have rendered this conclusion premature (24). Small case numbers make conclusions very tentative, but we have found no apparent increase in risk among patients with Down syndrome undergoing atlantoaxial or occipitoaxial fusion procedures in which the same techniques are used that are applied elsewhere (25) (Fig. 1C).

The authors of this chapter have never seen a "type I" odontoid fracture. Conversely, os odontoideum and os avis (ossiculum terminale) are relatively common in cases of atlantoaxial subluxation among both children and adults referred to our service for surgery (26). Good-quality plain films, usually supplemented with multiplanar computed tomographic (CT) images, are adequate for diagnosis. Although the differentiation between os avis (distal epiphyseal nonunion) and os odontoideum (middle epiphyseal nonunion) can be subtle, the differentiation from an acute fracture is rarely difficult. A smoothly marginated fragment and proximal dens stump make acute fracture unlikely (Fig. 2). After having observed a series of debilitating or fatal spinal cord injuries related to this form of atlantoaxial instability, we feel that all such cases should be offered prophylactic C1-2 fusion (27).

The technique for such fusions varies according to age, size, and associated pathology (28–30). In children in whom the odontoid dysplasia is the only bony anomaly and in whom cervical traction produces an anatomical reduction of the C1-2 dislocation, a posterior atlantoaxial fusion is suggested. In those weighing less than 35 kg, a Brooks technique with bilateral sublaminar titanium cables and autologous bone is used (Fig. 3A,B). In those heavier than 35 kg, the Brooks cables are supplemented with transarticular screws in the Magerl technique (31) (Fig. 3C). A single ipsilateral screw is used in those with unilaterally small or absent vertebral arteries (32). Most patients heavier than 50 kg will accept 4.0-mm screws in the C2 pars; 3.5-mm screws are used in smaller patients. The C2 pars is usually too small for even a 3.5-mm screw in patients weighing less than 35 kg. Screws smaller than 3.5 mm are biomechanically suspect and prone to fracture.

In patients with deficient posterior C1 rings, either congenitally or secondary to surgical damage, transarticular screws are used alone if the anatomy allows bilateral 4.0 screws. Small-diameter bilateral or unilateral posterior transarticular screws are supplemented with anterior transarticular screws (33). Patients with irreducible anterior C1 on C2 subluxation undergo transoral, transpharyngeal resection of the fusion masses and odontoid fragment, then osteotomy of the C1-2 joints followed by reduction and posterior fusion.

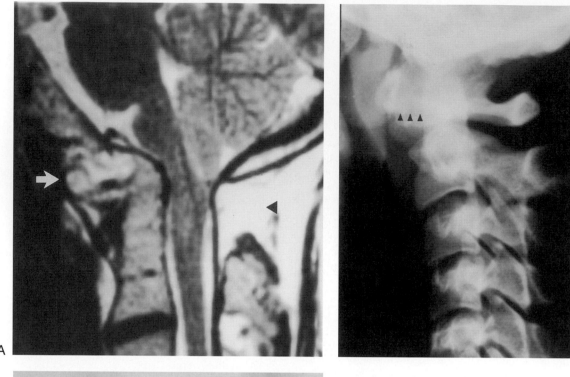

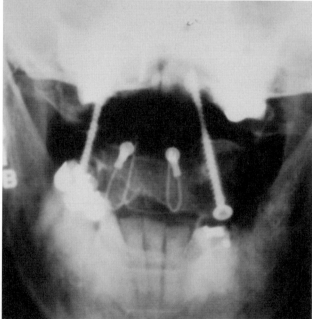

Fig. 1. A: Achondroplastic dwarf with deformation of the basiocciput, basilar invagination, and severe cervicomedullary junction stenosis despite C1 laminectomy (*arrowhead*). C1 is incorporated into the skull base, with the atlantodental interval widened to more than 1 cm (*white arrow*). **B:** Down syndrome with ligamentous laxity and atlantoaxial dislocation without fracture (*arrowheads*) in a 19-year-old patient. **C:** Postoperative radiograph of case in **B**. Brooks sublaminar cables and Magerl transarticular screws provided stable realignment without complication.

IATROGENIC SAGITTAL PLANE DEFORMITY IN CHILDREN. Laminectomy for the resection of intradural tumors or surgical management of syringomyelia is the most common cause of sagittal plane deformities of the cervical spine in children (34). Bell et al. (6) found clinically significant kyphotic or hyperlordotic anomalies in 53% of 89 children who had undergone this type of surgery. In their series and in the experience at the University of South Florida, hyperlordosis was more common in young children and was rarely seen in those more than 5 years old. Postlaminectomy kyphosis, on the other hand, may be seen at any age.

The substitution of various forms of laminoplasty instead of laminectomy in the management of children with intradural pathology may have decreased the incidence of postoperative deformity but has not eliminated the problem. Even with complete laminar replacement techniques, deformities develop in many children within 3 to 12 months after surgery. Such deficits appear to occur more commonly among those patients with neurological deficits. In the series of Bell et al. (6), the location and number of levels laminectomized did *not* correlate with the risk for postoperative deformity. In more recent laminoplasty series, similar observations have been made (35,36).

As with all forms of surgery to correct spinal deformity in children, the correction of cervical sagittal plane deformity is problematic. The fusion of growing vertebrae before the pubertal growth spurt is never an ideal solution. However, in the

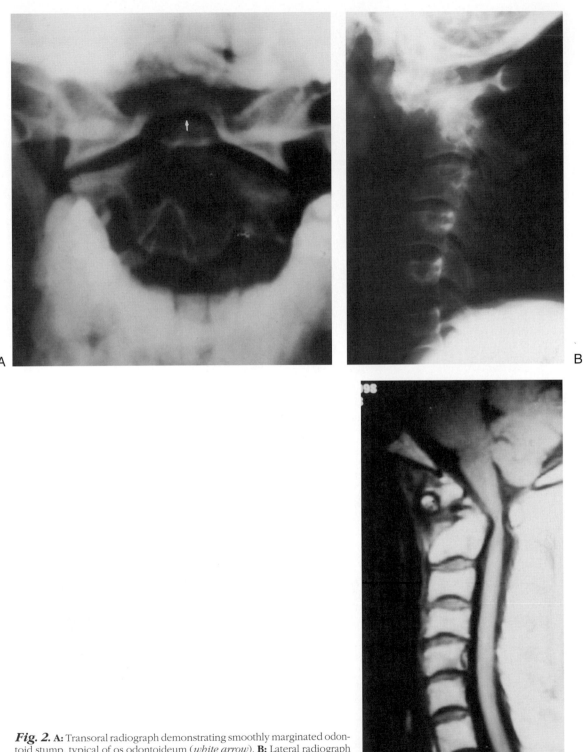

Fig. 2. **A:** Transoral radiograph demonstrating smoothly marginated odontoid stump, typical of os odontoideum (*white arrow*). **B:** Lateral radiograph revealing gross C1-2 dislocation. **C:** Sagittal magnetic resonance imaging (MRI) demonstrates obvious cord compression.

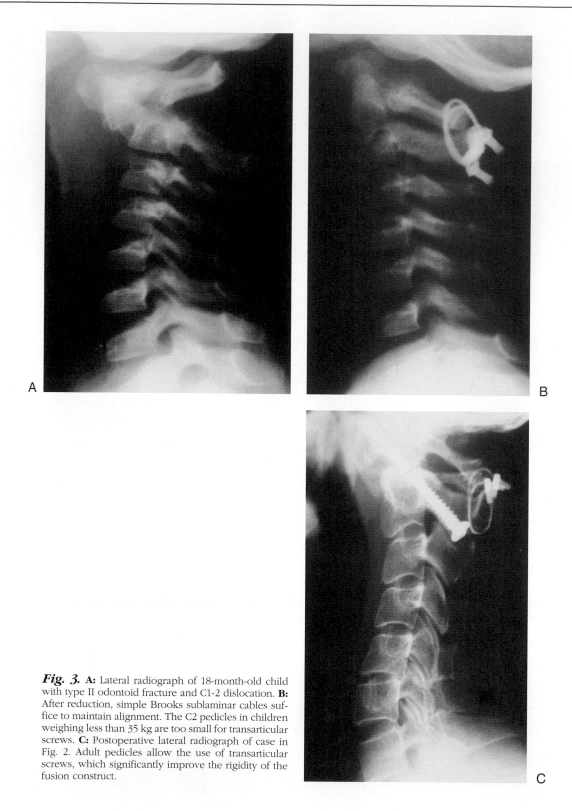

Fig. 3. **A:** Lateral radiograph of 18-month-old child with type II odontoid fracture and C1-2 dislocation. **B:** After reduction, simple Brooks sublaminar cables suffice to maintain alignment. The C2 pedicles in children weighing less than 35 kg are too small for transarticular screws. **C:** Postoperative lateral radiograph of case in Fig. 2. Adult pedicles allow the use of transarticular screws, which significantly improve the rigidity of the fusion construct.

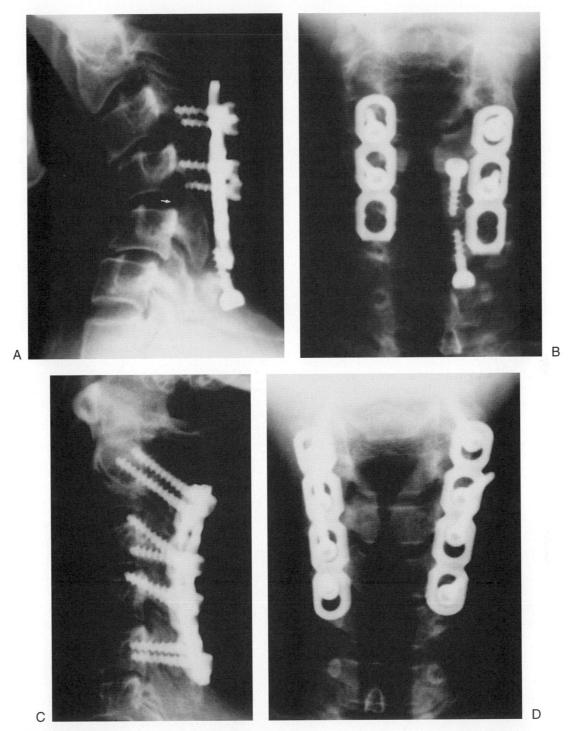

Fig. 4. **A,B:** A 28-year-old woman with kyphotic deformity status post C3-5 laminectomy for resection of ependymoma. Lateral mass plates centered on the wrong side of the pathological axis of rotation (*arrow*) and fixed with very short lateral mass screws have failed. **C,D:** Anteroposterior (AP) and lateral radiographs after repair with C2 pedicle screws and long subaxial lateral mass screws.

absence of any means to reconstruct the motion segment, fusion is usually the only alternative. The goals of fusion are to restore near-normal neutral stance alignment and standing balance without producing iatrogenic deformity and while fusing as few levels as possible. Normal lordotic alignment is far more easily restored in those whose deformity is diagnosed early. Depending on the age and growth rate at the time of original surgery, deformities in existence for more than 3 to 12 months may require anterior and posterior multilevel osteotomies if near-normal alignment is to be restored. Many pediatric surgeons choose *in situ* fusion as a less traumatic alternative. Conversely, deformities caught early can often be corrected with relatively simple short-segment anterior or posterior procedures (Fig. 4).

In either kyphotic or hyperlordotic deformities, preoperative cervical traction is very useful for surgical planning. Deformities that reduce to an acceptable alignment can often be treated with a simple posterior approach and the use of rigid or nonrigid tension band devices. Interspinous cables supplemented with lateral mass rods or plates from intact segment above to intact segment below are usually employed on our services. No bone grafts are placed in prepubertal children. In the absence of any usable posterior elements, lordotic lateral mass rods or plates sometimes suffice. Alternatively, anterior discectomy followed by restorative overdistraction with the use of interbody cages at two or three levels at the apex of the deformity may be effective (37).

The mechanism by which hyperlordosis develops in younger children after laminectomy is unclear. It has been proposed that a potential posterior fusion develops after the laminectomy. If anterior vertebral body growth persisted in the face of this posterior fusion, hyperlordosis would ensue. No data are available to support this theory. If the theory were correct, then no form of posterior fusion procedure would suffice to prevent or correct this deformity. An alternative would be multisegmental anterior discectomy followed by compression with anterior in-

strumentation. We have no experience with this approach. In prepubertal children, such an approach may risk conversion of the hyperlordotic deformity to a kyphosis.

Adult Deformity

SAGITTAL PLANE DEFORMITY IN ADULTS. Like the deformities of children, those of adults can be categorized according to whether they involve the upper cervical segments between the skull and the axis or are predominantly subaxial. This distinction is imprecise and not uniformly applicable but is based on common pathological entities and is convenient. Acute sagittal deformities, as seen in odontoid fractures, subaxial facet dislocations, and destructive lesions of the anterior column such as tumors or infections, are discussed elsewhere in this text. We limit the following discussion to chronic deformities in the sagittal and longitudinal planes.

Among adults, occipitoatlantoaxial deformities are most commonly associated with rheumatoid (or other autoimmune) arthritis, chronic untreated odontoid fractures, or congenital dysplasia of the bony elements of the occipitocervical junction. Subaxial sagittal plane deformity is most often seen as a result of chronic degenerative disc disease and spondylosis. Other causes include trauma (deformity developing after treatment of a burst fracture by closed means) and surgery (deformity developing after multisegmental laminectomy or anterior cervical discectomy without fusion). The typical cervical deformities seen with ankylosing spondylitis and the secondary cervical deformities associated with thoracolumbar scoliosis are discussed elsewhere in this text.

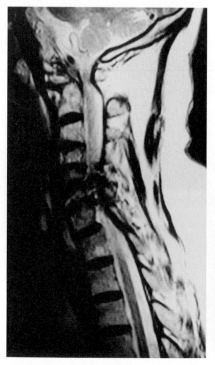
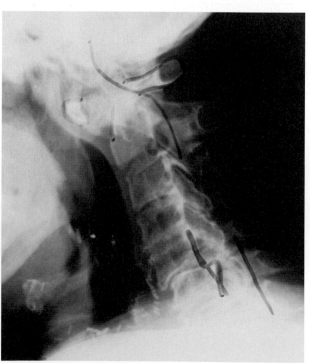

A   B

Fig. 5. Sagittal MRI (**A**) and lateral radiograph (**B**) of 61-year-old woman with psoriatic arthritis; C1-2 instability with anterior subluxation is combined with multisegmental subaxial instability and stenosis. This is a common picture during the middle stages of rheumatoid spondylosis and related conditions.

OCCIPITOATLANTOAXIAL DEFORMITY IN ADULTS.

Rheumatoid arthritis accounts for the majority of cases of occipitocervical junction deformity in most adult practices. Related conditions, such as psoriatic arthritis, often present with the same clinical picture (Fig. 5). In our practice, chronic C1-2 dislocations secondary to undiagnosed odontoid fracture in older patients and os odontoideum in younger adults are also quite common. Less common but not rare are the various forms of congenital bony dysplasias, which may result in sagittal plane deformity secondary to anomalous development of the skull base, atlas, or axis (Fig. 6). Adult cases of Down syndrome are not uncommon.

Although rheumatoid disease is discussed in a dedicated chapter elsewhere in this text, we nonetheless consider it here. The natural history of rheumatoid degeneration of the atlantoaxial complex provides an excellent context for a discussion of the biomechanical requirements for reconstruction after correction of sagittal deformity (38). Many other pathological entities can be corrected with similar techniques.

In rheumatoid disease, the initial pathological movement is usually anterior subluxation of C1 over C2, which occurs when inflammatory dissolution of the alar and transverse odontoid ligaments coupled with erosion of the C1-2 joints has progressed to the point of incompetence (39) (Fig. 5). Chronic pathological movement at the C1-2 junction leads to the formation of pannus, with further encroachment on the spinal canal at C1. An almost identical pathological picture may occur in chronic untreated odontoid fracture. In either case, the surgical management of the problem is straightforward if the condition is caught before the subluxation becomes a fixed malalignment and before longitudinal plane foreshortening ("cranial settling," "telescoping," "basilar invagination") has occurred.

In the absence of gross cord compression and clinical myelopathy, a C1-2 subluxation that reduces spontaneously or in traction may be very satisfactorily treated with simple posterior atlantoaxial fusion (40,41). A successful fusion leads to disappearance of the pannus surrounding the odontoid within 6 to 24 months. In the absence of vertebral artery anomalies, most such cases are anatomically aligned and then fixated by means of Brooks sublaminar cables and Magerl transarticular screws coupled with autologous bone grafts (42,43) (Fig. 3C).

Conversely, a chronic C1-2 subluxation that has become fixed in the malaligned position presents a greater surgical challenge. Regardless of whether the original insult is rheumatoid disease, trauma, Down syndrome, or another condition, a fixed anterior C1 on C2 subluxation entails sagittal imbalance, with a forward shift of the head, sigmoid cord deformation, and *dorsal* spinal canal encroachment by the posterior arch of the atlas. Resection of the C1 arch may provide some relief of cord encroachment but does nothing for the sagittal plane imbalance or cord deformation and may contribute to further instability of the already incompetent motion segment.

In most such cases on our services, a two-stage procedure is performed under a single anesthetic (44). In the first stage, a transoral, transpharyngeal approach is used to resect the anterior arch of the atlas, the dens, and any associated pannus, drill away any anterior fusion mass, and open the C1-2 facets. The patient is then rotated into the prone position (in traction) and realigned by direct traction on the posterior arch of the atlas. This maneuver is followed by sublaminar cable and transarticular screw instrumentation and fusion.

In late-stage rheumatoid disease, the cranium may "settle" across the grossly eroded lateral masses of C1 (45) (Fig. 7). The odontoid process or even the entire atlantoaxial complex may thus penetrate through the foramen magnum. Congenital anomalies, including platybasia, occipitalization of the atlas,

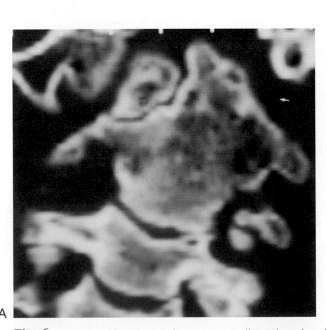
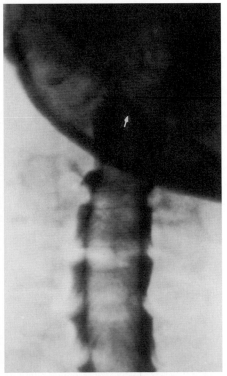

Fig. 6. A 37-year-old woman with severe torticollis and myelopathy secondary to congenital atlantoaxial dysplasia with incomplete hemivertebrae at both C1 and C2. **A:** Coronal computed tomography (CT) demonstrates absence of left side of the atlas (*arrow*) with axial and odontoid deformity. **B:** AP myelogram demonstrates fixed torticollis and cervicomedullary junction block (*arrow*). (*Figure continues.*)

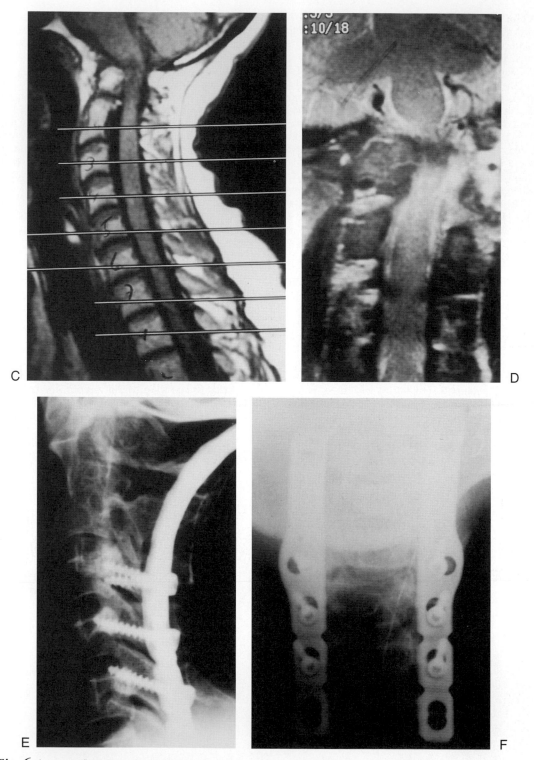

Fig. 6. (continued). **C,D:** Sagittal and coronal MRI documents obvious cord compression. **E,F:** Lateral and AP radiographs after transoral resection of aberrant anterior atlantoaxial elements; iliac strut graft from the clivus to the lower body of C2 and rigid posterior fixation from the occiput to C5. (Anomalous C2 pedicles precluded the use of pedicle screws.) Posterior hardware was removed at 18 months after surgery to restore subaxial motion. Note correction of coronal plane deformity.

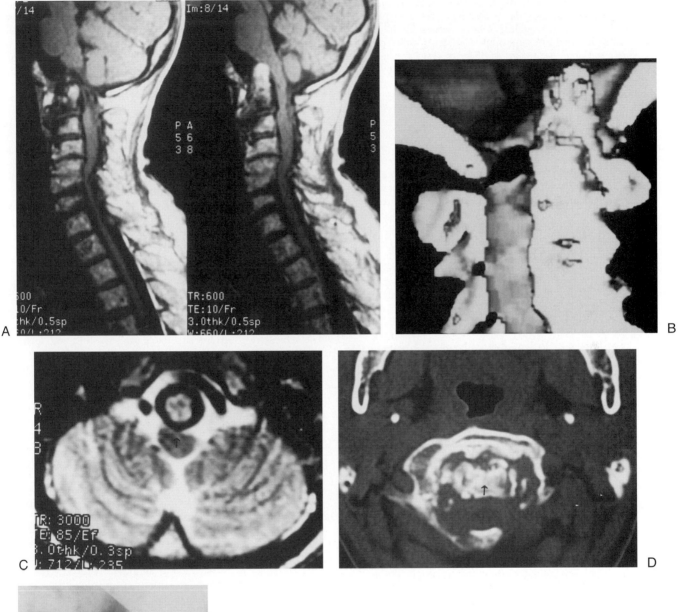

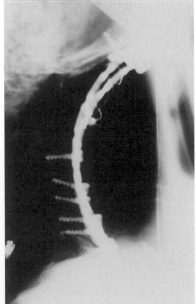

Fig. 7. Late-stage rheumatoid spondylosis in a 69-year-old woman. **A,B:** Sagittal MRI and three-dimensional CT reveal that the entire odontoid process and a large part of the C2 body are within the cranium. Subaxial kyphosis and stenosis are also apparent. **C:** Axial MRI shows distortion of the pontomedullary junction (*arrow*) by the dens. **D:** Axial CT reveals the lower body of C2 (*arrow*) within the C1 ring. **E:** Postoperative film after transpharyngeal resection of the anterior elements of C1 and C2-3 discectomy, clivus-to-C3 strut grafting, subaxial cervical laminectomy, correction of the longitudinal and kyphotic deformities, and rigid fixation of the occiput to T1 with T1 pedicle screws and multiple lateral mass screws.

dysplasia or hypoplasia of the atlas or axis, condylar dysgenesis, and others, may present a similar problem. In such cases, the deformity is no longer "sagittal." It is longitudinal and entails compression or foreshortening of the long axis of the spine. In rheumatoid patients, we make an effort to restore height and decompress the foramen magnum via traction. In many cases, several days of cervical traction will literally pull the odontoid and atlas remnants out of the head. In such cases, no ventral decompression is necessary, but *rigid* posterior occipitocervical instrumentation is mandatory if resettling is to be prevented postoperatively (46,47). Nonrigid techniques may fail in this setting, even when supplemented with rigid external orthoses (Fig. 8).

In rheumatoid patients in whom traction fails to restore height or decompress the foramen magnum, and in most patients with congenital anomalies of the occipitocervical junction, an anterior transpharyngeal procedure is necessary to resect pathological bony elements and pannus that have penetrated the skull and to resect eroded or anomalous anterior and lateral elements of the C1 and C2 vertebrae (48,49). If it is necessary to resect more than half of the C1-2 facets during the anterior procedure, we usually restore a weight-bearing column by means of a structural autologous graft extending from the lower clivus to the body of C2 or C3 (Fig. 6). The anterior procedure is followed by the same rigid posterior occipitocervical instrumentation mentioned above.

In the performance of rigid occipitocervical instrumentation, several anatomical details must be borne in mind (50) (Fig. 9). First, it must be noted that the suboccipital bone is usually of inadequate thickness to provide adequate screw purchase anywhere except in the midline. Second, we have found that lateral mass screws are often unable to resist the forces placed on them in such constructs, even when many are applied. The subaxial cervical lateral mass provides only 6 to 8 mm of purchase, even when the Magerl technique is used. Therefore, we usually fixate the cervical end of occipitocervical constructs with long, 4.0-mm C2 pars screws or C1-2 transarticular screws if the anatomy allows. Fixation to the C7 or T1 pedicles also works well if a longer construct is warranted. On our services, such constructs usually entail the use of custom-made devices. Rigid fixation may allow the correction of multiplanar deformities in cases of complex bony anomalies.

Successful sagittal plane restoration of the occipitocervical junction requires translation of the skull back into the center of balance of the spine at hand. Overall spinal alignment and subaxial cervical and thoracolumbar deformity must be considered in preoperative surgical planning. Posterior translation of the skull to restore perfect occiput-to-axis alignment would be counterproductive in the face of a subaxial hyperlordosis or swan-neck deformity. Anterior translation of the atlas in reference to the axis for the correction of chronic posterior odontoid subluxation may be counterproductive in the face of subaxial kyphosis. Overall balance is the key to success in the management of cervical deformity, just as in the management of deformity in other regions of the spine (51).

SUBAXIAL DEFORMITY IN ADULTS. No general agreement has been reached regarding the stage at which the loss of subaxial cervical lordosis becomes a clinical concern. Without doubt, many persons in the general population remain blissfully asymptomatic and unaware of their straight or frankly kyphotic cervical geometry. Conversely, many others suffer chronic neck pain with the same geometry. Although hard data are lacking, there can be little doubt that "bowstringing" the cord in a kyphotic, stenotic cervical canal may contribute to progressive myelopathy.

If we exclude the acute pathological processes mentioned above, most of the remaining subaxial sagittal deformities seen in adults are caused by chronic spondylosis with disc space collapse, facet degeneration, stenosis, and secondary loss of lordosis. Spondylolisthesis with anterior or posterior slip is commonly associated. Overall sagittal alignment may be straight, kyphotic, or doubly curved in a swan-neck deformity.

In a lesser number of cases, loss of lordosis may follow anterior or posterior surgical procedures. Deformity may follow laminectomy, anterior discectomy without fusion, or anterior discectomy and fusion complicated by graft resorption or extrusion (52,53). In many, if not most, such iatrogenic cases, the beginning of the deformity was evident before the surgery and progressed thereafter secondary to further destabilization inherent in the decompressive procedure. Unfortunately, many such cases are caught late after further degenerative change, ossification of ligaments, and partial autofusion have fixed the deformity in a rigid state (Fig. 10).

Regardless of the cause of the malalignment, the preoperative evaluation of such patients must include studies to evaluate cord and root compression on the one hand, and cervical alignment and motion on the other. In most cases, this means cervical magnetic resonance imaging (MRI) and simple flexion/extension dynamic radiography. In some circumstances, intrathecally enhanced computed tomography (CT) or dynamic MRI may be necessary to appreciate the pathology fully and plan the repair.

In cases in which a nearly normal lordotic posture is found on preoperative standing, extension, or supine neutral films, a single approach, either anterior or posterior, is feasible. The decision regarding which approach to use should be guided by the requirements for satisfactory decompression of the neural elements, the minimum number of segments that must be fused to be reasonably certain of postural correction, and any previous surgical procedures. Generally, posterior procedures are associated with more postsurgical pain and a slightly higher risk for cord injury, whereas anterior procedures are associated with a higher risk for chronic dysphagia or dysphonia. The choice must be individualized.

In cases of symptomatic loss of lordosis, kyphosis, or double-curve deformity in which the deformity never corrects on preoperative dynamic radiographs, a decision must be rendered regarding what an acceptable alignment may be. For many older patients who come to surgery for myelopathy, a straight or even slightly kyphotic alignment may be quite satisfactory. If a successful fusion is obtained, most will never complain of cervicalgia after surgery. On the other hand, most young people and those older patients in whom neck pain is a significant preoperative problem often continue to have pain after surgery, even with a successful fusion, if some lordosis is not reestablished.

Currently on our services, laminoplasty is usually substituted for laminectomy in patients under 50 years of age (54). In those older than 50, elective laminectomy is always accompanied by lateral mass fusion with lordotic rods or plates. In both age groups, anterior cervical discectomy or corpectomy is always reconstructed by means of rigid distraction cages stabilized with buttress plates. Since instituting these techniques, we have largely (but not completely) eliminated the problem of iatrogenic postsurgical kyphosis after elective first surgeries.

In patients with rigid, nonflexible deformities in whom sagittal imbalance and pain must be addressed, a 360-degree or 540-degree surgical approach is often needed (Figs. 10 and 11). Collapse and autofusion of the discs is often accompanied by autofusion of the facets; hence, anterior and posterior osteotomies are often necessary before corrective measures can be

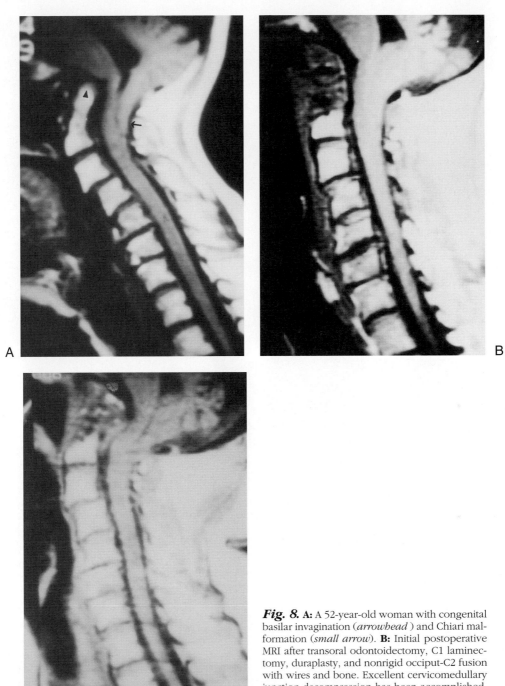

Fig. 8. **A:** A 52-year-old woman with congenital basilar invagination (*arrowhead*) and Chiari malformation (*small arrow*). **B:** Initial postoperative MRI after transoral odontoidectomy, C1 laminectomy, duraplasty, and nonrigid occiput-C2 fusion with wires and bone. Excellent cervicomedullary junction decompression has been accomplished. **C:** MRI 6 months later reveals recurrent cranial settling and cervicomedullary compression despite wire and bone fusion and 3 months in a halo orthosis after surgery. Rigid fixation devices prevent this complication.

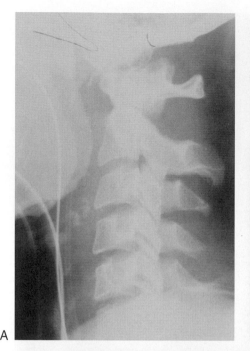
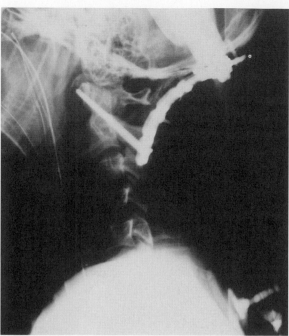

A

B

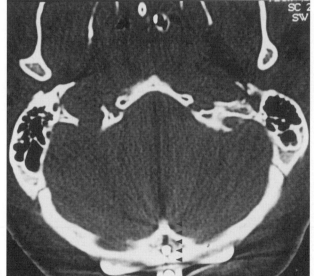

C

Fig. 9. An 18-year-old man with atlanto-occipital dislocation. **A:** Initial lateral radiograph demonstrating obvious dislocation. **B:** Postoperative radiograph after rigid fixation with occipital "T plate" and C1-2 transarticular screws. Halo ring that had been used for initial closed reduction and stabilization was removed after surgery. **C:** Axial CT through subocciput reveals that the midline occipital crest is the *only* part of the occipital bone that is consistently thick enough to hold highly stressed screws (*arrowheads*). **D:** Sequential coronal CT through C1 and C2 demonstrating deep purchase of transarticular screws.

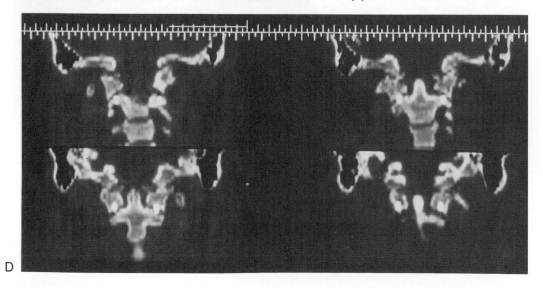

D

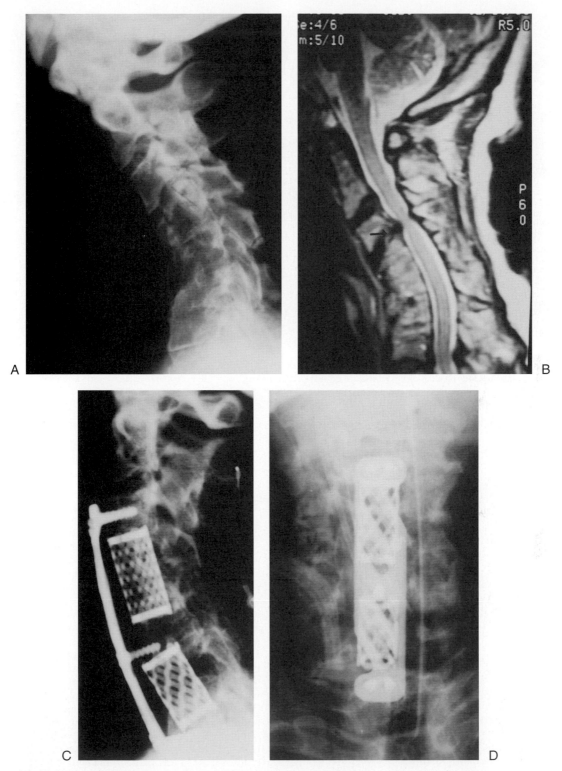

Fig. 10. A 35-year-old man 8 years after three-level anterior discectomy without fusion. **A:** Lateral radiograph reveals rigid 45-degree kyphotic deformity. **B:** Sagittal MRI demonstrates solid fusion mass through kyphosis and next segment failure (*arrow*) with C3-4 stenosis and cord compression. **C,D:** Postoperative radiographs after 540-degree correction. Initial facet subtraction laminectomy was followed by nonsequential corpectomies taken through the fused transverse foramina; anterior distraction and fusion with nonsequential cages and anterior plate were followed by posterior cable tension band to complete lordotic restoration.

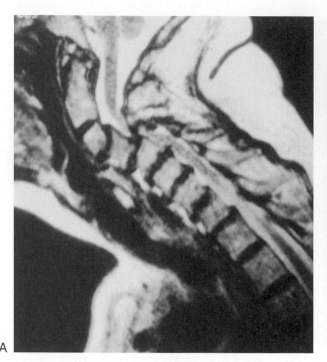

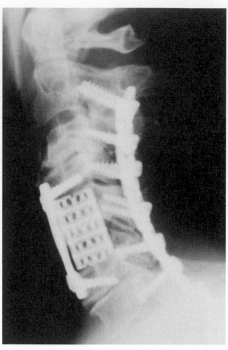

A   B

Fig. 11. A 67-year-old man with swan-neck deformity secondary to severe degenerative spondylosis. **A:** Lateral radiograph demonstrates double-curve deformity and severe multilevel stenosis. **B:** Postoperative radiograph after 360-degree procedure consisting of corpectomies of C5 and C6, followed by distraction and reconstruction with local bone in a cage and an anterior plate, followed by C3 to C7 laminectomy and restoration of near-normal lordosis with posterior plates.

applied to restore lordosis. In most cases, anterior osteotomy entails multisegmental discectomy or corpectomy. Not uncommonly, spontaneous or surgical fusion bone extends to the transverse processes; therefore, anterior resection must include the anterior and medial margins of the transverse foramina. This is easily accomplished, although care must be taken to protect the vertebral arteries and nerve root sheaths. In such cases, posterior osteotomy usually entails resection of the entire lateral masses of one, two, or three levels to restore intersegmental mobility and allow dorsal tension banding to restore lordosis.

We usually approach such cases in a stepwise fashion. The patients are placed in a prone position in traction so that the lateral mass resections (dorsal extension osteotomies) can be performed first. An interspinous cable or lordotic rods are then placed to assess the degree of correction now possible *if* no large ventral osteophytes or disc herniations are present. If significant ventral pathology is noted, no effort at correction is made at this stage. If correction is not possible because of anterior collapse with fusion *or* if significant ventral canal encroachment is present, the patient is closed and rotated to a supine position (still in traction). Anterior decompression and osteotomy are now accomplished (55). At this point, interbody distraction allows correction of anterior height. Two or three sequential interbody cages are used to maintain height. The cages (filled with autologous bone from the corpectomy) are fixed with *nonrigid* anterior buttress plates. The patient is then rotated to a prone position once again and reopened, and the final posterior fixation and bone graft are applied. Nearly anatomical alignment can be restored in many cases by means of these techniques, which have proved less traumatic for the patients than may be first imagined.

Technical Tips

In the correction of sagittal plane deformity in the subaxial spine, hardware limitations should be carefully considered. For anterior approaches, one should recall that the fusion failure rate is proportional to the number of fusion surfaces (56). Corpectomy struts fail less often than multisegmental discectomy grafts (57). We prefer to use cages rather than structural grafts in most cases. Cages eliminate the need for distant graft harvest, are more rigid and less likely to extrude or collapse than structural grafts, and are infinitely malleable to the requirements of a given case. We have also found that rigid anterior cervical plates are often counterproductive. In anterior-only procedures, we usually prefer dynamic anterior cervical plates or rods, which allow the cage to bear the weight without stress shielding (Fig. 12). We never use an anterior plate or rod fixated only at its terminal ends in constructs extending more than three motion segments (four vertebrae) unless a posterior fixation is also planned. In long-segment, anterior-only cases, a caudal end buttress plate is less likely to fail (Fig. 13).

In posterior subaxial constructs, the relative impotence of lateral mass screws must be remembered (58,59). If significant lordotic force is to be applied over lateral mass plates or rods, several tricks can be used to decrease the risk for screw failure. If the laminae and spinous processes are present, an interspinous cable greatly facilitates lordotic maneuvers and decreases the risk for terminal screw pullout on the lateral mass device. In the absence of suitable posterior elements, pedicle screws used in place of lateral mass screws at the terminal ends of the construct are far stronger and resistant to pullout (60–62). The C2 and T1 pedicles can usually be cannulated with 4.0- or

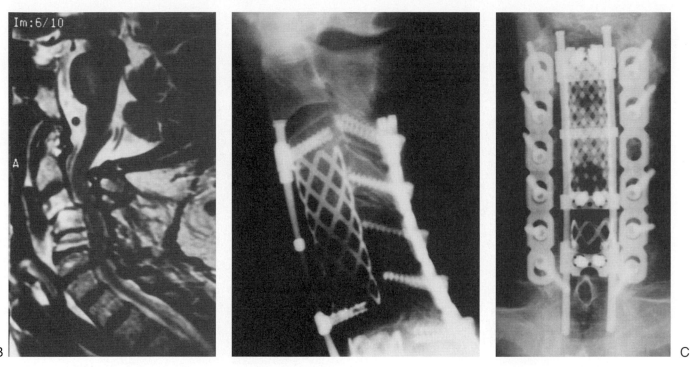

Fig. 12. **A:** Sagittal MRI reveals severe kyphotic deformity and cord compression. **B,C:** AP and lateral radiographs after C4 and C5 corpectomies, C6-7 discectomy, and anterior reconstruction with two cages stabilized by dynamic anterior rod device. This was followed immediately by laminectomy and posterior plate fixation. Note that despite cages and posterior plates, the anterior rod device is maximally compressed, even at 3 days after surgery. Rigid anterior plates do not prevent this phenomenon.

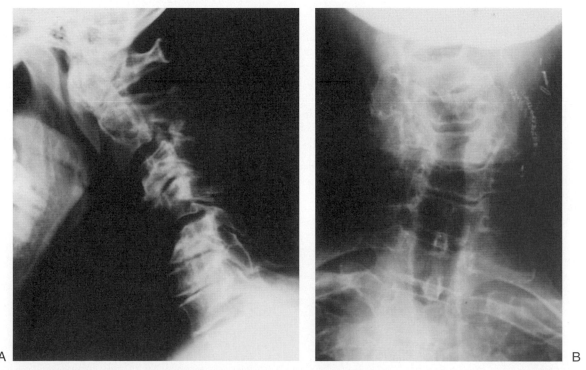

Fig. 13. **A,B:** AP and lateral radiographs demonstrate severe kyphotic and scoliotic deformities secondary to degenerative spondylosis in this 72-year-old woman. (*Figure continues.*)

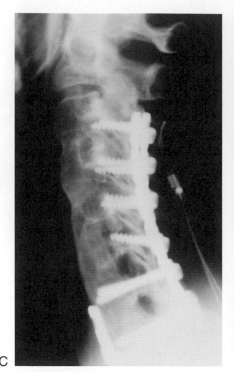
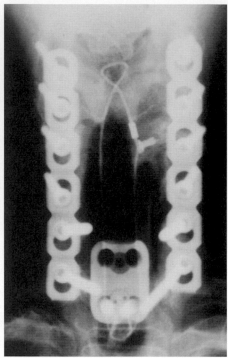

C

D

Fig. 13. (continued). **C,D:** Five-year postsurgical films after C4, C5, and C6 corpectomies and anterior reconstruction with an autologous iliac strut stabilized with a caudal "kick plate" followed by laminectomy and posterior lordotic plates and cable tension band. Note correction of deformity in both planes. We never use anterior cervical plates over more than three disc levels without a point of interval fixation.

4.5-mm screws. The C7 pedicles will accept 3.5-mm screws in many cases. The subaxial pedicles at C3 through C6 are usually too small to accept even 3.5-mm screws but can be used occasionally. Direct visualization of the pedicles after laminectomy makes this process a good deal more accurate.

Conclusions

The ability to correct fixed alignment in the cervical spine has been greatly facilitated by modern hardware. Unfortunately, *fixed* correction is still the best we can do. The restoration of motion and hence function remains only a goal. For many patients with sagittal plane deformity, the best therapy would have been prevention. Decompressive laminectomy and anterior discectomy without fusion may be procedures whose time has past. Similarly, rheumatoid patients should undergo fusion long before cranial settling and basilar invagination are allowed to transpire. No child or adult with os odontoideum should ever be allowed to suffer a neurological injury.

Although far from ideal, current technology has made possible significantly improved management strategies for most patients with existing or potential sagittal deformities. Biomechanically informed surgery may minimize or delay the progression of deformity, reduce the number of motion segments that must be fused, and prevent avoidable neurological injuries.

References

1. Saito T, Yamamuro T, Shikata J, et al. Analysis and prevention of spinal column deformity following cervical laminectomy. I. Patho-

genic analysis of postlaminectomy deformities. *Spine* 1991;16: 494–502.
2. Guigui P, Benoist M, Deburge A. Spinal deformity after multilevel cervical laminectomy for spondylotic myelopathy. *Spine* 1998;23: 440–447.
3. Cusick JF, Pintar FA, Yoganandan N. Biomechanical alterations induced by multilevel cervical laminectomy. *Spine* 1995;20: 2392–2398.
4. Mikawa Y, Shikata J, Yamamuro T. Spinal deformity and instability after multilevel cervical laminectomy. *Spine* 1987;12:6–11.
5. Albert TJ, Vaccuro A. Postlaminectomy kyphosis. *Spine* 1998;23: 2738–2745.
6. Bell DF, Walker JL, O'Conner G, et al. Spinal deformity after multiple-level cervical laminectomy in children. *Spine* 1994;19:406–411.
7. Isu T, Miyasaka K, Abe H, et al. Atlantoaxial dislocation associated with neurofibromatosis. Report of three cases. *J Neurosurg* 1983;58: 451–453.
8. Herman MJ, Pizzutillo PD. Cervical spine disorders in children. *Orthop Clin North Am* 1999;30:457–466.
9. Tandon V, Williamson JB, Cowie RA, et al. Spinal problems in mucopolysaccharidosis I (Hurler's syndrome). *J Bone Joint Surg Br* 1996; 78:938–944.
10. McLaughlin MR, Wahlig JB, Pollack IF. Incidence of postlaminectomy kyphosis after Chiari decompression. *Spine* 1997;22:613–617.
11. Nakagawa T, Yone K, Sakou T, et al. Occipitocervical fusion with C1 laminectomy in children. *Spine* 1997;22:1209–1214.
12. Menenzes AH, Ryken TC. Craniovertebral abnormalities in Down's syndrome. *Pediatr Neurosurg* 1992;18:24–33.
13. Pueschel SM, Scola FH, Tupper TB, et al. Skeletal abnormalities of the upper cervical spine in children with Down's syndrome. *J Pediatr Orthop* 1990;10:607–611.
14. VanDyke DC, Gahagan CA. Down syndrome. Cervical spine abnormalities and problems. *Clin Pediatr* 1988;27:415–418.
15. Pueschel SM, Scola FH. Atlantoaxial instability in individuals with Down syndrome: epidemiologic, radiographic, and clinical studies. *Pediatrics* 1987;80:555–560.
16. Pueschel SM, Scola FH, Pezzullo JC. A longitudinal study of atlanto-

dens relationships in asymptomatic individuals with Down's syndrome. *Pediatrics* 1992;89(6 Pt 2):1194–1198.

17. Berdon WE. Lateral cervical spine films in Down's syndrome. *Pediatr Radiol* 1996;26:748.

18. Uno K, Kataoka O, Shiba R. Occipitoatlantal and occipitoaxial hypermobility in Down's syndrome. *Spine* 1996;21:1430–1434.

19. Cremers MJ, Bol E, deRoos F, et al. Risk of sports activities in children with Down's syndrome and atlantoaxial instability. *Lancet* 1983;342: 511–514.

20. Brockmeyer D. Down syndrome and craniovertebral instability. Topic review and treatment recommendations. *Pediatr Neurosurg* 1999;31:71–77.

21. American Academy of Pediatrics. Atlantoaxial instability in Down's syndrome: subject review. An American Academy of Pediatrics report on sports medicine and fitness. *Pediatrics* 1995;96(1 Pt 1): 151–154.

22. Parfenchuck TA, Bertrand SL, Powers MJ, et al. Posterior occipitoatlantal hypermobility in Down syndrome: an analysis of 199 patients. *J Pediatr Orthop* 1994;14:304–308.

23. Gabriel KR, Mason DE, Carnago P. Occipito-atlantal translation in Down's syndrome. *Spine* 1990;15:997–1002.

24. Doyle JS, Laurman WC, Wood KB, et al. Complications and long-term outcome of upper cervical spine arthrodesis in children with Down's syndrome. *Spine* 1996;21:1223–1231.

25. Rizzolo S, Lemos MJ, Mason DE. Posterior spinal arthrodesis for atlantoaxial instability in Down syndrome. *J Pediatr Orthop* 1995; 15:543–548.

26. Ducker TB. Os odontoideum. *J Spinal Disord* 1993;6:364–365.

27. Nagashima C. Atlantoaxial dislocation due to agenesis of the os odontoideum or odontoid process. *J Neurosurg* 1970;33:270–280.

28. Smith MD, Phillips WA, Hensinger RN. Fusion of the upper cervical spine in children and adolescents. An analysis of 17 patients. *Spine* 1991;16:695–701.

29. Brockmeyer DL, York JE, Apfelbaum RI. Anatomical suitability of C1-2 transarticular screw placement in the pediatric patient. *J Neurosurg* 2000;92(1 suppl):7–11.

30. Brockmeyer D, Apfelbaum R, Tippets R, et al. Pediatric cervical spine instrumentation using screw fixation. *Pediatr Neurosurg* 1995; 22:147–157.

31. Wang J, Vokshoor A, Kim S, et al. Pediatric atlantoaxial instability: management with screw fixation. *Pediatr Neurosurg* 1999;30:70–78.

32. Wright NM, Lauryssen C. Vertebral artery injury in C1-2 transarticular screw fixation: results of a survey of the AANS/CNS section on disorders of the spine and peripheral nerves. *J Neurosurg* 1998;88: 634–640.

33. Hacker RJ. Screw fixation for odontoid fracture: a comparison of the anterior and posterior technique. *Nebr Med J* 1996;81:275–288.

34. Inoue A, Ikata T, Katoh S. Spinal deformity following surgery for spinal cord tumors and tumorous lesions: analysis based on an assessment of the spinal functional curve. *Spinal Cord* 1996;34: 536–542.

35. Nowinski GP, Visarius H, Nolte LP, et al. A biomechanical comparison of cervical laminoplasty and cervical laminectomy with progressive facetectomy. *Spine* 1993;18:1995–2004.

36. Sasai K, Saito T, Akagi S, et al. Cervical curvature after laminoplasty for spondylotic myelopathy—involvement of yellow ligament, semispinalis cervicis muscle, and nuchal ligament. *J Spinal Disord* 2000;13:26–30.

37. Toyama Y, Matsumoto M, Chiba K, et al. Realignment of posterior cervical kyphosis in children by vertebral remodeling. *Spine* 1994; 19:2565–2570.

38. Sherk HH. Atlantoaxial instability and acquired basilar invagination in rheumatoid arthritis. *Orthop Clin North Am* 1978;9:1053–1063.

39. Puttlitz CM, Goel VK, Clark CR, et al. Biomechanical rationale for the pathology of rheumatoid arthritis in the craniovertebral junction. *Spine* 2000;25:1607–1616.

40. Larsson SE, Toolanen G. Posterior fusion for atlanto-axial subluxation in rheumatoid arthritis. *Spine* 1986;11:525–530.

41. Grob D, Wursch R, Grauer W, et al. Atlantoaxial fusion and retrodental pannus in rheumatoid arthritis. *Spine* 1997;79:197–203.

42. Eleraky MA, Masferrer R, Sonntag VK. Posterior atlantoaxial screw fixation in rheumatoid arthritis. *J Neurosurg* 1998;89:8–12.

43. Paramore CG, Dickman CA, Sonntag VK. The anatomical suitability of the C1-2 complex for transarticular screw fixation. *J Neurosurg* 1996;85:221–224.

44. Crockard HA, Calder I, Ransford AO. One-stage transoral decompression and posterior fixation in rheumatoid arthritis. *J Bone Joint Surg Br* 1990;72:682–685.

45. Menezes AH, VanGilder JC, Clark CR, et al. Odontoid upward migration in rheumatoid arthritis. An analysis of 45 patients with "cranial settling." *J Neurosurg* 1985;63:500–509.

46. Pait TG, Al-Mefty O, Boop FA, et al. Inside-outside technique for posterior occipitocervical spine instrumentation and stabilization: preliminary results. *J Neurosurg* 1999;90(1 suppl):1–7.

47. Hurlbert RJ, Crawford NR, Choi WG, et al. A biomechanical evaluation of occipitocervical instrumentation: screw constructs and wire fixation. *J Neurosurg* 1999;90(1 suppl):84–90.

48. Crockard HA, Pozo JL, Ransford AO, et al. Transoral decompression and posterior fusion for rheumatoid atlanto-axial instability. *J Bone Joint Surg Br* 1986;68:350–356.

49. Dickman CA, Locantro J, Fessler RG. The influence of transoral odontoid resection on stability of the craniovertebral junction. *J Neurosurg* 1992;77:525–530.

50. Vale FL, Oliver M, Cahill DW. Rigid occipitocervical fusion. *J Neurosurg* 1999;91(2 suppl):144–150.

51. Stanley D, Laing RJ, Forster MC, et al. Posterior decompression and fusion in rheumatoid disease of the cervical spine: redressing the balance. *J Spinal Disord* 1994;7:439–443.

52. Johnson CE 2nd. Post-laminectomy kyphoscoliosis following surgical treatment for spinal cord astrocytoma. *Orthopedics* 1986;9: 587–594.

53. Lonstein JE. Post-laminectomy kyphosis. *Clin Orthop* 1977;Oct: 93–100.

54. Matsunaga S, Sakou T, Nakanisi K. Analysis of the cervical spine following laminoplasty and laminectomy. *Spinal Cord* 1999;37: 20–24.

55. McMaster MJ. Osteotomy of the cervical spine in ankylosing spondylitis. *J Bone Joint Surg Br* 1997;79:197–203.

56. Swank ML, Lowery GL, Bhat AL, et al. Anterior cervical allograft arthrodesis and instrumentation: multilevel interbody grafting or strut graft reconstruction. *Eur Spine J* 1997;6:138–143.

57. Eleraky MA, Llanos C, Sonntag VK. Cervical corpectomy: report of 185 cases and review of the literature. *J Neurosurg* 1999;90(1 suppl): 35–41.

58. Swank ML, Sutterlin CE 3rd, Bossons CR, et al. Rigid internal fixation with lateral mass plates in multilevel anterior and posterior reconstruction of the cervical spine. *Spine* 1997;22:274–282.

59. Seybold EA, Baker JA, Criscitello AA, et al. Characteristics of unicortical and bicortical lateral mass screws in the cervical spine. *Spine* 1999;24:2397–2403.

60. Kotani Y, Cunningham BW, Abumi K, et al. Biomechanical analysis of cervical stabilization systems. An assessment of transpedicular screw fixation in the cervical spine. *Spine* 1994;19:2529–2539.

61. Ludwig SC, Kramer DL, Vaccaro AR, et al. Transpedicle screw fixation of the cervical spine. *Clin Orthop* 1999;Feb:77–88.

62. Jones EL, Heller JG, Silcox DH, et al. Cervical pedicle screw versus lateral mass screws. Anatomic feasibility and biomechanical comparison. *Spine* 1997;22:977–982.

178. Sagittal Plane Deformity of the Thoracic Spine

Robert F. Heary and Christopher M. Bono

The thoracic spine is a common region for sagittal plane deformity. Various processes can cause either lordotic or kyphotic angulation. The etiology can be idiopathic, such as Scheuermann's kyphosis, or iatrogenic as in postlaminectomy kyphosis. Prevention is disease specific and is usually limited to early diagnosis. The treatment, both operative and nonsurgical, is determined by several factors, including the likelihood of progression, the degree of deformity, and functional impairment. Nonoperative treatment usually involves careful observation and/or judicious use of braces. For operative management, a rationale based on sound biomechanical principles of deformity correction is crucial. Particularly in the thoracic spine, specific anatomical limitations such as the rib cage and the great vessels as well as the severity of the curve will determine the best operative approach. Although various methods exist, selection of the appropriate fusion levels and techniques of stabilization is vital to achieve a mechanically balanced thoracic spine without compromising neurological function.

Etiology and Epidemiology

Congenital spinal deformities are rare. Curve direction is dependent on the location of the vertebral anomaly. Posterior defects, such as a hemivertebra, lead to disproportionately greater posterior versus anterior growth resulting in a hyperkyphosis (1). Similarly, anterior defects can result in hypokyphotic (lordotic) patterns (2). Congenital curvatures are caused by defects of either segmentation or formation and may be either kyphotic or lordotic. In general, defects in segmentation cause round or "smooth" deformities, while defects in formation more commonly result in a sharp angulatory gibbus (Fig. 1). Congenital lordosis is the most progressive, but the least common, congenital spinal deformity (2). It usually occurs secondary to a failure of formation and can lead to life-threatening pulmonary compromise if left untreated. Kyphosis is the second most common congenital thoracic deformity and it is more frequently caused by a defect in segmentation. Such defects lead to a round-back deformity that tends to progress slowly. Less frequently, congenital kyphosis is a result of failure in formation that causes a kyphotic gibbus. Kyphotic gibbi are significantly more progressive and have the highest incidence of paraplegia among spinal deformities (3).

Occurring in adolescents and young adults, Scheuermann's disease is characterized by progressive hyperkyphosis. The prevalence has been documented to be between 0.4% and 8.3%, with a two to one predisposition for males. In most congenital deformities, Scheuermann's kyphosis creates longer radius curves that extend over multiple segments (4). By definition, a minimum of 5 degrees or more of angular kyphosis is present in at least three consecutive vertebral levels (5). Though the specific etiology remains unknown, several investigators have hypothesized both biochemical and mechanical mechanisms. Metabolic influences, such as vitamin deficiency and malnutrition as well as abnormal levels of growth hormone, have been suggested (6). Bradford et al. (7) suggested that abnormal stresses along the anterior longitudinal ligament might cause pathological thickening leading to a bowstring effect of the thoracic spine. Others have postulated that microinjuries to the vertebral body growth plate lead to diminished anterior spinal growth (8–10).

Sagittal thoracic deformities can occur as the sequelae of commonly performed spinal procedures. By destabilizing the posterior elements, postlaminectomy kyphosis can result from an overly aggressive decompression. Deformity is more likely in younger patients and is more frequent in cephalad- versus caudad-level surgery (11). Yasouka and associates (11) suggested that in patients younger than 15 years of age, posterior destabilization may place large compressive forces on the anterior column that may have an inhibitory effect on the remaining growth potential of the vertebral apophyses. In support of this suggestion, Tachdjian and Matson (12) reported postoperative kyphosis in 26% of children after decompressive laminectomy for spinal tumor resection. Flat-back syndrome, depicted by pain associated with an iatrogenic diminution of the physiological sagittal spinal curvature, is a recognized complication of distractive instrumentation used to correct scoliotic deformities in the thoracic spine. Radiographic flattening of the thoracic or lumbar spine is present in 6% to 40% of cases after correction of scoliotic deformity (13,14).

Thoracic sagittal deformity is caused by numerous other etiologies. Kyphosis may develop in 10% to 100% of cases of spinal tumors treated with irradiation (15). Ninety percent of thoracic spinal trauma involves compression of the anterior column, which has a predisposition for kyphotic deformity (16). Kyphotic deformities occur in nearly all cases of unstable thoracic spine fractures and may be potentiated by spinal fusions that do not span an adequate number of vertebral motion segments (17). Ankylosing spondylitis is the most common cause of kyphosis secondary to inflammatory disease (6). In the elderly, uncontrolled osteoporosis predisposes patients to low-energy

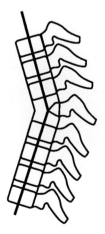

Fig. 1. A sharp angulatory gibbus is more common in congenital kyphosis secondary to failure of formation. Smoother "round-back" curves are indicative of defects in vertebral segmentation. (© 2002, Thomas H. Weinzerl.)

compression fractures, which commonly lead to thoracic round-back deformity.

Prevention

Prevention, when possible, is directed by the etiology of the disease. In most cases, early diagnosis is the primary means of prevention. Genetic counseling can be of benefit for specific congenital deformities with proposed hereditary patterns (18). More importantly, maternal folate intake prior to conception decreases the chance of congenital neural tube defects (19). Prenatal screening, including alpha-fetoprotein levels and ultrasound, is important in the early detection of spinal deformities such as myelomeningocele. In the infant, congenital spinal defects must be suspected when other anomalies are present. Genitourinary and cardiac malformations, present in 20% and 12% of patients, respectively, are among the most common anomalies in children with congenital spinal disorders.

Early diagnosis of Scheuermann's disease is helpful in preventing progression of a spinal curvature that, if undetected, may no longer be amenable to nonoperative measures. Postirradiation kyphosis is best prevented by exclusion of the spine from the radiation field (20). Though inevitable with the treatment of intraspinal tumors, it may be avoidable by careful planning when treating neoplastic disease of extravertebral structures.

Postlaminectomy kyphosis can be prevented or minimized by maintaining 50% of the facet joint integrity in nonfused cases (21). In children, deformity may develop as late as 6 years postoperatively. This necessitates meticulous long-term radiographic follow-up (12). Postoperative deformity may also occur secondary to either a failed arthrodesis or incorrect selection of fusion levels (17,22).

Biomechanical Principles

The thoracic spine normally has an average of 30 degrees of kyphosis, with an approximate range of 20 to 40 degrees (23). The apex of the normal thoracic curvature is at the level of the T6 or T7 vertebra. Normal kyphosis is produced primarily from anterior wedging of the vertebral bodies. Thus, anterior and posterior disc height should be comparable. In the thoracic spine, the facet joints are situated vertically midway between the coronal and sagittal planes, facilitating sagittal motion while limiting axial rotation (24). The rib cage is an integral component in the stability of the thoracic spine, providing an additional restraint to axial motion via costovertebral junctions (25).

In 1983, Denis (16) first described the three-column theory of stability for the thoracic and lumbar spines. In this theory, the anterior column consists of the anterior longitudinal ligament (ALL) and the anterior aspect of the vertebral body and disc. The middle column consists of the posterior longitudinal ligament (PLL) and the posterior aspect of the vertebral body and disc. The posterior bony neural arch, including the posterior ligamentous complex, is the posterior column. In the thoracic spine, the ribs articulate with the posterior vertebral body and transverse processes, thus adding stability to the middle and posterior elements. Disruption of any two of these columns implies mechanical instability (16).

The instantaneous axis of rotation (IAR) is the point about which the spine rotates in a specific plane of motion. Haher et

al. (26) investigated the location of the IAR with respect to the three columns of the spine. With flexion in an intact spine, the IAR is located at the anterior aspect of the disc, with compressive forces being transmitted in the anterior column and distractive forces posteriorly. In extension, the IAR is located at the posterior aspect of the disc, producing compressive forces in the middle column and distractive anterior vectors. Posterior instrumentation and lordogenic curves shift the IAR posteriorly. Likewise, the IAR migrates anteriorly with anterior instrumentation and kyphogenic curves.

The normal thoracic spine maintains sagittal balance. This can be assessed on a full-length lateral radiograph by dropping a plumb line from the seventh cervical vertebral body. Balance is realized if the line lies within 1 cm of the sacral promontory caudally (Fig. 2). Mechanically, this ensures that the weight borne by the spine is acting to maintain its anteroposterior position within space. Focal hyperkyphotic segments may be balanced by hyperlordosis in other segments. For example, a hyperkyphotic deformity of the thoracic spine may shift the weight-bearing line anteriorly. Therefore, sagittal balance can be preserved with a compensatory increase of lumbar lordosis, shifting the weight-bearing line back to the sacral promontory.

Deformity can progress past the point at which compensatory balance can be maintained. The weight-bearing line can no longer return to its stable position. This can result in a self-propagating sagittal imbalance. Corrective measures in deformity treatment attempt to restore the weight-bearing line to the anatomical axis. To illustrate this, one can compare a hyperkyphotic spine to the leaning tower of Pisa, Italy. The center of mass of the tower (spine) functions to maintain the vertical axis because the sum of the forces acting downward is within the axis of rotation at the base (sacrum). As the tower leans more,

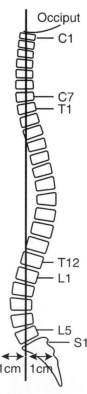

Fig. 2. Balance is realized if the line lies within 1 cm of the sacral promontory caudally. (© 2002, Thomas H. Weinzerl.)

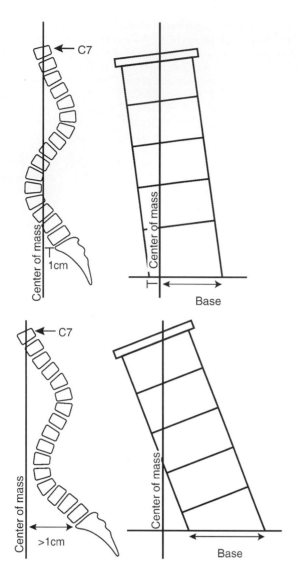

Fig. 3. To illustrate spinal balance, one can compare a hyperkyphotic spine to the leaning tower of Pisa, Italy. The center of mass of the tower (spine) functions to maintain the vertical axis because the sum of the forces acting downward is within the axis of rotation at the base (sacrum). As the tower leans more, the center of mass will eventually lie outside of the base, and the tower will fall. (© 2002, Thomas H. Weinzerl.)

the center of mass will eventually lie outside of the base, and the tower will fall (Fig. 3).

Deforming Forces

Sagittal deformities of the thoracic spine may arise from deformities of one or more of its components, either bony or soft tissue. Anterior column involvement may be present in the form of vertebral body or intervertebral disc wedging. Congenital anterior or posterior hemivertebrae may cause uneven sagittal growth of the immature spinal column. Posterior column insufficiency may be subsequent to trauma, neural arch defects, or wide decompressive laminectomies.

With long-standing deformities, spinal ligaments may act to maintain deformity. Fibrous structures become shortened and less elastic as a result of decreased motion and stress. In kyphotic deformities, the ALL can be stiff and contracted (4). In curves greater than 60 to 75 degrees, it can limit the passive correction by intraoperative positioning. As a result, ALL release or resection may be required to achieve a balanced fusion (27). The PLL, being the weakest of the spinal ligaments and closest to the IAR, contributes little to deformity maintenance (28).

Diagnosis and Imaging

PHYSICAL EXAM. The physical exam is an essential component in evaluating thoracic deformities. On inspection, a humpback deformity is an indication of a kyphotic deformity. Surface landmarks can be used to estimate the apex and extent of the curve. Skin inspection can detect abnormalities that will alert the practitioner to associated spinal lesions. An example of this are the café-au-lait spots seen in neurofibromatosis. In infants and children, midline tufts of hair over the low back may be evidence of neural tube defects. Shoulder height and pelvic obliquity should be observed as clues to the level of deformity and degree of compensation. Limb lengths must be measured to rule out associated extremity deformities. Passive flexion and extension can be helpful in assessing flexibility.

The overall functional level of the patient must be assessed. In kyphotic deformities greater than 90 degrees, respiratory function can be compromised, necessitating a formal evaluation of pulmonary function. Ambulatory status, especially in paralytic curves, influences the propensity for progression. Mental capabilities should also be noted for consideration of possible hygiene and wound care issues postoperatively.

A detailed neurological exam must be performed at the time of the initial visit. Occult spinal cord pathology must be ruled out preoperatively. A tethered cord syndrome or a diastematomyelia may be missed and may cause devastating neurological complications if they are not identified and addressed prior to deformity correction. The presence of upper-motor neuron signs is indicative of myelopathy. Bowel or bladder dysfunction can be baseline, as in myelomeningocele patients, or can indicate new-onset neurological compromise requiring neural decompression prior to or at the time of deformity correction. In an investigation of a tethered cord associated with intraspinal lipomas, the onset of bowel or bladder dysfunction was a negative predictor of neurological recovery (29).

PLAIN RADIOGRAPHY. High-quality radiographs of the thoracic spine are essential for evaluation and surgical planning. Lateral views demonstrate sagittal deformities. Anteroposterior radiographs are used to detect concomitant coronal or rotational deformity. The degree of deformity is determined on the lateral radiograph by the Cobb method. This is done by measuring the angle formed between parallel lines extended from the superior and inferior end plates of a kyphotic curve (Fig. 4). Using the Cobb method, kyphosis can be measured with reasonable consistency (30). Disc and vertebral body heights are easily measured to evaluate relative contributions to the deformity. Inspection of the vertebral bodies and disc spaces can reveal pathological lesions, including tumors, infections, or old fractures. Schmorl's nodes are central concavities of the vertebral end plates and are characteristic, but not pathognomonic, of Scheuermann's disease.

ADVANCED IMAGING. Computed tomography (CT) offers excellent visualization of bony detail. Axial images in the plane

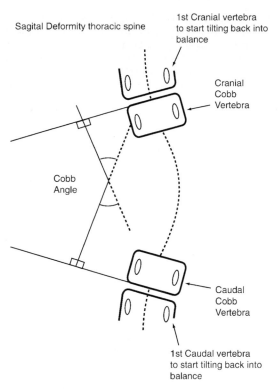

Sagital Deformity thoracic spine

1st Cranial vertebra to start tilting back into balance

Cranial Cobb Vertebra

Cobb Angle

Caudal Cobb Vertebra

1st Caudal vertebra to start tilting back into balance

Fig. 4. The degree of deformity is determined on the lateral radiograph by the Cobb method. This is done by measuring the angle formed between parallel lines extended from the superior and inferior end plates of a kyphotic curve. (© 2002, Thomas H. Weinzerl.)

of the vertebra enable inspection of the neural arch, as recognition of occult defects or lesions may be important in surgical planning. The space available for the cord (SAC) can also be measured for assessment of compressive lesions or stenosis. Magnetic resonance imaging (MRI) gives better visualization of the spinal cord and surrounding soft tissues than CT scans. In addition, MRI allows for multiplanar images in the sagittal plane. The presence of a spinal cord tumor, an intradural mass, a tethered spinal cord, and a syringomyelia can all influence management. Infection may be detected by either MRI or bone scans, with the former having higher specificity but equal sensitivity (31). Neoplastic lesions can be differentiated from nontuberculous infections by containment by the intervertebral disc space on MRI images (32).

Treatment: Nonoperative

Nonoperative treatment of sagittal deformities has limited utility. Hyperextension bracing or casting can be useful for kyphotic curves. Under-arm (Boston-type) braces end at the fourth thoracic vertebra cranially and are most useful for treating scoliotic rather than kyphotic deformities (33). Control of the upper thoracic spine has included use of mandibular pads (Milwaukee-type brace), but has been limited by associated dental malocclusion and abnormalities in the skeletally immature. Sternal pads (Jewett-type brace) can deliver posterior force to the upper thoracic spine without dental complication (34). Other major complications of bracing include curve progression secondary to noncompliance, and skin breakdown, especially in insensate patients.

Brace wear can be effective in curve prevention in spastic paralytic disorders (e.g., cerebral palsy). In flaccid paralytics, however, the lack of paraspinal muscle tone limits the efficacy of bracing, which often makes early operative stabilization of curves with 25 degrees or more the treatment of choice. Congenital curves are highly progressive and usually necessitate surgical intervention at initial presentation (2). Bracing has been largely ineffective in the management of postlaminectomy and postirradiation kyphosis (20). In posttraumatic deformities, bracing is indicated in skeletally immature patients. In the skeletally mature, most authors agree that operative stabilization offers the best chance for pain and deformity control (6).

A limited role for bracing has been established for the treatment of Scheuermann's disease in the adolescent patient. Sachs et al. (35) found bracing to effectively maintain correction in 69% of patients at 5-year follow-up. Consistent brace wear was associated with a better result, as were curves measuring less than 60 degrees. Kyphosis of greater than 74 degrees at initial presentation was associated with poor results. In contrast, Farsetti et al. (36) followed 20 patients for an average of 33 years after brace treatment. The authors noted that regardless of the initial correction obtained, all curves recurred to initial pretreatment measurements or greater at final radiographic evaluation. In adults, it is generally believed that brace treatment offers little benefit.

Treatment: Operative

Operative stabilization is useful in the correction of thoracic sagittal deformity. Surgery may involve initial correction, *in situ* stabilization, or removal of an offending lesion that will employ growth potential to achieve correction. Anterior and posterior approaches are common for fusions at one or both sites. Various surgical options exist for both. Corrective procedures address specific deforming elements, such as contracted ligaments or bony malformations, to restore mechanical balance. Stabilizing procedures include rigid fixation of the spine enabling solid bony fusion. Instrumentation is frequently used to obtain and maintain correction while fusion occurs. Instrumentation options are numerous, as selection is highly dependent on surgical preference and experience.

POSTERIOR SURGERY FOR KYPHOSIS. Congenital kyphosis can be addressed by posterior surgery alone. In children with absent to mild neurological deficits and with curves less than 50 degrees, posterior fusion can lead to excellent results (37). Ablation of the growth potential of the posterior elements with mild deformity (less than 50 degrees) enables continuing anterior column growth to slowly correct the kyphotic curve. Without instrumentation, Winter et al. (2) documented 100% fusion rates using hyperextension casting postoperatively followed by a scheduled second fusion at 6 months postoperatively. Acute correction is not necessary in these cases, as arrest of progression is the operative goal. In general, greater than 50 degrees of kyphosis is better treated with combined anterior and posterior procedures (2). With a sharp congenital gibbus deformity, posterior hemivertebra excision and both a single-level anterior and posterior fusion can achieve correction while maintaining cranial and caudal longitudinal spinal growth.

Indications for surgical stabilization of Scheuermann's kyphosis include intractable pain, progressive neurological deficit, progressive curves of 75 to 80 degrees, and less often cosmesis. Posterior surgery alone can be used if the curve passively reduces to at least 50 degrees. Correction can be achieved by compressing the posterior column without extensive bony resection. Multiple constructs have been used and advocated, with no distinct advantage of one system over another. Most commonly, systems employ segmental hook constructs with multilevel interlocking claws. The instrumented levels should include the upper Cobb vertebra measured cranially and extend to the first lordotic vertebra distal to the caudal Cobb vertebra (27). Fusion segments that fall short caudally can lead to distal junctional kyphosis that require secondary corrective procedures (22). In some instances, severe rigid kyphotic curves can be corrected by shortening the posterior column via bony resection (38). By resecting the superior and inferior aspects of adjacent lamina and facet joints, the surgeon creates a posterior column length deficit that may be compressed by segmental laminar hook instrumentation.

The anterior column can be osteotomized through a posterior approach to correct thoracic kyphosis. Michele and Krudger (39) developed the "eggshell" procedure, originally used for drainage of a vertebral body abscess. Through a posterior pedicle portal, the cancellous bone of the vertebral body is excavated. After "shelling out" the bone and posterior column resection, the posterior vertebral body wall is disrupted, allowing collapse of the middle column. With compressive posterior instrumentation, the kyphotic correction can be controlled and maintained. The procedure is technically demanding and should be reserved for surgeons with ample experience (40).

The function of the instrumentation is to maintain deformity correction while bony healing from the spinal fusion takes place. Regardless of the construct, the long-term operative goal is a solid bony arthrodesis of a corrected vertebral column. Techniques may vary from simple posterior to posterolateral fusion. Autogenous iliac crest bone graft, with or without augmentation with osteoinductive adjuncts, yields the highest fusion rates. Spinous processes, resected at the time of instrumentation, may be morselized for further graft material. Allograft, both fresh-frozen and freeze-dried, can also be used, but carry the theoretical risk of disease transmission. Both have no osteoprogenitor cells, while the fresh-frozen graft is significantly more osteoinductive than the freeze-dried specimen. In general, allograft bone placed posteriorly in an onlay fashion is less effective than autograft for achieving a long-term solid bony fusion.

POSTERIOR SURGERY FOR LORDOSIS. Lordosis surgery is infrequently performed. The vast majority of procedures are for congenital deformities. Lengthening osteotomies may be performed through the posterior elements for correction of congenital lordosis. Winter et al. (2) advocate this technique for severe deformities in patients with compromised pulmonary function. Distractive instrumentation constructs are then used to correct and maintain the posterior column length. Such techniques must be used in conjunction with an anterior fusion in the growing spine. Continued anterior spinal growth with posterior fusion has a corrective effect on the lordotic deformity.

ANTERIOR SURGERY FOR KYPHOSIS. Anterior surgery of the thoracic kyphotic spine enables the greatest amount of correction. In round-back kyphosis, curves greater than 50 degrees generally require an anterior soft tissue release and fusion supplemented with posterior fusion and stabilization. The surgeon must fuse both the anterior and posterior aspects of the spine to effectively prevent curve progression.

In Scheuermann's disease, most authors recommend anterior release prior to posterior fusion for curves of 75 to 80 degrees that do not passively correct to less than 50 degrees (27). The contracted ALL and anterior intervertebral discs contribute to the deformity. After release, the anterior column is destabilized and requires reconstruction. Fusion should extend from the most cranial Cobb vertebra to the first distal lordotic level and should be supplemented with posterior fusion and instrumentation that spans the same levels. Distal junctional kyphosis has been observed with inadequate fusion length in kyphotic deformities (22).

Stable anterior column reconstruction must follow anterior release. Normally, the anterior and middle columns bear 70% of the axial weight-bearing load of the vertebral column (41). To better maintain correction and diminish the tensile stresses placed on posterior fusion constructs, structural support should be implanted between or spanning the vertebral bodies. Important features of the support are high compressive strength and minimal subsidence. Rib autograft, corticocancellous sections of iliac crest, or femoral ring allograft have all been used as anterior strut grafts. The advantages of these materials are that they may be fully incorporated into the fusion, acting as both osteoconductive and osteoinductive agents. Over time, however, graft resorption can decrease the compressive strength before it is replaced with new bone. As an alternative, rigid metal cages have been developed to minimize the effects of resorption. Implantable titanium cages packed with autogenous graft can be cut to size and inserted into disc spaces. These devices do not resorb and are less likely to dislodge. Regardless of the method of reconstruction, we believe that maintenance of the vertebral end plate decreases the likelihood of subsidence. *In vitro* biomechanical studies have not unanimously supported this concept (42).

ANTERIOR SURGERY FOR LORDOSIS. In mild congenitally lordotic deformities, anterior fusion of the thoracic spine may be utilized to ablate the anterior vertebral growth potential (i.e., anterior epiphysiodesis). In the select skeletally immature patient, it may be performed alone without a posterior procedure. Lordotic deformities in the adult are rare but may also be addressed through an anterior approach. Flat-back deformities of the thoracic spine may require anterior closing wedge osteotomies in order to obtain a corrected kyphotic posture. In this situation, the deformity is corrected through shortening of the anterior column. The reduction can be further aided by distractive instrumentation posteriorly.

Pseudarthrosis is a major long-term complication of thoracic deformity surgery. It can manifest as hardware failure, loss of correction, and persistent pain. Pseudarthrosis rates as high as 41% have been reported for posterior fusion alone in the congenitally kyphotic spine (37). For posterior fusion alone in the adult kyphotic patient, nonunion rates of 6% to 9% have been documented, while combined front and back procedures have led to 100% union (7). Today, most authors agree that combined anterior and posterior fusion, whether staged or simultaneous, is biomechanically and clinically superior.

Summary

Thoracic sagittal deformities are a commonly encountered spinal entity and may be caused by a variety of etiologies, with idiopathic causes being the most common. Prevention is dependent on the etiology and focuses on early diagnosis before severe curve progression develops. Diagnosis is primarily clinical and radiographic, but may be aided by advanced imaging modalities. Treatment is directed toward producing a biomechanically balanced vertebral column that will maintain correction over time. Posterior approaches are best suited to mild and flexible curves, while combined anterior and posterior approaches offer the greatest degree of deformity correction and are often necessary in adults with rigid curves.

References

1. Gorup J, Brown C, Wong D, et al. Anterior thoracoscopic and posterior hemivertebral resection for congenital scoliosis. In: Devlin V, ed. *Spine: state of the art reviews*. Philadelphia: Lippincott-Raven, 1998:723–728.
2. Winter R, Lonstein J, Boachie-Adjei O. Congenital spinal deformity. In: Pritchard D, ed. *Instructional course lectures*. Rosemont, IL: American Academy of Orthopaedic Surgeons, 1996:117–127.
3. James J. Kyphoscoliosis. *J Bone Joint Surg* 1955;37B:414–426.
4. Riina J, Merola A, Cerabona F, et al. The role of anterior column surgery in the treatment of kyphosis. In: Devlin V, ed. *Spine: state of the art reviews*. Philadelphia: Hanley and Belfus, 1998:639–645.
5. Sorenson. 1969.
6. Holt R, Dopf C, Isaza J, et al. *The adult spine: principles and practice*. Philadelphia: Lippincott-Raven, 1997:1537–1578.
7. Bradford D, Moe J, Montalvo F, et al. Scheuermann's kyphosis. Results of surgical treatment by posterior spine arthrodesis in twenty-two patients. *J Bone Joint Surg* 1975;57A:439–448.
8. Hensigner R. Kyphosis secondary to skeletal dysplasia and metabolic disease. *Clin Orthop* 1977;128:113–128.
9. Kehl D, Lovell W, MacEwen G. Scheuermann's disease of the lumbar spine. *Orthop Trans* 1982;6:42.
10. Micheli L. Low back pain in adolescents. Differential diagnosis. *Am J Sport Med* 1979;7:362.
11. Yasouka S, Peterson H, Law E, MacCarty C. Pathogenesis and prophylaxis of postlaminectomy deformity of the spine after multiple level laminectomy. Difference between children and adults. *Neurosurgery* 1981;9:145–152.
12. Tachdjian M, Matson D. Orthopaedic aspects of intraspinal tumors in infants and children. *J Bone Joint Surg* 1965;47A:223–248.
13. Ye Q, Lin J, Shen J. Failure and complication following surgical treatment of scoliosis: analysis of 101 cases. *Chung Hua Wai Ko Tsa Chih* 1996;34:327–329.
14. Humke T, Grob D, Scheier H, et al. Cotrel-Dubousset and Harrington instrumentation in idiopathic scoliosis: a comparison of long-term results. *Eur Spine J* 1995;4:280–283.
15. Makipernaa A, Keikkila J, Merkantao J, et al. Spinal deformity induced by radiotherapy for solid tumors in children: a long-term follow up study. *Eur J Pediatr* 1993;152:197–200.
16. Denis F. The three columns of the spine and its significance in the classification of acute thoracolumbar spine injuries. *Spine* 1983;8:817–831.
17. Sasso R, Cotler H. Posterior instrumentation and fusion for unstable fractures and fracture dislocations of the thoracic and lumbar spine. *Spine* 1993;18:450–460.
18. Langer L, Moe J. A recessive form of congenital scoliosis different from spondylothoracic dysplasia. *Birth Defects Orig Artic Ser* 1975;11:83–86.
19. Morrow J, Kelsey K. Folic acid for prevention of neural tube defects: pediatric anticipatory guidance. *J Pediatr Health Care* 1998;12:55–59.
20. Otsuka N, Hey L, Hall J. Postlaminectomy and postirradiation kyphosis in children and adolescents. *Clin Orthop* 1998;354:189–194.
21. Abumi K, Panjabi M, Kramer K, et al. Biomechanical evaluation of lumbar spinal stability after graded facetectomies. *Spine* 1990;15:1142–1147.
22. Lowe T, Kasten M. An analysis of sagittal curves and balance after Cotrel-Dubousset instrumentation for kyphosis secondary to Scheuermann's disease. A review of 32 patients. *Spine* 1994;19:1680–1685.
23. Bernhardt M, Bridwell K. Segmental analysis of the sagittal plane alignment of the normal thoracic and lumbar spines and thoracolumbar junction. *Spine* 1989;14:717–721.
24. White A, Panjabi M. *Clinical biomechanics of the spine*. Philadelphia: Lippincott-Raven, 1990.
25. Oda I, Abumi K, Lu D, et al. Biomechanical role of the posterior elements, costovertebral joints, and rib cage in the stability of the thoracic spine. *Spine* 1996;21:1423–1429.
26. Haher T, O'Brien M, Felmly W, et al. Instantaneous axis of rotation as a function of the three columns of the spine. *Spine* 1992;17:S149–154.
27. Lowe T. Biomechanical aspects of the surgical treatment of kyphotic deformities. In: Haher T, Merola A. *Spine: state of the art reviews*. Philadelphia: Hanley and Belfus, 1996:433–454.
28. Pintar F, Yoganandan N, Myers T, et al. Biomechanical properties of human lumbar spine ligaments. *J Biomechanics* 1992;25:1351–1356.
29. Byrne R, Hayes E, George T, et al. Operative resection of 100 spinal lipomas in infants less than 1 year of age. *Pediatr Neurosurg* 1995;23:182–186.
30. Voutsinas S, MacEwen G. Sagittal profiles of the spine. *Clin Orthop* 1986;210:235–242.
31. Mazur J, Ross G, Cummings J, et al. Usefulness of magnetic resonance imaging for the diagnosis of acute musculoskeletal infections in children. *J Pediatr Orthop* 1995;15:144–147.
32. Hovi I, Lamminen A, Salonen O, et al. MR imaging of the lower spine. Differentiation between infectious and malignant disease. *Acta Radiol* 1994;35:532–540.
33. Chase A, Bader D, Houghton G. The biomechanical effectiveness of the Boston brace in the management of adolescent idiopathic scoliosis. *Spine* 1989;14:1989.
34. Colbert. 1987.
35. Sachs B, Bradford D, Winter R, et al. Scheuermann kyphosis. Follow-up of Milwaukee-brace treatment. *J Bone Joint Surg* 1987;69A:50–57.
36. Farsetti P, Tudisco C, Caterini R, et al. Juvenile and idiopathic kyphosis. *Arch Orthop Trauma Surg* 1991;110:165–168.
37. Winter R, Moe J, Lonstein J. The surgical treatment of congenital kyphosis: a review of 94 patients age 5 or older with 2 or more years follow-up in 77 patients. *Spine* 1985;10:224–231.
38. Ponte A. Scheuermann's kyphosis: posterior shortening procedure by segmental closing wedge resection. *Orthop Trans* 1995;19:603.
39. Michele A, Krudger F. A surgical approach to the vertebral body. *J Bone Joint Surg* 1949;31A:873–878.
40. Chewning S, Heinig C. Eggshell procedure. In: Bradford D. *Master techniques in orthopaedic surgery, the spine*. Philadelphia: Lippincott-Raven, 1997:199–208.
41. Haher T, Tozzi J, Lospinuso M, et al. The contribution of the three columns of the spine to spinal stability: a biomechanical model. *Paraplegia* 1989;27:432–439.
42. Hollowell J, Vollmer D, Wilson C, et al. Biomechanical analysis of thoracolumbar interbody constructs. How important is the endplate? *Spine* 1996;21:1032–1036.

179. Adult Thoracolumbar Scoliosis

**Stephen L. Ondra and
Sean A. Salehi**

Neurosurgery has traditionally dealt with diseases of the spine that resulted in neurological compression. Improved understanding of the pathophysiology and biomechanics of spine disease has led to a steady expansion in our ability to treat patients with complex disorders of the spine. This includes both problems of neurological compression and disorders that result in axial back pain or mechanical imbalance. Complementary to this increased understanding has been the development of new surgical techniques and instrumentation systems that allow us to place powerful stabilizing and corrective forces to the spine. This ability to change the biomechanics of the spine requires us to develop a deeper understanding of the pathophysiology of spine disease and the biomechanical forces at work in both disease and treatment. Implicit in this is an understanding of the long-term implications of both disease and treatment. It is with this change in the management of spinal diseases that the importance of considering and treating adult thoracolumbar scoliosis arises for the neurosurgeon. Principles of evaluation and management of adult spinal deformity are discussed in this chapter.

Scoliosis is defined as a coronal plane deformity of the spine that is greater than 10 degrees when measured by the Cobb angle method. It typically has a structural rotation at the apical motion segment (1) (Fig. 1). Adult degenerative scoliosis is a presentation of a spinal deformity of greater than 10 degrees in the coronal plane after the age of 20, or after having reached skeletal maturity. This deformity is typically exacerbated by degenerative changes in the spinal elements (2) (Fig. 2). The degenerative changes that result in the deformity progression also frequently result in back pain and neurological compression.

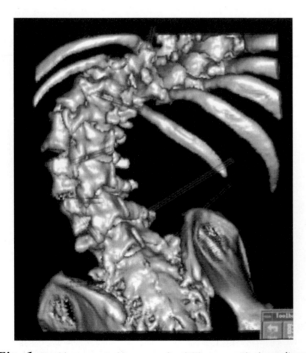

Fig. 1. Stealth computed tomography (CT) scan with three-dimensional reconstruction demonstrating the three-dimensional deformity seen in scoliosis.

To adequately treat the resulting pain syndromes, one must consider the biomechanical changes that are being created by both the deformity and the planned treatment. By understanding the interplay of these two biomechanical forces, an optimal long-term result can be obtained for the patient.

Demographics and Natural History

Adolescent idiopathic scoliosis is believed to be an inherited disease process that follows an autosomal-dominant pattern with incomplete penetrance. It is more prevalent in women, having an instance of approximately 7:1. This increased incidence in adolescent women leads to an increased incidence of degenerative scoliosis due to late progression of idiopathic curves in women. This is further accelerated by the higher incidence of osteoporosis in women. Presentations of de novo degenerative scoliotic curves are equal between men and women (3). There appears to be no exacerbation of either group due to pregnancy (4).

Degenerative curves of all types typically present after age 40. It is estimated that degenerative thoracolumbar scoliosis is present in between 1.9% and 3.9% of patients (5–7). Other studies have shown up to a 30% incidence in scoliosis in patients between the ages of 50 and 84 (8). This demonstrates the powerful influence that age plays on deformity due to degeneration of the vertebral column metabolic bone disease, degenerative disc disease, and degenerative joint disease (9,10). It is believed that the population of adult spinal deformity will actually increase with the relative aging of the population and the increasing incidence of both degenerative spine disease and osteoporosis. It is estimated that the average degenerative scoliotic curve will progress at a rate of 1 to 2 degrees per year. As a standard measurement error of 3 degrees is allowed, no curve should be considered progressive until it has progressed at least 5 degrees.

Thoracolumbar curves greater than 50 degrees are at highest risk of progression (11). In addition to the coronal curve measurement, the degree of axial rotation also has an effect. The greater the axial rotation, the greater the degeneration and higher rate of curve progression.

In the study by Collins and Ponsetti (12), it was estimated that 65% of all curves will progress by 5 degrees or more during the follow-up period.

Classification

The Scoliosis Research Society has divided idiopathic spinal deformity into a variety of basic categories. While idiopathic scoliosis is primarily diagnosed and treated in adolescents, adult degenerative scoliosis can result from a late progression of preexisting idiopathic curve. It may also develop de novo from degenerative disease of the spine or traumatic changes after skeletal maturity has already occurred. De novo degenerative

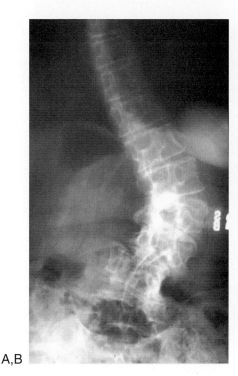
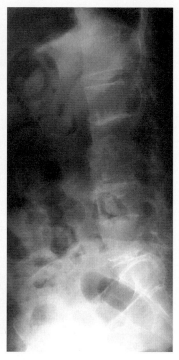

A,B

Fig. 2. Plain x-rays of a patient with advanced degenerative decompensation of a previously stable adolescent scoliosis. **A**: Note the disc height loss and large traction spurs. Lateral listhesis coexists with the severe rotatory deformity. **B**: There is also loss of lumbar lordosis.

scoliosis is a separate classification of spinal deformity and as such cannot be truly categorized into the King system (13). Late progression of a preexisting idiopathic curve is typically classified into one of the categories defined by King. The King classification defines five distinct curve patterns (Table 1). These patterns specifically apply to patients with preexisting idiopathic curves. Problems of pain and deformity are accelerated in all groups by degenerative disc disease, degenerative facet joint disease, and osteoporosis. While the King classification system has guided treatment in adolescents, the degenerative concerns of adults limit the value of this system.

All spinal deformity curves have two potential components. The structural portion of the curve is a rigid deformity that is not correctable by the patient's bending when observed on physical examination or in radiographic studies. The compensatory portion of the curve is a physiological curve that assists the patient in establishing better spinal balance for the rigid (structural) portion of the spinal deformity. It can be brought into more normal alignment with the remainder of the spine by having the patient bend and adjust position. Any classification system defines the curve in terms of the structural or rigid part of the deformity. This is the only aspect of the curve that requires treatment.

In adults, a portion of the curve that was previously physiological in adolescence often will become structural from longstanding uncorrected deformity and the progression of degenerative disease. This degenerative progression increasingly stiffens the spine, making the majority of adult curves true thoracolumbar rigid deformities. Additionally, the sagittal plane portion of the deformity becomes an increasing problem to adults with degenerative scoliosis, when compared to children and adolescents (9). Junctional kyphosis at the thoracolumbar junction is the rule in adult degenerative scoliosis. This results in a sagittal plane imbalance characterized by a loss of lumbar lordosis and thoracolumbar junction kyphosis. This throws the C7 plumb line anterior to the sacrum and requires the patient to increasingly flex at the hips to regain spinal-pelvic balance. This can result in hip flexor contraction and a characteristic posture and gait of flat-back syndrome due to loss of lumbar lordosis.

As in all types of spinal deformity, adult degenerative scoliosis should be characterized based only on the structural portion of the curve. If the adult curves do not fit easily into the King system, they should simply be characterized by stating the degree of curve measured by the method of Cobb and the apical and caudal vertebra used in that measurement for each rigid portion of the curve. The sagittal portions of the curve should also be stated. In this way, all adult curves can be classified by their component levels. Equally important is the ability provided by such measurements to assess progression of the curve on sequential films.

Symptoms of Scoliosis

Back, buttock, and leg pain are the overwhelming presenting symptoms in patients with adult degenerative scoliosis. It is estimated that 48% to 79% of adult patients will complain of pain as their primary symptoms (6,9,14). Lower extremity paresthesias, radiculopathy, sacroiliac joint pain, and muscle spasms are also common presentations. Complaint of pain in the thigh muscles from hip flexion is common in patients with a sagittal plane imbalance and is characteristic of flat-back syndrome. Additionally, patients may complain of gait disturbance due to sagittal plane imbalance. Some adults will also notice progress-

Table 1. Different Curve Patterns in Idiopathic Scoliosis According to the King Classification

King 1	Major lumbar, minor thoracic
King 2	Major thoracic, minor lumbar
King 3	Single thoracic curve
King 4	Thoracolumbar curve
King 5	Double thoracic curve

ing deformity of their back. It is rare that they will present with this condition and with exclusion of pain. As a general rule, the sagittal plane disturbance is far more troubling to adults than the coronal plane problems.

The prevalence of back and lower extremity radiating pain is common in the population. As such, it is essential that a careful history and physical examination be conducted. Eliciting factors such as location and duration of the pain, activities that increase or decrease pain, character and location of pain radiation, paresthesias, and urinary symptoms should be carefully reviewed. In this way the surgeon can assess if this is primary local degenerative pain or pain related to the deformity. Areas of muscle spasm and tightness should also be defined. Winter describes a characteristic pain pattern in scoliotic patients. Pain over the concavity of the scoliosis curve is thought to be due to facet degeneration, while pain over the convexity is felt to be due to muscle spasm. Pain in the midscapular and trapezius region in typically due to cervical rather than thoracolumbar pathology (15). Evaluation of posture and the possible coexistence of sacroiliac joint pathology should be evaluated. In this way, confusion as to the cause of the pain can be clarified (16). By understanding the true etiology of the pain, the risk of overtreating the problem can be minimized.

In Nachemson's (17) 30-year follow-up study, he found that patients with adult scoliosis did not have a greater incidence of spine pain than did the general population. He also concluded that low back pain in patients with scoliosis should receive the same conservative management as patients with nonscoliotic degenerative disease. Weinstein et al. (11) echoed Nachenson's finding when they reported that there was no relation between the severity of pain and the amount of scoliotic curve. These authors demonstrate the importance of remembering that not all pain in patients with scoliosis is due to the curve. In this way, the history, physical examination, and diagnostic testing can direct the physician to treating the proper source of the patient's symptoms to obtain maximum effectiveness and minimal morbidity.

Clinical Evaluation

Any patient being considered for reconstructive spinal surgery should undergo a careful assessment for the presence of associated adult degenerative scoliosis. The initial evaluation begins with a careful clinical examination. In addition to the standard neurological examination performed on patients with spinal disease, careful assessment of the spine, posture, and extremities should be performed. Patients should be dressed in a gown and ideally a standing examination is performed. The overall posture should be assessed from an anterior, posterior, and lateral perspective. From the anterior and posterior perspective, the shoulders and pelvis should be examined to see if there is any tilt that might indicate an underlying coronal scoliotic curve. The spine itself should also be examined and palpated to assess any evidence of curvature. From the lateral perspective, the overall posture and the sagittal plane should be assessed. This includes evaluating whether the head, shoulders, and pelvis fall into alignment, and whether the cervical and lumbar lordosis and the thoracic kyphosis are of normal contour. The hip posture should be evaluated to assess if there is rotation of the hips to compensate for an imbalance of the spine in the sagittal plane. The knee and hips should also be assessed; hip flexion may again be indicative of compensation for a spinal sagittal plane imbalance. The leg length should be assessed; a leg length discrepancy may be indicative of long-standing spinal imbalance. Lastly, gait should be assessed to evaluate the pa-

tient for a neurological change, and to evaluate an abnormal gait based on a structural basis.

Having completed the surface examination of the patient's skeletal structure and balance, a general neurological and medical evaluation should be performed. The neurological examination should assess evidence of radiculopathy or myelopathy. This will include careful motor, reflex, and sensory examinations. Evidence of a primary neuromuscular disease or neurocutaneous syndrome should also be assessed. The general medical evaluation should include a pulmonary and cardiovascular evaluation. Any patient with a significant thoracic kyphosis, coronal curve of greater than 70 degrees, or the clinical suggestion of pulmonary disease should undergo formal pulmonary function tests (PFTs).

Radiographic Evaluation

The most important diagnostic imaging in patients who are thought to have adult degenerative scoliosis is plain x-ray (16). All patients being considered for reconstructive surgery of the thoracolumbar spine should obtain standard anteroposterior (AP), lateral, and lateral flexion and extension spine films. A standard 36-inch cassette is essential to obtain useful images in patients with possible deformity. This is the only way to properly assess coronal and sagittal plane balance. If the patient has a spinal imbalance, right- and left-side bending films should be obtained in addition to the flexion/extension films. In this way, areas of the curve that correct with bending indicate that these are simple compensatory curves and may not need to be included fully in the fusion. Areas of the deformity curve that do not change with bending are structural and will require reconstruction and correction.

Follow-up plain x-rays give a wealth of information with regard to the progression of the curve (1). The lateral scoliosis film gives excellent assessment of sagittal plane balance. A plumb-line drop from C7 (or ideally the odontoid) should fall through the body of L1 and the body of S1. Normally this will be at the superior and posterior corner of the S1 vertebral body. This is called normal spinal balance in the sagittal plane (Fig. 3).

In general, the normal thoracic kyphosis is 35 to 45 degrees, with an average of 40 degrees. The normal lumbar lordosis has higher variability and may be 30 to 60 degrees, with a mean of 45 to 50 degrees. Any loss of lumbar lordosis (flat-back) or thoracic kyphosis results in the spine's plumb line being shifted anterior to the sacrum (Fig. 4). This is typically compensated for by rotation of the pelvis and flexion of the hips. In this way, the spine is returned to balance over the pelvis. This causes difficulty in patient ambulation and a tired, aching feeling in the thighs. An increase in thoracic kyphosis or lumbar hyperlordosis results in the plumb line falling posterior to the sacrum. In these cases, the patient will lean forward to try to restore spinal pelvic balance. In both cases, correction of the abnormal curve is required to restore normal spinal balance. When abnormalities have been of long-standing, often both thoracic and lumbar curves are abnormal. Correction of one will leave the patient out of balance or possibly worsen the spinal balance. Correction of both curves is necessary for restoration of spinal balance. Imbalance in the sagittal plane is much more debilitating to patients than coronal imbalance. As such, particular attention should be paid to understanding and correcting sagittal balance. The AP scoliosis film provides significant information regarding the scoliotic curve of a patient with adult degenerative scoliosis. The coronal curve is established in the same way as sagittal curves. The angle of deformity is typically measured

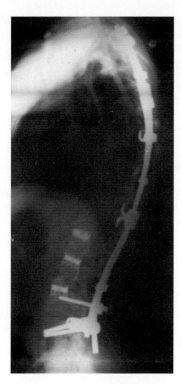

Fig. 3. Postscoliosis correction x-ray demonstrating restoration of normal sagittal balance.

in the method described by Cobb. In this method, a line is drawn parallel with the superior end plate of the apical vertebrae of the curve. An additional line is drawn parallel to the inferior end plate of the caudal vertebrae of the curve. Perpendicular lines are drawn to each of the end-plate lines. The angle of the curve is measured by assessing the angle defined by the intersection of these two lines. Angles should always be given with the apical and caudal vertebrae used to establish the angle listed in parenthesis next to the absolute number. In this way, intraobserver variability is minimized and accurate comparison to old films is enhanced.

The AP scoliosis films also allows establishment of coronal balance. A line drawn from C7 should fall through L1 and the middle of the sacrum. Any deviation from the sacral midline indicates a coronal imbalance. The stable vertebra of the curve is the vertebra bisected by the central sacral line. Rotation is typically measured using the Nash method. The neutral vertebra is the one that has both pedicles without rotation. The apical vertebra is the segment at the maximum deformity of the coronal curve.

Magnetic resonance imaging (MRI) is not always required in adolescents but is important in adult evaluation. MRI is essential in evaluating the patient for areas of spinal canal or foraminal compression. Disc hydration and degeneration can also be assessed in addition to evidence of herniation and neurological compression. In terms of the reconstruction, the most important aspect of the MRI is evaluation of disc hydration and degeneration. In general, a spinal reconstructive procedure should not be ended at the level of a severely degenerative or dehydrated disc (Fig. 5).

MRI may be difficult to assess in patients with severe scoliosis. Due to the rotation and angulation present, the amount of nerve root compression may be deceiving. In these cases, myelography and postmyelogram computed tomography (CT) can provide important and additional information that will help assess areas of neurological compression. Myelography and postmyelogram CT scanning are often helpful in assessing areas of neu-

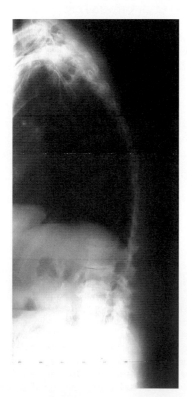

Fig. 4. Advanced degenerative changes in the disc spaces and facet joints have led to a loss of lumbar lordosis and a thoracolumbar junctional kyphosis. Both problems lead to a severe positive sagittal plane balance.

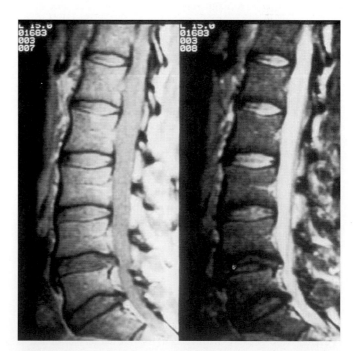

Fig. 5. Magnetic resonance imaging (MRI) shows degenerative disc disease with loss of height and hydration at the caudal two lumbar segments.

rological compression. The myelogram at times is easier to interpret than axial images in cases of deformity. Nerves can be evaluated for compression without the confusion of axial images that are distorted by the curve.

Discography has been used by some (18) to assess the disc status at the caudal or cephalad end of a reconstructive fusion. A negative discogram would indicate that it would be safe to conclude the fusion at this disc level, whereas a positive discogram would suggest extension of the fusion should be undertaken.

Bone density evaluation is also important in patients who have evidence of osteoporosis on plain x-ray. Bone density evaluation by DEXA bone scanning often provides important information regarding the quality of the bone and its ability to both hold instrumentation and withstand the corrective forces needed for deformity correction and stabilization. Osteoporosis will limit the ability of the spine to hold instrumentation and withstand the forces required for correction. Patients with poor bone mineral density may only be able to be fused *in situ*, as it is unlikely they can withstand the forces needed for correction. Additionally, patients with extremely poor bone mineral density may not be candidates for fusion at all. In these cases, alternative treatment measures may need to be considered.

Neurological and Medical Evaluation

Electromyography can be useful in assessing patients with degenerative scoliosis. These patients often have vague leg pain and multiple areas of central and foraminal stenosis. A positive electromyography may indicate which of the multiple abnormal foramen result in symptomatic neurological compression. While some authors have suggested that simple correction of deformity may obviate the need for decompression (19), we prefer to decompress any areas that are clearly symptomatic clinically or electrodiagnostically. Decompression limited to these areas, however, may limit the amount of decompression performed. This will preserve bone surface for fusion.

It is important in a patient with degenerative scoliosis who suffers from a thoracic hypokyphosis to undergo pulmonary function testing whether surgery is contemplated or not (12). We also routinely recommend a PFT for curves greater than 70 degrees, since the rate of pulmonary compromise in this group is high. In patients who complain of pulmonary symptoms and don't plan to undergo surgery, PFTs at regularly intervals may pick up subtle worsening of the pulmonary function. Also a preoperative PFT will help in postoperative care planning, for example maintaining postoperative intubation for a longer period as a safety precaution. This test is also important in an asymptomatic patient who has comorbid pulmonary conditions such as asthma, emphysema, or lung cancer, or cardiac disease. Pulmonary and cardiac evaluation is also important in establishing which patients will be able to withstand the physiological stress of surgery.

Nonsurgical Management

Patients who present with back pain, no clinical evidence of neurological compression, and with a curve less than 45 degrees should initially undergo a course of medical management (20). This includes nonsteroidal antiinflammatory agents and limited use of oral narcotics. In general narcotics should only be utilized for finite periods of time during periods of severe pain. Physical therapy is also useful in treating associated muscle spasm, improving body mechanics, and strengthening the supporting musculature of the spine. Massage can be included for muscle spasm. We find aquatic therapy especially helpful. It facilitates strengthening, stretching, and conditioning without axially loading the spine. The most important stretching is often in the hip flexors, which can release some of the hip flexor contraction that is commonly seen due to the flat-back syndrome and junctional kyphosis compensation.

In general, bracing is of no use in deformity stabilization or correction in adults (21). Some patients may benefit from a short course of brace stabilization until an acute pain exacerbation resolves. Long-term bracing is counterproductive due to the loss of muscle tone that can accompany it.

A program of weight loss combined with physical therapy will also significantly reduce the stress on the deformed degenerative spine. Patients with osteoporosis should also be considered for medications that may slow or reverse ongoing bone loss.

Minimally invasive management options consist primarily of injections. These include injections of painful degenerative facets, trigger-point injections for muscle spasm, and epidural steroid injections (20).

Surgical Management

Surgical indications for patients with adult scoliosis include severe and disabling back pain that fails to respond to maximal medical management, severe and unresponsive radiculopathy, and progression of physiological disturbances such as pulmonary dysfunction. Patients whose pain may or may not be manageable can also become surgical candidates based on mechanical evaluation and prediction of decompensation. Mechanical indications for surgery include the progression of sagittal or coronal plane imbalance of more than 5 to 10 degrees per year (2). Progressively unacceptable gait and sagittal imbalance as well as cosmetic issues may also enter into the decision to operate.

The age of the patient is less important than the patient's physiological health and predicted longevity. We have had excellent results in patients in their mid- to late 1970s who are otherwise healthy.

DECOMPRESSION ALONE. In patients with severe radiculopathy and well-controlled back pain, consideration can be given to decompression alone (17). Before considering this, one must carefully assess the patient's curve and stability. The surgeon must also consider how destabilizing the decompression will be and where in the curve will the mechanics be altered (22).

Curve decompensation and progression are at high risk if decompression is being done at the apex of the curve. Full laminectomies are also more destabilizing than hemilaminectomies due to the loss of muscle attachment and ligamentous support. When a foramenotomy is being performed, it has been suggested that not more than one third of the facet be removed. This is unrealistic and often ineffective in patients with scoliosis. In this group, the compression is often far lateral. Symptomatic radiculopathy is more common on the convex aspect of the curve. This is due to both degenerative changes and lateral disc bulging from the curve pressure. When radicular pain originates on the concave side it can result from foraminal stenosis. At times, the transverse process itself can have enough rotation to cause compression. As such, it is more common that full unilateral facetectomies are performed to relieve radiculopathy. In some cases transverse process resection is required. High-degree curves with significant rotation also have higher risk of decompensation when a decompression alone is carried out.

Other considerations include the bone density and quality, and the demand that the patient will physically place on the spine. In general, a very stiff spine on bending radiographs in a low-demand patient is at lower risk to decompensate than a more mobile spine in an active patient. If these factors are considered, a decompression for radiculopathy or neurogenic claudication may be appropriate.

POSTERIOR SEGMENTAL CORRECTION. In deformity of the spine, instrumentation provides both the corrective forces to reestablish spinal balance and internal fixation until fusion occurs. There have been many systems designed for the correction of scoliotic deformity (23–25). Initially, the Harrington rod system allowed some correction and stabilization of curves. The corrective force for this system was primarily provided by distraction. This resulted in frequent loss of sagittal plane balance and flat-back syndrome as well as a high rate of pseudarthrosis. Luque rods were another early system for deformity correction. It required multiple sublaminar wires and had a higher rate of postoperative correction loss due to the lack of rigid segmental control (26).

The introduction of posterior segmental instrumentation and correction by Cotrel and Dubousset revolutionized deformity correction. By controlling the spine across multiple segments with a combination of hooks, pedicle screws, and cables, powerful correction and immobilization forces can now be applied to the spine (27). Cotrel and Dubousset's concept is to control each critical segment of the spine with a bone fixation device (hook or pedicle screw). A rod is then bent to the desired sagittal and coronal contour. The spine is then brought to the rod segment by segment in a three-plane correction. This involves derotation and translation of the bone fixators to the rod.

The concept of segmental three-dimensional correction of the spine is the basis of all current deformity correction systems. It has resulted in improved rates of fusion and better maintenance of correction.

The most important step in spinal deformity correction is in the preoperative planning. Realistic goals should be set to achieve spinal balance and not simply straighten a portion of the spine. In patients who are relatively balanced and have no major cosmetic or pulmonary issue, an instrumented *in situ* posterior stabilization and fusion is a reasonable consideration. When deformity correction is needed to achieve balance, additional planning is needed.

In general, a 50% or greater correction of any segment is realistic in an adult. To achieve this, the typically rigid adult spine will need to be made mobile for correction. Once the areas for release have been decided, the pattern of corrective forces should be drawn out to consider all three planes of desired correction. This will provide a template for surgery that will allow achievement of both spinal balance and stabilization (Figs. 6 and 7).

Before corrective forces can be applied, the spine must be mobilized by release of partially fused ankylosed segments. This is done by performing osteotomies where corrective forces will be applied. In simple corrections in patients with preserved discs, posterior osteotomies alone may suffice. These are done in a wedge shape, with the larger part of the wedge on the convex side that is to be closed. Simple linear osteotomies can be done for sagittal plane correction. When large corrections

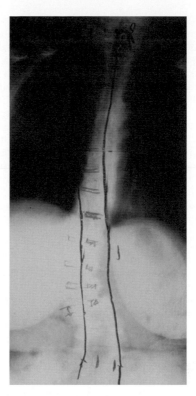

Fig. 6. Preoperative surgical plan for restoration of normal coronal plane balance in a patient with adult degenerative scoliosis.

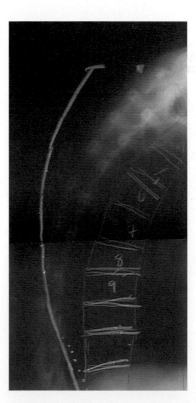

Fig. 7. Preoperative surgical plan for restoration of normal sagittal plane balance in a patient with adult degenerative scoliosis.

are needed or the spine is very rigid, an anterior discectomy and osteotomy may need to precede the posterior release and instrumentation. This is typically done by a thoracoabdominal approach on the convex side of the curve with discectomy and concave osteotomy. We typically utilize disc replacement cages placed eccentrically to the concave side to maintain the sagittal plane and allow coronal correction (Figs. 8 and 9).

There are some general guidelines for posterior segmental instrumentation constructs. In thoracolumbar correction, the construct should not end near the apex of a coronal or sagittal curve. This can result in a junctional deformity due to the mechanical stress. The construct should also not end at a spinal junction such as the thoracolumbar junction. If the construct is planned to T12, it should be extended to L1 or L2 to avoid a junctional decompensation. If the construct ends at L5, consideration should be given to extending to the sacrum, though some feel that if the L5/S1 disc is competent that the morbidity of extending the fusion to the sacrum exceeds the morbidity of lumbar sacral decompensation and the need for revision.

Fusions at L5/S1 have a variety of problems. There is a higher rate of instrumentation loosening and pseudarthrosis at L5-S1 (28). This risk can be reduced by obtaining rigid lumbosacral junction fixation. Interbody fusion devices placed at L5-S1, if possible, will decrease the stress on the caudal screws (Fig. 10). Bicortical fixation of the S1 screws should also be obtained. Consideration can also be given to additional screw placement at S2 or to the use of an intrasacral rod technique (Fig. 11). The use of ilial fixation by the Galveston technique and its modification can also be considered. While such techniques do improve stability, they alter pelvic motion and gait. They can also cause late pain due to rod loosening in the ilium from residual motion at the SI joint. We do not recommend their use in patients who are ambulatory, but we have found them quite helpful in nonambulators with paralytic scoliosis.

The rod should end at a stable vertebra at each end. Additionally, in adults the disc below the fusion should be assessed

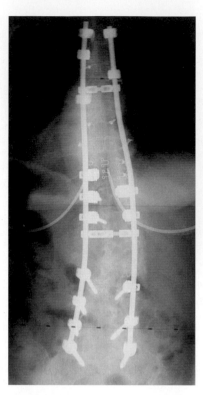

Fig. 9. Postcorrection, fusion, and instrumentation of an adult with degenerative scoliosis.

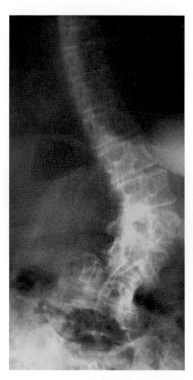

Fig. 8. Preoperative adult degenerative scoliosis demonstrating the coronal deformity.

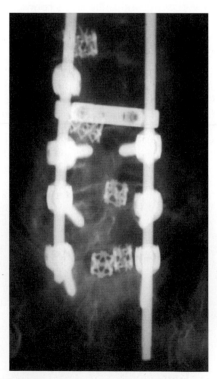

Fig. 10. The L4-5 and L5-S1 spaces are difficult to reach from the thoracoabdominal access route typically used for an anterior release for adult degenerative scoliosis. The rotation present often makes posterior lumbar interbody fusion (PLIF) techniques difficult. Anterior lumbar interbody fusion (ALIF) at these levels would require a third approach. TLIF cages are utilized here to provide anterior column support.

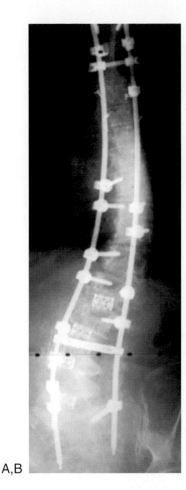
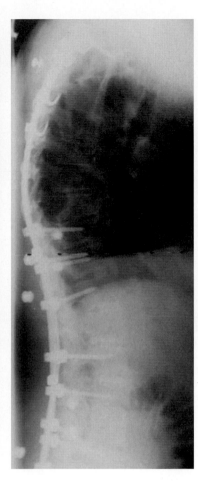

A,B

Fig. 11. **A,B**: Intrasacral rod placement can give added support to the caudal end of the construct. This minimizes the risk of caudal screw failure and pseudarthrosis in this high-risk area for failure.

to ensure that it is not degenerative. Ending a long deformity construct on a degenerative disc can lead to early failure of the segment adjacent to the fusion.

If possible, either the thoracolumbar or lumbosacral junctions should be left out of the fusion. This will allow patients a residual area of spinal motion that they can use to correct themselves over any residual imbalance in the reconstructed spine (Fig. 12). If both junctions must be included, as is all too often the case, extraordinary attention should be paid to optimizing the patient's reconstruction and balance in both the sagittal and coronal planes. With both junctions included in the reconstruction, the patient's only remaining compensating mechanism for balance is pelvic. If patients have significant hip disease, they will have no compensatory mechanisms.

Once the extent of the fusion has been determined, the pattern of segmental correction should be planned. In general, we prefer pedicle screws when possible due to their greater strength. Pedicle diameter in deformity can be highly variable even within the same spinal segment. Assessment of pedicle size to ensure that safe screw placement is possible is mandatory. This can be done with conventional CT, MRI, or CT obtained for image guidance. Segments that cannot accept pedicle screws can be controlled with hooks. General hook patterns should end in a claw construct (down-going hook at the top of the construct facing an up-going hook) at the ends of the rod. The intervening pattern should allow forces to be applied at the segments that are to be corrected. Typically, this will include the segments one or two levels above and below the apical vertebra, the stable vertebra, and a neutral vertebra at the ends. A combination of transverse process, pedicle, and

lamina hooks can be used. The hooks and screws can be supplemented with sublaminar cables at intervening levels.

In thoracolumbar curves, the hooks are placed to allow compression across the convex apex of the lumbar curve. This will help derotate the spine as well as correct the coronal plane. Since the compression is posterior to the instantaneous axis of rotation, it will also allow restoration or lordosis to the lumbar spine, which almost invariably is hypolordotic. The thoracic hooks are set up to allow distraction and derotation along the concave aspect of the thoracic curve. Again, this will help correct the coronal deformity, derotate the spine, and restore thoracic kyphosis.

The initial typical hook rod pattern is then set up to accept the first rod along the thoracic concave curve and the lumbar convex curve. The desired sagittal contour initially fits into these curves at 60 to 90 degrees to its desired end point. Once the rod is seated and loosely captured by the hooks and screws, it is turned back to its desired position and then fixed in place. This is the classic derotation maneuver. It restores balance in both sagittal and coronal planes (Figs. 13 and 14). Alternatively, equivalent results can be obtained by slowly translating the spine to the rod segmentally (5,28).

ANTERIOR SEGMENTAL CORRECTION. In recent years, the concept of single-stage anterior correction has gained popularity in treating adolescents and adults. Anterior correction allows for single-stage stabilization and correction with less blood loss and up to two or three fewer segments of fusion. Similar mechanical evaluation and principles of correction are applied

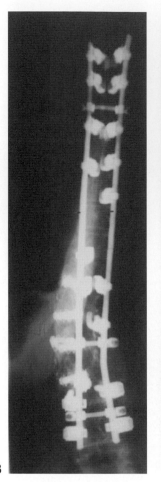
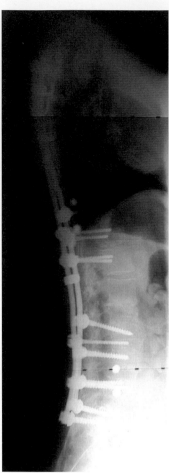

A,B

Fig. 12. Anteroposterior (AP) (**A**) and lateral (**B**) x-rays of scoliosis correction that stops short of the sacrum, allowing spinal and pelvic compensation mechanisms to correct any residual imbalance.

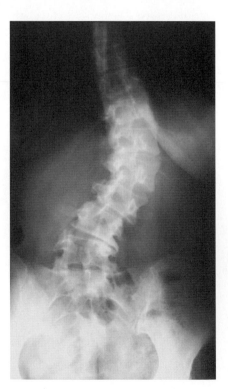

Fig. 13. Preoperative x-ray of a patient with adult degenerative scoliosis.

to the preoperative planning as were done in the posterior correction section.

This technique is possible if the posterior elements are not ankylosed, the correction can be accomplished within the limits of T8 to L4, and the curve does not exceed 60 degrees. Patients who do not fit these criteria should not be considered for a single-stage anterior correction. An anterior release is performed and disc replacement cages are placed in a fashion similar to the anterior release done for posterior correction. Bicortical vertebral body screws are then placed and the rod is coutoured to the desired correction. The rod is then placed and derotated. Final compression and distraction is performed with the knowledge that the rod is now anterior to the axis of rotation. As such, compression will result in mild loss of lordosis. If space permits, a second rod can be placed and cross-linked.

In general, the distal end of the fusion should include the stable vertebra and the neutral vertebrae, and it should be in the stable Harrington zone. It is desirable not to extend the construct below L4 so that the bending is not compromised. Also, as Hayes et al. (29) have shown in their biomechanics study of the lumbar spine after scoliosis correction, patients fused down to L3-L4 will have an increased incidence of retrolisthesis, increased translational motion, and low back pain as compared to higher levels of fusion (29). Such observations were not made when correction was done at a higher level than L3. In the case of a degenerative scoliosis where the patient is nonambulatory for any reason and the neutrality of L4-L5 is in question, a fusion down to the sacrum is recommended to assist with sitting and structural support to the spine. In cases where a fusion down to the sacrum is contemplated, we recommend simultaneous fusion of L4-5 and L5-S1 disc spaces using either

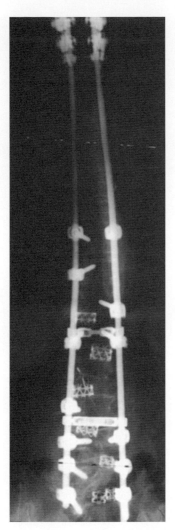

Fig. 14. Postoperative x-ray of a patient with adult degenerative scoliosis.

a posterior TLIF or an anterior approach for discectomy and placement of structural interbody cages. This added step is needed because of the nature of the lumbosacral junction, with its high rate of failure if only a posterior approach is used. Kostuik et al.'s (28) earlier results with Harrington rods had shown up to a 50% pseudarthrosis rate in the lumbosacral junction.

THORACOPLASTY. Though thoracoplasty puts the patient at risk for declining pulmonary function, especially in patients with poor preoperative pulmonary function, it has many other advantages (30,31). For one, the rib hump created from the spinal rotation in the axial plain will not completely resolve even after fusion. This will leave the patient with an unacceptable rib hump that is either not acceptable to the patient or is still causing symptoms such as pain when lying flat on a rib hump. In our institution we routinely perform thoracoplasty in a patient with acceptable pulmonary function who desires cosmesis or symptomatic relief from the rib hump. We use the same midline incision and perform a subfascial dissection down to the ribs in the apex of the curve. Subsequent to this, at least two ribs above and two ribs below the apex of the curve are identified and the proximal 7 to 10 cm are dissected off the

parietal pleura and cut. This releases the hump, and an immediate result is observed. Some surgeons may extend the rib resection more anterior, but in our experience this is not necessary since it requires a separate incision and will not accomplish much more in terms of cosmesis. The only time one may consider going more distally is when the surgeon desires more autogenous bone graft. Also, to prevent creating a ridge postoperatively, we routinely shave off the transverse processes of the involved vertebrae on the convex side.

If the pleura is accidentally opened, one may attempt closing it primarily, and obtain a chest x-ray prior to the closure of the incision. If the opening is large enough, a chest tube is then necessary until the pleura heals.

POSTOPERATIVE MANAGEMENT. In our institution, we place our patients into a thoracic lumbosacral orthosis (TLSO) for 3 months, allowing extra immobilization prior to solid bone fusion. After the 3-month period we place patients in a lumbosacral corset to remind them to limit their spine motion for an additional 6 weeks. In patients who have had fusion down to the sacrum or pelvis, a leg extension is used to limit the motion along the sacroiliac joint.

All of our patients postoperatively are taken to the neurospine intensive care unit, since all of them invariably have swollen airways and hence are still intubated and have required multiple blood transfusion intraoperatively.

All patients above 40 years of age are monitored for myocardial infarction (MI) and a careful fluid management is performed. Patients are kept sedated until they are ready to be extubated, the majority in less than 24 hours.

Postoperative AP and lateral plain radiographs of the spine are performed to ensure the stability of the construct. Regular postoperative laboratory tests such as hemoglobin, electrolytes, creatinine, and coagulation factors are done on a daily basis and adjusted subsequently.

As mentioned above, perioperative MI is always a consideration, and we always monitor the enzymes of patients at risk for this condition. Increased requirement for transfusion and massive fluid shifts during the surgery in an adult with low myocardial reserve predisposes the patient to some sort of cardiac events.

Pulmonary embolus is another untoward side effect of such surgeries. The length of the procedure and possible coagulopathy intraoperatively predisposes the patient to having a pulmonary embolus. We routinely use venous compression devices perioperatively and place patients on minidose heparin 24 hours after surgery. In patients with high risk of pulmonary embolus, e.g., obese, sedentary, or with a history of coagulopathy, a prophylactic caval filter is placed preoperatively. Routine lower extremity venous duplex is performed on a weekly basis while patients are still not ambulatory.

Ileus is a complication of spine surgery of some duration, especially if a retroperitoneal approach for an anterior fixation is used. In patients with ileus we routinely use a nasogastric tube to wall suction to decompress the gastrointestinal system and rest it.

Nutritional support is of paramount importance in patients postoperatively. In patients who for any reason cannot have any enteral feeding, hyperalimentation is used for 24 hours postsurgery due to the high metabolic demand of the body.

Physical therapy and occupational therapy is used postoperatively to readily mobilize the patients as soon as possible.

Results

There are a number of studies that find good to excellent results in terms of pain relief in 70% to 90% of patients (3,32–34). While

Table 2. Complications Associated with Scoliosis Correction

Neurological
  Paralysis
  Paraparesis
  Dural tear
  Pseudomeningeocele
  Blindness
Nonneurological
  Pulmonary embolus
  Myocardial infarction
  Pneumonia
  Wound infection
  Ileus
  Abdominal hernias
  Instrumentation failure
  Pseudarthrosis
  Hip pain

these results compare favorably with the surgical treatment for radicular and back pain from other causes, the magnitude of adult deformity surgery results in a significant complication risk. The rate of major and minor complications from adult deformity surgery can range from 20% to 47% (14,33) (Table 2). Most complications can be minimized by careful attention to nutrition, wound care, activity, venous thrombosis prophylaxis, and careful preoperative planning.

Most complications are relatively minor and transient and of limited long-term consequence. Major complications with serious sequelae occur at a high enough rate that both caution and experience should be employed when considering adult deformity correction. Further discussion on this topic is provided below.

Degeneration Beyond Fusion

It should be remembered that even though the caudal extent of fusion is determined as described above, one should also observe the discogram and MRI and extend the fusion beyond the disc space from where degeneration and symptoms may be emanating; this disc level and the vertebrae above are the caudal extension of the construct (2).

Also the fusion should never stop at the thoracolumbar junction because the chances of kyphosis progression tremendously increase. For example, in a King 2 curve, though the stable vertebrae might be T12, it should be extended down to at least L2 to include the junctional zone.

The crankshaft phenomenon will increase the likelihood of the disc degeneration in the adjacent disc level because of the fusion in the long constructs. Hence it is important to extend the fusion in a symptomatic patient who has had degeneration of the disc beyond the fusion level.

PSEUDARTHROSIS. In adult degenerative scoliosis, especially in an osteoporotic patient who has poor instrument–bone interface, a high rate of pseudarthrosis can be expected. Nuber and Schafer (14) found a 16.7% pseudarthrosis rate using a Harrington rod instrumentation system in 19 patients. However, in a study by Marchesi and Aebi (19), a 4% pseudarthrosis rate was observed in 27 patients using either a CDI system or AO internal fixator. This high rate of fusion in comparison to older studies

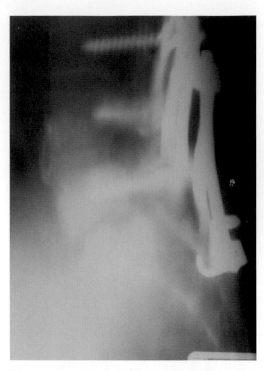

Fig. 15. This patient had three successive symptomatic pseudarthroses of a scoliosis construct. In this sagittal reconstruction, note the clear line of nonunion at L5-S1.

using the Harrington rod is due to the biomechanics properties of such a system.

A major risk factor for pseudarthrosis is fusion to the sacrum (Figs. 15 and 16). Saer et al. (35) had two pseudarthroses out of 17 patients who were fused down to the sacrum. Grubb et al. (9) reported a 17.5% pseudarthrosis rate after surgery, all occurring in patients fused to the sacrum. This rate can be reduced by combining the S1 pedicle screw fixation with a technique such as the Jackson intrasacral rod fixation. Also placement of cages through either an anterior approach or a posterior approach should reduce this high rate of pseudarthrosis.

A combined anterior and posterior approach to scoliosis surgery may decrease the rate of pseudarthrosis even further (14, 36). Byrd et al. (32), in a series of 26 patients with adult scoliosis, reported no cases of pseudarthrosis. Meticulous surgical principles such as resection of the soft tissue as much as possible and arthrodesis of the bony surface are of paramount importance. In our institutional experience, using an external orthosis for a period of 3 months is recommended to further decrease the rate of pseudarthrosis.

LOSS OF CORRECTION. Nuber and Schafer (14) in their series of 62 adult degenerative scoliosis patients corrected by either Harrington, Luque, or an anterior-posterior procedure had shown that the curve correction loss can be as high as 6.7 degrees in patients with Harrington rod instrumentation at 27 months follow-up, 4.2 degrees in the Luque rod instrumentation at 18 months follow-up, and 4.1 degrees in combined anterior-posterior procedure at 27 months.

Van Dam (31), using an anterior and posterior approach, reported only a 6% loss of curve as compared to an 8% to 14% loss for a posterior approach by other authors in the mid-1970s to mid-1980s.

These results show that either a segmental fusion technique

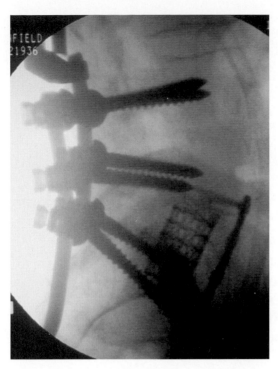

Fig. 16. Placement of a titanium cage and plate to prevent migration during the posterior reconstruction provided a durable solution for this patient.

or a combined procedure reduces the rate of curve correction loss. With better instrumentation such as CDI, one would expect better rates than previously reported.

WOUND INFECTION. Wound infection is minimized by meticulous surgical techniques and use of perioperative antibiotics. In patients who postoperatively develop wound infection with an intact fascial plain, local wound care is performed. For wounds that extend beyond the fascial plain, a second surgery to debride the wound and possibly placement of a flap by plastic surgeons over the instrumentation are done. We do not remove the hardware even if the infection is around the hardware. In our experience debridement of the devitalized tissue as described above followed by long-term intravenous and subsequently oral antibiotics controls the infection.

Conclusions

Changes in surgical techniques and instrumentation have given us unparalleled ability to stabilize and place corrective forces on the spine. When such power is applied correctly, we are able to treat many conditions that in the past had few options and often left patients debilitated with a deteriorating quality of life. When such power is applied incorrectly or poorly thought out, it can result in a disaster, leaving the patient worse off than before treatment.

It is this increase in technical ability that demands an equal increase in understanding of the pathophysiology and biomechanics of adult spine disease in general and scoliosis in particular. The understanding of spinal deformity treatment principles will help clinicians improve their understanding and treatment of all patients with spine disease.

As new techniques are developed that allow for manipulation of the biological environment of the spine and provide less invasive techniques for correction, it will be even more important to understand the underlying forces and disease.

References

1. Ogilvie JW. Adult scoliosis: evaluation and nonsurgical treatment [review]. *Instr Course Lect* 41:251–255, 1992.
2. Kostuik JP. Adult scoliosis: the lumbar spine. In: Bridwell KH, DeWald RL, eds. *The textbook of spinal surgery*, 2nd ed. Philadelphia: Lippincott-Raven, 1997.
3. Grubb SA, Lipscomb HJ, Suh PB. Results of surgical treatment of painful adult scoliosis. *Spine* 19(14):1619–1627, 1994.
4. Betz R, Bunnell W, Lambrecht-Mulier E, et al. Scoliosis and pregnancy. *J Bone Joint Surg* 69A:90, 1987.
5. Kostuik JP, Bentivoglio J. The incidence of low back pain in adult scoliosis. *Acta Orthop Belg* 47(4–5):548–559, 1981.
6. Kostuik JP, Bentivoglio J. The incidence of low-back pain in adult scoliosis. *Spine* 6(3):268–273, 1981.
7. Shands AR, Eisenberg HV. The incidence of scoliosis in the state of Delaware. *J Bone Joint Surg* 37(A):1243, 1955.
8. Robin GC, Span Y, Steinberg R, et al. Scoliosis in the elderly: a follow up study. *Spine* 7:355–359, 1982.
9. Grubb SA, Lipscomb HJ, Coonrad RW. Degenerative adult onset scoliosis. *Spine* 13(3):241–245, 1988.
10. Vanderpool DW, James JIP, Wynne-Davis R. Scoliosis in the elderly. *J Bone Joint Surg* 51A:446–455, 1969.
11. Weinstein SL, Zavala DC, Ponsetti I. Idiopathic scoliosis: long-term follow-up and prognosis in the untreated patients. *J Bone Joint Surg* 63A:702–712, 1983.
12. Collins DK, Ponsetti IV. Long-term follow-up of patients with idiopathic scoliosis not treated surgically. *J Bone Joint Surg* 51A: 425–445, 1969
13. King H, Moe JH, Bradford DS, et al. Selection of fusion levels in thoracic idiopathic scoliosis. *J Bone Joint Surg* 65A:1302–1313, 1983.
14. Nuber GW, Schafer MF. Surgical management of adult scoliosis. *Clin Orthop Rel Res* 208:228–237, 1986.
15. Winter RB, Lonstein JE, Denis F. Pain patterns in adult scoliosis. *Orthop Clin North Am* 19(2):339–345, 1988.
16. Epstein JA, Epstein BS, Jones MD. Symptomatic lumbar scoliosis with degenerative changes in the elderly. *Spine* 4(6):542–547, 1979.
17. Nachemson A. Adult scoliosis and back pain. *Spine* 4(6):513–517, 1979.
18. Kostuik JP. Recent advances in the treatment of painful adult scoliosis. *Clin Orthop Rel Res* 147:238–252, 1980.
19. Marchesi DG, Aebi M. Pedicle fixation devices in the treatment of adult lumbar scoliosis. *Spine* 17(suppl 8):S304, 1992.
20. van Dam BE. Nonoperative treatment of adult scoliosis [review]. *Orthop Clin North Am* 19(2):347–351, 1988.
21. Ascani E, Bartolozzi P, Logroscino CA, et al. Natural history of untreated idiopathic scoliosis after skeletal maturity. *Spine* 11:784–789, 1986.
22. Bener B, Ehni G. Degenerative lumbar scoliosis. *Spine* 4:548–552, 1979.
23. Dwyer AF, Newton NC, Sherwood AA. An anterior approach to scoliosis: a preliminary report. *Clin Orthop* 62:192–202, 1969.
24. Luque ER. Segmental spinal instrumentation for correction of scoliosis. *Orthopedics* 163:192–198, 1982.
25. Moe JH, Prucell GA, Bradford DS. Zielke instrumentation (VDS) for correction of spinal curvature. *Clin Orthop* 180:133, 1983.
26. Wegner DR, Carollo JJ, Wilkerson JA. Biomechanics of scoliosis correction by segmental spinal instrumentation. *Spine* 7(3):260–264, 1982.
27. Cotrel Y, Dubousset J, Guillaumat M. New universal instrumentation in spinal surgery. *Clin Orthop* 227:10–23, 1988.
28. Kostuik JP, Gleason TF, Errico TJ. The surgical correction of flat back syndrome (iatrogenic lumbar kyphosis). *Orthop Trans* 9:131, 1985.
29. Hayes MA, Tompkins SF, Herndon WA, et al. Clinical and radiolog-

ical evaluation of lumbosacral motion below fusion levels in idiopathic scoliosis. *Spine* 13(10):1161–1167, 1988.
30. Steel H. Rib resection and spine fusion in correction of convex deformity in scoliosis. *J Bone Joint Surg* 65A:920, 1983.
31. van Dam BE. Operative treatment of adult scoliosis with posterior fusion and instrumentation [review]. *Orthop Clin North Am* 19(2): 353–359, 1988.
32. Byrd A, Scoles PV, Winter RB, et al. Adult idiopathic scoliosis treated by anterior and posterior spinal fusion. *J Bone Joint Surg* 69A(6): 843–850, 1987.

33. Simmons ED Jr, Kowalski JM, Simmons EH. The results of surgical treatment for adult scoliosis. *Spine* 18(6):718–724, 1993.
34. van Dam BE, Bradford DS, Lonstein JE, et al. Adult idiopathic scoliosis treated by posterior spinal fusion and Harrington instrumentation. *Spine* 12(1):32–36, 1987.
35. Saer EH, Winter RB, Lonstein JE. Long scoliosis fusion to the sacrum in adults with nonparalytic scoliosis. An improved method. *Spine* 15(7):650–653, 1990.
36. Johnson J, Holt R. Combined use of anterior and posterior surgery for adult scoliosis. *Orthop Clin North Am* 19:361–366, 1988.

180. Adolescent Idiopathic Scoliosis

**Michael J. Rauzzino,
Christopher I. Shaffrey,
Russell P. Nockels,
Ajith Thomas, and
Gregory C. Wiggins**

Idiopathic scoliosis (IS) is the most common form of lateral deviation of the spine. IS is categorized according to the age of the patient at onset: infantile (0 to 3 years), juvenile (4 to 9 years), and adolescent (10 years to maturity). This chapter focuses on the most prevalent of the three—adolescent idiopathic scoliosis (AIS). The epidemiology and proposed mechanisms of AIS are reviewed, after which the clinical and radiographic evaluation of the patient and the natural history and classification of the various scoliotic curves are discussed. Lastly, treatment options and techniques are outlined.

Etiology and Epidemiology

The term *scoliosis* refers to a condition of lateral curvature of the spine. AIS is defined as a lateral curvature of the spine that develops near the onset of puberty for which no cause can be determined. It is always a diagnosis of exclusion and is differentiated from other forms of scoliosis, such as congenital scoliosis, which has a structural cause (i.e., a hemivertebra), and neuro-muscular scoliosis, in which the curvature results from a muscular imbalance (e.g., cerebral palsy). Based on the age of the patient at presentation, IS is categorized as infantile, juvenile, or adolescent (Table 1).

The prevalence of AIS depends on the magnitude of the curve used as a diagnostic criterion. A curve of 10 degrees, measured by the Cobb method, has been accepted as the smallest that can be considered diagnostic of AIS (1). If this criterion is used, 2% to 3% of adolescents (10 to 16 years) have scoliosis. As the magnitude of the curve on which the criterion is based increases, the prevalence decreases. AIS in which the curve is greater than 20 degrees has a prevalence of 0.3% to 0.5%, whereas the prevalence of AIS in which the curve is greater than 40 degrees is less than 0.1%. The majority of patients who are told that they have "scoliosis" have a minimal curve of less than 10 degrees and never require any form of treatment. The overall female-to-male ratio in AIS is 3.6:1. For small curves (~10 degrees), the distribution between the sexes is approximately equal, but as the magnitude of the curve increases, so does the female preponderance. The female-to-male ratio for AIS in which the curve is greater than 30 degrees is 10:1 (2) (Table 2).

The cause of AIS has not been clearly established. A number of theories have been proposed, but no one theory satisfactorily explains all aspects of AIS. Hereditary factors clearly play a role (3–5). In a metaanalysis of AIS in twins, the concordance was 73% in 37 sets of monozygotic twins and 36% in 31 sets of

Table 1. Classification of Scoliosis

Congenital scoliosis: Scoliosis resulting from congenitally anomalous vertebral development

Idiopathic scoliosis: A structural lateral spinal curvature for which no cause is established

Infantile scoliosis: Spinal curvature that develops during the first 3 years of life (0 to 3 years)

Juvenile scoliosis: Spinal curvature that develops between age 3 and puberty (3 to 10 years)

Adolescent scoliosis: Spinal curvature that develops at or about the onset of puberty (10 years to maturity)

Neuromuscular scoliosis: Scoliosis resulting from a known abnormality of the central nervous system or of the muscles and nerves

Table 2. Prevalence and Sex Distribution of Adolescent Idiopathic Scoliosis

Cobb angle (degrees)	Prevalence %	Female-to-male ratio
>10	2–3	1.4:1
>20	0.3–0.5	5.4:1
>30	0.1–0.3	10:1
>40	<0.1	NA

dizygotic twins (6). In these cases, the curves in the monozygotic twins were noted to develop and progress together. In a study of AIS in Boston, the incidence rates in first-, second-, and third-degree relatives were 11%, 2.4%, and 1.4%, respectively (7). If both parents have AIS, the risk to the offspring is 50 times greater than that of the normal population. Currently, the pattern of inheritance is presumed to be polygenic, an autosomal-dominant trait with incomplete penetrance. It has been noted that the age of mothers of patients with AIS is higher than that of mothers in the general population, and increased maternal age may be a risk factor for the disease.

Scoliosis occurs during periods of rapid growth, and such growth may be either a primary cause of AIS or a secondary trigger factor. It has been documented that girls with AIS are taller than nonscoliotic controls (8).

Changes in muscle have been studied (9). A greater proportion of type I fibers has been found on the convex side of a scoliotic curve, which suggests a muscle imbalance (10). Researchers using electron microscopy have noted differences in fiber size, target fibers, and internal nuclei on the convex versus the concave side of curves (11,12). Histochemical studies have also been performed. Results show decreased levels of adenosine triphosphatase and increased levels of intracellular calcium in both skeletal muscles and platelets in patients with AIS (13). Increased myoelectric amplitude and spontaneous activity have been noted in the muscles on the convex side of curves (14). Higher-amplitude myoelectric signals in the paraspinal muscles are found only in curves greater than 30 degrees, not in smaller curves or nonscoliotic controls (15).

Neuromuscular factors also play a role. Dysfunction of proprioceptive, vestibular, and visual systems has been noted in patients with AIS and may have a role in muscular imbalance. In a study of 150 patients with AIS, Yamamoto (16) noted that 79% had equilibrium dysfunction (versus 5% of nonscoliotic controls), which increased with progression of the scoliosis. This dysfunction was manifested in both the proprioceptive and optic reflex systems. Sahlstrand and Petruson (17) observed spontaneous and positional nystagmus in 50% of scoliotic patients but in only 3% of controls. An intrinsic developmental disturbance in the central nervous system involving central pattern generators in the spinal cord and causing a muscular imbalance, mainly in the spinal rotators associated with the ribs, has been reported (18).

The importance of the rib cage and the role of asymmetrical rib growth to the spinal column have also been studied. Scoliosis can be reliably produced in rabbits by resecting the costovertebral ligaments or dorsal rib heads. Other studies have shown that scoliosis induced in rabbits can be corrected by elongation or growth stimulation of ribs on the side of the convexity. According to the thoracic spinal theory proposed by Sevastik et al. (19), IS begins with overgrowth of the ribs (usually the left ribs) resulting from hypervascularity of the ipsilateral anterior hemithorax. The overgrowth alters the equilibrium of forces controlling the alignment of the normal spine and triggers the deformity in IS. This theory is useful for explaining the mode of origin of at least the most common form of IS, located in the thoracic spine.

In summary, the causes of IS remain elusive. Theories based on genetics, growth aspects, structural and biochemical changes in discs and muscles, and central nervous system changes have been entertained, but no single explanation has proved satisfactory, which suggests that the etiology is multifactorial. It is important for treating physicians to counsel their female patients of reproductive age who have AIS that their offspring are at increased risk for the development of scoliosis and should be monitored carefully.

Patient Evaluation

CLINICAL EXAMINATION. IS is a diagnosis of exclusion. A thorough medical history should be obtained from any patient with newly diagnosed scoliosis, and a rigorous physical examination should be performed to search for other causes of scoliosis. In taking the history, the examiner should inquire about when developmental milestones were attained and whether any siblings or relatives are affected. The age at menarche in female patients and voice change in male patients should be noted. A history of abnormalities of balance, gait, bowel/bladder function, hearing, vision, or any neurological symptoms, such as numbness or weakness, should be sought. The patient should be questioned regarding pain. Night pain may herald a pathological process, such as an osteoid osteoma (20).

The physical examination begins with a general inspection of the patient in the standing position. The patient's overall body habitus should be observed for disproportions, such as a discrepancy in leg length and ligamentous laxity. Obesity may mask early signs of spinal deformity. The skin should be examined for the cutaneous stigmata of occult spinal dysraphism (hairy patches, hyperpigmentation, dimples and pits, subcutaneous masses, or rudimentary appendages). Café-au-lait spots (particularly in the axilla), hyperpigmentation, or subcutaneous nodules may indicate neurofibromatosis. The relationship of the head and trunk to the pelvis, level of the shoulders, leg length, and lateral body profile must be recorded. A plumb line dropped from C7 should line up with the gluteal crease. The Adam forward-bend test can be used to reveal any shoulder asymmetry, rib hump, or lumbar prominence (20). The examiner should view the patient from three aspects: anterior, posterior, and lateral. An inclinometer is used during the forward-bend test to quantify the rib prominence and paralumbar prominence. A positive screen is defined as trunk rotation greater than 7 degrees in association with a scoliosis of 10 degrees and leads to a referral rate of 3% (21). If a discrepancy in leg length is noted, the forward-bend test should be performed with the patient in the sitting position. If a curve is found, manipulation and bending can be used to assess flexibility. When the neurological examination is performed, care must be taken not to miss subtle findings, such as asymmetrical reflexes or absent abdominal (umbilical) reflexes. Finally, physical maturity should be assessed and a Tanner rating assigned to determine the years of growth remaining. The maturation level is further corroborated by historical information obtained about menarche and by radiographic analysis of the hand and wrist for bone age.

RADIOGRAPHIC ASSESSMENT

General. The main goals of the radiographic evaluation are to assess the curve (location, magnitude of rotation, and flexibility) and the patient's skeletal maturity and to rule out any underlying structural pathology as a cause of the scoliosis. This information is essential for developing a treatment plan.

Curve Assessment. Standing scoliosis radiographs should be obtained on a 36-in film to include the cervicothoracic junction down to the middle of the pelvis. Films are obtained in the posterior-to-anterior (PA) direction to reduce radiation of the breasts. For the initial examination, frontal and sagittal radiographs should be obtained to assess the deformity in both planes; however, subsequent films can be in the frontal plane only so as to limit radiation exposure.

Curve magnitude is assessed by determining the Cobb angle

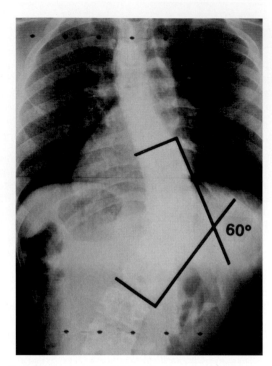

Fig. 1. Measurement of the Cobb angle. On a standing anteroposterior (AP) radiograph, perpendicular lines are drawn from the transverse axis of the upper and lower end vertebrae (each end vertebra being the last vertebra of a curve that tilts maximally toward the concavity of the curve). The angle formed by the intersection of the perpendicular lines defines the Cobb angle.

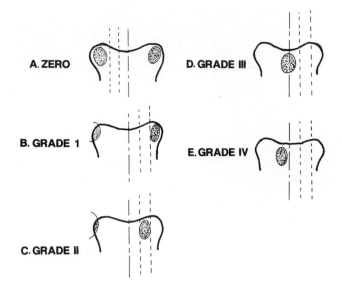

Fig. 2. The Nash and Moe method of evaluating vertebral rotation. On an AP film, two lines are drawn between the middle and lateral borders of the apical vertebral body of the convexity of the curve. **A:** Zero rotation. The pedicles are lined up at the edge of the vertebral bodies. **B,C,D:** Grades I through III rotation. The pedicle has moved into the first, second, and third sections, respectively. **E:** Grade IV rotation. The pedicle has rotated beyond the midpoint of the vertebra.

(22) (Fig. 1). Perpendicular lines are drawn from the transverse axis of the upper and lower end vertebrae (an end vertebra being the last vertebra of a curve that tilts maximally toward the concavity of the curve). The angle formed by the intersection of the perpendiculars is the Cobb angle.

Curve rotation is assessed either by the method of Nash and Moe according to a scale of five grades (0 through 4) or by the Pedriolle method as a measurement in degrees (21,23) (Figs. 2 and 3). This information is useful in determining which vertebrae are the neutral vertebrae; these are used to determine fusion levels.

Curve flexibility is assessed before any surgery is considered by supine bending. Traction films with the patient in a head halter and ankle traction also help in the assessment of curve flexibility. Knowing the degree of curve flexibility is necessary in deciding which levels need to be fused.

Curve classification is determined based on the location of the apical vertebra. In this classification, cervical curves have an apex between C1 and C6, cervicothoracic curves between C7 and T1, thoracic curves between T2 and T11, thoracolumbar curve between T12 and L1, lumbar curves between L2 and L4, and lumbosacral curves between L5 and S1. The direction of the apex, right or left, is also given in addition to the diagnostic category if known (Table 3). The most common curve pattern is a right thoracic curve with a left lumbar curve. However, a variety of curve patterns exist. In order of frequency, they include right thoracic, left lumbar, right thoracolumbar, double thoracic, and left thoracic, right thoracolumbar curves.

Scoliosis, kyphosis, and *lordosis* are terms used to describe deviations from normal spinal alignment. In the frontal plane, the spine is normally straight. In the sagittal plane, the thoracic region is kyphotic (range, 20 to 40 degrees), the lumbar region lordotic (range, 30 to 50 degrees), and the transition over the

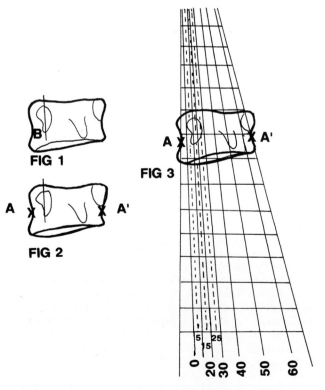

Fig. 3. The Pedriolle method of evaluating vertebral rotation of the apical vertebral body of the convexity of the curve. The largest dimension of the pedicle is marked (*A*), and a line is drawn between the two points marking the waist of each lateral border of the vertebra (*B, B'*). A torsiometer is superimposed over the lateral borders of the vertebral body as shown. The reading in this illustration is 10 degrees.

Table 3. Scoliotic Curves by Location

Cervical curve: Spinal curvature with an apex from C1 to C6
Cervicothoracic curve: Spinal curvature with an apex at C7 or T1
Thoracic curve: Scoliosis in which the apex of the curvature is between T2 and T11
Thoracolumbar curve: Spinal curvature with an apex at T12 or L1
Lumbar curve: Spinal curvature with an apex from L1 to L4
Lumbosacral curve: Spinal curvature with an apex at L5 or below

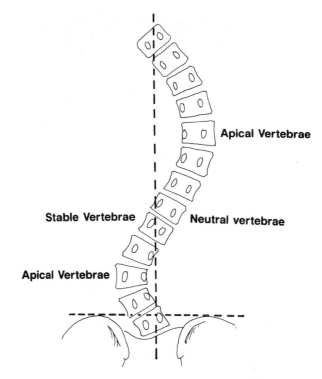

Fig. 4. Determination of the stable vertebra for surgical planning. The stable vertebra is the lowest vertebra with pedicles bisected by a perpendicular line drawn from the midpoint of the S1 pedicles.

thoracolumbar region relatively straight. Scoliosis, a curvature in the coronal plane, is also associated with transverse rotation and potentially a pathological lordosis or kyphosis. Therefore, the descriptive terms *lordoscoliosis* and *kyphoscoliosis* are frequently used to characterize the three-dimensional character of the deformity more precisely. When more than one pathological curvature exists along the length of the spine, a primary curve is designated based on size and rigidity, although a secondary curve, even if "compensatory," may be rigid or have a "structural" component (Table 4).

King and colleagues (24) developed an important classification system based on a review of frontal radiographs from 149 cases of AIS. A line was drawn on standing PA radiographs through the center of the sacrum perpendicular to the iliac crests. The vertebrae most nearly bisected by this line were designated the *stable* vertebrae (Fig. 4). This classification includes five curve patterns that are based on the number, flexibility, and deviation of curves from the midline (Fig. 5). A type I curve is an *S*-shaped double curve in which both the lumbar and thoracic curves cross the midline, but the lumbar curve is larger and less flexible than the thoracic curve. A type II curve is also an *S*-shaped double curve in which both the lumbar and the thoracic curves cross the midline, but here the thoracic curve is larger and less flexible. A type III curve is essentially a single major thoracic curve with an apex around T8 in which the lumbar curve does not cross the midline. A type IV curve is a long thoracolumbar curve with an apex near T10 and an end vertebra in the lumbar spine. A type V pattern is a double thoracic curve in which T1 tilts into the convexity of the upper thoracic curve, and the upper curve is structural when observed on side-bending films. Despite wide acceptance of this system, recent studies have shown that its intraobserver and interobserver reliability may be less than optimal.

Lenke and associates (25) have proposed a newer classifica-

Table 4. Scoliotic Curve Glossary

Primary curve: The first or earliest of several curves to appear, if identifiable.

Major curve: Term used to designate the larger (largest) curve(s), usually structural.

Minor curve: Term used to refer to the smaller (smallest) curve(s).

Structural curve: A segment of the spine with a fixed lateral curvature. Radiographically, it is identified in supine lateral side-bending views by the failure to correct. Structural curves may be multiple.

Compensatory curve: A curve, which can be structural, above or below a major curve that tends to maintain normal body alignment.

Fractional curve: A compensatory curve that is incomplete because it returns to the erect. Its only horizontal vertebra is caudad or cephalad.

Functional curve, nonstructural curve: A curve that has no structural component and that corrects or overcorrects on recumbent side-bending radiographic views.

tion for thoracic curves that is based on six types of curve patterns and their relationship to a center sacral vertebral line drawn on a standing 36-in PA radiograph. Type I is a primary thoracic curve. Type II is a double thoracic curve. Type III is a double major curve. Type IV is a triple major curve. Type V is a primary thoracolumbar curve. Type VI is a primary thoracolumbar curve with a secondary structural thoracic curve. The relationship of the lumbar curve to the center sacral vertebral line determines its magnitude and classifies the curve as type A (minimal), type B (moderate), or type C (large). A T5-12 sagittal plane modifier is used to include the degree of kyphosis ($-$, N, $+$) on the lateral radiograph (Fig. 6).

Skeletal Maturity. Skeletal maturity and hence the potential for further growth can be assessed by a variety of methods. A useful one involves the Risser sign (26), which is another radiographic means to estimate skeletal maturity and is based on the appearance and fusion of the iliac apophysis (Fig. 7). Ossification begins in the apophysis anteriorly and progresses in a posterior direction until the entire iliac wing is capped. Then the apophysis becomes fused to the body of the ilium. The Risser stages are numbered from 0 to 5; stage 0 is the stage before ossification of the iliac apophysis has begun. Stages 1 through 4 correspond to the sequential ossification of each quarter of the iliac crest, beginning with stage 1, in which ossification has taken place within the first 25% of the crest, and ending with stage 4, in which ossification has covered 75% to 100% of the crest. In stage 5, the apophysis is closed and fused to the ilium; stage 5 marks the end of growth. The appearance of the iliac ossification center signifies that puberty is under way in both boys and girls. Generally, spinal growth is complete once Risser stage 4 has been reached.

Occult Pathology. The incidence of spinal cord pathology in patients with presumed AIS has been reported to be between

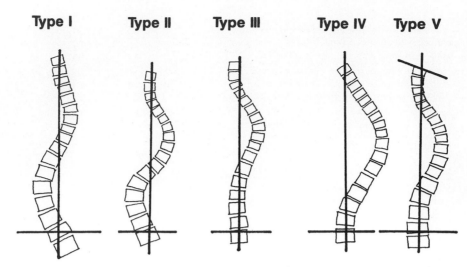

Fig. 5. King classification of thoracic scoliosis. Type I, *S*-shaped curve in which both the thoracic curve and the lumbar curve cross the midline. The lumbar curve is larger and less flexible than the thoracic curve. Type II, *S*-shaped curve in which both the thoracic curve and the lumbar curve cross the midline. The thoracic curve is larger and less flexible. Type III, thoracic curve in which the lumbar curve does not cross the midline. Type IV, long thoracic curve in which L4 tilts into the thoracic curve. Type V, double thoracic curve with T1 tilted into the thoracic curve. Upper thoracic curve is structural on side bending.

Curve Type

Type	Proximal Thoracic	Main Thoracic	Thoracolumbar / Lumbar	Curve Type
1	Non-Structural	Structural (Primary)	Non-Structural	Primary Thoracic
2	Structural	Structural (Primary)	Non-Structural	Double Thoracic
3	Non-Structural	Structural (Primary)	Structural	Double Major
4	Structural	Structural (Primary)	Structural	Triple Major
5	Non-Structural	Non-Structural	Structural (Primary)	Primary Thoracolumbar / Lumbar
6	Non-Structural	Structural	Structural (Primary)	Primary Thoracolumbar / Lumbar Secondary Structural Thoracic (Lumbar Curve > Thoracic by ≥ 10°)

STRUCTURAL CRITERIA

Proximal Thoracic: - Side Bending Cobb ≥ 25°
- T2 - T5 Kyphosis ≥ +20°

Main Thoracic: - Side Bending Cobb ≥ 25°

Thoracolumbar / Lumbar: - Side Bending Cobb ≥ 25°
- T10 - L2 Kyphosis ≥ +20°

LOCATION OF APEX
(SRS definition)

CURVE	APEX
THORACIC	T2 - T11-12 DISC
THORACOLUMBAR	T12 - L1
LUMBAR	L1-2 DISC - L4

Modifiers

Lumbar Spine Modifier	CSVL to Lumbar Apex
A	CSVL Between Pedicles
B	CSVL Touches Apical Body(ies)
C	CSVL Completely Medial

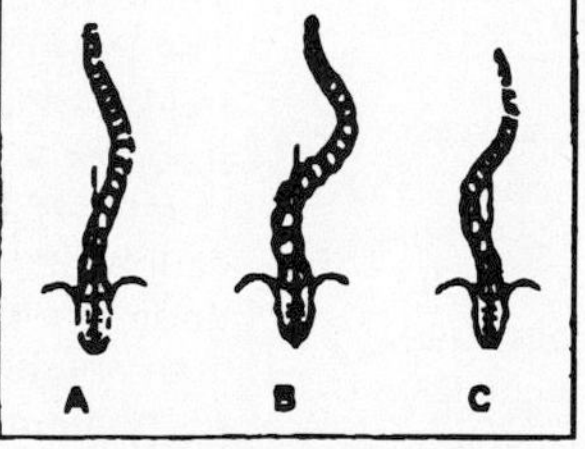

Thoracic Sagittal Profile T5 - T12		
–	(Hypo)	< 10°
N	(Normal)	10° - 40°
+	(Hyper)	> 40°

Curve Type (1-6) **+** Lumbar Spine Modifier (A, B, or C) **+** Thoracic Sagittal Modifier (-, N, or +)
Classification (e.g. 1 B +):_____

A

Fig. 6. Lenke system for the classification of thoracolumbar scoliosis. **A:** Curve types I through VI.

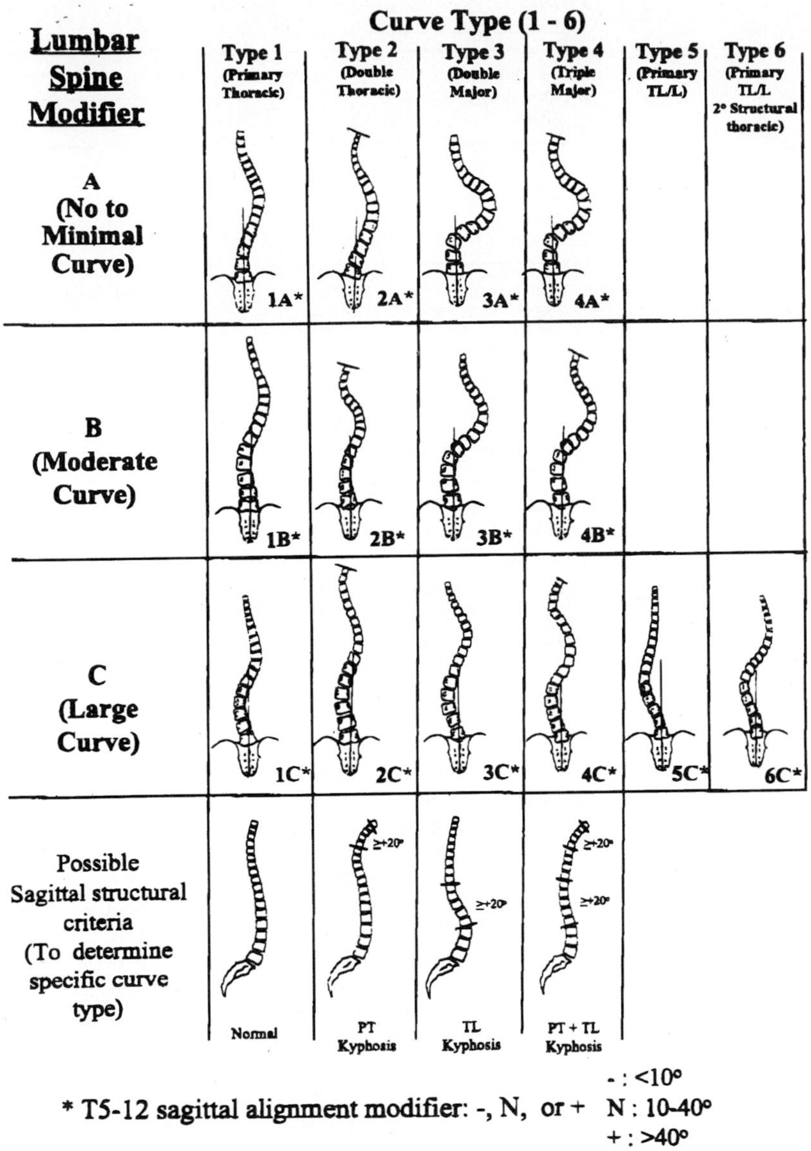

Fig. 6. (continued). **B:** Curve modifiers.

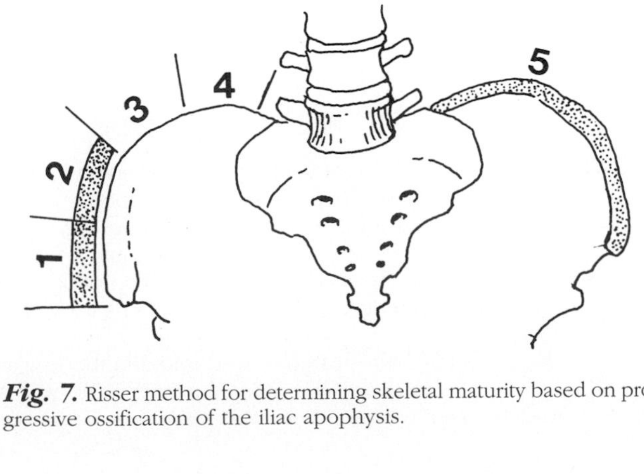

Fig. 7. Risser method for determining skeletal maturity based on progressive ossification of the iliac apophysis.

3% and 20% (27–29). For adolescent girls with normal neurological examination findings and a typical right thoracic curve pattern, it is usually not necessary to perform additional imaging [i.e., magnetic resonance imaging (MRI) or computed tomography (CT)]. It is important that the physician remember that a number of other conditions may result in scoliosis. Adolescents with occult spinal dysraphism (diastematomyelia, tethered cord, lipomyelomeningocele, dermoid and neurenteric cysts) may present with scoliosis. Patients with cutaneous stigmata, abnormal neurological findings, excessively large curves (>70 degrees), and atypical curves (left thoracic curves) merit additional imaging to exclude abnormal spinal pathology.

CLINICAL PRESENTATION. In AIS, the presence of deformity is the primary reason for referral because the patients are otherwise asymptomatic. Typically, AIS occurs in girls. The incidence in boys is approximately one-tenth that in girls. The patient usually presents when body asymmetry is noted, such as a trunk shift, uneven shoulders, rib prominence, breast asym-

Table 5. Factors That Positively Influence
Curve Progression in the Skeletally Immature Patient

Younger age at presentation
Premenarcheal status
Low Risser grade
Female sex
Double curves
Larger-magnitude curves

Table 7. Probability of Progression: Curve
Magnitude versus Age at Initial Detection

Curve magnitude at Detection (degrees)	Age at detection (y)		
	10–12	13–15	16
<19	25%	10%	0%
20–29	60%	40%	10%
30–59	90%	70%	30%
>60	100%	90%	70%

From Weinstein SL, Ponseti IV. Curve progression in idiopathic scoliosis. *J Bone Joint Surg Am* 65:447–456, 1983, with permission.

metry, or waist asymmetry. School screening has traditionally been a means of identifying these curves. Atypical cases such as left thoracic curves merit additional radiographic imaging, as noted above.

Natural History

The natural history of AIS can be assessed radiographically (curve progression) and by clinical outcome (pain, mortality).

CURVE PROGRESSION. The natural history of AIS as it pertains to curve progression was studied extensively by Weinstein and Ponseti, who followed the same group of 102 patients for more than 40 years (30). Before these studies, the prognosis for untreated curves was felt to be dismal because patients with all varieties of scoliosis (including neuromuscular scoliosis) were grouped together. Weinstein and Ponseti found six factors that influence the probability of curve progression in the skeletally immature female patient (Table 5): (a) chronological age (the younger the patient at the time of diagnosis, the higher the risk for curve progression); (b) menarche (the risk for progression is greater before the onset of menses); (c) Risser grade (a lower Risser grade is associated with greater curve progression); (d) female sex (girls are 10 times more likely to progress than boys); (e) double curves (which have a greater tendency to progress than single curves); and (f) curves of larger magnitude (which are more likely to progress) (Table 6). Nonpredictive factors are a positive family history, thoracic kyphosis, lumbar lordosis, and trunk imbalance (31).

Lonstein and Carlson reviewed 727 patients with IS and an initial curve of less than 30 degrees (32). All the patients were followed without any intervention. The overall progression rate was 23.2%, and the incidence of curve progression was related to the pattern and magnitude of the curve, the patient's age at presentation, the Risser sign, and the patient's menarcheal status. They noted that for a child with a small curve (<19 degrees), the risk for curve progression was more than 10 times

greater (22.6% vs. 1.6%) if the patient was skeletally immature (Risser grade 0 or 1). For a child with a larger curve (20 to 29 degrees), the risk was also increased (68% vs. 23%) if the patient was skeletally immature (Table 7). Thus, the worst prognosis for progression is in a skeletally immature patient who presents with a large curve. They did not find a correlation between sex and risk for progression.

During the adolescent years, curves typically progressed an average of 1 degree per month (30,33,34). Some curves progressed even after growth was finished, and curves in excess of 50 degrees were highly likely to progress even after skeletal maturity (30,35). Several risk factors have been determined for the progression of various curves, based mainly on the Cobb angle and degree of rotation of the apical vertebra (30,36). For example, an adult who has a thoracic curve with a Cobb angle larger than 50 degrees or a lumbar curve with a Cobb angle larger than 30 degrees is at significant risk for progression, and surgery should be considered (30,36) (Table 8).

In a more recent study, conducted by the Scoliosis Research Society (37), 159 girls with a mean age of 13 years (range, 10 to 15 years) who had AIS were followed prospectively until skeletal maturity or until the curve had increased 6 degrees or more. All patients had an initial curve of 25 to 35 degrees and an apical level between the eighth thoracic and first lumbar vertebrae, inclusively. The curves progressed at least 6 degrees in 80 patients. Predictive factors for progression included the patient's Risser sign, the apical level of the curve, and the degree of imbalance.

MORTALITY. Mortality rates for patients with AIS are comparable with those of age-matched controls (31). Kolind-Sorensten (38) reported that the mortality rate for patients with curves in the range of 40 to 100 degrees was comparable with that of the general population, but in patients with curves greater than 100 degrees, the mortality rate doubled. In a study of 194 patients with untreated AIS who were seen at the University of Iowa between 1932 and 1948, the mortality rate was 15%. Actuarial data for patients born in the same years as the scoliosis group indicated an expected mortality rate of 17%.

BACK PAIN. The incidence of back pain in patients with scoliosis is comparable with that in the general population (39–42). Horal (43) noted that patients with scoliosis did not represent a disproportionate incidence of disability pensions, and Nachemson (41) and Nilsonne and Lundgren (42) did not demonstrate any increase in clinical or financial problems related to IS in their studies.

Back pain in patients with AIS followed into adulthood was most likely to occur in those with curves greater than 50 degrees. Curves below any major deformity, such as a compensa-

Table 6. Probability of Progression According to Risser Grade and Curve Magnitude at Detection

Risser grade	Curve magnitude (degrees)	
	5–19	20–29
0–1	22%	68%
2–4	1.6%	23%

From Lonstein JE, Carlson JM. The prediction of curve progression in untreated idiopathic scoliosis during growth. *J Bone Joint Surg Am* 66:1061–1071, 1984, with permission.

Table 8. Progression Factors in Curves Greater than 30 Degrees at Skeletal Maturity

Lumbar	Thoracolumbar	Combined
Cobb angle >30 degrees	Cobb angle >30 degrees	Cobb angle >50 degrees
Apical vertebral rotation >30 degrees	Apical vertebral rotation >30 degrees	Apical vertebral rotation >30 degrees
Curve direction	Transitory shifts	
Transitory shifts		
Relation of L5 to interest line		

From Weinstein SL, Ponseti IV. Curve progression in idiopathic scoliosis. Long-term follow-up. *J Bone Joint Surg Am* 65:447–456, 1983, with permission.

tory lumbosacral fractional curve, were the most painful and disabling (44). Pain increased with age and the degree of scoliotic curvature and was felt to be caused by facet joint changes, radicular compression, and discogenic disease. Surgery was markedly beneficial in these patients, with 83% of surgical patients having obtained sufficient pain relief at an average follow-up of 5 years to have made surgery worthwhile.

PREGNANCY. The effects of pregnancy on curve progression were studied in a group of 175 patients with scoliosis who had had at least one pregnancy versus a similar group of 180 patients with scoliosis who had had no pregnancies (45). No difference in curve progression was noted between the two groups. Curve progression of 5 degrees was seen in 25% of patients in both groups, and curve progression of 10 degrees was noted in 5% of patients in both groups. The risk for progression was not affected by the age of the patient at the time of her first pregnancy, the number of pregnancies, or the curve stability. It was noted that scoliosis caused no problems during pregnancy except in four patients at the time of delivery. The rate of cesarean section was half that of the national average, and no cesarean section was directly related to a mother's scoliosis.

Bracing

Bracing is the mainstay of nonoperative treatment for AIS (46–50). The value of bracing with proper indications has been proved in numerous studies (51–67). A recent metaanalysis of nonoperative treatment for AIS showed bracing to be significantly better than either observation or electrical stimulation (47). Nonoperative treatments such as electrical stimulation and exercise have not been proved effective and should not be considered in the conservative approach to AIS. Bracing is expected to prevent progression of the curve until the patient's growth is complete and does not achieve significant curve correction on a long-term basis. Cosmesis, however, may be improved after a period of bracing. These considerations should be discussed thoroughly with patients and their families before any trial of bracing.

The efficacy of bracing must be studied in the context of the natural history of the disease (i.e., the risk for curve progression). The best published data come from a study of 747 untreated patients with AIS reported by Lonstein and Carlson (32). For example, if a patient is a skeletally mature adolescent girl (Risser grades 2 through 4) with a curve of less than 20 degrees, then the chance of her curve progressing is low (1.6%). It is apparent that bracing is unnecessary for this type of patient. Conversely, if a patient is a skeletally immature girl (Risser grade 0 or 1) with a curve measuring 20 to 29 degrees, then she is at high risk (68%) for progression, and her course may be modified by bracing. Knowing the natural history allows one to judge

the efficacy of treatment. For example, if 100 patients similar to the high-risk patient described above are braced and the progression rate is only 20%, compared with an expected progression rate of 68% in untreated patients, then the treatment can be considered successful.

Several studies have examined the efficacy of bracing in high-risk patients. Lonstein and Winter (63) reported 1,020 patients who had AIS treated with a Milwaukee brace. In this series, the high-risk, skeletally immature patients with a curve between 20 and 30 degrees had only a 40% rate of progression instead of the expected rate of 68%. Studies by Bassett et al. (53) and Durand and Salanova (55) reported similar success in this same population of patients, with progression rates of 28% and 21%, respectively.

In a prospective study by the Scoliosis Research Society (66), 247 girls who had AIS, a thoracic or thoracolumbar curve of 25 to 35 degrees, and a mean age of 12 years and 7 months were followed to determine the effect of (a) observation only, (b) an underarm plastic brace, or (c) nighttime surface electrical stimulation. Of the 111 girls braced with an underarm Boston brace for scoliosis of 25 to 35 degrees, the curve progressed in only 17 (15%). In comparison, a progression rate of 64% was noted for observation alone. The 64% progression rate for untreated high-risk patients is almost identical to that predicted by Lonstein and Carlson. Interestingly, the rate of progression in the group that received electrical stimulation alone was higher (67%) than the rate in the control group.

Based on the results of these studies, clear indications for the use of bracing in AIS have been developed, which are listed in Table 9 along with the contraindications for bracing.

MILWAUKEE BRACE. The Milwaukee brace was first designed by Blount and colleagues (68) for the treatment of postpoliomyelitis scoliosis. It consists of a plastic pelvic section, an anterior and two posterior uprights connected by a neck ring

Table 9. Indications for Bracing in Idiopathic Scoliosis

Curve magnitude (degrees)	Treatment
0–20	Observation only (at 6- to 12-month intervals)
20–30	Observe at 3-month intervals; brace if curve progresses to >5 degrees
30–45	Brace at presentation
>45	Consider surgery

Contraindications to bracing
Completion of growth
Severe thoracic lordosis (thoracic kyphosis = 0 degrees)
Progressive hypokyphosis while patient is braced
Morbid obesity
Patient's refusal to comply with bracing

superiorly, a throat mold anteriorly, and occipital pads posteriorly (63,69) (Fig. 8). The Milwaukee brace is the oldest and
most proven of all the braces used to treat scoliosis, and because
of its cervical superstructure, it is the only brace suitable for
curves with an apex at T8 or above (70). The authors noted
that the best predictor of the results of Milwaukee brace treatment was the initial response of the curve to the brace, especially during the first year of treatment. If the curve was reduced
in the brace to less than 50% of its initial measurement, the
chance of obtaining significant permanent correction was good.

BOSTON BRACE. The Boston brace is actually a system rather
than a single brace. It consists of a Boston thoracic brace, a
Boston thoracolumbosacral orthosis (TLSO), and a Boston lumbar brace. These braces come in various sizes and are padded
and fitted to the individual patient. Emans et al. (56) studied
295 patients treated with the Boston bracing system for curves
ranging between 20 and 59 degrees with a follow-up of at least
1 year. Of these patients, 88% had final correction of less than
15 degrees, but only 11% of the patients underwent surgery
during the period of bracing. The highest rates of correction
and control were obtained in major curves with an apex below
T8 and above L2. A strong correlation between best or initial
in-brace correction and follow-up correction was noted. In a
comparison study of the Boston system and the Charleston
brace, Katz et al. (60) found the Boston brace system to be
more effective than the Charleston brace.

WILMINGTON BRACE. The Wilmington brace, designed by
MacEwen in 1969, is a custom-fitted underarm thermoplastic
jacket made from an impression of a cast applied to the patient
(Fig. 9). Hanks et al. (58) studied 100 female patients treated
for IS with the Wilmington brace and noted a success rate of

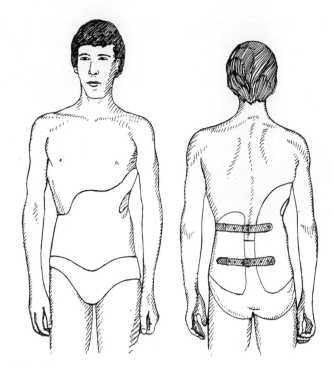

Fig. 9. Wilmington brace. Custom-molded underarm thoracolumbosacral orthosis (TLSO) effective for curves with an apex below T8.

81%. Ten patients (10%) underwent posterior spinal fusion for
curve progression.

Howard et al. (70) studied 170 patients who completed brace
treatment for AIS. The treatment groups consisted of 45 patients
with TLSOs (i.e., Wilmington braces), 95 with Charleston
braces, and 35 with Milwaukee braces. The TLSOs and Charleston braces were used on comparable curves, whereas the Milwaukee braces were used in a subgroup for which the other
brace designs were considered inappropriate (i.e., high thoracic
curves). Age, Risser stage, curve size, and duration of bracing
and observation did not differ between the groups. Mean progression of the curve during bracing was 1.1 degrees with the
TLSO, 6.5 degrees with the Charleston brace, and 6.3 degrees
with the Milwaukee brace. The proportion of patients with more
than 10 degrees of curve progression was 14% with the TLSO,
28% with the Charleston brace, and 43% with the Milwaukee
brace. The proportion of patients who underwent surgery was
18% with the TLSO, 31% with the Charleston brace, and 23%
with the Milwaukee brace.

CHARLESTON BRACE. The Charleston bending brace is a
custom-molded orthosis that holds the patient in maximal side-
bending correction. The patient is kept in a severely bent position that prevents ambulation, and therefore the brace is worn
only at night, for a minimum of 8 hours each day. It is more
attractive to patients because it is worn only at home. It has
been in use for a shorter period than the other types of braces,
and its indications and efficacy are less clear.

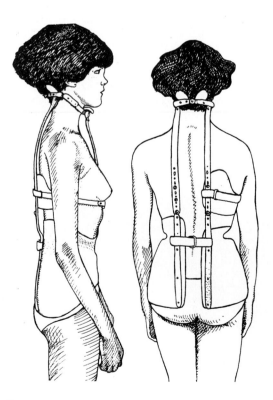

Fig. 8. Milwaukee brace. Note proper fitting with correction of lumbar
lordosis and adjustment of throat mold and occipital pads. It is effective
for most thoracic curves.

CHOICE OF BRACE. The choice of brace type is up to both
physician and patient. The Milwaukee brace, for which the most
clinical data are available to support its use, is highly effective.
However, it is somewhat cumbersome and cosmetically unap-
pealing. It is perhaps best limited to patients with curves in
which the apex is above T8, for whom other brace options are

less effective. TLSO braces such as the Boston and Wilmington braces are effective for thoracic curves below T7 and for thoracolumbar and lumbar curves. They also have a proven record of success, are more acceptable to the wearer than the Milwaukee brace, and are a first-line treatment option. The newer Charleston bending brace has the advantage of being the least socially traumatic to the wearer because it is worn only at night. Although studies have proved its usefulness, it is probably best reserved for patients with single curves of relatively small magnitude.

To be effective, bracing must be carried out properly. Braces should be (a) fitted properly (a 50% curve correction should be achieved with the brace at the initial fitting), (b) worn on a full-time basis (20 hours per day), and (c) worn for an extended period of time until growth stops (no further increase in height, at least 18 months since menarche, and a Risser grade of 4 or 5) (71).

Some authors advocate part-time bracing, noting that patients are often noncompliant anyway; however, data still support full-time bracing. In a metaanalysis of 37 peer-reviewed articles published between 1975 and 1993 in which 1,910 patients with IS were treated nonoperatively, Rowe et al. (47) noted the following mean proportions of success:

39.	Lateral electrical stimulation
78.	Observation only
138.	Bracing for 8 hours a day (part-time)
198.	Bracing for 16 hours a day (part-time)
0.93.	Bracing for 23 hours a day (full-time)

Surgical Decision Making

For those patients who present with large curves or whose curve progresses despite bracing, surgery offers both curve correction via instrumentation and a halt to curve progression with fusion. The decision-making process for surgical treatment is based on many factors. One of the most basic issues confronting the surgeon is proper identification of the curve type and accurate measurement of the curve. The choice of which curve(s) to fuse and the type of surgical approach to use (posterior, anterior, or a combination of the two) depends on the flexibility of the curve as noted on side-bending films. If a combined approach is indicated, then a decision is made either to stage the surgeries or to perform both in one session (Table 10). The goals of surgery should always be simple. It is hoped that the final result will be a patient with a well-balanced, cosmetically pleasing appearance who is functional and pain-free, both initially and later on into maturity (72,73) (Table 11).

DETERMINATION OF FUSION LEVELS. In 1983, King et al. (24) published their experience in the surgical treatment of 405

Table 10. Factors to Consider in Planning
Surgery for Scoliosis Correction

Skeletal age
Scoliosis magnitude
Scoliosis flexibility
Relative shoulder heights
Sagittal plane deformity
Stable vertebrae
Neutrally rotated vertebrae

Table 11. Basic Goals of Surgery for Deformity

Gain correction
Prevent progression
Maintain balance
Fuse as few levels as possible

patients with IS. They developed a classification system and treatment strategies that are still used today, particularly the concept of selective thoracic fusion for certain curves with both a thoracic and a lumbar component (King type II curve). Previously, Moe (74) had developed the concept of the "neutral" vertebra to define the extent of the curve and advocated fusion from the superior neutral vertebra to the inferior neutral vertebra. With their new classification scheme, King et al. stressed the importance of choosing as the inferior vertebra to fuse the most distal vertebra that was balanced over the sacrum. They developed the concept of the "stable vertebra"—the vertebra that is most nearly bisected by a vertical line drawn through the center of the sacrum after the pelvis has been leveled (Table 12). They noted that when a stable vertebra was selected to be the inferior level of fusion, a balanced and stable spine was virtually always achieved. If the neutral vertebra and the stable vertebra were one and the same, then the choice of fusion levels was simple. If, however, the stable vertebra was not the same vertebra as the neutral vertebra, the stable vertebra took precedence and was chosen to be the lowest fused vertebra. The lowest instrumented vertebra had to be as nearly parallel to the pelvis as possible (except in type II curves, in which it is best to have some residual tilt to allow the lumbar curve to accommodate). The top and bottom had to be within 10 degrees of neutral and fall within the stable zone of Harrington. The stable zone of Harrington is defined by drawing two vertical lines through the S1 pedicles perpendicular to the pelvis.

In a type I curve, the major lumbar curve (usually to the right) is larger and stiffer than the secondary thoracic curve (usually to the left). In the original series of King (75), it was suggested that this type of curve be treated with posterior fusion of both the lumbar and the thoracic curves down to the stable vertebra. In most cases, this approach is still used today. With the advent of improved anterior instrumentation systems, these lumbar curves can now be approached anteriorly in some cases (76). If the thoracic curve is flexible, then only the lumbar curve need be fused, and this can be approached anteriorly rather than posteriorly to spare lumbar levels (77). The importance of spar-

Table 12. Key Vertebrae Used to Determine Fusion Levels

Apical vertebra: The most rotated vertebra in a curve; the most deviated vertebra from the vertical axis of the patient.

End vertebra: The most cephalad vertebra of a curve whose superior surface, or the most caudad vertebra of a curve whose inferior surface, tilts maximally toward the concavity of the curve. It is used in the measurement of the Cobb angle.

Neutral vertebra: Vertebra with no transverse plane rotation, so that on the frontal plane anteroposterior radiograph, the spinous process is located midway between the pedicles. It is often found at the transition zone between two curves and is often the most tilted vertebra.

Stable vertebra The vertebra most nearly bisected by a line through the center of the sacrum on the frontal view. A line is drawn perpendicular to a line across the top of the sacrum or iliac crest that passes through the sacral spinous processes. It indicates that the vertebra is situated over the center of the sacrum.

Transitional vertebra: Vertebra that is neutral in relation to rotation, usually at the end of a curve.

Table 13. Back Pain Versus Level of Fusion

Level	Percentage with pain
L1	25
L2	30
L3	39
L4	62
L5	82
Control	53

From Cochran T, Irstam L, Wachemson A. Long-term anatomic and functional changes in patients with adolescent idiopathic scoliosis treated with Narrington rod instrumentation. *Spine* 8:576–584, 1983, with permission.

ing lumbar levels to preserve motion segments and reduce back pain in adulthood is well recognized (78). Cochran et al. (79) documented that the risk for the development of late back pain after fusion is directly related to the length of the fusion. They noted that if a fusion could be stopped before L4, then the risk for the development of back pain later in life was no greater than that in the general population (Table 13). Additionally, the anterior fusion allows discectomies to release segments and, in turn, increase correction. The surgeon can then involve fewer levels, and it is often necessary to fuse only the vertebrae within the curve instead of fusing to the stable vertebra. However, it is often necessary to insert structural allograft into the anterior disc spaces to prevent the development of kyphosis across the instrumented levels (Fig. 10).

The pattern of a King type II curve is the reverse of a type I pattern. The thoracic curve is the structural curve, being larger and stiffer than the lumbar curve. The literature is fairly controversial in terms of the recommended treatment (80–83). The major issue is whether it is necessary to include the lumbar

curve in the fusion. The most predictable trunk balance is achieved by instrumentation to the stable vertebra. However, in a double major curve (King types I and II), L4 may be the lower stable vertebra. Therefore, a dilemma exists because the weight of evidence suggests that early lumbar arthritis will develop when fusion is carried to L4. An attractive alternative would be to fuse only the thoracic curve selectively and allow the lumbar curve to correct with future growth.

King and colleagues (24) examined this issue and demonstrated that in certain cases selective thoracic fusion is the preferred treatment for King type II curves. They reported their experience in treating a series of 67 cases of AIS with a King type II curve pattern by selective lumbar posterior fusion. The magnitude of the unfused lumbar curve remained equal to or smaller than that of the corrected thoracic curve in 94% of their patients, and no patient required extension of fusion. Additionally, truncal decompensation was minimal; only one case of inferior junctional kyphosis greater than 10 degrees developed and did not require extension of fusion. No cases of superior junctional kyphosis developed when the fusion stopped at the T12 level. These investigators concluded that the concept of selective thoracic fusion in the King type II curve pattern appears to be valid. In a later article, King (75) pointed out the following as key to successful selective thoracic fusion in the type II group:

1. Properly identifying the stable and neutral vertebrae and stopping the fusion at the stable vertebra will ensure a centered and well-balanced fusion.
2. Avoiding overcorrection of the curve to anything beyond what was achieved on side-bending film.
3. Avoiding the so-called derotation maneuver with the Cotrel-Dubousset (CD) system because it can lead to lumbar decompensation if the rotation is translated into the lumbar curve.
4. Ending a fusion at T11 or T12 is acceptable if either is the

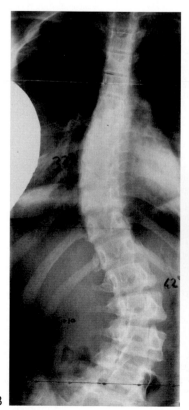
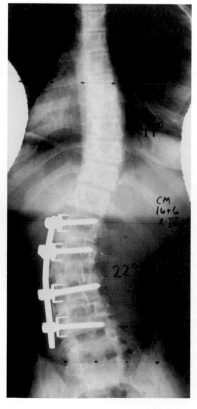

A,B

Fig. 10. C. M. is 15 + 10-year-old girl who initially presented with back asymmetry and a discrepancy in leg length. **A:** She had a King type I curve pattern with a left lumbar scoliotic curve of 62 degrees measured from T12 through L4 and a compensatory right thoracic curve of 37 degrees measured from T6 through T11. She was postmenarcheal and Risser grade 4. On radiographs obtained with the patient side bending to the left, the lumbar curve is almost completely corrected to 7 degrees. Her curve was 55 degrees on side bending to the right; however, her thoracic curve almost completely corrected to 14 degrees. If her curve had been inflexible, she would have required a T5 to L4 posterior instrumented fusion. Instead, because her thoracic curve was flexible, she could be treated with an anterior L1-4 segmental instrumented fusion. **B:** Postoperatively, she has a 22-degree curve measured between T12 and L4 and a 19-degree thoracic compensatory curve, and she remains pain-free.

stable vertebra. The dogma of not ending a fusion at the thoracolumbar junction to prevent junctional kyphosis has been obviated by the newer instrumentation systems.

It must be remembered that for a selective thoracic fusion, the lower lumbar curve must be flexible and the apex of the upper curve must not be translated past the midline. For large and stiff lumbar curves greater than 50 degrees, the lumbar component must be included to achieve adequate correction. Unfortunately, this means that the fusion usually must go to the L4 level. Fusion of both curves is best accomplished via a posterior approach. Selective fusion of the thoracic curve alone is usually accomplished posteriorly, although these cases are now also being approached anteriorly (76,84) (Fig. 11).

A type III curve is essentially a single thoracic curve. The thoracic curve is structural, and the curve of the lumbar vertebrae does not cross the midline and is very flexible. Forward bending produces a thoracic prominence but no lumbar prominence. This feature helps to distinguish the type III pattern from the type II pattern, in which a small lumbar prominence is present. The stable vertebra is usually L1 or L2. Posterior fusion is the usual treatment, according to the guidelines of fusing to the stable vertebra (75) (Fig. 12). Hypokyphosis is often associated with this curve. Pulmonary function may be diminished. The hypokyphosis can be addressed by a rod rotation maneuver. Anterior instrumentation may play a role in these curves because its kyphogenic effect works well with the thoracic hypokyphosis.

A type IV curve is a long thoracic curve with an apex in the thoracic spine near T10 and a lower end vertebra in the lumbar spine. The L4 body usually tilts into the curve. With posterior instrumentation, it is preferable to stop at L3, if possible, as noted above. It is especially important in these curves to attempt to maintain lumbar lordosis. In this setting, the CD instrumentation is preferable to the Harrington system (85,86). Anterior instrumentation with a short-segment construct may also be used for these curves (Fig. 13).

A type V curve is a double major thoracic curve. Type V curves are best treated posteriorly from stable vertebra to stable vertebra according to the criteria noted above (75). The most difficult aspect of managing a King type V curve is recognizing it and differentiating it from other types of curves. A common error in the surgical management of scoliosis is the failure to recognize the upper thoracic curve and include it in the fusion (75,77,87). A King type V curve is identified as two structural thoracic curves that lack flexibility on bending films. The first is usually a high left curve with its apex at T3, an upper end vertebra at T1 or T2, and a lower end vertebra at T5 or T6. The second is a lower right thoracic curve with an apex around T9, an upper end vertebra at T5 or T6, and a lower end vertebra at T11-L2. A positive "tilt" is seen when a line is drawn along the upper end plate of T1, higher on the left than on the right. If the left shoulder is elevated on presentation, then the upper curve must always be included because fusing the lower curve alone will only worsen the shoulder deformity. If the patient has balanced shoulders and a rigid right thoracic curve and a flexible left cervicothoracic curve, then it is usually safe to fuse the right curve only (Fig. 14).

Thoracolumbar and lumbar curves have an apex at either T12-L2 or in the lumbar spine. They are usually convex to the left and are well managed with anterior instrumentation (77). To help maintain lumbar lordosis and resist the kyphogenic effects of anterior systems, it is best to pack structural grafts in the open anterior disc spaces before compression. To prevent

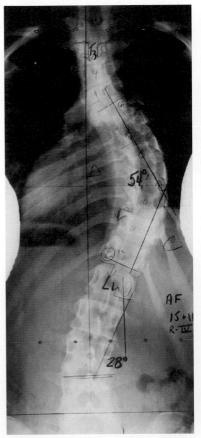
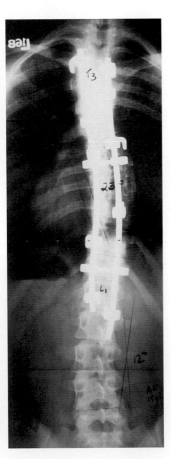

A,B

Fig. 11. A. F. is a 15+ 11-year-old girl, Risser stage 4, with a right thoracic King type II scoliosis curve pattern measuring 54 degrees and a left lumbar curve measuring 28 degrees (**A**). The curve improved to 43 degrees on right side bending and increased to 62 degrees on left side bending. The patient underwent posterior segmental instrumentation and fusion from T3 through L1 with thoracoplasty. The postoperative roentgenographic examination shows that she now has a 20-degree curve measured between T5 and T12 and a lumbar curve measuring 12 degrees (**B**).

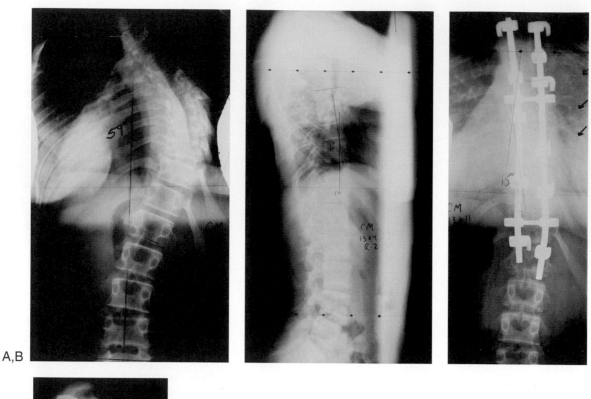

A,B

C

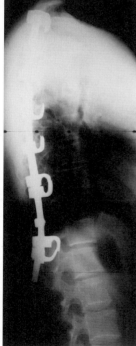

D

Fig. 12. C. M. is a 13+ 10-year-old girl, Risser grade 2 and 9 months postmenarcheal. She had a right King type III curve of 38 degrees between T6 and T11 and a thoracic hypokyphosis with an actual thoracic lordosis of −12 degrees (**A, B**). She was well balanced over the sacrum but had a prominent rib hump. She had been managed in a TLSO brace 23 hours a day but progressed from 38 to 59 degrees. Preoperative pulmonary function tests revealed a reduction of both the forced expiratory volume in 1 second (FEV$_1$) and the ratio of 1-second forced expiratory volume to vital capacity (FEV$_1$/VC) to 75% of normal. She underwent posterior segmental instrumentation and fusion from T3 through T12 with thoracoplasty. Postoperatively, she has a 13-degree curve measured between T6 and T12. Her thoracic hypokyphosis is also improved (**C, D**).

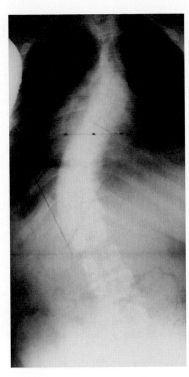

Fig. 13. A. H. is a 13+ 0 boy, Risser grade 3. He presented with a large left thoracolumbar King type IV scoliosis pattern with an apex at T10 and a curve of 56 degrees measured between T7 and L2.

Table 14. Considerations for Posterior Fusion

Advantages	Disadvantages
Gold standard of treatment	Risk for crankshaft phenomenon in skeletally immature patients
Excellent fusion rates	Potential for worsening of lumbar curve after surgery
Surgeon's familiarity and ease of procedure	Failure to correct thoracic hypokyphosis consistently
Good curve correction	Risk for junctional kyphosis below level of the instrumentation
Minimal complications	Prominent hardware
	?Late infection

long-term degenerative changes, it is important for the lowest instrumented vertebra to be nearly as parallel to the pelvis as possible and to preserve lumbar lordosis at all costs.

DETERMINATION OF SURGICAL APPROACH

Posterior Approach

OVERVIEW. The posterior approach to fusion in IS is the gold standard with which all other methods must be compared. It has a proven track record of success, with excellent fusion rates and good curve correction (Table 14). Harrington (88,89) first introduced distraction rods and hooks to manage scoliotic curves in 1960. His system was the first to achieve some fixation with some correction. Despite the usefulness of his distraction rod, the patients must wear casts postoperatively to prevent rod dislodgement and maintain correction. Frequently, surgery required distraction into the lumbar spine, causing loss of lordosis in the sagittal plane and the development of a debilitating "flat-back" syndrome in some patients (78). Luque (90) introduced the concept of segmental fixation; his rod with sublaminar wires achieved multiple points of fixation and allowed segmental correction. Enthusiasm for this technique waned when neurological deficits related to the passage of the sublaminar wires developed in some patients. This system is still frequently used to treat neuromuscular scoliosis.

More recently, several new systems have been developed to achieve posterior segmental instrumentation. The prototype is the CD system, which was first introduced in 1984 and is still in use today (86,91–93) (Fig. 15). The CD system was designed to provide bilateral segmental fixation of the spine, allow for selective distraction and compression at different levels, and improve spinal alignment in the coronal, sagittal, and axial planes. One advantage of the CD system is that more correction in the sagittal plane is achieved than with the older Harrington system (94). The CD system uses a series of hooks, screws, and rods to achieve better stable segmental fixation, which obviates the need for bracing postoperatively. The hooks vary in width, blade angle, and blade depth to accommodate changes in canal dimension throughout the length of the spine. A bifid hook may be used to gain purchase on the thoracic pedicles, whereas in other areas of the spine the hook blade is flat. The hook bodies can be open or closed. The open hook design allows the rod to be placed after the hooks are positioned on the strategic vertebra. The ability to "top load" the rod makes insertion much easier. Rod diameters and strengths can be varied to accommodate differences in body habitus. Rods of 1/4 in (6.5 mm) are used in most cases; however, for small adolescents or children, rods of 3/16 in (5.0 mm) are available and are used with lower-profile hook systems to reduce hardware promi-

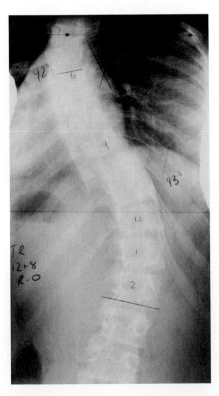

Fig. 14. T. R. is a 12+ 9-year-old girl with a King type V, 43-degree left thoracic curve measured between T2 and T9 and a 42-degree right thoracolumbar curve measured between T9 and L2. She is 1 month postmenarcheal and Risser grade 3.

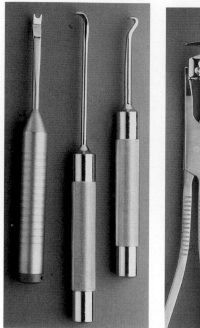

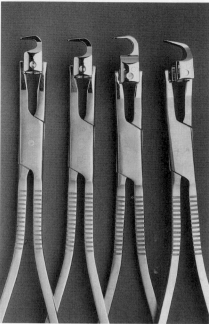

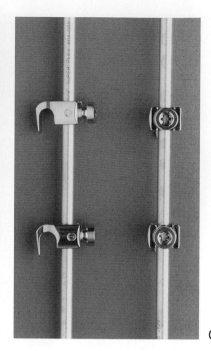

A,B

C

D

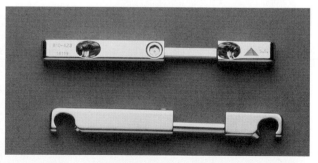

E

Fig. 15. The Cotrel-Dubousset system is a posterior instrumentation system allowing segmental fixation of the spine. **A:** From left to right, pedicle finder, transverse process finder, lamina finder. **B:** Standard and ramped lamina hooks on hook appliers. **C:** Hooks attached to ¼-in rod. Note breakaway caps to lower final profile. **D:** From left to right, rod template, ¼-in rod, rod holder, rod bender. **E:** Adjustable cross-links.

nence. Strength varies inversely with rod diameter, but the manufacturing technique and metal type also influence strength. Stainless steel is most commonly used for rod construction, but titanium, which is stronger, lighter, and more expensive, has become readily available. Titanium has the advantage of being compatible with MRI, so that its use in conjunction with canal decompression may be preferred. Titanium rods have more memory, are more difficult to contour, and are more prone to break if repeatedly bent or notched.

Another recent advance in posterior instrumentation is the use of pedicle screws to achieve solid fixation and prevent hardware pullout or loosening. A number of studies have demonstrated the efficacy and safety of including them in the construct (95). In 1993, Esses et al. (96) reported a series of 617 patients in whom 3,949 pedicle screws were applied with only 12 nerve root injuries (1.9%). In a 1996 study by Hamill et al. (97), treating King types I, II, and IV curves with a combination of pedicle screws and hooks was superior to hooks alone in regard to degree of correction achieved and degree of tilt in the lower instrumented vertebrae, with no major complications reported.

SURGICAL TECHNIQUE. In the posterior approach, the patient is positioned on a four-post scoliosis frame or Jackson table to allow the abdomen to hang freely, so that venous pressure and bleeding are reduced. All patients are asked to donate two units of their own packed red cells preoperatively. A cell saver system is routinely employed, and great care is taken at surgery to wring out all sponges and avoid blood loss. With these precautions taken, it is rare for a patient to require banked blood. All procedures are planned to include the use of somatosensory evoked potential (SSEP) monitoring, and the possibility of a wake-up test is explained to the family. Preoperative antibiotics are given and readministered as appropriate every 4 hours during the procedure. The entire back and iliac crests are prepared within the surgical field. The tissue dissection is the same along the entire length of the posterior spine, but the orientation and configuration of the vertebrae differ and must be studied. Exposure of the spine is carried out to the tips of the transverse processes. The principles of posterior fusion are the same ones used by any surgeon performing a routine fusion. Autologous bone is the gold standard of fusion substrates. The transverse processes are decorticated, and generous facetectomies are performed at all levels to be fused. It is important to perform the facetectomies and graft all uninstrumented levels before the rods are placed in position; otherwise, access to the facets will be blocked. If a hook and rod system is employed, hook sites are prepared after exposure and before the decortication to minimize blood loss.

Curve correction is achieved by distracting against the concavity of the curve and compressing across the apex of the convexity of the curve. The placement of points of fixation is planned to facilitate this process. Multiple points of fixation are desirable to maximize curve correction, particularly in stiff curves. Sagittal plane alignment must always be considered. For a typical King type II curve pattern (in which the thoracic curve is the structural curve), the concave rod is bent and inserted first. Distractive forces are applied across the thoracic concavity to increase thoracic kyphosis. The second rod is then inserted and compression is achieved across the apex, followed by additional distraction on the concave side.

Conversely, if the major curve is in the lumbar spine, the convex rod is inserted first and the hooks are compressed. This rod compression enhances lumbar lordosis and restores the physiological sagittal plane contour. Distraction is then performed across the thoracic portion of the second rod. Double major curves are treated by instrumenting the concave portion of the thoracic curve and the convex portion of the lumbar curve.

COMPLICATIONS. Despite the utility of the posterior approach and posterior instrumentation, a number of complications associated with these procedures have been noted and must be recognized by the surgeon during preoperative planning.

Crankshaft Phenomenon. A major deficiency of posterior fusion alone with either the CD or Harrington system is the development of the "crankshaft" phenomenon (98–101). First described by Dubousset and Cotrel (92), this occurs when the anterior column of the spine continues to grow in the presence of a solid posterior fusion. The spine is unable to elongate because of the tethering effect of the posterior fusion mass, and continued anterior growth causes sagittal deformity. The resultant deformity is always concave to the side of the fusion mass and convex to the side of the continued growth; a lordoscoliosis is produced with rotation in the direction of the original rotatory deformity. This process has been used to explain curve progression in preadolescent patients following posterior instrumentation and fusion. The main risk factor is skeletal immaturity with a still large potential for growth. This is measured by the Risser grade (0 through 2), status of the triradiate cartilage (open), and predicted degree of residual curve (>30 degrees)

after posterior correction. In a retrospective review of 86 immature patients who underwent posterior thoracic fusion for IS, Roberto et al. (100) found that the crankshaft effect developed in 75% of patients who were Tanner stage I, with open triradiate cartilage (progression >10 degrees) but in none of the patients who were Tanner stage IV. Because the crankshaft phenomenon is difficult to correct once it develops, it is recommended that patients with the risk factors listed above undergo either a spinal instrumentation without fusion and serial distraction until they mature or a combined anterior–posterior fusion.

Truncal Decompensation. A second problem associated with posterior segmental instrumentation systems such as the CD system is lumbar curve decompensation (worsening of the concomitant lumbar curve after thoracic fusion) (102–105). Choosing incorrect levels of instrumentation can result in persistent deformity or truncal decompensation when further spinal growth occurs. Truncal decompensation occurs when the capacity of the upper spine to correct exceeds the capacity of the lower, uninstrumented segment of the spine. In this situation, the lower spinal segment remains structurally deformed, with an oblique takeoff from the sacrum. This problem causes cosmetic deformity and theoretically predisposes the patient to arthritis secondary to asymmetrical loading of the vertebral segments.

King's success with selective thoracic fusion for type II curves was mainly achieved with the use of the Harrington instrumentation. Later, when the Harrington instrumentation was supplanted by newer systems, such as the CD system, numerous studies noted the development of coronal lumbar decompensation, particularly in patients with King type II curve patterns. Lenke and colleagues (82) reported their initial experience in 1992, noting coronal decompensation in 5 (10%) of 50 patients treated with posterior CD instrumented fusion for King type I or type III curves (82). In a later series of 76 patients, they saw no instances of coronal decompensation (86). They concluded that the problem could be avoided by accurately diagnosing and treating true King type II curves, avoiding a full 90-degree rod rotation, and avoiding overcorrection with the instrumentation. The "rod rotation maneuver" is the process of taking the lateral curve of the rod *in situ* and rotating it 90 degrees so that this curve is transmitted into kyphosis. The maneuver actually transmits forces into the lower curve, which can lead to decompensation (102). Overcorrection is defined as a postoperative curve correction greater than that achieved on the patient's own bending films.

Late Infection. A disturbing complication that has been recently linked with the use of posterior instrumentation systems is late infection (26,106,107). In one series, the incidence was as high as 10%, and it is unclear whether this was a consequence of micromotion of the implants, causing fretting corrosion, or of contamination of the implantation. Newer systems have been designed with improved closure methods to eliminate micromotion.

Anterior Approach

OVERVIEW. At approximately the same time that Harrington was developing posterior instrumentation for scoliosis correction in the United States, Dwyer in Australia was developing the first anterior system (108). Dwyer reasoned that better correction could be achieved by instrumenting the vertebral bodies after an anterior release and discectomy. Dwyer's anterior approach and the instrumentation (vertebral body screw, staple, and cable construct) he used were the prototype for subsequent systems. A newer system for anterior instrumentation of scoliotic deformities was proposed by Zielke, who substituted a single threaded rod and nuts for the cable and introduced a derotator to correct rotation.

Anterior systems are biomechanically attractive for several

Table 15. Considerations for Anterior Fusion

Advantages	Disadvantages
Better curve correction (biomechanical advantage)	?Higher pseudoarthrosis rates
Better correction of thoracic hypokyphosis	?Increased hardware failure
Prevention of crankshaft phenomenon	Potential for hyperkyphosis
Reduced risk for lumbar curve decompensation	Risk for thoracotomy complications
"Selective" fusion allows saving of distal segments	May require availability of second surgeon
Potential for decreased low-back pain by saving levels	
No prominent hardware	

reasons (Table 15). Up to 90% of the rotational stability of the spine lies in the anterior two thirds of the vertebral body and disc, which is why an anterior release is such an effective maneuver before fusion. Because the instantaneous axis of rotation of the vertebral column is located near the spinal canal, the moment arm for correction is far superior with a screw placed in the vertebral body through an anterior approach than with a posterior hook placed in the sublaminar space through a posterior approach. These biomechanical advantages do indeed translate clinically into improved curve correction, particularly in inflexible thoracic curves. Lenke et al. (85) reported the correction they obtained in both anterior and posterior fusions. Overall, 58% correction was achieved in the anterior group, versus only 38% correction in the posterior group. Part of the difference in curve correction was a consequence of the authors' attempt to avoid curve overcorrection in the posteriorly fused group, which can lead to later lumbar decompensation. The anterior group also had better spontaneous correction of the lumbar curve (56% vs. 37%). For King type II curves, the correction was more dramatic: 67% in the anterior group versus 27% in the posterior group. In a prospective series of 178 patients, Betz et al. (84) examined the results of anterior versus posterior instrumentation for thoracic AIS. One group of 78 patients underwent anterior instrumentation with vertebral body screws and flexible rods, and another 100 patients underwent posterior spinal fusion with multisegmented hook systems. The coronal correction and balance were equal in both groups, despite the fact that in the anterior group the majority of the curves (97%) were fused short to L1, whereas in the posterior group the fusions were longer, with only 18% fused short to L1, which saved an average of 2.5 lumbar levels.

Most patients with thoracic scoliosis have a loss of the normal thoracic kyphosis (hypokyphosis), and the anterior systems are by nature kyphogenic and more effectively restore normal kyphosis (90,109).

Anterior systems are ideally suited for thoracic or thoracolumbar scoliosis in which the thoracic curve is minimal or flexible (110–113) (Fig. 4). Curves can be corrected with the sparing of lumbar levels. In fusions involving the thoracolumbar spine, adequate lordosis must be maintained. As stated previously, anterior systems are kyphogenic by nature, and it is important to maintain intervertebral height through either rib autograft or the placement of autograft-packed anterior cages. Failure to maintain lordosis puts the patient at risk for flat-back syndrome.

SURGICAL TECHNIQUE. The use of monitoring, cell saver systems, and antibiotics are as described for the posterior approach. The patient is positioned in the lateral decubitus position with the convex side up. For double major curves, two separate surgical

approaches may be required: a thoracotomy for the thoracic curve and a thoracoabdominal approach on the opposite side for the thoracolumbar or lumbar curve.

Thoracic scoliosis generally requires a standard thoracotomy. The incision and rib resection are performed on the rib of a vertebra one or two segments above where the most rostral instrumentation is planned. For typical patients with IS, this is usually the fifth or sixth rib. Longer thoracic curves occasionally require a second, more caudal thoracotomy based on the 11th rib via the same or a separate incision. A typical thoracoabdominal approach requires that the incision planned from the angle of the rib be directed posteriorly to the costal cartilage of the 10th rib and then angled anteriorly and inferiorly. The number of lumbar segments that must be exposed determines the length of the abdominal incision. The thoracic portion of the curve is treated through the chest cavity, and the lumbar portion through a retroperitoneal approach. The vertebral discs to be spanned by the instrumentation must be exposed sufficiently to allow complete removal back to the posterior longitudinal ligament. Therefore, the psoas muscle is mobilized in the lumbar spine, and the segmental vessels frequently must be ligated to achieve the exposure. A large Cobb elevator is used to scrape the end plates clean of any remaining disc material. Following discectomy, the vertebral end plates are decorticated to expose bleeding surfaces for fusion. Gel foam is used temporarily after discectomy to control bleeding while the implants are inserted. It is important to excise the rib heads and the associated capsular ligaments to achieve effective destabilization of the rib and permit better correction. The vertebral body screws vary in diameter from 5.5 to 7.0 mm, and pullout strength increases in proportion to thread depth (diameter). The screws are inserted in the midlateral point of the vertebral body until a thread penetrates the far cortex to maximize holding power. Screw length can be measured before insertion and the direction gauged by looking across the disc space. With proper exposure, a finger can be placed on the far side of the vertebral body to avoid prominence of the tip. The end screws are placed first, followed by the intermediate screws for ease of alignment. In a rod rotation maneuver, the rod is placed within the screw heads and rotated to convert the scoliosis into lordosis. After rotation, the disc spaces visibly open anteriorly, and the space should be filled with bone graft after some temporary distraction between the screws. Rib graft harvested at the time of the surgical approach is the ideal bone source. Anterior titanium cages filled with bone graft can be used to improve sagittal plane correction and remove stress from the rod-and-screw construct. Vertebral compression and definitive tightening of the screws to the rod are then performed to stabilize the construct. The rods vary from 4.8 to 6.5 mm in diameter and may be strong enough that postoperative bracing or casting is unnecessary.

COMPLICATIONS. Despite the recent enthusiasm for treating thoracic scoliosis through an anterior approach, significant problems can be encountered. Surgical complications of a thoracotomy or retroperitoneal approach with diaphragmatic takedown include pneumothorax, a prolonged need for chest tube drainage, pulmonary contusion or embolus, and injury to major vessels or lymphatic structures (111,114–116).

In addition to the possibility of pulmonary compromise and other morbidity related to thoracotomy, the rates of pseudoarthrosis and hardware failure are higher than with posterior systems. Betz et al. (84) compared anterior and posterior systems and noted that the incidence of pseudoarthrosis was significantly greater in the anterior group (5% vs. 1%), as was implant breakage (31% vs. 1%). These authors also found that when the preoperative thoracic kyphosis was greater than 20 degrees, the anterior group fared less well. In these patients, anterior instrumentation and arthrodesis frequently resulted in overcor-

Table 16. Indications for Combined Anterior/Posterior Procedures

Prevention of crankshaft phenomenon in juvenile or skeletally immature adolescents

Large curves (>75 degrees) in skeletally mature or immature patients

Excessively rigid curves that do not correct on side-bending films to less than 60 degrees

Curves with severe thoracic lordosis (>−20 degrees)

Curves with severe thoracic kyphosis

Correction of thoracolumbar curves that require fusion to the sacrum

rection in the sagittal plane and the development of hyperkyphosis in 40% of them.

Combined Anterior and Posterior Approach. The combined approach is indicated in several situations in which neither the anterior nor the posterior approach alone will suffice (33). For the most complicated cases of deformity, such as children or adults with large, rigid curves and young children with significant deformity and significant amounts of growth remaining, a combined anterior and posterior approach is becoming the preferred treatment. Although surgical procedures for complex deformity via a combined approach are usually long and complicated, they usually achieve better correction, require the fusion of fewer spinal levels, reduce the incidence of pseudoarthrosis, and result in a better long-term outcome (117–122) (Table 16).

Possible candidates for a combined procedure include the following: (a) patients who are skeletally mature or immature and have large curves (>75 degrees); (b) patients who are skeletally immature and at high risk for the development of the crankshaft phenomenon after posterior surgery alone; (c) patients with smaller but excessively rigid curves that do not correct on side-bending films to less than 60 degrees; and (d) patients with a fixed thoracic kyphosis of more than 50 degrees. Generally, patients with a significant kyphosis require anterior structural support in addition to anterior release and bone grafting to minimize loss of correction. Severe kyphosis with neurological deficit requires an anterior decompression of the spinal cord in conjunction with the anterior and posterior reconstruction. Conversely, patients whose deformity is a severe thoracic lordosis (>20 degrees) usually require correction by anterior wedge osteotomy, followed by posterior instrumentation and fusion.

The combined anterior and posterior approach can be performed in a single operation or as a staged procedure. Traditionally, the anterior procedure was performed first and the patient was allowed to recover for 1 to 2 weeks before the posterior procedure. Complication rates of these procedures have been very high, ranging from 33% to 75%. Mandelbaum and associates (123) demonstrated that after the first procedure, patients are nutritionally deficient and in a state of catabolism before undergoing the second procedure, so that they are prone to complications. Studies by Powell et al. (124), Saer et al. (125), and Shufflebarger et al. (126) demonstrated the efficacy of the one-stage combined procedure. Hospital stays are shorter, so that costs are reduced; complications, including wound infections, are fewer; and less blood is lost.

Special Topics

THORACOPLASTY. The rib hump is often the most noticeable part of the cosmetic deformity in patients with AIS and can be the presenting characteristic that leads to the original diagnosis (127,128). The rib hump develops because the spinal deformity in scoliosis does not occur in isolation; the ribs and thoracic and abdominal viscera are also involved (129). The hump occurs on the convexity of the curve and is most prominent in the ribs attached to the apical vertebrae. The ribs on the convexity are displaced and rotated posteriorly with a sharp angulation that worsens as the lateral curvature of the spine progresses. The opposite occurs on the concave side of the curve, where the ribs are displaced and rotated anteriorly with a flattened angle. Both of these effects cause a decreased anteroposterior diameter of the chest wall, which leads to respiratory compromise and impaired pulmonary function. The term *thoracoplasty* refers to resection of the rib prominence for cosmetic purposes. The original operation for thoracoplasty was described by Volkmann in 1889. The operation was popularized again by Steel (130), who described his experience with 378 patients who underwent thoracoplasty in conjunction with posterior spinal fusion. Adults who had undergone scoliosis surgery as adolescents had a better functional level, better self-image, and less pain in comparison with a similar cohort that had been offered surgery but refused. The procedure was carried out through a separate incision over the prominence, and the ribs that were obtained were used as bone graft material. Shufflebarger et al. (131) described a variation of the procedure in which the ribs were taken internally through the thoracotomy in patients undergoing combined anterior and posterior procedures (Fig. 16).

The main complication of thoracoplasty is a decline in pulmonary function with the rib resections. This loss can be clinically significant, particularly within the first 3 months to 1 year. Steel (130) noted that patients did experience a slow return of pulmonary function during the next several years and felt that for those able to tolerate the procedure, the resultant cosmetic improvement outweighed the loss of pulmonary function.

All patients who are considered candidates for thoracoplasty should undergo preoperative pulmonary testing, with the general rule being that patients with less than 60% of predicted function are unsuitable for the procedure. Even if these guidelines are followed, the risk for a requirement for prolonged ventilatory support must be explained to the families preoperatively.

INTRAOPERATIVE MONITORING. The use of intraoperative monitoring during the correction of scoliotic curves has become the standard of care (132) (Table 17). Spinal cord monitoring involves the use of SSEPs, motor evoked potentials (MEPs), or both. An accurate determination of these parameters requires both a skilled neurophysiologist and an experienced anesthetist. The use of halogenated anesthetics and decreases in core temperature diminish the amplitude and latency of SSEPs. Brainstem evoked potentials may be used in conjunction with other modalities because they are less affected by halogenated anesthetics. SSEPs are sensitive but not specific; the false-positive rate is about 10%. A false negative (i.e., SSEPs are normal but the patient awakens with a neurological deficit) is a reportable event. If a reduction in signals of more than 50% occurs during or immediately after a correction maneuver, the corrective forces should be released and blood pressure and perfusion increased. If the signals do not return, the Stagnara wake-up test should be performed (133). SSEPs should also be carefully monitored when segmental vessels are ligated during the anterior approach. Neurological deficit after elective scoliosis surgery must be minimal. The Scoliosis Research Society has estimated that the risk for a new neurological deficit after posterior spinal fusion surgery is 0.72% (134).

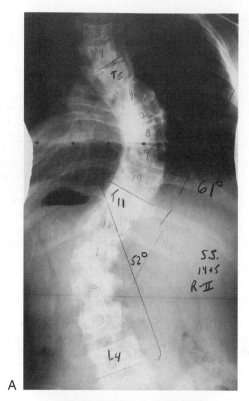

A

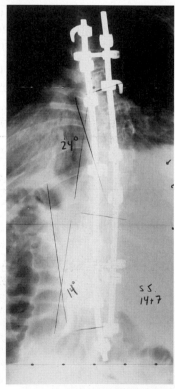

B

Fig. 16. S. S. is a 14+ 5-year-old girl with a King type II scoliosis who was initially managed in a 23/24-hour Boston brace. She had a severe right thoracic rib prominence and progressed rapidly despite bracing. Preoperatively, her right thoracic curve was 61 degrees measured from T5 to T11, and her left lumbar curve measured from T11 to L4 was 52 degrees (**A**). A thoracoplasty was performed to improve cosmesis and for correction and to obviate the need for a separate bone graft harvest. Her initial postoperative films demonstrate correction of her thoracic curve to 24 degrees and her lumbar curve to 14 degrees. Note rib removal for the thoracoplasty in the postoperative study (**B**).

Table 17. Intraoperative Considerations for Scoliosis Correction

Positioning to relieve pressure on abdomen, avoid peripheral nerve injury
Monitoring lines: arterial, peripheral, and central
Foley catheter
Spinal cord evoked potential monitoring
Cell saver
Controlled hypotension
Antibiotic coverage

BONE GRAFT MATERIALS. In patients with AIS, the goal of surgery is to achieve a bony fusion that will maintain correction and prevent further progression of the curve. A successful fusion involves many factors. Options for bone grafting include autograft, banked allograft, and synthetic allograft. Recently, the use of bone morphogenic proteins has been considered as an adjunct to bony fusion. Allograft bone has been shown to be less than optimal as a fusion substrate in adult posterolateral fusions, with fusion rates poorer than those obtained with autologous bone (135–137). The results in children are more encouraging. Stricker and Sher (138) reported the efficacy of freeze-dried cortical allograft as the sole fusion substrate in a series of 34 consecutive patients undergoing posterior instrumented fusion for IS, with no pseudoarthrosis noted at 34 months. In a retrospective series of 25 patients with scoliosis undergoing posterior fusion with the CD system, Blanco and Sears (139) noted a 100% fusion rate. Fabry (140) examined the use of autograft versus allograft bone in scoliosis by a multivariate statistical analysis that compared two matched groups of patients undergoing posterior arthrodesis for IS. He noted no difference in curve correction or pseudoarthrosis rates in the two groups, but he did see a statistically significant reduction in operation time and blood loss in the allograft group. Montgomery et al. (137) reported similar results in terms of blood loss and operating room time in a group of children undergoing posterior spinal arthrodesis with allograft for neuromuscular scoliosis.

Despite the encouraging data, we continue to advocate use of the patient's own bone as the ultimate substrate for fusion. Patients who undergo thoracotomy or thoracoplasty will have rib available for use that can be combined with allograft cubes of bone to obviate the need for iliac harvest. This is especially true in anterior approaches, in which the morselized rib can be used to fill titanium cages that provide structural support.

PSEUDOARTHROSES. In most cases of spinal surgery, a race between the fatigue life of the implants and the formation of a solid bony fusion takes place. One or more of the following symptoms and signs indicate the presence of a pseudoarthrosis: pain, progressive deformity, and metal failure (rod breakage or hook pullout). Imaging studies, such as CT or bone scans, can be used to confirm the diagnosis and the location of the pseudoarthrosis. If the signs of pseudoarthrosis are present, exploration and grafting of the defect are recommended. The defect is usually found in the area of tension. Treatment entails removal of all fibrous tissue, copious bone grafting, and instrumentation designed to produce compression across the site. Cultures are obtained as a matter of routine because of the clear association of infection with pseudoarthrosis.

INFECTION. Postoperative infections are undesirable complications that are best managed by prevention (141). In 1973,

Lonstein et al. (142) reported an overall infection rate of 9.3% in a series of adult and pediatric patients with scoliosis treated with Harrington instrumentation. The routine use of perioperative antibiotics kept the incidence of infection at approximately 1 to 3 per 100 for idiopathic cases, whereas the rate rose to approximately 4 to 10 per 100 for neuromuscular cases. In the 1985 series of Transfeldt et al. (143), in which prophylactic antibiotics were routinely used, the overall infection rate declined to 2.5% (2.6% in posterior procedures and 0.9% in anterior procedures). The use of instrumentation raised the rate of infection from 1.5% to 3.6%, and in patients who had previously undergone surgery, the rate rose to 6.8%.

Factors that predispose to infection include development of a hematoma, presence of preoperative dermatological conditions (especially acne in adolescents), concurrent infection (e.g., urinary tract infection), poor nutrition, and prolonged operative time. Copious irrigation and relaxation of retractors during the surgery are necessary to prevent infection.

Persistent fever above 101.5°F after the fifth day postoperatively may indicate an acute wound infection. Adequate evaluation includes a culture of all systems, including blood, urine, and lungs, and aspiration of the wound. A purulent aspirate or a persistent large hematoma should be treated aggressively by irrigation in the operating room. Parenteral antibiotics should follow prompt irrigation until cultures have been returned. If an established infection is found, removal of the loose bone graft is necessary. Most surgeons close over a drain, but other options include closure over a close suction–irrigation system or leaving the wound open for packing, with healing by secondary intention. The latter method is generally used when the other options fail. Similarly, the duration and route of antibiotic administration will vary. The most common schedule is parenteral administration for at least 3 weeks followed by oral administration for 3 weeks. The sedimentation rate is useful to follow; however, it may not normalize for several weeks after treatment of an acute inflammation. Therefore, undertreatment is unlikely if this parameter is used as a guide.

Delayed infections are now well recognized following spinal surgery. Patients present with back pain, signs of inflammation, or drainage months to years after spinal surgery. The most common organisms are *Staphylococcus epidermidis, Propionibacterium acne,* and other skin flora. These organisms of low virulence are thought to contaminate the wound at the time of surgery and remain subclinical for an extended period of time. Treatment should be according to the same guidelines that are used in acute infections. Aggressive irrigation and debridement followed by wound drainage is the first measure. Healing by secondary intention may be necessary if the initial attempt fails. Rarely will the hardware have to be removed to control a spinal infection, and every attempt to salvage the instrumentation should be made. Pseudoarthrosis is common following infection, and if it is symptomatic, it should be treated by autogenous grafting once the infection has been treated. Postoperative antibiotics should be utilized for several weeks following the grafting to reduce the chance of a recurrence.

Conclusions

AIS is a disease with a well-defined natural history and indications for treatment. Surgery has a definite role for patients whose curves are likely to progress. It has been shown that adults who underwent scoliosis surgery as adolescents have a better functional level, better self-image, and less pain in comparison with a similar cohort who were offered surgery but refused (144). Surgery to correct deformity in the modern era

is remarkably safe. In a retrospective review, Bridwell et al. (145) noted a 0.36% rate of major complications (only four major complications in 1,090 patients). Although excellent results have been obtained in most cases by means of posterior fusion with instrumentation alone, the use of anterior exposures has gained popularity in certain situations because of biomechanical advantages permitting better correction and the potential to save fusion levels. Hardware failure with anterior instrumentation and arthrodesis have been reduced by the newer, stronger instrumentation systems that have evolved. Overall, the basic tenets for surgeons are the same today as they were 40 years ago. The proper selection of surgical candidates, fusion levels, and operative approaches combined with meticulous surgical technique are the keys to successful outcomes. Earlier recognition of the disease through school screening has resulted in smaller curves at presentation and better outcomes. The average Cobb angle operated on by Dr. Moe in 1958 was about 71 degrees. In the 1992 study of Lenke et al. (82), the average Cobb angle operated on was only 54 degrees. Bracing still plays a significant role in management. Improved technology in terms of instrumentation systems has improved curve correction and patient satisfaction. Minimally invasive surgery and the use of genetically engineered bone morphogenic proteins are areas that will continue to be examined critically. The surgeon must be cognizant that the success or failure of any operation performed in childhood will be judged over a long life span. The outcomes of these patients will emerge as patients treated by pioneers in the field pass into maturity.

References

1. Martinez-Lozano AG. Terminology and definitions. In: Weinstein SL, ed. *The pediatric spine: principles and practice.* New York: Raven Press, 1994:1831–1832.
2. Weinstein SL. Adolescent idiopathic scoliosis: prevalence and natural history. In: Weinstein SL, ed. *The pediatric spine: principles and practice.* New York: Raven Press, 1994:463–478.
3. Bell M, Teebi AS. Autosomal dominant idiopathic scoliosis? [Letter]. *Am J Med Genet* 55:112, 1995.
4. Carr AJ. Adolescent idiopathic scoliosis in identical twins. *J Bone Joint Surg Br* 72:1077, 1990.
5. Inoue M, Minami S, Kitahara H, et al. Idiopathic scoliosis in twins studied by DNA finger printing: the incidence and type of scoliosis. *J Bone Joint Surg Br* 80:212–217, 1998.
6. Kesling KL, Reinker KA. Scoliosis in twins. A metaanalysis of the literature and report of six cases. *Spine* 22:2009–2014, 1997.
7. Risser JC, Norquist DM, Cockrell BR, et al. The effect of posterior spine fusion on the growing spine. *Clin Orthop* 46:127–139, 1966.
8. Wilner S. A study of height, weight, menarche in girls with idiopathic structural scoliosis. *Acta Orthop Scand* 46:84–89, 1975.
9. Oi T. Electromyographical studies on scoliosis. *J Jpn Orthop Assoc* 40:71–98, 1966.
10. Hadley-Miller N, Mims B, Milewicz DM. The potential role of the elastic fiber system in adolescent idiopathic scoliosis. *J Bone Joint Surg Am* 76:1193–1206, 1994.
11. Carr AJ, Ogilvie DJ, Wordsworth BP, et al. Segregation of structural collagen genes in adolescent idiopathic scoliosis. *Clin Orthop* 274:305–310, 1992.
12. Hsu JD, Slager U, Swank SM, et al. Idiopathic scoliosis: a clinical morphometric and histopathological correlation. *J Pediatr Orthop* 8:147–152, 1988.
13. Yarom R, Robin GC. Studies on spinal and peripheral muscles from patients with scoliosis. *Spine* 4:12–21, 1979.
14. Wong YC, Yau AC, Low WD, et al. Ultrastructural changes of the back muscles of idiopathic scoliosis. *Spine* 4:251–260, 1977.
15. Zetterberg C. *Paravertebral muscles in adolescent idiopathic scoliosis* [Doctoral Thesis]. University of Goteborg, Sweden, 1982.
16. Yamamoto H. A postural dysequilibrium as an etiological factor

in idiopathic scoliosis. Presented at the 17th annual meeting of the Scoliosis Research Society, Denver, Colorado, 1982.

17. Sahlstrand T, Petruson B. A study of labyrinthine function in patients with adolescent idiopathic scoliosis. I. An electro-nystagmographic study. *Acta Orthop Scand* 50:759–769, 1979.

18. Burwell Cole AG, Cook TA, et al. Pathogenesis of idiopathic scoliosis: the Nottingham concept. *Acta Orthop Belg* 58:33–51, 1991.

19. Sevastik B, Xiong B, Sevastik J, et al. Rib–vertebral angle asymmetry in idiopathic, neuromuscular and experimentally induced scoliosis. *Eur Spine J* 6:84–88, 1997.

20. McCarthy RE. Evaluation of the patient with deformity. In: Weinstein SL, ed. *The pediatric spine: principles and practice*. New York: Raven Press, 1994:185–224.

21. Lonstein JE. Patient evaluation. In: Bradford DS, Lonstein JE, Moe JH, et al., eds. *Moe's textbook of scoliosis and other spinal deformities*. Philadelphia: WB Saunders, 1987:47–88.

22. Cobb J. Outline for the study of scoliosis. *AAOS Instr Course Lect* 5:261–275, 1948.

23. Nash CLJ, Moe JH. A study of vertebral rotation. *J Bone Joint Surg Am* 51:223–229, 1969.

24. King HA, Moe JH, Bradford DS, et al. The selection of fusion levels in thoracic idiopathic scoliosis. *J Bone Joint Surg Am* 65:1302–1313, 1983.

25. Lenke LG, Betz RR, Harms J, et al. A new classification system of adolescent idiopathic scoliosis. Presented at the 32nd annual meeting of the Scoliosis Research Society, St. Louis, Missouri, September 25–27, 1997.

26. Richards BS. Delayed infections following posterior spinal instrumentation for the treatment of idiopathic scoliosis. *J Bone Joint Surg Am* 77:524–529, 1995.

27. Maiocco B, Deeney VF, Coulon R, et al. Adolescent idiopathic scoliosis and the presence of spinal cord abnormalities. Preoperative magnetic resonance imaging analysis. *Spine* 22:2537–2541, 1997.

28. Schwend RM, Hennrikus W, Hall JE, et al. Childhood scoliosis: clinical indications for magnetic resonance imaging. *J Bone Joint Surg Am* 77:46–53, 1995.

29. Winter RB, Lonstein JE, Heithoff KB, et al. Magnetic resonance imaging evaluation of the adolescent patient with idiopathic scoliosis before spinal instrumentation and fusion. A prospective, double-blinded study of 140 patients. *Spine* 22:855–858, 1997.

30. Weinstein SL, Ponseti IV. Curve progression in idiopathic scoliosis. Long-term follow-up. *J Bone Joint Surg Am* 65:447–456, 1983.

31. Weinstein SL, Zavala DC, Ponseti IV. Idiopathic scoliosis: long-term follow-up and prognosis in untreated patients. *J Bone Joint Surg Am* 63:702–712, 1981.

32. Lonstein JE, Carlson JM. The prediction of curve progression in untreated idiopathic scoliosis during growth. *J Bone Joint Surg Am* 66:1061–1071, 1984.

33. Rauzzino MJ, Shaffrey CI, Wagner J, et al. Surgical approaches for the management of idiopathic thoracic scoliosis and the indications for combined anterior–posterior technique. *Neurosurg Focus* 6: Article 6, 1999.

34. Weinstein S. Idiopathic scoliosis: natural history. *Spine* 11:780–786, 1986.

35. Ascani E, Bartolozzi P, Logroscino CA, et al. Natural history of untreated idiopathic scoliosis after skeletal maturity. *Spine* 11: 784–789, 1986.

36. Cordover AM, Betz RR, Clements DH, et al. Natural history of adolescent thoracolumbar and lumbar idiopathic scoliosis into adulthood. *J Spinal Disord* 10:193–196, 1997.

37. Peterson LE, Nachemson AL. Prediction of progression of the curve in girls who have adolescent idiopathic scoliosis of moderate severity. Logistic regression analysis based on data from the brace study of the Scoliosis Research Society. *J Bone Joint Surg Am* 77:823–827, 1995.

38. Kolind-Sorensen V. A follow-up study of patients with idiopathic scoliosis. *Acta Orthop Scand* 44:98–103, 1973.

39. Ginsburg HH, Goldstein L, Haake PW, et al. Longitudinal study of back pain in postoperative idiopathic scoliosis: long-term follow-up, phase IV. Presented at the annual meeting of the Scoliosis Research Society, Asheville, NC, September 14–16, 1995.

40. Nachemson AL. Long-term follow-up study of nontreated scoliosis. *Acta Orthop Scand* 39:466–476, 1968.

41. Nachemson AL. Adult scoliosis and back pain. *Spine* 4:513–517, 1979.

42. Nilsonne U, Lundgren KD. Long-term prognosis in idiopathic scoliosis. *Acta Orthop Scand* 39:456–465, 1968.

43. Horal J. The clinical appearance of low back disorders in the city of Gothenburg, Sweden. Comparisons of incapacitated probands with matched controls. *Acta Orthop Scand Suppl* 118:1–109, 1969.

44. Jackson RP, Simmons EH, Stripinis D. Incidence and severity of back pain in adult idiopathic scoliosis. *Spine* 8:749–756, 1983.

45. Betz RR, Bunnell WP, Lambrect-Muller E, et al. Scoliosis and pregnancy. *J Bone Joint Surg Am* 69:90–96, 1986.

46. Roach JW. Adolescent idiopathic scoliosis: nonsurgical treatment. In: Weinstein SL, ed. *The pediatric spine: principles and practice*. New York: Raven Press, 1994:497–510.

47. Rowe DE, Bernstein SM, Riddick MF, et al. A metaanalysis of the efficacy of nonoperative treatment for idiopathic scoliosis. *J Bone Joint Surg Am* 79:664–674, 1997.

48. Winter RB, Lonstein JE, Drogt J, et al. The effectiveness of bracing in the nonoperative treatment of idiopathic scoliosis. *Spine* 11:790–791, 1986.

49. Winter RB. The pendulum has swung too far. Bracing for adolescent scoliosis in the 1990s. *Orthop Clin North Am* 25:195–204, 1994.

50. Winter RB, Lonstein JE. To brace or not to brace: the true value of school screening. *Spine* 22:1283–1284, 1997.

51. Adams W, Bunnell WP. Psychological effects of the Wilmington brace in the treatment of scoliosis. *Orthop Trans* 13:91, 1989.

52. Bassett GS, Bunnell WP. Influence of the Wilmington brace on spinal decompensation in adolescent idiopathic scoliosis. *Clin Orthop* 223:164–169, 1987.

53. Bassett GS, Bunnell WP, MacEwen GD. The treatment of idiopathic scoliosis with the Wilmington brace: results in patients with a 20-degree to a 29-degree curve. *J Bone Joint Surg Am* 68:602–605, 1986.

54. Carr WA, Moe JH, Winter RB, et al. Treatment of idiopathic scoliosis in the Milwaukee brace: long-term results. *J Bone Joint Surg Am* 62:599–612, 1980.

55. Durand H, Salanova C. *Brace treatment of adolescent idiopathic scoliosis: results in 477 patients* [Doctoral Thesis]. University of Toulouse, France, 1991.

56. Emans JB, Kaelin A, Bancel P, et al. The Boston bracing system for idiopathic scoliosis: follow-up results in 295 patients. *Spine* 11: 792–801, 1986.

57. Federico DJ, Renshaw TS. Results of treatment of idiopathic scoliosis with the Charleston bending orthosis. *Spine* 15:886–887, 1990.

58. Hanks GA, Zimmer B, Nogi J. TLSO treatment of idiopathic scoliosis. An analysis of the Wilmington jacket. *Spine* 13:626–629, 1988.

59. Kahanovitz N, Levine DB, Landone J. The part-time Milwaukee brace treatment of juvenile idiopathic scoliosis: long-term follow-up. *Clin Orthop* 167:145–151, 1982.

60. Katz DE, Richards S, Browne RH, et al. A comparison between the Boston brace and the Charleston brace for adolescent idiopathic scoliosis. *Spine* 22:1302–1312, 1997.

61. Keiser RP, Shufflebarger HL. The Milwaukee brace in idiopathic scoliosis: evaluation of 123 completed cases. *Clin Orthop* 118: 19–24, 1976.

62. Keller RB. *Nonoperative treatment of adolescent idiopathic scoliosis*. Orthopaedic Instructional Course, 1986.

63. Lonstein JE, Winter RB. The Milwaukee brace for the treatment of adolescent idiopathic scoliosis: a review of one thousand and twenty patients. *J Bone Joint Surg Am* 76:1207–1221, 1994.

64. Moe JH, Kettleson D. Idiopathic scoliosis: analysis of curve patterns and preliminary results of Milwaukee brace treatment in 169 patients. *J Bone Joint Surg Am* 52:1509–1533, 1970.

65. Montgomery F, Willner S. Prognosis of brace-treated scoliosis. Comparison of the Boston and Milwaukee methods in 244 girls. *Acta Orthop Scand* 60:383–385, 1989.

66. Nachemson AL, Peterson L, et al. Effectiveness of treatment with a brace in girls who have adolescent idiopathic scoliosis. A prospective controlled study based on data from the brace study of the Scoliosis Research Society. *J Bone Joint Surg Am* 77:815–821, 1995.

67. Olafsson Y, Saroste H, Sodeolund V, et al. Boston brace in the treatment of idiopathic scoliosis. *J Pediatr Orthop* 15:524–527, 1995.

68. Blount WP, Schmidt AC, Bidwell RG. Making the Milwaukee brace. *J Bone Joint Surg Am* 40:526–528, 1958.
69. Andrew G, MacEwen GD. Idiopathic scoliosis: an 11-year follow-up study of the role of the Milwaukee brace in curve control and truncopelvic alignment. *Orthopedics* 12:809–816, 1989.
70. Howard A, Wright JG, Hedden D. A comparative study of TLSO, Charleston, and Milwaukee braces for idiopathic scoliosis. *Spine* 23:2404–2411, 1998.
71. Green NE. Part-time bracing of adolescent idiopathic scoliosis. *J Bone Joint Surg Am* 68:738–742, 1986.
72. Bridwell K. Surgical correction of adolescent idiopathic scoliosis: the basics and the controversies. *Spine* 19:1095–1100, 1994.
73. Shufflebarger HL. Surgical treatment of scoliosis. In: Welch WC, Jacobs GB, Jackson RP, eds. *Operative spine surgery.* Stamford, CT: Appleton & Lange, 1999:202–227.
74. Moe JH. Methods of correction and surgical techniques in scoliosis. *Orthop Clinic North Am* 3:17–48, 1972.
75. King HA. Selection of fusion levels for posterior instrumentation and fusion in idiopathic scoliosis. *Orthop Clin North Am* 19:247–255, 1988.
76. Betz RR, Harms J, Clements DH, et al. Anterior instrumentation for thoracic idiopathic scoliosis. *Semin Spine Surg* 9:141–149, 1997.
77. Bridwell K. Adolescent idiopathic scoliosis: surgical treatment. In: Weinstein SL, ed. *The pediatric spine: principles and practice.* New York: Raven Press, 1994:511–556.
78. Connolly PJ, Von Schroder HP, Johnson GE, et al. Adolescent idiopathic scoliosis. Long-term effect of instrumentation extending to the lumbar spine. *J Bone Joint Surg Am* 77:1210–1216, 1995.
79. Cochran T, Irstam L, Nachemson A. Long-term anatomic and functional changes in patients with adolescent idiopathic scoliosis treated with Harrington rod instrumentation. *Spine* 8:576–584, 1983.
80. King HA. Analysis and treatment of type II idiopathic scoliosis. *Orthop Clin North Am* 25:225–237, 1994.
81. Lenke LG, Bridwell KH, Baldus C, et al. Ability of Cotrel-Dubousset instrumentation to preserve distal lumbar motion segments in adolescent idiopathic scoliosis. *J Spinal Disord* 6:339–350, 1993.
82. Lenke LG, Bridwell KH, Baldus C, et al. Preventing decompensation in King type II curves treated with Cotrel-Dubousset instrumentation. Strict guidelines for selective thoracic fusion. *Spine* 17(8 suppl):S274–S281, 1992.
83. McCance SE, Denis F, Lonstein JE, et al. Coronal and sagittal balance in surgically treated adolescent idiopathic scoliosis with the King II pattern. A review of 67 consecutive cases having selective thoracic arthrodesis. *Spine* 23:2063–2073, 1998.
84. Betz RR, Harms J, Clements DH, et al. Comparison of anterior and posterior instrumentation for correction of adolescent idiopathic scoliosis. *Spine* 24:225–239, 1999.
85. Lenke LG, Betz R, Harms J, et al. Spontaneous curve correction following selective fusion in idiopathic scoliosis. Presented at the annual meeting of the North American Spine Society, New York, October 25–27, 1997.
86. Lenke LG, Bridwell KH, Blanke K, et al. Radiographic results of arthrodesis with Cotrel-Dubousset instrumentation for the treatment of adolescent idiopathic scoliosis. A five- to ten-year follow-up study. *J Bone Joint Surg Am* 80:807–814, 1998.
87. Lenke LG, Bridwell KH, O'Brien MF, et al. Recognition and treatment of the proximal thoracic curve in adolescent idiopathic scoliosis treated with Cotrel-Dubousset instrumentation. *Spine* 19:1589–1597, 1994.
88. Harrington PR. Surgical instrumentation for management of scoliosis. *J Bone Joint Surg Am* 42:1448, 1960.
89. Harrington PR. Technical details in relation to the successful use of instrumentation in scoliosis. *Orthop Clin North Am* 3:49–67, 1972.
90. Luque ER. Segmental spinal instrumentation for correction of scoliosis. *Clin Orthop* 163:192–198, 1982.
91. Cotrel Y, Dubousset J, Guillaumat M. New universal instrumentation in spinal surgery. *Clin Orthop* 227:10–23, 1988.
92. Dubousset J, Cotrel Y. Application technique of Cotrel-Dubousset instrumentation for scoliosis deformities. *Clin Orthop* 264:103, 1991.
93. Hopf DG, Eysel P, Dubousset J. Operative treatment of scoliosis with Cotrel-Dubousset-Hopf instrumentation. *Spine* 22:618–627, 1997.
94. Bridwell KH, Betz RR, Capelli AM, et al. Sagittal plane analysis in idiopathic scoliosis patients treated with Cotrel-Dubousset instrumentation. *Spine* 15:921–926, 1990.
95. Barr SJ, Schuette AM, Emans JB. Lumbar pedicle screws versus hooks: results in double major curves in adolescent idiopathic scoliosis. *Spine* 22:1369–1379, 1997.
96. Esses SI, Sachs BL, Breyzin V. Complications associated with the technique of pedicle screw fixation. A selected survey of ABS members. *Spine* 18:2231–2239, 1993.
97. Hamill CL, Lenke LG, Bridwell KH, et al. The use of pedicle screws fixation to improve correction in lumbar spine patients with idiopathic scoliosis. Is it warranted? *Spine* 21:241–249, 1996.
98. Dubousset J, Hering J, Shufflebarger H. The crankshaft phenomenon. *J Pediatr Orthop* 9:541–550, 1989.
99. Lee CS, Nachemson AL. The crankshaft phenomenon after posterior Harrington fusion in skeletally immature patients with thoracic or thoracolumbar idiopathic scoliosis followed to maturity. *Spine* 22:58–67, 1997.
100. Roberto RF, Lonstein JE, Winter RB, et al. Curve progression in Risser stage 0 or 1 patients after posterior spinal surgery for idiopathic scoliosis. *J Pediatr Orthop* 17:718–725, 1997.
101. Shuffelbarger H, Clark C. Prevention of crankshaft phenomenon. *Spine* 16:S409–S411, 1991.
102. Bridwell KH, McAllister JW, Betz RR, et al. Coronal decompensation produced by Cotrel-Dubousset "derotation" maneuver for idiopathic right thoracic scoliosis. *Spine* 16:769–777, 1991. (Study. *J Bone Joint Surg Am* 57:968–972, 1975.)
103. Mason DE, Carango PP. Spinal decompensation in Cotrel-Dubousset instrumentation. *Spine* 16:394–403, 1991.
104. Shufflebarger HL, Crawford AH. Is Cotrel-Dubousset instrumentation the treatment of choice for idiopathic scoliosis in the adolescent who has an operative thoracic curve? *Orthopedics* 11:1579–1588, 1988.
105. Thompson JP, Transfeldt EE, Bradford DS, et al. Decompensation after Cotrel-Dubousset instrumentation of idiopathic scoliosis. *Spine* 15:927–931, 1990.
106. Viola RW, King HA, Adler SM, et al. Delayed infection after elective spinal instrumentation and fusion. A retrospective analysis of eight cases. *Spine* 22:2444–2450, 1997.
107. Wimmer C, Gluch H. Aseptic loosening after CD instrumentation in the treatment of scoliosis: a report about eight cases. *J Spinal Disord* 11:440–443, 1998.
108. Dwyer AF. Experience of anterior correction of scoliosis. *Clin Orthop* 93:191–206, 1973.
109. Kaneda K, Shono Y, Satoh S, et al. Anterior correction of thoracic scoliosis with Kaneda anterior spinal system. *Spine* 22:1358–1368, 1997.
110. Halm HF, Liljenqvist U, Niemeyer T, et al. Halm-Zielke instrumentation for primary stable anterior scoliosis surgery: operative technique and two-year results in ten consecutive adolescent idiopathic scoliosis patients within a prospective clinical trial. *Eur Spine J* 7:429–434, 1998.
111. McAfee PC, Regan JJ, Zdeblick T, et al. The incidence of complications in endoscopic anterior thoracolumbar spinal reconstructive surgery: a prospective multicenter study comprising the first 100 consecutive cases. *Spine* 20:1624–1632, 1995.
112. Moe JH, Purcell GA, Bradford DS. Zielke instrumentation (VDS) for the correction of spinal curvature. Analysis of results in 66 patients. *Clin Orthop* 180:133–153, 1983.
113. Turi M, Johnston CE, Richards BS. Anterior correction of idiopathic scoliosis using TSRH instrumentation. *Spine* 18:417–422, 1993.
114. Grossfeld S, Winter RB, Lonstein JE, et al. Complications of anterior spinal surgery in children. *J Pediatr Orthop* 17:89–95, 1997.
115. McCarthy RE, Lonstein JE, Mertz JD, et al. Air embolism in spinal surgery. *J Spinal Disord* 3:1–5, 1990.
116. Weis JC, Betz RR, Clements DH, et al. Prevalence of perioperative complications after anterior spinal fusion for patients with idiopathic scoliosis. *J Spinal Disord* 10:371–375, 1997.
117. Andrew T, Piggot H. Growth arrest for progressive scoliosis: combined anterior and posterior fusion of the convexity. *J Bone Joint Surg Br* 67:193–197, 1985.
118. Bridwell K. Spinal instrumentation in the management of adolescent idiopathic scoliosis. *Clin Orthop* 335:64–72, 1997.
119. Byrd JA, Scoles PV, Winter RB, et al. Adult idiopathic scoliosis

treated by anterior and posterior spinal fusion. *J Bone Joint Surg Am* 69:843–850, 1987.

120. Dick J, Boachie-Adjei O, Wilson M. One stage versus two stage anterior and posterior spinal reconstruction in adults. *Spine* 17: S310–S316, 1992.
121. Floman Y, Micheli LJ, Penny JN, et al. Combined anterior and posterior fusion in seventy-three spinally deformed patients: indications, results and complications. *Clin Orthop* 164:110–122, 1982.
122. Holt RT, Johnson JR, Eldridge JC, et al. An analysis of 107 cases of single stage anterior and posterior spinal surgery. Presented at the annual meeting of the Scoliosis Research Society, Amsterdam, The Netherlands, September 17–22, 1989.
123. Mandelbaum B, Toto VT, McAfee PC, et al. Nutritional deficiencies after staged anterior and posterior spinal reconstructive surgery. *Clin Orthop* 234:5–11, 1988.
124. Powell ET, Krengel WF II, King HA, et al. Comparison of same-day sequential anterior and posterior spinal fusion with delayed two-stage anterior and posterior spinal fusion. *Spine* 19:1256–1259, 1994.
125. Saer E, McCarthy R, McCullough F. Anterior/posterior spine surgery done as one-stage vs. two-stage procedures. Presented at the annual meeting of the American Academy of Orthopaedic Surgeons, Washington, DC, February 20–25, 1992.
126. Shufflebarger HL, Grimm JO, Bui V, et al. Anterior and posterior spinal fusion. Staged versus same-day surgery. *Spine* 16:930–933, 1991.
127. Geissele QE, Ogilvie JW, Cohen M, et al. Thoracoplasty for the treatment of rib prominence in thoracic scoliosis. *Spine* 19: 1636–1642, 1994.
128. Owen R, Turner A, Banforth JSG, et al. Costectomy as the first stage of surgery for scoliosis. *J Bone Joint Surg Br* 68:91–95, 1986.
129. Manning CW, Prime FJ, Zorab PA. Partial costectomy as a cosmetic operation in scoliosis. *J Bone Joint Surg Br* 55:521–528, 1973.
130. Steel HH. Rib resection and spine fusion in correction of convex deformity in scoliosis. *J Bone Joint Surg Am* 65:920–925, 1983.
131. Shufflebarger HL, Smiley K, Roth HJ. Internal thoracoplasty. A new procedure. *Spine* 19:840–842, 1994.
132. Hall JE, Levine CR, Suhir KG. Intraoperative awakening to monitor spinal cord function during Harrington instrumentation and fusion. Description of procedure and report of three cases. *J Bone Joint Surg Am* 60:533–536, 1978.
133. Padberg AM, Wilson-Holden TJ, Lenke LG, et al. Somatosensory- and motor-evoked potential monitoring without a wake-up test during idiopathic scoliosis surgery. An accepted standard of care. *Spine* 15:1392–1400, 1998.
134. Stasikelis PJ, Pugh LI, Allen BL. Surgical correction in scoliosis: a metaanalysis. *J Pediatr Orthop* 2:111–116, 1998.
135. Jorgenson SS, Lowe TG, France J, et al. A prospective analysis of autograft versus allograft in posterolateral lumbar fusion in the same patient. A minimum of 1-year follow-up in 144 patients. *Spine* 19:2048–2053, 1994.
136. McCarthy RE, Peek RD, Morrissy RT, et al. Allograft bone in spinal fusion for paralytic scoliosis. *J Bone Joint Surg Am* 68:370–375, 1986.
137. Montgomery DM, Aronson DD, Lee CL, et al. Posterior spinal fusion: allograft versus autograft bone. *J Spinal Disord* 3:370–375, 1990.
138. Stricker SJ, Sher JS. Freeze-dried cortical allograft in posterior spinal arthrodesis: use with segmental instrumentation for idiopathic adolescent scoliosis. *Orthopedics* 20:1039–1143, 1997.
139. Blanco JS, Sears CJ. Allograft bone use during instrumentation and fusion in the treatment of adolescent idiopathic scoliosis. *Spine* 15; 22:1338–1342, 1997.
140. Fabry G. Allograft versus autograft bone in idiopathic scoliosis surgery: a multivariate statistical analysis. *J Pediatr Orthop* 11:465–468, 1991.
141. Theiss SM, Lonstein JE, Winter RB. Wound infections in reconstructive spine surgery. *Orthop Clin North Am* 27:105–110, 1996.
142. Lonstein J, Winter R, Moe J, et al. Wound infection with Harrington instrumentation and spine fusion for scoliosis. *Clin Orthop* 96: 222–233, 1973.
143. Transfeldt EE, Lonstein JE, Winter RB, et al. Wound infections in reconstructive spinal surgery. *Orthop Trans* 9:128, 1985.
144. Dickson JH, Mirkovic S, Noble PC, et al. Results of operative treatment of idiopathic scoliosis in adults. *J Bone Joint Surg Am* 77: 513–523, 1995.
145. Bridwell KH, Lenke LG, Baldus C, et al. Major intraoperative neurologic deficits in pediatric and adult spinal deformity patients. Incidence and etiology at one institution. *Spine* 23:324–331, 1998.

181. Late Deformity after Spinal Fusion

**Robert F. Heary and
Vishwanathan Rajaraman**

Since the first documented spinal fusion surgery in the United States, by Russell Hibbs (1) in 1911, these operations have helped many patients with a variety of spinal disorders. In general, they are extremely successful procedures associated with minimal morbidity. The techniques have evolved continually, and the last few decades have seen an exponential increase in research and development in the field of instrumentation. Consequently, the techniques and equipment used by present day spinal surgeons are vastly superior to what was available 20 years ago. However, the long history of fusion surgery has provided us with an opportunity to analyze critically its long-term effects on spinal growth in individual patients and also its effects on adjacent spinal elements.

A better understanding of biomechanics, coupled with advances in spinal imaging, has played a major role in delineating the causes and consequences of late deformity after spinal fusion. The techniques and instrumentation in use today were developed specifically to address the problem of late deformity.

Only long-term follow-up can confirm their effectiveness. This chapter presents an overview of late deformity in relation to a variety of spinal fusion operations and strategies for its prevention, and we briefly outline methods for correction. The indications, techniques, and selection of patients for the different types of fusion surgery are discussed elsewhere in this book.

Biomechanical Effects of Fusion

Long-term follow-up studies of children who had previously undergone spinal fusion for scoliosis demonstrated the importance of differential growth patterns between the anterior and posterior elements. Preservation of the centers of ossification is essential to ensure proportional growth during puberty and adolescence. Operations such as convexity epiphysiodesis, instrumentation without fusion, short fusion, and long instrumentation were all developed based on an understanding of the biomechanical effects of fusion. It has been only during the last two decades that the effects of spinal fusion on the rest of the spine have come under greater scrutiny. Several authors believe that a reduction in the number of mobile segments increases strain in the unfused segments, predisposing them to early degeneration (2–4). Others have demonstrated increased motion at spinal segments adjacent to fused segments. Hayes et al. (5) found an 80% incidence of retrolisthesis and a 30% incidence of translational motion at the unfused levels. Cochran and Nachemson (3) confirmed a similar finding of retrolisthesis in a series of 100 patients 5 years after Harrington instrumentation for scoliosis. Spondylolysis and spondylolisthesis have also been reported following surgery for scoliosis (6,7).

In addition to a loss of alignment, increased mobility between spinal segments causes reactive changes in the bones and soft tissues, which in turn lead to foraminal and central spinal stenosis. An increased incidence of spinal stenosis corresponding to segments of hypermobility adjacent to long-segment (4) and short-segment (8) spinal fusions has been reported. These clinical findings are not surprising, considering the results of biomechanical studies in the laboratory. Nagata et al. (9) demonstrated an increase in lumbosacral motion and facet loading following immobilization of the proximal segments, with the degree of increase proportional to the length of the immobilized segment. Balderston et al. (10), in a prospective study of magnetic resonance imaging (MRI) changes in the lumbosacral motion segments below scoliosis fusion 3 years after surgery, found T2-weighted signal abnormality in 25% and disc space narrowing in a third of the patients studied. Bohlman et al. (2) found a 9% incidence of symptomatic cervical spondylosis at adjacent levels following anterior cervical discectomy and fusion for cervical radiculopathy. On the other hand, Fuller et al. (11), in a cadaveric model, found uniform redistribution of motion and stress among the remaining, unfused segments of the cervical spine. More recent studies in the field of spinal fusion are beginning to consider these factors in developing strategies for levels and types of fusion (10,12).

Causes of Late Deformity after Spinal Fusion

The causes of late deformity after spinal fusion can be classified as follows:

1. Differential growth of the spine after spinal fusion in childhood
2. Iatrogenic causes
   a. Improper selection of hardware/levels in scoliosis surgery
   b. Inadequate fusion in scoliosis surgery
   c. Failure to appreciate the extent of damage in trauma/tumor/infection
   d. Poor surgical technique
3. Progression resulting from underlying disease

DIFFERENTIAL GROWTH PATTERN. The effect of spinal fusion on spinal growth has been an area of intense debate. Spinal growth originates from three areas: the cartilage overlying the articular processes, the vertebral end plates, and the neurocentral synchondrosis. Previously, the neurocentral synchondrosis was thought to close by the age of 8 years; however, recent evidence indicates that the center remains active into early adolescence (13). It was believed initially that the posterior spinal fusion mass possesses biological plasticity with a potential for longitudinal growth (14). Based on a study of body segment ratios before and after spinal fusion, Risser et al. (14) concluded incorrectly that the posterior fusion mass lengthens with time. Studies by Moe et al. (15) and Letts and Bobechko (16) clearly demonstrated an absence of longitudinal growth once posterior fusion is achieved.

The cause of the gradual deterioration of fusion results in children became apparent when Dubousset, in 1973, and later Hefti and McMaster (17) described the effects of unrestricted anterior spinal column growth in the presence of a posterior tether. In 1989, Dubousset et al. (18) coined the term *"crankshaft" phenomenon* to describe a progressive twisting of the anterior aspect around the fused posterior aspect of the spine, similar to the movement of an automobile crankshaft. Hefti and McMaster (17) accurately documented the rotational changes, apical deviations, and degree of loss of correction. The crankshaft phenomenon is difficult to measure objectively. Radiographic parameters, such as changes in the Cobb angle, rotational changes, lateral trunk shift, translation of apical vertebra, and changes in rib deformity, have all been used. Although some of these parameters may be affected by changes outside the fusion mass, the rest may not be affected equally by the crankshaft phenomenon. More recently, Sanders et al. (19) showed that the younger the child, the greater the risk for the development of a crankshaft phenomenon. This phenomenon is most obvious in cases of idiopathic scoliosis, but it has also been recorded in other types of scoliotic deformity, such as congenital (20) and neuromuscular (21) scoliosis treated by posterior fusion alone.

IATROGENIC CAUSES OF LATE DEFORMITY

Improper Selection of Hardware/Levels in Scoliosis Surgery. The management of scoliosis and other spinal deformities was revolutionized in the 1960s by the introduction of the Harrington rod compression–distraction system. This posterior instrumentation system for the correction of deformity gained wide popularity because of its ease of application and excellent correction of disfiguring scoliosis (22). However, 10- and 15-year follow-up of the scoliotic children treated with Harrington instrumentation revealed a high incidence of sagittal plane imbalance. It became increasingly apparent that distraction instrumentation in the lumbar spine invariably compromised the normal lumbar lordosis.

FLAT-BACK SYNDROME. If the loss of lumbar lordosis is severe enough to cause sagittal plane imbalance, a disabling symptom complex called *flat-back syndrome* develops. Clinically, it is characterized by low-back and midthoracic pain, cervical muscular strain, knee pain, forward inclination of the trunk, and an inability to stand erect (23). The typical patient with flat-back syndrome maintains a degree of hip and knee flexion in an attempt to compensate for the loss of sagittal plane balance and to diminish the pain associated with an upright posture. The most common cause of this loss of lumbar lordosis is the use of distraction instrumentation that extends to the lumbar segments. The degree of loss is proportional to the distal extent of the fusion (24–26). Kostuik and Hall (27), in a study of 45 adults who had undergone scoliosis fusion up to the sacrum, found a loss of lumbar lordosis in nearly half of them. Loss of lumbar lordosis can also follow other forms of surgery in the region (see below).

Inadequate Fusion in Scoliosis Surgery. With the recognition of the flat-back syndrome, spinal surgeons endeavored to preserve motion segments during fusion, especially in the lumbar region. Two major developments, the concept of segmental correction, developed and popularized by Luque, and then universal segmental spinal instrumentation systems, such as the Cotrel-Dubousset (CD) system, brought about a major shift in the management of scoliosis. These techniques made it possible to correct major structural scoliotic curves almost completely while leaving residual compensatory curves, which tend to be nonstructural or flexible, uncorrected. Although many compensatory curves correct spontaneously, some of them progress (28).

TRUNCAL DECOMPENSATION SYNDROME. Frontal plane decompensation in the upper trunk may occur when the lumbar component of a double major curve (King type II curve) is not included in the fusion (29). This mistake arises primarily because of failure to identify a double major curve (30,31). Other causes include maximal derotation maneuver and the inability of less flexible lumbar curves to adapt to the degree of thoracic correction. Lenke et al. (32) formulated strict guidelines regarding the importance of the relative apical translation of the thoracic to the lumbar curve to establish the feasibility of treating the thoracic curve selectively. Similarly, failure to provide sufficiently proximal fusion in patients with upper cervicothoracic curves (King type V curves) can lead to progressive shoulder imbalance (33).

Failure to Appreciate Extent of Damage in Trauma/Tumor/Infection.
Another iatrogenic cause of late deformity is the failure to appreciate the extent of bone loss or ligamentous injury.

DORSAL SURGERY. Distraction applied to reduce a thoracolumbar burst fracture, with ligamentotaxis to reduce fracture displacement, is not an uncommon procedure. As is being increasingly appreciated, in the absence of adequate anterior column support, these procedures fail because of progression to kyphosis (34). Based on a prospective 10-year study of more than 156 patients with thoracolumbar fractures, Farcy (23) further developed the concept of sagittal index and advocated anterior strut grafting if the index is greater than 35. Late kyphotic deformity of the cervical spine may result for similar reasons when anterior column bone or ligamentous injury is not appreciated at the time of posterior fusion (35).

VENTRAL SURGERY. Loss of correction after a ventral decompression and grafting procedure is often secondary to graft failure. Despite a structurally sound ventral strut graft, deformity will develop if posterior column integrity is not taken into consideration. This is especially apparent in the setting of trauma; deformity after surgery for trauma can be up to five times more frequent than deformity after surgery for degenerative conditions (36). Bell and Bailey (37) reported a 58% rate of mechanical complications eventually leading to kyphosis in their series, and 92% of these patients were shown to have dorsal instability on review. Similar concerns have been raised in the setting of osteomyelitis of the cervical vertebrae treated by ventral decompression and grafting (38).

Poor Surgical Technique.
With the use of modern spinal instrumentation systems, the major iatrogenic deformity is flatback syndrome in patients who have undergone fusion surgery for degenerative disease of the lumbar spine. This is caused by improper positioning (e.g., flexion of the hip) of the patient on the operating room table, use of an incorrect operating room table, or inadequate contouring of the rods or plates during surgery. It is essential to position the patient with the hips extended on the operating table to avoid an intraoperative loss of lumbar lordosis, which inevitably results in the postoperative development of a flat-back condition.

PROGRESSION RESULTING FROM UNDERLYING DISEASE. Late deterioration after technically adequate spinal fusion surgery has been well recognized in certain disease states.

Neurofibromatosis. The prevalence of spinal deformity in neurofibromatosis is reported to be between 10% and 77% (39). Structural scoliosis in neurofibromatosis is of two types—one mimicking idiopathic scoliosis and the other dysplastic or dystrophic. The latter has a characteristic radiological appearance with multiple areas of dystrophy. The cause of these changes is not settled, but theories include osteomalacia, endocrine disturbances, primary mesodermal dysplasia, infiltration of neurofibromatous tissue, and pressure effects of neurofibromas. Dystrophic curves occur most commonly in the thoracic spine, then in the thoracolumbar and cervical spine. Many authors have found that in such cases, despite solid arthrodesis after adequate surgery, curve progression still occurs (40,41). In a recent study, Wilde et al. (42) found that despite adequate fusion, deformity progressed in all their patients, with 40% of them experiencing curve deterioration of more than 20 degrees. The degree of worsening was correlated with peripheral skeletal dystrophy, among other variables. It is therefore believed that the disease process leads to progression even after adequate correction and fusion of the original deformity.

Rheumatoid Arthritis. Rheumatoid arthritis commonly affects the cervical spine, producing characteristic clinical and radiographic changes. In a small percentage of patients, it causes a progressive destruction of the joints and surrounding soft tissues that leads to subluxations, instability, and neural and vascular compromise. Clinically, patients present with radiculopathy, myelopathy, quadriparesis, and severe disability; even sudden death may occur (43,44). Cervical spinal involvement is seen in up to one third of patients hospitalized with rheumatoid arthritis. Although any of the synovial joints of the spine may be affected, the disease characteristically begins in the atlantoaxial complex. Synovitis in the atlas–dens joint and ligamentous destruction of the posterior zygapophyseal facet joints leads to early subluxation. Later, involvement of the occipitoatlantal complex and erosion of the zygapophyseal joints can lead to cranial settling. The increasing subluxation combined with inflammatory pannus formation may lead to progressive neural and vascular compromise. Neurological deterioration further compromises the muscular stabilizers and aggravates spinal instability. Subaxial subluxations develop later in the course of the disease and have been reported in 20% of patients (45).

Tuberculosis. Spinal tuberculosis, or Pott disease, is the most dangerous form of skeletal tuberculosis because of its ability to destroy bone and cause deformity and neurological deficit. Symptomatic skeletal tuberculosis is seen in 3% to 5% of patients with tuberculosis who are not infected by the human immunodeficiency virus (HIV), and the incidence is as high as 60% in the HIV-positive population (46). Most of these afflictions, without deformity or major neurological deficit, can be effectively managed medically. Surgical treatment is reserved for the drainage of paraspinous abscesses, correction of deformity caused by bony destruction, or relief of spinal cord compression. Several studies have revealed some worsening of the deformity irrespective of the method of treatment (46,47). However, the degree of kyphosis appears to stabilize at about 6 months after the initiation of effective chemotherapy (47,48). Because tuberculosis usually begins close to the growth plate of the vertebra and because multilevel radical surgery compromises the anterior growth potential of the spine, late deformity after fusion surgery for tuberculosis is not uncommon, especially in children (49).

Pyogenic Osteomyelitis. The majority of pyogenic infections of the spine are managed effectively with appropriate antibiotics. Spinal fusion surgery is especially indicated in the cervical spine in the presence of severe bony destruction. The results of surgical debridement, primary bone grafting, and antibiotic therapy are excellent, with most series reporting high rates of recovery and solid bony fusion with minimal kyphotic deformity (50,51). However, recent studies have revealed an increased incidence of graft complications and late deformity following anterior cervical fusion if the preoperative kyphotic angulation exceeds 21 degrees or the corpectomy involves two or more levels (38). These findings suggest an incompetence of the posterior ligamentous elements secondary to the inflammatory disease process that may not always be apparent on the initial radiological studies. For this reason, we routinely recommend that combined anterior and posterior (AP) fusion be performed in patients requiring corpectomy in two or more vertebrae for pyogenic vertebral osteomyelitis.

Incidence of Late Deformity in Specific Conditions

CONGENITAL SCOLIOSIS. Posterior fusion *in situ* has been considered the gold standard for the treatment of congenital scoliosis. The short- and long-term results are generally very good (16,52). The anterior growth potential of patients with congenital scoliosis is abnormal in comparison with that of patients with idiopathic scoliosis because of the presence of multiple segmentation and fusion defects. It is therefore not surprising that the incidence of delayed deformity and progression secondary to the crankshaft phenomenon is lower after correction for congenital scoliosis (20,52). In the series of Winter and Moe (52), 12 of 32 patients younger than 5 years showed progression after dorsal spinal fusion. This has raised the issue of AP fusion in children with a Risser grade of 0 (with open triradiate cartilage) (53). Another reason for the progression of deformity is a failure to appreciate associated intraspinal pathology and resultant neurological deficit (54).

IDIOPATHIC SCOLIOSIS. Dubousset et al. (18) reported a nearly 100% progression of curves in 40 patients who underwent posterior fusion before reaching Risser grade 1. Yamada et al. (55) reported progression of deformity secondary to true crankshaft phenomenon in only 12% of 53 patients studied. Recommendations for AP fusion have been based on the skeletal maturity of the patient (19,53,56). Thus, Shufflebarger and Clark (57) completely prevented the crankshaft effect by a combination of periapical anterior growth arrest and posterior fusion with instrumentation. More recently, Lee and Nachemson (58), in a study of 63 patients followed to maturity, found a 67% overall incidence of progression of deformity. However, the progression was moderate, with an average Cobb angle of 9 degrees and rotation of 7 degrees, which neither surgeon nor patient felt warranted routine combined AP fusion.

SCHEUERMANN KYPHOSIS. The primary treatment of this condition is nonoperative. In skeletally immature patients with kyphotic deformity of less than 80 degrees, treatment with bracing is always successful (59). Adults with deformity of greater than 75 degrees, disabling back pain, or progression may be candidates for surgical correction. Posterior fusion with instrumentation alone has been followed by loss of correction, failure

of instrumentation, and a high rate of pseudarthrosis (60). More recently, the need for anterior release, anterior support, and posterior shortening has been appreciated. The major postoperative complication after corrective surgery for this disorder is the development of junctional kyphosis, which is directly related to inappropriate selection of levels of fusion or attempted overcorrection of the kyphotic deformity (61). Both proximal and distal junctional kyphoses have been reported.

ADULTHOOD AND CHILDHOOD FRACTURES AND FRACTURE DISLOCATIONS. Before the wide availability of modern segmental spinal fusion systems, the idea of longer instrumentation and short fusion was quite popular. This allowed a better reduction and stabilization of the fracture, provided a longer lever arm, and at the same time avoided the ill effects of fusing multiple motion segments. The technique was not without problems, as many investigators reported progressive kyphosis after rod removal (62,63). Another, older method of treating thoracolumbar fractures was with Williams plates. Aho et al. (64), in a long-term follow-up study, reported an average loss of correction of 10 degrees and final late deformity of 17.4 degrees. Acaroglu et al. (65) reported 22 patients with late deformity following the initial surgical treatment of thoracolumbar fractures as adults. The chief reason for presentation was pain secondary to pseudarthrosis, kyphotic deformity, and new neurological deficits. The average time since first surgery was 4 years (range, 1 to 12 years). Successful correction of the deformity was achieved in every case by a combined AP fusion technique (see case illustration).

Another effect of spinal fusion is increased mobility of the adjacent levels. This has been shown in both lumbar and cervical spinal levels. Birney and Hanley (66) reported hypermobility of the adjacent spine in 3 of 23 young patients who underwent cervical arthrodesis. The exact opposite effect, of decreased motion secondary to extension of fusion mass, has also been reported. McGrory and Klassen (67) reported a 38% incidence of extension of fusion mass in a study of 42 children and adolescents who had been followed for a minimum of 7 years following cervical arthrodesis for trauma.

TUBERCULOSIS. A review of 10- and 15-year follow-up data from Medical Research Council studies revealed excellent overall results of chemotherapy and debridement or radical anterior surgery. With both these surgical approaches, an initial increase in kyphotic deformity occurred within the first 6 months of treatment, but no further deterioration developed during the next several years of follow-up (47,48). Radical anterior surgery resulted in better correction of deformity than debridement surgery. However, the results of such radical surgery in young children with residual growth potential have been conflicting (49,68). A study revealed worsening of the deformity secondary to inadequate remodeling of the anterior fusion block in cases of anterior radical operations, which did not occur after combined AP fusion operations (49).

RHEUMATOID ARTHRITIS. Studies with 5 and 10 years of follow-up have revealed progression of both radiographic and neurological findings in 15% to 50% of untreated patients (69, 70). It is therefore not surprising that several series of patients with rheumatoid arthritis treated by fusion and stabilization procedures have recorded deterioration of deformity, as a result of either inadequate fusion or involvement of other joints during disease progression (69,70). An appreciation of the progressive nature of the disorder has prompted a more aggressive management strategy in the last decade (71,72).

In a study of patients with rheumatoid arthritis, Agarwal et al. (71) noted that subaxial subluxation developed in 5.5% of their 55 patients who underwent C1-2 fusion for atlantoaxial subluxation. On the other hand, subaxial subluxation developed in 36% of their 22 patients with atlantoaxial subluxation and superior migration of the odontoid who underwent occipitocervical fusion. Overall, recurrent cervical instability developed in 15% of their 110 study patients with a previous fusion. These authors therefore concluded that early treatment of atlantoaxial subluxation, before the development of superior migration of the odontoid, decreases the chances of progression of cervical instability with resultant late deformity.

Management of Late Deformity

PREVENTION. Some of the preventive strategies should be self-evident according to the causes of late deformity. We concentrate here on some specific conditions.

Prevention of Flat-Back Syndrome (Loss of Lumbar Lordosis). During surgery for scoliosis, the general principle of fusion from stable vertebra to stable vertebra should be followed. Recording the apical vertebral translation and rotation and the lower limit of transition of the curve, in addition to the Cobb angle, helps to differentiate among the various types of curves. Extension of the fusion to the lower lumbar region should be avoided, if at all possible, because many compensatory lumbar curves correct spontaneously over time. The tendency is to spare as many lumbar motion segments as possible.

With the widespread availability and use of posterior segmental fusion instrumentation in the management of traumatic and degenerative lumbar disease, the potential for iatrogenic loss of lumbar lordosis is increased. This has been called *kyphotic decompensation syndrome* by some authors (12), to differentiate it from the loss that occurs after scoliosis surgery. Appropriate intraoperative positioning of the patient and radiographic confirmation of adequate lordosis before stabilizing the construct are vital in preventing this deformity. Operating room tables that allow for hip extension are the most effective method of maintaining lumbar lordosis. Adequate contouring of the rod or plates is also mandatory.

Prevention of Truncal Decompensation. Truncal decompensation is particularly a problem with the use of the powerful CD segmental correction system for scoliosis because most major curves can be almost completely corrected by this means. In an overzealous maneuver, however, one can easily cause frontal plane imbalance without being aware of it. Preoperative supine and side-bending films can help determine the degree of spontaneous correction of compensatory (nonstructural) curves that can be expected.

Prevention of the Crankshaft Phenomenon. Based on the available evidence, a definite case cannot be made for routinely using the AP fusion technique in the management of young children with scoliosis to prevent the crankshaft effect. However, in carefully selected cases, techniques such as apical fusion, convexity epiphysiodesis, and AP fusion can help minimize the effect of this phenomenon (53). The recent laboratory demonstration of the effectiveness of posterior transpedicular stabilization of anterior column growth appears promising (73). The use of pedicle screws can allow for simultaneous stabilization of the anterior and posterior regions of the spine via a single dorsal procedure. As a result, pedicle screw instrumentation has been increasingly utilized in the management of spinal deformity.

Prevention of Delayed Deformity in Infections and Trauma. A complete evaluation of the extent of injury with the use of computed tomography (CT) and MRI in addition to plain radiography is of paramount importance. One should be open to the possibility of further surgery based on what is found at the first operation. The importance of the sagittal index in the evaluation of thoracolumbar fractures and the degree of kyphosis in cervical injuries is becoming increasingly apparent. Likewise, an awareness of the need to perform AP fusions primarily in severe infections will lead to fewer problems of postoperative deformity.

TREATMENT

Treatment of Flat-Back Syndrome. The sagittal plane imbalance observed in flat-back and kyphotic decompensation syndromes covers a wide spectrum of deformity and symptomatology. Nearly half of all these patients can be effectively managed with physical therapy, removal of hardware, or both. Careful follow-up of this group, however, is essential because a certain number fail to maintain their sagittal balance and return with further back pain and failure of the discs below the level of original fusion (12). The remainder of them, with greater degrees of sagittal imbalance, require surgical realignment with anterior and posterior osteotomies and posterior instrumentation. LeGrone et al. (26) reported the results of corrective osteotomies and the use of Harrington instrumentation in compression in 55 patients. The average amount of sagittal plane correction was 4.2 cm, and at follow-up 47% of the patients still complained of "leaning forward." However, 95% of the patients thought that they had benefited from the corrective surgery. Farcy and Schwab (12) proposed that distal fusion to the sacrum could be spared if at least the last two discs (L4-5 and L5-S1) were intact on MRI or the sagittal malalignment was less than 4 cm.

Treatment of Truncal Decompensation. Soon after the CD system became available, reports of truncal decompensation following selective thoracic fusion were made. Therefore, Ibrahim and Benson (31) recommended reclassifying the King type II curve into two subtypes. Lenke et al. (32) suggested that the lumbar flexibility and the amount of deviation of the lumbar curve from the central sacral line play a critical role in the development of postoperative truncal decompensation. Others have warned about overcorrection of the thoracic curve because this tends to transmit rotational forces to the lumbar curve and aggravate the deformity by reducing its ability to correct spontaneously (74). Patients with minimal truncal decompensation can be followed periodically for curve progression. In more severe decompensation, an orthosis directed at the lumbar component of the curve can be attempted. Failure of conservative measures warrants extension of fusion to the distal stable vertebra of the lumbar curve.

Treatment of Shoulder Imbalance. In patients with progression of a cervicothoracic curve and associated shoulder asymmetry, the upper curve may have to be included in the instrumentation and the original shorter construct replaced with a longer one. Alternatively, a short rod can be used to instrument only the upper curve, with the site of the distal hook in the midportion of the original fusion mass. In either case, overdistraction must be avoided because undesired cervical kyphosis can result almost as easily as the residual scoliosis is corrected.

Conclusions

In this chapter, the various causes of late deformity following spinal fusion and the incidence, strategies for prevention, and management of certain specific deformities have been described. Newer strategies are being developed to address the issue of postfusion growth in children. Many of the iatrogenic causes can be prevented by the use of modern segmental instrumentation, adequate preoperative planning with attention to sagittal, coronal, and axial balance, and careful intraoperative positioning and meticulous surgical technique. At the same time, it is comforting to learn that the human spine has some capacity, at least in children, to remodel and self-correct surgeon-induced deformity (75). AP fusion can be very effective in correcting or preventing postfusion deformity. All risks, benefits, and alternatives must be carefully weighed before any surgical alternative aimed at preventing postfusion deformity is undertaken.

Case Illustration

A 51-year-old woman with a known history of osteoporosis, smoking, steroid-dependent reactive airway disease, and a complete hysterectomy with bilateral oophorectomies sustained a minor fall and fractures of the C7 and T3 vertebral bodies (Fig. 1). Three operations had been performed at an outside hospital before her transfer.

Surgery No. 1. A C7 corpectomy with allograft fusion of C6 through T1 and screw/plate stabilization. The surgery and postoperative course were uneventful.

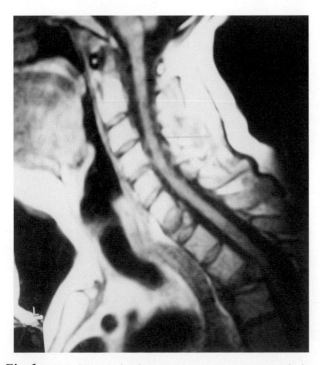

Fig. 1. A sagittal T1-weighted magnetic resonance imaging study demonstrates fractures of the C7 and T3 vertebral bodies. Height has been lost at both fracture sites, and the T3 fracture fragment abuts the spinal cord. No posterior ligamentous disruption is seen.

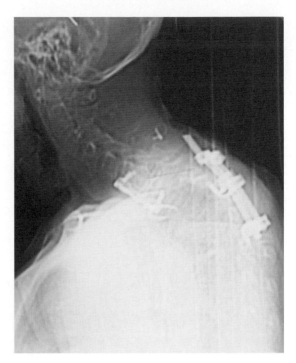

Fig. 2. Lateral radiograph of cervicothoracic junction after failure of a third operation. A loss of integrity of the posterior hardware led to a significant focal kyphotic deformity.

Surgery No. 2. A dorsal hook/rod stabilization and fusion of the upper thoracic spine for treatment of the T3 fracture. Postoperative hardware failure and resultant kyphosis developed.

Surgery No. 3. Revision of the dorsal upper thoracic instrumented fusion with modification of the hardware. An increasingly progressive kyphotic deformity developed (Fig. 2).

At this point, the patient was referred for evaluation for complex, reconstructive spinal surgery because the kyphosis had progressed to 95 degrees between the C5 and T8 levels (Fig. 3). A "chin-on-chest" deformity was present, with progressive airway compromise. The patient was placed on alendronate sodium, calcium supplementation, and estrogen replacement therapy.

Surgery No. 4. Posterior hardware removal with T2 laminectomy to provide a posterior "release." Postoperative skeletal traction for 2 weeks led to appreciable improvement (37 degrees) in the kyphotic deformity.

Surgery No. 5. AP upper thoracic fusions with posterior instrumentation. *Anterior* T3 corpectomy via a median sternotomy approach, fusion with structural autologous iliac bone graft. *Posterior* C7 through T7 instrumented fusion with pedicle screw/rod construct (Fig. 4).

The patient remained stable for 2 years, after which a pseudarthrosis developed at the upper aspect of the dorsal fusion, with hardware failure and progressive kyphotic deformity at the C5 through C7 levels. After skeletal traction for 4 days, the kyphosis improved significantly before the next surgical revision was undertaken.

Surgery No. 6. AP occipital–cervical–thoracic fusions with autologous structural iliac grafts anteriorly and autologous morselized iliac grafts posteriorly. AP instrumentation was utilized. *Anterior* removal of C6 through T1 screw/plate and four-level discectomy from C2-3 through C5-6; screw/plate stabilization of C2 through C6. *Posterior* removal of C7, T1, and T2 pedicle screws (right T2 screw had fractured); pseudarthrosis was pres-

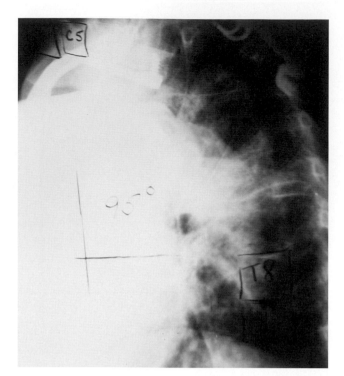

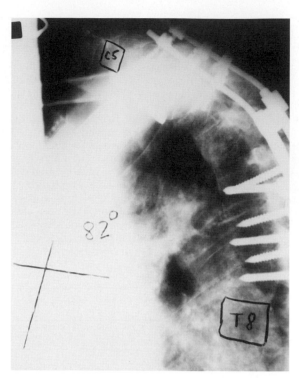

Fig. 3. Lateral radiograph of the cervicothoracic junction at initial evaluation. The angle between the C5 and T8 vertebral bodies measures 95 degrees. The patient had to lift her chin upward to maintain an adequate airway.

Fig. 4. Lateral radiograph of the cervicothoracic junction following a C7-T7 fusion with pedicle screw/rod stabilization. The C5-T8 angle improved to 82 degrees with this surgery. The T3 anterior corpectomy is fully incorporated.

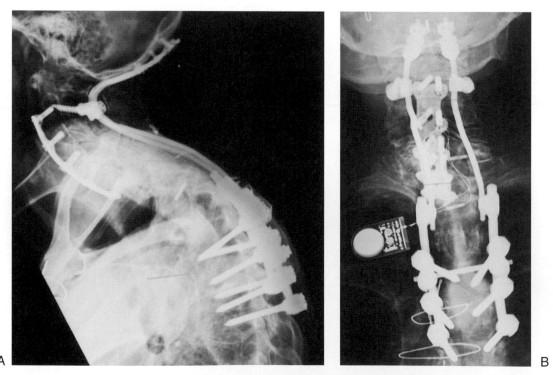

Fig. 5. A: Lateral radiograph of the occipital–cervical–thoracic region after an occiput-T7 fusion. The anterior column was reconstructed with structural iliac crest autografts and a screw/plate from C2-C6. The posterior fixation included screws in the occiput (6), C2 pedicles (2), and pedicles of T5-T7 bilaterally (6). **B:** Anteroposterior radiograph of the occipital–cervical–thoracic region. The implantable bone stimulator is seen in addition to wires from the prior transsternal surgery.

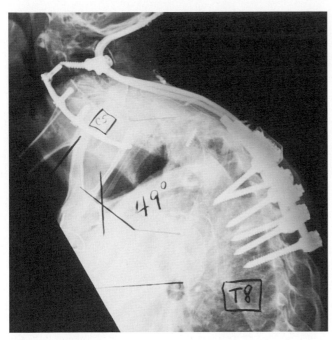

Fig. 6. Lateral radiograph of the occipital–cervical–thoracic region following halo/vest removal. The angle between C5-T8 measures 49 degrees (a 46-degree improvement over the angle before the initial complex reconstructive procedure).

ent at C7 through T2 level with stable fusion below T2; fusion from occiput to T3 with autologous onlay iliac cancellous graft; screw/rod stabilization with six bicortical screws into the midline bony keel of the occiput, two pedicle screws in C2, and connection of the rods into the stable inferior construct at the T3 level; placement of an implantable bone growth stimulator; placement of a halo/vest (Fig. 5).

SUMMARY. Because of numerous problems related to the patient's bone metabolism (osteoporosis, smoking, steroid use, complete hysterectomy), a nearly catastrophic kyphotic deformity developed that progressed steadily. A loss of the posterior muscular–ligamentous tension band led to failure of the dorsal fusion and the subsequent cascade of events. The patient has remained neurologically intact from the time of her initial injury through the postoperative period of her most recent spinal surgery (the sixth overall).

She is now fused from the occiput to the T7 level. Her angulation between C5 and T8 measures 49 degrees, which represents an improvement of 46 degrees over her initial evaluation angle of 95 degrees (Fig. 6). She now has an acceptable, albeit not ideal, sagittal and coronal alignment. This case illustrates the myriad of late complications that can occur following spinal fusion in a patient with severe metabolic bone disorders. In retrospect, this neurologically intact patient might have been better off with the use of a simple external orthosis for the fractures of the C7 and T3 vertebral bodies, which were not grossly unstable. The use of both anterior and posterior spinal reconstructive techniques was required to restore an acceptable spinal alignment.

References

1. Hibbs RA. An operation for progressive spinal deformities. *N Y Med J* 93:1013–1016, 1911.

2. Bohlman HH, Emery SE, Goodfellow DB, et al. Robinson anterior cervical discectomy and arthrodesis for cervical radiculopathy. *J Bone Joint Surg* 75A:1298–1307, 1993.

3. Cochran T, Nachemson A. Long-term anatomic changes in patients with adolescent idiopathic scoliosis treated by Harrington rod fusion. *Spine* 8:576–584, 1983.

4. Luk KDK, Lee RBI, Leong JYC, et al. The effect on the lumbosacral spine of long spinal fusion for idiopathic scoliosis. *Spine* 12:996-1000, 1987.

5. Hayes MA, Tompkins SF, Herndon WA, et al. Clinical and radiological evaluation of lumbosacral motion below fusion levels in idiopathic scoliosis. *Spine* 13:1161–1167, 1988.

6. Brunet JA, Wiley JJ. Acquired spondylolysis after spinal fusion. *J Bone Joint Surg Br* 66:720–724, 1984.

7. Friedman RJ, Micheli LJ. Acquired spondylolisthesis following scoliosis surgery. *Clin Orthop* 190:132–134, 1984.

8. Bowen SR, Branch CL Jr. The incidence and management of lumbar spinal stenosis adjacent to previous pedicle screw fixation. Presented at the 48th annual meeting of the Congress of Neurological Surgeons, Seattle, October 3–8, 1998.

9. Nagata H, Schendel MJ, Transfeldt EE, et al. The effects of immobilization of long segments of the spine on adjacent and distal facet force and lumbosacral motion. *Spine* 18:2471–2479, 1993.

10. Balderston RA, Albert TJ, Mckintosh T, et al. Magnetic resonance imaging analysis of lumbar disc changes below scoliosis fusions. A prospective study. *Spine* 23:54–59, 1998.

11. Fuller DA, Kirkpatrick JS, Emery SE, et al. A kinematic study of the cervical spine before and after segmental arthrodesis. Presented at the annual meeting of the Cervical Spine Research Society, New York, December 3, 1993.

12. Farcy JC, Schwab FJ. Management of flat back and related kyphotic decompensation syndromes. *Spine* 22:2452–2457, 1997.

13. Vital JM, Beguiristain JL, Algara C, et al. The neurocentral vertebral cartilage: anatomy, physiology and pathophysiology. *Surg Radiol Anat* 11:323–328, 1989.

14. Risser JC, Norquist DM, Cockrell BR, et al. The effect of posterior spine fusion on the growing spine. *Clin Orthop* 46:127–139, 1966.

15. Moe JH, Winter RB, Lonstein JA, et al. Clinical study of spine fusion in the growing child. *J Bone Joint Surg Br* 46:784, 1964.

16. Letts RM, Bobechko WP. Fusion of the scoliotic spine in young children: effect on prognosis and growth. *Clin Orthop* 101:136–145, 1974.

17. Hefti FL, McMaster MJ. The effect of the adolescent growth spurt on early posterior spinal fusion in infantile and juvenile idiopathic scoliosis. *J Bone Joint Surg Br* 65:247–254, 1983.

18. Dubousset J, Herring JA, Shufflebarger H. The crankshaft phenomenon. *J Pediatr Orthop* 9:541–550, 1989.

19. Sanders JO, Herring JA, Browne RH. Posterior arthrodesis and instrumentation in the immature spine in idiopathic scoliosis. *J Bone Joint Surg Am* 77:39–45, 1995.

20. Terek RM, Wehner J, Lubicky JP. Crankshaft phenomenon in congenital scoliosis: a preliminary report. *J Pediatr Orthop* 11:527–532, 1991.

21. Jackson L, Banta JV, Smith BA. Crankshaft phenomenon in neuromuscular scoliosis. Paper No. 58, presented at the annual meeting of the Scoliosis Research Society, Dublin, September 1992.

22. Harrington PR. The history and development of Harrington instrumentation. *Clin Orthop* 93:110–112, 1973.

23. Farcy JC. Iatrogenic thoracolumbar spine deformity. In: Farcy JC, ed. *Complex spinal deformities: state of the art reviews*. Philadelphia: Hanley & Belfus, 1994:673–680 (vol 8).

24. Aaro S, Ohlen G. The effect of Harrington instrumentation on the sagittal configuration and the mobility of the spine in scoliosis. *Spine* 8:570–575, 1983.

25. Kostuik JP, Maurais GR, Richardson WJ, et al. Combined single stage anterior and posterior osteotomy for correction of iatrogenic lumbar kyphosis. *Spine* 13:257–266, 1988.

26. LeGrone MO, Bradford DS, Moe JH, et al. Treatment of symptomatic flat back after spinal fusion. *J Bone Joint Surg Am* 70:569–580, 1988.

27. Kostuik JP, Hall B. Spinal fusion to sacrum in adults with scoliosis. *Spine* 8:489–500, 1983.

28. Kalen V, Conklin M. The behavior of the unfused lumbar spine following selective thoracic fusion for idiopathic scoliosis. *Spine* 15:271–274, 1990.

29. Richards BS, Birch JG, Herring JA, et al. Frontal plane and sagittal

plane balance following Cotrel-Dubousset instrumentation. *Spine* 14:733–737, 1989.

30. Bridwell KH, McAllister JW, Betz R, et al. Coronal decompensation produced by Cotrel-Dubousset derotation maneuver for idiopathic right thoracic scoliosis. *Spine* 16:769–777, 1991.

31. Ibrahim K, Benson L. Cotrel-Dubousset instrumentation for double major right thoracic left lumbar scoliosis: the relation between frontal balance, hook configuration and fusion levels. *Orthop Trans* 15: 114, 1991.

32. Lenke LG, Bridwell KH, Baldus C, et al. Preventing decompensation in King type II curves treated with Cotrel-Dubousset instrumentation. Strict guidelines for selective thoracic fusion. *Spine* 17(8 suppl): S274–S281, 1992.

33. Wenger DR, Mubarak SJ. Managing complications of posterior spinal instrumentation and fusion. In: Garfin SR, ed. *Complications of spine surgery.* Baltimore: Williams & Wilkins, 1989:127–143.

34. McLain RF, Sparling E, Benson D. Early failure of short-segment pedicle instrumentation for thoracolumbar fractures. *J Bone Joint Surg Am* 75:162–167, 1993.

35. An HS, Coppes MA. Posterior cervical fixation for fracture and degenerative disc disease. *Clin Orthop* 335:101–111, 1997.

36. Cloward RB. Treatment of acute fractures and fracture dislocations of the cervical spine by vertebral body fusion. *J Neurosurg* 18:201, 1961.

37. Bell GD, Bailey SI. Anterior cervical fusion for trauma. *Clin Orthop* 128:155–158, 1977.

38. Eichbaum E, Rezai A, Woo H, et al. Surgical management of cervical pyogenic osteomyelitis. Presented at the meeting of the North American Spine Society, 1998.

39. Crawford AH, Gabriel KR. Dysplastic scoliosis: neurofibromatosis. In: Bridwell KH, DeWald RL, eds. *The textbook of spinal surgery,* 2nd ed. Philadelphia: Lippincott–Raven Publishers, 1997:277–298.

40. Holt RT, Johnson JR. Cotrel-Dubousset instrumentation in neurofibromatosis spine curves. A preliminary report. *Clin Orthop* 245: 19–23, 1989.

41. Hsu LCS, Lee PC, Leong JCY. Dystrophic spinal deformities in neurofibromatosis: treatment by anterior and posterior fusion. *J Bone Joint Surg Br* 66:495–499, 1984.

42. Wilde PH, Upadhyay SS, Leong JCY. Deterioration of operative correction in dystrophic spinal neurofibromatosis. *Spine* 19:1264–1270, 1994.

43. Menezes AH, Van Gilder JC, Clark CR, et al. Odontoid upward migration in rheumatoid arthritis. An analysis of 45 patients with "cranial settling." *J Neurosurg* 63:500–509, 1985.

44. Smith HP, Challa VR, Alexander E. Odontoid compression of the brainstem in a patient with rheumatoid arthritis. A case report. *J Neurosurg* 53:841–845, 1980.

45. Santavirta S, Konttinon YT, Sandelin J, et al. Operations for the unstable cervical spine in rheumatoid arthritis: sixteen cases of subaxial subluxations. *Acta Orthop Scand* 61:106–110, 1990.

46. Moon M. Spine update: tuberculosis of the spine, controversies and a new challenge. *Spine* 22:1791–1797, 1997.

47. Medical Research Council Working Party on Tuberculosis of the Spine. A ten-year assessment of a controlled trial comparing debridement and anterior spinal fusion in the management of tuberculosis of the spine in patients on standard chemotherapy in Hong Kong. *J Bone Joint Surg Br* 64:393–398, 1982.

48. Upadhyay SS, Sell P, Saji JM, et al. Surgical management of spinal tuberculosis in adults. Hong Kong operation compared with debridement surgery for short- and long-term outcome of deformity. *Clin Orthop* 302:173–182, 1994.

49. Schulitz K, Kothe R, Leong JCY, et al. Growth changes of solidly fused kyphotic bloc after surgery for tuberculosis. Comparison of four procedures. *Spine* 22:1150–1155, 1997.

50. Colmenero JD, Jimenez-Mejias ME, Sanchez-Lora FJ, et al. Pyogenic, tuberculous and brucellar vertebral osteomyelitis: a descriptive and comparative study of 219 cases. *Ann Rheum Dis* 56:709–715, 1997.

51. Emery SE, Chan DPK, Woodward HR. Treatment of hematogenous pyogenic vertebral osteomyelitis with anterior debridement and primary bone grafting. *Spine* 14:284–291, 1989.

52. Winter RB, Moe JH. The results of spinal arthrodesis for congenital spinal deformity in patients younger than five years old. *J Bone Joint Surg Am* 64:419–432, 1982.

53. Lapinsky AS, Richards BS. Preventing the crankshaft phenomenon by combining anterior fusion with posterior instrumentation. Does it work? *Spine* 12:1392–1398, 1995.

54. Arai S, Ohtsuka Y, Ohki I, et al. Scoliosis associated with syringomyelia. *Orthop Trans* 17:105–106, 1993.

55. Yamada H, Transfeldt EE, Ogilvie JW, et al. The crankshaft phenomenon in adolescent idiopathic scoliosis—fact or fiction. Presented at the annual meeting of the Scoliosis Research Society, Dublin, September 18, 1993.

56. Dubousset J, Katti E, Seringe R. Epiphysiodesis of the spine in young children for congenital spinal deformation. *J Pediatr Orthop* 1:123, 1991.

57. Shufflebarger HL, Clark CE. Prevention of the crankshaft phenomenon. *Spine* 16:S409–S411, 1991.

58. Lee CS, Nachemson AL. The crankshaft phenomenon after posterior Harrington fusion in skeletally immature patients with thoracic or thoracolumbar idiopathic scoliosis followed to maturity. *Spine* 22: 58–67, 1997.

59. Lowe T. Current concepts review: Scheuermann disease. *J Bone Joint Surg Am* 72:940–945, 1990.

60. Bradford DS, Moe JH, Montalvo FJ, et al. Scheuermann's kyphosis. Results of surgical treatment by posterior spine arthrodesis in twenty-two patients. *J Bone Joint Surg Am* 57:439–448, 1975.

61. Lowe TG, Kasten MD. An analysis of sagittal curves and balance after Cotrel-Dubousset instrumentation for kyphosis secondary to Scheuermann's disease. A review of 32 patients. *Spine* 19: 1680–1685, 1994.

62. Myllynen P, Bostman O, Riska E. Recurrence of deformity after removal of Harrington's fixation of spine fractures. Seventy-six cases followed for two years. *Acta Orthop Scand* 59:497–502, 1988.

63. Willen J, Lindhal S, Norwall A. Unstable thoracolumbar fractures: comparative clinical study of conservative treatment and Harrington instrumentation. *Spine* 10:111–122, 1985.

64. Aho AJ, Savunen TJA, Makela PJ. Operative fixation of fractures of the thoracic and lumbar vertebrae by Williams plates with reference to late kyphosis. *Injury* 19:153–158, 1988.

65. Acaroglu ER, Schwab FJ, Farcy JP. Simultaneous anterior and posterior approaches for correction of late deformity due to thoracolumbar fractures. *Eur Spine J* 5:56–62, 1996.

66. Birney TJ, Hanley EN. Traumatic cervical spine injuries in childhood and adolescence. *Spine* 14:1277–1282, 1989.

67. McGrory BJ, Klassen RA. Arthrodesis of the cervical spine for fractures and dislocations in children and adolescents. *J Bone Joint Surg Am* 76:1606–1616, 1994.

68. Upadhyay SS, Saji MJ, Sell P, et al. The effect of age on the change in deformity after radical resection and anterior arthrodesis for tuberculosis of the spine. *J Bone Joint Surg Am* 76:701–708, 1994.

69. Pellicci PM, Ranawat CS, Tsairis P, et al. A prospective study of the progression of rheumatoid arthritis of the cervical spine. *J Bone Joint Surg Am* 63:342–350, 1981.

70. Santavirta S, Konttinen YT, Laasonen E, et al. Ten-year results of operations for rheumatoid cervical spinal disorders. *J Bone Joint Surg Br* 73:116–120, 1991.

71. Agarwal AK, Peppelman WC, Kraus DR, et al. Recurrence of cervical spine instability in rheumatoid arthritis following previous fusion: can disease progression be prevented by early surgery? *J Rheumatol* 19:1364–1370, 1992.

72. Boden SD, Dodge LD, Bohlmann HH, et al. Rheumatoid arthritis of the cervical spine: a long-term analysis with predictions of paralysis and recovery period. *J Bone Joint Surg Am* 75:1282–1297, 1993.

73. Kioschos HC, Asher MA, Lark RG, et al. Overpowering the crankshaft mechanism. The effect of posterior spinal fusion with and without stiff trans-pedicular fixation on the anterior spinal column growth in immature canines. *Spine* 21:1168–1173, 1996.

74. Thompson JP, Transfeldt EE, Bradford DS, et al. Decompensation after Cotrel-Dubousset instrumentation of idiopathic scoliosis. *Spine* 15:927–931, 1990.

75. Toyama Y, Matsumoto M, Chiba K, et al. Realignment of postoperative cervical kyphosis in children by vertebral remodeling. *Spine* 19:2565–2570, 1994.

182. Cervical Pseudoarthrosis

**Edward C. Benzel and
Christopher D. Kager**

Pseudoarthrosis is defined as a failure of full bony healing in which an abnormal union is formed by fibrous tissue. With a heightened awareness of this problem, including potential causes and strategies for avoidance, surgeons may obtain increased rates of fusion and, it is hoped, improved clinical outcomes. In this chapter, we present a review of cervical pseudoarthrosis, including contributing factors and imaging modalities in addition to strategies for prevention, revision, and augmentation.

Factors Contributing to Pseudoarthrosis

SMOKING. Cigarettes and other tobacco products have clearly been shown to have a deleterious effect on spinal fusion (1–4). A twofold to fourfold higher rate of pseudoarthrosis has been reported in smokers. This effect may be primarily produced through the systemic absorption and effects of nicotine. Thus, any tobacco product (including cigarettes, cigars, and chewing tobacco) in addition to aids for smoking cessation, such as nicotine gum, may contribute to pseudoarthrosis.

Nicotine has been shown in animal studies to inhibit the revascularization of bone grafts and then eventual fusion. Indeed, the fusion mass that does form may be biomechanically inferior (2,5). Nicotine also inhibits the expression of a wide range of cytokines, including those associated with neovascularization and osteoblast differentiation (6). Therefore, the effects of nicotine appear to involve more than just local vasoconstriction. It has also been proposed that decreased arterial levels of oxygen in smokers may contribute to lower rates of fusion. Other mechanisms of the negative effects of smoking on bony fusion have been proposed but not thoroughly studied (7). Furthermore, clinical studies have been reported in which these findings correlate with poor patient outcome (8).

Physicians can have a powerful effect in helping patients to quit using tobacco (4). They should counsel their patients regarding all the health risks of tobacco, in addition to its deleterious effect on spinal fusion. They should urge any patient who smokes to quit using tobacco, and the patient should also be referred to an appropriate smoking cessation program if the physician or the patient feels this would be useful. These discussions should be repeated at each office visit and clearly documented in the medical record. Some surgeons routinely refuse to perform elective spinal fusions on current tobacco users. The cessation of tobacco use can be documented with blood or urine chemistries.

MEDICATIONS

Corticosteroids. Experimentally, corticosteroids have clearly been shown to inhibit spinal fusion (9). The use of corticosteroids is particularly harmful in the first 2 to 3 weeks following a fusion procedure. This effect probably is primarily a consequence of interference with the first stage of bony healing, the inflammatory response. Inhibition at this point results in failure of sufficient vascular ingrowth to support bony incorporation

and remodeling. In addition, long-term steroid use may lead to osteoporosis, which has a negative impact on spinal fusion (see below).

Nonsteroidal Antiinflammatory Drugs. Nonsteroidal antiinflammatory drugs (NSAIDs) have been shown to inhibit spinal fusion significantly at doses typically given for pain control (10, 11). They act by inhibiting cyclooxygenase enzymes and therefore diminishing prostaglandin production. Prostaglandins, however, are intimately involved in the modulation of bone metabolism, and both clinical and laboratory studies indicate that prostaglandins preferentially favor bone anabolism. Many alternatives for pain control are available. A pain management consultation may be sought if pain control becomes problematical in the postoperative period. Because of their antiplatelet effects, NSAIDS should also be avoided before surgery.

Chemotherapy. Chemotherapeutic drugs have cytotoxic and immunosuppressive effects that deleteriously affect bone fusion. Ideally, patients should not be on chemotherapeutic drugs at the time of surgery or in the first 2 weeks postoperatively. Although this is not always possible, it is important to recognize the potentially adverse effects of chemotherapy (12).

RADIATION. Radiation therapy is often utilized following surgical decompression and fusion procedures for spinal neoplasms. Radiation impairs bone healing by inhibiting cellular proliferation and producing a vasculitis that inhibits vascular ingrowth to the graft (13,14). The effect on bone fusion appears to be time- and dose-sensitive, with a maximal effect occurring during the first 1 or 2 weeks postoperatively and with total radiation doses exceeding 4,000 cGy (14). It appears prudent to begin radiation therapy after 2 weeks postoperatively (to allow both bone fusion and wound healing) and tailor the radiation to a maximally effective but not excessive dose.

SYSTEMIC FACTORS

Rheumatoid Arthritis. Rheumatoid arthritis, which has an incidence of approximately 1%, affects women twice as often as men. This disease process is characterized by inflammatory synovitis in joints throughout the body, including the cervical spine. Osteoporosis and immunosuppression as a primary effect of the disease both impair bone fusion. Also, these patients are frequently taking corticosteroids. Steroids and other cytotoxic/immunosuppressive medications should be discontinued for as long as is safely possible before an elective spinal fusion procedure is undertaken. With care, spinal fusion rates above 90% have been reported in this population (15–17).

Osteoporosis. Osteoporosis is defined as a bone mineral density that is more than 2.5 standard deviations below the mean of young, healthy persons. Osteoporosis is a major public health threat for 28 million Americans, 80% of whom are women. In the United States today, 10 million persons already have osteoporosis, and 18 million more have a low bone mass, so that they are at increased risk for this disease (18). The overall incidence increases with age and is much higher in postmenopausal women. The practical effect of weakened bone in spinal fusion

1965

procedures is a loss of structural support, potentially leading to early and even catastrophic construct failure. This in turn may cause neurological deficits, spinal deformity, and pseudo-arthrosis. One strategy to combat the effects of osteoporosis is to use more extensive constructs (e.g., anterior and posterior constructs) and to span multiple levels beyond the area of bone grafting. Optimizing the treatment of osteoporosis before spinal fusion is advised.

Diabetes Mellitus. Diabetes causes far-reaching systemic effects that interfere with normal bone healing and fusion. Impairment of the microcirculation hampers ingrowth of the blood supply to bone grafts. Impairment of the immune system in diabetes interferes with the inflammatory stage of bone fusion. Diabetes appears to be more likely to be associated with a poor clinical outcome in patients who are insulin-dependent.

Obesity. Although anecdotal reports have cited obesity as a risk factor for pseudoarthrosis, the only study that directly addressed this issue did not find a correlation (19). Nonetheless, patients should be counseled that obesity may place them at a higher risk for other complications of surgery (20).

Malnutrition. Malnutrition has a negative impact on fracture healing (21), blunts the immune response, and impairs wound healing. Data suggest that a large percentage of patients (particularly older patients) undergoing elective lumbar spinal surgery are malnourished (22). It is recommended that close attention be paid to the perioperative nutritional status of patients undergoing spinal fusion surgery. Patients with suboptimal nutritional parameters should be given nutritional supplementation and replenishment before elective surgery.

TECHNICAL FACTORS

Preparation of the Site. In any fusion procedure, careful preparation of the surfaces is required. All cartilage, ligament, and disc material should be removed from the end plates and all soft tissue removed from the graft. However, care must be taken to remove cartilage from the end plate in such a way that subchondral bone is exposed but cancellous bone is not entered, so that a weakened surface will not lead to excessive subsidence. The shapes of the surfaces must be matched to ensure a maximal area of contact. This provides a greater area in which fusion can occur, resists subsidence, and imparts stability to the construct. During fusion procedures, the use of bone wax should be avoided because it interferes with vascular ingrowth and bony healing.

Allograft versus Autograft. In comparisons of fusion rates following spinal fusion procedures, autograft appears to have an advantage over allograft but entails the potential for donor site morbidity, inadequate volume, and poor bone quality. The choice of autograft or allograft should be made on a case-specific and patient-specific basis. For example, in single-level discectomy, the fusion rates for allograft and autograft are essentially equivalent (16,23–26), but in multilevel anterior cervical procedures, pseudoarthrosis rates appear higher with allograft (27). The method of preparation of the allograft also likely affects fusion rates; fusion rates with fresh-frozen allograft are superior to those obtained with freeze-dried or ethylene oxide-sterilized grafts.

Imaging of Pseudoarthrosis

Various radiographic studies have been evaluated for the assessment of spinal pseudoarthrosis and are discussed below.

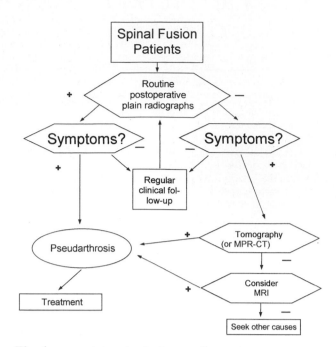

Fig. 1. Proposed algorithm for the cost-effective diagnostic evaluation of patients following spinal fusion. Anteroposterior (AP) and dynamic lateral radiographs at 3, 6, 12, and 24 months after surgery.

A rational plan for the postoperative evaluation of fusion is necessary. By taking into consideration the strengths and weaknesses of each modality, one can formulate a logical series of steps to be followed. Hilibrand and Dina (28) have developed a succinct flow chart to be utilized in evaluating pseudoarthrosis (Figs. 1 and 2).

ROENTGENOGRAPHY/TOMOGRAPHY. Plain radiographs are the postoperative images generally obtained following fusion procedures. Anteroposterior (AP) and lateral projections are the usual views and may provide details of bone graft consolidation or incorporation. However, these views are generally considered inadequate to determine the presence of pseudoarthrosis definitively, particularly in the thoracic and lumbar spine. In an intertransverse fusion, resorption of graft material without consolidation may signal nonunion. On a lateral view of internal fixation devices (i.e., pedicle screws), a radiolucency surrounding the implant ("halo") may signify nonunion; failure of these devices may also be indicative of nonunion. It has been suggested that radiolucent lines within the fusion mass on AP or lateral views are diagnostic of nonunion. However, in one study (29), plain radiographic findings correlated with intraoperative findings only 68% of the time. Most of the disagreements were caused by false-negative errors in which the plain radiographs appeared to show solid fusion. Plain radiographs, therefore, may be quite specific in diagnosing a nonunion but of low sensitivity. Flexion–extension lateral radiographs have also been utilized with varying success in determining solid lumbar fusions (30,31).

Following anterior cervical fusions, lateral radiographs may demonstrate bridging trabecular bone as early as 6 weeks after surgery. In late postoperative radiographs, regression of uncovertebral spurs may be indicative of solid interbody fusion. Flexion–extension lateral radiographs are generally relied on for the long-term assessment of cervical fusion (32–35); however, these studies did not confirm fusion with surgical exploration.

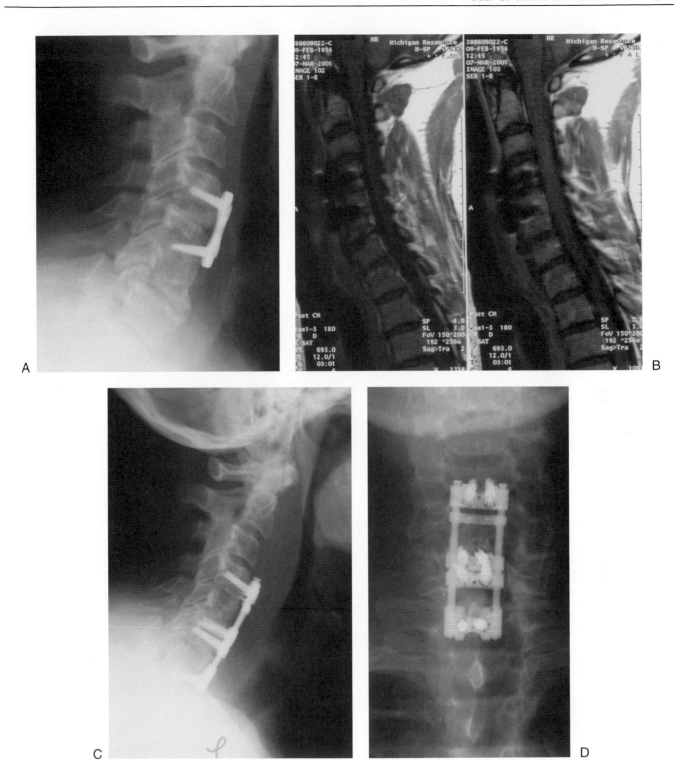

Fig. 2. A 47-year-old man, after undergoing three separate anterior cervical discectomies and fusions (C4-5, C5-6, C6-7), presented with progressive axial neck pain and limited cervical mobility. **A:** Lateral cervical spine radiograph shows likely pseudoarthrosis at both C4-5 and C6-7. Also note loss of cervical lordosis. **B:** Preoperative magnetic resonance imaging confirms likely pseudoarthroses. **C,D:** Postoperative AP and lateral radiographs. Note revisions of C4-5 and C6-7, which were confirmed pseudoarthroses intraoperatively; the fusion at C5-6 was solid. Also note restoration of cervical lordosis.

Various forms of conventional tomography are utilized in the evaluation of pseudoarthrosis. However, the availability of conventional tomography is on the wane as the field of radiology has moved toward computed tomography (CT) and magnetic resonance imaging (MRI). Excellent correlation between conventional tomography and surgical findings in thoracolumbar fusion has been reported but is unsubstantiated (30). Tomography may also be useful in the evaluation of cervical fusion. In any region of the spine, metallic implants can produce artifact that obscures the findings of tomography.

COMPUTED TOMOGRAPHY. CT allows rapid, high-resolution spiral scanning with multiplanar reconstruction, and it may be the imaging test of choice following plain radiography in evaluating pseudoarthrosis. Again, metal implants are a source of artifact and degrade CT images. Previous studies (30) have suggested that CT may be no more accurate than plain radiography in diagnosing pseudoarthrosis. However, one of these studies utilized only axial CT images without reconstruction, and the other study was limited by the amount of artifact generated by metallic implants. It may be that current CT software and thinner slice scans improve accuracy by minimizing artifact; other studies (36,37) have documented the excellent ability of CT to evaluate pseudoarthrosis.

MAGNETIC RESONANCE IMAGING. Several studies have investigated the utility of MRI in evaluating spine fusion. Lang et al. (38) described the T1 and T2 signal changes seen with normal posterolateral lumbar fusions and pseudoarthrosis; the accuracy of predicting pseudoarthrosis was 83%. In anterior cervical fusions, MRI demonstrates a gradual change in marrow signal in the interbody graft in the first 2 years following fusion. How this relates to the diagnosis of pseudoarthrosis is unclear. Metallic implants (stainless steel and titanium) degrade MR images; certain methodologies are utilized to minimize this effect.

NUCLEAR IMAGING. Bone scintigraphy, especially single photon emission computed tomography (SPECT), is being increasingly utilized in the evaluation of potential spinal pseudoarthrosis. In these nuclear studies, postoperative spinal fusion is characterized by diffusely increased uptake of the radioactive tracer in the area of fusion. Pseudoarthrosis, on the other hand, is characterized by areas of focally increased uptake. Some studies have documented the ability of SPECT to identify pseudoarthrosis reliably (39). However, in a large review of 940 articles on bone imaging with SPECT, Littenberg et al. (40) found only weak evidence in 13 relevant articles that SPECT is useful in detecting pseudoarthroses after failed spinal fusion. Another prospective study demonstrated that SPECT alone is inaccurate in diagnosing pseudoarthrosis when surgical exploration is used as the gold standard (41). The sensitivity and specificity of this modality are therefore questionable in these and other studies (40,42). However, SPECT may provide added detail in questionable cases.

Cervical Pseudoarthrosis

The clinical syndrome of a failed cervical fusion consists primarily of mechanical neck pain and (possibly) referred pain, including radicular or occipital pain. True radiculopathy may be indicative of inadequate initial decompression, or of progressive neurological compression from the effects of a pseudoarthrosis. These two distinct entities may be difficult to distinguish. Hardware failure is also potentially indicative of pseudoarthrosis (43) because most cervical instrumentation eventually fails if fusion does not occur.

To determine the natural history of pseudoarthrosis, in addition to risk factors and treatment outcomes, Phillips et al. (34) performed a retrospective study of the long-term clinical outcomes in 48 patients with radiographically documented pseudoarthroses after anterior cervical discectomy and fusion. Of the 48 patients, 32 were symptomatic at last follow-up or at the time of reoperation. Of the 48 patients with pseudoarthroses, 16 (33%) remained asymptomatic at a mean of 5.1 years after anterior cervical discectomy and fusion. A younger age at the time of initial surgery increased the likelihood that the pseudoarthrosis would become symptomatic. Following multilevel anterior cervical discectomy and fusion, the most caudal operated level accounted for 82% of the pseudoarthroses.

ANTERIOR CERVICAL PSEUDOARTHROSIS. Following anterior cervical discectomy or corpectomy, anterior cervical plating may be efficacious in preventing pseudoarthrosis, maintaining sagittal alignment, and preventing the need for further operations. A recent large series showed that the use of anterior cervical plating following anterior cervical discectomy and fusion decreased the pseudoarthrosis rate from 11.8% to 3.6% (44). Although not every study has reached this conclusion (26), most studies of multilevel cervical fusions support the use of anterior cervical plating (45,46).

A recent article reported the efficacy of pseudoarthrosis revision with autogenous iliac crest bone grafting and anterior cervical plating; 81% of these patients went on to solid arthrodesis (47). Another study also documented the efficacy of anterior revision of the pseudoarthrosis with iliac crest allograft and anterior cervical plating; a 100% fusion rate was achieved in 19 patients (39). In the study of Phillips et al. (34), cited previously, a solid fusion was achieved in 14 of 16 patients who underwent anterior repair of the pseudoarthrosis, and fusion was achieved in all six patients who underwent surgery via a posterior approach for anterior pseudoarthrosis. Excellent clinical outcomes were obtained in 19 of the 20 patients in whom fusion was achieved with a second cervical operation. A 1997 study (48) analyzed 35 patients treated for failed anterior cervical discectomy and fusion; all patients underwent repeated surgery via an anterior approach. Cervical corpectomy was performed if kyphosis was present. Excellent results were obtained in 83% of patients. Caspar and Pitzen (49) reported an important series of 41 patients with "failed cervical spine surgery" (pseudoarthrosis, graft fracture or dislocation, and kyphotic angulations) who underwent anterior reoperation, fusion, and anterior plating. Of the 37 patients for whom follow-up was available, 31 improved clinically, and a stable bony fusion with optimal anatomical alignment was achieved in all 37 patients.

It is our practice to reexplore failed fusions from an anterior approach. In this way, direct debridement and revision of the previous fusion attempt and correction of any deformity are possible. Anterior cervical plating is also used to take advantage of the previously discussed properties of plating. We utilize multiple points of fixation, so that this a three-point construct, better able to resist deformation. When appropriate, an anterior cervical plating system allowing controlled dynamism is used. This allows the graft to see loads but prevents excessive settling. During anterior cervical cases that require correction of deformity, two other strategies are used. We place a large roll under the patient's shoulders and a foam donut under the head. After the anterior decompression, removal of the foam donut restores lordosis to the cervical spine and helps to correct the deformity.

The second technique is prior contouring of the anterior cervical plate to an appropriate lordosis. After the anterior decompression has been performed and the grafts applied, the contoured anterior cervical plate is placed. Screws are then used to secure the ends of the plate and placed in the intervening vertebral bodies, so that the intervening vertebral bodies are brought to the plate. Excellent success rates have been achieved with this strategy.

Several studies alternatively evaluated the utility of posterior cervical lateral mass instrumentation and fusion in the salvage of anterior cervical pseudoarthrosis. Brodsky et al. (50) reported an 88% rate of satisfactory clinical results in patients who underwent reoperation via a posterior fusion, versus 59% in patients who underwent anterior reoperation and fusion. Lowery et al. (51) evaluated 44 patients with symptomatic anterior cervical pseudoarthrosis, of whom 20 underwent anterior pseudoarthrosis repair and anterior plating, 17 posterior cervical fusion and lateral mass plating, and 7 both anterior revision and posterior lateral mass plating. A solid radiographic fusion was achieved in all 7 patients undergoing a circumferential procedure, and a solid fusion was achieved in 16 (94%) of 17 patients who had posterior repairs. However, a solid fusion was obtained in only 45% of the patients after anterior repair alone. Another study reported 100% fusion rates and excellent pain relief in 19 patients following posterior nerve root decompression and fusion after failed anterior cervical fusion (32). Posterior spinous process wiring has also been used for symptomatic nonunion after anterior cervical discectomy, and fusion with radiographic union was achieved in all 14 patients reported (52).

POSTERIOR CERVICAL PSEUDOARTHROSIS. Posterior cervical lateral mass plating and fusion are being increasingly utilized in degenerative and traumatic lesions of the subaxial cervical spine. The reported pseudoarthrosis rate is 0% to 1.4%, which makes it quite uncommon. Few reports detail strategies utilized to prevent or revise posterior cervical pseudoarthroses. It is our practice, after a posterior cervical pseudoarthrosis has been diagnosed, to reexplore the posterior cervical fusion, debride the nonunion, reinstrument or extend the instrumentation if necessary, and fuse with autograft if available. Another potential strategy is to augment the fusion, as discussed below.

Fusion Augmentation

Certain strategies are now available that can aid in preventing pseudoarthrosis or be utilized in treating a failed fusion. Two methods of augmenting fusions are electrical stimulation and the use of bone growth factors.

ELECTRICAL STIMULATION. Although the first report on the use of electrical stimulation for bony nonunion dates from 1841, the first report on the efficacy of electrical stimulation in augmenting a spinal fusion was published in 1974 by Dwyer and Wickham (53). Currently, two types of electrical stimulation are in wide use: direct current electrical stimulation (DCES) and pulsed electromagnetic field (PEMF). In DCES, implantable metallic leads are placed in direct contact with bony surfaces, and in PEMF, noninvasive external coils are used to generate an electromagnetic field across an area of attempted fusion. Excellent reviews of the development of this technology (including mechanisms of action and clinical studies) are available (54). Most clinical studies have found a benefit of electrical stimulation (increases in fusion rates ranging from 10% to 28%) (55–57) in lumbar fusions; however, no clinical studies of its use in cervical fusion procedures have been published. The devices currently available cost between approximately $3,800 and $5,000; thus, an informed decision should be made regarding their use.

GROWTH FACTORS. A recent explosion of reports has heralded the arrival of bone morphogenetic proteins (BMPs) as an adjunct to spinal fusion. Many excellent reviews have documented the development of the use of these osteoinductive growth factors in augmenting fusion (58–60). Most of the studies have been in animal models, and several have demonstrated that BMP-containing allograft or synthetic carrier medium is as effective as or superior to autograft bone in promoting spinal fusion. In the limited number of human trials utilizing BMPs to treat nonunions in the appendicular skeleton, the results have been promising (60). Prospective, randomized trials investigating the use of BMPs in augmenting spinal fusions, including pseudoarthroses, are ongoing. When commercially available for human use, the cost of BMPs may be prohibitively high and thus preclude their routine use.

Conclusions

Pseudoarthrosis following cervical spinal fusion procedures is a challenging clinical problem. With attention to the risk factors and technical factors that contribute to this outcome, its incidence should diminish. The imaging of pseudoarthrosis is complex, and a management scheme has been presented. Good strategies are available for the surgical treatment of cervical pseudoarthrosis, including the use of fusion augmentation, which is likely to develop further in the future.

References

1. Hadley MN, Reddy SV. Smoking and the human vertebral column: a review of the impact of cigarette use on vertebral bone metabolism and spinal fusion. *Neurosurgery* 1997;41:116–124.
2. Silcox DH, Daftari T, Boden SD, et al. The effect of nicotine on spinal fusion. *Spine* 1995;20:1549–1553.
3. Boden SD, Sumner DR. Biologic factors affecting spinal fusion and bone regeneration. *Spine* 1995;20:102S–112S.
4. Rechtine GR, Frawley W, Castellvi A, et al. Effect of the spine practitioner on patient smoking status. *Spine* 2000;25:2229–2233.
5. Daftari TK, Whitesides TE, Heller JG, et al. Nicotine on the revascularization of bone graft. An experimental study in rabbits. *Spine* 1994;19:904–911.
6. Theiss SM, Boden SD, Hair G, et al. The effect of nicotine on gene expression during spine fusion. *Spine* 2000;25:2588–2594.
7. Bose B. Anterior cervical instrumentation enhances fusion rates in multilevel reconstruction in smokers. *J Spinal Disord* 2001;14:3–9.
8. Glassman SD, Anagnost SC, Parker A, et al. The effect of cigarette smoking and smoking cessation on spinal fusion. *Spine* 2000;25:2608–2615.
9. Sawin PD, Dickman CA, Crawford NR, et al. The effects of dexamethasone on bone fusion in an experimental model of posterolateral lumbar spinal arthrodesis. *J Neurosurg* 2001;94 (Supp):76–81.
10. Boden SD, Schimandle JH. Biologic enhancement of spinal fusion. *Spine* 1995;20:113S–123S.
11. Glassman SD, Rose SM, Dimar JR, et al. The effect of postoperative nonsteroidal anti-inflammatory drug administration on spinal fusion. *Spine* 1998;23:834–838.

12. Pelker RR, Friedlaender GE, Panjabi MM, et al. Chemotherapy-induced alterations in the biomechanics of rat bone. *J Orthop Res* 1985;3:91–95.

13. Emery SE, Hughes SS, Junglas WA, et al. The fate of anterior vertebral bone grafts in patients irradiated for neoplasm. *Clin Orthop* 1994; 300:207–212.

14. Bouchard JA, Koka A, Bensusan JS, et al. Effects of irradiation on posterior spinal fusions. A rabbit model. *Spine* 1994;19:1836–1841.

15. Chan DP, Ngian KS, Cohen L. Posterior upper cervical fusion in rheumatoid arthritis. *Spine* 1992;17:268–272.

16. Santavirta S, Konttinen YT, Laasonen E, et al. Ten-year results of operations for rheumatoid cervical spine disorders. *J Bone Joint Surg Br* 1991;73:116–120.

17. Zoma A, Sturrock RD, Fisher WD, et al. Surgical stabilisation of the rheumatoid cervical spine. A review of indications and results. *J Bone Joint Surg Br* 1987;69:8–12.

18. Osteoporosis prevention, diagnosis, and therapy. *JAMA* 2001;285: 785–795.

19. Andreshak TG, An HS, Hall J, et al. Lumbar spine surgery in the obese patient. *J Spinal Disord* 1997;10:376–379.

20. Wimmer C, Gluch H, Franzreb M, et al. Predisposing factors for infection in spine surgery: a survey of 850 spinal procedures. *J Spinal Disord* 1998;11:124–128.

21. Rhoades JE, Kasinkas W. Influence of hypoproteinemia on the formation of callus in experimental fracture. *Surgery* 1942;11:38.

22. Klein JD, Hey LA, Yu CS, et al. Perioperative nutrition and postoperative complications in patients undergoing spinal surgery. *Spine* 1996;21:2676–2682.

23. Cloward RB. The anterior approach for removal of ruptured cervical disc. *J Neurosurg* 1958;15:602.

24. Grossman WC, Peppelman WC, Baum JA, et al. The use of freeze-dried fibular allograft in anterior cervical fusion. *Spine* 1992;17:565.

25. Zdeblick TA, Ducker TB. The use of freeze-dried allograft for anterior cervical fusions. *Spine* 1991;16:726.

26. Alvarez JA, Hardy RW. Anterior cervical discectomy for one- and two-level cervical disc disease: the controversy surrounding the question of whether to fuse, plate, or both. *Crit Rev Neurosurg* 1999; 28:234–251.

27. Zhang ZH, Yin H, Yang K, et al. Anterior intervertebral disc excision and bone grafting in cervical spondylotic myelopathy. *Spine* 1983; 8:16.

28. Hilibrand AS, Dina TS. The use of diagnostic imaging to assess spinal arthrodesis. *Orthop Clin North Am* 1998;29:591–601.

29. Kant AP, Daum WJ, Dean SM, et al. Evaluation of lumbar spine fusion: plain radiographs versus direct surgical exploration and observation. *Spine* 1996;20:2313–2317.

30. Brodsky AE, Kovalsky ES, Khalil MA. Correlation of radiologic assessment of lumbar spine fusions with surgical exploration. *Spine* 1991;16:S261–S265.

31. Frymoyer JW, Hanley EN, Howe J, et al. A comparison of radiographic findings in fusion and nonfusion patients ten or more years following lumbar disc surgery. *Spine* 1979;4:435–440.

32. Farey ID, McAfee PC, Davis RF, et al. Pseudarthrosis of the cervical spine after anterior arthrodesis. Treatment by posterior nerve-root decompression, stabilization, and arthrodesis. *J Bone Joint Surg Am* 1990;72:1171–1177.

33. Hilibrand AS, Yoo JU, Carlson GD, et al. The success of anterior cervical arthrodesis adjacent to a previous fusion. *Spine* 1997;22: 1574–1579.

34. Phillips FM, Carlson G, Emery SE, et al. Anterior cervical pseudarthrosis. Natural history and treatment. *Spine* 1997;22:1585–1589.

35. White AA, Southwick WO, Deponte RJ, et al. Relief of pain by anterior cervical spine fusion for spondylosis. *J Bone Joint Surg Am* 1973; 55:525–534.

36. Herzog RJ, Marcotte PJ. Assessment of spinal fusion. Critical evaluation of imaging techniques. *Spine* 1996;21:1114–1118.

37. Lang P, Genant HK, Chafetz N, et al. Three-dimensional computed tomography and multiplanar reformations in the assessment of pseudarthrosis in posterior lumbar fusion patients. *Spine* 1988;13: 69–75.

38. Lang P, Chafetz N, Genant HK, et al. Lumbar spinal fusion. Assessment of functional stability with magnetic resonance imaging. *Spine* 1990;15:581–588.

39. Coric D, Branch CL, Jenkins JD. Revision of anterior cervical pseudarthrosis with anterior allograft fusion and plating. *J Neurosurg* 1997; 86:969–974.

40. Littenberg B, Siegel A, Tosteson AN, et al. Clinical efficacy of SPECT bone imaging for low back pain. *J Nucl Med* 1995;36:1707–1713.

41. Albert TJ, Pinto M, Smith MD, et al. Accuracy of SPECT scanning in diagnosing pseudoarthrosis: a prospective study. *J Spinal Disord* 1998;11:197–199.

42. McMaster MJ, Merrick MV. The scintigraphic assessment of the scoliotic spine after fusion. *J Bone Joint Surg Br* 1980;62:65–72.

43. Lowery GL, McDonough RF. The significance of hardware failure in anterior cervical plate fixation. Patients with 2- to 7-year follow-up. *Spine* 1998;23:181–187.

44. Geck MJ, Wang JC, Delamarter RB. Anterior cervical discectomy and fusion with and without plates in 205 patients: clinical results, pseudoarthrosis rates, and adjacent segment disease. Presented at the 68th annual meeting of the American Academy of Orthopaedic Surgeons, paper No. 260, San Francisco, March 2, 2001.

45. Wang JC, McDonough PW, Endow KK, et al. Increased fusion rates with cervical plating for two-level anterior cervical discectomy and fusion. *Spine* 2000;25:41–45.

46. Epstein NE. Anterior cervical diskectomy and fusion without plate instrumentation in 178 patients. *J Spinal Disord* 2000;13:1–8.

47. Tribus CB, Corteen DP, Zdeblick TA. The efficacy of anterior cervical plating in the management of symptomatic pseudoarthrosis of the cervical spine. *Spine* 1999;24:860–864.

48. Zdeblick TA, Hughes SS, Riew KD, et al. Failed anterior cervical discectomy and arthrodesis. Analysis and treatment of thirty-five patients. *J Bone Joint Surg Am* 1997;79:523–532.

49. Caspar W, Pitzen T. Anterior cervical fusion and trapezoidal plate stabilization for re-do surgery. *Surg Neurol* 1999;52:345–352.

50. Brodsky AE, Khalil MA, Sassard WR, et al. Repair of symptomatic pseudoarthrosis of anterior cervical fusion. Posterior versus anterior repair. *Spine* 1992;17:1137–1143.

51. Lowery GL, Swank ML, McDonough RF. Surgical revision for failed anterior cervical fusions. Articular pillar plating or anterior revision? *Spine* 1995;20:2436–2441.

52. Siambanes D, Miz GS. Treatment of symptomatic anterior cervical nonunion using the Rogers interspinous wiring technique. *Am J Orthop* 1998;27:792–796.

53. Dwyer AF, Wickham GG. Direct current stimulation in spinal fusion. *Med J Aust* 1974;1:73–75.

54. Kahanovitz N. Spine update. The use of adjunctive electrical stimulation to enhance the healing of spine fusions. *Spine* 1996;21: 2523–2525.

55. Kane WJ. Direct current electrical bone growth stimulation for spinal fusion. *Spine* 1988;13:363–365.

56. Mooney V. A randomized double-blind prospective study of the efficacy of pulsed electromagnetic fields for interbody lumbar fusions. *Spine* 1990;15:708–712.

57. Goodwin CB, Brighton CT, Guyer RD, et al. A double-blind study of capacitively coupled electrical stimulation as an adjunct to lumbar spinal fusions. *Spine* 1999;24:1349–1357.

58. Helm GA, Alden TD, Sheehan JP, et al. Bone morphogenetic proteins and bone morphogenetic protein gene therapy in neurological surgery: a review. *Neurosurgery* 2000;46:1213–1222.

59. Boden SD. Biology of lumbar spine fusion and use of bone graft substitutes: present, future, and next generation. *Tissue Eng* 2000; 6:383–399.

60. Zlotolow DA, Vaccaro AR, Salamon ML, et al. The role of human bone morphogenetic proteins in spinal fusion. *J Am Acad Orthop Surg* 2000;8:3–9.

183. Lumbosacral Pseudoarthrosis and Instrumentation Failure

David W. Cahill, Fernando Vale, and Michael V. Hajjar

Traditional, uninstrumented *posterolateral* lumbar fusion procedures failed 20% to 60% of the time (1–5). The risk for failure was related to many factors, some case-specific, some patient-specific, and some universal. The advent of posterior segmental instrumentation with pedicle fixation appears to have decreased the overall failure rate of posterolateral fusions toward the lower end of the previous range (about 20%) (1–3,5–8). However, this is still not an inconsequential frequency.

The failure rate of anterior and posterior lumbar interbody fusion with threaded cages is substantial (at least 20%) when it is applied as a stand-alone procedure (9–11). The failure rate of stand-alone posterior lumbar interbody fusion (PLIF) procedures exceeds 50% under certain circumstances.

Lumbar fusion failures are most likely to occur in some of the same demographical groups that are most likely to need such surgery. Heavy laborers and smokers have a very high incidence of degenerative disc disease and spondylosis. Fusion failure rates approach 50% for smokers as a whole (12,13). Postmenopausal women with osteoporosis are prone to age-related spondylosis, stenosis, and compression fractures, any or all of which may lead to surgery. Like smokers, they have a high rate of fusion failure. Patients who have had previous lumbar operations are more likely to fail reoperative fusions (14). Patients who use nonsteroidal antiinflammatory drugs (NSAIDs) for their underlying degenerative arthritis are more likely to fail lumbar fusions (15). The groups of patients that are least likely to suffer lumbar fusion failures are the groups that are least likely to require such surgery (i.e., young, healthy nonsmokers who do not use NSAIDs or steroids, have never had a previous operation, and whose disease is limited to a single segment)!

Sadly, a finite incidence of pseudoarthrosis appears inescapable with the use of current surgical techniques. However, there are many ways in which a surgeon can minimize the risk in any given case. These include careful patient selection, preoperative and postoperative conditioning, and the appropriate use of various technical operative options of procedure and hardware. In the following pages, we attempt to describe the various factors contributing to lumbar fusion failure and suggest clinical algorithms for minimizing risk.

Biomechanical Factors Contributing to the Risk for Fusion Failure

The two most caudal lumbar motion segments (L4-5 and L5-S1) are subjected to the greatest tangential shear stresses applied to any spinal level. The normal lumbar lordosis places the disc spaces and corresponding facet joints at a variable angle, which may average 45 degrees relative to the gravitational load vector in an upright standing position. While bearing the weight of the head, neck, upper extremities, and torso, these segments remain mobile and hence are subjected to multiaxial stresses applied sagittally, coronally, axially, and longitudinally. It should come as no surprise that these levels are often the first to fail (16).

A successful fusion construct bridging the lumbosacral motion segments must resist motion in all planes, restore the weight-bearing capacity of damaged structures, and maintain or restore a nearly "normal" standing lordosis in the sagittal plane. A neutral or at least balanced coronal and axial alignment must also be established. Fusions may fail because of failure to restore weight-bearing capacity, failure to restore lordosis, or failure to restore coronal and axial balance, or because of unrelated factors discussed below.

An additional biomechanical problem arises from the junctional nature of the lumbosacral articulation. Under normal circumstances, the lumbar spine is quite mobile, especially in the sagittal plane. The sacrum, by contrast, is a fixed structure mounted rigidly between the iliac bones, forming the pelvic keystone. Consequently, any construct that crosses the lumbosacral junction is subjected to greater stress at its sacral end. Because the fulcrum of the beam lies at the lumbosacral junction, increasing the length of the construct at the lumbar end progressively increases the stresses applied across the lumbosacral junction and hence the risk for sacral-end hardware failure and pseudoarthrosis. The anatomy of the sacrum precludes caudal extension of the construct below the S2 segment; therefore, a posteriorly balanced construct is not an option. Sacral screw fracture is the most common mode of failure of cantilevered, posterior-only, pedicle screw-fixated constructs (Fig. 1).

The biomechanics of the lumbosacral region are significantly altered in several commonly encountered pathological conditions. As discs degenerate and collapse (with or without the help of surgeons), the relative load-bearing axis in the lumbosacral spine shifts posteriorly, producing additional stresses on the facet joints. In turn, degeneration and hypertrophy of the facet joints causes canal or foraminal stenosis, and they may eventually become incompetent enough that sagittal dislocation (spondylolisthesis) develops. Surgical procedures that resect hypertrophic joint elements, intersegmental ligaments (supraspinous, interspinous, flavum, facet capsules, posterior longitudinal), or disc remnants further destabilize the already damaged motion segment and hence increase the strength and rigidity requirements for any subsequently implanted hardware. Accurately judging the degree of instability preoperatively improves the surgeon's chance of choosing a successful fusion construct.

In patients with spondylolisthesis, the entire spine is shifted anteriorly on the cephalic side of the slip. The sagittal center of gravity is usually corrected by hyperlordosis of the lumbar segments above the slip. It is our practice to attempt to realign such cases by reducing the dislocation to restore sagittal balance. The hardware requirements to reduce and maintain reduction in such cases, however, are significantly greater than those for *in situ* fusion. In most cases, reduction requires radical bilateral discectomy in addition to posterior element resection. Successful reconstruction therefore requires circumferential repair. Conversely, *in situ* fusion in which the disc and posterior longitudinal ligament are left intact can usually be accomplished with a posterior-only construct.

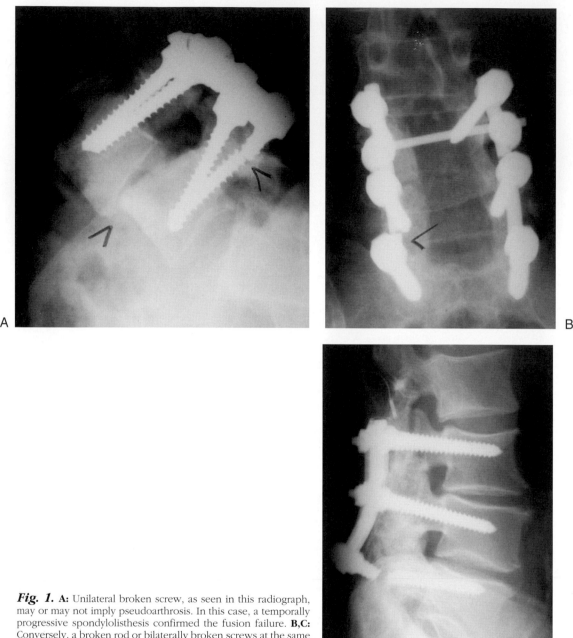

Fig. 1. A: Unilateral broken screw, as seen in this radiograph, may or may not imply pseudoarthrosis. In this case, a temporally progressive spondylolisthesis confirmed the fusion failure. **B,C:** Conversely, a broken rod or bilaterally broken screws at the same level virtually always imply a pseudoarthrosis.

Mechanisms of Failure

In the intact and healthy lumbar spine, 80% to 90% of the load is borne by the anterior and middle columns and transmitted through the discs. The remaining 10% to 20% of the load is borne by the posterior column via the facet joints. No load is normally transmitted through the transverse processes. In posterolateral lumbar fusion procedures, grafted bone is expected to cross the 2- to 4-cm gaps between transverse processes. In doing so, it bears no load. It must then form fusion masses robust enough to resist the forces applied across the lumbosacral spine 2 to 4 cm *anterior* to the center of mass. It is remarkable that *any* posterolateral lumbar fusion succeeds!

A variety of metabolic factors are well-known to increase the risk for fusion failure. It has been established both clinically

and in the laboratory that nicotine is toxic to growing bone. *Smokers* are both more likely to have degenerative disc disease and spondylosis and more likely to experience fusion failure (50% rate of pseudoarthrosis for lumbar fusions in smokers in some series) (12). Postmenopausal women and others with *osteoporosis* have a variety of spinal ailments that are best treated by fusion. Fusions in these patients often fail because of screw pullout, induced pedicle or body fracture, or the poor quality of autogenous bone graft (17). *Diabetics* and those with collagen-vascular diseases often have pseudoarthrosis secondary to infection or presumed microvascular failure, which leads to graft resorption without repair. Patients who have undergone *irradiation* to the operated area often experience fusion failure because of the same microvascular impairment (18). Steroidal drugs and more recently *NSAIDs* decrease fusion rates both in the laboratory and the clinic (15,18). A variety of *chemothera-*

peutic agents used against malignant diseases quite likely also work against growing bone (18). *Obesity* increases the stresses applied across any lumbar fusion construct and hence the risk for failure, although it is questionable whether obesity is an independent risk factor like smoking, diabetes, and *a sedentary life style.*

Obviously, some of the foregoing factors can be eliminated by the surgeon before surgery (smoking, deconditioning, NSAIDs), whereas others usually cannot (osteoporosis, diabetes). Still others can sometimes be modified to advantage (steroid use, timing of irradiation, chemotherapy schedule). The wise surgeon will decrease as many risk factors as possible both before and after the operation.

Unfortunately, the fusion failures commonly encountered today are often unrelated to any of the foregoing risk factors. Instead, the failures result from the surgeon's misunderstanding or misjudgment of the biomechanical requirements for repair of the pathology in the case at hand. Generally, many factors contribute to the failure of a given case. Poor patient selection (failure to eliminate risk factors), poor choice of hardware or fusion construct, and poor technique are the usual culprits.

Diagnosis of Lumbosacral Pseudoarthrosis

Although valid outcome studies are lacking, it has been established that fusion success shows little correlation with clinical outcome. Busy spinal surgeons see many patients with successful fusions but persistent pain, and simultaneously many others with asymptomatic pseudoarthrosis. In yet another large category are the patients whose fusion status is indeterminate. The diagnosis of pseudoarthrosis is often difficult.

In either posterior or anterior lumbar fusions, the presence of radiopaque metal hardware may either clarify or obscure the diagnosis. In cases of posterior segmental instrumentation, screw fracture or pullout, hook pullout, or wire breakage commonly signals underlying fusion failure. If both screws or both hooks at a single level have failed, pseudoarthrosis is relatively certain. Conversely, if only one of two anchors at a given level has failed, the diagnosis of underlying fusion failure is less certain. The exploration of constructs with unilaterally failed hardware often reveals solid fusion despite hardware failure.

The presence of intact posterior hardware by no means implies successful fusion. Conversely, radiopaque hardware often obscures underlying fusion bone, so that radiographic assessment of the fusion status is difficult or impossible. Posterolateral fusion masses beneath such hardware are often obscured on both plain films and computed tomography (CT). Magnetic resonance imaging (MRI) of bone is rarely beneficial.

Similarly, metal interbody devices such as threaded cages may either help or hinder the diagnosis of pseudoarthrosis. Cages that are mobile, extruded, or surrounded by a radiographic "halo" make the diagnosis of pseudoarthrosis obvious. However, cages that remain well positioned in the interbody space do not guarantee fusion. In the absence of bridging, trabecular bone surrounding such devices, fusion success cannot be radiographically established by plain films or CT. Radiolucent interbody devices make the assessment of fusion status much easier and more precise.

By plain radiography or CT, the presence of robust posterolateral bone masses also does not ensure fusion. Such masses may be discontinuous or detached from the underlying spine on exploration. The fusion status is more accurately assessed in the absence of hardware or after its removal (Fig. 2).

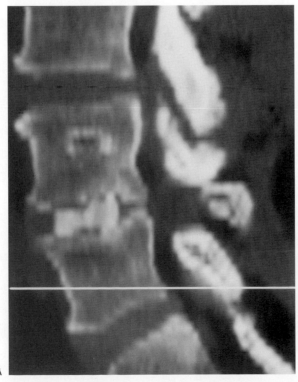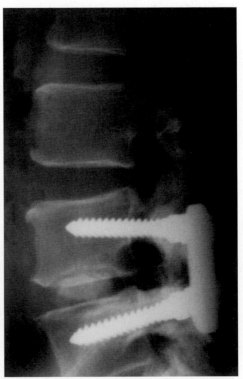

A   B

Fig. 2. **A:** Failed allograft anterior lumbar interbody fusion (ALIF). Sagittal computed tomographic (CT) reconstruction reveals halo around graft. **B:** Posterior segmental instrumentation and autograft fusion immediately after surgery. Interbody graft went on to solid fusion 1 year later.

Static radiographic assessment may suggest the diagnosis of fusion failure if an obvious change in alignment has occurred since the time of surgery. A new or progressive spondylolisthesis usually implies fusion failure. Dynamic (flexion–extension) radiographs are sometimes very helpful if movement across the operated segment is obvious. However, the absence of movement does not guarantee underlying fusion.

In patients whose symptoms persist 12 months or more after lumbar fusion surgery, we obtain static and dynamic plain films first. If the fusion status is unclear after this evaluation, MRI and CT are performed to assess soft-tissue and bony pathology, respectively. If the fusion status is still unclear, we then obtain an isotope bone scan with single photon emission computed tomography (SPECT). Although the SPECT findings are usually abnormal for the first year after a fusion procedure, they normalize once successful fusion has transpired. SPECT findings that are persistently abnormal at the site of a previous fusion at 2 years after surgery usually portend pseudoarthrosis. Unfortunately, normal SPECT findings do not ensure fusion (Fig. 3).

Most cases of fusion failure can be diagnosed by one of the means listed above; occasionally, however, thorough radiographic assessment fails to establish fusion success or failure. Surgical reexploration then becomes the only remaining option. At the time of such exploration, it is mandatory to remove all posterior hardware and excise all soft tissues and scar to expose the underlying bony spine. We use intersegmental distractors to assess either the posterior or anterior fusion status. The appearance of the dorsal surface of the fusion masses may be quite misleading, obscuring the underlying pseudoarthrosis until distractive forces are applied between the underlying vertebrae.

Management of Lumbar Pseudoarthrosis

Lumbar pseudoarthrosis repair is guided by several factors. These include the approach used in the failed procedure (anterior, posterior, circumferential), the type of instrumentation used in the failed procedure, and the type of graft material previously used (autograft iliac cancellous bone, autograft laminar fragments, allograft bone, or various commercially available allograft "matrices") (19).

The removal of unseated hooks, broken wires or cables, and extruded screws is usually straightforward and uncomplicated (Fig. 4). In the removal of a malpositioned hook or broken wire, care must be exercised to protect the underlying dural tube and exiting nerve roots. The removal of broken screws is somewhat more difficult but is greatly facilitated by the use of a variety of commercially available instruments for screw removal; these usually involve reverse-threaded sleeve saws or conical metal bits. We usually attempt to remove all remaining screw shafts, although this may be unnecessary if the involved vertebra is not to be reinstrumented.

Virtually all data available to this point suggest that allograft bone is rarely successful when used for posterolateral fusion in the lumbar spine (20). Whether newly available allograft matrices, which ostensibly include various growth factors, will be more successful remains to be demonstrated. Allograft fusion rates are clearly higher in interbody constructs, although still well below autograft fusion rates in our experience and that of others. Hence, we always attempt to use *good-quality, cancellous, iliac crest autograft* in any reoperation for fusion failure,

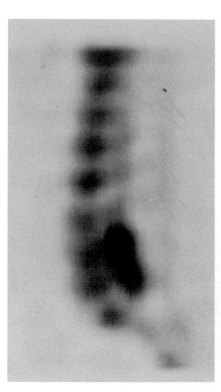

Fig. 3. Single photon emission computed tomography 2 years after failed posterolateral fusion. Hardware was intact, and no movement was seen on dynamic radiographs.

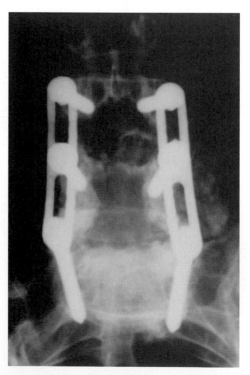

Fig. 4. Absence of posterior elements makes posterior reconstruction mandatory. In this case, the procedure was accomplished via a single posterior approach in which the failed level was salvaged with radiolucent cages to reduce the slip and provide a weight-bearing strut; this was followed by segmental instrumentation.

whether anterior or posterior. In patients whose iliac wings have been previously harvested, *"buffy coat" preparations* obtained from autologous blood via a cell saver may be useful to provide autologous growth factors to improve bone growth. No currently approved *recombinant or nonrecombinant bone morphogenetic protein preparations* are yet available, although this situation may soon change. Whether the supplementation of sparse autograft with commercially available *allograft matrix preparations* is of benefit has not been established.

With or without instrumentation, fusion failure rates are higher for posterior lumbar fusions than for interbody constructs (21). The only exception to this rule may be PLIF procedures performed with cages and without posterior segmental instrumentation. The approach to failed posterior fusions should be guided by the following considerations:

1. Spinal alignment or lack thereof
2. Canal or foraminal compromise
3. Presence or absence of previous posterior or interbody hardware
4. Disc height and integrity (previous discectomy?)
5. Presence or absence of posterior bony elements and facet joints

In the presence of previous discectomy, spontaneous disc rupture, degenerative disc collapse, or other anterior interbody pathology, reoperation and repeated posterior-only instrumentation are associated with a high risk for failure. Unless the involved discs are perfectly normal (a very rare case indeed), reoperations for lumbar pseudoarthrosis in our hands virtually always also involve an interbody fusion (Fig. 5).

In the presence of canal or foraminal compromise or malalignment (spondylolisthesis or scoliosis), a posterior or circumferential approach is usually required for repair. Broken posterior hardware or an absence of posterior elements (laminae, facets) usually also mandates a posterior or circumferential ap-

proach for repair. Conversely, in cases with near-normal alignment, no canal or foraminal compromise, *intact* posterior segmental instrumentation, and no previous interbody fusion, an anterior interbody approach with distractive cages and autograft may be associated with less morbidity and be more successful. Unfortunately, such cases are a minority of today's failures.

In the absence of cage extrusion or malalignment, *stand-alone PLIF failures* can usually be salvaged with the addition of posterior segmental instrumentation applied in compression over the existing interbody devices and supplemented with autograft bone posterolaterally (22,23). *Failed anterior lumbar interbody fusion (ALIF) procedures* in which the alignment and cage or graft position remain intact can be salvaged by the same technique. However, the most common and most difficult lumbosacral fusion failures are those in which both posterior segmental and interbody reconstruction is required because of malalignment, disc incompetence, failed interbody device, canal or foraminal compromise, previous posterior element resection or fracture, or some combination of the above factors. These cases present the greatest surgical challenge.

Once all failed posterior hardware and all scar and granulation tissue have been removed and residual fusion bone has been exposed, it is necessary to expose the normal remaining lateral masses and transverse processes. It may be necessary to remove significant amounts of unfused bone dorsal to the underlying spine to decorticate and prepare a new graft bed successfully. If the failed procedure was not instrumented, pedicle screws are placed bilaterally above and below each disc level to be fused. If the failed procedure was instrumented, new screws with a larger diameter are placed in the absence of pedicle fractures.

At this point, dissection of the spinal canal and exiting nerve roots is undertaken. Careful epidural dissection usually allows exposure of the disc spaces, which are then opened or re-

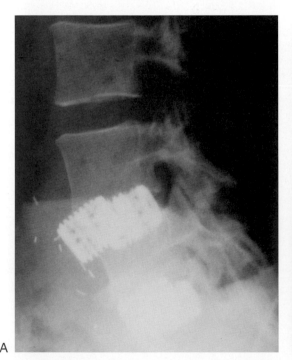
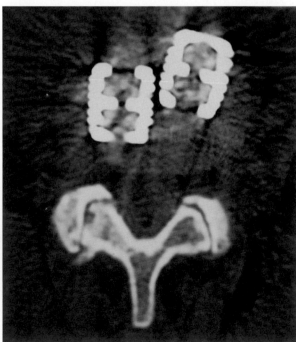

A   B

Fig. 5. Lateral radiographs (**A**) and axial CT (**B**) following two-level ALIF with cages. Extruded left L4-5 cage makes the diagnosis of fusion failure clear. (*Figure continues.*)

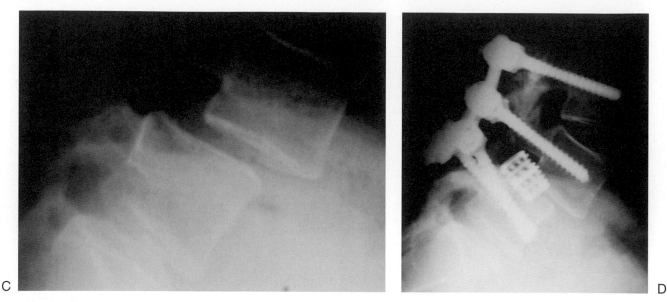

C   D

Fig. 5. (continued). Preoperative lateral radiograph (**C**) demonstrates spondylolisthesis at L4-5. Three months after surgery, lateral radiograph (**D**) demonstrates recurrent slip with dorsal cage extrusion into the canal.

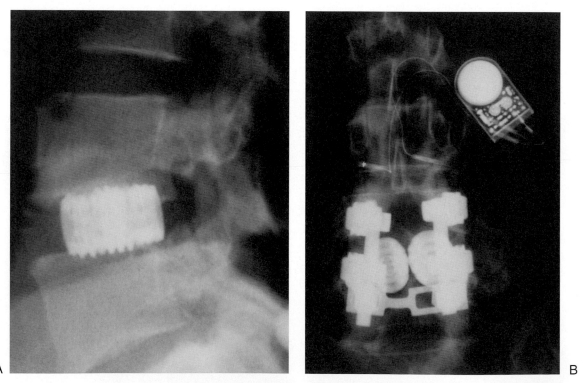

A   B

Fig. 6. **A:** Pseudoarthrosis after L4-5 ALIF with stand-alone cages. Lateral radiograph demonstrates lucency around the cages. **B:** The case was salvaged with simple posterior instrumentation and autograft fusion immediately after surgery. Interbody graft went on to solid fusion 1 year later.

opened to accomplish bilateral radical discectomy. If necessary, malpositioned PLIF devices are removed, and sagittal plane malalignment is corrected by interbody or pedicular distraction if possible. If alignment can be reduced to grade 0 or grade 1 status, PLIF is accomplished with either transverse or longitudinal cages and autograft. This is followed by posterior segmental instrumentation in lordotic compression and posterolateral autografting.

If the disc spaces cannot be safely accessed posteriorly because of extreme scarring, if previously placed PLIF devices cannot be safely removed, or if sagittal plane malalignment cannot be reduced to a grade 0 or 1 status, then dissection is discontinued. The wound is temporarily closed, and the patient is rotated into the supine position. Anterior dissection then allows discectomy, removal of failed interbody devices, realignment if necessary, and ALIF with distractive cages and autograft. The patient is then returned to the prone position for completion of the posterior segmental instrumentation and grafting.

An accumulating body of class II and III data suggest that *electronic bone growth stimulators* may improve fusion success rates in patients who are undergoing reoperation or have other significant risk factors (24,25) (Fig. 6). Experience in our institution during the past 5 years supports those data. Such devices are available as implantable systems or as externally worn belts or corsets. The preponderance of published data favors implantable systems. The advantage of implantable devices is that patient compliance is not an issue; the disadvantage is that the batteries must usually be removed (under a local anesthetic) after 6 to 12 months. Costs are similar. We currently implant electronic bone growth stimulators in all patients undergoing reoperation for failed lumbar fusion.

Conclusions

The availability of interbody cages and pedicle screw instrumentation has greatly improved the surgeon's ability to repair failed lumbar fusions. Ironically, the use of such cages as standalone devices in the face of significant collateral instability has greatly increased the number of failed lumbar fusions in need of repair. It is likely that a more biomechanically informed approach to lumbar fusion surgery, coupled with new advances in bone growth factor research, materials science, and osteoporosis prevention, will decrease the need for reoperative surgery in the future.

References

1. Lorenz M, Zindrick M, Schwargler P, et al. A comparison of single-level fusion with and without hardware. *Spine* 1991;16(8 suppl): S455–S458.
2. Bernhardt M, Swartz DE, Clothiaux PL, et al. Posterolateral lumbar and lumbosacral fusion with and without pedicle screw internal fixation. *Clin Orthop* 1992;284:109–115.
3. Grubb SA, Lipscomb HJ. Results of lumbosacral fusion for degenerative disc disease with and without instrumentation. Two- to five-year follow-up. *Spine* 1992;17:349–355.
4. Axelsson P, Johnson R, Stromquist B, et al. Posterolateral lumbar fusion. Outcome of 71 consecutive operations after 4 (2–7) years. *Acta Orthop Scand* 1994;65:309–314.
5. Schwab FJ, Nazarian DG, Mahmud F, et al. Effects of spinal instrumentation on fusion of the lumbosacral spine. *Spine* 1995;20: 2023–2028.
6. Temple HT, Kruse RW, van Dam BE. Lumbar and lumbosacral fusion using Steffee instrumentation. *Spine* 1994;19:537–541.
7. Ricciandi JE, Pfwrger PC, Isaza JE, et al. Transpedicular fixation for the treatment of isthmic spondylolisthesis in adults. *Spine* 1995;20: 1917–1922.
8. Wood GW II, Boyd RJ, Carothers TA, et al. The effect of pedicle screw/plate fixation on lumbar/lumbosacral autogenous bone graft fusions in patients with degenerative disc disease. *Spine* 1995;20: 819–830.
9. Agassi S, Reierdin A, May D. Posterior lumbar interbody fusion with cages: an independent review of 71 cases. *J Neurosurg* 1999;91(2 suppl):186–192.
10. Ray CD. Threaded titanium cages for lumbar interbody fusions. *Spine* 1997;22:667–679.
11. Greenough CG, Taylor LJ, Fraser RD. Anterior lumbar fusion results, assessment techniques and prognostic factors. *Eur Spine J* 1994;3: 225–230.
12. Brown CW, Orme TJ, Richardson HD. The rate of pseudoarthrosis (surgical nonunion) in patients who are smokers and patients who are nonsmokers: a comparison study. *Spine* 1986;11:942–943.
13. Jenkins LT, Jones AL, Harms JJ. Prognostic factors in lumbar spinal fusion. *Contemp Orthop* 1994;29:173–180.
14. Laverman WC, Bradford DS, Ogilvie JW, et al. Results of lumbar pseudoarthrosis repair. *J Spinal Disord* 1992;5:149–157.
15. Dimar JR, Ante WA, Zhang YP, et al. The effects of nonsteroidal anti-inflammatory drugs on posterior spinal fusions in the rat. *Spine* 1996;21:1870–1876.
16. Traynelis VC, Goel VK, Gillaertson LG. Biomechanics of the thoracolumbar spine. In: Menezes AH, Sonntag VK, eds. *Principles of spinal surgery*. New York: McGraw-Hill, 1996:85–108.
17. Vardiman AB, Morgan HW, D'Alise MD. Nonunion. In: Benzel EC, ed. *Spine surgery*. New York: Churchill Livingstone, 1999: 1475–1485.
18. Dickman CA, Maric Z. The biology of bone healing and techniques of spinal fusion. *BNI Quarterly* 1994;10:2–8.
19. Albert TJ, Pinto M, Denis F. Management of symptomatic lumbar pseudoarthrosis with anteroposterior fusion. A functional and radiographic outcome study. *Spine* 2000;25:123–130.
20. Cook SD, Dalton JE, Prewette AB, et al. *In vivo* evaluation of demineralized bone matrix as a bone graft substitute for posterior spinal fusion. *Spine* 1995;20:877–886.
21. Suk SE, Lee CK, Kim WJ, et al. Adding posterior lumbar interbody fusion to pedicle screw fixation and posterolateral fusion after decompression in spondylolytic spondylolisthesis. *Spine* 1997;22: 210–219.
22. McAfee PC, Cunningham BW, Lee GA, et al. Revision strategies for salvaging or improving failed cylindrical cages. *Spine* 1999;24: 2147–2153.
23. Enker P, Steffee AD. Interbody fusion and instrumentation. *Clin Orthop* 1994;300:90–101.
24. Simmons JW. Treatment of failed posterior lumbar interbody fusion on the spine with pulsing electromagnetic fields. *Clin Orthop* 1985; 193:127–132.
25. Kane WI. Direct current electrical bone growth stimulation for spinal fusion. *Spine* 1988;13:363–365.

184. Revision Strategies for Interbody Spinal Surgery: A Revision Algorithm

Stephen E. Heim, J. J. Abitbol,
Kevin T. Foley, Reginald Knight,
Hallett Mathews, Stephen L. Ondra,
Chester Sutterlin, and
Thomas Zdeblick

The recent evolution of threaded interbody fusion cages has presented a significant new form of segmental fixation (interbody fixation devices) for application to the lumbar and lumbosacral spine. These interbody constructs are metallic (titanium alloy) or femoral allograft designs at this time. They serve as carriers for autogenous graft material while restoring segmental stability to the involved motion segment.

The biomechanics of these devices greatly surpass those of the interbody spacers used historically (e.g., femoral ring composite grafts, tricortical wedges, and various "containment devices" for cancellous bone), which have not offered significant stability in flexion/extension or torsion. In fact, a number of biomechanical studies have shown this recent class of construct to compare quite favorably with the segmental pedicular fixation/posterior lumbar interbody fusion (PLIF) constructs (1–3). The interbody spacers historically have been utilized as a component of an overall construct employing segmental posterior instrumentation. On the other hand, when applied effectively, the threaded interbody cages confer a degree of stability to the diseased motion segment so as to function as stand-alone constructs. The biomechanics of the interbody cage constructs,

in general, is based on a significantly narrowed preoperative disc space. The act of reconstituting the anterior column height restores the annular tension—a key factor in the proper construct mechanics (Fig. 1). It is in such an application that the favorable comparison to pedicular fixation/PLIF constructs is obtained.

Inappropriate size and/or placement of the threaded interbody constructs may result in poor tensioning of the annulus fibrosis and may not result in a biomechanically stable motion segment as a stand-alone construct. In these instances, supplemental stabilization techniques may be required. In fact, as was separately reported by McAfee et al. (4) and ourselves (5), this failure to obtain adequate distraction of the annulus fibrosis has been among the most common reasons for failure of the procedure. This has been particularly evident in cages inserted via the PLIF approach. Also, the use of local bone (e.g., from a laminectomy) rather than cancellous iliac autograft has consistently been associated with failure of the procedure.

Complications may arise intraoperatively from the process of surgical approach and application of the interbody cages, as well as postoperatively with infection, loss of fixation, or pseud-

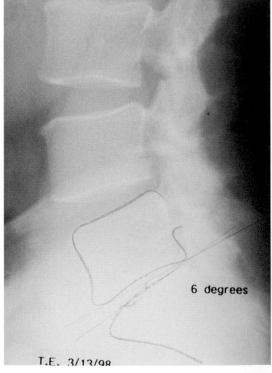
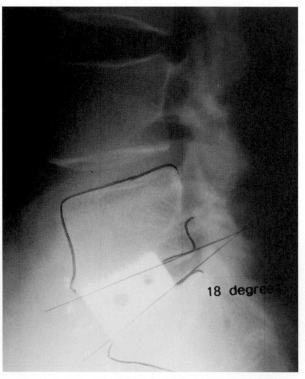

6 degrees

18 degrees

A T.E. 3/13/98

B

Fig. 1. **A**: Markedly narrowed preoperative disc space. **B**: Anterior column height and annular tension restored by interbody fixation device.

arthrosis. Preoperative planning and patient selection remain critically important in reducing these risks. In terms of preoperative planning, great care must be exercised in the process of templating the cage size and placement. Selection of the appropriate cage size requires templating off of the adjacent normal height disc space. Once the appropriate cage length and diameter have been determined in this manner, the placement of the bilateral cages within the disc space is templated on both the anteroposterior and the lateral radiographs. Axial computed tomography (CT) or magnetic resonance imaging (MRI) can also be of use in this process. It is at this point that cage fit problems should be apparent or at least anticipated. The most common problem seen involves undersized cages in height (sagittal component). This prevents adequate tension by the annular fibers and results in loss of fixation and high rates of pseudarthrosis. Equally problematic is insufficient consideration of the axial diameter needed to accommodate the cage height (diameter × 2 + interval between cages). This may result in total cage width exceeding the end-plate width. Cages can then crack out laterally and/or impinge on a nerve root exiting the foramen. The popularity of these devices demands consideration of the problems and revisions that are needed.

The algorithms in Tables 1 through 8 resulted from the overall experience of the authors. They represent the authors' collective experience in addressing potential complications with interbody constructs.

References

1. Brodke DS, Dick JC, Zdeblick TA, et al. Biomechanical comparison of posterior lumbar interbody fusion including a new threaded titanium cage. Presented at the annual meeting of the North American Spine Society, San Diego, 1993.
2. Sutterlin CE, Bianchi JR, Reilly T, et al. *Threaded cortical dowel construct stiffness testing.* Technical monograph, University of Florida Tissue Bank, 1997.
3. Zdeblick TA, Warden KE, Zou D, et al. Anterior spine fixators. A biomechanical in vitro study. *Spine* 18(4):513–517, 1993.
4. Heim S, Abitbol JJ, Foley K, et al. *Revision strategies for interbody spinal surgery: a revision algorithm* (monograph). 1988.
5. McAfee P, Cunningham B, Fedder I. Revision strategies for salvaging or improving failed cylindrical cages. Proceedings of the North American Spine Society, San Francisco, 1998.

Table 1. Undersized Threaded Interbody Construct

I. Avoidance
  A. Patient selection
    1. Significant disc space narrowing
    2. Restore anterior column height: preoperative templating off of adjacent manual disc height to select appropriate TIC length and diameter
    3. Planned surgical approach: ability to place the appropriate templated TIC safely
      Anterior approach: mobilization of vascular structures
      Posterior approach: risk of neurological/dural injury, risk of further motion segment destabilization by the extent of bone resection for cage insertion
  B. Disc space distraction to the point that the annulus fibrosis is tensioned; verify that the final distraction plug size remains appropriate for the TIC size to be inserted
  C. Intraoperative fluoroscopic monitoring: used not only for the determination of the appropriate TIC orientation, but also for demonstration of the correct amount of end-plate engagement by each TIC
  D. If the disc space distracts further than templated, make an adjustment to the next TIC size; ensure that the TIC placement and the end-plate engagement is satisfactory prior to completing procedure

(Table continues)

REVISING AN UNDERSIZED THREADED INTERBODY CONSTRUCT

TIC Position Satisfactory
- Bilateral Posterolateral Grafting with segmental instrumentation
- Monitor TIC position radiographically with the routine (2 week, 3-6-12-24 month) follow-up of the posterolateral graft and instrumentation
  - TIC Migration
    - Remove
  - No Migration

TIC Unsatisfactory

- **Anterior Prominence (Vascular Impingement)**
  - Revision (Anterior Approach)
    - Metallic Cage
      - Remove Impinging Cage
    - Threaded Cortical Bone Dowel
      - Remove Impinging Threaded Cortical Bone Dowel (Consider re-contouring only if exposure is prohibitive)
    - If space permits, replace with appropriate larger cage
    - Check contralateral cage—if spatially feasible within the volume of the disc space, also revise with appropriate larger cage
    - Consider Supplemental Segmental Fixation pending assessment of construct stability

- **Posterior Prominence (Symptomatic)**
  - Revision (Posterior Approach)
    - Metallic Cage
    - Threaded Cortical Bone Dowel
      - If only a portion of a single allograft cortex is prominent, consider partial excision rather than complete removal, otherwise remove Symptomatic TIC
    - Remove Symptomatic TIC
    - If space permits, replace with appropriate larger TIC
    - Check contralateral (asymptomatic) TIC position (see TIC Position Satisfactory)
    - Add Supplementary Segmental Posterior Fixation with Bilateral Posterolateral Grafting

- **Lateral Prominence (Symptomatic)**
  - Revision (Posterior-less commonly a lateral approach)
    - Metallic Cage
    - Threaded Cortical Bone Dowel
      - If less than an entire allograft cortex is prominent, consider partial excision rather than complete removal. Otherwise, go to next box
    - Remove Symptomatic TIC
    - If space permits, replace with appropriate larger TIC—in proper position within the disc space
    - Check contralateral (asymptomatic) TIC (see TIC Position Satisfactory)
    - Add Supplementary Segmental Posterior Fixation & Bilateral Posterolateral Grafting

*TIC = Threaded Interbody Construct

Table 2. Single Midline Threaded Interbody Construct

1. Avoidance
   A. Patient positioning
      1. Ensure neutral rotation and ability to visualize the posterior vertebral cortices of the involved motion segment—anteroposterior (AP)/lateral fluoroscopy
      2. Verify that the patient position remains neutral at conclusion of the exposure of the involved disc space
   B. Exposure
      1. Must have a true sagittal plane of exposure for proper working cannula alignment
      2. Mobilize the vascular structures to allow a clearly visible margin of annulus fibrosis to be present medial and lateral to the working cannula (right and left discal entry sites)
      3. Avoid extraneous cautery marks on the annulus fibrosis—there should be only a midline and the right and left discal entry sites present
      4. At each step, visualize all three annular cautery marks prior to proceeding with that step
      5. Repeat AP fluoroscopy if any question is present regarding the location of the midline or right and left discal entry sites
II. Biomechanics of a single midline TIC
   A. Graph (Fig. 2): A single vs. bilateral threaded interbody construct placement in flexion/extension and right/left side bending
III. Issues relating to a single midline TIC
   A. Suboptimal biomechanics
   B. Limited surface area of end-plate engagement
   C. Usually unable to fit a second TIC adjacent to the midline implant
   D. The degree of end-plate reaming in the midline can severely compromise the medial support of TIC if repositioned to the right and left potentially discal entry sites
   E. If a second TIC is fit adjacent to the midline TIC, particular attention must be paid to TIC length, angle, and fixation

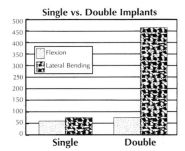

SINGLE MIDLINE THREADED INTERBODY CONSTRUCT

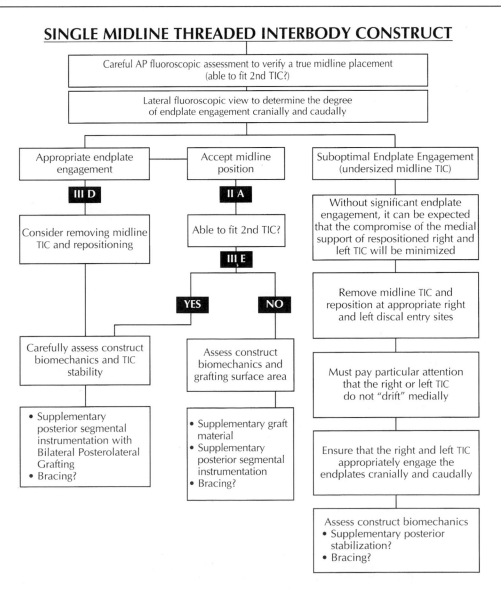

Table 3. Lateral Threaded Interbody Construct Placement with Neurological Deficit

I. Avoidance
  A. Patient positioning
    1. Ensure neutral rotation and ability to visualize the posterior vertebral body cortices of the involved motion segment—AP/lateral fluoroscopy
    2. Verify that patient position remains neutral throughout the procedure
  B. Exposure
    1. Must have a true neutral plane of exposure for proper working cannula alignment
    2. Mobilize the vascular structures to allow a clearly visible margin of the annulus fibrosis medial and lateral to the working cannula at each discal entry site
    3. Avoid extraneous cautery marks on the annulus fibrosis—there should be only a midline, right, and left discal entry site visible
    4. At each step, visualize all three annular cautery marks prior to proceeding with that step
    5. Repeat AP fluoroscopy if any question is present regarding the location of the midline or right/left discal entry sites
II. Address early
  A. Revise prior to fusion occurring to minimize bony destruction during revision
  B. Reposition TIC
    Relocate to proper position
    Larger diameter TIC without additional distraction
    Carefully assess TIC purchase and construct stability
  C. Adjust TIC depth or length
    Consider switching to a shorter cylindrical TIC
  D. TIC removal
    Supplementary graft (structural or nonstructural) to restore surface area contact
    Supplementary fixation—anteriorly or posteriorly depending on spinal level
III. TIC
  A. TIC composition opens the opportunity to remodel/recontour a prominent margin of the TIC
  B. Upon remodeling/recontouring the TIC, construct biomechanics must be carefully considered (the amount of remodeling or recontouring, i.e., bone removal, is to be considered)

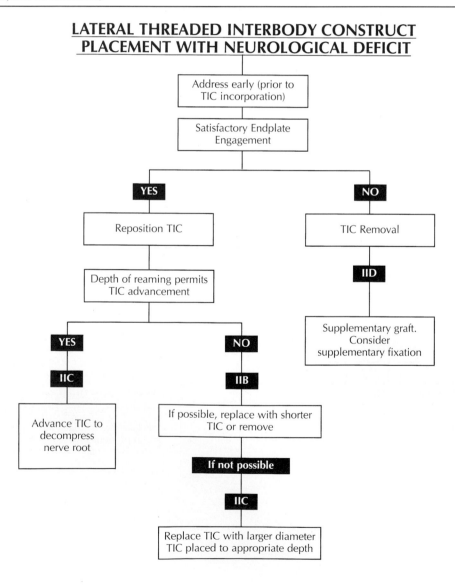

LATERAL THREADED INTERBODY CONSTRUCT PLACEMENT WITH NEUROLOGICAL DEFICIT

Table 4. Lateral Threaded Interbody Construct Placement with Nerve Root Irritation (Minimal or No Deficit)

I. Avoidance
    A. Patient positioning
        1. Ensure neutral rotation and ability to visualize the posterior vertebral body cortices of the involved motion segment—AP/lateral fluoroscopy
        2. Verify that patient position remains neutral throughout the procedure
    B. Exposure
        1. Must have a true neutral plane of exposure for proper working cannula alignment
        2. Mobilize the vascular structures to allow a clearly visible margin of the annulus fibrosis medial and lateral to the working cannula at each discal entry site
        3. Avoid extraneous cautery marks on the annulus fibrosis—there should be only a midline, right, and left discal entry site visible
        4. At each step, visualize all three annular cautery marks prior to proceeding with that step
        5. Repeat AP fluoroscopy if any question is present regarding the location of the midline or right/left discal entry sites
II. Quality of fixation
    A. Satisfactory: permits monitoring of neural symptoms
    B. Unsatisfactory:
        Revise early—prior to TIC incorporation
        Suboptimal fixation risks later TIC migration; progressive motion segment subluxation and compromises potential incorporation success

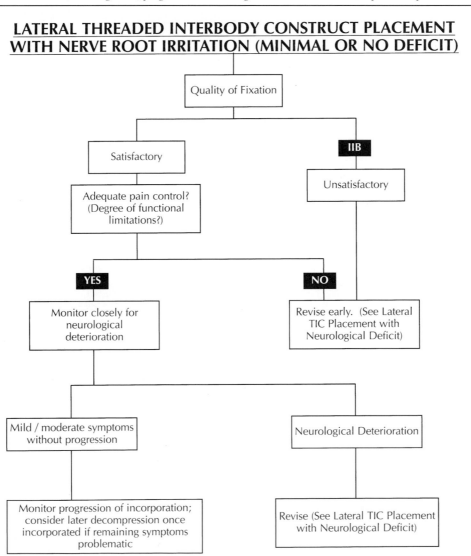

LATERAL THREADED INTERBODY CONSTRUCT PLACEMENT WITH NERVE ROOT IRRITATION (MINIMAL OR NO DEFICIT)

Table 5. Anteriorly Prominent Threaded Interbody Construct

I. Avoidance
  A. Patient positioning
    1. Ensure neutral rotation and ability to visualize the posterior vertebral body cortices of the involved motion segment—AP/lateral fluoroscopy
    2. Verify that patient position remains neutral throughout the procedure
  B. Exposure
    1. Must have a true neutral plane of exposure for proper working cannula alignment
    2. Mobilize the vascular structures to allow a clearly visible margin of the annulus fibrosis medial and lateral to the working cannula at each discal entry site
    3. Avoid extraneous cautery marks on the annulus fibrosis—there should be only a midline, right, and left discal entry site visible
    4. At each step, visualize all three annular cautery marks prior to proceeding with that step
    5. Repeat AP fluoroscopy if any question is present regarding the location of the midline or right/left discal entry sites
II. Assess the degree of prominence
  A. If there is any question of vascular impingement, correct implant position at the time of surgery
      Metallic cage: either adjust depth of insertion (avoid stripping cage) or replace with a shorter cage
      Threaded cortical bone dowel: adjust depth of insertion (avoid stripping); replace with shorter threaded cortical bone dowel or remodel/recontour TIC (consider TIC biomechanics)

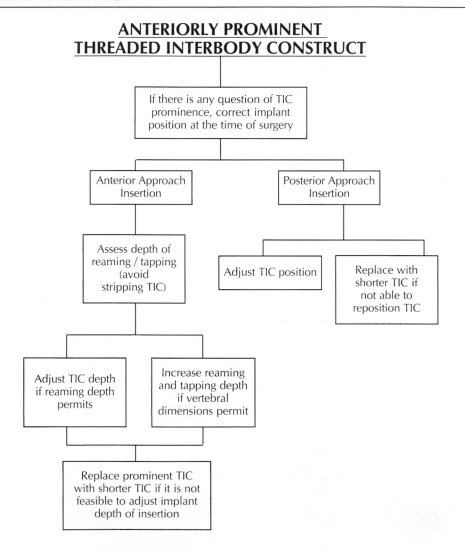

ANTERIORLY PROMINENT THREADED INTERBODY CONSTRUCT

If there is any question of TIC prominence, correct implant position at the time of surgery

Anterior Approach Insertion

Posterior Approach Insertion

Assess depth of reaming / tapping (avoid stripping TIC)

Adjust TIC position

Replace with shorter TIC if not able to reposition TIC

Adjust TIC depth if reaming depth permits

Increase reaming and tapping depth if vertebral dimensions permit

Replace prominent TIC with shorter TIC if it is not feasible to adjust implant depth of insertion

Table 6. Posteriorly Prominent Threaded Interbody Construct

I. Avoidance
  A. Careful accurate preoperative templating
  B. Intraoperative fluoroscopic visualization and careful assessment of images
      Must be certain that the patient positioning permits visualization of the posterior vertebral body prior to starting the procedure
  C. Do not conclude procedure until implant position is certain and well demonstrated on AP and lateral images
II. Posteriorly prominent TIC
  A. Symptomatic neural deficit
    1. Treat early
    2. Fixation quality appropriate
       Reposition TIC
    3. Fixation quality inadequate
       Remove TIC
       Consider replacement with appropriate large diameter TIC
       Replace with additional bone graft (structural vs. nonstructural) and supplementary fixation
  B. Asymptomatic
    1. Fixation quality appropriate
       Monitor TIC position and incorporation closely
       If further TIC migration occurs (without symptomatology) add supplementary fixation
    2. Fixation quality inadequate
       Revise early
       Consider replacement with appropriate larger diameter TIC
       TIC removal and replacement with additional graft material (structural vs. nonstructural) and supplementary fixation

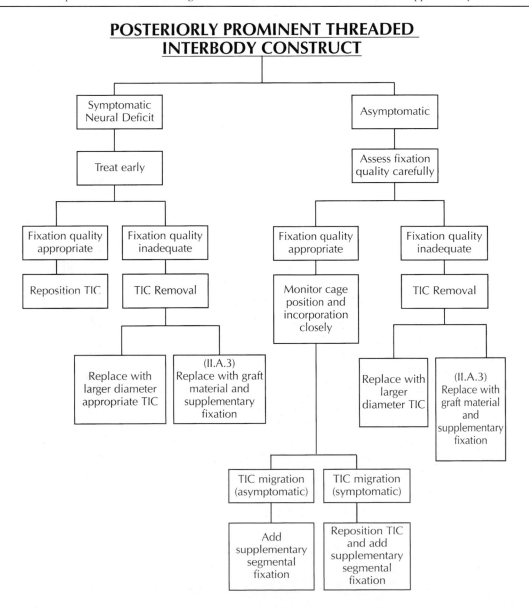

POSTERIORLY PROMINENT THREADED
INTERBODY CONSTRUCT

Table 7. Stripped Threaded Interbody Construct

I. Avoidance
  A. Careful preoperative planning/templating
    Implant length
    Depth of reaming and tapping
  B. Patient positioning to ensure the ability to visualize the posterior vertebral cortices of the involved motion segment on lateral fluoroscopy
  C. Intraoperative fluoroscopic monitoring
    Depth of reaming/tapping (save images of final reaming/tapping depth)
    Assessment of implant depth compared to the saved final reaming/tapping depth images
  D. Attention to changes in the torque of insertion during TIC placement
II. Stripped cylindrical TIC
  A. Replace with a larger TIC
  B. Do not distract further
    Further distraction would loosen the contralateral TIC
    Save fluoroscopic image of the reaming/tapping depth and compare to position of the advancing TIC

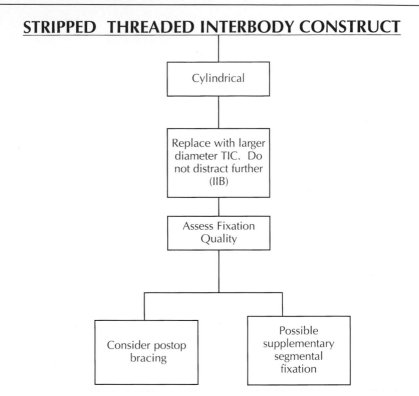

STRIPPED THREADED INTERBODY CONSTRUCT

Table 8. Pseudarthrosis

I. Diagnosis
  A. Mechanical symptomatology/examination
  B. Plain radiographs
    1. End-plate engagement
    2. Implant migration
      a. Safe—no neurological or visceral/vascular impingement
      b. At risk—see relevant scenario
    3. Resorption
      a. Degree of bony destruction?
      b. Revisability?
  C. Flexion/extension radiographs
    1. Demonstrable motion
    2. Demonstrable translation of implants?
  D. Bony union
    1. Thin-slice computed tomography (CT) (1.0-mm sections) with sagittal and coronal reconstruction
II. Implant position
  A. Acceptable
    1. Revision with segmental posterior instrumentation/posterolateral graft
    2. Monitor TIC position through follow-up radiographs for the incorporation of the bilateral posterolateral grafts
  B. Unacceptable—see revision scenario
    1. Revision with segmental posterior instrumentation and posterolateral graft
    2. Monitor TIC position through follow-up radiographs for the incorporation of the bilateral posterolateral grafts

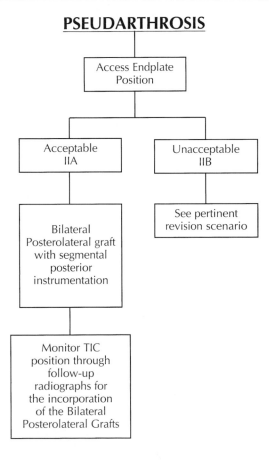

185. Atlantoaxial Rotational Subluxation

**Erol Veznedaroglu and
Leslie N. Sutton**

Atlantoaxial rotation was first described in 1907 by Corner (1) and has since remained shrouded in controversy and confusion. Contributing to the confusion are the numerous terms applied to the condition, including *rotatory subluxation, rotatory dislocation,* and *rotatory fixation of the atlantoaxial joint.* Atlantoaxial rotational subluxation (AARS) usually affects children and follows minor trauma or an infection of the nasopharynx. Adult cases generally develop after more severe trauma (2). In addition, numerous systemic diseases have been implicated. Ligamental laxity in patients with Down syndrome is associated with a relatively high incidence of vertebral anomalies. Approximately 20% of patients with Down syndrome have atlantoaxial instability (3). Even minor trauma should alert the clinician to the development of associated complications in this group of patients. Patients who undergo surgery of the head and neck are also at increased risk for torticollis. Whether this is a consequence of positioning, inflammation of the ligaments, or a combination thereof is unclear. In addition, a multitude of rare entities may present as torticollis, including fibrodysplasia ossificans progressiva, juvenile fibromatosis, Morquio syndrome, juvenile rheumatoid arthritis, calcified discitis, and tumors affecting the bone and spinal cord (4).

Fielding and Hawkins (5) distinguished rotatory subluxation from fixation and categorized four types based on their series of 17 cases of irreducible atlantoaxial fixation. Recently, new insight has been gained into the pathophysiology and causes of this enigmatic disease. The advent of modern imaging techniques has made it possible to develop new diagnostic criteria, and valuable information has been acquired related to diagnosis, treatment, and prognosis.

Anatomy

To understand the pathophysiology and mechanical basis of rotational subluxation, it is imperative to understand the anatomy of the occipitoatlantoaxial complex. White and Panjabi offer an excellent biomechanical analysis of this complex (6, 7). Four planes of motion are possible in the occipital-C1-2 (OC1-2) complex: flexion, extension, rotation, and lateral bending. The occipitoatlantal complex allows flexion and extension, with the atlantoaxial joint responsible for most of the rotation. Synovial joints facilitate the necessary movements of the OC1-2 complex, in which intervertebral discs would be restrictive.

The atlas (C1) articulates with the occipital condyles via a concave surface on the C1 lateral masses. These joints form a so-called roller-in-groove joint, suitable for flexion and extension. The horizontally aligned facets of the atlantoaxial articulation are another unique anatomical feature, allowing free rotation without bony obstruction. The ligamentous structures also are vital to the stability of this region and are involved in the pathology (Fig. 1). The most important and strongest of these is the transverse ligament. The horizontal component of the cruciate ligament, it adheres to the anteromedial aspect of the lateral masses of the atlas and wraps around the posterior surface of the dens. The dens is separated anteriorly from the C1

ring and posteriorly from the transverse ligament by synovial bursae. The transverse ligament also serves to inhibit anterior translation of C1 on C2. Other ligaments that are key to the occipitoatlantoaxial complex are the tectorial membrane, paired alar ligaments, cruciate ligament, and apical dental ligament. The tectorial membrane is a direct continuation of the posterior longitudinal ligament. It attaches the body of C2 to the clivus, inhibiting flexion of the basion beyond the tip of the dens and extensive extension. The paired alar ligaments, which bind the lateral masses of the atlas to the dens, inhibit lateral bending and excessive rotation; excessive rotation in one direction is inhibited by the contralateral alar ligament (8). The rotation of C0-1 is very limited, with a mean of 4 degrees noted (range, 0 to 8 degrees) (9). Werne (10) has shown that sectioning of these ligaments results in complete occipitoaxial dislocation.

C2 remains stationary during rotation of C1 on C2 of up to 20 degrees; after C1 rotates more than 20 degrees, C2 begins to rotate in the same direction. This is anatomically explained by the force of the alar ligaments pulling on the dens. However, an angular separation between C1 and C2 is always present, up to a maximum of 47 degrees (6,7). This is instrumental in both pathophysiology and diagnosis.

Pathophysiology

The pathophysiology of AARS is varied and may be traumatic, postinfectious/surgical (Grisel syndrome), secondary to other predisposing diseases (Down syndrome, Morquio syndrome, collagen-vascular disease, Chiari malformation, brainstem tu-

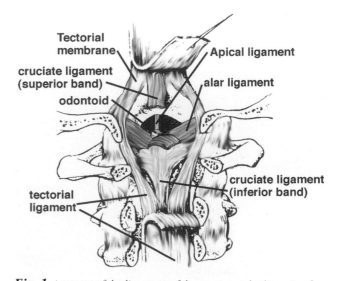

Fig. 1. Anatomy of the ligaments of the craniovertebral junction from a posterior view. The tectorial membrane has been divided.

mors), or idiopathic. A definite tendency of AARS to affect children has been noted, and congenital forms of childhood torticollis are common. Congenital muscular torticollis is usually seen by 10 days of age and is associated with a characteristic rubbery mass in the sternocleidomastoid. This usually resolves with muscle-stretching exercises (4). Grisel syndrome is a nontraumatic subluxation of the atlantoaxial joint that develops following an infection in the head and neck region. First described by Sir Charles Bell in 1830, it bears the name of the French physician Grisel, who reported two cases 100 years later (11). The condition has been described following tonsillectomy, surgery of the mastoid and nasopharynx, repair of choanal atresia, ventriculojugular shunt, and cleft palate repair; it also arises spontaneously (2,4,5,11). Grisel syndrome primarily affects children, although adult cases have been reported (12). It is believed that Grisel syndrome is caused by ligamentous instability following an inflammatory process (11). Parke and colleagues (13) have provided a convincing anatomical rationale for this theory. The authors describe lymphovenous anastomoses that appear to drain the posterosuperior pharyngeal region, creating a conduit for spread to the ligaments of the atlantoaxial complex. The anatomical differences between the pediatric and adult cervical spine also help to explain why the incidence is higher in children. In the study of Sullivan et al. (12), 77% of cases were in children less than 13 years of age; these authors demonstrated how the facet joints in the high cervical region are more horizontally oriented in children than in adults (12). In a cadaveric study, Kawabe et al. (14) also found a steeper incline of the lateral mass of C2 in children than in adults. Interestingly, this group found folds in the upper cervical joints of all the cadaveric children, whereas no such folds were found in the cadavers of persons more than 62 years of age. They indicated that the folds appear to atrophy with age and may pose an anatomical substrate for locking of the C1-2 joints.

Clinical Diagnosis

As discussed, the incidence of atlantoaxial dislocation is higher in children. Furthermore, the incidence of fracture in children under the age of 13 seems to be lower, whereas fracture, particularly of the dens, appears to be more common in children over 13 years of age (15). Regardless, a correct diagnosis and prompt treatment are vital to prevent neurological injury and deformity. The classical presentation of rotatory fixation is the "cock robin" position, lateral flexion with rotation to the opposite side (likened to a robin listening for a worm), with the shoulder on the chin side elevated and that side of the face flattened (Fig. 2). Patients are usually neurologically intact, although some may have occipital pain caused by irritation of the greater occipital nerve, which emerges between C1 and C2. The goal in AARS is to distinguish a torticollis of muscular origin from that of a fixed subluxation. Clinically, a compensatory counterrotation of the axis in a nonvoluntary, reflex attempt to return the head and visual axis back to midline in AARS is known as the *Sudek sign* (16). In contradistinction, the spinous process of the axis is turned in the direction of the rotation in muscular torticollis. Another useful diagnostic clue is found by examining the sternocleidomastoid muscle. In muscular torticollis, the shortened sternocleidomastoid is in spasm, whereas in torticollis secondary to rotatory subluxation, the lengthened sternocleidomastoid (chin side) is in spasm as if to correct the strain (2,5). It must be emphasized that although the clinical examination is helpful in the diagnosis, dynamic computed tomography (CT) of the OC1-2 complex, discussed in the following section, is essential in diagnosis.

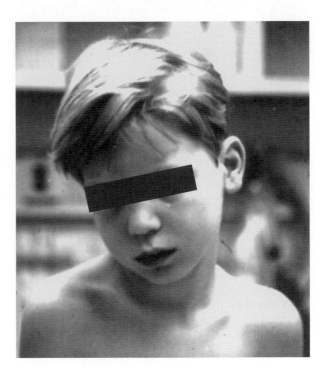

Fig. 2. The typical "cock robin" position of a child with a rotatory subluxation. The head is rotated, flexed, and laterally deviated.

Fielding and Hawkins (5) categorized four types of atlantoaxial rotation and fixation:

Type I. Rotatory fixation with anterior displacement of 3 mm or less. This is the most common form; the ligaments are intact. The dens acts as a pivot, and rotation is within normal physiological range. Treatment is expectant with nonsteroidal antiinflammatory drugs (NSAIDs) and a cervical collar; traction is rarely needed.

Type II. Rotatory fixation with anterior displacement of 3 to 5 mm. This is the second most common form, with disruption of the transverse ligament. One lateral mass of the atlas is anteriorly displaced while the opposite acts as a pivot. Treatment is expectant, with traction in a halter often required.

Type III. Rotatory fixation with anterior displacement of more than 5 mm. It is associated with deficiency of both the transverse and secondary ligaments. Both lateral masses are displaced. Treatment is with traction and surgery for those in whom realignment is not achieved.

Type IV. Rotatory fixation with posterior displacement. This type is rare and usually associated with severe trauma or preexisting disease.

The inciting trauma is typically minor (17), and although fatalities have been documented, they are extremely rare (1,18).

Radiographic Diagnosis

The diagnosis of rotatory subluxation and fixation has evolved gradually. Until the advent of CT, plain films were often misleading and difficult to interpret in the absence of clear pathology. Although the evaluation of all cases of torticollis or suspected C1-2 instability should begin with a series of plain films, including anteroposterior (AP), lateral, and open-mouth views,

an abnormal C1-2 relationship or other pathology is detected only with dynamic CT. Although Fielding and Hawkins (5) proposed asymmetry of the lateral masses on open-mouth radiographs, it has been shown that asymmetry may be present in the absence of abnormality (18). Indeed, the literature on the normal rotational behavior of the atlantoaxial complex is contradictory (7,19,20,21). In a study of 10 human cervical spines to evaluate this discrepancy, Sutherland and colleagues (19) concluded that the variation is so wide that the odontoid–lateral mass interspace is not a reliable indicator of atlantoaxial instability. In AARS, the C1-2 complex rotates as a unit to the opposite side of the chin (Fig. 3). Three-dimensional reconstructions show this in detail (Fig. 4). AP projections may reveal rotation of the C2 spinous process to the same side as the chin while the lower segments are in counterrotation to reorient the visual axis, the so-called Sudeck sign; this is helpful if present, but not reliable. Rinaldi et al. (22) were among the first to describe the use of dynamic CT, which is performed by obtaining axial images of the C0-C1-C2-C3 complex in three positions: (a) presenting position, (b) head turned maximally in direction of rotation, (c) head turned as far as patient comfort allows in the opposite direction. It was proposed that a diagnosis of rotatory fixation could be made if the C1 and C2 posterior arches did not change in the above-mentioned positions.

Since the advent of CT, many criteria have been proposed for the diagnosis of AARS (2,23,24). In general, it stands to reason that if the angle of the C1-2 complex does not move in any of the dynamic positions, then a diagnosis of AARS can be made. However, Li and colleagues argued that a spectrum of abnormal rotational deformities that are not fixed are missed by this loose

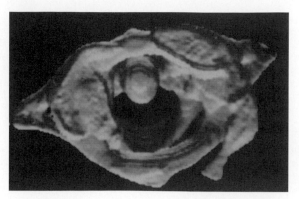

Fig. 4. CT with three-dimensional reconstructions of a patient with rotatory subluxation. The fixed rotational deformity of C1 on C2 is clearly seen.

criterion (25). Based on 20 pediatric cases, they proposed a new diagnostic criterion based on the normal C1-2 motion curve. They incorporated this new diagnostic criterion into five categories based on the angles of C1, C2, and C1-2. The patient is scanned in three positions: presenting (P), midline (Po), and maximally turned away from the side of deformity (P−). They classified AARS into two subtypes based on the biomechanical information: type I "fixed" and type II "nonfixed" AARS. In type I, the C1-2 angle does not change during attempts to correct the torticollis. Type II is "nonfixed" in that a reduction of the C1-2 angle occurs during attempts to correct the deformity. They further categorized this type into type IIA, in which the C1-2 angle decreases but C1 never crosses C2, and type IIB, in which C1 does cross C2, but at an abnormal angle of C1.

Evaluation and Treatment

A general plan for the evaluation and treatment of rotatory subluxation is presented in Figs. 5 and 6. Any patient presenting with torticollis should undergo a routine cervical spinal series, including AP, lateral, and open-mouth views, to assess for fracture, subluxation, and congenital abnormalities. Concomitantly, NSAIDs should be started. If plain films are noncontributory, then the clinician should proceed with dynamic CT to assess for fixation or abnormal rotation of the atlantoaxial complex.

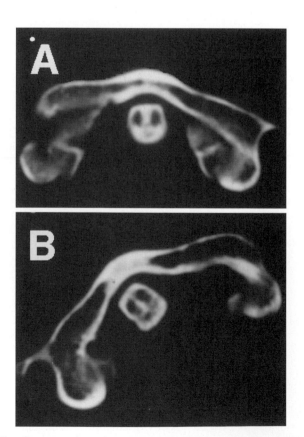

Fig. 3. Dynamic computed tomography (CT) of the C1-2 complex. **A:** The patient is in attempted neutral, and the arch of C1 is rotated with respect to the odontoid. **B:** On rotation, C1 and C2 rotate together, which distinguishes rotatory subluxation from voluntary rotation.

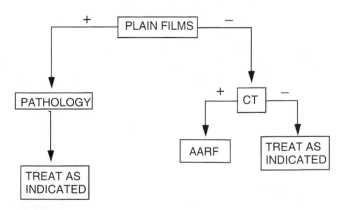

Fig. 5. Scheme for evaluating the patient with acute torticollis suggestive of rotatory subluxation.

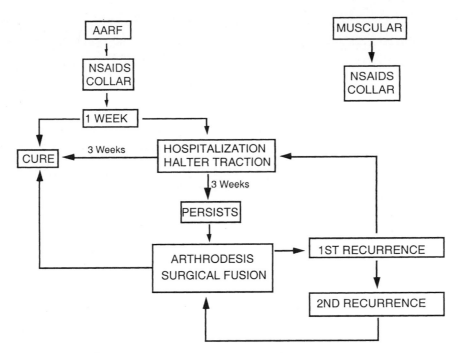

Fig. 6. Suggested management of rotatory subluxation and recurrences.

At this point, if the CT results are nondiagnostic, a cervical collar should be placed, with the antiinflammatory medications continued and CT repeated in 1 week. A negative study warrants only supportive treatment, with a cervical collar and NSAIDs, and close follow-up. Torticollis that has been present for a week or less usually reduces with immobilization and bed rest. This may take up to 6 weeks. If the torticollis continues after this time period with the use of NSAIDs, hospitalization and halter traction are required (2,5,25). A starting weight of 5 lb should be used, with increments of 5 lb until the desired reduction is obtained. Generally, 10 lb per vertebral level is the maximum weight allowed. However, skin breakdown becomes a problem with increasing weight and time of traction. The success of reduction appears to be related to the duration of subluxation, with more desirable results achieved in patients who have had rotation for less than 1 month. Traction may be attempted for up to 3 weeks; however, the likelihood of reduction is slim, and arthrodesis should be advocated at this point. Indeed, in the series of Fielding and Hawkins (5), the diagnosis was delayed in all the patients, and arthrodesis of C1-2 was required after preoperative traction for an average of 15 days. The mean follow-up was 4.2 years; 11 patients remained asymptomatic with a normal head position. The risks of manipulative reduction are greatest with long-standing fixation. In any manipulative reduction, close and continuous monitoring of the patient's neurological status is imperative. Cervical immobilization should be carried out for 4 to 6 weeks after reduction to prevent recurrence and allow the ligaments to heal.

Recurrence

Like successful reduction, the recurrence of rotatory subluxation appears to be related to the duration of torticollis. Phillips and Hensinger (2) treated 23 patients with AARS. Reduction was achieved in 11 patients seen within a week of symptom onset, eight of whom required traction. Reduction was accomplished in five patients seen between 1 week and 1 month with traction lasting from 3 to 23 days. No recurrences were noted in this group. Seven patients were seen more than 1 month after the onset of torticollis. Of these, only one required arthrodesis for failure of reduction (mean follow-up of 1 year). However, four of the remaining six had a recurrence, and two required arthrodesis. The five patients who had recurrences were older and had had a longer hospital stay, and four of the five had had torticollis for more than 1 month (2). No manipulative or intraoperative reductions were performed.

Patients with a recent history of torticollis are more likely to experience resolution with bed rest and expectant management alone. A first recurrence warrants halter traction with 12 weeks of cervical immobilization after reduction. A second recurrence, or a recurrence after halo immobilization, requires a C1-2 fusion. Hettiaratchy and colleagues (26) proposed open reduction in the operating room with a limited fusion and subsequent halo immobilization. They argue that this approach preserves flexion–extension and rotation; however, the occipitoatlantal joint affords only a fraction of these movements. Further, open reduction under anesthesia is controversial, and the argument is made that a more extensive fusion would obviate the need for halo immobilization for 3 months. Nakagawa and colleagues (27) proposed occipitocervical fusion with C1 laminectomy to treat atlantoaxial instability and dislocation. They reported solid bone fusion, maintenance of the reduced position, and preservation of the normal curvature of the cervical spine, height and width of the vertebral bodies, and AP diameter of the spinal canal in eight patients with a mean follow-up of 5.9 years. Posterior C1-2 fusion is usually performed for unstable or fixed rotatory subluxation. The fusion may be extended to the occiput in cases that cannot be reduced in which sublaminar wires may be unsafe or decompressive C1 laminectomy is needed. Extension to the occiput with rigid instrumentation in children may have the added benefit of avoiding external halo immobilization with minimal additional loss of motion.

References

1. Corner EM. Rotatory dislocations of the atlas. *Ann Surg* 1907;45: 9–26.
2. Phillips WA, Hensinger RN. The management of rotatory atlantoaxial subluxation in children. *J Bone Joint Surg* 1989;71A:664–668.
3. Hreidarsson S, Magram G, Singer H. Symptomatic atlantoaxial dislocation in Down syndrome. *Pediatrics* 1982; 69:568–571.
4. Sutton LN, Schut L, Bruce DA, et al. Acquired torticollis in childhood. *Concepts Pediatr Neurosurg* 1985; 5:13–25.
5. Fielding JW, Hawkins RJ. Atlantoaxial rotatory fixation. *J Bone Joint Surg* 1977;59A:37–44.
6. White AA, Panjabi MM. The clinical biomechanics of the occipitoatlanto-axial complex. *Orthop Clin North Am* 1978;9:867–878.
7. White AA, Panjabi MM. *Clinical biomechanics of the spine,* 2nd ed. Philadelphia: JB Lippincott Co, 1990.
8. Anderson MJ, Schutt AH. Spinal injury in children: a review of 156 cases seen from 1959 through 1978. *Mayo Clin Proc* 1980;55: 499–504.
9. Dvorak J, Panjabi M, Gerber M, et al. CT functional diagnostics of the rotatory instability of upper cervical spine. Part I: An experimental study on cadavers. *Spine* 1987;12:197–205.
10. Werne S. Studies in spontaneous atlas dislocation. *Acta Orthop Scand Suppl* 1957;23:1–150.
11. Grisel P. Enucleation de l'atlas et torticollis nasopharyngien. *Presse Med* 1930;38:50–53.
12. Sullivan CR, Bruner AJ, Harris LE. Hypermobility of the cervical spine in children: a pitfall in the diagnosis of cervical dislocation. *Am J Surg* 1958;95:636.
13. Parke WW, Rothman RH, Brown MD. The pharyngovertebral veins: an anatomical rational for Grisel's syndrome. *J Bone Joint Surg* 1984; 66A:568–574.
14. Kawabe N, Hirotani H, Tanaka O. Pathomechanism of atlantoaxial rotatory fixation in children. *J Pediatr Orthop* 1989;9:569–574.
15. Lui TN, Lee ST, Wong CW, et al. C1-C2 fracture dislocations in children and adolescents. *J Trauma* 1996;40:408–411.
16. Sudeck P. Ueber drehnungsverrenkung des atlas. *Dtsch Chir* 1923; 183:289–303.
17. Birney TJ, Hanley EN. Traumatic cervical spine injuries in childhood and adolescence. *Spine* 1989;14:1277–1282.
18. Coutts MB. Atlanto-epistropheal subluxations. *Arch Surg* 1934;29: 297–311.
19. Sutherland JP, Yaszemski MJ, White AA. Radiographic appearance of the odontoid lateral mass interspace in the occipitoatlantoaxial complex. *Spine* 1995;20:2221–2225.
20. Shapiro R, Youngberg AS, Rothman SLG. The differential diagnosis of traumatic lesions of the occipito-atlanto-axial segment. *Radiol Clin North Am* 1973;11:505–526.
21. Jofe MH, White AA, Panjabi MM. Clinically relevant kinematics of the cervical spine. In: The Cervical Spine Research Society Editorial Committee, ed. *The Cervical Spine.* Philadelphia: JB Lippincott Co, 1989:57–63.
22. Rinaldi I, Mullins WJ, Delaney WF, et al. Computerized tomographic demonstration of rotational atlanto-axial fixation. *J Neurosurg* 1979; 50:115–119.
23. Kowalski HM, Cohen WA, Cooper P, et al. Pitfalls in the CT diagnosis of atlantoaxial rotatory subluxation. *AJR Am J Roentgenol* 1987;149: 595–600.
24. Ono K, Yonenobu K, Fuji T, et al. Atlantoaxial rotatory fixation: radiographic study of its mechanism. *Spine* 1985;10:602–608.
25. Li V, Pang D. Atlantoaxial rotatory fixation. In: Pang D, ed. *Disorders of the pediatric spine.* New York: Raven Press, 1995:531–553.
26. Hettiaratchy S, Chou N, Sabin I. Nontraumatic atlanto-occipital and atlantoaxial rotatory subluxation: case report. *Neurosurgery* 1998; 43:162–165.
27. Nakagawa T, Yone K, Sakou T, et al. Occipitocervical fusion with C1 laminectomy in children. *Spine* 1997;22:1209–1214.

186. Achondroplasia

Vishal Sarwahi, Gregory A. Coté, and John F. Sarwark

Achondroplasia is the most common of the skeletal dysplasias, with an estimated incidence of 1 in 25,000 births. It is characterized by abnormal endochondral bone formation, which is caused by a mutation in the fibroblast growth factor receptor-3 gene that leads to maldevelopment of the skeletal system. The phenotype of this most frequent form of short-limb dwarfism is distinctive and easily identified at birth by deformities of the midface, vertebrae, and long bones. Mild to moderate hypotonia is common, and motor milestones are usually delayed. Intelligence is normal unless hydrocephalus or other central nervous system (CNS) complications arise. Some type of neurological dysfunction develops in most persons with achondroplasia later in life. Neurological signs in the leg develop in nearly 80% of these patients by the sixth decade (1). Despite the remarkable degree of maldevelopment in achondroplasia, the mean life expectancy of achondroplastic persons is only 10 years less than that of the general population. However, the mortality of achondroplastic children is considerable in the first few years of life. A mortality rate of up to 7.5% has been reported in the first year of life, and of about 2.5% between the ages of 1 and 4 years (2). The overall standardized mortality ratio in comparison with the general population is 2.27, and mortality is increased at all ages (2). These figures illustrate the importance of thorough monitoring of achondroplastic infants, even in the absence of abnormal signs or symptoms, through a multidisciplinary approach to management.

Physical Features

Men and women with achondroplasia stand approximately 4 feet tall. Despite being classified as one of more than 100 short-stature syndromes, achondroplasia cannot be reliably diagnosed in a neonate by simply measuring the body length. A thorough physical examination and radiographic findings are important to diagnose achondroplasia soon after birth. A relatively normal trunk in combination with shortening of the proximal segment of the extremities (rhizomelia) and trident hands are characteristic features. The head is disproportionately enlarged relative to the limbs because the membranous bones are unaffected. For this reason, hydrocephalus, which is seen in

30% of these patients, may be suspected (3). The hydrocephalus is a communicating type and is caused by altered dynamics of the cerebrospinal fluid (CSF), which improve with growth. Frontal bossing, prominent mandibles, conspicuous depression of the nasal bridge, and hypoplasia of the midface complete the "achondroplasia facies."

Hyperextensibility of most joints, especially the knees, is common. Extension and rotation are limited at the elbow. Rhizomelia (meaning "root limbs") leads to a decrease in elbow extension, which may also be caused by joint abnormality. Posterolateral dislocation of the radial heads may be present. The hands do not reach below the greater trochanter, a severely limiting feature for these patients. The clavicles develop normally, so that the shoulders have a broad appearance. The anteroposterior (AP) diameter of the chest is decreased, and ribs may flare out in infancy. A dorsolumbar gibbus is typically present at birth but usually gives way to exaggerated lumbar lordosis when the child begins to ambulate. The posture is distinctive, characterized by a protruding abdomen, prominent buttocks, a flat chest with flaring ribs, and exaggerated lumbar lordosis. Tibial bowing is seen in 10% of cases by 5 years of age. This continues to develop into adulthood, and nearly 40% of the patients are affected at some time (1). The hind foot is in varus.

Radiographic Features

The primary dysfunction in achondroplasia is defective endochondral bone formation; intramembranous ossification remains unaffected. Therefore, the trunk length is within the normal limits of the general population, whereas the limbs are dramatically short. The most characteristic radiographic feature of achondroplasia is a progressive narrowing of the interpedicular distances from the lower thoracic vertebrae to the sacrum, seen on AP spinal roentgenography. This is secondary to the short and stubby pedicles present from birth. Spinal roentgenography also demonstrates a decreased size of the vertebral bodies and a reduced diameter of the posterior vertebral arches. In addition, the size and the shape of the foramen magnum are significantly altered. These findings are discussed in detail later in the chapter.

Roentgenography of the skull demonstrates midface hypoplasia, frontal prominence, an enlarged calvaria, and shortening of the skull base. A dorsolumbar kyphosis is seen with associated changes. The proximal limb segments are shortened (rhizomelia), and the long bones have flared metaphyses with mushroom-shaped epiphyses. All the metacarpals grow to an equal length, and the fibulae are disproportionately long. Rhizomelia limits elbow extension, long fibulae cause genu varum, and the equally sized metacarpals produce a "starfish hand." The fibula is longer perhaps because of normal appositional growth at its ends. The difference in length of long bones has no histological basis. Tibial bowing is seen by the age of 5 years and continues to develop throughout childhood and into adult life. The triradiate cartilage, which grows by endochondral ossification, is affected and forms horizontal acetabular roofs. Growth of the iliac apophysis is unaffected and normal, and relatively large, square iliac wings ("elephant ears" pelvis) develop. The pelvis is typically broad and short with short sciatic notches. The width of the pelvic inlet is greater than its depth, giving it a "champagne glass" appearance. The sacrum displays an exaggerated horizontal tilt. Greater trochanteric overgrowth produces a coxa vara appearance. Interestingly, congenital dysplasia of the hip is not reported.

Genetics

Achondroplasia is inherited in an autosomal-dominant fashion. Homozygosity is usually lethal to the neonate, and thus 80% of the cases are secondary to a random mutation. A paternal age of more than 36 years has an effect on mutations (4). The risk for a second affected child in cases of mutation is negligible. Achondroplastic parents, however, transmit the gene 50% of the time to their children. Homozygotes have a severe disorder of the skeleton that leads to early death from neurological and respiratory complications. The responsible gene for achondroplasia has been localized on the short arm of the fourth chromosome, 4p16.3, by linkage analysis (5–7). This correlates with the location of the fibroblast growth factor receptor-3 gene (FGFR3), which is a tyrosine kinase transmembrane receptor for fibroblast growth factors. In mice, the FGFR3 homologue is expressed in cartilage; it directs chondrocyte migration and inhibits terminal chondrocyte differentiation and calcification of the cartilage matrix (8). Studies have confirmed that more than 90% of achondroplastic patients have a guanine-to-adenine transition in a single site of the FGFR3 gene (8–10). This remarkable specificity for one particular nucleotide helps to explain the lack of heterogeneity in the achondroplasia phenotype. It also allows for simple detection on polymerase chain reaction analysis and now provides a method for prenatal diagnosis.

Growth and Development

Fowler et al. (11) summarized the issues well, stating that ". . . abnormal development does not mean maladaptive and [that] different development is not defective development." Delays and aberrance in these children are secondary to their anatomical constraints. Generalized hypotonia is present from birth and leads to significant delays in motor development. Children with achondroplasia begin sitting independently at approximately 9 months and start walking independently around 18 months. It is unclear if hypotonia represents an underlying neurological deficit or if this delay is of constitutional origin. Cervical cord compression is seen on imaging studies at the level of the foramen magnum and is a result of congenital stenosis.

Intelligence is not normally compromised in achondroplasia. All incidents of an abnormally low intelligence quotient have been linked to hydrocephalus or some other CNS complication. Small studies, however, do report lower levels in 10% to 16% of cases (12,13). This prevalence of mental retardation is greater than that in the general population. Ruiz-Garcia et al. (14) suggested that subnormal intelligence may be more frequent in achondroplasia than is reported. Hecht et al. (12) found that cognitive development was average and did not correlate with motor development, which was typically delayed. It is noteworthy that decreased mental capacity correlated with evidence of respiratory dysfunction detected by polysomnography.

As the child begins to sit up, a more severe thoracolumbar kyphosis may develop. Furthermore, as the child begins to ambulate, a lumbar lordosis usually evolves. This hyperlordosis of the lumbar spine is compensatory; the disproportionately large head, congenitally misshapen vertebrae, and weak spinal ligaments are other contributing factors. The hip flexion contractures present are probably secondary to lordosis. The abnormal axial loading of the lower spine is an outcome of these mechanical factors, which can have significant neurogenic implications later in life.

In recent years, several studies have demonstrated significant short-term benefits of growth hormone therapy without adverse effects. Shohat et al. (15) investigated the effects of treatment with recombinant human growth hormone in achondroplasia. They found significant increase in the growth rate of only the lower segments during the first year of treatment, but no increase in body disproportion was noted. Responsiveness to growth hormone decreased during the second year of treatment. Weber et al. (16) reported that responses vary. Patients with a relatively low height velocity before treatment seem to derive greater benefit. Little evidence is available of the effect of growth hormone therapy on the final height of achondroplastic patients. The final height in adult men is 118 to 145 cm and in adult women 112 to 136 cm (17). It has been recommended that children remain within 1 standard deviation of the mean weight-for-height curves for achondroplastic patients (18). Long-term data are unavailable, and currently the Committee on Genetics does not include growth hormone therapy as a standard of care for achondroplastic patients.

Medical Complications

Several organ systems are involved throughout the life of a person with achondroplasia. CNS complications include megalencephaly, hydrocephalus, cervicomedullary stenosis, spinal stenosis, and impairment of intellectual development. The incidence of respiratory problems and sleep apnea is greater in these children than in the general population. Studies have shown that as many as 85% of persons with achondroplasia have some type of respiratory anomaly. Most difficulties are caused by respiratory system maldevelopment, such as a small thoracic cage or an obstructed upper airway (12,19–23). The rib cage circumference in this population falls below the third percentile, and a small rib cage is seen in patients with or without respiratory problems. The hypoplastic midface and prominent mandibles lead to thrusting of the tongue, which in turn causes feeding and respiratory problems in infants. The eustachian tubes are small and short; this anomaly leads to frequent otitis media childhood and potential hearing problems in adulthood. The complications can also delay speech development. Speech is reportedly delayed in 18.6% of achondroplastic patients, and 10.9% have articulation defects (1). An underdeveloped midface and prominent mandibles cause dental malocclusion in more than 50% of patients, and children should be evaluated for this problem around 5 or 6 years of age (1).

As many as 60% of achondroplastic patients exhibit some degree of obesity (18,24). The hunger and satiation centers in the brain "presume" that the body is of average size. This problem must be assertively managed throughout life because obesity can exacerbate the orthopedic and respiratory problems associated with achondroplasia. It can also contribute to early cardiovascular mortality.

Women undergo early menopause, and fibroids tend to develop. The pelvic outlet is severely narrowed, so that cesarian section is required for delivery. Because of their spinal stenosis, spinal anesthesia is contraindicated.

Recommendations of the International Symposium on Achondroplasia (25,26) include the following: measurement of growth and head circumference according to growth curves standardized for achondroplasia; careful neurological examina-

tion, including computed tomography (CT), magnetic resonance imaging (MRI), somatosensory evoked potential (SSEP) measurement, and polysomnography; surgical enlargement of the foramen magnum in cases of severe stenosis; management of frequent middle ear infections and dental crowding; measures to control obesity starting in early childhood; growth hormone therapy, which is still under evaluation, as is surgical lengthening of bones; tibial osteotomy or epiphysiodesis of the fibular growth plate to correct bowing of the legs; lumbar laminectomy for spinal stenosis, which typically manifests in early adulthood; delivery by cesarean section in pregnant women with achondroplasia; and prenatal detection of affected fetuses by ultrasonography.

Spinal Problems

The most significant clinical effect of cartilage growth failure occurs in the spine. An absolute reduction in the coronal and sagittal diameters is seen from the foramen magnum to the sacrum. Developmentally, this is explained by the assumption that the centrum of the vertebra is an epiphysis shared by the paired long bones forming the sides of the primitive canal (27). Failure of longitudinal growth of these elements at the neurocentral synchondrosis results in short and stubby pedicles, which cause stenosis. Also, the pedicle thickness increases in a caudal direction (the L5 pedicle can be three times thicker than the L1 pedicle). Mechanical compromise of the spinal canal also occurs in the sagittal plane with thoracolumbar kyphosis. Thus, generalized stenosis, a small foramen magnum, thoracolumbar kyphosis, and increased compensatory lumbar lordosis may distort the spinal canal dimensions in achondroplastic patients.

CERVICOMEDULLARY STENOSIS

Incidence. Cervical myelopathy has been recognized as a complication of achondroplasia since 1901, and it frequently affects young children. The concerns about compression of the cervicomedullary junction (CMJ) have arisen from published estimates of mortality rates in the infantile age group. These have varied from 2.7% to 7.5%. The rate of sudden unexpected death is three times that of sudden infant death syndrome (SIDS) in the normal population and is believed to be secondary to respiratory or CMJ compression. Unlike death in SIDS, death can occur in these children while they are sleeping in a sitting position (3). Reid et al. (22) followed 26 patients prospectively and found that 85% had respiratory symptoms and that 35% had evidence of CMJ compression. Most of the respiratory problems were secondary to restrictive lung disease caused by a diminished chest size or upper airway obstruction. In only three patients were the respiratory symptoms caused by cord compression, and all three showed marked improvement after decompression. They estimated an incidence of CMJ compression of approximately 14% in their study group. Hunter et al. (1) noted apnea in 10.9% of children by 4 years of age and in 16.1% of patients overall. They also reported that 6.8% of their patients underwent surgical decompression by 4 years of age, whereas 16.5% of patients overall had this surgery.

Almost 25% to 35% of patients in the craniocervical studies carried out by Ruiz-Garcia et al. (14) had cord compression at the CMJ, whereas 60% had stenosis only. Imaging studies show a very high rate of compression, which may or may not be evident clinically. On the other hand, some authors have suggested that a thorough neurological examination is neither completely sensitive nor specific in identifying compression (22). Many children have developed satisfactorily without surgery of the foramen magnum, and some showed marked improvement after the operation. The challenge is to identify those patients whose condition will not improve without surgery.

Pathoanatomy. The foramen magnum anatomically consists of the exoccipital, supraoccipital, and basioccipital bones. These grow by enchondral ossification, which in these patients is compromised. The compromise leads to a short basicranium, short clivus, shallow posterior fossa, narrow foramen magnum, and abnormal craniovertebral relationship. An abnormal location and premature fusion of the posterior basal synchondrosis also contribute to the small diameter of the foramen magnum. Narrowing of the coronal axis is more marked and more contributory to reduction on cross section. The sagittal dimensions are less affected. On CT, 96% of children have a cross-sectional area of the foramen magnum that is 3 standard deviations below the normal mean (28). The size of the foramen magnum in the average achondroplastic adult is equivalent to that of a 2-year-old in sagittal diameter and that of a newborn in transverse diameter.

The relative anterior placement of the foramen magnum further exacerbates the stenosis. The result is an upward displacement of the brainstem, so that the cervical cord lies at the foramen, and hyperextension of the brainstem in a neutral head position. Autopsy studies have shown acute and chronic extrinsic compression of the cord and medulla. Findings at surgery include forward extension of the squamous portion of the occiput, thickening of the posterior rim of the foramen magnum, the presence of dense fibrotic epidural bands in front of the posterior ring of C1, and varying degrees of cord compression.

Natural History. No comprehensive study of the natural course of achondroplasia is available. For this reason, various criteria have been applied for operative intervention in the face of assumed symptomatology resulting from CMJ compression. The rate of intervention has been reported to be as high as 34.6% to 42.2% (1). The degree of risk for sudden death, indications for surgery, and frequency of surgery are controversial. Pauli et al. (21) reported surgery in 5 of 53 patients studied prospectively. They felt that hyperreflexia/clonus, a small foramen magnum, and central hypopnea were the best identifiers (97% accuracy in combination) of high-risk patients. Rimoin (29) contested these findings and reported that only 9 of his 200 patients required surgery. The mortality rate in his series was 0.5% and would have been at most 5% if all nine who underwent surgery had died in the absence of intervention. He warned that more patients are being operated on for presumed "life-threatening" CMJ compression than the mortality rate would suggest. Hunter et al. (1) reported surgery in 6.8% of children by 4 years of age. They emphasized that because of the progression of neurological symptoms, the apparent indication for intervention manifests later, in adulthood, and they estimated that 17% of patients eventually require surgical decompression.

Most infants with achondroplasia are hypotonic, acquire gross motor skills slowly, sit without support late (at 9 to 12 months), and ambulate after 1 1/2 years of age. Nearly all of them gain normal tone and strength and achieve age-related motor skills by 2 to 3 years of age. Rimoin (29) stated that almost all patients with hypotonia, clonus, and hyperreflexia eventually attain normal motor development and neurological status. Follow-up MRI shows that posterior impingement of the cord at the level of the foramen magnum decreases with age and may eventually disappear. He stated that narrowing of the cord on MRI may persist permanently with an intact neurological status. Narrowing of the cord may persist even after surgery. Surgery, however, leads to a rapid and marked improvement in neurological function. Thus, it is important to identify high-risk patients whose condition will not improve spontaneously and are at risk for sudden death or paraparesis in the absence of intervention.

High-Risk Patients. The clinical findings that can be used to identify high-risk patients are subtle and nonspecific. These include quadriparesis, paraparesis, asymmetries, hypertonia, opisthotonus, delay of motor milestones for longer than expected in achondroplasia, difficulties in swallowing, respiratory compromise, and apnea. Hypotonia, if persistent, must be viewed with suspicion. Asymmetries are not common in achondroplasia and if present should be investigated. Pauli et al. (21) stated that a patient with simultaneous hyperreflexia/clonus, a small foramen magnum, and central hypopnea must be evaluated for cord compression. However, each of these findings is of less significance individually. They found hyperreflexia/clonus in 12% and central hypopnea in 40% of their nonsurgical cases.

Rimoin (29) considered surgical inpatients with severe floppiness who had significant truncal and limb hypotonia, significant apnea, findings of intracord lesions on T2-weighted MRI, or total lack of CSF flow anteriorly and posteriorly. He noted significant sweating and failure to thrive in this subgroup of patients. However, excessive sweating has been reported as a nearly universal feature in achondroplasia and is probably of no diagnostic significance. Keiper et al. (3), reporting their prospective experience with 11 infants, found all to be asymptomatic with normal examination findings on first evaluation. All underwent MRI on initial evaluation, and two underwent surgery immediately based on the MRI findings. Opisthotonus developed later in two of the remaining patients, and they underwent surgery. These authors recommend that all neonates undergo a neurological examination and MRI. SSEP measurement must be performed if the MRI shows compression, and sleep studies if the history suggests sleep apnea. It has also been suggested that monitoring for sleep apnea be carried out to detect abnormalities until 2 to 3 years of age, at which time natural resolution of the compression can be expected (30).

Investigations

MAGNETIC RESONANCE IMAGING. Whereas CT is ideal for evaluating osseous structures, MRI provides an accurate assessment of the CMJ. In children with achondroplasia, ossification of the occipital bone around the foramen magnum is delayed, and ventral compression results from cartilaginous overgrowth of the odontoid. Most patients have significant anterior–posterior narrowing between the tip of the dens and the posterior rim of the foramen magnum. This is often exaggerated by a thickened dura and transverse ligament. MRI thus offers an advantage over CT in that it shows the soft-tissue component of the area of stenosis better and so the actual compression. Other advantages of MRI are that nonionizing radiation is used, imaging can be performed in the sagittal, coronal, and axial planes, and no contrast is required. MRI allows an evaluation of CSF dynamics and shows intrinsic cord changes. It is important to realize that notching or indentation of the cord at the level of foramen magnum is of no clinical significance. Keiper et al. (3) recommended a prospective MRI measurement of all neonates between the transverse ligament at the tip of the dens and the posterior rim of the foramen magnum. All their patients had a sagittal diameter of less than 1 cm, and three of the four patients who underwent surgery had a diameter of less than 0.7 cm at this level. Yamada et al. (31), using sagittal images, calculated the ratio of the brainstem diameter at the foramen magnum to the diameter at the pontomedullary junction and to the diameter at the C3 level, where it was normal. They decided on surgery based on this ratio, clinical symptoms, and age of the patient.

SOMATOSENSORY EVOKED POTENTIALS. Boor (32), in a study of 30 patients, showed that all patients with clinical symptoms had abnormal SSEPs. The sensitivity for cervical cord compression was 89%, and the specificity for myelomalacia was 92%. Nelson et al. (33) postulated that SSEPs, which are a parameter of the dorsal column response, have good sensitivity in detecting early cord compression because the lip of the foramen magnum indents the cord posteriorly. However, this has not been considered a significant finding. Reid et al. (22) found normal SSEPs in all patients without persistent compression, but several of their patients with cord involvement had normal findings. Pauli et al. (21) reported a high false-positive rate. Ruiz-Garcia et al. (14) evaluated amplitude, interpeak values, and total latencies in 37 of their 39 patients. They considered the values abnormal if they were more than 3 standard deviations from age-related values and formulated a grading system. Of the asymptomatic patients, 43% had "slightly" abnormal values. They recommended neuroimaging for patients with "severely" abnormal findings based on their grading system.

SLEEP STUDIES. Sleep apnea is often seen in infants with achondroplasia and has been implicated in SIDS. Respiratory compromise may be caused by several factors. These include upper airway obstruction secondary to midfacial hypoplasia and the effects of a diminutive rib cage and brainstem compression on central respiratory mechanisms. A prevalence of 75% to 80% has been reported for chronic pneumopathy (34), which irrespective of cause results in chronic hypoxemia and sleep disorders. Sleep studies can therefore detect any tendencies to sleep apnea, hypoxemia, or hypercapnia. Polysomnography, including overnight monitoring of the sleep state, heart rate, oxygen saturation, chest and abdominal impedance, nasal and oral air flow, and end-tidal levels of carbon dioxide, is carried out. Pauli et al. (35) reported frequent central hypopneic episodes in their patients and found desaturation in the range of 80% to 85%. They stated that central hypopnea is characteristic of achondroplasia. Reid et al. (22) and Francomano et al. (36) documented central apnea in patients with achondroplasia. Seizures and apneusis breathing have also been reported.

Treatment. Decompressive surgery provides clear benefits, with marked and immediate improvement seen. Decompression of the posterior fossa is carried out and may be combined with C1 laminectomy. Duraplasty may be required if the dura is violated during the division of epidural bands. Surgery is performed preferably with the patient prone. Decompression is performed with a high-speed burr and should extend laterally to the medial surfaces of the occipital condyles on both sides. Overly aggressive bone removal cephalad must be avoided to prevent "cerebellar sag." The entire horizontal portion forming the posterior rim of the foramen magnum must be removed along with the posterior arch of C1 to complete the decompression. The fibrous epidural bands must be lysed. Adequate decompression is confirmed by intraoperative ultrasonography and clinically by visualizing a pulsatile cord. In doubtful cases, the dura must be opened and additional adhesions lysed. The dura is patched with fascial or cadaveric lyophilized dural grafts. The need for duraplasty is assessed according to the individual case. Bone decompression must be sufficient to prevent regrowth with age.

The rate of surgical complications varies with age and will probably decrease as experience is gained. Pauli et al. (21) reported the sole complication of CSF leak in 10 operated patients. Keiper et al. (3) reported no complications, and their patients were asymptomatic at an average of 4.6 years of follow-up. Ryken and Menezes (37) had one complication, and Ruiz-Garcia et al. (14) reported three poor outcomes with eventual death among seven patients who underwent surgery. Reid et al. (22) had one death and multiple complications in nine operated cases.

Ventriculomegaly and Hydrocephalus. These patients usually have ventriculomegaly, and up to 30% have symptomatic hydrocephalus (3). Some children have only megacephaly, others have true hydrocephalus, and yet others have dilated ventricles without hydrocephalus (38). The fact that *FGFR3* transcripts are present in fetal and adult brain may be relevant to the megacephaly. The mechanism for hydrocephalus includes venous hypertension resulting from impaired CSF absorption secondary to a stenotic jugular foramen, impaired passage of CSF through the foramina of Luschka and Magendie secondary to a stenotic foramen magnum, and obstruction of the basal cisterns by the brainstem. Most authors agree that the large subarachnoidal space and ventriculomegaly are caused by abnormal CSF dynamics (3,31). Diversionary shunts are performed when necessary but are not needed in most cases. Hunter et al. (1) found that 10.5% had a ventricular shunt, all but one of which had been performed before the teenage years. Hydrocephalus in almost all cases is of the communicating type. A comparison of head circumference and development, including gait, with parameters for achondroplasia identifies patients with symptomatic hydrocephalus. It has been recommended that ultrasonography be performed at birth and at 2, 4 and 6 months to establish ventricular size and detect hydrocephalus (39).

DORSOLUMBAR KYPHOSIS

Incidence. More than 90% of infants with achondroplasia have kyphosis at less than 1 year of age, which resolves spontaneously over a period of time. However, nearly 10% to 15% have a fixed-angulation kyphosis of the dorsolumbar junction as adults (40–42). This angular kyphosis may be severe and cause neurological problems. Kopits (42) reported the frequency of kyphosis in different age groups: 97% before the age of 1 year, 87% between 1 and 2 years, 39% between 2 and 5 years, and 11% between 5 to 10 years. Persistent kyphosis was seen in 11% of cases by Wynne-Davies et al. (43), 14.3% by Nelson (27), and 9.2% by Bailey (44). Beighton and Bathfield (45) noted a significantly higher incidence of kyphosis in a population of South African blacks. They postulated that their method of carrying babies on their backs increased spinal flexion and exacerbated the kyphosis. Avoidance of this position in their opinion could decrease or prevent this deformity.

Pathoanatomy. Hypotonia of the trunk is present in all infants with achondroplasia. This, in combination with a very large head (weighing approximately 14% more than normal) and generalized ligamentous laxity, result in a *C*-shaped posture during sitting. These forces create an abnormal axial loading stress on the end plates of the vertebrae, which during a period of time respond by remodeling. The *C*-shaped flexible slump of the spine is replaced, in few cases, by an angular deformity that becomes fixed over time. Draping of the cord and anterior spinal vessels over this "knuckle" can cause ischemic changes.

Natural History. Kyphosis of the dorsolumbar junction is seen in nearly all infants with achondroplasia. It resolves in most children at the time they achieve independent ambulation. As a child begins to stand, hip flexion contracture causes the lumbar spine to assume a lordotic position. This probably leads to flattening of the kyphosis to allow truncal balance. However, an estimated 10% of these children have persistent kyphosis that becomes rigid and requires surgical treatment. Preventive action in this group can probably decrease the need for surgery, as is discussed later.

Radiographic Features. All patients have localized kyphosis with preservation of the disc space. It is characterized by anterior wedging and posterior displacement of the vertebra at the apex of the curve, which causes a beaked appearance of the vertebral body. The deformity is accentuated in erect and sitting positions. The early kyphosis is flexible, and cross-table roentgenograms obtained with the patient lying down reveal the degree of flexibility. It has been suggested that angular wedging or beaking indicates a risk for progression or persistence of the deformity (40). Such wedging develops only after the first year of life.

MRI shows the conus lying at or above the apex of the curve, with draping or stretching of the cord and cauda equina over the deformity. The signal intensity of the disc spaces is usually normal, although the discs may be herniated and aggravate the kyphosis further. The intensity of the cord signal may be abnormal, depending on the intrinsic changes.

Preventive Treatment. The initial treatment is observation based on the natural history. In the past, suggestions were made to keep the infant from sitting up; however, firm data showing that positioning change directly affects kyphosis were missing. In cases in which kyphosis was seen to be progressive or persistent, a thoracolumbar spinal orthosis (TLSO) and stretching of the hip flexion contractures were advised, and surgery was recommended if spontaneous resolution did not occur or brace correction failed.

Kopits (42) reported experience with 76 children who were braced. Bracing was performed between the ages of 8 and 26 months in patients with vertebral wedging on roentgenograms. Improvement or stabilization of the kyphosis was noted after bracing for an average 29 months in 84.2% of the patients. In 1997, Pauli et al. (40) reported 66 infants with kyphosis who were part of a prospective study. The parents of those children who were less than 1 year of age were counseled to use hard-backed seating devices and prevent unsupported sitting and sitting at an angle of more than 60 degrees from the horizontal. Roentgenograms were obtained to document flexibility of the spine and anterior wedging. Children with kyphosis of more than 30 degrees, significant wedging, or retrograde displacement of the apical vertebra were braced in a modified TLSO. Bracing was continued until the anterior column height of the vertebra was restored, the child started walking independently, or the residual kyphosis became rigid. Only 20 of their patients required bracing according to their criteria. In all of them, a median residual kyphosis of 8 degrees was noted after an average 15 months. Progression was not noted subsequently in any of these cases, and the authors found bracing to be effective when initiated before 3 years of age. In this series, 35% of the patients had rib cage deformities, which were considered minor and regressed after the completion of brace wear. They also found that the children whose parents were counseled had significantly less residual kyphosis, and fewer of them required bracing. They recommended that those patients not requiring bracing according to their criteria nevertheless be followed every 4 to 6 months until the age of 3 years. They concluded that the neurological risk for angular kyphosis, seen in 10% to 15% of achondroplastic adults and adolescents, could be eliminated by this regimen.

Surgery. Tolo (46) presented experience with 17 patients who underwent surgery for kyphosis of the dorsolumbar junction. The median kyphosis was 85 degrees (range, 42 to 152 degrees), and the patients were from 3 to 39 years of age. Only seven of them had preoperative symptoms. All underwent ante-

rior and posterior fusion except for one, who had anterior fusion only. Neurological improvement was seen postoperatively, and no cases of pseudarthrosis developed. One patient had a postoperative neurological deficit. In five patients, laminectomy for stenosis was performed at the same session. Parisini et al. (47) reported 11 cases. The average age of the patients in their group was 35 years, and seven patients had severe cord compromise. They performed laminectomies and stated that fusion was not necessary after extensive laminectomy. No discectomies were performed to avoid destabilizing the spine, and posterior fusion without laminectomy was considered equally futile. They believed that anterior surgery alone could have some adverse effect on the cord and reported one case with severe deficit. However, they stated that combined anterior and posterior fusion and decompression with or without instrumentation were the best means of treating this deformity. Early surgery was advocated to prevent neurological complications.

Dubousset and Masson (41) stated that posterior fusion alone was not sufficient. Even in the absence of pseudarthrosis, stretching developed because of the lack of anterior fusion. Combined anterior and posterior fusion was considered adequate, with fusion performed at L4 to allow forward flexion. Tolo (48) recommended surgery by the age of 5 years for curves of more than 40 degrees and vertebral wedging. A combined anterior and posterior fusion in one stage with cord monitoring was performed, and Drummond button wires were used posteriorly to hold the correction. A body cast was used for 6 months.

We have performed anterior and posterior spinal fusion at an early age for rigid deformities greater than 60 degrees. Anterior surgery consists of discectomy, release of the anterior longitudinal ligament, curettage of the end plates, and the use of rib and allograft. Because we consider release of the anterior longitudinal ligament an important step, especially with large, rigid curves, we do not perform thoracoscopic procedures. The use of anterior cages with bone graft augments the correction and provides a durable fusion. In cases of neurological impairment, anterior decompression must be adequate to relax the "draped-over" cord. We do not favor the use of wires alone posteriorly because of our experience of late follow-up failures with such techniques in other settings. The wires break with time, and the curve may progress further. Stenosis precludes the use of hooks and sublaminar cables. Much of the correction is achieved by anterior release. In laminectomies, pedicle screws are used posteriorly and inserted by the anatomical free-hand approach. A freer is placed on the medial wall of the pedicle to detect any breach of the medial cortex during tapping and insertion of the screw. Further confirmation is obtained with the ball-tipped probe and roentgenography. Preoperative CT is essential to evaluate pedicle size. Implants do not encroach on the spinal canal. Intraoperative direct electromyelography is used to confirm the adequacy of pedicle screw placement and rule out nerve root impingement. Postoperatively, the child is prescribed a well-molded TLSO with or without thigh extension. The child is allowed to walk and wears the brace full-time for 6 months.

SPINAL STENOSIS

Incidence. Stenosis is the most common spinal problem in achondroplasia. Although the lumbar canal is stenotic from birth, lower-extremity symptoms are unusual before adolescence and are most common in middle adulthood. Symptomatic stenosis develops in more than half of patients with achondroplasia. Fortuna et al. (49) found a mean age at onset of symptoms of about 30.5 years in a review of cases from the literature and their own cases during a period of 24 years.

Hall (25) reported in a survey of Little People of America that stenotic symptoms were present in 20% to 30% of patients. Of these, 10% were considered candidates for surgery. Bethem et al. (50) reported that 7 of their 30 cases had claudication or paralysis secondary to stenosis. Kopits (42) reported that 70% of children between 4 and 10 years of age in his experience had leg pain. This was probably related to altered knee mechanics with fibular overgrowth in the growing children. Most reports confirm that symptoms are seen in older patients. Nelson (27) reported an age-related increase in symptoms. Hunter et al. (1) also reported a worsening of symptoms with increasing age. Only 20% of their patients who were less than 12 years old had symptoms, whereas 50% of their adult patients had problems. Fewer than 10% of patients younger than 10 years had neurological signs. This percentage increased to 20% in the second decade and to 80% by the fifth decade.

Pathoanatomy. Because of a congenital defect of enchondral ossification, synostosis of the vertebral body ossification center and posterior arch occurs prematurely. This leads to short and stumpy pedicles (30% to 40% thicker than normal), thick laminae, and short vertebral bodies. The posterior aspect of the vertebral body is concave anteriorly at the level of the pedicles, which helps maintain adequate anteroposterior space. However, because the interpedicular distance is short (one-third smaller than normal), the cross-sectional area is reduced to one-third to one-half that seen in the normal population. The trefoil shape of the canal is also abnormal. It is essential to understand that these are bony abnormalities, and hypertrophied soft tissues can constrict the canal further. Backward projection of the vertebral end plates and discs into the spinal canal gives rise to the characteristic myelographic appearance. The dye pool opposite the vertebral body is normal, whereas in the disc area it is minimal or absent. The short pedicles cause the nerve root foramen to narrow anteroposteriorly (it is 1 to 2.8 mm smaller than normal), and the posteriorly projecting disc spaces and end plates compromise the foramina further. The lumbar enlargement of the spinal cord occurs at T10, where the normal increase in the area of the central canal does not take place. In achondroplasia, this feature creates a critical site for compromise and is of surgical relevance in a determination of the proximal extent of laminectomy.

The average area of L1 is reduced by 39% and that of L5 by 27%, yet the presenting symptoms are reported in adulthood. Fortuna et al. (49) profiled 35 patients and found 17% with associated herniated disc, 60% with degenerated spondyloarthropathy, and 23% with associated vertebral wedging and kyphosis. Changes related to aging, such as osteophytes, facet hypertrophy, and disc degeneration resulting in a loss of disc height, further narrow the canal and nerve root foramina. Patients with significant dorsolumbar kyphosis tend to have early symptoms because exaggerated compensatory lumbar lordosis compromises the canal.

Clinical Features. The symptoms and signs reflect the underlying pathology and dynamics of the canal. The changes in circulation in the microvascular, the movement of nerves in the constricted canal, and tension on the dural sac and nerves secondary to kyphosis, narrowing of the spinal canal, and age-related changes all contribute to the clinical picture. The most common symptom is the vague pain or aching of the legs after prolonged walking that is associated with neurogenic claudication. The pain is not time-specific but is related to the distance walked and is relieved by sitting. The symptoms and signs of neurological weakness resulting from canal dynamics are thus best elicited by having the patient walk for some time. With prolonged walking, distended veins encroach on the free space; demands on the blood supply and the accumulation of metabolites are increased because of the altered circulation in the mi-

crovascular. The capacity of the spinal canal in lordosis is half of that in a flexed position, which, coupled with bulging discs and thickened ligamenta flava, exacerbates the stenosis. This explains the relief of symptoms obtained by sitting or stooping forward and helps differentiate neurogenic claudication from vascular claudication.

Fortuna et al. (49) reported 35 patients with symptomatic stenosis and reviewed their clinical profiles. They found weakness of the lower limbs in 82.8% of cases, low back pain radiating to the lower limbs in 14.3%, sphincter disturbances in 40%, and sexual disturbances in 5.7%. Lutter and Langer (51) devised a classification system for achondroplastic patients based on the presentation and neurological impairment in spinal stenosis. They proposed four patterns, which are useful in the prognosis and in understanding the progress of the signs and symptoms.

Type I. Symptoms progress after an insidious onset. Back pain associated with sciatica and paresthesia is seen initially. Motor, sensory, and reflex changes occur later and can lead to an inability to walk and urinary incontinence. Patients usually have paraparesis at the time of surgery. Kyphosis is very common, and the prognosis is better in the absence of dorsolumbar kyphosis.

Type II. This is the most common presentation. Neurological findings are absent initially, but progressive paraparesis and sensory loss eventually develop. The presenting feature is intermittent claudication with leg pain and weakness, which are aggravated by activity and relieved by rest. Kyphosis is absent, and 60% of patients have a good recovery with laminectomy.

Type III. Symptoms and signs are secondary to disc prolapse. Evidence of root tension, root compression, or root inflammation is present. Good results are generally the rule, and this group can be compared with patients who have herniated nucleus pulposus.

Type IV. Acute back and leg pain with paraplegia or paralysis is seen on presentation. Poor results with little or no neurological improvement are frequent. Kyphosis is common.

Investigations

ROENTGENOGRAPHY. Plain x-ray films show interpedicular narrowing. The lateral roentgenogram shows dorsolumbar kyphosis and may also show traction spurs and osteophytes. The presence of dorsolumbar kyphosis and an interpedicular distance of less than 20 mm at L1 and less than 16 mm at L5 have been associated with severe symptoms at presentation and a poor prognosis (52).

MYELOGRAPHY/COMPUTED TOMOGRAPHY-MYELOGRAPHY. With the advent of MRI, myelography and CT–myelography are less often performed. Myelography, apart from being less sensitive than MRI, is a technically demanding and invasive procedure and can cause complications in achondroplasia. In view of the dorsolumbar kyphosis, withdrawal of minimal amounts of CSF from the lumbar spine can worsen the neurological status. Thus, the cisterna or upper cervical region is the preferred area for needle placement.

MAGNETIC RESONANCE IMAGING. In patients with achondroplasia, it is preferable to study the whole spine in view of the stenosis at the cervical, lumbar, and thoracic levels. It is important to realize that stenosis is present throughout the spine and therefore MRI findings must be clinically correlated. In cases with previous surgery, any recurrence of symptoms at the same level must be carefully studied. The possibility of a disc prolapse must be ruled out, apart from compression by scar tissue. Gadolinium-enhanced MRI can help differentiate between the two.

OTHER METHODS. A urodynamic study including a cystometrogram may be needed if urinary symptoms are present. Bladder involvement is an early sign of neural involvement, especially with low-level compression. A postvoid residual urine estimate can help in the diagnosis of bladder dysfunction. Cystometrography preoperatively has been advised in adult patients because a bladder problem may become more apparent postoperatively.

Surgery. Laminectomies are carried out to at least one or two levels above the level of compression. The usual extent is from the lower thoracic spine to the sacrum. Disc herniation is managed in the usual manner. Additional bone must be removed for better exposure. This extensive surgery is necessary to avoid stenosis at adjacent levels. We prefer spinal cord monitoring. The decompression is performed from the sacrum to at least the dorsolumbar junction. Partial removal of arthritic facets is carried out for adequate decompression, especially in the lateral recess. Foraminotomy is carried out on both sides, especially in cases with nerve root impingement. It is vital to remember that the canal is stenotic and that epidural fat is absent because of chronic compression. Thus, rongeurs are avoided, and a burr is used to thin out the lamina just medial to the facet joint. The shell of the inner cortex is carefully scored with a curette, and the loose piece of lamina can then be lifted off. The ligamentum flavum is elevated carefully from the dura. The dura is thin, and tears are not uncommon; they must be repaired. Intractable tears are managed by using muscle to obliterate the dead space, and closure is then carried out in layers. Pseudomeningocele is a known complication and can cause compressive symptoms.

Fusion is usually not needed. Despite the extensive surgery, instability is uncommon; however, patients should be followed on a long-term basis. In cases of laminectomy over a kyphotic segment, fusion is recommended. A severe deformity must be managed by anterior release. Posterior instrumentation may be needed, and pedicle screws are preferred.

RESULTS. Fortuna et al. (49) reviewed 35 cases with myeloradicular symptoms who had undergone laminectomies for stenosis. All patients with kyphosis had major neurological problems and poor surgical results, irrespective of the duration of their symptoms. Patients with severe preoperative neurological deficit secondary to stenosis or disc prolapse but no kyphosis also had poor results, irrespective of age, duration of symptoms, or timing of the intervention. In the remaining cases, the prognosis was better when surgery was performed within 3 years of the onset of symptoms.

Pyeritz et al. (53) reported a long-term retrospective study of laminectomies in achondroplasia. Their follow-up was 8 years, and 22 patients were reviewed. Improvement was noted postoperatively in 20 patients; the number decreased to 12 at 5 years and to one at 8 years of follow-up. Better results were seen in the absence of cervical stenosis and with a shorter duration of symptoms.

References

1. Hunter AGW, Bankier A, Rogers JG, et al. Medical complications of achondroplasia: a multicentre patient review. *J Med Genet* 35:705–712, 1998.
2. Hecht JT, Francomano CA, Horton WA. Mortality in achondroplasia. *Am J Med Genet* 41:454–464, 1987.
3. Keiper GL Jr, Koch B, Crone KR. Achondroplasia and cervicomedullary compression: prospective evaluation and surgical treatment. *Pediatr Neurosurg* 31:78–83, 1993.
4. Stoll C, Roth M-P, Bigel P. A reexamination of paternal age effect on the occurrence of new mutations for achondroplasia. In: Papadatos CJ, Bartsocas CS, eds. *Skeletal dysplasias.* New York: Alan R Liss, 1982:419–426.
5. Velinov M, Slaugenhaupt SA, Stoilov I, et al. The gene for achondroplasia maps to the telomeric region of chromosome 4p. *Nat Genet* 6:318–321, 1994.
6. Le Merrer M, Rousseau F, Legeai-Mallet L, et al. A gene for achondroplasia–hypochondroplasia maps to chromosome 4p. *Nat Genet* 6:314–317, 1994.
7. Francomano CA, Ortiz de Luna RI, Hefferon TW, et al. Localization of the achondroplasia gene to the distal 2.5 Mb of human chromosome 4p. *Hum Mol Genet* 3:787–792, 1994.
8. Rousseau F, Bonaventure J, Legeai-Mallet L, et al. Mutations in the gene encoding fibroblast growth factor receptor-3 in achondroplasia. *Nature* 371:252–254, 1994.
9. Shiang R, Thompson LM, Zhu Y-Z, et al. Mutations in the transmembrane domain of *FGFR3* cause the most common genetic form of dwarfism, achondroplasia. *Cell* 78:335–342, 1994.
10. Bellus GA, Hefferon TW, Ortiz de Luna RI, et al. Achondroplasia is defined by recurrent G380R mutations of *FGFR3. Am J Hum Genet* 56:368–373, 1995.
11. Fowler ES, Glinski LP, Reiser CA, et al. Biophysical bases for delayed and aberrant motor development in young children with achondroplasia. *J Dev Behav Pediatr* 18:143–150, 1997.
12. Hecht JT, Thompson NM, Weir T, et al. Cognitive and motor skills in achondroplastic infants: neurologic and respiratory correlates. *Am J Hum Genet* 41:208–211, 1991.
13. Yamada H, Nakamura S, Tajima M, et al. Neurological manifestations of pediatric achondroplasia. *J Neurosurg* 54:49–57, 1981.
14. Ruiz-Garcia M, Tovar-Baudin A, Del Castillo-Ruiz V, et al. Early detection of neurological manifestations in achondroplasia. *Childs Nerv Syst* 13:208–213, 1997.
15. Shohat M, Tick D, Barakat S, et al. Short-term recombinant human growth hormone treatment increases growth rate in achondroplasia. *J Clin Endocrinol Metab* 81:4033–4037, 1996.
16. Weber G, Prinster C, Meneghel M, et al. Human growth hormone treatment in prepubertal children with achondroplasia. *Am J Med Genet* 61:396–400, 1996.
17. Horton WA, Rotter RI, Rimoin DL, et al. Standard growth curves for achondroplasia. *J Pediatr* 93:435–438, 1978.
18. Hunter AGW, Hecht JT, Scott CI Jr. Standard weight for height curves in achondroplasia. *Am J Med Genet* 62:255–261, 1996.
19. Waters KA, Everett F, Sillence D, et al. Breathing abnormalities in sleep achondroplasia. *Arch Dis Child* 69:191–196, 1993.
20. Zucconi M, Weber G, Castronovo V, et al. Sleep and upper airway obstruction in children with achondroplasia. *J Pediatr* 129:743–749, 1996.
21. Pauli RM, Horton VK, Glinski LP, et al. Prospective assessment of risks for cervicomedullary-junction compression in infants with achondroplasia. *Am J Hum Genet* 56:732–744, 1995.
22. Reid CS, Pyeritz RE, Kopits SE, et al. Cervicomedullary compression in young children with achondroplasia: value of comprehensive neurologic and respiratory evaluation. *J Pediatr* 110:522–530, 1987.
23. Mogayzel PJ Jr, Carroll JL, Loughlin GM, et al. Sleep-disordered breathing in children with achondroplasia. *J Pediatr* 132:667–671, 1998.
24. Hecht JT, Hood OJ, Schwartz RJ, et al. Obesity in achondroplasia. *Am J Med Genet* 31:597–602, 1988.
25. Hall J. The natural history of achondroplasia. In: Nicoletti B, Kopits SE, Ascani E, et al., eds. *Human achondroplasia: a multidisciplinary approach.* New York: Plenum Press, 1988:3–9.
26. Horton WA, Hecht JT, Hood OJ, et al. Growth hormone therapy in achondroplasia. *Am J Med Genet* 42:667–670, 1992.
27. Nelson MA. Kyphosis and lumbar stenosis in achondroplasia. *Basic Life Sci* 48:305–311, 1988.
28. Wang H, Rosenbaum AE, Reid CS, et al. Pediatric patients with achondroplasia: CT evaluation of the craniocervical junction. *Radiology* 164:515–519, 1987.
29. Rimoin DL. Cervicomedullary junction compression in infants with achondroplasia: when to perform neurosurgical decompression [Editorial]. *Am J Hum Genet* 56:824–827, 1995.
30. Wassman ER Jr, Rimoin DL. Cervicomedullary compression with achondroplasia [Letter]. *J Pediatr* 113:411, 1988.
31. Yamada Y, Ito H, Otsubo Y, et al. Surgical management of cervicomedullary compression in achondroplasia. *Childs Nerv Syst* 12:737–741, 1996.
32. Boor R. Abnormal subcortical somatosensory evoked potentials indicate high cervical myelopathy in achondroplasia. *Eur J Pediatr* 158:662–667, 1999.
33. Nelson FW, Goldie WD, Hecht JT, et al. Short-latency somatosensory evoked potentials in the management of patients with achondroplasia. *Neurology* 34:1053–1058, 1984.

34. Mador MJ, Tobin MJ. Apneustic breathing. A characteristic feature of brainstem compression in achondroplasia? *Chest* 97:877–883, 1990.
35. Pauli RM, Scott CI, Wassman ER Jr, et al. Apnea and sudden unexpected deaths in infants with achondroplasia. *J Pediatr* 104:342–348, 1984.
36. Francomano CA, Carson B, Seidler A, et al. Morbidity and mortality in achondroplasia: efficacy of prospective evaluation and surgical intervention. *Am J Hum Genet* 53-A(suppl):112, 1993.
37. Ryken TC, Menezes AH. Cervicomedullary compression in achondroplasia. *J Neurosurg* 81:43–48, 1994.
38. Dennis JP, Rosenberg HS, Alvord EC Jr. Megalencephaly, internal hydrocephalus and other neurological aspects of achondroplasia. *Brain* 84:427–445, 1961.
39. Committee on Genetics. Health supervision for children with achondroplasia. *J Pediatr* 95:443–451, 1995.
40. Pauli RM, Breed A, Horton VK, et al. Prevention of fixed, angular kyphosis in achondroplasia. *J Pediatr Orthop* 17:726–733, 1997.
41. Dobousset J, Masson JC. Spinal disorders: kyphosis and lumbar stenosis. *Basic Life Sci* 48:299–303, 1988.
42. Kopits SE. Thoracolumbar kyphosis and lumbosacral hyperlordosis in achondroplastic children. *Basic Life Sci* 48:241–255, 1988.
43. Wynne-Davies R, Walsh WK, Gormley J. Achondroplasia and hypoachondroplasia: clinical variation and spinal stenosis. *J Bone Joint Surg Br* 63:508–515, 1981.
44. Bailey JA. Orthopaedic aspects of achondroplasia. *J Bone Joint Surg Am* 52:1285–1301, 1970.
45. Beighton P, Bathfield CA. Gibbal achondroplasia. *J Bone Joint Surg Br* 63:328–329, 1981.
46. Tolo VT. Surgical treatment of kyphosis in achondroplasia. In: Nicoletti B, Kopits SE, Ascani E, et al., eds. *Human achondroplasia: a multidisciplinary approach*. New York: Plenum Press, 1988: 257–259.
47. Parisini P, Greggi T, Casadei R, et al. The surgical treatment of vertebral deformities in achondroplastic dwarfism. *Chir Organi Mov* 81: 129–137, 1996.
48. Tolo VT. Spinal deformity in skeletal dysplasia conditions. In: Bridwell KH, De Wald RL, eds. *The textbook of spinal surgery,* 2nd ed. Philadelphia: Lippincott–Raven Publishers, 1997.
49. Fortuna A, Ferrante L, Acqui M, et al. Narrowing of thoracolumbar spinal canal in achondroplasia. *J Neurol Sci* 33:185–196, 1989.
50. Bethem D, Winter RB, Lutter L, et al. Spinal disorders of dwarfism. *J Bone Joint Surg Am* 63:1412–1425, 1981.
51. Lutter LD, Langer LO. Neurologic symptoms in achondroplastic dwarfs—surgical treatment. *J Bone Joint Surg Am* 59:87–92, 1977.
52. Kahanovitz N, Rimoin DL, Sillence DO. The clinical spectrum of lumbar spine disease in achondroplasia. *Spine* 7:137–140, 1982.
53. Pyeritz RE, Sack GH, Udvarhelyi GB. Thoracolumbosacral laminectomy in achondroplasia: long-term results in 22 patients. *Am J Med Genet* 28:433–444, 1987.

187. Adult Complications of Spinal Dysraphism

David G. McLone

A large number of children with dysraphism have been aggressively treated and now approach adulthood either as normal individuals or with a stable deficit; however, they will remain at risk throughout life.

More children are crippled by myelomeningocele than by poliomyelitis, muscular dystrophy, or traumatic paraplegia. At least 75% of children born with this disease can be expected to reach young adulthood. As a consequence, many physicians, including those who treat primarily adult patients, must now confront this disease and help determine the proper management. Until recently, little solid information has been available regarding the long-term prognosis of children with myelomeningocele, and even less about the late problems they will face as adults.

Spinal lipomas are a common cause of spinal cord tethering. Recently, the prophylactic surgical removal of spinal lipomas has been questioned, especially those of the conus medullaris. Unfortunately, few statistically significant series have been reported. A total of 213 children with spinal lipomas underwent surgery at the Children's Memorial Hospital in Chicago, in whom 270 procedures were carried out, between 1975 and 1995. The status of these children was retrospectively reviewed to determine the differences in outcome between patients who underwent prophylactic surgery before the onset of symptoms and those who underwent surgery after the onset of symptoms (1).

It has fallen to the pediatric neurosurgeon to review the current knowledge of outcomes and late complications in adult patients with spinal dysraphism and make this information available to physicians and patients who must decide difficult issues. This chapter presents our experience with the outcomes and late complications of treatment in a large (>1,500) population of children born with this complex disease and addresses a few of the remaining controversies (2–5).

Outcome

Between 1947 and 1956, 89% of English children born with a myelomeningocele died before the age of 6 months. Laurence (6) reviewed the outcome of 407 children cared for at a large children's hospital just before effective shunting devices became available. In this group, the myelomeningocele was repaired in only 160 (39%) of the 407 children. Clinical evidence of hydrocephalus was noted in 73% of them. Intracranial infection was the single most common cause of death. In the study of Laurence, a newborn infant with myelomeningocele had a 29% chance of living to the age of 12 years. Infants who survived to the age of 4 months had a 51% chance of living to the age of 12 years. Those who survived to the age of 1 year had a 77% chance of surviving to the age of 12 years. The mortality rate began to level off at about 48 months. Similar leveling of the mortality rate has been observed in recent studies.

Between the mid-1950s and 1985, effective methods were developed for treating hydrocephalus. As patient survival improved, Lorber and Salfield (7) applied selection criteria to divide children with a myelomeningocele into two groups: those with a poor prognosis and those with a good prognosis. Long-term follow-up of this selected series of patients indicated that the overall mortality of the two groups approached 70%, mostly because of the selection process itself. The mortality in the group with a poor prognosis was nearly 100%. The mortality in the group with a good prognosis, selected to be the "best" possible survivors, was 14%.

Bowman and McLone (2) treated all patients with myelomeningocele without applying any selection criteria and studied two cohorts. The overall mortality for the initial cohort, comprising 118 unselected patients followed for 20 years after closure of the back, was 23%. Survival curves for the second cohort, comprising 100 children, were identical to those for the first group. In these studies, 2% of the children did not survive to leave the hospital despite initial closure of the back and shunting procedures. A total of 10% had died by the end of 5 years. The most common cause of death in the early years was hindbrain dysfunction associated with stridor, apneic spells, and reflux aspiration. In the first cohort, comprising 118 patients, 11 of the deaths were caused by hindbrain dysfunction. Death was caused by central nervous system (CNS) infection in 1%. Two children died before discharge from the hospital (2%). One additional patient died after 48 months when complications developed during a urological procedure at another hospital.

Fifty-five patients presented with a lipoma of the filum terminale and 158 with a lipoma of the conus medullaris. In the filum terminale group, 28 were asymptomatic at the initial operation, and 27 presented with symptoms. Of the asymptomatic children with a lipoma of the filum terminale, none worsened after surgery, and all remained asymptomatic throughout follow-up (mean follow-up, 3.4 years). Benefits were also observed for the symptomatic patients in this group; no cases of further deterioration were noted, and the clinical status of five patients returned to normal. In the conus group, 71 patients were asymptomatic at initial surgery, and 87 presented with symptoms. The condition of 9 of the 71 children with a lipoma of the conus medullaris who underwent prophylactic surgery later deteriorated (mean follow-up, 6.2 years), and these children required a second untethering operation, which resolved all symptoms in four cases. Thus, the condition of 5 of the 71 deteriorated, whereas 66 (93%) of the children remained normal throughout the period of follow-up. On the other hand, of the 87 patients who underwent surgery after the onset of symptoms, the condition of 36 (41%) deteriorated further, and they required subsequent reoperation. In these 87 children, the final outcome at the end of follow-up (mean follow-up, 6.6 years) was as follows: the condition of 20 (23%) had deteriorated in comparison with the initial presentation, 44 (51%) remained at initial clinical baseline, and 23 (26%) improved or returned to normal clinical status. Prophylactic surgery in the case of asymptomatic infants with a spinal lipoma showed a clear benefit. A good outcome was also observed when surgery was carried out after the onset of symptoms. Prophylactic surgery had a better general outcome by actuarial calculations when only patients with a follow-up of more than 5 years were considered. Deterioration occurred in 5 (16.7%) of the children with a follow-up of more than 5 years, whereas 25 (83.3%) remained normal. Furthermore, in patients who underwent prophylactic surgery, not only was the incidence of deterioration requiring reoperation smaller, but the time interval between initial surgery and the need for reoperation was longer than in the patients who underwent surgery after the onset of symptoms. Spinal lipomas should be managed surgically as soon as possible on a prophylactic basis, with careful and constant follow-up to permit prompt reintervention in cases with deterioration (1).

HINDBRAIN DYSFUNCTION. Nearly all patients born with a myelomeningocele have occasional problems of hindbrain dysfunction (8). Of the first 118 patients, 32% had serious sequelae of hindbrain dysfunction, and 11% died of hindbrain dysfunction. These represented 73% of all deaths in the myelomeningocele group; therefore, hindbrain dysfunction is now the major cause of death in children with myelomeningocele.

In the first cohort, comprising 118 patients, 13 had severe problems (apnea, cyanosis, gastric reflux with aspiration) during the neonatal period and required repeated hospitalizations and surgical procedures to manage the sequelae. One of the 13 children was born with vocal cord paralysis. In the other 12, problems developed during the neonatal period. Four of the 13 underwent posterior cervical decompression to treat progressive respiratory pauses and apnea. Two of these four died. One still requires a tracheostomy, and one has recovered. Of these 13 patients, 11 (85%) ultimately died.

HYDROCEPHALUS. In the study of the natural history of myelomeningocele by Laurence (6), hydrocephalus was evident clinically in 73% of the children. Shunting was attempted in 53 (13%) of the 407 patients but probably was not effective in any case. The hydrocephalus was arrested in 8 (15%) of the 53 children.

In the study of Bowman and McLone (2), 85% of the 118 children in the first cohort showed clinical evidence of hydrocephalus and required shunting; 15% were not shunted. In this group, however, not all the children were evaluated radiologically. In the second cohort, comprising 100 children, routine ultrasonography of the head detected ventricular dilation in 95%. Shunts were required in 90% of these 100 children; 10% were not shunted. In a third cohort, comprising nearly 100 patients, a pattern similar to that seen in the second cohort has emerged. Thus, it would appear that approximately 10% of patients with myelomeningocele do not require shunt diversion of the cerebrospinal fluid (CSF).

In the entire cohort of 285 patients, ventricular enlargement developed in 264 (93%) of the patients (9). Of the 264 with enlarged ventricles, 245 (93%) were shunted. Thus, 86% of the entire group received shunts. The size of the ventricles varied after shunting: 40% of the patients had slit ventricles, 20% had ventricles of normal size, and 40% had enlarged ventricles. Intelligence quotient (IQ) did not correlate with ventricular size except in extreme cases. No differences in IQ were noted among any of the groups based on ventricular size until the ventricles were 4+ dilated after shunting (<1 cm of the cortical mantle). Only 14% of the surviving children with 4+ ventricles have an IQ above 80, whereas 70% of all the other children have an IQ above 80. The shunt revision rate in the children with slit ventricles is twice that of the other groups combined.

INTELLIGENCE QUOTIENT. In the study of Laurence (6), half the children who survived with moderate to severe hydrocephalus had an IQ above 85. Several children were well above average. In the past decade, several studies have claimed a significant reduction in IQ when the myelomeningocele is associated with hydrocephalus severe enough to require a shunt. Soare and Raimondi (10) evaluated 173 unselected children with a myelomeningocele. The mean IQ of those with myelomeningocele alone was 102. The mean IQ of children with myelomeningocele and hydrocephalus was 87, a significant difference. Put differently, 87% of those with myelomeningocele alone had an IQ above 80, whereas only 63% of those with myelomeningocele and hydrocephalus had an IQ above 80. If allowances are made for the heterogeneity of patient populations, differences in treatment regimens, and variations in the tests used to evaluate IQ, it appears valid to conclude that the IQ can be expected to be significantly lower when the myelomeningocele is associated with hydrocephalus. However, an uncontrolled variable affected the results.

As previously reported, the mean IQ of those who did not require a shunt was 102. The mean IQ of those patients who were shunted but remained infection-free was 95. This value is not significantly different from the IQ of the nonshunted group. Those children who were shunted in whom a CNS infection subsequently developed had a mean IQ of only 73 (11). This value is significantly different from those for the other two groups. Put differently, of those who did not require shunting, 87% had an IQ above 80. Of those who were shunted in whom a CNS infection later developed, only 31% had an IQ above 80. Thus, our data indicate that hydrocephalus alone is not a significant limiting factor in ultimate intellectual growth, but CNS infection is. Control of shunt infection must be a major concern for all physicians treating patients with myelomeningocele.

The IQ is not the sole predictor of performance. Studies have demonstrated that as many as one half of children with myelomeningocele may have some learning disability (12). The degree of learning disability in our first two cohorts has yet to be determined. Recent evidence indicates that this problem is really an attention deficit with hyperactivity. Fortunately, it responds remarkably well to methylphenidate (Ritalin).

Routine assessment of a child's intellectual function is valuable not only in projecting future competitiveness but also in providing an indication of shunt function. We have seen a number of children with subtle shunt malfunctions that were discovered on medical psychological evaluation.

Today, 50% of the young adult survivors are either in college or have graduated.

URINARY CONTINENCE.
Before 1975, many children with myelomeningocele underwent a series of urinary diversion procedures intended to minimize the loss of renal function resulting from infection. Because of the consequences of these procedures, including the odor of urine, these children became social pariahs. Since 1975, clean intermittent catheterization and pharmacotherapy have made it possible for such children to develop social continence of urine; they can avoid incontinence in social functions and behave like other children by maintaining a schedule of self-catheterization (or parent-performed catheterization) in the bathroom. They do not have normal neuromuscular control of urination, but they can engage in normal social behavior.

In our series, nearly 85% of the adults have been able to achieve social continence of urine. Urinary diversions are now rare. More than 100 patients in our total clinical population have undergone reimplantation procedures ("undiversions") during the last 10 years. A small number of selected children have been treated with artificial sphincters. As a result, they no longer exude an objectionable odor of urine. The children are accepted by their peers and can be placed in regular schools and educated with the mainstream of society.

In five (7%) of the patients in the lipoma group, symptoms remained stable or improved in some cases, but not all. Symptoms did not worsen after the second operation. The symptoms that improved greatly, with parameters returning to initial clinical baseline after the second operation, were the following: foot deformity, or fibula-deviated foot (1 case), weakness (2 cases), spasticity (1 case), pain (1 case), gait difficulty (2 cases), urinary incontinence (3 cases), and urinary retention (1 case). The following symptoms remained stable: scoliosis (2 cases), foot deformity (1 case), weakness (1 case), and incontinence (2 cases).

Life-long monitoring of urinary function is critical in this population. Infection, high pressure, and reflux can insidiously degrade renal function.

COMMUNITY AMBULATION AND SCHOOLING.
Patients are designated "community ambulators" if they can move about the community without the use of a wheelchair. Because of their motor deficits, many patients require reciprocal braces, canes, and walkers to help them maintain an erect posture and be community ambulators. As these children become older, however, their increase in their body weight may exceed their increase in motor strength, so that they face progressive difficulty in walking. Many ultimately become wheelchair-bound.

As adults, most patients with myelomeningocele who have thoracic level function require a wheelchair to be mobile. Nevertheless, we do not approve of placing these children in a wheelchair immediately. Rather, we start them in the erect position and then "graduate" them to a wheelchair if necessary. Electing to use a wheelchair must not be seen as a failure. Rather, the children choose to use a wheelchair to conserve energy for other activities of daily living. Socially, it is more important that these patients be able to move about the community to accomplish their business than that they do so with a brace rather than a chair.

Complete ambulation data are available for 73 survivors in our first cohort of 118 patients with myelomeningocele. Ambulation was precluded in 13 children with severe CNS involvement in the form of significant mental retardation, hypotonia, or both. These children are unlikely to become competitive and independent. In the children without such CNS involvement, the community ambulation rate is 89%. This rate represents 50% of all surviving children and 50% of the original cohort of 118. Community ambulation was achieved by 100% of the patients with sacral or lower lumbar myelomeningocele. Community ambulation was achieved as children by 63% of those with higher lesions. Use of the reciprocating brace has markedly increased the number of children with thoracic level function who ambulate. However, it is likely that the number of thoracic level ambulators will decrease with time and that the wheelchair will become the preferred method of locomotion for such patients in the community.

Almost all patients treated aggressively as children remain ambulatory as adults. For all patients with dysraphism, life-long monitoring of lower-extremity motor function is essential. The causes of deterioration are treatable.

COMPETITIVE INDIVIDUALS.
An IQ of 80 or higher makes it likely that a child will be able to compete successfully in society as an adult and become a self-supporting, tax-paying citizen. Persons with an IQ below 80 are unlikely to become competitive. Our data indicate that approximately 25% of unselected children with myelomeningocele will survive in a noncompetitive condition. Mental retardation, hindbrain dysfunction, and hypotonia are the most common causes of an inability to compete successfully.

Adult survivors are presenting the medical community with a new challenge. Our medical and surgical colleagues who principally treat adult patients have not often been exposed to the growing population of adolescents before seeing them for the first time as young adults. They may then lack the special expertise developed by those of us who "grew up" with these patients. This is especially true of specialists in gynecology and obstetrics.

It is also obvious that in addition to efforts to fill the medical needs of these patients, major programs should be directed toward job training and employment.

Late Complications

A gradual deterioration in neurological function was for a long time assumed to be the natural history of children with a myelomeningocele. This assumption has been proved wrong. It is now quite clear that neurological deterioration should not occur, at least into adulthood, provided that the late complications of myelomeningocele are sought and treated diligently. These major late complications include Chiari II malformation (13,14), tethering by scarring of the spinal cord to the closure (15,16), and hydromyelia leading to scoliosis, spasticity, and loss of function.

CHIARI II MALFORMATION. In a few patients, the hindbrain dysfunction associated with Chiari II malformation continues to present problems through childhood into adolescence and early adulthood. Pain at the base of the skull and neck posteriorly, nystagmus, weakness in the upper extremities, lower cranial nerve symptoms, and either hypotonia or spasticity are common features of this problem. Early recognition and treatment can preserve function and occasionally prevent sudden death. These symptoms almost always indicate a shunt malfunction. Therefore, optimal function of the shunt must first be determined before posterior cervical decompression is considered. Posterior cervical decompression, when indicated, is much more likely to be effective in correcting symptoms in this age group than in newborns.

Late progressive scoliosis and spasticity may insidiously destroy a patient's ability to function. Scoliosis develops proximal to the level of the myelomeningocele and is not associated with vertebral anomalies. The role that Chiari II malformation and cervical compression play in this late deterioration is not clear. Hydromyelia (see below) usually communicates with the ventricular system, and the hydromyelia can often be managed by restoring ventricular shunt function. A shunt malfunction is the first problem to be ruled out when hydromyelia is present and certainly must be corrected before cervical decompression is undertaken. Resolution of the neurological deterioration resulting from decompensated hydromyelia after cervical decompressive laminectomy and plugging of the obex has been reported (17). This procedure is based on the hydrodynamic theory and usually ineffective.

Many patients with progressive scoliosis, spasticity, or both show little evidence of hindbrain compression and no hydromyelia. We also see segmental hydromyelia or syringomyelia and occasional holocord hydromyelia, which does not appear to communicate with the ventricular system.

When scoliosis fails to respond to a shunt revision, release of a tethered cord is indicated, even if evidence of hindbrain compression and hydromyelia is found on magnetic resonance imaging (MRI).

HYDROMYELIA. *Hydromyelia* signifies dilation of the central canal of the spinal cord, just as *hydrocephalus* signifies dilation of the ventricles of the brain. In patients with myelomeningocele, CSF has been shown to pass from the ventricles to the central canal via the iter of the central canal at the level of the obex. Thus, hydromyelia may be a consequence of untreated or inadequately treated hydrocephalus.

The most common symptoms of hydromyelia include rapidly progressive scoliosis, weakness of the upper extremities, spasticity, and an ascending motor loss in the lower extremities.

In patients with myelomeningocele, an incidence of hydromyelia ranging from 50% to 80% has been reported. This wide variation probably reflects variations in how well the hydrocephalus was controlled and how diligently the diagnosis was sought, and also the difficulty of making the diagnosis accurately before the advent of computed tomography (CT) and MRI. In our series, CT and MRI demonstrated hydromyelia in 40% of the cases studied.

Several methods are available to investigate the causes of late deterioration in spinal cord function (18–21). MRI is the diagnostic tool of choice. In patients with symptomatic hydromyelia, even when the findings on head scans are unchanged from those on previous examinations, it must be determined that the shunt is actually working properly before other forms of therapy are undertaken. In several of our cases, we revised the shunt without noting any changes on CT and were rewarded with dramatic improvement or stabilization of the scoliotic curve. When the MRI is diagnostic, we presently favor a minimyelogram with CT and only low concentrations of contrast, not fluoroscopy, to determine the presence of either a tethered cord or hydromyelia.

Kyphoscoliosis is often present in patients with myelomeningocele. It is very often progressive in patients with retethering of the cord by scar or with hydromyelia. Therefore, kyphoscoliosis should be viewed as a symptom of an underlying problem. Hydromyelia must be sought specifically in any patient with very rapidly progressive scoliosis. In these cases, effective treatment of the hydromyelia is often associated with regression of the curvature. It is hoped that with aggressive treatment of tethered cord and hydromyelia, the incidence of kyphoscoliosis will be reduced to less than 20%.

Once persistence of hydromyelia despite a functioning shunt has been demonstrated, and if hindbrain compression is detected on MRI, then posterior cervical decompression is indicated if clinical evidence of hindbrain compression is also present. We prefer posterior cervical decompression and rarely placement of a shunt from the fourth ventricle to the subarachnoid space. If this procedure fails or if clinical or MRI evidence of hindbrain compression is lacking, we place a shunt from the central canal to the pleural cavity.

Aggressive treatment of the hydromyelia at the onset of scoliosis is mandatory. We were able to improve or stabilize the curve in 80% of cases.

Progressive lordosis is often associated with a tethered cord. In the absence of a vertebral anomaly, thoracic or upper lumbar scoliosis with a low lumbar or sacral level myelomeningocele is almost invariably the result of a treatable lesion. Occasionally, the cause is hydromyelia; more often, it is a tethered cord.

In adults, maturation of the spinal column makes spinal curvature less likely, and therefore deterioration in bladder, bowel, and lower-extremity function is more likely.

RETETHERING OF THE SPINAL CORD. Limitation of movement at the distal end of the spinal cord can produce a variety of symptoms consequent to deterioration of cord function. Fixation or tethering of the end of the spinal cord allows intermittent "bow stringing" of the spinal cord between the normal cephalic attachment and the point of the tether in both myelomeningocele and spinal cord lipoma. The distal cord vasculature is attenuated by stretching, so that the distal spinal cord is subjected to intermittent ischemia that leads to myelomalacia. We believe that middle and upper levels of the spinal cord are compressed anteriorly against the apices of the thoracic curved vertebral column, and deterioration resulting from chronic cord compression can lead to scoliosis.

The most common symptoms of cord tethering in patients with a myelomeningocele or lipoma of the spinal cord are a deterioration in bladder function, subtle atrophy, pain, progressive foot deformities, ascending motor loss, and scoliosis. Commonly, the pain radiates to the legs, especially during exercise. Pain, sensory loss, and motor loss often do not follow dermatomal patterns. The patient may exhibit lordosis and a bent-knee posture on standing. Hip dislocation in a patient previously doing well may be the first sign of neurological deterioration. Bladder and bowel dysfunction or a change in the catheterization pattern may signal an urgent situation requiring immediate attention.

In addition to these signs of cord tethering, patients with myelomeningocele often exhibit subtle changes in muscle tone, usually spasticity and muscle functional loss. These changes are often insidious and can be detected only with a scheduled routine of close follow-up observation. Routine examinations of muscle function have proved very useful for the early detection of this problem. Other investigators have reported that routine measurement of somatosensory evoked potentials reliably detects early spinal cord deterioration.

We have operated on and followed closely several hundred cases of retethering of the spinal cord after primary repair of a myelomeningocele. Thirty-three of these cases were part of the first cohort of 118 patients, so that the incidence of retethering appears to be at least 33% in patients repaired by our technique (22,23). We believe that the incidence of retethering may be related to the type of initial repair. Tight closure that restricts the underlying neural elements creates a serious risk for both immediate ischemic cord damage and later retethering of the spinal cord. Loose or patulous closure provides a generous CSF compartment in which the cord can float away from the surgical scar. In addition, when it is possible to roll the neural placode into a tube with the use of pial–pial sutures, one can sequester the raw tissue of the neural placode deep to the glistening pia of the "remade" cord and reduce the raw surface most likely to scar to a vertical middorsal suture line. In our experience, both factors help to reduce the incidence of rescarring and certainly make release much easier.

Of the 100 patients with retethering of the cord, 38% had associated hydromyelia and 16% had an inclusion (epi)dermoid tumor. Progressive scoliosis was the presenting symptom in 50%, motor loss in 51%, and spasticity in 40%. Pain was the principal complaint in two patients.

Following release, the scoliosis improved in 53%, stabilized in 14%, and progressed in 33%. Spasticity improved or decreased in 64% and remained stable in 36%. Bladder and bowel function improved in 25%, and pain was relieved in 100% of the patients. Motor improvement was noted in 57%, although motor function was worse in three patients; the legs of one were significantly weaker after release, but the scoliosis improved markedly. We are at present hoping to develop better methods to manage spasticity.

A frequent difficulty is that neither Chiari II malformation or tethered cord can be excluded, or both conditions are contributing to the problem. We have simultaneously decompressed the cervical spinal cord and untethered the cord at the same operation in these cases. If the patient's condition precludes a double procedure, we would at present release the tethered cord first.

Retethering in patients with lipoma remains a problem throughout life. Retethering is much more frequent in children and adults who were treated late after symptoms developed.

OTHER CAUSES OF LATE COMPLICATIONS. It must be stressed again that subtle shunt malfunction can mimic any of these conditions and can cause all the signs of deterioration already mentioned. It is therefore essential to establish first that the shunt is indeed functioning properly. Other treatable causes of late deterioration in neurological function include syringobulbia, inclusion (epi)dermoids, arachnoid cysts, missed thick filum terminale, and diastematomyelia.

The clinical presentation of syringobulbia is essentially the same as the late manifestations of Chiari II malformation. Although it has not been reported in other series, we have now seen three cases. MRI demonstrates the lesion well, and intraoperative ultrasonography localizes the cavity within the brainstem (24). We have managed syringobulbia with laser fenestration and placement of a small tube from the cavity to the subarachnoid space. Dramatic, almost immediate improvement has occurred in children managed by this method.

Arachnoid cysts produce symptoms similar to those of tethered cord. MRI is less effective than the mini-myelogram in identifying the lesion. Once the cyst has been identified, the outer membrane is totally or partially removed and the cavity is made to communicate with the subarachnoid space.

Diastematomyelia and a thick filum terminale are the result of incomplete evaluation at the time of initial repair of the myelomeningocele. The symptoms are those of a tethered cord and an asymmetrical neurological deficit in the lower extremity. CT with myelography or MRI should delineate both these problems. The treatment is the same as for either of these lesions in the absence of a myelomeningocele. In addition, it is usually necessary to untether the distal spinal cord at the closure site.

The signs and symptoms of an inclusion (epi)dermoid cyst are difficult to separate from those of a tethered cord because the two are almost invariably associated.

Summary

Late deterioration is common in patients with dysraphism. Most and possibly all deterioration can be prevented or corrected. Late deterioration is not simply part of the natural history of these diseases.

Only through close follow-up by trained observers can problems be anticipated and discovered early. Regularly scheduled evaluations of intellectual, musculoskeletal, and urinary systems are essential.

The medical and surgical needs of adults with these complex diseases represent a major challenge to that part of the medical community that sees only adults. It is likely that many of the problems of childhood will follow these patients into adult life. Psychiatric and reproductive issues remain a great unknown. Shunt malfunction remains the killer of the young adult with a myelomeningocele. Often, such malfunction is missed by neurosurgeons until the patient's condition rapidly deteriorates, at which time survival is unlikely or irreversible damage has been sustained. Pediatric surgical specialists must work with their adult counterparts to ensure the quality survival of this large population now reaching adulthood.

When the clinician is familiar with the signs and symptoms of the various causes of deterioration and is armed with ultrasonography, myelography, CT, and MRI, the most likely cause can be identified and a treatment plan outlined.

References

1. La Marca F, Grant JA, Tomita T, et al. Spinal lipomas in children: outcome of 270 procedures. *Pediatr Neurosurg* 1997;26:8–16.
2. Bowman R, McLone DG. Spina bifida outcome: a twenty-five year perspective *Pediatr Neurosurg* 2001;34:114–120.
3. McLone DG. Treatment of myelomeningocele: arguments against selection. *Clin Neurosurg* 1986;33:359–370.

4. McLone DG. The handicapped newborn: diagnosis, prognosis and outcome—the neonatal view. *Issues Law Med* 1986;2:15–24.

5. McLone DG. Results of treatment of children born with a myelomeningocele. *Clin Neurosurg* 1983;30:407–412.

6. Laurence KM. The natural history of spina bifida cystica: detailed analysis of 407 cases. *Arch Dis Child* 1964;39:41.

7. Lorber J, Salfield S. Results of selective treatment of spina bifida cystica. *Arch Dis Child* 1981;56:822–830.

8. Caldarelli M, Di Rocco E, McLone DG. Chiari II malformation: clinical manifestations and indications for decompression. In: McLaurin R, ed. *Spina bifida: a multidisciplinary approach*. New York: Praeger Publishing, 1986:174–181.

9. Storrs BB. Ventricular size and intelligence in myelodysplastic children. *Concepts Pediatr Neurosurg* 1988;8:51–57.

10. Soare PL, Raimondi AJ. Intellectual and perceptual motor characteristics of treated myelomeningocele children. *Am J Dis Child* 1977; 131:199–204.

11. McLone DG, Czyzewski D, Raimondi A, et al. Central nervous system infections as a limiting factor in the intelligence of children with myelomeningocele. *Pediatrics* 1982;70:338–342.

12. Agnes P, McLone DG. Learning disabilities in children with a myelomeningocele (*personal communication*).

13. Fernbach SK, McLone DG. Derangement of swallowing in children with myelomeningocele. *Pediatr Radiol* 1985;15:311–314.

14. Tomita T, McLone DG. Acute respiratory arrest: a complication of malfunction of the shunt in children with myelomeningocele and Arnold-Chiari malformation: a report of three cases. *Am J Dis Child* 1983;137:142–144.

15. McLone DG, Naidich TP. Spinal dysraphism: experimental and clinical. In: Holtzman RNN, Stein BM, eds. *The tethered spinal cord*. New York: Thieme-Stratton, 1985:14–28.

16. McLone DG, Naidich TP. Myelodysplasia and tethered spinal cord. In: Tachdjian MO, ed. *Pediatric orthopaedics*. Philadelphia: WB Saunders, 1989.

17. Park TS, Hoffman HJ, Hendrick EB, et al. Experience with surgical decompression of the Arnold-Chiari malformation in young infants with myelomeningocele. *Neurosurgery* 1983;13:147–152.

18. Naidich TP, Harwood-Nash DC, McLone DG. Radiology of spinal dysraphism. *Clin Neurosurg* 1983;30:341–365.

19. Naidich TP, Maravilla K, McLone DG. The Chiari II malformation. In: McLaurin R, ed. *Spina bifida: a multidisciplinary approach*. New York: Praeger Publishing, 1986:164–173.

20. Naidich TP, McLone DG, Fulling KII. The Chiari II malformation: part IV. The hindbrain deformity. *Neuroradiology* 1983;25:179–197.

21. Naidich TP, McLone DG, Harwood-Nash D. Spinal dysraphism. In: Newton TH, Potts DG, eds. *Computed tomography of the spine and spinal cord. Modern neuroradiology*, vol 1, Clavadel Press, San Francisco 1983:299–355.

22. McLone DG. Technique for closure of myelomeningoceles. *Childs Brain* 1980;6:65–73.

23. Reigel D, McLone DG. Myelomeningocele: operative treatment and results—1987. *Concepts Pediatr Neurosurg* 1988;8:41–50.

24. Shkolnik A, McLone DG. Intraoperative real-time ultrasonic guidance of intracranial tube placement in infants. *Radiology* 1982;144: 573–576.

188. Transoral Approach to the Upper Cervical Spine and Skull Base

Stephen L. Ondra and
Geoffrey P. Zubay

A variety of pathological conditions arise anterior to the spinal cord at the craniovertebral junction. Access to this area is made difficult by the pharynx, vascular anatomy, and lower cranial nerves. The pathological conditions that commonly affect the region include both benign and malignant disorders. These range from posterior displacement of the odontoid by rheumatoid pannus to a variety of primary and metastatic malignancies.

The upper anterior cervical spine and skull base can be accessed via a transoral, direct lateral, or transcervical approach. The latter two approaches are dealt with in other chapters. The transoral route is the one most commonly used for extradural pathology that lies between the lower third of the clivus and the C2-3 disc space in the sagittal plane and within 1.5 to 2.0 cm of the midline. Pathology located beyond these anatomical parameters is, in our opinion, better dealt with via either of the other two approaches. We prefer the transcervical approach for lesions arising within the dura because of the difficulty of transoral dural closure and the morbidity associated with a cerebrospinal fluid (CSF) to the pharyngeal fistula (1).

Preoperative Evaluation

The radiographic assessment should include magnetic resonance imaging (MRI) and usually computed tomography (CT). This combination assists in delineating the extent of bony deconstruction and soft-tissue tumor. The extent of a lesion should be carefully assessed to ensure that decompression can be carried out within the anatomical limits of whichever approach is to be used.

Attention should also be given to mouth opening. A minimum of 2.5 cm is needed to obtain adequate exposure and access to the posterior pharynx (2). Conditions such as rheumatoid arthritis, which are commonly associated with the types of pathology treated transorally, often limit mouth opening.

A tracheostomy is rarely required for this approach. We typically perform a simultaneous tracheostomy only if a problem affecting swallowing or ventilation is present before surgery, such as lower cranial nerve palsy, vocal cord paralysis, or swallowing dysfunction.

We utilize fiberoptic oral intubation rather than transnasal intubation. Although the latter is often convenient for the prolonged intubation typically required in this procedure because of airway edema, we find that it frequently obstructs our view, particularly in the region of the soft palate. This problem can lead to the need for a larger split of the soft or hard palate and the increased morbidity that attends such exposure. Aerobic and anaerobic cultures of the nasopharynx are obtained in the office. Antibiotics are utilized only if a pathological flora is present. We also utilize broad-spectrum antibiotics if a CSF leak occurs. Antibiotics are continued for 7 days after the leak has been closed.

Although fluoroscopy remains the mainstay of intraoperative imaging, we have recently begun to use image guidance to augment and confirm the resection of pathology. Image guidance typically involves the placement of cranial fiducials and scanning of the fiducials and pathology. Accurate intraoperative registration demands stable anatomy. An alternative method is to utilize fluoroscopic image guidance techniques. These can be helpful in cases of mobile anatomy at the craniovertebral junction.

Operative Technique

The patient is positioned on an operating table that will accommodate anteroposterior and lateral fluoroscopy. The head is padded in a foam head holder. We typically avoid Mayfield pin fixation. If a posterior fusion is not planned as part of the procedure, the head is placed on a foam pad, or a neutral head position can be maintained with 5 to 10 lb of Gardner Wells skull traction. If an occipital cervical fusion is planned as part of the procedure, we typically place the patient in halo fixation before surgery. In this way, optimal head positioning for both daily function and swallowing can be assessed before fusion. After intubation, the anterior posts can be removed until completion of the operation to facilitate access.

After fiberoptic oral intubation is carried out and examination stability is confirmed, the patient is placed under general anesthesia. We typically use somatosensory monitoring because of the upper cervical cord and brainstem compression typically associated with such lesions.

A pharyngeal throat pack (vaginal packing of 1.0- or 0.5-in gauze) is placed manually into the upper pharynx below the caudal extent of the pathology. A suture is affixed to the throat pack before insertion to facilitate retrieval postoperatively. This prevents blood, bone, preparative solutions, and other material from being swallowed or potentially aspirated. A 10% povidone solution is used to prepare the mouth and pharynx.

After draping, a Crockard retractor system is utilized for access (Figs. 1 and 2). A soft plastic mouth guard is fitted on the upper teeth blade and seated against the upper dentition. The ratcheted tongue blade is then seated to the posterior aspect of the tongue, and the system is ratcheted open to expose the posterior pharynx. Care should be taken that the posterior tongue is retracted but the tongue blade does not press on the pharynx. After the retractor is placed, we use the operating microscope to help with lighting, vision, and magnification.

The superior and inferior exposure is now assessed (Fig. 3), typically with fluoroscopy. If the apex of the pathology can be reached by elevating the palate, the palatal retractors are placed without splitting the soft palate. The endotracheal tube can also be retracted. If the apex cannot be reached by retracting the soft palate, the palate must be split in the midline. First, a solution of lidocaine and 1:200,000 epinephrine is injected, then the soft palate is incised in the midline. This midline split will deviate to the right or left when the uvula is reached. In rare cases, the soft tissue over the hard palate can also be incised and a small portion of the bone removed to extend the reach cephalad. Once the soft palate is split and hemostasis is obtained, the retractors are placed.

The midline of the spine is identified and injected with the same local anesthetic and epinephrine solution. A midline incision in the posterior pharyngeal mucosa is made from just above to just below the area of dissection and resection. The longus colli and longus capitis muscles are dissected free with

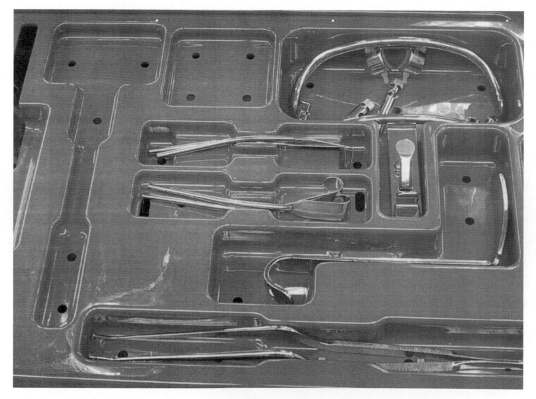

Fig. 1. Crockard retractor instrument tray for transoral access to the upper cervical spine.

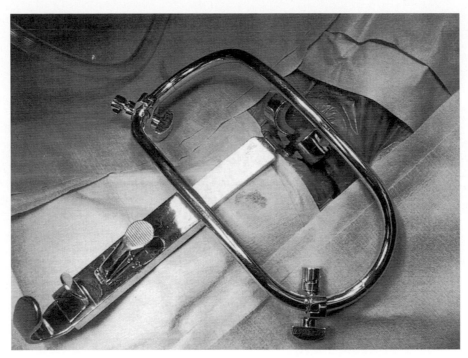

Fig. 2. Crockard retractor inserted into mouth and oral pharynx.

a combination of subperiosteal retractors and Bovie electrocautery. The pharyngeal retractor is placed during this process to facilitate exposure. A subperiosteal dissection is carried out for at least 1.0 cm to each side of the midline. If the pathology demands, this can be extended on one or both sides to a distance of 1.5 cm. Lateral dissection beyond 1.5 cm or, in cases of optimal anatomy, 2.0 cm risks injury to such posterior pharyngeal structures as the carotid artery, eustachian tubes, and vertebral artery (1,2).

After exposure is complete, resection begins. We typically use a high-speed gas-powered drill to remove bone. If pathology has not eroded C1, we begin with this. After removal of the C1 arch to 1.0 cm on each side of midline, the remainder of the pathology can be addressed. If the odontoid is to be resected, removal should begin at the apex, with gradual complete removal of the C2 body. In this way, a free-floating odontoid that is difficult to handle and remove is avoided. We prefer to identify the odontoid apex and lateral walls clearly before resection. A Penfield dissector is used to assess the odontoid tip and right and left base to its posterior edge (Figs. 4 and 5). In this way, the completeness of dissection is not in doubt. Fluoroscopy is very helpful to ensure that the apex is completely removed. Care should also be taken to ensure that lateral bone is completely removed. In the case of odontoidectomy,

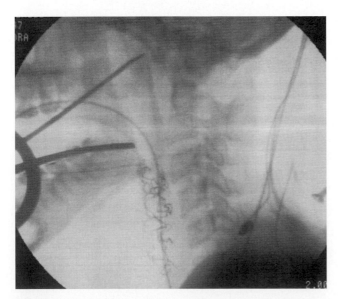

Fig. 3. Penfield dissector inserted after the soft palate has been elevated to assess whether access to the odontoid apex is possible without splitting the soft palate.

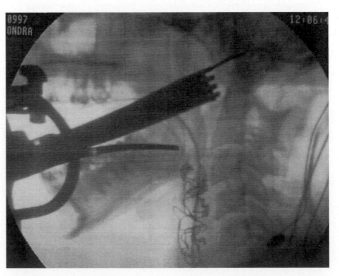

Fig. 4. Apex of the odontoid assessed with Penfield dissector.

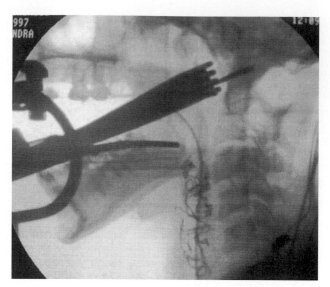

Fig. 5. Lateral aspect of the odontoid base assessed to its posterior margin.

we prefer complete definition of the entire odontoid to include the lateral borders before resection.

After bony exposure, the pathology is removed (Fig. 6). Fluoroscopy or imaging is performed to ensure that the resection is complete. The dura is fully decompressed of both pathology and areas of bony compression. The tectorial membrane is also removed. The dura should be pulsatile to ensure that it is fully decompressed.

If a CSF leak is encountered, it should be repaired immediately. Attempts at repair with suture can be difficult, and few surgeons have much experience with this. More often, a combination of fibrin glue, tight closure, and CSF diversion for 4 to 7 days is used and typically is successful.

Closure is accomplished in layers. The muscle is closed in one or two layers with 2-0 polyglycolic suture in a simple interrupted manner. Long vascular or cardiac (Castro) needle holders are helpful. Instrument ties are needed unless the patient

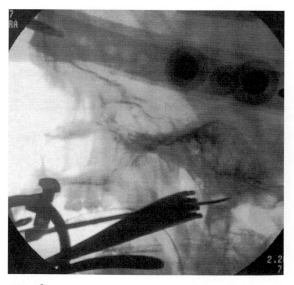

Fig. 6. Base of resection assessed with a Penfield dissector.

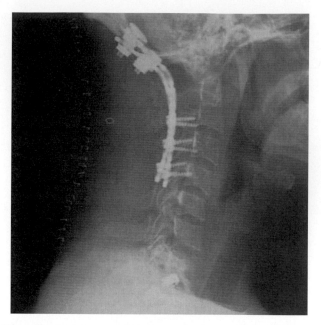

Fig. 7. Occipitocervical fusion and instrumentation following transoral odontoid resection.

has a short pharynx. The mucosa is closed with 2-0 or 3-0 polyglycolic suture in a simple interrupted manner. The tongue blade is relaxed enough to withdraw the throat pack. A feeding tube is inserted through the nose and into the esophagus and stomach. It should pass the pharyngeal closure under direct vision to ensure that it does not injure or compress the dura.

If the soft palate has been opened, it is now closed. The posterior mucosal wall is closed with 3-0 polyglycolic suture. The same suture can be used to close any muscular layer. The anterior inferior palate mucosa is then closed in a simple manner with the same 3-0 suture. All the sutures are placed about 5.0 mm apart.

The Crockard retractor is removed. The feeding tube is sewn into the nasal septum with 0 monofilament suture. Care should be taken not to tie tightly to the septum. The endotracheal tube is secured to an upper tooth with a wire or suture. These steps are performed to ensure that neither of the tubes is removed inadvertently.

If a posterior fusion is required, typically this can be carried out in the same sitting (Fig 7). All patients with rheumatoid arthritis, and many others, require this. If the situation is unclear, the patient should be kept in a collar and undergo flexion and extension fluoroscopy 5 to 7 days postoperatively to establish stability (1–3).

Postoperative Care

The patient is kept intubated until swelling of the tongue and pharynx has resolved to the point at which the patient can ventilate easily without a tube. This typically takes 2 to 4 days. In older patients, it may take longer. When extubation is planned, an ear, nose, and throat and an anesthesia consult should be available. A fiberoptic scope is placed down the tube to facilitate reinsertion if necessary. In case of airway emergency, a tracheostomy can be performed. Standard intubation should be avoided before of the risk to the pharyngeal wound and underlying dura.

The patient is sedated throughout the period of intubation. Mouth care consists of cleaning the teeth and gums two to three times daily with a nystatin solution. Instructions are posted not to insert dental care or suction beyond the teeth or anterior third of the tongue. It is important that the entire staff responsible for care be made aware of the risk for injury to the posterior pharynx.

Nutrition is maintained with enteral feedings via the nasogastric feed tube for 1 week. If wound healing is proceeding normally, a full liquid diet is begun at the end of the first week to 10 days. At the end of 2 weeks, a dental soft diet is begun. If the wounds are well healed, a regular diet is begun in 3 to 4 weeks.

Complications

The most common complication is wound dehiscence (1). If this occurs, debridement and primary repair should be performed immediately. Typically, an ear, nose, and throat consult is involved in wound revision. Wound breakdown of the pharynx is typically visible. Breakdown of the palate is associated with regurgitation into the nasopharynx during swallowing, or a change in voice tone.

Infection and abscess are surprisingly rare (1,2). They are associated with fever, airway difficulty, or new difficulty in swallowing. This is a surgical emergency and requires immediate drainage.

Dural tears and CSF leakage are managed with fibrin glue and CSF diversion, as discussed earlier. Arterial injury can be packed. In carotid injury, if the pressure must be reduced, neck compression can be performed. If needed, an injured vessel can be embolized or occluded.

If neurological deterioration develops, the patient should undergo imaging to rule out retained pathology, bony compression, or abscess.

Associated Procedures

If access cannot be obtained via the transoral root and the pathology lies in the midline, an adjunct to extend the midline incision should be considered. This includes a Leforte I extended maxillotomy (drop-down maxillotomy), mandible dislocation, or median glossotomy and midline mandibulotomy (4, 5). These procedures allow extension superiorly or inferiorly. They also significantly increase morbidity. When the pathology is limited to the C1-2 region, the less morbid anterior transcervical or direct lateral exposure should be considered (6–8).

Conclusions

The transoral approach provides quick and relatively easy access to extradural lesions that lie within 1.5 cm of the midline between the lower third of the clivus and C2-3. The retractor systems designed for this exposure have significantly shortened the procedure and improved access. Careful attention should be given to the comorbidity often associated with such pathology. The presence of comorbidity typically means that an occipital cervical fusion will accompany this procedure.

Recovery is relatively rapid after the first week. Postoperative complications are typically associated with wound breakdown and less commonly infection.

References

1. Menezes AH. Complications of surgery at the craniovertebral junction: avoidance and management. *Pediatr Neurosurg* 1992;17: 254–266.
2. Menezes AH, VanGilder JC. Transoral–transpharyngeal approach to the anterior craniocervical junction: a 10-year experience with 72 patients. *J Neurosurg* 1988;69:895–903.
3. Dickman CA, Locantro J, Fessler RG. The influence of transoral odontoid resection on stability of the craniovertebral junction. *J Neurosurg* 1992;77:525–530.
4. James D, Crockard HA. Surgical access to the base of skull and upper cervical spine by extended maxillotomy. *Neurosurgery* 1991;29: 411–416.
5. Maloney F, Worthington P. The origin of the LeForte I maxillary osteotomy: Cheevers operation. *J Oral Surg* 1984;39:731–734.
6. McDonnell DE, Harrison S. Transcervical approach to the upper cervical spine. In: *Principles of spinal surgery*. New York: McGraw-Hill, 1996.1307–1323.
7. Shucart WA, Borden JA. Lateral approaches to the cervical spine. In: *Principles of spinal surgery*. New York: McGraw-Hill, 1996: 1325–1332.
8. Shucart WA, Kleriga E. A lateral approach to the upper cervical spine. *Neurosurgery* 1980;6:278–281.

189. Anterolateral Approach to the Craniocervical Junction and Rostral Cervical Spine

John R. Vender,
Steven J. Harrison, and
Dennis E. McDonnell

The management of lesions in the region of the craniocervical junction (CCJ) can present a significant therapeutic challenge. When the appropriate surgical approach to this region is being selected, several factors must be considered. Most importantly, predominantly ventral pathology is often best addressed via an anterior or anterior lateral surgical approach. Stability of the region must also be ascertained. Instability may be the result of pathological involvement of the ligamentous and osseous structures in the region, or it may occur secondarily as a result of surgical decompression. In either event, stabilization with fusion and instrumentation must be planned before the decompressive procedure.

The transoral approach to the CCJ has gained widespread popularity (1–12). This technique provides straightforward access to the C1 arch and odontoid process. However, the approach has several limitations. The rostral–caudal extent of the exposure is significantly limited, and if access to more caudal cervical segments is needed, then the transoral approach is not adequate. Also, with optimal lateral dissection, the operative field remains relatively narrow, and the treatment of lesions any distance from the midline can be challenging. Individual patient factors, such as the opening angle of the mandible and extent of the hard palate, can also significantly limit a straightforward transoral approach, so that a more involved cranial base procedure is required. Furthermore, although intradural surgery via the transoral route has been reported, the contaminated oral cavity and difficulties in dealing with a cerebrospinal fluid (CSF) fistula are relative contraindications to the transoral approach for intradural lesions (13–15).

In up to 75% of patients who undergo transoral odontoidectomy, particularly if the middle third of the anterior arch of the atlas is also included, the region is unstable, and supplemental fusion with instrumentation is required (16–18). Although a limited number of reports have described the placement of anterior fusion and instrumentation constructs via the transoral approach (19,20), the preferred method of arthrodesis remains a posterior occipitocervical fusion. This can be performed either during the same surgical setting or at a later time. In either case, a second surgical exposure is required. Also, with incorporation of the occiput, occipitocervical mobility is sacrificed.

The high anterior cervical, retropharyngeal approach to the CCJ has been described previously (21–29). Via this approach, wide bilateral exposure is possible. With some modification of the dissection, the entire cervical spine can be exposed. Also, a C1-3 fusion can be performed during the same surgical setting with only a minimal increase in operative time. In this way, the need for a second, posterior procedure is obviated, and occipitocervical mobility is preserved. Although the approach has not become as widely popular as the transoral procedure, with careful attention to the anatomical layers of the upper cervical region and a wide, sharp, cadaveric dissection, it can be safely mastered by most spine surgeons.

Preoperative Assessment

Many patients requiring surgery in the region of the CCJ are significantly compromised preoperatively, both medically and neurologically. In many cases, the patient is chronically debilitated or using steroids. It is essential to communicate clearly to the patient and family the extent of this undertaking. Patients should expect a long convalescence regardless of the surgical technique selected. Preoperatively, the nutritional, immunological, and neurological status must be optimized. An evaluation for the presence of chronic infections must be carried out, and any such infections treated, before surgery is undertaken. In some cases, parenteral or enteral nutritional support must be implemented preoperatively. Placement of a feeding tube (if not already present) will be necessary before the cervical spine surgery. The feeding tube is usually maintained for 3 months, at which time it can be discontinued if the patient is taking adequate oral nutrition. The patient must also anticipate a prolonged intubation. Previously, a tracheostomy was placed before the high anterior cervical approach was begun. In our recent experience, however, we have been able to utilize endotracheal tubes successfully, with delayed extubation on approximately the fifth postoperative day. A halo orthosis is also required, and patients are advised that this will have to be worn for a minimum of 3 months.

High Anterior Retropharyngeal Approach

PERIOPERATIVE PREPARATION. Patients undergo fiberoptic, awake intubation. After intubation, neurophysiological monitors are placed for the evaluation of somatosensory evoked potentials and motor evoked potentials. If intradural surgery is anticipated, a lumbar drain can be placed preoperatively before final positioning to facilitate CSF drainage during the procedure and assist with CSF diversion postoperatively. Because most patients require halo immobilization postoperatively, a halo head ring is placed after the induction of anesthesia and is affixed to the operating table. A three-pin Mayfield head holder can also be used. The surgical side is selected to allow access to the side of greatest pathology if the lesion is asymmetrical. For midline or symmetrical lesions, a left-sided approach is routinely selected by the authors. The head is extended 15 degrees and rotated 30 degrees away from the side of surgery. With appropriate extension and rotation of the head, the angle of the mandible is elevated up and away from the surgeon's line of sight. If autograft fascia or fat may be required, the patient's thigh can be prepared on the side of the surgical approach. If autograft cancellous bone is required, the ipsilateral lower abdominal quadrant is also prepared to allow access to the iliac crest. In most cases, a central venous catheter and radial arterial line are placed. Prophylactic antibiotics providing gram-positive coverage and stress-dose steroids (if necessary) are administered.

DISSECTION OF SOFT TISSUE. A horizontal skin incision is created 2 cm inferior and parallel to the mandible. Care must be taken to avoid injuring the marginal mandibular branch of the facial nerve. The incision begins 1 cm from the midline contralateral to the surgical side and extends to the posterior border of the anterior belly of the ipsilateral sternocleidomastoid muscle. Subcutaneous tissues are extensively dissected free from the underlying platysma muscle to create two subcutaneous flaps that can be easily retracted (Fig. 1). With the platysma widely exposed, an incision is created vertically in the midline raphe. After this midline fascial raphe (linea alba) has been opened, the platysma muscle is transected horizontally in line with the original skin incision. With dissection of the deep surface of the platysma, both flaps of muscle can be retracted from the surgical field (Fig. 2). At every subsequent step of the cervical dissection, it is important to identify the fascial investment of each individual structure (30). With wide, sharp dissection of each of the fascial planes, adequate exposure of the retropharyngeal space is possible with minimal retraction. With elevation of the platysma muscle, the inferior margin of the submandibular gland is visualized. Careful dissection of the fascial capsule of the submandibular gland mobilizes the structure. The gland is elevated with the aid of a self-retaining retractor in a cephalic direction. Care must be taken not to injure the glandular stroma to avoid the risk for wound sialorrhea. The facial artery and vein can be identified posterior, lateral, and deep to the submandibular gland. With dissection and mobilization of the facial artery and vein, it is possible to retract these structures superolaterally. On occasion, it is necessary to ligate the facial vein. After the facial artery and vein have been mobilized, the tendon of the digastric muscle is identified running

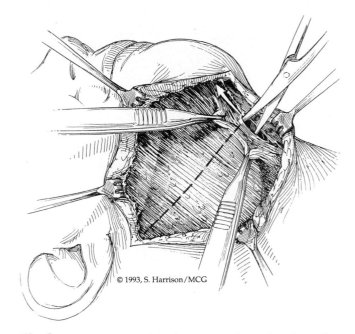

Fig. 2. The medial extent of the platysma muscle is split in the midline from the mental symphysis to the superior notch of the thyroid cartilage. The muscle is then transected along the line of the original skin incision (*dotted line*).

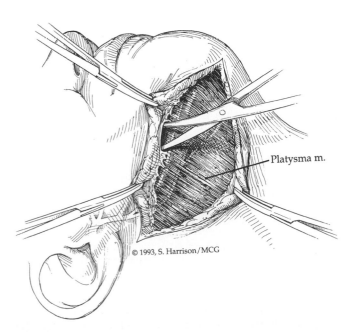

Fig. 1. The skin incision is 2 to 3 cm below and parallel to the mandible. Subcutaneous tissues are dissected from the underlying platysma muscle.

parallel to the skin incision deep to the inferior margin of the submandibular gland (Fig. 3). This tendon is tethered by a fascial sling to the hyoid bone. With transection of the fascial sling, the tendon is freed. With additional dissection of the undersurface of the anterior and posterior bellies, the digastric muscle can be retracted rostrally. The next structure to be identified is the hypoglossal nerve, which is deep and slightly inferior to the digastric tendon. The hypoglossal nerve runs parallel to the digastric tendon. With dissection of the fascial planes around the hypoglossal nerve, the nerve can also be safely mobilized rostrally. Deep to the hypoglossal nerve are the hyoglossal muscles. At this point in the dissection, the greater wing of the hyoid bone is visible. Occasionally, this bone must be palpated to be identified. The fascia overlying the hyoid bone is incised along the bone laterally to the carotid sheath. The carotid artery can then be gently retracted laterally to provide access to the lateral retropharyngeal space (Fig. 4). At this point in the dissection, care must be taken to avoid injury to the superior laryngeal nerve. Although this nerve runs deep to the internal carotid along the middle pharyngeal constrictor muscles in a course oriented toward the superior wing of the hyoid and adjacent to the superior pharyngeal constrictor muscle, it can be injured by excessive retraction. Wide dissection of each subsequent tissue plane minimizes the amount of force necessary for exposure of the retropharyngeal space and thereby reduces the risk for injury to the superior laryngeal nerve. If more caudal dissection and exposure of the cervical spine are required, then this nerve must be identified, isolated, mobilized, and retracted from the surgical field. The pharyngeal muscles are retracted medially with a deep right angle retractor. The areolar tissue of the retropharyngeal space is opened sharply with scissors and bipolar electrocautery. The anterior tubercle of C1 and the anterior surfaces of the C2 and C3 vertebral bodies are easily palpated through the remaining soft tissue. It is critical during this part of the procedure to remember the orientation of the patient's spine with rotation of the head. The ipsilateral lateral mass of C1 is higher, in some cases, than the anterior tubercle and may

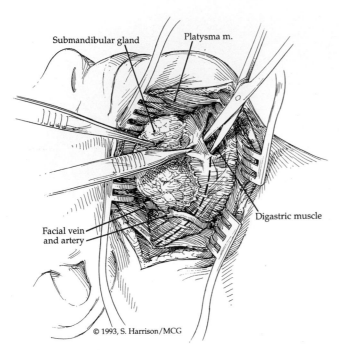

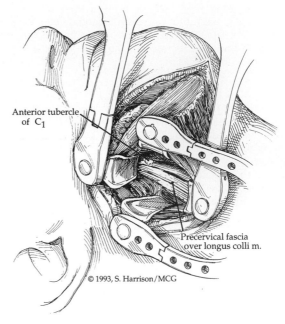

Fig. 3. The submandibular gland is elevated, and the fascial plane deep to the gland is opened. The digastric muscle and tendon are then visualized. The facial artery and vein are seen at the lateral extent of the exposure.

Fig. 5. With retraction of the lateral pharyngeal wall, the anterior tubercle can be seen. The convergence of the longus colli muscles at the anterior C1 tubercle is demonstrated. Of note is the minimal distortion of the C1-2 anatomy. However, with elevation of the ipsilateral C1 lateral mass, care must be taken to identify the C1 tubercle accurately.

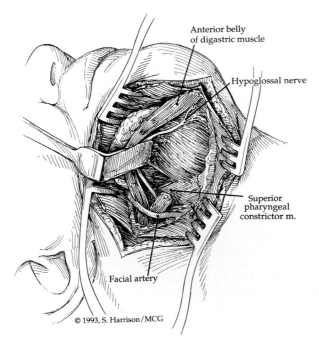

Fig. 4. After sectioning of the fascial band overlying the digastric tendon and careful dissection of the fascial investments of the digastric muscle and hypoglossal nerve, these structures can be safely retracted rostrally. The lateral pharyngeal wall and superior pharyngeal constrictor muscles can then be visualized.

actually be palpated instead of the anterior tubercle (Fig. 5). If the lateral mass is mistaken for the anterior tubercle, the remaining soft-tissue dissection will be misdirected. The longus colli and longus capitis muscles are freed from their insertion on the ventral surface of the vertebral bodies. With a standard high anterior cervical, retropharyngeal approach as described, the C2-3 disc space is located in the caudal portion of the dissection. Also, with palpation of the C1 arch, a surgical level can be determined. On occasion, with a prominent soft-tissue mass, an intraoperative roentgenogram or fluoroscopic image is helpful to confirm orientation at this point. Freeing the soft tissue from the ventral surface of the upper cervical spine is facilitated by use of the KTP laser. A self-retaining retractor can then be fixed to the superior surface of the anterior arch of C1 and retracted rostrally with rubber bands attached to the surgical drapes.

CORPECTOMY. After the vertebral bodies have been exposed and the surgical orientation has been confirmed, the odontoid process and body of C2 can be removed with a 5-mm round cutting burr. The cutting burr is utilized until only a thin cortical shell of bone remains. The corpectomy can then be completed with a 3-mm diamond burr, Kerrisen rongeurs, or curettes. It is important to begin removing bone at the apex of the dens and proceed caudally to reduce the risk for disconnecting the dens from the C2 vertebral body. If this should happen, the mobile dens may cause injury to the underlying neural tissues during the final bone removal. Significant epidural veins are encountered during the corpectomy. These are often very difficult to control with bipolar electrocautery but can be easily managed with Avitene, cottonoids, and patience. It is usually unnecessary to remove the arch of C1 to complete the C2 corpectomy. In isolated cases, the inferior, posterior portion of the anterior arch can be thinned to allow better visualization. Care

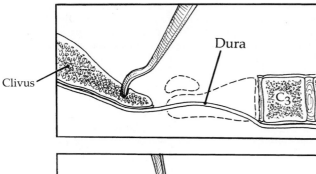

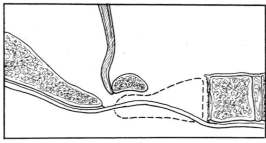

Fig. 6. The C2 corpectomy defect is noted (*dotted lines*) in both diagrams. On completion of the decompression, the dura can be seen to be bulging into the corpectomy defect. The C2-3 disc has been completely removed, and the C3 vertebral body has been freed of its cartilaginous end plate. In the top diagram, the arch of C1 has also been removed, and the self-retraining retractor has been inserted into a notch in the caudal portion of the clivus. The bottom diagram depicts the more typical location of the retractor on the rostral surface of the anterior arch of C1.

must be taken, however, to not undermine the structural integrity of the C1 arch, particularly if a C1-3 arthrodesis is planned.

A complete discectomy of the C2-3 intravertebral disc is also performed. Attention must be given to complete removal of the cartilaginous end plate of C3. Occasionally, a dental mirror is helpful in visualizing the posterior portions of this end plate because the end plate of C3 angles away from the surgeon's line of sight.

On occasion, the anterior arch of C1 is involved in the pathological process and must be removed along with C2. In these rare cases, the arch of C1 can easily be removed before the C2 resection. After resection of C1, the clivus can be identified rostral to the odontoid process. A notch can be created in the clivus with a 3-mm cutting burr to receive the self-retaining retractor that will allow rostral exposure during the remainder of the surgery (Fig. 6).

EPIDURAL SPACE. After the corpectomy has been completed, the laser is again helpful in resecting the ligamentous structures in the epidural space. By means of careful dissection with a small dissecting tool, the transverse ligament can be elevated from the ventral dural surface. The ligament is then incised sharply in the midline and dissected laterally, where it is cut and removed from the epidural space. Again, attention must be given to the venous structures in the lateral recesses of the exposure. Frequently, significant amounts of reactive pannus tissue can be resected most efficiently with the laser. Decompression of these soft-tissue elements must be extended into the lateral epidural space. On completion of an adequate decompression, the dura will be noted to be bulging and pulsating into the corpectomy defect.

INTRADURAL SURGERY. If an intradural lesion is present, the dura can be opened at this time. This is usually performed with a midline incision under microscopic visualization. The microscope is particularly helpful during this procedure for both magnification and illumination. After the dura has been opened, the lumbar drain can also be opened to reduce the CSF present in the wound. Intradural lesions can be easily dealt with via this approach. In the case of most ventrally located intradural masses, the lower cranial nerves can be identified deep and lateral to the abnormality. The dura can then be closed primarily with a running Neurolon suture, or an autogenous or allograft patch can be placed. This also is secured to the dura with a running nylon suture. After suture closure of the dura, the suture lines are reinforced with fibrin–thrombin glue (31).

C1-3 ARTHRODESIS. In most cases, the authors perform a C1-3 arthrodesis with anterior cervical plating (32). Various options are available for arthrodesis, including allograft or autograft ilium and allograft humerus. The authors prefer to use allograft humerus because the circumferential cortical bone confers greater structural integrity to the graft. The distance from the inferior surface of the arch of C1 to the superior end plate of C3 is carefully measured with calipers. The humerus is then fashioned with a notch on its cephalic end such that the distance between the base of the notch and the inferior edge of the graft is equal to the C1-3 distance. The graft extends 1 to 1.5 cm above the notch. In addition, it is important to measure the width and depth of the corpectomy defect and compare this with the diameter of the humeral allograft. Occasionally, some shaving with a cutting burr is necessary to decrease the diameter of the graft. The cancellous cavity of the graft can then be cleared of residual trabecular bone with a cutting burr and filled with morcellated autograft. If the C2 vertebral body is not involved in the pathological process, then the C2 body alone will provide adequate bone graft material. If the C2 body cannot be used or is inadequate in volume, and if the patient has no systemic disorder of bone, then cancellous autograft can be harvested from the iliac crest. If autograft is not an option, crushed cancellous allograft bone mixed with demineralized bone matrix putty has been used with success. After hemostasis has been ensured in the epidural space, the notched end of the humeral allograft is inserted around the anterior arch of C1. The inferior end of the graft is then seated onto the superior end plate of C3. Often, a 1-cm-wide curved osteotome can be used as a lever to aid in positioning the inferior end of the graft. The osteotome is inserted over the superior end plate of C3 with the concave portion of the blade oriented inferiorly. As the graft is tapped into position, gentle elevation of the osteotome will distract the C1-3 interval and guide the inferior portion of the allograft into the defect (Fig. 7). Occasionally, a small degree of beveling of the posterior, inferior surface of the humeral allograft is necessary to facilitate this maneuver. Such beveling, if necessary in rare cases, must be minimized to avoid the risk for decreasing purchase on the C3 body.

ANTERIOR CERVICAL INSTRUMENTATION. An anterior cervical plate is utilized to secure C1-3. It is imperative that a plate of adequate length be selected. This can be challenging because after placement of the allograft, the anterior arch of C1 is no longer visible. With the aid of a lateral fluoroscope or lateral roentgenograms, a plate of appropriate length can be identified. Ideally, the top of the plate should end at the level of the top of the arch of C1 when the tops of the inferior-most screw holes are at the level of the C3 end plate. Two bicortical screws are placed into C1. Guide holes are drilled through the anterior notch of the graft and through both cortices of C1.

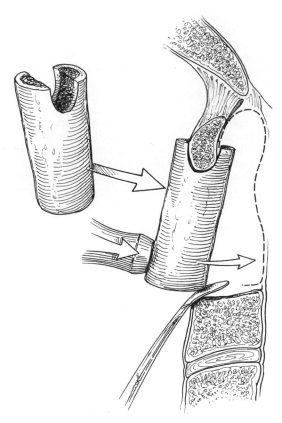

Fig. 7. The notched end of the humeral allograft is seated onto the undersurface of C1. The curved osteotome over the superior end plate of C3 facilitates placement of the inferior end of the graft.

These cortical surfaces can be felt easily as the drill passes through them. Lateral fluoroscopic images can also help, although they may be disoriented. It is not necessary to engage the posterior notch of the graft. Two bicortical screws are then placed into the vertebra of C3. The authors believe that the bicortical purchase adds extra biomechanical strength to this construct. After the C1 and C3 screws have been placed, one or two additional screws are inserted through the midportion of the plate through the anterior cortex of the graft. These screws help stabilize the graft by increasing resistance to rotational forces (Fig. 8). Pin and screw placement is facilitated if a fluoroscope is utilized during this portion of the procedure because numerous roentgenograms may be required.

ARTHRODESIS AND INSTRUMENTATION AFTER REMOVAL OF C1 AND C2.
If the anterior arch of C1 is structurally inadequate or if it has been removed because it is involved in the pathological process, two options are available for arthrodesis. An allograft humerus can be fashioned to incorporate the clivus rostrally and the superior end plate of C3 caudally. A plate can then be affixed to the clivus and the anterior surface of C3. In most instances, however, this construct is of questionable stability, and the authors have opted to perform a posterior occipitocervical fusion.

ARTHRODESIS AND INSTRUMENTATION INVOLVING MORE CAUDAL SPINAL SEGMENTS.
If additional, more caudal vertebral bodies are also removed because of ventral compression below the level of C2, then a longer strut can

be fashioned. In some cases with compression secondary to unresectable ventral masses (e.g., multiple intradural neurofibromas), no arthrodesis is placed. A bone graft in these instances will only reconstruct the compression that was relieved by the original corpectomy. In these rare cases, the patient is maintained in traction, and a posterior cervical fusion is performed within the next several days.

CLOSURE. Before wound closure, it is essential to ascertain that hemostasis has been achieved. This is confirmed with gentle elevation of the blood pressure or Valsalva maneuvers. The wound is then flooded with saline solution, and air is injected into a nasogastric tube placed into the pharyngeal region by the anesthesiologist. If no bubbles are seen in the wound, the pharyngeal wall is deemed intact. At this time, the exposure is closed as in any anterior cervical procedure. The precervical fascia is approximated with absorbable sutures. The platysma muscle and subcutaneous tissues are reapproximated as separate layers. A subcuticular closure of the skin edges can then be performed. The placement of wound drains is optional and has not been found to be necessary.

POSTOPERATIVE CARE. Patients are transported to the neurological critical care unit postoperatively. They remain intubated for a minimum of 3 days after surgery to allow edema in

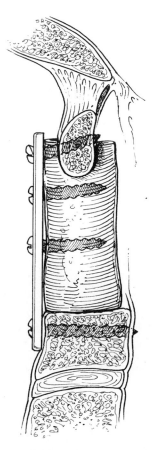

Fig. 8. The placement of bicortical screws into the anterior arch of C1 and the C3 vertebral body securely fixes the anterior cervical plate. The upper screws do not have to engage the posterior portion of the allograft. Two additional screws have been placed through the ventral cortex of the allograft to help stabilize the graft.

the pharynx and retropharyngeal space to resolve. Weaning of mechanical ventilatory support, however, should begin immediately after reversal of anesthesia to reduce the degree of respiratory muscle deconditioning. This is particularly important for patients who had neuromuscular impairment preoperatively. Enteral nutrition is begun immediately postoperatively and maintained for several weeks. Although nasojejunal tubes are occasionally adequate, we prefer obtaining surgical enteric access after the induction of anesthesia and before the start of the cervical surgery. As the patient's oral intake improves, the use of enteral feeds can be gradually tapered. The tube is easily removed, usually 2 to 4 weeks after surgery.

If a lumbar drain was placed preoperatively because of a need for intradural surgery, or postoperatively for inadvertent dural injury, CSF drainage is continued for 5 days postoperatively. Any method acceptable to the individual surgeon for controlling CSF drainage is adequate; however, we have been using a pump-regulated drainage strategy (33). In adult patients, the optimal rate of drainage appears to be 12 to 14 mL of CSF per hour. Drainage is continued for 3 to 5 days postoperatively.

The halo head ring that was placed in the operating room before surgery is connected to a halo vest. The patient is maintained in the halo orthosis for 3 months. At that time, the halo posts are loosened and a flexion and extension roentgenogram is obtained. If radiographic evidence is found that fusion is not complete, halo bracing is continued, and this maneuver is postponed for an additional 6 weeks. If radiographic evidence of fusion is present and the patient maintains alignment during flexion and extension, the halo can be removed, and the patient is placed in a rigid cervical collar for an additional 6 weeks. If evidence of radiographic fusion is not present at 18 weeks, or if evidence of movement is noted during flexion and extension despite apparent radiographic fusion, the patient is replaced in the halo and an elective posterior occipitocervical fusion is performed. In our series to date, adequate fusion was not achieved via the anterior construct in only one patient, who required a posterior fusion.

CSF fistula occurred in six patients. In three cases, the patients had undergone resection of intradural tumors. In all cases, CSF diversion was adequate to control the fistula, and no patients required reexploration at the cervical site. In two cases, lumbar drains were placed to treat persistent CSF leaks. Wound infection of the superficial cervical tissues occurred in one patient. This was treated with irrigation, debridement, and placement of a closed irrigation drainage system. The hardware and graft did not have to be removed. Most patients reported dysphagia in the immediate postoperative period. In all but one case, this cleared spontaneously within 1 to 2 weeks of surgery. One death on the first postoperative day was caused by myocardial infarction. In all cases, neurological function after decompression was unchanged or improved in comparison with the preoperative baseline.

Solid fusion was achieved in 9 of the 10 patients treated with anterior fusion constructs. One fusion failure occurred. In this patient, who had advanced rheumatoid arthritis and had been taking steroids for a prolonged period, the anterior arch of C1 was mechanically inadequate to support the fusion construct. The strut graft migrated ventrally through the anterior arch of C1. This was noted clinically when, after an initial improvement, the patient's neurological function regressed to the preoperative baseline. The anterior construct was removed, and the patient underwent an occipitocervical fusion. During the original surgery, a small portion of the inferior portion of the arch of C1 had been resected to facilitate removal of the reactive tissues. The reduction of atlantal bone combined with advanced disease and abnormal bone structure rendered the anterior arch of C1 structurally inadequate to resist the translational forces applied to it. This case of fusion failure emphasizes the importance of minimizing resection of the arch of C1 and intraoperatively determining the suitability of the arch of C1 for anterior arthrodesis. In cases of a congenitally small or abnormal arch or an arch heavily involved in the pathological process, or in the rare cases in which excessive resection of the arch of C1 is required for adequate decompression, the decision to proceed with posterior stabilization is warranted.

Results

Twenty-nine patients have undergone high anterior cervical, retropharyngeal corpectomies. In two patients, additional corpectomies were performed caudal to C2. An anterior arthrodesis with anterior cervical plating was performed in the 10 patients most recently undergoing C2 corpectomy. No patient required removal of the C1 arch as part of the original corpectomy. Before the anterior fusion and instrumentation technique, patients underwent stabilization posteriorly with the Locksley intersegmental tie bar technique (28). Lesions affecting the CCJ are outlined in Table 1.

Table 1. Lesions of the Craniocervical Junction

Pathology	No. patients
Rheumatoid arthritis	6
Pathological fracture of C2	6
Access to ventral foramen magnum region tumors/upper cervical spinal cord tumors	5
Os odontoideum with basilar impression	5
Chronic C2 fracture, nonunion	4
Acute C2 fracture with herniated C2-3 disc	1
Odontoid agenesis	1
Segmentation anomalies with medullary compression	1

Conclusions

The high anterior cervical, retropharyngeal approach to the upper cervical spine provides the surgeon with wide access bilaterally from the clivus to C3. With minimal modification of the dissection, more caudal segments of the cervical spine can be exposed. In addition, via this approach, intradural surgery can be performed safely and arthrodesis with instrumentation can be applied successfully. The option of anterior arthrodesis with instrumentation during the same procedure can spare the patient a second operation and preserve occipitocervical mobility. As always, clinical judgment must be used to determine those cases in which anterior arthrodesis would be suboptimal. This approach avoids the contaminated space of the oral cavity and allows the surgeon greater versatility in dealing with CSF fistula and intradural lesions. If the surgeon understands the anatomical structures in the upper cervical region and uses sharp, wide, cadaveric dissection, the upper cervical spine can be exposed with relative ease. This procedure can be accomplished with instruments widely available at most centers performing spinal surgery and can be mastered by most spine surgeons.

References

1. Apuzzo MLJ, Wise MH, Heiden JS. Transoral exposure of the atlantoaxial region. *Neurosurgery* 1978;3:201–207.

2. Crockard H. The transoral approach to the base of the brain and upper cervical cord. *Ann R Coll Surg Engl* 1985;67:321–325.

3. Crockard HA, Pozo JL, Ransford AO, et al. Transoral decompression and posterior fusion for rheumatoid atlanto-axial subluxation. *J Bone Joint Surg Br* 1986;68:350–356.

4. Di Lorenzo N. Craniocervical junction malformation treated by transoral approach. A survey of 25 cases with emphasis on postoperative instability and outcome. *Acta Neurochir* 1992;118:112–116.

5. Hadley MN, Spetzler RF, Sonntag VKH. The transoral approach to the superior cervical spine. A review of 53 cases of extradural cervicomedullary compression. *J Neurosurg* 1989;71:16–23.

6. Harkey HL, Crockard HA, Stevens JM, et al. The operative management of basilar impression in osteogenesis imperfecta. *Neurosurgery* 1990;27:782–786.

7. Jain V, Behari S, Banerji D, et al. Transoral decompression for craniovertebral osseous anomalies: perioperative management dilemmas. *Neurol India* 1999;47:188–195.

8. Kingdom T, Nockels R, Kaplan M. Transoral–transpharyngeal approach to the craniocervical junction. *Otolaryngology* 1995;113:393–400.

9. Menezes A, VanGilder J, Graf C, et al. Craniocervical abnormalities: a comprehensive surgical approach. *J Neurosurg* 1980;53:444–455.

10. Pasztor E, Vajda J, Piffko P, et al. Transoral surgery for craniocervical space-occupying processes. *J Neurosurg* 1984;60:276–281.

11. Rock JP, Tomecek FJ, Ross L. Transoral surgery: an anatomic study. *Skull Base Surg* 1993;3:109–116.

12. Spetzler RF, Selman WR, Nash CL Jr, et al. Transoral microsurgical odontoid resection and spinal cord monitoring. *Spine* 1979;4:506–510.

13. Bonkowski JA, Gibson RD, Snape L. Foramen magnum meningioma: transoral resection with a bone baffle to prevent CSF leakage. *J Neurosurg* 1990;72:493–496.

14. Crockard HA, Sen CN. The transoral approach for the management of intradural lesions at the craniovertebral junction: review of 7 cases. *Neurosurgery* 1991;28:88–98.

15. Goel A. Transoral approach for removal of intradural lesions at the craniocervical junction [Letter]. *Neurosurgery* 1991;29:155–156.

16. Dickman C, Locantro J, Fessler R. The influence of transoral odontoid resection on stability of the craniovertebral junction. *J Neurosurg* 1992;77:525–530.

17. Dickman CA, Crawford NR, Brantley AGU, et al. Biomechanical effects of transoral odontoidectomy. *Neurosurgery* 1995;36:1146–1153.

18. Menezes A, VanGilder J. Transoral–transpharyngeal approach to the anterior craniocervical junction. Ten-year experience with 72 patients. *J Neurosurg* 1988;69:895–903.

19. Kandziora F, Kerschbaumer F, Starker M, et al. Biomechanical assessment of transoral plate fixation for atlantoaxial instability. *Spine* 2000;12:1555–1561.

20. Kerschbaumer F, Kandziora F, Klein C, et al. Transoral decompression, anterior plate fixation and posterior wire fusion for irreducible atlantoaxial kyphosis in rheumatoid arthritis. *Spine* 2000;25:2708–2715.

21. De Andrade JR, MacNab I. Anterior occipito-cervical fusion using an extrapharyngeal exposure. *J Bone Joint Surg Am* 1969;51:1621–1626.

22. Lesoin F, Autricque A, Franz K, et al. Transcervical approach and screw fixation for upper cervical spine pathology. *Surg Neurol* 1987;27:459–465.

23. McAfee PC, Bohlman HH, Riley LJ Jr, et al. The anterior retropharyngeal approach to the upper part of the cervical spine. *J Bone Joint Surg Am* 1987;69:1371–1383.

24. McDonnell DE. Anterio-lateral cervical approach to the cranio-vertebral junction (atlas-axis-clivus). In: Rengachary SS, ed. *Neurosurgical operative atlas*. Baltimore: Williams & Wilkins, 1991:147–164.

25. McDonnell DE. Anterolateral cervical approach to the craniovertebral junction. In: Rengachary SS, Wilkins RH, eds. *Neurosurgical operative atlas*, vol 1. Baltimore: Williams & Wilkins, 1991:147—164.

26. McDonnell DE, Harrison SJ. Anterolateral cervical approach to the craniovertebral junction. In: Wilkins RH, Rengachary SS, eds. *Neurosurgery*. New York: McGraw-Hill, 1996:1641–1653.

27. McDonnell DE, Harrison SJ. High cervical retropharyngeal approach to the craniovertebral junction. *Perspect Neurol Surg* 1996;7:121–141.

28. Vender JR, McDonnell DE. Management of lesions involving the cranio-cervical junction. *Neurosurg Q* 2001 11:151–171.

29. Whitesides TE, McDonald AP. Lateral retropharyngeal approach to the upper cervical spine. *Orthop Clin North Am* 1978;9:1115–1127.

30. Grodinsky M, Holyoke E. The fascia and fascial spaces of the head, neck, and adjacent regions. *Am J Anat* 1938;63:267–408.

31. Shaffrey CI, Spotnitz WD, Shaffrey ME, et al. Neurosurgical applications of fibrin glue: augmentation of dural closure in 134 patients. *Neurosurgery* 1990;26:207–210.

32. Vender JR, Harrison SJ, McDonnell DE. Fusion and instrumentation at C1-C3 via the high anterior cervical approach. *J Neurosurg (Spine)* 2000;92:24–29.

33. Houle P, Vender JR, Fountas K, et al. Pump-regulated lumbar-subarachnoid drainage. *Neurosurgery* 2000;46:929–932.

190. Special Consideration for the Cervicothoracic Junction and Upper Thoracic Spine

David W. Cahill, D. Mark Melton, and Michael V. Hajjar

Each of the junctional areas of the spine (occipitocervical, cervicothoracic, thoracolumbar, and lumbosacral) presents unique challenges to the reconstructive spine surgeon. Fortunately, the incidence of pathology leading to the need for reconstruction of the occipitocervical and cervicothoracic junctions is relatively low; in contrast, pathological problems are commonly encountered at either end of the lumbar spine (1).

At the cervicothoracic junction, technical problems arise from five anatomical and physiological features. The first challenge is posed by the differences in size and shape of the subaxial cervical versus upper thoracic vertebrae (2). The second challenge is presented by the curve reversal from the upper thoracic kyphosis to the lower cervical lordosis. The third difficulty stems from the mobile nature of the normal subaxial cervical spine versus the immobile nature of the rib-fixed thoracic spine. The fourth difficulty is that posed by the anatomical structures surrounding the cervicothoracic junction and the concomitant difficulties associated with lateral and anterior transcavitary approaches. Finally, these characteristics create reconstructive problems that are not easily overcome with the routine anterior and posterior hardware currently available for use on either the cervical or thoracic spine. In the following pages, each of these challenges is discussed individually, along with the means by which they can be met and overcome.

Variations in Size and Shape

The vertebrae of the lower subaxial cervical spine are small. They have no functional transverse processes. More precisely, the transverse processes are anteriorly translocated and modified into the transverse foramina; these contain the vertebral arteries, injury to which can pose a significant neurological risk (3–6). In addition, the normal enlargement of the cervical spinal cord associated with the second-order control mechanisms for the upper extremities causes a decrease in the ratio of canal diameter to cord diameter, so that little room is left for the safe placement of sublaminar hooks or cables (Fig. 1A).

The "lateral masses" or "facet pillars" of the subaxial cervical spine are also small. If the Magerl technique for placing lateral mass screws is used, purchase is rarely more than 7 or 8 mm (7) (Fig. 1B). Screw diameter is usually limited to 3.5 or 4.0 mm. Large patients may occasionally accept 4.5-mm screws at the upper end of the junction. C7, however, usually has very small, transitional lateral masses, often too thin for any useful screw purchase (8–13) (Fig. 2).

The cervical pedicles are similarly quite small. From C3 to C6, the pedicle forms the medial wall of the transverse foramen. It is often less than 4 mm in minimum diameter and may be almost entirely cortical in composition (14–17). Although the cervical pedicles from C3 to C6 may accept screws in some cases, the risks for pedicle fracture, vertebral artery injury, and nerve root injury are high (Fig. 3). Conversely, the C7 pedicles are usually large enough to accept 4.0-mm screws, although not 5.0-mm screws (2–4).

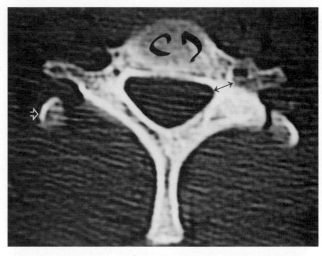

Fig. 2. This C7 vertebra has a vestigial mass on the right and bilateral vestigial transverse foramina that do not contain vertebral arteries. Lateral mass screw placement would be tenuous at best. Conversely, the C7 pedicles can easily accommodate 3.5-mm screws.

Anteriorly, the vertebral bodies of C6 and C7 are usually too small to accept a strut graft or cage any larger than 16 mm in anteroposterior (AP) depth or 20 mm in width (left to right dimension) (3,18). Smaller struts are usually required in young people and women (Fig. 4).

Taken together, these anatomical restrictions limit the dimensions of the anterior and, more importantly, posterior hardware that can be used on the cephalic side of the cervicothoracic junction, so that the devices are mostly smaller than those generally used in the thoracic spine.

On the caudal side of the junction, the upper thoracic vertebrae vary significantly from T1 to T5 (2,19). Although transverse foramina and vertebral arteries are lacking, the transverse processes are usually robust, obscuring the costovertebral junctions when viewed from behind. The spinal cord is relatively small

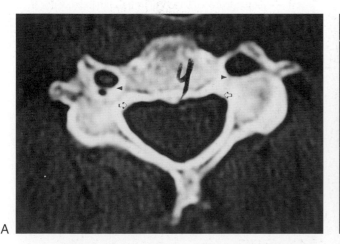

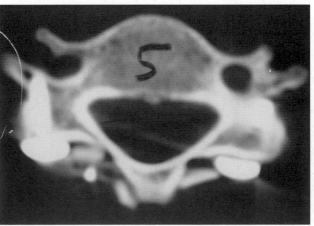

A   B

Fig. 1. **A:** Axial computed tomography (CT) of mid-subaxial vertebra (C4). Note that the pedicles are less than 3 mm in minimum diameter and that transverse foramina are the lateral pedicle wall; spinal canal is the medial wall. **B:** Axial CT of C5 vertebra with typical lateral mass screw. Note bone purchase is only 8 mm, even with use of the Magerl technique.

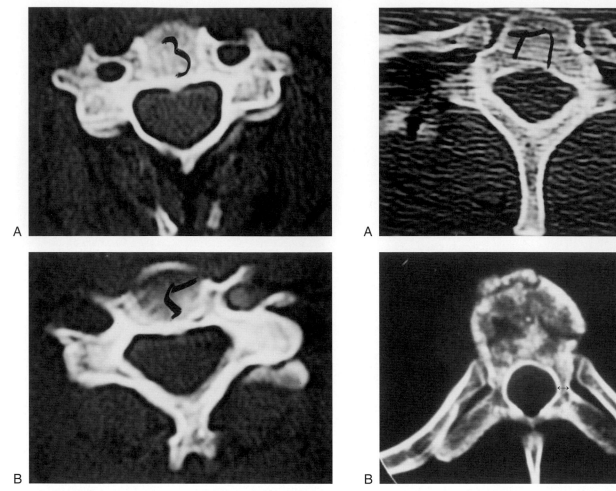

A

B

Fig. 3. **A:** Axial CT of a typical C3 vertebra. Pedicles are 60 degrees off the axial meridian and 3 mm at minimum width. **B:** Axial CT of a typical C5 vertebra. In this case, the pedicles are entirely cortical and without marrow cavities.

Fig. 5. **A:** Typical T1 vertebra has large pedicles easily accommodating 4.5- to 5.0-mm screws. **B:** Typical T3 vertebra with pedicles far too small to accept 5.0-mm screws but with robust laminae and transverse processes.

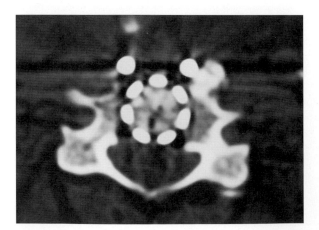

Fig. 4. C5 vertebra in a woman. The interbody cage in this case is a 14-mm cylinder. In a small person, no larger strut can be accommodated.

in the canal, so that lamina-fixated devices are somewhat safer (Fig. 5B).

The pedicles of T1 are usually larger, easily accepting 4.5- or 5.0-mm screws in most adults (20) (Fig. 5A). Unfortunately, the pedicle diameter decreases progressively from T1 to T6, with the pedicles from T3 to T6 rarely large enough to accept a 5.0-mm screw (21,22). On the positive side, the laminae and facet pillars of the upper thoracic vertebrae are relatively robust, and in combination with the similarly substantial transverse processes, they are quite amenable to the placement of hook-fixated devices (23) (Fig. 6).

Anteriorly, the bodies of the upper thoracic vertebrae are usually too narrow in the sagittal (AP) plane to accept more than one transverse screw. Rigid anterolateral devices are not a viable option because of this size limitation (24). The presence of the transverse foramina on the other side of the junction also limits their use (Fig. 6).

Because of these restrictions, it is often difficult to create a suitable biomechanical construct for bridging the cervicothoracic junction (25,26). In general, the hardware commonly used anterolaterally or posteriorly in the thoracic spine is too large to use in the cervical spine, whereas the hardware commonly used anteriorly or posteriorly in the cervical spine is too small to resist the forces applied across an unstable junction.

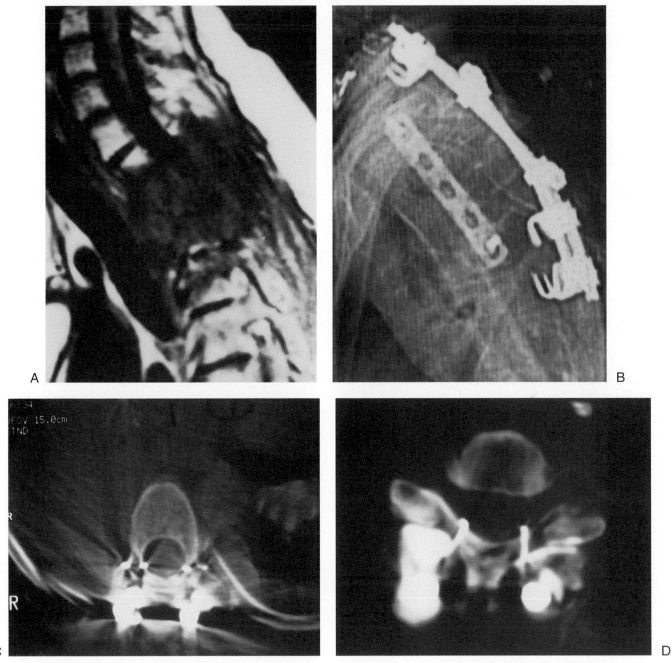

Fig. 6. A 29-year-old woman with Pancoast tumor invading T2, T3, and T4. **A:** Preoperative sagittal magnetic resonance imaging (MRI). **B:** Postoperative lateral radiograph after circumferential resection of T2, T3, and T4, then anterior reconstruction with a fibular strut stabilized with a lateral plate and fixated posteriorly with hook and cable rods. (Lateral thoracotomy allowed simultaneous resection of primary lung tumor. This case is from 1990; today, we use an anterior cage and cervical end pedicle screws.) The anteroposterior (AP) diameter of the upper thoracic vertebrae is usually sufficient for only a single transverse screw. Rigid anterolateral devices are therefore precluded. (We currently usually use staple-fixated single rods in this circumstance.) Sublaminar hooks work well in the upper thoracic spine, where the cord diameter is small and the risk low. In this case, they form the down-going side of the caudal end claw. **C:** Upper thoracic pedicles are usually too small for screws but very suitable for pedicle hooks, as seen here on the up-going side of the caudal end claw. **D:** When cervical end pedicle screws are not feasible, traditional sublaminar wires can be used to fixate rods at the cervical end, as seen here at C6.

Joining Mobile to Immobile Segments

The elliptical cylinder formed by the upper thoracic spine, ribs, and sternum is a relatively rigid container designed to protect the all-important engine components mounted within (8). Conversely, the lower subaxial cervical spine is quite flexible in the sagittal plane and somewhat mobile in the coronal plane. The hinge or pivot point of the junction is highly stressed, with the primary failure made in flexion (see further discussion below) (27).

Relatively focal pathologies, such as C7-T1 facet dislocations, have a well-defined fulcrum or pathological axis of rotation. Diffuse pathologies, such as tumor resections at multiple levels, do not leave a single pivot point but spread the points of maximum stress to the poles of an anterior, weight-bearing construct. The most stressed segment in such constructs is at the lower pole of the anterior construct, if the lengths of the upper and lower portions of the posterior construct are approximately equal. Increasing the relative length of the cephalic (cervical) portion of the construct shifts the pathological axis of rotation cephalad, toward the upper pole of the anterior strut.

Obviously, preservation of mobility in the thoracic spine is unimportant and the length of the thoracic component of bridging constructs largely irrelevant. Too long on the thoracic side is harmless; too short can be disastrous.

Conversely, preservation of movement on the cervical side is surely desirable, and minimization of the number of cervical segments included in the construct is clearly a goal. Nonetheless, the primary pathological vector in such cases is flexion. Failure to obtain adequate purchase on the cephalic side of the axis of rotation risks catastrophic failure of the construct. The goals of adequate purchase and preservation of motion cannot be reconciled with current hardware. The number of cervical motion segments that must be sacrificed depends on the overall length of the anterior reconstructive construct and on whether any cervical segments have been resected anteriorly. For example, a simple acute C7-T1 facet dislocation can generally be repaired with a sacrifice of movement only at C7-T1 (Fig. 7 A,B), whereas a tumor in which the C7 and T1 bodies must be resected often requires a posterior construct extending to C4 (three levels above the upper end of the anterior strut) (Fig. 7 C,D).

On the positive side of this problem is the fact that the greatest stresses placed across all such posterior constructs are at the caudal pole, again because flexion is the primary mode of failure. Strong fixation of the lower pole in the posterior thoracic spine is usually straightforward.

Curve Reversal

Like all the junctional areas of the spine below the occiput, the cervicothoracic junction is normally sigmoid in the sagittal plane. The kyphosis on the thoracic side reverses to lordosis on the cervical side. Almost all the pathological processes that affect the junctional region result in relative hyperkyphosis. Most of the traumatic conditions are caused by flexion–compression injuries. Tumors and infections usually destroy the anterior column first, so that collapse and kyphosis develop. Even degenerative diseases such as ankylosing spondylitis usually result in kyphotic deformity. Hence, in most such cases, restoration of a posterior tension or compression band is required at minimum, and restoration of anterior height and weight-bearing capacity is also often required.

Ambulatory patients present with a high "hunchback" deformity and secondary cervical hyperlordosis above the level of the pathology. Nonambulatory patients use multiple pillows in bed because their heads do not contact the mattress during recumbency. In severe cases, hyperlordosis of the upper cervical spine is not sufficient for patients to be able to see ahead while sitting or standing.

When the patient is prone on an operating table, the head is well below the shoulders, and the table usually must be modified to allow mobile support during the procedure. When the patient is supine, the back of the head must be supported, and the available space between the chin and chest is often minimal.

The correction of kyphotic deformity and restoration of normal cervical lordosis are more difficult than the correction of kyphotic deformity limited to the thoracic spine. Relatively weak or nonrigid bony purchase on the cervical side and concerns about the risks for cervical spinal cord injury with overly aggressive efforts at correction conspire to make curve correction from a single posterior approach less than adequate except in the simplest of cases. Restoration of a sigmoid configuration often requires both anterior and posterior osteotomy procedures, a combination of careful anterior distraction with posterior compression. Compression forces applied across the posterior construct are often limited by the relative weakness of the fixation on the cervical side. External manipulation of the head outside the drapes is often necessary.

In older adults, the normal thoracic kyphosis may approach 45 degrees. Hence, even after correction of a cervicothoracic flexion deformity, an anterior strut graft seated on a normal upper end plate of an upper thoracic vertebrae may lie 30 to 45 degrees from the vertical in the sagittal plane. Unlike subaxial cervical grafts, which tend to fail by ventral extrusion of the lower pole of the graft, grafts that bridge the cervicothoracic junction tend to fail by extrusion of the lower pole into the spinal canal. An anterior cervical type of buttress plate is not adequate to prevent this disaster when used alone (see further discussion below).

Limitations of the Approach

Unlike the approaches to the cervical, lumbar, and even lower thoracic regions, where bony impediments to accessing the spine laterally or anteriorly are minimal, the approaches to the cervicothoracic junction are considerably more difficult. The small, elliptical bony cage formed by the upper ribs and sternum impairs access anteriorly. The scapulae and shoulder girdles impair access laterally. Even posterior midline approaches are more difficult than elsewhere because of the positioning problems created by the flexion deformity of the neck, mentioned above, and the subcutaneous prominence of the bony posterior elements (and, hence, any applied posterior hardware), so that pain and wound breakdown are of concern in many cases.

ANTERIOR LIMITATIONS. With the exception of barrel-chested persons, approaches as low as the T1-2 disc space can usually be accomplished without extraspinal bone work. The presence of the aortic arch makes a true anterior approach below the T4-5 disc space difficult or impossible in most people. Anterior access to the T2, T3, and T4 vertebrae usually requires some form of sternotomy (28). Once the bony obstacles have been overcome, careful handling of the trachea, esophagus,

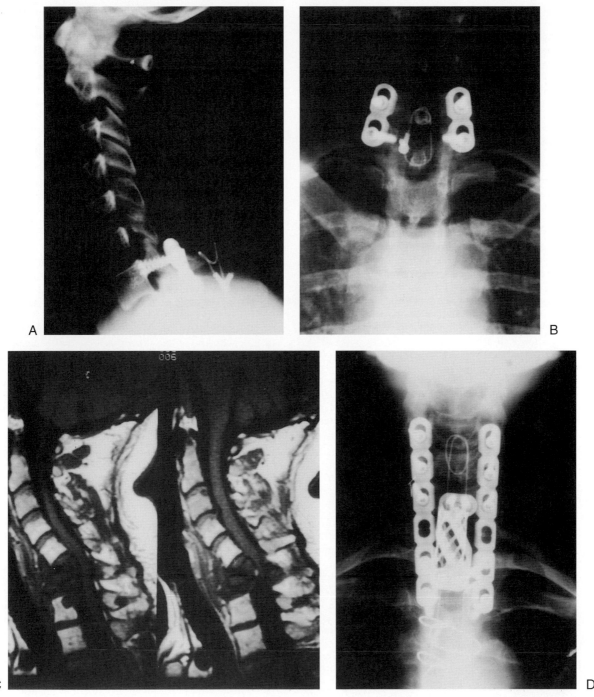

Fig. 7. **A,B:** Postoperative radiographs after reduction of bilateral facet dislocation at C7-T1. Simple posterior construct consisting of T1 pedicle screws, C7 lateral mass screws, and interspinous cable is quite sufficient in the absence of posterior element fractures or ventral pathology. **C,D:** Conversely, in this metastatic tumor involving C6, C7, and T1 **(C)**, a circumferential reconstruction is mandatory, even in the absence of posterior element involvement. Anterior buttress plate fixation is inadequate to prevent late kyphotic collapse **(D)**.

great vessels, recurrent laryngeal nerves, and thoracic duct is necessary (29–33).

Once the anterior aspect of the lower cervical and upper thoracic spine is exposed, many neophytes are very surprised by the obliquity of the thoracic spine as it disappears from the surgeon's view behind the aorta and heart. In a significant flexion deformity, the displaced cephalic part of the spine may completely obscure the normal caudal thoracic spine below the dislocation. Resection of overlapping vertebral bodies is often necessary to visualize and prepare the caudal graft recipient site. As noted above, the seating of the caudal end of bridging cervicothoracic strut grafts or cages is critical to prevent dorsal displacement into the spinal canal with loading (Fig. 8).

LATERAL LIMITATIONS. The upper thoracic spine can also be accessed laterally via a parascapular thoracotomy (34). However, the arms, shoulder girdle, and scapula may impede such an approach. Significant risks for shoulder dysfunction secondary to parascapular muscle transection or to lower trunk brachial plexus injury are inherent in this approach. Another problem arises in that the exposure gained is oblique and limited to T1-2 at its upper most extent, even when the shoulder girdle is well mobilized. Lateral bridging hardware to the cervical spine is rarely feasible with this approach. The approach is most useful when C7 can be preserved and access below T4 is necessary. The entire thoracic spine is easily available through this procedure (Fig. 6).

In summary, the anatomical limitations imposed by the upper thorax and shoulder girdle mean that neither true lateral nor true anterior approaches are feasible. Oblique approaches from either direction are straightforward, but care must be exercised to obtain proper positioning during realignment and graft placement.

Hardware Limitations

Because of the variations in size, shape, and function of cervical vertebrae versus those of the thoracic vertebrae, hardware has been developed that is intended for use in either but not both. Many companies now offer devices for joining their posterior cervical systems to their posterior thoracic systems (Fig. 8), but no device specifically designed to bridge the cervicothoracic junction is available. We address the limitations of the available types of hardware individually in the following paragraphs.

ANTERIOR HARDWARE. A single-level C7 or T1 corpectomy in which the posterior elements are normal can usually be stabilized with an anterior cervical plate alone. An anterior plate alone is inadequate for any more extensive procedure. As noted above, anterior strut grafts are oblique and very likely to fail at the cervicothoracic junction. In grafts that extend for two or more vertebral segments, an anterior cervical plate should be used as no more than a buttress for the graft. Stabilization of the construct must be applied posteriorly (35) (Fig. 8).

Similarly, in an upper thoracic resection performed via a parascapular thoracotomy in which the T1 vertebra is spared, a single lateral rod can sometimes be applied via transverse screws. Such rods are stronger than anterior cervical plates, but they do not resist rotational and seesaw failure. These also should be stabilized posteriorly.

POSTERIOR HARDWARE. The forces applied across the cervicothoracic junction are significant and cannot, in general, be adequately resisted by unconstrained hardware applied to the cervical lateral masses (Fig. 8). Hence, on the cervical side of the construct, pedicle screw fixation or sublaminar cable fixation is preferable (36–38). As noted above, the pedicles above C7 are often, if not usually, too small to accept even 4.0-mm screws. Sublaminar cables are not rigid, tend to loosen over time, and can injure the spinal cord (39). Hence, on the cervical side of such constructs, some combination of pedicle screws, sublaminar cables, lateral mass screws, and interspinous cables must often suffice. Lateral mass screws alone, even when many are placed, are rarely adequate. In weighing strength requirements against risk, the best combination is cervical pedicle screws with interspinous cables. Unfortunately, the cases in which this technique is feasible are the exception rather than the rule.

On the thoracic side, 5.0-mm thoracic-type pedicle screws are usually feasible only at T1 or at T1 and T2. Some combination of hooks must usually be used for T3 through T6. Although hooks are less rigid than screws, they resist pullout well and are far stronger than the purchase obtained by any combination of devices at the cervical end of the construct. Unconstrained cervical plates or rods may bridge the cervicothoracic junction fixated on both sides with 3.5- or 4.0-mm cervical-type screws. Experience has taught that such fixation is inadequate to resist the loads imposed after mobilization.

Cervical lateral mass plates or rods, preferably fixated at least in part with lower cervical pedicle screws, may be joined to thoracic rods with currently available junctional devices (40). Single thoracic rods may also be extended to the cervical spine and fixated with sublaminar cables in a more traditional approach. The former approach is more difficult, not as strong, and less risky; the latter simpler, less rigid, and more dangerous (Fig. 6).

Surgical Approaches

Pathological processes that affect the cervicothoracic junction include trauma and posttraumatic deformity, congenital dysplasias such as hemivertebrae, tumors, infections, and rarely degenerative disc and joint disease. A few of the problems can be successfully dealt with from a single anterior or posterior approach. More commonly, however, a circumferential reconstruction is required. In the following sections, we discuss our current approaches to representative entities, beginning with the one that is simplest to repair.

POSTERIOR-ONLY RECONSTRUCTION. Acute traumatic facet dislocations at C7-T1 are uncommon and potentially missed on initial workup in the trauma bay (41–44). The patients are often neurologically intact or have only root-related symptoms that are frequently mistaken for shoulder trauma. The C7-T1 region is notoriously difficult to visualize on plain lateral radiographs, both at the time of initial workup and subsequently with the intraoperative fluoroscope.

Except in patients who have severe ligamentous disruption (they usually present with paraplegia), closed reduction with traction tongs is often unsuccessful. Our current approach is to attempt closed reduction with weights that are rapidly escalated to 70 to 100 lb. Patients who are intact are given sedatives and muscle relaxants, and 12 to 24 hours is allowed for reduction. Those with partial or complete deficits are taken to the operating room if reduction has not occurred by 2 hours after admission. Magnetic resonance imaging may be performed before and after surgery to assess disc status.

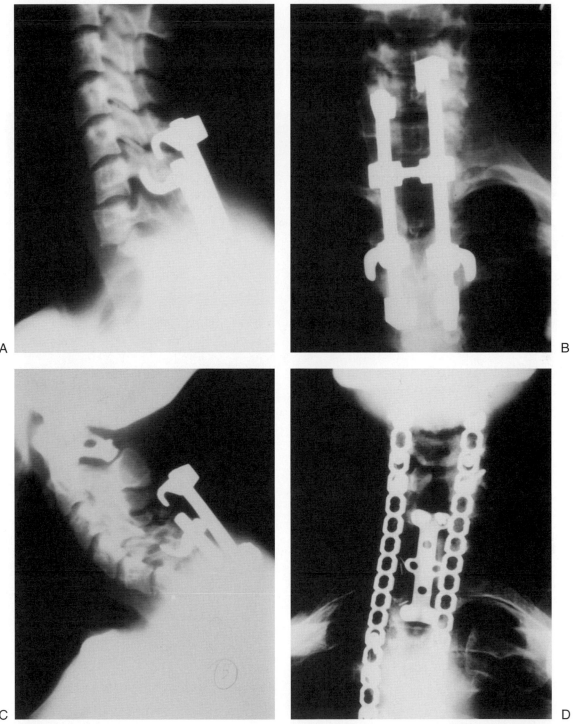

Fig. 8. This 19-year-old male football player underwent a T1 corpectomy via a suprasternal approach and T1 laminectomy for a benign tumor. The sequence of events presented here emphasizes the risks of cervicothoracic reconstruction. **A,B:** AP and lateral radiographs after the first surgery, performed at the referring institution. T1 corpectomy was followed by a nonfixated fibular strut graft. The T1 laminectomy was followed by fixation; this construct consisted of two thoracic rods held with up-going T4 sublaminar hooks clawed to T3 transverse process hooks at the caudal end. At the rostral end, the right rod has a down-going C6 sublaminar hook, and the left rod has an up-going C6 sublaminar hook. A single cross-link is between the rods. Not only does this construct place two sublaminar hooks of thoracic size in the C6 canal; it also does not resist failure by tilting across the nonfixated anterior strut. **C:** Unfortunately, this is precisely what happened, as seen here after the graft failed by anterior tilting and the nonrigid hook fixation at the upper end failed. **D:** The surgeons reoperated, performing an additional corpectomy of C7. The patient was not placed in traction for realignment preoperatively or intraoperatively. A fibular graft from C6 to T2 was now fixated, with an anterior plate fixed at C6 and T2 but not to the graft. The posterior fixation now consisted of very long cervical lateral mass plates fixated with nonconstrained lateral mass screws at C5, C6, and C7 **(D)** (C7 had been resected anteriorly) and 3.5-mm cervical screws in the pedicles of T3, T4, and T5. The posterior construct failed within 24 hours of surgery and a similar construct was created, this time even longer and now fixated at the upper end with lateral mass screws at C3, C4, and C5, as seen here. (*Figure continues*)

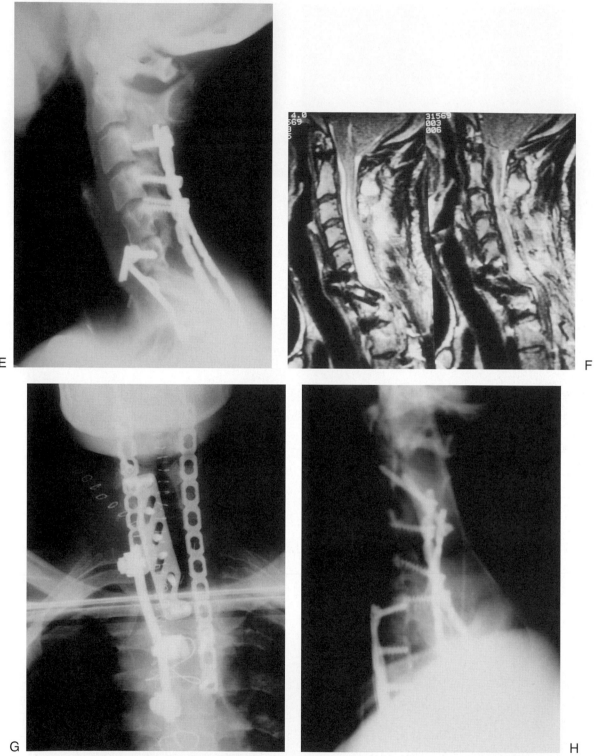

Fig. 8. (continued). **E,F:** Where this nonrigid and nonconstrained construct failed, the graft extended into the spinal canal, leading to immediate and complete quadriplegia. Lateral radiograph **(E)** reveals broken anterior plate and canted fibula graft. MRI **(F)** documents cord injury. It is this tendency to extrude dorsally at the caudal pole that makes graft-to-anterior plate fixation advisable for grafts spanning the cervicothoracic junction; in contrast, purely cervical grafts usually extrude ventrally at the caudal pole. Cages are now preferable to strut grafts for many reasons, including the fact that cage-to-plate fixation does not weaken the graft, as is the case with bone struts. **G,H:** After referral to our institution, the case was once again revised, this time with use of an autologous, large-diameter iliac strut, an anterior plate screwed to four vertebrae and to the graft, and posterior fixation consisting of cervical plate-to-thoracic rod hardware. The cervical plates at the upper end were fixed with long C2 pedicle screws and as many lateral mass screws as we could fit into this multiply reoperated spine. A junctional device allowed fixation of the left cervical plate to a claw-fixed thoracic rod. For lack of such a device on the other side, 4.5-mm thoracic pedicle screws were used in a lateral mass plate on the right. Today, junctional devices would have been used on both sides.

With rare exception, however, C7-T1 facet dislocations can be reduced easily when the patient is prone, in traction, on the operating frame. Once reduction has been achieved, simple cervical lateral mass plates or rods fixated with pedicle screws at C7 and T1 and supplemented with an interspinous cable are quite adequate for repair (Fig. 7 A,B). In cases with posterior element fractures, the lateral mass plates or rods are extended one or two levels caudally to shift the construct axis of rotation away from the damaged joints (45). When intact patients are reduced under anesthesia, intraoperative evoked potentials are often recommended, although we have generally found them noncontributory. It should be noted that late posttraumatic deformities can rarely be corrected through this simple approach.

ANTERIOR-ONLY APPROACHES. Primary or metastatic tumors involving the anterior elements of either C7 or T1 (but not both) can usually be treated by corpectomy followed by strut or cage grafting and anterior plating. As long as the posterior elements are intact and uninvolved, no posterior construct is necessary (46). Conversely, if a tumor or infection spans two or more vertebrae crossing the junction, circumferential reconstruction is mandatory (see below).

Single-level discectomy or corpectomy for ruptured discs or spondylosis can also be performed via an anterior-only approach.

CIRCUMFERENTIAL RECONSTRUCTION THROUGH A SINGLE POSTERIOR APPROACH. With tumors that involve only the upper thoracic side of the junction or with congenital anomalies, such as a hemivertebra of T2 or T3, a complete spondylectomy can be accomplished through a single midline

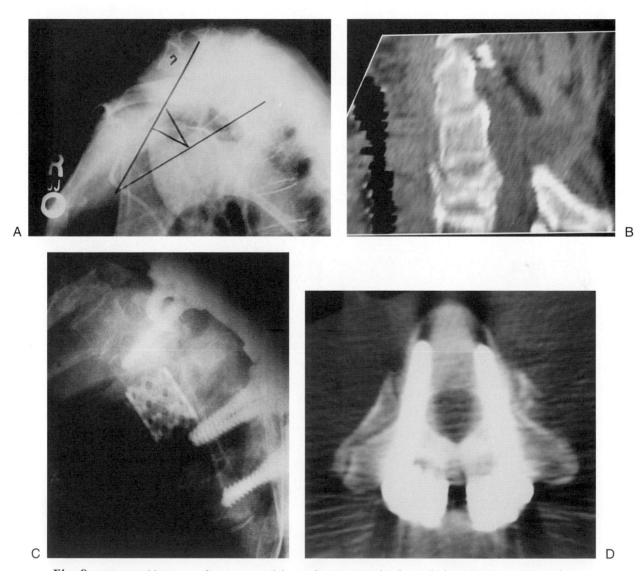

Fig. 9. A 72-year-old woman after an automobile accident. **A:** Lateral radiograph demonstrates exaggerated upper thoracic kyphosis. **B:** Sagittal CT reveals T2 fracture. **C:** Lateral radiograph after complete spondylectomy through a single dorsal approach. Anterior column reconstruction with restoration of height was accomplished by placing an interbody cage via posterolateral approach. Patient was a left-upper-extremity amputee. Cage placement was from the amputated side, where T1 or T2 root sacrifice was not a risk. Posterior reconstruction was accomplished with a 5-mm pedicle screw in the left T1 pedicle, a down-going transverse process hook on the right side of T1 (no risk taken with the remaining T1 root), and bilateral pedicle screws placed in unusually large T3 and T4 pedicles **(D)**. The pedicles at T3 and T4 are usually too small for 5-mm screws.

posterior approach (47,48). Anterior reconstruction is then accomplished via posterolateral insertion of the weight-bearing device through the cavity created by resection of the proximal ribs on one or both sides. This is followed by the posterior placement of semirigid rods (Fig. 9). This procedure poses little risk at T2 and below, but at T1 and above, the C8 and T1 nerve roots, and hence hand function, are very much at risk. (For details of the procedure, see reference 48).

THREE HUNDRED SIXTY-DEGREE PROCEDURES. For tumors and infections involving two or more vertebrae spanning the cervicothoracic junction, we generally employ an anterior then posterior sequence. Anterior exposure is accomplished via median sternotomy (49,50). Simple median sternotomy is quick, simple, and easily repaired, and this procedure is performed thousands of times annually for coronary artery bypass surgery. Additionally, it is largely painless and does not require disarticulation of the clavicle. In our opinion, the manubrioclavicular approaches commonly advocated are rarely, if ever, indicated (51–53). Such procedures are painful, far more time-consuming, and often associated with chronic postoperative shoulder pain and dysfunction.

After resection of the involved vertebrae, an autologous, curved, full-thickness iliac strut or longitudinal cage is carefully seated and gently compressed with an anterior cervical rod or plate device; the strut or cage is fixed to the plate to prevent dorsal displacement. The wound is then closed, and the patient is rotated to a prone position on the turning frame.

Posterior instrumentation is placed and extended at least three levels above and below the ends of the anterior graft (Fig. 10). The options for fixation at the cervical and thoracic ends have been discussed. Low-profile hardware is especially desirable in thin persons and in those who have been or will be irradiated.

FIVE HUNDRED FORTY-DEGREE APPROACHES. For patients with fixed, rigid (i.e., congenital or late posttraumatic) deformities, anterior and posterior osteotomies are usually necessary if near-normal alignment is to be restored. In most cases, our preference is to perform the posterior osteotomies or laminectomies or dorsal arch resections first. The patient is then rotated to a supine position for the transsternal approach so that anterior osteotomies, discectomies, or corpectomies can be completed to achieve reduction and realignment. These procedures are followed by anterior grafting and plating, as described above. Finally, the patient is returned to the prone position for posterior instrumentation. In most cases, we prefer to perform all three stages under a single anesthetic because the risk for another dislocation and anterior graft displacement is high in the absence of posterior compression hardware.

In all cases in which circumferential osteotomies functionally separate the upper and lower bony spinal segments, careful control of both ends is mandatory to prevent worsened dislocation and deformity, overdistraction, and cord injury. Whether placed through a single posterior approach or through combined approaches, short temporary retaining rods fixated with simple hooks are often useful in maintaining alignment while the bony resection and grafting are completed.

In most repairs of cervicothoracic deformity, the greatest risk is undercorrection of the flexion deformity secondary to inadequate anterior distraction. Such distraction can be very difficult in long-segment anterior resections and in spondylectomies performed via a single posterior approach. In older patients, the force required to restore anterior column height is often more than their osteoporotic end-vertebrae can withstand. In such cases, circumferential spondylectomy and foreshortening of the spine may allow better correction of kyphosis (54). This is more easily accomplished after upper thoracic than after cervicothoracic corpectomies.

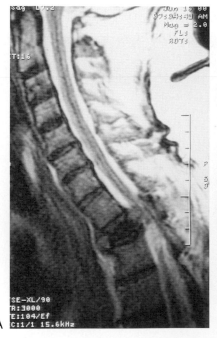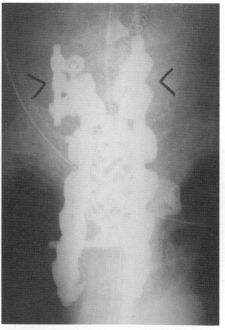

Fig. 10. **A:** Sagittal MRI of a 52-year-old man with metastatic tumor in T2. Note anterior and posterior involvement. The patient had extensive metastatic disease and was becoming paraplegic despite radiation therapy. **B:** Posteroanterior radiograph after total spondylectomy performed via single posterior approach. Posterior reconstruction was accomplished via C7 and T1 pedicle screws and cervical rod interconnected to hook-fixated thoracic rod on the left. On the right, the thoracic rod was extended up to the cervical spine and fixed with sublaminar hooks. Each approach has advantages and disadvantages. See text.

Summary

The five factors analyzed in this chapter conspire to make repairs across the cervicothoracic junction more difficult and less successful than those at any other junctional zone. Modern hardware has made occipitocervical, thoracolumbar, lumbosacral, and even spinopelvic reconstruction both easier and more often successful. Fortunately, pathology at the cervicothoracic junction is comparatively rare. The procedures described above are uncommonly performed and probably should be kept in the hands of those who specialize in complex spine reconstruction.

Nonetheless, evolutionary improvements in hardware never cease. Our understanding of the biomechanical requirements for repair of a given problem has advanced far beyond that of our predecessors. Incremental advances such as cervical pedicle screws and cervicothoracic junctional devices are clear evidence of progress. Although far from perfect, today's reconstructive options are better than yesterday's. We look forward to tomorrow's.

References

1. An HS, Vaccaro A, Cotler JM, et al. Spinal disorders at the cervicothoracic junction. *Spine* 1994;19:2557–2564.
2. An HS, Wise JJ, Xu R. Anatomy of the cervicothoracic junction: a study of cadaveric dissection, crypmicrotomy, and magnetic resonance imaging. *J Spinal Disord* 1999;12:519–525.
3. Bailey AS, Staescu S, Yeasting RA, et al. Anatomic relationships of the cervicothoracic junction. *Spine* 1995;20:1431–1439.
4. Boyle JJ, Singer KP, Milne N. Morphological survey of the cervicothoracic junctional region. *Spine* 1996;21;544–548.
5. Stanescu S, Ebraheim NA, Yeasting R, et al. Morphometric evaluation of the cervico-thoracic junction. Practical considerations for posterior fixation of the spine. *Spine* 1994;19:2082–2088.
6. Xu R, Ebraheim NA, Tang G, et al. Location of the vertebral artery in the cervicothoracic junction. *Am J Orthop* 2000;29:37–40.
7. Seybold EA, Baker JA, Criscitello AA, et al. Characteristics of unicortical and bicortical lateral mass screws in the cervical spine. *Spine* 1999;24:2397–2403.
8. Wellman BJ, Follett KA, Traynelis VC. Complications of posterior articular mass plate fixation of the subaxial cervical spine in 43 consecutive patients. *Spine* 1998;23:193–200.
9. Ebraheim NA, Klausner T, Xu R, et al. Safe lateral-mass screw lengths in the Roy-Camille and Magerl techniques. An anatomic study. *Spine* 1998;23:1739–1742.
10. Xu R, Haman SP, Ebraheim NA, et al. The anatomic relation of lateral mass screws to the spinal nerves. A comparison of Magerl, Anderson, and An techniques. *Spine* 1999;24:2057–2061.
11. Ebraheim NA, Tremains MR, Xu R, et al. Lateral radiologic evaluation of lateral mass screw placement in the cervical spine. *Spine* 1998;23:458–462.
12. Heller JG, Carlson GD, Abitbol JJ, et al. Anatomic comparison of the Roy-Camille and Magerl techniques for screw placement in the lower cervical spine. *Spine* 1991; 16(10 suppl):S552–S557.
13. Xu R, Haman SP, Klausner T, et al. The anatomic relation of lateral mass screw placement in the lower cervical spine: an anatomic study. *J Spinal Disord* 1998;(3):237–240.
14. Panjabi MM, Duranceau J, Goel V, et al. Cervical human vertebrae. Quantitative three-dimensional anatomy of the middle and lower regions. *Spine* 1991;16:861–869.
15. Panjabi MM, Shin EK, Chen NC, et al. Internal morphology of human cervical pedicles. *Spine* 2000;25:1197–1205.
16. Xu R, Kang A, Ebraheim NA, et al. Anatomic relationships between the cervical pedicles and the adjacent neural structures. *Spine* 1999;24:451–454.
17. Ludwig SC, Kramer DL, Vaccaro AR, et al. Transpedicle screw fixation of the cervical spine. *Clin Orthop* 1999;359:77–88.
18. Majd ME, Vadhva M, Holt RT. Anterior cervical reconstruction using titanium cages with anterior plating. *Spine* 1999;24:1604–1610.
19. Panjabi MM, Duranceau J, Goel V, et al. Thoracic human vertebrae. Quantitative three-dimensional anatomy. *Spine* 1991;16:888–901.
20. Heller JG, Shuster JK, Hutton W. Pedicle and transverse process screws of the upper thoracic spine. Biomechanical comparison of loads to failure. *Spine* 1999;24:654–658.
21. Ebraheim NA, Xu R, Ahmad M, et al. Projection of the thoracic pedicle and its morphometric analysis. *Spine* 1997;22:233–238.
22. Kothe R, O'Halloran JD, Liu W, et al. Internal architecture of the thoracic pedicle. An anatomic study. *Spine* 1996;21:264–270.
23. Ebraheim NA, Xu R, Ahmad M, et al. The quantitative anatomy of the thoracic facet and the posterior projection facet. *Spine* 1997;22: 1811–1817.
24. Ebraheim NA, Xu R, Ahmad M, et al. Anatomic considerations of anterior instrumentation of the thoracic spine. *Am J Orthop* 1997; 26:419–424.
25. Coe JD, Warden KE, Sutterlin CE III, et al. Biomechanical evaluation of cervical spinal stabilization methods in a human cadaveric model. *Spine* 1989;14:1122–1131.
26. Oda I, Abumi K, Lu D, et al. Biomechanical role of the posterior elements, costovertebral joints, and rib cage in the stability of the thoracic spine. *Spine* 1996;21:1423–1429.
27. Shea M, Edwards WT, White AA, et al. Variations of stiffness and strength along the human cervical spine. *J Biomech* 1992;25: 689–690.
28. Lazennec JY, Roy-Camille R, Guerin-Surville H, et al. Partial cervicosternotomy: a useful approach to the cervicothoracic junction. *Ital J Orthop Traumatol* 1993;19:19–23.
29. Nazzaro JM, Arbit E, Burt M. "Trap door" exposure of the cervicothoracic junction. *J Neurosurg* 1994;80:338–341.
30. Xu R, Grabow R, Ebraheim NA, et al. Anatomic considerations of a modified anterior approach to the cervicothoracic junction. *Am J Orthop* 2000;29:37–40.
31. Darling GE, McBroom R, Perrin R. Modified anterior approach to the cervicothoracic junction. *Spine* 1995;20:1519–1521.
32. Gieger M, Roth PA, Wu K. The anterior cervical approach to the cervicothoracic junction. *Neurosurgery* 1995;37:704–710.
33. Kurz L, Pursel SE, Herkowitz HN. Modified anterior approach to the cervicothoracic junction. *Spine* 1991;16(10 suppl):S542–S547.
34. Hernigou P, Duparc F. Lateral exposure of the cervicothoracic spine for anterior decompression and osteosynthesis. *Neurosurgery* 1994; 35:1121–1125.
35. Sapkas G, Papadakis S, Katonis P, et al. Operative treatment of unstable injuries of the cervicothoracic junction. *Eur Spine J* 1999;8: 279–283.
36. Chapman JR, Anderson PA, Pepin C, et al. Posterior instrumentation of the unstable cervicothoracic spine. *J Neurosurg* 1996;84:552–558.
37. Albert TJ, Klein GR, Joffe D, et al. Use of cervicothoracic junction pedicle screws for reconstruction of complicated spine pathology. *Spine* 1998;23:1596–1599.
38. Jones EL, Heller JG, Silcox DH, et al. Cervical pedicle screws versus lateral mass screws. Anatomic feasibility and biomechanical comparison. *Spine* 1997;22:977–982.
39. Zindrick MR, Knight GW, Bunch WH, et al. Factors influencing the penetration of wires into the neural canal during segmental wiring. *J Bone Joint Surg Am* 1989;71:742–750.
40. Jeanneret B. Posterior rod system of the cervical spine: a new implant allowing optimal screw insertion. *Eur Spine J* 1996;5:350–356.
41. Vanden Hoek T, Propp D. Cervicothoracic junction injury. *Am J Emerg Med* 1990;8:30–33.
42. Nichols CG, Young DH, Schiller WR. Evaluation of the cervicothoracic junction injury. *Ann Emerg Med* 1987;16:640–642.
43. Evans DK. Dislocations at the cervicothoracic junction. *J Bone Joint Surg Br* 1983;65:124–127.
44. Pick RY, Segal D. C7-T1 bilateral facet dislocation: a rare lesion presenting with the syndrome of anterior spinal cord injury. *Clin Orthop* 1980;(150):131–136.
45. Sapkas G, Papadakis S, Katonis P, et al. Operative treatment of unstable injuries of the cervicothoracic junction. *Eur Spine J* 1999;8: 279–283.
46. Marchesi DG, Boos N, Aebi M. Surgical treatment of tumors of the cervical spine and first two thoracic vertebrae. *J Spinal Disord* 1993; 6:489–496.

47. Akeyson EW, McCutcheon IE. Single-stage posterior vertebrectomy and replacement combined with posterior instrumentation for spinal metastasis. *J Neurosurg* 1996;85:211–220.
48. Cahill DW, Kumar R. Palliative subtotal vertebrectomy with anterior and posterior reconstruction via a single posterior approach. *J Neurosurg* 1999;90(1 suppl):42–47.
49. Gokaslan ZL, York JE, Walsh GL, et al. Transthoracic vertebrectomy for metastatic spinal tumors. *J Neurosurg* 1998;89:599–609.
50. Lehman RM, Grunwerg B, Hall T. Anterior approach to the cervicothoracic junction: an anatomic dissection. *J Spinal Disord* 1997;10: 33–39.

51. Rusca M, Carbognani P, Bobbio P. The modified "hemi-clamshell" approach for tumors of the cervicothoracic junction. *Ann Thorac Surg* 2000;69:1961–1963.
52. Korst RJ, Burt ME. Cervicothoracic tumors: results of resection by hemi-clamshell approach. *J Thorac Cardiovasc Surg* 1998;115: 286–294.
53. Sar C, Hamzaoglu A, Talu U, et al. An anterior approach to the cervicothoracic junction of the spine (modified osteotomy of manubrium sterni and clavicle). *J Spinal Disord* 1999;12:102–106.
54. Shimada Y, Abe E, Sato K. Total *en bloc* spondylectomy for correcting congenital kyphosis. *Spinal Cord* 2000;38:382–385.

191. Posterior Approaches to the Thoracic Spine

**Adetokunbo A. Oyelese,
Daniel H. Kim, and
Richard G. Fessler**

Approaches for surgical intervention in pathological processes within the thoracic spine are greatly dependent on the locus of pathology. Neoplastic lesions (primary and metastatic), vascular malformations, discogenic disease, bacterial and tuberculous infections as well as traumatic vertebral fractures typically result in neurological compromise by compression of the ventral aspect of the spinal cord. An exceptional vulnerability of the spinal cord in the thoracic region exists because of (a) a markedly decreased spinal cord to canal ratio, (b) the existence of a susceptible watershed area extending from T4 to T9 as the result of a tenuous vascular supply, and (c) tethering of the spinal cord anteriorly by the dentate ligament and laterally by exiting nerve roots markedly limiting spinal cord mobility in this region. Surgical intervention in this region must thus be undertaken with great care and consideration, with the goal being safe and effective resection of the offending lesion with preservation of neurological function (Table 1).

Posterior approaches to the thoracic spinal cord such as the laminectomy are commonly performed procedures that provide easy access to the posterior aspects of the spinal canal and cord. These approaches to the thoracic spine are particularly useful in decompression for thoracic spinal stenosis from facet and ligamentum hypertrophy. In addition, posterior spinal approaches are useful in the resection of dorsally based lesions such as posterior epidural abscesses, meningiomas, hematomas, and posterior column spinal fractures while providing access for posterior stabilization of the thoracic spine. However, cumulative experience over the years has revealed that anteriorly based pathological processes are neither adequately nor safely decompressed via a posterior approach such as a laminectomy (1–5). Indeed, irreversible, devastating neurological impairment such as paresis or paraplegia occurred in as many as 34% of patients undergoing herniated disc resection via this approach (6).

The difficulty in employing a laminectomy in the decompression of anteriorly based thoracic spinal lesions lies in the inadequate visualization of the anterior spinal elements when using this posterior approach (7). Additionally, retraction and manipulation of the highly vulnerable thoracic spinal cord within a markedly limited space is unavoidable. It was thus necessary to develop additional approaches that provided improved visualization of the anterior spinal elements and eliminated the need for retraction and manipulation of the thoracic spinal cord.

Posterolateral approaches, beginning with the costotransversectomy, which was developed around the turn of the 20th century for decompression of Pott's disease (8), have sought to meet these goals. The costotransversectomy was later modified by Capener (9) to provide greater exposure of the lateral and anterior spinal elements in a procedure known as the lateral rhachiotomy. The lateral rhachiotomy formed the basis for Larson et al.'s (10,11) later development of the lateral extracavitary approach, a procedure allowing simultaneous access to the anterolateral and posterior spinal elements. A further modification of this procedure by Fessler and associates (12) referred to as the lateral parascapular extrapleural approach allowed access to lesions at the cervicothoracic junction and upper thoracic spine.

The laminectomy is a simple operation that provides access to the posterior spinal elements. The first successful laminectomy is credited to Alban G. Smith, a general surgeon who in 1828 performed a posterior decompression on a patient paralyzed from a lamina fracture suffered after falling from a horse (13). As experience with this surgical approach to the thoracic spine grew, it became evident that the laminectomy provided inadequate and indeed unsafe access to the more commonly occurring anteriorly based lesions in this spinal region (3). The need for safe access to the anterior spinal elements that were more commonly involved in thoracic spinal pathology led to the evolution of safer posterior and posterolateral approaches including the transpedicular approach, the costotransversectomy, and lateral extracavitary approaches.

The transpedicular approach pioneered by Patterson and Arbit (14) employs a posterior midline approach like the laminectomy. However, unlike the laminectomy, it involves the partial removal of the pedicle and facet joint on the side of interest, thus offering added exposure of and access to the lateral spinal elements (14,15). A trough is created ventral to the spinal cord into which material compressing the spinal cord may be safely

Table 1. Surgical Intervention in the Thoracic Spine

Approach	Indications	Contraindications	Advantages	Disadvantages
Posterior				
Laminectomy	Posterior lamina fractures or epidural hematomas; spinal stenosis from ligament and facet hypertrophy	Anteriorly located compressive lesions such as disc herniations or tumors	Easy to perform; allows for posterior instrumentation	May result in spinal instability and severe neurological compromise when used in the decompression of anterior lesions
Transpedicular	Posterior and posterolateral lesions including disc herniations	Anterior pathology requiring spinal retraction; central and intradural disc herniations	Access is readily gained to the posterolateral thoracic spinal elements with minimal dissection and postoperative morbidity	Spinal instability may result from pedicle and facet disruption; inadequate for decompression of anterior spinal elements
Transfacet	As above	As above	Less pedicle disruption than with the transpedicular approach; less postoperative pain, instability	As above
Posterolateral				
Costotransversectomy	Accessible anterolateral spinal lesions	Anterior lesions with significant midline or vertebral body involvement	Involves less surgery than does a transthoracic approach; posterior stabilization can be performed	Visualization of anterior spinal elements and anterior instrumentation are difficult
Lateral extracavitary	Anterolateral lesions including those involving the vertebral body	Extensive trauma; multiple medical complications	Good visualization of anterolateral spinal cord; allows simultaneous posterior and anterior instrumentation	Extensive surgery

curetted, decompressing the spinal cord. This approach has been shown to be excellent for thoracic disc herniations in that it provides adequate exposure and visualization of the lateral spinal elements, permitting safe decompression while avoiding the extensive surgery involved in an anterior or transthoracic approach. Moreover, in contrast to the costotransversectomy and lateral extracavitary approaches, it does not involve rib resection. A recent modification of this approach by Stillerman and associates (16) known as the transfacet pedicle-sparing approach provides similar exposure with less pedicle and facet resection. The modified approach is purported to diminish postoperative pain resulting from facet and pedicle disruption while preserving the integrity of the thoracic spine and decreasing iatrogenic postoperative spinal instability.

The costotransversectomy was first described by Menard (8) in 1894 for the decompression of tuberculous abscesses (Pott's disease) of the spine. It was subsequently employed by Hulme (17) in the excision of thoracic herniated discs. This approach, which involves the resection of the transverse process and medial aspect of the ribs, provides exposure of the posterior and lateral aspects of the thoracic vertebrae. Today it is used in vertebral body and disc biopsies, discectomies, limited anterolateral thoracic spinal cord and vertebral body decompression, as well as anterior spinal fusions. The limited exposure of ventral spinal elements, however, makes this approach less than ideal for resection of the more problematic ventral intradural disc herniations (6) and other anteriorly based lesions causing cord compression.

Larson and associates (10) developed a lateral extracavitary approach that provides excellent exposure of anterior and lateral spinal elements at many thoracic spinal levels, allowing for simultaneous anterior decompression, fusion, and posterior stabilization through a single incision. Subsequently, Fessler and co-workers (12) modified this procedure to enable improved exposure of the upper thoracic spine with a lateral parascapular extrapleural approach. This posterolateral approach

to the spine can achieve exposure of all anterior and posterior vertebral elements from inferior C7 to L5.

This chapter discusses the surgical technique for posterior approaches to the thoracic spine, including the laminectomy, transpedicular, and costotransversectomy approaches. It also discusses the indications and contraindications for each method, the relevant surgical anatomy and preoperative assessment and other considerations in patients undergoing the procedure. The lateral extracavitary approach (Fig. 1D) is described in Chapter 192 and thus is not discussed here.

Indications and Contraindications

As described earlier, the thoracic laminectomy is a simple, commonly used approach for posterior-based spinal pathology. Thoracic laminectomies are indicated for the decompression of posterior lamina fractures causing spinal cord entrapment, evacuation of posterior epidural abscesses or hematomas, and posterior stabilization procedures (Fig. 1A). Laminectomies have the advantage of involving less surgery and allowing for repair of inadvertent durotomies occurring posteriorly. However, a laminectomy should not be employed in isolation for lesions producing anterior spinal cord compression, as this has been shown to result in worsening neurological function (3,5, 18). Moreover, laminectomies in isolation for anterior spinal pathology may result in worsening spinal instability (19).

The transpedicular approach may be employed for accessible lesions involving the anterolateral thoracic cord elements and in cases where anterior stabilization is not required. It has the advantages of providing limited access to the lateral vertebral body (Fig. 1B), entailing less surgery, and permitting simultane-

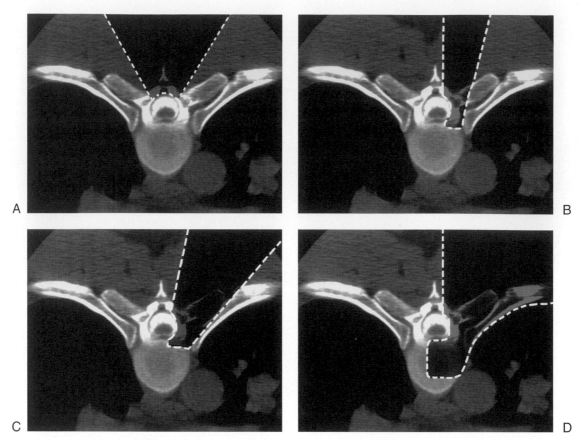

Fig. 1. The extent of bony resection and access provided to the anterolateral spinal cord. **A:** Bony resection in a standard laminectomy. Access is gained only to the posterior spinal elements. **B:** With the transpedicular and transfacet approaches, the pedicle and facets are partially removed providing access to the lateral aspects of the spinal cord. **C:** The costotransversectomy approach involves resection of one or more ribs, thereby providing greater access to the lateral spinal cord as well as limited access to the anterior spinal cord. **D:** The lateral extracavitary employs a greater extent of rib resection in addition to partial resection of the vertebral body for access to the anterior spinal elements. This approach allows for simultaneous anterior tumor resection and posterior instrumentation.

ous posterior instrumentation. There is, however, a limited exposure of the lateral and anterior spinal elements using this approach, and thus a risk of inadequate decompression of central and intradural disc herniations and other anterior lesions. This approach should not be used in cases involving marked spinal deformity or extensive vertebral body fracture. Spinal deformity may potentially result from facet and pedicle disruption in cases where instrumentation is not performed (15).

The costotransversectomy approach, which provides improved access to the posterolateral and lateral aspects of the thoracic spine, particularly in the upper regions, is useful for performing anterior decompression of the spinal cord, disc space, or vertebral bodies as well as limited anterior instrumentation for stabilization (Fig. 1C). This approach has the advantage over anterior spinal approaches of avoiding a thoracotomy. However, it does not permit complete decompression of anterior spinal elements.

Preoperative Evaluation

The preoperative evaluation should include a thorough systemic and neurological workup. A goal of the preoperative evaluation should also be to identify coexistent medical illnesses

that may significantly impact morbidity from the procedure under consideration.

Appropriate radiographic imaging should be obtained, including plain film x-rays, magnetic resonance imaging (MRI) scans, and possibly postmyelogram computed tomography (CT) scans if indicated. Plain film radiographic studies should include anteroposterior (AP) and lateral views and are essential in the demonstration of traumatic or pathological vertebral fractures, osteomyelitic lesions, and metastatic lytic lesions. In most cases a spinal CT scan or MRI or both in combination is indicated. A CT scan in isolation gives excellent detail as to the extent of bony involvement in fractures, infections, and malignancy but is less sensitive in the evaluation of thecal sac and nerve root compression, or intradural lesions. If the clinical presentation or examination is suggestive of such a lesion, the patient should be evaluated using MRI studies or myelography with postmyelogram CT scan. Myelography followed by CT scan can demonstrate the presence of intraaxial or extraaxial lesions as well as disc herniations and retropulsed bony fragments from fractures. These may appear as an indentation or a complete blockade of the myelographic dye column in the spinal canal. While sagittal MRI scans may tend to exaggerate certain pathology such as disc herniations, this diagnostic tool, when used with the administration of contrast material, is extremely useful in the evaluation of intramedullary neoplastic lesions, spinal vascular malformations, as well as paravertebral and intraspinal abscesses without the associated risks of myelography.

Relevant Surgical Anatomy

A thorough knowledge and understanding of the pertinent anatomy of the thoracic region is essential for surgical approaches to this region. We briefly review here the relevant surgical anatomy of the thoracic spine as it pertains to the bony structures including the vertebrae and ribs, the ligamentous structures, and the musculature of the thoracic spine.

OSTEOLOGY

Thoracic Vertebrae. The thoracic spine consists of 12 vertebrae that increase in size with caudal progression, and articulate with the ribs of the thoracic cage. Each vertebra consists of a *body*, which has a concavo-convex, cylindrical profile and almost equivalent anteroposterior and transverse dimensions. The *vertebral canal* is bordered on either side by *pedicles*, which tend to be less divergent than those in the cervical region forming a smaller, rounder vertebral foramen for the smaller thoracic spinal cord. The *laminae* are short, thick, and broad, and overlap from a cranial to caudal direction, fusing at the midline to from the *spinous processes*, which also slant inferiorly. Paired *superior articular (apophyseal) processes* are found at the pediculolaminar junctions projecting posteriorly while the *inferior articular processes* project inferiorly from the lamina with their facets directed anteriorly. Also arising from the pediculolaminar junctions are paired, large *transverse processes* projecting posterolaterally with *costotubercular facets* on their apices for articulation with the tubercles of their corresponding ribs. Paired *superior and inferior costocapitular demifacets* exist on the respective surfaces of the vertebral body also for rib articulation. The vertebral body and spinous process consist of an extensive cancellous bony interior encased in a thin shell of compact bone, while the pedicles and articular and transverse processes are composed of mainly compact bone.

Ribs. The thoracic cage is formed by 12 pairs of ribs articulating with the vertebral column posteriorly and the sternum or costal cartilages anteriorly. The 11th and 12th rib are termed floating ribs as they have free, nonarticulating anterior ends. The posterior or vertebral end of the second through the 10th rib has a head, neck, and tubercle. On the head are two articular facets separated by a transverse crest. The more inferior and larger facet articulates with the corresponding vertebral body, the superior facet with the body of the superior vertebra, and the crest attaches to the intervertebral disc above. The neck lies anterior to the transverse process while the tubercle articulates with the transverse process via an articular facet. Costovertebral and costotransverse joints join the ribs to the vertebral column.

Costovertebral Articulation. With the exception of the first and 10th through 12th ribs, the head of each typical rib articulates with its corresponding vertebral body, the superior vertebral body, and the intervertebral disc space between a synovial joint. A fibrous capsule connects the costal heads to the articular surfaces of the demifacets of the inferior and superior vertebral bodies and the intervertebral disc. Superior, inferior, and intermediate radiate ligaments attach the anterior parts of the costal heads to the superior and inferior vertebral bodies and the intervertebral disc, respectively. An intraarticular ligament attaches the transverse crest between the costal articular facets to the intervertebral disc and bisects the synovial joint into two compartments.

Costotransverse Articulation. Articulation of the costal tubercle with the transverse process of the corresponding vertebra occurs in the first through 10th ribs via a joint maintained by three different groups of ligaments surrounded by a fibrous capsule. The lateral costotransverse ligament extends from the posterior tubercle to the apex of the transverse process. The medial or capsular costotransverse ligament articulates the posterior neck of the rib with the anterior surface of the transverse process. The anterior and posterior superior costotransverse ligaments extend from the superior border of the neck to the inferior border of the transverse process of the vertebral body immediately superior. Laterally, the anterior ligaments blend with the internal intercostal membrane and are crossed by the intercostal vessels and nerve. The dorsal rami of the thoracic spinal nerves and associated vessels pass between the superior costotransverse ligament and a more medial accessory ligament.

MUSCULATURE. The muscles of the back can be divided into two broad categories: the *extrinsic* back muscles, which include superficial and intermediate layers, and the *intrinsic* back muscles, composed of superficial, intermediate, and deep muscle groups. The extrinsic back muscles attach the upper limb to the axial skeleton and are involved in respiration and movements of the upper limb. The intrinsic back muscles, in contrast, are concerned with posture and movements of the vertebral column.

Superficial Extrinsic Back Musculature. This group, which includes the trapezius, latissimus dorsi, levator scapulae, and the rhomboids major and minor, serves to attach the upper limb to the axial skeleton and is involved in its movement.

The trapezius is a broad, flat, triangular-shaped muscle and is the first muscle encountered after skin incision (Fig. 2A). It originates from the medial third of the superior nuchal line, external occipital protuberance, ligamentum nuchae, and the spinous processes of C7 through T12 vertebrae. Its superior fibers insert on the lateral third of the clavicle, the middle fibers onto the acromion and spine of the scapula, and the inferior fibers on the base of the scapula spine via an aponeurosis. The nerve supply is derived from the spinal root of the accessory nerve [cranial nerve (CN) XI] and ventral rami of C3 and C4 and the blood supply from the dorsal scapula artery. The trapezius serves to elevate, rotate, and retract the scapula.

The latissimus dorsi is a wide, fan-like muscle extending from T6 to the iliac crest. It originates on the spinous processes of the inferior six thoracic vertebrae and the inferior portion of the thoracolumbar fascia and inserts into the intertubercular groove of the humerus (Fig. 2A). This muscle derives its nerve supply from the thoracodorsal nerve and serves to extend, adduct, and medially rotate the humerus at the shoulder joint.

The rhomboid major and minor muscles lie deep to the trapezius and pass inferolaterally from the vertebrae to the scapula (Fig. 2A). The rhomboid major has its origin in the spinous processes of the T2 to T5 vertebrae, whereas the rhomboid minor originates on the ligamentum nuchae and the spinous processes of C7 and T1. Both insert onto the medial border of the scapula, the rhomboid major below and the minor above the scapula spine. They derive their nerve supply from the dorsal scapular nerve and serve to retract and rotate the scapula.

The levator scapulae muscle is a strap-like muscle whose inferior third lies deep to the trapezius and the superior two thirds deep to the sternocleidomastoid. It originates on the

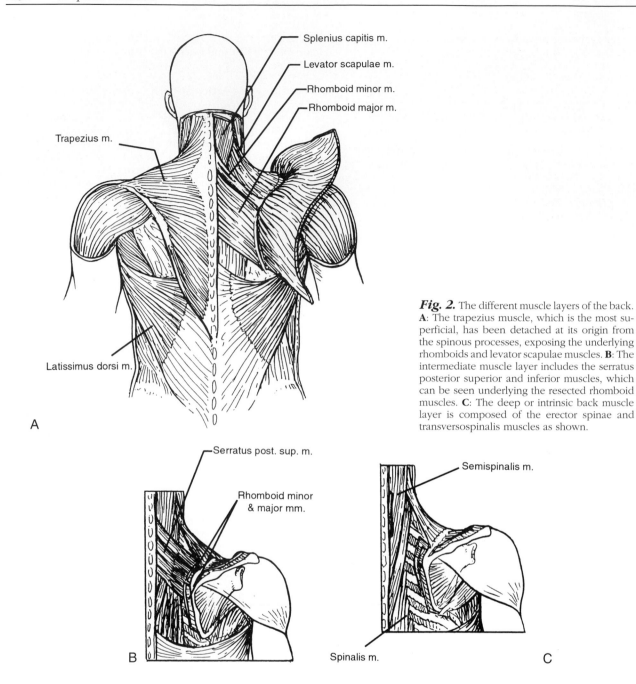

Splenius capitis m.

Levator scapulae m.

Rhomboid minor m.

Rhomboid major m.

Trapezius m.

Latissimus dorsi m.

A

Fig. 2. The different muscle layers of the back. **A**: The trapezius muscle, which is the most superficial, has been detached at its origin from the spinous processes, exposing the underlying rhomboids and levator scapulae muscles. **B**: The intermediate muscle layer includes the serratus posterior superior and inferior muscles, which can be seen underlying the resected rhomboid muscles. **C**: The deep or intrinsic back muscle layer is composed of the erector spinae and transversospinalis muscles as shown.

Serratus post. sup. m.

Rhomboid minor & major mm.

Semispinalis m.

Spinalis m.

B

C

transverse processes of the first four cervical vertebrae and inserts onto the superior medial border of the scapula. It is supplied by the dorsal scapula nerve, and helps elevate and rotate the scapula.

Intermediate Extrinsic Back Musculature. This layer is composed of the serratus posterior muscles including the superior and inferior divisions. The superior division arises from the ligamentum nuchae and the spinous processes of C7 through T3, running inferolaterally to insert into the superior border of ribs two through five (Fig. 2B). The inferior division arises from the spinous processes of T11 through L2, and runs superolaterally to insert into the angles of the inferior three ribs. The intermediate muscles are innervated by intercostal nerves and are thought to participate in stabilization of the ribs during respiration.

Intrinsic Back Musculature. These muscles are concerned with the maintenance of posture and movements of the verte-

bral column and are thus true back muscles. They lie deep to the superficial or extrinsic muscle layer and the thoracolumbar fascia. Upon removal of this fascia, the deep musculature can be seen as paired longitudinal bands on either side of the spinous processes (Fig. 2C). Three layers of intrinsic back muscles are described based on their depth from the surface and the direction of their fibers: (a) a superficial layer with fibers passing superolaterally, (b) an intermediate layer with fibers running longitudinally and parallel to the axis of the vertebral column, and (c) a deep layer with fibers passing superomedially.

Superficial Intrinsic Back Musculature. This group comprises two muscles, the splenius capitis and splenius cervicis originating from the inferior half of the ligamentum nuchae and the spinous processes of C7 to T6. The splenius capitis inserts onto the mastoid process of the temporal bone and onto the lateral third of the superior nuchal line, whereas the splenius cervicis inserts onto the transverse processes of the superior two to four cervical vertebrae.

Intermediate Intrinsic Back Musculature. This muscle group is composed of the large erector spinae muscle located on either side of the vertebral column and extending vertically and parallel to the spinous processes, from the pelvis to the skull. The erector spinae muscles originate in a dense aponeurotic band from the sacrum and divides into three muscular columns—the iliocostalis, longissimus, and spinalis muscles—in the superior lumbar region.

The iliocostalis muscle, comprising the lumborum, thoracis, and cervicis, is the most lateral of the erector spinae muscle group and inserts onto the ribs. The longissimus muscle is the middle column and the longest, inserting onto the transverse processes of the thoracic and cervical vertebrae and the mastoid process of the temporal bone. The medial-most column is the spinalis muscle arising from the spinous processes in the superior lumbar and inferior thoracic region and inserting onto spinous processes in the superior thoracic region. The erector spinae muscles serve to extend the vertebral column or bend it laterally.

Deep Intrinsic Back Musculature. The deep intrinsic back muscles run from the transverse processes to the spinous processes of the vertebrae and are thus collectively referred to as the *transversospinalis* muscles. This group comprises the semispinalis, multifidus, and rotatores muscles. The semispinalis is the most superficial and inserts onto the thoracic and cervical spinous processes (semispinalis thoracis and cervicis, respectively) spanning approximately five segments. The superior portion of this muscle (semispinalis capitis) inserts into the occipital bone. The multifidus muscle comprises many bundles arising from a dense aponeurosis overlying the erector spinae and from the transverse processes of the thoracic and cervical vertebrae inserting onto the inferior portion of the spinous processes. This muscle group lies deep to the semispinalis and stabilizes and rotates the vertebral column. The deepest of the intrinsic muscles is the rotatores group. These short small muscles run between the spinous and transverse processes the entire length of the vertebral column one segment at a time. They serve to stabilize, extend, and rotate the vertebral column.

Surgical Technique

LAMINECTOMY

Positioning. After induction of general endotracheal anesthesia, the patient is positioned prone. This may be difficult in patients with chronic obstructive pulmonary disease (COPD) and ascites. Positioning should be optimized to provide adequate exposure of the thoracic spine, reduce epidural venous bleeding intraoperatively by avoiding abdominal compression, and allow for unrestricted movement of the thoracic cage to permit easy ventilation and to maintain the upper extremities in an anatomical configuration to avoid joint and nerve (brachial plexus) injury. Care must also be taken to provide adequate support for the head and avoid compression injury to the ocular structures. We have consistently positioned our patients prone on a Wilson frame, although some surgeons prefer to use bolsters placed under the pectoral and iliac regions. The frame should be flexed and the supports adequately spaced to reduce abdominal compression. A disadvantage of the standard Wilson frame is its interference with the acquisition of radiographic

images for localization. As such we have utilized a radiolucent Wilson frame in the positioning of our patients.

For upper thoracic approaches (T1 to T5), the arms may be tucked at the patient's side and adhesive tape used to retract the shoulders toward the feet. The head should be fixed in a three-point Mayfield headrest or horseshoe headrest for upper thoracic approaches and the table placed in slight reverse Trendelenburg position with the neck and the feet in flexion. Positioning for lower thoracic exposures requires the same cautionary measures for protection of crucial organs. The arms are abducted and flexed at no greater than 90 degrees at the shoulder and elbow joints. The arms, elbows, and axillae are padded liberally. Care is taken not to hyperextend the shoulder joint to avoid injury to the lower brachial plexus.

Compression stockings and sequential compression devices should be placed on the patient's legs prior to induction of general anesthesia. If the surgery is expected to last longer than 2 hours, as in fusion procedures, a Foley catheter should be inserted prior to positioning. The genitalia in male patients and breasts in female patients must always be checked to ensure that they are free of compression.

EXPOSURE OF THE SPINAL COLUMN. After positioning of the patient, the thoracic region is prepared and draped in sterile fashion. We use an iodinated saline solution followed by alcohol and then Duraprep in our skin preparation. A wide area of skin is prepared extending beyond the desired exposure and then covered with iodinated adhesive drape. Prophylactic intravenous antibiotic is given at this time as well as intravenous steroid medication when indicated. Surface and bony landmarks are identified for localization of level. Useful landmarks include the C7 spinous process (vertebra prominens), the spine and inferior angle of the scapula (T3 and T7, respectively) and the 12th rib (Fig. 3). A cross-table AP roentgenogram should always be obtained prior to skin incision in single-level, microscopic procedures for accurate localization of the desired level, as surface landmarks may often be misleading. One or two spinal needles are inserted into the skin overlying the spinous processes of interest for localization on x-ray. For instrumentation procedures, intraoperative fluoroscopy should be utilized for localization as well as for placement of instrumentation hardware.

Once the desired level is identified, a sterile marking pen is used to mark out an incision line along the midline. The extent of the incision is tailored to the particular pathology and the

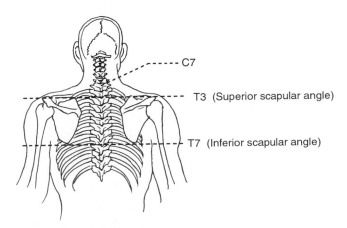

Fig. 3. Useful bony landmarks include the C7 spinous process (vertebra prominens), the superior scapular angle (corresponding to T3), and the inferior scapular angle (corresponding to T7).

number of laminae to be removed. The skin is then infiltrated with a solution of local anesthetic [lidocaine (Xylocaine)] containing epinephrine, and a midline skin incision is made through the previously marked skin. Cutaneous bleeders are coagulated using a bipolar or Bovie electrocautery with care being taken to avoid injury to the skin surface. A small self-retaining retractor is used for skin retraction. The incision is carried down through the subcutaneous tissues to the fascial layer with the Bovie on coagulation mode. The first structures encountered following incision of the skin and underlying subcutaneous tissues are the trapezius muscle (and its attachment to the spinous processes via the ligamentum nuchae) in the upper thoracic region and the thoracolumbar fascia in the lower thoracic region. The spinous processes are identified by palpation once this layer is reached and, using a Cobb elevator to provide gentle traction on the fascia and paraspinal muscles, a subperiosteal dissection of the paraspinal muscles is carried out at the desired level. It is crucial that once the tip of the spinous process is identified, the tip of the Bovie is applied directly to the bone with gentle traction on the paraspinal muscles using the Cobb elevator. This technique will allow for a subperiosteal stripping of the paraspinal muscles away from the bone and greatly minimize bleeding. Subperiosteal stripping of the paraspinal muscles must be performed carefully to avoid injury to the neurovascular supply of the muscles or the muscles themselves. A longer incision reduces the need for excessive traction, diminishing postoperative pain from spasm.

Due to the high degree of oblique "shingling" of the thoracic vertebral laminae, the spinal canal and thecal sac are well protected and the spinous process may then be followed down to the lamina and out laterally to the facet with care taken to avoid injury to the facet capsule, as this tends to produce significant postoperative pain. Hemostasis of muscle bleeders should be meticulously achieved. A technique found to be useful in hemostasis as well as facilitating the subperiosteal dissection involves the use of a sponge that is tightly packed into the space between the lamina and muscle tissue, using a Cobb elevator to push the sponge against the bone, stripping the muscle away. Larger self-retaining retractors may be used to hold the muscle tissue and expose the thoracic laminae. Intraoperative radiographic confirmation of position is imperative prior to removal of any bone.

RESECTION OF BONE. The exposed spinous processes and laminae may be removed using an Addson rongeur or Horsel bone cutter with avoidance of twisting motions. A Kerrison rongeur may then be used to widen the laminectomy. With the use of this latter instrument, the plane between the lamina and ligamentum flavum should first be defined with a fine cupped, angled curet. The footplate of the rongeurs should always be angled upward against the lamina with absolutely no pressure placed on the thecal sac, as injury can easily occur to the spinal cord in this region. Alternatively, a high-speed cutting drill such as a Midas AM-8 may be used in creating a trough by thinning the bone on either side of the lamina at the junction with the facet joints. After defining the plane between the lamina and ligamentum flavum with an angled, cupped curet, a Kerrison rongeur is then used to take down the remainder of the bone, and the entire posterior arch may be removed as one piece. For multilevel laminectomies, a Midas B1 or B5 drill footplate may be inserted under the lamina of the inferior extent of the laminectomy, and several laminae can be resected in one piece. The latter maneuver allows the laminae to be replaced at the end of the case as a laminoplasty. This is of greater significance in the pediatric population, with the spine still in growth, for preservation of stability and prevention of kyphosis.

Bony bleeding is stopped with the use of bone wax, and epidural venous bleeding is controlled with bipolar electrocautery. Exposure of the dura is accomplished by removal of the ligamentum flavum. This tough, fibrous ligament composed of yellow, elastic fibers arises on the anterior surfaces of adjacent lamina, extending from the zygapophysial capsules to the midline where the lamina fuse to form the spinous process. The ligament extends from the anterior surface of the lamina of the superior vertebra to the posterior surface and upper margin of the lamina of the inferior vertebra. The ligamentum flavum is sharply incised with a no. 15 scalpel blade while holding it up under traction with a pair of Cushing forceps. The incision is carefully carried through until the epidural fat is visualized. The plane between the epidural fat and the ligament is developed by blunt dissection, and the ligament is then transected sharply with the scalpel or with a Kerrison rongeur. The laminectomy is widened by undercutting the facet joints. This may be accomplished by use of a Kerrison rongeur after the bone has been thinned out with a high-speed drill. The dura is protected during this maneuver with a cottonoid pad, avoiding excessive traction or pressure. If a laminoplasty is performed, the dorsal arch is replaced and the lamina is stabilized and reattached with mini–bone plates.

As mentioned in previous sections, the posterior laminectomy approach is excellent in providing access to posteriorly based spinal lesions. Figure 4 shows sagittal (Fig. 4A) and axial (Fig. 4B) views of an MRI scan obtained in a patient with a dorsal spinal meningioma of the upper thoracic spine. This lesion was resected via a laminectomy. However, laminectomies are contraindicated as a means of decompressing the spinal cord from anteriorly based pathology. In one study it was noted that 50% of patients undergoing laminectomy for thoracic disc herniation deteriorated or experienced no benefit from the procedure (3). This is particularly true of central disc herniations. However, a thoracic disc herniation may on occasion occur far laterally, and a posterior laminectomy approach provides safe access to the lesion. In this case the laminectomy should be extended laterally to the facet joint, and a lateral approach to the herniated disc material should be achieved with care taken to ensure that the thecal sac is neither compressed nor deformed to any degree.

TRANSPEDICULAR APPROACH. As with laminectomies, the transpedicular approach begins with a midline incision. The considerations given to positioning and preparation are thus essentially similar to those described in the previous section. With the patient in the prone position, a midline incision is made over the spinous processes of interest after adequate localization. A subperiosteal dissection of the fascia and paravertebral muscles is then carried out exposing the spinous processes and lamina on either side. The dissection is extended on the side of the lesion to expose the facet joints and the transverse process. Hemostasis is achieved, and the artery arising over the transverse process is carefully coagulated with bipolar electrocautery.

Upon exposure of the facet joint and transverse process at the desired level, an operative microscope is brought into the operative field to provide increased illumination and visualization of critical structures. A high-speed drill with a cutting burr (e.g., Midas AM-8) is used to perform a window laminotomy and partial medial facetectomy by drilling the inferior and medial aspect of the lamina and facet joint. The laminotomy is widened (using a Kerrison rongeur or diamond-tipped drill upon encountering the dural sac) to the lateral edge of the dural sac. With the dural sac protected and under microscopic visualization, the superior and medial borders of the caudal vertebral body are identified by palpation using a cupped angled curet. Care is taken to ensure that there is no retraction or

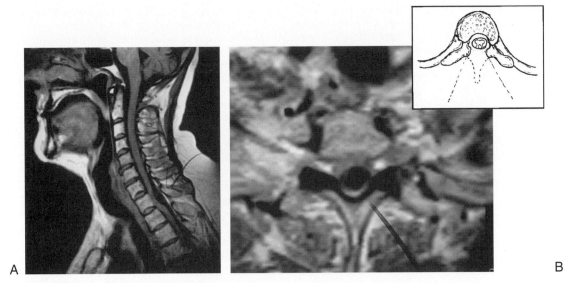

Fig. 4. A: T1-weighted sagittal magnetic resonance imaging (MRI) scan of the upper thoracic spine showing a posteriorly located meningioma in a 55-year-old man. **B**: Axial T1-weighted images of the same lesion (*arrow*) showing the dorsal location. The lesion was resected via a simple laminectomy with no neurological sequelae.

pressure applied to the dural sac. A few millimeters of the pedicle is then removed with a high-speed diamond-tipped drill until it is flush with the vertebral body (the medial transverse process may also be removed at its point of attachment to the lateral pedicle if the entire pedicle is to be resected, although this is not essential). Exposure of the rostral aspect of the vertebral body as well as the adjacent intervertebral disc space is thus gained.

Soft lesions such as herniated disc free fragments may now be removed by gentle curettage, and the disc space may be entered lateral to the thecal sac below the exiting nerve root. The contents of the disc space are extricated using pituitary rongeurs. To minimize injury to the spinal cord, bony or hard adherent material should be delivered with a down-biting angled curet into a cavity created ventral to the cord in the poste-

rior aspect of the vertebral body. Special down-biting angled curets with slender necks designed specifically for this procedure have been utilized by Le Roux et al. (15) for anterior decompression of central disc herniations. In their series, 20 patients with herniated discs operated on utilizing the transpedicular approach all showed postoperative improvement without intraoperative or postoperative complications. Upon adequate anterior decompression of the spinal cord, a laminectomy can be safely completed by removal of first the lateral and then the medial lamina elements. Figure 5 shows sagittal (Fig. 5A) and axial (Fig. 5B) MRI of a left-sided T11-12 disc herniation that was safely excised via a transpedicular approach.

A modification of this procedure known as the transfacet pedicle-sparing approach was developed by Stillerman and col-

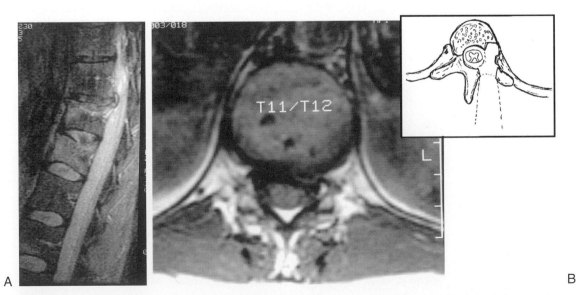

Fig. 5. A: Sagittal T2-weighted MRI scan of a disc herniation at the T11-12 level. **B**: On axial imaging it is noted that the herniation lateralizes to the left. This disc herniation was resected via a transpedicular approach (**inset).**

leagues (16) as an alternative to radical pedicle and facet resection while providing comparative access to and visualization of the spinal elements. Using the same approach as for a transpedicular procedure, a high-speed drill is used in performing a partial medial facetectomy under fluoroscopic and microscopic guidance. Access to the lateral portion of the disc capsule is gained through the neural foramen. Removal of disc material is then performed under microscopic visualization.

COSTOTRANSVERSECTOMY. After induction of general endotracheal anesthesia, the patient is placed in either a lateral decubitus position or a modified lateral decubitus position, elevated 30 degrees from the prone position. A gelatin roll is placed in the axilla and below the shoulders. Additional supports are placed under the abdomen and chest wall to prevent increased pressure producing excessive venous bleeding. A pillow is placed between the legs and the knees are flexed. The patient is secured to the table with straps and heavy adhesive tape. The skin is then prepared and draped in the standard fashion with the posterior iliac crest included in the prepped field if autologous bony fusion is a consideration.

A right-sided approach is used for access to centrally based pathology such as a disc herniation, or in the absence of lateralizing signs to avoid injury to the artery of Adamkiewicz, which typically originates from the intercostal arteries of the lower left thoracic region. Localization of the level is accomplished intraoperatively by inserting a spinal needle into the skin overlying the structures of interest and obtaining a cross-table roentgenogram. Local anesthetic solution containing epinephrine is injected into the skin prior to making the incision for anesthesia and hemostasis. A variety of skin incisions may be utilized depending on the level of the lesion. These include (a) a midline incision over the spinous processes, and (b) a curvilinear incision starting and ending approximately 3 cm lateral to the spinous processes and curving 6 to 8 cm form the midline. Hemostasis is meticulously achieved with a Bovie or bipolar electrocautery.

The incision is carried through the subcutaneous tissue to the level of the posterior superficial muscle layer. Depending on the level, the trapezius and then the thoracolumbar fascia or latissimus dorsi and rhomboid major and minor muscle are encountered and divided in line with the skin incision and retracted medially. This dissection exposes the erector spinae and transversospinalis muscles, which then may be divided in line with the incision or dissected in the plane between the iliocostalis laterally and the longissimus medially and elevated off the posterior surface of the transverse process and ribs with a Cobb elevator. With exposure of the desired rib or ribs, a subperiosteal dissection is performed using a Doyen subperiosteum elevator. Care is taken to separate and preserve the intercostal neurovascular bundle on the inferior surface of the rib.

The rib is cut at a distance of approximately 8 cm from the costotransverse joint using a rib cutter and elevated by rotation with a bone clamp. The medial border of the rib remnant is beveled to prevent injury to the pleura. The costotransverse and capsular ligaments are then divided sharply with a knife. Upon resection of the ligaments, the rib may be disarticulated in its entirety or divided at its neck with later removal of the head and the vertebral transverse process. A bone rongeur or osteotome is used to remove the transverse process at its attachment to the superior facet and pedicle if the rib head is separately resected. Following removal of the rib, the intercostal neurovascular structures are once again identified and followed through their entrance into the spinal canal—the intervertebral foramen. Every attempt should be made to preserve these structures, although the muscular branches from the intercostal artery may be ligated or cauterized if necessary. The parietal pleura and sympathetic trunk are separated from the anterolateral surface of the vertebral body by blunt dissection as well as from the surfaces of the inferior and superior ribs. The pleura is then depressed with a malleable ribbon or a large Deaver retractor.

The pedicles forming the intervertebral foramen are resected using a Kerrison rongeur. Alternatively, a high-speed drill may be used for resection of the pedicle, although this should be done only under microscopic magnification for added illumination and visualization. The lateral aspect of the dural sac is exposed with removal of the pedicle, and ventral pathology such as a herniated disc may be visualized. The midportion of the disc space is incised and the disc space contents are extricated using a pituitary rongeur and a variety of fine-cupped curets. Fragments directly underlying the thecal sac are depressed into the intervertebral space for later retrieval. Anterolaterally based neoplastic or infectious lesions may also be resected or biopsied via this exposure. Additional exposure is achieved by resection of more ribs.

Lesions invading the lateral aspect of the thoracic spinal cord can be safely resected via a costotransversectomy (Fig. 6). Addi-

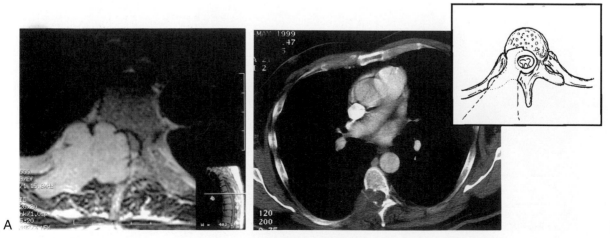

Fig. 6. **A**: A laterally based neoplastic lesion invading the spinal canal. **B**: As this lesion was located primarily on the lateral aspect of the spine, it was approached and resected via a costotransversectomy (**inset**).

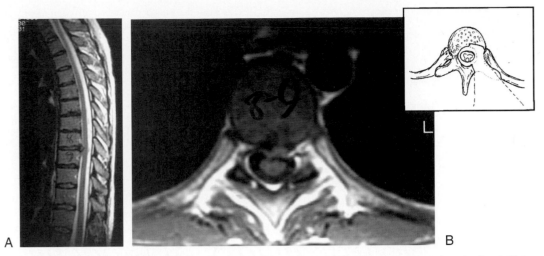

Fig. 7. Central disc herniation seen on T2-weighted sagittal (**A**) and axial (**B**) MRI scan at the T8-9 level. This was excised via a costotransversectomy approach.

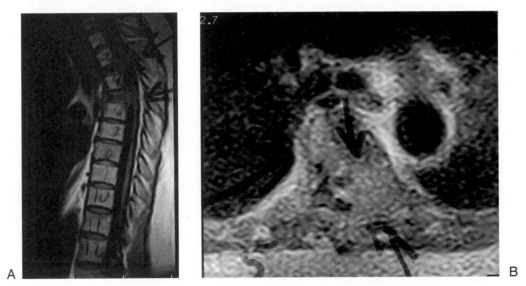

Fig. 8. A: Sagittal MRI scan showing metastatic invasion of the T3 and T5 vertebral bodies. Note the kyphosis of the thoracic spine. **B**: Ventral spinal cord compression from this tumor is clearly demonstrated on axial images. This lesion was considered too extensive for resection via a costotransversectomy and was thus resected with the lateral extracavitary approach.

tionally, some central disc herniations have been excised through this approach (Fig. 7). Large anteriorly based lesions involving the vertebral body and requiring reconstruction such as depicted in Fig. 8 should not be resected via a costotransversectomy. Such lesions would be more appropriately and safely resected via a lateral extracavitary approach.

References

1. Arce CA, Dohrmann GJ. Herniated thoracic disks. *Neurol Clin* 1985; 3:383–92.
2. Bennett MH, McCallum JE. Experimental decompression of spinal cord. *Surg Neurol* 1977;8:63–7.
3. Arseni C, Nash F. Thoracic intervertebral disc protrusion. A clinical study. *J Neurosurg* 1960;17:418–30.
4. Doppman JL, Girton M. Angiographic study of the effect of laminectomy in the presence of acute anterior epidural masses. *J Neurosurg* 1976;45:195–202.
5. Perot PL Jr, Munro DD. Transthoracic removal of midline thoracic disc protrusions causing spinal cord compression. *J Neurosurg* 1969; 31:452–8.
6. Fessler RG, Sturgill M. Review: complications of surgery for thoracic disc disease. *Surg Neurol* 1998;49:609–18.
7. Dickman CA, Theodore N, Hurlbert JR, et al. Thoracic disc [letter; comment]. *J Neurosurg* 1996;85:187–8; discussion 189–90.
8. Menard V. Causes de la paraplegie dans le maladie de Pott, son traitment chirurgical par l'ouverture directe du foyer tuberculeaux des vertebres. *Rev Orthopaed* 1894;5:47–64.
9. Capener N. The evolution of lateral rhachotomy. *J Bone Joint Surg* 1954;36B:173–9.
10. Larson SJ, Holst RA, Hemmy DC, et al. Lateral extracavitary approach

to traumatic lesions of the thoracic and lumbar spine. *J Neurosurg* 1976;45:628–37.

11. Maiman DJ, Larson SJ, Luck E, et al. Lateral extracavitary approach to the spine for thoracic disc herniation: report of 23 cases. *Neurosurgery* 1984;14:178–82.

12. Fessler RG, Dietze DD Jr, Millan MM, et al. Lateral parascapular extrapleural approach to the upper thoracic spine. *J Neurosurg* 1991; 75:349–55.

13. Patchell RA, Tibbs PA, Young AB, et al. Alban G. Smith and the beginnings of spinal surgery. *Neurology* 1987;37:1683–4.

14. Patterson RH Jr, Arbit E. A surgical approach through the pedicle to protruded thoracic discs. *J Neurosurg* 1978;48:768–72.

15. Le Roux PD, Haglund MM, Harris AB. Thoracic disc disease: experi-

ence with the transpedicular approach in twenty consecutive patients. *Neurosurgery* 1993;33:58–66.

16. Stillerman CB, Chen TC, Day JD, et al. The transfacet pedicle-sparing approach for thoracic disc removal: cadaveric morphometric analysis and preliminary clinical experience [see comments]. *J Neurosurg* 1995;83:971–6.

17. Hulme A. The surgical approach to thoracic intervertebral disc protrusions. *J Neurol Neurosurg Psychiatry* 1960;23:133–7.

18. Terry AF, McSweeney T, Jones HW. Paraplegia as a sequela to dorsal disc prolapse. *Paraplegia* 1981;19:111–7.

19. Yoganandan N, Maiman DJ, Pintar FA, et al. Biomechanical effects of laminectomy on thoracic spine stability. *Neurosurgery* 1993;32: 604–10.

192. Lateral Extracavitary Approaches to the Thoracolumbar Spine

Daniel H. Kim,
Adetokunbo A. Oyelese, and
Richard G. Fessler

Surgical approaches to the anterior vertebral structures of the thoracic and lumbar spine present unique challenges to surgeons operating in these regions. In the upper thoracic spine, for instance, narrowing of the thoracic cage creates intimate associations between the lungs, superior mediastinal structures, and the vertebral column. The result is a reduction in available space for surgical exposure in addition to an increased depth field while placing many critical structures directly in the surgical field. Anterior approaches to the lumbar spine, in contrast, are complicated by the diaphragmatic insertions onto the vertebrae and the presence of the great vessels on the anterolateral aspect of the vertebral bodies. It is thus not surprising that a myriad of surgical procedures have been described for achieving exposure of the anterior vertebral elements in the thoracolumbar spine.

As described in Chapter 191, thoracic spinal lesions present a unique challenge as they typically result in anterior compression of the spinal cord. Access to these anteriorly located lesions is complicated by the extreme vulnerability of the spinal cord within this region to manipulation during surgery. Three anatomical considerations underlie the vulnerability of the thoracic cord during surgical manipulation: a small spinal canal to cord ratio; a tenuous vascular supply particularly between T4 and T9; and ventral and lateral tethering by dentate ligaments and exiting nerve roots, respectively, rendering the spinal cord relatively immobile.

Acceptable approaches to this spinal region must thus allow the surgeon to (a) adequately and safely decompress anteriorly located lesions without any manipulation or retraction of the thecal sac; (b) directly visualize the ventral spinal cord and dura, making possible the resection of intradural pathology; and (c) minimize the risk of spinal instability while permitting instrumentation and stabilization procedures, should they be indicated. Early data revealed posterior decompressive procedures such as the laminectomy to be inadequate in the treatment of anterior thoracic spinal lesions as both spinal instability and neurological deterioration frequently ensued (1–7). Unsatisfac-

tory results with the posterior approach led to the evolution of safer surgical approaches in the thoracic spine.

At the turn of the 20th century Menard (8) described an approach to the anterior elements of the thoracic spine that he termed the costotransversectomy. This approach, as described in Chapter 191, was utilized in the decompression of Pott's disease and was subsequently employed by Hulme (9) in the excision of herniated thoracic discs. The costotransversectomy involved resection of a short segment of rib and the adjacent transverse process to expose the posterolateral aspects of the vertebral body. While providing adequate exposure of the mid- and lower thoracic spine, it had limited use in the upper thoracic region because of the relationship between the scapula and the insertions of the levator scapulae, rhomboid, and trapezius muscles.

Capener (10) in 1954 modified the costotransversectomy procedure renaming it the "lateral rhachotomy," an approach providing additional exposure of the mid- to lower thoracic spine vertebral elements via a semilunar incision with lateral reflection of the trapezius muscle and division of the erector spinae muscle. These modifications to the costotransversectomy permitted excellent exposure of the mid- to lower thoracic spine. However, exposure of the upper thoracic spine was inadequate using this procedure. Additionally, exposure of the mid- to lower lumbar spine was technically complex using this approach.

Anterior approaches to the lower spine in the modern era have been described by Hodgson and Stock (11) with their development of the retroperitoneal approach. The success of anterior approaches to the thoracic spine lies in part in that they permit complete decompression of anterior pathology and stabilization of the spine, should this be indicated, with good results. The extensive surgeries involved with anterior approaches were not without significant morbidity, however. Until recently, anterior approaches to the thoracic spine were preferentially utilized by surgeons, with anterior and posterior fixation being performed in staged procedures when required.

In 1976, Larson and associates (12) reported a modification of the lateral rhachotomy that provided excellent exposure of the mid- to lower thoracic spine and the lumbar spine with somewhat less morbidity. Their modifications included the use of a "hockey-stick" incision rather than a semilunar incision and mobilization of the erector spinae musculature medially and laterally. Rather than transecting these muscles, they were reflected contralaterally over the spinous processes. This approach was still limited in the upper thoracic spine, however.

Subsequently, Fessler and co-workers (13) modified this procedure to enable improved exposure of the upper and thoracic spine. By identifying the fascial plane separating the trapezius and rhomboid muscle from the erector spinae and reflecting these laterally as an independent myocutaneous flap, excellent exposure can be obtained down to the inferior aspect of C7. With this simple modification, referred to as the lateral parascapular extrapleural approach, the posterolateral approach to the spine can achieve exposure of all anterior vertebral elements from L5 to inferior C7.

Indications and Contraindications

The lateral extracavitary approach (LECA) has been used successfully in a myriad of pathological processes of the anterior thoracic or lumbar spine and is indicated in lesions resulting in biomechanical instability or neurological dysfunction (14). Such lesions may be neoplastic (benign or malignant, metastatic disease), infectious (such as osteomyelitis, Pott's disease, and anterior epidural abscesses), degenerative, or traumatic in nature. In general, any significant disease process resulting in myelopathy from anterior spinal cord compression or anterior instability is a reasonable indication for the LECA. This is because, in contrast to most anterior and posterior approaches to the thoracolumbar spine, the LECA allows for excellent simultaneous exposure of the anterior, lateral, and posterior spinal elements. Circumferential decompression and simultaneous posterior or segmental instrumentation of multiple segments between C7 and L5 is therefore possible through a single incision. Thus, the LECA has found common use in the management of pathological or traumatic fractures that require anterior decompression and or reconstruction (13,15–17).

The LECA is not recommended, however, in patients with a limited life expectancy secondary to a severe systemic illness including metastatic malignancy and severe cardiac or pulmonary disease. The procedure should not be performed in patients with severe diffuse vertebral bone disease who may require postdecompressive stabilization as they would be rendered unstable. Another contraindication would be extensive exposures likely to require intra- or postoperative blood transfusions in patients averse to accepting blood products.

Preoperative Evaluation

The preoperative evaluation should include a thorough systemic and neurological workup. In addition to a complete history and physical examination, a meticulous neurological evaluation should be performed. Blood work should include a complete blood count with differential, electrolyte, and renal profiles, as well as liver profile and erythrocyte sedimentation rate. Testing for serum calcium, alkaline phosphatase, and serum protein electrophoresis may be helpful in evaluating for disease processes such as multiple myeloma. Antinuclear antibody and rheumatoid factor analysis may be useful in the evaluation of rheumatoid arthritis. Prostatic specific antigen and serum acid phosphatase levels should be obtained where metastatic prostatic disease is suspected. Systemic illnesses such as severe cardiac or pulmonary disease, which may complicate the intraoperative or postoperative course, should be identified prior to surgery.

The preoperative workup must also include appropriate radiographic imaging—specifically, plain film x-rays, magnetic resonance imaging (MRI) scans, and possibly postmyelogram computed tomography (CT) scans tailored to the specific diagnosis. Additional radiographic studies such as radionucleotide bone scintigraphy, chest and abdominal CT scans, and plain film x-rays may be of benefit in the workup of malignancy or infection. Some authors consider it important to localize the artery of Adamkiewicz preoperatively using spinal angiography (18). Knowledge of the laterality of this artery has been employed by some surgeons in determining the side of surgical approach (18,19). The artery of Adamkiewicz is present on the left side in 60% of patients, entering the spinal canal between T9 and T12 75% of the time, between T7 and T8 15% of the time, and between L1 and L2 10% of the time (19–21). Rare cases of spinal cord ischemia from sacrifice of this artery have been reported.

Plain film radiographic studies should include anteroposterior (AP) and lateral views and are useful in the demonstration of traumatic or pathological vertebral fractures, osteomyelitic lesions, and metastatic lytic lesions. Fractures are demonstrated on plain film x-rays as vertebral collapse, loss of alignment, and widening of the pedicles. Osteomyelitis or discitis may initially appear as a narrowing of the disc space. Destructive changes, which appear as lytic areas in the anterior aspect of the vertebral body adjacent to the disc and end plate, may be seen at 3 to 6 weeks. Bony metastases are usually defined by vertebral collapse, unilateral erosion of a pedicle, osteoblastic lesions. and "fish-mouthing" (i.e., superior and inferior end-plate concavity of the vertebral body).

In most cases obtaining a spinal CT or MRI scan or both is indicated. A CT scan alone gives excellent detail as to the extent of bony involvement in fractures, infections, and malignancy but is less useful in the evaluation of thecal sac, nerve root, or intradural involvement of most lesions. Thecal sac or nerve root encroachment is better assessed using MRI studies or myelography with postmyelogram CT scan. Myelography followed by CT scan can demonstrate the presence of intraaxial or extraaxial lesions as well as disc herniations and retropulsed bony fragments from fractures. These lesions may appear as an indentation or a complete blockade of the myelographic dye column in the spinal canal. Sagittal MRI scans may tend to exaggerate certain pathology such as disc herniations. However, when used in conjunction with contrast administration, this diagnostic tool is extremely useful in the evaluation of intramedullary neoplastic lesions, spinal vascular malformations, as well as paravertebral and intraspinal abscesses without the associated risks of myelography.

Surgical Technique

ANESTHESIA AND POSITIONING. General anesthesia has been utilized for all patients with a combined protocol of ethane inhalant and intravenous sufentanil. Three separate intubation methods have been assessed and utilized in patients undergoing the LECA: (a) routine single-lumen endotracheal intubation,

(b) double-lumen endotracheal intubation, and (c) single-lumen endotracheal intubation with high-frequency ventilation. A major disadvantage of routine, single-lumen endotracheal intubation is that the ipsilateral lung expands and contracts within the surgical field during the critical periods of the procedure, potentially obscuring the field of view and increasing the potential for injury to the pleural elements. Double-lumen endotracheal intubation requires a significantly lengthier anesthesiology preparation time and is associated with a higher complication rate. However, it offers the added advantage of allowing temporary unilateral deflation of the ipsilateral lung during critical periods of corpectomy and decompression. Single-lumen endotracheal intubation with high-frequency ventilation allows for retraction of the lung out of the surgical field with minimal reinflation during the corpectomy and decompression while permitting simultaneous ventilation of the remainder of the ipsilateral lung. The latter technique appears to be ideal for procedures involving the upper thoracic spine. Single-lumen endotracheal intubation is adequate for exposures of the low thoracic and lumbar spine not requiring extrapleural manipulation. However, in patients undergoing a surgical procedure between C7 and T6, the high-frequency ventilation technique should be employed.

Prior to positioning large-bore intravenous access lines, arterial lines and a Foley catheter should be placed. All patients should be fitted with full-length pneumatic stockings prior to induction of general anesthesia and postoperatively. The patient is positioned prone on chest rolls with the arms tucked to the side or positioned above the head (Fig. 1A), although some surgeons prefer the three-quarter prone position (15). Where the surgical approach is to C7-T6, the ipsilateral chest roll is positioned somewhat medially on the chest, allowing the shoulder to fall ventrally and carry the scapula with it. This enables the scapula to fall out of the surgical field upon release of the rhomboids and trapezius. Intravenous antibiotics and a steroid bolus (10 mg dexamethasone) are given where not contraindicated prior to making the incision. Monitoring of somatosensory evoked potentials (SSEPs) should be performed continuously throughout the operation. Midazolam administration has been shown to cause a decrease in amplitude and a delay in SSEPs

(22) and thus should be avoided during induction of anesthesia where these are being monitored.

SKIN INCISION AND MUSCULOCUTANEOUS FLAP. The entire posterior aspect of the neck and back from the nuchal line to the intergluteal fold is prepared and draped for surgery. A midline "hockey-stick" incision is marked out with a sterile marking pen (Fig. 1A). Useful landmarks including the spinous process of C7 and portions of the scapula corresponding to T3 and T7, respectively, are depicted in Fig. 1B. A case of a patient presenting with a compressive lesion involving the T3 vertebral body is shown in Fig. 2. Sagittal and axial MRI images (Fig. 2A,B) and bone scan studies (Fig. 2C) demonstrate the metastatic involvement. This patient's tumor was resected using the LECA.

After the incision has been marked out, the skin is infiltrated with a solution of local anesthetic containing epinephrine. The extent of the incision is tailored to the specific exposure desired. Multilevel corpectomies require a minimum incision extending three spinous processes above to three spinous processes below the level of the lesion. This extended incision allows for adequate mobilization of the paraspinal muscles out of the surgical field and is necessary for posterior reconstruction. Exposures for thoracic disc excision, in contrast, only require an incision extending one to two levels above and below the level of the lesion. The curved portion of the hockey-stick incision is extended inferiorly and laterally to the midscapular line on the side of the lesion. This incision is carried to the thoracodorsal fascia with minimal subcutaneous dissection.

The thoracodorsal fascia is then incised along the spinous processes. A subperiosteal dissection of the trapezius and rhomboid muscles off the spinous processes in the upper thoracic regions is then performed, leaving the interspinous ligament intact. By identifying each of the muscle layers as they are dissected, a plane of loose areolar tissue can be located between these shoulder muscles and the erector spinae muscles—the thoracoscapular space (Fig. 3). Blunt dissection of this plane enables the trapezius and rhomboid muscles to be reflected together toward the medial border of the scapula as a myocuta-

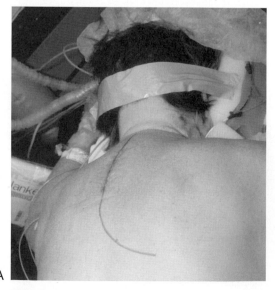

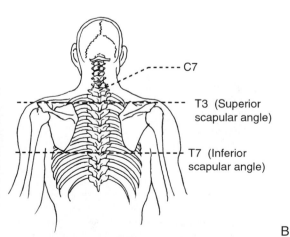

Fig. 1. **A**: The patient is placed in the prone position on bolsters. A "hockey-stick" incision is then made extending over the desired level with the incision length tailored to the particular lesion. **B**: Useful bony landmarks include the spine of C7, the superior scapular spine (T3), and the inferior scapular spine (T7).

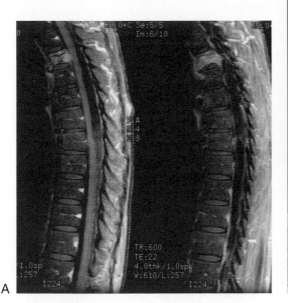

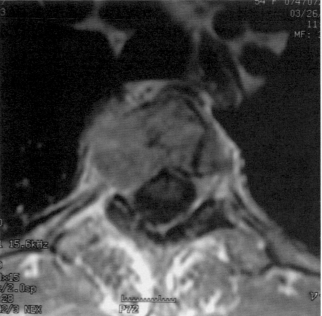

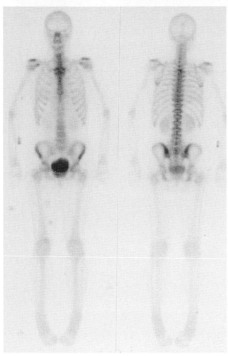

Fig. 2. **A**: T1-weighted, contrast-enhanced magnetic resonance imaging (MRI) scan of the upper thoracic spine showing a metastatic melanoma involving the T3 vertebral body in a 54-year-old woman. **B**: Axial T1-weighted images of the same lesion demonstrating the anterior location of the tumor. This patient's tumor was resected via a lateral extracavitary approach (LECA). **C**: Radionucleotide bone scan showing involvement of the T3 vertebral body with metastatic melanoma.

neous flap (Fig. 4A). Often, the inferior fibers of the trapezius must be transected to reflect this flap. Tagging of the transected edges with sutures allows for reapproximation of these fibers at the conclusion of the operation. Immediately anterior to the inferior trapezius muscles the superior fibers of the latissimus dorsi muscle are exposed. Reflection of the musculocutaneous flap is limited by the superior and lateral extents of the skin incision and the medial border of the scapula.

Mobilization of the trapezius-rhomboid complex is unnecessary in the mid- to lower thoracic and lumbar spine as the thoracodorsal fascia does not cover a large muscle mass but rather forms an aponeurosis extending from the spinous processes to the lateral insertions of the trapezius. Incision of this aponeuro-

sis immediately exposes the paraspinal (erector spinae) muscles. The consequence of this specific anatomical relationship is that a musculocutaneous flap cannot be developed in this region. A large potential space for seroma formation is created and must be obliterated during closure. Additionally, the skin flap edges in this region are at higher risk of necrosis from diminished blood flow than in the upper thoracic spine.

Following mobilization of the trapezius and rhomboid muscles (or trapezius aponeurosis), the erector spinae muscles are mobilized medially (Fig. 4A) (off the spinous processes and laminae) and laterally (off the facet complexes and transverse processes). Retraction of this muscle mass posteriorly and medially over the spinous processes provides excellent exposure of

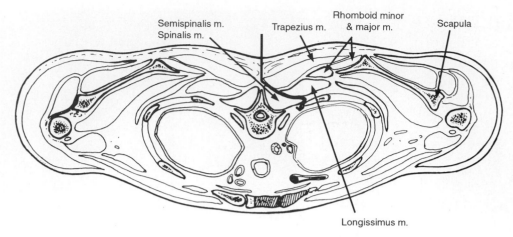

Fig. 3. The plane of dissection utilized in the lateral extracavitary approach is depicted (*curved arrow*). A midline incision is made and the dissection is carried through the "thoracoscapular space" between the superficial back muscles and the erector spinae muscles to expose the posterior rib cage.

the posterior rib cage (or external oblique muscle) and posterior vertebral elements (Fig. 4B). For surgery between C7 and T6, the scapula will fall anteriorly and laterally out of the surgical field.

RIB RESECTION. The posterior aspect of the thoracic cage is opened by removing between one and four ribs, depending on the specific pathological process anticipated. Single-level thoracic disc herniations rarely require resection of more than one rib; however, multilevel metastatic lesions of the spine may require the resection of three or more ribs. Complete exposure of a single vertebral element requires resection of the corresponding rib and the rib below it. Thus, to expose the T3 vertebral body, the third and fourth ribs must be removed (Fig. 5A). These ribs are resected at the point where they angle and begin to run anteriorly, generally 6 to 8 cm lateral to the costovertebral junction (Fig. 5B). An additional rib may be removed should further exposure be required, with the side of approach and the location of the pathology determining the rib to be removed.

Intraoperative fluoroscopy is used to verify the appropriate ribs and/or vertebral bodies for resection. Two methods have been used for rib resections. The first method, employed in total rib removal, involves a periosteal dissection of the intercostal muscles and neurovascular bundles off the ribs. The costotransverse and costovertebral ligaments are incised to free the rib head and neck. The posterior rib is cut laterally as described earlier, with care taken to protect the cut end to prevent pleural injury. Further sharp dissection using a periosteal elevator and a Mayo scissors frees the rib from its ligamentous attachment to the vertebral body. The rib is then removed and soaked in antibiotic solution for possible use as an intervertebral strut or posterior fusion graft.

The second method enables the surgeon to use the resected rib as a vascularized rib graft. In this technique, the neurovascular bundle is identified and dissected bluntly from the rib head and neck but allowed to remain attached to the next several centimeters of the rib. Lateral to that area, the neurovascular bundle is again stripped from the rib. The rib is then cut laterally as described above. After identifying the intercostal nerve and

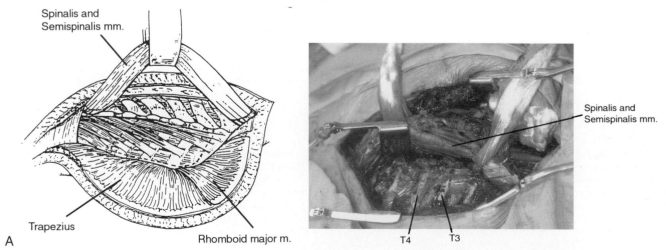

Fig. 4. A: Schematic depicting elevation of myocutaneous flap and medial retraction of the paraspinal muscles with exposure of the posterior rib cage. B: Intraoperative photo showing dissection at the T3-4 level with elevation of the myocutaneous flap containing the trapezius and rhomboid muscles. The underlying transversospinalis muscles are retracted medially with the aid of a sponge. The third and fourth ribs are shown.

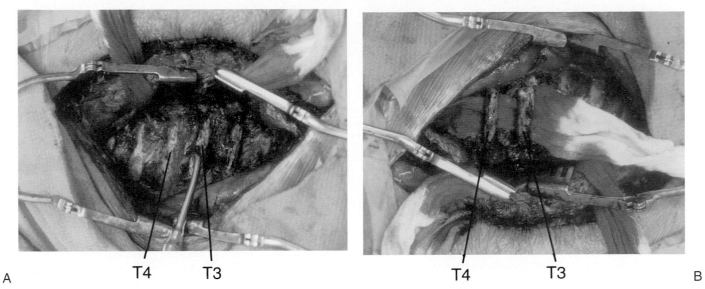

A   T4   T3   T4   T3   B

Fig. 5. **A**: The posterior rib cage at the desired level is exposed by retraction of the paraspinal muscles. The third and fourth ribs shown here must be excised for access to the T3 vertebral body. **B**: The ribs to be resected are verified using intraoperative fluoroscopy. A subperiosteal dissection of the rib is performed and the rib is resected approximately 6 to 8 cm from its junction with transverse process using a Doyen rib resector.

dissecting free of the intercostal artery, vein, and rib, the rib head is dissected as described above. The resected vascularized rib can then be reflected on its pedicle cephalad or caudally out of the immediate operative field (with care taken not to kink the artery) and used later in reconstruction.

The intercostal muscles are then removed, and if necessary the intercostal veins can be sacrificed. The intercostal nerves can either be retracted or ligated and transected depending on the amount of exposure required. If they are transected, the ligating sutures should be left long and used for gentle retraction on the lateral aspect of the dura.

LATERAL VERTEBRAL AND THECAL SAC EXPOSURE. By tracing the intercostal nerves and arteries to the intervertebral

foramen, the superior and inferior pedicles can be identified. The rami communicantes and radicular arteries and veins can then be identified and the rami communicantes followed to the sympathetic chain. After coagulation of the rami communicantes and the radicular vasculature, a subperiosteal dissection can be utilized in the mobilization and reflection of the sympathetic chain anterolaterally along with the pleura or periosteum. This will expose the lateral vertebral body and, in the case of a neoplastic or osteomyelitic process, clearly demonstrate the pathology. Corpectomy is preceded by exposure of the lateral thecal sac by removal of the pedicles (and transverse processes and laminae if necessary) cephalad and caudal to the pathology. A clear visualization of the nerve roots and lateral dura is thus provided throughout the remainder of the procedure (Fig. 6A, B).

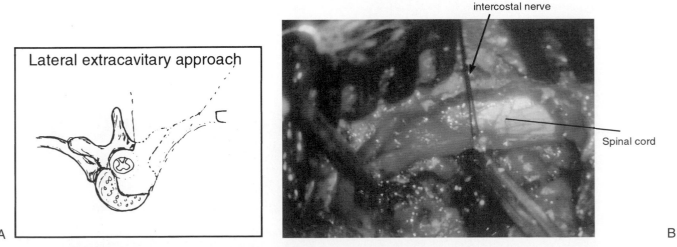

Lateral extracavitary approach

A

Ligature on T3 intercostal nerve

Spinal cord

B

Fig. 6. **A**: Following rib removal, a laminectomy can be performed with exposure of the anterolateral aspect of the T3 vertebral body. **B**: This intraoperative photograph demonstrates exposure of the thecal sac and resection of the tumor anteriorly. The intercostal nerve is shown ligated.

CORPECTOMY AND VERTEBRAL RECONSTRUCTION.
The pathological process is removed via complete corpectomy
using either curettage or a high-speed drill. Simple discectomies
can be performed using routine curettage and a pituitary rongeur. The anterior longitudinal ligament and if possible the posterior longitudinal ligament should be preserved, as they serve
as protective barriers to the thecal sac and anterior mediastinal
structures. Vertebral reconstruction is performed using a rib
graft, vascularized rib graft, or allograft bone in cases of
compression fractures or infection. In cases of primary or metastatic spinal tumors, we prefer Steinmann pins and methylacry-
late, although grafting may be performed in cancer patients
with a longer predicted life expectancy (Fig. 7). If the intercostal
nerves have been cut, they are ligated proximal to the dorsal
root ganglion and transected. This proximal transection may
reduce the frequency of neuroma formation and the incidence
of postoperative neuralgia.

Posterior spinal fixation is performed using segmental stabilization such as that which can be achieved with the Texas Scottish Rite Hospital or the Cotrel-Dubousset instrumentation system (16) (Fig. 8). In the high thoracic region where the normal
kyphosis causes the center of gravity to be located significantly
anterior to the midvertebral body, the segmental stabilization
must be extended into the lower cervical spine. The extensive
exposure provided by the LECA enables the surgeon to perform
anterior decompression and posterior segmental stabilization
in the same operative procedure (Fig. 9). Autologous iliac graft
is used for posterior spinal fusion.

WOUND CLOSURE. Prior to wound closure, the operative
field is filled with saline to check for evidence of air leak. Although rare (less than 1% in our experience), if an air leak is
present, a 22- or 24-French chest tube should be placed and
brought out percutaneously in a posterolateral position below
the incision. The greatest risk of air leakage exists in patients
with extensive adhesions from previous surgeries, radiation
therapy, or infiltrative tumors. The wound is then copiously
irrigated with antibiotic solution and inspected for evidence
of hemorrhage. Two no. 5 Hemovac drains are placed, one

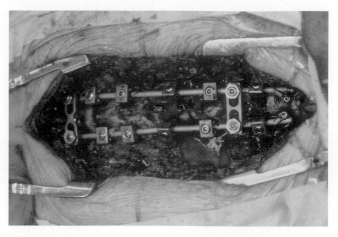

Fig. 8. Posterior instrumentation is performed via the same incision
upon completion of tumor resection and anterior reconstruction.

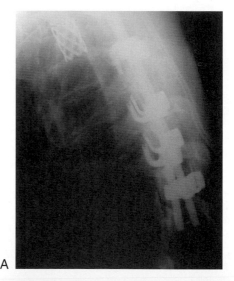

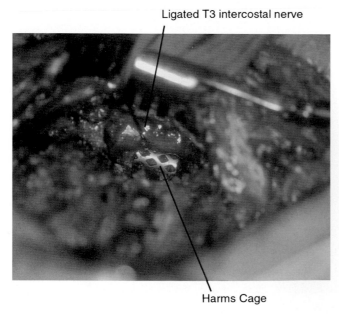

Ligated T3 intercostal nerve

Harms Cage

Fig. 7. Intraoperative photo showing anterior instrumentation with
a Harms cage in place.

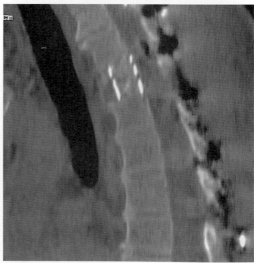

Fig. 9. **A**: Fluoroscopic image showing placement of a Harms cage
anteriorly and posterior instrumentation with lamina and transverse
process hook construct using dual titanium rods and cross-links. **B**:
Postoperative computed tomography (CT) scan demonstrating patent
spinal canal. Note anterior artifact from the Harms cage.

alongside the vertebral reconstruction and brought out percutaneously below the incision posterolaterally (or parascapularly, if a chest tube was inserted), and the other adjacent to the posterior spinal fixation and brought out percutaneously below the incision near the midline.

A layered closure is performed. The paraspinal muscle mass is returned to its anatomical position and the thoracodorsal and/or deep cervical fascia are reapproximated at the midline. The respective muscle layers from each side are reapproximated at the midline and the superficial and deep fascial layers are replaced in separate layers, taking care to obliterate potential dead spaces between layers. The skin is stapled closed and an occlusive dressing is applied.

Postoperative Care

Multilevel corpectomy procedures take between 6 and 8 hours on average, and a thoracic discectomy using this approach generally takes less than 4 hours. Total blood loss may average from approximately 400 cc for a discectomy to 1,500 cc for a multilevel corpectomy. Intraoperative utilization of a cell saver in the absence of contraindicating factors such as malignancy or infection limits blood loss. Blood loss is typically replaced with a combination of packed red blood cells, 5% albumin, and crystalloid. If the procedure is unusually long or the patient receives large volumes of fluid intraoperatively, the endotracheal tube should be left in place overnight and the patient should be monitored in the intensive care unit for neurological, hemodynamic, or respiratory changes. The patient can then be extubated on the day following surgery and transferred to a regular hospital bed.

The Hemovac drains placed are connected to pancake suction or low-intermittent wall suction (10 to 20 pounds per square inch) and the quantity and quality of drainage noted. We prefer to continue prophylactic IV antibiotic therapy while drains are left in place. If leakage of cerebrospinal fluid is encountered any time during surgery, gravity drainage is preferred. Drains can be removed 48 to 72 hours after surgery. Patients are generally allowed to sit without bracing on the day following surgery; however, patients undergoing corpectomy and reconstruction should be fitted with a thoracic lumbosacral orthosis (TLSO) before being allowed to walk more than short distances. For corpectomies involving L5, a thigh extension to the brace is used while a cervical extension is added for high thoracic regions. The braces are used for 3 to 6 months.

Potential Operative Complications

One clear advantage of the LECA is the ability to perform decompressive and reconstructive procedures via a single incision and surgical operation. There is thus a theoretical reduction in morbidity by avoiding a second surgical procedure. Nonetheless, several types of complications, albeit relatively rare, have been described in association with this procedure. As with any major surgical procedure requiring an extensive incision and operative time, there are risks of wound infection, dehiscence, pneumonia, urinary tract infection, and decubitus ulcer occurring more commonly in patients with paraplegia. Excessive blood loss requiring transfusion (and its associated risks), myocardial infarction, stroke, deep venous thrombosis, and pulmonary embolism are other potential complications to consider.

With meticulous hemostasis during the initial dissection and the decompressive and instrumentation portions of the procedure, as well as use of a cell saver, excessive blood loss and the need for a transfusion can be reduced. The risk of deep venous thrombosis is reduced by the use of pneumatic compressive devices and stockings.

Surgical complications more specific to this procedure include pneumothorax, pseudarthrosis, failure of instrumentation, progressive instability, delayed compression fracture, osteomyelitis, and meningitis. In addition, neurological complications (secondary to injury) such as paraplegia, bowel and bladder incontinence, Horner's syndrome, anesthesia dolorosa, and subarachnoid-pleural fistula formation may occur. Additionally, there is a risk of injury to nearby structures such as the aorta, vena cava, thoracic duct, sympathetic chain, lung, pleura, and shoulder. Neuroma formation may occur following nerve transection resulting in debilitating pain syndromes. The overall risk of suffering any of the above complications from this procedure is on average less than 10%, with the incidence of death or worsening neurological function being less than 1% (3,17, 18). The associated risk is greater in patients with extensive systemic/malignant disease.

References

1. Yoganandan N, Maiman DJ, Pintar FA, et al. Biomechanical effects of laminectomy on thoracic spine stability. *Neurosurgery* 1993;32: 604–10.
2. Perot PL Jr, Munro DD. Transthoracic removal of midline thoracic disc protrusions causing spinal cord compression. *J Neurosurg* 1969; 31:452–8.
3. Fessler RG, Sturgill M. Review: complications of surgery for thoracic disc disease. *Surg Neurol* 1998;49:609–18.
4. Doppman JL, Girton M. Angiographic study of the effect of laminectomy in the presence of acute anterior epidural masses. *J Neurosurg* 1976;45:195–202.
5. Bennett MH, McCallum JE. Experimental decompression of spinal cord. *Surg Neurol* 1977;8:63–7.
6. Arseni C, Nash F. Thoracic intervertebral disc protrusion. A clinical study. *J Neurosurg* 1960;17:418–430.
7. Arce CA, Dohrmann GJ. Herniated thoracic disks. *Neurol Clin* 1985; 3:383–92.
8. Menard V. Causes de la paraplegie dans le maladie de Pott, son traitement chirurgical par l'ouverture direcre du foyer tuberculeaux des vertebres. *Rev Orthopaed* 1894;5:47–64.
9. Hulme A. The surgical approach to thoracic intervertebral disc protrusions. *J Neurol Neurosurg Psychiatry* 1960;23:133–137.
10. Capener N. The evolution of lateral rhachotomy. *J Bone Joint Surg* 1954;36B:173–9.
11. Hodgson A, Stock F. Anterior spinal fusion. *Br J Surg* 1956;446: 266–275.
12. Larson SJ, Holst RA, Hemmy DC, et al. Lateral extracavitary approach to traumatic lesions of the thoracic and lumbar spine. *J Neurosurg* 1976;45:628–37.
13. Fessler RG, Dietze DD Jr, Millan MM, et al. Lateral parascapular extrapleural approach to the upper thoracic spine. *J Neurosurg* 1991; 75:349–55.
14. Dietze DD Jr, Fessler RG. Lateral parascapular extrapleural approach to spinal surgery. *Compr Ther* 1992;18:34–7.
15. Benzel EC. The lateral extracavitary approach to the spine using the three-quarter prone position. *J Neurosurg* 1989;71:837–41.
16. Benzel EC, Kesterson L, Marchand EP. Texas Scottish Rite Hospital rod instrumentation for thoracic and lumbar spine trauma [see comments]. *J Neurosurg* 1991;75:382–7.
17. Dietze DD Jr, Fessler RG. Thoracic disc herniations. *Neurosurg Clin North Am* 1993;4:75–90.

18. Maiman DJ, Larson SJ, Luck E, et al. Lateral extracavitary approach to the spine for thoracic disc herniation: report of 23 cases. *Neurosurgery* 1984;14:178–82.
19. Champlin AM, Rael J, Benzel EC, et al. Preoperative spinal angiography for lateral extracavitary approach to thoracic and lumbar spine [see comments]. *AJNR* 1994;15:73–7.
20. Tartaro A, Simonson TM, Maeda M, et al. Preoperative spinal angiog-
raphy for lateral extracavitary approach to thoracic and lumbar spine [letter; comment]. *AJNR* 1995;16:1947–8.
21. Turnbull IM. Microvasculature of the human spinal cord. *J Neurosurg* 1971;35:141–7.
22. Lauer K, Munshi C, Larson S. The effect of midazolam on median nerve somatosensory evoked potentials. *J Clin Monit* 1994;10: 181–4.

193. Retroperitoneal Approaches to the Lumbosacral Spine

**Karin R. Swartz and
Gregory R. Trost**

Posterior fusion of the spine was first described in 1911 by Albee (1), who used it to stabilize the spine of a patient with spinal tuberculosis. Anterior fusion was described two decades later in 1932, when Capener (2) performed an anterior lumbar interbody fusion. The need for access to the spine or, more importantly, access to the retroperitoneal contents and vasculature led specifically to a variety of transperitoneal and retroperitoneal surgical approaches. In 1806, Abernethy (3) described a flank retroperitoneal approach to the aorta that he felt decreased adhesions, third spacing, pain, and respiratory problems in comparison with the contemporary transabdominal approach. In 1982, Fraser (4) adapted this approach to develop a muscle-splitting but still retroperitoneal version for spinal fusion in which surgical trauma to the patient was diminished. With the advent of modern endoscopic techniques, further advances in the execution of closed laparoscopic transabdominal/endoscopic retroperitoneal approaches are ongoing (5).

Anatomy

The anatomical issues are numerous, regardless of anterior approach. Beginning with the external landmarks of the lower abdomen, a rule of thirds applies (6,7). The umbilicus is at approximately the level of the L3-4 interspace; if a line is dropped inferiorly to the symphysis pubis, the distance can be divided into thirds to estimate the lumbar level. The junction of the upper and middle thirds is L4-5, and the junction of the middle and lower thirds is L5-S1 (Fig. 1).

The musculature of the abdominal wall consists of four muscle groups: external oblique, internal oblique, transversus abdominis, and rectus abdominis. The latter lies medially along the anterior abdominal wall. Laterally, the three muscular layers—external oblique, internal oblique, and transversus abdominis—are thicker and better developed and more easily identified. Medially, they thin out into flat fascial layers immediately adjacent to the underlying peritoneum. The sheath of the rectus abdominis is formed by aponeuroses of all three of the lateral muscles. Above the umbilicus, they split medially around the rectus abdominis. Below the umbilicus, the aponeuroses do not split, only passing anterior to the rectus; no posterior rectus sheath is found below this level (Fig. 2).

Once the preperitoneal fat has been passed, the abdominal peritoneal wall appears as a thin, blue membrane. The abdominal viscera, with omental investments, can be gently retracted to expose the posterior peritoneal wall. The visceral contents of the retroperitoneal space include the kidneys (right slightly lower than left), adrenal glands, pancreas, and the small intestine (duodenum and proximal jejunum). The psoas muscles are important landmarks and easily identified in the retroperitoneal space. The genitofemoral nerve traverses anteriorly along the body of the psoas on either side, and the lumbar nerve roots exit at the lateral margin of the muscle. Care must be taken when the psoas is manipulated or retracted; the muscle should not be penetrated because penetration can lead to complications related to nerve injury (Fig. 3).

The sympathetic chain (Fig. 4) runs in the paraspinous mus-

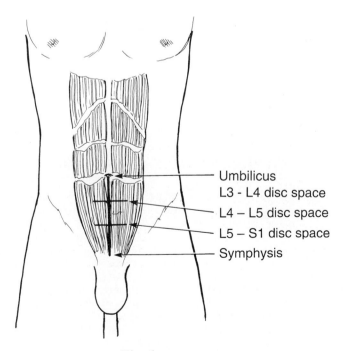

Umbilicus
L3 - L4 disc space
L4 – L5 disc space
L5 – S1 disc space
Symphysis

Fig. 1. Rule of thirds.

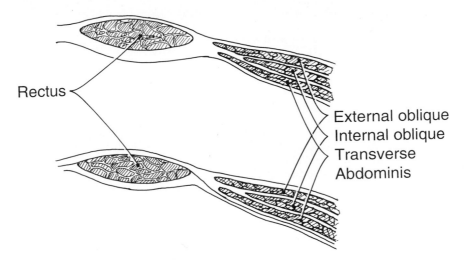

Fig. 2. Axial retroperitoneum.

cles; frequently and unavoidably, it is damaged by stretch, electrocautery, or sharp dissection. When the lumbar sympathetic nerves are injured, the patient complains of a contralateral cold foot; actually, it is the ipsilateral circulation that is affected, being abnormally warm secondary to loss of sympathetic vasoconstriction (7). The superior hypogastric plexus lies along the anterior surface of the aorta and continues into the pelvis over the bifurcation, where it may be a plexiform mesh of nerves or a single presacral nerve. It usually courses over the left common iliac artery and left internal iliac artery onto the ventral surface of the sacrum (6–8). For L5-S1 exposures, it is often best to enter this area at a point medial to the left internal iliac vessels and gently sweep right to left en bloc (8). If the preaortic sympathetic plexus is damaged (i.e., by electrocautery on the anterior surface of the L5-S1 disc), retrograde ejaculation may result.

Normally, the plexus is responsible for closure of the bladder neck during ejaculation. This is a rare complication and almost always temporary. It does not lead to impotence (6–8) because functioning of the vas deferens and seminal secretion remain intact.

The lymphatics course along the iliac nodes toward the lumbar nodes on either side of the aorta, oftentimes intertwining with the venous system; they join with the intestinal trunks to form the cisterna chyli at the level of L1-2, which lies posterior to the sympathetic chain. The cisterna narrows to form the thoracic duct, which traverses the right side of the thorax adjacent to the aorta, crosses to the left side of the thorax, and eventually empties into the left internal jugular or subclavian vein (9).

The ureter is a peristaltic cylinder, often adherent to the undersurface of the peritoneum (8), or it may be found coursing over the psoas and genitofemoral nerve in an inferomedial di-

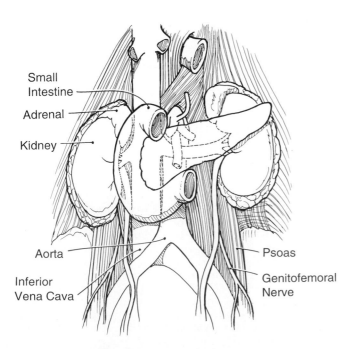

Fig. 3. Retroperitoneal anatomy.

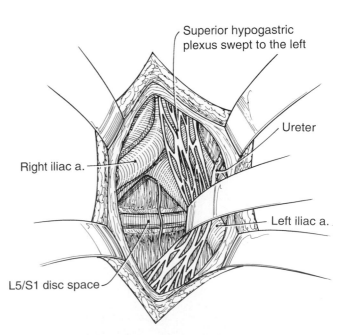

Fig. 4. Superior hypogastric plexus.

rection toward the bladder, crossing under the testicular/ovarian vessels and over the proximal external iliac vessels as it enters the pelvis.

Knowledge of vascular anatomy and common anomalous configurations is important. The inferior vena cava (IVC) lies posterior to the aorta on the right of midline, formed by the juncture of several ascending vessels. Included among these are the iliac and segmental veins, the ascending lumbar vein, which obstructs a full view at L4-5, and the iliolumbar vein. A vein ranging from 4 to 8 mm in diameter can branch off either the IVC as a large L5 segmental vein or off the left iliac vein as the iliolumbar vein. It courses posterolaterally, acting as a tether for the IVC. The iliolumbar vein must be identified and ligated in any dissection that requires left-to-right mobilization of the IVC. If the IVC is avulsed, large volumes of blood can be lost rapidly. The left iliac vein encumbers L5-S1 approaches; it courses in the bifurcation of the aorta, often appearing as a flat and avascular structure overlying the L5-S1 interspace. Occasionally, it is bulbous, large, and difficult to retract. It can vary in appearance and location and therefore is vulnerable. The middle sacral vessels are usually small branches off the left iliacs that cross the L5-S1 disc space; these should be ligated and dissected when the L5-S1 disc space is accessed (7,8,10).

The course of the aorta is in the midline (Fig. 5), slightly to the left of and anterior to the IVC, until it divides into the common iliac arteries, which are anterior and lateral to the iliac veins as they course toward the legs. Vertebral bodies correlate with arterial branches: L1 with the superior mesenteric artery rostrally and the renal and middle suprarenal arteries laterally; L2 with the testicular or ovarian artery laterally; L3 with the inferior mesenteric artery rostrally; L4-5 with the bifurcation of the aorta; and L5-S1 with the bifurcation of the common iliac arteries into the internal and external iliac arteries (8,10–12).

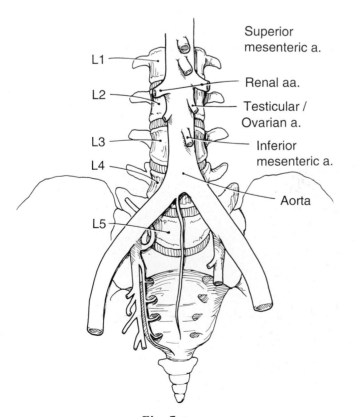

L1
L2
L3
L4
L5

Superior mesenteric a.

Renal aa.

Testicular / Ovarian a.

Inferior mesenteric a.

Aorta

Fig. 5. Aorta.

The sacral arteries are dorsal and unpaired, becoming an issue at the L5-S1 disc space (see above).

Indications

The indications for retroperitoneal approaches are many and widely debated (13). In general, most feel that a retroperitoneal approach is often the most direct, least painful, and fastest, and it results in less blood loss. Spinal deformities, including congenital and posttraumatic abnormalities, are often amenable to an anterior/retroperitoneal approach. It may be possible to address conditions such as degenerative disc disease, spondylolisthesis, spondylolysis, retrolisthesis, facet disturbances, hemivertebrae, instability resulting from fractures or dislocations, and failure of previous posterior operations (6,10,11, 13–16) through a retroperitoneal approach. Sympathectomy (8), infections (6,13,16,17), and certain tumors can also be approached retroperitoneally; intradural tumors are difficult to expose adequately in a retroperitoneal approach (8,13,16).

Preoperative Planning

In addition to determining the need for surgery based on the history, physical examination findings, and results of radiographic studies, a surgeon must choose the approach. The side ipsilateral to the pathology is often chosen, but if feasible, an approach from the left minimizes the amount of retraction required and the risk for injury to vessels; dissecting the aorta off the spine is easier than dissecting the more variable and oftentimes more friable IVC (6–8,16,17). The arrangement of the operative suite, including accommodations for fluoroscopy or other cross-table imaging devices and for electrophysiological monitoring, if desired, must be planned well in advance to minimize crowding of the surgical team.

Retroperitoneal Approaches

The major advantage inherent in a retroperitoneal approach is that the peritoneum is not violated, so that the possibility of trauma to the abdominal contents is diminished. Also, anterior dissection near the great vessels for exposure is unnecessary because a more lateral trajectory is used (Fig. 6).

RETROPERITONEAL FLANK APPROACH. A traditional retroperitoneal flank approach can be ideal to access the more proximal levels of the lumbar spine in unilateral approaches to L1 through L4 (8). Full exposure of L5 is quite challenging with this approach, but it is an excellent choice in patients with prior intraperitoneal surgery or peritoneal dialysis, skin problems that might limit an anterior skin incision, or a horseshoe kidney (10). Positioning is direct lateral, with the shoulders and pelvis perpendicular to the table to maintain the position in which the patient is to be fused. The patient may be placed over the break in the table to allow lateral flexion, which increases the distance between the costal margin and iliac crest. If possible, choose left side up to avoid liver retraction and manipulation of the IVC. Flex the ipsilateral hip to relax the psoas and thereby simplify

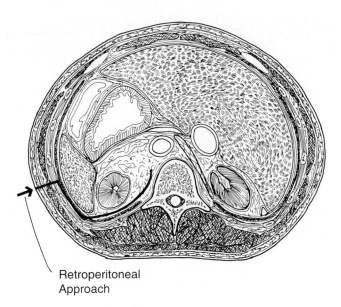

Retroperitoneal
Approach

Fig. 6. Axial retroperitoneum.

exposure and limit the risk for injury to the lumbar plexus. An axillary roll is also placed, and all pressure points are padded for protection. The patient is secured in this final position with 3-in. adhesive tape across the shoulder and greater trochanter; the iliac crest is left exposed for grafting purposes (Fig. 7). The skin incision is oblique for L1 through L5; it is carried down through the oblique muscles from the anterior border of the rectus muscle and extends posteriorly through to the paravertebral musculature. Takedown of the diaphragm may assist exposure of higher levels. Ribs may be transected or disarticulated posteriorly for additional exposure, with care taken not to enter the pleural space. Dissection through each of the three layers of abdominal muscles, with appropriate tags, is performed, followed by opening of transversalis fascia. The peritoneal cavity is identified and reflected anteromedially by blunt dissection, as is the ureter. If the peritoneum is entered, it should be repaired immediately. The psoas is mobilized laterally to expose the vertebral body after protection of the sympathetic trunk. The senior author prefers to mobilize the psoas with electrocautery. The segmental vessels are identified and suture-ligated in the midportion of the vertebral bodies. Ligating the vessels in this location allows satisfactory collateral flow of blood within the spinal canal. The anterior and posterior limits of the vertebral bodies are identified, as is the location of the spinal canal and vertebral foramina. Disc removal, bony resection, and lesion removal are performed. Grafting and instrumentation are performed as necessary. A meticulous layered closure of the oblique muscles with heavy absorbable suture is required. A closed suction drain may be left in the retroperitoneum if desired.

ENDOSCOPIC RETROPERITONEAL APPROACH.

Endoscopy has been used in an attempt to minimize surgical trauma further during anterior access to the spine. McAfee et al. (17) have described an approach that entails a shorter hospital stay than does the open retroperitoneal approach (average of 3 days). Positioning is lateral decubitus, with no Trendelenburg required. Three 12-mm portals are created: one for working, one for a trochar, and one for retraction of the psoas major off the spine posteriorly; a fourth portal for suction may be needed. The working portal may also be elongated, up to 5 cm, to ac-

commodate tools, but then the benefit of insufflation is lost with a large portal. The retroperitoneal space is dissected bluntly with a finger, by balloon insufflation, or with an optical dissecting trochar (Optiview; Ethicon Endosurgery, Cincinnati, Ohio). The intended disc level is exposed in the technique described above and verified with roentgenography. The respective midportions of the adjacent vertebral bodies are exposed, and then the retroperitoneal contents, perinephric fascia, and transversalis fascia are retracted anteriorly. The anterior longitudinal ligament is not disrupted in a lateral retroperitoneal approach. Many surgeons are comforted by the fact that the side opposite to the reaming and instrumentation is the psoas, not the thecal sac, as is true in an anteroposterior trajectory. Of added benefit, with a lateral approach, the risk of pushing disc material into the spinal canal is relatively small. The major drawback is the difficulty of accessing the lower lumbar spine; partial removal of the iliac crest may be needed to obtain orthogonal positioning. The large mass of the psoas, harboring the lumbosacral nerve roots, can also be obstructive, and it must be gently mobilized laterally. Careful observation of the location of the ureter at all times is key to avoiding complications.

RETROPERITONEAL PERIRECTUS APPROACH.

The retroperitoneal perirectus approach is the least invasive of the approaches to the lumbosacral spine, with the best cosmesis (6). Anterior lumbar interbody fusion (ALIF) is becoming an important surgical technique, and the perirectus or mini-ALIF

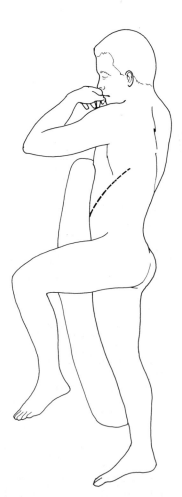

Fig. 7. Flank retroperitoneal approach.

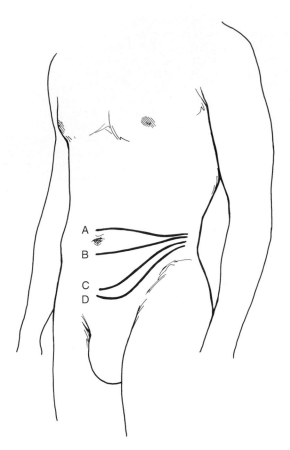

Fig. 8. Retroperitoneal incisions. **A:** L2-3. **B:** L3-4. **C:** L4-5. **D:** L5-S1.

approach is used. An access surgeon, whether a general or vascular surgeon, should be present for the case. The patient is placed in a supine position, with kidney rests at the level of the iliac crest or a blanket roll in the small of the back to allow at least partial restoration of the lumbar lordosis.

Depending on the level, the incision is begun 2 to 3 cm lateral to the left of midline; it is extended 4 to 5 cm along the Langer lines of the natural skin creases, transversely for a single level and curvilinearly for multiple levels or in obese patients (Fig. 8). A vertical incision may also be attempted, again begun 2 to 3 cm lateral to the midline. The incision is carried down to the rectus sheath with electrocautery, and Gelpi retractors are placed into the wound for exposure. The rectus sheath is then incised transversely to expose the rectus abdominis muscle and tagged with hemostats. A rectus fascial Z-plasty (medial and lateral ends are reflected 2 cm inferiorly and superiorly, respectively) is performed (Fig. 9A). The rectus abdominis muscle proper is separated from the anterior rectus sheath with electrocautery. Care is taken to avoid the inferior epigastric vessels. A Richardson retractor is placed under the lateral edge of the rectus muscle to retract in a midline direction. Overlying the peritoneum, above the semilunar line (refer to preceding discussion of anatomical features), are the transversalis fascia and posterior rectus sheath. With a No. 10 blade, the transversalis layer is divided in a feathering fashion, and the cut edges are grasped with hemostats (Fig. 9B). Bluntly, with Kittner wands, the peritoneum is teased off the transversalis fascia and carried dorsomedially. The psoas muscle is first encountered, with the landmark genitofemoral nerve. For L5 through S1, work must be performed between the iliac vessels, within the bifurcation. With a broad Deaver retractor placed on the medial side of the

right iliac vessels, retraction is carried in a rightward fashion; a broad nerve root retractor is placed medial to the left iliac vessels to retract leftward. After radiographic films have confirmed the level, the middle sacral vessels should be identified at the bifurcation of the aorta and the IVC. They are ligated and transected, as is the iliolumbar vein (Fig. 9C). For L4-5, retraction of vascular structures is to the right; the left ureter should be swept to the right along with the peritoneum. Desirable aspects of this approach include the following: pain is minimal because the abdominal wall musculature is not cut; a direct view of the spine is obtained; vascular structures are safely mobilized; no endoscopic instrumentation is needed; wide choices for graft construct techniques are available.

For the upper lumbar spine, transpleural–retroperitoneal approaches have been described for the thoracolumbar hinge (18); these are not described here.

Complications

Complications of the retroperitoneal approach can in may instances be minimized by appropriate patient selection. Poor candidates include patients who have previously undergone radiation therapy or retroperitoneal surgery and those with retroperitoneal sarcoma or long-standing vertebral body infection; all can obliterate the retroperitoneal space (7).

Operative complications involve injury to specific structures, and almost all can be avoided if the surgeon thoroughly understands and properly identifies the anatomical structures. Injury to the lymphatics can result in clear drainage of the wound, which is nonserous in nature. Advocated treatment is expectant; fluoroscopic placement of a 14F catheter at the site of the lymphatic vessel injury as determined by lymphangiography allows the surgical wound to heal without the need for direct debridement or repair. In some instances, a diet low in fat and rich in medium-chain triglycerides may be of benefit. Lymphatic complications during spinal surgery are rare despite the presence of a rich network of lymphatics surrounding the vertebral column; patients fast before surgery to reduce the already low level of lymphatic flow, and the presence of complex collaterals alleviates the undoubtedly frequent minor lymphatic injuries that occur during anterior surgery (9).

Rectus sheath hematoma can be avoided by meticulous hemostasis during dissection, although it has also been reported after prolonged bouts of forceful coughing. It typically involves the inferior epigastric artery at the arcuate line, where the aponeuroses of the external oblique, internal oblique, and transversus muscles pass anterior to the rectus muscle mass, and where the inferior epigastric vessels reach the rectus sheath from the transversalis fascia (19).

Vascular lacerations or contusions are most commonly created inadvertently during the discectomy (8). Being prepared for anomalies and possible obstructions to access with appropriate preoperative studies can dramatically reduce the risk for injury; frequently overlooked are degenerative changes, old fractures, and "spondylotic claws" that can cause dense adhesions of vessels to the anterior surface of the disc spaces (6,7, 17,20). Also, an awareness of the position of instruments in relation to the bony anatomy minimizes the unintended inclusion of vessels within instrument jaws. If vessels are lacerated during the course of surgery, the application of pressure proximally and distally as rapidly as possible facilitates direct repair of the injured vessels (6).

Neural injury can occur at any point in the case. Lengthy and painful postoperative dysesthesias can be avoided if the surgeon knows where the ilioinguinal and iliohypogastric

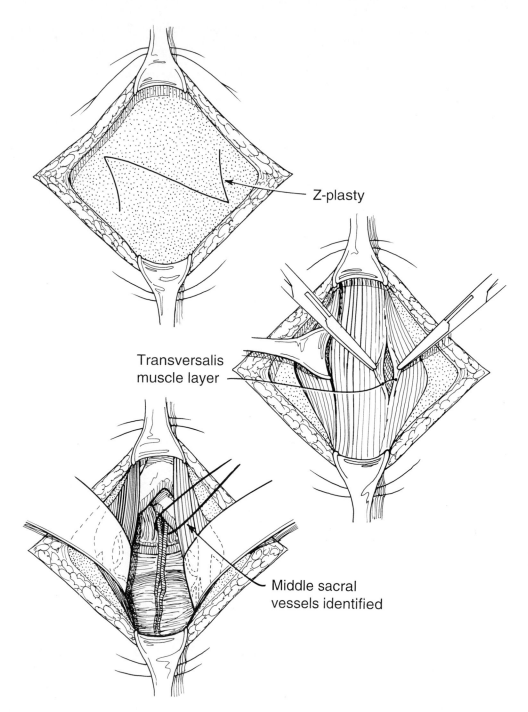

Fig. 9. Retroperitoneal perirectus approach. **A:** Recuts facial Z-plasty. **B:** Division of the transversalis fascia. **C:** Identification of middle sacral vessels at the bifurcation of the aorta and the inferior vena cava.

nerves cross subcutaneously. Preoperative review of the retroperitoneal landmarks, including the genitofemoral nerve as it crosses the psoas, the lumbar and sacral plexuses, and the pathways of the sympathetic nerves, is encouraged (20). Sympathetic injury with resultant retrograde ejaculation is relatively infrequent after either transperitoneal open (6%) or laparoscopic procedures (5%) (17,21); it is less common after retroperitoneal approaches to the spine (4%) (open or endoscopic) (22). A cold foot usually suggests an ipsilateral warm foot secondary to lack of sympathetic vasoconstrictive input, but vascular occlusion cannot be overlooked because the threat of arterial plaque embolization is not negligible (20).

Hardware failure, whether graft displacement, migration, subsidence, pseudarthrosis, or nonunion, is not a great problem in anterior fusion. However, much of the early literature was based on patients who underwent anterior fusion after posterior fusion had been performed (6,13,17,20,23). Vertebral fracture during placement of the graft constructs is still a concern (17, 20).

Peritoneal adhesions and visceral injury are matters of concern both intraoperatively and postoperatively (7,14,20); they occur frequently in repeated operations, whether transabdominal or retroperitoneal. Likewise, ureter laceration or contusion (20) is more common in repeated operations, but again, the surgeon must anticipate the anatomical path. Generally, it is not necessary to cut any longitudinal structure in the retroperitoneal space (7).

As with any surgery, infection, pulmonary embolism, and blood loss are considerations; specific to abdominal procedures are intestinal ileus and incisional hernia (12,14,17,20).

Complications at the bone graft donor site occur in up to 25% of cases (6,7,16,20); these include infection, hernia, hematoma, damage to the lateral femoral cutaneous nerve (meralgia paresthetica), pain at the bony defect site, perforation of the peritoneum, and even pelvic fracture. With fibular grafts, damage to the lateral aspect of the leg and the traversing nerves, vessels, and muscles can be prevented by staying close to bone.

When patients are properly chosen, outcomes are good/satisfactory according to surgeon and patient assessments of the ability to return to work and perform the activities of daily living. The most recent reports indicate good fusion rates, citing 75% to 100% regardless of the approach used (13,17,23,24); however, many of these studies have been small and of short duration (follow-up <2.5 years in most cases), and good clinical comparisons of the operations have not been made. Some data do not suggest a difference in fusion or healing rates between smokers and nonsmokers; allograft and autograft in lumbar interbody fusion union appear to be at least equal (20).

References

1. Albee FH. Transplantation of a portion of the tibia into the spine for Pott's disease: a preliminary report. *JAMA* 1911;57:885–886.
2. Capener N. Spondylolisthesis. *Br J Surg* 1932;9:374.
3. Abernethy J. *Surgical observations.* London: Longman, 1806: 209–231.
4. Fraser RD. A wide muscle-splitting approach to the lumbosacral spine. *J Bone Joint Surg Br* 1982;64:44–46.
5. Obenchain TG. Laparoscopic lumbar diskectomy: case report. *J Laparoendosc Surg* 1991;1:145–149.
6. Guyer RD, Fulp T. Perirectus retroperitoneal approach for anterior lumbar interbody fusion. In: Zdeblick TA, ed. *Anterior approaches to the spine,* 1st ed. St. Louis: Quality Medical Publishing, 1999: 203–217.
7. Watkins R. Anterior lumbar interbody fusion surgical complications. *Clin Orthop* 1992;284:47–53.
8. Sturgill M, Fessler RG, Woodard EJ. The lumbar and sacral spine. In: Benzel ED, ed. *Spine surgery: techniques, complication avoidance, and management,* 1st ed. New York: Churchill Livingstone, 1999: 169–191.
9. Hanson D, Mirkovic S. Lymphatic drainage after lumbar surgery. *Spine* 1998;23:956–958.
10. Rechtine GR, McAllister EW. Flank retroperitoneal approach to the lumbar spine. In: Zdeblick TA, ed. *Anterior approaches to the spine,* 1st ed. St. Louis: Quality Medical Publishing, 1999:193–201.
11. Sicard GA, Reilly JM. Left retroperitoneal approach to the aorta and its branches: part I. *Ann Vasc Surg* 1994;8:212–219.
12. Slabaugh PB, Winter RB, Lonstein JE, et al. Lumbosacral hemivertebrae: a review of 24 patients, with excision in eight. *Spine* 1980;5: 234–244.
13. Mayer HM. A new microsurgical technique for minimally invasive anterior lumbar interbody fusion. *Spine* 1997;22:691–699.
14. DeWald CJ, Millikan KW, Hammerberg KW, et al. An open, minimally invasive approach to the lumbar spine. *Am Surg* 1999;65: 61–68.
15. Sacks S. Anterior interbody fusion of the lumbar spine. *J Bone Joint Surg Br* 1965;47:211–223.
16. Siddiqi SN, Fehlings MG. Ventral and ventrolateral spine decompression and fusion. In: Benzel ED, ed. *Spine surgery: techniques, complication avoidance, and management,* 1st ed. New York: Churchill Livingstone, 1999:267–284.
17. McAfee PC, Regan JJ, Geis WP, et al. Minimally invasive anterior retroperitoneal approach to the lumbar spine: emphasis on the lateral BAK. *Spine* 1998;23:1476–1484.
18. Burgos J, Rapariz JM, Gonzalez-Herranz P. Anterior endoscopic approach to the thoracolumbar spine. *Spine* 1998;23:2427–2431.
19. Graham JM, Kozack JA, Reardon MJ. Rectus sheath hematoma after anterior lumbar fusion. *Spine* 1991;16:1377.
20. Gill K. Technique and complications of anterior lumbar interbody fusion. In: Lin PM, Gill K, eds. *Lumbar interbody fusion.* Rockville, MD: Aspen, 1989:95–106.
21. Tiusanen H, Seitsalo S, Osterman K, et al. Retrograde ejaculation after anterior interbody lumbar fusion. *Eur Spine J* 1995;4:339–342.
22. Christensen FB, Bunger CE. Retrograde ejaculation after retroperitoneal lower lumbar interbody fusion. *Int Orthop* 1997;21:176–180.
23. Newman MH, Grinstead GL. Anterior lumbar interbody fusion for internal disc disruption. *Spine* 1992;17:831–833.
24. Kozak JA, Heilman AE, O'Brien JP. Anterior lumbar fusion options: technique and graft materials. *Clin Orthop* 1994;300:45–51.

194. Anterior Approaches to the Lumbosacral Spine

Steve Klafeta and Russell P. Nockels

Use of the anterior approach in the lumbosacral spine, although necessary in attaining access to ventral pathology and implementing anterior stabilization, is coupled with an increase in surgical morbidity compared with posterior approaches. Many spinal surgeons are not skilled in these approaches and require a vascular or general surgeon to perform them. This combined effort is both more timely and convenient, especially if a complication should occur that would necessitate the skills of these other surgeons. Although the spinal surgeon may not be involved in the approach, it is important to know the anatomical nuances of the region, advantages and disadvantages of each approach, and all complications involved in every aspect of the operation.

Transperitoneal approaches to the spine were first utilized in the early 1900s for Pott's disease. In the 1920s, the retroperitoneal route was used for sympathectomies. Since then, the indications for anterior exposure of the spine have greatly increased. Spondylolisthesis, instability secondary to fracture or dislocation, infection, tumor, scoliosis, and failed posterior lumbar surgery (including pseudarthrosis) are a few of the generally accepted indications. More controversial reasons are disc degeneration or herniation and discogenic pain. In 1991, Obenchain (1) reported the first laparoscopic lumbar discectomy, and more recently surgeons are developing endoscopic retroperitoneal techniques to the spine (2,3).

The majority of retroperitoneal approaches are from the left for several reasons. The liver is difficult to mobilize anteriorly compared with the spleen, and the aorta is less friable than the inferior vena cava. Due to a thicker wall, the aorta is easier to retract and repair if lacerated. The kidneys are retroperitoneal organs located anterior to the diaphragm at their superior aspect. Inferiorly, the kidneys are anterior to the quadratus lumborum and the psoas muscles. The ureters are also retroperitoneal throughout their entire course and are closely approximated to the parietal peritoneum. The ureters are approximately 5 mm in diameter and travel to the pelvis posterior to the ovarian and testicular vessels. They cross the pelvic brim anterior to the iliac arteries. Their close association with the peritoneum allows for easy mobilization during retroperitoneal approaches. If a redo operation is needed, ureteral stents can be placed for confident identification of the ureters during this more difficult dissection. In the approach to the lower thoracic and upper lumbar spine, the diaphragm needs to be mobilized. The posterior aspect of the diaphragm is attached to the 12th rib, L1 transverse process, and via the crura to the anterior vertebral bodies. This configuration allows for the medial and lateral arcuate ligaments to pass over the psoas muscle and quadratus muscle, respectively. The left crus attaches to L1 through L2 and the right crus to L1 through L3.

During the exposure of the anterior spine, it is necessary to sacrifice one or more segmental branches of the aorta. The artery of Adamkiewicz, or great radicular artery, is at risk during this maneuver. Paraplegia after anterior spinal surgery secondary to cord ischemia is reported, but more commonly discussed by vascular surgeons during aortic grafting procedures. The origin of the great radicular artery is at T9 to T12 in 75% and L1 to L2 in 10%. It arises from the left in 78%, and the diameter is 1.2 to 2.5 mm (4,5). Some surgeons advocate preoperative spinal angiogram to identify this artery. Benzel (6) discusses the importance of collateral supply to the great radicular artery, and sacrificing segmental branches of the aorta is well tolerated if performed proximal to the collateral supply. Ischemic complications of the cord occur when the great radicular artery is ligated at the level of the neuroforamina, because at this point it is an end artery.

The lumbar plexus arises from the neuroforamina of L1 through L4 and is located posterior to the psoas muscle and anterior to the quadratus lumborum muscle. The genitofemoral nerve arises from L1 and L2 and passes through the substance of the psoas muscle to exit anteriorly at the level of L3. This nerve is at risk when the psoas is divided to gain better lateral exposure of the spine. The innervation by the genitofemoral nerve is the cremaster muscle, which is responsible for the cremasteric reflex, and sensory to the anterior thigh. Injury to the lumbar plexus can occur with dissection lateral or posterior to the psoas muscle. To prevent damaging the lumbar plexus, dissection should not extend lateral to the pedicle. Accomplishing this is more difficult when tumor or osteomyelitis can obscure the planes between the pedicle and the psoas muscle.

The sympathetic nerves arise from the cell bodies in the intermediolateral nucleus from T1 through L2. The sympathetic chains are located on both sides of the vertebral bodies in a groove formed by the psoas muscle.

The hypogastric plexus is located in the retroperitoneal space anterior to the L5 body and the sacral promontory between the common iliac arteries. These nerves are an extension of the sympathetic chain and innervate the internal vesical sphincter, vas deferens, and the seminal vesicles. The majority of the plexus courses with the left iliac vessels, so dissection of the L5-S1 disc space should be from right to left. The importance

of this anatomy relates to sexual function of the male. Injury to this plexus during an L5-S1 discectomy can result in retrograde ejaculation secondary to dysfunction of the bladder sphincter, thus resulting in functional sterility (7).

Parasympathetic fibers from S2 through S4 join the hypogastric plexus deep in the pelvis to form the pelvic and prostatic plexus. The parasympathetic portion of this plexus is responsible for erectile function of the penis via the large and small cavernous nerves. These fibers are generally safe in anterior lumbosacral surgery, and therefore impotence should not be a complication (7).

Surgical Approaches

There are many approaches, and the decision to do one over another is dependent on several factors. Preoperative planning that takes into account all imaging [plain radiographs, computed tomography (CT), magnetic resonance imaging (MRI), myelogram, angiogram], the pathology involved, the location, and patient variables are important. Some authors recommend preoperative spinal angiograms to locate the artery of Adamkiewicz since segmental branches from the aorta have to be sacrificed during the exposure (6). With low thoracic and thoracolumbar junction pathology, the decision to proceed via a transpleural or retropleural thoracotomy versus retroperitoneal transdiaphragmatic route needs to be made. Generally, there is more morbidity with violating both the peritoneal and pleural spaces. Occasionally, more than one approach is needed, such as anterior releases in scoliosis correction. A retroperitoneal route can be employed for the majority of lumbar interspaces but is difficult for the L5-S1 disc space, for which a midline transperitoneal approach should be used. The majority of surgeons use a left-sided approach, because the liver is difficult to retract in a retroperitoneal approach, and the aorta is easier to mobilize than the vena cava. In scoliosis surgery, the side of approach should allow the convexity of the curve to be facing up so that the disc spaces are open to the surgeon. Patient factors can be pivotal in the decision. Preoperative pulmonary function testing may reveal that a patient would not tolerate a thoracotomy and chest tube, necessitating a retroperitoneal/retropleural approach. Also, the history of previous abdominal operations, peritonitis, or radiation therapy may dictate a change in the approach or side of approach.

Many components are crucial to the success of the operation, such as the availability of fluoroscopy, operative table and frames that are radiolucent, spinal cord monitoring, all necessary instrumentation and tools, and autologous or banked blood. When the spinal surgeon is performing the approach, a thoracic, general, or vascular surgeon should be available in case a complication arises that the spinal surgeon is not comfortable handling. All patients should receive a mechanical bowel prep and appropriate preoperative antibiotics to reduce intestinal flora in case a visceral injury occurs.

Thoracolumbar Junction

The standard approach to the thoracolumbar junction is transthoracic. The exposure is extensive; however, it increases morbidity. These procedures require the violation of two body cavities, an incision in the diaphragm, and a chest tube. The chest tube delays early mobilization and increases the risk of infection. Retropleural techniques that have been developed obviate the need for a chest tube, but at the expense of exposure (8,9).

TRANSTHORACIC. The entire thoracic spine can be exposed via this approach. The approach is from the left, because the aorta can be retracted more safely than the vena cava. The patient is in the lateral decubitus position with an axillary roll under the right arm. The flexion point in the table should be at the level of pathology. A selective bronchial intubation with a double-lumen tube should be performed to aid in lung deflation for increased exposure. Generally, the rib to be resected dictates the location of the incision. The rib located two levels above the pathology is resected for transpleural exposures and only one level above for retropleural exposures. Resecting the rib at the level of interest in the midaxillary line is another method for planning the incision. Removal of the rib is performed in a subperiosteal fashion 4 cm from the head of the rib, and it is saved for grafting.

In the transpleural approach, after the parietal pleura is opened and the lung retracted, an incision in the mediastinal pleura is made over the spine. At the midportion of the vertebral body, the two intercostal vessels above and below the level are ligated. This allows for maximal displacement of the aorta. The pleura does not need to be closed at the completion of the operation, but a chest tube is necessary.

When performing the retropleural approach, the rib is resected and the intercostal muscles divided, leaving the parietal pleura intact. Blunt dissection is used to free the pleura from the posterior aspect of the ribs and the muscles posteriorly toward the spine. The intercostal vessels are in this plane and are easily ligated. Following the nerves to the spine will identify the neuroforamina. The watershed arterial supply to the spinal cord enters via the foramen. To avoid damaging these vessels, electrocautery should not be used near the foramen, especially between T9 and L2 (4–6).

RETROPLEURAL RETROPERITONEAL. The incision for this exposure is centered over the 11th rib and curves caudally to the anterior iliac spine (9). The 11th and 12th ribs are removed subperiosteally for graft. The parietal pleura is left intact and dissected from the underside of the ribs and intercostal muscles. T10 is the rostral limit of this exposure because the pleura behind the mediastinum is difficult to dissect. Segmental vessels are ligated in the midline, allowing for retraction of the aorta. The attachments of the diaphragm to the 11th and 12th ribs are divided. The lateral arcuate ligament is followed medially to the insertion on the L1 transverse process. Dividing the attachment to the L1 transverse process frees both the medial and lateral arcuate ligaments. Finally, detaching the crus from the spine allows the diaphragm to be mobilized. Every insertion of the diaphragm that is separated during the approach must have a cuff of tissue preserved for reattachment of the diaphragm at the end of the procedure. The retroperitoneal dissection is performed in the standard fashion and is discussed in the approach to the midlumbar spine, below. A chest tube is not necessary if the pleura was left intact (8).

TRANSPLEURAL RETROPERITONEAL. The advantage of proceeding in a transpleural direction is unlimited exposure to the thoracic spine. The incision is along the rib located two levels above the desired spinal level and travels inferiorly to the anterior iliac spine. The approach to the thoracic spine is described in the transthoracic approach, above. The diaphragm is released from the thoracic wall with a 2-cm cuff for reattach-

ment. The retroperitoneal technique is discussed in the following section.

Midlumbar Spine

RETROPERITONEAL. This approach allows for exposure of L1 through L5. The patient is placed in the lateral decubitus position with the right side down. Care must be taken not to injure the spleen during the retroperitoneal dissection. Attempting to approach from the right is difficult secondary to the position of the liver. The left leg is flexed at the knee to release the tension of the psoas muscle, thereby maximizing its retraction. There should be an axillary roll to prevent pressure on the brachial plexus, and the table should be flexed to open the flank. The skin incision depends on the level desired. To approach L1 to L2 the incision is below the 12th rib, for L4 to S1 the incision is just superior to the iliac wing, and for L2 to L4 the incision is located in between. The muscle is divided with electrocautery exposing the transversalis fascia. This fascia is carefully incised, preserving the peritoneum. Blunt dissection is used to reflect the peritoneum anteriorly, exposing the psoas muscle and the great vessels. The psoas is retracted laterally to expose the spine. After localization of the appropriate level using fluoroscopy, the segmental arteries off the aorta are isolated and divided. This prevents avulsion or inadvertent injury to the arteries during the discectomy. Large segmental arteries and the artery of Adamkiewicz identified by preoperative angiography should be spared (6). The genitofemoral nerve exits the anterior portion of the psoas at the level of L3 and can be easily injured. The exposure of L4 through L5 requires mobilization of the iliac vessels. The left iliolumbar vein is easily avulsed during this exposure and should be sacrificed prior to retraction of the vessels (10). Attaining exposure to the L5-S1 disc is very difficult with the iliac wing. The major disadvantage to this approach, according to some surgeons, is the inability to extend the table, as in the supine position, and attain adequate distraction of the disc space. With this distraction, the interbody device or bone graft is held in compression after the extension is relieved. A technique to overcome this shortcoming in the lateral position is to apply pressure to the spine at the level of the discectomy, thus distracting the disc space for insertion of the graft.

TRANSPERITONEAL. See next section.

Lumbosacral Junction

TRANSPERITONEAL. This is the senior author's preferred approach to the L5-S1 disc space. Positioning is supine with a lumbar roll to increase the extension of the lumbar spine. A table that can rotate into the Trendelenburg position helps with retraction of abdominal contents and brings the L5-S1 disc space into a perpendicular plane. Three different incisions can be used: midline vertical, left paramedian, and Pfannenstiel. The abdomen is opened and the contents retracted superiorly and laterally. The posterior peritoneum is then opened over the sacral promontory. Some surgeons advocate injecting the area with saline to improve the dissection planes. To avoid injuring the hypogastric plexus, the peritoneum is incised sharply on the right and retracted to the left using blunt dissection only.

Electrocautery in this area is believed to injure the delicate plexus resulting in retrograde ejaculation. It is usually necessary to ligate the left iliolumbar vein during mobilization of the iliac vessels. If not ligated, this vessel is easily avulsed during retraction. To gain access to the L5-S1 disc space the middle sacral vessel needs to be sacrificed. An L4-5 discectomy can be accomplished in patients with a prefixed iliac bifurcation.

RETROPERITONEAL. There are two variations of this approach: anterior and lateral. In the anterior approach, an anterior paramedian incision is made and the abdominal musculature opened, preserving the peritoneum. Positioning is similar to the transperitoneal approach. This technique allows the peritoneum, abdominal contents, and ureter to be retracted to the right. The operation continues as described above. This approach can be used to access the sacral iliac joint, with an incision over the iliac spine and dissection posterior to the iliacus muscle. The lateral retroperitoneal approach to the sacrum is limited by the iliac crest and access to only one side of the sacrum; therefore, it is necessary to mobilize the iliac vessels for visualization of the disc space.

Complications

In the recent past, many spine surgeons have been reluctant to approach the thoracolumbar spine anteriorly because it is so invasive. The rate of morbidity associated with these approaches is high, even in the most experienced hands. The majority of complications are of a general surgical nature and related to the approach rather than the spinal portion. The complications to all anterior approaches are similar, such as urinary infections and retention, atelectasis, pneumonia, wound infections and dehiscence, incisional hernias, pneumothorax, deep vein thrombosis, pulmonary embolus, and death. Intraperitoneal approaches have the potential for bowel injury, intraabdominal adhesions with future small bowel obstructions, and prolonged ileus. The retroperitoneal route is popular, because the risk of these complications is reduced. However, ureteral injury and splenic injury can occur with retroperitoneal approaches. Other reported complications of anterior spinal surgery include retroperitoneal fibrosis, partial sympathectomy, arterial thrombosis, and paraplegia secondary to spinal cord ischemia.

Regan et al. (11) reported a review of the literature concerning the complication rate in 942 anterior lumbar interbody fusion procedures. The rate of ileus, deep vein thrombosis, incisional hernia, and atelectasis was 4% each in this review. Patients complaining of a warm leg (a symptom of sympathetic nerve injury), thrombophlebitis, and urinary retention were each between 8% and 10%. Faciszewski et al. (12) reviewed 1,223 cases, with the majority being anterior-posterior combined spinal fusions with a complication rate of 40%. Despite this high overall complication rate, the risk of serious complications, such as death, paraplegia, and deep wound infections was 0.3%, 0.2%, and 0.6%, respectively. The risk of vessel injury in this series was 0.8%, much lower than previously reported incidences, which were as high as 18% for anterior incisions. All approaches used in this series were lateral. The reported incidence of postthoracotomy pain syndrome in this series was 9.2%.

Westfall et al. (13) reported their data on 85 patients with anterior thoracolumbar spine procedures. Their series included three deaths, due to sepsis, adult respiratory distress syndrome

(ARDS), carcinoma, and 29 patients were continued on mechanical ventilation postoperatively. Of 16 patients who had restrictive lung disease detected through preoperative pulmonary function testing, only three were on a ventilator postoperatively. Other complications included urinary infections, atelectasis, pneumonia, pleural effusion, pneumothorax, empyema, ileus, wound infection, urinary retention, and pseudarthrosis.

Rajaraman et al. (14) reported a meticulous list of general surgical complications at a rate of 40% in 60 procedures. Their group had a vascular injury rate of 6.6% (all venous), sympathetic dysfunction of 10% (patient complains of cold leg opposite to the side of the approach), sexual dysfunction 5%, ileus, pancreatitis, deep vein thrombosis, wound dehiscence, and one colonic injury.

The incidence of retrograde ejaculation has been reported to range from 1% to 24%. Vascular surgeons report a rate of 10% retrograde ejaculation in patients undergoing aortic graft procedures. Most vascular surgeons believe that bilateral sympathetic injury must occur to cause retrograde ejaculation. Impotence is also commonly listed a complication, but it has not been attributed to any organic causes. Flynn and Price (7) reported sexual complications in 4,500 anterior procedures at the rates of 0.42% for sterility and 0.44% for impotence.

Minimally Invasive Approaches

With the advent of endoscopic advances in general surgery, there has been a push to apply this technology to spinal surgery for decreased postoperative pain, shorter hospital stay, and cosmetic concerns. The techniques have been both the traditional transperitoneal laparoscopy and newer endoscopic retroperitoneal approaches. Regan et al. (11) report a series of laparoscopic lumbar fusions compared with conventional approaches, in which hospital stay and blood loss were decreased in laparoscopic cases but operative time and complication rates were increased. In this series, complication rates were 14% in open versus 19% in laparoscopic operations, with a conversion to open operation rate of 10% because of bleeding or anatomical concerns. The authors offered several pearls from their experience in laparoscopic procedures: trocar insertion should be done under direct vision, the vena cava and iliac veins can be flattened from insufflation and need to be visualized at all times, and at the completion of the procedure the insufflation pressure should be lowered to check for bleeding.

A retroperitoneal endoscopic approach has been developed by McAfee et al. (2) for anterior spinal fusions. A single port is placed in the midaxillary line at the level of pathology and, using a dissecting trocar with a camera, penetrates the muscular abdominal layers to enter the preperitoneal fat. The trocar is used to form the potential space until the psoas is visualized. At this point a dissection balloon is filled with 1 L of saline to enlarge the potential space. Three to four ports are used to complete the discectomy or corpectomy. Using this technique, the authors were able to perform fusions between L1 and L5. Onimus et al. (15) describe an endoscopic anterior retroperitoneal approach to the L4-5 and L5-S1 disc spaces. Experience with these approaches is limited, and comparison with standard laparoscopic procedures and traditional approaches will need to be done in the future to determine their true efficacy.

References

1. Obenchain TG. Laparoscopic lumbar discectomy. *J Laparoendosc Surg* 1991;1:145–149.

2. McAfee PC, Regan JJ, Geis WP, et al. Minimally invasive anterior retroperitoneal approach to the lumbar spine. *Spine* 1998;23: 1476–1484.

3. Muhlbauer M, Pfisterer W, Eyb R, et al. Minimally invasive retroperitoneal approach for lumbar corpectomy and anterior reconstruction. *J Neurosurg (Spine)* 2000;93:161–167.

4. Alleyne CH Jr, Cawley CM, Shengelaia GG, et al. Microsurgical anatomy of the artery of Adamkiewicz and its segmental artery. *J Neurosurg* 1998;89:791–795.

5. Anderson TM, Mansour KA, Miller JI Jr. Thoracic approaches to anterior spinal operations: anterior thoracic approaches. *Ann Thorac Surg* 1993;55:1447–1452.

6. Benzel EC, eds. *Surgical exposure of the spine: an extensile approach*. American Association of Neurological Surgeons, 1995.

7. Flynn JC, Price CT. Sexual complications of anterior fusion of the lumbar spine. *Spine* 1984;9:489–492.

8. Kostuik JP. Surgical approaches to the thoracic spine. In: Frymoyer JW, ed. *The adult spine: principals and practice*, 2nd ed. Philadelphia: Lippincott-Raven, 1997.

9. Kim M, Nolan P, Finkelstein JA. Evaluation of 11th rib extrapleural-retroperitoneal approach to the thoracolumbar junction. *J Neurosurg (Spine)* 2000;93:168–174.

10. Watkins RG. *Surgical approaches to the spine*. New York: Springer-Verlag, 1983.

11. Regan JJ, Yuan H, McAfee PC. Laparoscopic fusion of the lumbar spine: minimally invasive spine surgery. *Spine* 1999;24:402–411.

12. Faciszewski T, Winter RB, Lonstein JE, et al. The surgical and medical perioperative complications of anterior spinal fusion surgery in the thoracic and lumbar spine in adults. *Spine* 1995;20:1592–1599.

13. Westfall SH, Akbarnia BA, Merenda JT, et al. Exposure of the anterior spine. *Am J Surg* 1987;154:700–704.

14. Rajaraman V, Vingan R, Roth P, et al. Visceral and vascular complications resulting from anterior lumbar interbody fusion. *J Neurosurg (Spine)* 1999;91:60–64.

15. Onimus M, Papin P, Gangloff S. Extraperitoneal approach to the lumbar spine with video assistance. *Spine* 1996;21:2491–2494.

195. Posterior Approaches to the Lumbar Spine

Peter K. Dempsey and Charles A. Fager

Surgery of the lumbar spine is one of the most commonly performed neurosurgical procedures, comprising over 50% of many practices. Various techniques have evolved to attempt to modify the basic decompressive procedure. The trend now is for minimally invasive techniques to decrease cost and improve patient satisfaction. This chapter discusses the surgical procedures for both disc herniation and the treatment of neurogenic claudication and spinal stenosis. We describe various posterior approaches to the lumbar spine and comment on their value in treating patients with lumbar spine disease. The emphasis is on patient selection and surgical technique.

History

Mixter and Barr (1), who described the first surgical treatment of lumbar disc herniation in 1934, noted for the first time that compression of a radicular nerve by a disc resulted in sciatica and that relief of the compression through a laminotomy and disc resection resulted in relief of pain. With the advent of the microscope in the 1960s, microdiscectomy became popular. This technique permitted removal of a ruptured disc through an incision measuring 1 to 2 cm in length (2). Proponents hailed the shortened length of stay in the hospital and quick return to work, whereas critics (3) worried about inadequate decompression. Regardless of the technical aspects of the procedure, the goal remains the same: relief of nerve root compression.

Standard Lumbar Discectomy

PATIENT SELECTION. The successful outcome of any surgical procedure for pain relief is directly proportional to proper

selection of the patient. Poorly selected patients will have poor outcomes regardless of the technique used. The ideal patient for a lumbar discectomy has a complaint of unilateral leg pain often associated with sensory changes in a dermatomal distribution. Adequate time should be given for the condition to heal itself. Most patients with sciatica or other lumbar radiculopathy become pain free in 4 to 6 weeks (4). Physical therapy over a 4- to 6-week period is often employed; however, it is unclear whether it is the therapy or the time that results in the patient's improvement. Nonsteroidal medications are also prescribed, with variable success. Other treatments, such as chiropractic manipulation, epidural steroid injections, and aquatherapy, have no proven benefit in the treatment of nerve root compression (5). Usually, reassurance from a physician that the patient's nerve root is not in peril and that the problem may be self-limiting is all that is required. It is surprising how many patients are seen in our surgical practice without ever having heard these words from primary care physicians.

The clinical history and physical examination are the two studies upon which to base a decision for surgery. In patients with radicular pain that fails to improve over a 4- to 6-week period, radiographic evaluation with magnetic resonance imaging (MRI) is the method of choice to confirm the diagnosis of disc herniation. It is the patient's relief of pain, not improvement seen on MRI, that is the goal of the operation. Care must be taken to correlate the patient's symptoms with the MRI findings. Not uncommonly, a large disc herniation present on MRI does not coincide with the patient's symptoms. The presence of a disc herniation or the "bulging" or "protruding" disc at times reported by radiologists on MRI does not mandate surgery. We have examples of large disc ruptures, managed nonsurgically, that are no longer apparent on follow-up MRI.

PATIENT PREPARATION. Preoperative evaluation is similar to that of other surgical procedures. Laboratory studies are obtained based on patient age according to the American Society of Anesthesiologists (ASA) criteria. We routinely do not order laboratory studies on healthy men younger than 40 years of age. Women in this age category require a hematocrit and hemoglobin. In patients 40 years or older, an electrocardiogram is obtained, and above age 60 years, radiography of the chest is obtained. It is not beneficial to order coagulation profiles.

Patients are admitted on the morning of surgery, and general anesthesia is used for most patients. Given strong patient preference, the standard discectomy can be performed under regional anesthesia. However, the position often becomes uncomfortable for the awake patient.

The value of perioperative antibiotics has been evaluated extensively, and they appear to be beneficial (6,7). We routinely use a second-generation cephalosporin, with one dose administered before operation and three doses given postoperatively.

Informed consent is obtained by the physician when the decision for surgery has been made. Risks, such as bleeding, infection, and injury to the nerve root, are explained. The most important risk to explain is the possibility that the patient may not feel improved after the operation. Many times, patient expectations are too high, and the patient needs to understand that a period of time is required before full improvement is realized. It is also important to stress that not everyone improves with surgery (8,9).

Patient education is an important part of the preoperative preparation. If patients know what to expect, they fare better after the operation. Each patient is given an instruction booklet before operation, and the physician or an assistant explains what will occur during the surgical procedure and in the postoperative period. On the day of the procedure, patients are told they will be ambulating on the day of surgery and discharged the following day. This is the same information they were given in the office.

OPERATIVE PROCEDURE. The operating room table is set up with the foot portion flexed 90 degrees and the table extension placed perpendicular to the foot portion, parallel to the floor (Fig. 1). Patients are positioned with their knees resting on the table extension, and a roll is placed under the chest, which lies on the main portion of the table. A support placed

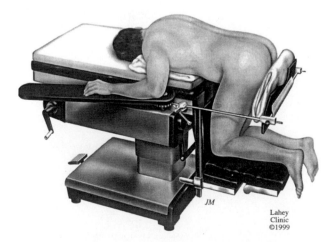

Fig. 1. The patient is positioned for lumbar disc surgery by keeping the abdomen free to reduce venous congestion. This can usually be accomplished with a support for the buttocks and padding beneath the chest and pelvis on each side. (Reprinted with permission of Lahey Clinic, Burlington, MA.)

across the buttocks permits the abdomen to be dependent and minimizes epidural venous bleeding during the procedure. Padding is placed on either side to keep the patient immobile. The back is prepared with an iodine solution.

Because discectomy is usually a unilateral procedure, extreme care must be taken to ensure that the proper side is being operated on. Each surgeon should develop a protocol for avoiding this mishap. In our preoperative area, the surgeon asks the patient which leg is painful. The circulating nurse also asks the patient which side is being operated on, and this information is written on a board in the operating room. The imaging studies are hung in the room at the start of surgery, and the surgeon confirms which side is being operated on. Despite all of these measures, it is still possible to operate on the wrong side. Only a concerted effort on the part of the surgeon to concentrate on this part of the procedure will prevent this problem from occurring.

To plan for the incision, the spinal level is estimated using surface landmarks. The ischial spines, palpated just lateral to the midline in the region of the lumbosacral junction, usually indicate the L5-S1 level. The iliac crest is located slightly above the L4-5 interspace. In a patient without much subcutaneous tissue, these levels can usually be found. Another method for preincisional localization is to place a spinal needle in the interspinous space and obtain a lateral radiograph before starting the procedure. After the level has been determined, a 3- to 4-cm linear incision is made along the midline. Soft tissue is dissected down to the fascia using a small, flat periosteal elevator to retract the tissue and a monopolar electrocautery to divide the tissue. The fascial layer is well demarcated during the opening to assist with a tight closure at the conclusion of the procedure. The muscles are taken off the spinous processes and lamina with either periosteal elevators or a monopolar electrocautery. Care is taken to keep the dissection against the spinous processes and lamina at all times. The plane between the laminas must be respected to avoid inadvertent entry into the spinal canal. Certain electrocautery units are a blend of both cutting current and coagulating current. This permits adequate hemostasis while also providing tissue dissection. In many instances, a lateral radiograph is obtained at this time to confirm the proper level. However, many surgeons do not perform intraoperative localization, preferring to rely on identification of the sacrum as seen during the procedure and on a preoperative radiograph. Operations above the L5-S1 level require a longer incision. However, if intraoperative localization is not confirmed, lateral and posteroanterior radiographs must be available in the operating room for proper identification of the relationship of the sacrum to the lumbar spine. Plain radiographs of the lumbar spine should be obtained for every patient who is scheduled for surgery for accurate assessment of the presence or absence of a transitional vertebrae. Whether this film is obtained intraoperatively or preoperatively is not the issue. The important concept is that the MRI or computed tomography (CT) scan must be compared with a plain roentgenogram to determine the presence of a transitional vertebra.

After the proper level has been determined, the paraspinal muscles and soft tissue are dissected laterally until the facet is exposed. This also enables visualization of the two adjacent laminas over the level of disc herniation. A self-retaining retractor with a blade on one side (for retracting the paraspinal soft tissue) and a post with a sharp point on the opposite side (to anchor the retractor in the spinous process or interspinous ligament) permit adequate soft tissue retraction. These retractors are available in various lengths to accommodate patients of different sizes. A curet is used to develop the opening between the superior lamina and the ligamentum flavum. The curet is preferred in many procedures in the spine, keeping the blunt side of the instrument toward the dura. This serves to separate

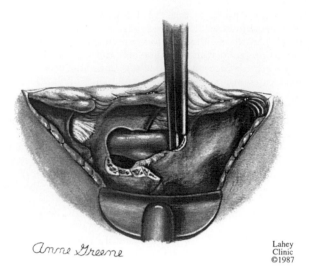

Fig. 2. Resection of the inferior lamina permits exposure of the nerve root as it arises from the thecal sac. (Reprinted with permission of Lahey Clinic, Burlington, MA.)

the dura from the overlying ligament and bone. A rongeur is then used to perform partial resection of the lamina, keeping the foot of the rongeur above the ligamentum flavum. This should prevent accidentally catching the dura in the instrument. The ligamentum flavum is not continuous throughout the spine and, as the lamina is removed superiorly, eventually the ligamentum flavum is opened and the spinal canal is entered. On occasion, the ligament must be opened sharply. In these instances, a number 11 blade is used to incise the ligament parallel to the fibers, with care taken not to extend too deeply with the blade lest the dura be opened.

After the ligament has been opened, bony resection is carried out laterally, permitting additional removal of the ligament (Figs. 2 and 3). As dissection proceeds inferiorly and laterally, the pedicle of the adjacent inferior vertebral body is encountered. This landmark is critical for determining the location of the nerve root and is the principal "navigation device" in the spine. Exposure of the pedicle ensures identification and thus

adequate decompression of the nerve root. In the case of a large paramedian disc fragment that may be obstructing the spinal canal or producing a cauda equina syndrome, the laminectomy should be extensive enough to provide adequate decompression before attempting excision of the disc.

With gentle inspection and retraction of epidural fat, the nerve root is now exposed. There appears to be no benefit to preserving epidural fat, and if it obscures the root, it should be removed. Often the root is found to be elevated by the underlying disc fragment. The root is moved medially, with care given to avoid traction on the nerve. Epidural veins can be adherent to the root and must be coagulated with bipolar electrocautery and divided before adequate root retraction is achieved. Prolonged use of the bipolar electrocautery in the spinal canal may lead to thermal injury of the root. The preferred method of achieving hemostasis is identification of the bleeding vessel and a short burst of the bipolar electrocautery. If the disc herniation is not readily apparent at this point, the root must be explored thoroughly. Often, the fragment is contained within the axilla of the root or perhaps it has migrated out laterally into the foramen.

Uncommonly, the herniation is a true "free" fragment, that is, it has ruptured free of the annulus and can be removed without opening the disc annulus. More often, the disc remains sequestered in the annulus. The annulus is sharply opened with a number 11 blade, and a blunt hook is used to tease the fragment out. Gentle retraction on the fragment is essential, with a teasing motion from side to side used to attempt to remove the fragment in one piece. After a large fragment has been removed, additional disc material is taken from the disc space using small pituitary rongeurs to reduce the chance of a postoperative recurrence (Figs. 4 and 5). The depth of the instrument must be monitored constantly so that the instrument is not placed too deeply within the disc space. The great iliac vessels lie in close proximity to the anterior border of the vertebral body. Inadvertent puncture of these vessels can lead to rapid hypotension, shock, and even death (10,11) (Fig. 6). Three different rongeurs are used for intradiscal exploration. A small rongeur with a single tooth, another with a fenestration, and a third that is angled upward assist in reaching across the disc

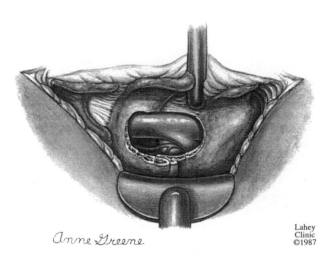

Fig. 3. Further resection of the lamina and medial portion of the facet exposes the nerve root in the foramen as well as the disc fragment. (Reprinted with permission of Lahey Clinic, Burlington, MA.)

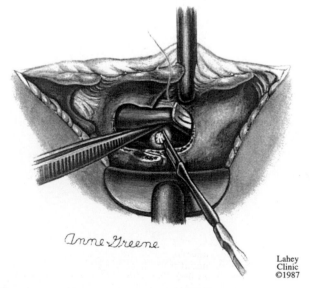

Fig. 4. The annulus over the fragment is sharply opened. (Reprinted with permission of Lahey Clinic, Burlington, MA.)

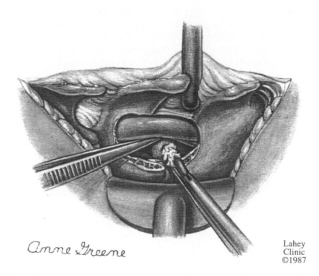

Fig. 5. Rongeurs are used to remove disc material from beneath the annulus and ligament. (Reprinted with permission of Lahey Clinic, Burlington, MA.)

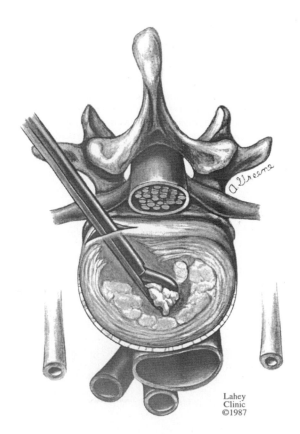

Fig. 6. Deep blind grasping at disc tissue far beyond view of the extracting instrument should be avoided to prevent anterior penetration and possible damage to iliac vessels or ureter, a potential risk more serious than that of recurrent rupture. (Reprinted with permission of Lahey Clinic, Burlington, MA.)

space. A curet with a "down-facing" foot can be used to elevate the root and thecal sac off a fragment and push the fragment down into the disc space where it can easily be removed.

Thorough exploration around the thecal sac and nerve root is essential. It must be remembered that the goal of the operation is decompression of the neural elements. A small, flat-bladed elevator can be used to palpate beneath the nerve root and thecal sac as well as down to the foramen. Not uncommonly, a large fragment has been found, hidden under the nerve root, during "one last look" before closing.

The use of the operating microscope for lumbar discectomy engenders much debate in neurosurgical circles. The use of a particular tool does not necessarily define the operation. A true microdiscectomy employs an incision of 2 to 3 cm in length, whereas a "standard" discectomy is usually 4 to 6 cm long. The length of the incision is not the critical issue. It is the adequacy of the nerve root decompression that results in patient satisfaction. In our experience, no difference exists in outcome, length of stay, or wound healing complications among surgeons who use a microscope and those who perform a standard discectomy.

After thorough inspection has occurred and no further disc material remains compressing the root, a small foraminotomy is performed to provide for longitudinal decompression of the nerve root. The wound is irrigated with antibiotic-containing solution until hemostasis is achieved. Often, further bipolar electrocauterization of epidural veins is needed along with the use of bone wax in the regions of laminotomy and bone removal.

The incision is closed in layers, using absorbable sutures. Recently, we have changed to absorbable skin closure to reduce one postoperative visit for suture removal. A solution of long-acting anesthetic (0.25% bupivacaine) is injected into the subcutaneous layer before skin closure. This practice helps in the postoperative management of pain.

Patients are ambulated on the day of surgery. With proper preoperative education, most patients can be discharged on the day of surgery, or the following day. Some older male patients have had difficulty urinating after same-day discharge and have required a return to the hospital for placement of a bladder catheter.

In the postoperative period, patients are encouraged to return to their usual activities as soon as possible. The only restriction is to avoid lifting anything over 10 to 15 pounds in the first few weeks after surgery. After 4 weeks, this restriction is lifted. Patients with non–labor-intensive jobs are encouraged to return to work as soon as possible, whereas those whose jobs require strenuous activity are kept out of work for 4 weeks.

FAR LATERAL DISCECTOMY. Extension of disc material into the lateral foramen is an uncommon occurrence (12,13). The clinical picture is unusual in that it is the more rostral nerve root that is affected by the disc rupture. MRI, particularly the far lateral parasagittal images and axial images, permits easy identification of this problem, whereas it may have been missed on myelography. The goal of the surgical approach for a far lateral disc herniation is identification of the nerve root within and outside the foramen. Some surgeons recommend removal of the facet joint to facilitate exposure of the root from its exit from the thecal sac. A more efficient approach that does not compromise the facet to the same degree is lateral facetectomy. The standard midline incision is made somewhat longer to aid in exposure. The lamina and facet are identified. Soft tissue exposure is continued over and lateral to the facet down to the level of the transverse process. This is a convenient landmark for locating the pedicle. The transverse process arises from the vertebral body at the level of the pedicle. Knowledge of this

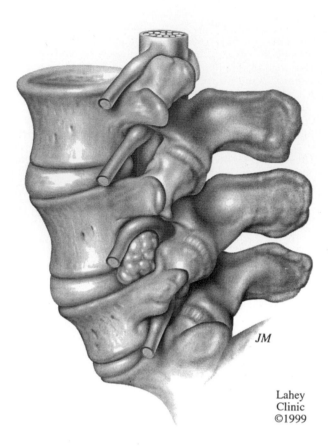

JM

Lahey
Clinic
©1999

Fig. 7. Surgical approach to lateral disc rupture, exposing the lateral aspect of the foramen. (Reprinted with permission of Lahey Clinic, Burlington, MA.)

anatomy permits identification of the pedicle and thus the nerve root exiting beneath the pedicle. After the transverse process has been exposed, the operating microscope can be used to assist in completing the exposure. The root must be found before attempting to remove the disc; otherwise injury to the root or ganglion may occur. After the root has been found, the annulus can be incised and disc material removed (Fig. 7).

SURGERY FOR RECURRENT DISC HERNIATION. Some patients will require a repeat operation for recurrent disc herniation, and reoperation can often be a daunting task. Once again, patient selection is the primary determinant to a successful outcome. Patients who did not respond well to surgery after one attempt may not benefit from further operation. On the other hand, the patient who had a successful first operation and several years later experienced a recurrence can be expected to benefit from repeat surgery.

Distinction should be made between the residual disc fragment and a recurrent disc fragment. The real incidence of either condition is probably not known because most patients do not undergo imaging studies immediately after surgery. The patient who experiences no improvement in preoperative pain in the immediate postoperative period may have a residual disc fragment. A residual disc herniation can occur despite finding a large disc at the time of surgery.

The key to successful repeat surgery for disc herniation is finding the unoperated normal anatomy. Reexploration should be started where familiar landmarks are seen. Often this requires extending the incision beyond the initial approach. After normal tissue planes have been identified, exploration into the previous site can begin. The presence of scar tissue and its adherence to the thecal sac and nerves roots obscures the normal landmarks. Preoperative imaging can be a guide as to the amount of bone removed during the initial operation. In addition, the location of the pedicle and its relationship to the prior surgery and the intended disc fragment can be identified. During surgery, the pedicle becomes the landmark on which to base the exploration. Only by following this method can inadvertent injury to the thecal sac and nerve root be avoided.

After the spinal canal has been entered, a plane can be developed between the scar tissue and the dura. Surprisingly, in many instances the scar can be peeled off the dura, permitting elevation of the nerve root. Additional bony decompression is often helpful in providing better visualization without having to retract the nerve root.

The disc fragment may also be contained within scar tissue and is often not easily removed. The fragment can become encased in fibrous tissue, which is then adherent to the root. In this situation, the disc space can be entered and any loose material removed. The plane between root and scar can then be identified, and, after ensuring the root is protected, the scar tissue can be sharply incised. Care must be taken to avoid excessive traction on the nerve root. This may result in worsening symptoms after surgery.

Standard Lumbar Laminectomy

PATIENT SELECTION. Patients with lumbar spinal stenosis differ from those with a ruptured disc. They tend to be older, with slowly progressive symptoms. The pain is often bilateral in the lower extremities. A typical history for the neurogenic "claudicator" is a history of discomfort originating in the lower back and extending into the buttocks and down into the posterior thighs to the level of the knees. It usually does not travel below the knees. Discomfort often improves while sitting and can be lessened by leaning forward while walking, such as leaning forward on a shopping cart. The diagnosis must be differentiated from vascular claudication and degenerative disease of the hip. Often noninvasive vascular studies or plain films of the hips are helpful in differentiating between these entities.

MRI is the most valuable modality for confirming the diagnosis of spinal stenosis. The T2-weighted sagittal images give a clear indication of canal diameter and identify the involved levels. The stenosis may be a result of disc bulging or protruding into the canal, ligamentous hypertrophy, or facet arthropathy, or most often a combination of all three. On occasion, patients will have an element of scoliosis, which makes interpretation of MRI in the sagittal plane difficult. In these instances, myelography with CT has been useful. Radiographic documentation of canal narrowing and thecal sac compression along with a clinical history of neurogenic claudication is sufficient to offer the patient surgery. Other tests, such as electromyogram (EMG) or nerve conduction studies, are of no value. Likewise, in the absence of contrast material, CT is often too indistinct to confirm the diagnosis of stenosis.

The preoperative evaluation for a laminectomy may be more extensive than that for a discectomy. The patient population tends to be older with more medical problems, and operative intervention is on a larger scale, particularly when multiple segments are to be decompressed. Unlike with discectomy, a blood bank specimen is often necessary because transfusion is occasionally needed during or after this operation. Patients are instructed about the procedure and what to expect in the immediate postoperative period. Elderly patients requiring support services should be identified and those services arranged before admission. These services decrease hospital length of stay and facilitate easier transition after the operation.

The goal of the treatment of spinal stenosis is similar to that of discectomy: decompression of the nerve roots.

OPERATIVE PROCEDURE. Patients are positioned in a fashion similar to that for discectomy, although older patients with hip and knee prostheses are sometimes operated on in the prone position on chest rolls as opposed to the knee-chest position. Unlike for discectomy, patients undergoing laminectomy often benefit from a Foley catheter placed after induction of anesthesia.

A larger area of skin is prepared because the incision is longer. After the fascia in the midline has been opened, the paraspinal muscles are bilaterally dissected off the spinous processes and laminas. In patients with significant facet arthropathy, it may be difficult to obtain the lateral soft tissue exposure. The tissue may need to be removed lateral to the facets to have adequate exposure. Self-retaining retractors are placed to hold the muscles, and a lateral radiograph is obtained to confirm the appropriate level. A large rongeur is used to remove the spinous processes and to thin out the lamina. Many surgeons prefer a drill to remove the remaining lamina; however, with care, a rongeur with a footplate can be used to perform the laminectomy. It is essential to use a narrow dissector under the lamina to free up the ligament from the bone before using the rongeur. In addition, the footplate of the rongeur is angled upwardly so as to avoid catching the dura. Another technique to avoid dural injury is to watch the dura itself while using the rongeur. If the dura has adequately been dissected free from the ligament on bone, no movement of the dura should be seen when placing the rongeur.

Removal of the bony lamina often does not result in adequate decompression. The hypertrophied ligament between the two adjacent laminas must also be removed. This often results in a portion of the lamina of the inferior or superior vertebral segment also being resected. After decompression has been achieved in the midline, it must be expanded laterally to expose the nerve roots as they exit into the foramina. This is a crucial part of the procedure because it is decompression of these roots that is the goal of the surgery. A Penfield dissector is used to palpate the pedicle at each level and separate the dura from the ligament. The angled rongeur can then remove the ligament and the medial aspect of the facet. It is sometimes helpful to undermine the facet, leaving the more superficial portion intact while opening up the deeper portion immediately above the nerve root (Fig. 8). On occasion, with aggressive bony resection, the entire medial aspect of the facet may be removed. This should not compromise stability of the spine; however, care should be taken to avoid a similar problem on the opposite side. Each pedicle and its corresponding exiting nerve root must be seen clearly. A long dissector is extended into the foramen, and the root is palpated through the foramen to ensure adequate decompression. This procedure is followed bilaterally at each level.

After decompression has been ensured, the wound is irrigated with antibiotic-laced saline solution, and hemostasis is achieved. Bone wax may need to be applied to bleeding bone, and Gelfoam or Surgicel placed into the lateral gutters to control epidural venous bleeding. Given the large amount of soft tissue dissection and the large amount of exposed bone, a drain is often used. Led out through a stab incision, the drain is connected to a self-contained suction device and left in place for 24 hours.

The paraspinal muscle is reapproximated with absorbable

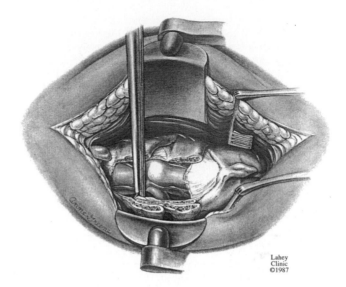

Fig. 8. Bone is removed beyond the lateral margin of dura mater, taking away the residual lateral shelf of ligamentum and continuing this lateral excision with removal of medial facet elements. Such posterolateral exposure requires minimal retraction of the dura mater and cauda equina. (Reprinted with permission of Lahey Clinic, Burlington, MA.)

sutures. This is accomplished to eliminate any dead space and prevent hematoma formation. The fascia is closed in an interrupted fashion, and the skin is closed in layers.

Patients are ambulated on the day of or the day after surgery. Hospital stay is generally 2 days.

Many patients with spinal stenosis will have evidence of degenerative listhesis on preoperative imaging, with canal narrowing occurring as a result of facet arthropathy and disc protrusion. An important component of the history in these patients is the presence or absence of lower back pain. Patients with a complaint of back pain along with symptoms of neurogenic claudication may have instability of the lumbar spine. Flexion/extension lateral radiographs can confirm the presence of lumbar instability if motion is seen. In patients with a complaint of lower back pain and evidence of instability on imaging, fusion is often recommended. In the absence of back pain, adequate decompression can usually be achieved without fusion and without removal of the disc. Fusion is not required in most of our patients.

Leakage of Cerebrospinal Fluid

Occasionally, during routine surgery for lumbar disc herniation or spinal stenosis, a tear in the dura resulting in leakage of cerebrospinal fluid (CSF) will occur. This often happens using the rongeur when the dura is caught between the footplate of the rongeur and the bone. Compression of the instrument results in a dural perforation. If the tear is readily seen, an attempt should be made to close it primarily. Typically, a 4-0 or 5-0 nylon or other nonabsorbable suture is used. Care should be taken not to permit any of the neural elements to herniate through the rent in the dura or to catch the rootlets in the suture. If the tear is not readily seen, it should be left alone because further extensive decompression to locate the leak is probably not warranted. If a repair has been made, a muscle patch is often placed over the tear to facilitate a fibrotic reaction.

Often, a small Silastic drain, such as that used in ventriculostomy, is placed in the epidural space and led out beneath the fascia through a separate incision. The fascia is closed very tightly, as is the subcutaneous layer and skin. The drain is left at the level of the hip and not put to suction. The patient remains in bed for 2 days and then is slowly mobilized with the drain in place. After 4 days, the drain is removed and the exit site sutured. This practice permits the fascial layer to heal for several days without the formation of a meningocele beneath it.

If CSF leakage from the wound occurs during the postoperative period, an initial attempt at fortifying the skin closure is made, often using a running locked suture. If this fails to control the leak, reexploration of the wound in the operating room may be required.

Residual/Recurrent Pain

In most instances, patients will experience immediate relief of pain after surgery. However, in some patients, the pain is unchanged. The possible causes of this include incompletely removed disc material or inadequate decompression. In some situations, immediate imaging is indicated to plan for acute reexploration. An example is the patient who had a clear-cut radiographic finding before surgery and in whom insignificant abnormalities were seen at surgery, that is, a large disc herniation was present on preoperative MRI, but no large disc was seen at operation. The more common eventuality is the patient who has an initial improvement after surgery but returns with the same or similar lower extremity pain within weeks of the operation. In this patient, contrast-enhanced MRI is obtained to rule out recurrent disc herniation. In the absence of this specific finding, further surgery is not recommended.

Conclusions

Lumbar spine surgery is a straightforward means of relieving persistent, incapacitating pain in the lower extremities. When the procedure is performed properly in the carefully selected patient, the results can be gratifying for both patient and surgeon. Adherence to the basic principles of adequate exposure of the nerve roots and ensuring complete decompression of the neural elements result in a satisfactory outcome with minimal complications.

References

1. Mixter WJ, Barr JS. Rupture of the intervertebral disc with involvement of the spinal canal. *N Engl J Med* 1934;211:210–215.
2. Williams RW. Microlumbar discectomy: a conservative surgical approach to the virgin herniated lumbar disc. *Spine* 1978;3:175–182.
3. Fager CA. Lumbar microdiscectomy: contrary opinion. *Clin Neurosurg* 1986;33:419–456.
4. Long DM. Nonsurgical therapy for low back pain and sciatica. Clin Neurosurg 1989;35:351–359.
5. Carette S, Leclaire R, Marcoux S, et al. Epidural corticosteroid injections for sciatic due to herniated nucleus pulposus. *N Engl J Med* 1997;336:1634–1640.
6. Haines SJ. Antibiotic prophylaxis in neurosurgery: The controlled trials. *Neurosurg Clin North Am* 1992;3:355–358.
7. Horwitz NH, Curtin JA. Prophylactic antibiotics and wound infections following laminectomy for lumbar disc herniation. *J Neurosurg* 1975;43:727–731.
8. Junge A, Frohlich M, Ahrens S, et al. Predictors of bad and good outcome of lumbar spine surgery. A prospective clinical study with 2 years' follow up. *Spine* 1996;21:1056–1065.
9. Pappas CT, Harrington T, Sonntag VK. Outcome analysis in 654 surgically treated lumbar disc herniations. *Neurosurgery* 1992;30:862–866.
10. Salander JM, Youkey JR, Rich NM, et al. Vascular injury related to lumbar disk surgery. *J Trauma* 1984;24:628–631.
11. Sagdic K, Ozer ZG, Senkaya I, et al. Vascular injury during lumbar disk surgery. Report of two cases: a review of the literature. *Vasa* 1996;25:378–381.
12. Reulen HJ, Müller A, Ebeling U. Microsurgical anatomy of the lateral approach to extraforaminal lumbar disc herniations. *Neurosurgery* 1996;39:345–351.
13. Hassler W, Brandner S, Slansky I. Microsurgical management of lateral lumbar disc herniations: Combined lateral and interlaminar approach. *Acta Neurochir (Wien)* 1996;138:907–911.

196. Laminoforaminotomy for Radiculopathy

Evan M. Packer, Donald A. Smith, and David W. Cahill

Posterior approaches for decompression of cervical nerve roots were first popularized in the early 1940s by Spurling and Scoville (1), and later by Frykholm (2), and gained wide acceptance in the 1950s and 1960s as the primary surgical treatment for lateral cervical disc herniation. These techniques have had proven efficacy and safety over time, although they have been utilized less frequently by neurosurgeons since the introduction of anterior approaches to the cervical spine. Nonetheless, posterior approaches retain popularity because of the ease of surgical exposure and the opportunity they afford to decompress nerve root pathology while still preserving a normal motion segment. Laminoforaminotomy has been effective in the relief of cervical radiculopathy due to acute lateral disc herniations or foraminal stenosis caused by cervical spondylotic disease (3–9). It may be a particularly attractive alternative to an anterior procedure in patients who have undergone a prior radical neck dissection and/or radiation therapy.

Pain referred to the shoulder or arm is generally more responsive to surgery than is midline (axial) pain. Those patients presenting with significant motor deficit or suffering from "intractable pain" despite an appropriate course of conservative treatment are considered for operation. The primary symptoms and the objective neurological examination should be concordant (10). A definitive neuroimaging study [magnetic resonance imaging (MRI), myelogram, or myelo–computed tomography (CT)] should define pathology in the lateral spinal canal or neural foramen consistent with the patient's signs and symptoms. If clinical localization and neuroimaging studies do not portray a coherent picture, the advisability of operation is in doubt. Laminoforaminotomy is also poorly suited to the treatment of midline pathology (11), which is better addressed via laminectomy, laminoplasty, or an anterior procedure. Preoperative workup should include plain x-rays of the cervical spine with flexion-extension views to exclude unsuspected instability at the operated or adjacent levels, knowledge of which could alter the scope of the procedure.

Surgical Procedure

Laminoforaminotomy is usually performed under general endotracheal anesthesia. Multiple positioning techniques have been described, including the "Concorde," park bench, prone, and sitting positions. The sitting position has many adherents, and certainly dependent drainage of blood from the operative field is advantageous (7). The risk of clinically significant air embolism is very low in laminoforaminotomy if appropriate precautions are undertaken. Nonetheless, we prefer the straight prone position, which in our hands has a faster setup time and enables greater involvement of the surgical assistant. The patient is initially induced while supine on a radiolucent turning table. The neck is stabilized in 10 pounds of tong or halter traction. The head and face are supported on a soft foam cushion with wide cutouts around the mouth, nose, and orbits as the patient is turned prone onto padded bolsters. The orbits must be free of any compression and it is imperative that they be reinspected once the patient is established in the prone position. A cross-table lateral x-ray is made to confirm satisfactory spinal alignment and to localize the skin levels for subsequent incision. In husky individuals visualization caudal to C4-5 can be problematic. Localization in such cases may be facilitated by depression of the shoulders through traction tapes or light wrist restraints. Obese patients may present a challenge to successful radiographic localization. In these cases it is sometimes necessary to expose dorsal elements rostral to the target segment for radiographic identification or to directly visualize the characteristic appearance of the C2 spinous process. Access to the target level is most convenient when the approach corridor parallels the orientation of the cervical laminae. Because the cervical laminae slope caudally, the skin incision is optimally centered one to two levels inferior to the target segment, straddling the tips of the associated spinous processes. In slender individuals an incision of 2 to 3 cm in length will suffice for the exposure of a single level. Intravenous antibiotics are administered for wound prophylaxis prior to commencing operation, and the operative field is prepped and draped according to custom. We prefer to infiltrate the proposed incision site with a mixture of lidocaine and epinephrine to assist with hemostasis. If paraspinal muscles are infiltrated as well, it is important to aspirate first to ensure against intravascular injection.

Although a paramedian approach for laminoforaminotomy has been described, we have not found it to be of particular advantage (12,13). We favor a simple midline incision that is opened sharply and then deepened to expose fascia. The fascia

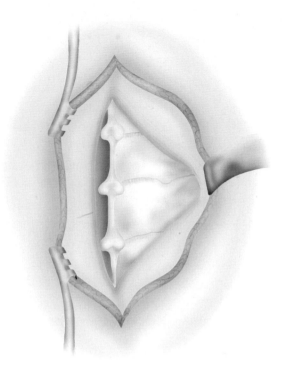

Fig. 1. The required exposure for laminoforaminotomy demonstrates the necessary visualization of the spinous processes, laminae, and facet complexes.

has an avascular midline raphe, which is entered and dissected to expose the tips of the spinous processes. Either image guidance techniques or a lateral x-ray with a radiographic marker in the field are employed at this point to reconfirm accurate localization. Further soft tissue dissection is limited to the symptomatic side. The paraspinal muscles are reflected in a subperiosteal plane to uncover the spinous processes, laminae, and facet complex, which bracket the target disc and neural foramen. At this point, a self-retaining post-and-blade retractor is inserted to maintain exposure (Fig. 1).

The facet complex is exposed laterally to allow accurate definition of the junction between the laminae and the associated lateral mass. The more rostral lamina will slightly overhang the caudal lamina, and the nerve root will exit the lateral spinal canal directly beneath this area of shingling. Bone removal commences on the lateral aspect of the rostral and caudal lamina using a high-speed drill under constant irrigation. We prefer to perform this and subsequent dissection under loupe magnification, although the operating microscope is an excellent alternative, especially in a teaching environment. About 5 mm of bone are burred away from the rostral and caudal laminae in a centrifugal fashion until the underlying ligamentum flavum is exposed. The ligamentum is first dissected and then elevated with a nerve hook so that it may be safely avulsed with a small Kerrison punch (Fig. 2).

The nerve root is usually accompanied by radicular vessels, fat, and loose connective tissue, which may sometimes obscure its identification. If the anatomy is not obvious by this point, it is most convenient to isolate the nerve root at its point of departure from the thecal sac medially. With the nerve root identified, the medial one third to one half of the facet complex can be thinned down with a drill until only a thin shell of cortical bone and investing ligament remains (Fig. 3). A small curet or fine

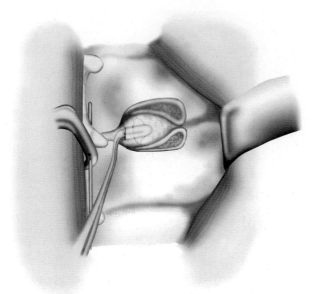

Fig. 2. With the exposure and bony work completed, a nerve hook is used to dissect the ligamentum flavum from its surrounding structures.

Kerrison rongeur is used to remove these last remnants and decompress the dorsal aspect of the nerve root within the proximal foramen. At this point an approximately 1-cm disc of bone has been removed, centered on the junction of the lateral laminae with the medial facet complex (Fig. 4). This degree of bone and joint removal has not been associated with spinal instability in our experience or in that of others (14,15). The exiting nerve root is visible over several millimeters as it courses from the

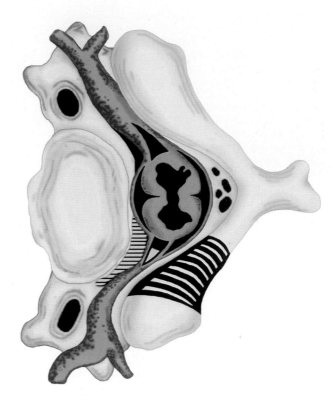

Fig. 4. An axial view of the cervical spine is shown, with the *black-barred* region demonstrating the section of bone removal required for the procedure. The *thinly striped* area shows the origin of posterolateral pathology that laminoforaminotomy is best suited to treat.

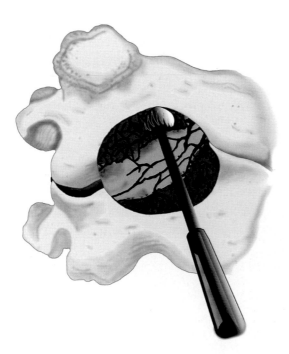

Fig. 3. A high-speed burr is employed to remove the necessary amount of bone for visualization of the nerve root. Bone has been removed from the lamina, as well as the superior and inferior articular processes.

thecal sac, through the lateral spinal canal, and into the neural foramen.

Careful review of the preoperative imaging studies will allow the operator to anticipate the pathology to be encountered at the neural foramen. A laterally herniated disc fragment will present ventral to the nerve root and will be revealed by cautious elevation of its axilla. Before this maneuver is attempted, the course of the root should be probed laterally into the neural foramen to ensure that it is not tethered by a dorsal osteophyte projecting from the inferior or superior articulating processes. This can be performed with a Woodson-type elevator, which should pass freely into the foramen. After the nerve root is dissected free of any soft tissue adhesions, a blunt nerve hook is passed ventrally and swept through 360 degrees to ascertain the existence of any compressive pathology at the level of the disc space. The axilla of the nerve root is then gently elevated, allowing direct inspection of the disc space (Fig. 5). Retraction is never applied medially against the spinal cord.

A free disc fragment is readily mobilized with a microdissector and retrieved with a small pituitary rongeur (Fig. 6). Subligamentous disc herniation is more common and is revealed as a palpably soft bulge contained beneath the intact posterior longitudinal ligament (PLL). Extraction of a subligamentous disc herniation will require opening of the PLL. This is done with an incision directed inferiorly and laterally away from the nerve root axilla and the thecal sac. Loose disc material can then be milked out through the ligamentous incision with a 3-0 cervical curette. No effort is made to enter the disc space per se or to perform a midline or subtotal discectomy. The need to resect significant midline pathology is a strong indication for an anteriorly directed procedure.

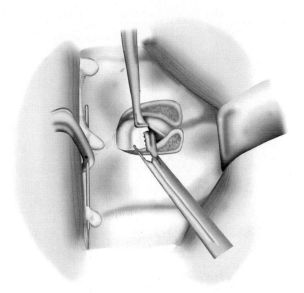

Fig. 5. Once the nerve root is well visualized and detethered from surrounding structures, it can be gently elevated superiorly. A herniated subligamentous disc can be seen once this mobilization is complete.

In the spondylotic spine, cervical nerve roots are also subject to ventral compression by so-called hard discs. These represent osteophytes that erupt from the margins of the vertebral end plates at the insertion points of Sharpey's fibers into the periosteum and at the uncovertebral joints. These may be trimmed back using 3-0 curets or a fine drill under continuous irrigation as the root is cautiously mobilized and protected. Frequently the "bone spurs" associated with cervical spondylosis affect multiple disc spaces, underscoring the necessity of accurate clinical localization of the affected nerve root. Sometimes this cannot be defined with complete confidence, and occasionally multiple nerve roots may become symptomatic simultaneously.

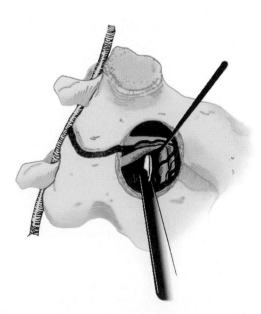

Fig. 6. After mobilization with a microdissector, a free fragment of disc is removed with the pituitary rongeur.

In a series of 736 consecutive dorsal foraminotomies, multilevel procedures were performed in 13% (6). Although spinal stability does not appear to be significantly compromised by single-level laminoforaminotomy (14,15), we have been reluctant to advocate contiguous multilevel procedures or bilateral same-level laminoforaminotomy without supplemental posterior stabilization. In such circumstances we often advise an anterior operation.

Whether operating for a "soft" disc herniation or performing a laminoforaminotomy for spondylosis, the adequacy of the decompression should be terminally confirmed by probing the ventral canal with a blunt nerve hook and by the ready acceptance of a Woodson elevator (or similar instrument) into the neural foramen. Bleeding in the epidural space is secured through accurate use of low-power bipolar cautery or by packing with small pledgets of resorbable hemostatic materials. Bone bleeding is controlled with wax. The wound is closed in an anatomically layered fashion according to preference. A wound drain is rarely needed. Postoperative care is routine, and a soft cervical collar is provided optionally as a comfort measure. Most patients are discharged within 24 hours and some may be treated on an outpatient basis (16). Recently endoscopic techniques have been adapted to enable posterior cervical foraminotomy and discectomy through a minimally invasive, "stab wound" exposure (17,18).

Discussion

The efficacy of laminoforaminotomy in the treatment of cervical radiculopathy has never been subjected to a scientifically valid clinical trial (19). Nonetheless, there are numerous case series attesting to the value of this procedure in the relief of radiculopathy due to both acute disc herniation and cervical spondylosis (4,6–9,20–22). These are vulnerable to the usual criticisms leveled against retrospective reports: unknown referral and selection biases, poorly characterized outcome measures, lack of blinded and independent patient assessment, limited follow-up, and absence of a concurrent control group. Such reports as these generally relate "successful" outcomes in 78% to 97% of patients undergoing laminoforaminotomy (6,23). These results are in general accord with those reported for similarly indicated anteriorly directed procedures (24–27). "Success," however, is seldom defined or measured with rigor.

Laminoforaminotomy is straightforward procedure employing surgically familiar exposures and techniques. Besides simplicity, its other main virtue is preservation of the motion segment at the operated level. It averts fusion-specific problems such as graft dislodgment, pseudarthrosis, donor-site morbidity, and construct failure. In our hands laminoforaminotomy has been less applicable to cases of multilevel or bilateral radiculopathy, or to cases of myeloradiculopathy for which decompression of the central canal may be crucial. However, in the appropriately selected patient with single-level or noncontiguous multilevel radiculopathy who has failed "conservative" management or who presents with a significant weakness, laminoforaminotomy remains a valid surgical option and alternative to an anteriorly directed procedure.

References

1. Spurling RG, Scoville WB: Lateral rupture of the cervical intervertebral discs. *Surg Gynecol Obstet* 1944;38:350–358.

2. Frykholm R: Cervical nerve root compression resulting from disc degeneration and root sleeve fibrosis. *Acta Chir Scand* 1951;160: 1–149.
3. Murphey F, Simmons JCH, Brunson B: Surgical treatment of the laterally ruptured cervical disc: Review of 648 cases, 1939–1972. *J Neurosurg* 1973;35:679–683.
4. Aldrich F: Posterolateral microdiscectomy for cervical monoradiculopathy caused by posterolateral soft disc cervical disc sequestration. *J Neurosurg* 1990;72;370–377.
5. Krupp W, Schattke H, Muke R: Clinical results of the foraminotomy as described by Frykholm for the treatment of lateral cervical disc herniation. *Acta Neurochir* 1990;107:22–29.
6. Henderson CM, Hennessy RG, Shuey HM, et al.: Posterior-lateral foraminotomy as an exclusive operative technique for cervical radiculopathy: a review of 846 consecutively operated cases. *Neurosurgery* 1983;13:504–512.
7. Zeidman SM, Ducker TB: Posterior cervical laminoforaminotomy for radiculopathy: report of 172 cases. *Neurosurgery* 1993;33:356–362.
8. Odom GL, Finney W, Woohall B: Cervical disk lesions. *JAMA* 1958; 166:23–38.
9. Davis RA: A long-term outcome study of 170 surgically treated patients with compressive cervical radiculopathy. *Surg Neurol* 1996; 46:523–530.
10. Spurling R: *Lesions of the cervical intervertebral disc.* Springfield, IL: Charles C. Thomas, 1956.
11. Fager CA: Posterior surgical tactics for the neurological symptoms of cervical disc and spondylotic lesions. *Clin Neurosurg* 1978;25: 218–244.
12. Hunt WE, Miller CA: Management of cervical radiculopathy. *Clin Neurosurg* 1986;33:485–502.
13. Ducker TB, Zeidman SM: The posterior operative approach for cervical radiculopathy. *Neurosurg Clin North Am* 1993;4:61–74.
14. Zdeblick TA, Zou D, Warden KE, et al.: Cervical stability after foraminotomy: a biochemical in vitro analysis. *J Bone Joint Surg* 1992;74: 22–27.
15. Raynor RB, Pugh J, Shapiro I: Cervical facetectomy and it effect on spine strength. *J Neurosurg* 1985;63:278–282.
16. Tomarcas CR, Blacklock TB, Parker WD, et al.: Outpatient surgical treatment of cervical radiculopathy. *J Neurosurg* 1997;87:41–43.
17. Fontanella A: Endoscopic microsurgery in herniated cervical discs. *Neurol Res* 1999;21:31–8.
18. Roh SW, Kim DH, Cardoso AC, et al.: Endoscopic foraminotomy using MED system in cadaveric specimens. *Spine* 2000;25:260–264.
19. Kumar GR, Maurice-Williams RS, Bradford R: Cervical foraminotomy: an effective treatment for cervical spondylotic radiculopathy. *Br J Neurosurg* 1998;12:563–568.
20. Fager CA: Management of cervical disc lesions and spondylosis by posterior approaches. *Clin Neurosurg* 1977;24:488–507.
21. Silveri CP, Simpson JM, Simeone FA, et al.: Cervical disk disease and the keyhole foraminotomy: proven efficacy at extended long-term follow up. *Orthopedics* 1997;20:687–692.
22. Murphey F, Simmons JCH, Brunson B: Ruptured cervical discs; 1939–1972. *Clin Neurosurg* 1973;20:9–17.
23. Woertgen C, Holzschuh M, Rothoel RD, et al.: Prognostic factors of cervical disc surgery: a prospective, consecutive study of 54 patients. *Neurosurgery* 1997;40:724–729.
24. Bertalanffy H, Eggert H: Clinical long-term results of anterior discectomy without fusion for treatment of cervical radiculopathy and myelopathy; a follow-up of 164 cases. *Acta Neurochir (Wien)* 1988; 90:127–135.
25. Hadley MN, Sonntag VK. Cervical disc herniations; the anterior approach to symptomatic interspace pathology. *Neurosurg Clin North Am* 1993;4:45–52.
26. Lunsford LD, Bissonette DJ, Janetta PT, et al.: Anterior surgery for cervical disc disease. Part I: treatment of lateral cervical disc herniation in 253 cases. *J Neurosurg* 1980;53:1–11.
27. Bohlman HH, Emery SE, Goodfellow DB, et al.: Robinson anterior discectomy and arthrodesis for cervical radiculopathy; a long-term follow up of 122 patients. *J Bone Joint Surg* 1993;75:1298–1307.

197. Cervical Laminectomy and Laminoplasty

Elizabeth A. Vitarbo and Allan D. O. Levi

Cervical spondylotic myelopathy represents a heterogeneous group of disorders first recognized in the 1950s. Since that time, there has been a growing body of evidence supporting its diverse clinical symptomatology and attendant pathophysiological changes. A clear understanding of pathology, prognosis, and the role of surgical intervention is critical for all neurosurgeons, as it is one of the most frequently encountered disorders requiring neurosurgical care.

Pathophysiology

Cervical spondylotic myelopathy (CSM) typically results from variable combinations of congenital canal stenosis [sagittal anteroposterior (AP) diameter <12 mm], degenerative osteophyte formation, hypertrophy of uncovertebral and facet joint complexes, ligamentous hypertrophy, and instability. There may be ossification of the posterior longitudinal ligaments and ligamentum flavum, which may alter the biomechanics, with resultant management implications addressed below. The final common denominator of these changes is a reduction in spinal canal area, ultimately leading to spinal cord compression.

While the majority of patients (70% to 85%) older than 65 years have radiographic evidence of multisegmental cervical spondylosis, only a small percentage become symptomatic (1). The precise contributions of static and dynamic forces to disease progression remain controversial. Experimentally, the importance of dynamic forces in disease progression is supported by the finding that the severity of histopathological changes is proportional to the incidence of pathophysiological stresses (hyperflexion, hyperextension, instability) at the site of spinal cord compression (2). Additionally, clinical evidence exists that those exhibiting radiographic evidence of instability treated conservatively did worse than those without gross instability (3).

Clinical Presentation

Hand symptoms and gait changes are often the earliest and most subtle symptom. Tripping and mild unsteadiness are common, as are complaints of lower extremity spasticity and subjective weakness. Sensory manifestations are logically dependent on the location. Some degree of posterior column involvement is the most consistent finding.

Bowel and/or bladder dysfunction associated with CSM is reported in approximately 20% of cases (4,5). Bowel and bladder dysfunction are rarely the presenting manifestations of CSM. In addition to the above, upper motor neuron inhibition commonly results in hyperactive reflexes. Pathologically hyperactive reflexes are common below the level of compression.

Management

While acute deterioration has been reported with CSM, the disease is often relatively chronic in nature and progressive. Deterioration is most commonly stepwise, with episodic acute exacerbations superimposed on established symptoms or deficits, leading to progressive disability. A significant subset of patients exhibit slow, steady progression, devoid of quiescent periods. Again, although Epstein and Epstein (6) have reported a 36% rate of clinical improvement and a 38% rate of disease stabilization with conservative management, Clark and Robinson (7) found disease regression and neurological improvement to be rare. Though conflicting evidence exists, the majority of available evidence suggests that CSM is largely a surgical disease in the presence of symptoms, appropriate radiographic evidence, and supportive studies.

The mainstay of conservative therapy is immobilization together with antiinflammatory medications, in an attempt to address modifiable sources of static and dynamic cord compression.

Once surgical intervention is decided upon, the principal decision regarding surgical management is whether an anterior or posterior approach should be employed. An anterior decompressive procedure and fusion is the most appropriate surgical procedure in the presence of anterior compressive factors limited to one or two vertebral body levels. This procedure most directly addresses the pathology, and facilitates fusion with the use of bone graft, with or without the addition of instrumentation.

Decompressive laminectomy effectively enlarges the functional spinal canal area, thus allowing the spinal cord to move away from compressive elements and expand. It does so at the expense of posterior stabilizing structures. Depending on the age of the patient, preoperative spinal alignment, the levels of decompression, and the period of time passed since surgery, development of spinal instability and gradual kyphotic deformity may be observed. Given these concerns, together with the considerable population suffering from multilevel compressive pathology necessitating posterior decompression, Asian surgeons developed the "laminoplasty" procedure in the late 1970s (8,9), with numerous modifications since that time (10–15). This procedure, by leaving the posterior stabilizing structures *in situ*, is believed to mitigate the development of kyphosis, and, with subsequent bone fusion, stabilize the cervical spine with improved outcome. While evidence exists to both support and refute these claims, it is now acknowledged that patients with preoperative kyphotic alignment are unlikely to do well with either procedure, and are best managed with an anterior surgery.

Surgical Techniques

While the patient is in the supine position with the neck minimally extended, endotracheal intubation is performed after administration of a general anesthetic. In selected cases, the surgeon may be especially concerned about the risk of spinal cord injury with any extension of the cervical spine because of the severity of the stenosis and spinal cord compression. An awake fiberoptic intubation with the aid of a bronchoscope can then be performed to reduce the risk of hyperextension of the neck and also permits the surgeon to repeat the neurological exam after placement of the endotracheal tube. In very selected cases, one may prefer to also turn the patient in the prone position awake, as this represents yet another instance in which inadvertent movements of the neck may occur and result in neurological deterioration. Some neurosurgeons have advocated the routine use of methylprednisolone prophylaxis as a neuroprotective agent prior to the start of surgery, the rationale being that provision of this drug in the setting of a potential spinal cord injury situation may reduce the severity of injury. As no data have been presented to suggest that it is effective as a neuroprotective agent in cervical decompressive surgery, its routine use cannot be recommended.

Neurophysiological monitoring options include somatosensory evoked potentials (SSEPs), motor evoked potentials (MEPs), and electromyograms (EMGs). The value of the routine use of such monitoring is often questioned as it has been difficult to demonstrate that the information provided can actually change what the surgeon does during the surgery. However, some retrospective studies have demonstrated the positive predictive value of such tests in determining outcome (16,17). The stimulating and recording electrodes are placed and secured and baseline recordings are obtained prior to turning the patient. A number of options exist for holding the head during surgery in the prone position. We use the Mayfield three-pin headrest, which allows the surgeon to easily control the degree of flexion and extension of the cervical spine as well as reducing the possibility of pressure on the patient's eyes. The patient is then transferred onto the operating table in the prone position, with the head secured in a slightly flexed position. Tape can be applied to the superior and dorsolateral aspects of both shoulders, and secured to the caudal region of the operating table to assist with intraoperative radiographic visualization of the lower cervical levels as required. After the operative field is prepped and draped, the midline is infiltrated with commercially available 1% lidocaine with epinephrine to minimize skin bleeding. A midline incision is made and monopolar or bipolar electrocautery is used to control soft tissue bleeding. The midline fascia is then incised with monopolar electrocautery, and subperiosteal dissection is used to reflect the soft tissue structures off the spinous processes and lamina and mesial portions of the facets bilaterally, taking care to preserve the facet capsules.

CERVICAL LAMINECTOMY. After confirming operative levels with an intraoperative radiograph, the spinous processes are removed with a Horsely or a Leksell rongeur. A sharp curet is then used to mobilize the ligamentum flavum off the lamina to be resected, and a small Kerrison punch is used to remove all interspinous and interlaminar soft tissue at the cephalad and caudad borders of the decompression. A high-speed air drill is then brought into the operative field. Using a small drill bit (e.g., AM-8 bit, Medtronic Sofamor Danek, Memphis, TN), sagittal troughs are made in the outer cortex of each lamina, just medial to the facet joint. With great care, these troughs are carried down through the inner cortex as well, such that the posterior arch is attached only by soft tissue structures after this procedure is completed. Kocher clamps are then used to grasp and stabilize the posterior arches at the cephalad and caudad extremes, and to exert countertraction against the ligamentum flavum. A second surgeon then visualizes the epidural space and gradually frees the ligamentum from its lateral attachments, thus mobilizing it and associated laminar segments, with the use of a Kerrison punch. At this point, the neural foramina may be decompressed as indicated. If foraminotomies are performed, great care must be taken to limit resection of the facet complex to less than 50%, especially if bilateral. More aggressive resection of the facet joints will further destabilize the spine and may necessitate an instrumented fusion.

One may choose to add instrumentation and bone graft to fuse the spine after a laminectomy. Several options exist, including facet wiring techniques as well as posterolateral fusion (18) using lateral mass screws and/or cervical pedicle screws (19). It has been argued that the addition of rigid stabilization to the cervical laminectomy allows one to remove the dynamic factors, which contribute to the pathophysiology of CSM. Several series have published good results with this technique (18); however, at least one surgeon has described the risks of screw pullout, accelerated adjacent level disease, and the possibility of cervicothoracic kyphosis if the fusion is not extended up to C2 and down to C7 or T1 with lateral mass or pedicle screws (20).

OPEN-DOOR EXPANSILE CERVICAL LMAINOPLASTY.
Cervical laminoplasty is usually recommended in patients who have multilevel cervical spondylosis and stenosis typically extending over three to four levels. Patients generally have a normal cervical lordosis and/or a relatively straight cervical spine. A posterior decompressive procedure is avoided in the presence of significant kyphosis. The majority of patients are recommended to undergo decompression from an open-door cervical laminoplasty from C3 to C7 with partial laminectomies of C2 and T1 and fusion with rib allograft at C3, C5, and C7, supplemented by vertebral autograft. The decompression extends somewhat rostral and caudal to the maximum levels of compression so that the spinal cord does not migrate back and become entrapped or kinked at the rostral or caudal levels (lamina) of the decompression.

The initial portion of this procedure is identical to that described above. Soft tissue dissection and retraction of the extensor cervical muscle groups and exposure of the cervical lamina and mesial facets are obtained from the inferior portion of C2 to the superior limits of T1. The inferior third of the C2 lamina and the superior third of the T1 lamina are removed using a combination of a high-speed air drill and a 2-mm Kerrison punch to visualize the underlying dura at this level. We also remove the spinous processes of C3 to C7 inclusively with a Horsely and morselize the bone for subsequent autografting.

The next segment of the procedure involves doing osteotomies of cervical lamina three to seven. In so doing, one creates an "open" side and a "hinged" side of the above lamina (Fig. 1). In general the side with the greatest compression and/or the most clinically symptomatic is the open side. If one is planning to do foraminotomies in addition to the laminoplasty, the open side is best placed on the side of the intended foraminotomies. A high-speed air drill with a small bit is used to create troughs at the level of the lamina-facet junction from C3 to C7. Drilling proceeds through the outer and inner cortical margins of the lamina on the side to be opened. On the hinge side, drilling proceeds through the outer cortical margin and cancellous bone; however, the inner cortex is not violated. After the drilling is complete, bone allografts are prepared for purposes of stabilizing canal expansion. We prefer to use rib allografts for this purpose. Again using the drill, three separate grafts are

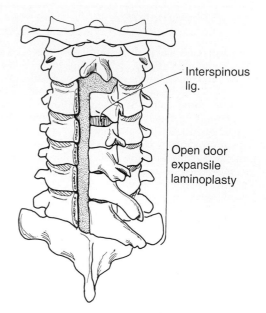

Fig. 1. Diagram depicting left open-door expansile laminoplasty after troughs have been drilled and the lamina of C3 to C7 have been greenstick fractured upward. The next step is to insert the rib allografts to help support the position of the lamina (Fig. 2).

cut, each approximately 8 to 16 mm in length. Grooves are then made transversely along the cut surfaces of the rib grafts, approximating the thickness of the cut laminae. After the grafts have been prepared, attention is turned to "opening the door." Initially, two small curets are introduced into the open gap produced by drilling the laminae, and advanced just deep to the outer cortex. By pulling the curets upward, the laminar facet gap on the open side is slowly enlarged and thus results in a greenstick fracture along the previously created trough on the hinged side. Minimal advances are made before moving to other laminae, in an effort to open all the involved laminae as a functional unit. The goal is to expand the AP diameter of the canal by approximately 4 mm. Great care must be taken to achieve this goal without fracturing the inner cortex of the hinge side. Once this is accomplished, the rib allografts are placed in the gap, which has been created at the C3, C5, and C7 levels, with the cut edges of the lamina resting in the cut groove of the rib. If done properly, the grafts should fit snugly in the gap, there should be slight "closing" force securing the graft position, and the inner cortex of the hinge side should be intact (Fig. 2). We then use the morselized spinous process autograft and place it over the decorticated bone surfaces of the facet and lamina on the hinged side to provide some "stiffness" to the construct.

Should the patient suffer from radiculopathy as well as myelopathy, one can add one or several foraminotomies to the laminoplasty procedure. Typically the foraminotomy is initiated once the lamina has been elevated and the ligamentum flavum excised. The mesial one third to one half of the facet over the exiting nerve root is drilled with a high-speed drill. The opening can be widened with 1- or 2-mm angled Kerrison punches.

Should rigid stabilization be required, facet cables with or without rib allograft can be inserted. Lateral mass screws attached to a plate or a rod can also be applied. It is sometimes difficult to position the rib allografts to hold open the lamina once additional hardware is placed, but it can be done. Other variations of the approach include the use of the spinous process autograft instead of the rib allograft to hold open the lamina. Some surgeons prefer to stabilize the rib allograft with mini-

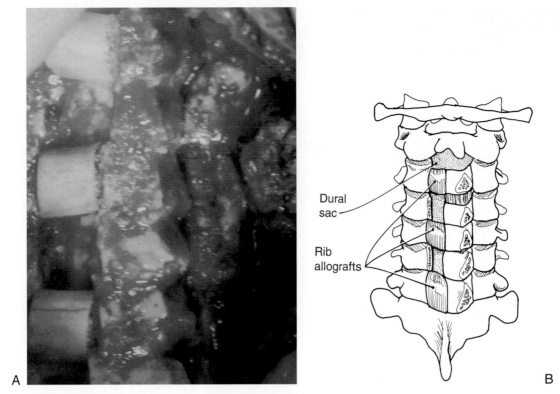

Fig. 2. A: Intraoperative photograph of C3-7 left open-door laminoplasty, with stabilizing rib allografts at C3, C5, and C7 as described in text. **B**: Artistic rendering of the pertinent structures shown in **A**, specifically noting exposed facet joints, allografts maintaining the gap between the mesial facet and the reflected lamina, and the underlying dural sac.

plates to the adjacent lamina and facet on the open side (21) or sutures. The lamina can be split in the midline with a T-handled "Gigli-like" saw and the allograft spacers positioned between the greenstick fractured hemilaminae (22).

In our experience, an open-door expansile cervical laminoplasty (without additional stabilization procedures) takes approximately 90 minutes to complete, with an average blood loss of 200 cc. The complication rate is low (see below), particularly when compared to decompressive operations that attempt to achieve the same number of levels of decompression and stabilization when tackled from the front (23). It is ideally suited for the elderly myelopathic, osteoporotic patient with multiple levels of stenosis and little or minimal neck pain. In the young patient, particularly if there is significant axial neck pain, an anterior procedure may be better suited. In patients with acute traumatic central cord syndrome without evidence of radiographic instability, an expansile laminoplasty is a surgical option (24).

Complications

The complication rate for posterior decompressive procedures is low (25) and includes, but is not limited to, infection, cerebrospinal fluid leak, hemorrhage, spinal cord injury, nerve root injury, and the risk of the general anesthetic. Specific complications associated with the laminoplasty procedure itself historically include "sinkage" of the open door. With the addition of stabilizing structures, such as rib allograft, the risk is minimal. Delayed C5 nerve root weakness occurs at a reported rate of 4.6% to 13.3% (12,26,27). Though it is transient in most cases,

recovery may require up to 6 years (27). Axial neck and shoulder girdle pain can be problematic and usually responds to an aggressive course of physical therapy. However, axial neck pain and malalignment have little impact on ultimate outcome and JOA scores (26,28–30), unless associated with a decreased cervical curve index of >10 (27,31).

An additional concern regarding laminectomy is the development of the "postlaminectomy membrane" (32). This entity has been implicated in arachnoiditis and restenosis, and may theoretically result in clinical deterioration (21). These findings have not been reported following laminoplasty.

Numerous studies have demonstrated that postlaminectomy kyphotic deformity and instability can be problematic particularly in the younger patient (33–35). Incidence rates as high as 43% have been reported (12,21,36). It may occasionally develop following cervical laminoplasty (37).

Overall, recovery rates of approximately 50% are consistently reported following laminoplasty (10,26,27,29), though improvement has been reported in as many as 75% of patients (38). With respect to spondylotic radiculopathy, a retrospective study found outcomes were best following anterior decompression (92%), and only slightly worse (86%) following laminoplasty (39). Laminectomy was associated with the poorest outcome (66%) (39).

Discussion

While management decisions must take into account a number of factors and are highly individualized, the following repre-

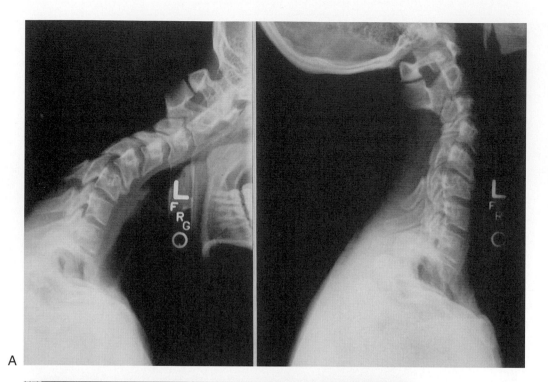

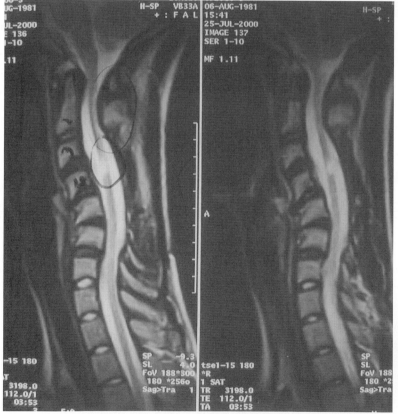

Fig. 3. A 17-year-old girl underwent a three-level cervical laminectomy for myelopathy. Her initial pathology consisted of a bulging C3, C4 disc superimposed on a congenital spinal stenosis. She developed a progressive midcervical kyphosis within 2 years. **A**: C-spine x-ray demonstrates a relatively fixed deformity on flexion extension views measuring 55 degrees. **B**: The patient has intrinsic changes within the cord as seen on T2-weighted magnetic resonance imaging at the level of the previous compression.

sents some general guidelines and our interpretation of critical literature.

The anterior approach plays an important role in the management of a number of cervical spine disorders. Regarding CSM, the anterior approach directly addresses the predominant pathology, i.e., osteophytes, and facilitates fusion utilizing bone graft placed under compressive forces and can be supplemented by titanium anterior cervical plates. The anterior approach is also preferable in the presence of kyphotic deformity (23,40), which is associated with poorer results following posterior decompressive procedures (39).

Posterior decompression is typically indicated when multisegment pathology needs to be addressed, and when predominantly posterior pathology exists. Additionally, in the case of ossification of the posterior longitudinal ligament (OPLL), significant adhesion between the posterior longitudinal ligament (PLL) and the underlying dura results in additional risk of dural laceration when approached anteriorly (41). Laminectomy has traditionally been used for decompression, and continues to be the procedure of choice for many clinicians in North America. It is a relatively safe, effective, and quick procedure that generally produces disease stabilization, if not improvement. Decompression does occur, but at the expense of the posterior stabilizing structures. Loss of cervical lordosis or development of kyphosis is seen in as many as 43% of patients (12,21); however, clinically significant malalignment and instability are less common (4,15). Additionally, radiographic "failures" do not necessarily translate into clinical failures. The crucial implication of kyphosis is its potential role in subsequent clinical deterioration, as kyphotic alignment of the spine can result in secondary ventral cord compression and is associated with a poorer outcome (42). While this risk may be relatively insignificant in a patient who is otherwise debilitated with limited life expectancy, it is a very significant risk in a younger patient requiring earlier treatment due to underlying congenital canal stenosis (Fig. 3).

Given the relatively high incidence of multilevel OPLL presenting in a younger patient population than CSM, Asian surgeons were long ago faced with the concerns of delayed kyphosis, instability, and postlaminectomy membrane following multilevel laminectomy, and the clinical implications of such. Additionally, as noted above, dural adhesions make anterior approaches more difficult (41). Expansile laminoplasty was developed to address these concerns. Theoretically, by minimizing "violation" of posterior structures, one can successfully enlarge the spinal canal while largely preserving posterior stabilizing structures, thus reducing postoperative deformity or instability, and alleviating the need to perform additional fusion. While the procedure was first described by Oyama (8,9), it did not become popularized until several years later. Initial procedures were cumbersome and lengthy, requiring complex reconstruction of the posterior arch (9). Numerous modifications since that time have resulted in simplified, faster procedures with improved stability (10-15,21). The importance of preserving spinoligamentous complexes in order to mitigate kyphosis has been recognized, and resulted in "tissue-sparing" techniques (11,26,28,31,43–46). However, such preservation is also recognized to significantly increase the closing force on the elevated laminae (47).

To combat the problem of delayed closure, a variety of techniques have been employed. These primarily involve the use of "spacers" to buttress the created gap or the use of sutures to "attach" the remaining spinous process to the facet or soft tissue structures of the hinge side. We prefer the former, utilizing rib allograft, with the "closing forces" of the hinge maintaining firm positioning of the graft, which facilitates an intersegmental fusion. Further stability may be obtained, in addition to

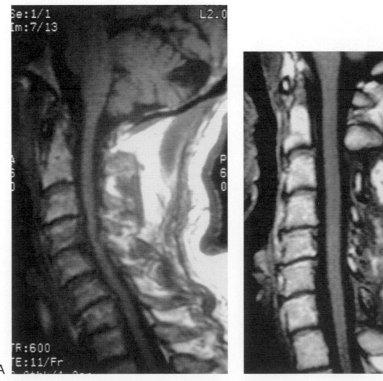

Fig. 4. A: A preoperative T1-weighted MRI revealing multilevel (C4-7) cervical spondylosis and significant spinal cord compression, particularly at C4 and C5, in an elderly patient. **B**: Postoperative MRI following C3-7 open-door expansile laminoplasty, demonstrating significant enlargement of the cervical spinal canal, without residual cord compression.

or in lieu of the above techniques, using onlay bone grafting at the hinge site(s) (36).

Animal studies have supported the potential benefits of laminoplasty over laminectomy. In one study, laminectomies or laminoplasties were performed at C3-5 in goats, with monthly radiographic follow-up over a 6-month period. Results were compared with controls, confirming that, radiographically, laminoplasties were biomechanically superior in maintaining alignment (48). An additional study in rabbits found that, while postoperative range of motion was similar between groups, laminectomy was associated with increased angle deformity and poorer outcome (49).

Clinically, studies have shown that clinical improvement directly correlates to degree of canal expansion (Fig. 4). However, excessive expansion as well as an irregular canal area (50) may be associated with additional problems. It appears that optimal canal expansion approximates 4 to 5 mm in the sagittal AP diameter (12), correlating to approximately 50% increase canal area (51), and facilitating a 3-mm posterior shift of the spinal cord (52). However, decreased lordosis correlates with decreased volume expansion following laminoplasty, as well as decreased posterior migration of the cord (51). While improvement certainly occurs with less substantial enlargement, more aggressive enlargement is not advisable. Retrospective studies indicate that increased canal diameters (beyond the above) are associated with an increased incidence of postoperative complications, specifically C5-6 paresis. Presumably, this is due to traction on the nerve roots, as the C5 level frequently represents the apex of the lordotic curve, and exhibits the most significant "migration." While numerous studies suggest this is a transient phenomenon in most cases, it is obviously distressing for the patient, who may take as long as 6 years to recover sufficiently (27). Far more critical than canal expansion is subsequent cord expansion, with studies showing a direct correlation between JOA scores and spinal cord area (53).

Both clinically and radiographically, limited range of motion (ROM) is frequently observed following laminoplasty. Studies suggest that approximately 50% ROM is lost following laminoplasty, particularly extension (12,22,35,54–56). This correlates well with radiographic evidence of spontaneous bony fusion (36,54). It has been proposed that this is actually beneficial, in that it ameliorates ongoing mechanical stress or injury without being "rigid" and inducing stress and degeneration of adjacent levels. While numerous studies have shown no correlation between limited ROM and recovery rates or outcome, this may represent a biomechanical etiology for the postoperative axial pain, which can be problematic. However, it is important to remember that the majority of studies pertain to patients undergoing decompression for OPLL, which itself is associated with increased rigidity and thus may overestimate the restricted ROM attributable to the laminoplasty procedure.

Conclusions

While the laminoplasty procedure was designed to address some of the concerns of multilevel decompressive laminectomy, it is not without its own complications. Historically, "sinkage" of the open door was a concern, but this is now rare with the addition of stabilizing structures. However, axial neck pain, shoulder girdle/C5-6 weakness, and decreased ROM continue to be particularly problematic. Additionally, while numerous studies suggest malalignment and instability are more common following laminectomy (34,35), both may develop following laminoplasty, occasionally at rates comparable to those seen with laminectomy (37). Overall, recovery rates of approximately 50% are consistently reported following laminoplasty, with axial pain and malalignment having little impact on ultimate outcome and JOA scores (26,28–30), unless associated with a decreased cervical curve index of >10 (27,31). Outcomes are comparable to (14), if not better than (39), those associated with laminectomy. Laminoplasty, however, may be preferable in patients with poor bone quality, as well as younger patients with multilevel compression in the setting of lordotic alignment, as these patients are most at risk to develop delayed malalignment or instability.

References

1. Gokaslan ZL, Cooper PR. Treatment of disc and ligamentous diseases of the cervical spine by the anterior approach. In: Youmans JR, ed. *Youman's neurological surgery*, 4th ed. Philadelphia: WB Saunders, 1996:2253–2261.
2. Hukuda S, Ogata M, Katsuura A. Experimental study on acute aggravating factors of cervical spondylotic myelopathy. *Spine* 1988;13:15–20.
3. Barnes MP, Saunders M. The effect of cervical mobility on the natural history of cervical spondylotic myelopathy. *J Neurol Neurosurg Psychiatry* 1984;47:17–20.
4. Hukuda S, Mochizuki T, Ogata M, et al. Operations for cervical spondylotic myelopathy. A comparison of the results of anterior and posterior procedures. *J Bone Joint Surg* 1985;67B:609–615.
5. Epstein N, Epstein J, Carras R. Cervical spondylostenosis and related disorders in patients over 65: current management and diagnostic techniques. *Orthotransactions* 1987;11.
6. Epstein JA, Epstein WE. The surgical management of cervial spinal stenosis, spondylosis and myeloradiculopathy by means of the posterior approach. In: The Cervical Spine Research Society, eds. *The cervical spine*, 2nd ed. Philadelphia: JB Lippincott, 1989:625–643.
7. Clark E, Robinson PK. Cervical myelopathy: a complication of cervical spondylosis. *Brain* 1956;79:483.
8. Yue WM, Tan CT, Tan SB, et al. Results of cervical laminoplasty and a comparison between single and double trap-door techniques. *J Spinal Disord* 2000;13:329–335.
9. Oyama M, Hattori S, Moriwaki N, et al. A new method of posterior decompression. *Centr Jpn J Orthop Traumatic Surg* 1973;16:792–794.
10. Kokubun S, Sato T, Ishii Y, et al. Cervical myelopathy in the Japanese. *Clin Orthop* 1996;129–138.
11. Kurokawa T. Enlargement of the spinal canal by sagittal splitting of spinal processes. *Bessatsu Seikeigeka* 1982;2:234–240.
12. Hirabayashi K, Watanabe K, Wakano K, et al. Expansive open-door laminoplasty for cervical spinal stenotic myelopathy. *Spine* 1983;8:693–699.
13. Itoh T, Tsuji H. Technical improvements and results of laminoplasty for compressive myelopathy in the cervical spine. *Spine* 1985;10:729–736.
14. Nakano N, Nakano T, Nakano K. Comparison of the results of laminectomy and open-door laminoplasty for cervical spondylotic myeloradiculopathy and ossification of the posterior longitudinal ligament. *Spine* 1988;13:792–794.
15. Tsuji H. Laminoplasty for patients with compressive myelopathy due to so-called spinal canal stenosis in cervical and thoracic regions. *Spine* 1982;7:28–34.
16. Bouchard JA, Bohlman HH, Biro C. Intraoperative improvements of somatosensory evoked potentials: correlation to clinical outcome in surgery for cervical spondylitic myelopathy. *Spine* 1996;21:589–594.
17. Calancie B, Harris W, Broton JG, et al. "Threshold-level" multipulse transcranial electrical stimulation of motor cortex for intraoperative monitoring of spinal motor tracts: description of method and comparison to somatosensory evoked potential monitoring. *J Neurosurg* 1998;88:457–470.
18. Kumar VG, Rea GL, Mervis LJ, et al. Cervical spondylotic myelopathy: functional and radiographic long-term outcome after laminectomy and posterior fusion. *Neurosurgery* 1999;44:771–777; discussion 777–778.

19. Abumi K, Kaneda K, Shono Y, et al. One-stage posterior decompression and reconstruction of the cervical spine by using pedicle screw fixation systems. *J Neurosurg* 1999;90:19–26.

20. Cahill D. Multisegmental cervical laminectomy and cervical fusion using plates and screws with C2 pars and C7 or T1 pedicle screws. Joint Section on Disorders of the Spine and Peripheral Nerves (AANS/CNS) 14th Annual Meeting, Rancho Mirage, CA, 1998.

21. O'Brien MF, Peterson D, Casey AT, et al. A novel technique for laminoplasty augmentation of spinal canal area using titanium miniplate stabilization. A computerized morphometric analysis. *Spine* 1996;21:474–483; discussion 484.

22. Edwards CC 2nd, Heller JG, Silcox DH 3rd. T-Saw laminoplasty for the management of cervical spondylotic myelopathy: clinical and radiographic outcome. *Spine* 2000;25:1788–1794.

23. Macdonald RL, Fehlings MG, Tator CH, et al. Multilevel anterior cervical corpectomy and fibular allograft fusion for cervical myelopathy. *J Neurosurg* 1997;86:990–997.

24. Uribe J, Vanni S, Jagid J, et al. Acute traumatic central cord syndrome: Experience using early surgical decompression with open door expansile cervical laminoplasty. Joint Section on Disorders of the Spine and Peripheral Nerves (AANS/CNS), 17th annual meeting, Phoenix, AZ, 2001.

25. Lee TT, Green BA, Gromelski EB. Safety and stability of open-door cervical expansive laminoplasty. *J Spinal Disord* 1998;11:12–15.

26. Hidai Y, Ebara S, Kamimura M, et al. Treatment of cervical compressive myelopathy with a new dorsolateral decompressive procedure. *J Neurosurg* 1999;90:178–185.

27. Satomi K, Nishu Y, Kohno T, et al. Long-term follow-up studies of open-door expansive laminoplasty for cervical stenotic myelopathy. *Spine* 1994;19:507–510.

28. Sasai K, Saito T, Akagi S, et al. Cervical curvature after laminoplasty for spondylotic myelopathy—involvement of yellow ligament, semispinalis cervicis muscle, and nuchal ligament. *J Spinal Disord* 2000;13:26–30.

29. Mochida J, Nomura T, Chiba M, et al. Modified expansive open-door laminoplasty in cervical myelopathy. *J Spinal Disord* 1999;12:386–391.

30. Fujimura Y, Nishi Y, Chiba K, et al. Multiple regression analysis of the factors influencing the results of expansive open-door laminoplasty for cervical myelopathy due to ossification of the posterior longitudinal ligament. *Arch Orthop Trauma Surg* 1998;117:471–474.

31. Kimura I, Shingu H, Nasu Y. Long-term follow-up of cervical spondylotic myelopathy treated by canal-expansive laminoplasty. *J Bone Joint Surg* 1995;77B:956–961.

32. Morimoto T, Okuno S, Nakase H, et al. Cervical myelopathy due to dynamic compression by the laminectomy membrane: dynamic MR imaging study. *J Spinal Disord* 1999;12:172–173.

33. Herman JM, Sonntag VK. Cervical corpectomy and plate fixation for postlaminectomy kyphosis. *J Neurosurg* 1994;80:963–970.

34. Matsunaga S, Sakou T, Nakanisi K. Analysis of the cervical spine alignment following laminoplasty and laminectomy. *Spinal Cord* 1999;37:20–24.

35. Inoue A, Ikata T, Katoh S. Spinal deformity following surgery for spinal cord tumors and tumorous lesions: analysis based on an assessment of the spinal functional curve. *Spinal Cord* 1996;34:536–542.

36. Shikata J, Yamamuro T, Shimizu K, et al. Combined aminoplasty and posterolateral fusion for spinal canal surgery in children and adolescents. *Clin Orthop* 1990:92–99.

37. Tanaka J, Seki N, Tokimura F, et al. Operative results of canal-expansive laminoplasty for cervical spondylotic myelopathy in elderly patients. *Spine* 1999;24:2308–2312.

38. Lee TT, Manzano GR, Green BA. Modified open-door cervical expansive laminoplasty for spondylotic myelopathy: operative technique, outcome, and predictors for gait improvement. *J Neurosurg* 1997;86:64–68.

39. Herkowitz HN. A comparison of anterior cervical fusion, cervical laminectomy, and cervical laminoplasty for the surgical management of multiple level spondylotic radiculopathy. *Spine* 1988;13:774–780.

40. Orr RD, Zdeblick TA. Cervical spondylotic myelopathy. Approaches to surgical treatment. *Clin Orthop* 1999:58–66.

41. White AA 3rd, Panjabi MM. Biomechanical considerations in the surgical management of cervical spondylotic myelopathy. *Spine* 1988;13:856–860.

42. Kawakami M, Tamaki T, Iwasaki H, et al. A comparative study of surgical approaches for cervical compressive myelopathy. *Clin Orthop* 2000:129–136.

43. Hoshino Y, Kurokawa T, Machida H. Long term results of the double door laminoplasty by longitudinal splitting of spinous process. *Rinsho Seikeigeka* 1992;27:257–262.

44. Fujimura Y, Nishi Y. Atrophy of the nuchal muscle and change in cervical curvature after expansive open-door laminoplasty. *Arch Orthop Trauma Surg* 1996;115:203–205.

45. Hirabayashi K, Toyama Y, Chiba K. Expansive laminoplasty for myelopathy in ossification of the longitudinal ligament. *Clin Orthop* 1999:35–48.

46. Kamioka Y, Yamamoto H, Tani T, et al. Postoperative instability of cervical OPLL and cervical radiculomyelopathy. *Spine* 1989;14:1177–1183.

47. Tsuzuki N. A novel technique for laminoplasty augmentation of spinal canal area using titanium miniplate stabilization: a computerized morphometric analysis. *Spine* 1997;22:926–927.

48. Baisden J, Voo LM, Cusick JF, et al. Evaluation of cervical laminectomy and laminoplasty. A longitudinal study in the goat model. *Spine* 1999;24:1283–1288; discussion 1288–1289.

49. Fields MJ, Hoshijima K, Feng AH, et al. A biomechanical, radiologic, and clinical comparison of outcome after multilevel cervical laminectomy or laminoplasty in the rabbit. *Spine* 2000;25:2925–2931.

50. Kimura S, Homma T, Uchiyama S, et al. Posterior migration of cervical spinal cord between split laminae as a complication of laminoplasty. *Spine* 1995;20:1284–1288.

51. Baba H, Uchida K, Maezawa Y, et al. Three-dimensional computed tomography for evaluation of cervical spinal canal enlargement after en bloc open-door laminoplasty. *Spinal Cord* 1997;35:674–679.

52. Sodeyama T, Goto S, Mochizuki M, et al. Effect of decompression enlargement laminoplasty for posterior shifting of the spinal cord. *Spine* 1999;24:1527–1531; discussion 1531–1532.

53. Morio Y, Yamamoto K, Teshima R, et al. Clinicoradiologic study of cervical laminoplasty with posterolateral fusion or bone graft. *Spine* 2000;25:190–196.

54. Seichi A, Takeshita K, Ohishi I, et al. Long-term results of double-door laminoplasty for cervical stenotic myelopathy. *Spine* 2001;26:479–487.

55. Kawaguchi Y, Matsui H, Ishihara H, et al. Axial symptoms after en bloc cervical laminoplasty. *J Spinal Disord* 1999;12:392–395.

56. Kohno K, Kumon Y, Oka Y, et al. Evaluation of prognostic factors following expansive laminoplasty for cervical spinal stenotic myelopathy. *Surg Neurol* 1997;48:237–245.

198. Anterior Cervical Discectomy with and without Fusion

Mark R. McLaughlin and Hae-Dong Jho

Anterior and cervical discectomy with or without fusion was first pioneered by Cloward (1) and Smith and Robinson (2) in the 1950s. Since that time this procedure has become a well-accepted technique for the treatment of cervical spondylosis with resultant radiculopathy or myelopathy (3–12). Variations of the anterior technique have been reported (13–17). Although there is significant debate within the spine community regarding the choice of an anterior or posterior approach to cervical radiculopathy (18), as well as the necessity of fusion and/or instrumentation for single level discectomy (19–22), this controversy is beyond the scope of this chapter. Suffice it to say that anterior cervical discectomy with or without fusion is a highly effective surgical technique for the treatment of cervical disc disease that has failed conservative therapy (3,4,9,10,23). This chapter reviews the indications and risks of the procedure and details the operative technique of anterior cervical discectomy and fusion.

Risks

Potential risks specific to anterior cervical discectomy include vascular injury to the carotid or vertebral arteries. Carotid injury is extremely rare; however, ischemic events due to manipulation of the carotid have been reported. The risk of injury to the vertebral artery is also small using the anterior approach, but this complication has been reported with a greater frequency than carotid injury (24,25). The vertebral artery is at risk for injury when the surgeon is performing the most lateral portion of the foraminotomy (26,27).

Infection rates with the anterior cervical discectomy are less than 1% (4). More common risks associated with the anterior cervical approach include mild dysphagia, which usually resolves within a week or two after the surgery. Hoarseness secondary to injury of the recurrent laryngeal nerve occurs in approximately 1% of patients (4). This nerve is at more significant risk with exposure at lower levels, typically at C6-7 or C7-T1, because of its more oblique course to the larynx. Because of this risk, some have advocated a left-sided approach to decrease the incidence of nerve injury as the recurrent laryngeal nerve runs more closely to the trachea and is less likely to be injured. We have not found a right-sided approach to be a significant problem with hoarseness, and have found that blunt dissection using a Kittner dissector or peanut tends to decrease injury to this nerve.

Other risks include, pseudarthrosis manifested as persistent neck pain. The incidence of pseudarthrosis for single-level anterior cervical discectomy with fusion ranges from 2% to 8% in the literature (21,22). The incidence increases with multilevel discectomy (22,28). There is some evidence to suggest that rigid internal fixation for multilevel fusions will increase the fusion rate and decrease the graft migration rate, as well as hasten a patient's return to work (21,29).

Surgical Technique

POSITIONING. In the preoperative setting, it is important to assess a patient's degree of cervical extension. This is particularly important in patients with myelopathy, as positioning a patient in hyperextension may create more severe spinal cord compression and possible injury. The patient is placed in a supine position with the head in a soft doughnut in gentle extension. An intravenous (IV) bag is placed under the neck for support and stabilization. It is our preference to avoid the use of esophageal monitors as they cause increased rigidity of the esophagus, resulting in more difficult retraction. In multilevel procedures esophageal monitors can cause mucosal injuries by prolonged pressure exerted by the medial to lateral retractors. During exposure we utilize partial muscle paralysis (one twitch out of a train of four). This level of pharmacological paralysis offers good muscle relaxation, yet still allows for observing nerve root irritation during the decompression.

After the patient is placed in appropriate extension, the anterior cervical region is palpated to allow the surgeon a mind's-eye view of the appropriate level of incision. We prefer utilizing a right-sided approach for right-handed surgeons. Although there is a reported slightly higher incidence of recurrent laryn-

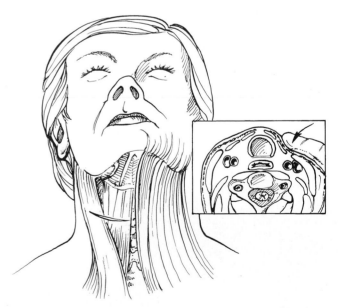

Fig. 1. With the patient in the supine position and the head placed in gentle extension, the transverse incision is planned within a skin crease in the neck. Usually there are two skin creases that can be utilized. The cricothyroid space usually marks the C5-6 interspace, and the level of the incision can be planned off of this. Alternatively, the carotid tubercle can be palpated. Palpation of the carotid tubercle should be avoided in elderly patients, as carotid embolic events potentially can be precipitated. **Inset:** The avascular plane and route of dissection down to the prevertebral space. Dissection is medial to the carotid sheath and lateral to the trachea and esophagus.

geal nerve irritation, it has been our experience that this is minor, and minimized by utilizing blunt dissection as much as possible.

Typically, the cricothyroid membrane marks the C5-6 interspace. The carotid tubercle can also be palpated; however, we tend to avoid using this landmark particularly in older patients for fear of precipitating carotid embolic events. Once the appropriate level is identified based on external landmarks, a transverse incision planned within the skin crease approximately 4 to 5 cm in length. The incision is based one third over the sternocleidomastoid and two thirds toward the midline (Fig. 1).

EXPOSURE. After prepping and draping, the incision is carried down through the subcutaneous tissues to the platysma muscle. The platysma muscle is transected transversely and undermined superiorly and inferiorly (Fig. 2). It should be noted in any significant venous structure anterior to the platysma and should be coagulated and divided early to allow for adequate exposure.

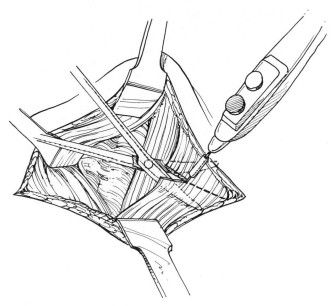

Fig. 3. The omohyoid muscle is typically encountered at the C5-6 level and can be retracted superiorly or inferiorly depending on the level of exposure. In wide exposures the omohyoid can be transected, allowing a much more relaxed exposure for long cephalad and caudal dissections. The avascular plane between the carotid sheath laterally and the esophagus and trachea medially can be dissected with gentle finger dissection to expose the prevertebral fascia.

Once the platysma has been undermined, the investing sheath of sternocleidomastoid is opened with Metzenbaum scissors and the avascular plain between the carotid sheath laterally and the trachea and esophagus medially is dissected. This is carried down to the prevertebral fascia. The omohyoid muscle is encountered usually at the C5-6 level and can be either retracted inferiorly for superior approaches or superiorly for inferior approaches. In patients with a large omohyoid or in multilevel exposures, the muscle can be transected without any subsequent deficit. It does not need to be reapproximated at closure (Fig. 3).

The prevertebral fascia is identified and opened with a Metzenbaum scissors (Fig. 4). This is then dissected bluntly superiorly and inferiorly with Kittner dissectors to expose the appropriate interspace and vertebral bodies.

An intraoperative radiograph is obtained to identify the correct level. Typically, we utilize a spinal needle cut to expose 1 cm of metal beyond the plastic hub. This needle is attached to a straight hemostat. Utilizing this technique, the surgeon can get a good estimate of the depth of the vertebral bodies based on the intraoperative localizing film with fixed length of the 1-cm cut spinal needle. This aids both in the decompression and in the choice of screw length if a fusion is desired.

The Caspar retractor system (Aesculap, San Francisco, CA) is then placed to retract the longus coli muscles and expose the appropriate disc space (30) (Fig. 5). When upper cervical exposures are required, the Thompson-Farley retractor system can be utilized (Thompson Surgical Instruments, Traverse City, MI) (31). It is best to suture the medial lateral retractor to the skin of the anterior cervical region to keep the retractor in good position. Then a superior and inferior retractor is placed and the disc space is completely exposed.

Once the appropriate disc spaces are identified and exposed, the anterior osteophytes are gardened with a Leksell rongeur (Fig. 6). The disc space is delineated with monopolar electrocautery. The medial portion of the uncovertebral joints should

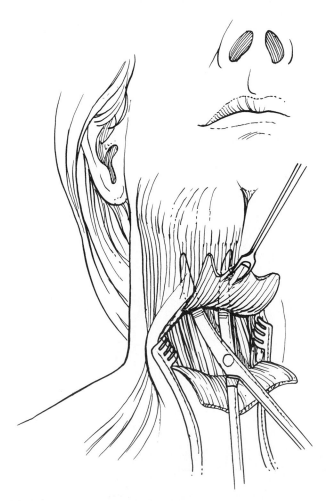

Fig. 2. Generous releasing dissection in the subplatysmal plane is critical for obtaining adequate exposure. This subplatysmal plane should be dissected superiorly and inferiorly so that when the retraction blades are placed, there is no additional tension on the external structures and adequate exposure of the disc space can be obtained. Dissection of the subplatysmal plane will expose the sternocleidomastoid passing obliquely through the field. The investing sheath of the sternocleidomastoid is identified and opened sharply. The avascular plane can then be dissected with a Metzenbaum scissors or finger dissection.

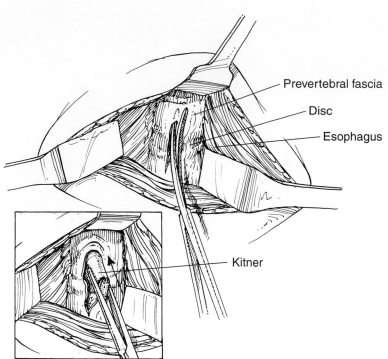

Prevertebral fascia

Disc

Esophagus

Kitner

Fig. 4. The prevertebral fascia is identified as a transparent membrane with longus coli muscle bellies located on the lateral borders. Prevertebral fascia can be opened with a Metzenbaum scissors and the disc space can be identified. Using a monopolar cautery device, the longus coli muscles are undermined and mobilized in a subperiosteal fashion. A marker is placed and a localizing film is obtained.

be exposed bilaterally so that the gentle early up-slope of the joint can be seen. This is important to accurately visualize the midline. The longus coli muscles are dissected in a subperiosteal fashion laterally with an insulated monopolar.

The vertebral bodies adjacent to the symptomatic disc space are exposed, dissected, and cleaned of all soft tissues to allow for accurate placement of distraction pins within the central portion of the vertebral body.

DISCECTOMY. Distraction pins are then placed in the appropriate vertebral bodies and a Caspar distractor is positioned.

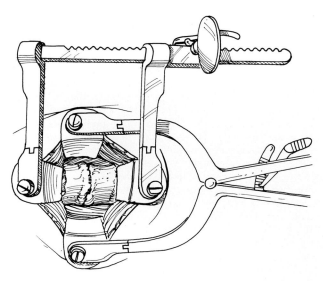

Fig. 5. Once the correct level is identified, mediolateral retractor blades are placed with the teeth incorporating the longus coli muscles. Then, a superior/inferior retractor is also placed with blunt blades to allow for adequate disc space exposure.

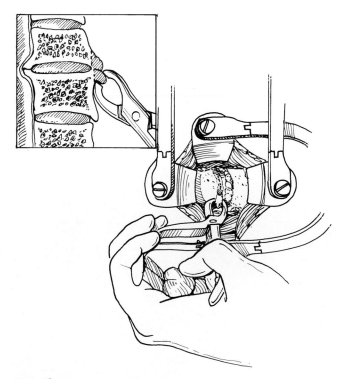

Fig. 6. Anterior osteophytes are removed using a Leksell rongeur to create flat surface areas on the anterior vertebral body faces. This step is critical for accurate identification of the mid-vertebral body and for optimally placing the bone graft and plate if a fusion is intended.

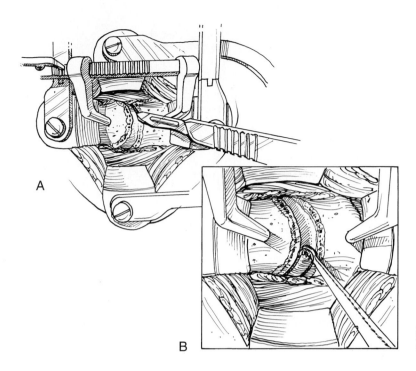

Fig. 7. A,B: An annulotomy is performed with a no. 15 blade knife, and the anterior portion of the disc is removed with curets and a Kerrison rongeur.

Gentle distraction is then dialed into the distractor. An annulotomy and partial discectomy is performed, and then gentle distraction is placed on the disc space (Fig. 7). The anterior rim of the superior vertebral body is removed with a Kerrison rongeur or with a Midas Rex high-speed drill (Medtronic Sofamor Danek, Memphis, TN). This will create a better working channel to see the posterior portions of the disc and posterior longitudinal ligament (Fig. 8). A complete discectomy is then performed utilizing a combination of small and medium curets. The posterior osteophytes are then drilled off (Fig. 9). After the discectomy and osteophytectomy is completed, the posterior vertebral wall is identified with the use of a forward-angled curet that dissects the posterior longitudinal ligament off of the dorsal vertebral body rim.

Distraction can be increased after the discectomy; however, it is important not to overdistract this interspace, as this will result in significant postoperative neck pain. The posterior longitudinal ligament is then elevated using a right-angled nerve hook and then cut sharply, exposing the epidural space. The posterior longitudinal ligament is then removed with a Kerrison rongeur, and foraminotomies are performed bilaterally. A more generous decompression should be directed to the symptomatic side. If a right-handed surgeon performs the discectomy on a patient with right-sided symptoms, it is important for the surgeon to come to the opposite side of the table to approach the right neural foramina. This will allow the surgeon to get an optimal foraminotomy at this level. Once adequate spinal cord and nerve root decompression is obtained, patients not undergoing fusion are ready for closure.

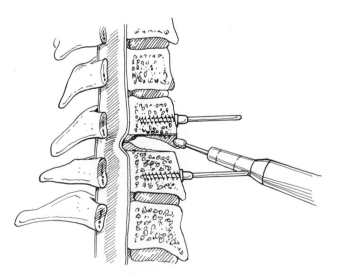

Fig. 8. Using a high-speed drill, the superior vertebral end plate is then prepared creating a parallel plane with the inferior vertebral body. This will allow for good graft position as well as better visualization of the posterior osteophytectomy.

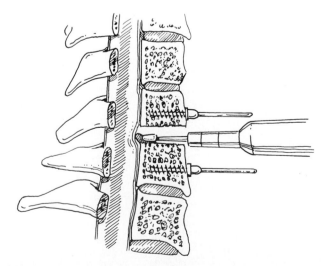

Fig. 9. Posterior osteophytes are then removed with a high-speed drill to complete the bony decompression.

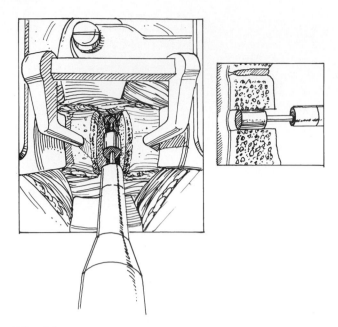

Fig. 10. Using the Cornerstone drill bits (Medtronic Sofamor Danek, Memphis, TN), parallel end plates are created for graft site preparation.

FUSION. If a fusion is planned, the end plates need to be prepared more aggressively than with a standard discectomy. Using a Midas Rex, the ventral portion of the superior vertebral body should be drilled and customized to create a parallel surface area with relation to inferior vertebral body (Fig. 10). The dorsal osteophytes of both the superior and inferior vertebral bodies need to be removed as well. The goal of end-plate and osteophyte removal is to achieve parallel surface areas for maximal interface and stability with the interbody graft to be placed.

If the patient is a smoker or has multiple risk factors for pseudarthrosis, harvested iliac crest autograft should be considered. For all other patients, we prefer to use allograft banked fibula or Cornerstone (Medtronic Sofamor Danek). Once the end plates are prepared, the distraction is released and then redialed into an even pressure that gently restores cervical lordosis at this level. We prefer to release the distraction and then redial the distractor to get a good idea of what size graft is necessary.

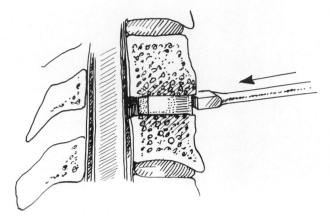

Fig. 12. Once the graft is countersunk, the distraction pins are moved.

Once the distraction is adequately obtained, the interbody distance is measured and a graft is customized to fit this interspace. The graft is then packed with locally harvested bone fragments or demineralized bone matrix and mortised into position (Fig. 11). Typically the graft is countersunk approximately 2 mm. It is important to keep the allograft and the anterior portion of the vertebral bodies as this provides more structural support and will prevent subsidence of the graft (Fig. 12).

While there is some evidence that suggests two-level anterior cervical discectomy patients will benefit from rigid internal fixation, there is significant debate regarding single-level disease (21,29). Because rigid internal fixation with the use of an anterior cervical plate allows patients the ability to recover without the use of a hard collar, it is an option for single-level disease (Fig. 13). It has been our practice to offer patients the option of having a hard cervical orthosis for 6 weeks after a fusion or to undergo placement of an anterior cervical plate. Future studies will elicit the overall benefits and risks of single-level instrumentation.

CLOSURE. For single-level anterior cervical disease, anterior cervical discectomy with or without fusion, a drain is usually not necessary. For multilevel discectomies and depending on the extent of exposure, occasionally a Jackson-Pratt drain is

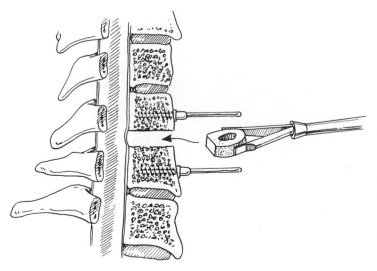

Fig. 11. If a fusion is desired, the distraction pins are released and then redialed to the appropriate distraction to reestablish cervical lordosis. A graft packed with locally harvested autograft from the gardening of the anterior spine is then tamped into position.

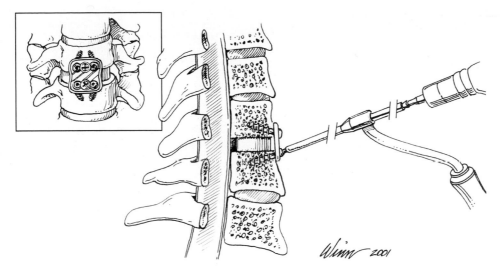

Fig. 13. If desired, an anterior cervical plate can then be affixed to the spine using 14-mm screws. If a plate is utilized, it is important to use the shortest plate possible so that the superior and inferior portion of the plate does not encroach upon other intervening motion segments.

necessary. Otherwise, after the discectomy, the wound is irrigated with antibiotic solution and if a fusion or instrumentation is performed, a second intraoperative x-ray is obtained to verify graft position and plate fixation. The distraction pins are then removed and the holes are waxed to prevent any bone bleeding. The esophagus is carefully inspected to verify no disruption of the esophageal wall. If there is any concern regarding an esophageal injury, methylene blue can be injected via a nasogastric (NG) tube placed to verify the integrity of the esophageal wall.

The platysma is then reapproximated with interrupted 3-0 absorbable sutures and the subcutaneous tissues are closed in a similar fashion. The skin is closed with a running 5-0 subcuticular absorbable monofilament suture. Steri-Strips are applied. If the fusion has been performed without plate fixation, then a hard cervical collar is placed. For patients with discectomy alone or for patients with fusion and supplemental plating, no collar is necessary.

Postoperative Care

Patients can be discharged based on the surgeon's and patient's preference. Diet is rapidly advanced and the patients are restricted only mildly in their activities. Typically, recommend no lifting over 10 lb for 4 to 6 weeks. They can ambulate ad lib. Postoperative x-rays are usually obtained at 3 months and at a year if a fusion has been performed.

Conclusions

Anterior cervical discectomy with or without fusion and instrumentation is an excellent procedure for the treatment of cervical radiculopathy and/or myelopathy. It is important to correlate the patient's history and neurological examination with the findings on radiological imaging. Occasionally, patients will have two levels that are symptomatic, but typically only one nerve root is involved. The surgeon should pay careful attention to

both the neural foramina as well as the disc herniations. Many mild to moderate central disc herniations can seem quite large, but are asymptomatic. A patient with even mild foraminal stenosis may have severe symptoms of radiculopathy. With careful attention to patient selection and surgical technique, surgeons will find anterior cervical discectomy with and without fusion to be one of the most patient- and surgeon-gratifying procedures they perform.

References

1. Cloward RB: The anterior approach for removal of ruptured cervical disks. *J Neurosurg* 15:602–617, 1958.
2. Smith GW, Robinson RA: The treatment of certain cervical spine disorders by anterior removal of the intervertebral disc and interbody fusion. *J Bone Joint Surg* 40A:607–624, 1958.
3. Epstein JA: Management of cervical spinal stenosis, spondylosis, and myeloradiculopathy. *Contempt Neurosurg* 7:1–6, 1985.
4. Hadley MN, Sonntag VKH: Cervical disc herniations. In: *Neurosurgical clinics of North America*, VKH Sonntag, ed. Philadelphia: WB Saunders, 4(1):45–52, 1993.
5. Johnson RM, Murphy MJ, Southwick WO: Surgical approaches to the spine. In: Rothman RH, Simeone FA, eds. *The spine, 3rd ed.* Philadelphia: WB Saunders, 1607–1738, 1988.
6. Lunsford LD, Bissonette DJ, Jannetta PJ, et al.: Anterior surgery for cervical disc disease. Part 1: treatment of lateral disc herniation in 253 cases. *J Neurosurg* 53:1–11, 1980.
7. Martins AN: Anterior cervical discectomy with and without interbody bone graft. *J Neurosurg* 44:290–294, 1976.
8. Robertson JT: Anterior removal of cervical disc without fusion. *Clin Neurosurg* 20:259–261, 1973.
9. Robinson RA, Walker AE, Ferlic DC, et al.: The results of anterior interbody fusion of the cervical spine. *J Bone Joint Surg* 44A:1569–1587, 1962.
10. Scoville WB, Dohrmann GJ, Corkill G: Late results of cervical disc surgery. *J Neurosurg* 45:203–210, 1976.
11. Whitecloud TS: Anterior surgery for cervical spondylotic myelopathy: Smith-Robinson, Cloward and vertebrectomy. *Spine* 13:861–863, 1988.
12. Wilson DH, Campbell DD: Anterior cervical discectomy without bone graft. *J Neurosurg* 47:551–555, 1977.
13. Comey CH, McLaughlin MR, Moossy J: Anterior thoracic corpectomy without sternostomy: a strategy for malignant disease of the upper thoracic spine. *Acta Neurochir (Wien)* 139:712–718, 1997.

14. Geiger M, Roth PA, Wu JK: The anterior cervical approach to the cervicothoacic junction. *Neurosurgery* 37:704–719, 1995.

15. Jho HD: Microsurgical anterior cervical microforaminotomy for radiculopathy: a new approach to cervical disc herniation. *J Neurosurg* 84:155–160, 1996.

16. Lesoin F, Biondi A, Jomin M: Foraminal cervical herniated disc treated by anterior discoforaminotomy. *Neurosurgery* 21:334–338, 1987.

17. Maurice-Williams RS, Dorward NL: Extended anterior cervical discectomy without fusion: a simple and sufficient operation for most cases of cervical degenerative disease. *Br J Neurosurg* 10:261–266, 1996.

18. Epstein JA, Epstein NE: The surgical management of cervical spinal stenosis and myeloradiculopathy by means of the posterior approach. In: The Cervical Spine Research Society Editorial Committee, eds. *The cervical spine*, 2nd ed. Philadelphia: Lippincott, 625–643, 1989.

19. Hankinson HL, Wilson CB: Use of the operating microscope in anterior cervical discectomy without fusion. *J Neurosurg* 43:452–456, 1975.

20. Paramore CG, Dickman CA, Sonntag VK: Radiographic and clinical follow-up review of Caspar plates in 49 patients. *J Neurosurg* 84:957–961, 1996.

21. Shapiro S. Banked fibula and the locking anterior cervical plate in anterior cervical fusions following cervical discectomy. *J Neurosurg* 84:161–165, 1996.

22. Zdeblick RA, Hughes SS, Riew KD, et al.: Failed anterior cervical discectomy and arthrodesis: analysis and treatment of thirty-five patients. *J Bone Joint Surg* 79A:523–532, 1997.

23. Gore DR, Sepic SB, Gardner GM, et al.: Neck pain: a long-term follow-up of 205 patients. *Spine* 12:1–5, 1987.

24. Golfinos JG, Dickman CA, Zabramski JM, et al.: Repair of vertebral artery injury during anterior cervical decompression. *Spine* 19: 2552–2556, 1994.

25. Smith MD, Emery SE, Dudley A, et al.: Vertebral artery injury during anterior decompression of the cervical spine: a retrospective review of ten patients. *J Bone Joint Surg* 75B:412–415, 1993.

26. Ebraheim NA, Lu J, Biyani A, et al.: Anatomic considerations for uncovertebral involvement in cervical spondylosis. *Clin Orthop* 334: 200–206, 1997.

27. Pait TG, Killefer JA, Arnautovic KI: Surgical anatomy of the anterior cervical spine: The disc space, vertebral artery, and associated bony structures. *Neurosurgery* 39:769–776, 1996.

28. Phillips FM, Carlson G, Emery SE, et al.: Anterior cervical pseudoarthrosis: natural history and treatment. *Spine* 22:1585–1589, 1997.

29. McLaughlin MR, Purighalla V, Pizzi FJ: Cost advantages of two-level anterior cervical fusion with rigid internal fixation for radiculopathy and degenerative disease. *Springer Neurol* 48:560–565, 1997.

30. Caspar W, Barbier DD, Klara PM: Anterior cervical fusion and Caspar plate stabilization for cervical trauma. *Neurosurgery* 25:491–502, 1989.

31. Bores LF: Instrumentation, technique and technology: Thompson-Farley spinal retraction system. *Neurosurgery* 33:159–163, 1993.

199. Cervical Vertebrectomy and Fusion

Michael A. Leonard and Paul R. Cooper

Vertebrectomy and fusion are important techniques for the management of degenerative, infectious, traumatic, and neoplastic disease of the cervical spine. Although these conditions share many features in common, each requires a slightly different approach to achieve satisfactory decompression and stabilization. Neoplastic lesions will be only briefly mentioned here and will be discussed in more detail in Chapter 167.

Indications for Vertebrectomy

DEGENERATIVE CONDITIONS. Degenerative conditions comprise the most common indication for cervical vertebrectomy. Within this category are two clinical entities: cervical spondylosis and ossification of the posterior longitudinal ligament (OPLL). The pathogenesis of cervical spondylosis has been clarified in a number of publications but the etiology of OPLL remains obscure (1–4). However, patients who have congenitally small cervical spinal canals possess a predisposition toward developing symptoms from either of these conditions. Several authors have noted that cervical spinal canal width above 13 mm is rarely associated with symptomatic spondylosis, with the reported incidence rising as the canal width narrows (4–7).

Cervical Spondylosis. Patients with myelopathy from cervical spondylosis typically present later in life, usually in the sixth to

eighth decades. Magnetic resonance imaging (MRI) or computed tomography (CT) scan demonstrates compression at and adjacent to the disc space from osteophytes. Frequently osteophytic compression of the spinal cord occurs at two or more contiguous levels. While these patients may be decompressed by multilevel anterior cervical decompressions and fusions (ACDFs), cervical vertebrectomy has several advantages. Because osteophytes may extend well above and below the disc space, after decompression there is frequently little bone left in the vertebral body that lies between two decompressed levels (e.g., C5 vertebral body after C4-5 and C5-6 osteophytectomy). Placement of bone grafts may result in fracture of the small amount of intervening vertebral body. Attempts to spare bone removal from this body can lead to incomplete decompression of osteophytes. In addition, successful long-term stabilization after the placement of grafts at two adjacent levels requires fusion at four bone–graft interfaces with an increase in pseudarthrosis rate compared to single-level fusion.

Vertebrectomy followed by bone grafting and plating is more rapidly performed than multilevel ACDF and is more likely to result in successful fusion. Placement of an anterior cervical plate reduces the incidence of pseudarthrosis, and prevents graft extrusion. Several authors have confirmed that a construct utilizing a single graft and plate is more stable than multiple grafts (5,8,9).

Ossification of the Posterior Longitudinal Ligament (OPLL). In contrast to the spinal cord compression caused by spondylosis, OPLL characteristically extends behind the verte-

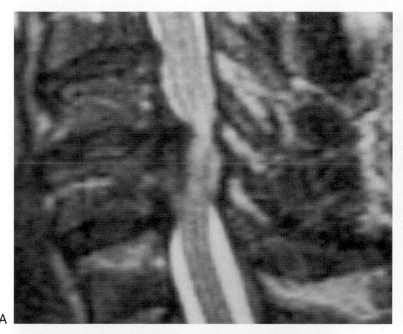

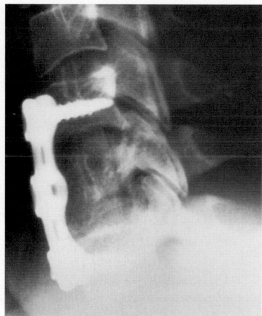

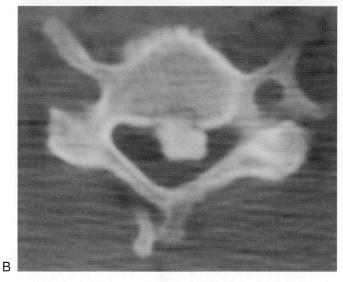

Fig. 1. Sagittal T2-weighted magnetic resonance imaging (MRI) scan (**A**) and axial computed tomography (CT) scan (**B**) demonstrating significant ossification of the posterior longitudinal ligament (OPLL) with spinal cord compression behind the C6 vertebral body. Postoperative film (**C**) demonstrates the C6 vertebrectomy with reconstruction using iliac crest bone graft and an anterior cervical plate.

bral body, frequently at multiple levels, and is not confined to the disc space (Fig. 1). Adequate decompression from an anterior approach is rarely possible without vertebrectomy.

INFECTION. Infections of the cervical spine can be caused by bacterial, granulomatous, fungal, or parasitic organisms (7, 10–13). The incidence of spinal infections appear to be increasing due to the growing number of immunosuppressed patients and intravenous drug users (11). Pyogenic infections are most commonly caused by *Staphylococcus aureus* followed by streptococci and gram-negative species (14). Although spinal tuberculosis (Pott's disease) is considerably less common than infections caused by pyogenic organisms, the incidence of spinal infections caused by mycobacteria also appears to be increasing (15).

Patients who present early will have predominantly a discitis with little bone destruction and no spinal cord compression. As the infection progresses, it erodes the end plates of the adjacent vertebral bodies and, if left untreated, destroys the vertebral body, causing spinal deformity and instability (Fig. 2). Neurological deficit results from spinal cord compression by a partially destroyed vertebral body retropulsed into the spinal canal, by kyphotic deformity, or by epidural pus and granulation tissue.

TRAUMA. Vertebrectomy is indicated in patients with trauma when the spinal cord is compressed by a retropulsed vertebral body or when the vertebral body compression and coexisting posterior ligamentous injury result (or are likely to result) in kyphotic deformity (Fig. 3).

Patients who present with an incomplete spinal cord injury or a deteriorating neurological exam and demonstrable spinal cord compression on their imaging studies should be decompressed as soon as possible. In either of these instances, cervical traction can reduce the spinal deformity and canal compromise and alleviate compression of the spinal cord. If the patient's neurological exam begins to improve or stabilizes from these measures, and follow-up radiological studies demonstrate an improvement, then surgical intervention can be scheduled in

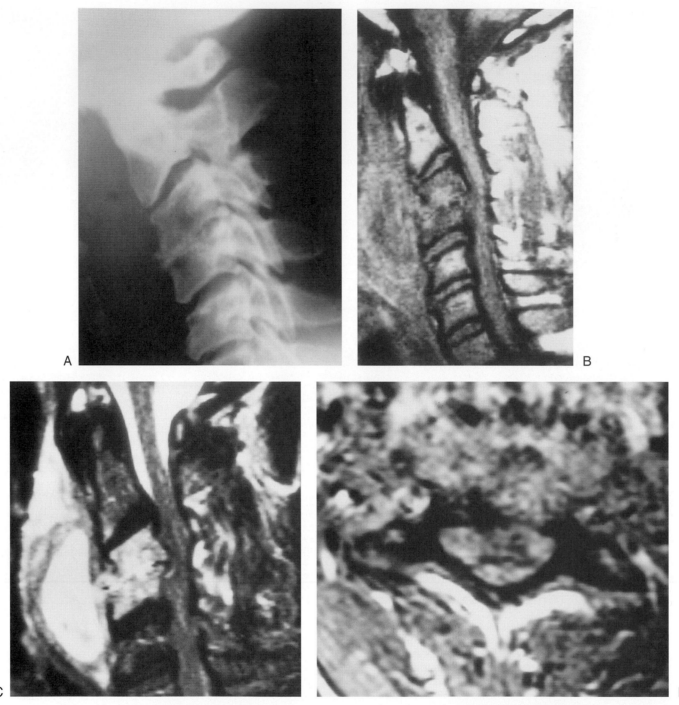

Fig. 2. Lateral plain film (**A**) of a patient with C3-4 discitis osteomyelitis. Sagittal T1- (**B**) and T2- (**C**) weighted MRI scans showing significant involvement of both the C3 and C4 vertebral bodies. Note the extensive retropharyngeal abscess. Axial image (**D**) through the region of maximal spinal cord compression shows significant epidural spread of the infectious process.

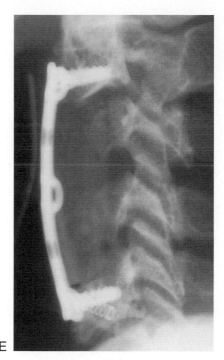

Fig. 2. (continued). Postoperative film (**E**) demonstrates the C3 and C4 vertebrectomy, with reconstruction utilizing iliac crest bone graft and an anterior cervical plate from C2 to C5.

a less emergent fashion. However, if the patient fails to improve, or worsens, surgical intervention should proceed as expeditiously as possible.

It is unusual for more than a single vertebral body to be involved, and a single-level vertebrectomy, bone grafting, and anterior cervical plating will almost always result in spinal cord decompression and stabilization. For patients who also demonstrate severe posterior ligamentous disruption, a posterior stabilization with lateral mass plates should also be performed after the anterior procedure to preclude graft and plate complications and delayed kyphotic deformity at the operated level.

Contraindications to Vertebrectomy

Graft dislodgment, collapse, and telescoping as well as plate loosening increase with the number of levels resected. For this reason, in patients with spinal cord compression from degenerative disease requiring vertebrectomy at more than two levels, we now prefer to perform decompression with laminectomy followed by stabilization with lateral mass plates.

In patients with neoplastic disease or infection, there is little choice but to resect the involved vertebrae, regardless of the number involved. Fortunately, it is unusual for either of these conditions to involve more than two vertebral bodies. If three or more vertebrae must be resected, bone grafting and anterior plating are followed by posterior cervical plating. We have found that the use of supplemental posterior plating virtually eliminates plate and graft complications in this situation.

Preoperative Imaging Evaluation

We consider the preoperative diagnostic triad of plain films, CT, and MRI to be essential for intelligent planning of the operative procedure, minimizing postoperative complications.

PLAIN FILMS. Plain films are especially important in patients with destructive lesions and trauma to demonstrate alignment, and the level of bone injury or destruction. Narrowing of the disc space with changes in the adjacent end plates or vertebral bodies is pathognomonic of an infectious process, whereas destruction of one or more vertebral bodies with disc space preservation is most consistent with a neoplastic process.

COMPUTED TOMOGRAPHY. CT with bone windows and sagittal reformatting is the most useful study for delineating bony pathology. In patients with neoplastic disease or osteomyelitis, CT will define quite accurately the extent of bone removal necessary for adequate decompression and secure placement of a graft. In patients with trauma it will identify occult fractures of adjacent vertebral bodies or posterior elements that will be important in deciding the number of vertebral bodies to be resected and the necessity for supplemental posterior instrumentation. In patients with OPLL and spondylosis, sagittal reformatting will provide the best assessment of the bony anatomy of compression. If MRI cannot be obtained or is contraindicated, CT following the administration of intravenous contrast may be useful in defining the extent of tumor or granuloma compressing the spinal cord.

MAGNETIC RESONANCE IMAGING. MRI is the imaging study of choice to identify neural compression by bone or soft tissue but is less useful in delineating bony anatomy than is CT. It is the best study for defining soft tissue compression of the spinal cord by tumor or infection. In patients with multilevel degenerative disease signal change within the spinal cord is indicative of the site of compression, causing neurological signs or symptoms.

Perioperative Preparation

CORTICOSTEROIDS. We utilize corticosteroids in patients with spinal cord injury from acute trauma according to a previously published protocol (16). Corticosteroids are also administered to patients with neurological deficit from neoplastic disease and infection. In patients with neurological deficit from degenerative disease, we do not give corticosteroids unless the deficit is rapidly progressive.

ANTIBIOTICS. Prophylactic antibiotics are given to all patients as the operative incision is made. In patients with spinal osteomyelitis, if a bacteriological diagnosis has been made by cultures from extraspinal sources of infection, appropriate antibiotics should be given preoperatively. In the absence of a positive culture in patients with osteomyelitis, antibiotics are started only after obtaining cultures at surgery.

INTUBATION AND OPERATIVE POSITIONING. All patients are intubated using fiberoptic techniques with the neck

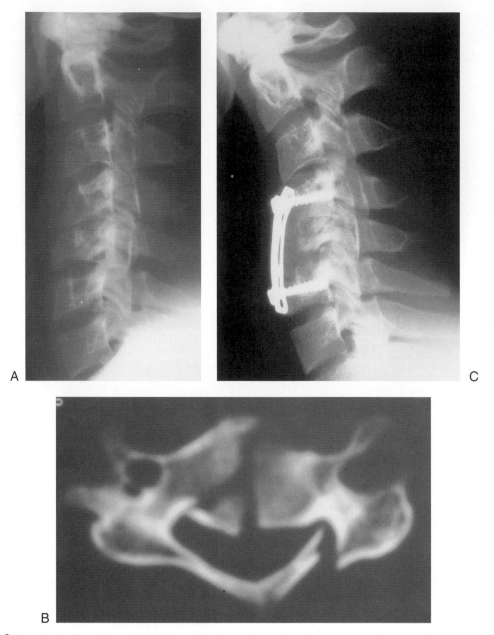

Fig. 3. Lateral plain film (**A**) and axial CT scan (**B**) of a patient with a C5 compression fracture with retropulsed bone fragments and canal compromise. Postoperative film (**C**) demonstrates C5 vertebrectomy with reconstruction utilizing iliac crest bone graft and an anterior cervical plate.

in a neutral position. Operation with the neck in extension facilitates exposure, particularly in operations on the upper cervical spine. In patients with cervical spine trauma (with the exception of patients with ankylosing spondylitis), extension is generally the position of safety. In patients who tolerate preoperative extension of the neck, a folded towel or foam padding is placed under the shoulders to increase extension. Cervical traction is utilized for patients with trauma and those with neoplastic disease or osteomyelitis with spinal instability, but the traction weight must be reduced to 5 lb before muscle relaxants and general anesthesia are given to prevent distraction injury to the spinal cord.

Adhesive tape is then placed over the medial and lateral aspects of the arms and forearms and fixed to the end of the operating table to pull the shoulders down and allow visualiza-

tion of the lower cervical spine on intraoperative imaging studies. A foot board is placed to prevent the patient from being pulled inferiorly by the shoulder traction.

The C-arm fluoroscopy is utilized to determine the alignment of the cervical spine, and confirm that the cervical vertebrae to be resected or plated can be visualized. The intended skin incision is marked slightly superior to the midpoint of level(s) of bony resection. Thus if the C5 and C6 vertebral bodies are to be resected, the skin incision is made just below the middle of the C5 vertebral body.

EVOKED POTENTIAL MONITORING. We utilize intraoperative somatosensory and motor evoked potential monitoring, although its usefulness as a means of preventing (rather than predicting) neurological deterioration is unclear. Although some authors contend that there is a significant difference in outcome when patients managed with intraoperative evoked potential monitoring are compared with those who did not have monitoring, none of these studies was controlled and any claims as to the efficacy of monitoring in improving neurological outcome must be regarded with skepticism (17–19).

Operative Technique

OPERATIVE INCISION. A transverse skin incision made beginning at the midline and carried to the medial border of the sternocleidomastoid muscle will provide adequate exposure for a one- or two-level vertebrectomy. A vertical incision along the medial border of the sternocleidomastoid muscle is less desirable from a cosmetic point of view but may provide better exposure if a three-level vertebrectomy is contemplated.

In a very small percentage of patients the right recurrent laryngeal nerve is aberrant and may be injured during exposure. It is never aberrant on the left and for that reason a left-sided incision is utilized in obtaining exposure for lower cervical vertebrectomies. If spinal cord compression is predominantly from one side, a contralateral incision is preferred because the surgeon's line of vision is directed to the side opposite the incision.

In patients with known carotid occlusion, the incision should be made ipsilateral to the occluded carotid artery to avoid compression of the ipsilateral functioning carotid artery by self-retaining retractors. In patients with recurrent laryngeal nerve injury from prior surgery or other causes, the skin incision should be made ipsilateral to the injured nerve as even temporary or partial dysfunction of the remaining recurrent laryngeal nerve can result in airway obstruction.

SOFT TISSUE DISSECTION. After the subcutaneous tissue is incised, the platysma muscle is cut perpendicular to its fibers the full length of the skin incision. The platysma is then undermined and a plane is dissected both rostrally and caudally for several centimeters between the platysma muscle and the superficial cervical fascia to facilitate rostral and caudal exposure. The superficial cervical fascia is then opened sharply. Using blunt finger dissection, the plane between the sternocleidomastoid muscle and carotid artery laterally and the trachea and esophagus medially is developed. Avoidance of sharp dissection at this stage of the operation is crucial and will avoid injury to the carotid artery and esophagus. The carotid artery is retracted laterally with a hand-held retractor. A second hand-held retractor retracts the esophagus medially and the assistant is directed to press the retractor blades against the anterior aspect of the vertebral bodies. The prevertebral fascia is opened sharply. Orientation in relationship to the midline is obtained by observing the longus coli muscles on either side of the midline. Anterior osteophytes or other bony abnormalities visualized at operation may be compared to the CT scan for further confirmation of the midline. The midline is marked, a needle is placed in a disc space, and the correct level if confirmed using fluoroscopy.

The medial borders of the longus coli muscles are freed from their attachment to the vertebral bodies using the bipolar forceps both for hemostasis and dissection. The longus coli should be mobilized one vertebral body above and below the area of intended bone and disc resection and at least 3 cm in a medial-lateral direction to permit adequate bone resection and placement of the bone graft and anterior plate.

Sharp self-retaining retractor blades, such as those marketed by Sofamor Danek (Memphis, TN) for this purpose, are placed underneath the medial aspect of the longus coli muscles and the retractor is spread to gain medial-lateral exposure. A second set of retractors with dull blades is placed to gain rostral and caudal exposure.

BONE AND DISC REMOVAL. The disc spaces above and below the vertebral bodies to be resected are identified and the correct levels confirmed using fluoroscopy. The anterior longitudinal ligament and anterior annulus are incised and excised. Careful examination of the MRI and bone windows on the CT scan is essential to define the location and extent of bone removal that will be necessary. In the midcervical spine the distance from the medial border of the foramen transversarium to the medial border of the same structure contralaterally is approximately 3 cm.

In patients with spondylosis or OPLL it may be necessary to remove as much as 2 cm of bone in a transverse direction to achieve adequate decompression. In patients undergoing vertebrectomy for neoplastic disease or infection, bone resection of a similar extent may sometimes be necessary. Resection of 2 cm of bone will leave only 5 mm from the most lateral extent of bone removal to the medial border of the foramen transversarium. It is thus essential that the midline be accurately identified. In patients with destructive lesions, it is important to note if the medial bony margin of the foramen transversarium has been destroyed to avoid vertebral artery injury during removal of pathological soft tissue.

We begin bone resection with the high-speed drill with a 6-mm extra-rough diamond burr. Once the outline of the bone resection is made to a depth of 2 to 3 mm, the risk of injury to any soft tissue structures by the drill is reduced, and a 6-mm cutting burr is used. The operating microscope is brought into the field and the cutting burr is used to resect bone until the posterior cortical bone is reached, after which the diamond burr is used. Alternatively a rough diamond burr may be used for the entire bone resection. This burr resects bone almost as rapidly as the cutting burr but is hemostatic during resection of vascular cancellous bone and it will not snag soft tissues. Because the diamond burr produces considerable heat during drilling, it must be irrigated continuously to avoid thermal trauma to the spinal cord.

The last bits of bone are removed using fine curets. Kerrison rongeurs must never be used to remove bone unless the bone has already been mobilized anteriorly away from the spinal cord. In patients with spinal cord compression by tumor or osteomyelitis, the amount of drilling needed may be minimal and decompression may be achieved by resection of soft tissue with curets, pituitary forceps, or a nerve hook. In patients with osteomyelitis or neoplasm, aggressive removal of all affected bone is essential. Bone grafts will not be held in place by soft bone, and screws placed in such bone will loosen.

When the most posteriorly located bone or soft tissue is removed the surgeon should reconnoiter and make certain that adequate bone removal has been performed in all directions. The surgeon's line of vision is directed to the side contralateral to the skin incision, thus there is a tendency to remove more bone on the contralateral side than the ipsilateral one. Rotating the operating table toward the surgeon or redirecting the operating microscope toward the side ipsilateral to the incision will help expose this "blind" side and avoid asymmetrical bone removal. The operating microscope may be briefly moved out of the field and the extent of bone removal in relation to the midline determined. As the drilling proceeds, further confirmation of bone removal in relation to the midline can be obtained by observing the upward swing of the uncovertebral joints. Bone should be removed to this point but not further laterally.

After vertebral body resection is complete, remaining disc above and below the site of vertebrectomy is removed using curets. The cortical bone of the vertebrae adjacent to those resected is removed with the high-speed drill in preparation for bone grafting. The posterior longitudinal ligament (PLL) is then opened using a nerve hook to expose the dura. The posterior layer of the PLL is rarely adherent to the dura in patients with spondylosis or tumor and should be resected to the edge of the bony removal.

BONE GRAFTING. A piece of tricortical iliac crest autograft or allograft is used for bone grafting. Allograft has the advantage of decreasing operative time and avoiding the morbidity of a second incision, and it is our choice for vertebrectomies.

Fibular allograft is preferred by some surgeons. It is particularly desirable for multilevel vertebrectomies when sufficiently long pieces of tricortical allograft are unavailable or of the wrong configuration. We do not use fibula as it is mostly cortical bone and tends to telescope into the cancellous bone of the adjacent vertebrae and it takes longer to fuse than iliac crest.

The iliac crest graft should be no deeper in its anteroposterior dimension than 13 mm, although in children or adults with very small vertebral bodies this dimension may have to be smaller. After longitudinal distraction is carried out using the Caspar distraction instruments or by having the anesthesiologist apply manual distraction to the head or the cervical traction apparatus, the graft is impacted into place (Fig. 4). After placement of the graft the evoked potentials are assessed to rule out spinal cord dysfunction from overdistraction or intrusion of the graft into the spinal canal.

ANTERIOR CERVICAL PLATING. Several authors have described notching of the graft and adjacent vertebral bodies to prevent graft dislodgment (20–23). Although they report excellent results with this technique, we prefer to use anterior cervical plates in all patients who have had cervical vertebral body resection at one or more levels to prevent graft displacement, to share load bearing with the graft, to prevent the development of kyphotic deformity, and to obviate the need for cumbersome external orthoses.

Anterior osteophytes that interfere with plate placement should be removed, and the plate should be contoured so that the ends of the plate lie flush with the surface of the vertebral bodies. The correct-length plate is chosen utilizing the C-arm fluoroscopy. The ends of the plate should not overlie adjacent disc spaces or unfused adjacent vertebral bodies (Fig. 5). The plate is placed in the midline, care being taken not to skew either end away from the midline. The screws should be directed to the center of the vertebral body as seen on fluoroscopy. If the lower end of the plate and screws cannot be seen on fluoroscopy, the disc space just below the lower body to be fused is identified and the correct length of the plate and screw placement are estimated. Bicortical screw penetration is not necessary, and, for the most part, we use screws 14 mm in length.

A variety of plating systems are commercially available, most of which provide excellent fixation. All systems designed in the last 5 to 10 years utilize screws that lock to the plate; older systems without this locking feature should not be used, as screw back-out may result in disastrous perforation of the esophagus or other soft tissue structures.

An important choice in selecting a plating system is whether to use a plate with constrained or unconstrained screws. Constrained screws cannot move in relation to the plate. If the graft collapses, the screws cannot toggle. This places additional stress on the screws and plate, which may result in breakage of either the screw or plate, particularly with long constructs. The Cervical Spine Locking Plate (Synthes, Paoli, PA) and the Orion Plate (Sofamor Danek) are examples of constrained systems.

Unconstrained screws can "toggle" and the angle that the screw makes with the plate can change if the graft settles or telescopes into the adjacent vertebral bodies. An example of

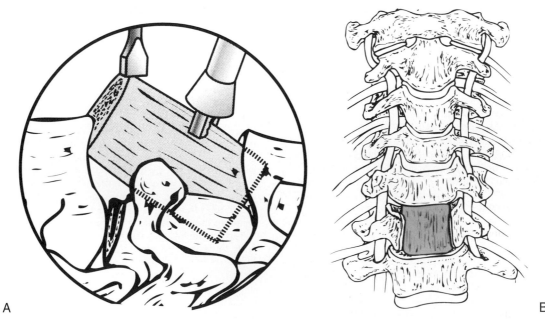

A   B

Fig. 4. **A**: Insertion of bone graft after vertebrectomy is complete. **B**: Bone graft in place. (Reproduced with permission of Sofamor Danek, Memphis, TN.)

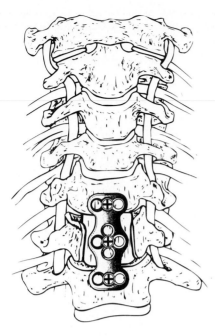

Fig. 5. An anterior cervical plate over bone graft. (Reproduced with permission of Sofamor Danek, Memphis, TN.)

this is the Atlantis Plate (Sofamor Danek), which may be utilized with constrained or unconstrained screws. In theory, hardware failure is less likely to occur with unconstrained screws. In practice either system is adequate and hardware breakage is unusual.

With a semiconstrained system such as the A-line plate (Surgical Dynamics, Norwalk, CT) the screws will not move unless they are subjected to considerable stress, which occurs with collapse or telescoping of the graft into adjacent vertebral bodies. In many ways this feature incorporates the best characteristics of both constrained and unconstrained systems. In addition, the screws used with the A-line plate can be directed rostrally or caudally 13 degrees to the perpendicular, a particular advantage if the screws are to be placed in a thin sliver of vertebral body that has been partially resected.

SPECIAL CONSIDERATIONS

Ossification of the Posterior Longitudinal Ligament (OPLL). In OPLL the PLL is calcified and frequently stuck to the dura, which may also be calcified. When the calcified PLL is adherent to the dura and no plane can be identified, a thin piece may be left in place provided that it does not produce mass effect and it is detached from all bony connections that would prevent it from moving anteriorly. Occasionally the dura is replaced by a calcified mass that must be resected to remove pressure from the spinal cord. In this event the area of dural resection is covered with a piece of Gelfoam and the patient is placed on spinal drainage postoperatively for a period of 3 or 4 days.

Osteomyelitis. In patients with osteomyelitis, resection of the thickened and inflamed PLL is usually indicated to reduce the mass effect against the dura. Although it is infrequent to find pus or granulation tissue posterior to the PLL, the PLL itself may be adherent to the dura as a result of inflammation. If a plane between the dura and PLL is not immediately evident, resection

of the PLL should be terminated, as entrance of viable organisms into the subarachnoid space can be disastrous.

Although placement of foreign bodies is usually avoided in the presence of infection, we have had extensive experience with the use of spinal instrumentation in the presence of infection and removal has only rarely been necessary (15,24). For this reason we advocate the use of anterior cervical plates in the presence of infection in a fashion identical to that described for noninfectious conditions.

Neoplastic Disease. In patients with residual neoplastic disease who are radiated, fusion may not occur after bone grafting or residual tumor may grow into the bone graft. For this reason we have increasingly performed vertebral body reconstruction with methylmethacrylate (MMA) rather than bone graft. In such circumstances MMA has several advantages: it is easily and rapidly inserted, it is strong and cannot be invaded by tumor, and it is unaffected by radiation therapy.

After vertebrectomy we insert a Steinmann pin into the center of the intact vertebral bodies adjacent to the vertebrectomy. The ends of the pins extend into the vertebrectomy defect. Semisolid MMA is poured into the vertebrectomy defect, and when it hardens it is held in place by the pins. This technique is discussed in more detail in another chapter of this volume. Alternatively the MMA may be held in place by an anterior cervical plate. We would emphasize that vertebral body reconstruction with MMA is never appropriate after vertebrectomy for degenerative disease, trauma, or infection.

Postoperative Management

A Jackson-Pratt drain is placed in the prevertebral space in all patients and is removed after 24 hours. In patients with dural tears, gravity drainage is utilized and suction is avoided. Patients are encouraged to ambulate the day after surgery and are instructed to wear a hard collar for 6 weeks.

COMPLICATION AVOIDANCE AND MANAGEMENT. The postoperative complications associated with cervical vertebrectomy are summarized in Table 1. Most series report a significant complication rate of 10% to 20% (25–27). A discussion of all the potential complications and their avoidance is beyond the

Table 1. Possible Complications of Cervical Vertebrectomy

Cervical wound infection/hematoma
Esophageal perforation
Tracheal injury
Recurrent laryngeal nerve injury
Thoracic duct injury
Pneumothorax
Horner's syndrome
Vascular injury (carotid artery, vertebral artery, internal jugular vein)
Dysphagia (esophageal dysmotility)
Bone graft donor-site complications (pain, hematoma, infection)
Postoperative airway obstruction
Graft complications
Hardware complications
Pseudarthrosis
Spinal cord injury
Nerve root injury
Dural tear

scope of this chapter. However, if the following rules are adhered to complications will be minimized: (a) use of a left-sided approach when possible, (b) soft tissue dissection below the superficial cervical fascia using blunt dissection only, (c) clear knowledge of the location of the midline and avoidance of bone removal lateral to the uncovertebral joint, (d) use of the operating microscope for bone removal and avoidance of Kerrison rongeurs or other space-occupying instruments to remove bone or osteophytes, (e) meticulous graft shaping and countersinking, (f) midline plate placement and plating only fused levels with plates ending proximal to adjacent disc spaces, (g) screw placement as close to the center of the vertebral body as possible, (h) use of meticulous hemostasis and wound drainage, and (i) use of supplemental posterior plating in patients with more than two-level vertebral resections or in those with preoperative instability or kyphotic deformity.

Conclusions

Cervical vertebrectomy is an important technique for the treatment of a wide variety of pathological processes involving the cervical spine. Careful preoperative determination of the diagnosis and the levels involved, as well as meticulous technique, is the best way to maximize surgical outcome while minimizing the associated complications. Further advances in surgical technique and instrumentation should continue to improve the outcome of all patients with pathology of the cervical spine.

References

1. Bohlman HH, Emery SE. The pathophysiology of cervical spondylosis and myelopathy. *Spine* 1988;3(7):843–846.
2. Murakami N, Muroga T, Sobue I. Cervical myelopathy due to ossification of the posterior longitudinal ligament: a clinicopathologic study. *Arch Neurol* 1978;35(1):33–36.
3. Nagashima C. Cervical myelopathy due to ossification of the posterior longitudinal ligament. *J Neurosurg* 1972;37(6):653–660.
4. Payne EE. The cervical spine. An anatomico-pathological study of 70 specimens with particular reference to the problem of cervical spondylosis. *Brain* 1960;80:571–592.
5. Adams CB, Logue V. Studies in cervical spondylotic myelopathy. II. The movement and contour of the spine in relation to the neural complications of cervical spondylosis. *Brain* 1971;94(3):568–586.
6. Wolf BS, Malis L. The sagittal diameter of the bony cervical spinal canal and its significance in cervical spondylosis. *J Mt Sinai Hosp* 1956;23:283–292.
7. Hashimoto I, Tak YK. The true sagittal diameter of the cervical spinal canal and its diagnostic significance in cervical myelopathy. *J Neurosurg* 1977;47(6):912–916.
8. White AAD, Panjabi MM. Biomechanical considerations in the surgical management of cervical spondylotic myelopathy. *Spine* 1988; 13(7):856–860.
9. Kaufman HH, Jones E. The principles of bony spinal fusion. *Neurosurgery* 1989;24(2):264–270.
10. Waldvogel FA, Papageorgiou PS. Osteomyelitis: the past decade. *N Engl J Med* 1980;303(7):360–370.
11. Price RW. Infections in AIDS and in other immuno-compromised patients. In: Kennedy PGE, Jr., ed. *Infections of the nervous system.* London: Butterworth, 1987:248–273.
12. Lifeso RM, Weaver P, Harder EH. Tuberculous spondylitis in adults. *J Bone Joint Surg* 1985;67A(9):1405–1413.
13. Fang D, Leong JC, Fang HS. Tuberculosis of the upper cervical spine. *J Bone Joint Surg* 1983;65B(1):47–50.
14. Osenbach RK, Hitchon PW, Menezes AH. Diagnosis and management of pyogenic vertebral osteomyelitis in adults. *Surg Neurol* 1990;33(4):266–275.
15. Rezai AR, et al. Modern management of spinal tuberculosis. *Neurosurgery* 1995;36(1):87–97; discussion 97–98.
16. Bracken MB, et al. A randomized, controlled trial of methylprednisolone or naloxone in the treatment of acute spinal-cord injury. Results of the Second National Acute Spinal Cord Injury Study (see comments). *N Engl J Med* 1990;322(20):1405–1411.
17. Morota N, et al. The role of motor evoked potentials during surgery for intramedullary spinal cord tumors. *Neurosurgery* 1997;41(6): 1327–1336.
18. Kothbauer K, Deletis V, Epstein FJ. Intraoperative spinal cord monitoring for intramedullary surgery: an essential adjunct (see comments). *Pediatr Neurosurg* 1997;26(5):247–254.
19. Epstein NE, Danto J, Nardi D. Evaluation of intraoperative somatosensory-evoked potential monitoring during 100 cervical operations. *Spine* 1993;18(6):737–747.
20. Saunders RL. Anterior reconstructive procedures in cervical spondylotic myelopathy. *Clin Neurosurg* 1991;37:682–721.
21. Awasthi D, Voorhies RM. Anterior cervical vertebrectomy and interbody fusion. Technical note. *J Neurosurg* 1992;76(1):159–163.
22. Simmons EH, Bhalla SK. Anterior cervical discectomy and fusion. A clinical and biomechanical study with eight-year follow-up. *J Bone Joint Surg* 1969;51B(2):225–237.
23. Whitecloud TS III. Fibular strut graft in reconstructive surgery of the cervical spine. *Spine* 1976;1:33–43.
24. Rezai AR, et al. Contemporary management of spinal osteomyelitis. *Neurosurgery* 1999;44(5):1018–1025; discussion 1025–1026.
25. Kojima T, et al. Anterior cervical vertebrectomy and interbody fusion for multi-level spondylosis and ossification of the posterior longitudinal ligament. *Neurosurgery* 1989;24(6):864–872.
26. Seifert V. Anterior decompressive microsurgery and osteosynthesis for the treatment of multi-segmental cervical spondylosis. Pathophysiological considerations, surgical indication, results and complications: a survey. *Acta Neurochir* 1995;135(3–4):105–121.
27. Selecki BR. Complications and limitations of anterior decompression and fusion of the cervical spine (Cloward's technique). *Med J Aust* 1972;1(6):281–282.

200. Thoracic Discectomy and Corpectomy via the Anterior Approach

Amory J. Fiore, Peter D. Angevine, and Paul C. McCormick

Clinically significant herniated intervertebral discs in the thoracic spine are rare. Their prevalence in the general population is estimated to be 1 in 1,000,000. Of herniated discs that come to clinical attention, approximately 0.25% to 0.75% are in the thoracic spine and only 0.2% to 4% of disc operations are for thoracic discs (1). Population studies, however, indicate that a significant proportion of the population harbors asymptomatic herniated discs in the thoracic region.

Diagnosis of herniated thoracic discs prior to modern imaging was difficult. The presenting symptoms of a herniated thoracic disc are protean, resulting in a delay of proper diagnosis. Thoracic pain, radicular pain, stiffness and spasticity, and bowel and bladder dysfunction may all be present in various combinations.

The anatomy of the thoracic spine makes it difficult to use the surgical approaches employed to remove the more common herniated intervertebral lumbar disc. In contrast to the lumbar region, the spinal canal is narrower. Most significant, however, is the presence not of free-floating nerve roots but rather the spinal cord. The spinal cord in the thoracic region also has a tenuous vascular supply, making it particularly sensitive to ischemic injury secondary to traction when trying to reach an anteriorly located disc from a posterior approach.

To avoid the historically poor clinical outcomes of thoracic laminectomy for discectomy, posterolateral and anterolateral approaches have been developed. The modern era of ventral approach to the thoracic spine began in 1969 with the independent papers of Perot and Munro (2) and Ransohoff et al. (3). The safety and efficacy of the transthoracic transpleural approach to the thoracic spine has been well established in the years since then. A variation on the transpleural route, the retropleural approach, has been developed and refined by McCormick (4) to avoid the potential morbidity of opening the pleural and directly retracting the lung. Both approaches provide wide anterior exposure to the majority of the thoracic spine, allowing for safe decompression of the spinal cord and, when necessary, extensive resection of vertebral bodies with proper fusion.

Indications for the Anterior Approach

Both the transpleural and retropleural approaches offer ventral access to the thoracic spine and to the thoracolumbar junction. Exposure can be obtained as high as T3 and, by modifying the dissection to free diaphragmatic attachments, as low as L1. The trajectory of the access is ventral and slightly lateral, which provides early visualization of the dura without having to work through the involved vertebral body or disc in order to define the dural limits.

Although discs in the thoracic region can be resected via posterolateral approaches, there are features of some discs that make them difficult to resect from any approach other than ventral. With the close tolerances of the relatively small thoracic spinal canal and the susceptibility of the thoracic cord to retraction injury, posterolateral approaches are often reserved for lateral discs. Central and centrolateral herniations, which may represent 70% to 94% of thoracic discs, are more easily removed anteriorly, especially if there is extensive calcification (5).

A significant proportion (65% in one series) of thoracic discs are calcified (5). These hard discs are not easily removed with a lateral approach. Their firm consistency puts the cord and dura at risk during extraction if the trajectory of removal is not directly away from the spinal canal. Dural tears encountered during the removal of hardened discs are difficult to repair primarily without the wide exposure of the ventral approaches. Chronic, calcified discs may erode through the dura, presenting the surgeon with intradural fragments that must be retrieved. Removal of intradural disc fragments through the limited exposure of the posterolateral approaches is technically challenging.

The most common indication for corpectomy in the thoracic spine is metastatic disease with pathological fracture or spinal cord compression, or both. Traumatic burst fracture is also a common indication for decompression of the thoracic spinal canal and fusion of the anterior column. General guidelines for operative intervention include fracture with greater than 40% loss of vertebral body height, greater than 50% canal compromise, major kyphotic deformity, or significant neural deficit. Although a ventral approach is important to ensure the adequate decompression of neural elements and the creation of anterior stability in these cases, a posterior approach may also be necessary to reestablish the integrity of the entire spine. The anterior and posterior procedures may be done concurrently or in separate operations.

The transpleural and retropleural approaches provide similar exposure. There are, however, situations in which one approach may be preferable to the other. The retropleural approach has the advantage of avoiding direct retraction on an exposed lung. This may decrease the risk of pulmonary contusion. The great vessels (aorta and vena cava) are less of a hindrance with the retropleural approach as the operative trajectory is more lateral. On the other hand, the transpleural exposure may be more amenable to cranial-caudal exposure for procedures that require exposure of more than one or two vertebral levels. Reoperations may be easier with either the transpleural or retropleural approach depending on the nature of the original surgery. A history of pleurodesis or pleuritis makes the transpleural approach more difficult due to the presence of scar tissue.

The main contraindication for a transthoracic approach, either retropleural or transpleural, is compromised pulmonary function. Preoperative evaluation of the patient for adequate pulmonary reserve is essential. In the case that the patient's pulmonary status is adequate but marginal, the retropleural approach with its avoidance of direct retraction trauma to the lung may provide a safer approach.

The posterolateral thoracotomy may be modified to reach lesions above T3. The approach is similar to that used by thoracic surgeons to resect Pancoast tumors (6). Depending on the nature of the pathology and patient-specific anatomical factors, an extended cervical approach with resection of the manubrium and medial clavicle can be used to approach high thoracic spine lesions. The retropleural approach should not be used above T3 as division of the sympathetic chain in that region may result in a Horner's syndrome.

In the last decade thoracoscopy has been developed as an alternative to open anterior approaches to the thoracic spine. In the hands of experienced neurosurgeons trained in the specialized techniques necessary for these procedures, thoracoscopic surgery may offer anterior exposure with reduced perioperative morbidity. As techniques are developed and disseminated, the indications for thoracoscopic procedures may increase (7).

Surgical Technique

PREOPERATIVE PLANNING AND POSITIONING. The side of approach is determined by a combination of factors, including the level and location of the pathology. An ipsilateral approach provides the most direct surgical route to lateralized pathology. Many surgeons are more comfortable approaching the upper thoracic spine from the right, thereby avoiding the heart and the great vessels. For the mid- and lower thoracic spine, a left-sided approach has the advantage of mobilization of the aorta rather than the inferior vena cava, which is less resistant to injury (1). Another consideration in the lower thoracic spine is the artery of Adamkiewicz, which is found between T9 and L2 in 85% of specimens and enters from the left in 80% (8). The medullary arteries, including Adamkiewicz, are not placed at risk if cautery is not used in the neural foramina. This will obviate the need for routine preoperative angiography.

It is important to evaluate preoperatively the level of the lesion and determine a suitable method for confidently localizing that segment in the operating room. The level of pathology is often determined preoperatively by the radiologist and surgeon using the sacrum or odontoid as a reference. These fixed landmarks may not be available in the operating room, either on the scans or with fluoroscopy. The most caudal rib can serve as a fixed reference if care is taken to establish its level, radiographic appearance, and relation to the pathological segment. Knowing the number of ribs and the number of nonribbed lumbar vertebrae as well as the appearance of the lumbosacral region (with particular attention to the presence of a transitional vertebra) will help to determine the operative level.

If an epidural catheter is to be used for postoperative analgesia, it should be placed prior to positioning and induction. The patient is placed on the operating table in a lateral position. A beanbag is placed under the patient to prevent pressure points and add stability. A soft roll is placed under the dependent axilla. The lower leg is flexed at the knee and hip for additional stability. A pillow is placed between the legs. Thoracolumbar lesions should be centered over the table break. A double-lumen endotracheal tube allows the anesthesiologist to deflate the ipsilateral lung to increase exposure for upper thoracic (above T6) lesions. The setup should allow the operating table to be lowered completely during the procedure.

PROCEDURE

Incision. The rib level is confirmed with intraoperative fluoroscopy or x-ray. For a retropleural approach to upper- and midthoracic lesions the incision is made over the rib of the involved level (the T10 rib for a T9-10 disc). In the upper thoracic spine, a hockey-stick incision is made along the medial and inferior border of the scapula. The muscular attachments of the scapula are released and it is rotated superiorly. A standard, approximately 12-cm incision is used for approaches to lesions from T5 to T10. It begins 4 cm lateral to the posterior midline, follows the appropriate rib, and ends at the posterior axillary line (4, 9) (Fig. 1).

In a transpleural approach the incision is made somewhat more anteriorly and generally two rib levels above the pathological segment. It begins just lateral to the paraspinal muscles on the posterior thorax and extends as necessary anteriorly, following the rib contour (10).

Exposure. Once the proper level has been confirmed and the incision made, the rib is exposed with subperiosteal dissection. The intercostal muscles are detached along an 8- to 10-cm length of rib. The exposed rib is resected and saved for autograft use, and the cut ends are waxed. In the rib bed a distinct tissue layer, the endothoracic fascia, is identified. This layer is continuous with the inner periosteum of the ribs and thoracic vertebral bodies. It contains the intercostal nerves and vessels, the thoracic sympathetic chain, thoracic duct, and the azygous vein (4).

The endothoracic fascia is sharply incised and the parietal pleura is exposed. In a retropleural approach, the pleura is bluntly dissected free from the endothoracic fascia with a Kittner clamp. Any small tears are repaired primarily with suture. For a lesion above T6 the ipsilateral lung should be deflated. The ribs are then spread with a crank retractor; a table-mounted retractor is placed to retract the lung gently. The opening in the endothoracic fascia is extended proximally to the rib head, and the pleural dissection is extended to the spinal column. Pleural tears can be minimized by freeing the pleura rostral and caudal to the operative level. The ligaments attaching the rib to the vertebra, the costotransverse and radiate ligaments, are divided. Any remaining soft tissue attachments are divided and the rib head is disarticulated and removed.

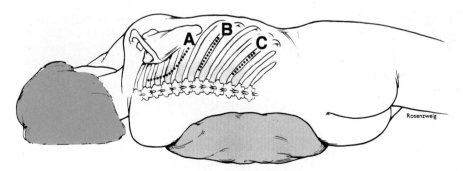

Fig. 1. Patient position and location of incisions for retropleural thoracotomy. Incision *A* is used for upper thoracic lesions, and incisions *B* and *C* for midthoracic and thoracolumbar lesions, respectively.

For a transpleural approach, the parietal pleura is incised in the rib bed after the endothoracic fascia is opened. If the lung remains inflated, it is covered with a moistened laparotomy pad and gently retracted medially and ventrally. Proximally, the parietal pleura will again need to be incised overlying the vertebral body. The periosteum is dissected off the vertebral body with a Cobb elevator taking care to preserve the segmental vessels. Working laterally gains exposure of the radiate ligaments, which are divided. The rib head is either drilled or disarticulated to expose the disc space, foramen, and pedicle (11) (Fig. 2).

Discectomy. The endothoracic fascia is incised over the involved disc space. This divides the sympathetic chain, which rarely has any clinically significant result in the thoracic spine. The fascia and vertebral periosteum are reflected rostrally and caudally away from the disc space. Contained in the fascia are the intercostal vessels, which overlie each vertebra at midbody. For a single-level discectomy these vessels can be preserved.

Curets and nerve hooks are used to define the pedicle margins. The disc is incised and removed with rongeurs and curets (Fig. 3). A high-speed drill is used to remove the end plates. The bony dissection is extended into the adjacent vertebral bodies. The pedicle is removed with the drill and with Kerrison rongeurs. This exposes the lateral spinal canal before dissection of the posterior vertebral body. With the dura clearly visible, the corpectomy is extended approximately 1.5 cm rostrally and caudally from the disc space. It should be extended 3 to 3.5 cm medially from the lateral margin of the vertebral body (Fig. 4).

At this point, only a thin shell of posterior vertebral body and the posterior longitudinal ligament (PLL) remains. The PLL often contains disc material and must be removed completely to accomplish an adequate decompression. It is sharply divided with a reverse-angled curet, and the remaining bone and ligament is pushed into the corpectomy defect with curets and removed. The vector of force must always be away from the spinal canal. This portion of the resection is done quickly, as epidural venous bleeding can be significant. The bleeding is controlled with bipolar cautery after the decompression is complete. The final step in a single-level discectomy is to drill appropriately sized

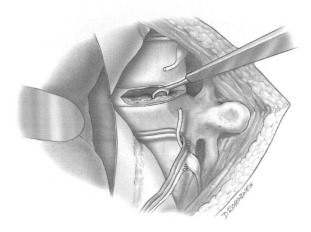

Fig. 3. The sympathetic chain is divided and the disc is evacuated.

troughs for the rib autograft interbody strut and tap the graft into place (Fig. 5).

Corpectomy. To perform a one-level corpectomy, the initial exposure includes an additional rib (for a T9 corpectomy, the 9th and 10th ribs are resected). The initial exposure and dissection is as for a discectomy. The intercostal vessels that overlie the involved segment cannot be preserved and are divided close to the midline between ligatures. Distal muscular and osseous branches will reconstitute flow in these vessels and maintain spinal cord blood flow (4). The segmental vessels rostral and caudal to the involved level may also need to be divided to mobilize the great vessels sufficiently (10).

The discs rostral and caudal to the pathological vertebra are incised and removed as described above. By removing the discs on either side of the pathological vertebral body first, the blood loss is minimized. The rostral end plate on the normal vertebra above the involved segment and the caudal end plate of the vertebra below are left intact (10). Rongeurs, curets, and a drill are used to complete the corpectomy. As for the discectomy, care must be taken to lever the posterior portion of the vertebral

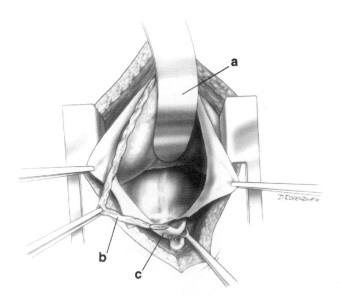

Fig. 2. With a malleable retractor (*a*) on the lung, the neurovascular bundle (*b*) is freed and partially mobilized from the underlying fascia. The proximal rib (*c*) is removed to expose the pedicle and disc space.

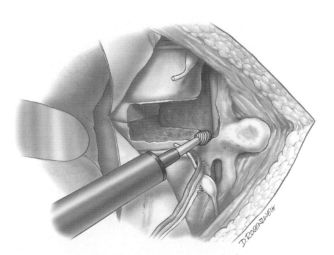

Fig. 4. Using a high-speed drill, the pedicle and adjacent end plates are removed, exposing the lateral dura.

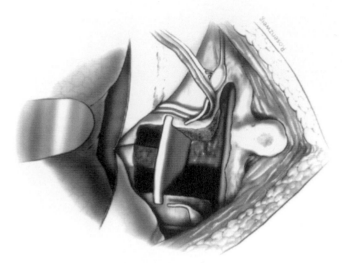

Fig. 5. Decompression is completed, the dura is inspected, and the resected rib is used as a strut autograft.

body into a previously made defect, thereby protecting the posterior neural structures (Fig. 6).

Closure. The endothoracic fascia is replaced in its original position over the vertebral body. For a transpleural approach, the pleura is approximated and a chest tube is left in the pleural space. An airtight pleural closure is not necessary, as the muscles will become repleuralized while the chest tube prevents buildup of pleural air. If no pleural tears occur during a retropleural approach, closed chest drainage is not necessary. If significant intrathoracic air remains at the end of the procedure or if significant pleural violation occurred, a chest tube should be placed. The pleural integrity can be tested by having the anesthesiologist deliver positive pressure.

The ribs adjacent to the resection are reapproximated with

suture to reduce the chest wall deformity. It is critical to avoid ensnaring the intercostal nerves that run inferior to each rib to prevent postthoracotomy neuralgia. One way to ensure this is to drill a hole in the inferior rib through which the suture is threaded.

Thoracolumbar Junction (T11-L1). The steeper rostrocaudal orientation of the ribs at the thoracolumbar junction necessitates an incision along the rib two levels above the involved segment. If the incision is made along the rib of the pathological segment, the rostral ribs will overlie the operative field and make exposure difficult. The incision and rib resection may be extended anteriorly by 2 to 4 cm to give additional exposure. Exposure is also facilitated by centering the pathological level over the table break.

The rib is removed and the lateral endothoracic fascia, if present, is opened. The retroperitoneal and retropleural spaces are united by sharply dissecting the pleural surface of the diaphragm from the T11 and T12 ribs with periosteal dissectors. Medially the detachment continues by freeing the arcuate ligaments from the psoas and quadratus muscles. Care must be taken to preserve the subcostal nerve as it runs laterally beneath the lateral arcuate ligament on the surface of the quadratus lumborum muscle. The ipsilateral crus of the diaphragm is divided on the vertebral body, completing the mobilization of the hemidiaphragm. The proximal rib head at the involved segment is resected as for higher levels. The psoas muscle attaches to the T12 rib and this insertion may need to be released. At this point, discectomy or corpectomy proceeds as described above.

Closure involves reestablishment of the diaphragmatic attachments. The arcuate ligaments are sutured to the psoas and quadratus lumborum muscles. As with a thoracotomy performed at higher levels, the pleura is carefully inspected. Small tears are repaired with suture. A chest tube should be left if larger tears occurred or if there is significant air in the pleural space. The layers are closed with absorbable suture.

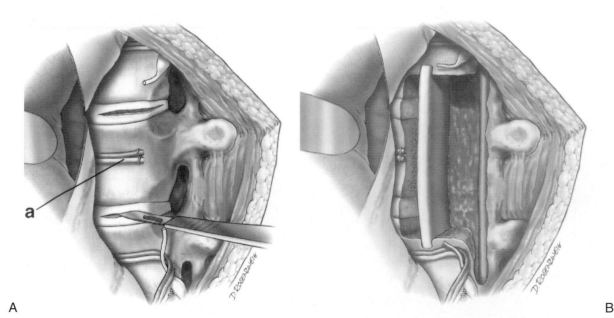

A   B

Fig. 6. **A**: Initial stages of corpectomy. The segmental vessels have been divided proximal to the foramen (*a*), the sympathetic chain is divided, and the discs are being incised. **B**: Completion of corpectomy. The rib is fashioned into a strut graft spanning the corpectomy defect.

Complications

Although the retropleural and transpleural approaches to the thoracic spine provide excellent exposure of bony and neural structures for discectomy and corpectomy, there are several potential complications. In one large retrospective series, the complication rate of the transthoracic approach was as follows: pleural effusion, 3%; pneumothorax, 1.8%; and postthoracotomy pain syndrome lasting greater than 6 months, 9.2% (12). These complications can be avoided with attention to detail and meticulous technique. Pneumothorax is possible any time a thoracotomy is performed. This is avoided in the transpleural approach by the routine placement of a chest tube during closure and careful management postoperatively according to standard principles. A chest tube does not need to be placed routinely during a retropleural approach as long as the pleura remains intact and any small tears are repaired with suture. The pleural closure should be tested as described above and a chest tube placed if there is a significant air leak.

A cerebrospinal fluid (CSF) leak is a potentially difficult problem to treat should it occur, especially if it progresses to a CSF-pleural fistula with pulmonary effusion. By removing the pedicle early in the procedure and identifying the dura in the lateral spinal canal, dural tears can be minimized. If a dural tear occurs, or if a durotomy is necessary to retrieve an intradural disc fragment, the dura should be closed primarily with 6-0 suture. A spinal drain may be placed postoperatively for CSF diversion while the dural closure heals.

There are some reports of anterior fixation devices placed from the left causing traumatic arterial aneurysms. Fixation devices should be placed anterolaterally if possible to prevent this complication (10).

While dividing the sympathetic chain in the mid- and lower thoracic region is generally without clinical sequelae, dividing the high thoracic sympathetic chain may result in a Horner's syndrome. The retropleural approach, therefore, should not be used above the T3 level. An extended cervical approach or a modified posterolateral thoracotomy may be used to approach high thoracic lesions anteriorly.

Injury to the spinal cord vasculature and a potentially disastrous spinal cord infarction can be avoided by not using cautery in the foramen and therefore protecting the medullary vessels. The intercostal neurovascular bundle needs to be divided only during a corpectomy; it may be easily preserved during discectomy by simply reflecting the endothoracic fascia away from the resection site.

Conclusions

The anterior approaches to the thoracic spine, retropleural and transpleural, provide unparalleled ventral and lateral access to the spine for discectomy and corpectomy. This exposure is necessary for early identification of neural and vascular structures that need to be preserved. Understanding the anatomy of the region and potential complications of these approaches is critical to a safe, effective procedure.

References

1. Errico TJ, Stecker S, Kostuik JP. Thoracic pain syndromes. In: Frymoyer JW, et al. *The adult spine: principles and practice.* Philadelphia: Lippincott-Raven, 1997.
2. Perot PL, Munro DD. Transthoracic removal of midline thoracic disc protrusions causing spinal cord compression. *J Neurosurg* 1969;31:452–458.
3. Ransohoff J, Spencer F, Siew F, et al. Transthoracic removal of thoracic disc. Report of three cases. *J Neurosurg* 1969;31:459–461.
4. McCormick PC. Retropleural approach to the thoracic and thoracolumbar spine. *Neurosurgery* 1995;37:908–914.
5. Stillerman CB, Chen TC, Couldwell WT, et al. Experience in the surgical management of 82 symptomatic herniated thoracic discs and review of the literature. *J Neurosurg* 1998;88:623–633.
6. Paulson DL. Carcinomas in the superior pulmonary sulcus. *J Thorac Cardiovasc Surg* 1975;70:1095–1104.
7. Rosenthal D, Dickman CA. Thoracoscopic microsurgical excision of herniated thoracic discs. *J Neurosurg* 1998;89:224–235.
8. Krauss WE. Vascular anatomy of the spinal cord. *Neurosurg Clin North Am* 1999;10:9–15.
9. Birch BD, Desai RD, McCormick PC. Surgical approaches to the thoracolumbar spine. *Neurosurg Clin North Am* 1997;8:471–485.
10. Kostuik JP. Surgical approaches to the thoracic and thoracolumbar spine. In: Frymoyer JW, et al. *The adult spine: principles and practice.* Philadelphia: Lippincott-Raven, 1997.
11. Stillerman CB, McCormick PC, Benzel EC. Thoracic discectomy. In: Benzel EC, ed. *Spine surgery: techniques, complication avoidance, and management.* New York: Churchill Livingstone, 1999.
12. Faciszewski T, Winter RB, Lonstein JE, et al. The surgical and medical perioperative complications of anterior spinal fusion surgery in the thoracic and lumbar spine in adults. *Spine* 1995;20:1592–1599.

201. Lumbar Microdiscectomy

Perry A. Ball

Lumbar microdiscectomy is a modification of the standard technique of laminotomy and discectomy performed to relieve sciatica caused by a herniated lumbar intervertebral disc. The cornerstone of the procedure is the use of the operating microscope for magnification and illumination, which makes possible a smaller incision and more precise handling of tissues.

The operating microscope was introduced into neurological surgery in the 1960s to address intracranial lesions. Although use of the operating microscope during lumbar discectomy was reported by Yasargil (1) and Caspar (2), it was Williams (3,4) who was largely responsible for the eventual acceptance of this technique to perform surgery in the lumbar spine. Interestingly, Williams first used the operating microscope for cases of recurrent disc herniation or failed prior surgery; he felt the improved visualization would facilitate dissection around scar tissue. Experience in these challenging cases led to his using the microscope to treat first-time herniations, in the hope that less tissue dissection would prevent some of the scarring seen at repeated operations (5). With time, use of the operating microscope during lumbar discectomy became widely accepted, and series

Table 1. Studies Comparing Microdiscectomy with Standard Laminotomy and Discectomy

Retrospective, nonrandomized studies	
Wilson and Harbaugh, 1981 (14)	Shorter hospitalization and faster return to work in microsurgical group; similar clinical outcomes
Nyström, 1987 (9)	Shorter hospitalization, faster return to work, and better pain relief in microsurgical group; similar clinical outcomes
Silvers, 1988 (11)	Shorter hospitalization in microsurgical group; similar clinical outcomes
Kahanovitz et al., 1989 (17)	Shorter hospitalization in microsurgical group; similar clinical outcomes
Barrios et al., 1990 (18)	Shorter hospitalization and faster return to work in microsurgical group; similar clinical outcomes
Andrews and Lavyne, 1990 (6)	Less pain medication used and faster return to work in microsurgical group
Caspar et al., 1991 (7)	Shorter hospitalization, fewer complications, better clinical outcomes in microsurgical group
Prospective, nonrandomized study	
Abromovitz and Neff, 1991 (23)	No clear advantage to use of microscope
Prospective, randomized study	
Tullberg et al., 1993 (12)	No differences in length of hospitalization, timing of return to work, clinical outcomes

with excellent results have been published through the years (6–18). However, acceptance has not been universal, and the procedure also has its critics, who argue that the trade-off for a smaller incision is the risk for less visualization and the possibility of missed pathology (19,20).

The operating microscope offers some clear advantages. With loupe magnification, a three-dimensional appreciation of the surgical field is possible only if the incision is at least as wide as the distance between the pupils of the eyes, which is on average about 7 cm. With the operating microscope, the incision can be reduced to about 3 cm while three-dimensional vision is maintained (21). With a smaller incision, less muscle dissection is needed to reach the surgical target, so that recovery may be faster. The brilliant illumination possible with the operating microscope is aimed directly in the line of sight. Another advantage is that the surgeon and the assistant share the same view of the operative field.

The operating microscope also presents some disadvantages. A learning curve is involved, and the scope must be repositioned to change the line of site. The field of view is more restricted than with loupe magnification, so pathology can be missed. Also, the risk for infection may be higher. The microscope is covered by a sterile drape, but the eyepieces are exposed, and the drape can be contaminated by personnel in the operating room who are not scrubbed. Wilson and Harbaugh (14) noted a 2% rate of infection in microsurgical discectomies, which is about twice the expected rate for elective clean procedures.

Numerous studies have compared microdiscectomy with standard laminectomy, and these are summarized in Table 1. Studies comparing microdiscectomy with historical controls undergoing standard laminotomy and discectomy have in general shown similar rates of pain relief but have consistently shown shorter hospital stays in the microsurgery patients (6,7,9,11,14,17,18). These results must be interpreted with caution, however, because the length of a hospital stay is determined by multiple factors, and economic pressures in recent years to reduce the length of hospital stays have been tremendous. Reports of both the standard (22) and the microsurgical procedure (16) being performed on an outpatient basis have been published. A prospective, multicenter, nonrandomized study showed no clear benefit to the use of the microscope (23). The one prospective, randomized study showed no differences in length of hospitalization, return to work, or pain relief at 1 year (12). If little clear evidence is available to support the superiority of the microscope in lumbar discectomy, why should surgeons bother to use it? The answer is that it is a matter of surgeon preference; many surgeons find that the magnification and illumination offered by the microscope facilitate surgery.

Indications

The indication for lumbar discectomy is radicular pain secondary to radiographically confirmed compression of a lumbar nerve root by a herniated intervertebral disc in a patient who has failed conservative management. It is important to point out that patient selection is critical to the result of surgery. In the classical analysis of the causes of failure of discectomy procedures of Fager and Freidberg (24), improper indications for surgery were a major cause of poor results. The temptation to think that because an operation is performed through a smaller incision with less surgical trauma it is therefore appropriate for patients with less clear indications for surgery is a mistake that should be avoided.

The large majority of lumbar disc herniations occur in the posterolateral direction, and in general, these can be satisfactorily approached by microdiscectomy. However, certain situations that are apparent on imaging studies require some modification of the surgical approach. Occasionally, a disc migrates under the posterior longitudinal ligament in either a cranial or caudal direction; such migration is most apparent on magnetic resonance imaging (MRI) performed in the sagittal plane. In this situation, a large part of the disc herniation lies outside the disc space, so that it is necessary to extend the skin incision and laminotomy opening in either a superior or inferior direction. It may even be necessary to explore the root above or below the one that crosses the disc space in question. A small incision is appropriate for most patients; however, in some obese patients, the deep layer of subcutaneous fat makes attempting a procedure through a 3-cm incision unwieldy, and the skin incision must be extended. Some patients, especially older ones, have a degree of facet joint hypertrophy and consequently stenosis of the lateral recess where the nerve root exits the canal into the neural foramen. In these patients, it may be difficult to access the disc herniation or satisfactorily decompress the nerve root without extending the bone removal laterally to include removal of the medial portion of the facet joint. Williams (4) has argued that with such modifications, the procedure is no longer "microlumbar discectomy"; however, this argument is essentially a matter of semantics; the operating microscope is still used, as are the principles of tissue handling to minimize trauma.

Furthermore, microdiscectomy is not the preferred procedure in certain situations. When a large central disc herniation is present, especially in the setting of cauda equina syndrome, it is probably safer in terms of nerve root retraction to perform a laminectomy and approach the disc bilaterally. About 10% of disc herniations are lateral to the neural foramen, and these require an altered approach directed at the extraforaminal space.

Operation

PROPHYLAXIS. Evidence indicates that the use of preoperative antibiotics may reduce the rate of infection in spinal surgery (25). Ideally, these should be given before the incision is made. A first-generation cephalosporin, such as cefazolin, with good activity against staphylococci is a reasonable choice. In patients allergic to cephalosporins or with a history of a serious allergic reaction to penicillin, an alternative is vancomycin.

Deep venous thrombosis is a risk associated with any surgical procedure, but the risk does not appear to be particularly high in lumbar disc surgery. This is probably because of the short operative times involved and rapid postoperative mobilization. A study of patients undergoing lumbar laminotomy or laminectomy with only mechanical prophylaxis, such compression stockings, showed no incidence of pulmonary embolism or deep venous thrombosis that required anticoagulation (26).

ANESTHESIA. General anesthesia is preferred for this procedure. The main drawback of spinal anesthesia is that when patients are awake, it is difficult for them to remain completely still, and they often shift their upper torso to some degree. If positional shifting occurs during manipulation of the nerve root, the result can be catastrophic. Infusion of local anesthetic is another alternative, but in this situation, it is difficult to provide adequate anesthesia to the periosteum of the lamina.

POSITIONING. The patient should be positioned to minimize pressure on the abdomen. Elevated abdominal pressure results in elevated pressure in the epidural venous system and thus increased bleeding during the procedure. Some surgeons choose to place the patient in a prone position, with bolsters from the rib cage to the iliac crests, or to use a positioning frame, such as the Wilson frame. The knee–chest or kneeling position allows the abdomen to hang freely and has been shown to result in less blood loss than the prone position (27). In either case, the patient's arms should be positioned with the shoulder abducted at 90 degrees and the elbow flexed. Care should be taken to avoid pressure on the ulnar nerve at the elbow. The head can be supported either by turning the neck to the side or keeping it in a neutral position, but in either case, great care should be taken to avoid pressure on the eyes when the face is padded.

INCISION. To minimize the size of the skin incision, it is best to localize the level before the incision is made. In some thin persons, localization can be accomplished by palpation. The first palpable interspace above the posterior superior iliac spines is usually L5-S1. In doubtful cases, a spinal needle can be inserted though the skin down to the level of the tips of the spinous processes, a lateral radiograph obtained, and the level confirmed. It is usually easier for the surgeon to stand on the

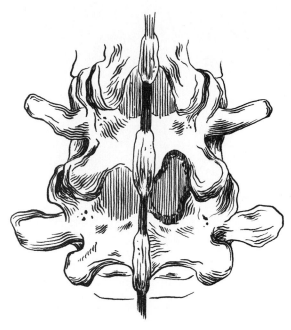

Fig. 1. Approximate extent of laminotomy performed.

side of the disc herniation. The skin incision should be long enough to provide adequate visualization and dissection of the superior and inferior laminae. For most patients, the appropriate length is 2 to 3 cm (Fig. 1). The subcutaneous fat can be dissected with electrocautery down to the level of the lumbodorsal fascia. After the fascia is opened sharply on the side of the disc herniation, the paraspinal musculature is visible. This muscle is then dissected of its attachment to the spinous processes and the hemilaminae. Dissection can be performed with electrocautery or a periosteal elevator. At this point, is worthwhile to obtain a localizing radiograph to confirm the level of the dissection; a towel clip can be placed on a spinous process for this purpose. Confirmation should be obtained even if a spinal needle was used before the incision because dissection at the wrong level is a risk in this procedure (3,14). It is not clear whether the small incision size makes this more likely. If the radiograph demonstrates that the level is incorrect, the skin incision must be extended and the dissection carried out at the appropriate level.

DISSECTION. Exposure is facilitated with the use of a self-retaining retractor. Williams retractors, which are available in a variety of sizes, have a post on one side, which is placed against the superior spinous process, and a blade on the other, which is placed against the paraspinous musculature.

At this point, the operating microscope is draped in a sterile fashion and introduced into the field. Most surgeons find that for procedures on the lumbar spine, a 300-mm focal length for the objective lens provides a satisfactory working space between the field and the microscope. The magnification can be varied, but magnification of between two and six times provides acceptable visualization and depth of focus. The field of view at this point is the superior hemilamina, the inferior hemilamina, and the ligamentum flavum between them. In the original description of Williams (3), the ligament was opened without any bone removal. This is often relatively easily accomplished at the L5-S1 level, where the interlaminar space is quite wide, but at more rostral levels, the interlaminar space is narrower, so

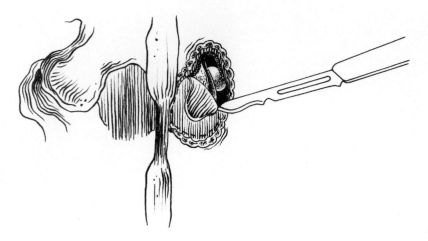

Fig. 2. Opening the ligamentum flavum with a blade.

that access to the level of the disc space is easier if a laminotomy is performed on the superior hemilamina. This is started by dissecting the leading edge of the lamina from the underlying ligament with a curette and then using a Kerrison punch angled at 45 degrees to perform the laminotomy. The amount of bone that must be removed can be estimated from the preoperative sagittal MRI. If the disc herniation does not extend beyond the disc space either rostrally or caudally, removal of about one fourth of the lamina will provide adequate visualization. A reasonable landmark is the insertion of the ligamentum flavum.

The ligamentum flavum is now opened by grasping it with toothed forceps and dividing its fibers vertically with a No. 15 blade (Fig. 2). Epidural fat usually comes into view as the ligament is divided, but in some persons, the dura lies directly underneath the ligament, so that great care must be exercised as the ligament is divided. Once an opening into the epidural space has been achieved, the cut surface of the ligament is grasped with forceps, and the opening in the ligament can be extended with the blade laterally and inferiorly. The ligament is then divided along the superior edge of the inferior hemilamina and removed. At this juncture, a Penfield No. 4 dissector is placed into the epidural space to probe laterally. The remaining lateral portion of the ligament has a distinctive thin edge, which has been referred to as the *falciform* (28) or *shelving* (29) portion of the ligament. It is necessary to remove this edge to access the nerve root, and removal is most easily accomplished with a Kerrison punch biting laterally. However, it is important first to probe carefully under the falciform edge with the Penfield dissector. Occasionally, the nerve root is displaced upward by the disc herniation and lies against this portion of the ligament, and the root can be injured with the Kerrison if it is not dissected free of the ligament. Once the falciform edge of the ligament has been removed, the nerve root should be visible at the lateral edge of the operative field. If the nerve root is not clearly visible at this point, it may be necessary to use the Kerrison to remove the medial portion of the facet. The lateral surface of the nerve is defined with the Penfield dissector and the nerve root retracted medially. A higher than expected incidence of dural tears and cerebrospinal fluid leaks during nerve root manipulation has been reported during lumbar microdiscectomy (10,13). If the durotomy can be clearly visualized, sutured repair should be attempted. More often, it is difficult to determine the location of the durotomy. In this situation, the patient is kept at bed rest for 24 hours before mobilization.

A nerve root retractor can now be substituted for the Penfield dissector, and the disc herniation should be visible (Fig. 3). If the herniation has extruded through the posterior longitudinal ligament, the fragment can be grasped with a pituitary rongeur and removed. However, an intact ligament has a glistening surface, which is divided with a blade in cruciate fashion. The underlying disc herniation is then grasped with the pituitary rongeur. The amount of disc material that should be removed has been the subject of controversy; some authors argue that an extensive removal should be attempted to prevent recurrence of herniation (10,28), whereas others argue that it is necessary to remove only the herniated portion of the disc (3,4,30). If it has been decided to attempt a more aggressive disc removal, the pituitary rongeur is passed into the disc space and the disc material removed. It is important not to advance the rongeur more that 3 cm into the disc space to avoid passing the instrument through the anterior longitudinal ligament and injuring structures in the retroperitoneum, such as the iliac vessels and bowel. If profuse bleeding from the disc space or unexplained hypotension develops, injury of a great vessel should be suspected. This devastating complication carries a high mortality rate (31) and must be addressed promptly. The would should be packed, the patient returned to a supine position, and immediate consultation from a general surgeon obtained.

At the conclusion of the disc removal, the nerve root should be probed and shown to be free of compression out into the neural foramen. If an additional portion of the medial facet must be resected to achieve that goal, resection can be performed

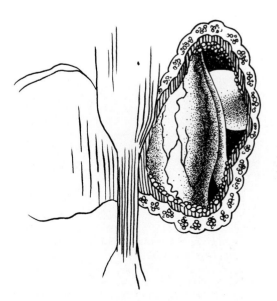

Fig. 3. Dura with underlying disc herniation.

at this point with a Kerrison punch. Some surgeons place a fat graft at this point over the opening in the ligament in an attempt to prevent postoperative scarring, but it is not clear that this technique offers any benefit (32). The wound should be thoroughly irrigated, the lumbodorsal fascia and subcutaneous layer approximated with interrupted absorbable sutures, and the skin closed with a running absorbable stitch.

The patient is encouraged to ambulate as soon as possible after awakening from anesthesia and should notice a reduction in radicular pain from the preoperative level. If the radicular pain persists, an imaging study should be obtained to ensure that the procedure has been carried out at the correct level and that disc material has not been retained. The patient can be discharged on the following day and is encouraged to walk frequently but discouraged from prolonged sitting or heavy lifting for 6 weeks.

References

1. Yasargil MG. Microsurgical operation of herniated lumbar disc. *Adv Neurosurg* 1976;4:81.
2. Caspar W. A new surgical procedure for lumbar disc herniation causing less tissue damage through a microsurgical approach. *Adv Neurosurg* 1976;4:74–77.
3. Williams RW. Microlumbar discectomy: a conservative approach to the virgin herniated lumbar disc. *Spine* 1978;3:175–182.
4. Williams RW. Microlumbar discectomy: a 12-year statistical review. *Spine* 1986;11:851–852.
5. Williams RW. Introduction: a personal history of spinal microsurgery. In: McCulloch JA, Young PH, eds. *Essentials of spinal microsurgery*. Philadelphia: Lippincott–Raven Publishers, 1998.
6. Andrews DW, Lavyne MH. Retrospective analysis of microsurgical and standard lumbar discectomy. *Spine* 1990;15:329–335.
7. Caspar W, et al. The Caspar microsurgical discectomy and comparison with conventional standard lumbar disc procedure. *Neurosurgery* 1991;28:78–87.
8. Goald HJ. Microlumbar discectomy: follow-up of 147 patients. *Spine* 1978;3:183–185.
9. Nyström B. Experience of microsurgical compared with conventional technique in lumbar disc operations. *Acta Neurol Scand* 1987;76:129–141.
10. Rogers LA. Experience with limited versus extensive disc removal in patients undergoing microsurgical operations for ruptured lumbar discs. *Neurosurgery* 1988;22:82–85.
11. Silvers HR. Microsurgical versus standard discectomy. *Neurosurgery* 1988;22:837–841.
12. Tullberg T, Isacson J, Weidenhielm L. Does microsurgical removal of lumbar disc herniation lead to better results than the standard procedure? Results of a one-year randomized study. *Spine* 1993;18:24–27.
13. Wilson DH, Kenning J. Microsurgical lumbar discectomy: preliminary report of 83 consecutive cases. *Neurosurgery* 1979;4:137–140.
14. Wilson DH, Harbaugh R. Microsurgical and standard removal of the protruded lumbar disc: a comparative study. *Neurosurgery* 1981;8:422–486.
15. Zahrawi F. Microlumbar discectomy. *Spine* 1988;13:358–359.
16. Zahrawi F. Microlumbar discectomy: is it safe as an outpatient procedure? *Spine* 1994;19:1070–1074.
17. Kahanovitz N, Viola K, McCulloch J. Limited surgical discectomy and microdiscectomy: a clinical comparison. *Spine* 1989;14:79–81.
18. Barrios C, et al. Microsurgical versus standard removal of the herniated lumbar disc. *Acta Orthop Scand* 1990;61:399–403.
19. Fager CA. Lumbar microdiscectomy: a contrary opinion. *Clin Neurosurg* 1986;33:419–456.
20. Saunders RL. Microsurgical lumbar discectomy: a dissenting view. In: Schmidek HH, Sweet WH, eds. *Operative neurosurgical techniques: indications, methods, and results*. New York: Grune & Stratton, 1982:1319.
21. McCulloch JA. Focus issue on lumbar disc herniation: macro- and microdiscectomy. *Spine* 1996;21:45S–56S.
22. Newman MH. Outpatient conventional laminotomy and disc excision. *Spine* 1995;20:353–355.
23. Abramovitz JN, Neff SR. Lumbar disc surgery: results of the prospective lumbar discectomy study of the Joint Section on Disorders of the Spine and Peripheral Nerves of the American Association of Neurological Surgeons and the Congress of Neurological Surgeons. *Neurosurgery* 1991;29:301–308.
24. Fager CA, Freidberg SR. Analysis of failures and poor results of lumbar spine surgery. *Spine* 1980;5:87–94.
25. Rubinstein E, et al. Perioperative prophylactic cephazolin in spinal surgery. *J Bone Joint Surg Br* 1994;76:99–102.
26. Ferree BA. Deep venous thrombosis following lumbar laminotomy and laminectomy. *Orthopedics* 1994;17:35–38.
27. Böstman O, et al. Blood loss, operating time, and positioning of the patient in lumbar disc surgery. *Spine* 1990;15:360–363.
28. Wilson DH, Harbaugh R. Microsurgical lumbar disc excision. In: Schmidek HH, Sweet WH, eds. *Operative neurosurgical techniques: indications, methods and results*. New York: Grune & Stratton, 1982.
29. Hudgins WR. Comment. *Neurosurgery* 1988;22:85.
30. Spengler DM. Lumbar discectomy: results with limited disc excision and selective foraminotomy. *Spine* 1982;7:604–607.
31. Montorsi W, Ghiringhelli C. Genesis, diagnosis and treatment of vascular complications after intervertebral disk surgery. *Int Surg* 1973;58:233–235.
32. MacKay M, et al. The effect of interposition membrane on the outcome of lumbar laminectomy and discectomy. *Spine* 1995;20:1793–1796.

202. Anterior Screw Fixation of Odontoid Fractures

Christopher M. Uchiyama and Ronald I. Apfelbaum

Odontoid process fractures are the most common fractures of the axis, accounting for one fifth of all cervical spine fractures (1). Anderson and D'Alonzo (2) classified odontoid fractures into types I, II, and III. Type I fractures involve the apex of the odontoid, are rare, and were previously thought to represent stable fractures. Scott et al. (3), however, reported a case of a type I odontoid fracture causing death due to associated atlanto-occipital and atlantoaxial subluxation. They proposed that type I fractures herald an underlying instability of the craniocervical junction and may not be as stable as previously believed. Type III odontoid fractures extend into the body of C2 and heal with fusion success rates greater than 80% with rigid external immobilization (4–10). Type II fractures traverse the base of the odontoid process and are the most common odontoid fractures encountered in clinical practice (1,2). A type II variant termed IIa (11) is associated with a comminuted fracture at the base of the odontoid process and is considered markedly unstable. Type II fractures can potentially cause catastrophic spinal cord injury due to the resulting atlantoaxial instability. Type II fractures usually assume one of three orientations: horizontal, anterior-oblique (superior-posterior to inferior-anterior direction), and posterior-oblique (superior-anterior to inferior-posterior direction). There may be associated anterolisthesis or retrolisthesis of the fractured odontoid process relative to the C2 body.

Management of type II odontoid fractures has been controversial, and treatment options have historically included no treatment; immobilization with a hard collar, halo vest, or Minerva jacket; posterior cervical fusion; and anterior odontoid screw fixation (reviewed in ref. 12). Conflicting reports in the literature regarding the effectiveness of external immobilization vs. surgical treatment of type II odontoid fractures have led some to advocate a trial of rigid external immobilization as the primary treatment (10), while others have recommended early surgical stabilization in all patients (9,13,14), or in selected patients who meet specific criteria (4–8). An evidence-based management approach is a potential means of resolving the controversy regarding the treatment of type II fractures in order to establish standardized treatment paradigms. Although this literature review process for developing practice guidelines has been helpful in some areas (15), a comprehensive review for the specific purpose of developing clinical treatment guidelines for type II odontoid fractures has not identified a superior management approach (12).

Despite that latter conclusion, it was noted that "fusion" success rates achieved with anterior screw fixation was slightly higher in comparison to other methods for treating type II odontoid fractures. Since the major issue regarding treatment of type II odontoid fractures is stabilization of atlantoaxial instability, one can argue that a stable, bony union across the fracture site per se is an appropriate outcome to guide rational treatment. Therefore, anterior screw fixation in fact may be the treatment of choice.

A major disadvantage of external mobilization is a high nonunion rate, particularly in individuals with specific risk factors. Hadley et al. (1) found a 67% nonunion rate in nonsurgically treated patients with more than 6 mm of odontoid process displacement in any direction. Apuzzo et al. (16) found an 88% nonunion rate in patients older than 40 years of age who had more than 4 mm of odontoid displacement treated with external immobilization. Dunn and Seljeskog (5) found a 70% to 78% nonunion rate in nonsurgically treated patients who were older than 65 years of age and had retrolisthesis of the odontoid process. Furthermore, halo-vest immobilization has been described as being analogous to holding a snake at both ends and trying to prevent movement between those two ends. Under fluoroscopy, we have witnessed patients with atlantoaxial instability move from significant retrolisthesis to anterolisthesis with each respiratory excursion despite halo-vest immobilization.

Anterior screw fixation of the odontoid is an attractive surgical treatment that is almost exclusively used for traumatic type II and selected rostral type III odontoid fractures. It provides immediate stability without the need for autogenous or allogeneic bone graft, and in contrast to posterior cervical fusion constructs, preserves C1-2 rotation. This is significant because 50% of rotation occurs at C1-2 (17). Odontoid screw fixation was first described by Nakanishi (18) and Bohler (19), and subsequent modifications of the technique have been reported by Lesoin et al. (20), who described an approach requiring an extensive neck dissection, and by Geisler et al. (21), who treated nine patients with a low anterior cervical approach. Apfelbaum

(22–24) has described an anterior odontoid screw fixation method that utilizes a small, transverse anterior cervical incision and a standard Cloward approach to the prevertebral space, which should be familiar to all spine surgeons who perform anterior cervical discectomy procedures. Successful stable union rates ranging from 79% to 100% have been reported by various authors using anterior odontoid screw fixation methods (25–29). It has been our practice to offer anterior odontoid screw fixation as the initial treatment of choice for recent type II and selected rostral type III odontoid fractures.

Anterior Odontoid Screw Fixation Method

PATIENT SELECTION. Appropriate patient selection is important for optimizing outcome when considering anterior screw fixation of the odontoid. Type II and selected type III fractures should be less than 6 months old and an intact C1 ring and transverse ligament is required. Disruption of the transverse ligament can be assessed with magnetic resonance imaging (MRI) or inferred from computed tomography (CT) studies showing avulsion fractures or hemorrhage at the site of ligamentous attachment to the atlas. Other contraindications for anterior screw fixation include pathological fractures of the odontoid, and potential hardware infection risks in the retropharyngeal space from coexisting penetrating injuries of the oropharynx, esophagus, or trachea.

Past contraindications to odontoid screw fixation have included obese, barrel-chested or large-breasted individuals whose upper torso could interfere with the low trajectory needed for optimal screw placement. An angled drill handpiece allows the surgeon to overcome that obstacle, and we do not consider those individuals to be poor candidates for the operation. Severe osteoporosis is a relative contraindication for screw fixation because excessive leverage of the drill, tap, or screw against the osteopenic bone can cause unwanted fractures, particularly in the anterior face of the C2 body.

A method for treating chronic, nonunited odontoid fractures with anterior screw fixation has been previously described (22–24). However, our follow-up on these cases, as discussed later in this chapter, has not yielded satisfactory results, and we rarely offer anterior screw fixation to these patients.

SURGICAL TECHNIQUE. The following description of surgical technique is based on the senior author's method of odontoid screw fixation (22–24). A set of instruments consisting of specialized retractors and a guide tube system (Aesculap Instrument Corp., South San Francisco, CA, and Aesculap AG, Tuttlingen, Germany) has been developed that greatly facilitates this procedure.

Under lateral fluoroscopic guidance, the patient is placed in the supine position with the neck extended as much as tolerable without displacing the odontoid process posteriorly into the spinal canal. Optimal reduction and realignment of the fractured dens with respect to the body of C2 should be attempted manually when possible under fluoroscopy to maximize the bony surface area available for healing across the fracture site, and to facilitate satisfactory passage of the screw within the odontoid peg. In patients with a retrolisthesed odontoid process, extension of the head is deferred until later in the procedure when the C2-3 complex has been engaged by the drill guide, and can be displaced posteriorly relative to C1 and the odontoid process to restore normal alignment. The head is im-

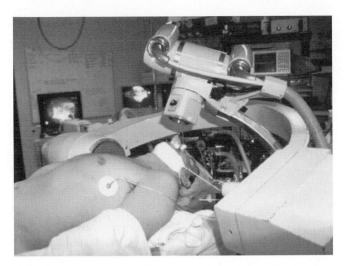

Fig. 1. Patient positioning for anterior odontoid screw fixation. Two C-arm fluoroscopy units are used to obtain anteroposterior (AP) and lateral views of cervical spine during surgery. (From Apfelbaum RI. Anterior screw fixation of odontoid fractures. In: Rengechary SS, Wilkins RH, eds. *Neurosurgical operative atlas*, vol 2. Baltimore: Williams & Wilkins, 1992:189–199, with permission.)

mobilized with 5 to 10 lb of halter, tong, or halo traction. If available, the most efficient method of intraoperative imaging is with the use two separate C-arm fluoroscopy units positioned in a manner to obtain simultaneous open mouth and lateral projections during surgery (Fig. 1). A radiolucent mouth gag (e.g., wine bottle cork placed between teeth) is placed to allow visualization of C1-2 via the open mouth projection using one C-arm unit, and the second C-arm unit is positioned to obtain the appropriate lateral view. If only one C-arm is available, it should be positioned and draped to allow frequent rotation in both the anteroposterior (AP) and lateral plane. However, this can be cumbersome, time-consuming, and may require multiple re-drapings of the C-arm unit to preserve a sterile field.

High-quality fluoroscopy units with image storage and display capabilities are required for this operation. We use the OEC fluoroscopy system (OEC Medical Systems, Inc., Salt Lake City, UT) at our institution. The ability of holding one image on one screen and comparing it to a new image is desirable during screw fixation. One can compare the saved AP and lateral images of the trajectory created by the drill or tapping instrument and use these to guide precise placement of the odontoid screws through the same tracts.

The neck is prepared and draped in the usual manner as in any standard anterior cervical discectomy procedure. A horizontal skin incision is made at approximately the level of C5-6. Alternatively, fluoroscopic visualization of a radiopaque object [e.g., Kirschner wire (K-wire)] placed adjacent to the neck and oriented for optimal screw trajectory can be used to estimate the appropriate level of the incision. Dissection of natural tissue planes is performed using a standard Cloward or Smith-Robinson method. The anterior longitudinal ligament is incised in the midline over approximately 1½ vertebral bodies, and the two bellies of the longus colli muscles are elevated bilaterally using periosteal elevators or monopolar electrocautery. Caspar retractor blades are secured beneath the longus colli muscles to create the prevertebral working space. The specialized lateral retractor system is also used later in the procedure to secure a third, angled retractor blade. Blunt dissection is performed with a Kittner sponge held with a tonsil clamp using a gentle sweeping, side-to-side motion in the prevertebral space *anterior* to

the unelevated, intact longus colli muscles, which remain cephalad to the retracted longus colli muscles. Careful progression up to the anterior C1-2 region in this manner creates a working channel in the prevertebral space extending from C1-2 to the incision site. This working channel is further exposed with the appropriate angled retractor that mates to the previously placed lateral retractors (Fig. 2).

In preparation for placement of the odontoid screw, a screw entry site must be carefully selected under biplanar fluoroscopy. In the AP plane, a midline location is chosen if one screw is to be placed. If two screws will be placed, a paramedian location 2 to 3 mm off of the midline is chosen for passage of the first screw. (A discussion of the one-screw vs. two-screw method follows later in this chapter.) In the lateral plane, the entry site is at, or slightly posterior to, the anterior inferior lip of the C2 body. A K-wire is then impacted in the entry site approximately 3 to 4 mm (Fig. 3A). A manual 8-mm hollow overdrill is placed over the K-wire and rotated to create a shallow working trough through the superior anterior face of C3 and through the anterior C2-3 annulus (Fig. 3B–D). Note that no bone is removed from C2. Next, a guide tube system consisting of an inner and outer guide tube assembly is passed over the K-wire (Fig. 4A,B). Fixation spikes on the distal end of the outer guide tube is oriented toward the spine, and the entire guide tube assembly is carefully advanced over the K-wire to the region of C2-3. The spikes are then impacted into the C3 body. The orientation of the guide tubes should approximate the trajectory of the screw in both AP and lateral projections. Once secured, the inner guide tube is further advanced through the trough created through the C2-3 annulus until it contacts the screw entry site at C2 (Fig. 4C). The K-wire is removed and a powered 3-mm drill bit is inserted through the drill guide. An angled drill hand piece helps accommodate a low trajectory (Fig. 5). A pilot hole is drilled through the body of C2 and aimed toward the tip of the odontoid using biplanar fluoroscopic guidance.

It should be noted that adequate fracture reduction prior to screw placement may improve the strength of the final construct since laboratory studies have suggested that interdigitation of the fractured ends provides additional stability in excess of the isolated strength of an odontoid screw (30). If preoperative closed reduction has not been satisfactorily achieved, it is possible to improve alignment of the fractured odontoid process at this stage of the procedure. Since the guide tube system is anchored to C2-3 by the fixation spikes, it can be used to translate C2-3 relative to the C1–odontoid process complex either anteriorly or posteriorly. The realignment of an antero- or retrolisthesed odontoid process can thus be perfected as the drill bit is advanced through the fracture site. After advancing through the fracture site, drilling should continue until the full thickness of the apical odontoid cortex has been pierced. Penetration through the apical cortex is safe since the direction of drilling is not toward the spinal cord, but toward the clivus where a safety zone is provided by the apical ligaments. The odontoid process is constrained by its periosteal attachments to the alar and apical ligaments and will not be displaced by drilling or by any of the subsequent steps. A fluoroscopic image can then be saved of the realigned atlas–odontoid peg complex with the drill bit engaged through the distal odontoid peg, and this image can be used as a guide for subsequent realignment during the tapping and screw placement steps to follow.

Biplanar fluoroscopy should be used liberally at this point since drilling is a critical step of the procedure. Advancing the drill bit slowly and with frequent monitoring of AP and lateral trajectories will optimize final screw placement and maximize success. In past years, it was difficult to correct a trajectory once drilling had begun. We have now switched from a 2-mm to a 3-mm diameter drill bit, and consequently the more stable, larger caliber drill bit permits minor changes in trajectory en route to

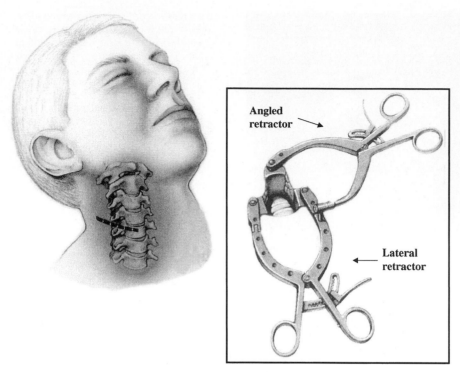

Fig. 2. A standard horizontal skin incision is made as shown and exposure of the prevertebral space performed with lateral retractors. Following cephalad soft tissue dissection anterior to the longus colli muscles, a special angled retractor that mates to the lateral retractor is used to create a working tunnel toward C2-3. (From Apfelbaum RI. Anterior screw fixation of odontoid fractures. In: Rengechary SS, Wilkins RH, eds. *Neurosurgical operative atlas*, vol 2. Baltimore: Williams & Wilkins, 1992:189–199, with permission.)

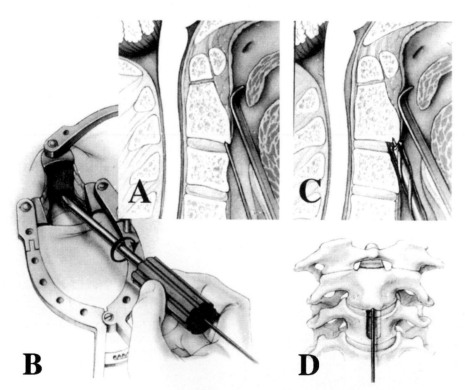

Fig. 3. Preparation of odontoid screw entry site. **A**: In the lateral view, a Kirschner wire (K-wire) is placed at, or just posterior to, the anterior inferior lip of the C2 body. In the AP projection, a midline entry site is chosen for single-screw placement and paramedian locations for the two-screw method (refer to text). **B–D**: After impacting the K-wire into the C2 body, a hollow overdrill is placed over the K-wire and used to create a trough through the anterior C2-3 annulus. (Modified from Apfelbaum RI. Anterior screw fixation of odontoid fractures. In: Rengechary SS, Wilkins RH, eds. *Neurosurgical operative atlas*, vol 2. Baltimore: Williams & Wilkins, 1992:189–199, with permission.)

Outer drill guide **Inner drill guide**

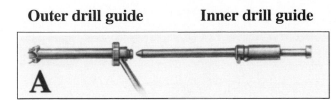

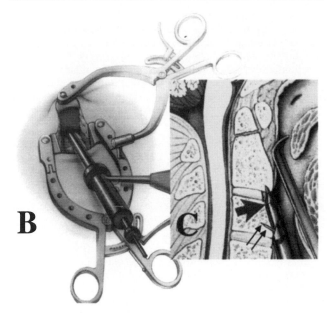

Fig. 4. **A**: Outer and inner drill guide system. Note the fixation spikes on the distal end of the outer drill guide. **B**: The outer/inner drill guide assembly is passed over the K-wire to the screw entry site. **C**: Biplanar fluoroscopy should be used to confirm satisfactory positioning of the drill guide prior to impacting the fixation spikes (*small double arrows*) into the body of C3. Once the outer drill guide is secured, the inner drill guide (*large arrow*) is advanced such that the distal end contacts the inferior body of C2. The K-wire is then removed. (Modified from Apfelbaum RI. Anterior screw fixation of odontoid fractures. In: Rengechary SS, Wilkins RH, eds. *Neurosurgical operative atlas*, vol 2. Baltimore: Williams & Wilkins, 1992:189–199, with permission.)

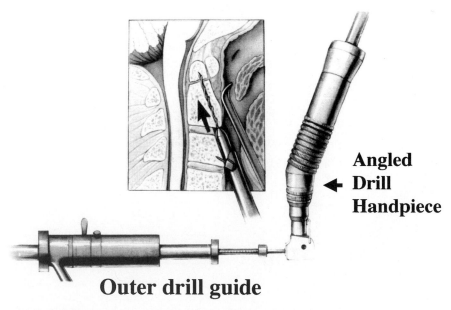

Angled Drill Handpiece

Outer drill guide

Fig. 5. A 3-mm powered drill bit is carefully advanced under biplanar fluoroscopy across the fracture site and must penetrate through the apical cortex of the odontoid process. An angled handpiece facilitates a low trajectory and overcomes obstacles related to patient body habitus such as obesity or a barrel chest. (Modified from Apfelbaum RI. Anterior screw fixation of odontoid fractures. In: Rengechary SS, Wilkins RH, eds. *Neurosurgical operative atlas*, vol 2. Baltimore: Williams & Wilkins, 1992:189–199, with permission.)

the odontoid apex. Creating the optimal drill path should be performed without error during this step. Attempting to salvage a full-length, poorly created drill hole by drilling a new, different trajectory may be detrimental with regard to later screw placement or bony purchase, especially in osteopenic individuals.

Once the drill has penetrated the outer cortex of the apical odontoid peg, a screw length can be determined by reading the calibrations on the drill shaft. The depth markings indicate the distance between the tip of drill bit to the tapered distal end of the inner guide. Thus, for accurate estimation of the screw length that will be required, the inner drill guide should abut the inferior edge of C2. If this is not possible, the measured depth of drill penetration should be shortened accordingly by subtracting the distance between the planned screw entry site in C2 and the tip of the inner drill guide as seen on the lateral fluoroscopic view. Additionally, if a significant gap at the fracture site is present, this must be factored into choosing an appropriate shorter screw length since this gap should close when the odontoid peg is drawn back to the C2 body during screw placement.

The drill and the inner drill guide are removed and a tap is placed through the outer drill guide (Fig. 6). Tapping should continue through the entire length of the drilled pathway to avoid splitting of the dense cortical bone of the odontoid process during final screw placement.

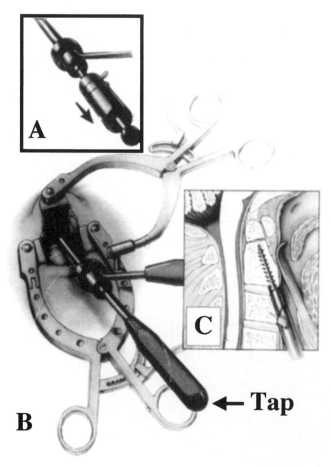

Fig. 6. **A**: After drilling is completed, the inner drill guide is removed. **B**: The tapping instrument is placed through the remaining outer drill guide and the full length of the drilled path is tapped under fluoroscopy (**C**). (Modified from Apfelbaum RI. Anterior screw fixation of odontoid fractures. In: Rengechary SS, Wilkins RH, eds. *Neurosurgical operative atlas*, vol 2. Baltimore: Williams & Wilkins, 1992:189–199, with permission.)

A partially threaded 4.0-mm cortically threaded lag screw (Aesculap AG, Tuttlingen, Germany) of the appropriate length is placed through the outer drill guide and placed under biplanar fluoroscopic guidance. It should penetrate the distal odontoid cortex, and in acute fractures should easily allow closure of the gap at the fracture site by drawing the odontoid process closer to the C2 body. If a second screw is used, the entry site is carefully selected on the contralateral side 3 to 4 mm away from the first entry site. A fully threaded cortical screw should be used since no additional lag effect should be expected.

After obtaining hemostasis, the retractors can be removed and stability of C1-2 can be confirmed by controlled, intraoperative flexion-extension under fluoroscopy. Standard closure is performed in layers of the sternocleidomastoid fascia, platysma, and dermal layers using absorbable sutures. The skin edges are reapproximated with sterile adhesive skin tapes. No drains are required if good hemostasis has been achieved.

POSTOPERATIVE MANAGEMENT. The decision to immobilize the patient postoperatively with a hard collar is an individual one made by the treating surgeon. We routinely do not use a hard collar unless the patient has osteopenic bone, is at risk for falls, or requires one for comfort. In the typical patient with an acute, traumatic odontoid fracture with no additional serious injuries or medical conditions, hospital stays typically range from 1 to 3 days following surgery. Osteoporotic patients should be treated with vitamin D and calcium if their dietary intake is insufficient, and in the osteoporotic, postmenopausal woman, concomitant hormone replacement, alendronate, nasal calcitonin, or raloxifene should be considered if not contraindicated.

Assessment of bony union, stability, and neurological status in our patients is performed at postoperative intervals of approximately 4 to 6 weeks, 3 months, 6 months, and yearly as necessary. Lateral, open mouth and flexion-extension films are obtained to evaluate screw position, fracture alignment, and bone healing. In some cases CT imaging through the C1-2 region may be necessary to assess bony union.

One of four different outcomes can be expected postoperatively: anatomical bony fusion, nonanatomical bony fusion, stable fibrous union, and nonunion. The presence of anatomical bony fusion is based on anatomical alignment of the fracture fragment, trabeculation across the fracture site, and lack of C1-2 motion on flexion-extension films. Nonanatomical bony fusion is nonanatomical alignment of the fractured fragment but with other fusion criteria present. A stable fibrous union is defined as the presence of a visible fracture line but absence of motion on flexion-extension films. In patients with a stable, fibrous union, additional surgical stabilization is not usually warranted. A nonunion is instability noted on dynamic radiographs and requires revision via a posterior C1-2 fusion.

Results

Results of anterior odontoid screw fixation on 147 patients with type II and selected type III odontoid fractures at the University of Utah ($n = 94$) and the National Institute of Traumatology, Budapest, Hungary ($n = 53$), has been reviewed (29). The mean age at surgery was 50.1 years (range 15 to 92 years) and included 98 males (67%) and 49 females (33%); 133 patients were available for follow-up with a mean follow-up period of 18.2 months; 117 patients had surgery performed within 6 months from the time of initial injury with the majority (102 of 117) undergoing surgery within 1 month of injury. Successful bony fusion was seen in 88% of patients (85% with anatomical bony fusion and 3% with nonanatomical bony fusion). An additional 3% of patients demonstrated a stable fibrous union, which combined with the bony fusion group to give an overall stabilization rate of 91%. No differences were seen in the outcomes of patients who had surgery within 1 month of injury versus those operated 3 to 6 months from the time of injury. Similar outcomes were also seen in elderly patients with no significant differences in patients in their 7th, 8th, or 9th decade of life (29).

Our analysis of 16 patients with remote fractures (greater than 6 months old) revealed a poor bony fusion rate of 25% and a high nonunion rate of 31% when treated with anterior screw fixation. Therefore, these patients are no longer routinely offered anterior screw fixation at our institution. They should be treated with posterior cervical fusion methods with C1-2 transarticular screws and a standard Brooks (31) or Sonntag-Dickman (32) fusion construct. The rare exception might be a younger patient with a large odontoid process that has not fused to the arch of C1 and/or the clivus, and where a small gap exists between the C2 body and fractured odontoid process. If such an individual desired an opportunity to preserve C1-2 rotation, was willing to accept at least a 50% chance of failure, and, in the event of failure, understood the need for a subsequent posterior cervical fusion, anterior odontoid screw fixation could be offered as the initial surgical treatment.

Discussion

Our successful stabilization results with anterior odontoid screw fixation are similar to those reported in the literature (25–28), and support the efficacy of anterior screw fixation for the treatment of type II and selected type III odontoid fractures.

The decision to place one vs. two odontoid screws (Figs. 7 and 8) is made at the surgeon's discretion and has been the subject of past debate. The theoretical advantage of placing two screws is increased resistance to torsional stress, but this specific biomechanical parameter has not been investigated. One biomechanical study comparing the one and two-screw techniques in fresh human cadaveric specimens showed no significant differences in load-to-failure testing (33). The only difference seen with the two-screw fixation method was increased stiffness in extension loading. Both the one-screw and two-screw techniques restored stability to approximately 50% of an unfractured odontoid specimen. These laboratory data, therefore, suggest that the two-screw technique has only a slight biomechanical advantage over the one-screw method, and this difference is likely irrelevant in the clinical setting. This is supported by a report by Jenkins et al. (27), who found no significant difference in successful union rates using one or two screws.

Several reasons for failure of anterior odontoid screw fixation have been identified. These include severely osteopenic patients, fractures greater than 6 months old, and associated fractures extending into the C2 body. Type II fractures with an anterior-oblique orientation had a lower success rate than fractures oriented in a horizontal or posterior-oblique direction (29). Finally, failure to penetrate the apical cortex of the dens with the tip of the screw has resulted in screws backing out (Fig. 9). Thus, adequate engagement of the apical cortical bone is essential regardless of whether one or two screws are placed.

Conclusions

We advocate early surgical treatment with direct anterior screw fixation of the odontoid rather than external immobilization or posterior cervical fusion and consider it the initial treatment of choice for traumatic type II and selected type III odontoid fractures less than 6 months old. This method can be easily learned by surgeons who routinely perform anterior cervical discectomy procedures, and is greatly facilitated by specialized instruments designed for this purpose. Anterior screw fixation provides immediate stabilization, preserves C1-2 rotation, and eliminates the need for bone graft. If necessary, individuals who fail anterior screw fixation can be salvaged with a standard posterior C1-2 fusion, and patients should be counseled of this possibility prior to undergoing odontoid screw fixation.

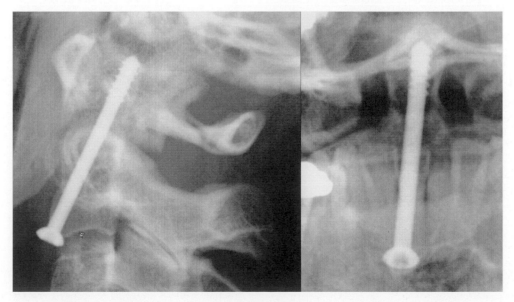

Fig. 7. Lateral and AP views demonstrating single anterior odontoid screw fixation.

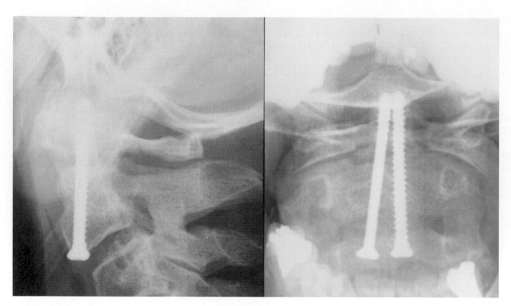

Fig. 8. Lateral and AP views demonstrating double anterior odontoid screw fixation method. Note the partially threaded lag screw, which is first placed to close the gap between the fractured ends. The second fully threaded screw is then placed on the contralateral side.

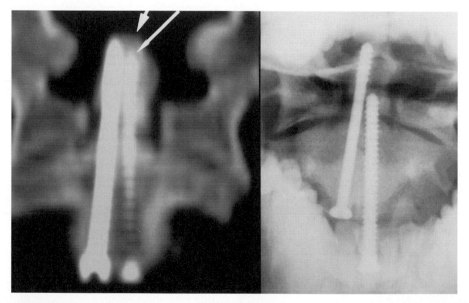

Fig. 9. Example of odontoid screw failure. **Left**: The tip of the lag screw has satisfactorily engaged the apical cortex of the dens. The second screw tip (*long arrow*) was not adequately placed and did not engage the distal cortex (*short arrow*). **Right**: The poorly placed screw backed out as seen on a subsequent postoperative film, while the contralateral screw remains firmly fixed. This illustrates the importance of screw penetration through the apical cortex of the dens and is an avoidable cause of odontoid screw failure.

References

1. Hadley MN, Dickman CA, Browner CM, et al. Acute axis fractures: a review of 229 cases. *J Neurosurg* 1989;71:642–647.
2. Anderson LD, D'Alonzo RT. Fractures of the odontoid process of the axis. *J Bone Joint Surg* 1974;56A:1663–1674.
3. Scott EW, Haid RW, Peace D. Type I fractures of the odontoid process: implications for atlanto-occipital instability. Case report. *J Neurosurgery* 1990;72:488–492.
4. Clark CR, White AA. Fracture of the dens. A multicenter study. *J Bone Joint Surg* 1985;67:1340–1348.
5. Dunn ME, Seljeskog EL. Experience in the management of odontoid process injuries: an analysis of 128 cases. *Neurosurgery* 1986;18:306–310.
6. Ekong CEU, Schwartz ML, Tator CH, et al. Odontoid fracture: management with early immobilization using the halo device. *Neurosurgery* 1981;9:631–637.
7. Fujii E, Kobayashi K, Hirabayashi K. Treatment in fractures of the odontoid process. *Spine* 1988;13:604–609.
8. Hadley MN, Browner CM, Sonntag VK. Axis fractures: a comprehen-

sive review of management and treatment in 107 cases. *Neurosurgery* 1985;17:281–290.

9. Maiman DJ, Larson SJ. Management of odontoid fractures. *Neurosurgery* 1982;11:471–476.

10. Ryan MD, Taylor TKF. Odontoid fractures: a rational approach to treatment. *J Bone Joint Surg* 1982;64B:416–421.

11. Hadley MN, Browner CM, Liu SS, et al. New subtype of acute odontoid fractures (type IIA). *Neurosurgery* 1988;22:67–71.

12. Traynelis VC. Evidence-based management of type II odontoid fractures. *Clin Neurosurg* 1997;44:41–49.

13. Schiess RJ, DeSaussure RL, Robertson JT. Choice of treatment of odontoid fractures. *J Neurosurg* 1982;57:496–499.

14. Wilson TAS Jr, McWhorter JM. *Atlantoaxial injuries*. Baltimore: Williams & Wilkins, 1992.

15. Brain Trauma Foundation. *Guidelines for the management of severe head injury*. Park Ridge, IL: American Association of Neurological Surgeons, 1995.

16. Apuzzo MLJ, Heiden JS, Weiss MH. Acute fractures of the odontoid process: an analysis of 45 cases. *J Neurosurg* 1978;48:85–91.

17. White AA, Panjabi MM. *Clinical biomechanics of the spine*, 2nd ed. Philadelphia: JB Lippincott, 1990:610–611.

18. Nakanishi T. Internal fixation of the odontoid fracture (Japanese). *Cent Jpn J Orthop Traumatic Surg* 1980;23:399–406.

19. Bohler J. Anterior stabilization for acute fractures and non-unions of the dens. *J Bone Joint Surg* 1982;64A:18–27.

20. Lesoin F, Autricque A, Franz K. Transcervical approach and screw fixation for upper cervical spine pathology. *Surg Neurol* 1987;27:459–465.

21. Geisler FH, Cheng C, Poka A, et al. Anterior screw fixation of posteriorly displaced type II odontoid fractures. *Neurosurgery* 1989;25:30–38.

22. Apfelbaum RI. Anterior screw fixation of odontoid fractures. In: Rengechary SS, Wilkins RH, eds. *Neurosurgical operative atlas*, vol 2. Baltimore: Williams & Wilkins, 1992:189–199.

23. Apfelbaum RI. *Anterior screw fixation of odontoid fractures*. Tuttlingen, Germany: Aesculap AG, 1993.

24. Apfelbaum RI. Screw fixation of odontoid fractures. In: Wilkins R, Rengechary S, eds. *Neurosurgery*. New York: McGraw-Hill, 1996:2965–2973.

25. Rainov NG, Heidecke V, Burkert W. Direct anterior fixation of odontoid fractures with a hollow spreading screw system. *Acta Neurochir (Wien)* 1996;138:146–153.

26. Etter C, Coscia M, Jaberg H, et al. Direct anterior fixation of dens fractures with a cannulated screw system. *Spine* 1991;16(suppl):S25–S32.

27. Jenkins JD, Coric D, Branch DL. A clinical comparison of one- and two-screw odontoid fixation. *J Neurosurg* 1998;89:366–370.

28. Subach BR, Morone MA, Haid RW, et al. Management of acute odontoid fractures with single screw anterior fixation. *Neurosurgery* 1999;45:812–820.

29. Apfelbaum RI, Lonser RR, Veres R, et al. Direct anterior screw fixation for recent and remote odontoid fractures. *J Neurosurg* 2000;93:227–236.

30. Doherty BJ, Heggeness MH, Esses SI. A biomechanical study of odontoid fractures and fracture fixation. *Spine* 1993;18:178–184.

31. Brooks A, Jenkins E. Atlanto-axial arthrodesis by the wedge compression method. *J Bone Joint Surg* 1978;60A:279–284.

32. Sonntag VKH, Dickman CA, Vardiman A. Anterior odontoid screw fixation. In: Menezes A, Sonntag V, eds. *Principles of spinal surgery*. New York: McGraw-Hill, 1996:1039–1049.

33. Sasso R, Doherty BJ, Crawford MJ, et al. Biomechanics of odontoid fracture fixation. *Spine* 1993;18:1950–1953.

203. Posterior Atlantoaxial and Occipitocervical Fixation and Fusion Techniques

**Jonathan J. Baskin,
Paul J. Apostolides,
Curtis A. Dickman, and
Volker K. H. Sonntag**

The craniovertebral junction (CVJ) is composed of the occipital bone, the first two cervical vertebrae (atlantoaxial complex), and their soft tissue articulations. Traumatic disruption of these osseous elements, their tethering ligaments, or both can cause immediate instability of this most rostral region of the axial skeleton. Alternatively, these bony and soft tissue structures can be compromised over a more insidious course. Patients with degenerative, inflammatory, infectious, developmental, or neoplastic processes involving the CVJ typically have progressive clinical symptoms related to worsening mechanical incompetence and compression of the upper cervical spinal cord and lower brainstem. The surgical management of patients with instability of the CVJ must therefore achieve both neural decompression and structural stabilization. Technical considerations related to the latter topic are the primary concern of this chapter.

Most contemporary spine surgeons use stabilization techniques that rely on titanium-based materials (magnetic resonance imaging compatible) to establish immediate rigid internal fixation of the occipitocervical junction and the C1-2 complex. These techniques have significantly increased the frequency of arthrodesis compared to earlier methods that used only onlay autologous bone to promote fusion in this particularly mobile region of the spine. The use of internal rigid fixation limits the need for routine postoperative external bracing with a halo orthosis. Consequently, convalescence is more comfortable, and patients can resume productive activities more rapidly after surgery.

Hardware fatigue and its eventual failure are time-dependent certainties without a solid arthrodesis. Therefore, regardless of the particular instrumentation used, meticulous attention to the biological and mechanical principles that influence the fusion response is crucial to attain a successful clinical outcome. This chapter focuses on our preferred method of performing posterior atlantoaxial arthrodesis using a combination of transarticular facet fixation and interspinous wiring, and on our preferred method of occipitocervical fusion using a contoured, threaded Steinmann pin or titanium grooved rod that is anchored with suboccipital and sublaminar wires. Alternative methods of stabilizing the occipitocervical junction with screw plates are also noted.

Indications

Atlantoaxial fusion is indicated for patients with C1-2 instability. Occipitocervical fusion is indicated for patients with occipitocervical instability, including those with rheumatoid settling, primary basilar invagination, occipitoatlantal dislocation, or primary or metastatic neoplastic disease that involves the CVJ. Occipitocervical fusion can also be used as a "salvage" procedure for a failed C1-2 arthrodesis or for complex atlantoaxial fractures in which interspinous wiring or transarticular screw fixation is unfeasible or contraindicated.

Operative Technique

PREOPERATIVE PREPARATION AND POSITIONING.
Typically, patients with occipitocervical or atlantoaxial instability arrive in the operating room wearing an external cervical orthosis (hard collar or halo vest). Intravascular access is secured, and a prophylactic dose of antibiotic (cefuroxime 1.5 g,

or cefazolin 2 g) is administered. General anesthesia is induced and the patient is intubated, often using an awake fiberoptic technique to minimize the risk of neurological injury from an inadvertent occipitocervical or atlantoaxial dislocation. Paralytic medications are not used with the anesthetic agents to avoid exacerbating instability of the CVJ. Clinical evidence of spinal cord or nerve root irritation can then also be observed during the procedure.

Intraoperatively, somatosensory, motor, and brainstem auditory evoked potentials are monitored. Baseline waveforms are often recorded before the patient is rotated into the prone position. If patients have severe preoperative myelopathy or instability or if the evoked potentials change significantly during surgery, methylprednisolone may be administered in accordance with the North American Spinal Cord Injury Study (NASCIS III) guidelines. Postoperatively, the steroid is discontinued if the patient's neurological examination is stable.

If the patient is wearing a cervical collar, the Mayfield headholder (Codman, Inc., Raynham, MA) is applied before prone positioning. If the patient is wearing a halo brace, the Mayfield adaptor is connected to the halo ring to fixate the patient to the operating table (Fig. 1). A lateral cervical radiograph is obtained after the patient is positioned to assess the atlantoaxial or craniovertebral alignment. Intraoperative fluoroscopy is used if closed manipulation of the vertebral column is required before the procedure begins or for performing open reduction before instrumentation is placed. For atlantoaxial arthrodesis, transarticular screws are inserted under direct, continuous fluoroscopic guidance.

Autologous bone is the substrate of choice to promote posterior cervical arthrodesis. Allograft bone is unreliable for achieving a posterior cervical arthrodesis. The donor site must be prepared in a sterile fashion at the start of the procedure, and

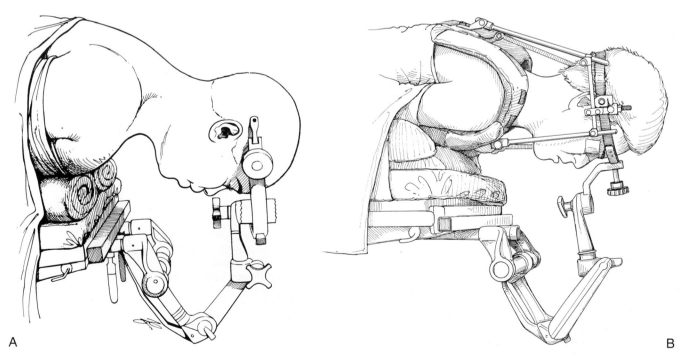

A   B

Fig. 1. **A**: Patients are placed in the prone position and secured to the surgical table using the Mayfield headholder (Codman, Inc., Raynham, MA). Patients with craniovertebral instability are positioned while wearing a hard cervical collar to minimize the risk of a harmful loss of reduction. **B**: The Mayfield halo adaptor is used to stabilize patients wearing a halo brace. The posterior aspect of the halo vest can be removed to allow access to the iliac crest for autologous bone graft material. The posterior bars of the halo apparatus can be removed from the surgical field. Alternately, they function well as hand rests for surgeons during the procedure. (With permission from Barrow Neurological Institute.)

it must be accessible after draping. Interspinous wiring of the C1-2 complex relies on a bicortical strut graft fashioned from a tricortical graft obtained from the posterior iliac crest. We have seldom found a surgical drain to be necessary at this site if meticulous attention is directed toward hemostasis. Iliac crest bone (cortical and cancellous grafts) is preferred for occipitocervical fusion. Autologous rib provides an excellent alternative to the iliac crest for onlay corticocancellous bone. With its use fusion rates have been comparable to those associated with iliac crest grafts, and morbidity at the donor site is minimal (1).

SKIN INCISION AND SOFT TISSUE DISSECTION. The surgical exposures necessary for performing posterior atlantoaxial and occipitocervical fusions are similar. The rostral aspect of exposure is the external occipital protuberance. The minimum extent of caudal dissection includes the complete exposure of the dorsal elements of the first three cervical vertebrae. Further caudal dissection may be necessary if additional fixation points are warranted to maximize the stability of the construct. Soft tissue dissection is limited to the levels of craniovertebral instability to avoid the inadvertent fusion or potential destabilization of normal motion segments.

The patient's hair is shaved in the occipitocervical midline from the inion to over the spinous process of C5. After a standard sterile preparation, the inscribed midline incision is infiltrated with 0.5% lidocaine with epinephrine for hemostasis. The skin and subcutaneous tissues are incised down to the dorsal cervical fascia, and this plane is developed laterally to facilitate closure. The avascular midline plane between the cervical paraspinal muscles is dissected using monopolar cauterization to expose the underlying occipital squama and the spinous processes of the cervical vertebrae.

Sharp dissection and cauterization are used to elevate this muscle laterally in a subperiosteal plane along the occipital bone and cervical laminae. Adequate soft tissue retraction and bony exposure provide unimpeded visualization of the foramen magnum and the upper three cervical laminae bilaterally as far as the lateral aspect of their respective facet joints (Fig. 2). For occipitocervical fusion procedures, the occipital bone is exposed slightly more to allow the Steinmann pin to be seated and the appropriate burr holes to be placed for suboccipital wire passage. During the course of dissecting and retracting soft tissues, meticulous care should be exerted to avoid dislocation of unstable vertebral segments.

ATLANTOAXIAL FIXATION AND FUSION. At our institution, the treatment of choice for atlantoaxial instability entails a combination of interspinous wiring (2) and transarticular facet screw placement (3). The immediate rigid three-point internal fixation provided by this construct eliminates the need for a routine postoperative halo orthosis.

Not all patients with C1-2 instability are candidates for both techniques, however. Interspinous wiring requires the presence of intact posterior elements at C1 and C2. These structures can be compromised as a consequence of trauma, degenerative processes, or the laminectomy performed for neural decompression. If interspinous wiring is impossible, the C1-2 complex can be stabilized by the isolated placement of transarticular screws or by performing an occipitocervical fusion that extends to the adjacent vertebrae. Finally, anteriorly placed C1-2 transarticular screws are available as a salvage procedure to secure atlantoaxial stability when circumstances prevent placement of posterior fixation devices (4).

Prospective analysis has demonstrated that almost 20% of patients harbor regional anatomy that contraindicates transarticular screw placement on at least one side (5), usually due to a

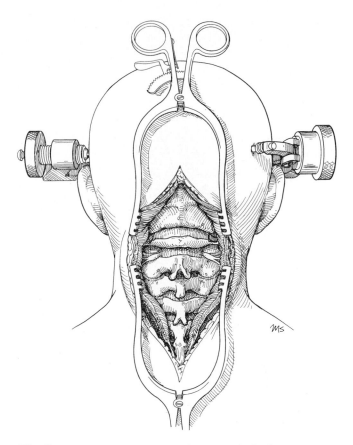

Fig. 2. The posterior midline surgical exposure for both occipitocervical and atlantoaxial fusion techniques. For occipitocervical fusion, slightly more of the occipital bone needs to be exposed to allow placement of burr holes for suboccipital wire passage. (With permission from Barrow Neurological Institute.)

unilateral anomaly. Of 94 patients in this same study, the anatomy of three (3.2%) was unsuitable bilaterally for transarticular screw placement. Thus, when C1-2 transarticular screws are contemplated, the workup should include fine-cut computed tomographic scans in the plane of the transarticular screw with sagittal reconstructions. These studies permit the width of the pars interarticularis and the proximity of the vertebral artery to the proposed screw course to be assessed. Other contraindications to unilateral placement of a transarticular screw include fractures of the C1 lateral mass or C2 pars interarticularis. The inability to realign C1 on C2 before surgery also precludes transarticular screw placement and is associated with a high risk for vertebral artery injury.

In addition to the risks for neurovascular injury, screw malpositioning is also associated with a high risk for screw fracture. If both interspinous wiring and transarticular screw placement are deemed feasible, the latter procedure is performed first. A single transarticular screw in conjunction with interspinous atlantoaxial wiring confers sufficient stability to obtain excellent fusion outcomes after immobilization in a hard collar (6).

As noted, fluoroscopy is used to direct patient positioning to achieve an appropriate atlantoaxial reduction and to estimate the proper trajectories for drill and screw passage. Cervical flexion is usually required to facilitate transarticular screw placement. However, the degree of flexion needed to insert the screw from within the operative wound is sometimes impossible to achieve due to the associated risk of dislocating the atlantoaxial junction. Rather than extending the skin incision and muscle

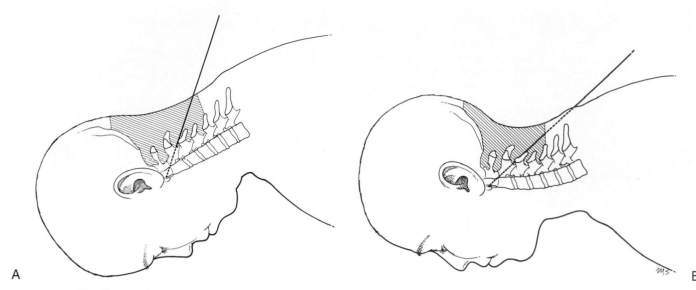

A   B

Fig. 3. Some element of cervical flexion is necessary to achieve the proper trajectory for transarticular screw placement. The *shaded area* illustrates the typical extent of soft tissue dissection (inion to the C5 spinous process). **A**: In some circumstances, adequate flexion can be performed safely so that the transarticular screw can be inserted from within the surgical site. **B**: The more common percutaneous technique used to compensate when a lesser degree of cervical flexion is possible. (With permission from Barrow Neurological Institute.)

dissection caudally, the screws are delivered percutaneously along the necessary trajectory through the pars interarticularis of C2 and the lateral mass of C1 (Fig. 3). Before the patient is draped, the locations of the stab incisions for percutaneous placement are estimated using fluoroscopy and must be included within the sterile field.

The key anatomical landmarks for transarticular screw placement include the posterior elements and facet joints between C1-2 and C2-3. The C1-2 facet is directly visualized by using a Penfield dissector to gently retract the C2 nerve root and its associated venous plexus rostrally. The medial border of the pars interarticularis of C2 is also visualized directly to ensure that screw placement does not violate its medial border and encroach upon the vertebral canal. In preparation for subsequent interspinous wiring, soft tissues between the posterior elements of C1 and C2 are removed using curets and rongeurs before any instrumentation is placed.

TRANSARTICULAR SCREW PLACEMENT. We prefer a cannulated screw technique for C1-2 fixation using the Universal Cannulated Screw System (Sofamor Danek, Memphis, TN). A long, thin Kirschner (K)-wire is used to drill the initial path across the C1-2 facet. The wire fixates the adjacent unstable segments and guides screw placement. Because its diameter is narrow, the K-wire can be repositioned to optimize screw location without sacrificing potential screw purchase.

The atlas and axis must be realigned before the transarticular screw is placed. If the atlas has been dislocated anteriorly, open manipulation can be performed by applying tension to a sublaminar wire at the C1 level (which can later be used for interspinous wiring). An Allis clamp applied to the C2 spinous process can further facilitate open reduction of C1 on C2. The screw entry point is 2 to 3 mm above the caudal edge of the C2 inferior facet and 2 to 3 mm lateral to the medial border of the C2-3 facet (Fig. 4). A high-speed drill is used to penetrate the cortical bone at the entry point to help seat and direct the K-wire.

The screw trajectory is estimated with fluoroscopy by holding

a long instrument adjacent to the patient's neck and thorax. If screw insertion cannot proceed directly through the incision and percutaneous delivery is necessary, a tunneling instrument (i.e., a tissue sheath and stylet) is passed carefully through the paraspinal soft tissues and positioned adjacent to the C2-3 facet. The C2 pars interarticularis and C1-2 facet joint should be visualized directly to achieve the proper mediolateral screw trajectory during K-wire and screw insertion.

The stylet is removed from the tissue sheath and the K-wire drill guide is inserted. A 50-cm long, 1.2-mm diameter, end-threaded K-wire is attached to a reversible pneumatic drill and passed through the drill guide to the screw entry point. The medial surface of the C2 pars interarticularis is defined with a

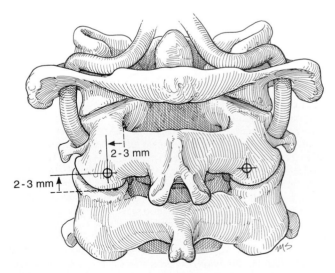

Fig. 4. The entry point for transarticular screw placement is depicted. The anatomy of individual patients may require this entry point to be modified to avoid intercepting the vertebral artery. (With permission from Barrow Neurological Institute.)

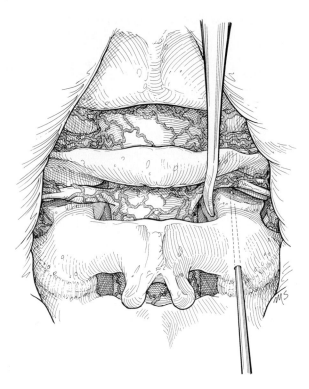

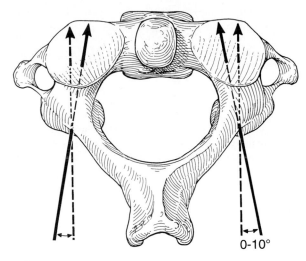

Fig. 6. The transarticular screw is placed along the longitudinal axis of the pars interarticularis. Slight medial angulation may be necessary to avoid the vertebral artery. Overcompensation can cause the screw to encroach on the vertebral canal. (With permission from Barrow Neurological Institute.)

Fig. 5. Before the transarticular screws are placed, the most medial aspect of the C2 pars interarticularis is visualized. The C1-2 facet joint is also visualized by rostral displacement of the C2 nerve root and its accompanying venous plexus. A Kirschner (K)-wire has been placed through the entry point (see Fig. 4) and is about to cross the C1-2 facet joint. (With permission from Barrow Neurological Institute.)

no. 4 Penfield dissector (Fig. 5). The C2 nerve root and venous plexus are retracted upward to provide direct visualization of the C2 pars and the posterior aspect of the C1-2 facet joint. The K-wire is aimed between 0 and 10 degrees medial to the point of screw entry through the central axis of the pars interarticularis (Fig. 6). Lateral fluoroscopic monitoring is used to adjust the trajectory of the K-wire so that its tip is aimed at the middle of the C1 tubercle (Fig. 7). The anterior C1 tubercle is a crucial landmark for directing transarticular screw placement. Other investigators have reported an association between screw malposition and an absent C1 tubercle (7). Thus, we attempt to preserve at least a portion of this structure during a transoral odontoidectomy in the event that transarticular screw fixation will be necessary later.

Once the proper screw trajectory has been determined, the K-wire is drilled through the C2 pars interarticularis, across the posterior edge of the C1-2 facet joint, and into the lateral mass of C1 under fluoroscopic guidance. To avoid creating excessive torque on the K-wire that could cause it to bend or break, the position of the drill guide and sheath should not be altered after the K-wire begins to engage the bone. If its trajectory is suboptimal, the K-wire should be removed completely, by reversing the drill direction, and be reinserted along a new tract through a new entry point on the bone surface. Screws placed too ventrally can penetrate C1 anteriorly and enter the pharynx. Screws placed too rostrally can cross the occipitoatlantal joint and injure the hypoglossal nerve or produce a painful occipitocervical joint. Screws placed too laterally can injure the vertebral arteries, and screws placed too medially can injure the spinal cord.

After the K-wire is positioned satisfactorily in the bone, a

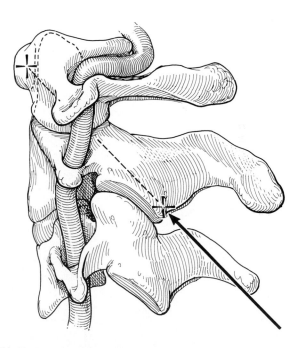

Fig. 7. The trajectory for C1-2 transarticular screw placement. A key landmark for deriving the trajectory is the anterior tubercle of the atlas. Failure to visualize this structure before the screw is placed under fluoroscopic guidance has been correlated with a substantially increased risk of positioning the screw suboptimally. (With permission from Barrow Neurological Institute.)

second K-wire of identical length is inserted into the tissue sheath until it contacts the bone surface. The difference between the ends of the K-wires is then measured with a ruler to determine the appropriate screw length. A fully threaded screw or an end-threaded screw can be used for fixation. In general, the widest diameter (3.5 vs. 4.0 mm), self-tapping cannulated screw that the patient's anatomy will accommodate should be used to fixate the C1-2 complex. If the patient's bone is soft, the self-tapping, self-drilling screw can be inserted directly over the K-wire. If the bone is normal, it often needs to be tapped before the screw is inserted. If the bone is hard, a pilot hole is made with a cannulated 2.0- or 2.5-mm drill and then tapped. The screw is placed over the K-wire and inserted into the bone using a hollow screwdriver (Fig. 8). The surgeon must carefully avoid advancing the K-wire while preparing the pilot holes or inserting the screws. The end of the K-wire should protrude beyond the end of the tap and screwdriver handles and be anchored by the surgical assistant with a needle holder. As the screw engages the bone, the positions of the K-wire and screw are monitored fluoroscopically. When the screw crosses the joint space into the lateral mass of C1, the surgeon typically feels a characteristic stiffness as the atlas and axis lock together.

Once the screw has crossed the atlantoaxial articular surface and is satisfactorily seated within the distal bone, the K-wire is removed using the pneumatic drill. The screw head should be recessed slightly into the bone to prevent the screw from levering against the C2-3 joint space. An overtightened screw can shear through its thread track and destroy its purchase in the bone. The final position of the screw is verified with fluoroscopy in the anteroposterior and lateral planes. The contralateral screw is inserted in an identical manner. Suspicion of a vertebral artery injury during the initial screw insertion precludes placement of a contralateral screw. Of note, the successful application of frameless stereotactic navigational technology to spinal surgery currently enables transarticular screw insertion with enhanced accuracy and without the need for intraoperative fluoroscopy.

INTERSPINOUS WIRING. A variety of posterior atlantoaxial wiring techniques have been described and each has its advocates (8). We believe that the advantage of the interspinous wiring method, as described by Sonntag's group (2,8) resides in its combination of excellent biomechanical characteristics for resisting rotational and translational forces and the safety of requiring sublaminar wire passage at only a single level (C1). A partial invagination of the posterior C1 ring into the foramen magnum can impede passage of the sublaminar wire. In that instance, rather than shave down (and weaken) the rostral aspect of the dorsal C1 arch, the foramen magnum is enlarged to provide adequate room for safe sublaminar passage. The adjacent edges of the posterior caudal C1 arch and rostral C2 spinous process and lamina are decorticated with a high-speed drill or Kerrison rongeur. The inferior surface of the C2 laminae is notched bilaterally to seat the wires at the spinolaminar junction (Fig. 9).

A tricortical bone graft (approximately 4 cm long × 3 cm high) is obtained from the posterior iliac crest. A bicortical, curved strut graft is created by removing the rounded cortical margin with a Leksell rongeur. The strut graft is sized to fit between the posterior arches of C1 and C2 under compression and to re-create the normal height of the C1-2 complex. The inferior margin of the bone graft is notched at its midpoint so that it straddles the C2 spinous process. After the graft has been contoured adequately, it is removed from the field until the sublaminar wire is positioned.

A braided sublaminar cable, positioned under direct visualization of the epidural space, is used for interspinous wiring. The cable is passed beneath the posterior C1 arch in the midline where the epidural space is widest (Fig. 10). Sublaminar wire passage is facilitated by passing the blunt end of a large needle attached to a 2-0 Vicryl suture under the posterior C1 arch, tying it to the cable loop, and passing both under the C1 arch with a simultaneous feeding-pulling technique (Fig. 11). Complications associated with sublaminar wire passage are related to

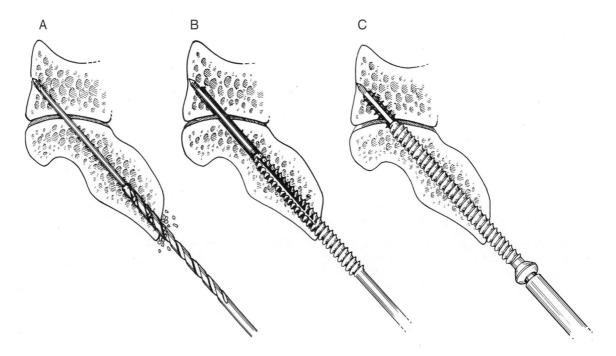

Fig. 8. **A**: After the K-wire has crossed the C1-2 joint and has obtained adequate purchase of the C1 lateral mass, a pilot hole is drilled with a cannulated drill bit. After the screw course has been tapped (**B**), the cannulated screw is placed (**C**). (With permission from Barrow Neurological Institute.)

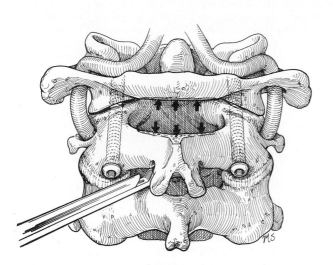

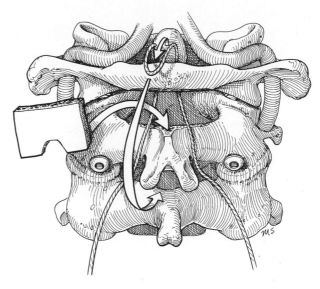

Fig. 9. Interspinous fusion is performed after the transarticular screws have been placed. The adjacent surfaces of the C1-C2 posterior elements are decorticated to enhance the likelihood of integrating the autologous strut graft. A Kerrison rongeur is used to notch the spinolaminar junction bilaterally at the caudal aspect of the C2 level to allow seating of the braided interspinous wires. (With permission from Barrow Neurological Institute.)

Fig. 10. A sublaminar wire is looped ventral to the posterior ring of C1. It is passed in a caudal-to-rostral fashion with care exerted to avoid compressing the underlying dura. The autologous strut graft is then positioned between the lamina of C1 and C2, and the sublaminar loop is doubled back over the C2 spinous process (Sonntag fusion). (With permission from Barrow Neurological Institute.)

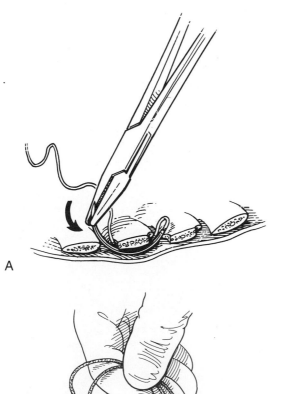

Fig. 11. Sublaminar wire passage. **A:** The blunt end of a needle is passed retrograde along the sublaminar course. The suture is pulled through and the needle is removed. **B:** The suture is tied to the cable loop, and both are simultaneously "fed and pulled" to avoid developing slack in the wire that could compress the spinal cord. (With permission from Barrow Neurological Institute.)

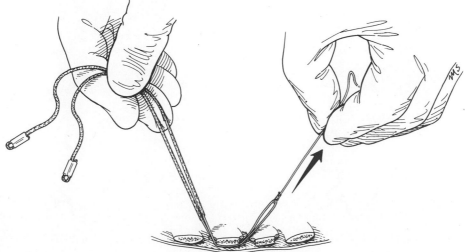

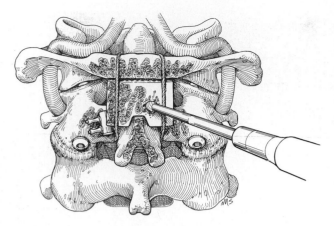

Fig. 12. After the interspinous wire has been tightened and crimped, the dorsal elements of C1-2 and the autologous graft are decorticated to maximize the surface area of exposed cancellous bone. (With permission from Barrow Neurological Institute.)

allowing the wire to bow ventrally and compress the spinal cord. Every effort is therefore expended to ensure that the wire hugs the undersurface of the lamina during passage and maintains a low profile.

The graft is repositioned between the atlas and axis. The loop of cable is passed over the posterior C1 ring, over the dorsal surface of the graft, and secured in the notches beneath the C2 spinous process. The free ends of the cable are positioned anteriorly to the graft and are also seated beneath the notched C2 spinous process. The cable is tightened and crimped with the bone graft secured between the surrounding cables and posterior elements of C1 and C2. At the time of cable tightening, careful observation is required to ensure that the wire does not

cut through the laminae of C1 or C2. The surfaces of the dorsal atlantoaxial complex and bone graft are decorticated with a high-speed air drill (Fig. 12). Continuous irrigation is employed to minimize the risk of thermal injury to the fusion bed that could cause bone resorption or otherwise impede arthrodesis. Morselized, cancellous bone graft from the iliac crest is compressed against the fusion surfaces. Curets, osteotomes, or drills can also be used to remove the articular surfaces of the C1-2 facets, which can then be packed with autologous cancellous bone to further promote arthrodesis.

OCCIPITOCERVICAL FIXATION AND FUSION. Occipitocervical fusion is performed to treat occipitoatlantal instability or atlantoaxial instability that is either not amenable to or has failed previous efforts at arthrodesis. Several metal implants are available for fixating the occipitocervical junction. These include threaded/grooved titanium or steel rods, smooth steel templates, a titanium frame, and a variety of screw plates (Fig. 13). At our institution, a fully threaded, $^5/_{32}$-diameter, grooved titanium rod is preferred to anchor the occipitocervical fusion mass (9). The grooved rod helps resist compaction or "telescoping" of the fusion construct, which can lead to vertical migration of the dens into the foramen magnum. Regardless of the surgeon's preference for implant, however, the cables or screws used to secure the device should be made of the same metal to avoid accelerated corrosion, early fatigue, and instrument failure.

We rely on a unique rod bender (BendMeister, Sofamor Danek, Memphis, TN) that permits easily reproducible contouring of the pins with smooth primary and secondary curves (10). In contrast, other methods of rod shaping (table vises, bending irons, French benders) can produce sharp angles and notch rods, thereby creating stress risers and diminishing the biomechanical strength of the metal. Smooth curves distribute forces more uniformly on the rod and help to optimize its strength and to increase its resistance to breaking. Use of the rod bender

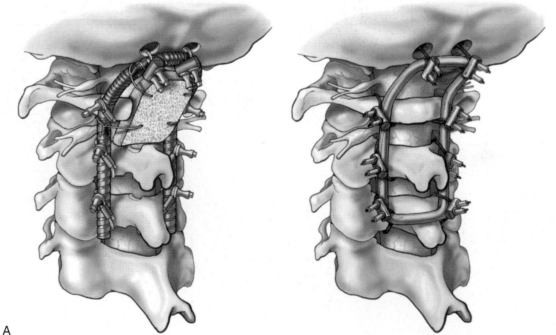

A   B

Fig. 13. Metal implants available for occipitocervical fixation. **A:** Grooved titanium rod. **B:** Hartshill rectangle.

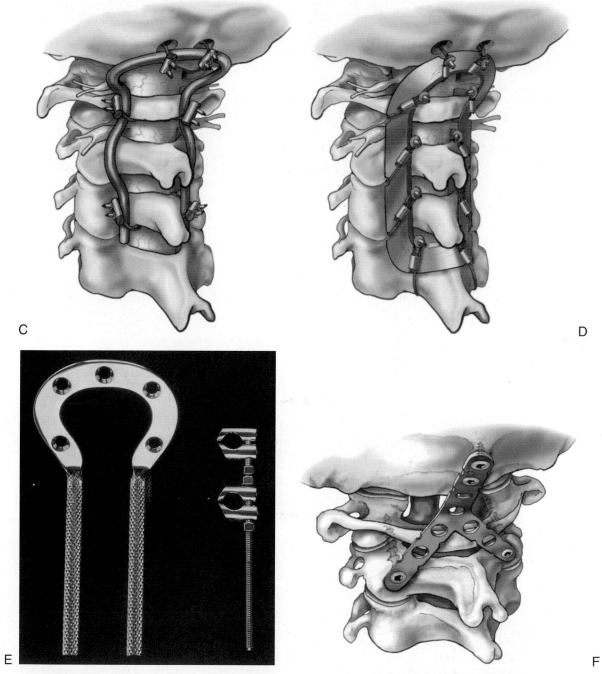

Fig. 13. (continued). **C**: Ransford loop. **D**: Codman titanium frame. **E**: Cotrel-Dubousset rod/screw plate (note transverse connector for rod stabilization). **F**: Grob Y screw plate (note transarticular or C2 pars screw placement possibilities).

(*Figure continues*)

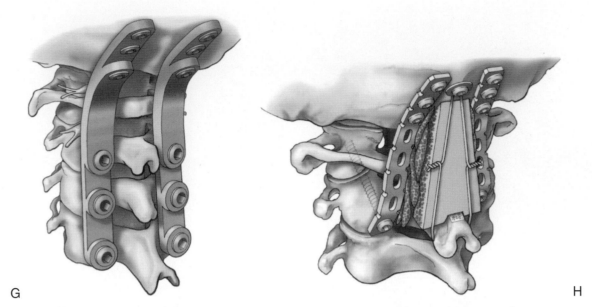

G

H

Fig. 13. (continued). **G**: Roy-Camille screw plate. **H**: Magerl technique. (**A–D** and **F–H** with permission from Barrow Neurological Institute. **E** with permission from Thieme New York.)

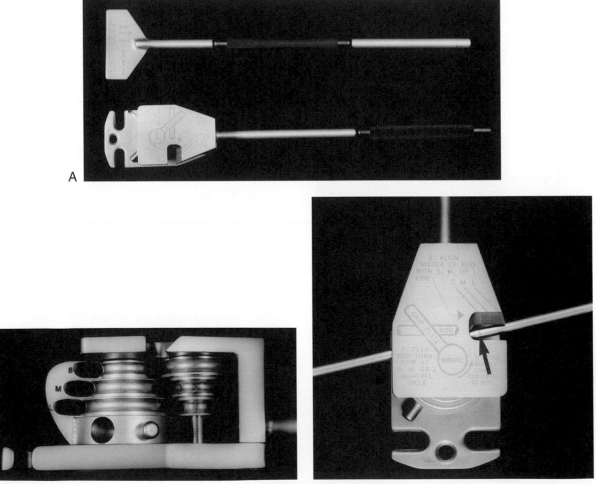

A

B

C

Fig. 14. **A**: The BendMeister Rod Bender has two components including a Rod Bender-Handle (*top*) and the Rod Bender proper (*bottom*). **B**: Lateral view of the Rod Bender bending mandrel with the options for small (S), medium (M), and large (L) radii of curvature. **C**: Surface of the rod bender with instructions for creating a primary curve in a pin. (From Apostolides PJ, Karahalios DG, Sonntag VKH. Use of the BendMeister Rod Bender for occipitocervical fusion. Technical note. *Neurosurgery* 1998;43:389–391, with permission.)

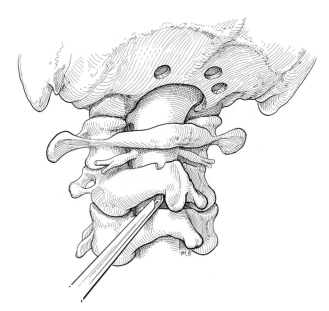

Fig. 15. Preparation for occipitocervical fusion. Suboccipital burr holes are placed for wire passage out through the foramen magnum. The most medial aspect of the lamina to receive a sublaminar wire is notched to facilitate wire passage. (With permission from Barrow Neurological Institute.)

further simplifies the performance of occipitocervical fusion procedures because only one size titanium rod or Steinmann pin is needed in the operating room at the time of custom sizing (Fig. 14). In contrast, reliance on precontoured loops or rectangles requires the availability of multiple implant sizes and shapes (degrees of curvature) for any one patient.

In devising an occipitocervical fusion construct, achieving adequate rigidity must be balanced against minimizing the number of cervical motion segments sacrificed for that purpose ("as long as necessary, but as short as possible"). The number of levels that should be incorporated in a particular occipitocervical fusion is influenced by the degree of preoperative instability. For patients with occipitocervical instability, intact posterior laminar elements, and no anterior compressive pathology or basilar invagination, we perform the fusion procedure through the axial level (occiput C1-2). Patients who require an anterior decompressive transoral odontoidectomy usually require a subsequent occipitocervical fusion. These patients often require additional points of fixation to stabilize their fusion construct sufficiently, as do patients with evidence of basilar invagination. We usually immobilize these patients with a fusion mass that extends to C3 or C4. For patients with incompetent posterior elements, either as a result of traumatic injury or as a requirement for posterior decompression of the vertebral canal, we typically extend the occipitocervical fusion at least two levels below the unstable segment. If the lamina of a particular level is incompetent, facet wires can be used to anchor the titanium rod. Comparatively, sublaminar wires have greater strength to resist pulling out and provide more rigid immobilization than facet wires. Thus, they are the preferred fixation method. Occipitocervical screw plates provide an option for fixation that does not require sublaminar wire passage. They are especially useful if cervical laminae are incompetent or absent (Fig. 13F–H).

All soft tissues in the region of the proposed fusion site should be removed, including the occipitoatlantal membrane between the foramen magnum and C1 and the interspinous ligaments and ligamentum flavum between C1-2 and C2-3. The posterior rim of the foramen magnum can be enlarged with a high-speed air drill to facilitate suboccipital epidural wire passage for anchoring the titanium rod to the skull base. Three burr holes are placed within the occipital bone approximately 1 cm away from the margin of the enlarged foramen magnum and off the midline. The burr holes are waxed, and the dura is dissected away from the inner table of the skull toward the foramen magnum. If the foramen magnum is relatively inaccessible because the patient's anatomy is anomalous or cervical flexion is limited, three sets of burr holes can be placed around the periphery of the foramen magnum, between which the suboccipital wires are passed. The laminae to be wired are often notched as medially as possible to facilitate wire passage (Fig. 15).

Suboccipital wires are passed between the occipital burr holes and foramen magnum in whichever direction appears to be easiest. The tip of the wire is bent into a blunt loop to help avoid violation of the dura. Using the technique described for interspinous wiring of the atlantoaxial complex, sublaminar

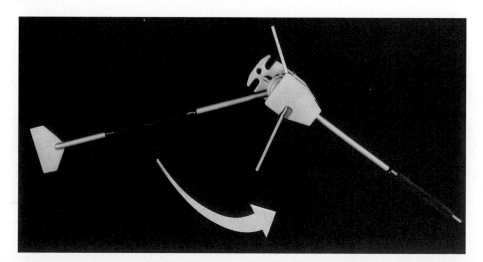

Fig. 16. Insertion of the handle into the Rod Bender with counterclockwise rotation and creation of a primary curve. (From Dickman CA, Apostolides PJ, Karahalios DG. Surgical techniques for upper cervical spine decompression and stabilization. *Clin Neurosurg* 1997;44:137–160, with permission.)

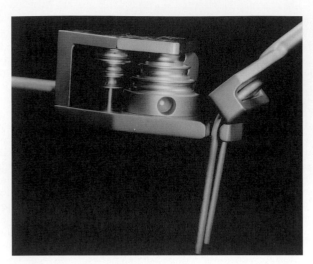

Fig. 17. At its end, the Rod Bender has a bending hole that holds the rod after its primary curve has been created. The secondary curve is formed using the paddle end of the Rod Bender-Handle. (From Dickman CA, Apostolides PJ, Karahalios DG. Surgical techniques for upper cervical spine decompression and stabilization. *Clin Neurosurg* 1997; 44:137–160, with permission.)

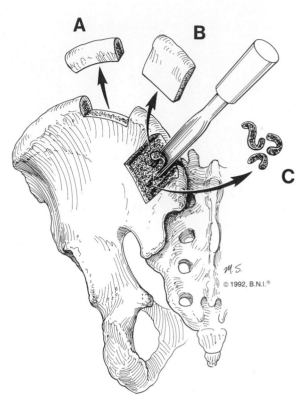

Fig. 19. Autologous iliac crest bone. Bone harvest is usually contained within 6 to 8 cm lateral to the sacroiliac joint to avoid injury to the cluneal nerves. The sacroiliac joint itself is left intact to avoid causing pelvic pain or instability. A tricortical bone graft (**A**) is harvested for the infraspinous C1-2 fusion and wiring procedure. The tricortical bone segment is modified to a bicortical strut graft and is sized to fit the interspinous space between C1-2 using a Leksell rongeur. Osteotomes can be used to cut a window in the posterior iliac crest to yield a unicortical plate (**B**) and cancellous bone (**C**) for occipitocervical fusion. (With permission from Barrow Neurological Institute.)

wires are passed as medially as possible to minimize the risks of neurological injury or cerebrospinal fluid leaks. Sublaminar wires are positioned at the most lateral aspects of the laminae when the construct is in final position.

A wide diameter ($\frac{5}{32}$-inch), threaded stainless steel Steinmann pin or titanium grooved rod is contoured to the anatomy of the patient's CVJ. The pin must be shaped precisely to maximize the area of metal–bone interface, which creates the most stable fixation construct. A sterile, malleable, endotracheal tube stylet is used to model the shape of the CVJ and to serve as a template for contouring the pin.

A primary U-shaped curve (Fig. 16) and smooth secondary curves (Fig. 17) are made with the BendMeister Rod Bender. When placed into the wound, the pin should lie flush against the occiput and laminae. Gaps between the pin and bone sur-

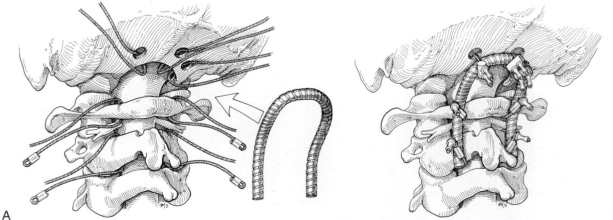

Fig. 18. A: Sublaminar and suboccipital wires have been positioned, and the contoured, grooved pin is seated flush against the osseous craniovertebral surfaces. The sublaminar wires were passed medially within the vertebral canal and then carefully mobilized laterally for fixation. Three suboccipital burr holes have been placed with the epidural wires brought through the foramen magnum. **B:** Final construct of Steinmann pin with suboccipital and sublaminar wires. (With permission from Barrow Neurological Institute.)

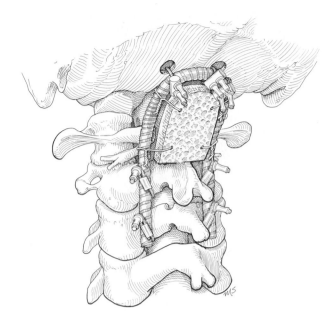

Fig. 20. In the case of a C1 laminectomy, a unicortical graft can be sutured or wired to the Steinmann pin to function as a template for osseous integration and to preserve the decompression of the craniovertebral junction. (With permission from Barrow Neurological Institute.)

faces suboptimally fixate the unstable segments and can allow excessive motion that can lead to instrument failure and nonunion. The ends of the pin are cut so that they do not extend beyond the lowest segment to be fused. Failure to do so risks causing leverage on the hardware that can destabilize the fixation construct or unintentionally incorporate an additional motion segment within the fusion mass.

The pin is wired against the occiput and cervical laminae or facets (Fig. 18). The occiput, facet joints, and posterior arches of the cervical levels to be fused are decorticated with curets and a high-speed air drill to maximize the surface area for bone incorporation. Generous amounts of autologous, cancellous, iliac crest bone grafts are compressed against the levels to be fused (Fig. 19). If a suboccipital craniectomy or cervical laminectomy is required to decompress the neural elements, a unicortical plate of iliac crest bone can be sutured or wired to the central portion of the rod to act as a template for the fusion and to preserve the neural decompression (Fig. 20). A routine multilayered wound closure is performed.

Orthoses and Postoperative Follow-Up

After both atlantoaxial and occipitocervical fusion procedures, patients are usually maintained in a hard cervical collar. Patients are evaluated at 2- to 4-week intervals to assess their clinical progress and the healing of their fusion. After 10 to 12 weeks, dynamic radiographs with cervical flexion and extension are obtained to assess the stability of the construct. Patients with C1-2 instability who cannot have transarticular screws placed routinely have their interspinous wiring supplemented with a halo brace. Poor bone quality (rheumatoid arthritis), significant ligamentous instability (occipitoatlantal dislocation), and other

individual patient characteristics that negatively impact the anticipated success of bone healing, such as malnutrition, cigarette smoking, metabolic disorders, exogenous steroid use, or a history of previously unsuccessful fusion attempts, are potential indications for halo bracing after rigid internal fixation to optimize the chances for fusion.

Complications

The potential risks associated with atlantoaxial or craniovertebral stabilization techniques include infection; bleeding requiring transfusion with the associated possibilities of transfusion reactions or infection (hepatitis or HIV); medical complications (myocardial infarction, pneumonia, urinary tract infection, or deep venous thrombosis); high cervical myelopathy due to craniovertebral manipulation or sublaminar wire passage with its associated requirements for tracheostomy and placement of a feeding tube; lower cranial nerve injury; stroke related to injury of the vertebral artery; intracranial hemorrhage related to suboccipital wire passage; dural tear with a cerebrospinal fluid leak; suboccipital numbness; hardware failure with breakage of the screws, wires, or pin; and failure to obtain bony arthrodesis. Risks of surgery also include those related to donor-site morbidity such as infection, hematoma, cosmetic deformity, and prolonged pain or numbness.

The predominant concern regarding these procedures is to avoid a vertebral artery or spinal cord injury. A survey of 101 neurosurgeons who had placed transarticular screws in 1,318 patients (2,492 screws placed) reported the risk for vertebral artery injury at 2.2% per screw. Only two patients with either a known or suspected vertebral artery injury manifested neurological deficits. Only one patient, who sustained bilateral vertebral artery injuries, died (11). The well-recognized risk of myelopathy related to cervical sublaminar wire placement (12) can be minimized by carefully passing wires in a "push-pull" method as described and by exposing the dura widely so it can be visualized for distortion during wire passage.

Conclusions

Combining transarticular screw placement and interspinous wiring represents an excellent technique for rigidly fixating C1-2. Occipitocervical fixation with titanium or steel implants and suboccipital and sublaminar wires confer immediate rigid internal fixation in patients with occipitocervical instability. The procedures are technically demanding. Absolute familiarity with the regional anatomy is mandatory for surgeons planning to perform these procedures. The great variability in CVJ anatomy among patients, particularly at C1-2, requires patients to undergo a thorough radiographic workup to ensure accurate preoperative planning. The outcomes of arthrodesis with these techniques are excellent, and morbidity rates are low in experienced hands. Regardless of the internal fixation technique used, careful preoperative planning and adherence to time-proven surgical principles are fundamental to achieving successful arthrodesis.

Acknowledgment

This chapter was adapted from Baskin JJ, Apostilides PJ, Dickman CA. Posterior atlantoaxial and occipitocervical fixation and fusion techniques. In: Tornetta P III, O'Brien M, Sandhu H, eds. *Techniques in fracture surgery.* Philadelphia: Mosby Year Book, *in press.* With permission from Mosby Year Book.

References

1. Sawin PD, Traynelis VC, Menezes AH. A comparative analysis of fusion rates and donor-site morbidity for autogeneic rib and iliac crest bone grafts in posterior cervical fusions. *J Neurosurg* 1998;88:255–265.
2. Dickman CA, Sonntag VKH, Papadopoulos SM, et al. The interspinous method of posterior atlantoaxial arthrodesis. *J Neurosurg* 1991;74:190–198.
3. Marcotte P, Dickman CA, Sonntag VKH, et al. Posterior atlantoaxial facet screw fixation. *J Neurosurg* 1993;79:234–237.
4. Apostolides PJ, Dickman CA, Sonntag VKH. Anterior atlantoaxial facet screw fixation. In: Dickman CA, Sonntag VKH, Spetzler RF, eds. *Surgery of the craniovertebral junction.* New York: Thieme, 1998:735–738.
5. Paramore CG, Dickman CA, Sonntag VKH. The anatomical suitability of the C1-2 complex for transarticular screw fixation. *J Neurosurg* 1996;85:221–224.
6. Song GS, Theodore N, Dickman CA, et al. Unilateral posterior atlanto-axial transarticular screw fixation. *J Neurosurg* 1997;87:851–855.
7. Madawi AA, Casey AT, Solanki GA, et al. Radiological and anatomical evaluation of the atlantoaxial transarticular screw fixation technique. *J Neurosurg* 1997;86:961–968.
8. Sonntag VKH, Dickman CA. Posterior atlantoaxial wiring techniques. In: Dickman CA, Sonntag VKH, Spetzler RF, eds. *Surgery of the craniovertebral junction.* New York: Thieme, 1998:783–794.
9. Apostolides PJ, Dickman CA, Golfinos JG, et al. Threaded Steinmann pin fusion of the craniovertebral junction. *Spine* 1996;21:1630–1637.
10. Apostolides PJ, Karahalios DG, Sonntag VKH. Use of the BendMeister rod bender for occipitocervical fusion. Technical note. *Neurosurgery* 1998;43:389–391.
11. Wright NM, Lauryssen C. Vertebral artery injury in C1-2 transarticular screw fixation: results of a survey of the AANS/CNS Section on Disorders of the Spine and Peripheral Nerves. American Association of Neurological Surgeons/Congress of Neurological Surgeons. *J Neurosurg* 1998;88:634–640.
12. Geremia GK, Kim KS, Cerullo L, et al. Complications of sublaminar wiring. *Surg Neurol* 1985;23:629–635.

204. Posterior Interspinous Wiring and Lateral Mass Plates

**Geoffrey P. Zubay and
Stephen L. Ondra**

Over the past century there have been numerous advances in surgical techniques used to stabilize the spine. The earliest reported use of instrumentation was reported by Wilkins (1). He used a carbonized wire looped around the pedicles of T12 and L1 to internally fixate an unstable segment of the spine in 1887. In 1891, Hadra (2) described the use of an interspinous wire to stabilize the cervical spine in cases of traumatic and inflammatory cervical instability. Later in the early 20th century, Albee and Hibbs reported on their experiences laying autologously harvested bone over the posterior elements of the spine to achieve biological fusion in the treatment of instability related to Potts disease (1).

Not until the later half of the twentieth century would the crucial concept in spinal instrumentation and fusion be understood and described. Harrington coined the problem as "the race between instrumentation failure and the acquisition of spinal fusion." This concept was revolutionary and most succinctly described the role of internal fixation—to achieve temporary immobilization and stabilization of a compromised segment of the spine until bone fusion could occur. With advances in instrumentation techniques and a more complex understanding of the biomechanics involved, success rates have improved significantly. Now there are numerous techniques readily available to the surgeon to fixate the cervical spine from both anterior and posterior approaches in the treatment of subaxial cervical spine disease. Choosing the appropriate methodology requires a thorough and complete understanding of the disease processes that result in subaxial cervical instability and of the limitations of the different applied techniques.

Stabilization of the subaxial cervical spine is frequently achieved using posterior fixation techniques. Interspinous wiring, Luque rods and rectangles, sublaminar wires and clamps, and lateral mass plates are the most common techniques used today. Each technique has its appropriate application and its associated limitations. Understanding the biomechanics of the cervical spine and the mechanics of each type of fixation construct is important if one is to successfully use these fixation techniques.

Biomechanics of the Subaxial Cervical Spine

White and Panjabi (3) most adequately described the goals of spinal stabilization: (a) to restore stability to the structurally compromised spine; (b) to maintain alignment after correction of deformity; (c) to prevent progression of a deformity; and (d) to alleviate pain. Anterior and posterior techniques in the cervical spine can achieve these results readily when applied appropriately.

Posterior approaches to the subaxial cervical spine are typically used to restore stability and prevent untoward deformity progression. In contrast, in the cervical spine, deformity correction is a goal difficult to achieve with posterior fixation techniques alone. Commonly used posterior techniques are interspinous wiring, facet wiring, sublaminar clamps, and lateral mass screws. Each technique affords its own set of advantages and disadvantages, which are the product of the technique's individual biomechanical properties and limitations; therefore, understanding the basic biomechanical principles involved is the first step in understanding the appropriate indications for the use of these fixation techniques.

THE NORMAL CERVICAL SPINE. The primary role of the spine is to support load and in the process of bearing this load protect the spinal cord. *In utero*, there are two primary curves in the spine, the thoracic kyphosis and the sacral curvature, which are relatively fixed curves. With the assumption of the upright posture, the cervical lordosis and lumbar lordosis develop and are hence known as secondary curves. Because these curves develop in order to maintain sagittal balance during the upright posture, the vertebral bodies do not undergo structural changes to accommodate the curvature as they do in the thoracic spine and sacral spine, where the individual bodies have a wedge-shaped appearance. In contrast to the thoracic and sacral curvatures, the cervical and lumbar curves are compensatory in nature and hence are relatively mobile.

The typical cervical spine affords approximately 60 to 75 degrees of flexion and extension (4). This range of motion is afforded by the integrity of the intervertebral discs. Sagittal translation may occur 2 to 3 mm at each level in the cervical spine. Motion in this vector is limited by virtue of the facet joints and posterior ligamentous tension band. In contrast to the rest of the spine, lateral bending is prominent in the cervical spine. Above C6, 10 to 12 degrees of lateral bending occurs at each segment; below C6, 4 to 8 degrees of lateral bending is allowed (4).

THE UNSTABLE CERVICAL SPINE. Injuries to the cervical spine impair the normal load-bearing features of the cervical spine. These injuries may be iatrogenic, traumatic, degenerative, or infectious in nature. When the normal compensatory mechanisms of the spine are exceeded, derangements of normal alignment may occur, resulting in compromise of the spinal cord. Surgical fixation and fusion have as their goal to either prevent the genesis of deformity as a result of spinal column injury or restore normal alignment resulting from compromise of the normal load-bearing features of the spine. Deciding when surgery is indicated to stabilize the subaxial cervical spine requires an understanding of the structural mechanics of the normal and injured cervical spine. Several investigators have attempted to simply this matter by devising clinical and radiographic models for interpreting when injuries to the spine are destabilizing and which injuries are likely to result in progressive deformity.

Denis (5) developed a three-column model of the spine to evaluate the stability of the thoracolumbar spine. In his model compromise of two or more columns of support leads to instability. His model has been modified and applied to numerous treatment algorithms. For the cervical spine, White and Panjabi (3) developed a similar set of radiographic and clinical criteria that has been used as a predictor of subaxial cervical spine instability. Although these algorithms are useful in determining which injuries will be accompanied by radiographic instability, neither has been tested in predicting clinical outcomes when surgical and nonsurgical means are used to treat such injuries. These algorithms are useful as far as they can serve as a guideline for decision making when assessing different injuries. In practice, instability is frequently assessed based primarily on radiographic studies such as plain radiographs, flexion-exten-

sion radiographs, computed tomography (CT), and magnetic resonance imaging (MRI).

When instability is present, a treatment modality needs to be applied. Many unstable injuries to the cervical spine can be treated with just an external orthotic immobilization device. Unilateral facet fractures, ligamentous injuries, and simple body fractures can often be treated successfully with bracing alone. Bracing immobilizes the spine until spontaneous healing of the injured segment is able to occur. When injuries are more complex, bracing may be unable to provide adequate immobilization of the injured segment, putting the spinal cord at risk for further injury and preventing proper healing of the injury from occurring. These more complex injuries may require surgery for adequate restoration of spinal stability until proper healing can occur.

Surgery provides short-term stability with internal hardware fixation and long-term stability with surgically stimulated bone fusion. Successful surgical fixation depends on (a) identifying the injured component of the spine, (b) repairing the injured component, (c) decompressing any compromised neural elements, and (d) correcting any deformity that has resulted from the injured component. By doing so, the surgeon achieves the restoration of normal spinal balance and stability, and prevents the genesis or progression of deformity.

In the subaxial cervical spine, there are numerous techniques available to the surgeon. Techniques are applied from either an anterior or posterior approach. The approach limits which component of the cervical spine the surgeon can access for treatment. Therefore, posterior subaxial cervical spine fixation techniques are typically used to treat conditions that result in compromise of the posterior elements of the subaxial cervical spine. Correspondingly, posterior techniques are limited in their ability to effectively treat conditions that originate in the anterior column of the cervical spine. Understanding the advantages and limitations of posterior subaxial fixation techniques requires an understanding of the anatomical requirements and the biomechanical properties of different fixation techniques.

Interspinous wiring techniques use a wire to loop around the spinous process of two adjacent or multiple segments of the cervical spine. Interspinous wiring techniques help to recreate the posterior tension band when it is compromised. The application of interspinous wires requires that the bony components of the posterior spinal column be intact. Because of how the wire is applied, the wire is able to only effectively resist flexion.

Laminar and facet wires can also be used. These are alternative techniques of applying wires to the posterior cervical spine. Because these wires are applied bilaterally they may provide better resistance to rotational or torsional forces. Nevertheless, simple wiring techniques offer little stability with regard to extension, lateral bending, or lateral rotation. Because wires are assembled as a rigid loops, narrowing of the interanchor distance with extension introduces laxity resulting in adequate immobilization, which may prevent delayed bone fusion and result in the development of pseudarthrosis. Laminar clamps and hooks suffer from similar limitations by their fixed interanchor distance.

The use of Luque rods or rectangles in conjunction with sublaminar wires and interspinous wires can provide greater stability. By using wires or cables to segmentally fixate the spine to a rod, greater stability is achieved by limiting the degrees of freedom when forces from extension, lateral bending, and rotation occur.

The most rigid biomechanical system that can be applied from a posterior approach is the lateral mass plating system. Lateral mass plates afford numerous advantages. Because these plates are assembled by placing screws in the lateral masses, the structural integrity of the lamina and spinous processes is not required for their assembly. When assembled, the system biomechanically behaves as a three-point bending model or a nonfixed moment arm cantilever beam fixation system providing stability to lateral bending, rotation, and extension in contrast to a simple tension band fixation system that can only effectively resist flexion. In fact, biomechanical studies have demonstrated that lateral mass plate fixation increases segmental stability in flexion by 92% and in extension by 60%, while interspinous wiring alone increases segmental stability in flexion only by 33% and fails to provide any substantial stability in extension (6,7).

All these techniques are typically applied in no-load conditions. Preloading the construct with compressive forces in an attempt to reduce a deformity predisposes the construct to failure. Segmental failure may occur with fracture of a spinous process, lamina, or lateral mass. Global failure may occur with subsidence or progression of kyphosis. Because posterior constructs are typically assembled in no-load conditions, deformity reduction needs to be achieved before assembly of the construct. When deformity correction needs to be performed, frequently anterior approaches are required to achieve the needed results. Because subaxial cervical deformity frequently is the result of abnormal kyphosis, correction will often require reconstruction of the anterior column. If reduction of a kyphosis is attempted with a posterior approach alone, excessive loading on the posterior construct may lead to hardware failure. Correction of an abnormal kyphosis with a load-bearing strut anteriorly helps reduce load on the posterior hardware because of load-sharing principles.

Indications for Performing Posterior Techniques

When surgery needs to be performed to stabilize the subaxial cervical spine, numerous techniques are at the disposal of the surgeon. Choosing when to use posterior fixation techniques depends on the understanding of the biomechanical needs of the patient. These needs are a product of the underlying pathology; therefore, understanding the different pathological processes that can be successfully treated by posterior techniques is essential. The underlying pathological process can result from trauma, degenerative disease, iatrogenic causes, and acquired causes such as tumor and infection.

TRAUMA. Trauma is the most common cause of instability in the subaxial cervical spine. Instability can result from ligamentous injury, structural injury, or a combination of the two. Traumatic instability arising from only compromise of the posterior interspinous ligamentous tension band can usually be treated with an external orthosis while the healing process occurs. In some patients, reconstructing the posterior tension band with either wiring techniques or lateral mass plates may be indicated to expedite mobilization of the patient and prevent deformity progression. Which patients with such ligamentous injuries require surgical fixation to achieve stability during the healing process has not been determined.

Some patients present with more complex ligamentous injuries that may disrupt the articular facet joints in the absence of any acute fractures. These patients typically present with unilateral or bilateral perched or locked facets. Facet dislocations rarely can be treated with immobilization alone. They typically require emergent reduction to reestablish normal alignment and to relieve any associated neural compression. Some

believe that reduction and stabilization is best achieved with posterior fixation techniques. However, because unilateral and bilateral locked facets are associated with a 42% and 62% incidence, respectively, of associated anterior disc herniation, locked or perched facets are frequently treated by anterior techniques, which afford initial disc space decompression prior to open reduction of the deformity (8).

Fractures that involve the articular fact joints, lamina, and pedicles are frequently accompanied by significant ligamentous injuries. Subsequently, adequate immobilization and healing in an external orthosis may not be possible (9,10). When the anterior column is not significantly compromised and anterior load sharing is not an issue, surgery using posterior techniques is optimal. Wiring techniques are frequently not usable because they require intact posterior elements for their appropriate assembly. When the facets are relatively spared from injury, laminar and spinous process fractures can be fixated using facet wires or lateral mass screws. Lateral mass screws are more versatile because even when the facets are compromised at the injured level, they can be assembled to bridge the deformity. In contrast, wiring constructs typically need to be assembled at each level of fixation.

When fractures involve the anterior column of support, the vertebral body, posterior techniques are rarely adequate alone. Compromise of the anterior column from trauma often leads to impairment of the normal anterior load-bearing features of the subaxial cervical spine and may place undue stress and strain on posterior constructs. Anterior approaches allow reconstruction of the compromised anterior column. When injuries are significant, posterior techniques may be used in conjunction with anterior techniques to augment their stability.

DEGENERATIVE DISEASE. Degenerative disease can lead to posterior articular facet arthropathy, spondylosis, and intervertebral disc space degeneration. When such disease processes lead to stenosis-related neural compression that is not primarily anterior in origin, the cervical spinal cord may be adequately decompressed by posterior approaches. If bilateral compromise of the facet joints is necessary during the surgical decompression, posterior stabilization and fusion may be afforded by lateral mass screws or facet wires to re-create the compromised posterior tension band. To achieve decompression of a nerve root from a posterior approach, typically 8 to 10 mm of the nerve root needs to be exposed, which frequently requires resection of as much as 60% to 70% of the adjacent facet joint (11). When greater than 50% of the facet joint is compromised, biomechanical studies have shown that the facet joint becomes incompetent (11). This may explain the high incidence of postlaminectomy kyphosis in children and adults. Prevention can be achieved with posterior fixation techniques.

IATROGENIC INSTABILITY. Postlaminectomy kyphosis is a common problem. Its incidence in children has been cited as high a 95% and in adults as high as 20% (1,12). Once kyphosis has developed, correction of the kyphotic angulation prior to stabilization is frequently the goal of surgery. Correction of kyphosis is best achieved by anterior approaches and has been adequately described in the literature (13). Resection of the apex of the kyphosis with a multilevel corpectomy typically allows adequate deformity correction (12,13). Appropriate stabilization may require posterior fixation in addition to anterior fixation.

While treatment of postlaminectomy kyphosis may require a combined approach, prevention of postlaminectomy kyphosis is best achieved by posterior fixation techniques alone. When wide posterior decompressive laminectomies are performed in the cervical spine, lateral mass plates and screw and rod constructs can be used to reconstruct the compromised posterior column, preventing the development of pathologic kyphosis.

ACQUIRED INSTABILITY. Infection and tumor can compromise the structural elements of the subaxial cervical spine. Often, surgical treatment requires the aggressive resection of the affected components to achieve good results. During the resection of tumor- or infection-related components, the spine is frequently destabilized both anteriorly and posteriorly. Subsequently, many patients undergoing such surgical procedures will require anterior and posterior fixation techniques to restore stability to the spine.

Preoperative and Intraoperative Considerations

To optimize surgical outcomes, several preoperative and intraoperative issues should be considered. The surgeon can optimize his outcomes by obtaining adequate preoperative imaging, using proper positioning and monitoring techniques, and using appropriate exposure techniques.

IMAGING. Preoperative imaging is of utmost importance. Static plain radiographs help to define the anatomical alignment of the spine. Repeat lateral radiographs when the patient is positioned prone in the operating room should be performed to ensure that adequate alignment exists prior to fixation. Preoperative MRI should be performed in patients undergoing procedures as sublaminar wiring. Significant spinal stenosis may be a contraindication for the placement of such wires because of the possible canal compromise. Preoperative CT scanning should also be performed not only to delineate the nature of the bony derangement or injury but also to ensure that adequate bone exists for fixation. Small lateral masses or aberrant vertebral arteries identified by CT scanning may contraindicate the use of lateral mass screws.

POSITIONING AND MONITORING. General anesthesia is generally used with orotracheal intubation. When strict cervical spine precautions need to be maintained during intubation, awake fiberoptic techniques should be used. This helps to minimize any unwanted displacements to the cervical spine during intubation and allows direct monitoring of the patient's neurological status during intubation (14).

Prior to positioning of the patient, baseline somatosensory evoked potentials should be obtained by the electrophysiologist to ensure that attenuated or delayed potentials are not the result of positioning. The patient's head is then fixated in three points with a Mayfield head holder in a bicoronal orientation. The patient is then rolled to the prone position with all pressure points adequately padded and with strict cervical alignment being maintained by the surgeon during the position change prior to securing the Mayfield to the operating table.

When the cervical spine is grossly unstable, the neck can be secured in a halo preoperatively. The patient is then intubated in the halo using awake fiberoptic techniques. Baseline evoked potentials are obtained. The patient is then rolled to the prone position in the halo. The halo ring can be secured to the operating table using a special adapter. Once secured to the operating

table, the posterior aspect of the halo device can be disassembled to allow access to the posterior cervical spine.

Once the position change is completed and the patients head is secured to the operating room table, a repeat set of evoked potentials is obtained by the electrophysiologist. If there are any changes in the evoked potentials, consideration should be given to changing the patient's position or returning the patient to the supine orientation with awake testing of neurological function.

SURGICAL EXPOSURE. The patient's neck and hip should be surgically prepped. To facilitate exposure, the base of the hairline will frequently need to be shaved. A midline exposure following the relatively avascular nuchal line is then performed. Hemostasis is achieved with the bovi electrocautery and the bipolar electrocautery. Exposure should be limited to the regions to be fixated. Care should be taken to preserve the soft tissue and ligamentous bands surrounding the adjacent segments to avoid any untoward compromise of their stability. Harvest of autologous bone from the hip is advocated for all cases. Appropriate long-term fusion is best optimized with the used of autologously harvest cancellous bone. All sites where autologously harvested bone is applied should be decorticated with a high-speed drill to reduce long-term complications related to the development of pseudarthrosis or inadequate fusion.

Techniques

There are numerous techniques used to fixate the subaxial cervical spine from a posterior approach. Each technique has advantages and disadvantages. Understanding how different techniques are applied elucidates these points. Because of the biomechanical superiority of lateral mass plating systems and lateral mass screw rod techniques, many of these techniques are not frequently used today; however, when anatomical constraints preclude the use of lateral mass plating systems, these other techniques may be a good alternative.

WIRING TECHNIQUES. Numerous wiring techniques have been developed over the years. There are essentially three types of wiring techniques: interspinous wiring, sublaminar wiring, and facet wiring. Each has advantages and disadvantages. Because of potential compromise of the spinal cord during the passage of sublaminar wires in the subaxial cervical spine, this technique is used less frequently today.

Wiring techniques are easy to perform. Most current wiring techniques are performed using braided cables. Braided cables are typically composed of two strands of 22-gauge wire. These cables have the advantage of being more flexible and having greater strength than individual wires of the same gauge. Many wires today are available in titanium alloys, which help to produce less artifact during conventional imaging techniques.

POSTERIOR INTERSPINOUS WIRING. Posterior interspinous wiring is infrequently used alone to fixate the subaxial cervical spine. Its use requires intact posterior elements. The spine is surgically prepared by exposure of the spinous processes. A tricortical bone graft is harvested from the hip and shaped to fit in the interspinous space. To promote fusion, the regions where the bone graft comes in contact with the spinous processes are decorticated. The graft is then placed under mild compression with a wire looped around the spinous adjacent spinous processes. Because the wire has minimal elastic properties, tension across the points of fixation requires that the distance between the spinous processes remains fixed. Theoretically, the interspinous bone graft helps prevent complications related to a decrease in the interanchor distance, which could result in failure of the wire. Nevertheless, the construct demonstrates poor stability with regard to rotational and lateral bending stresses. Consequently, interspinous wiring techniques are rarely applied as a stand-alone construct in multisegment fixations.

There are a variety of techniques used to assemble interspinous wires. Rogers (15) originally described the technique in 1942. During Rogers' wiring, transverse holes are made through the bases of the two adjacent spinous processes. A single cable is then looped through the base of the more rostral spinous process. The other end of the cable is then passed through the base of the more caudal spinous process and looped around the inferior aspect of the base of the spinous process. The cable is then tightened and crimped together.

The Whitehall modification is a simpler wiring technique (16). Transverse holes are made at the base of the spinous processes to be fixated, excluding the most caudal spinous process. At each level, a single cable is then passed through the transverse hole in the base of the superior spinous process and looped around the inferior margin of the spinous process below completing a simple loop (Fig. 1). If more than one level is to be fixated, the loops are made at each adjacent level in an overlapping fashion.

The Benzel-Kesterson modification is a more complex wiring technique that uses a tricortical bone graft harvested from the hip (17). Holes are made in the bases of two adjacent spinous processes to allow passage of a cable to complete a simple loop connecting the two spinous processes. A second cable is then passed underneath the first cable in the interspinous process space, and a loop is completed posterior to the interspinous cable securing two pieces of tricortical bone graft on both sides of the spinous processes.

The Bohlman triple-wire technique is a modification of the Rogers technique (18). Two adjacent spinous processes are first secured using the Rogers wiring technique. Two separate cables are then individually passed through the base of each of the spinous processes. On either side of the spinous processes, the two wires are used to buttonhole a bone graft before securing the bone graft to the underlying spinous processes and lamina.

Facet wires can also be used to fixate adjacent segments of the subaxial cervical spine. Facet wires have the advantage of not requiring completely intact posterior elements. There are essentially two types of facet wiring techniques used: oblique facet wiring as described by Cahill et al. (19) in 1983, and facet wiring as described by Callahan et al. (20).

Oblique facet wiring is a technique that can be used to secure two adjacent segments of the subaxial cervical spine. In its original description, the technique was used to secure a segment with posterior element fractures but intact facets to an intact caudal segment in the cervical spine. To perform the technique, the facets between the two levels to be fixated are prepared by opening the facet capsules and removing the articular cartilage. A hole is then made through both inferior articular processes of the rostral vertebral body. The holes are used to pass individual cables that are then both looped around the spinous process of the caudal vertebrae (Fig. 2). Because the technique spares the facet joints of the vertebral body caudal to the injured segment, it does not predispose the caudal segment to iatrogenic instability.

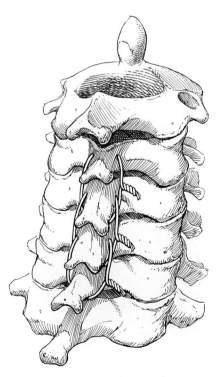

Fig. 1. An interspinous wiring construct using the Whitehall interspinous wiring modification. Note that the holes placed transversely through the base of each spinous process are made at each level excluding the most caudal level of fixation. The illustration demonstrates how the wires at each level are passed through the hole in the superior spinous process and looped around the base of the inferior spinous process. (Courtesy of Barrow Neurological Institute, Phoenix, AZ.)

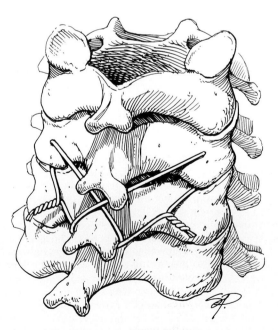

Fig. 2. Facet wiring, as described by Cahill, can be used to fixate two adjacent segments. Holes are made through the inferior articular process of the rostral body. Wires are then passed through the inferior articular facet process and looped around the spinous process of the caudal body bilaterally. (Courtesy of Barrow Neurological Institute, Phoenix, AZ.)

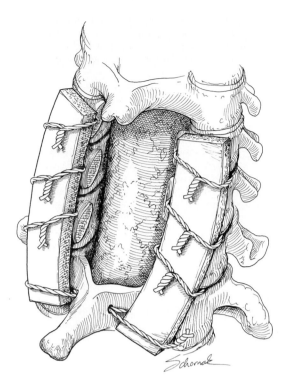

Fig. 3. Facet wiring techniques can be used to secure an overlying rib graft bilaterally as described by Callahan. (Courtesy of Barrow Neurological Institute, Phoenix, AZ.)

Callahan et al. described an alternative means of wiring facet joints. Their technique was originally described as a way to fuse the spine postlaminectomy to prevent subsequent kyphosis. In their technique the facets at the exposed levels are prepared by opening the joint capsules and removing the articular cartilage. Holes are made through the inferior articular processes at each level. The holes used to pass cables, which are then secured to an overlying rib graft (Fig. 3). The original technique is disadvantaged by violating the facet capsules at the most caudal level of the construct, potentially destabilizing the adjacent segment. One could alternatively use oblique facet wiring at the caudal level of the construct to avoid a destabilizing injury to the adjacent level.

LUQUE INSTRUMENTATION. When multiple segments need to be fixated, stainless steel pediatric Luque L rods and rectangles may be used. The Luque rectangle provides better torsional stability and is the preferred hardware construct. The rectangle is shaped to bridge the segments of the subaxial cervical spine to be fused from the posterior approach. The rod should not extend beyond the segments of the spine that are to be fused. Prior to its application, an attempt should be made to shape the rod to restore the normal cervical lordosis. The rectangle is then fixated to the spine posteriorly using wires attached to the spine at as many levels as possible. Sublaminar wires, interspinous wires, and facet wires can all be used.

The spine is prepared in the usual fashion. The patient is positioned prone with the head typically supported in the correct orientation using a Mayfield head holder. A midline posterior cervical exposure is performed following the relatively avascular plane of the nuchal line. Exposure should include the lateral aspects of the adjacent lateral masses at each level to be included in the fixation.

The interspinous ligament is disrupted at the rostral and caudal points of the segment of the cervical spine to be fixated to accommodate placement of the Luque rectangle. The rectangle should be shaped to meet as many points of contact with the underlying posterior elements of the cervical spine as possible. The rectangle should also be contoured to restore the normal cervical lordosis as much as is permitted.

The rectangle is then secured to the spine at as many points as possible using facet or sublaminar wires. When such wires cannot be placed, interspinous wires may be used in substitution.

Sublaminar wires are placed in the usual fashion. Each segment is prepared by separating the underlying ligament from the overlying lamina. A suture may then be carefully passed underneath the lamina. A double-ended cable is then bent in half, and one end of the suture is secured at the midpoint of the cable. The suture may then be used to help passage of the wire through the sublaminar space while tension is being applied to both ends of the wire simultaneously. This will prevent buckling of the wire during passage, which could result in compression of the underlying spinal cord. The wires are then looped around the bars of the overlying rectangle prior to being sequentially tightened.

Alternatively, facet wires can be used. Facet wires are applied in the manner previously described. Holes are made in the inferior articular process of each facet to allow passage of the wire or cable. It is recommended that at the most caudal level in the construct, the facet not be violated to prevent destabilization of the adjacent level. Facet wires and cables are then looped around the Luque rectangle and sequentially tightened to the appropriate tension.

Although a seemingly simple task, tightening the wires in a multilevel construct can be fraught with complications: overtightening wires and cables can lead to inadvertent fractures; tightening wires on one side of the construct can lead to the introduction of undesired torsional strain to the spine before fixation is completed; and tightening of one wire can result in loosening of an adjacent wire. To reduce such complications, wires should be tightened in a sequential fashion. Systems that allow wires or cables to be tightened with temporary stays is preferred, so that all wires can be gradually tightened to the optimal tension before being crimped and fastened.

COMPRESSION CLAMPS AND HOOK ROD CONSTRUCTS. When intact lamina and facet joints are present, clamps and hooks can be used instead of wires to help fixate the subaxial cervical spine. The best-known clamp device is the Halifax clamp. The use of this clamp was first described by Tucker (21) in 1975 for a posterior C1-2 arthrodesis. This device is applied typically over one motion segment bridging two adjacent intact lamina. Application requires only exposure of the lamina and the medial aspects of the adjacent facet joints. Prior to application, the posterior surfaces of the lamina are denuded with an air-powered drill, and an autologous bone graft is typically placed between the adjacent lamina to allow the clamp to be applied under compressive forces and to fix the interanchor distance. The interlaminar bone graft helps prevent hardware failure resulting from forces that may reduce the interanchor distance (Fig. 4). Clamps are typically applied bilaterally to reduce multiplanar instability and to prevent the introduction of any torsional strain with hardware application.

Alternatively opposing sulaminar hooks may be assembled to allow the application of similar compressive forces. The hooks are fixed to vertically oriented rods that are contoured to match the cervical lordosis. Hooks are rarely applied unilaterally because of complications related to the development of torsional strain. The application of bilateral hooks connected

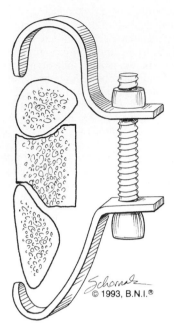

© 1993, B.N.I.®

Fig. 4. A sagittal view of the spine showing the relationship of a clamp device to the adjacent lamina and how an interlaminar bone graft helps to fix the interanchor distance when the clamp is secured. This is an important principle that is also used when applying sublaminar and interspinous wires to help fix the interanchor distance. (Courtesy of Barrow Neurological Institute, Phoenix, AZ.)

to rods and the use of cross-connectors provides the construct with adequate stability to torsional strain. Hooks are never assembled in a pure distraction mode because of the cervical spine's propensity to develop an abnormal kyphotic angulation.

Although hooks and clamps are more rigid constructs than constructs using wiring techniques, they suffer from similar biomechanical limitations. The absence of direct fixation to the spine and the reliance on a fixed interanchor distance to maintain tension in the construct make hooks and clamps prone to failure from an inability to resist extension effectively. A reduction of the interanchor distance with extension introduces laxity to the system, potentially leading to hardware failure. Although less biomechanically stable than lateral mass screws and plates, hooks and clamps have a role when anatomical limitations preclude the application of screws into the lateral masses.

LATERAL MASS PLATES. Lateral mass plates are the preferred technique because they do not require intact spinous processes or lamina for their application. They also provide superior stability with regard to torsion and flexion. Because of their superior biomechanical properties, the use of an external orthosis may be obviated postoperatively.

Lateral mass plates are not without disadvantages. Because of how the screws are placed in the lateral masses, there is the potential for injury to the adjacent nerve roots and the vertebral artery. Using the appropriate screw trajectory and assisted fluoroscopic guidance of screws helps to minimize the risk of these potential complications. Furthermore, because the construct's stability depends on the adequacy of the screw's purchase, patients with poor bone quality may not be able to achieve adequate results because of an inadequate screw bone interface. Screw pullout is a frequent mode of failure. To avoid screw pullout, the longest possible screws should be used, overdrill-

ling of holes with heated drills should be minimized, and tapping the hole with too large a tapping screw should be avoided. When the screw's purchase is compromised as in osteopenic patients, methylmethacrylate may be injected into the hole to augment its purchase.

To place lateral mass screws, a posterior exposure is performed in a fashion similar to that described for the Luque rectangle. Complete exposure of the entire lateral mass and facet joint should be achieved to optimally expose the required landmarks for screw placement at each level of fixation (Fig. 5A).

There are numerous described techniques used for placing screws safely into the lateral masses of the cervical spine. The original technique described by Roy-Camille et al. (6) describes placing screws in a trajectory through the midpoint of the lateral mass directed anteriorly and 10 degrees laterally. Since then, there have been numerous other techniques described for inserting lateral mass screws. Each technique differs based on its entry point and trajectory. Jeanneret et al. (22) described placing screws through the midpoint of the lateral mass directed 20 degrees cephalad and 10 degrees laterally. Magerl et al. (23) described using an entry point slightly medial and rostral to the midpoint of the lateral mass with a screw directed 25 degrees laterally and parallel to the facet joint in the sagittal plane. Anderson et al. (24) described using an entry point 1 mm medial to the midpoint of the lateral mass, with the screw directed 10 degrees laterally and 30 to 40 degrees rostrally in the sagittal plane. An et al. (23) described using an entry point 1 mm medial to the midpoint of the lateral mass with the screw directed 30 degrees laterally and 15 degrees rostrally in the sagittal plane. Which technique affords the lowest complication rate and the best screw purchase is clear. One anatomical study comparing different techniques on cadaveric specimens demonstrated a lower risk of nerve root damage due to overpenetration in drilling or insertion of too long of a screw (25).

All techniques for placing lateral mass screws are based on similar principles. Aiming cephalad helps to avoid penetration of the facet joint and potential injury to the underlying nerve root (Fig. 5B). Aiming laterally helps to avoid penetration of the foramen transversarium housing the vertebral artery (Fig. 5C). Anatomical studies demonstrate that the vertebral artery is typically located between 13 and 16 mm anterior to the posterior cortex of the adjacent lateral mass. Therefore, using screws smaller than 16 mm and aiming laterally is advocated to avoid complications related to vertebral artery injury (26,27).

Holes may be made with a hand drill or a powered drill. Use of a powered drill may impair the screw's purchase. Air-powered drills tend to produce significant yawl, which may unintentionally increase the size of the screw hole. Also heat transfer during drilling may impair the quality of the surrounding bone. Additionally the use of self-tapping screws or the use of a tap one size smaller than the size of the screw to be placed may help optimize the screw bone interface, increasing the screw's pullout strength. Typical screws used are 3.5 to 4.5 mm wide and 13 to 19 mm long. Although using a shorter screw reduces the risk of nerve root injury and vertebral artery injury, using a longer screw is preferred so a bicortical purchase through the lateral mass can be achieved.

When points of fixation need to be achieved at C7 or lower, pedicle screws are preferred because the lateral mass tends to be small at these levels. Placement of pedicle screws at C7 or lower is achieved using the inferior aspect of the facet joint as a landmark. Usually a point 1 mm inferior to the joint is used as an entry point (28). Because of potential complications related to adjacent root and cord injury, a small adjacent laminotomy to enable direct visualization of the adjacent pedicle is advised. This helps to ensure the screw is placed in an optimal orientation and trajectory.

Prior to placement of screws, an arthrodesis is performed.

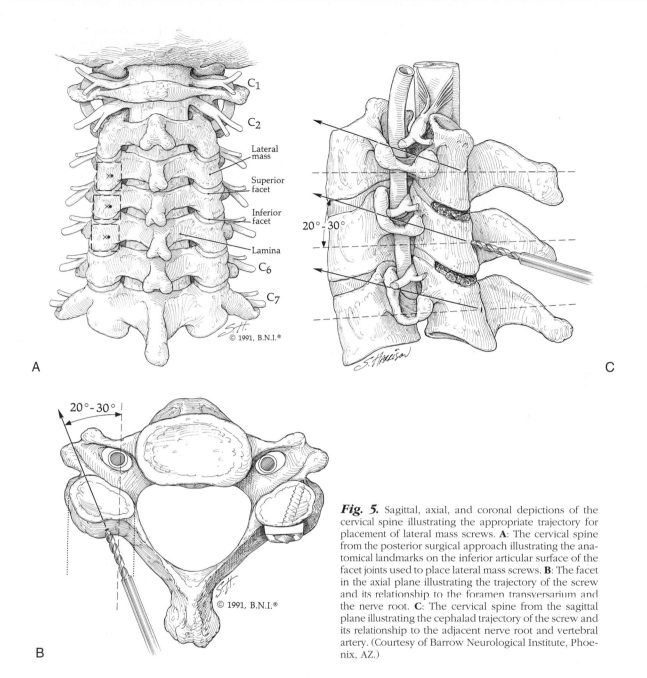

Fig. 5. Sagittal, axial, and coronal depictions of the cervical spine illustrating the appropriate trajectory for placement of lateral mass screws. **A**: The cervical spine from the posterior surgical approach illustrating the anatomical landmarks on the inferior articular surface of the facet joints used to place lateral mass screws. **B**: The facet in the axial plane illustrating the trajectory of the screw and its relationship to the foramen transversarium and the nerve root. **C**: The cervical spine from the sagittal plane illustrating the cephalad trajectory of the screw and its relationship to the adjacent nerve root and vertebral artery. (Courtesy of Barrow Neurological Institute, Phoenix, AZ.)

Arthrodesis is best achieved by removing the articular cartilage in the facet joints, decorticating the facet joint surfaces, and packing the joint with autologously harvested cancellous bone. Although some authors argue that when the primary condition is related to a traumatic fracture, an autologous bone fusion does not need to be performed, we do not recommend this.

Lateral mass screws may be used to either secure a rod or plate to the spine. Lateral mass plates are more commonly used (Fig. 6). Plates typically come in a variety of sizes to accommodate the variable alignment of screw holes. Plates are contoured to contact the underlying spine at as many points as possible. The plate should be contoured to maintain cervical lordosis. Because of difficulties related to aligning screw holes with the premanufactured plate, some advocate drilling holes in the lateral masses after placing the contoured plate over the spine to optimize screw plate alignment. Furthermore, some investigators argue that when screws are secured to the plate the lateral

mass may be pulled to the plate because of the fixed contour of the plate resulting in adjacent foraminal stenosis (29).

Newer systems use malleable rods. These systems allow easier assembly of the construct because the rod can be contoured in both the sagittal and coronal plane to accommodate the variable location of screws. Systems that use rods may also be stronger because the screw–rod interface is a more rigid interface, akin to a pedicle screw construct. Whereas lateral mass plates function more like a posterior tension band construct, screw and rod constructs may function more like a rigid cantilever beam fixation system. Furthermore, the screw and rod constructs are more versatile during their assembly; for example, rods can be extended into the proximal thoracic spine for direct connection to thoracic pedicle screws, cross-connectors that augment torsional stability can be easily integrated with the construct, and some systems have laminar hooks that can be integrated with the construct. Biomechanical testing still

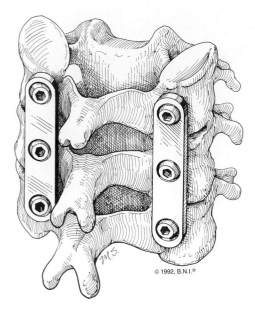

© 1992, B.N.I.®

Fig. 6. An assembled lateral mass plate construct in the cervical spine. (Courtesy of Barrow Neurological Institute, Phoenix, AZ.)

needs to be done to elucidate whether these newer systems are biomechanically superior.

Conclusions

Fixation of the subaxial cervical spine can be readily achieved with a variety of techniques. One can use wires, cables, clamps, plates, and rods to achieve stability of the subaxial cervical spine. All techniques have their appropriate indications and relevant contraindications. Understanding these limitations is important in the appropriate application of the above-described techniques. Frequently one may use a combination of the above techniques to improve results. For example, sublaminar wires can be used to help decrease load and stress experienced by screws at segmental points of fixation. Similarly, hooks placed at the termini of screw and rod constructs may help reduce the propensity for failure related to screw pullout. Being familiar with each technique ensures that the surgeon has more options at his disposal during surgery to accommodate the individual needs of the patient.

It must be emphasized that all methods of achieving internal fixation are only temporary means of stabilizing the cervical spine. Long-term stability is afforded only when a solid bone fusion is achieved. Successful fusion is not only a function of the stability of the fixation technique but also a direct function of the application of proper arthrodesis techniques. Adequate preparation of the spine for arthrodesis and the liberal use of autologously harvested bone is essential for long-term successful fusion.

References

1. Heller JG, Silcox DH: Postlaminectomy instability of the cervical spine. In: Frymoyer JW, ed. *The adult spine: principles and practice*, 2nd ed. Philadelphia: Lippincott-Raven, 1997.
2. Hadra BE: Wiring the vertebrae as a means of immobilization in fractures and Pott's disease. *Trans Am Orthop Assoc* 4:206, 1891.
3. White AA, Panjabi MM: Biomechanical considerations in the surgical management of the spine. In: White AA, Panjabi MM, eds. *Clinical biomechanics of the spine*. Philadelphia: J.B. Lippincott, 1990.
4. Yoganandan N, Halliday AL, Dickman CA, et al.: In: Benzel EC, ed. *Practical anatomy and fundamental biomechanics in spine surgery*. New York: Churchill Livingstone 1999:93–118.
5. Denis F: The three column spine and its significance in the classification of acute thoracolumbar spinal injuries. *Spine* 8:817–831, 1983.
6. Roy-Camille R, Saillant G, Mazel C: Internal fixation of the unstable cervical spine by posterior osteosynthesis with plates and screws. In: Cervical Spine Research Society, eds. *The cervical spine*, 2nd ed. Philadelphia: JB Lippincott, 1989:390–396.
7. Wellman BJ, Follett KA, Traynelis VC: Complications of articular mass plate fixation of the subaxial cervical spine in 44 consecutive patients. *Spine* 23(2):193–200, 1998.
8. Rizzolo SJ, Vaccaro AR, Cotler JM, et al.: Intervertebral disc injury complicating cervical spine trauma. *Spine* 16S:187–189, 1991.
9. Bucholz RD, Cheung KC: Halo vest versus spinal fusion for cervical injury: evidence from an outcome study. *J Neurosurg* 70:884–892, 1989.
10. Sonntag VKH, Hadley MN: Nonoperative management of cervical spine injuries. *Clin Neurosurg* 34:630–649, 1988.
11. Raynor RB, Pugh J, Shapiro I: Cervical facetectomy and its effect on spine strength. *J Neurosurg* 63:278–282, 1985.
12. Bell DF, Walker JL, O'Connor G, et al.: Spinal deformity after multiple level cervical laminectomy in children. *Spine* 19:406–411, 1994.
13. Herman JM, Sonntag VKH: Cervical corpectomy and plate fixation for postlaminectomy kyphosis. *J Neurosurg* 80:963–970, 1994.
14. Sawin PD, Todd MM, Traynelis VC, et al.: Cervical spine motion with direct laryngoscopy and orotracheal intubation: an in vivo cinefluoroscopic study of subjects without cervical pathology. *Anesthesiology* 85:26–36, 1996.
15. Rogers WA: Treatment of fracture dislocations of the cervical spine. *J Bone Joint Surg* 24A:245–258, 1942.
16. Whitehall R, Reger SI, Fox E, et al.: The use of methylmethacrylate cement as an instantaneous fusion mass in posterior cervical fusions. A canine in vivo experimental model. *Spine* 9:246–252, 1984.
17. Benzel EC, Kesterson L: Posterior cervical interspinous compression wiring and fusion for mid to low cervical spine injuries. *J Neurosurg* 70:893–899, 1989.
18. Bohlman HH: Acute fractures and dislocations of the cervical spine. An analysis of three hundred hospitalized patients and review of the literature. *J Bone Joint Surg* 61A:1119–1142, 1979.
19. Cahill DW, Bellegarrigue R, Ducker TB: Bilateral facet to spinous process fusion. A new technique for posterior fusion after trauma. *Neurosurgery* 13:1–4, 1983.
20. Callahan RA, Johnson RM, Margolis RM, et al.: Cervical facet fusion for control of instability following laminectomy. *J Bone Joint Surg* 59A:991–1002, 1977.
21. Tucker HH: Technical report: method of fixation of subluxed or dislocated cervical spine below C1-2. *Can J Neurol Sci* 2:381–382, 1975.
22. Jeanneret B, Magerl F, Ward EH, et al.: Posterior stabilization of the cervical spine with hook plates. *Spine* 16(suppl 3):S56–S63, 1991.
23. An HS, Gordin R, Renner K: Anatomic considerations for plate-screw fixation of the cervical spine. *Spine* 16:552–557, 1991.
24. Anderson PA, Hanely MB, Grady MS, et al.: Posterior cervical arthrodesis with AO reconstruction plates and bone graft. *Spine* 16(suppl 3):S72–S79, 1991.
25. Xu R, Haman SP, Ebraheim NA, et al.: The anatomic relationship of lateral mass screws to the spinal nerves. A comparison of the Magerl, Anderson, and An techniques. *Spine* 24:2057–2061, 1999.
26. Ebraheim NA, Klauser T, Xu R, et al.: Safe lateral mass screw lengths in the Roy Camille and Magerl techniques. An anatomical study. *Spine* 23:1739–1742, 1998.
27. Heller JG, Carlson GD, Abitbol JJ, et al.: Anatomic comparison of the Roy Camille and Magerl techniques for screw placement in the lower cervical spine. *Spine* 16(suppl 10):S552–S557, 1991.
28. Sawin PD, Sonntag VKH: Techniques of posterior subaxial cervical fusion. *Oper Tech Neurosurg* 1(2):72–83, 1998.
29. Heller SG, Silcox DH, Sutterlin CE III: Complications of posterior cervical plating. *Spine* 20:2442–2448, 1995.

205. Cervical Graft Options

**Frank Feigenbaum and
Fraser C. Henderson**

The concept of bone grafting is by no means recent, with early attempts beginning over 500 years ago in the Arab, Peruvian, and Aztec cultures. The first successful attempt at fusion to be recorded in English-language medical literature was performed in 1878 by MacEwan, a student of Lister. Later, in 1911, Albee (1) reported on the transplantation of a portion of the tibia into the spine for Pott's disease. These pioneers, and others such as Barth, Marchand, and Axhausen, have advanced our understanding of fusion to the currently held view that transplanted bone undergoes a process of revascularization and substitution by autologous elements. In 1965, Urist (2) ushered the concept of fusion into the molecular realm by proposing the theory of osteoinduction, in which morphogenetic proteins stimulate perivascular mesenchymal cells to disaggregate, migrate into the area of an implant, reaggregate, proliferate, and differentiate into cartilage and bone.

The Biology of Fusion

Incorporation of a nonvascularized autologous (autogeneic) bone graft involves successive phases of hematoma formation, inflammatory response induction, host blood vessel ingrowth, and formation of fibrovascular stroma by fibroblastic cells. Autogenous bone grafts and some graft substitutes, such as coralline hydroxyapatite, are considered *osteoconductive* because they facilitate fusion by providing a structural scaffolding or framework for vascular ingrowth. Fresh autogenous bone is also, to a certain extent, *osteogenic* as it provides a limited supply of living cells. While the majority of cells within grafted bone do not survive, some osteoblasts, osteocytes, periosteal cells, and osteoclasts do survive by diffusion of nutrients from the surrounding host tissue. Processed and banked allograft provides no such osteogenic potential.

The ability of graft-derived factors to stimulate the ingrowth of bone forming elements, and to induce osteoprogenitor cell differentiation is called *osteoinductivity*. This phenomenon appears to be largely the result of noncollagenous proteins, collectively termed bone morphogenetic proteins (BMPs), which are found in extremely small quantities in bone mineral, extracellular matrix, and cytoplasm. BMP is inactivated by exposure to temperatures greater than 60°C, dehydration, irradiation, alkalinity, and chemicals such as hydrogen peroxide (3).

As precursors to bone formation penetrate the graft, the *morphogenetic phase* begins. This phase is characterized by cell disaggregation, migration into the graft, reaggregation, and proliferation (4). As a result, fibroblast-like mesenchymal cells recruited from the host aggregate in the graft scaffolding, proliferate, and undergo cytodifferentiation into chondroblasts, chondrocytes, osteoblasts, and osteocytes.

Primary membranous bone is then formed near the graft–host interface. Small osteoid seams form near trabeculae, and variable amounts of cartilage form between pieces of bone graft, leading to subsequent enchondral ossification. Presumably, the pattern of cartilage and bone formation reflects differing oxygen gradients within the graft. Chondroid tissue grows where blood supply is poor, and bone forms where blood supply is adequate.

In the second week, the inflammatory process diminishes and fibrous granulation tissue invades the graft bed. Blood vessels grow into the Volkmann's canals of cancellous bone over weeks, and penetrate into cortical bone over months. As the graft becomes progressively more vascularized, cartilaginous and cancellous regions undergo a process of gradual dissolution and replacement, termed *creeping substitution*. Decortication of host cortical bone improves the flow of nutrients and osteoprogenitor cells into the graft and is critical in facilitating creeping substitution.

A *woven bone* matrix consisting of collagenous macromolecules and calcium phosphate is then secreted by trabeculae-bound osteoblasts. As woven bone is produced, there is gradual growth of trabeculae from the periphery into the central necrotic zone of the graft (5). The trabeculae thicken at the expense of intervening connective tissue to produce primary spongiosa, or "spongy bone." Osteoblasts trapped within newly formed bone undergo transformation into osteocytes interconnected by a network of canaliculi.

In the middle, or *reparative phase*, of bone fusion, vascularization increases, necrotic bone is resorbed, and differentiation of osteoprogenitor cells into osteoblasts and chondroblasts continues. The rate of vascularization within cancellous and cortical regions of a graft differs because the more porous nature of cancellous bone allows for rapid invasion of blood vessels. Additionally, the larger number of surviving endosteal cells in cancellous bone may contribute to formation of end-to-end vascular anastomoses.

Experimentally, it can be demonstrated that cortical bone grafts undergo a prolonged bone *resorption phase* that causes a reduction in graft strength. Animal studies have demonstrated that fibular grafts initially weaken over the first 6 to 24 weeks, and return to normal strength by 2 years (6). At the cellular level, this phase is typified by increased osteoclastic activity stimulated, in part, by BMP released from devitalized bone.

In the late, or *remodeling phase*, small portions of the cortical rim surrounding the fusion undergo remodeling. Trabeculae continue to grow from the rim into the center of the graft, thereby increasing the volume of spongiosa bone. The marrow volume increases, largely at the expense of grafted cancellous bone. Despite activity within cancellous portions of the graft, most of the grafted cortical bone remains unremodeled donor tissue.

Eventual remodeling occurs primarily in response to loading forces placed on the graft. The primary lattice of trabeculae laid down in the spongiosa bone becomes thickened around vascular channels, forming primitive haversian systems. Scattered points of bone then undergo osteoclastic erosion, and form long cylindrical cavities called lacunae. Osteoclastic activity in the lacunae then decreases, and osteoblastic activity resumes with the laying down of concentric lamellae of bone in secondary haversian systems. This process of internal bone destruction and reconstruction continues over several generations of haversian systems. At any time, a cross section through mature bone will show osteons in various stages of development.

The events of allograft incorporation are similar to those for autografts. New bone formation tends to occur peripherally at the host–graft interface, with lesser amounts of new osteoid formation occurring within the necrotic center. Strictly speaking, the assessment of a successful fusion requires the presence of lamellar bone and definitive haversian systems. Bone that is not stressed remains disordered and is more likely to fracture. A concern with rigid spine instrumentation is the effect of "stress shielding," which shields grafted bone from intervertebral stress forces, and causes weakening by preventing the formation of definitive haversian systems.

Immunogenicity

Immunogenicity plays a critical role in the incorporation of grafted bone, particularly when allogeneic bone is used. After placement of a bone graft, its incorporation will continue along one of three paths: acceptance as genetically similar, acceptance as having only minor disparity, or rejection. Up to 10% of allogeneic grafts are immunogenically incompatible, although it is uncertain how many of these grafts fail to fuse as a result of their incompatibility.

Presumably, the difference in incorporation rate between allograft and autograft relates in part to the immunogenic disparities between grafted material and host.

The importance of immunohistocompatibility has been demonstrated in animal studies where allografts are more successfully incorporated between closely matched dogs than in those where major histocompatibility barriers exist (7). Despite the fact that allograft material is freeze-dried to reduce its antigenicity, weakly reactive antigens such as cell surface glycoproteins, bone collagen, and noncollagenous proteins remain. Other immunogenic entities, such as osteocytes and osteoblasts within lacunae, are partially sequestered from the immune reactive T cells and the cytotoxic antibodies of the host. Using microtoxicity studies, Friedlaender (8) was able to demonstrate the presence of graft-specific anti–human leukocyte antigen (HLA) antibodies in 21% of recipients of corticocancellous grafts within 4 to 7 weeks of surgery (8). Suffice to say, immunohistocompatibility responses, though generally ignored by clinicians, probably play a significant role in the successful incorporation of allogeneic bone graft.

Autograft Versus Allograft

When should autograft be used as opposed to allograft? When properly prepared by disc removal and decortication, the compressive environment found in the intervertebral space is conducive to the incorporation of both autologous and allogeneic bone. While successful fusion is largely determined by the condition of the recipient site and host systemic factors, slightly higher rates of fusion have been obtained with autologous grafts (83% to 97%) versus allografts (79% to 92%) (9,10). Presumably, autologous bone grafts are slightly superior as they are more immune compatible with the host. They also possess a higher osteogenic potential since they contain viable cells, undenatured matrix, and active osteoinductive factors.

In comparison, the osteogenic properties of allogeneic bone are substantially diminished, largely due to the processing it undergoes to reduce immunogenicity after harvest. Allogeneic bone is thoroughly rinsed with high-pressure water and ethylene oxide or antibiotic solution, freeze-dried in a vacuum for 10 days at −80°C, and often exposed to 30 cGy of radiation. Due to the damage to collagenous proteins, this process impacts on structural integrity of the graft by causing a 10% loss in compression strength and 70% loss of torsional strength (11). Additionally, freeze-dried allogeneic bone is brittle and must be rehydrated before use to restore its elasticity. Failure to do so may cause graft fracture after implantation. After processing, allografts can be stored for up to 5 years provided that vacuum packaging is maintained.

Despite the apparent superiority of autograft, there are important advantages to the use of allogeneic grafts. Such advantages include the avoidance of graft harvest related morbidity, and reduction in both operative time and length of hospital stay due to earlier patient mobilization (10). Furthermore, allogeneic grafts may be preferable when the patient is very young, osteopenic, or known to have bone metastases. Smoking adversely affects the success rate of fusion, particularly that of allograft (9).

Graft Alternatives

RIB GRAFT. Autogenous rib harvest can provide a ready source of long, curved grafts that are well suited for cervical spine fusion. In the author's experience, rib graft harvesting is simple, efficient, and safe. The low morbidity of rib grafting is well documented in the literature. In one series of 28 patients with 31 rib grafts, patients were mobilized within 24 hours. There were no instances of pneumothorax, wound infection, long-term pain, or unacceptable scarring (12). In another series of 300 patients, donor-site morbidity was reported in 3.7% of patients, including pneumonia, persistent atelectasis, and superficial wound dehiscence (13). This morbidity rate compares favorably with the 25% morbidity rate associated with iliac crest graft harvest (13). Furthermore, some studies cite higher rates of fusion with rib graft (98%) when compared with iliac crest graft (94%) (13). The superior rate of successful fusion with rib grafts is thought to be due to its higher BMP content (13). While rib grafts are generally employed in posterior fusion, they are also useful in lateral and anterior fusions. Two ribs wired side to side make an excellent graft for fusion following anterior corpectomy.

Rib graft material can be obtained with the patient supine, prone, or lateral. With the patient prone, a 6-cm incision is made in the subscapular region along Langer's lines to minimize postoperative scarring (Fig. 1A). The incision is carried through the subcutaneous tissues to the trapezius muscle. An attempt is made to leave each muscular layer intact, minimizing the muscle dissection necessary to gain adequate exposure. The lateral third of the trapezius muscle is divided, and the rest retracted medially. The accessory nerve is found under the midportion of the muscle and preserved.

The latissimus dorsi is split along the grain of the muscle fibers, which run upward and laterally at the level of the 8th rib. While a few fibers of this muscle attach to the scapula, the bulk of the latissimus should run below the angle of the scapula, then ascend to insert upon the humerus. Injury to the long thoracic nerve, which causes adduction of the arm, should be avoided by retracting the latissimus fibers superomedially and inferolaterally. The nerve descends along the posterior axillary line and swings inferomedially to innervate the bulk of the latissimus muscle. Division of the latissimus muscle is performed only if further exposure is needed. It is useful to have an assistant retract the muscle with an army-navy retractor.

The ribs to be dissected are then palpated through the overlying serratus posticus inferior fascia, muscle, and periosteum. These layers are divided with electrocautery and elevated with an Alexander periosteal elevator along the upper and lower edges of the rib. The opposite end of the Alexander is then applied closely to the rib to elevate the external intercostal muscle, the underlying middle intercostal membrane, and the inter-

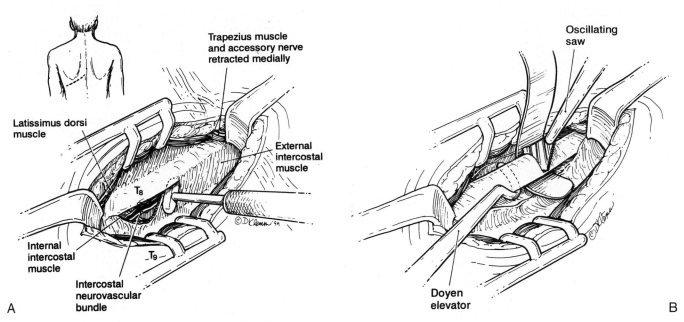

Fig. 1. **A**: Rib exposure. **B**: Rib graft harvest.

costal vein, artery, and nerve. Maintaining a subperiosteal plane helps to avoid injury to the pleura.

A Doyen rib raspatory completes the stripping of tissue from the rib throughout the length required (Fig. 1B). The rib is cut using Stille rib shears or a sagittal saw. The author generally removes two adjacent rib segments through the same incision. In children, however, adjacent ribs should not be taken due to the risk of delayed spinal deformity.

A spatula should be used to protect the pleura when sewing or using the sagittal saw. If a tear in the pleura is incurred, a primary closure should be performed while placing the lungs under continuous positive airway pressure to help maintain lung expansion. A no. 10 red rubber catheter can be placed through the tear into the pleural cavity until the conclusion of the surgery, then carefully removed. The wound is then flooded with saline and a Valsalva maneuver performed to demonstrate the absence of air leakage. If a chest tube is necessary, it should be placed through a separate incision.

From the anterior approach, ribs can be harvested in women through an inframammary incision, or in men through an anterior axillary incision, where the ribs are relatively more superficial.

ILIAC CREST GRAFT HARVEST

Anterior Iliac Crest Approach. With the patient supine, exposure of the iliac crest is facilitated by placing padding under the hip. The medial boundary of the iliac crest (anterior superior iliac spine) is determined by palpation. A 4-cm skin incision is made paralleling the palpated iliac prominence beginning at least 3 cm lateral to the anterior superior iliac spine (Fig. 2A). Injury is thereby avoided to the insertions of both the inguinal ligament and sartorius muscle, and to the lateral femoral cutaneous nerve, which occasionally exits the pelvis over the iliac crest (14). With lean individuals having prominent iliac crests, incisional tension and postoperative wound dehiscence can be avoided by placing the incision on a parallel line 1 to 2 cm inferior to the palpated iliac prominence.

After the skin and subcutaneous tissues are dissected, the fascia directly overlying the iliac crest is divided and reflected away from the iliac crest using a periosteal elevator. After placing a self-retaining retractor, the iliacus muscle underlying the graft is carefully dissected free. In so doing, the muscle and abdominal wall are retracted medially to prevent peritoneal perforation. The ilioinguinal and iliohypogastric nerves lie near the dissection within the fascia over the iliacus muscle and should be carefully avoided. Avoid excessive muscle dissection to minimize blood loss and prevent weakening of the hip musculature.

With an oscillating saw, two perpendicular cuts are made in the exposed anterior ilium to a depth of 2 cm (Fig. 2B). There should be an adequate margin between these cuts and the anterior superior iliac spine to prevent weakening and fracture of the ilium. A curved osteotome and mallet are then used to gently cleave the tricortical bone graft free at its base.

Meticulous hemostasis must be obtained by cauterizing bleeding vessels and waxing exposed bone edges. Failure to do so may result in substantial blood loss, postoperative pain, and wound breakdown. If desired, the cosmetic integrity of the bone defect can be reconstituted with antibiotic-impregnated methylmethacrylate. The fascial layer is then reapproximated tightly using interrupted 0-Vicryl sutures to prevent herniation of abdominal musculature. A medium-size drain is placed above the fascial layer through a separate incision and the superficial layers are closed.

Final modifications in graft dimensions are made with the oscillating saw or high-speed drill. The graft can be stored in cold saline for a short time, but it is best to perform the harvest near the end of the surgical procedure to limit cell death and possible contamination.

Posterior Iliac Crest Approach. With the patient prone, the medial (posterior superior iliac spine) and lateral (iliac crest) boundaries of the ilium are palpated. An incision is made over the iliac prominence beginning at the posterior superior iliac crest and extending laterally no more than 8 cm. Injury to the cluneal nerves coursing over the posterior iliac crest is thereby

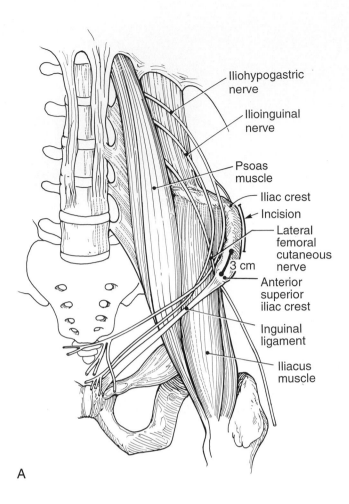

A

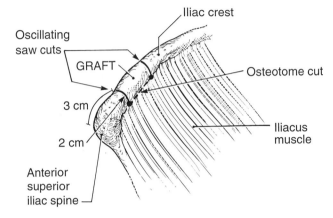

Fig. 2. **A**: Anterior iliac crest anatomy. **B**: Graft harvest. (© 2002, Thomas H. Weinzerl.)

B

avoided (9) (Fig. 3). The subcutaneous tissues are dissected and retracted to expose the fascial layer overlying the iliac crest.

Beginning at the posterior superior iliac spine, the fascia is divided proceeding laterally over the iliac crest. The iliacus muscle underlying the graft is dissected away carefully to prevent peritoneal perforation. Similarly, overlying gluteus musculature is stripped away carefully to avoid damage to the gluteal artery. Ligamentous structures are preserved to prevent destabilization of the sacroiliac joint.

As in the anterior approach, two perpendicular cuts can be made into the iliac crest to a depth of 2-cm using an oscillating saw. The sciatic notch is avoided medially to prevent injury of the superior gluteal nerve and vessels, ureter, and sacroiliac ligaments. In the event of gluteal vessel injury, the sciatic notch can be unroofed in order to ligate the gluteal artery. If this is not possible, the patient can be turned to the supine position for transabdominal vessel control and ligation. Blind attempts at stopping bleeding without adequate exposure are likely to cause further injury to nearby structures and, potentially, death from blood loss.

A curved osteotome and mallet are used to gently sever the bone graft at its base, and meticulous hemostasis is obtained. It is also possible to remove the outer table of the ilium harvesting cortical-cancellous bone and cancellous bone, preserving the inner table if nonstructural graft is needed. This is more common in posterior procedures. Wound closure and drain placement are similar to those of the anterior approach. The potential complications of the anterior and posterior approaches are listed in Table 1.

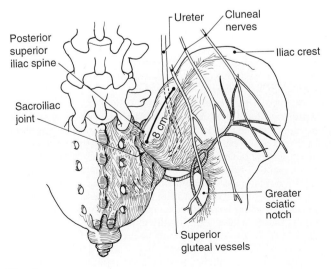

Fig. 3. Posterior iliac crest anatomy. (© 2002, Thomas H. Weinzerl.)

Table 1. Potential Complications of Iliac Crest Graft Harvest

Anterior approach
  Persistent postoperative pain
  Later femoral cutaneous nerve injury (dysesthesia, meralgia paresthetica)
  Ilioinguinal nerve injury
  Cosmetic deformity
  Infection/osteomyelitis
  Tension dehiscence of wound
  Iliac crest fracture
  Peritoneal perforation
  Fascial hernia
  Weakening due to excessive muscular dissection
Posterior approach
  Persistent postoperative pain
  Superior cluneal nerve injury
  Gluteal vessel injury
  Infection
  Ureteral injury
  Peritoneal perforation
  Fascial hernia
  Sacroiliac joint destabilization

Bone Graft Substitutes

DEMINERALIZED BONE MATRIX. Several patented procedures now exist for the demineralization of allogenic bone. This process serves to expose osteoinductive proteins and remove infectious elements. While experiments have shown that demineralized bone (DMB) products have osteoinductive potential in some animals, DBM has not demonstrated the ability to induce new bone formation without the presence of autogenous graft in humans. In this respect, humans are similar to dogs and monkeys in that they lack the ability to form new bone in a DMB matrix. However, DMB does serve as an excellent "bone graft extender." On occasions when we have reexplored graft sites where DBM was used in conjunction with autogenous bone, a more solid and homogeneous appearance of the graft was found.

DBM has also been found to be an excellent "carrier" substrate in experimental studies with monkeys, where its use with bone protein extracts provides a stronger and stiffer fusion than that of autograft (5). Other advantages to DBM include its lack of immunogenicity and low risk of disease transmission.

POROUS (Coralline) HYDOXYAPATITE. Hydroxyapatite (HA) is a hydroxylated derivative of calcium phosphate that normally constitutes 65% of bone matrix. Through a patented hydrothermal process, the calcium carbonate of specific marine coral can be converted to HA suitable for use in grafting.

As a graft substitute, coralline HA offers a negligible risk of disease transmission and is antigenically inert (15). Unlike allograft, it is reabsorbed very slowly, thereby allowing a greater time period for incorporation into the host. The inherent interconnected porosity of coralline HA mimics that of bone (16), an important attribute since studies have shown that graft porosities of 100 to 500 μm are essential for osteoconduction. Despite its high porosity, coralline HA possesses similar strength to posterior iliac crest coticocancellous graft when placed under compression. However, like all ceramics, coral is more brittle and relies on the ingrowth of bone for incorporation. In long bones, coralline HA appears to heal radiographically within 4 to 5 months and enjoys a 95% incorporation rate at 12 months (17).

Coralline HA can serve as a carrier for osteoinductive proteins, such as bovine-derived growth factor extract, which it binds tightly. Such a combination prevents heterotopic calcification and promotes accelerated absorption as new bone is formed (17). Histometric studies have demonstrated that coralline HA is resorbed at a rate of 5% to 10% per year, and that it possesses an osteoinduction index (volume fraction of new bone growth into the coral graft) of 55%. These attributes qualify coralline HA as an osteoconductive vehicle for new bone growth.

A major limitation to the use of coralline HA is its inability to function alone as a graft substitute in most posterolateral spinal applications. However, it has been used alone successfully in more vascular environments, such as the tibial femoral metaphysis (17). Also, when mixed 1:1 with autogenous iliac crest bone graft, it serves as an excellent graft extender.

Animal and human studies have demonstrated the relative efficacy of coralline HA in interbody and corpectomy sites. In the goat model, coralline HA was less effective than autograft for cervical fusion following discectomy (18). The importance of limiting motion at the coral host interface to achieve fusion was stressed. Others have demonstrated excellent fusion rates with coralline HA. In a retrospective, nonrandomized study, a 100% incorporation rate was established radiographically in 25 patients who underwent fusion with coralline HA and anterior plate stabilization following anterior cervical discectomy (19).

SYNTHETIC HYDROXYAPATITE IMPLANTS. A number of synthetic, or noncoralline, HA implants are currently available for use in the cervical spine following discectomy. They are durable, biomechanically stable, and possess a chemically determined porosity designed to provide maximum strength. Unlike autogeneic grafts, they do not collapse, thereby maintaining spinal alignment after implantation. Kim et al. (20) used synthetic HA in 64 cases, and a single instance of implant dislocation was the only complication.

However, synthetic HA implants offer no osteoinductivity and little osteoconductivity. Their success relies on the growth of bone around the implant rather than through it. Despite their extremely slow rate of bioabsorption and the lack of substantial bone growth into the ceramic, synthetic HA implants offer a reasonable alternative to the use of autogeneic graft.

Recombinant Human Bone Morphogenetic Protein-2 (rhBMP-2)

While still in the experimental phase of development, studies in goats and monkeys have demonstrated the efficacy of rhBMP-2 in promoting bone fusion following discectomy in the cervical and lumbar spine. Similarly, the use of collagen soaked in rhBMP-2 results in accelerated arthrodesis and significantly higher fusion rates (21). The ease with which arthrodesis might be performed using BMP is alluring, but to date, the safety and efficacy of rhBMP-2 in humans has not been established.

Conclusions

Our understanding of bone fusion is increasing rapidly, as is the number of surgical grafting options. However, the large number of options available should not draw the surgeon away from first considering whether fusion is really necessary. The benefits of fusing adjacent cervical spine segments always come at a price: cervical spine biomechanics are altered, degenerative changes are accelerated at adjacent motion segments, and normal range of motion is hindered. We suggest a critical analysis of each case to determine whether fusion will be in the long-term best interests of the patient.

References

1. Albee FH. Transplantation of a portion of the tibia into the spine for Pott's disease. *JAMA* 57:885–886, 1911.
2. Urist MR. Bone: formation by autoinduction. *Science* 150:893–899, 1965.
3. Urist MR. Bone morphogenetic protein, bone regeneration, heterotopic ossification and the bone bone-marrow consortium. In: Peck WA, ed. *Bone and mineral research*, vol 6. Amsterdam: Elsevier, 57–112, 1989.
4. Urist MR, Delange RJ, Finerman GAM. Bone cell differentiation and growth factors. *Science* 220:680–686, 1983.
5. Boden SD, Schimandle JH, Hutton WC. The use of an osteoinductive growth factor for lumbar spinal fusion. Part II: study of dose, carrier and species. *Spine* 20:2633–2644, 1995.
6. Burchardt H, Glowczewskie FP, Enneking WF. Allogenic segmental fibular transplants in azathioprine immunosuppressed dogs. *J Bone Joint Surg* 59A:881, 1977.
7. Goldberg VM, Powell A, Schaffer JW, et al. Bone grafting: role of histocompatibility in transplantation. *J Orthop Res* 3:389–404, 1985.
8. Friedlaender GE. Immune responses to osteochondral allografts. Current knowledge and future directions. *Clin Orthop Rel Res* 174:58–68, 1983.
9. Bishop RC, Moore KA, Hadley MN. Anterior cervical interbody fusion using autogeneic and allogeneic bone graft substrate: a prospective comparative analysis. *J Neurosurg* 85:206–210, 1996.
10. Zdeblik TA, Ducker TB. The use of freeze-dried allograft bone for anterior cervical fusions. *Spine* 16:726–729, 1991.
11. Pelker RR, Friedlander GE, Markham TC. Biomechanical properties of bone allografts. *Clin Orthop* 174:54–57, 1983.
12. Scouteris CA, Sotereanos GC. Donor morbidity following harvesting of autogenous rib grafts. *J Oral Maxillofac Surg* 47:808–812, 1989.
13. Sawin PD, Traynellis VC, Menezes AH. A comparative analysis of fusion rates and donor site morbidity for autogeneic rib and iliac crest bone grafts in posterior cervical fusions. *J Neurosurg* 2: 255–265, 1998.
14. Kurz LT, Garfin SR, Booth RE. Harvesting autologous iliac bone grafts: a review of complications and techniques. *Spine* 14: 1324–1331, 1989.
15. Mooney V, Holmes R. A new bone graft substitute. In: Uthoff HK, ed. *Current concepts of external fixation of fractures*. Berlin: Springer-Verlag, 425–431, 1982.
16. White E, Shors EC. Biomaterials aspects of Interpore-200 porous hydroxyapatite. *Dent Clin North Am* 30:49–67, 1986.
17. Boden SD, Martin GJ Jr, Morone M, et al. The use of coralline hydroxyapatite with bone marrow, autogenous bone graft, or osteoinductive bone protein extract for posterolateral lumbar spine fusion. *Spine* 24:320–327, 1999.
18. Zdeblic TA, Cooke ME, Kunz DN, et al. Anterior cervical discectomy and fusion using a porous hydroxyapatite bone graft substitute. *Spine* 19:2348–2357, 1994.
19. Thalgott JS, Fritz K, Giuffre J, et al. Anterior interbody fusion of the cervical spine with coralline hydroxyapatite. *Spine* 24:1295–1299, 1999.
20. Kim P, Wakai S, Matsuo S, et al. Bisegmental cervical interbody fusion using hydroxyapatite implants: Surgical results and long-term observation in 70 cases. *J Neurosurg* 88:21–27, 1998.
21. Zdeblic TA, Ghanayem AJ, Rapoff AJ, et al. Cervical interbody fusion cages. An animal model with and without bone morphogenetic protein. *Spine* 23:758–766, 1998.

206. Anterior Cervical Plating

**Charles A. Wolff,
Michael P. B. Kilburn, and
Mark N. Hadley**

The use of anterior cervical plate and screw constructs as adjuncts to anterior cervical spine fusion procedures has gained increasing popularity in recent years and can be of important anatomical and biomechanical benefit to selected patients. This chapter describes the surgical technique of plate and screw insertion and discusses the indications, potential benefits, and potential pitfalls of its use.

Historical Perspective

Wolfgang Caspar (1) of Austria described in 1981 his experience with the use of a metallic anterior cervical plate as an internal fixation device to facilitate bony fusion and reconstruction following anterior cervical spinal procedures. He advocated spanning an intervertebral space at which an anterior cervical fusion

procedure had been performed following discectomy or vertebrectomy, with a contoured stainless steel internal fixation plate, affixed to the vertebral segments above and below with bicortical screws, to provide strength to the operated spinal segments and to promote bony fusion. While other surgeons also experimented with this concept and various devices, primarily in Europe, Caspar was the first to describe their application and potential in detail, and is credited with popularizing their use in contemporary clinical practice. Today, dozens of anterior cervical fixation plate/screw devices are commercially available and are utilized hundreds to thousands of times each day in North America.

Use and Utilization

Advocates and manufacturers of anterior cervical internal fixation plate/screw implants argue that their application is safe,

Table 1. Complications of Anterior Cervical Plating

Authors	Year	Number treated	Number of complications	Percent complications
Gassman and Seligson	1983	13	2	15.4
Lesoin et al.	1984	145	2	1.4
De Olivera	1987	40	1	2.5
Tippets and Apfelbaum	1988	28	1	3.6
Caspar et al.	1989	260	17	6.5
Suh et al.	1990	13	1	7.7
Aebi et al.	1991	86	1	1.2
Ripa et al.	1991	92	3	3.3
Kostuik et al.	1993	42	7	16.7
Connolly et al.	1996	25	4	16.0
Shapiro	1997	195	1	0.5
McLaughlin et al.	1997	64	1	1.6
Bose	1998	97	11	11.3
Heidecke et al.	1998	96	12	12.5

effective, and efficacious. While this is true in general, it is not universally true and correct in all clinical settings.

Whatever the clinical circumstance, the safety of inserting an anterior cervical plate and securing it to two vertebral bodies is not 100%; the added risk of its use is not zero. There is considerable experience with the use of anterior cervical internal fixation devices reported in the neurosurgical literature (2–23). While it is difficult to disassociate the potential complications of anterior cervical spinal surgery—recurrent laryngeal nerve palsy, wound infections, postoperative radiculopathy, and myelopathy—from the exposure, decompression, and fusion portions of the procedure, many complications that have occurred following these procedures have been attributed to plate/screw application specifically. Dural laceration and/or neurological injury (root or cord) from overpenetration of bicortical screws, vertebral body fracture, screw back-out, esophageal perforation, screw fracture, plate fracture or migration, and injury to an adjacent disc space or vertebra are examples. While the incidence of these complications is relatively low, they have been reported even in the most straightforward of cases (Table 1) (8, 10–12,14,15,17–20,24–33).

When properly utilized and correctly applied, anterior cervical plate/screw constructs are effective internal fixators of the treated cervical spinal segments. Utilized as an adjunct to cervical spinal reconstruction following attempted bony stabilization at an intervertebral disc space following diskectomy, or bridging one or more vertebral bodies following vertebrectomy, the addition of an anterior cervical plate/screw fixation device provides significant biomechanical buttress and support to the cervical spine. Biomechanical studies indicate that anterior cervical plate constructs can add substantial stiffness to the cervical spine following attempted fusion procedures, particularly in flexion and extension, and virtually eliminate the need for postoperative external fixators and orthoses (34–39).

Four types of plate-screw systems exist and differ with respect to rigidity at the plate-screw interface. A nonconstrained system allows nonrigid binding of the screw to the plate and allows for the greatest freedom of screw trajectory with maximal potential graft loading. For long-term stability, however, a nonconstrained system requires bicortical screw purchase. The potential pitfalls of a nonconstrained system include an increased likelihood of screw back-out when bicortical purchase is suboptimal, and toggle of the plate on the screws with resultant loos-

ening of the construct. The constrained system design produces a rigid screw-plate interface, which does not yield except at failure. The rigidity of the system limits the variability of screw trajectory and may stress shield the graft, potentially reducing the likelihood of successful arthrodesis. A semiconstrained system provides semirigid binding of the screw to the plate, which provides for a greater range of screw trajectory than the constrained system, but potentially increases the potential for toggle of the plate on the screws. Modern semiconstrained systems have a very low propensity for screw back-out. Last, a dynamic screw-plate interface system allows for controlled intersegmental movement, maintains the weight sharing capacity of the graft, and eliminates some of the less desirable attributes of both the nonconstrained and constrained systems. Screw attachment mechanisms that decrease the probability of screw back-out include the establishment of bicortical purchase, a screw head with an expanding bushing or expanding head that when tightened will lock to the plate, or a secondary locking screw that locks the bone screw to the plate. Alternatively a cam lock that fixes each screw to the plate has also been shown to be successful in preventing screw back-out (34–38).

Increasing clinical experience with a variety of anterior cervical plate/screw constructs suggests that their use can improve cervical spine fusion success rates, particularly for traumatic cervical injuries or when two or more intervertebral disc spaces have been treated (3,4,12,14,17,18,20,24,27–33,40–42). The effectiveness of the use of anterior cervical plate/screw devices following single-level anterior cervical discectomy and fusion procedures has not been established, despite their widespread use in this setting. Fusion success rates for single-level procedures are invariably high without the addition of a plate, particularly if autograft bone is used as the fusion substrate (Table 2) (2,5,33,39–41,43–47). Use of an internal fixation plate can prevent graft collapse and angulation, which invariably occurs after interbody fusion, more effectively maintaining lordosis, alignment, and disc space/nerve root decompression. Despite this rationale, to date the addition of an anterior cervical plate to a single-level fusion procedure has not been convincingly proven to statistically significantly improve upon the already high fusion success rates or patient outcomes associated with single-level fusion without internal fixation (24,29,31,33,41,46).

Irrespective of the indications that have led to the use of an anterior cervical plate/screw internal fixator in an individual patient, its effectiveness cannot be realized without careful surgical exposure techniques, without bone as a biological fusion substrate, and without proper placement and application of the device. The failure rate of anterior cervical plate-screw constructs ranges between 1% and 10% in most clinical series (Table

Table 2. Fusion Success Rate Without Anterior Plating

Author	Year	Number treated	Percent fusion
Zdeblick and Ducker	1991	41 auto (s)	95
		19 allo (s)	95
		18 auto (m)	83
		8 allo (m)	38
Bishop et al.	1996	60 auto (s)	97
		32 allo (s)	87
		23 auto (m)	100
		17 allo (m)	89
Connolly et al.	1996	18	83.3
Caspar et al.	1998	210	94.3
Wang et al.	2000	28	75.0

(s), single level; (m) multiple level.

Table 3. Anterior Cervical Plate Hardware Failure

Author	Year	Number treated	Number with failure	Percent failure
Gassman and Seligson	1983	13	1	7.7
Lesoin et al.	1984	145	4	2.8
Tippets and Apfelbaum	1988	28	0	0.0
Brown et al.	1988	13	3	23.1
Caspar et al.	1989	260	1	0.4
Suh et al.	1990	13	1	7.7
Ripa et al.	1991	92	1	1.1
Aebi et al.	1991	86	2	2.3
Kostuik et al.	1993	42	2	4.8
Connolly et al.	1996	25	3	12.0
Katsuura et al.	1996	44	0	0.0
Shapiro	1997	195	5	2.6
McLaughlin et al.	1997	39	2	5.1
Vaccaro et al.	1998	45	9	20.0
Caspar et al.	1998	146	2	1.4
Bose	1998	97	19	19.6
Heidecke et al.	1998	96	3	3.1
Wang et al.	2000	32	0	0.0

3) (8,10,11,15,17–20,22,24,27–33). Instrumentation failure is most often related to poor or misapplication of the construct or poor bony fusion/reconstruction techniques.

Proponents of anterior cervical plate-screw devices insist that their use is safe and effective. When properly applied for a variety of indications, most investigators agree that the devices can be safely inserted with little additional risk, and that their application can be quite effective, particularly at multiple cervical levels or when allograft bone is used as the fusion substrate (Fig. 1) (12,14,17,20–24,26,28–33,41,42,47,48). It is the efficacy of their use that generates the most controversy, particularly in the circumstance of a single-level interspace fusion, their most common application. Opponents of their universal use have questioned if the devices are efficacious and cost-effective for a single-level anterior fusion procedure, in light of the additional expense of the device, the additional operating room time required to insert it, and the additional risk associated with its use (albeit small), especially when the fusion success rate is 95% or better without its use. Investigators who use them routinely respond yes, and point out that while yet statistically unproven, anterior cervical plate-screw constructs do improve fusion success rates even at a single level (30,31,33,40,41). They note that their use precludes autograft iliac crest harvest (obviating the important potential individual patient morbidity of 3% to 15%) (46,47), and that patients are not required to wear a collar postoperatively (17,27–31,33,41). Advocates of plate-screw constructs following anterior cervical spine fusion procedures argue that patients are more satisfied earlier, and return to work more rapidly than those with similar disease treated with fusion but without internal fixation (33). These latter claims are the most difficult to substantiate. If, indeed, their accuracy could be validated in properly performed, blinded, randomized outcome studies, then the efficacy of the routine use of anterior cervical plate-screw constructs following anterior cervical spinal fusion procedures would be known. Until those data are available, surgeons must rely on good judgment and good surgical technique to guide their use of these devices in selected patients.

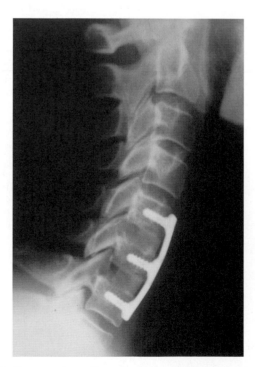

Fig. 1. Postoperative radiograph of a constrained anterior cervical plate system used in a multiple-level decompression, reconstruction, and fusion procedure.

Operative Management

We utilize several adjuncts in the operating room to optimize the success of anterior cervical spinal procedures in our patients. Our major concern is for the patient's spinal cord. Individuals with cervical spinal instability will have been immobilized preoperatively. We utilize the halo ring-vest orthosis to provide immobilization of the patient's cervical spine following trauma, and following closed reduction of both acute traumatic injuries and chronic progressive cervical deformities. Depending on patient pathology, the degree of underlying cord compression, and the severity of the patient's preoperative neurological condition, we will communicate to our anesthesia colleagues the need for fiberoptic intubation, Bullard intubation, or standard techniques. We individualize the decision to administer intravenous methylprednisolone to the patient at induction. Patients with profound cord compression, and rapidly progressive myelopathy, particularly those with signal change within their spinal cord substance on preoperative magnetic resonance imaging (MRI) studies are offered the North American Spinal Cord Injury Study (NASCIS II) protocol of 30 mg/kg intravenous methylprednisolone loading dose, followed by a 23-hour infusion of 5.7 mg/kg (49).

We ask the anesthesiologist to help maintain perfusion of the spinal cord by maintaining a mean systemic blood pressure of 85 mm Hg. This rarely requires the administration of pressors, but often requires extra attention throughout the procedure, and may require the use of an arterial line for minute-to-minute real-time monitoring. When performing an anterior cervical plating procedure following anterior cervical spinal fusion and reconstruction, we utilize low-dose pulsed intraoperative lateral-view fluoroscopy for spot-check analysis of vertebral column realignment, positioning of the fusion substrate, and the length and contour of the internal fixation plate. Screw position and depth of penetration are also visualized in this way for optimal insertion angulation and depth, and to avoid screw penetration of the vertebral end plates. During the initial dissection over the ventral aspects of the vertebral segments being treated, spot-check lateral fluoroscopy can confirm the level and, importantly, can help prevent the disruption of Sharpey's fibers and the uninvolved disc spaces cephalad and caudad to the pathological levels. We use it sparingly, but strategically, to maximize our efforts with each patient.

Finally, realignment of the cervical spine and restoration of sagittal balance are important goals of the reconstruction procedure. In addition to halo ring-vest use as indicated in selected patients, we routinely use two other adjuncts to optimize the re-creation of anatomical cervical lordosis prior to proceeding with internal fixation. Properly angled intervertebral distraction posts, one placed into the body above and the other into the body below, can, when distracted, help re-create lordosis. We will also ask the anesthesiologist to insert rolled surgical towels beneath the patient's neck to provide upward, dorsal support once we have provided a ventral release. These positioning techniques, in addition to the placement of a wedge-shaped intervertebral bone graft and adding a slight bend to the anterior cervical fixation plate, can optimize the achievement of sagittal realignment during these procedures.

Surgical Treatment

The anterior approach to the cervical spine has been described in detail in Chapters 198 and 199 in this textbook. For this section, we describe those techniques that help facilitate and accomplish the successful application of an anterior cervical plate and screw construct after anterior cervical discectomy/vertebrectomy and bony reconstruction.

We approach the anterior cervical spine from the patient's right side unless extenuating circumstances preclude this route of access. Once the patient is properly positioned in the supine position on the operating room table, we place several rolled surgical towels under the patient's neck to help maintain cervical lordosis. We place a rolled cloth doughnut under the base of the patient's head and tape the head to the cephalad-most portion of the operating room table, creating a sling under the patient's chin, thus lifting it upward and causing modest neck extension and providing modest immobilization. These maneuvers are not intended to hyperextend or to force the neck into an undesirable position, but can be important adjuncts in the attempt to re-create cervical lordosis prior to the internal fixation portion of the operative procedure.

We make a 2½- to 3-cm skin incision in a skinfold in the right neck, centered over the anterior border of the sternocleidomastoid muscle, for procedures involving two to three vertebral levels (one or two disc spaces). A curvilinear, almost sigmoid-shaped incision is made along the anterior border of the sternocleidomastoid muscle if three disc spaces and four vertebral levels are to be treated. The precise level for each incision is determined by spot-check intraoperative fluoroscopy, centered over the middle of the operative field to avoid an incision either too high or too low. A centered incision can be very important when attempting to appropriately direct screws through a plate over three cervical vertebral levels through a small, cosmetically attractive incision.

We open the platysma longitudinally and the superficial cervical fascia along the anterior margin of the sternocleidomastoid muscle. Thereafter, we use blunt dissection only, down to the ventral surface of the cervical spine. Digital blunt dissection, a hand-held lipped edge esophageal retractor, and Kittner dissection allow nontraumatic exposure down to the adventitial fascia overlying the ventral vertebral bodies. We utilize unipolar cautery to dissect the medial margins of the longus colli musculature, dissecting laterally and bilaterally to the ventral-lateral

edges of the vertebral bodies being treated. Dissecting the longus musculature in this way allows accurate determination of the mid- and lateral portions of each vertebral segment, and allows solid placement of toothed lateral retraction blades under the medial muscle margins. Effective self-retaining retraction in this way provides terrific exposure for both the decompression/fusion portion of the procedure and the internal fixation component that follows. Also, this combination of careful, gentle, blunt dissection and retraction below and of the longus colli musculature minimizes the potential complication of a recurrent laryngeal nerve palsy.

When exposing the ventral surfaces of the vertebral bodies we work longitudinally, top to bottom, rather than horizontally, side to side, to avoid compromise of Sharpey's fibers and/or the disc spaces at the most rostral and caudal extents of the exposure. Spot-checking with lateral intraoperative fluoroscopy can also help direct the rostral and caudal extent of the dissection, to avoid unnecessary exposure of levels not to be included in the treatment plan. We utilize distraction posts and a ratchet-type, self-retaining distraction device to allow unrestricted exposure to the interspace (discectomy) or intervertebral space (vertebrectomy). Distraction posts also provide rostral-caudal distraction of the soft tissues, obviating the need for rostral-caudal retraction blades. They allow distraction at the interspace for better exposure and decompression, they can help to re-create cervical lordosis if placed properly, and they allow distraction for snug placement of the intervertebral graft followed by intervertebral graft compression upon distractor release and post removal.

The superior post should be placed midposition in the superior vertebral body in the midline, angled slightly upward, screwed completely down flush with the ventral surface of the vertebral body. The inferior post should be placed just below the midportion of the lower vertebral body, in the midline, angled parallel with the superior end plate. Distraction at this interspace, once the annulus has been incised, with the posts in this configuration will distract the interspace, will help to maintain (or re-create) cervical lordosis, and will be positioned such that the inferior post is out of the operative "line of sight" as the surgeon works within the depths of the interspace. If working at more than one interspace, we place distraction posts in each vertebral body, individually treating each interspace in turn. If performing a vertebrectomy, we place posts only in the most superior and inferior vertebral bodies. Once the decompression and grafting portions of the operation are complete, the distraction posts are removed in preparation for the anterior cervical plating portion of the procedure.

We have utilized a variety of anterior cervical fixation plates over the years. We prefer titanium, rather than stainless steel constructs, mainly to avoid image artifact on subsequent MRI studies. We prefer unicortical screws that affix to the anterior cervical plate, rather than bicortical screws, but utilize both for selected occasions. Irrespective of the type of screw fixation, the internal fixation plate must be of appropriate size, length, and contour. Petite females, the young, and individuals with smaller, narrower, less stout vertebral bodies, particularly higher in the cervical spine, require a less broad anterior cervical plate. There are several varieties from different manufacturers. They all appear to function well. The key is to get the anterior cervical plate exactly ventral and in the midline as straight up and down as possible (Figs. 2 to 5). Occasionally a plate will be placed in a less than ideal position, too far toward one side or the other. In this circumstance the off-center screw could cause injury if it is placed "too wide" and/or it may not serve its purpose because of poor purchase in the vertebral body. A narrower, less broad plate in this circumstance can help reduce placement errors. Thorough dissection of the ventral aspects of the vertebral bodies being treated, as previously mentioned,

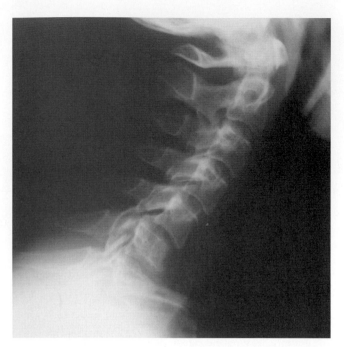

Fig. 2. Lateral radiograph of acute C5-6 fracture-dislocation injury.

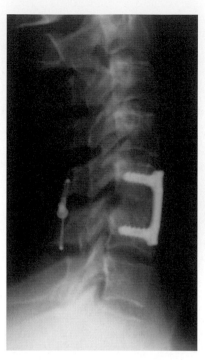

Fig. 4. Postoperative lateral radiograph of dorsal and ventral internal fixation devices used as adjuncts to realignment and bony fusion following traumatic injury. Note restoration of alignment and lordosis.

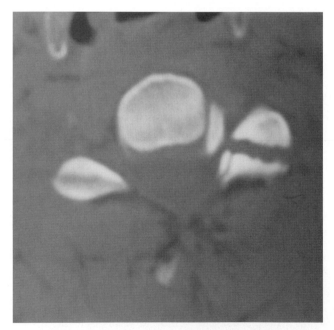

Fig. 3. Axial computed tomography (CT) scan shows a left C5-6 facet fracture.

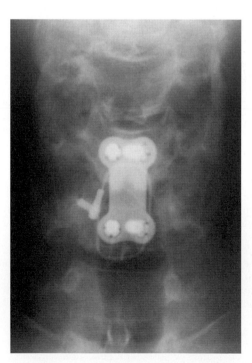

Fig. 5. Postoperative anteroposterior (AP) radiograph shows proper midline positioning of an anterior cervical internal fixation plate.

can help the surgeon identify the lateral edges of each vertebral segment and therefore the "midline," and assist with optimal plate placement.

The length of the anterior cervical plate is important. On several occasions we have been required to treat "pseudarthrosis" following an anterior cervical fusion and internal fixation procedure, only to identify that the inferior screws were originally placed through the inferior vertebral end plate, or into the caudal disc space. This form of pseudarthrosis and plate failure would likely have been avoided with a shorter internal fixation plate with the inferior screws solidly into the caudal vertebral body. We utilize spot-check lateral fluoroscopy to help select the appropriate plate length, 1 to 2 mm short of the superior end plate of the cephalad level and 2 mm short of the inferior end plate of the caudal vertebral level. If fluoroscopy is not utilized or if the inferior aspect of the construct cannot be visualized with fluoroscopy, careful direct inspection can identify the inferior end plate without compromise of Sharpey's fibers or the annulus below. In this circumstance also, attentive dissection during the initial exposure can keep the surgeon out of trouble and prevent him/her from plating "too long." While it appears to occur less often, the surgeon also wants to avoid plating too high. Careful dissection with or without spot-check lateral fluoroscopy helps to avoid this circumstance as well.

Screw placement can impact on the long-term success of the fusion and internal fixation procedure; therefore, care must be taken to apply them correctly. Screws must be solidly placed within the vertebral body without penetration of the end plate and/or compromise of the adjacent disc space. We angle the superior screws upward, parallel with the superior end plate of the superior vertebral body. Middle screws (if used) are angled as parallel as possible to the vertebral end plates. Inferior screws must not compromise the inferior vertebral end plate. We place these parallel with the vertebral end plate as well, although it is more difficult to achieve inferiorly due to the overlying soft tissues. We triangulate each pair of screws, placing them convergent toward the under portion of the vertebral body for greatest biomechanical advantage. When anterior cervical plates are utilized following vertebrectomy and strut fusion, we do not place screws into the interposition graft, as this may weaken the graft.

We use unicortical screws that lock to the anterior cervical plate (by one mechanism or another) almost without exception. The rare cases when we utilize bicortical screws include anterior cervical plate application into the second cervical vertebra and, even rarer, when attempting a salvage procedure after removal of a unicortical locking screw-plate system. In the former instance, we can better contour bicortical screw-plate systems to the unique ventral surface of C2 and the proximal dens, and can better direct two or more screws into C2. Bicortical screws have a smaller diameter, can be convergently placed closer together, and can achieve terrific purchase of C2, particularly when the body of C2 itself is small and screws are required at the base of the dens or higher (Figs. 6 to 8). Prebent locking screw-plate systems typically allow fewer options for variable screw placement compared to most bicortical screw-plate systems.

Occasionally when we treat pseudarthrosis and internal fixation failure, we can remove the locking screw-plate system, resect the failed graft substrate, decompress the thecal sac and roots, and have enough vertebral body left above and below to fuse and re-instrument without having to go above and/or below to the next vertebral level(s) to provide adequate substrate for internal fixation. In those circumstances in which another cancellous screw locking screw-plate system is inappropriate, bicortical screws can be effectively utilized to provide anchors for the anterior cervical plate.

Whenever bicortical screws are used, we always employ in-

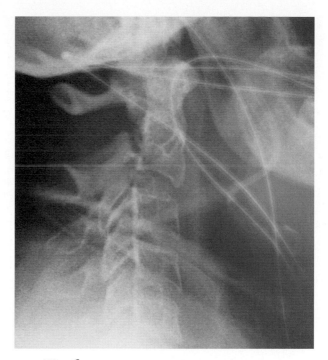

Fig. 6. Lateral radiograph of a C2-3 fracture injury.

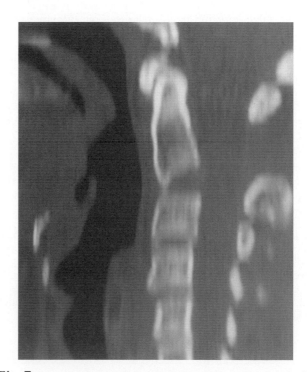

Fig. 7. CT reconstruction shows marked C2-3 disruption and instability despite immobilization in halo immobilization device.

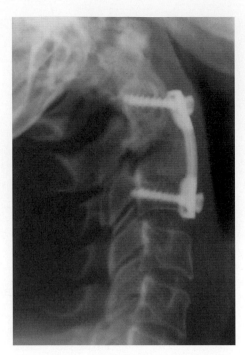

Fig. 8. Postoperative lateral radiograph shows realignment and internal fixation with fusion of a C2-3 injury. We prefer nonconstrained, bicortical screw-plate fixation system at these levels. Intraoperative fluoroscopy is an important adjunct when utilizing bicortical screws.

traoperative fluoroscopy to guide their insertion and to avoid overpenetration, either by the pilot drill bit, the tap if one is used, or the screws themselves. The pilot drill should just barely pass through the dorsal vertebral body cortical surface, and screw penetration should be one to two threads (1 to 2 mm) maximum, through that cortical surface.

Conclusions

Anterior cervical plate-screw internal fixators can be important adjuncts to successful anterior cervical spinal fusion procedures. Their application is straightforward. Little additional operative time is required to insert them. Their use typically obviates the need for a postoperative orthosis. They are not, however, without risk for potential complications, their efficacy has not been established for single-level interbody fusion procedures (their most common application), and they do represent an additional cost to the patient. Careful patient selection, meticulous surgical technique, and several of the operative adjuncts and techniques described above can optimize their utility in an individual patient.

References

1. Caspar W. Die ventrale interkorporale stabilisierung mit der HWS Trapez-Osteosyntheseplatte: Indikation. Technik. Ergebnisse. *Z Orthop* 119:809–810, 1981.
2. Aronson NI. The management of soft disc protrusions using the Smith-Robinson approach. *Clin Neurosurg* 20:253, 1973.
3. Bremer AM, Nguyen TQ. Internal metal plate fixation combined with anterior interbody fusion in cases of cervical spine injury. *Neurosurgery* 12:649–653, 1983.
4. Hermann HD. Metal plate fixation after anterior fusion of unstable fracture dislocations of the cervical spine. *Acta Neurochir (Wien)* 32:101–111, 1975.
5. Riley LH Jr, Robinson RA, Johnson KA, et al. The results of anterior interbody fusion of the cervical spine. Review of ninety-three consecutive cases. *J Neurosurg* 30:127–133, 1973.
6. Bohler J, Gaudermak T. Anterior plate stabilization for fracture dislocations of the lower cervical spine. *J Trauma* 20:203–205, 1980.
7. Orozco Delcious R, Liovet Tapies J. Osteointesis en las fractures de raquis cervical. *Rev Ortop Traumatol* 14:285–288, 1997.
8. Ripa DR, Kowall MG, Meyer PR Jr, et al. Series of ninety-two traumatic cervical spine injuries stabilized with anterior ASIF plate fusion technique. *Spine* 16:546–555, 1991.
9. Aebi M, Mohler J, Zach GA, et al. Indication, surgical technique, and results of 100 surgically-treated fractures and fracture-dislocations of the cervical spine. *Clin Orthop* 203:244–257, 1986.
10. Aebi M, Zuber K, Marchesi D. Treatment of cervical spine injuries with anterior plating: Indications, techniques, and results. *Spine* 16(suppl):S38–S45, 1991.
11. Brown JA, Havel P, Ebraheim N, et al. Cervical stabilization by plate and bone fusion. *Spine* 13:236–240, 1988.
12. Cabanela ME, Ebersold MJ. Anterior plate stabilization for bursting teardrop fractures of the cervical spine. *Spine* 13:888–891, 1988.
13. Caspar W. Anterior stabilization with trapezial osteosynthetic plate technique in cervical spine injuries. In: Kehr P, Weidner A, eds. *Cervical spine*, vol 1. New York: Springer-Verlag, 198–204, 1987.
14. DeOliveira JC. Anterior plate fixation of traumatic lesions of the lower cervical spine. *Spine* 12:324–329, 1987.
15. Gassman J, Seligson D. The anterior cervical plate. *Spine* 8:700–707, 1983.
16. Morscher E, Sutter F, Jenny H, et al. Die vordere Verplattung der Halswirbelsaule mit dem Hohlschrauben-Plattensystem aus Titanium. *Chirurg* 57:702–707, 1986.
17. Tippets RH, Apfelbaum RI. Anterior cervical fusion with the Caspar instrumentation system. *Neurosurgery* 22:1008–1013, 1988.
18. Lesoin F, Cama A, Lozes G, et al. The anterior approach and plates in lower cervical post-traumatic lesions. *Surg Neurol* 21:581–587, 1984.
19. Suh PB, Kostuik JP, Esses SI. Anterior cervical plate fixation with the titanium hollow screw plate system: a preliminary report. *Spine* 15:1079–1081, 1990.
20. Caspar W, Barbier DD, Klara PM. Anterior cervical fusion and Caspar plate stabilization for cervical trauma. *Neurosurgery* 25:491–502, 1989.
21. Randle MJ, Wolf A, Levi L, et al. The use of anterior Caspar plate fixation in acute cervical spine injury. *Surg Neurol* 36:181–189, 1991.
22. Kostuik JP, Connolly PJ, Esses SI, et al. Anterior cervical plate fixation with the titanium hollow screw plate system. *Spine* 18:1273–1278, 1993.
23. Harkey HL. Synthes cervical spine locking plate (Mosher plate). *Neurosurgery* 32:682–683, 1993.
24. Connolly PJ, Esses SI, Kostuik JP. Anterior cervical fusion: outcome analysis of patients fused with and without anterior cervical plates. *J Spinal Disord* 9:202–206, 1996.
25. Cauthen JC, Kinard RE, Vogler JB, et al. Outcome analysis of noninstrumented anterior cervical discectomy and interbody fusion in 348 patients. *Spine* 23(2):188–192, 1998.
26. Garvey TA, Eismont FJ, Roberti LJ. Anterior decompression, structural bone grafting, and Caspar plate stabilization for unstable cervical spine fractures and/or dislocations. *Spine* 17(suppl):S431–435, 1992.
27. Shapiro S. Banked fibula and the locking anterior cervical plate in anterior cervical fusions following cervical discectomy. *J Neurosurg* 84:161–165, 1996.
28. Heidecke V, Rainov NG, Burkert W. Anterior cervical fusion with the Orion locking plat system. *Spine* 23(16):796–1803, 1998.
29. Bose B. Anterior cervical fusion using Caspar plating: analysis of results and review of the literature. *Surg Neurol* 49:25–31, 1998.
30. Wang JC, McDonough PW, Endow KK, et al. Increased fusion rates with cervical plating for two-level cervical discectomy and fusion. *Spine* 25(1):41–45, 2000.
31. Katsuura A, Hukuda S, Imanaka T, et al. Anterior cervical plate used

in degenerative disease can maintain cervical lordosis. *J Spinal Disord* 9(6):470–476, 1996.

32. Vaccaro AR, Falatyn SP, Scuderi GJ, et al. Early failure of long segment anterior cervical plate fixation. *J Spinal Disord* 11(5):410–415, 1998.

33. McLaughlin MR, Purighalla V, Pizzi FJ. Cost advantages of two-level anterior cervical fusion with rigid internal fixation for radiculopathy and degenerative disease. *Surg Neurol* 48:560–565, 1997.

34. Sutterlin CE III, McAfee PC, Warden KE, et al. A biomechanical evaluation of cervical spinal stabilization methods in a bovine model: Static and cyclical loading. *Spine* 13:795–802, 1988.

35. Griffith SL, Zogbi SW, Guyer RD, et al. Biomechanical comparison of anterior instrumentation for the cervical spine. *J Spinal Disord* 8(6):429–438, 1995.

36. Grubb MR, Currier BL, Shih J-S, et al. Biomechanical evaluation of anterior cervical spine stabilization. *Spine* 23(8):886–892, 1998.

37. Ryken TC, Clausen JD, Traynelis VC, et al. Biomechanical analysis of bone mineral density, insertion technique, screw torque, and holding strength of anterior cervical plate screws. *J Neurosurg* 83: 324–329, 1995.

38. Clausen JD, Ryken TC, Traynelis VC, et al. Biomechancial evaluation of Caspar and Cervical Spine Locking Plate systems in a cadaveric model. *J Neurosurg* 84:1039–1045, 1996.

39. Simmons EH, Bhalla SK, Butt WP. Anterior cervical discectomy and fusion. A clinical and biomechanical study with eight-year follow-up. *J Bone Joint Surg* 51B:225–237, 1969.

40. Seifert V, Stolke D. Multisegmental cervical spondylosis: Treatment by spondyloectomy, microsurgical decompression, and osteosynthesis. *Neurosurgery* 29:498–503, 1991.

41. Caspar W, Geisler FH, Pitzen T, et al. Anterior cervical plate stabilization in one- and two-level degenerative disease: Overtreatment or benefit? *J Spinal Disord* 11:1–11, 1998.

42. Johnston FG, Crockard HA. One-stage internal fixation and anterior fusion in complex cervical spinal disorders. *J Neurosurg* 82:234–238, 1996.

43. Robinson RA, Walker AE, Ferlic DC, et al. The results of anterior interbody fusion of the cervical spine. *J Bone Joint Surg* 44A: 1569–1586, 1962.

44. Murphy MA, Trimble MB, Piedmonte MR, et al. Changes in the cervical foraminal area after anterior discectomy with and without a graft. *Neurosurgery* 34:93–96, 1994.

45. Gore DR, Sepic SB. Anterior cervical fusion for degenerated or protruded discs: a review of one hundred forty-six patients. *Spine* 9: 667–671, 1984.

46. Bishop RC, Moore KA, Hadley MN. Anterior cervical interbody fusion using autogenic and allogenic bone graft substrate: a prospective comparative analysis. *J Neurosurg* 85:206–210, 1996.

47. Zdeblick TA, Ducker TB. The use of freeze-dried allograft bone for anterior cervical fusions. *Spine* 16(7):726–729, 1991.

48. Rechtine GR, Cahill DW, Gruenberg M, et al. The Synthes cervical spine locking plate and screw system in anterior cervical fusion. *Tech Orthop* 9:86–91, 1994.

49. Bracken MB, Shepard MJ, Collins WF, et al. A randomized controlled trial of methylprednisolone or naloxone in the treatment of acute spinal cord injury. *N Engl J Med* 322:1405–1411, 1990.

207. Anterior Instrumentation for the Thoracolumbar Spine

Gregory R. Trost

The anterior approach to the thoracolumbar spine is indicated in the treatment of trauma, tumor, and infection. It has become the first choice of many surgeons to treat disease processes involving the vertebral bodies of the thoracic and lumbar spine. Instrumentation has been developed that can be applied to the anterior spine for the purpose of stabilization, so that treatment is possible without a concomitant posterior approach, and motion segments are potentially spared. These devices have evolved during the past several years.

In 1966, Dwyer introduced an anterior instrumentation system in which screws and cables were used to provide stabilization in cases of scoliosis. This system worked by applying tension across the segments to be fused (1,2). A number of failures occurred, with subsequent pseudarthrosis (3–5). Zielke et al. (6) modified this device by replacing the cable with a threaded rod. Unfortunately, a number of failures occurred that resulted in loss of correction, progression of kyphosis, and pseudarthrosis (7–10). The Dunn device was introduced in 1984 for anterior thoracolumbar stabilization (11). This device was noted to be prominent, and vascular complications were subsequently reported (12). The Kostuik-Harrington device was also associated with a significant number of failures (13). It was noted to have less rigidity than posterior Harrington rods or Luque wire.

The modern devices were developed to avoid the shortcomings of their predecessors. The newer devices are rigid, with at least one screw or bolt being affixed to the longitudinal member at each vertebral body in a constrained fashion. Each of the devices discussed in this chapter resists motion in multiple axes. The current systems attempt to have a low profile. The plate systems are lower in profile than the rod systems, so that vascular complications are decreased when the devices are optimally placed. The current systems provide a mechanism for the reduction of kyphosis in addition to allowing for compression of the bone graft. Additionally, the implants are constructed of titanium or titanium alloys so that they are compatible with magnetic resonance imaging (MRI).

This chapter discusses the most widely used anterior thoracolumbar instrumentation systems in the author's opinion. The plate systems detailed include the following: Zplate II ATL (Sofamor Danek, Memphis, Tennessee); Anterior Thoracolumbar Locking Plate (Synthes, Paoli, Pennsylvania); Profile (DePuy Motech, Warsaw, Indiana); and M2 Anterior Plate (DePuy Acromed, Boston, Massachusetts). Two rod systems are discussed: the VentroFix (Synthes) and the Kaneda SR (DePuy Acromed).

General Comments

When pathology in the thoracic and lumbar spine is treated, the approach to the spine is usually from the left. The position of the aorta should be checked on preoperative imaging studies. Occasionally, the aorta lies to the left of midline, so that an approach from the right side is required. The anatomical structures at risk with the right-sided approach include the relatively fragile inferior vena cava and the liver. Ideally, no instrumentation should abut or impinge on any vascular structure.

The preoperative images should be evaluated for a variety of anatomical details in addition to the position of the great vessels. The position of the spinal canal in relation to the rib heads can be a valuable piece of information when the entry points for screws are being planned.

On occasion, the position of the spinal canal is quite anterior, so that the risk for inadvertent screw placement and subsequent canal compromise is increased. The length of the screws can be approximated from the preoperative images. The vertebral bodies become smaller in the upper thoracic spine. The surgeon must know the shortest screw length available in the instrumentation system that will be used. The shape of the vertebral bodies may change as the upper thoracic spine is approached, becoming smaller anteriorly. This limits the space available for the placement of instrumentation.

The position of the patient must be straight lateral. The area of pathology may be positioned over a break in the table to facilitate graft placement. After the graft is placed, the table is straightened and the instrumentation is placed.

Zplate II

The Zplate II is a recently released modification of the original Zplate manufactured by Sofamor Danek. The plate is designed with holes on one end for the bolt and screw and slots on the opposite end (Fig. 1). The plate is usually applied from the left side with the slots in the cephalic position. It can be placed from the right with the slots positioned caudally.

Different plate configurations have been designed for use in the various regions of the spine. All components are made of titanium. The Zplate II ATL is straight in the sagittal plane and is used for fixation from T9 to L4. The plates are available in lengths from 4 to 13 cm in 1-cm increments, with 6.5-, 7.5-, and 8.5-cm lengths also available. The bolt diameter is 7.5 mm, and the screw diameter is 6.5 mm. The bolts range in length from 30 to 55 mm and the screw length from 30 to 60 mm. The Zplate II anterior thoracic fixation system has sagittally curved plates to match the thoracic kyphosis and is applied from T3 to T9. The thoracic plate is available in sizes from 4 to 13 cm in 1-cm increments. The bolt and screw diameters are 5.5 and 4.5 mm, respectively. The lengths range from 15 to 45 mm for bolts and 20 to 55 mm for screws. Both plate designs are radially curved

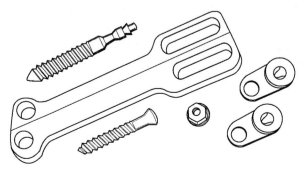

Fig. 1. Zplate II components. The plate features slots on the rostral end with a sliding stabilizer for the posterior bolts.

to match the contour of the vertebral bodies. The posterior slot has an integral sliding stabilizer for the bolt (Fig. 1).

The bolts and screws are self-tapping and are intended to be placed in a bicortical fashion. Taps are available if their use is desired. The screws are generally 5 mm longer than the bolts. Washers, with a hole for the bolt head and a hole for the screw, are specific for particular ends of the plate. The hole in the washer for the screw has a slot that allows the hole to expand so that the screw can pass through it (Fig. 1). This feature prevents screw backout.

INSERTION TECHNIQUE. The instrumentation is applied following vertebral resection. The bolts are placed first. The entry sites for the Zplate II ATL bolts are located 8 mm from the spinal canal and 8 mm from the superior end plate of the rostral vertebra and inferior end plate of the caudal vertebra. For the anterior thoracic fixation system, the entry sites are 4 to 5 mm from the corresponding landmarks. The appropriately sized awl is passed through the awl guide, which angulates 10 degrees away from the spinal canal. The bolts are placed bicortically and should parallel the end plate. The interface between the bolt and plate allows for some variability in bolt placement.

The bolts are used for distraction during reduction and graft placement. The distractor is applied to the machine thread portion of the bolts. The distractor is outside the vertebral resection site, allowing full access to the end plates of the vertebrae.

The provided template or, alternatively, measurement of the distance between the bolts with the calipers is used to determine the appropriate size of the plate. When the anterior thoracic fixation system is used, the kyphosis in the plate must match the kyphosis in the thoracic spine. If the plates are placed from the right side, the slots should be positioned inferiorly.

The plate is then placed over the bolts. The shortest plate possible should be applied to minimize impingement on the superior end plate and allow maximal compression. The bolt post in the slot end must pass through the integral stabilizer. Because the plate must be seated completely on the bolt heads, removal of bone from the lateral prominence of the vertebral end plates may be required.

The variable and slot washers are placed over the bolt posts and aligned with the slot and hole for the screws. Nuts are applied to the bolt posts, and the nut in the hole end of the plate is provisionally tightened with finger pressure only. The nut on the slot end bolt post is also tightened. Care must be taken not to overtighten this nut because this bolt must be allowed to slide along the plate during compression. The nut driver should not be removed.

Compression is then performed. The shoe of the compressor is placed around the base of the nut driver in the slot end of the plate. While compression is applied, the nut is tightened and torqued to 80 to 100 in-lb. Countertorque must be applied during final tightening. The inferior nut is then finally tightened by means of the same technique.

The superior and inferior anterior screw sites are prepared with the screw-positioning guide, which is placed in the retaining rings of the variable and slot washers. The screws are angled between 0 and 10 degrees posteriorly. To engage the opposite cortex, the screws must be 5 mm longer than the implanted bolts. The screws pass through the retaining rings on the variable and slot washers and seat firmly against the plate. If screw removal is necessary, placing an instrument in the gap can expand the retaining ring.

The posts are broken off the bolts with use of the post breakoff wrench. The wrench is turned in a clockwise direction until

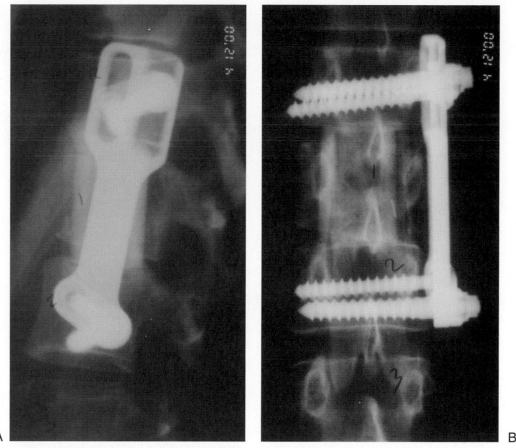

Fig. 2. Anteroposterior (**A**) and lateral (**B**) views of a completed construct. All bolts and screws are placed bicortically. Sagittal and coronal alignments are normal following a burst fracture in this patient with a significant preoperative kyphotic deformity.

the post extension has broken. Fig. 2 is a postoperative radiograph demonstrating the completed construct.

Profile

The Profile anterior spinal fixation system is designed for use from the upper thoracic through the lumbar spine. Separate plates are available for use in the thoracic spine and thoracolumbar spine. The thoracolumbar plates are available in lengths from 50 to 120 mm, and the thoracic plates are available in lengths from 40 to 110 mm. Both plates have posterior cutouts that allow visualization of the graft and posterior decompression site.

The thoracolumbar plates feature slots posteriorly (Fig. 3). The undersides of the slots have teeth to match the teeth on the bolt heads (Fig. 4). There are three anterior screw holes, two placed inferiorly and one superiorly (Fig. 3). A diagonal slot along the intermediate portion of the plate allows for placement of a screw into the graft regardless of the position of the graft in relation to the plate.

The thoracic plate has three screw holes on either end. It is curved to match the kyphosis of the thoracic spine. A diagonal slot is also present in the intermediate portion of the plate. The thoracic plate is designed for use above T10.

The posterior bolts are designed for use with the thoracolumbar plate. The bolts are designed for bicortical use and are not self-tapping, but they can be used unicortically in good-quality bone. The bolts are 7 mm in diameter and range in length from 25 to 60 mm. Locking teeth on the bolt heads interface with the plate (Fig. 4). This feature allows secure fixation between the bolt and plate and also allows for fine adjustment. The bolts use a dual-locking mechanism; an outer nut fixates the plate rigidly to the bolt, and an inner screw prevents loosening of the nut.

Locking screws are provided for the anterior portion of the thoracolumbar plate and exclusively for the thoracic plate. Their length ranges from 20 to 60 mm, and their diameter is 6.0 mm. The screws are self-tapping and are intended for unicortical

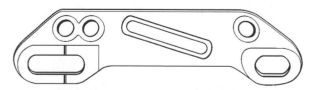

Fig. 3. The Profile plate features slots for bolts and holes for screws. Posterior cutouts allow visualization of the spinal canal. The line etched across the inferior, longer slot aids in determining which screw hole to use, as discussed in the text.

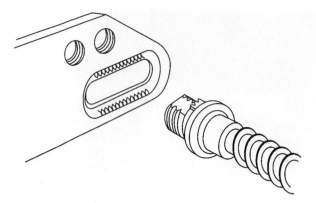

Fig. 4. The underside of the plate has teeth to match teeth on the bolts.

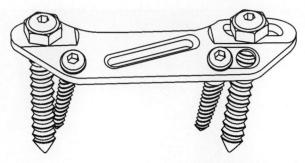

Fig. 6. The bolts are secured with an outer nut and an inner screw.

use. The screws feature a single-lead thread that changes to a triple-lead thread that allows locking of the screw to the plate (Fig. 5). The screw threads through the plate.

INSERTION TECHNIQUE. The manufacturer describes two techniques for placement of the plate. In the first, a template is used after the graft is placed. The template acts as an awl/drill guide to ensure parallel placement of the bolts. Removal of the lateral prominence of the vertebral end plates may be required to allow the template to sit flat on the lateral surface of the vertebral bodies.

In the second technique, the bolts are placed before the bone graft. The bolts can then be used as distraction points during graft placement. The entry site for the bolts is located in line with the junction of the pedicle with the vertebral body. A free hand guide is used to ensure parallel placement of the bolts.

A bolt post is threaded into the bolt in a counterclockwise direction. The bolts are inserted until the collar is firmly against the bone, but not countersunk. If the graft has not been previously placed, one can distract against the bolts and place the graft.

A plate is selected that will not impinge on the adjacent vertebrae. It is seated onto the bolts with the cutout facing posteriorly and the short slot cephalad. If a right-sided approach is used, the short slot will be located caudally. The teeth should be engaged between the plate and the bolts. The cephalic nut is tightened. Compression can be applied before the inferior nut is tightened.

The screws are placed anteriorly. The screw at the caudal end is placed in the hole that does not oppose the bolt. A line is etched on the plate that assists in determining which screw hole should be used. If any portion of the nut crosses this etched line, the alternate hole must be used. A drill guide is attached

to the plate at the appropriate hole. A screw that is 5 mm shorter than the bolt is appropriate. The screws are not intended for bicortical purchase. The screw is locked to the plate when it is flush.

The outer nuts are torqued and the inner screws placed (Fig. 6). The inner screws are applied in a counterclockwise fashion. These screws prevent loosening of the nuts.

Only screws are used in the thoracic plate. The graft must be placed before the plate. A plate of the appropriate size is selected. The screws are place as previously described with use of the drill guides to ensure parallel placement. At least two screws must be placed at each level. Three screws may be used if feasible.

Screws may be placed into the graft through the diagonal slot in the intermediate part of the plate if desired. Screws 4 mm in diameter with lengths of 15, 20, 25, and 30 mm are available. This screw is designed to prevent migration or backout.

Anterior Thoracolumbar Locking Plate

The Anterior Thoracolumbar Locking Plate is indicated for use from T10 through L5. The plate is made of commercially pure titanium and is applied only after the bone graft has been placed. The system allows compression of the bone graft through the use of temporary screws placed through the dynamic compression plate holes (Fig. 7). Plate lengths from 57 to 103 mm are available.

The 7.5-mm-diameter screws are intended for unicortical purchase only. A machine thread on the proximal screw locks the screw to the plate. Lengths range from 30 to 55 mm in increments of 5 mm. The screws are placed in a triangulated fashion for further resistance to pullout.

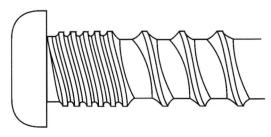

Fig. 5. The thread on the proximal screw locks the screw to the plate.

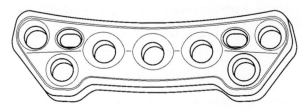

Fig. 7. The Anterior Thoracolumbar Locking Plate has dynamic compression holes for the temporary screws. The holes are ramped, so that as the screws are tightened, they slide in the dynamic compression plate holes and cause compression.

INSERTION TECHNIQUE. Following corpectomy and graft placement, the plate is placed on the lateral vertebral surface in a position ensuring that no screw will violate the spinal canal. The holes for the temporary screws are drilled with a 2.5-mm bit placed through the dynamic compression plate drill guide in the dynamic compression plate hole. An automatic stop at 30 mm corresponds to the length of the 4.0-mm-diameter temporary screws. The screw is placed, but not completely tightened. The second temporary screw is placed in a similar fashion. The temporary screws are sequentially tightened until satisfactory compression has been accomplished.

Drill guides are placed at the posterior screw holes. This ensures that screw placement will be perpendicular to the plate. A 5.0-mm drill is used to drill holes for the posterior screws. The bit is 30 mm in length. An appropriately sized screw is selected; it should be recalled that only unicortical purchase is recommended.

The temporary screws are now removed. If the temporary screws are not removed, they will interfere with the placement of the anterior screws. Placement of the anterior screws is similar to that of the posterior screws.

M2 Anterior Plate

The M2 Anterior Plate is designed for use throughout the thoracic and thoracolumbar spine. The plates are made of medical-grade titanium (Ti6A14V) and are available in lengths from 40 to 100 mm in 10-mm increments. Anterior and posterior nested slots are located on the rostral and caudal ends of the plates. The posterior slots, three in number, can accommodate either screws or bolts. The anterior nested slots, two in number, accommodate only screws. Therefore, the system is designed to be used as a two-bolt–two-screw construct or a four-screw construct. The anterior and posterior slots are both angled 8 degrees from the center line.

The M2 bolt is 5.5 mm in diameter and is available in lengths from 25 to 55 mm in 5-mm increments (Fig. 8B). They are not self-tapping and are intended to be placed bicortically. The bolt has an integral nut with a machine-threaded section above it. The integral nut is designed to sit in a longitudinal slot on the underside of the plate along the posterior slots (Fig. 8A).

The screws are 4.75 mm in diameter and are available in lengths similar to those of the bolts (Fig. 8C). Bicortical placement is recommended. The rounded head allows for up to 15 degrees of angulation through the nested slots.

INSERTION TECHNIQUE. The M2 Anterior Plate is placed after decompression and graft placement. A plate is selected that will not impinge on the adjacent disc spaces. Templates are available for each size of plate. The template must rest on the vertebral bodies, so that removal of the lateral prominence of the vertebral end plates may be necessary.

The length of the posterior bolt or screw is determined from the preoperative radiographic studies or by direct measurement intraoperatively. A 3.2-mm adjustable drill bit is used to create holes for the posterior anchors. The length of the drill bit is set 10 mm longer than the anticipated bolt/screw length to accommodate for the thickness of the template. A hole is selected that will allow for approximately one nest of compression. After the first hole is drilled, a pin is placed through it to maintain the position of the template while the second hole is prepared. The posterior holes are then tapped with the 5.50-mm tap, and a

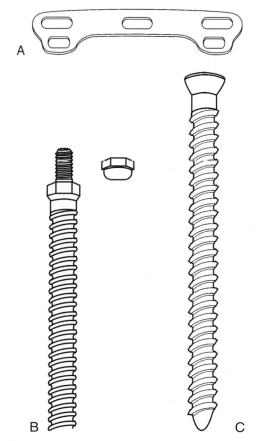

Fig. 8. The M2 Anterior Plate has nested slots on each end, three posteriorly and two anteriorly. **A**: The underside of the plate features a slot into which the integral nut (**B**) fits. **C**: Screws can be used in all holes of the plate.

bolt of the appropriate length is inserted so that the integral nut will fit into the longitudinal slot on the undersurface of the plate.

The plate is placed onto the bolts with the integral nut in the longitudinal slot on the plate undersurface. This ensures that the bolt will not move during nut tightening. The nuts are applied to the machine-threaded portion of the bolts, compression is applied, and the nuts are finally tightened.

Anterior screws are placed after drilling and tapping. Bicortical purchase is recommended. If bicortical purchase is not obtained, the screw should be removed and replaced with one that penetrates the opposite cortex.

If screws are to be used in the posterior slots, a 4.75-mm tap is used. The screws are placed through the plate into the prepared holes.

Kaneda SR

The Kaneda SR is a dual-rod stabilization system used to treat abnormalities from T10 to L3 (Fig. 9). As many as four motion segments can be spanned with this type of construct. Quarter-inch rods are used as the longitudinal members with this system.

Spiked plates are secured to the vertebral bodies (Fig. 10). They are available in small (15 × 26 mm), medium (18.5 ×

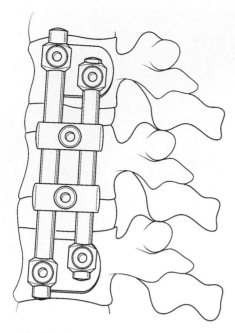

Fig. 9. The Kaneda SR is a dual-rod system.

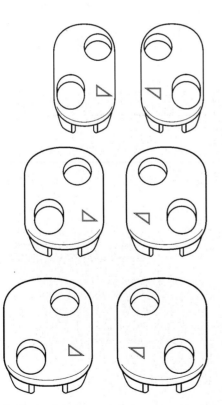

Fig. 10. The four-spike plates are designed as pairs with markings to designate anterior, posterior, rostral, and caudal.

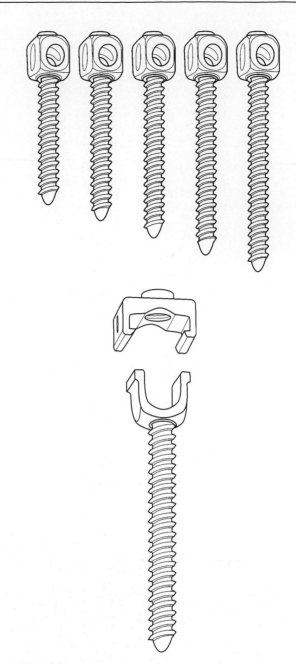

Fig. 11. The screws come in open and closed configurations.

25 mm), and large (20.5 × 27 mm) sizes. The plates are designed as pairs, with rostral and caudal components. Each spinal plate is marked with anterior and posterior designations in addition to the appropriate rostral and caudal designations. These plates assist in screw alignment and interfere with screw migration.

The 6.25-mm screws come in open, top-loading, and closed varieties (Fig. 11). Only one open screw can be used with any single plate. The lengths range from 30 to 60 mm in 5-mm increments. The screws have a cancellous thread and should be placed in a bicortical fashion.

Transverse couplers are used to connect the rods (Fig. 12). At least two should be used with each construct. These couplers assist in resisting torsional loads. They come in widths from 13 to 16 mm in 1-mm increments.

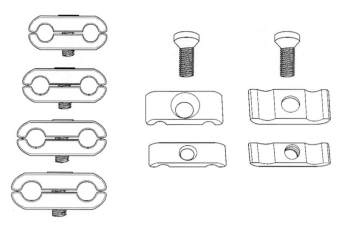

Fig. 12. The transverse couplings help resist torsional loads.

INSERTION TECHNIQUE. Bony resection is completed before placement of the Kaneda SR. The four-spike plates are placed on the vertebral bodies and impacted. The plate that provides maximal coverage of the lateral vertebral bodies with the four spikes completely placed in bone is selected. All components of the system must be placed at least 1 cm from any vascular structure. When the plates are correctly placed, the anterior rod is longer than the posterior rod. Plates may be placed at intervening vertebral bodies if the construct is long.

The correct screw length can be determined as previously discussed. The posterior screw is angulated 10 degrees from the spinal canal and is parallel to the end plate. It is very important that the screw pairs, both posterior and both anterior screws, be parallel. The anterior screws should be parallel to the vertebral end plate and posterior vertebral cortex. The screws

recess into the spiked plate when completely driven. Screws should be placed in a bicortical fashion. The screws may be used for deformity correction before the rods are placed.

Rod length is determined by measuring the distance between the ends of the connectors. The rods should extend approximately 2 mm beyond the end of each connector. Each rod is then passed through the screw heads or top-loaded if open screws are used. One set screw for each rod is tightened. Compression is applied, and the second set screw is tightened. The set screws are torqued to a minimum of 60 in-lb.

The transverse connectors are applied with a self-retaining wrench. The bolt is loosened, and the two portions of the transverse coupler are rotated until they are perpendicular to each other. The lower portion is introduced between the rods and rotated into its final position. The coupler is placed into its final position on the construct, and the lower portion is engaged with the rod with gentle upward pressure. The bolt is tightened and torqued. A second connector is placed near the other end of the construct.

All set screws are once again torqued to a minimum of 60 in-lb following completion of the construct. Fig. 13 depicts a completed construct.

VentroFix System

The VentroFix System is a second example of a dual-rod system designed for anterior use from T8 to L5 (Fig. 14). The instrumentation is applied after decompression and graft placement.

Three clamp designs are available that allow fixation to either the left or right side of the spine (Fig. 15). Two of the clamps have holes that are offset in relation to one another for use on opposite ends of the construct, whereas the third clamp design

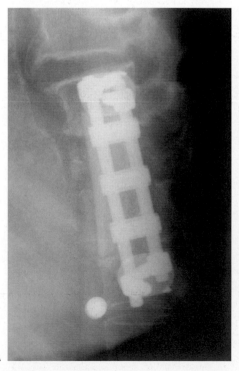

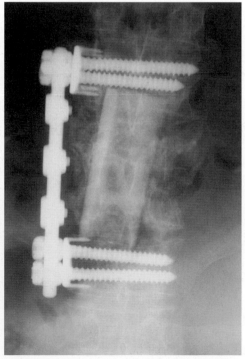

A   B

Fig. 13. Anteroposterior (**A**) and lateral (**B**) postoperative radiographs of a patient who underwent two-level corpectomy and reconstruction with the Kaneda SR.

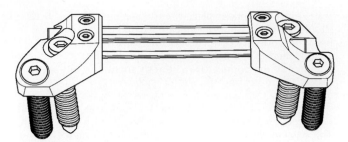

Fig. 14. The VentroFix is a dual-rod system that requires only unicortical fixation.

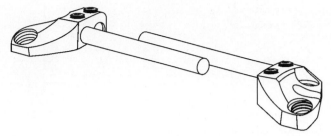

Fig. 16. The rods are placed in the closed holes and secured. They are then placed through the open holes to complete the construct.

has holes that are placed in line with each other. The third clamp is intended for use when a portion of the vertebral body is missing or removed. Each clamp has one closed and one open hole for rod placement.

The 7.5-mm-diameter screws are available in lengths from 30 to 55 mm in 5-mm increments. The screws are self-tapping and intended for unicortical purchase. A machine-threaded section on the proximal screw allows the screw to be locked to the clamp.

Rods 6 mm in diameter are utilized and come in precut lengths of 50, 75, 100, 125, and 150 mm. The rods can be cut to intermediate lengths as desired. A parallel connector is available if the construct length exceeds that of the available rods.

INSERTION TECHNIQUE. The construct is placed following decompression and graft placement. The length of the construct is determined with a rod template. Rods are cut to the appropriate length. The clamps are selected.

The rods are placed into the closed hole on each clamp and secured. The free end of each rod is then placed through the open hole of the opposing clamp (Fig. 16). The construct is adjusted to the desired length and set screws are tightened. The rods should not protrude more than 5 mm from the end of the clamp.

A drill guide is threaded into the posterior hole of each clamp. The construct is placed onto the lateral aspect of the spine in the desired position. Holes are drilled and the posterior screws are placed. The anterior screws are placed in a similar fashion. The construct is compressed and set screws are secured.

Final Comments

Various types of instrumentation are available for use in the anterior thoracolumbar spine. Many of these systems have been recently released or are modifications of previous systems. No study is available comparing the current devices.

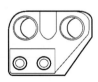

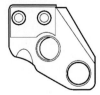

Fig. 15. The three configurations of the VentroFix clamps. Each clamp has one closed hole and one open hole for the rod.

References

1. Dwyer AF, Newton NC, Sherwood AA. An anterior approach to scoliosis: a preliminary report. *Clin Orthop* 1969;62:192–202.
2. Dwyer AF, Schafer MF. Anterior approach to scoliosis: results of treatment in fifty-one cases. *J Bone Joint Surg Br* 1974;56:218–224.
3. Hsu LC, Zuchermann J, Tang SC, et al. Dwyer instrumentation in the treatment of adolescent idiopathic scoliosis. *J Bone Joint Surg Br* 1982;64:536–541.
4. Kohler R, Galland O, Mechin H, et al. The Dwyer procedure in the treatment of idiopathic scoliosis: a 10-year follow-up review of 21 patients. *Spine* 1990;15:75–80.
5. Luk KDK, Leong JCY, Reyes L, et al. The comparative results of treatment in idiopathic thoracolumbar and lumbar scoliosis using the Harrington, Dwyer, and Zielke instrumentations. *Spine* 1989;14:275–280.
6. Zielke K, Stunkat R, Beaujean F. Ventrae derotations spondylodese. *Arch Orthop Unfall Chir* 1976;85:257–277.
7. Horton WC, Holt RT, Johnson JR, et al. Zielke instrumentation in idiopathic scoliosis: late effects and minimizing complications. *Spine* 1988;13:1145–1149.
8. Moskowitz A, Trommanhauser S. Surgical and clinical results of scoliosis surgery using Zielke instrumentation. *Spine* 1993;18:2444–2451.
9. Trammel TR, Benedict F, Reed D. Anterior spine fusion using Zielke

instrumentation for adult thoracolumbar and lumbar scoliosis. *Spine* 1991;16:307–316.

10. Wojcik AS, Webb JK, Burwell RG. An analysis of the effect of the Zielke operation on S-shaped curves in idiopathic scoliosis: the use of EVAs showing that correction of the thoracic curve occurs in its lower part: significance of the thoracolumbar spinal segment. *Spine* 1989;14:625–631.

11. Dunn HK. Anterior stabilization of thoracolumbar injuries. *Clin Orthop* 1984;189:116–124.

12. Jendrisak MD. Spontaneous abdominal aortic rupture from erosion by a lumbar fixation device: a case report. *Surgery* 1986;99:631–633.

13. Kostuik JP. Anterior fixation for burst fractures of the thoracic and lumbar spine with or without neurological involvement. *Spine* 1988; 13:286–93.

208. Hook and Rod Fixation of the Thoracic and Lumbar Spine

Michael Steinmetz, Eldan Eichbaum, and Edward C. Benzel

History

The era of hook and rod instrumentation began with the work of Paul Harrington. In the 1950s, Dr. Harrington was the orthopedic surgeon responsible for the care of patients suffering with polio at the City-County Hospital in Houston, Texas (1). Treatment goals in these patients with spinal deformity were to halt (and possibly correct) the scoliotic curvature, and subsequently prevent life-threatening complications such as cardiopulmonary compromise. For these patients, early treatment consisted of casting or surgery, which at the time was very dangerous. Harrington, understanding the shortcomings of nonoperative strategies, began to utilize surgical approaches to halt the progression of the scoliotic curvature in these cardiopulmonary compromised patients.

Harrington considered an internal fixation system. The first consisted of facet screw fixation (1), followed by a system consisting of hooks and a threaded rod adjusted by nuts. Further modifications led to the development of stainless steel rods and hooks placed in both compression and distraction. The initial deformity correction was excellent, but frequent early construct failures, such as instrument fracture and hook dislodgment, led to loss of correction. This experience confirmed the tenet that a bony fusion was essential for stable correction. Harrington published his results first in 1962 and after further revisions, the Harrington instrumentation system was popularized

These early experiences led to the development of universal spinal instrumentation (USI). The new systems are universal in that they have the capability to stabilize and manipulate the entire spinal column. They allow the application of multiple corrective forces on the same rod and the utilization of multiple points of fixation. This permitted the preservation of motion segments, the enhancement of fusion rates, and the minimization of instrumentation failure (2). The newer constructs permitted the customization of an implant, based on the pathology, location, quality of bone, and spinal biomechanics (2).

Relevant Anatomy

When considering the use of spinal instrumentation, knowledge of the variable anatomy of the spine is essential. This is not only important regarding surgical technique, but also for consideration of implant selection, mode of application, and location of placement.

Both the width and depth of the vertebral bodies increase while descending caudally, with the exception of C6 and the lower lumbar levels where the size decreases (3,4). In the thoracic region, the dorsal vertebral height is greater than the ventral height, whereas the opposite occurs in the lumbar spine. This leads to a structural and physiological kyphosis in the thoracic spine and a lordosis in the lumbar region.

The thoracic vertebrae warrant special mention. They are an integral part of a rugged, osteoligamentous complex that includes the ribs and sternum (5). This configuration is extremely stable. The rib articulates with both the vertebral body and transverse process, and there are associated ligaments with each articulation.

The facet joints are apophyseal joints with a loose capsule and a synovial lining (6). The facet joints change from essentially a coronal configuration in the cervical and thoracic region to a sagittal orientation in the lumbar spine (Fig. 1). This facet orientation allows for pedicular hook placement in the thoracic spine, but precludes pedicle hook placement in the lumbar spine. Furthermore, the coronal orientation of the facets in the thoracic spine allows greater lateral bending, while limiting movement in the sagittal plane. In the lumbar spine, the sagittal orientation permits flexion and extension, but resists lateral rotation.

The most important factor regarding sublaminar hook placement is the spinal canal diameter. This diameter is narrowest in the thoracic and greatest in cervical region. In the case of spinal stenosis, the extramedullary space may be markedly diminished. This narrow spinal canal diameter in the thoracic spine places laminar hooks at higher risk for neural element injury. Therefore, many surgeons prefer pedicle hooks.

The size of the pedicle increases as the spine is descended. The sagittal pedicle width increases from the cervical to the thoracic region, and then decreases as the lumbar spine is descended (Fig. 2). The transverse pedicle width increases from the cervical to the lumbar spine (4,7,8) (Fig. 3). This makes the lumbar spine a favored site for pedicle screw instrumentation. Nevertheless, the mechanical strength of the pedicle and its close proximity to the facet joints make the pedicle an important anchor site in the thoracic spine (2). Aiding hook placement in the thoracic spine is the more coronal orientation of the facets.

The transverse processes arise from the junction of the pedicle and lamina. In the mid- to lower thoracic region they are of substantial size and project in a lateral and dorsal orientation

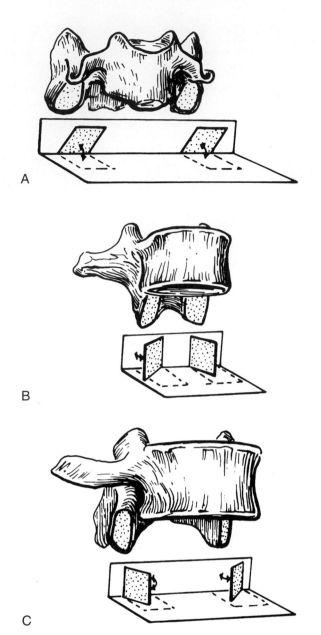

Fig. 1. The relative coronal orientation of the facet in the cervical region (**A**). This changes to an intermediate orientation in the thoracic region (**B**). The relative sagittal orientation in the lumbar region (**C**). (From Benzel EC: *Biomechanics of spine stabilization. Principles and clinical practice.* New York: McGraw-Hill, 1995:1–269, with permission.)

(6). In this region, they are relatively easy to isolate and can be used for hook purchase, although not as strong as the lamina or pedicle. In the lower thoracic spine, the transverse processes are more atretic and are not useful for hook placement. In the lumbar spine, the transverse processes project in a ventral and ventrodorsal direction (6). Because of their large size they may be used for hook purchase.

Biomechanics

In the era of spinal instrumentation, a sound understanding of the biomechanics of the normal and pathological spine is

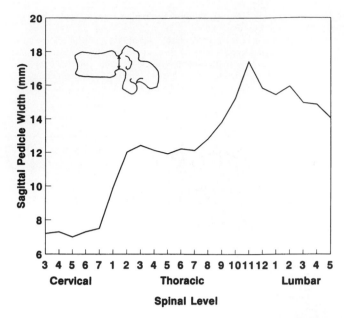

Fig. 2. Sagittal pedicle width vs. spinal level. (From Benzel EC: *Biomechanics of spine stabilization. Principles and clinical practice.* New York: McGraw-Hill, 1995:1–269, with permission.)

essential, since this knowledge influences clinical decision making and subsequent outcome. This section focuses on dorsal hook and rod constructs that apply compression, distraction, and/or three-point bending fixation. With USI strategies, these forces can be applied at multiple levels along the construct.

Dorsal Distraction Fixation

Isolated distraction is rarely achieved. When multiple spinal levels are placed in distraction via a dorsal implant, an associ-

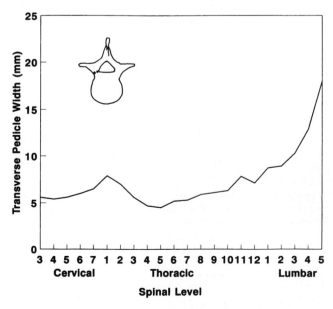

Fig. 3. Transverse pedicle width vs. spinal level. (From Benzel EC: *Biomechanics of spine stabilization. Principles and clinical practice.* New York: McGraw-Hill, 1995:1–269, with permission.)

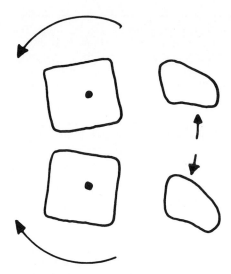

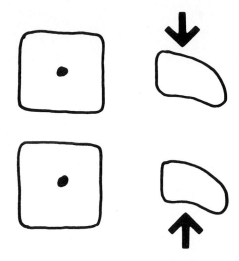

Fig. 4. A distraction force placed dorsal to the instantaneous axis of rotation (IAR) produces a flexion bending moment. (From Benzel EC: *Biomechanics of spine stabilization. Principles and clinical practice.* New York: McGraw-Hill, 1995:1–269, with permission.)

Fig. 5. The direction of forces used with dorsal tension-band fixation. (From Benzel EC: *Biomechanics of spine stabilization. Principles and clinical practice.* New York: McGraw-Hill, 1995:1–269, with permission.)

ated three-point bending moment is often observed (6). Simple distraction may be achieved by applying the force at only one motion segment. The Knodt rod may be used for this type of force application. This force application is dorsal to the instantaneous axis of rotation (IAR). This results in a flexion bending moment (6) (Fig. 4). The IAR is defined as the point about which a spinal segment rotates. A dorsally applied distraction force opens the neuroforamina, but rarely corrects the spinal deformity (9). It may also lead to the exaggeration of a kyphosis or the straightening of a lordosis, with a resultant flat back, with or without chronic pain. Due to these complications and its limited utility, it is rare to use dorsal distraction solely. Some surgeons apply dorsal distraction forces in the hope of reducing a vertebral fracture via ligamentotaxis. To achieve enough force for this to occur, a longer three-part bending construct is usually required.

By placing hooks at multiple levels, USI can provide multisegmental rigid distraction (6). This leads to increased stability and a decreased chance of instrumentation failure. This high efficacy and low complication rate are related to the "sharing" of the load by multiple fixation sites. Finally, hooks may be placed in a "claw" configuration, thus increasing stability and decreasing the chance of failure.

Tension-Band Fixation

Placing a dorsal implant into a compression mode produces tension-band fixation. The forces are applied dorsal to the IAR and result in extension of the spine via the application of a bending moment (Fig. 5). The absence of ventral neural element compression must be assured prior to the application of tension-band fixation forces. Otherwise, placing the spine in compression may lead to the protrusion of disc or bone fragments into the spinal canal and the worsening of a neurological deficit. Kyphotic deformities may be corrected with tension-band fixation force application if the IAR is well enough forward of the points of dorsal compression force application. Of note is that if the facet joints are disrupted, tension-band fixation may

result in excessive extension, leading to dorsal neural element impingement.

The bending moment applied at the site of pathology treated by a tension-band spinal implant is defined by the product of the compressive force applied at the rostral and caudal termini of the construct (at the instrument-bone interface) and its perpendicular distance from the IAR (10) (Fig. 6). Therefore, the bending moment applied to the spine by a tension-band fixator is dependent on the distance of force application to the IAR, but independent of construct length. Tension-band fixation al-

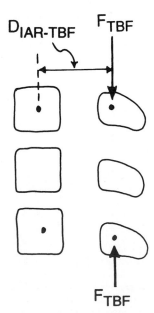

Fig. 6. The forces applied by a tension-band fixation construct are described by the equation ($M_{tbf} = F_{tbf} D_{iar-tbf}$) where M_{tbf} is the bending moment, F_{tbf} is the compression force applied at the upper and lower termini of the construct at the instrument–bone interface, and $D_{iar-tbf}$ is the perpendicular distance from the IAR to the tension-band fixation applied-force vector. (From Benzel EC: *Biomechanics of spine stabilization. Principles and clinical practice.* New York: McGraw-Hill, 1995: 1–269, with permission.)

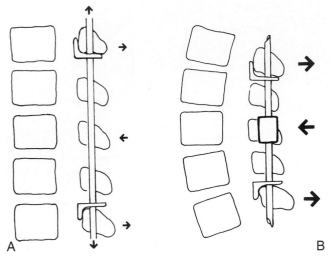

Fig. 7. Dorsal instrumentation used in distraction placed dorsally directed forces at the construct terminae and a ventrally directed force at the fulcrum leading to a three-point bending moment (**A**). A sleeve placed at the fulcrum may be used to increase the ventrally directed force, thereby aiding in the reduction of a kyphotic deformity (**B**). (From Benzel EC: *Biomechanics of spine stabilization. Principles and clinical practice.* New York: McGraw-Hill, 1995:1–269, with permission.)

lows for the use of short constructs that apply relatively small forces to the spine. This leads to a diminished overall stiffness (6).

Three-Point Bending Fixation

Three-point bending is defined by its dorsally directed forces at the terminae of the construct that are opposed by a ventrally directed force at the fulcrum (Fig. 7A). This complex force application allows for the correction of kyphoses or retropulsed bone and/or disc fragments (6). A sleeve may act to increase the ventrally applied force (Fig. 7B).

The bending moment at the fracture site by three-point bending fixation is equal to the product of the distances from both terminal hook-bone interfaces and the ventrally applied force at the fulcrum, divided by the sum of the distances from the fulcrum to the hook-bone interfaces (6) (Fig. 8). As opposed

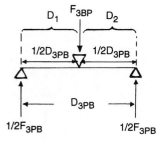

Fig. 8. If a three-point bending construct is symmetrically placed, that is, if the length of the construct above the fulcrum is equal to that below the fulcrum, then $D1$ is equal to $D2$, both of these are equal to $2\ D_{3pd}$, and the situation is described by the equation $[M_{3pd} = (\frac{1}{2}D_{3pd})^2\ F_{3pd}/D_{3pd} = 0.25\ D_{3pd}\ F_{3pd}/D_{3pd} = 0.25\ D_{3pd} \times F_{3pd}]$ where M_{3pd} is the bending moment at the fracture site, F_{3pd} is the ventrally directed force applied at the fulcrum, and D_{3pd} is the length of the construct. (From Benzel EC: *Biomechanics of spine stabilization. Principles and clinical practice.* New York: McGraw-Hill, 1995:1–269, with permission.)

to tension-band fixation, the forces applied by three-point bending fixators are perpendicular to the spine. Therefore, the bending moment applied to the spine is directly proportional to construct length. In other words, the length of the construct is directly proportional to the strength of the force application. If more substantial moments are required, a longer construct is desirable.

Three-point bending fixation requires fixation at only three levels. USI implants may be placed multisegmentally to help ensure increased stability and diminish the chance of failure.

The Systems

USI implants are versatile and allow for the placement of multiple corrective forces at a variety of points along the construct. They also allow short segment fixation, thus preserving motion segments. Despite these advantages, these systems are expensive and there is a steep learning curve regarding their application.

There are numerous hook-rod systems available today. There are variations in hooks, rods, and coupling devices. The Cotrel-Dubosset (CD) system has a wide variety of hooks, both open and closed (Fig. 9). The system is top-loading and top-tightening. Unique to the CD system is a knurled rod and the necessity of stripping the locking screw on final tightening, which makes removal difficult (11). Newer renditions, however, have been developed. The ISOLA system provides open and closed hooks. This system offers hooks of varying sizes (Fig. 10). The closed hook uses a drop-entry technique and the open hook is top loading (2); both are top tightening. Unique to ISOLA is the ability of the hook-rod angle to change with tightening, which acts to increase bony engagement (12) (Fig. 11). The Texas Scottish Rite Hospital system consists of hooks that are side loading and side tightening. This system has a large variety of hooks (Fig. 12). Unique to this system is the three-point sheer clamp coupler (the strongest hook rod connector available) (13) and the transverse connector (Fig. 13), which allows for the most rigid quadrilateral construct available (14).

Today there are many more than the three aforementioned systems, with subtle and not so subtle differences. This variety of implants allows for surgeon preference and for an ease of application based on experience, location, or spinal pathology.

Surgical Indications

Indications for complex spinal instrumentation include traumatic, degenerative, neoplastic, iatrogenic, and infectious etiologies. Spinal instrumentation may be placed ventrally, dorsally, or both, depending on the mechanism of injury and the degree of spinal column instability. Spinal stability has been defined as the ability of the spine to resist physiological loads and prevent excessive motion, spinal deformity, neurological injury, and/or chronic pain (15). Several definitions and gradations of spinal instability have been described (16–19). In clinical practice, the three-column spinal theory of Denis is the most widely accepted (Fig. 14). He defines instability as greater than two-column involvement (20,21).

Indications for dorsal thoracic and thoracolumbar fusion and instrumentation include ventral, dorsal, and combined ventral/dorsal instability, especially when translational deformity is present. In general, dorsal instrumentation provides a stronger

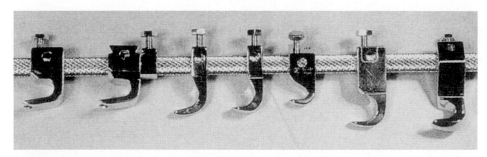

Fig. 9. The Cotrel-Dubosset (CD) system utilizes a knurled rod and offers open and closed hooks. (From Benzel EC, ed. *Spinal instrumentation*. AANS, 1994, with permission.)

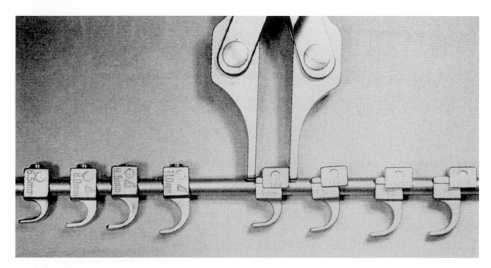

Fig. 10. The ISOLA system offers hooks of varying sizes and shapes in open and closed varieties. (From Benzel EC, ed. *Spinal instrumentation*. AANS, 1994, with permission.)

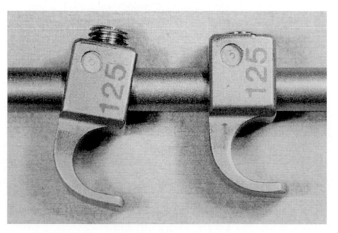

Fig. 11. Tightening the insert screw results is the hook rotating 15 degrees relative to the rod. This drives the blade under the bone and improves fixation strength. (From Benzel EC, ed. *Spinal instrumentation*. AANS, 1994, with permission.)

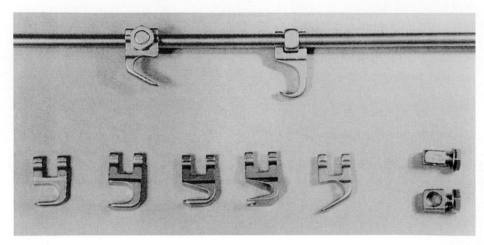

Fig. 12. The Texas Scottish Rite Hospital (TSRH) system offers a wide variety of hooks in different sizes and shapes. They are secured to the rod by the three-point sheer clamp. (From Benzel EC, ed. *Spinal instrumentation.* AANS, 1994, with permission.)

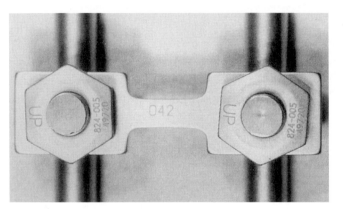

Fig. 13. The TSRH cross-link is coupled to the rod with an eyebolt lock-nut combination. (From Benzel EC, ed. *Spinal instrumentation.* AANS, 1994, with permission.)

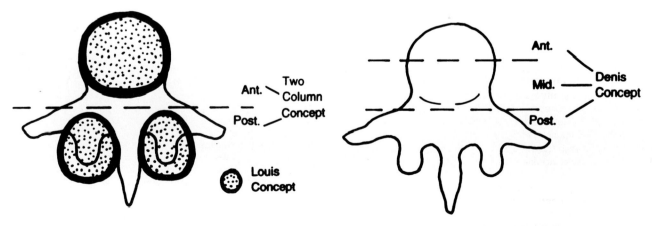

Fig. 14. The two-column concept described by Louis on the left, and the three-column theory described by Denis on the right. (From Benzel EC: *Biomechanics of spine stabilization. Principles and clinical practice.* New York: McGraw-Hill, 1995:1–269, with permission.)

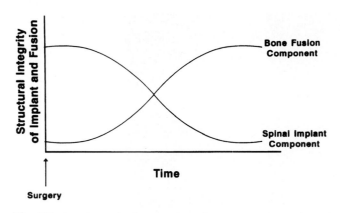

Fig. 15. The relationship between bone fusion acquisition and spinal implant integrity changes with time following surgery. (From Benzel EC, ed. *Spinal instrumentation.* AANS, 1994, with permission.)

construct compared to ventral instrumentation. This is because dorsal instrumentation provides increased translational and torsional force resistance via the use of a long moment arm. The moment arm applied to the site of pathology is proportional to the length of the construct. Furthermore, multiple fixation points facilitate deformity correction, load sharing, and pullout resistance. The loss of multiple motion segments and the associated problems of reduced motion, facet arthropathy, and chronic pain syndromes often complicate these advantages of multisegmental fixation.

In theory, spinal instrumentation affords immediate internal spinal stabilization, facilitating fusion and allowing for early patient mobilization. Early mobilization, in turn, both hastens recovery and decreases the risk of extraspinal complications. The establishment of a solid arthrodesis remains the ultimate goal of any instrumentation construct because the failure to achieve a solid arthrodesis will invariably lead to instrumentation failure (Fig. 15).

Instrumentation Construct Design

The nuances of construct design are beyond the scope of this chapter, but some principles should be discussed. The determination of hook placement is based on several variables, including the spine region, pathology, the biomechanical forces desired, and surgeon preference. A claw configuration is the strongest type of hook construct. It involves two ipsilateral hooks facing one another at the same level or at consecutive levels, most commonly placed at the terminal ends of a dorsal construct (Fig. 16). Usually sublaminar hooks rostral to the pathological level (or deformity) face rostrally, whereas hooks caudal to the pathological level face caudally. Pedicle hooks always face rostrally, and transverse process hooks face caudally. Transverse process hooks are usually used in tandem with a pedicle hook.

Of equal importance to the decision regarding the segmental levels to be instrumented, one must also determine the levels to be fused. The advantages of both "instrumenting and fusing long" include a greater lever arm for deformity reduction and stabilization, as well as multiple points of fixation, thus minimizing the chance of construct failure. The disadvantages of this construct include immobilization of multiple normal spinal levels, thus sacrificing future function for an improved mechanical advantage. In the rigid thoracic spine, this may be relatively

unimportant, but in the flexible lumbar spine this can be severely debilitating. Short segment fixation preserves motion segments, but creates significantly higher bone/implant stresses, thereby promoting construct failure.

Finally, some surgeons prefer to employ the concept and technique of fusion/instrumentation mismatch. This involves a long instrumentation construct in which only the pathological levels are fused. In this situation, most surgeons recommend implant removal at about 1 year postoperatively to allow for a successful strong fusion, while minimizing complications (e.g., facet arthropathy, pain syndromes, permanent motion segment immobilization).

Technique

EXPOSURE. After the induction of anesthesia, the patient is carefully turned from the supine to the prone position, preferably onto a radiolucent operating room table. This should be done with adequate assistance, especially when spinal precautions are necessary. Appropriate padding is provided for the hip, the brachial plexus, and both the lower and upper extremities. The abdomen is allowed to fall ventrally to decrease intraabdominal pressure and venous engorgement. This minimizes intraoperative blood loss.

A generous incision is drawn on the back. This should allow for adequate rostral and caudal exposure, as well as lateral exposure if necessary. The incision may be midline, paramedian, or midline with lateral extension (i.e., hockey stick), depending on the approach planned (Fig. 17). An incision is also drawn over the iliac crest unilaterally or bilaterally for autologous bone graft harvest. After generous sterile preparation and draping, the skin may be injected subcutaneously with a lidocaine/epinephrine mixture (1%/1:200,000), and incised with a sharp knife through the dermis to the subcutaneous fat. Monopolar cautery is then used for hemostasis and subsequent dissection. Monopolar cautery and a periosteal elevator are used to dissect the paraspinous muscles from medial to lateral, exposing the spinous processes, laminae, facet joints, and transverse processes. Care is taken not to violate the facet capsule with the electrocautery, especially in nonpathological segments. This can be accomplished by either monopolar cautery dissection over the capsule or blunt dissection using a pair of periosteal elevators and sponge.

The frequent intermittent release of the self-retaining retractors decreases muscle ischemia, minimizing muscle necrosis, postoperative infections, and wound healing difficulties. Also, cell saver suction may be valuable, except in patients with infection or cancer. Bone and epidural bleeding may be brisk, but most often occurs with a slow, persistent ooze. Furthermore, bone wax is relatively contraindicated in fusion procedures. Therefore, Gelfoam and/or Surgicel is standard for bony hemostasis.

If no obvious deformity is present to ensure the correct spinal level, an intraoperative plain radiograph is performed. An anteroposterior (AP) radiograph is taken to localize the level in the upper and midthoracic spinal column, whereas a lateral radiograph is performed for lower thoracic or thoracolumbar localization. Ribs are counted in the AP projection, while vertebral bodies from the sacrum are counted on the lateral projection. C-arm fluoroscopy is often used in cases involving pedicle screw constructs, but may also be used for intraoperative localization. Preoperative plain radiographs are mandatory, not only to correlate pathology with other imaging modalities, such as computed tomography (CT) or magnetic resonance imaging (MRI), but also to correlate with intraoperative radiographs.

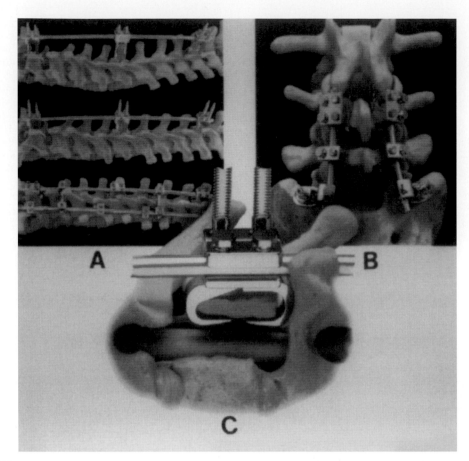

Fig. 16. Example of a claw configuration. The claw is usually placed at the caudal and rostral ends of the construct. (From Benzel EC, ed. *Spine surgery: techniques, complication avoidance, and management.* New York: Churchill-Livingstone, 1999, with permission.)

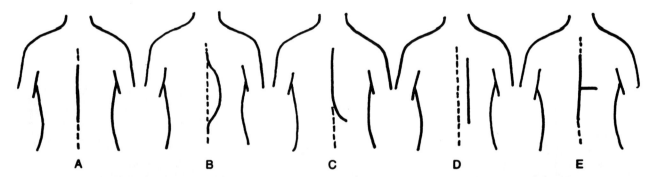

Fig. 17. Skin incisions that may be used for dorsolateral exposure of the thoracic or lumbar spine. **A**: Dorsal midline. **B**: Semilunar. **C**: Hockey stick. **D**: Straight paramedian. **E**: T-shaped. (From Benzel EC, ed. *Spine surgery: techniques, complication avoidance, and management.* New York: Churchill-Livingstone, 1999, with permission.)

Dorsal element preparation for hook placement and the preparation of the fusion bed is then performed. Spinal decompression, if required, should be performed prior to dorsal element preparation. Dorsal hook placement may be sublaminar, abutting the pedicle, or abutting the transverse process. Preoperative construct planning guides the decision regarding the designated dorsal element(s) for hook placement.

HOOK INSERTION. The spinal laminae provide solid sites for hook placement. They have the greatest bone/metal interface, decreasing the risk of hook pullout or migration, and have the strongest purchase and the greatest strength for deformity correction and/or stabilization of the spinal column. Lumbar or sacral hook placement is well accepted, but thoracic hook placement rostral to the conus medullaris is more controversial (specifically in neurologically intact or incomplete individuals) because of the relatively narrow thoracic spinal canal and its tenuous blood supply. The risk of neurological injury with sublaminar hook placement is present, but very low.

LAMINAR HOOKS. Laminar hook insertion is initiated with laminotomies of the rostral half of the lamina below and the caudal half of the lamina above the level of hook placement. Removal of the spinous process to its base is frequently necessary to facilitate hook and dorsal rod placement throughout the length of the construct. After removal of the ligamentum flavum, and occasionally a portion of the medial facet, the completed laminotomy resembles a rectangle (Fig. 18). This laminotomy must be large enough to allow for adjacent hook placement. To aid in pullout resistance and because the lumbar lamina is large, a pedicle screw may be used in conjunction. A laminar tester may be used to measure the laminar size and contour, but this is not required. The maximization of the bone–implant interface is optimal. Therefore, the widest possible hook should be inserted. If the hook does not fit the contour of the lamina, then either the lamina may be further contoured to fit the hook, or, depending on the system used, another hook may be inserted. Attaching the hooks to the rod may be performed after placing all hooks initially, or by using a sequential tightening technique (22).

Briefly, one must begin at either terminus, securing the first hook to the end of the rod and then sequentially attaching each successive hook to the rod until the unilateral construct is complete. It is of extreme importance to apply dorsally directed forces to the rod at all times to avoid hook migration ventrally. Each hook is securely tightened upon insertion and compressed onto its respective lamina. Biomechanical forces (e.g., distraction, compression) may be placed sequentially or after completion of hook attachment. Prior to hook attachment, the rod must be measured, cut, and contoured to fit the spinal curve or to apply specific desired biomechanical forces during deformity correction (the desired spinal curve). This step is repeated for the adjacent hook-rod construct, and subsequently the rods are interconnected with two cross-fixators. Cross-fixation increases the stability of the implant by resisting torsional and translational forces, as well as by minimizing hook pullout.

PEDICLE HOOKS. The most common site for hook insertion in the thoracic spine is the pedicle, caudal to the inferior facet and rostral to the rostral facet. The coronal orientation of the thoracic facet joints promotes this strategy, whereas the sagittal orientation of the thoracolumbar facet joints precludes it. Furthermore, lateral placement helps avoid spinal cord compression, minimizing the chance of neural element injury.

Either a high-speed drill resects the caudal-medial quadrant of the caudal facet or an osteotome is used (Fig. 19). The hook is then inserted pointing rostrally, engaging the pedicle. Adequate bone resection maximizes pedicle purchase, whereas too much bone removal may cause pedicle fracture, and too little bone removal precludes adequate pedicle purchase. Bifid hooks promote pedicle purchase, but nonbifid hooks may also provide a strong purchase, due to the close approximation of the inferior and superior facet complex.

TRANSVERSE PROCESS HOOKS. Transverse process hooks are also commonly placed in the thoracic spine. This is due, in part, to the relatively large transverse processes. The ventral-rostral orientation of these transverse processes promotes hook insertion, most commonly caudally directed. This is performed after stripping off the costotransverse ligament, usually in con-

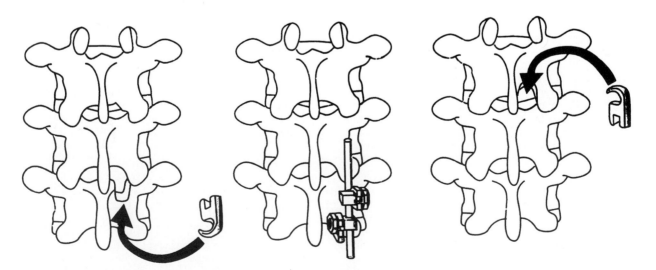

Fig. 18. Technique for laminar hook insertion. A pedicle screw may be used with the lumbar hook to aid in pullout resistance. (From Benzel EC, ed. *Spine surgery: techniques, complication avoidance, and management.* New York: Churchill-Livingstone, 1999, with permission.)

A

B

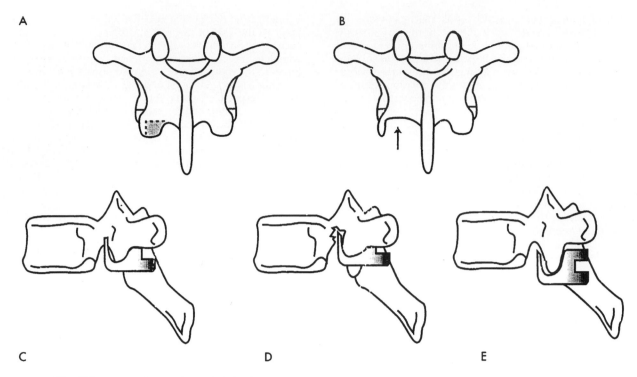

C   D   E

Fig. 19. **A–E:** Technique for pedicle hook insertion. (From Benzel EC, ed. *Spine surgery: techniques, complication avoidance, and management.* New York: Churchill-Livingstone, 1999, with permission.)

junction with a rostrally facing pedicle hook, creating a claw configuration. The transverse processes in the thoracolumbar region are rudimentary and the facet joints are sagittally oriented, precluding transverse process or pedicle hook insertion.

Once the construct is completed, bone graft harvest should be performed. The bone harvested during preparation of the spine may be used as graft material, but is usually not of great enough quality or quantity to function as "stand-alone" graft material. Iliac crest cortical and cancellous bone is an excellent source of bone graft, and is readily harvested from either the same or a separate incision. The caudal length of the incision dictates whether a separate incision is required for the graft harvest site. Once a large portion of the dorsal iliac crest is exposed, thin unicortical (matchstick) strips are created with a straight osteotome (or oscillating saw) and mallet. These sticks are carefully removed, and the exposed cancellous bone is gouged and collected into a container with normal saline. Care is taken not to cut too deeply into the ilium. Prior to cutting and removal of the graft, all soft tissue should be stripped off the bone graft bed to maximize the chances of fusion. Following completion of the harvest, a copious amount of antibiotic fluid is irrigated into the wound and a large piece of Gelfoam is placed firmly on the cancellous bone. The wound is then closed in layers.

FUSION BED PREPARATION. The fusion bed is prepared using a high-speed air drill, curet, or osteotome to decorticate to healthy bleeding bone. The transverse processes are most commonly decorticated in the thoracic spine due to their large size, strength, and distance from the spinal canal. The lamina and facet complexes are excellent recipients of bone graft, but frequently are not available due to bony destruction from the pathological process and/or the decompression. Decortication should not be so extensive as to weaken the recipient bone.

The wound is then copiously irrigated with 2 to 3 L of antibiotic solution.

The harvested cancellous bone and the spinous process/lamina nonstructural cortical bone graft are then morselized and kept separately. This graft material may be combined with a demineralized bone matrix, containing bone morphogenic protein (e.g., Grafton, Osteofil). This increases osteoblast production and enhances fusion rates. These substances also improve the handling ability of the graft material. The graft material is then placed bilaterally, spanning the desired levels of fusion. The harvested iliac crest bone is placed initially, since this is superior graft material, followed by the spinous process/lamina bone. Ideally, the unicortical strips are placed with their cancellous half positioned against the graft bed, spanning at least one motion segment.

Wound closure is then initiated with the release of the retractors and meticulous paraspinous muscle hemostasis. Prior to closure, some surgeons prefer to place large drains in the subfascial space, tunneled through a distant stab incision. A large absorbable suture is used for fascial closure and the closure of the more superficial layers up to the skin (i.e., Vicryl O, OO). The skin may be secured with either staples or a monofilament suture.

Complications

The potential complications of spinal surgery are increased with the use of instrumentation. Besides the common complications such as dural laceration and cerebrospinal fluid leak, the risk of blood loss, infection, and neural element injury are increased with the use of instrumentation. Complications associated with dorsal hook rod instrumentation systems include hook pullout, neural element injury due to hook insertion or construct failure, and fusion failure.

Hook pullout most frequently occurs at the rostral terminus of a construct. In a construct that uses three-point bending forces to reduce a deformity, the incidence of failure may be minimized by using a terminal claw configuration. In general, claw configurations increase the bone/implant interface and are used with an increased construct strength, thus decreasing the risk of hook pull-out and immobilization of fewer motion segments.

Sublaminar hooks are associated with the risk of neural element compression during insertion or following the placement of the implant. Sublaminar hook insertion must be performed with extreme care under a meticulously prepared lamina, adhering closely to the ventral laminar surface. Preoperative neuroimaging should alert the surgeon to the presence of spinal stenosis. Sublaminar hooks should be immediately secured to the rod, with the surgeon placing dorsally directed forces on the construct at all times. Three-point bending forces, by definition, create a ventrally directed force at the midpoint of the construct. Hence, sublaminar hooks used as intermediate points of fixation in these constructs are at risk for spinal canal encroachment and neural element injury. Finally, pedicle hooks may also migrate and encroach on the spinal cord in the canal or nerve root in the neuroforamen. Although this is not common, strategies to avoid this include meticulous bony removal to ensure the snug fit of the hook between the facet complexes. Bifid pedicle hooks improve pedicle purchase, but may also fracture the pedicle, rendering it (and the construct) weaker. Multiple hook trials in the facet complex should decrease the incidence of this complication.

To minimize complications, spinal decompression and implant insertion must be performed with great care. Meticulous adherence to surgical and sterile technique with the frequent release of retractors and the liberal use of irrigation should aid in decreasing infection rates and construct failures. Also, meticulous hemostasis is of extreme importance in decreasing potential complications in these complicated procedures.

Conclusions

Dorsal hook-rod instrumentation is indicated in individuals with spinal instability, especially with dorsal spinal column involvement, with or without ventral column involvement. Dorsal hook-rod instrumentation constructs afford superior strength, compared to ventral constructs, especially in rotation and translation. The three regions for hook insertion (sublaminar, pedicle, or transverse process) have advantages and disadvantages. Due to the relatively narrow spinal canal and the tenuous blood supply of the thoracic spine, many surgeons prefer not to utilize sublaminar hooks. In our opinion, however, sublaminar hooks may be placed safely throughout the thoracic spine and provide substantial strength for deformity correction and stability.

Many universal spine systems are available for use throughout the spinal column. Once their insertion technique is mastered, the implant may be placed safely and relatively quickly. Meticulous adherence to bone preparation, hemostasis, and sterile technique will minimize common complications. The careful insertion of the hooks with extreme caution using a constant dorsally directed force should minimize neural element injury.

References

1. Harrington PR: The history and development of Harrington instrumentation. *Clin Orthop* 93:110–112, 1973.
2. Stillerman CB, Gruen JP, Roy R: Thoracic and lumbar fusion: techniques for posterior stabilization. In: Menzes AH, Sonntag VKH, eds. *Principles of spinal surgery*. New York: McGraw-Hill 1996: 1199–1225.
3. Berry JL, Moran JM, Berg WS, et al.: A morphometric study of human lumbar and selected thoracic vertebrae. *Spine* 12:362–366, 1987.
4. Panjabi MM, Duranceau J, Coel V, et al.: Cervical human vertebrae: quantitative three-dimensional anatomy of the middle and lower regions. *Spine* 16:861–869, 1991.
5. Haber TR, Felinly WT, O'Brian M: Thoracic and lumbar fractures: diagnosis and management. In: Bridwell KH, DeWald RL, eds. *The textbook of spinal surgery*, 2nd ed. New York: Lippincott-Raven, 1997:1763–1839.
6. Benzel EC: *Biomechanics of spine stabilization. Principles and clinical practice*. New York: McGraw-Hill, 1995:1–269.
7. Krag MH, Weaver DL, Beynnon BD: Morphometry of the thoracic and lumbar spine related to transpedicular screw placement for surgical spine fixation. *Spine* 13:27–32, 1988.
8. Zindrick MR, Wiltse LL, Dournik A, et al.: Analysis of the morphometric characteristics of the thoracic and lumbar pedicles. *Spine* 12: 160–166, 1987.
9. Nasca RJ, Littlefield PD: Knodt rod distraction instrumentation in lumbosacral arthrodesis. *Spine* 15:1356–1359, 1990.
10. Benzel EC: Biomechanics of lumbar and lumbosacral spine fractures. In: Rea GL, ed. *Spinal trauma: current evaluation and management*. American Association of Neurological Surgeons 1993: 165–195.
11. Bridwell KH: Spinal instrumentation in the management of adolescent scoliosis. *Clin Orthop* 335:64–72, 1997.
12. Flores E, Rengachary SS, Hitchon PW: ISOLA instrumentation. In: Hitchon PW, Tragneis VC, Regachary SS, eds. *Techniques in spinal fusion and stabilization*. New York: Thieme, 1995:209–218.
13. Benzel EC, Baldwin NG, Ball PA: Texas Scottish Rite Hospital hook-rod fixation. In: Hitchon PW, Tragneis VC, Regachary SS, eds. *Techniques in spinal fusion and stabilization*. New York: Thieme, 1995: 229–240.
14. Johnston EC, Ashman RB, Coron JD: Mechanical effects of cross-linking rods in Cotrel-Dubousset instrumentation. Presented at the Scoliosis Research Society combined with the British Scoliosis Society, 21st annual meeting, September 21–25, 1986, Hamilton, Bermuda.
15. White AA, Punjabi MM: *Clinical biomechanics of the spine*. Philadelphia: JB Lippincott, 1978.
16. Benzel EC: The anatomic basis of spinal instability. *Clin Neurosurg* 41:224–241, 1993.
17. Farfan HF, Gracovetsky S: The nature of instability. *Spine* 9:714–719, 1984.
18. James KS, Wenger KH, Schlegel JD, et al.: Biomechanical evaluation of the stability of thoracolumbar burst fractures. *Spine* 19(15): 173–190, 1994.
19. Posner I, Edwards WT, Hayes WC: A biomechanical analysis of the clinical stability of the lumbar and lumbosacral spine. *Spine* 7: 374–389, 1982.
20. Denis F: Spinal instability as defined by the three-column spine concept in acute spinal trauma. *Clin Orthop* 189:65–76, 1984.
21. Denis F: The three-column spine and its significance in the classification of acute thoracolumbar spinal injuries. *Spine* 8:817–831, 1983.
22. Benzel EC, Ball PA, Baldwin NG, et al.: The sequential hook insertion technique for universal spine instrumentation application. *J Neurosurg* 17:608–611, 1993.
23. Stillerman CB, Gruen JP, Universal spinal instrumentation. In: Benzel EC, ed. *Spinal instrumentation*. American Association of Neurological Surgeons, Illinois: 1994.
24. Benzel EC, ed. *Spine surgery: techniques, complication avoidance, and management*. New York: Churchill-Livingstone, 1999.

209. Anterior Lumbar Interbody Fusion and Vertebral Replacement

Jeffery E. Masciopinto

The surgical decision-making process in reconstructive spine surgery should always incorporate the principles of adequate neural decompression, mechanical stabilization, and maximal preparation for fusion. The choice of surgical approach, therefore, should consider the location of compressive pathology, and subsequently allow for maximal immediate structural stability with adequate bone graft contact for fusion. Disease processes that involve the vertebral body or disc and cases of angular deformity often are best approached from an anterior trajectory. This chapter reviews the pertinent anatomy and approach decision making with an emphasis on pathophysiological considerations, surgical technique, and graft and instrumentation choices.

To maximize surgical success and minimize complications in anterior lumbar surgery, a familiarity with the prevertebral structures is essential. In addition, an understanding of the three-dimensional anatomy of the lumbar spine is crucial. Most importantly, the surgeon must be prepared for the different perspectives of the lumbar vertebral body, pedicles, foramen, and nerve roots that are present with the varying patient positions based on the approach employed. The retroperitoneal and anterior approaches to the lumbar spine have been covered in detail in other chapters; however, the cogent anatomy is briefly reviewed here.

Biomechanics of Anterior Lumbar Reconstruction

Anterior reconstruction of the lumbar spine represents a teleologically satisfying method of surgically establishing stability. Approximately 70% of the lumbar spine's inherent stability is derived from the vertebral body, disc, and anterior longitudinal ligament. Therefore, surgery designed to stabilize the spine should focus on maximizing the stability of this region. In particular, when the pathology has destroyed the structural integrity of the anterior column, such as in cases of tumor, trauma, or spondylolisthesis, the surgical approach must allow for re-creating anterior stability. In addition, when treating discogenic pathology, interbody fusion may provide for a more effective means of attaining initial stability and engraftation surface area, and thereby of improving fusion rates.

To effectively stabilize the lumbar spine, a combination of meticulous surgical technique and proper implant selection should be used. From a technical perspective, adequate decompression and end-plate preparation with maximal discectomy create the optimal environment for stabilization and fusion. Overly aggressive end-plate decortication can lead to a weakened construct, and incomplete discectomy reduces fusion surface area (1). In addition, proper size graft or implants should be placed into the defect while distracted, and therefore they remain under compression to create a load-bearing construct (2). Implant geometry and end-plate contact area also significantly affect mechanical stability and may influence fusion rates as demonstrated by Tsantrizos et al. (3) in their analysis of five different interbody constructs. This study found all devices increased the neutral zone, but had varying effects on

lateral bend stiffness. It has been demonstrated that threaded devices provide better rotational stability than bone grafts, and the device end-plate interface friction increases overall construct stability (4,5). While stand-alone anterior constructs are often performed, and have anecdotal support in the literature, clear evidence-based efficacy is lacking. There is good evidence from the literature that circumferential instrumentation enhances construct strength in all degrees of motion (6,7). In addition, the use of anterior and posterior stabilization often necessitates fusing fewer motion segments than in posterior-alone approaches. For these reasons, posterior augmentation of anterior constructs is often warranted, particularly when the treated pathology has created significant preoperative instability.

A secondary biomechanical effect of anterior interbody fusion can be seen at the junctional levels above and below the fused segment. Chow et al. (8) demonstrated in a cadaveric model that in a single-level fusion, the level above and below moved through a broader range of motion than in an intact spine, but that the discs experienced no increased loading. It is hypothesized that the increased stiffness of anterior constructs may overload adjacent segments and hasten junctional zone failure at an increased rate compared to the less stiff posterior fusion. While class I evidence for the use of anterior spinal reconstruction is lacking, a keen understanding of the biomechanical principles of spine fusion allows for the targeting of surgical procedures to the pathology present and attainment of surgical goals.

Anterior Lumbar Interbody Fusion: Pathophysiology and Indications

Anterior interbody fusion is applied to numerous lumbar spinal pathologies, including discogenic back pain, spondylolisthesis, pseudarthrosis, deformity, and infection. This technique offers biomechanical advantages and can be applied for first-time treatment of the above pathologies, or in salvage operations when the posterior approach has failed or if the posterior anatomy is distorted congenitally or iatrogenically. In native cases, where lack of neural compression obviates the need for posterior decompression, the anterior approach offers the advantage of sparing significant surgical trauma to the posterior musculature and ligaments. As a corollary, in situations where the posterior elements are lacking, such as myelodysplasia, or when the posterior elements are missing or devascularized from previous surgery, the anterior approach provides a fresh bony surface for successful engraftation. However, it must be kept in mind that the anterior approaches have the potential for complications to the vascular, neural, and intraabdominal anatomy.

Spondylolisthesis

Prior to the advent of instrumentation techniques, the treatment of spondylolisthesis involved bony fusion alone, and the anterior approach was utilized for stabilization as early as the 1920s. The term *spondylolisthesis* is derived from the Greek roots *spondylo*, or vertebra, and *olisthesis*, to slip or slide. The accepted categories based on the inherent spinal pathology are the dysplastic, isthmic, degenerative, traumatic, and pathological types (9). In addition, the amount of slippage can be classified by the method described by Meyerding (10) based on the position of the posterior cortex of the displaced segment relative to the intact segment (Fig. 1). In all cases, the slippage occurs because of insufficiency of the posterior elements creating excessive forces across the anterior column, allowing for a ventral displacement of the superior vertebral body. This phenomenon occurs most commonly at the L4-5 and L5-S1 levels secondary to the ventrally directed slip angle forces found at these levels (Fig. 2). The type of posterior pathology that creates the instability plays an important role in surgical decision making. For example, the glacial changes that lead to spondylolisthesis in spondylolysis or degenerative slips may allow for anterior stabilization alone, because the posterior elements may be relatively stable as demonstrated on flexion extension radiographs (11–19). However, in situations where the posterior elements have acutely failed, such as in trauma or pathological spondylolisthesis, or if the slip is increased on flexion extension radiographs, augmentation of anterior reconstruction with posterior fusion with or without instrumentation improves initial stability and may affect ultimate clinical outcome favorably (11,16).

The indications for surgery in patients with spondylolisthesis remain controversial, and no class I information is found in the literature. The basic tenets of spine surgery must be considered in deciding on what operation to perform on which patient and when. Customizing the need for decompression, with or without stabilization and arthrodesis, to each patient's clinical complaints and pathological anatomy will always maximize the chance for clinical success. Asymptomatic spondylolisthesis does not need to be addressed surgically unless there is defined progression to greater than 50% (grade III) slippage or the presence of mobile grade IV slippage. The treatment of symptomatic spondylolisthesis depends on many factors, including assess-

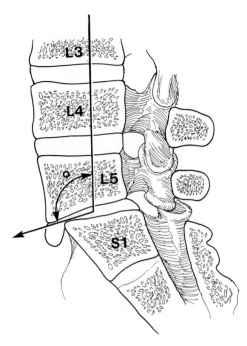

Fig. 2. The slip angle of the lower lumbar levels is greater than the cephalad levels, creating more ventral force vectors. (© 2002, Thomas H. Weinzerl.)

ment of radiculopathy, mechanical pain, and secondary gain/psychosocial issues. Certainly in cases with severe neural compression centrally, a combined anterior posterior or posterior alone approach is most reasonable. However, in situations with mechanical pain only and absence of central stenosis, an anterior-alone reconstruction may be appropriate.

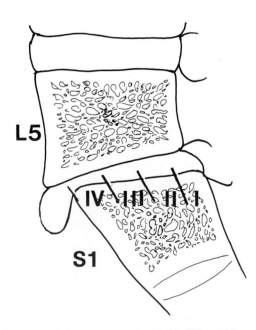

Fig. 1. The classification of lumbar spondylolisthesis is based on the position of the posterior cortex of the cephalad vertebral body in relation to the posterior cortex of the caudal vertebral body. (© 2002, Thomas H. Weinzerl.)

Discogenic Back Pain

According to the National Center for Health Statistics, low back pain is one of the most common ailments associated with physician visits in the United States, accounting for 14% of physician visits or 13 million new patient visits per annum. Unfortunately, because of the wide range of possible etiologies, an exact diagnosis is often not made. However, careful history taking, physical exam, and diagnostic testing can lead to more specific diagnosis and treatment plans. The diagnosis of discogenic back pain is possible with application of the surgeon's understanding of the pathophysiology involved and appropriate diagnostic means.

Discogenic back pain is produced by a failure of the mechanical integrity of the disc or a change in the biochemical milieu of the disc leading to an unresolved pain syndrome. Zdeblick (20) categorized discogenic syndromes into three anatomic categories: internal disc disruption (IDD), degenerative disc disease (DDD), and segmental instability. This schema correlates radiographic findings to the clinical syndrome. IDD refers to the patient with normal plain radiographs, and findings on magnetic resonance imaging (MRI) described as "black disc disease," with or without evidence of annular tears. It is postulated that the abnormal disc may elicit biochemical intermediaries, which irritate annular or end-plate pain fibers, and create back pain (21). In a similar fashion, DDD with the inherent loss of

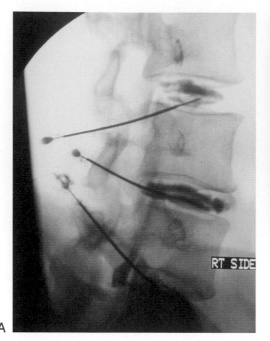 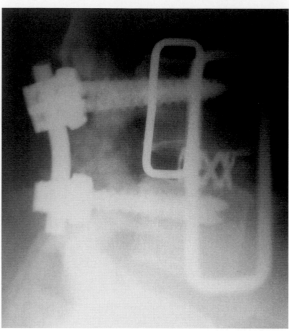

A   B

Fig. 3. A: A 40-year-old woman with mechanical back pain and degenerative disc changes at L4-5. Three-level lumbar discography shows P2 concordant pain at L4-5, and grade III disc disruption. Control levels are a P0 (painless) clinical response. **B**: Postoperative x-rays after the patient underwent an anterior discectomy, cage reconstruction, and posterior fixation.

disc height and presumed micromotion or gross instability irritates end-plate nerve endings, creating pain (22). Removing inciting disc pathology and providing long-term stabilization are the targets of surgical intervention.

The diagnosis of discogenic back pain is first and foremost a clinical diagnosis based on a history consistent with mechanical back pain, and the exclusion of other etiologies, typically without significant evidence of neural compression. Once the clinical diagnosis has been made, supplementary anatomical information obtained by MRI and discography can be correlated to the symptoms. In addition, relief of pain with a trial of lumbar corset bracing has been advocated as a positive preoperative diagnostic assessment (18). MRI provides important adjunctive information to the clinical diagnosis by localizing possible pain generators to specific lumbar levels. It is imperative to remember that the majority of abnormal discs identified by MRI are asymptomatic, and it is incumbent on the surgeon to attempt exact localization prior to planning surgical intervention. This process can be aided by the use of pressure discography. To obtain useful information from discography, abnormal and control levels should be injected to standard pressures, and subjective pain scores and follow-up imaging should correlate to the pathological level or levels (Fig. 3). Dilemmas occur when abnormal radiographic levels do not correlate with subjective pain; this scenario should create significant caution in recommending fusion (23,24). When a solid diagnosis of discogenic low back pain can be localized to specific lumbar levels, and conservative measures have failed, anterior interbody fusion may allow for consistently good surgical results, especially when compared to intertransverse fusion alone (15).

Corpectomy

The disease processes that require corpectomy and reconstruction offer fewer dilemmas with regard to diagnosis and surgical indications and planning. Pathologies that destroy the anterior column or create instability with or without neural impingement are the most common indications for corpectomy. The most common etiologies of anterior column instability include trauma, infection, and tumor. The basic surgical strategy should include neural decompression, removal of pathological tissue, and reconstruction. In general, the approach should focus on the site of the lesion when dealing with neural compression, particularly when dealing with infection and tumor. Historically, if ventral pathology is creating canal stenosis, laminectomy alone has been found to be an insufficient treatment both for relief of neurological symptoms and for reasons of stability. It is crucial to assess posterior stability prior to surgical intervention, and frequently if three-column insufficiency is present, an anterior and posterior approach is warranted.

Anatomy Approaches and Techniques

The unique anatomy of the anterior lumbar spine and those structures encountered during exposure present relatively unfamiliar territory to those most familiar with posterior lumbar approaches. A mastery of the relevant neurovascular structures and the three-dimensional anatomy of the vertebral bodies and foramina is crucial in surgical planning and safe execution. The anatomical structures found in the retroperitoneal space include the aorta and vena cava with their bifurcations to the common iliac vessels, the segmental lumbar arterial and venous branches, the middle sacral inferior mesenteric branches, and the hypogastric plexus and sympathetic trunk. In addition, the position of the ureters and the lumbar nerve roots located in the psoas muscle must be considered.

The relationship of the aortic bifurcation and the origin of the vena cava to the lower lumbar spine create various permutations. In general, the aorta lies to the left and anterior to the more posterior and right position of the vena cava. The Y-shaped aortic bifurcation most commonly lies over the body of L4 and less commonly overlies the L4-5 disc space or the L3-4 disc. The origin of the vena cava most commonly overlies the L5 vertebral body, and less commonly over the L4-5 disc space or L4 vertebral body. The segmental lumbar bundles traverse the midvertebral body to the intervertebral foramen. The middle sacral artery arises from the region of the aortic bifurcation and courses vertically over the L5 vertebral body and the L5-S1 disc space. The sympathetic trunks lie in the region of the lateral vertebral bodies. The superior hypogastric plexus is most commonly formed from communicating rami of the sympathetic trunks bilaterally as well as the celiac and mesenteric plexi. The plexus typically forms over the inferior aorta and extends over the L5-S1 disc space and the sacrum medially prior to separating and coursing to the pelvis to join the inferior hypogastric plexus to innervate the bladder and ejaculatory mechanism in males. However, in the minority of cases it can prematurely coalesce into trunks either unilaterally or bilaterally.

Discectomy

The choice of incision and approach for anterior lumbar discectomy depends on the level to be operated, the number of levels, and the patient's body habitus. The point of bifurcation of the aorta and vena cava can be grossly ascertained from preopera-

tive MRI or computed tomography (CT) scans and may help in surgical planning (25). In general, the L5-S1 disc can be accessed from a ventral approach, the L4-5 and L3-4 discs from either a ventral or lateral retroperitoneal approach, and the higher lumbar discs from the lateral retroperitoneal approach. In multilevel procedures, a lateral approach is most commonly used except when L4-5 and L5-S1 are the targeted levels. Typically, a general or vascular surgeon's experience with the exposure provides a level of comfort for the spine surgeon and provides guaranteed emergency backup in case of vascular injury. Therefore, a general surgeon is often consulted to provide assistance with anterior procedures. The lower lumbar discs (L3-S1) can be accessed from a ventral midline or paramedian exposure with a transperitoneal or retroperitoneal approach. For L5-S1 either a vertical incision initiated in the subumbilical region and extending to 2 to 3 cm above the pubis or a transverse Pfannenstiel incision centered two finger breaths above the pubis will allow adequate exposure. For L4-5 and L3-4 discectomies, a vertical incision centered two thirds below the umbilicus for L4-5 and two thirds above the umbilicus for L3-4 will suffice. For upper lumbar discectomies and corpectomies, the lateral retroperitoneal approach is recommended. For exposure of L2-4, a curvilinear incision begins at the midpoint between the iliac crest and rib cage extending to a point above the umbilicus, or for L4-5 or L5-S1 targets the same incision should be carried to a point just below the umbilicus (L4-5) or just above the pubis (L5-S1) (Fig. 4). Though published data are lacking, many surgeons are experimenting with less invasive laparoscopic or "minilaparotomy" approaches with success, and retractor systems designed for these applications are available (26,27). The specifics of these approaches are found in other chapters in this text.

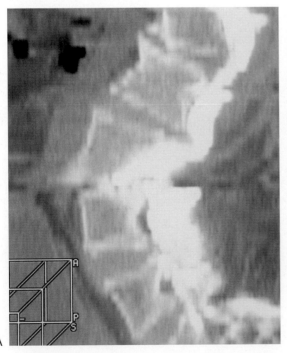
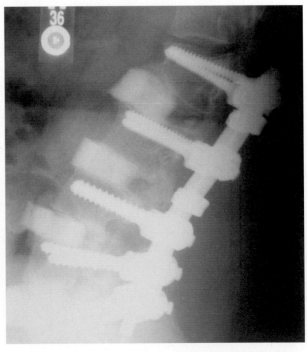

Fig. 4. **A**: Preoperative sagittally reconstructed computed tomography (CT) of a 36-year-old achondroplastic dwarf with prior L2-S1 laminectomy, back pain, and recurrent stenosis. **B**: Postoperative x-ray after anterior retroperitoneal multilevel discectomy, femoral ring allograft reconstruction, and posterior instrumentation. Note how the anterior approach allows for reconstruction of disc height and improved sagittal balance.

Ventral Approaches and Techniques to L3-S1

Upon approaching the ventral spine, the major vessels should be identified, and the disc space localized via radiograph. L5-S1 typically lies below the notch of the bifurcation, and therefore it is easiest to mobilize the vessels laterally. The hypogastric plexus should be mobilized bluntly, and hemostasis performed with bipolar cautery as opposed to monopolar to avoid damage to the plexus. The middle sacral vessels are isolated and divided. At the higher levels, the approach is dictated by the anatomy. At L4-5, if the bifurcation is above the disc space, the vessels can often be mobilized laterally, as with L5-S1. However, at L4-5 when the bifurcation is low, or at L3-4, it is necessary to mobilize the vessels to allow for them to be retracted to the right. This requires isolation and division of the L5 and L4 segmental vessels. The aorta should then be mobilized sufficiently to allow for visualization of the midline. When the dissection is complete, the vessels can be retracted with the aid of a table-mounted general surgery retractor, or by placing Steinmann pins medial to the vessels and impacting them into the vertebral bodies. The annulus is then incised in such a way as to allow it to be returned to an anatomical position when the procedure is complete to provide for a vascular pedicle and protect the vasculature from graft contact. Despite some manufacturer recommendations, a complete discectomy should be performed with the use of curets, ring curets, and flat-bladed instruments until bleeding end-plate bone is exposed. It is crucial to reach this point without penetrating the end plate, to maximize fusion surface for engraftation without weakening the end plate and risking graft subsidence.

Once the discectomy is completed, reconstruction is performed with attention to restoration of lordosis, maximization of endplate/graft surface contact, creating compression across the graft or implant and stabilization. All grafts or implants should be placed into a distracted interspace, with the goal of re-creating a normal disc space height. This allows for maximal restoration of lordosis as well increased foraminal diameter (28–31).

A myriad of graft and implant choices exist and have been utilized for anterior interbody fusion. Initially, autologous iliac crest bone was used for its structural characteristics and fusion capacity. Later, allograft femoral rings were used with similar fusion rates (32–36). These grafts are placed using interbody distraction, and despite the lack of integral fixation, often are used in a stand-alone fashion. More recently, systems to place machined bone products and metallic implants have been designed to provide for interbody distraction and a degree of fixation. These devices include lordotic and ridged femoral rings, vertically placed titanium mesh cages, and horizontally placed threaded interbody devices. These devices may provide for more consistent disc space distraction, and have been shown to have increased initial stability when compared to standard graft constructs (4,7,37–39). These devices are typically packed with autologous bone graft; however, early trials using bone morphogenetic proteins have been promising (40). While a number of retrospective reports as to the efficacy of anterior lumbar interbody fusion (ALIF) exist, controlled trials are lacking. In addition, debate continues as to the need for supplemental posterior fixation by traditional means (pedicle screws) or newer concepts such as transarticular fixation.

Corpectomy

Incision choice for lumbar corpectomy follows similar guidelines as mentioned above for discectomy, except that the ventral approaches are rarely used. Adequate access to the lower half of L1 can be attained via a lateral incision; however, it is difficult to perform a L1 corpectomy or instrumentation to L1 without taking down a portion of the diaphragm. Once the vertebral body is identified, an attempt should be made to mobilize the vascular structures at least to the midline if not slightly beyond. This requires ligation and transection of the segmental vessels of the involved levels and often a level above and below. Following this, the psoas muscle should be bluntly dissected dorsally until the vertebral foramen can be palpated with an instrument. This allows for adequate bony exposure and orients the surgeon to the anatomy to prevent nerve root injury as well as defining the lateral spinal canal. The periosteum is then incised, and a subperiosteal dissection of the vertebral body beyond the midline is performed, while sparing the anterior longitudinal ligament. The disc spaces above and below the involved level are then incised, and initial discectomies are performed. Rongeurs and a high-speed drill are then used to remove the anterior vertebral body. In trauma, a cortical rim of bone can be left anteriorly and to the far side, while in infection or tumor cases an attempt should be made to remove as much of the body as possible. As the dissection is carried posteriorly, knowledge of the position of the posterior cortex, tumor invasion of the canal, or traumatic fracture fragments will allow for a careful approach to the spinal canal and thecal sac. It is beneficial to identify the canal at a position that is anatomically normal, and then proceed to reduce the fragment or tumor that has invaded the floor of the canal. Typically, intracanal fragments can be pulled anteriorly with curets; however, it is sometimes necessary to drill the fragment to free it from impingement. In addition, it is beneficial in traumatic cases to distract across the affected vertebral body and allow ligamentotaxis to reduce the fragment into the vertebral body defect. The entire canal should be decompressed from pedicle to pedicle to ensure complete neural decompression. The posterior longitudinal ligament should be preserved in trauma, but extradural inspection should be performed in cases of infection or tumor.

Reconstruction

After corpectomy, anterior column reconstruction should be approached with the intent of providing immediate stability and to maximize fusion potential. Pertinent to these goals, graft choice and the use of instrumentation are crucial. Graft choices include autologous iliac crest, long bone allograft (femur or humerus), cage devices packed with autograft and synthetic materials (Fig. 5). Biomechanical studies have demonstrated that constructs with maximal end-plate contact surface area and some surface texture (such as cages), are inherently more stable than smaller smooth surfaced constructs (i.e., iliac crest) (5). As with interbody constructs, grafts should be placed under vertebral distraction to allow for compressive forces across the graft. In addition, when instrumentation is used, attention should be given to graft placement to the maximal load-sharing position. For example, with lateral anterior plating, the graft should be placed beyond the midline contralateral to the plate, and more midbody or slightly anterior if posterior instrumentation is applied (Fig. 6). In general, instrumentation should be considered to augment the anterior column reconstruction. From a purely biomechanical perspective, the literature demonstrates that anterior reconstruction with posterior instrumentation is more stable than anterior instrumentation alone (6,41, 42). Figure 7 demonstrates two different techniques for anterior and posterior reconstruction and stabilization. However, from a clinical perspective, many reports exist of successful anterior

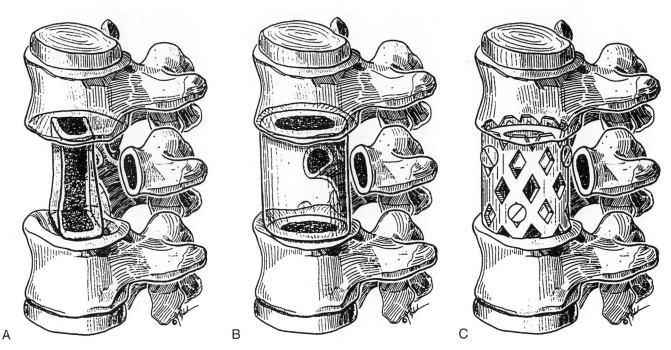

Fig. 5. Examples of three types of reconstructions after anterior corpectomy. **A**: Autologous tricortical graft. **B**: Femoral allograft. **C**: Titanium cage packed with autograft.

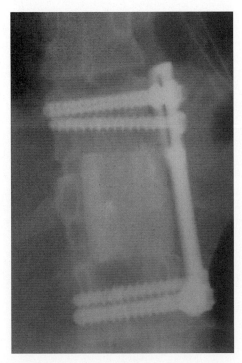

Fig. 6. Postoperative x-ray demonstrating results after anterior T12 corpectomy and femoral allograft reconstruction, with lateral plating with Z-plate (Sofamor Danek, Memphis, TN) for a traumatic T12 burst fracture. Note how the femoral allograft provides maximum end-plate contact, increasing the fusion area and providing inherent construct stability.

reconstruction and instrumentation (43,44). No class I information exists in the literature as to improved clinical outcomes assessing the variables of graft or instrumentation choice.

Outcomes

INTERNAL DISC DISRUPTION. There are no prospective or randomized studies supporting the use of anterior interbody fusion for IDD; however, a number of retrospective outcome-based studies are available. Study populations typically consisted of patients with mechanical low back pain who failed conservative therapy, and with abnormal MRI scanning and positive discography. Christensen et al. (18) note preoperative bracing to be a statistically significant predictor of operative success. Fusion rates varied from 52% to 91%, and typically predicted greater clinical success (20,33). Clinical success varied from 34% to 80% with poor results as high as 47% (23,24,33, 45–49). Vamvanij et al. (50) describe a significantly improved outcome when posterior facet screws are used in conjunction with an anterior threaded cage fusion versus anterior cage alone. Negative predictors of clinical success include prior surgery, multilevel fusion, secondary financial gain issues, and psychological dysfunction (18,20,47). The results of the use of anterior interbody fusion to salvage pseudarthrosis after posterior fusion attempts are varied, but the trend is toward poor outcomes (32,36,51,52). Reports of the use of anterior interbody fusion for isthmic spondylolisthesis is less prolific, with the trend in small series toward good results in 75% and 90% of patients (11–13). Assessment of revision rates for initial interbody fusion is not available in the literature.

CORPECTOMY. There are very few published reports on the outcome of anterior corpectomy reconstruction. However,

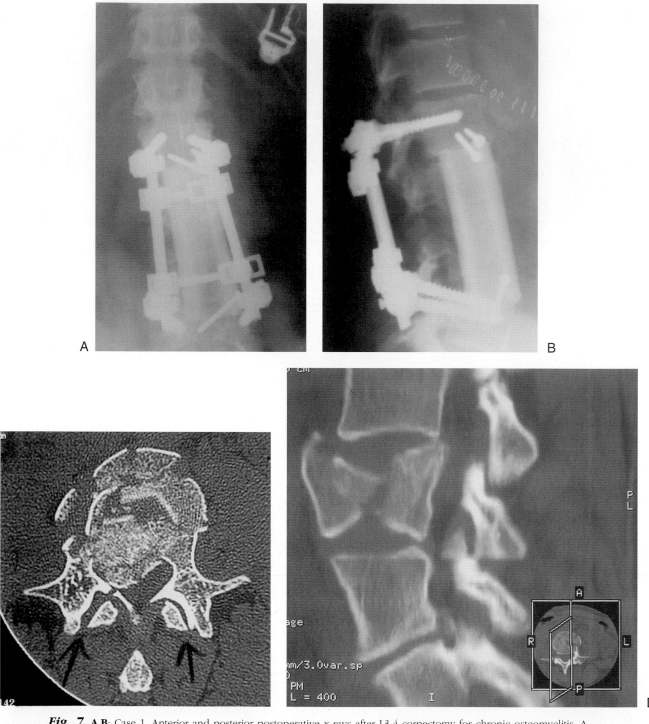

Fig. 7. A,B: Case 1. Anterior and posterior postoperative x-rays after L3-4 corpectomy for chronic osteomyelitis. A femoral shaft allograft was used for anterior reconstruction, with toenail screws used to anchor the graft during repositioning for posterior instrumentation. **C–F**: Case 2. Axial (**C**) and sagittally (**D**) reconstructed CT images of a traumatic L4 burst fracture.

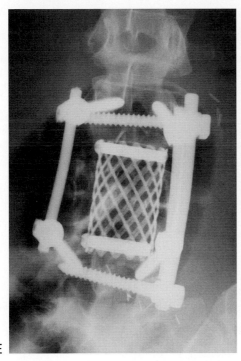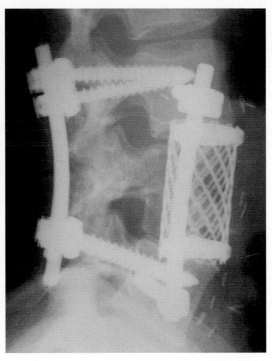

E   F

Fig. 7. (continued) Anterior (**E**) and posterior (**F**) postoperative x-rays after an anterior retroperitoneal approach were used to perform L4 corpectomy with titanium mesh cage reconstruction. An anterior rod was used to allow for maximal compression across the construct. Note how the L5 screw begins anterior to the vertebral body to avoid contact with the iliac vessels, and the screws are positioned to allow subsequent pedicle screw placement at L3 and L5.

Ghanayem and Zdeblick (43) and Kaneda et al. (53), in separate reports, demonstrate excellent fusion rates and clinical outcomes.

these procedures expand the surgeon's armamentarium for dealing with complex spine problems.

Complications

Major complications from anterior approaches to the lumbar spine are rare, and the safety of this approach has been verified in a number of large retrospective series (54–56). The incidence of major vascular injury or thrombosis has been reported mainly on an anecdotal basis (54,57–60). Likewise, rates of injury to other abdominal structures are extremely low (61–63). However, it is generally agreed upon that the incidence of permanent retrograde ejaculation is traditionally underreported at 1% to 5% (64,65). Tiusanen et al. (64) found this complication in 7 of 40 men, leading them to recommend against routine use of the anterior approach for low lumbar pathology in males of reproductive age. These unique nonspine complications must be understood and communicated to the patient prior to recommending anterior surgical spine operations.

Conclusions

Understanding correct surgical indications and mastering the techniques required for anterior lumbar fusion surgery are important skills for all advanced spine surgeons to master. With an understanding of the biomechanics and surgical techniques,

References

1. Riley LH 3rd, Eck JC, Yoshida H, et al. Laparoscopic assisted fusion of the lumbosacral spine. A biomechanical and histologic analysis of the open versus laparoscopic technique in an animal model. *Spine* 1997;22(12):1407–1412.
2. Kozak JA, Heilman AE, O'Brien JP. Anterior lumbar fusion options. Technique and graft materials. *Clin Orthop* 1994;300:45–51.
3. Tsantrizos A, Andreou A, Aebi M, et al. Biomechanical stability of five stand-alone anterior lumbar interbody fusion constructs. *Eur Spine J* 2000;9(1):14–22.
4. Tencer AF, Hampton D, Eddy S. Biomechanical properties of threaded inserts for lumbar interbody spinal fusion. *Spine* 1995; 20(22):2408–2414.
5. Lee SW, Lim TH, You JW, et al. Biomechanical effect of anterior grafting devices on the rotational stability of spinal constructs. *J Spinal Disord* 2000;13(2):150–155.
6. Oda I, Cunningham BW, Abumi K, et al. The stability of reconstruction methods after thoracolumbar total spondylectomy. An in vitro investigation. *Spine* 1999;24(16):1634–1638.
7. Oxland TR, Lund T. Biomechanics of stand-alone cages and cages in combination with posterior fixation: a literature review. *Eur Spine J* 2000;9(suppl 1):S95–101.
8. Chow DH, Luk KD, Evans JH, et al. Effects of short anterior lumbar interbody fusion on biomechanics of neighboring unfused segments. *Spine* 1996;21(5):549–555.
9. Wiltse LL, Newman PH, MacNab I. Classification of spondylolisthesis and spondylosis. Clin Orthop 1976;117:23–29.
10. Meyerding HW. Spondylolisthesis. Surg Gynecol Obstet 1932;54: 371–377.

11. Kim NH, Lee JW. Anterior interbody fusion versus posterolateral fusion with transpedicular fixation for isthmic spondylolisthesis in adults. Comparison of clinical results. *Spine* 1999;24(8):812–816; discussion 817.

12. Kim NH, Kim DJ. Anterior interbody fusion for spondylolisthesis. *Orthopedics* 1991;14(10):1069–1076.

13. Takahashi K, Kitahara H, Yamagata M, et al. Long-term results of anterior interbody fusion for treatment of degenerative spondylolisthesis. *Spine* 1990;15(11):1211–1215.

14. Fraser RD. Interbody, posterior, and combined lumbar fusions. *Spine* 1995;20(24 suppl):167S–177S.

15. Greenough CG, Peterson MD, Hadlow S, et al. Instrumented posterolateral lumbar fusion. Results and comparison with anterior interbody fusion. *Spine* 1998;23(4):479–486.

16. Kim SS, Denis F, Lonstein JE, et al. Factors affecting fusion rate in adult spondylolisthesis. *Spine* 1990;15(9):979–984.

17. Kim NH, Kim DJ. Anterior interbody fusion for spondylolisthesis. *Orthopedics* 1991;14(10):1069–1076.

18. Christensen FB, Karlsmose B, Hansen ES, et al. Radiological and functional outcome after anterior lumbar interbody spinal fusion. *Eur Spine J* 1996;5(5):293–298.

19. Penta M, Fraser RD. Anterior lumbar interbody fusion. A minimum 10-year follow-up. *Spine* 1997;22(20):2429–2434.

20. Zdeblick T. Discogenic back pain. In: Rothman R, Simeone F, eds. 4th ed. *The spine*, Philadelphia: WB Saunders, 1999:250.

21. Coppes MH, Marani E, Thomeer RT. Innervation of the annulus fibrosus in low back pain. *Lancet* 1990;336:189–190.

22. Suseki K, Takahashi Y, Yakahashi K, et al. Sensory nerve fibres from lumbar intervertebral discs pass through the rami communicantes. A possible pathway for discogenic low back pain. *J Bone Joint Surg* 1998;80B(4):737–742.

23. Derby R, Howard MW, Grant JM, et al. The ability of pressure-controlled discography to predict surgical nonsurgical outcomes. *Spine* 1999;24(4):364–371; discussion 371–372.

24. Knox BD, Chapman TM. Anterior lumbar interbody fusion for discogram concordant pain. *J Spinal Disord* 1993;6(3):242–244.

25. Capellades J, Pellise F, Rovira A, et al. Magnetic resonance anatomic study of iliocava junction and left vein positions related to L5-S1 disc. *Spine* 2000;25(13):1695–1700.

26. McAfee PC, Regan JJ, Geis WP, et al. Minimally invasive anterior retroperitoneal approach to the lumbar spine. Emphasis on the lateral BAK. *Spine* 1998;23(13):1476–1484.

27. Lazennec JY, Pouzet B, Ramare S, et al. Anatomic basis of minimal anterior extraperitoneal approach to lumbar spine. *Surg Radiol Anat* 1999;21(1):7–15.

28. Voor MJ, Mehta S, Wang M, et al. Biomechanical evaluation of posterior and anterior lumbar interbody fusion techniques. *J Spinal Disord* 1998;11(4):328–334.

29. Kumar A, Kozak JA, Doherty BJ, et al. Interspace distraction and graft subsidence after anterior lumbar fusion with femoral strut allograft. *Spine* 1993;18(16):2393–2400.

30. Chen D, Fay LA, Lok J, et al. Increasing neuroforaminal volume by anterior interbody distraction degenerative lumbar spine. *Spine* 1995;20(1):74–79.

31. Soini J. Lumbar disc space heights after external fixation and anterior interbody fusion: a prospective 2-year follow-up of clinical and radiographic results. *J Spinal Disord* 1994;7(6):487–494.

32. Buttermann GR, Glazer PA, Hu SS, et al. Revision of failed lumbar fusions. A comparison of anterior auto and allograft. *Spine* 1997;22(23):2748–2755.

33. Newman MH, Grinstead GL. Anterior lumbar interbody fusion for internal disc disruption. *Spine* 1992;17(7):831–833.

34. Arthornthurasook A. Anterior lumbar discectomy: a study of iliac and fibular bone grafts. *J Med Assoc Thai* 1992;75(5):273–277.

35. Wimmer C, Krismer M, Gluch H, et al. Autogenic versus allogenic bone grafts in anterior lumbar interbody fusion. *Clin Orthop* 1999;(360):122–126.

36. Cohen DB, Chotivichit A, Fujita T, et al. Pseudoarthrosis repair. Autogenous iliac crest versus femoral ring allograft. *Clin Orthop* 2000;(371):46–55.

37. Sandhu HS, Turner S, Kabo JM, et al. Distractive properties of a threaded interbody fusion device. A model. *Spine* 1996;21(10):1201–1210.

38. Nasca RJ, Montgomery RD, Moeini SM, et al. Intervertebral spacer as an adjunct to anterior lumbar fusion. Six-month implantation in baboons. *J Spinal Disord* 1998;11(2):136–141.

39. Leong JC, Chow SP, Yau AC. Titanium-mesh block replacement of the intervertebral disk. *Clin Orthop* 1994;300:52–63.

40. Sandhu HS. Anterior lumbar interbody fusion with osteoinductive growth factors. *Clin Orthop* 2000;371:56–60.

41. Vahldiek MJ, Panjabi MM. Stability potential of spinal instrumentation in tumor vertebral replacement surgery. *Spine* 1998;23(5):543–550.

42. Kanayama M, Ng JT, Cunningham BW, et al. Biomechanical analysis of anterior versus circumferential spinal reconstruction for various anatomic stages of tumor lesions. *Spine* 1999;24(5):445–450.

43. Ghanayem AJ, Zdeblick TA. Anterior instrumentation in the management of thoracolumbar fractures. *Clin Orthop* 1997;335:89–100.

44. Miyakoshi N, Abe E, Shimada Y, et al. Anterior decompression with single segmental spinal interbody fusion for lumbar burst fracture. *Spine* 1999;24(1):67–73.

45. Linson MA, Williams H. Anterior and combined anteroposterior fusion for lumbar disc preliminary study. *Spine* 1991;16(2):143–145.

46. Gill K, Blumenthal SL. Functional results after anterior lumbar fusion at L5-S1 in patients with normal and abnormal MRI scans. *Spine* 1992;17(8):940–942.

47. Greenough CG, Taylor LJ, Fraser RD. Anterior lumbar fusion: results, assessment techniques and prognostic factors. *Eur Spine J* 1994; 3(4):225–230.

48. Olsen D, McCord D, Law M. Laparoscopic discectomy with anterior interbody fusion of L5-S1. *Surg Endosc* 1996;10(12):1158–1163.

49. Tiusanen H, Seitsalo S, Osterman K, et al. Anterior interbody lumbar fusion in severe low back pain. *Clin Orthop* 1996;(324):153–163.

50. Vamvanij V, Fredrickson BE, Thorpe JM, et al. Surgical treatment of internal disc disruption: an outcome study on fusion techniques. *J Spinal Disord* 1998;11(5):375–382.

51. Lauerman WC, Bradford DS, Ogilvie JW, et al. Results of lumbar pseudarthrosis repair. *J Spinal Disord* 1992;5(2):149–157.

52. Barrick WT, Schofferman JA, Reynolds JB, et al. Anterior lumbar fusion improves discogenic pain at levels of prior posterolateral fusion. *Spine* 2000;25(7):853–857.

53. Kaneda K, Taneichi H, Abumi K, et al. Anterior decompression and stabilization with the Kaneda device thoracolumbar burst fractures associated with neurological deficits. *J Bone Joint Surg* 1997;79A(1):69–83.

54. McAfee PC, Regan JR, Zdeblick T, et al. The incidence of complications in endoscopic anterior thoracolumbar spinal reconstructive surgery. A prospective multicenter study comprising the first 100 consecutive cases. *Spine* 1995;20(14):1624–1632.

55. Faciszewski T, Winter RB, Lonstein JE, et al. The surgical and medical perioperative complications of anterior fusion surgery in the thoracic and lumbar spine in adults. A review of 1223 procedures. *Spine* 1995;20(14):1592–1599.

56. Rajaraman V, Vingan R, Roth P, et al. Visceral and vascular complications resulting from anterior lumbar interbody fusion. *J Neurosurg* 1999;91(1 suppl):60–64.

57. Tanaka M, Nakahara S, Tanizaki M. Aortic pseudoaneurysm in the L3-L4 disc space after lumbar disc surgery. A case report. *J Bone Joint Surg* 1998;80B(3):448–451.

58. Raskas DS, Delamarter RB. Occlusion of the left iliac artery after retroperitoneal exposure of spine. *Clin Orthop* 1997;338:86–89.

59. Marsicano J, Mirovsky Y, Remer S, et al. Thrombotic occlusion of the left common iliac artery after an anterior retroperitoneal approach to the lumbar spine. *Spine* 1994;19(3):357–359.

60. Khazim R, Roos N, Webb JK. Progressive thrombotic occlusion of the left common iliac artery anterior lumbar interbody fusion. *Eur Spine J* 1998;7(3):239–241.

61. Guingrich JA, McDermott JC. Ureteral injury during laparoscopy-assisted anterior lumbar fusion. *Spine* 2000;25(12):1586–1588.

62. Rajaraman V, Heary RF, Livingston DH. Acute pancreatitis complicating anterior lumbar interbody fusion. *Eur Spine J* 2000;9(2):171–173.

63. Jurbala BM, Kelly JD 4th, Dempsey DT, et al. Gastroparaspinal fistula: a late postoperative complication of a spinal fusion. *Orthopedics* 1997;20(10):985–987.

64. Tiusanen H, Seitsalo S, Osterman K, et al. Retrograde ejaculation after anterior interbody lumbar fusion. *Eur Spine J* 1995;4(6):339–342.

65. Christensen FB, Bunger CE. Retrograde ejaculation after retroperitoneal lower lumbar interbody fusion. *Int Orthop* 1997;21(3):176–180.

210. Posterior Lumbar Interbody Fusion: Historical and Technical Overview

David S. Jones, Steven D. Wray, and Charles L. Branch, Jr.

Despite an increase in the popularity of spinal fusion during the past decade, its role in the management of degenerative conditions of the lumbar spine remains controversial. Applicable in a variety of degenerative, traumatic, and congenital disorders, posterior lumbar interbody fusion (PLIF) combines a traditional posterior approach to discectomy and neural decompression with an interbody fusion. PLIF allows for direct visualization, decompression of neural elements, total discectomy, restoration of disc space height, and elimination of abnormal motion by the creation of a solid arthrodesis. The addition of segmental internal fixation following PLIF provides immediate stability and enhances fusion rates.

History and Development

The concept of lumbar interbody fusion was first introduced by Mercer in 1936 (1). Later, Cloward (2) successfully performed PLIF with iliac crest wedges and presented his early results at various meetings between 1945 and 1951. Lin (3) used the "unigraft" concept to modify Cloward's technique, filling the disc space with cancellous bone strips in addition to cortical grafts. Lin's goal was for the cancellous bone to appear as dense as the cortical bone on radiographs, thereby facilitating more rapid fusion. Despite this work, PLIF was met with little enthusiasm initially, presumably because of the technical difficulties involved and the inability to duplicate clinical outcomes and fusion rates. Many authors described various modifications of the PLIF technique, including the use of autologous iliac crest bone grafts, allograft bone, dowel-shaped grafts, keystone grafts, tricortical grafts, bone chips, metallic implants, carbon fiber implants, and threaded fusion cages (4–13).

Indications

Improvements in surgical technique and instrumentation and a better understanding of the theoretical advantages of PLIF have greatly expanded successful applications of the procedure. Spinal fusion is typically indicated when segmental instability causes clinical symptoms. However, what determines segmental instability continues to be debated, particularly in degenerative conditions of the spine. Kirkaldy-Willis and Farfan (14) suggested that progressive degenerative changes in the spine lead to a loss of normal integrity of the functional spinal unit. Frymoyer et al. (15) defined segmental instability as a "loss of motion stiffness such that force application to that motion segment produces greater displacement than would be seen in a normal structure, resulting in a painful condition and the potential for progressive deformity." In practice, the determination of clinical instability and therefore the decision to fuse rest on a careful consideration of both clinical symptoms and radiographic findings. Translation of more than 4 mm or angular motion of more than 10 degrees between adjacent end plates on lateral flexion and extension radiographs is generally accepted as indicative of instability (16).

The global indication of Cloward (2) for PLIF was "the treatment of low back pain with or without sciatica due to lumbar disc disease." Others, attempting to refine the indications for PLIF, have created lengthy lists of more specific conditions, but none has significantly narrowed the scope of Cloward's indications. Included in the list of indications for PLIF are spondylolisthesis, recurrent disc herniation, failed back surgery syndrome, bilateral or massive midline disc herniation, segmental instability, symptomatic spinal stenosis, degenerative disc disease with posturally related back pain, and disc herniation in patients with physically demanding occupations (5,6,17).

Planning

Although carefully performed lumbar spine fusions from either the posterior interbody, posterolateral, or anterior approach yield high rates of fusion and clinical success in appropriate patients, it is our opinion that the familiarity of the surgical exposure, the potential for neural decompression, and the capacity to preserve or restore disc space height make the PLIF technique superior to other techniques for lumbar fusion.

Several PLIF techniques are currently available to the spine surgeon. Although a detailed description of the merits of each is beyond the scope of this chapter, we briefly describe four basic techniques.

NONINSTRUMENTED ALLOGRAFT/AUTOGRAFT POSTERIOR LUMBAR INTERBODY FUSION. Cloward (2) achieved high rates of fusion and clinical success with his original PLIF technique. He performed wide laminectomies and facetectomies and radical discectomies to place as much allograft as possible in the intervertebral space. An interlaminar spreader was used to facilitate exposure and provide distraction for graft insertion. The cortical end plate was perforated or removed to create bleeding surfaces, and four bicortical or tricortical iliac crest grafts were inserted into the disc space. Cloward (2) favored the placement of large grafts at the expense of facet integrity, stating that it is "not necessary to preserve the facets" because one is "fusing a larger area, the vertebral bodies."

Lin (3) later modified the Cloward PLIF technique, stressing adherence to four biomechanical principles to enhance the rate of osteosynthesis. These principles are the following: (a) preservation of the posterior portion of the motion segment; (b) near-total discectomy; (c) partial decortication of the end plate; and (d) use of the "unigraft" concept, in which four to six unicortical autogenous peg grafts are tightly inserted in the disc space, so that the retraction complications associated with the large Cloward grafts are avoided. In both the Cloward and Lin techniques and in subsequent modifications, radical discectomy and meticulous end plate preparation were important, but technically demanding, concepts.

THREADED FUSION CYLINDER POSTERIOR LUMBAR INTERBODY FUSION. In an attempt to simplify the PLIF procedure further, standardized threaded fusion cages were developed. The first commercially available cages included Ray threaded fusion cages (Surgical Dynamics, Norwalk, Connecticut) and BAK threaded fusion cages (Spine Tech, Minneapolis, Minnesota). Threaded fusion cages are hollow titanium alloy cylinders that can be filled with autograft bone. They are available in a variety of sizes. Theoretically, they provide immediate stability to a spinal segment by distracting the intact annular fibers, which in turn compress the implant. Early reports of these devices advocated their stand-alone use without additional internal fixation (12). The assessment of fusion on postoperative imaging of fusion cage levels is notoriously difficult, and the degree of neural retraction required for posterior insertion is associated with postoperative neurogenic pain. Additionally, the application of fusion cages may be restricted to a limited patient population. Contraindications include osteoporosis, spondylolisthesis of grade II or higher, degeneration at adjacent levels, three or more levels of instrumentation, and disc space height greater than 12 mm because of inability to obtain adequate cage purchase (12).

Threaded allograft dowels are an alternative to titanium threaded fusion cages. The dowels are hollow, threaded cortical grafts that are packed with cancellous bone before insertion. Biomechanically, bone dowels appear to be comparable with titanium cages initially, although their deterioration or resorption rates may vary. Because these are bone grafts, it may be easier to assess the fusion mass on postoperative imaging.

CARBON FIBER RECTANGULAR CAGE POSTERIOR LUMBAR INTERBODY FUSION. Brantigan interbody fusion cages (DePuy AcroMed, Cleveland, Ohio) are made of a radiolucent, carbon fiber-reinforced polymer that allows radiographic visualization of the fusion mass. These rectangular cages are packed with autogenous bone graft and impacted into a prepared disc space. They have an open design to increase bone graft-to-end plate surface contact, and their stiffness matches that of bone. The design theoretically reduces stress shielding by transferring compressive load to the graft while maintaining disc space height. Meticulous discectomy and end plate preparation with a variety of tools are required with this technique. Brantigan cages are indicated for a posterior approach in patients with degenerative disc disease at one or two lumbar levels whose condition requires an interbody fusion combined with posterolateral fusion and pedicle screw fixation.

IMPACTED ALLOGRAFT/AUTOGRAFT POSTERIOR LUMBAR INTERBODY FUSION. With the Tangent posterior discectomy and grafting instrumentation set (Sofamor Danek, Memphis, Tennessee), a cutting chisel device is used to prepare the disc space and cortical end plates to receive a preformed cortical allograft. Tapping the chisel into the disc space at an angle that parallels the cortical end plates creates a fusion surface mirroring the dimensions of the preformed allograft. Disc space height is restored without significant dural retraction. Cancellous autograft bone is packed into the disc space between two allograft struts. The cortical bone provides mechanical strength, and the cancellous bone promotes rapid fusion. Significantly less nerve root retraction is required for this technique, so that it may be less likely to cause the root retraction problems associated with threaded fusion cages.

Overview of Techniques

In all PLIF procedures, regardless of technique, the preparation, positioning, and initial exposure are similar to those used in patients undergoing discectomy or decompression alone. The spine is exposed through a dorsal midline incision, and a combination of sharp dissection and monopolar cautery is used to reflect the paraspinous musculature in a subperiosteal fashion to expose the facets and transverse processes at the involved levels. An attempt is made to preserve the spinous processes, supraspinous ligament, and interspinous ligaments because these provide an element of posterior stability.

Intraoperative radiographs or fluoroscopy can be used to confirm the spinal segment. After careful dissection of the soft tissue from the involved lamina, the initial bilateral laminotomies, medial facetectomies, and foraminotomies are performed as in simple decompression of a lateral recess stenosis with Kerrison rongeurs, osteotomes, or a high-speed air-powered drill. Bone removed during the decompression can be saved for later use as autograft. Bone removal is continued laterally to the medial border of the pedicle. This provides adequate exposure so that the disc space and end plates may be prepared with minimal neural retraction. The neural elements should be freely mobile, especially in patients with previous lumbar surgeries, because dural adhesions may prevent safe dural retraction and lead to dural lacerations or nerve root injury.

Careful attention is paid to epidural hemostasis. The epidural vasculature is coagulated with bipolar cautery and then divided. The posterior longitudinal ligament and posterior annulus are incised bilaterally, and various disc rongeurs and curettes are used to perform the initial discectomy. The main goal of this step is to remove extruded disc fragments, decompress the neural elements, and provide entry into the disc space for distraction. If significant disc space collapse is present, complete discectomy may be difficult until the disc space is distracted. The remainder of the procedure depends on the specific PLIF technique to be used, and these are discussed briefly.

NONINSTRUMENTED POSTERIOR LUMBAR INTERBODY FUSION AS DESCRIBED BY CLOWARD AND LIN. A near-total discectomy is performed with rongeurs, curettes, and disc space shapers. A radical discectomy is important because it provides a greater surface area for graft contact with the vertebral bodies. Any osteophytes are removed with a chisel.

A chisel, curette, or osteotome is used for partial decortication of the end plate. It is important to ensure good graft contact with bleeding cancellous bone to facilitate revascularization of the graft material and more rapid osteosynthesis. Lin (18) believes that total decortication is "not necessary, nor is it desirable" because it may lead to graft subsidence into the soft cancellous vertebral bodies. Instead, "islands" of decortication are created to ensure a rich blood supply to the graft.

The disc space is then filled with bone graft material. The selection of graft material is important, and many authors have reported successful outcomes and high fusion rates with various grafts, including autologous iliac crest grafts, allograft bone, dowel-shaped grafts, keystone grafts, tricortical grafts, and bone chips (2,6,7,17,19). Cloward (2) used a large punch and hammer to insert iliac crest bone plugs into the interspace, ensuring that the cancellous portion of the grafts was in contact with the bleeding surfaces of the vertebral bodies. The neural elements were retracted gently to prevent injury, and as many bone plugs as possible were driven into the interspace. Lin (18) favors the "unigraft" concept, in which four to six unicortical autogenous peg grafts are tightly inserted, with the cortical bone of the peg graft parallel to the longitudinal axis of the body. Autogenous cancellous bone strips are then tightly packed between the peg grafts. Bone grafts are countersunk approximately 5 mm below the posterior vertebral margin. A small notch created in this location during end plate preparation may help prevent posterior extrusion of the graft. Cloward and Lin do not recommend routine use of segmental internal fixation.

POSTERIOR LUMBAR INTERBODY FUSION WITH THREADED FUSION CAGES. Threaded fusion cages are hollow titanium cylinders that are filled with autogenous cancellous bone. Templates representing various cage diameters and lengths are available; these can be placed over imaging studies during preoperative planning to determine the appropriate cage size. Proper cage selection and placement are critical because an undersized cage will seldom fuse, and an oversized cage increases the risk for neural retraction injury. Fluoroscopy is recommended because it allows rapid sequential images that can be used to assess proper cage trajectory during insertion. In general, the midline of the bilaterally inserted cages should be at the level of the medial border of the pedicle. Threaded fusion cages should be inserted parallel to the end plates, and they should obtain 3 mm of bony purchase in each end plate.

BAK cages utilize plugs to distract the disc space. Once this is accomplished, a toothed drill tube and protective sheath are anchored into the vertebral bodies to enable effective disc space preparation. Great care is taken to protect the dura and nerve roots during placement of the drill tube to prevent neural entrapment. The exiting nerve root at the superior level may be at increased risk because it is often difficult to visualize. A hand drill is used to ream the disc space of any remaining disc material, and the disc space is then tapped. A BAK cage is packed with cancellous bone and inserted into the disc space under fluoroscopic guidance. The procedure is then repeated on the opposite side.

Ray cages utilize a Tang retractor to distract the disc space and guide end plate preparation and cage insertion. Proper retractor placement is critical. The prongs of the retractor are placed into the interspace, and the retractor is impacted into position. The medial prong should be at or near the midline to ensure proper positioning of the cage. The Tang retractor must be parallel to the vertebral end plates so that the prongs do not penetrate the either end plate. The hand drill is used to drill the end plate to a preset depth and remove remaining disc material. The hole is tapped, and the cage is inserted under fluoroscopic guidance. The cage should be countersunk approximately 3 mm below the posterior margins of the vertebral bodies. The procedure is then repeated on the opposite side, and the cages are filled with graft material.

POSTERIOR LUMBAR INTERBODY FUSION WITH BRANTIGAN CAGES. In the Brantigan cage technique, disc space spreaders are used to achieve disc space distraction. Disc space shavers are then used to remove remaining disc material. After placement of a retractor to protect the neural elements, an implant channel is prepared with reamers and broach instruments of the appropriate size. Trial implants can be inserted to verify the fit and depth of the prepared rectangular channel. Cancellous bone is packed into the cage, and the implant is tapped into place with an insertion tool. The cage should be placed as far laterally in the interspace as possible. Additional bone graft is packed into the disc space around the cages, and the interbody fusion is supplemented with bilateral posterolateral fusion and transpedicular fixation.

POSTERIOR LUMBAR INTERBODY FUSION WITH THE TANGENT TECHNIQUE. With the Tangent instrumentation system, sequentially placed disc space distractors are used to restore disc space height. After careful dural retraction with the nerve root protector, a rotating cutter is used to remove residual disc material. The remaining soft tissue and end plate coverings are then removed with a round scraper. A cutting chisel provides final end plate preparation. The size of the cutting chisel can be estimated during preoperative planning with templates or by using the height restored with the disc space distractor. The chisel is impacted parallel to the end plates to a depth of 30 mm and then removed with a slap hammer. The procedure is then repeated on the opposite side. Once the entire disc space has been prepared, two preformed allograft wedges are impacted into the previously created tracts with an inserter. The grafts should lie 2 to 3 mm below the posterior rims of the adjoining vertebral bodies. Locally harvested cortical–cancellous autograft bone is packed into the disc space around the allograft bone. Segmental internal fixation is routinely used with this technique.

SEGMENTAL INTERNAL FIXATION. Regardless of the PLIF technique used, the nerve roots and neural foramina should be inspected after the grafts are in place to ensure adequate decompression. All soft tissue is removed from the facets of the involved levels to promote pedicle localization and plate seating. Several methods are available to localize the pedicle screw entry points, but adequate knowledge of the lumbar spinal anatomy is essential. Pedicle probes, fluoroscopic guidance, or image guidance may be used as an adjunct to pedicle screw placement. The surgeon must be well versed in the use of pedicle screw systems, the location of the pedicle screw entry zones, and the placement of the screw within the pedicle. Improper placement can result in neurological injury and screw breakage (20). The choice of screw length and diameter is based on the patient's anatomy as assessed on preoperative imaging studies. The cortical bone overlying the pedicle screw entry zone is removed, and a pedicle probe is used to localize and follow the intramedullary canal of the pedicle. The pedicle is tapped, and a probe is used to ensure that the wall of the pedicle has not been penetrated. Screws of appropriate diameter and length are then inserted. Once plates have been secured to the screws, any remaining autologous bone graft may be placed posterolaterally over the transverse processes to enhance the fusion surface.

Postoperative Care

Postoperative radiographs are obtained to verify the integrity of the construct. The patient is maintained at bed rest until the first postoperative day, at which time prophylactic antibiotics and bladder catheterization are discontinued. Early ambulation in an external orthosis such as a corset is encouraged on the first postoperative day.

Problems and Complications

Significant complications of the PLIF procedure can occur, so that some may be led to consider an alternative but potentially less effective technique. Surgeons experienced with the PLIF technique generally concur that it is technically demanding and requires a thorough knowledge of the regional anatomy and careful attention to detail (6,18,20).

Several authors have listed potential complications associated with PLIF (6,9,18,20). These include pseudoarthrosis, graft resorption and collapse, graft retropulsion, wound infection, neural injury, dural laceration, and excessive hemorrhage. Meticulous surgical technique with identification and protection of the neural elements is mandatory. In patients who have undergone previous lumbar surgeries, dissection and lysis of epidural scar before nerve root or dural retraction can prevent neural injury. Reasonable hemostasis can usually be achieved, but the use of a blood-recycling unit may prevent the potential complications associated with blood transfusion. The addition of segmental internal fixation entails further risks: loss of fixation in osteopenic vertebrae, screw breakage, and increases in infection, neural injury, blood loss, operative time, cost, and morbidity and mortality (19,21).

Lin (18) reviewed PLIF complications and their avoidance in five collected series involving more than 2,000 patients. The rate of symptomatic graft retropulsion ranged from 0.3% to 2.4%. Lin also noted a 1.6% complication rate in series comprising 60 to 700 patients, and a 9% rate in series comprising 3 to 60 patients, figures that suggest a correlation between the complication rate and the experience of the surgeon.

The incidence of clinically significant pseudoarthrosis is difficult to determine, although most authors report a fusion rate of 85% to 90%. The addition of rigid segmental fixation as an adjunct to fusion can substantially lower pseudoarthrosis rates (16). Steffee and Sitkowski (22) reported a 100% successful fusion rate in 67 patients who underwent PLIF with segmental fixation for various indications. Interestingly, radiographic pseudoarthrosis rates do not always correlate with poor outcomes, and successful fusion rates do not always correlate with good outcomes (16,19).

Results

Few prospective, randomized trials have compared results of the PLIF technique with results of other fusion techniques, decompression without fusion, or nonsurgical treatment. Therefore, it is difficult to establish a set of indications in which PLIF, in comparison with other management options, is most likely to have a successful outcome.

Reported rates of successful fusion range from 50% to 94% (3,11,23–25), and reported satisfactory clinical outcomes range from 54% to 94% (26). Turner and colleagues (27) performed a metaanalysis of the results of lumbar spinal fusion. They reviewed 47 articles that included at least 12 months of follow-up data for at least 30 adults who had undergone fusion. In a series of five studies, PLIF was found to have an overall 75% clinical success rate and a 95% fusion rate. Table 1 compares these results with those of other fusion techniques. No significant differences in clinical success rates were noted between

Table 1. Outcomes According to Fusion Technique Based on a Metaanalysis of the Literature

	No. of studies	Success rate (%)	Fusion rate (%)
Posterior	9	66	88
Posterolateral	19	68	89
Anterior interbody	5	67	73
PLIF	5	75	95

PLIF, posterior lumbar interbody fusion.
From Turner JA, Herron L, Deyo RA. Meta-analysis of the results of lumbar spinal fusion. *Acta Orthop Scand* 64:120–122, 1993, with permission.

16 studies that reported the use of no instrumentation (67%) and 12 studies that reported the use of instrumentation with all fusions (71%).

Branch and Branch (7) reviewed 46 cases of PLIF for recurrent disc herniation with a mean follow-up of 12 months and an average of 1.4 previous operations. A satisfactory outcome was documented in 76% of the patients, a percentage that compared favorably with those in similar patients treated with laminectomy alone (satisfactory outcome in 40%) or with laminectomy and lateral fusion (satisfactory outcome in 66%). If PLIF can be performed safely and quickly with satisfactory fusion rates, it can effectively decompress the neural elements and eliminate the potential need for repeated operations at fused levels.

One potential long-term consequence of segmental fusion in patients with degenerative spinal conditions is increased mechanical stress at adjacent levels, which may lead to accelerated degeneration and instability at those levels. Lehmann et al. (28) found a 45% incidence of instability in adjacent segments at an average follow-up of 33 years. Further lumbar spine operations may be required to treat symptomatic degeneration at adjacent levels.

Conclusions

Controversy regarding the use of fusion to manage degenerative conditions of the lumbar spine is ongoing. Clinical experience that has been acquired during more than four decades seems to validate the PLIF technique as a safe and efficacious procedure applicable in a variety of degenerative lumbar conditions. Evidence also indicates that for recurrent lumbar disc herniations or spondylolisthesis, PLIF may be superior to repeated discectomy or decompression alone. Generally, one can expect a clinical success rate of 75% and fusion rates above 90%. Advantages of the PLIF technique include a familiar posterior approach, decompression of the neural elements, and restoration of disc space height with a load-bearing graft. The addition of segmental fixation can provide immediate postoperative stability, correct anatomical deformities, and enhance fusion rates.

References

1. Mercer W. Spondylolisthesis: with description of a new method of operative treatment and notes of 10 cases. *Edinb Med J* 43:545–572, 1936.
2. Cloward RB. The treatment of ruptured intervertebral discs by vertebral body fusion. I. Indications, operative technique, aftercare. *J Neurosurg* 10:154–168, 1953.
3. Lin PM. Technique and complications of posterior lumbar interbody fusion. In: Lin PM, Gill K, eds. *Lumbar interbody fusion.* Rockville, MD: Aspen Publications, 1989:171–199.
4. Jaslow IA. Intercorporal bone graft in spinal fusion after disc removal. *Surg Gynecol Obstet* 82:215–218, 1946.
5. Branch CL Jr. The case for posterior lumbar interbody fusion. *Clin Neurosurg* 43:252–267, 1996.
6. Branch CL Jr. Posterior lumbar interbody fusion. In: Hardy RW Jr, ed. *Lumbar disc disease,* 2nd ed. New York: Raven Press, 1993: 187–200.
7. Branch CL, Branch CL Jr. Posterior lumbar interbody fusion: the keystone technique. In: Lin PM, Gill K, eds. *Lumbar interbody fusion.* Rockville, MD: Aspen Publications, 1989:211–219.
8. Briggs H, Milligan PR. Chip fusion of the low back following exploration of the spinal canal. *J Bone Joint Surg Am* 26:125–130, 1944.
9. Brodke DS, Dick JC, Kunz DN, et al. Posterior lumbar interbody

fusion. A biomechanical comparison, including a new threaded cage. *Spine* 22:26–31, 1997.

10. Christoferson LA, Selland B. Intervertebral bone implants following excision of protruded lumbar discs. *J Neurosurg* 42:401–405, 1975.

11. Collis JS. Total disc replacement: a modified posterior lumbar interbody fusion. Report of 750 cases. *Clin Orthop* 193:64–67, 1985.

12. Onesti ST, Ashkenazi E. The Ray threaded fusion cage for posterior lumbar interbody fusion. *Neurosurgery* 42:200–205, 1998.

13. Wiltberger BR. Intervertebral body fusion by the use of the posterior bone dowel. *Clin Orthop* 3S:69–79, 1964.

14. Kirkaldy-Willis WH, Farfan HF. Instability of the lumbar spine. *Clin Orthop* 165:110, 1982.

15. Frymoyer JW, Newberg A, Pope MH, et al. Spine radiographs in patients with low-back pain. *J Bone Joint Surg Am* 66:1048–1055, 1984.

16. Sidhu KS, Herkowitz HN. Spinal instrumentation in the management of degenerative disorders of the lumbar spine. *Clin Orthop* 335:39–53, 1997.

17. Hutter CG. Spinal stenosis and posterior lumbar interbody fusion. *Clin Orthop* 193:103–114, 1985.

18. Lin PM. Posterior lumbar interbody fusion technique. Complications and pitfalls. *Clin Orthop* 193:90–102, 1985.

19. Lin PM, Cautilli RA, Joyce MF. Posterior lumbar interbody fusion. *Clin Orthop* 180:154–168, 1983.

20. Matsuzaki H, Tokuhashi Y, Matsumoto F, et al. Problems and solutions of pedicle screw plate fixation of lumbar spine. *Spine* 15:1159–1165, 1990.

21. Stonecipher T, Wright S. Posterior lumbar interbody fusion with facet screw fixation. *Spine* 14:468–471, 1988.

22. Steffee AD, Sitkowski DJ. Posterior lumbar interbody fusion and plates. *Clin Orthop* 227:99–102, 1988.

23. Hutter CG. Posterior intervertebral body fusion. A 25-year study. *Clin Orthop* 179:86–96, 1983.

24. Blume HG. Unilateral lumbar interbody fusion (posterior approach) utilizing dowel grafts. In: Lin PM, Gill K, eds. *Lumbar interbody fusion*. Rockville, MD: Aspen Publications, 1989:201–209.

25. Rish BL. A critique of posterior lumbar interbody fusion: 12 years' experience with 250 patients. *Surg Neurol* 31:281–289, 1989.

26. Simmons JW. Posterior lumbar interbody fusion (PLIF). In: Frymoyer JW, et al., eds. *The adult spine. Principles and practices*. New York: Raven Press, 1991:1961–1987.

27. Turner JA, Herron L, Deyo RA. Meta-analysis of the results of lumbar spinal fusion. *Acta Orthop Scand* 64:120–122, 1993.

28. Lehmann TR, Spratt KF, Tozzi JE, et al. Long-term follow-up of lower lumbar fusion patients. *Spine* 12:97–104, 1987.

211. Bone Harvest Techniques, Supplementation, and Alternatives

Wendy J. Spangler, Mark Adams, and Curtis A. Dickman

Fusion with bone graft has become an integral part of spine surgery. Autologous and allogeneic bone grafts are used in fusions at all levels of the spine and ultimately play a more important role than the instrumentation involved in fusion procedures. In fact, in many cases, bone is even used as an instrument. Many different types of bone grafts can be obtained, the most common being tricortical, bicortical, and cancellous. Autogenous cancellous bone is the most successful grafting material because of its osteogenic, osteoconductive, and osteoinductive properties. Cortical grafts are less ideal because cortical bone has fewer osteoblasts and osteocytes and offers less surface area than does cancellous bone. It provides a barrier to vascular ingrowth and bony remodeling. Mechanically, however, cortical bone is stronger than cancellous bone.

Autografts are often preferred to allografts because they are sterile, nonreactive, live, and genetically identical to the host. Potential complications, however, are associated with harvesting, and the quality or quantity of the grafts can be inadequate. With allografts, vascularization can be delayed, bone formation can be slow, and considerable resorption can occur, or the graft can become infected or be rejected. The distinct advantage of allograft is the lack of morbidity associated with harvesting.

Iliac Crest Grafts

Local trauma to tissue should be minimized to maximize vascularization at a fusion site. Bipolar coagulation and copious irrigation during drilling can minimize thermal injury to bone. All periosteum and soft tissue, which can induce a fibrous interface and hence nonunion, must be meticulously removed from the bone graft and fusion bed. Fusion sites should be decorticated to expose the bone marrow. Bone grafts should fit precisely into the fusion site to maximize the surface area of bone-to-bone contact. Dead space within the fusion bed should be eliminated. Fixation enhances union rates in the grafted segment by minimizing excessive movement and the formation of fibrous tissue.

HARVESTING ANTERIOR GRAFTS. Anterior iliac crest bone grafts should be harvested at least 3 cm behind the anterior superior iliac spine (Fig. 1). Disruption of the ilioinguinal ligament and a potential avulsion fracture of the bone anterior to the harvest site are thereby avoided. A linear incision is made parallel to the iliac crest directly over the harvest site. Monopolar or blunt dissection proceeds subcutaneously down to the fascial layer. The fascia and periosteum over the iliac crest are opened via a linear incision with the use of monopolar cauterization, and subperiosteal dissection is performed. A cuff of fascia and periosteum is left intact for a secure closure. Medial and lateral subperiosteal dissection is continued with the use of a Cobb periosteal elevator until the tricortical graft site has been exposed. Again, care is exerted to avoid injury to the ilioinguinal nerve, lateral femoral cutaneous nerve, blood vessels, and viscera (Fig. 2).

The exposed bone graft can be harvested with oscillating saws or osteotomes. The medial and lateral exposures of the

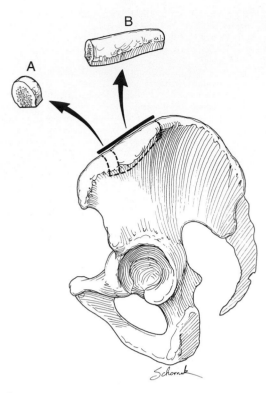

Fig. 1. Tricortical bone grafts harvested from the anterolateral ileum for (**A**) single-level interbody fusion or (**B**) multiple-segment vertebral body reconstruction. (From the Barrow Neurological Institute, with permission.)

iliac crest are usually packed with sponges to avoid injury to the muscles and inadvertent entry into the peritoneal cavity. When the graft will be used for mechanical weight bearing, oscillating saws are preferred for harvesting because osteotomes can create microfractures that weaken the graft. A posterior ledge of cortex can be left intact.

Once the graft has been harvested, bone wax or Gelfoam (Upjohn, Kalamazoo, Michigan) is placed along the graft site for hemostasis. Drains are rarely needed with this technique. The wound is closed in multiple layers; the fascial and periosteal layers should be reapproximated carefully with interrupted sutures.

HARVESTING POSTERIOR GRAFTS. A posterior approach can be used to obtain tricortical grafts, cortical matchstick grafts, corticocancellous plates, or cancellous bone strips (Fig. 3). Grafts are obtained from the medial 6 to 8 cm of the iliac crest to avoid injury to the superior cluneal nerves and the resulting buttock numbness or painful neuromas (Fig. 4).

A curved skin incision begins at the posterior iliac spine and extends superolaterally. Dissection proceeds carefully to preserve the anatomical tissue planes, especially the fascial and periosteal layers. Monopolar cauterization and Cobb periosteal elevators are used to expose the medial and lateral cortical surfaces. Care is taken to maintain the dissection subperiosteally to avoid branches of the gluteal artery, which can retract into the muscle and cause brisk bleeding. Maintaining the dissection lateral and cephalic to the posterior iliac spine avoids the sacroiliac joint medially and the sciatic notch inferiorly. If a tricortical graft is needed, the anterior surface of the iliac crest should be dissected carefully to avoid injury to the ureter lying within the retroperitoneal fat pad.

Grafts are obtained with a combination of oscillating saws, osteotomes, sharp curettes, and bone gouges. Bone wax and

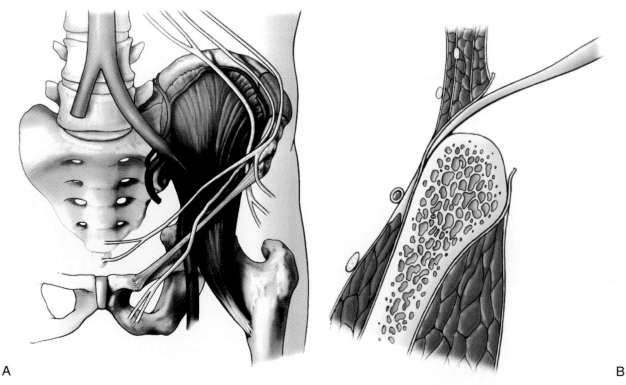

A   B

Fig. 2. Graft exposure over the anterolateral iliac crest (**A**) with subperiosteal dissection (**B**) avoids the iliohypogastric, ilioinguinal, and lateral femoral cutaneous nerves. (From the Barrow Neurological Institute, with permission.)

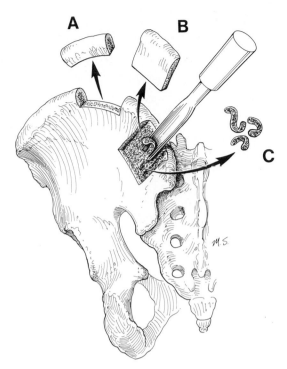

Fig. 3. Tricortical graft (**A**), corticocancellous plate (**B**), and cancellous bone strips (**C**) harvested from the posterior ileum. (From the Barrow Neurological Institute, with permission.)

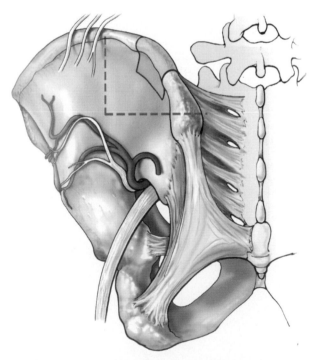

Fig. 4. The posterior iliac crest bone dissection is kept above the plane of the posterior superior iliac spine. The sacroiliac ligaments are avoided medially, the sciatic nerve caudally, the gluteal vessels caudally and submuscularly, the superior cluneal nerves laterally, and the ureter anteriorly. (From the Barrow Neurological Institute, with permission.)

Gelfoam are used to achieve hemostasis along the graft site. Although bone wax provides excellent hemostasis, it can inhibit bone healing and preclude obtaining grafts from the same site in the future. Gelfoam may therefore be preferred. After a graft has been harvested, a suction drain can be placed if oozing from the graft donor site persists. Typically, the drain can be removed on the first postoperative day. Meticulous closure of the periosteal and fascial layers is key to prevent herniation of the abdominal contents and reduce postoperative muscle pain. The wound is closed in multiple layers to ensure obliteration of dead space and optimal healing.

Alternative Autologous Graft Sites

Although iliac crest is the preferred site for autologous bone graft, autologous bone can also be obtained from the rib, fibula, and calvarium. Rib grafts can be used as struts or as sources of cancellous bone. Straight or curved segments can be used for spinal fusion and also for internal fixation of the occiput and cervical spine. Because the mechanical strength of such segments is limited, they should not be used to reconstruct major spinal deformities without internal fixation devices. To harvest the graft, a linear incision is made in the skin parallel to the rib directly over its surface (Fig. 5). The outer surface of the rib is exposed by incising the overlying muscles and periosteum. Blunt dissection with a Doyen rib dissector is used to detach the intercostal muscles and the parietal pleura intact from the undersurface of the rib. The ends of the rib graft are then transected sharply with a rib cutter or an oscillating saw. The rib cutter is less ideal than an oscillating saw because it can crush, splinter, and weaken the ends of the ribs. Bone edges are smoothed and waxed to prevent pleural puncture and hence pneumothorax. Once hemostasis has been obtained, the wound is closed in multiple layers. Postoperative chest radiographs are obtained to ensure that a pneumothorax has not developed.

Fibula grafts are obtained from the middle third of the fibula shaft (Fig. 6). This approach avoids injury to the peroneal nerve at the proximal head and preserves ankle function distally with no overall functional consequences. Fibula provides excellent strut grafts but relatively little cancellous bone. It is used primarily for anterior reconstruction of vertebral body defects, especially in the cervical spine. To obtain the graft, an incision is oriented parallel to the fibula over the lateral surface of the lower leg.

Nonvascularized grafts can be obtained after subcutaneous and muscle dissection of the fibula with subperiosteal exposure circumferentially. If a muscular cuff is left around the graft, along with the nutrient vessels, a vascularized graft can also be obtained. A vascular pedicle of the peroneal artery and vein, along with the nutrient vessels, can be preserved for anastomosis. The bone is transected proximally and distally to the measured length with a Gigli saw or an oscillating saw. The wound can then be closed in a routine multilayered fashion. For vascularized grafts, the vessels can be anastomosed with the superior thyroid artery and vein or other accessible large vessels in the anterior cervical spine. Posteriorly, the graft can be anastomosed to the occipital artery. Typically, vascularized grafts are incorporated more rapidly if the anastomoses remain patent. Because of the increased time involved with harvest and fusion, however, vascularized grafts tend to be reserved for special circumstances.

Calvarial bone grafts are useful in children whose iliac crest and fibula have not yet ossified (Fig. 7). Full-thickness grafts can be obtained from the middle occipital bone and used for

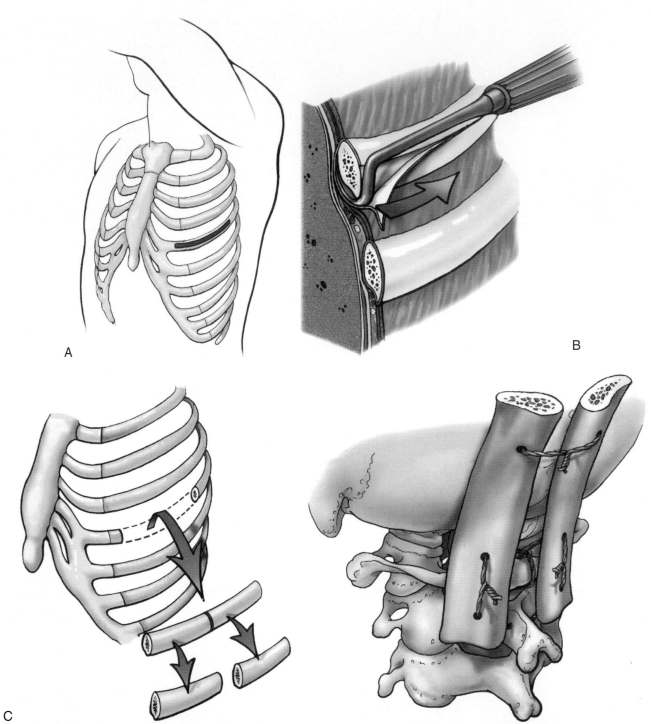

Fig. 5. A: Rib exposure over a curved segment. **B:** Extrapleural periosteal dissection of the neurovascular bundle and muscle attachments from the rib. **C:** The ribs are sharply cut with a cutting tool. **D:** Occipitocervical fusion with ribs wired to the occiput and cervical laminae. (From the Barrow Neurological Institute, with permission.)

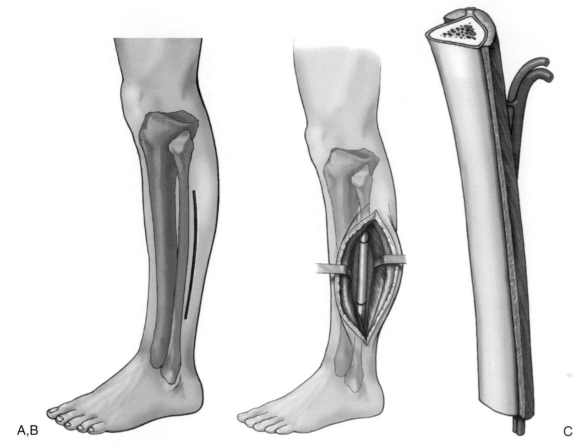

A,B   C

Fig. 6. **A:** Exposure of the fibula over its middle third. **B:** Periosteal incisions proximally and distally along the fibula with isolation of peroneal vessels and preservation of a muscle cuff and margin of periosteum around the graft. **C:** Harvesting the vascularized graft with preserved muscle cuff and vascular pedicle, which is anastomosed to vessels within the host site. (From the Barrow Neurological Institute, with permission.)

cervical fusion. One or two burr holes are drilled to expose the dura, and the atlanto-occipital membrane is sharply dissected from the edge of the foramen magnum. The bone graft can be cut with a craniotome. The dura is carefully separated from the bone before the craniectomy is removed. Split-thickness grafts can be obtained from parietal bones. A bicoronal or *C*-shaped incision is made at the vertex to expose paramedian craniotomy flaps. The midline bone is left intact over the superior sagittal sinus if bilateral craniectomies are performed. The top half of the graft is reattached to the skull with wires or miniplates, and the scalp is closed routinely with galeal and skin sutures. The split-thickness grafts can then be contoured to the desired shape and fixated to the spine.

Bone Graft Alternatives and Supplementation

Despite their drawbacks, autogenous bone grafts have long been the gold standard for arthrodesis. Cadaveric allografts remain the preferred alternative when autogenous bone is not available (1). Fibular allografts are commonly used for cervical

arthrodesis; occasionally, tibial, humeral, or femoral strut grafts are used in the thoracolumbar spine. Autografts and allografts have similar rates of fusion when used for single-level discectomies in the cervical spine. For multilevel fusions, however, allografts have a higher rate of failure than autografts (2,3). Bone banks procure allografts via established standards. They are sterilely harvested, processed, and freeze-dried or stored fresh-frozen. Serology is tested, autopsy specimens are evaluated, and donors are screened to minimize the risk for infection. The risk for transplanting human immunodeficiency virus (HIV) in bone has been estimated to be less than 1 per 1 million. Immunogenicity is also reduced by treating allografts with ethylene oxide, freezing, or freeze-drying.

Methylmethacrylate has been used in place of bone grafts for spinal reconstruction. However, it is less than ideal because it does not promote bone healing and is not osteoconductive, osteoinductive, or osteogenic. It resists compression but fails under tension and must be anchored to bone. It becomes encapsulated and can elicit a foreign-body response. It never becomes biologically incorporated. Methylmethacrylate should therefore be reserved for patients who are expected to place little mechanical stress on the fusion or who have a short life expectancy.

Pulsed electromagnetic fields promote bone healing by triggering angiogenesis. However, few clinical or basic science

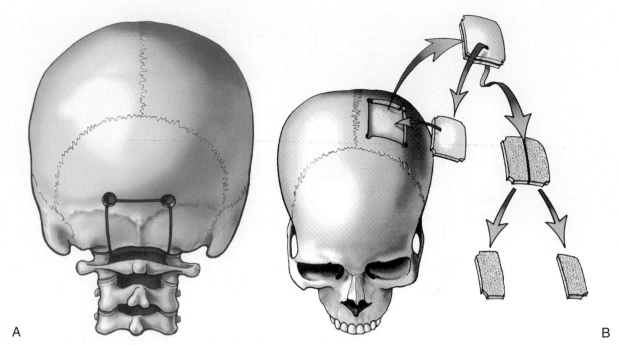

Fig. 7. A: A full-thickness, rectangular bone graft harvested from the occiput with a craniotome. **B:** A split-thickness calvarial graft harvested from the parietal bone. The full-thickness graft is removed with a craniotome and divided with a microreciprocating saw. The upper layer is reattached with miniplates, and the grafts from the lower layer are sized and wired to the spine. (From the Barrow Neurological Institute, with permission.)

studies have evaluated electromagnetic stimulation in the context of spinal fusion, and its efficacy is not yet established.

Augmenting autologous fusion has moved into the realm of molecular biology. Experimentally, the degree and strength of fusion have been enhanced by using a variety of osteoinductive proteins. Studies have demonstrated the effectiveness of hydroxyapatite combined with recombinant human bone morphogenetic protein type 2 (rhBMP-2) and rhOP-1 in promoting bone fusion and healing in animal models (4–8). The best-defined is BMP, an osteoinductive glycoprotein extracted from bone matrix that induces mesenchymal cells to differentiate into bone cells. BMP has tremendous potential for stimulating bone healing and promoting spinal fusion. In the future, it may obviate the need for autologous bone grafts.

References

1. Cloward RB. Gas-sterilized cadaver bone grafts for spinal fusion operations—a simplified bone bank. *Spine* 1980;5:4–10.

2. Holmes R, Mooney V, Bucholz R, et al. A coralline hydroxyapatite bone graft substitute—preliminary report. *Clin Orthop* 1984;188: 252–262.

3. Rish BL, McFadden JT, Penix JO. Anterior cervical fusion using homologous bone grafts. A comparative study. *Surg Neurol* 1976;5: 119–121.

4. Sheehan JP, Kallmes DF, Sheehan JM, et al. Molecular methods of enhancing lumbar spine fusion. *Neurosurgery* 1996;39:548–554.

5. Sandhu HS, Kanim LEA, Toth JM, et al. Experimental spinal fusion with recombinant human bone morphogenetic protein-2 without decortication of osseous elements. *Spine* 1997;22:1171–1180.

6. Urist MR. Bone transplants and implants. In Urist MR, ed. *Fundamentals and clinical bone physiology*. Philadelphia: JB Lippincott Co, 1980:331–368.

7. Urist MR, Dawson E. Intertransverse process fusion with the aid of chemosterilized autolyzed antigen-extracted allogeneic (AAA) bone. *Clin Orthop* 1981;154:97–113.

8. Urist MR, Mikulski A, Lietze A. Solubilized and insolubilized bone morphogenetic protein. *Proc Natl Acad Sci U S A* 1979;76: 1828–1832.

212. Minimally Invasive Surgery in the Cervical Spine: Posterior Cervical Microendoscopic Laminoforaminotomy for Decompression or Discectomy

Steven D. Chang, Daniel H. Kim,
Sung W. Roh, and
Richard G. Fessler

In the last decade neurosurgical research has made significant progress in the development of less invasive techniques for cervical spine surgery. There are three reasons for this progress. First, neurosurgeons have been increasingly interested in using less invasive surgical methods, particularly as their understanding of spine biomechanics evolves. Second, corporate research investment has yielded advances in medical instrument design and has stimulated the development of ancillary minimally invasive technologies. Third, prevailing health care trends have required physicians to develop and apply medical procedures that reduce patients' postoperative hospitalization by shortening their recovery times. Minimally invasive surgery is a product of these influences.

Cervical spine surgery typically involves treatment of degenerative and/or herniated disc disease and spinal stenosis, using either an anterior or posterior approach, depending on the pathology. Traditional surgical techniques are useful and reliable, but it seems likely that less invasive methods can achieve the same, if not better, results for a variety of cervical disease processes. Furthermore, it is likely that new techniques will become available in the future and will continue to improve traditional surgical techniques and refine the current less invasive ones. As with other subspecialties in neurosurgery, treatment of the spine is constantly evolving.

This chapter reviews a microendoscopic technique used to perform cervical laminoforaminotomy for decompression or discectomy. While this technique is still under development, it has the potential to be very successful in treating diseases of the cervical spine. Although conventional cervical spine approaches are not likely to be abandoned, microendoscopic decompression/discectomy is a promising alternative for some neurosurgical patients. This chapter discusses the indications, instruments, technique, results, and potential complications of microendoscopic decompression/discectomy.

Indications

The primary surgical indication for microendoscopic decompression is similar to that of an open cervical microdiscectomy—neural foraminal stenosis with impingement on a cervical nerve root at the neural foramen. This is generally a manifestation of degenerative disease of the cervical spine and common symptoms include radicular pain, paresthesias or numbness in a dermatomal distribution, motor weakness attributable to the nerve root in question, or any combination of these symptoms. If several neural foramina are stenosed, patients may have symptoms characteristic of multiple cervical nerve root involvement. The primary indication for posterior microendo-

scopic discectomy (MED) is a lateral posterior herniated disc fragment impinging on a cervical nerve root at the neural foramen. Patients often have a stenotic neural foramen that becomes further compromised by a disc herniation. Patients with free disc fragments (soft discs) may benefit from microendoscopic decompression alone, but a microendoscopic discectomy with resection of the disc fragment is the more appropriate procedure in the majority of cases.

Contraindications to performing posterior microendoscopic decompression or discectomy are pathologies that should be treated using anterior surgical procedures. These include midline cervical discs or osteophytes, resulting in compression of neural elements. Relative contraindications include previous posterior cervical spine surgery in which postsurgical scar tissue may hinder adequate identification of normal anatomy through the endoscope.

Instruments

Successful microendoscopic decompression/discectomy requires using a standard instrument set for an open posterior cervical discectomy, including suction, bipolar and Bovie units, Gelfoam, cottonoids, irrigation, as well as specialized instruments designed to be used with the microendoscope. The instruments and equipment for the MED system (Sofamor Danek, Memphis, TN) may be grouped as the introducer set, the video and endoscope, and the surgical instruments. The introducer set includes a guidewire (0.062 × 12 inches), and three dilators measuring 5.3, 10, and 14.5 mm in diameter (Fig. 1). There is

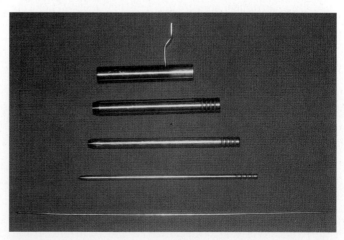

Fig. 1. The guidewire (*bottom*), the three sequential dilators, and the tubular retractor (*top*).

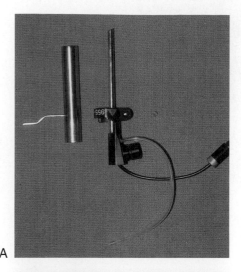

A

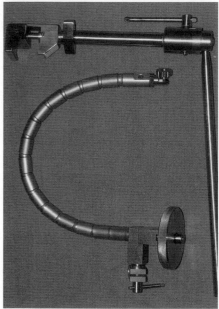

B

Fig. 2. The tubular retractor system (**A**) attached to the flexible arm system (**B**). The endoscope is shown within the tubular retractor.

also a 16-mm tubular retractor and a flexible arm assembly (Fig. 2) that can be attached to the operating room table.

The procedure requires the use of standard video equipment, including a color monitor, video integrator system, VHS or super-VHS recorder, a color video printer (if images are desired), and an endoscope (Fig. 3). A V-mount camera head is attached to a MED coupler, and the coupler is attached to the MED endoscope by way of the endoscope boss, using a locking ring mechanism. A light cable is attached to the light port of the MED endoscope. The endoscope's specifications of the MED system are a working length of 100 mm, a 25-degree angle of view, a 90-degree field of view, and a 5- to 50-mm variable depth of field.

Microinstruments for microendoscopic decompression or discectomy include those used in any standard open posterior cervical spine surgical procedure: bone decompression instruments, such as 1-, 2-, and 3-mm Kerrison rongeurs and a high-speed microdrill; straight and angled 2- and 3-mm pituitary rongeurs for soft tissue removal; curved or straight tip microscissors and straight microknives; nerve root retractors, ball probes,

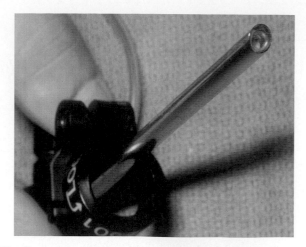

Fig. 3. The microendoscopic discectomy (MED) endoscope showing its size relative to the operating surgeon's hand.

nerve hooks, and a Penfield no. 4 dissector; and cauterizing instruments, such as the bayonet bipolar forceps and Bovie cautery with extension.

Surgical Technique

The surgical approach to a posterior foraminotomy has been previously described in detail in a number of reports (1–4), and a similar approach is used for microendoscopic decompression or discectomy. Prior to surgery, intravenous access is obtained and intravenous antibiotics are administered. Arterial lines and central venous access are generally not indicated. The patient is positioned prone with the head secured in three-point fixation or placed on a horseshoe head holder; if necessary, the hair over the suboccipital scalp and neck is shaved. The operating room should be of adequate size to accommodate the fluoroscopy unit and monitor, as well as the video monitor. All equipment should be arranged according to the surgeon's preference. Special attention should be placed on the position of the monitors so that the operating surgeon does not have to turn away from the operative field as he or she works. The fluoroscopy arm should be positioned in such a way that it can be moved out of the way cranially between imaging uses without compromising sterility of the surgical field.

Following a sterile skin preparation, the incision line is marked out. Under lateral fluoroscopic control, a 22-gauge spinal needle is inserted through the skin 1 cm off the midline at the appropriate disc space level. After making a small stab incision with a no. 15 blade, the guidewire is inserted under fluoroscopy (Fig. 4) to the inferior edge of the superior lamina at the level to be decompressed, or to where a discectomy is to be performed. The skin incision is then extended cranially or caudally to accommodate the dilators. The smallest dilator is then placed over the guidewire and docked on the superior lamina between the spinous process and the facet joint. Once the cannula is docked to the lamina, the guidewire is no longer needed and should be removed. Lateral fluoroscopy confirms the position of this initial cannula with respect to the disc space. Sequentially larger cannulated dilators are inserted through the posterior neck musculature to the junction of the lamina and the lateral mass. A 16-mm tubular retractor is then inserted over the largest dilator, the dilators are removed, and position is once

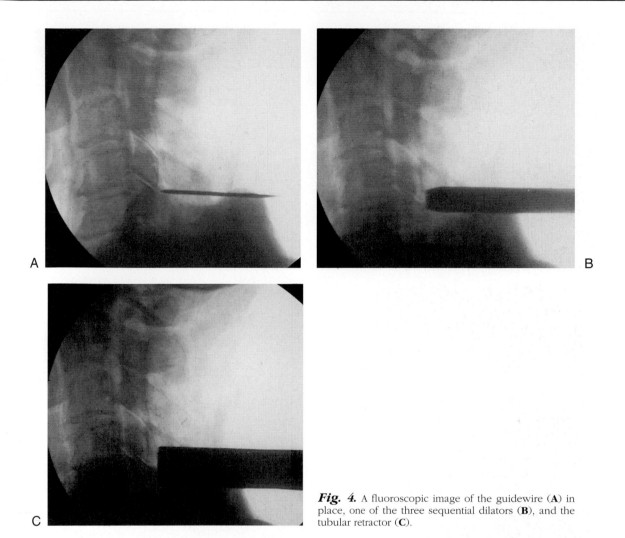

Fig. 4. A fluoroscopic image of the guidewire (**A**) in place, one of the three sequential dilators (**B**), and the tubular retractor (**C**).

again confirmed by fluoroscopy to ensure that the tip of the retractor is positioned just above the inferior edge of the lamina. The tubular retractor is fixed to the flexible self-retaining arm assembly, which is attached to the operating room table to secure its position. The endoscope is then inserted onto the tubular retractor, the magnification is adjusted, and the endoscope is fixed to the flexible arm assembly with a ring clamp. The endoscope can be positioned anywhere within a 360-degree arc on the retractor, and can be advanced or withdrawn to allow for variable magnification. If the distal endoscopic tip is either fogged or obstructed by debris, it may be cleaned with anti-fog solution and dry gauze.

Image orientation is a key step in microendoscopic procedures. When the endoscope is first inserted, the orientation of the video image is not likely to correspond to the orientation of the underlying anatomy. To achieve the correct image orientation, place the tip of a surgical instrument, such as a Penfield no. 4, into the visual field and rotate the camera until the video image matches the anatomical position.

The tip of the tubular retractor is then adjusted so that the superior and inferior laminar edges and the medial facet joint are visible. A small curved curet is then used to identify the inferior edge of the superior lamina and the medial edge of the lateral mass (Fig. 5). Soft tissue overlying the intralaminar space is removed with a pituitary rongeur. Bipolar and Bovie electrocautery should be used to provide meticulous hemostasis and to remove any obstructing soft tissue. Curets are then used to

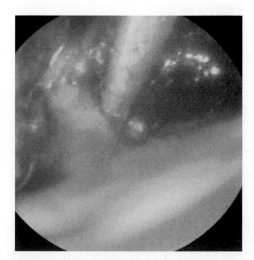

Fig. 5. A curet is used to identify the laminar edges.

detach the ligamentum flavum from the laminar edges. Bone removal of the inferior-lateral portion of the superior lamina is performed using 1- or 2-mm, 45-degree angled Kerrison rongeurs or a high-speed drill (Fig. 6). The superior edge of the inferior lamina is then removed and, after using a microprobe to confirm the location of the pedicles, the medial facet joint is also removed. The ligamentum flavum covering the nerve root can then be removed using a combination of curets and Kerrison punches. It is not necessary to remove the ligamentum flavum overlying the posterior thecal sac. A small probe or blunt nerve hook is then used to identify the location of the neural foramen laterally, and decompression continues, exposing the nerve root exiting the thecal sac. To ensure maximum decompression, the nerve root must also be freed by dissecting superiorly and inferiorly. Exploration of the neural foramen with a small probe confirms adequate decompression. Epidural venous bleeding is not uncommon, and is controlled using either bipolar coagulation, if single veins can be isolated, or with gentle Gelfoam or Surgicel packing, if the bleeding is diffuse.

If a discectomy is to be performed, the nerve root is identified and then dissected free from the surrounding tissue. Using either a nerve root retractor or a Penfield no. 4 dissector, it is then mobilized either medially for a herniated disc at the shoulder of the nerve root, or superiorly for a disc herniation in the axilla of the nerve root. Inspection around the nerve root is performed using either a small ball probe or dissector, and epidural veins are coagulated with bipolar cautery. If a soft disc fragment is located, it is removed with a small pituitary rongeur (Fig. 7). If an annulotomy is required to remove the herniated disc, it can be performed using a microknife, all the while protecting the nerve root with a retractor under direct visualization. Both the axilla and the shoulder of the nerve root must be carefully explored to ensure that disc material is not left behind. If a small disc protrusion is encountered, it can be gently teased out with either a pituitary rongeur or small dissector. Microprobes are used to confirm resection of the surgical disc fragment and adequate decompression of the nerve root.

Upon completion of the procedure, the disc space is irrigated with copious antibiotic irrigation. The tubular retractor is removed and the fascial layer closed with a single absorbable suture. The skin is closed with an absorbable subcuticular 4-0 suture and Steri-Strips, and a bandage is then applied. The patient is carefully removed from head fixation or the horseshoe

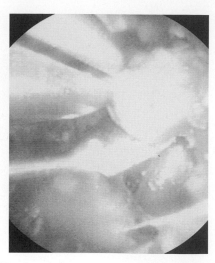

Fig. 7. A pituitary rongeur is used to remove disc material.

headrest, and rolled over to a supine position on a bed prior to transport to the recovery room.

Surgical Results

Roh et al. (5) treated a series of four patients using a microendoscopic foraminotomy technique, either with or without accompanying discectomy. These patients presented with cervical radiculopathy that failed to improve with medical therapy, and all patients had documented foraminal stenosis or lateral located disc fragments. All four procedures were without complications. The first two patients remained overnight in the hospital following the procedure. Currently, patients are discharged the same day of the surgery. All four patients significantly recovered their neurological function, and they reported a marked reduction in pain during a subsequent 3-month follow-up period.

The overall clinical outcome for patients undergoing traditional open posterior foraminotomies is excellent (3,4), with a 96% incidence of relief from significant arm pain and a 98% incidence of resolution from preoperative motor deficits. We anticipate that, as the series of patients undergoing microendoscopic decompression or discectomy increases, we will observe similar excellent and promising results.

Complications

The ability to maintain hemostasis while using the endoscope is the primary difficulty with this procedure. Specially designed straight and curved-tip microbipolars are useful in cauterizing bleeding epidural veins. While no complications were noted in the Roh et al. (5) microendoscopic foraminotomy series, potential complications remain the same as those for posterior traditional foraminotomies or microdiscectomies. As with other posterior foraminotomy approaches, other surgical complications are rare. Wound infections have a reported incidence of 0.4% (3) and are minimized by treating patients preoperatively with antibiotics. Prolonged postsurgical paresis is also uncommon.

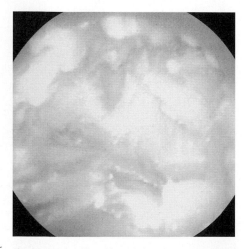

Fig. 6. A high-speed drill can be used to decompress the lamina and medial facet.

Transient paresthesias, numbness, radiculitis, and paresis are more common, but still occur infrequently.

Conclusions

Microendoscopic decompression or discectomy is a minimally invasive surgical technique available to patients presenting with cervical spine disease. While it is unlikely that traditional treatments for cervical spine pathology will be completely replaced in the near future, microendoscopic methods have the potential to successfully treat some neurosurgical patients, providing them with excellent results. As with the introduction of any new or novel surgical treatment, neurosurgeons must carefully and objectively monitor and scrutinize their patients' clinical outcomes. Only then will they be able to decide which is the best treatment regimen for their patients.

References

1. Aldrich F. Posterolateral microdiscectomy for cervical monoradiculopathy caused by posterolateral soft cervical disc sequestration [see comments]. *J Neurosurg* 1990;72:370–377.
2. Fager CA. Posterolateral approach to ruptured median and paramedian cervical disk. *Surg Neurol* 1983;20:443–452.
3. Williams RW. Microcervical foraminotomy. A surgical alternative for intractable radicular pain. *Spine* 1983;8:708–716.
4. Henderson CM, Hennessy RG, Shuey HM Jr, et al. Posterior-lateral foraminotomy as an exclusive operative technique for cervical radiculopathy: a review of 846 consecutively operated cases. *Neurosurgery* 1983;13:504–512.
5. Roh SW, Kim DH, Cardoso AC, et al. Posterior cervical laminoforaminotomy using microendoscopic discectomy (MED) system in live porcine animals and early clinical report of four patients. *Spine* 2000; 25:260–264.

213. Minimally Invasive Spine Surgery

Rabih G. Tawk and John C. Liu

The recent trend toward minimally invasive surgery (MIS) of the spine is the consequence of rapid improvements in video-assisted endoscopic technology, reductions in postoperative pain and recovery time, and the current emphasis on delivering cost-effective care (1–6). MIS represents the result of evolving advances in surgical technique.

The definition of MIS is not well established in the literature; however, the term should be used for any surgical intervention that entails relatively little trauma to tissues. MIS includes procedures that address lesions as directly as possible with minimal manipulation of other, normal tissue.

Historically, endoscopic surgery began with the invention of the cystoscope by Philip Bozzini in 1806 (7), who developed the first endoscopic instrument, consisting of a candle attached to a thin cannula that allowed illumination (8). He was the first to look into the hollow cavities of the human body by conducted light (9). In 1853, Desormeaux was the first to introduce the use of a lens to focus a direct light source to obtain a clear image (10,11).

Because of visualization problems, the applications of endoscopy remained limited until the 1950s, when cold-light fiberglass illumination was used by Hopkins and Kanapy (12). In the 1970s, medical engineering set the stage for progress in fiberglass and fiberoptic technology, which allowed heat to be dissipated and led to the development of the cold-light system. Later on, the development of endoscopic video cameras and improvements in surgical instrumentation further enhanced the applications of endoscopy.

In the last few years, minimally invasive techniques have improved dramatically, so that they are now valuable alternatives to open procedures for the effective treatment of spine-related conditions. They have revolutionized many surgical specialties.

In comparison with traditional methods, MIS can reach the surgical site with less violation of normal tissue. Spinal endoscopic techniques are demanding, and surgeons must develop the skills necessary to use sophisticated new devices. Whereas soft herniated discs do not present any particular problems, calcified discs, incidental durotomy, and vascular injury still entail major risks and represent potential problems.

Cervical Spine

Recent advances in endoscopic technology have led to initial trials in the management of cervical disc disease (13).

PERCUTANEOUS NUCLEOTOMY. Although this technique has been used to treat lumbar disc disease, the experience in cervical disc herniation is restricted to a small number of cases (14). Limited data are available on its use in the treatment of cervical disc herniation. The selection criteria are poorly defined (14), and reported success rates are variable, with remarkably short follow-up periods (15–17).

The goal of this technique is to reduce pressure within the disc by removing the nucleus pulposus. A 2- to 3-cm incision is made parallel to the sternocleidomastoid muscle. The anterior spine is exposed by opening the plane between the carotid sheath laterally and the trachea and esophagus medially. Discography of the diseased disc is performed after placement of the needle within the annulus. The working cannula is directed into the disc interspace, and the nucleus pulposus is removed.

Whereas grasping and cutting instruments are used in the manual technique, Onik described the automated technique, which consists of a nucleotome formed by a cutting/aspiration probe. The potential benefits of the manual technique may be that a more thorough excision of the disc material is achieved by hand than with automated suction (14). The combination of chemonucleolysis followed by automated nucleotomy was reported in 22 patients. When they were followed for a period of at least 1 year, 19 patients showed good or excellent results (17).

Although this therapeutic modality does not allow complete excision of a herniated disc (18), minor reduction of the intradiscal pressure may relieve irritation of the nerve root and thereby alleviate radicular pain (19–21).

MICROENDOSCOPIC DISCECTOMY. Among the various current minimally invasive techniques, the microendoscopic discectomy (MED) system is newly developed for the cervical spine, and both anterior and posterior approaches have been reported.

Posterior Foraminotomy. Posterior foraminotomy is considered an effective procedure in selected cases of posterolateral disc herniation and cervical foraminal stenosis. The feasibility of this approach with use of the MED system has been demonstrated in animal models (22). Another cervical foraminotomy study was undertaken in both a cadaveric model and in three clinical cases, including one case of a multiple-level procedure. It provided exceptional visualization and facilitated the patient's postoperative recovery (23).

The major disadvantage of posterior approaches is that the patient experiences significant postoperative neck discomfort (23). Compared with the open procedure, MED requires less dissection of paraspinous muscle. Transmuscular dilation by means of the endoscopic tubular working channel can minimize postsurgical pain and provide rapid postoperative recovery (22). Minimal medial facetectomy also eliminates the need for fusion and preserves a functioning motion segment (13,22,24,25).

Patients are placed in a sitting position, which is commonly used for traditional keyhole foraminotomy (23), to decrease the epidural bleeding often encountered with cervical foraminotomies. The skin incision is made 5 mm off the midline, and the trajectory to the facet is followed with the use of a spinal needle under fluoroscopic guidance. The paraspinous muscles are split by using a flat-blade nasal speculum. Once the bone of the lamina–facet border is reached, the rigid endoscope is brought into the field. Laminotomy is performed, and after identification of the superior and inferior pedicles, the foraminal decompressive procedure is achieved by using both Kerrison punches and the endoscopic drill.

In clinical cases, no difficulty was encountered in controlling sites of bleeding. Experience with lumbar MED indicates that hemostasis can at times be challenging. This remains an important issue because the epidural venous plexus surrounding the cervical nerve roots can be the source of significant bleeding (26).

Preliminary results clearly suggest that MED may provide a viable technique for cervical hemilaminectomy and foraminotomy. Roh et al. (13) reported similar technique in a cadaveric model and demonstrated that the amount of bone removal and exposure was equal to that in the standard keyhole method. In another study, they reported a significantly greater degree of vertical diameter decompression and a higher percentage of facet removal than with the open technique (22).

OTHER APPLICATIONS IN THE CERVICAL SPINE

Anterior Cervical Discectomy with Fusion. Anterior cervical discectomy with fusion as described by Smith-Robinson is considered a minimally invasive procedure. It allows fusion with or without instrumentation, and minimal muscle dissection

is required. It is associated with less postoperative pain and fast recovery, and the patient may be discharged the same day.

Microsurgical Anterior Foraminotomy. Because fusion often occurs, even if not performed, after an anterior cervical discectomy, thereby eliminating the functioning motion segment (27–29), a new technique was developed to accomplish direct nerve root decompression by microsurgical anterior foraminotomy, in which the motion segment is preserved. The approach is similar to anterior cervical discectomy, but retraction exposes the ipsilateral longus colli muscle rather than the midline anterior disc. The nerve root is decompressed under an operating microscope from its origin to the point at which it passes behind the vertebral artery laterally (30). The longus colli muscle is excised on its medial portion to expose the uncovertebral joint and the medial parts of the upper and lower transverse processes. The uncinate process is removed to gain appropriate access to decompress the nerve root. This procedure was designed to preserve the disc as much as possible. The long-term outcome of the motion segment and the potential risk for damaging the vertebral artery remain to be defined. Similar anterior approaches (27,31,32) were reported previously, but none has stood the test of time.

Thoracic Spine

Thoracoscopic surgery of the spine has become a well-established and valuable surgical approach. Microsurgical approaches for the treatment of disease located in the ventral spine by means of video-assisted thoracic surgery (VATS) allow access to the disc spaces, paravertebral soft tissues, spinal cord, spinal nerves, and sympathetic chain with minimal invasion (33). Thoracoscopy minimally disrupts the soft tissues and avoids retraction while permitting surgery to be performed in a wide space (34). It has demonstrated clinical utility for discectomy, anterior release of spinal deformities, corpectomy, and spinal reconstruction (35–38). It can also be used effectively for sympathectomy, biopsy, tumor resection, debridement of infection, internal fixation, and intrathoracic nerve sheath tumor resection (3,38–43). However, it is a very technically demanding procedure, and extensive skills and dedicated practice in the laboratory are required to master the new psychomotor skills if the procedure is to be performed safely (34).

It is unlikely that a truly randomized, prospective study in which thoracotomy is compared with thoracoscopic discectomy will be carried out (44); therefore, conclusions are based on nonrandomized studies. In comparison with thoracotomy, thoracoscopy provides identical visualization and exposure of the spine with less pain, fewer pulmonary problems, less blood loss, less chest tube drainage, shorter hospitalization, and fewer complications. It is also associated with reductions in the use of pain medications, intercostal pain, and post-thoracotomy syndrome (3,36,45). In comparison with posterolateral approaches, it provides more complete visualization and access to the ventral spine and spinal cord and enables more complete resection of midline and calcified discs (34).

GENERAL PRINCIPLES AND TECHNIQUE. Thoracoscopy is performed under general anesthesia and with single-lung ventilation. The patient is placed on a radiolucent operating table in the right or left lateral position, depending on the location and eccentricity of the abnormality and the regional anatomy. A Trendelenburg or reverse Trendelenburg position is used for appropriate visualization of the lower or upper thoracic spine, respectively. The patient is anteriorly tilted; this position allows the ipsilateral lung to fall away from the dorsal spine without insertion of a lung retractor.

Single-lung ventilation on the nonoperative side is achieved with a double-lumen endotracheal tube; the ipsilateral lung must be deflated. If resorptive atelectasis does not occur, carbon dioxide insufflation for brief periods at a pressure of 8 cm H_2O can be performed to facilitate lung collapse. To minimize postoperative atelectasis, the deflated lung can be reinflated intraoperatively for 5 to 10 minutes for every hour of operative time (46).

Portals are placed at a distance from the spinal lesion to provide a panoramic view and a larger space for the operative field and to avoid instrument crowding or "fencing." Appropriate orientation of the instruments and camera facing the spine is of primary importance; thus, the surgeon should be standing on the ventral side of the patient and facing the monitors. Endoscopes provide depth perception and facilitate precise dissection around the spinal cord, nerve roots, and vertebrae (36). However, even the latest three-dimensional technology still depends on televised projection, in which the depth of the field does not compare with that of direct or microscopic vision (44).

To avoid perforating the diaphragm, the sixth or seventh intercostal space in the midaxillary line is the safest place for the first thoracoscopic portal (38). Other portals are placed under thoracoscopic visualization to avoid instrument-induced injuries. They can be placed in the anterior, middle, and posterior axillary lines, triangulated and centered around the abnormality (36).

Once the first portal is made, it is of primary importance to rule out and release pleural adhesions to prevent lung damage. The anterior axillary line is used when visualization of the spinal canal is of concern, and the midaxillary line is used for scoliosis surgery, in which the spine is rotated toward the apex of the curve.

RELEVANT ANATOMICAL CONSIDERATIONS. The ribs articulate with the vertebral body (VB) at the same level and the VB above except for ribs 1, 11, and 12, which articulate only with the lower vertebra. The proximal end of the rib and the disc space are collinear, and this relation helps to orient the surgeon during the procedure. The head covers the disc posterolaterally and overlies a portion of the neural foramen of the same level. Resection of rib heads exposes the pedicles, neural foramen, and disc spaces.

The neurovascular bundle traveling with the sixth rib contains the sixth intercostal nerve, which then passes under the pedicle of T6 just below its articulation with the rib. The apex of the aortic arch is usually found at approximately T4, and the descending aorta travels along the anterior VBs just to the left of midline. Lying posterior and medial to the aorta is the thoracic duct. The azygos system runs to the right of midline and is especially important in the operative approach because it offers more space behind the aorta in comparison with the left side. With abduction of patient's arm, access can be gained to the upper thorax. Above T4-5, the mediastinum and aortic arch generally preclude a safe left-sided approach (47).

In the middle thoracic spine, exposure can be obtained from either side according to the location and nature of the abnormality and the position of the thoracic duct, artery of Adamkiewicz, azygos vein, aorta, and other anatomical structures.

In the lower thoracic spine, the left side is easier to expose because the left hemidiaphragm is lower than its counterpart on the right side, under which the liver is located (36). At the level of T12-L1, the diaphragm presents an operative corridor.

Its release and the dissection of retroperitoneal tissue may prove beneficial (47).

The segmental vessels course along the midbody of each vertebra halfway between each of the disc spaces. It is important for the surgeon to realize that the segmental vessels lying along the VBs may supply the spinal cord and that reasonable attempts to preserve these vessels should be made. Each thoracic vertebra has a concavity relative to the spinal canal, and the pedicles emanate from the superior portion of the body, much higher than in the cervical or lumbar regions. The disc space is typically much narrower than in the lumbar spine, affording a relatively small operative window. The pedicle is a key landmark overlying the lateral aspect of the spinal canal (36,47).

The ribs are counted rostrally to caudally to the disc space of interest. Accurate location is then confirmed by placing a long tool or a needle through the portal into the disc space and obtaining plain radiographs or fluoroscopic visualization. The first rib forms a more acute angle than the second rib and is often not visualized, but it can be palpated. The second rib is the most cephalic identifiable visual landmark (35).

Endoscopic clips are used to ligate segmental vessels where they directly communicate with great vessels, and bleeding from any vascular bundle is controlled with bipolar cauterization. If the aorta has been displaced laterally and interferes with access to the disc space, it can be mobilized anteriorly after several sets of segmental vessels have been ligated (34).

ADVANTAGES. The advantages of thoracic endoscopic surgery include excellent visualization of critical anatomical structures (8). In comparison with thoracotomy, it avoids sequelae such as a decrease in functional residual capacity and atelectasis secondary to chest wall splinting from pain (48,49); it is associated with less blood loss, less use of narcotics, a shorter period of chest tube drainage, and a smaller incidence of intercostal neuralgia (46). Cosmetically, it is more appealing because long scars are not created, and because it is a less invasive surgical modality, the damage to other tissues that occurs during thoracotomy is avoided, so that earlier mobilization and rehabilitation are facilitated. Although performed through tiny incisions, it provides direct visualization of the entire ventral surface of the dura and spinal cord (50) with a decreased potential for infection. It facilitates a more complete resection of midline and calcified discs in comparison with posterior and posterolateral approaches (46).

The procedure allows grafting to be performed, and being less traumatic, it results in improved shoulder girdle function and less morbidity (45). It is an appropriate alternative for patients with severe lung disease who cannot tolerate the physiological effects of thoracotomy secondary to chest wall splinting from pain. Another advantage over thoracotomy is the relatively easier access to the thoracic spine above T4.

Visualization is provided to the entire operating team, so that greater participation is possible.

In comparison with posterior techniques, anterior approaches provide a more direct approach to all but laterally oriented disc herniations.

DISADVANTAGES. The chief disadvantages of thoracoscopy are related to the inability to perform single-lung ventilation in patients with severe pulmonary disease and the need to use long instruments that may hinder surgical control. Because of the steep learning curve and unfamiliar surgical techniques that are involved, this procedure is relatively impractical for surgeons who do not perform it frequently (44). Bilateral lung

Table 1. Complications of Thoracoscopy

Atelectasis
Air leak from lung[a]
Pleural effusion, hemothorax, chylothorax
Infection
Intercostal neuralgia
Subcutaneous emphysema
Neurological deterioration
Retained disc fragments
Excessive epidural blood loss
Conversion to open thoracotomy
Disc level misidentification
Transient paraparesis
Penetration of right hemidiaphragm
Intrathoracic breakage of instruments

[a] Can be repaired by endoscopic stapler.

compromise is frequent in patients with multiple injuries, so that they are poor candidates for ipsilateral lung collapse.

This technique may not be feasible if the patient has previously undergone a thoracotomy and has dense lung adhesions. Prior pleurodesis, empyema, or hemothorax can also preclude its use (50).

The use of double-lumen endotracheal tubes may not be feasible in small children because of the difficulty of maintaining oxygen saturation.

Cleaning bone dust from the endoscope significantly interrupts the progress of the procedure (44). Vascular injuries can be problematical, and incidental durotomy may require open repair or lumbar drainage of the cerebrospinal fluid. The complications of thoracoscopy are listed in Table 1.

INDICATIONS. The efficacy, indications, and limitations of this procedure have not been established in the literature. However, thoracoscopy is generally indicated for patients in whom an anterior approach is required (3,42,51–53).

VATS has been useful in biopsy of VB tumor, osteomyelitis, and paravertebral abscess. It has proved useful in the treatment of disc herniations, compression fractures, VB lesions, osteomyelitis, and paravertebral abscess, and in such procedures as vertebrectomy for infection and tumor, sympathectomy, decompression of the spinal cord, and release the anterior spinal ligament for reduction of deformities (2,37,42,54,55). It has also been used in fusion, spinal reconstruction (33), and hemivertebra resection (38).

In experienced hands, VATS can be used successfully in repeated operations on thoracic discs despite the presence of pleural adhesions, scar tissue, and anatomical destruction at the operative site (50).

As technical approaches evolve, factors that will have to be considered include training and experience of the surgeon; types of symptoms; anatomical relationships of the herniation, spinal cord, nerve root, and bone; and consistency of the herniation (soft or calcified).

CONTRAINDICATIONS. Generally, VATS is contraindicated in patients who cannot tolerate single-lung ventilation or have acute respiratory distress. Pleural symphysis and extensive pleural adhesions resulting from previous surgical procedures or empyema preclude successful access to the spine.

Previous tube thoracostomy or thoracotomy is considered a relative contraindication.

THORACOSCOPIC DISCECTOMY. The spinal level is identified by placing a needle into the disc space. Anteroposterior (AP) views are required because lateral views do not provide the perspective needed to count ribs and vertebrae accurately (36).

Once the appropriate level has been identified, the parietal pleura is opened over the disc space. After adequate cauterization, the rib head and proximal 2 to 3 cm are removed. Adjacent segmental vessels are usually not divided because they are located in the midportion of the vertebral body. Nevertheless, they can be dissected free, ligated, and sacrificed if necessary to expose the lateral surface of the pedicle and neuronal foramen.

The pedicle is a key landmark; once identified, it can be removed to obtain lateral exposure of the dura and spinal cord for a safe procedure (36). It can be resected with Cobb periosteal elevators, curved curettes, Kerrison rongeurs, rib cutters, or drills. The rib corresponding to the lower vertebra should be removed, except at the T11-12 level, where removal is not necessary because the rib insertion is below the disc space.

A pyramid-shaped cavity is created in the dorsolateral vertebral bodies and disc space to provide a means of access, and this is sufficient for small or moderately soft discs. This cavity is essential, allowing sufficient room for removal of the compressive disc material away from the epidural space. The working space minimizes the need to bring tools into the compressed epidural space. It should be wide enough for adequate visualization and exposure of the entire ventral dura across the spinal canal to the medial border of the contralateral pedicle. With large, ossified discs, much more room is needed, and even corpectomy for appropriate exposure (34). Calcified disc materials, osteophytes, and vertebral end plates can be removed with curettes, microdissectors, drills, or disc rongeurs.

Patients with previous thoracic disc surgery and retained disc material can be approached from the contralateral side. When corpectomy is required for exposure, fusion is considered for reconstruction (36); however, routine thoracic discectomy does not appear to destabilize the spine, so that fusion is not required (56).

After adequate hemostasis, one or two chest tubes are placed and left in place until the output is less than 100 mL/d. Chest radiographs should be obtained in the recovery room for appropriate assessment.

ANTERIOR RELEASE OF SPINAL DEFORMITY. In cases of scoliosis, anterior discectomy is performed to increase the mobility of the spine and degree of correction (5,37,38,54,57). This procedure is typically carried out by combined anterior release then posterior reduction and internal fixation of the deformity. Thoracoscopy allows anterior releases over multiple levels as the scope is switched between port sites to ensure optimal visualization and instruments are aligned with the disc being removed. The release of stiff scoliotic deformities or thoracic kyphosis makes it possible to restore the physiological curvature, and bone grafting is a key to maximizing correction, reducing the pseudarthrosis rate and preventing further progression of the curvature (58–61).

The advantages of anterior release are that it can be performed relatively quickly in trained hands and that graft is inserted under the same anesthetic. The indications are the same as for conventional surgery. During the last several years, thoracoscopy has been used to perform anterior release, internal costoplasty (62), and epiphysiodesis to prevent crankshaft phenomenon (63,64).

In most series of surgery for deformity, procedures were carried out in the lateral decubitus position, as in open thoracotomy (38,54,65). For scoliosis, four or more ports were placed in the anterior or midaxillary line, whereas for kyphotic deformities, three portals were enough, and most authors performed a spine fusion at the same time as the disc release (66). The concave approach generally is not technically feasible, and very large deformities may be better addressed through an open thoracotomy because of the small distance between the chest wall and the spine (64).

Technique. After a longitudinal incision of the pleura, blunt dissection of the segmental vessels is carried out. The anterior longitudinal ligament is sectioned at each level, and the intervertebral discs are entered by cauterizing the annulus fibrosus. Discectomy is performed, and resection is completed for five or six levels until anterior instability is achieved.

Classically, after the posterior procedure has been completed, an anterior approach is used for interbody fusion and definite correction of the abnormality and for stabilization. Portals are reinserted through the previous intercostal incisions, and autologous blocks of bone graft are inserted in the interspaces. The pleura is closed to decrease postoperative drainage from the operative site, so that earlier removal of the chest tube is possible.

The first two cases in which scoliosis was corrected endoscopically via an entirely anterior approach have been reported, with excellent results (67). The authors were able to insert screws just anterior to the head of the ribs in each of six vertebrae and attach a connecting rod through four 1-cm incisions. Multiple small incisions facilitated the placement of screws because incisions could be placed anteriorly or posteriorly and at any level to ensure that screws were inserted parallel to the vertebral end plates. However, this benefit was offset by the ability to feel the screw penetrating the opposite cortex during open thoracotomy. The potential risks included screw penetration to the spinal canal if it angled posteriorly, or it could come out anteriorly if it angled too much in the other direction. The main advantage of this technique was that fusion of fewer vertebrae was required, and mobility was spared at several intervertebral levels (67). It was also assumed that correction via an entirely anterior approach produced better results and prevented development of the crankshaft phenomenon (68). The spine is easier to access in kyphotic deformities than in scoliosis, and a larger number of discs can be released with a smaller number of portals.

Dickman (69) also reported one case of endoscopic correction, in which he used an anterior screw/rod system from T5 to T9. He was able to correct the curve from 85 to 55 degrees. At 1.5 years of follow-up, a solid fusion had developed, and the correction was maintained at 58 degrees. Another experimental system has also been reported to decrease the Cobb angle and could be successfully adapted for clinical use (70).

CORPECTOMY. Corpectomy is very similar to discectomy and is performed for many conditions, such as infections, tumors, and fractures. The proximal rib heads are removed and saved for later fusion. Discectomy of the levels above and below helps to define the superior and inferior boundaries of resection (33). This is followed by decortication of the vertebral end plates. A trough is created in the center of the VB and expanded to a large cavity to create the working space. After adequate dissection, visualization and palpation of the contralateral pedicle ensure that the decompressive pathology has been completely removed (47).

VERTEBRAL RECONSTRUCTION. Once the fusion bed has been prepared by removing the disc material and cartilaginous end plates from the distal ends of the vertebrectomy site, an allograft or autograft strut is used to create a fusion across the defect (47). Thoracoscopic reconstruction can be achieved with use of the resected ribs, a tricortical iliac crest fragment, or a whole-shaft humerus allograft. Methylmethacrylate can also be used for reconstruction; it is injected under fluoroscopic guidance into a Silastic tube and anchored deeply into the adjacent normal vertebrae to prevent loosening (36). It is essential to prevent its heating effects on neural tissue and extrusion by means of sterile water irrigation and careful observation. Internal reconstruction can be achieved by using cages filled with autologous bone or by fixation with thoracic screws and Z-plate (35,36).

ENDOSCOPIC TRANSPEDICULAR THORACIC DISCECTOMY. Particularly in the thoracic spine, the disc is located at the level of the facet joint, and the rostral edge of the pedicle is close to the intervertebral disc. This is why the facet joint must be removed either partially or totally to expose the intervertebral disc laterally. The approach was first described by Patterson and Arbit (71).

Endoscopic transpedicular thoracic discectomy is performed through a 2-cm transverse skin incision made 1 cm lateral to the midline. Under endoscopic or microscopic visualization, the medial portion of the facet, the very lateral portion of the lamina, and the rostral third of the pedicle are removed (72). The very lateral margin of the spinal cord dura mater is exposed, and a 70-degree endoscope is used to visualize the ventral aspect of the dura matter directly.

THORACOLUMBAR JUNCTION. Endoscopic treatment of the thoracolumbar junction (T11-L2) poses a great challenge, but access by a team of laparoscopic and spine surgeons obviates the need for major surgery to open the retroperitoneum and thoracic cavity (73,74). The complications of conventional open surgery can be minimized or even avoided by means of thoracoscopic access with splitting of the diaphragm (75), an endoscopic retroperitoneal approach (76,77), or a combination of both methods (78). The T11-12 disc is more easily accessed from the left side of the thoracic cavity because the diaphragm is lower on that side, and the aorta is in the midline at that level. When L1 fractures are approached from the abdomen, the titanium plate is fixed on T12, which requires splitting of the diaphragm. Burgos et al. (76) developed an animal model that was confirmed in cadavers and then in clinical cases. The technique combines an initial thoracoscopic approach with a subsequent retroperitoneal endoscopic approach. No significant complications occurred, but a potential weakness is in closure of the diaphragm.

When carbon dioxide is used in the retroperitoneum, the gas may escape into the thoracic cavity. However, this situation can be managed easily by adjusting the ventilatory parameters without increased risk to the patient (74).

SYMPATHECTOMY. Endoscopic thoracic sympathectomy is mainly indicated for palmar and axillary hyperhidrosis. It was first performed in 1949 by Kux (79), and various techniques have subsequently been described (68,72,80–87). The procedure has gained wide acceptance, with an efficacy of 95% to 100% (1,86–89), as a permanent treatment of hyperhidrosis after failure of medical therapy. Although general anesthesia is required, it can be performed on an outpatient basis (90,91).

The prevalence of hyperhidrosis is 0.6% to 1.0% (89), and the condition has a marked impact on professional and social life; it can cause people to avoid shaking hands and may lead to emotional problems. The excessive sweating is from eccrine glands, located primarily in palmar, plantar, and axillary regions, that are innervated by fibers of the sympathetic system.

The upper arm is elevated above the chest, and the ipsilateral elbow is flexed at 90 degrees to remove the scapula from the operative field. The endoscopic portal is placed in the fourth intercostal space along the posterior axillary line; one or two other trocars can be used and are inserted in third and fifth intercostal spaces along the anterior axillary line. Within the upper thorax, the chain lies against the neck of the ribs (47). The controversy regarding the extent of ganglion ablation necessary to obtain sympathetic denervation of the hand and axilla is considerable (89). Ablation of the second and third sympathetic ganglia is sufficient for palmar hyperhidrosis, and the fourth and fifth are also resected if axillary hyperhidrosis is present (1,42,85,86,88,89,92). If the stellate ganglion is left untouched (usually located over the first rib), the risk for postoperative Horner syndrome is negligible (89).

Failures are extremely rare (<1%) (46) and have been attributed to an inability to recognize the nerve of Kuntz, which can be seen shimmering through the pleura lateral to the main stem and bypassing the sympathetic chain to the upper extremity. Other causes of failure are incomplete resection, the presence of intermediate ganglia in the communicating rami and spinal nerves (89,93), and regeneration (94) (one reported case with conclusive evidence of regeneration). Failure can be avoided (46) or predicted (95) by monitoring the ipsilateral palmar temperature, and adequate sympathectomy is achieved if the temperature rises by more than 1°C. Excessive palmar sweating for a day or two during the first week has been seen (89) and was attributed to a final transmitter release.

Upper thoracic sympathectomy has also been used to treat other conditions, but the results have been less durable, temporary, and less satisfying (89). These include Raynaud disease (96,97), other vasospastic disorders/acrocyanosis and causalgia (98), angina pectoris (99–102) (in which symptoms were reduced and time to onset of symptoms was increased), long QT syndrome (103–106), ischemia of the upper extremity, hyperthyroidism (46), social phobia (107), essential hypertension, bronchial asthma, peptic ulcer, and reflex sympathetic dystrophy (108). In thoracoscopic splanchnic sympathectomy, the sympathetic chain and splanchnic branches are divided from level IV to levels X–XI (109), and the use of this technique to manage severe pain in chronic pancreatitis and pancreatic cancer has been described (110–113).

Complications. Side effects that have been reported (1,2,42, 46,81,85,86,88,89,92) include compensatory sweating primarily affecting the trunk and lower extremities (the most common side effect, occurring in 30% to 74% of patients), Horner syndrome, transient gustatory sweating, pleural tears, vascular tears, pneumothorax or hydrothorax, injury to the thoracic duct, intercostal neuralgia, infection, atelectasis, sensory loss, bradycardia, nasal obstruction (114), and injury to the phrenic nerve and brachial plexus.

PERCUTANEOUS VERTEBROPLASTY. Percutaneous vertebroplasty (PVP) was first described in 1987 by Galibert et al. (115), who injected polymethylmethacrylate to prevent crushing of a C2 vertebra partially destroyed by an aggressive hemangioma. In this technique, a trocar is introduced into the anterior third of the VB by the transpedicular route (115,116). In alternative approaches, including the parapedicular and posterolateral approaches, cement leakage may be more likely to occur, especially when the trocar is being removed (117). The patient should be maintained in a recumbent position to prevent weight bearing while the cement hardens. Polymethylmethacrylate typically sets within 20 minutes, and approximately 90% of its

ultimate strength is attained within 1 hour of injection (117). Despite the fact that their efficacy has never been validated, antibiotics are usually given 30 minutes before the procedure to prevent infection. For patients who are known to be immunocompromised, antibiotics may also be administered in the cement (117).

When PVP is performed as an outpatient procedure, the patient is observed for 1 to 3 hours in the recovery room. PVP offers rapid relief from the pain associated with vertebral compression fractures and is evolving as a standard of care for this condition (118). Pain relief is reported after 4 to 24 hours and is not proportional to the amount of injected cement. Less than complete fill of the VB usually provides good pain relief (119–121). Although early PVP was performed via a bipedicular injection, a recent study found that unipedicular injections that achieve fill across the midline can substantially restore strength (117). The proposed mechanisms of pain relief, which are poorly understood, include thermal necrosis, chemotoxicity of intraosseous pain receptors, and mechanical stabilization (95).

The primary indication for PVP is to increase strength and relieve the pain associated with vertebral compression fractures in patients with osteoporosis or osteopenia (116,122–124). Indications are being extended to other entities, such as vertebral involvement in osteolytic metastasis (121,122,125–129), lymphoma (126), Langerhans histiocytosis (130), myeloma (125, 126), and even cervical disease, treated through a transoral approach (131). This is mainly for the nonsurgical treatment of tumor-induced osteolysis in metastatic bone disease, and the indications should be dictated by a multidisciplinary team approach (117) and according to the patient's localized and general condition. PVP can be used to treat several fractures at the same time and can be combined with internal fixation with a screw/rod system to correct kyphosis or scoliosis (116).

Infrequent serious complications are mainly related to posterior, paravertebral, and discal leakage, which can be decreased with the use of careful fluoroscopic guidance and meticulous radiological technique. Visualization of the cement during injection and careful monitoring for extravasation are key for a safe PVP. Other reported complications are transient fever, transient worsening of pain, rib fractures, radiculopathy, cement accumulation in the inferior vena cava/azygos vein (116,125,132), pulmonary embolism, infection (132), and spinal cord compression. The rate of complications varies with the indication; in osteoporotic patients, it is 1% to 2%, and most of the complications are transient and not related to the nervous system (118, 119,133,134). In patients with malignant tumors, the rate of complications is higher because of VB destruction and resulting cement leak. An initially slow introduction of cement with avoidance of pressure peaks may reduce the risk for leakage (116).

Transient radiculopathy has been reported in 3% to 6% of cases, and these patients have been managed successfully with steroids and antiinflammatory medications (121,132,134,135). Persistent radiculopathy has occurred in 2% to 3% of cases, and surgery was required for cement removal. Because of this neurological complication, some authors converted the classical percutaneous approach to an open surgical procedure to obtain direct visual control of neural structures and remove spilled cement immediately; thus, the danger of compressive, chemical, and thermal effects on neural elements during the polymerization of methylmethacrylate was eliminated.

Biomechanical studies have shown that PVP increases vertebral strength and restores VB stiffness, but it does not restore VB height. In a follow-up of 48 months, pain was significantly decreased after 1 month; no progression of vertebral deformity was noted, but the risk for vertebral fracture was significantly increased (odds ratio, 2.27) in the vicinity of the cemented vertebra (136). Increased activity on bone scans performed before treatment has been shown to be highly predictive of a positive clinical response to PVP (137). Inflatable bone kyphoplasty (tamp) in osteoporotic cadaveric VBs resulted in significant (97%) restoration of vertebral body height versus 30% restoration with PVP (138).

Lumbar Spine

One of the major driving forces in surgery is the desire to achieve maximal benefit with minimal intervention. In the treatment of lumbar disc disease, this desire has resulted in the development of many MIS techniques and approaches. Advances in these approaches can be considered either in relation to the spine or in relation to the nature of the surgical procedure. The posterior approaches have evolved with the use of the posterolateral percutaneous portal, and the anterior approaches with either transperitoneal or retroperitoneal techniques. With the development of endoscopic tools and retractor technology, both approaches are changing rapidly (139). Each one offers particular advantages and entails particular disadvantages, and the choice of which to use is determined by the individual patient's anatomy (140). Moreover, the wide range of therapeutic options available allows the surgeon to base decisions on the primary pathology.

GENERAL PRINCIPLES AND RELEVANT ANATOMICAL CONSIDERATIONS.

In an anterior approach, it is of great importance to identify the location of the vascular bifurcation before any procedure to determine the surgical suitability relative to the aortic bifurcation and the disc space (141). This can be evaluated preoperatively with magnetic resonance imaging (MRI) and computed tomography (CT), and intraabdominal ultrasonography can be used during surgery if difficulties arise. Before surgery, the VB size and disc space height are determined. A corresponding intervertebral fusion cage size is determined. Nonsteroidal agents are discontinued at least 1 week before the intervention to minimize blood loss and promote healing and fusion, and the bowel is prepared the night before.

Because it is not possible to ascertain the rate of presacral nerve injury leading to retrograde ejaculation and infertility, patients should be informed of this risk, and many surgeons will not consider a transperitoneal approach in young male patients.

The position of the ureter must constantly be considered in both transperitoneal and retroperitoneal approaches (78). The right ureter courses over the right iliac artery and vein and can be identified by the peristalsis associated with probing of this structure, whereas the left ureter lies deep to the sigmoid colon in the retroperitoneal space (142). The middle sacral vein is used to identify the midline.

When lesions are compatible with infection or tumor, the use of carbon dioxide insufflation should be avoided because pressure can force tumor cells or bacteria into the bloodstream (143–146).

As a general rule, in the lateral position, the segmental vessels should always be ligated and divided before the intervertebral disc is exposed in the anterior half of the VB so as to maintain collateral circulation to the neuroforamen and spinal cord (78); it is important to use two vascular clips on the high-pressure side of the vessels. If major vascular damage has occurred, conversion to an open procedure is always possible; the operating room must be equipped for standard open surgery, and the assistance of an experienced vascular surgeon may be helpful.

This means that a vascular surgeon is included as a member of the surgical team or is on standby.

MINIMALLY INVASIVE METHODS OF BONE HARVESTING.

To decrease the morbidity of the traditional open harvesting procedures, the iliac bone graft can be harvested with a minimally invasive, *T*-shaped, 10-mm trocar (78). An incision in the lateral aspect of the abdomen, midway between umbilicus and pubis, is used both for bone harvesting and as a lateral retraction portal. The removal of autogenous bone graft from the external table of the ilium reduces postoperative morbidity at the donor site (147). Moreover, when autologous bone is harvested regionally from a neighboring VB, the procedure is anatomically safe and biomechanically acceptable (148).

ANTERIOR APPROACHES

Laparoscopy. Laparoscopy was used mainly by urological and gynecological surgeons until the 1980s; the first laparoscopic appendectomy was performed by Semm (149). Only recently have minimal access techniques been applied in spinal procedures; the first laparoscopic procedure on the spine was a lumbar discectomy at the L5-S1 level, reported in 1991 by Obenchain (150). Zucherman et al. were the first to perform instrumented interbody fusion laparoscopically with the use of BAK cages (6).

The pain associated with an anterior procedure is caused by the incision of the oblique abdominal muscles, and laparoscopy was an attempt to decrease the morbidity of the flank approach while offering the advantages of a traditional anterior approach.

General advances in laparoscopic surgery and the advantages of traditional anterior lumbar interbody fusion (ALIF), including restoration of disc height and exposure for safe nerve decompression, provided a basis for this technique to address anterior column abnormality with a low rate of surgical morbidity (141). When the patient is supine, laparoscopy is straightforward, and dissection in the retroperitoneal space can be closely monitored. Surgical time and blood loss with laparoscopic ALIF are directly related to the learning curve, and in all current studies, surgical time and blood loss have decreased as technical competence has advanced.

As in any intraabdominal procedure, the ureter, abdominal viscera, and large and small intestine can be damaged, and great care must be taken. The complications of laparoscopy are listed in Table 2. The limitations are related to the difficulty of access-

Table 2. Complications of Laparosopy

Vascular injuries[a]
Recurrence of previous nerve root pain
Implant malposition[b]
Implant migration
Retrograde ejaculation[c]
Peripheral sympathetic denervation[c]
Hypotension, hypoxemia, and hypercarbia
Iliofemoral deep-vein thrombosis
Small-bowel obstruction resulting from adhesions
Bladder lacerations and cautery burns of the intestine
Superficial wound infection at the bone graft site

[a] They were treated successfully, most by open conversion, and no impact on other outcome parameters was identified.
[b] It tends to occur laterally beyond the midpedicular line, so that foraminal stenosis develops.
[c] Both conditions may be secondary to neuropraxia rather than to division.

ing proximal levels, and to the presence of adhesions in patients with a history of trauma or previous surgery (139,151).

Previous anterior spinal surgery and significant previous peritoneal disease or surgery are contraindications to laparoscopic spinal surgery. Previous laparoscopic pelvic or abdominal surgery is not a contraindication (139).

surgical technique. The patient is supine on a radiolucent table, which aids intraoperative imaging. Abduction and flexion of the hips relax the tension on the aortoiliac and iliocaval vessels. The patient is placed in a steep Trendelenburg position to allow a more perpendicular approach to the disc and to retract the intestines toward the diaphragm and away from the lumbosacral region.

Through a small incision made in the periumbilical region, carbon dioxide is insufflated until a pressure of 10 to 15 mm Hg is achieved. Although a variety of portal strategies are possible, generally four laparoscopic ports are established as standard. The midline port in the region of the umbilicus is used for the endoscope. The working portal for instrumenting the L5-S1 disc is determined by fluoroscopy on a lateral view. It should be in the midline, at the point where the axis of the disc meets the surface. An 18-mm portal is inserted through which the interbody implant is placed. Two or more commonly three subsidiary working ports, for suction/irrigation and retractors, can be introduced laterally. The right and left lower-quadrant ports should be placed lateral to the epigastric vessels, and an additional port in the left abdomen can be placed to assist exposure if needed. At the L4-5 level, and for more proximal levels, exposure is technically more demanding, and the camera portal is placed supraumbilically.

The small bowel is retracted cephalad, and the sigmoid colon is retracted to the left and secured to the abdominal wall by the epiploic appendix. Care must be taken to identify and protect the right ureter as it crosses the right external iliac artery.

The parietal peritoneum is identified over the sacral promontory and divided under direct vision to expose the extraperitoneal connective tissue, and with the use of endoscopic vascular retractors, exposure of the L5-S1 disc is complete. The middle sacral artery and vein located in the midline are ligated with hemostatic clips, and the common iliac vessels are displaced laterally. In male patients, because of the potential risk for plexal injury and resultant transient or permanent retrograde ejaculation, great care must be taken. Cautery is to be avoided, and the presacral plexus is displaced laterally by blunt dissection. After the intervertebral disc is removed, removal of the end plate follows with exposure of bleeding cancellous bone. When the disc space is reamed, a tendency to a lateral drift is noted because of the convexity of the exposed annulus, and great care must be taken.

Depending on the level of the aortic bifurcation and the inferior vena cava, L5-S1 dissection usually takes place between the bifurcation, and L4-5 dissection can be either inferior to the bifurcation or lateral to the common iliac artery. The left common iliac vein usually overlies the left part of the annulus over the typical position for the left cage. The right iliac vein is rarely in the way and does not usually require significant mobilization (152). If the ureter is in the dissection field, it can be mobilized and protected.

The approach to the L4-5 disc is more technically demanding, and the vessels should be retracted medially from left to right (153). After the peritoneum is opened at the base of the sigmoid mesocolon, the left iliac artery and vein are mobilized. Dissection is carried down the left side of the aorta and left common iliac artery. To allow mobilization of these structures and the inferior vena cava overlying the L4-5 or L3-4 disc, the iliolumbar vein and one or two lumbar arteries should be mobilized and divided (139,142,152). The iliac veins must be carefully mobilized because they can be made densely adherent to the annulus

by inflammatory adhesions (152). Occasionally, a patient may have a high bifurcation, so that the L4-5 disc can be removed from within the bifurcation (153).

When vessel retraction is started, the vessels should be protected, and great care must be taken because the vessels tend to creep back toward the midline and into the operative field.

Initial pilot holes are created in the annulus at either side of the midline to accommodate the implants (142). Initial drilling is performed to enlarge the holes, and subsequently the remaining disc is evacuated. Distraction plugs of increasing size are placed into one hole until the original disc height has been restored and tension of the posterior longitudinal ligament is achieved.

Minimally Invasive Retroperitoneal Approach. Currently, the minimally invasive retroperitoneal approach is used by general, vascular, and urological surgeons in a variety of conditions, especially inguinal hernias. It is also used to perform lumbar sympathectomies. This approach is technically difficult because the retroperitoneal space is only a virtual cavity that must be developed by the surgeon. The conventional retroperitoneal approach is an invasive procedure in which considerable trauma to tissue is caused just to gain access to the surgical target area (154–156). Muscle-sparing retroperitoneal approaches have been described in an effort to decrease the morbidity associated with incising the oblique musculature during a flank approach (157,158). In cases of single-level ALIF, the pararectus or endoscopically assisted approaches have been reported to reduce surgery-related morbidity (6,141,159–161). The minimally invasive retroperitoneal approach provides access to at least three VBs, allowing corpectomy and spinal reconstruction (162). Just as in conventional retroperitoneal surgery, a microscope can be used, especially if the goal is to access the spinal canal.

The minimally invasive retroperitoneal approach offers several advantages over conventional anterior transperitoneal approaches and eliminates the risk for small-bowel obstruction and postoperative intraperitoneal and abdominal adhesions (78,163,164). These risks, and the complications attributed to carbon dioxide pneumoperitoneum, are reduced in a retroperitoneal approach (141,165–167). The overall morbidity of the procedure is lower than that associated with traditional open retroperitoneal or laparotomy techniques (78).

Anterior Paramedian Muscle-Sparing Approach. The muscle-sparing retroperitoneal approach allows direct visualization and access to the lumbar spine. A traditional technique and familiar instrumentation are used, but the small, transverse skin incision remains below the underwear line. This is especially useful in spondylolisthesis and cases of vertebral fracture requiring anterior column support, in which the approach provides excellent exposure with little risk (153). Also, a wide variety of strut devices can be used. Postoperative recovery is quicker and postoperative mobility greater than with the flank approach, and pain and ileus are notably decreased (157,158).

The safety of this technique was demonstrated in 28 patients with severe spinal deformity or instability who required both anterior and posterior spinal fusion and in whom one, two, or three intervertebral segments were fused. No vascular, visceral, or surgical complications were related to the surgical approach (153). The cases included 20 of spondylolisthesis, 7 of segmental instability, and 1 of flat-back syndrome. Zdeblick and David (168) reported the safety and efficacy of this technique in a prospective study in which they compared it with laparoscopic fusion for L4-5.

technique. The patient is placed in a supine position, and fluoroscopy is used in the AP and lateral planes to mark a 7-cm transverse (one level) or 9-cm slightly oblique (two levels) incision (168). The anterior rectus sheath is divided 1 cm superiorly and 1 cm inferiorly at the lateral border of the rectus muscle. The rectus abdominis is retracted toward the midline to expose the posterior sheath (above the arcuate line), and less commonly the arcuate line or preperitoneal space. The posterior rectus sheath–arcuate line is divided in a vertical direction and the preperitoneal space is identified. It is then extended bluntly, and the peritoneum is separated medially to expose the retroperitoneal space (153). After identification of the psoas muscle, the left ureter, peritoneum, and abdominal contents are mobilized across the midline.

Dewald et al. (153) made a skin incision along the natural skin creases, and the rectus fascia was incised transversely. They used a 2-cm inferior longitudinal extension medially adjacent to the midline, and a superior extension laterally at the confluence of the anterior rectus fascia, oblique muscles, and transversalis fascia. This approach easily allowed exposure of one to two levels, and by lengthening the superior longitudinal extension proximally, three levels were easily exposed.

Lateral Retroperitoneal Approach. Retroperitoneal endoscopic spinal surgery does not require a Trendelenburg position, entrance into the peritoneum, carbon dioxide insufflation, or anterior dissection near the great vessels to provide safe exposure for spinal surgery (78). The complications of the retroperitoneal approach are listed in Table 3. The three techniques used to dissect the retroperitoneal space are finger dissection, balloon insufflation, and use of an optical, transparent dissecting trocar (169). McAfee et al. reported a prospective series of 18 patients with a mean follow-up of 24.3 months. They were able to perform anterior decompression or stabilization via endoscopy by using two parallel transverse cages that restored the height of the neural foramen. The desired amount of lordosis was achieved by inserting a larger anterior cage, distraction plug, or bone dowels.

The advantages and disadvantages of the lateral retroperitoneal approach are listed in Table 4.

TECHNIQUE. The patient is placed in a right lateral decubitus position and rotated dorsally 20 to 30 degrees. This position facilitates exposure of the lumbar spine because gravity retracts the abdominal contents anteriorly. A left-sided is preferable to a right-sided approach because it is easier to dissect the aorta off the spine than to dissect the more friable inferior vena cava (78). The operating table is tilted under fluoroscopic control to achieve a parallel projection of the vertebral end plates of the level to be approached. The skin incision is centered above the projection of the center of the disc space or over the targeted vertebra in the midaxillary line. Once the trocar has penetrated, it is used to create a potential retroperitoneal space until the psoas major muscle is identified. A dissection balloon can be filled with normal saline solution or air to dissect the retroperitoneal layer. Alternatively, carbon dioxide insufflation can be forced into the retroperitoneal cavity up to a pressure of 20 mm Hg to create a working space. Once the retroperitoneal space is enlarged, two other portals are inserted at the anterior axillary

Table 3. Complications of the Retroperitoneal Approach

Genitofemoral nerve palsy[a]
Psoas hematoma[b]
Lumbar sympathectomy
Peritoneal perforation
Thrombophlebitis
Urinary retention

[a] Most commonly transient.
[b] Gives rise to femoral neuralgia.

Table 4. Advantages and Disadvantages of the Lateral Retroperitoneal Approach

Advantages	Disadvantages
No need for manipulation of the common iliac vein and artery.	A large mass of the psoas muscle containing lumbosacral nerve roots may have to be mobilized laterally.
Facilitates exposure of the lumbar spine. With the straight lateral position, it is easier to be perpendicular to the disc space and spine.	At L4-5 level, it may be necessary to remove part of the iliac crest, or place the docking portals through the iliac wing to be orthogonal to the L4-5 disc space.
The anterior and posterior longitudinal ligaments are not violated.	
Drilling, reaming, tapping, and cage insertion are directed toward the contralateral psoas muscle instead of the neurological structures.	
Obviates the risk for small-bowel obstruction and intraperitoneal adhesions.	
Lower incidence of retrograde ejaculation.	

line, opposite to the surgical field. The transversalis fascia, perinephric fascia, and retroperitoneal contents are retracted anteriorly.

The disc space height is restored by using a distraction plug placed from side to side. A drill tube is placed over the distraction plugs, and therefore the center of the distraction plug corresponds to the center of the BAK interbody fusion cages or endoscopic bone dowels (170). The surgeon can use longer cages in the transverse axis, and supplemental lateral plating may be provided to enhance stability and therefore improve the fusion rate. Occasionally, for longer strut grafts, the 10-mm working portal is extended as much as 5 cm, and an endoscopically assisted, mini-laparotomy type of retroperitoneal exposure facilitates corpectomy and spinal instrumentation. This technique is advantageous because airtight seals are not required and the standard thoracoscopic instruments can be used on the lumbar spine (78).

For approaching L1 or L2, a 1-cm incision is made at the anterior portion of rib 12, which is partially removed. The left diaphragmatic crura are transected, and phrenotomy is not required (162).

This approach allows complete decompression of the dural sac and the nerve roots at the entrance to the vertebral foramen under direct, three-dimensional microscopic visualization (162). It is important to decompress the spinal canal all the way across to the base of the opposite pedicle, and decompression is accomplished only when the opposite pedicle is palpated or visualized (78).

Olinger et al. (74) addressed the safety of this approach in 12 patients who underwent anterior fusion for fractures from levels T12 to L5. They notched the diaphragm insertion at the vertebral body to reach T12. Muhlbauer et al. (162) demonstrated the feasibility of lumbar corpectomy and anterior reconstruction via a minimally invasive retroperitoneal approach through a 5-in skin incision made parallel to the external oblique muscle and centered over the targeted vertebral body, and they used a recently introduced self-retaining retractor system for fusion (171).

FUSION IN MINIMALLY INVASIVE SURGERY. Although fusion was initially described in 1911 for posterior stabilization in cases of spinal tuberculosis (172,173), minimally invasive approaches for lumbar fusion are in their infancy. The posterolateral microendoscopic discectomy (MED) onlay is evolving, and laparoscopic ALIF has been recently described (6,174,175).

The advantages of ALIF in concert with the benefits of laparoscopic techniques fostered an interest in laparoscopic discectomy with interbody fusion as an approach to issues including anatomical interference and historical evidence of collapse with percutaneous interbody soft grafting techniques (141). Another major advantage was the ability to perform fusion without affecting the facet joints of the vertebra above, as often happens in a posterior approach. Partly for this reason, and despite being new, ALIF with the use of threaded devices has become a commonly performed procedure for many conditions, including degenerative disc disease, internal disc disruption, and pseudarthrosis (168).

Because of a stronger emphasis on the restoration of height and stability in the anterior column, where 80% of the axial load occurs, the use of anterior interbody fusion devices has increased (176,177). Experimentally, it was found that if posterolateral fusion increased spinal stiffness by 40%, in comparison, stiffness increased by 80%, so that virtually all motion through the disc space was eliminated when the anterior interbody fusion technique was used (178).

One unique advantage of cages is that they can be implanted via a minimally invasive anterior or posterior approach, and the risk for collapse and resorption associated with autogenous bone grafts is avoided (179–181).

POSTERIOR APPROACHES

Percutaneous Nucleotomy. Since the 1970s, various methods of nucleotomy have been developed and used clinically (182). These procedures are based on a variety of intradiscal diagnostic and therapeutic methods that can be performed via a needle or cannula, including discography, percutaneous manual discectomy, automated percutaneous discectomy, chemonucleolysis, endoscopic and microscopic discectomy, and laser percutaneous discectomy.

Theoretically, percutaneous nucleotomy works by centrally decompressing the nucleus pulposus. The decreased pressure in the center of the disc results in a fall of intradiscal pressure, with consequent migration of the herniation away from the nerve root. The success rate of any percutaneous procedure based on the concept of central disc decompression depends highly on the selection of patients with pathology that is amenable to such an approach (183). Patients with extruded or sequestered disc fragments generally are not candidates for these techniques, and the presence of bony lateral stenosis is a relative contraindication to most percutaneous disc procedures (176, 184). Their use for far lateral lumbar disc herniation has been described previously (185,186). Less invasive techniques to address this particular pathology have been investigated recently (147,184,187).

Automated Percutaneous Lumbar Discectomy. Despite the initial enthusiasm for this technique, its efficacy has been questioned (188,189), and currently it is considered primarily of historical interest. In reported series, the success rate varies according to the selection criteria. APLD is potentially efficacious only in patients whose herniations are still contained by the annulus or the posterior longitudinal ligament; MRI can help to exclude obviously migrated fragments and large disc extrusions (183). A lower success rate can be expected if during discography contrast material flows behind the posterior longitudinal liga-

ment, indicating a complete tear of the annulus but not a complete extrusion. CT discography, perhaps the definitive procedure for selecting patients for APLD, demonstrates complete tears of the annulus and posterior longitudinal ligament; the free flow of contrast material into the epidural space indicates those herniations that are extrusions. Clinically, patients who are candidates for APLD have classical symptoms of a radiculopathy with sciatica. Patients with vague or equivocal symptoms and bulging discs are not good candidates.

Chemonucleolysis. The complications associated with this technique have severely curtailed its broad acceptance, and it has fallen out of use. Among these complications are headaches after injection, systemic reactions, anaphylaxis, injection outside the nucleus pulposus, and associated transverse myelitis.

Percutaneous Laser Disc Decompression. In percutaneous laser disc decompression, the pressure within a herniated intervertebral disc is reduced through the application of laser energy. Despite its proven safety and efficacy, this technique is currently being evaluated and is not in widespread use (190). No general anesthesia is required, no scarring results, rehabilitation time is reduced, the procedure can be repeated, and open surgery is not precluded should it become necessary.

Clinical results vary widely. Success rates range from 50% to 84% (191,192) and depend highly on patient selection. At 5-year follow-up, one study showed recovery or markedly diminished sciatica in 78% of the patients (193). Clinical signs and symptoms of segmental instability were detected in 24%. Recently, endoscopic laser foraminoplasty has been reported to be useful for monosegmental, unilateral, and lateral recess stenosis (194). Although these techniques are promising, they have yet to be standardized and subjected to extensive trials.

Standard Microendoscopic Discectomy. In contrast to automated percutaneous techniques, endoscopy allows direct visualization of the herniation, so that the safety and efficacy of the procedure are increased (187). Advances in instrumentation have made possible a "working channel" through which various tools can be utilized under endoscopic visualization to remove contained or extruded disc material safely. This approach offers a particular advantage in that it combines endoscopic and standard open microsurgical techniques and minimizes paraspinous muscle trauma (186). The access to the foramen and disc space, through a paramedial approach, is familiar to most spine surgeons (the same as that used for discography). The procedure can be performed on an outpatient basis under epidural anesthesia (186,187). It has been used successfully in the management of posterolateral lumbar disc herniations located from L2-3 to L5-S1, with encouraging early results (195–198).

TECHNIQUE. The patient is placed in a prone position with the abdomen free and the spine flexed to aid exposure. The entry point is 1.5 to 2 cm off midline. Under fluoroscopic control, a needle is used to localize the disc level. A small stab wound is made, and the guidewire is directed toward the inferior edge of the superior lamina. The skin incision is extended, and sequential cannulated dilators are inserted over the wire. The initial dilator is directed to the region between the spinous process and facet complex, just above the inferior edge of the lamina. The tubular retractor is passed over the largest dilator down to the lamina and held by the flexible arm. After introduction of the endoscope, the laminar edge is identified, and laminotomy and medial facetectomy are accomplished. Once the nerve root has been identified, it is retracted medially, and the herniated disc is then removed with a pituitary rongeur. Lateral recess or foraminal stenosis can be addressed in this fashion.

This procedure is essentially the same as the standard open microdiscectomy, but it causes less muscular damage.

Far Lateral Disc Microendoscopic Discectomy. Foley et al. (184) determined the feasibility of performing far lateral discectomy with an incision made 4.5 to 5 cm off midline. The K-wire is directed toward the junction of the transverse process and pars interarticularis of the superior vertebra. The initial dilator is docked onto the junction of the cephalic transverse process and the pars, and a 16-mm tubular retractor is used that is held by an articulated arm.

Lew et al. (187) also reported the safety and efficacy of this technique in a series of 47 patients with far lateral or foraminal herniations. Access is obtained through a triangular working zone bounded superiorly by the nerve root, inferiorly by the transverse process, and medially by the superior facet (199). The needle entry site is 8 to 12 cm off midline, and the needle is directed to the level of facet joint. On AP and lateral projections, the needle is in the correct position when it is parallel to the disc space, midway between the end plates, proximal to the annulus, with the tip lateral to the medial border of the pedicles.

Currently, many techniques are being evaluated, and it is difficult to recommend them for widespread use (176). These include foraminotomy performed as an MIS technique and endoscopic laser foraminoplasty, which has proved useful for unilateral lateral recess stenosis (194). Given the small size of these series and the lack of control groups, it is impossible to draw any statistical conclusions from a comparison of MED with open techniques (184). Moreover, MED for far lateral disc herniations is technically demanding and is not recommended until the surgeon has acquired expertise in using it for more typical disc herniations.

Percutaneous Pedicle Screw Fixation. Percutaneous fixation of the lumbar spine eliminates the need for a large midline incision and significant paraspinous muscle dissection. It was first described by Magerl (200); Mathew and Long were the first to describe and perform a wholly percutaneous lumbar pedicle fixation. Plates were used as the longitudinal connectors, and in all cases, they were placed either externally or beneath the skin (200,201).

Recently, Foley et al. (174) reported the Sextant technique in a series of 12 patients. Successful fixation was performed in 10 patients with spondylolisthesis and in two patients with nonunion of a prior interbody fusion. These investigators have modified an existent multiaxial lumbar pedicle screw system. Screws are placed percutaneously with the use of cannulated extension sleeves that allow remote manipulation and engagement of the screw-locking mechanism. The rod insertion device, linked to the sleeves, allows placement of a precut, precontoured rod through a small stab wound. Because extensive retraction of soft tissue and muscle is avoided, it is much easier to achieve the required medial angulation. Screw placement is guided by virtual fluoroscopy, which combines an image-guided surgical computer and a C-arm. The images are automatically calibrated with FluoroNav software, so that it is possible to choose the entry points for the pedicles to be instrumented.

Intradiscal Electrothermal Therapy. Intradiscal electrothermal therapy (IDET) has been shown to be safe and effective in managing chronic disabling discogenic pain that fails to respond to aggressive conservative modalities (202–204). With this technique, thermal therapy is targeted to the annulus of the disc by means of a navigable intradiscal catheter (205). The targeted thermal energy coagulates nerve tissue (206), shrinks collagen fibrils, and cauterizes granulation tissue (207–209).

The pathophysiology of low-back pain in general and chronic discogenic pain in particular is complex (202), and chronic, unremitting low-back pain is one of the most difficult clinical problems (210). The disc is a nociceptively innervated structure capable of generating pain (211–218). In degenerative and "painful" discs, it has been found that free nerve endings grow in areas of the disc deeper than the outer third of the annulus fibrosis (211).

Internal disc disruption (IDD) is a common cause of disabling low-back pain in young, healthy adults (202). It is characterized by a degraded nucleus pulposus with radial fissures extending into the peripheral annulus fibrosus (219,220) that are not features of degradation. Discogenic lumbar pain can occur in the absence of nerve root compression and CT or myelographic abnormalities (221), and in some 20% to 30% of patients, IDD may be indicated by a high-intensity signal in the posterior annulus (222–224). This correlation provides the diagnostic criterion for painful lumbar IDD, which is distinct from a full-thickness tear or disc herniation (203). A strong correlation has been found between disruption of the outer annulus and reproduction of pain on discography (225); the painful disc must exhibit a radial fissure reaching at least the outer third of the annulus fibrosus, but the outer perimeter of the annulus must be intact. This condition accounts for 40% of cases of chronic low-back pain of unknown origin (226). Pain may be referred to the lower limb, but the patient has no features of radiculopathy (203).

THERMAL CATHETER PROTOCOL. Under fluoroscopic guidance and local anesthesia, IDET is performed with a 17-gauge needle inserted into the center of the disc. The catheter is introduced and navigated adjacent to the inner posterior annulus (210), inserted between the lamellae within the annulus fibrosus, and deflected circumferentially. Electrothermal heat is gradually increased along the active portion of the catheter during a period varying from 13 to 17 minutes to reach 80° to 90°C for approximately 4 minutes. The 90°C catheter creates annular temperatures of 60° to 65°C, and heating typically reproduces the patient's pain. Antibiotics are administered intradiscally for prophylaxis against disc infection (202); a local anesthetic can be given for postoperative analgesia, and Omnipaque can be used to verify the intradiscal injection (203).

This technique has yielded impressive preliminary results (205,209), and attempts at treating IDD by fusion have been less satisfying (203). In most patients, a clinically meaningful and statistically significant reduction in pain and an improvement in function were achieved, as assessed by multiple tools to measure outcome (227,228). Inclusion criteria in these clinical trials were chronic and intense back pain limiting function, lack of response to conservative treatment, normal findings on neurological examination, absence of nerve root tension signs or compressive lesions on MRI, and concordant reproduction of pain and typical symptoms with provocative discography (202). In some studies, discography had to reproduce concordant pain at low pressure (dye volume ≤1.25 mL) at one or more levels while pain was absent in adjacent control levels (210).

Improved clinical outcomes were observed at 6 months (229–231) with minimal morbidity (202). With longer follow-up periods of 16 months and a mean duration of preoperative symptoms of 60 months, a 71% rate of improvement was seen (210). Patients typically began to display signs of improvement in the second or third month and continued to improve up to the sixth month (209); response was maintained at 6 and 12 months.

Results have varied between authors, and degrees of improvement have varied on different scales (210). The follow-up periods were too short to assess the efficacy of this major spinal procedure, and no evidence is available regarding long-term effects. Studied criteria such as relief of pain and return to work were not sufficiently compelling (227,228). Furthermore, preliminary results should be interpreted in the context of the likelihood of spontaneous improvement in this population (218).

IDET is much less invasive than other techniques. Other available sources of thermal energy/radiofrequency cannot access the broad expanse of the posterior annular wall (232), and intradiscal laser energy is hazardous to bone and nerve tissue (207,208).

Human and animal studies have demonstrated that collagen thickening and remodeling occur without the development of scar tissue at this level of heat (207,208). Trousier et al. (233) showed that a bipolar radiofrequency electrode can destroy a portion of the nucleus pulposus in cadaver spine. When IDET was studied in cadavers, a decrease in spinal segment motion was seen without destabilization of the spinal segment (234).

Because IDET appears to be a promising and cost-effective minimally invasive treatment, randomized, double-blinded, controlled trial must be undertaken comprising a significant sample size, and histological and biochemical studies will be required to answer many of the remaining questions.

Future Considerations

BONE MORPHOGENETIC PROTEINS AND FUSION. In an effort to eliminate the need to harvest bone graft from the iliac crest and reduce the incidence of nonunion, the search for bone graft substitutes has intensified. Numerous experimental studies have now been performed demonstrating the potential efficacy of bone morphogenetic proteins (BMPs) in the induction of spinal arthrodesis (235–240). Since 1993, the efficacy of recombinant human bone morphogenetic protein-2 (rhBMP-2) has been demonstrated in spinal fusion models in rabbits, dogs, sheep, goats, and rhesus monkeys (238,241–244). Fusion rates were significantly higher with rhBMP-2 than with autografts, and the fusion mass was stronger biomechanically (238,240).

Based on primary results in both animal and human studies, the use of rhBMP-2 as a means of replacing harvested autograft and changing the extent of internal fixation appears likely (245). Molecules of rhBMP are not rejected and do not elicit a host response, as do some xenogeneic materials, and they are entirely free of infectious agents and contaminants (244). BMPs also increase the rate of bone induction at the center of the graft, a region that heals with difficulty and has been implicated as a cause of nonunion (246). As a chemotactic factor, rhBMP-2 initiates the recruitment of progenitor and stem cells. As a growth factor, it stimulates both angiogenesis and the proliferation of stem cells from surrounding mesenchymal tissues. As a differentiation factor, it promotes the maturation of stem cells into chondrocytes, osteoblasts, and osteocytes (245).

The results of using osteogenic protein-1 (OP-1, BMP-7) as a coating on implants and in conjunction with a carrier material indicate that it may enhance the osseous integration of metal implants and can induce significant new bone formation at the implant–bone interface (247). Interestingly, Sandhu et al. (239) demonstrated that rhBMP-2 can lead to long-term spinal arthrodesis without decortication of the adjacent spinal elements.

Early clinical results of lumbar fusion with threaded intervertebral implants filled with rhBMP-2 have been favorable (244). The first clinical demonstration of the efficacy of rhBMP-2 in 14 patients with single-level disease came from a multicenter trial. Of the 11 patients treated with rhBMP-2 (1.5 mg/mL), 10 achieved fusion by 3 months, and all of them achieved fusion by 6 months. Of the three control patients treated with autogenous bone graft, only two had achieved fusion after 12 months. CT showed new bone growth through and anterior to the cages at 6 and 12 months after surgery. Preliminary data from a clinical trial in which threaded allograft bone dowels containing rhBMP-2 was used suggested evidence of healing by 3 months after surgery and strong graft incorporation without lucency by 6 months (244).

In vivo gene therapy is another approach that is currently being investigated. Osteogenic genes are inserted into cells in tissue culture, and the genetically altered cells are subsequently implanted into the paraspinal region of experimental animals. The cellular implants express and secrete bone morphogens, which in turn induce an osteogenic response (248). With further development, BMP gene therapy should be able to induce bone formation in virtually every region of the spine in a minimally invasive fashion (246). The technique may be used in the future to promote bony union between transverse processes, facets, laminae, spinous processes, and VBs. It would provide clear advantages in the treatment of numerous degenerative processes in which a percutaneous delivery of bone growth agents could result in spinal fusion without major instrumentation procedures.

ARTIFICIAL DISC TECHNOLOGY AND NUCLEAR IMPLANTS. In a move toward less invasiveness and better restoration of physiological and mechanical properties, artificial discs and prosthetic nuclei have been developed. In contrast to most artificial discs, which require open surgery for removal of the end plates and fixation of the implant to the VBs, the prosthetic nucleus can be implanted by means of an endoscopic technique that requires only a small incision in the annulus (249). With replacement of only the nucleus, the function of the remaining disc tissues (annulus and end plates) is preserved. Another major advantage is that no fixation component is required because the implant is not designed to be affixed to the vertebrae, and in case of failure, the implant can be removed and the disc replaced or fused.

The major limitation of this technique is that it can be used only in patients in whom disc degeneration is at an early or intermediate stage because a competent natural annulus must be present. It is not suitable for discs with a significant loss of height, and it is not appropriate in cases of lateral recess stenosis (176,249). The reason for this is that when a disc loses height, the collagen fibers may take on new structural characteristics and be difficult to stretch.

Preliminary investigations of nuclear implants have shown a restoration of segmental mobility (250–252). Many implants have been introduced but have not met the basic requirements for biocompatibility and mechanical strength that must be filled before entry into clinical trials. Recently, in an effort to minimize implant extrusion and improve artificial disc technology with minimally invasive methods, a new system featuring a polymer formulation, delivery balloon, and polymer injection gun has been developed (253).

Conclusions

Given the current trend toward MIS, the techniques described above should be assessed on a case-by-case basis, and ultimately, the surgical approach should be tailored to the patient's disorder and the surgeon's experience. Endoscopic surgery offers a reliable and minimally invasive technique for the management of appropriately selected patients, but its availability should not lead to an excessive extension of its indications.

Throughout the development of minimally invasive techniques, the importance of careful, supervised training, including practice on animal, cadaveric, and simulation models, has been emphasized (139). Results should be those of standard open procedures. At the present time, it can be concluded that in comparison with traditional methods, MIS offers several advantages. As the quality of endoscopic equipment evolves and its availability increases, it is likely that MIS will assume a more prominent place in the rapidly changing field of spinal surgery (23).

Multicenter studies are now required to identify more precisely the indications for MIS and to compare it with conventional techniques.

References

1. Claes G, Drott C, Gothberg G. Thoracoscopy for autonomic disorders. *Ann Thorac Surg* 1993;56:715–716.
2. Coltharp WH, Arnold JH, Alford WC Jr, et al. Videothoracoscopy: improved technique and expanded indications. *Ann Thorac Surg* 1992;53:776–778.
3. Dickman CA, Karahalios DG. Thoracoscopic spinal surgery. *Clin Neurosurg* 1996;43:392–422.
4. Southerland SR, Remedios AM, McKerrell JG, et al. Laparoscopic approaches to the lumbar vertebrae. An anatomic study using a porcine model. *Spine* 1995;20:1620–1623.
5. Rosenthal D, Rosenthal R, de Simone A. Removal of a protruded thoracic disc using microsurgical endoscopy. A new technique. *Spine* 1994;19:1087–1091.
6. Zucherman JF, Zdeblick TA, Bailey SA, et al. Instrumented laparoscopic spinal fusion. Preliminary results. *Spine* 1995;20:2029–2034.
7. Bozzini P. Lichtleiter, eine Erfindung zur Anschung innerer Theile und Krankheiten nebst Abbidung. *Pract Arzekunde* 1806;24:107.
8. Kaushik D, Rothberg M. Thoracoscopic surgery: historical perspectives. *Neurosurg Focus* 2000;9:Article 10.
9. Bush RB, Leonhardt H, Bush IM, et al. Dr. Bozzini's Lichtleiter. A translation of his original article (1806). *Urology* 1974;3:119–123.
10. Rosenthal DJ, Dickman CA. The history of thoracoscopic spine surgery. In: Dickman CA, Rosenthal DJ, Perin NI, eds. *Thoracoscopic spine surgery*. New York: Thieme Medical Publishers, 1999:1–5.
11. Smythe WR, Kaiser LR. History of thoracoscopic surgery. In: Kaiser LR, Daniel TM, eds. *Thoracoscopic surgery*. Boston: Little, Brown and Company, 1993:1–16.
12. Kanapy NS. *Fiber optics. Strong concepts of classical optics*. 1958:553–596.
13. Roh SW, Kim DH, Cardoso AC, et al. Endoscopic foraminotomy using a microendoscopic discectomy system in cadaveric specimens. *Neurosurg Focus* 1998;4:Article 2.
14. Kotilainen E. Percutaneous nucleotomy in the treatment of cervical disc herniation: report of three cases and review. *Minim Invasive Neurosurg* 1999;42:152–155.
15. Courtheoux F, Theron J. Automated percutaneous nucleotomy in the treatment of cervicobrachial neuralgia due to disc herniation. *J Neuroradiol* 1992;19:211–216.
16. Zhou YC, Zhou YQ, Wang CY. Percutaneous cervical discectomy for treating cervical disc herniation—a report of 12 cases. *J Tongji Med Univ* 1994;14:110–113.
17. Hoogland T, Scheckenbach C. Low-dose chemonucleolysis combined with percutaneous nucleotomy in herniated cervical disks. *J Spinal Disord* 1995;8:228–232.
18. Kotilainen E. Microinvasive lumbar disc surgery. A study on patients treated with microdiscectomy or percutaneous nucleotomy for disc herniation. *Ann Chir Gynaecol Suppl* 1994;209:1–50.
19. Hijikata S. Percutaneous nucleotomy. A new concept technique and 12 years' experience. *Clin Orthop* 1989;238:9–23.
20. Monteiro A, Lefevre R, Pieters G, et al. Lateral decompression of a pathological disc in the treatment of lumbar pain and sciatica. *Clin Orthop* 1989;238:56–63.
21. Kotilainen E, Alanen A, Erkintalo M, et al. Magnetic resonance image changes and clinical outcome after microdiscectomy or nucleotomy for ruptured disc. *Surg Neurol* 1994;41:432–440.
22. Roh SW, Kim DH, Cardoso AC, et al. Endoscopic foraminotomy using MED system in cadaveric specimens. *Spine* 2000;25:260–264.
23. Burke TG, Caputy A. Microendoscopic posterior cervical foraminotomy: a cadaveric model and clinical application for cervical radiculopathy. *J Neurosurg* 2000;93(1 suppl):126–129.
24. Williams RW. Microcervical foraminotomy. A surgical alternative for intractable radicular pain. *Spine* 1983;8:708–716.
25. Zdeblick TA, Zou D, Warden KE, et al. Cervical stability after foraminotomy. A biomechanical *in vitro* analysis. *J Bone Joint Surg Am* 1992;74:22–27.
26. Kubo Y, Waga S, Kojima T, et al. Microsurgical anatomy of the lower cervical spine and cord. *Neurosurgery* 1994;34:895–890.
27. Hakuba A. Trans-unco-discal approach. A combined anterior and lateral approach to cervical discs. *J Neurosurg* 1976;45:284–291.
28. Hankinson HL, Wilson CB. Use of the operating microscope in anterior cervical discectomy without fusion. *J Neurosurg* 1973;43:452–456.
29. Martins AN. Anterior cervical discectomy with and without interbody bone graft. *J Neurosurg* 1976;44:290–295.
30. Hae-Dong J. Microsurgical anterior cervical foraminotomy for radiculopathy: a new approach to cervical disc herniation. *Neurosurg Focus* 1998;4:Article 1.
31. Lesoin F, Biondi A, Jomin M. Foraminal cervical herniated disc treated by anterior discoforaminotomy. *Neurosurgery* 1987;21:334–338.
32. Snyder GM, Bernhardt AM. Anterior cervical fractional interspace decompression for treatment of cervical radiculopathy. A review of the first 66 cases. *Clin Orthop* 1989;246:92–99.
33. Visocchi M, Masferrer R, Sonntag VK, et al. Thoracoscopic approaches to the thoracic spine. *Acta Neurochir (Wien)* 1998;140:737–743.
34. Rosenthal D, Dickman CA. Thoracoscopic microsurgical excision of herniated thoracic discs. *J Neurosurg* 1998;89:224–235.
35. Dickman CA, Mican CA. Multilevel anterior thoracic discectomies and anterior interbody fusion using a microsurgical thoracoscopic approach. Case report. *J Neurosurg* 1996;84:104–109.
36. Dickman CA, Rosenthal D, Karahalios DG, et al. Thoracic vertebrectomy and reconstruction using a microsurgical thoracoscopic approach. *Neurosurgery* 1996;38:279–293.
37. Horowitz MB, Moossy JJ, Julian T, et al. Thoracic discectomy using video-assisted thoracoscopy. *Spine* 1994;19:1082–1086.
38. McAfee PC, Regan JR, Zdeblick T, et al. The incidence of complications in endoscopic anterior thoracolumbar spinal reconstructive surgery. A prospective multicenter study comprising the first 100 consecutive cases. *Spine* 1995;20:1624–1632.
39. Kao MC, Tsai JC, Lai DM, et al. Autonomic activities in hyperhidrosis patients before, during, and after endoscopic laser sympathectomy. *Neurosurgery* 1994;34:262–268.
40. Landreneau RJ, Dowling RD, Ferson PF. Thoracoscopic resection of a posterior mediastinal neurogenic tumor. *Chest* 1992;102:1288–1290.
41. Lyons MK, Gharagozloo F. Video-assisted thoracoscopic resection of intercostal neurofibroma. *Surg Neurol* 1995;43:542–545.
42. Robertson DP, Simpson RK, Rose JE, et al. Video-assisted endoscopic thoracic ganglionectomy. *J Neurosurg* 1993;79:238–240.
43. Weder W, Schlumpf R, Schimmer R, et al. Thoracoscopic resection of benign schwannoma. *Thorac Cardiovasc Surg* 1992;40:192–194.
44. Johnson JP, Filler AG, McBride DQ. Endoscopic thoracic discectomy. *Neurosurg Focus* 2000;9:Article 11.
45. Ferson PF, Landreneau RJ, Dowling RD, et al. Comparison of open versus thoracoscopic lung biopsy for diffuse infiltrative pulmonary disease. *J Thorac Cardiovasc Surg* 1993;106:194–199.
46. Dickman CA, Detweiler PW, Porter RW. Endoscopic spine surgery. *Clin Neurosurg* 2000;46:526–553.
47. Vollmer DG, Simmons NE. Transthoracic approaches to thoracic disc herniations. *Neurosurg Focus* 2000;9:Article 8.
48. Logas WG, el-Baz N, el-Ganzouri A, et al. Continuous thoracic epidural analgesia for postoperative pain relief following thoracotomy: a randomized prospective study. *Anesthesiology* 1987;67:787–791.
49. Tarhan S, Moffitt EA, Sessler AD, et al. Risk of anesthesia and surgery in patients with chronic bronchitis and chronic obstructive pulmonary disease. *Surgery* 1973;74:720–726.

50. Dickman CA, Rosenthal D, Regan JJ. Reoperation for herniated thoracic discs. *Neurosurg Focus* 1999;6:Article 5.
51. Dwyer AF. Experience of anterior correction of scoliosis. *Clin Orthop* 1973;93:191–214.
52. Dwyer AF, Schafer MF. Anterior approach to scoliosis. Results of treatment in fifty-one cases. *J Bone Joint Surg Br* 1974;56:218–224.
53. Lobosky JM, Hitchon PW, McDonnell DE. Transthoracic anterolateral decompression for thoracic spinal lesions. *Neurosurgery* 1984;14:26–30.
54. Mack MJ, Regan JJ, Bobechko WP, et al. Application of thoracoscopy for diseases of the spine. *Ann Thorac Surg* 1993;56:736–738.
55. Kaiser LR. Video-assisted thoracic surgery. Current state of the art. *Ann Surg* 1994;220:720–734.
56. Broc GG, Crawford NR, Sonntag VK, et al. Biomechanical effects of transthoracic microdiscectomy. *Spine* 1997;22:605–612.
57. Nymberg SM, Crawford AH. Video-assisted thoracoscopic releases of scoliotic anterior spines. *AORN J* 1996;63:561–562, 565–569, 571–575.
58. Johnson JR, Holt RT. Combined use of anterior and posterior surgery for adult scoliosis. *Orthop Clin North Am* 1988;19:361–370.
59. Byrd JA 3rd, Scoles PV, Winter RB, et al. Adult idiopathic scoliosis treated by anterior and posterior spinal fusion. *J Bone Joint Surg Am* 1987;69:843–850.
60. Kostuik JP, Israel J, Hall JE. Scoliosis surgery in adults. *Clin Orthop* 1973;93:225–234.
61. Simmons ED Jr, Kowalski JM, Simmons EH. The results of surgical treatment for adult scoliosis. *Spine* 1993;18:718–724.
62. Mehlman CT, Crawford AH, Wolf RK. Video-assisted thoracoscopic surgery (VATS). Endoscopic thoracoplasty technique. *Spine* 1997;22:2178–2182.
63. Gonzalez Barrios I, Fuentes Caparros S, Avila Jurado MM. Anterior thoracoscopic epiphysiodesis in the treatment of a crankshaft phenomenon. *Eur Spine J* 1995;4:343–346.
64. Papin P, Arlet V, Marchesi D, et al. Treatment of scoliosis in the adolescent by anterior release and vertebral arthrodesis. *Rev Chir Orthop Reparatrice Appar Mot* 1998;84:231–238 (in French).
65. Regan JJ. Percutaneous endoscopic thoracic discectomy. *Neurosurg Clin N Am* 1996;7:87–98.
66. Arlet V. Anterior thoracoscopic spine release in deformity surgery: a meta-analysis and review. *Eur Spine J* 2000;9(suppl 1):S17–S23.
67. Picetti G 3rd, Blackman RG, O'Neal K, et al. Anterior endoscopic correction and fusion of scoliosis. *Orthopedics* 1998;21:1285–1287.
68. Dohin B, Dubousset JF. Prevention of the crankshaft phenomenon with anterior spinal epiphysiodesis in surgical treatment of severe scoliosis of the younger patient. *Eur Spine J* 1994;3:165–168.
69. Dickman CA. Thoracoscopic correction and placement of anterior instrumentation for scoliotic deformity. *Neurosurg Focus* 1999;7:Article 2.
70. Ebara S, Kamimura M, Itoh H, et al. A new system for the anterior restoration and fixation of thoracic spinal deformities using an endoscopic approach. *Spine* 2000;25:876–883.
71. Patterson RH Jr, Arbit E. A surgical approach through the pedicle to protruded thoracic discs. *J Neurosurg* 1978;48:768–772.
72. Hae-Dong J. Endoscopic transpedicular thoracic discectomy. *Neurosurg Focus* 2000;9:Article 4.
73. Huang TJ, Hsu RW, Liu HP, et al. Video-assisted thoracoscopic treatment of spinal lesions in the thoracolumbar junction. *Surg Endosc* 1997;11:1189–1193.
74. Olinger A, Hildebrandt U, Mutschler W, et al. First clinical experience with an endoscopic retroperitoneal approach for anterior fusion of lumbar spine fractures from levels T12 to L5. *Surg Endosc* 1999;13:1215–1219.
75. Buhren V, Beisse R, Potulski M. Minimally invasive ventral spondylodesis in injuries to the thoracic and lumbar spine. *Chirurg* 1997;68:1076–1084.
76. Burgos J, Rapariz JM, Gonzalez-Herranz P. Anterior endoscopic approach to the thoracolumbar spine. *Spine* 1998;23:2427–2431.
77. Olinger A, Hildebrandt U, Pistorius G, et al. Laparoscopic 2-level fusion of the lumbar spine with Bagby and Kuslich implants. *Chirurg* 1996;67:348–350.
78. McAfee PC, Regan JJ, Geis WP, et al. Minimally invasive anterior retroperitoneal approach to the lumbar spine. Emphasis on the lateral BAK. *Spine* 1998;23:1476–1484.
79. Kux E. The endoscopic approach to the vegetative nervous system and its therapeutic possibilities. *Dis Chest* 1951;20:139–147.
80. Kux M. Thoracic endoscopic sympathectomy in palmar and axillary hyperhidrosis. *Arch Surg* 1978;113:264–266.
81. Banerjee AK, Edmonson R, Rennie JA. Endoscopic transthoracic electrocautery of the sympathetic chain for palmar and axillary hyperhidrosis. *Br J Surg* 1990;77:1435.
82. Adams DC, Poskitt KR. Surgical management of primary hyperhidrosis. *Br J Surg* 1991;78:1019–1020.
83. Lin CC. A new method of thoracoscopic sympathectomy in hyperhidrosis palmaris. *Surg Endosc* 1990;4:224–226.
84. Claes G, Gothberg G. Endoscopic transthoracic electrocautery of the sympathetic chain for palmar and axillary hyperhidrosis. *Br J Surg* 1991;78:760.
85. Byrne J, Walsh TN, Hederman WP. Endoscopic transthoracic electrocautery of the sympathetic chain for palmar and axillary hyperhidrosis. *Br J Surg* 1990;77:1046–1049.
86. Edmondson RA, Banerjee AK, Rennie JA. Endoscopic transthoracic sympathectomy in the treatment of hyperhidrosis. *Ann Surg* 1992;215:289–293.
87. Malone PS, Duignan JP, Hederman WP. Transthoracic electrocoagulation (T.T.E.C.)—a new and simple approach to upper limb sympathectomy. *Ir Med J* 1982;75:20–21.
88. Ahn SS, Machleder HI, Concepcion B, et al. Thoracoscopic cervicodorsal sympathectomy: preliminary results. *J Vasc Surg* 1994;20:511–517.
89. Drott C, Gothberg G, Claes G. Endoscopic procedures of the upper-thoracic sympathetic chain. A review. *Arch Surg* 1993;128:237–241.
90. Reardon PR, Preciado A, Scarborough T, et al. Outpatient endoscopic thoracic sympathectomy using 2-mm instruments. *Surg Endosc* 1999;13:1139–1142.
91. Hsia JY, Chen CY, Hsu CP, et al. Outpatient thoracoscopic limited sympathectomy for hyperhidrosis palmaris. *Ann Thorac Surg* 1999;67:258–259.
92. Weale FE. Upper thoracic sympathectomy by transthoracic electrocoagulation. *Br J Surg* 1980;67:71–72.
93. Robertson DP. Thoracic sympathectomy. *J Neurosurg* 2000;92(1 suppl):124.
94. Singh B, Moodley J, Haffejee AA, et al. Resympathectomy for sympathetic regeneration. *Surg Laparosc Endosc* 1998;8:257–260.
95. Bostrom MP, Lane JM. Future directions. Augmentation of osteoporotic vertebral bodies. *Spine* 1997;22(24 suppl):38S–42S.
96. Trignano M, Boatto R, Mastino GP, et al. Video-thoracoscopic sympathectomy in the treatment of Raynaud's disease and palmar hyperhidrosis [in Italian]. *Minerva Chir* 2000;55:17–23.
97. Shnitko SN, Plandovskii VA. Thoracoscopic removal of upper thoracic sympathetic ganglia in treatment of Raynaud disease. *Khirurgiia (Mosk)* 1999;4:60–61.
98. Di Lorenzo N, Sica GS, Sileri P, et al. Thoracoscopic sympathectomy for vasospastic diseases. *JSLS* 1998;2:249–253.
99. Khogali SS, Miller M, Rajesh PB, et al. Video-assisted thoracoscopic sympathectomy for severe intractable angina. *Eur J Cardiothorac Surg* 1999;16(suppl 1):S95–S98.
100. Ushijima T, Akemoto K, Kawakami K, et al. Endoscopic transthoracic sympathectomy for angina pectoris: a case report. *Kyobu Geka* 1997;50:962–964.
101. Tygesen H, Claes G, Drott C, et al. Effect of endoscopic transthoracic sympathecotmy on heart rate variability in severe angina pectoris. *Am J Cardiol* 1997;79:1447–1452.
102. Claes G, Drott C, Wettervik C, et al. Angina pectoris treated by thoracoscopic sympathecotomy. *Cardiovasc Surg* 1996;4:830–831.
103. Reardon PR, Matthews BD, Scarborough TK, et al. Left thoracoscopic sympathectomy and stellate ganglionectomy for treatment of the long QT syndrome. *Surg Endosc* 2000;14:86.
104. Yamashita K, Tomiyasu S, Fujie T, et al. Endoscopic resection of the thoracic sympathetic trunk for the treatment of frequent syncopal attack of idiopathic long QT syndrome. *Masui* 1999;48:399–403.
105. Cheng TO. Left cardiac sympathetic denervation for long QT syndrome. *Int J Cardiol* 1997;62:281.
106. Chen L, Qin YW, Zheng CZ. Left cervicothoracic sympathetic ganglionectomy with thoracoscope for the treatment of idiopathic long QT syndrome. *Int J Cardiol* 1997;61:1–3.
107. Telaranta T. Treatment of social phobia by endoscopic thoracic sympathicotomy. *Eur J Surg Suppl* 1998;580:27–32.
108. Honjyo K, Hamasaki Y, Kita M, et al. An 11-year-old girl with reflex

sympathetic dystrophy successfully treated by thoracoscopic sympathectomy. *Acta Paediatr* 1997;86:903–905.

109. Lonroth H, Hyltander A, Lundell L. Unilateral left-sided thoracoscopic sympathectomy for visceral pain control: a pilot study. *Eur J Surg* 1997;163:97–100.

110. Wong GY, Sakorafas GH, Tsiotos GG, et al. Palliation of pain in chronic pancreatitis. Use of neural blocks and neurotomy. *Surg Clin North Am* 1999;79:873–893.

111. Moodley J, Singh B, Shaik AS, et al. Thoracoscopic splanchnicectomy: pilot evaluation of a simple alternative for chronic pancreatic pain control. *World J Surg* 1999;23:688–692.

112. Noppen M, Meysman M, D'Haese J, et al. Thoracoscopic splanchnicolysis for the relief of chronic pancreatitis pain: experience of a group of pneumologists. *Chest* 1998;113:528–531.

113. Kusano T, Miyazato H, Shiraishi M, et al. Thoracoscopic thoracic splanchnicectomy for chronic pancreatitis with intractable abdominal pain. *Surg Laparosc Endosc* 1997;7:213–218.

114. Lai YT, Yang LH, Chio CC, et al. Complications in patients with palmar hyperhidrosis treated with transthoracic endoscopic sympathectomy. *Neurosurgery* 1997;41:110–115.

115. Galibert P, Deramond H, Rosat P, et al. Preliminary note on the treatment of vertebral angioma by percutaneous acrylic vertebroplasty. *Neurochirurgie* 1987;33:166–168.

116. Wenger M, Markwalder TM. Surgically controlled, transpedicular methyl methacrylate vertebroplasty with fluoroscopic guidance. *Acta Neurochir (Wien)* 1999;141:625–631.

117. Mathis JM, Barr JD, Belkoff SM, et al. Percutaneous vertebroplasty: a developing standard of care for vertebral compression fractures. *AJNR Am J Neuroradiol* 2001;22:373–381.

118. Mathis JM, Eckel TS, Belkoff SM, et al. Percutaneous vertebroplasty: a therapeutic option for pain associated with vertebral compression fracture. *J Back Musculoskel Rehab* 1999;13:11–17.

119. Jensen ME, Evans AJ, Mathis JM, et al. Percutaneous polymethylmethacrylate vertebroplasty in the treatment of osteoporotic vertebral body compression fractures: technical aspects. *AJNR Am J Neuroradiol* 1997;18:1897–1904.

120. Mathis JM, Petri M, Naff N. Percutaneous vertebroplasty treatment of steroid-induced osteoporotic compression fractures. *Arthritis Rheum* 1998;41:171–175.

121. Cotten A, Dewatre F, Cortet B, et al. Percutaneous vertebroplasty for osteolytic metastases and myeloma: effects of the percentage of lesion filling and the leakage of methyl methacrylate at clinical follow-up. *Radiology* 1996;200:525–530.

122. Gangi A, Kastler BA, Dietemann JL. Percutaneous vertebroplasty guided by a combination of CT and fluoroscopy. *AJNR Am J Neuroradiol* 1994;15:83–86.

123. Lapras C, Mottolese C, Deruty R, et al. Percutaneous injection of methyl-methacrylate in osteoporosis and severe vertebral osteolysis (Galibert's technic). *Ann Chir* 1989;43:371–376.

124. Nguyen JP, Djindjian M, Pavlovitch JM, et al. Vertebral hemangioma with neurologic signs. Therapeutic results. Survey of the French Society of Neurosurgery. *Neurochirurgie* 1989;35:299–303, 305–308.

125. Cortet B, Cotten A, Boutry N, et al. Percutaneous vertebroplasty in patients with osteolytic metastases or multiple myeloma. *Rev Rhum Engl Ed* 1997;64:177–183.

126. Cotten A, Duquesnoy B. Vertebroplasty: current data and future potential. *Rev Rhum Engl Ed* 1997;64:645–649.

127. Kaemmerlen P, Thiesse P, Jonas P, et al. Percutaneous injection of orthopedic cement in metastatic vertebral lesions. *N Engl J Med* 1989;321:121.

128. Laredo JD, Bellaiche L, Hamze B, et al. Current status of musculoskeletal interventional radiology. *Radiol Clin North Am* 1994;32:377–398.

129. Cotten A, Boutry N, Cortet B, et al. Percutaneous vertebroplasty: state of the art. *Radiographics* 1998;18:311–323.

130. Cardon T, Hachulla E, Flipo RM, et al. Percutaneous vertebroplasty with acrylic cement in the treatment of a Langerhans cell vertebral histiocytosis. *Clin Rheumatol* 1994;13:518–521.

131. Tong FC, Cloft HJ, Joseph GJ, et al. Transoral approach to cervical vertebroplasty for multiple myeloma. *AJR Am J Roentgenol* 2000; 175:1322–1324.

132. Chiras J, Depriester C, Weill A, et al. Percutaneous vertebral surgery. Technics and indications. *J Neuroradiol* 1997;24:45–59.

133. Barr JD, Barr MS, Lemley TJ, et al. Percutaneous vertebroplasty for pain relief and spinal stabilization. *Spine* 2000;25:923–928.

134. Weill A, Chiras J, Simon JM, et al. Spinal metastases: indications for and results of percutaneous injection of acrylic surgical cement. *Radiology* 1996;199:241–247.

135. Deramond H, Depriester C, Galibert P, et al. Percutaneous vertebroplasty with polymethylmethacrylate. Technique, indications, and results. *Radiol Clin North Am* 1998;36:533–546.

136. Grados F, Depriester C, Cayrolle G, et al. Long-term observations of vertebral osteoporotic fractures treated by percutaneous vertebroplasty. *Rheumatology (Oxford)* 2000;39:1410–1414.

137. Maynard AS, Jensen ME, Schweickert PA, et al. Value of bone scan imaging in predicting pain relief from percutaneous vertebroplasty in osteoporotic vertebral fractures. *AJNR Am J Neuroradiol* 2000; 21:1807–1812.

138. Belkoff SM, Mathis JM, Fenton DC, et al. An *ex vivo* biomechanical evaluation of an inflatable bone tamp used in the treatment of compression fracture. *Spine* 2001;26:151–156.

139. O'Dowd JK. Laparoscopic lumbar spine surgery. *Eur Spine J* 2000; 9(suppl 1):S3–S7.

140. Regan JJ, Aronoff RJ, Ohnmeiss DD, et al. Laparoscopic approach to L4-L5 for interbody fusion using BAK cages: experience in the first 58 cases. *Spine* 1999;24:2171–2174.

141. Mathews HH, Evans MT, Molligan HJ, et al. Laparoscopic discectomy with anterior lumbar interbody fusion. A preliminary review. *Spine* 1995;20:1797–1802.

142. Regan JJ, Yuan H, McAfee PC. Laparoscopic fusion of the lumbar spine: minimally invasive spine surgery. A prospective multicenter study evaluating open and laparoscopic lumbar fusion. *Spine* 1999; 24:402–411.

143. Hewett PJ, Thomas WM, King G, et al. Intraperitoneal cell movement during abdominal carbon dioxide insufflation and laparoscopy. An *in vivo* model. *Dis Colon Rectum* 1996;39(10 suppl): S62–S66.

144. Jacobi CA, Ordemann J, Bohm B, et al. The influence of laparotomy and laparoscopy on tumor growth in a rat model. *Surg Endosc* 1997;11:618–621.

145. Jacobi CA, Ordemann J, Bohm B, et al. Does laparoscopy increase bacteremia and endotoxemia in a peritonitis model? *Surg Endosc* 1997;11:235–238.

146. Kruitwagen RF, Swinkels BM, Keyser KG, et al. Incidence and effect on survival of abdominal wall metastases at trocar or puncture sites following laparoscopy or paracentesis in women with ovarian cancer. *Gynecol Oncol* 1996;60:233–237.

147. Kambin P, Gennarelli T, Hermantin F. Minimally invasive techniques in spinal surgery: current practice. *Neurosurg Focus* 1998; 4:Article 8.

148. Steffen T, Downer P, Steiner B, et al. Minimally invasive bone harvesting tools. *Eur Spine J* 2000;9(suppl 1):S114–S118.

149. Nagy AG, Poulin EC, Girotti MJ, et al. History of laparoscopic surgery. *Can J Surg* 1992;35:271–274.

150. Obenchain TG. Laparoscopic lumbar discectomy: case report. *J Laparoendosc Surg* 1991;1:145–149.

151. Heini PF, Krahenbuhl L, Schwarzenbach O, et al. Laparoscopic assisted spine surgery. *Dig Surg* 1998;15:185–186.

152. Lieberman IH, Willsher PC, Litwin DE, et al. Transperitoneal laparoscopic exposure for lumbar interbody fusion. *Spine* 2000;25: 509–514.

153. Dewald CJ, Millikan KW, Hammerberg KW, et al. An open, minimally invasive approach to the lumbar spine. *Am Surg* 1999;65: 61–68.

154. Bolesta MJ, Bohlman HH. Surgical management of injuries to the thoracic and lumbosacral spine. In: Findlay G, Owen R, eds. *Surgery of the spine,* vol 2. Oxford: Blackwell Science, 1992: 1115–1129.

155. Found EM Jr, Weinstein JN. Surgical approaches to the lumbar spine. In: Frymoyer JW, ed. *The adult spine: principles and practice,* vol 2. New York: Raven Press, 1991:1523–1534.

156. Rechtine GR, McAllister EW. Flank retroperitoneal approach to the lumbar spine. In: Zdeblick TA, ed. *Anterior approaches to the spine.* St. Louis: Quality Medical Publishing, 1999:193–201.

157. Allen BT, Bridwell KH. Paramedian approach to the anterior lumbar spine. In: Bridwell KH, DeWald RL, eds. *The textbook of spinal surgery,* 2nd ed. Philadelphia: Lippincott–Raven Publishers, 1997: 267–275.

158. Selby DK, Henderson RJ, Blumenthal S, et al. Anterior lumbar fusion. In: White AH, Rothman RH, Ray CD, eds. *Lumbar spine surgery: techniques and complications.* St. Louis: Mosby, 1987.

159. de Peretti F, Hovorka I, Fabiani P, et al. New possibilities in L2-L5 lumbar arthrodesis using a lateral retroperitoneal approach assisted by laparoscopy: preliminary results. *Eur Spine J* 1996;5:210–216.

160. McAfee PC, Bohlman HH, Yuan HA. Anterior decompression of traumatic thoracolumbar fractures with incomplete neurological deficit using a retroperitoneal approach. *J Bone Joint Surg Am* 1985;67:89–104.

161. Onimus M, Papin P, Gangloff S. Extraperitoneal approach to the lumbar spine with video assistance. *Spine* 1996;21:2491–2494.

162. Muhlbauer M, Pfisterer W, Eyb R, et al. Minimally invasive retroperitoneal approach for lumbar corpectomy and anterior reconstruction. Technical note. *J Neurosurg* 2000;93(1 suppl):161–167.

163. Lajer H, Widecrantz S, Heisterberg L. Hernias in trocar ports following abdominal laparoscopy. A review. *Acta Obstet Gynecol Scand* 1997;76:389–393.

164. Levrant SG, Bieber EJ, Barnes RB. Anterior abdominal wall adhesions after laparotomy or laparoscopy. *J Am Assoc Gynecol Laparosc* 1997;4:353–356.

165. Olsen D, McCord D, Law M. Laparoscopic discectomy with anterior interbody fusion of L5-S1. *Surg Endosc* 1996;10:1158–1163.

166. Regan JJ, McAfee PC, Guyer RD, et al. Laparoscopic fusion of the lumbar spine in a multicenter series of the first 34 consecutive patients. *Surg Laparosc Endosc* 1996;6:459–468.

167. Regan JJ, McAfee PC, Mack MJ, eds. *Atlas of endoscopic spine surgery.* St. Louis: Quality Medical Publishing, 1995.

168. Zdeblick TA, David SM. A prospective comparison of surgical approach for anterior L4-L5 fusion: laparoscopic versus mini anterior lumbar interbody fusion. *Spine* 2000;25:2682–2687.

169. Geis WP, Kim HC, Brennan EJ, et al. Robotic arm enhancement to accommodate improved efficiency and decreased resource utilization in complex minimally invasive surgical procedures. In: Sieberg H, Weghorst S, Morgan K, eds. *Health care in the information age.* Cincinnati, OH: IOS Press and Ohmsha, 1966:471–481.

170. Bagby GW. Arthrodesis by the distraction–compression method using a stainless steel implant. *Orthopedics* 1988;11:931–934.

171. Mayer HM. A new microsurgical technique for minimally invasive anterior lumbar interbody fusion. *Spine* 1997;22:691–699; discussion 700.

172. Albee FH. Transplantation of a portion of the tibia into the spine for Pott's disease: a preliminary report. *JAMA* 1911;57:885–886.

173. Hibbs RA. An operation for progressive spinal deformities: a preliminary report of three cases from the service of the orthopaedic hospital. *N Y Med J* 1911;93:1013–1016.

174. Foley KT, Gupta SK, Justis JR, et al. Percutaneous pedicle screw fixation of the lumbar spine. *Neurosurg Focus* 2001;10:Article 10.

175. Foley KT, Smith MM. Microendoscopic discectomy. *Tech Neurosurg* 1997;3:301–307.

176. Benz RJ, Garfin SR. Current techniques of decompression of the lumbar spine. *Clin Orthop* 2001;384:75–81.

177. Schlegel KF, Pon A. The biomechanics of posterior lumbar interbody fusion (PLIF) in spondylolisthesis. *Clin Orthop* 1985;193:115–119.

178. Lee CK, Langrana NA. Lumbosacral spinal fusion. A biomechanical study. *Spine* 1984;9:574–581.

179. Dennis S, Watkins R, Landaker S, et al. Comparison of disc space heights after anterior lumbar interbody fusion. *Spine* 1989;14:876–878.

180. Sandhu HS, Turner S, Kabo JM, et al. Distractive properties of a threaded interbody fusion device. An *in vivo* model. *Spine* 1996;21:1201–1210.

181. Soini J. Lumbar disc space heights after external fixation and anterior interbody fusion: a prospective 2-year follow-up of clinical and radiographic results. *J Spinal Disord* 1994;7:487–494.

182. Siebert W. Percutaneous nucleotomy procedures in lumbar intervertebral disk displacement. Current status [in German]. *Orthopade* 1999;28:598–608.

183. Onik GM. Percutaneous diskectomy in the treatment of herniated lumbar disks. *Neuroimaging Clin N Am* 2000;10:597–607.

184. Foley KT, Smith MM, Rampersaud YR. Microendoscopic approach to far-lateral lumbar disc herniation. *Neurosurg Focus* 1999;7:Article 5.

185. Bonafe A, Tremoulet M, Sabatier J, et al. Foraminal and latero-foraminal hernia. Mid-term results of percutaneous techniques nucleolysis-nucleotomy [in French]. *Neurochirurgie* 1993;39:110–115.

186. Kambin P, O'Brien E, Zhou L, et al. Arthroscopic microdiscectomy and selective fragmentectomy. *Clin Orthop* 1998;347:150–167.

187. Lew SM, Mehalic TF, Fagone KL. Transforaminal percutaneous endoscopic discectomy in the treatment of far-lateral and foraminal lumbar disc herniations. *J Neurosurg* 2001;94(2 suppl):216–220.

188. Chatterjee S, Foy PM, Findlay GF. Report of a controlled clinical trial comparing automated percutaneous lumbar discectomy and microdiscectomy in the treatment of contained lumbar disc herniation. *Spine* 1995;20:734–738.

189. Kahanovitz N. Percutaneous diskectomy. *Clin Orthop* 1992;284:75–79.

190. Choy DS. Percutaneous laser disc decompression (PLDD): twelve years' experience with 752 procedures in 518 patients. *J Clin Laser Med Surg* 1998;16:325–331.

191. Casper GD, Mullins LL, Hartman VL. Laser-assisted disc decompression: a clinical trial of the holmium:YAG laser with side-firing fiber. *J Clin Laser Med Surg* 1995;13:27–32.

192. Liebler WA. Percutaneous laser disc nucleotomy. *Clin Orthop* 1995;310:58–66.

193. Kotilainen E, Valtonen S. Long-term outcome of patients who underwent percutaneous nucleotomy for lumbar disc herniation: results after a mean follow-up of 5 years. *Acta Neurochir (Wien)* 1998;140:108–113.

194. Knight MT, Vajda A, Jakab GV, et al. Endoscopic laser foraminoplasty on the lumbar spine—early experience. *Minim Invasive Neurosurg* 1998;41:5–9.

195. Ditsworth DA. Endoscopic transforaminal lumbar discectomy and reconfiguration: a postero-lateral approach into the spinal canal. *Surg Neurol* 1998;49:588–597; discussion 597–598.

196. Haag M. Transforaminal endoscopic microdiscectomy. Indications and short-term to intermediate-term results. *Orthopade* 1999;28:615–621.

197. Stucker R, Krug C, Reichelt A. Endoscopic treatment of intervertebral disk displacement. Percutaneous transforaminal access to the epidural space. Indications, technique and initial results. *Orthopade* 1997;26:280–287.

198. Yuan HA, Garfin SR, Dickman CA, et al. A historical cohort study of pedicle screw fixation in thoracic, lumbar, and sacral spine fusions. *Spine* 1994;19(suppl 20):2279S–2296S.

199. Kambin P, Gellman H. Percutaneous lateral discectomy of the lumbar spine: a preliminary report. *Clin Orthop* 1983;174:127–132.

200. Magerl FP. Stabilization of the lower thoracic and lumbar spine with external skeletal fixation. *Clin Orthop* 1984;189:125–141.

201. Lowery GL, Kulkarni SS. Posterior percutaneous spine instrumentation. *Eur Spine J* 2000;9(suppl 1):S126–S130.

202. Singh V. Intradiscal electrothermal therapy: a preliminary report. *Pain Physician* 2000;3:367–373.

203. Karasek M, Bogduk N. Twelve-month follow-up of a controlled trial of intradiscal thermal anuloplasty for back pain due to internal disc disruption. *Spine* 2000;25:2601–2607.

204. Barendse GA, van Den Berg SG, Kessels AH, et al. Randomized controlled trial of percutaneous intradiscal radiofrequency thermocoagulation for chronic discogenic back pain: lack of effect from a 90-second 70 C lesion. *Spine* 2001;26:287–292.

205. Derby R, Eek B, Chen Y, et al. Intradiscal electrothermal annuloplasty (IDET): a novel approach for treating chronic discogenic back pain. *Neuromodulation* 2000;3:82–88.

206. Letcher FS, Goldring S. The effect of radiofrequency current and heat on peripheral nerve action potential in the cat. *J Neurosurg* 1968;29:42–47.

207. Hayashi K, Thabit G 3rd, Bogdanske JJ, et al. The effect of nonablative laser energy on the ultrastructure of joint capsular collagen. *Arthroscopy* 1996;12:474–481.

208. Hayashi K, Thabit G 3rd, Vailas AC, et al. The effect of nonablative laser energy on joint capsular properties. An *in vitro* histologic and biochemical study using a rabbit model. *Am J Sports Med* 1996;24:640–646.

209. Saal JS, Saal JA. Management of chronic discogenic low back pain

with a thermal intradiscal catheter. A preliminary report. *Spine* 2000;25:382–388.

210. Saal JA, Saal JS. Intradiscal electrothermal treatment for chronic discogenic low back pain: a prospective outcome study with minimum 1-year follow-up. *Spine* 2000;25:2622–2627.

211. Coppes MH, Marani E, Thomeer RT, et al. Innervation of "painful" lumbar discs. *Spine* 1997;22:2342–2350.

212. Bogduk N, Tynan W, Wilson AS. The nerve supply to the human lumbar intervertebral discs. *J Anat* 1981;132(pt 1):39–56.

213. Groen GJ, Baljet B, Drukker J. Nerves and nerve plexuses of the human vertebral column. *Am J Anat* 1990;188:282–296.

214. Nakamura S, Takahashi K, Takahashi Y, et al. Origin of nerves supplying the posterior portion of lumbar intervertebral discs in rats. *Spine* 1996;21:917–924.

215. Yamashita T, Minaki Y, Oota I, et al. Mechanosensitive afferent units in the lumbar intervertebral disc and adjacent muscle. *Spine* 1993;18:2252–2256.

216. Yoshizawa H, O'Brien JP, Smith WT, et al. The neuropathology of intervertebral discs removed for low-back pain. *J Pathol* 1980;132: 95–104.

217. Morinaga T, Takahashi K, Yamagata M, et al. Sensory innervation to the anterior portion of lumbar intervertebral disc. *Spine* 1996; 21:1848–1851.

218. Bogduk N, Long DM. The anatomy of the so-called "articular nerves" and their relationship to facet denervation in the treatment of low-back pain. *J Neurosurg* 1979;51:172–177.

219. Bogduk N. The lumbar disc and low back pain. *Neurosurg Clin N Am* 1991;2:791–806.

220. Bogduk N. *Clinical anatomy of the lumbar spine and sacrum,* 3rd ed. Edinburgh: Churchill Livingstone, 1997:202–212.

221. Crock HV. Internal disc disruption. A challenge to disc prolapse fifty years on. *Spine* 1986;11:650–653.

222. Aprill C, Bogduk N. High-intensity zone: a diagnostic sign of painful lumbar disc on magnetic resonance imaging. *Br J Radiol* 1992; 65:361–369.

223. Ito M, Incorvaia KM, Yu SF, et al. Predictive signs of discogenic lumbar pain on magnetic resonance imaging with discography correlation. *Spine* 1998;23:1252–1260.

224. Schellhas KP, Pollei SR, Gundry CR, et al. Lumbar disc high-intensity zone. Correlation of magnetic resonance imaging and discography. *Spine* 1996;21:79–86.

225. Vanharanta H, Sachs BL, Ohnmeiss DD, et al. Pain provocation and disc deterioration by age. A CT/discography study in a low-back pain population. *Spine* 1989;14:420–423.

226. Schwarzer AC, Aprill CN, Derby R, et al. The prevalence and clinical features of internal disc disruption in patients with chronic low back pain. *Spine* 1995;20:1878–1883.

227. Deyo RA, Battie M, Beurskens AJ, et al. Outcome measures for low back pain research. A proposal for standardized use. *Spine* 1998; 23:2003–2013.

228. Gatchel RJ, Polatin PB, Mayer TG, et al. Use of the SF-36 health status survey with a chronically disabled back pain population: strengths and limitations. *J Occup Rehabil* 1998;8:237–246.

229. Derby R. Intradiscal electrothermal annuloplasty. Presented at the annual meeting of the North American Spine Society, San Francisco, California, 1998.

230. Karasek M, Karasek D, Bogduk N. A controlled trial of the efficacy of intradiscal electrothermal treatment for internal disc disruption. Presented at the annual meeting of the North American Spine Society, Chicago, Illinois, 1999.

231. Maurer P. Thermal lumbar disc annuloplasty: initial clinical results. Presented at the annual meeting of the North American Spine Society, Chicago, Illinois, 1999.

232. Houpt JC, Conner ES, McFarland EW. Experimental study of temperature distributions and thermal transport during radiofrequency current therapy of the intervertebral disc. *Spine* 1996;21: 1808–1812; discussion 1812–1813.

233. Troussier B, Lebas JF, Chirossel JP, et al. Percutaneous intradiscal radio-frequency thermocoagulation. A cadaveric study. *Spine* 1995; 20:1713–1718.

234. Lee J, Lutz GE, Campbell D, et al. Stability of the lumbar spine after intradiscal electrothermal therapy. *Arch Phys Med Rehabil* 2001;82:120–122.

235. Boden SD, Moskovitz PA, Morone MA, et al. Video-assisted lateral intertransverse process arthrodesis. Validation of a new minimally invasive lumbar spinal fusion technique in the rabbit and nonhuman primate (rhesus) models. *Spine* 1996;21:2689–2697.

236. Cook SD, Baffes GC, Wolfe MW, et al. The effect of recombinant human osteogenic protein-1 on healing of large segmental bone defects. *J Bone Joint Surg Am* 1994;76:827–838.

237. Morone MA, Boden SD, Hair G, et al. The Marshall R. Urist Young Investigator Award. Gene expression during autograft lumbar spine fusion and the effect of bone morphogenetic protein 2. *Clin Orthop* 1998;351:252–265.

238. Sandhu HS, Kanim LE, Kabo JM, et al. Effective doses of recombinant human bone morphogenetic protein-2 in experimental spinal fusion. *Spine* 1996;21:2115–2122.

239. Sandhu HS, Kanim LE, Toth JM, et al. Experimental spinal fusion with recombinant human bone morphogenetic protein-2 without decortication of osseous elements. *Spine* 1997;22:1171–1180.

240. Schimandle JH, Boden SD, Hutton WC. Experimental spinal fusion with recombinant human bone morphogenetic protein-2. *Spine* 1995;20:1326–1337.

241. Boden SD, Martin GJ Jr, Horton WC, et al. Laparoscopic anterior spinal arthrodesis with rhBMP-2 in a titanium interbody threaded cage. *J Spinal Disord* 1998;11:95–101.

242. Hecht BP, Fischgrund JS, Herkowitz HN, et al. The use of recombinant human bone morphogenetic protein 2 (rhBMP-2) to promote spinal fusion in a nonhuman primate anterior interbody fusion model. *Spine* 1999;24:629–636.

243. Holliger EH, Trawick RH, Boden SD, et al. Morphology of the lumbar intertransverse process fusion mass in the rabbit model: a comparison between two bone graft materials—rhBMP-2 and autograft. *J Spinal Disord* 1996;9:125–128.

244. Sandhu HS. Anterior lumbar interbody fusion with osteoinductive growth factors. *Clin Orthop* 2000;371:56–60.

245. Subach RB, Haid RW, Rodts GE, et al. Bone morphogenetic protein in spinal fusion: overview and clinical update. *Neurosurg Focus* 2001;10:Article 3.

246. Helm GA, Alden TD, Sheehan JP, et al. Bone morphogenetic proteins and bone morphogenetic protein gene therapy in neurological surgery: a review. *Neurosurgery* 2000;46:1213–1222.

247. Cook SD, Rueger DC. Osteogenic protein-1: biology and applications. *Clin Orthop* 1996;324:29–38.

248. Gazit D, Turgeman G, Kelley P, et al. Engineered pluripotent mesenchymal cells integrate and differentiate in regenerating bone: a novel cell-mediated gene therapy. *J Gene Med* 1999;1:121–133.

249. Bao Q-B, Yuan HA. Artificial disc technology. *Neurosurg Focus* 2000;9:Article 14.

250. Lee CK, Langrana NA, Parsons JR, et al. Development of a prosthetic intervertebral disc. *Spine* 1991;16(6 suppl):S253–S255.

251. Eysel P, Rompe J, Schoenmayr R, et al. Biomechanical behaviour of a prosthetic lumbar nucleus. *Acta Neurochir (Wien)* 1999;141: 1083–1087.

252. Zollner J, Rompe JD, Eysel P. Biomechanical properties of synthetic lumbar intervertebral disk implants. *Z Orthop Ihre Grenzgeb* 2000; 138:459–463.

253. Felt CJ, Bourgeault CA, Baker MW. Articulating joint repair. US Patent No. 5,888,220, March 30, 1999.